D1764912

ZOONOSES

ZOONOSES

Biology, Clinical Practice, and Public Health Control

S. R. PALMER,
LORD SOULSBY, and
D. I. H. SIMPSON

1998

Oxford   New York   Tokyo

OXFORD UNIVERSITY PRESS

1998

Oxford University Press, Great Clarendon Street, Oxford OX2 6DP

Oxford   New York

Athens   Auckland   Bangkok   Bogota   Bombay   Buenos Aires
Calcutta   Cape Town   Dar es Salaam   Delhi   Florence   Hong Kong
Istanbul   Karachi   Kuala Lumpur   Madras   Madrid   Melbourne
Mexico City   Nairobi   Paris   Singapore   Taipei   Tokyo   Toronto   Warsaw
and associated companies in
Berlin   Ibadan

Oxford is a trade mark of Oxford University Press

Published in the United States
by Oxford University Press Inc., New York

A catalogue record for this book is available from the British Library

Library of Congress Cataloging in Publication Data

Zoonoses/[edited by] S. R. Palmer, Lord Soulsby, and D. I. H. Simpson.
Includes bibliographical references and index.
1. Zoonoses.   I. Palmer, Stephen R.   II. Soulsby, E. J. L.   III. Simpson, David Ian Hewitt.
RC113.5.Z673   1998   616.9′59–dc21   97–30387

ISBN 0 19 262380 X (Hbk)

Typeset by EXPO Holdings, Malaysia

Printed in Great Britain by
The Bath Press, Avon

CONTENTS

PART 2   VIRAL ZOONOSES

Wendy Gibson, School of Biological Sciences, University of Bristol, Bristol BS8 1UG, UK

James Hope, BBSRC and MRC Neuropathogenesis Unit, Institute for Animal Health, Ogston Building, West Mains Road, Edinburgh EH9 3JF, Scotland, UK

Colin R. Howard, Department of Pathology and Infectious Diseases, Royal Veterinary College, Royal College Street, London NW1 0TU, UK

T. J. Humphrey, Public Health Laboratory Service Food Microbiology Research Unit, Public Health Laboratory, Church Lane, Heavitree, Exeter EX2 5AD, UK

P. A. Jenkins, Formerly of the Mycobacterium Reference Unit, Public Health Laboratory Service, University Hospital of Wales, Heath, Cardiff CF4 4XW, UK

M. A. Karmali, The Hospital for Sick Children, Toronto, Ontario, Canada

A. A. King, Central Veterinary Laboratory, Surrey, KT15 3NB, UK

Milan Labuda, Institute of Zoology, 84206, Bratislava, Slovakia

Colin J. Leake, Disease Control and Vector Biology Unit, Department of Infectious and Tropical Diseases, London School of Tropical Medicine and Hygiene, London, WCIE 7HT, UK

Inger Ljungström, Parasitology Laboratory, Swedish Institute for Infectious Disease Control and Microbiology and Tumour Biology Center (MTC), Karolinska Institute, S-105 21, Stockholm, Sweden

G. Lloyd, Centre for Applied Microbiology and Research, Wiltshire, SP4 O5G, UK

Sheelagh Lloyd, Department of Clinical Veterinary Medicine, University of Cambridge, Madingley Rd, Cambridge CB3 0ES, UK

M. B. McEvoy, Public Health Laboratory Service Communicable Disease Surveillance Centre, London NW9 5EQ, UK

P. McKenna, Belgian Zoonosis Workgroup, Queen Astrid Military Hospital, Bruynstraat 2, B-1120 Brussels, Belgium

J. McLauchlin, Public Health Laboratory Service Food Hygiene Laboratory, Central Public Health Laboratory, London NW9 5HT, UK

Thomas J. Marrie, Room 5014 A.C.C., Victoria General Hospital, 1278 Tower Road, Halifax, Nova Scotia B3H 2Y9, Canada

Philip Davis Marsden, Núcleo de Medicina Tropical UnB, Caixa Postal 4516 Asa Norte CEP 70.919-970 Brasília, DF, Brasil

R. T. Mayon-White, Oxfordshire Health Authority, Oxford OX3 9D2, UK

Thomas P. Monath, OraVax Inc., 38 Sidney St, Cambridge MA 02139; and Department of Tropical Public Health, Harvard School of Public Health, Boston MA 02115, USA

P. Morgan-Capner, Public Health Laboratory, Royal Preston Hospital, PO Box 202, Preston PR2 9HG, UK

Darwin Murrell, United States Department of Agriculture, Beltsville Area, 10300 Baltimore Avenue, Beltsville, Maryland 20705-2350, USA

S. Nelson, The Hospital for Sick Children, Toronto, Ontario, Canada

T. J. Nolan, Laboratory of Parasitology, School of Veterinary Medicine, University of Pennsylvania, 3800 Spruce Street, Philadelphia, Pennsylvania 19104, USA

Patricia A. Nuttall, Institute of Virology and Environmental Microbiology, Oxford, OX1 3SR, UK

Andrew Pearson, Nosocranial Infection Surveillance Unit 8 HLS Central Public Health Laboratory, Colindale, London NW9 5HT, UK

C. J. Peters, Special Pathogens Branch, National Center for Infectious Diseases, Centers for Disease Control and Prevention, Atlanta, GA 30333, USA

Michel Plommet, Directeur de recherche honoraire, INRA, France

David J. Pombo, Division of Infectious Diseases, University of Utah Medical Centre, 50 North Medical Drive, Salt Lake City, Utah 84132, USA

Edoardo Pozio, Laboratory of Parasitology, Instituto Superiore di Sanitá, Viale Regina Elena 299, I-00161 Rome, Italy

Paul Prociv, Department of Parasitology, The University of Queensland, QLD 4072, Australia

Didier Raoult, Unité des Rickettsies, CNRS UPRES-A 6020, Faculté de Médecine, 27 Boulevard Jean Moulin, 13385 Marseille Cedex 05, France

Hugh W. Reid, Moredun Research Institute, 408 Gilmerton Road, Edinburgh EH17 7JH, Scotland, UK

M. G. Roberts, Agresearch, Wallaceville Animal Research Centre, PO Box 40063, Upper Hutt, New Zealand

R. L. Salmon, Public Health Laboratory Service Communicable Disease Surveillance Centre (Welsh Unit), Abton House, Wedal Road, Roath, Cardiff CF4 3QX, UK

G. A. Schad, Laboratory of Parasitology, School of Veterinary Medicine, University of Pennsylvania, 3800 Spruce Street, Philadelphia, Pennsylvania 19104, USA

Daniel J. Sexton, Department of Medicine, Division of Infectious Diseases, Duke University School of Medicine, Durham, North Carolina 27710, USA

M. Sillis, Public Health Laboratory, Bowthorpe Road, Norwich, Norfolk, NR2 3TX, UK

M. B. Skirrow, Public Health Laboratory, Gloucestershire Royal Hospital, Gloucester GL1 3NN, UK

Robert M. M. Smith, Public Health Laboratory Service Communicable Disease Surveillance Centre (Welsh Unit), Abton House, Wedal Road, Roath, Cardiff CF4 3QX, UK

E. J. L. Soulsby, Department of Clinical Veterinary Medicine, University of Cambridge, Madingley Road, Cambridge CB3 0ES, UK

A. H. Sparkes, The Feline Centre, Division of Companion Animals, Department of Clinical Veterinary Science, School of Veterinary Science, University of Bristol, Langford House, Langford, Bristol BS18 7DU, UK

Deborah J. Stenzel, Analytical Electron Microscopy Facility, Queensland University of Technology, George Street, Brisbane, Queensland 4001, Australia

R. Swanepoel, University of the Witwatersrand, South Africa

M. G. Taylor, Department of Infectious and Tropical Diseases, London School of Hygiene and Tropical Medicine, London WCIE 7HT, UK

Daniel Thomas, Public Health Laboratory Service Communicable Disease Surveillance Centre (Welsh Unit), Abton House, Wedal Road, Roath, Cardiff CF4 3QX, UK

R. C. A. Thompson, WHO Collaborating Centre for the Molecular Epidemiology of Parasitic Infections and Institute for Molecular Genetics and Animal Disease, Division of Veterinary and Biomedical Sciences, Murdoch University, Murdoch, Western Australia, 6150.

E. J. Threlfall, Laboratory of Enteric Pathogens, Central Public Health Laboratory, 61 Colindale Avenue, London NW9 5HT, UK

P. C. B. Turnbull, Centre for Applied Microbiology and Research, Salisbury, SP4 OJ9, UK

A. Vaheri, Department of Virology, University of Helsinki, Haartmaninkatu 3, Fin- 00014, Helsinki, Finland

G. van der Groen, Department of Infection and Immunity, Division of Microbiology, Institute of Tropical Medicine, Nationalestraat 155, B-2000 Antwerp, Belgium

N. Van der Mee-Marquet, Laboratory de Microbiologie, Faculté de Médecine, Hôpital Trousseau, 37044 Tours, France

Jean-Michel Verger, INRA, Centre de Tours-Nouzilly, 37380 Nouzilly, France

Derek Wakelin, Department of Life Science, University of Nottingham, University Park, Nottingham NG7 2RD, UK

Dennis J. White, New York State Department of Health, 672 Corning Tower Building, Empire State Plaza, Albany, New York 12237, USA

Marion L. Woods, Division of Infectious Diseases, University of Utah Medical Centre, 50 North Medical Drive, Salt Lake City, Utah 84132, USA

S. E. Wright, Moredun Research Institute, Edinburgh, Scotland, EH17 7JH, UK

PREFACE

DEFINITIONS

Zoonoses are defined by the World Health Organization as 'Diseases and infections which are naturally transmitted between vertebrate animals and man' (WHO 1959), but there has been debate on this definition. Some believe there is not sufficient evidence in all accepted zoonoses for natural transmission, even though epidemiological evidence would appear to be strong. Others point out the desirability of including 'unnatural' opportunistic infections of severely immunosuppressed patients by organisms of invertebrate origin. Some would include intoxications, such as snake and spider venoms or botulism. The definition excludes the deliberate transmission of human infectious agents to animals, usually for experimental purposes.

Zoonoses cover a broad range of diseases with very different clinical and epidemiological features and control measures. The fundamental reason for grouping these diseases together is that successful control requires joint veterinary and medical efforts. While the concept of 'zoonoses' is anthropocentric (Nelson 1960), the epidemiological study and their control is not. However, too frequently the medical and veterinary aspects of a zoonotic disease are studied separately, and funding for work often is derived from separate sources. In many cases, the infection in animals is unapparent or mild, causing little or no animal health or economic concern, so that winning resources to study the veterinary sources is often difficult. This book is aimed at developing the co-ordinated medico-veterinary approach to investigation and control.

CLASSFICATION OF ZOONOSES

Various classifications of the zoonoses have been proposed largely based on epidemiological features and whether the reservoir hosts are man or lower vertebrate animals. Hence the term anthropozoonoses refers to infections transmitted to man from lower animals and zooanthroponoses to infections transmitted from man to lower vertebrates. Where infections can be maintained in both man and animals and transmitted in either direction, the term amphixenoses has been applied. However, such terms have led to confusion and sometimes have been used indiscriminately. They will not be used in this volume.

For teaching purposes Schwabe (1964) has suggested that a classification based on the type of life cycle of the infecting agent may be useful and proposes four categories:

(1) Direct zoonoses: transmission is by direct contact, by contact with a fomite or mechanical vector, the agent undergoing little or no propagative changes or development during transmission (e.g. rabies, brucellosis).
(2) Cyclo-zoonoses: requiring more than one species or vertebrate host, but not invertebrate host, to complete the developmental cycle of the agent (e.g. echinococcosis).

(3) Meta-zoonoses: transmission is by invertebrate vector in which the agent develops and/or multiples and there is an extrinsic incubation period before an infective stage is produced (e.g. arbovirus infection, plague, schistosomosis).

(4) Sapro-zoonoses: both a vertebrate host and a non-animal developmental site or reservoir is required. Organic matter, including food, soil, and plants, is considered non-animal (e.g. larva migrans, mycoses).

NOMENCLATURE OF DISEASES

There have been several attempts to standardize the nomenclature of diseases caused by parasitic infections (reviewed by Kassai *et al.* 1988). The disease entity is usually designated by adding the suffixes *-iasis* or *-osis* after the proper name, but this has varied to include *-asis* and *-iosis*. Whitlock (1955) had previously proposed that the suffix *-iasis* be applied to parasitic infections where clinical manifestations were not apparent and *-osis* where they were. One difficulty in accepting such a proposal is that as pathophysiological measurements of parasitic disease become more capable of measuring clinical effects, the point where *-iasis* becomes *-osis* is increasingly difficult to decide. However, Whitlock's proposal has not met with general favour. The most recent proposal, increasingly accepted by scientific organizations, journals and international bodies is the 'Standardized Nomenclature of Animal Parasitic Diseases (SNOAPAD)' (Kassai *et al.* 1988) which consists of adding the suffix *-osis* to the name of the parasite (e.g. echinococcosis, fasciolosis, sarcocystosis, trypanosomosis). The SNOAPAD recommendations, which are considered as a logical approach to nomenclatures of disease, are adopted in this volume. Nevertheless, there are some workers who feel very strongly that this change is unacceptable and, with the agreement of the editors, have continued to use the *-iasis* suffix, (e.g. Chapter 43).

There are several diseases where *-osis* has not been added to the taxon and their names are either specifically descriptive of the diseases or are named after the discoverer or in honour of a person (e.g. plague, yellow fever, Chagas disease, Rocky mountain spotted fever, hydatid disease, malaria, visceral larva migrans, cat-scratch disease). These names are well established but even so they do not necessarily specifically indicate the disease-producing agent and it is likely that more specific designations will be applied in the future.

TRENDS IN ZOONOSES

The close association of people with their animals in large areas of the world and often in unsatisfactory sanitary conditions continues to promote the opportunity for zoonotic infections. Animals continue to provide a substantial contribution to the energy requirements of agriculture in terms of converting poor-quality cellulose to first-class protein, in the provision of draught power by cultivation of crops and transport, and the provision of fuel. The need to care for these valuable animals, which represent a major capital investment to the peasant farmer, exposes millions of rural people to contact with zoonotic disease. The tropical parts of the world are high-risk areas, especially where the zoonotic infection is arthropod-borne.

The situation may become acutely worse when political or social instability occurs and normal sanitary arrangements are disrupted, disease control programmes discontinued, and medical and veterinary services cease to function.

Certain occupational groups may be at greater risk such as the rural agriculturist or pastoralist and including forest workers, hunters, and wildlife workers. Such groups may accentuate the problem through the expansion of rural and even urban settlement into undeveloped woodland, marginal land, or waste land.

While it might be thought that zoonoses are essentially a rural problem, the urban dimension must also be considered important in several respects. Wildlife can become established in suburban and recreation areas, in some cases encouraged by householders, which may enhance these as a source of zoonotic infection (e.g. foxes and *Echinococcus multilocularis*). However, the companion animal in the urban scene is an important source of zoonotic diseases, especially of parasitic infections. The population of dogs and cats as companion animals continues to grow, and it has been estimated in the United Kingdom that of the 22.56 million households at least 50 per cent own a companion dog or cat. In 1994 the companion animal populations in the United Kingdom were 6.65 million dogs and 7.18 million cats. Increasingly, the dangers of zoonotic diseases associated with these companion animals are recognized and national and local laws and regulations are enacted to control where animals can be taken and the fouling of the environment.

A new dimension of zoonotic diseases has been manifest by the growing numbers of immunosuppressed people, either through the use of immunosuppression in therapy as in transplantation, or through immunosuppressive diseases, particularly in the acquired immunodeficiency syndrome (AIDS). Infections which in the normal individual are inapparent, or at most, minor, self-limiting conditions, may become life threatening during immunosuppression or in AIDS patients (e.g. toxoplasmosis, cryptosporidiosis). There are increasing reports of unusual opportunistic zoonotic infections in immunosuppressed patients, such as *Microsporidium* spp and *Pleistophora*, a fish parasite (Eckert 1989).

With the possible advent of xenotransplantation, fears have been expressed that unknown infectious agents (viruses, prions, etc.) of a donor animal (pig) could be transmitted to the human recipient to cause clinical disease or even an epidemic.

These latter instances of infections being transmitted to human patients may not be regarded strictly as zoonoses since they would not meet the criterion of being 'naturally transmitted'. Should such infections become more commonplace then the definition of a zoonoses may require reconsideration.

Finally we should point out that many of the newly emerging or re-emerging infections which are causing concern, and for which global surveillance systems are being developed, are zoonoses. Important recent examples include Ebola virus in Africa, and Hantavirus in the United States of America, *Escherichia coli* O157 in Japan, the new equine morbillivirus in Australia, and brucellosis in the Middle East.

ZOONOTIC INFECTIONS REVIEWED

This volume deals with the major zoonoses; however, it does not attempt to be all-inclusive in its coverage. Minor or occasional infections in man with animal infectious agents have been excluded.

REFERENCES

Eckert, J. (1989). New aspects of parasitic zoonoses. *Veterinary Parasitology*, **32**, 37–55.

Kassai, T., Cordero Del Campillo, M., Euzeby, J., Gaafar, S., Hiepe, Th., and Himonas, C. A. (1988). Standardised Nomenclature of Animal parasitic diseases (SNOAPAD). *Veterinary Parasitology*, **29**, 299–326.

Nelson, G. S. (1960). Schistosome infections as Zoonoses in Africa. *Transactions of the Royal Society of Tropical Medicine and Hygiene*, **54**, 301–324.

Schwabe, C. N. (1964). *Veterinary medicine and human health.* William and Wilkins, Baltimore.

Whitlock, J. H. (1955). Trichostrongylosis in sheep and cattle. *Proceedings 92nd Annual meeting American Veterinary Medical Associations*, pp. 123–31.

World Health Organization (1959). *Zoonoses:* Second report of the Joint WHO/FAO Expert Committee.

ACKNOWLEDGEMENTS

The editors wish to express their sincere thanks to all the authors for their expertise, commitment and patience; and to Mrs Ruth Coomber and Mrs Hilary Fairney for their invaluable administrative assistance.

PART 1   BACTERIAL, CHLAMYDIAL AND RICKETTSIAL ZOONOSES

1 ANTHRAX

P. C. B. Turnbull

SUMMARY

Anthrax is primarily a disease of herbivorous mammals caused by the bacterium *Bacillus anthracis*, a Gram-positive, aerobic spore-forming bacillus, but few mammals are totally resistant to anthrax. Man generally acquires the disease directly or indirectly from animals by handling meat, hides, wool, hair, bones, etc. from infected animals. Animals are normally thought to contract anthrax by ingestion of spores from contaminated soil, but, in certain countries, fly bites may be involved. Anthrax remains common in various countries of Africa and Asia but, although relatively rare in Europe, America, and Australasia, occasional incidents still occur. Control depends on appropriate animal husbandry. In endemic areas the best approach is routine annual vaccination; in other countries, isolation of an affected area for 3 or more weeks after the last case, combined with vaccination of the remaining members of the affected herd or flock and appropriate clean-up measures, usually proves effective. In all instances, destruction of the carcass by heat treatment (incineration or rendering) is an essential part of effective control.

HISTORY AND BACKGROUND

Anthrax has been a scourge of man and animals since the first written history of disease. It was one of the plagues of Egypt in the time of Moses (*c.* 1250 BC) and was known in Asia Minor at the time of the Siege of Troy (*c.* 1200 BC). Accounts of its symptoms in the writings of Homer (*c.* 1000 BC), Hippocrates (*c.* 400 BC), Varro (116–27 BC), Virgil (70–19 BC), and Galen (*c.* AD 200) show that it was well known to the Greeks and Romans. It featured in Hindu literature of around 500 BC. In Europe, it was covered in a tenth-century collection of veterinary writings, the 'Hippiatrika', and again in an eleventh-century work, 'The Medicine of Quadrupeds' and major episodes were recorded in reports in 996 and 1090 in France; in 1552, 1898, and 1613–17 in Italy; in 1709–12 in Germany, Hungary, and Poland; in the early 1800s in Russia, Holland, and England; and again in Russia the mid-1800s (Salmon 1896; Wilson and Miles 1946; Klemm and Klemm 1959).

The large number of synonyms for anthrax reflect the historical familiarity with the different syndromes before it was realized they were manifestations of one aetiological agent (Christie 1987). The earliest scientific (as opposed to historical) reports are the descriptions of malignant pustule by Maret in 1752, Dym in 1769 and Fournier in 1769, and the description of the disease in animals by Chabert in 1780 (Wilson and Miles 1946).

The nineteenth-century work on anthrax has more than usual significance in that a major turning point in the history of medicine began with research on anthrax. It was the first disease of man and animals shown to be caused by a micro-organism and it was the disease on which much of the original work on bacteria and vaccines was done, and from which many of the well-known principles of pathogenic microbiology were derived. Particularly notable milestones were:

(1) the demonstration of the disease's infectiousness by Berthelemy in 1823, Eilert in 1836, and a number of others in the 1850s;

(2) the demonstration by Davaine in 1863–64 of its transmissibility, and by Tiegel and Klebs in 1864 that the infectivity of infectious material was lost on filtration through clay filters;

(3) the first observation of the bacillus by Delafond in 1838;

(4) the recognition between 1860 and 1880 that the one agent could produce different manifestations, ranging from malignant pustule to woolsorter's disease;

(5) Robert Koch established his famous postulates in 1877 by proving that *Bacillus anthracis* (so named by Cohn in 1875) was the cause of anthrax; and

(6) Pasteur's well-known pioneering work on vaccines included his demonstration in 1881 of protection against anthrax using history's second bacterial vaccine (Wilson and Miles 1946; Klemm and Klemm 1959; Parvizpour 1978; Choquette and Broughton 1981).

Pasteur's vaccine was used worldwide for some 50 years but many attempts at developing better alternatives were made in the 1920s and 1930s, culminating in Sterne's successful live spore vaccine which was largely responsible for making anthrax controllable across the world. This remains the livestock vaccine in use in most countries today.

In industrialized countries, improved factory hygiene and working conditions, together with non-living vaccines which became available in the 1950s and 1960s, have made occupational anthrax a very rare event. Nevertheless, areas endemic for anthrax remain, particularly in Africa and Asia, and the disease continues to occur in these areas in smaller or larger epizootics affecting livestock and wildlife, and associated epidemics in humans.

Since anthrax spores can persist for many decades where they fall, and can travel well in or on contaminated products of animal origin, no part of the world can afford to relax its vigilance against the possible unexpected outbreak at any time.

THE AGENT

TAXONOMY

Bacillus anthracis belongs to the genus *Bacillus*, the Gram-positive aerobic or facultatively anaerobic spore-forming, rod-shaped bacteria. Unlike most other *Bacillus* species, it is non-motile. It is frequently convenient to class it informally within the '*B. cereus* group' which comprises *B. cereus, B. anthracis, B. thuringiensis,* and *B. mycoides*. Until recently, it was long the subject of debate whether these are all variants of *B. cereus* or separate species in their own rights. Apart from

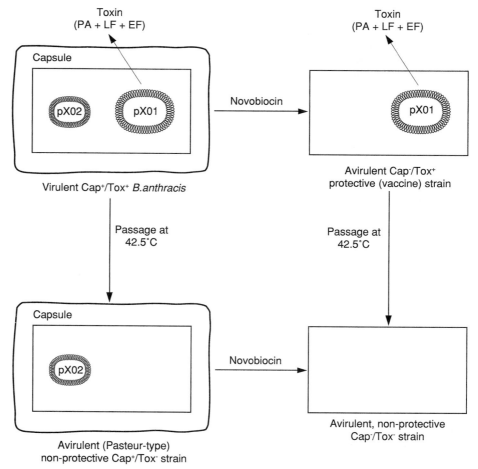

Fig. 1.1 Genetics of virulence factor production by *Bacillus anthracis*. Plasmids pX01 and pX02 code, respectively, for the toxin and the capsule. Loss of pX01 produces an avirulent, non-protective derivative; loss of pX02 results in a derivative of greatly reduced virulence that is capable of protection and is the basis of current livestock vaccines and human vaccines in Russia and China.

virulence, which can be lost by *B. anthracis* (Fig. 1.1), the only consistent phenotypic characters by which *B. anthracis* may be distinguished from *B. cereus* are lack of motility, absence of haemolysis on blood agar, and susceptibility to penicillin and the anthrax γ phage. However, genetic techniques are now providing clearer evidence that *B. anthracis*, with or without its virulence factors, can be reliably distinguished from the other members of the *B. cereus* group (Henderson *et al.* 1994).

MOLECULAR AND GENETIC ASPECTS OF PATHOGENESIS

The two known virulence factors of *B. anthracis* are the poly-γ-D-glutamic acid polypeptide capsule which protects it from phagocytosis by the host's defence cells and the toxin produced in the exponential phase of growth.

The toxin consists of three synergistic but separable proteins produced in the log phase of growth and termed protective antigen (PA), lethal factor (LF), and oedema factor (EF). Individually, these are non-toxic but intravenous administration of PA and LF together is lethal to mice and rats, while intradermal injection of PA and EF together in guinea-pigs or rabbits results in localized oedema. This had led to some workers referring to PA+LF as lethal toxin and PA+EF as oedema toxin, which is convenient and appropriate for structure–function studies of the separate entities, but it appears that in the natural state all three toxin components are always produced simultaneously.

The currently favoured model (Leppla 1991) of *in vivo* toxin action is shown in Fig. 1.2

EF is a calmodulin-dependent adenylate cyclase which, by catalysing the abnormal production of the cyclic-AMP, produces the altered water and ion movements that lead to the characteristic oedema of anthrax. By site-directed mutagenesis experiments, the ATP and calmodulin-binding regions on the EF molecule have been identified precisely (Little *et al.* 1994). The role of EF in the anthrax infection may be to prevent mobilization and activation of the polymorphonuclear leucocytes and thereby prevent the phagocytosis of the bacteria (Leppla 1991).

Evidence from studies on LF is consistent with it being a calcium- and zinc-dependent metalloprotease (Klimpel *et al.* 1994; Kochi *et al.* 1994). Although its precise mode of action is unknown as yet, it is accepted that the LF+PA complex is the major cause of tissue damage and death (Leppla 1991). Recent research suggests that the systemic shock and death characteristic of anthrax result primarily from the effects of high levels of cytokines, principally interleukin-1, produced by macrophages that have been stimulated by LF+PA;

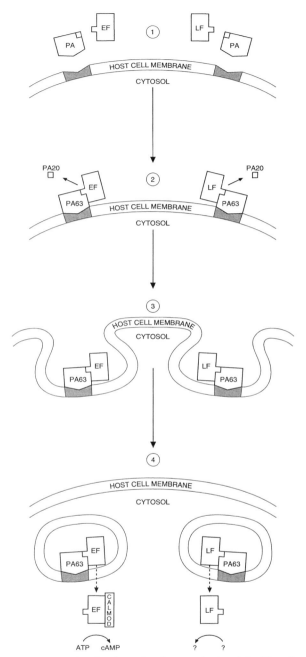

Fig. 1.2 Mode of action of anthrax toxin (model of Leppla 1991). Protective antigen (PA) binds to host cell-surface receptors (1) and is cleaved by a cell-surface protease, releasing a 20 kDa piece (2). This exposes a secondary receptor for the lethal factor (LF) and oedema factor (EF) components of the toxin, which compete to bind to it (2). The complex is internalized by receptor-mediated endocytosis (3) and acidification of the resulting vesicle leads to the transfer of LF/EF across the vesicular membrane into the cytosol where they effect their catalytic actions (4). Recently it has been reported (Milne *et al.* 1994) that PA and LF or PA and EF probably undergo internationalization in heptmeric complexes. (Reproduced from the *Oxford Textbook of Medicine*, 3rd edn, by kind permission.)

and macrophage depletion and reconstitution studies in mice have shown that microphages mediate, and are essential to, the action of lethal toxin *in vivo* (Hanna *et al.* 1993).

The genes for the virulence factors, capsule, and toxin, lie on two large plasmids. The three toxin genes, *pag, lef,* and *cya*, encoding PA, LF, and EF respectively, are located on the 170–185 kbp (119 MDa) plasmid, pX01, and have all been cloned and sequenced, revealing secreted proteins of 735 amino acids (PA; equivalent to 82.7 kDa), 776 amino acids (LF, 90.2 kDa) and 767 amino acids (EF, 88.8 kDa). Similarly, cloning and sequencing of the genes involved in capsule synthesis, which reside on a 90–95 kbp (60 Mda) plasmid, pX02, have revealed three cistrons designated *capA, capB,* and *capC*, which code for three membrane-associated enzymes mediating the polymerization of D-glutamic acid via the *B. anthracis* cell membrane. Coding for elaboration of both toxin proteins and capsule is under bicarbonate or CO_2 regulation ('bicarbonate' representing a mixture of CO_2, H_2CO_3, HCO_3^- and CO_3^{2-} in equilibrium) (Uchida *et al.* 1993). In the case of the toxin at least, bicarbonate control is through gene transcription, probably under the command of a negative regulatory gene encoding a repressor which binds to DNA and blocks some part of transcription in the absence of bicarbonate (Uchida *et al.* 1993). All three toxin genes (*pag, lef,* and *cya*) are coordinately required by HCO_3^- and temperature (Sirard *et al.* 1994).

Loss of either pX01 or pX02 and consequent loss of the ability to produce toxin or capsule leads to loss of virulence. This evidently can occur naturally (Turnbull *et al.* 1992*b*). pX01$^+$/pX02$^-$ strains form the basis of anthrax vaccines (see below).

MOLECULAR EPIDEMIOLOGY

The highly conserved nature of *B. anthracis* as a species has meant that, to date, it has defied attempts at devising a method for strain differentiation for epidemiological purposes, although some progress is being made using certain DNA fingerprinting approaches (Henderson *et al.* 1994; Henderson 1996).

As the only readily obtainable or identifiable entities truly specific to *B. anthracis* and not shared by other *Bacillus* species, the toxin antigens form the best basis at present for enzyme immunoassays for anti-anthrax antibodies (Turnbull *et al.* 1992*a*). Antibodies to the purified toxin antigens are the basis for new diagnostic systems on the principle that the presence of the toxin indicates the presence of the bacterium. Similarly, gene probes under development for rapid anthrax detection systems are primarily based on sequences within the genes encoding the toxin antigens or the

capsule precursors. However, the toxin agents are exponential phase vegetative cell metabolites. So since *B. anthracis* is invariably in its spore form when in the environment, attempts are constantly being made to identify spore-related antigens specific to *B. anthracis* which would lend themselves to more rapid detection assays.

DISEASE MECHANISMS

Infection normally commences by entry of the spore into the body by one of a number of routes (Fig. 1.3) and is followed by germination and multiplication locally or after transport to the regional lymph nodes where systemic infection is initiated, with involvement of the spleen soon after.

In the local cutaneous infection, multiplication and production of the toxin results in the characteristic eschar invariably accompanied by extensive oedema.

In the systemic disease, the bacilli multiply in the spleen and lymph nodes with few or no symptoms until a sudden, presumably toxin-induced, breakdown of the organs results in an explosive release of the toxin and huge numbers of the bacilli. This leads to abrupt onset of hyperacute illness with fever commencing a few hours before the final and rapid sequence of disorientation, shock, coma, and death.

The precise causes of death are undetermined but contributing factors are undoubtedly:

(1) the massive abnormal fluid movements induced cytotonically by the oedema factor and cytotoxically by the lethal factor directly and possibly also indirectly through release of vasoactive mediators producing vascular leakage; and conceivably

(2) hypoxia from the massive terminal bacteraemia which reaches 10^7–10^9 bacilli/ml of blood in susceptible species.

That the toxin is the main cause of death has been demonstrated experimentally in animals 'sterilized' late in infection by antibiotic treatment; also more resistant species, such as pigs, die with very low bacteraemic levels.

It is an unexplained phenomenon that, in laboratory animals, there appears to be an inverse relationship between susceptibility to infection and susceptibility to the toxin. Guinea-pigs, which are highly susceptible to infection, are quite resistant to the toxin, while the opposite is the case in rats. It would appear that the toxin is not highly potent in primates. Klein *et al.* (1962) observed that, of three 8 lb rhesus monkeys challenged with 200, 250, and 400 rat lethal doses (in 200, 250, and 400 ml volumes), the animal receiving 200 ml survived; those challenged with 250 and 400 ml died 60 and 30 hours later, respectively. With respect to rat lethal doses, Ezzell *et al.* (1984) established that 8 μg LF + 40 μg PA kills Fischer rats in 40 minutes.

GROWTH AND SURVIVAL

Bacillus anthracis is generally regarded as an obligate pathogen; its continued existence in the ecosystem appears to depend on a multiplication phase within an animal host (Fig. 1.3) and its environmental presence reflects contamination from an animal source at some time in the past rather than self-maintenance within the environment.

Much is made of the possible role of 'microcycling' in the environment and the theory on this proposed by Ness (1971) has been discussed elsewhere (Titball *et al.* 1991). However, our own experimental data (Turnbull *et al.* 1989, 1991; Bowen and Turnbull 1992; Lindeque and Turnbull 1994) have indicated that the nutritional level required for multiplication of germinated spores is far higher than is likely to be found in normal environments and that, should germination occur, the likely outcome is rapid death of the emergent bacillus. Consequently, we believe that environmental microcyling of *B. anthracis* is probably exceedingly rare.

The vegetative form of *B. anthracis* appears to be surprisingly fragile; survival of the species depends on rapid sporulation of bacilli shed by the dying animal on exposure to the air (Fig. 1.3) but the sporulation success rate never exceeds 0.1 per cent, and is usually considerably less than this (Lindeque and Turnbull 1994). However, once sporulated it is well established that the sports can survive for many decades and the time interval between infection of one host and infection of the next can be many years or decades.

HOSTS

Anthrax is primarily a disease of herbivores, although few mammals or birds are thought to be totally resistant to it. Man is really an incidental host and is fairly resistant to infection, generally acquiring it directly or indirectly from infected herbivores.

The disease remains enzootic in several countries of Africa and Asia where the value of a carcass following sudden death as meat for local consumption and as hide, hair, wool, and/or bones for sale greatly outweighs the perceived merits of burying or burning it. Consequently the cycle of infection in humans and animals continues to occur both locally and in distant non-endemic regions to which the animal products are transported.

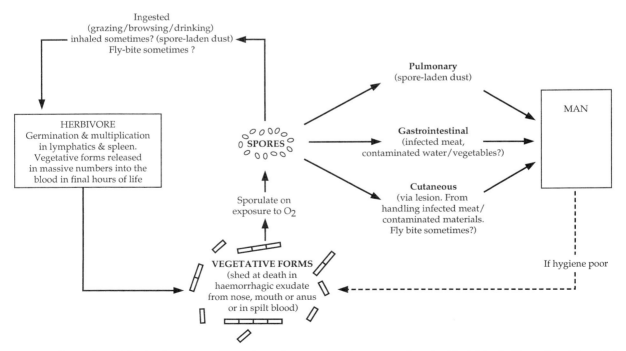

Fig. 1.3 The cycle of infection in anthrax. The primary hosts are herbivores; man is an incidental host. (Reproduced from the *Oxford Textbook of Medicine*, 3rd edn, by kind permission.)

Anthrax remains a major natural culling agent in herbivorous wildlife in certain parts of Africa and, possibly, Asia (see below).

CLINICAL MANIFESTATIONS AND DIAGNOSIS IN ANIMALS

Sudden death in a herbivore without prior symptoms or following a brief period of fever and disorientation should lead to suspicion of anthrax, and bloody fluid exuding from the nose, mouth, or anus of the dead animal is particularly suggestive. In pigs and carnivores, local oedemas, particularly in the neck region, are pathognomonic signs.

At death in most susceptible species, the blood contains 10^7–10^9 bacilli/ml, provided the animal has not been treated (numbers may also be lower in immunized animals which succumb to the disease). Pigs are noted for being an exception and the bacterium may be undetectable in blood at death.

The blood of an anthrax victim clots poorly and usually the small volume of blood necessary for diagnostic smear and culture can be drawn with a syringe from a vein in the reasonably fresh carcass. Where that is not possible, a small piece of tissue, traditionally (but not necessarily) an ear clipping because of its high capillary content, preferably with signs of blood on it, can be excised and used to make a smear and for culture.

Smears should be stained with polychrome methylene blue (M'Fadyean's stain); large numbers of blue–black-staining bacilli, often square ended and in short chains, surrounded by a clearly demarcated pink capsule is fully diagnostic. Specimens for culture should be submitted to the appropriate diagnostic laboratory.

If anthrax is suspected, the carcass should generally not be opened; contamination of the environment by spilled body fluids is thereby avoided. In pigs, where confirmation may depend on obtaining the relevant lymph node (submandibular, suprapharyngeal, or mesenteric) for culture, appropriate precautions should be taken before dissection to avoid environmental contamination.

For differential diagnosis, blackleg, botulism, toxicosis (e.g. toxic plants, heavy metals, snake bite), lightning strike, and peracute babesiosis may cause symptoms similar to those of anthrax.

CLINICAL MANIFESTATIONS AND DIAGNOSIS IN HUMANS

Traditionally, anthrax can take three forms in humans depending on the route of entry of the spores. Of the three—cutaneous, pulmonary, and intestinal—cutaneous is by far the most common.

In cutaneous anthrax, entry of the infecting *B. anthracis* takes place through a lesion in the skin. About 3–5 days later (range 2–12 days; Professor M. Doganay, Erciyes University, Kayseri, Turkey, personal communication), a small pimple appears. (Salmon (1896) recorded the personal observation of the development of a pustule 12 hours after inoculation of an abrasion on the knuckle of a groom by the strap of a new horse brush). Over the next 2–3 days, the centre of the pimple ulcerates to become a dry, black, firmly adherent scab, surrounded by a ring of vesicles. This is the typical anthrax eschar. Despite its angry appearance, there is little pain; pain and pus only develop if there is secondary infection of the lesion. The lesions vary greatly in size from about 2 cm to several centimetres across and are always accompanied by marked to massive oedema which may spread a long way from the lesion. The oedema from lesions on the face or neck may become life-threatening. In uncomplicated cases, the eschar begins to resolve about 10 days after the appearance of the initial papule; resolution takes 2–6 weeks, regardless of treatment, but usually leaves little trace. Infection may spread from skin lesions to the bloodstream causing an overwhelming septicaemia. In the 15-year period 1899–1913, well before the availability of a human vaccine or effective treatment, of 318 cases of industrial cutaneous anthrax in Britain, 40 (12.5 per cent) were fatal (Anon 1918). Today, we might expect that untreated, fewer than 20 per cent of cutaneous cases would be fatal.

Diagnosis of cutaneous anthrax is made by M'Fadyean-stained smears and/or culture of pre-treatment specimens of vesicular fluid obtained from under the edge of the eschar. For differential diagnosis, boil, orf, primary syphilitic chancre, erysipelas, plague, glanders, and tropical ulcer should be considered.

In pulmonary (due to inhalation of spores) and intestinal (due to ingestion of contaminated meat) forms of anthrax, illness begins insidiously with mild symptoms of slight fever, malaise, and gastroenteritis lasting one to a few days. This phase ends with the abrupt onset of severe illness with fever and chills quickly to prostration, shock, collapse, and death within a few hours. There is no practical way of confirming diagnosis before the onset of the acute phase and recognition of the likely cause of illness usually depends on knowledge of the patient's probable exposure to anthrax spores. It is thought that milder or subclinical infections do occur. It may be possible to observe the capsulated bacilli in M'Fadyean-stained smears of blood or faeces after onset of the acute phase. After death, the approach to diagnosis is the same as for animals (above).

An occasional complication of any of the other forms of anthrax is meningitis. The cerebrospinal fluid may be blood stained and the capsulated bacilli ma be visible on M'Fadyean-stained smears. Anthrax meningoencephalitis is seen with some frequency in Tamil Nadu, India (George *et al.* 1994).

Second infections in the same individual are rare but not unheard of (Heyworth *et al.* 1975; Anon 1982; Christie 1987).

INDUSTRIAL ANTHRAX

Human anthrax is frequently differentiated into non-industrial or industrial anthrax, depending on whether the diseases is acquired directly from animals or indirectly during the handling and processing of contaminated animal products. Non-industrial anthrax usually affects people who work with animals or animal carcasses, such as farmers, abattoir workers, knackers, butchers, and veterinary personnel, and is almost always cutaneous, although occasionally intestinal if, as occurs in developing countries, the owners skin, butcher, and eat the meat. Industrial anthrax, occurring as a result of handling and processing contaminated hair, wool, hides, bones, or other animal products, is usually cutaneous but has a higher chance of being pulmonary through inhalation of spore-laden dust. In the period 1899–1913, of 354 reported cases of industrial anthrax in Britain, 36 (10.2 per cent) were pulmonary (Anon 1918). (In contrast, between 1961 and 1980, of 122 occupationally exposed individuals with anthrax in Britain, only one pulmonary case was recorded CDSC (1982).)

PATHOLOGY

In most countries, autopsies of animals or humans known or suspected to have died of anthrax are forbidden. Inadvertent autopsies and experimental infections in contained facilities reveal a consistent picture; dark unclotted blood, markedly enlarged and haemorrhagic spleen and affected lymph nodes, and petechial haemorrhages of other viscera. In intestinal anthrax, the intestinal mucosa is dark red with glassy oedema and areas of necrosis at the site of the eschar.

The principal lesions of anthrax are those of oedema, haemorrhage, and necrosis. The microscopic picture of the cutaneous lesion is one of extensive cellulitis with much oedema, some necrosis, cellular infiltrators consisting of mononuclear, neutrophilic, and eosinophilic cells, haemorrhage, and a large number of bacilli. The oedema is the predominant change; much more so than the inflammatory cell infiltrate (study in the rhesus monkey, *Macaca mulatta*, Gleiser 1967).

Most of the detailed studies on the pathology of anthrax were done in the 1940s, 1950s, and 1960s. At that time, authors (Young *et al.* 1946; Barnes 1947; Ross 1955, 1957; Widdicombe *et al.* 1956; Gleiser 1967; Gleiser *et al.* 1968; Dalldorf *et al.* 1971) were universally agreed that the anthrax bacilli multiplied more rapidly in the lymph nodes than in other tissues, and that the nodes acted as centres for the proliferation and dissemination of the bacilli, leading to septicaemia and death (Widdicombe *et al.* 1956). Thus, if the primary site of infection is the skin, there is oedema, cellular infiltration and multiplication of the bacilli, and the regional lymph nodes become enlarged, haemorrhagic, and contain the bacilli. In inhalation anthrax, there is less involvement at the site of invasion and changes in lung parenchyma, such as hyperaemia, oedema, and cellular infiltration, are mild or absent (Young *et al.* 1946). The bacilli do not multiply in the lung itself but cause a massive infection of the mediastinal lymph nodes; the alveolar lining acts merely as a portal of entry of the bacilli, and multiplication and subsequent bacteriaemia only take place after infection of the lymph nodes draining the lungs (Barnes 1947). There was no evidence that inhaled anthrax spores reached the bloodstream direct from the lung. A proportion of spores are killed by the macrophages in transit (Ross 1957).

The earliest histological changes in the lymph nodes and spleen are necrosis of germinal centres. As infection proceeds, the nodes become oedematous and then haemorrhagic; veins and capillaries within the nodes become filled with thrombi composed of leucocytes, platelets, fibrin, and bacteria (Dalldorf *et al.* 1971). On occasion pneumonia does result from oedema and haemorrhage and thrombosis of the pulmonary vascular bed, though it is not clear if this represents primary infection or re-infection.

The basic disease mechanism is vascular injury with oedema, haemorrhage, and thrombosis. Vascular injury is the result of the toxin acting directly on the endothelial cell membranes, making them highly permeable to plasma and causing adhesion of the leucocytes and platelets with widespread intravascular thrombosis (Dalldorf *et al.* 1971).

Gleiser (1967) found a marked difference in the response in the lung to aerosol infection when comparing susceptible species, as represented by the sheep and rhesus monkey, with more resistant hosts, represented by the dog and the pig. In the latter, discrete, intensely haemorrhagic, fibrinous, and cellular lesions completely obliterated the normal pulmonary architecture. The centre of the lesion was massive haemorrhage; surrounding this was a zone comprised of dense masses of fibrin which occluded alveoli, bronchioles, and vessels. Intermingling with the fibrin at the periphery was a dense accumulation of neutrophils, plasma cells, monocytes, and large macrophages. Bacilli could not be demonstrated in these lesions. Such intense fibrinous and cellular responses were not observed in the sheep and rhesus monkey, which only showed a mild cellular and fibrinous response. The pathogenesis and pathology of anthrax in the pig has recently been re-examined (Redmond *et al.* 1997).

The histological appearance in the meningitic form seen in nine monkeys was again oedema, haemorrhage, and thrombosis of many small cerebral veins. These veins and the subarachnoid space contained thousands of anthrax bacilli (Dalldorf *et al.* 1971).

The intense reaction in the more resistant hosts was seen as representing their ability to isolate or 'wall off' the invading organisms. The lesions found in the lungs of dogs and pigs indicated that only local foci of infection had developed, the organisms, having been contained by the massive deposits of fibrin and activity of the cellular infiltrations. The ability of the host to respond in this manner must be one possible reason for the lack of systemic infection. Such lesions have not been observed in highly susceptible hosts such as the sheep, which show only minimal cellular changes in response to the large numbers of organisms seen in their lungs, probably representing their complete inability to cope with the infection (Gleiser 1967).

TREATMENT

Penicillin or its relatives are the best antimicrobials. Isolates resistant to penicillin have only been reported on two or three occasions and resistance does not seem to be readily transmissible. *Bacillus anthracis* is also sensitive to many other broad-spectrum antibiotics, including tetracyclines, chloramphenicol, gentamicin, and erythromycin, which may be used if the isolate is reported as resistant to penicillin or the patient is allergic to it.

It has been the experience of some veterinarians that tetracycline treatment is not always fully effective, although tests in monkeys showed that doxycycline gave good protection when administered prophylactically (Friedlander *et al.* 1993). The fluoroquinolone, ciprofloxacin, was also effective in this capacity. Antibiotics are not active against the spores of *B. anthracis*, however, and it appears that inhaled spares are only cleared slowly from the lungs (Friedlander *et al.* 1993). Thus antibiotic prophylaxis against known exposure to substantial numbers of inhaled anthrax spores may have to be prolonged (several weeks) and should be supplemented by vaccination so that immunity has been built up by the time the antibiotics are withdrawn.

In livestock in Britain, when a case of anthrax occurs in a herd of flock, the herd or flock is observed closely and antibiotics are administered at the first sign of fever among any other members of the herd of flock. This is normally an effective procedure.

PROGNOSIS

Because, until recently, there has not been a way of diagnosing mild or subclinical cases of anthrax in animals, the tendency has been to regard anthrax as inevitably fatal. The development of specific serological tests have made it possible to examine this more closely (Turnbull *et al.* 1993). The evidence from these is that low numbers of seropositives may be expected in any group of herbivores (most susceptible to anthrax) exposed to a source of infection, indicating that a small proportion of the group may suffer mild or subclinical infection and survive. In contrast, relatively high proportions of exposed carnivores (relatively resistant to anthrax) have antibodies, indicating that relatively few of those infected die of the disease.

The resistance of humans to anthrax is said to be intermediate between that of true herbivores and carnivores. Limited data from cutaneously or orally exposed but untreated individuals again suggest that mild or subclinical infection is not uncommon (Heyworth *et al.* 1975; Turnbull *et al.* 1993). The proportion of cutaneous cases might be expected to result in death if untreated is in the order of 10–20 per cent. Data on infectious dose on which to base assessments of risk from environments contaminated with anthrax spores have been compiled by Watson and Keir (1994).

Timely treatment is obviously paramount in fulminant anthrax infections. The cause of death is toxaemia and, while antibiotic treatment may effectively kill all the infecting *B. anthracis*, if administered too late, toxic death may still ensue. It is failure to recognize the symptoms early enough, rather than resistance to treatment in pulmonary and intestinal forms of anthrax, that leads to their high fatality rates.

EPIDEMIOLOGY

OCCURRENCE

According to reports received by the Office International des Epizooties (OIE), although few countries are truly enzootic for anthrax, most have some cases of the disease in their livestock in any one year (Fig. 1.4). Countries experiencing relatively increased incidence are those in sub-Saharan Africa, the Indian subcontinent and Indonesia, certain provinces of China, parts of Turkey, and various countries of the former USSR.

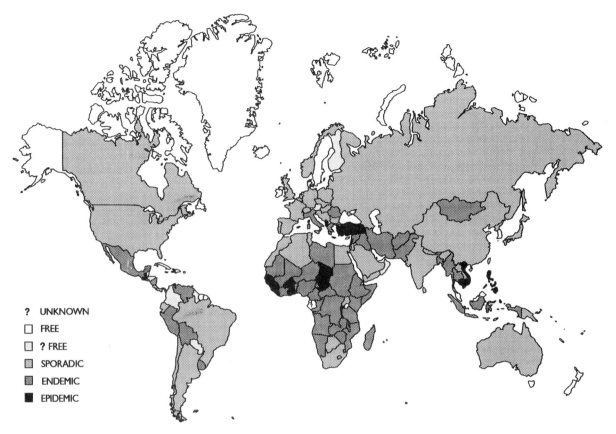

Fig. 1.4 Global incidence of anthrax. Collated from the 1992 FAO–WHO–OIE Animal Health Yearbook. (Computergraphics produced and kindly supplied by Dr M. E. Hugh-Jones, Director, WHO Collaborating Center for Reference and Training in Remote Sensing and Geographical Systems for Veterinary Public Health, School of Veterinary Medicine, Louisiana State University, USA.)

The incidence of the disease has declined dramatically in Britain over the past century (Fig. 1.5). This is due to:

(1) improved factory hygiene;
(2) the development in 1937 of an effective livestock vaccine which significantly reduced the incidence of the disease throughout the world, and hence the levels of contamination in animal products imported into this country;
(3) the increased use of man-made alternatives to animal products;
(4) the first stages of the processing of hides are now being carried out in the country of origin; and
(5) the human vaccine may have contributed to a reduction in industrial cases of anthrax.

More detailed information on notifications of anthrax in the United Kingdom and elsewhere in recent years is given the *Proceedings of the International Workshop on Anthrax* (Turnbull 1990).

Nevertheless, because of the ability of the anthrax spore to persist for decades, and because of the increasing rarity with which the disease is seen, there is a danger of complacency. Specialized leather and woollen industries continue to depend on hides and wool from particular species or breeds that can only be raised in countries that are still endemic; similarly, sun-dried bones from animals that die naturally in tropical Asia have qualities for charcoal production that cannot be reproduced in temperate Europe or North America. The demand in developed countries for bonemeal for feeds and fertilizers exceeds domestic availability and continues to depend on extensive importation, again often from endemic areas.

Most industrial processes kill anthrax spores, so final products such as woollen goods, leather, and charcoal are free of spores. Similarly, many manufacturers in developed countries consider it standard good practice to heat-treat bonemeal before placing it on the market. However, effluent from the early stages of processing, such as the initial wash, many carry anthrax

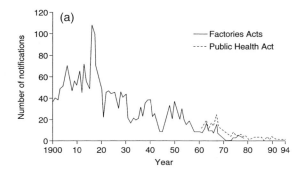

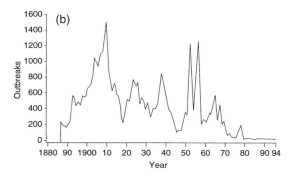

Fig. 1.5 Notifications of human (a) and livestock (b) anthrax in the UK since 1900. (Data kindly supplied by CDSC (a) and the MAFF Notifiable Diseases Unit, Tolworth (b).)

spores into the environment, for example through sewage sludge spread on fields, where they may infect livestock. Figure 1.6 is a diagrammatic representation of what we perceive to be the potential cycle of anthrax in Britain and, probably, other industrialized countries today.

TRANSMISSION IN ANIMALS

Epidemics are of the point source type; animal to animal transmission appears to be a rare event, although in some countries it is believed that such transmission is mediated by biting flies; there is experimental support for this possibility.

Although one of the oldest diseases in terms of human records, much is still not understood about how animals acquire anthrax and the factors influencing this. In large wild mammals, it would appear to be one of nature's culling agents; the disease only became a 'nuisance' when man began to domesticate animals. Among the unknowns are why it usually strikes spasmodically within groups of individuals which appear to be equally exposed, while at other times it causes large, unpredicted epizootics. There is little doubt that outbreaks are influenced climatically but, as reviewed by Lindeque and Turnbull (1994), the rules appear to differ in different parts of the world.

Some age/sex differences have been noted by authors from time to time but such differences appear to be of minor importance. An early study (Weinstein 1938) indicated that differences could not be readily attributable to the circulating sex hormones.

Very little experimental information is available to throw light on the anomalies of natural anthrax. Experimental anthrax is usually concerned with elucidating the effect of artificial scenarios, such as aerosol or parenteral LD_{50} determinations for vaccine protection purposes, usually to answer military defence-related concerns. Such oral feeding studies as have been done indicate that very high doses are required to initiate clinical infection, even in susceptible species—far higher than are likely to be encountered by livestock in endemic or spasmodic areas. The belief is that it only takes one spore reaching the right site to initiate infection and the high experimental dose is a

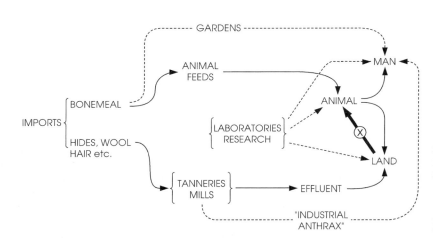

Fig. 1.6 The perceived cycle of anthrax into and within the UK and, probably, other industrialized countries. 'X' represents the stage at which the spores can persist for many years awaiting a new host. (Reproduced, with modification, from the *PHLS Microbiology Digest* (1992), volume 9, by kind permission.)

reflection of the many factors working against the occurrence of that event.

TRANSMISSION IN HUMANS

Human-to-human transmission is exceedingly rare, probably because of the high infectious dose, but exceptions have been recorded (Heyworth *et al.* 1975) (This author was told, when visiting a mission hospital in Zimbabwe in 1987, of a case of anthrax in a nursing orderly contracted while dressing the lesion of a patient.) As indicated earlier, man normally contracts anthrax directly or indirectly from animals. Since cutaneous anthrax normally occurs from infection through a lesion in the skin, exposed regions of the body are most frequently affected and the site of infection often reflects the occupation of the patient. Workers who carry hides or carcasses on their shoulders are liable to infection on the back of the neck; handlers of other animal materials or products tend to be infected on the hands, arms, or wrists. As with animals, biting flies are thought to be capable of transmitting anthrax to humans in some countries.

The fact that, in some countries, the value of meat from animals that have died unexpectedly outweighs the perceived risks of serious illness from eating it has already been mentioned, and gastrointestinal illness is contracted as a result of this in these countries. Traditions by which meat from such an animal may not be disposed of if the owner is away but must be held (dried) until he returns further exacerbate the problem, especially as increasing mobility is occurring in formerly isolated communities.

Man appears to be relatively resistant to infection. The best documented evidence of this comes from studies in the 1960s in mills in which unvaccinated workers 'chronically exposed' to anthrax had annual case rates of 0.6–1.4 per cent (Brachman *et al.* 1962). In a study of two such mills, *B. anthracis* was recovered from the nose and pharynx of 14 per cent of healthy workers; in another study (Dahlgren *et al.* 1960), workers were inhaling 600–1300 spores during the working day with no ill effect, although a well-documented outbreak of pulmonary anthrax occurred in one mill with a similar level of contamination (Plotkin *et al.* 1960). High exposure but low infection rates are evident today among humans in certain parts of Africa.

Some estimate of risk of infection in humans can be obtained from primate experiments. A parenteral LD_{50} of 3000 spores was reported in rhesus monkeys (Lincoln *et al.* 1967). Reported inhalation LD_{50}s in monkeys range from 4130 to 760 000 (Watson and Keir 1994). To base risk assessments for inhalation anthrax on an LD_{50} of 4000 for man is highly conservative since:

(1) dose may be dependent on body weight;
(2) humans are thought to be more resistant than monkeys, possibly related to their being more carnivorous;
(3) reports of inhalation LD_{50}s in species regarded as highly susceptible to anthrax are generally also in the order of tens of thousands;
(4) the probability of the spores reaching the lungs falls off greatly as inhaled particle size exceeds 5 μm; and
(5) case rates in pre-vaccination days were low in workers known to be inhaling spores in at-risk occupations.

As with cutaneous anthrax, the risk of inhalation anthrax anthrax can be greatly reduced by appropriate industrial hygiene, protective clothing, including protective breathing gear, vaccination, and medical awareness in the event of illness, leading to prompt treatment.

PREVENTION AND CONTROL

Control of anthrax for both humans and livestock lies in breaking the cycle of infection depicted in Fig. 1.3. Well-supervised disposal of carcasses from the occasional case of anthrax which occurs in cattle, sheep, horses, or pigs, and of materials contaminated from the carcasses, followed by disinfection of affected premises, and immediate vaccination of other members of the affected herd, ensure good containment and control of the disease.

In Britain, treatment is used as a control measure (in some countries this approach is not permitted). Following the first incident of anthrax in a herd, the remaining members of the herd are monitored carefully for symptoms of illness; any animal showing signs of elevated temperature or increased respiration rate is given immediate antibiotic treatment. In less-developed countries with limited communications and resources of fuel for incineration or rendering, shortages of disinfectants or antibiotics, and a reluctance to waste meat, the only approach is mass vaccination of livestock.

Although official recommendations in most countries are that anthrax carcasses be buried or burnt, the legacy of contaminated land apparent today from burials in the past (often decades ago) shows that incineration is the only truly satisfactory option. Some countries prefer rendering, although the problem of preventing contamination of environment and equipment during transport and loading into the rendering plant has to be addressed in this approach. Mobile blow-torch incinerators are available, but even with these, complete destruction of a bovine carcass can take more than 24 hours. A universal solution to the problem of anthrax carcass disposal is proving hard to devise.

Disinfection of rooms, animal houses, vehicles, and other equipment is best done with 5–10 per cent formaldehyde (15–30 per cent formalin), although it may be more practical to steam clean the surfaces or equipment and formalin treat the washings. Obviously neutralization of the formalin needs to be addressed also. Decontamination of soil at burial sites of infected animals can pose intractable problems. Chlorine solutions have to be very strong to be effective against anthrax spores. The topic of disinfection and decontamination for anthrax is treated in more detail elsewhere (Turnbull *et al.* 1993).

CONTROL IN WILDLIFE

Anthrax has probably been a major cause of mortality in herbivorous mammals, at least in warmer climates, throughout history, and, until recently, an equilibrium existed between these animals and *B. anthracis*, which probably played the role of one of nature's main culling agents at times of overpopulation. Problems have arisen in recent years because this equilibrium has been upset through reduction in the ranges of the animals and restriction of their natural migration patterns in the face of increasing human encroachment on their lands. This has led to overpopulation and overgrazing of the areas remaining available to the animals.

Applying control criteria designed for domestic animals is probably not appropriate or applicable. The legislation in most countries which requires incineration or burial of anthrax carcasses is generally impractical for wildlife, due to:

(1) the lack of personnel to carry out the work, or fuel to do the burning; and
(2) the fact that, for every carcass observed, many undoubtedly are not observed.

It remains debatable whether anthrax vaccine should become a routine part of game management, even in an enzootic area, and it is arguable that this could constitute unwarranted interference with natural processes. The ecological consequences of random mass vaccination in such environments is unpredictable. However, nowadays wildlife ranges are frequently artificially confined spaces and, since natural processes cannot always operate as they should, a management programme may have to involve a certain level of anthrax control activities. The possibility of an outbreak getting out of control or of endangering a particular species (rhino being a particularly good example) must be kept in mind and contingency plans should be ready.

At present, immunization depends on the use of the livestock vaccine which requires either direct dart gun administration or immobilization of the animals followed by administration with a syringe. Either way is expensive, traumatic for the animals and, at best, can only give cover to a small core of susceptible animals. Also it must be remembered that the duration of effectiveness of the vaccine is thought to be only about a year. Considerations are being given to development of suitable oral vaccines for this purpose, although numerous obstacles must be overcome before oral vaccines (there may have to be several for application under different circumstances and to different target species) satisfying all safety, environmental contamination, and efficacy criteria, and of delivery systems that guarantee uptake by the majority of targeted animals (but not non-targeted ones), are developed.

VACCINES

Credit for the development of the vaccine that turned anthrax from a global scourge to a relatively minor problem in most parts of the world belongs to Dr M. Sterne, whose live spore livestock vaccine developed in the 1930s is still used in most countries where anthrax is encountered. The vaccine consists of approximately 10^7 spores/ml of his strain $34F_2$ in 50 per cent glycerine-saline with about 0.5 per cent saponin, which acts as an adjuvant by causing irritation and inflammation at the vaccination site. The strain was a rough, avirulent descendant of an isolate from a case of bovine anthrax. It was subsequently shown to have lost plasmid pX02, thereby being unable to produce the capsule. It still produces the toxin and protects by inducing humoral and cell-mediated immunity to the protective antigen.

Although theoretically avirulent because it is acapsular, the Sterne vaccine does retain a residual virulence and occasional casualties in sheep, goats, laboratory, and other animals occur. As a result, the live vaccine was not considered suitable for human use in Western countries (live vaccines are used in Soviet countries in China) and acellular vaccines were developed in the 1950s in the United Kingdom and in the 1960s in the United States. The British vaccine consists of an alum-precipitated cell-free filtrate of Sterne strain cultures grown in such a way as to maximize the content of protective antigen.

Since control of anthrax depends on control of the disease in animals, the human vaccine is only for use in protecting persons in at-risk occupations. Much of the research within the field of anthrax in the past 15 years has centred around putative modern alternatives to the rather old human vaccine formulations.

The improved understanding of anthrax toxin at the molecular level in the past few years has led to a number of alternative ideas and approaches for improving anthrax vaccines in the future (Turnbull 1991). These range from subunit formulations consisting of purified PA mixed with an effective adjuvant, through live vaccines comprised of mutant strains which are fully antigenic but also fully avirulent, and recombinant vaccines in which another host expresses the PA, to oral vaccines consisting either of a suitable recombinant salmonella or microencapsulated PA. Regardless of the approach taken, the aim is to deliver protective antigen with an appropriate cellular immune stimulant. So far, however, it has not been possible to take promising formulations to clinical trials and, in consequence, the old vaccines remain in use. The obstacles, both scientific and regulatory, to getting any of these 'on the shelf' in the foreseeable future appear formidable.

REFERENCES

Anon (1918). Report of the Departmental Committee appointed to inquire as to precautions for preventing danger of infection from anthrax in the manipulation of wool, goat hair, and camel hair. Vol. III. Summary of evidence and appendices, p. 116. HMSO, London.

Anon (1982). Communicable disease report, 82/15. PHLS Communicable Disease Surveillance Centre, London.

Barnes, J. M. (1947). The development of anthrax following the administration of spores by inhalation. *British Journal of Experimental Pathology*, **28**, 385–94.

Bowen, J. E. and Turnbull, P. C. B. (1992). The fate of *Bacillus anthracis* in unpasteurized and pasteurized milk. *Letters in Applied Microbiology*, **15**, 224–7.

Brachman, P. S., Gold, H., Plotkin, S. A., Fekety, F. R., Werrin, M., and Ingraham, N. R. (1962). Field evaluation of a human anthrax vaccine. *American Journal of Public Health*, **52**, 632–45.

CDSC (1982). PHLS Communicable Disease Surveillance Centre Anthrax surveillance 1961–80. *British Medical Journal*, **284**, 204.

Choquette, L. P. E. and Broughton, E. (1981). In *Infectious diseases of wild mammals*, (ed. J. W. Davis, L. H. Karsted, and D. O. Trainer), (2nd edn), pp. 288–96. Iowa State University Press, Ames, Iowa.

Christie, A. B. (1987). Anthrax. In *Infectious diseases: epidemiology and clinical practice*, (ed. A. B. Christie), (4th edn), pp. 983–1003, Churchill Livingstone, London.

Dahlgren, C. M., Buchanan, L. M., Decker, H. M., Freed, S. W., Phillips, C. R., and Brachman, P. S. (1960). *Bacillus anthracis* aerosols in goat hair processing mills. *American Journal of Hygiene*, **72**, 6–23.

Dalldorf, F. G., Kaufmann, A. F., and Brachman, P. S. (1971). Woolsorter's disease. *Archives of Pathology*, **92**, 418–26.

Ezzell, J. W., Ivins, B. E., and Leppla, S. H. (1984). Immunoelectrophoretic analysis, toxicity, and kinetics of *in vitro* production of the protective antigen and lethal factor components of *Bacillus anthracis* toxin. *Infection and Immunity*, **45**, 761–7.

Friendlander, A. M., *et al.* (1993). Postexposure prophylaxis against experimental inhalation anthrax. *Journal of Infectious Diseases*, **167**, 1239–42.

George, S., Mathai, D., Balraj, V., Lalitha, M. K., and Jacob John, T. (1994). An outbreak of anthrax meningo-encephalitis, *Transactions of the Royal Society for Tropical Medicine & Hygiene*, **88**, 206–7.

Gleiser, C. A. (1967). Pathology of anthrax infection in animal hosts. *Federation Proceedings*, **26**, 1518–21.

Gleiser, C. A., Gochenour, W. S., and Ward, M. K. (1968). Pulmonary lesions in dogs and pigs exposed to a cloud of anthrax spores. *Journal of Comparative Pathology*, **78**, 445–9.

Hanna, P. C., Acosta, D., and Collier, R. J. (1993). On the role of macrophages in anthrax. *Proceedings of the National Academy of Sciences, USA*, **90**, 10198–201.

Henderson, I. (1996). Fingerprinting *Bacillus anthracis* strains. *Proceedings of the International Workshop on Anthrax, 19–21 September 1995*, (ed. P. C. B. Turnbull). Salisbury Medical Bulletin, No. 87, Special supplement, 55–8.

Henderson, I., Duggleby, C. J., and Turnbull, P. C. B. (1994). Differentiation of *Bacillus anthracis* from other *Bacillus cereus* group bacteria with the PCR. *International Journal of Systematic Bacteriology*, **44**, 99–105.

Heyworth, B., Ropp, M. E., Voos, U. G., Meinel, H. I., and Darlow, H. M. (1975). Anthrax in the Gambia: an epidemiological study. *British Medical Journal*, **4**, 79–82.

Klein, F., Hodges, D. R., Mahlandt, B. G., Jones, W. I., Haines, B. W., and Lincoln, R. E. (1962). Anthrax toxin: causative agent in the death of rhesus monkeys. *Science*, **138**, 1331–3.

Klemm, D. M. and Klemm, W. R. (1959). A history of anthrax. *Journal of the American Veterinary Medical Association*, **135**, 458–62.

Klimpel, K. R., Arora, N., and Leppla, S. H. (1994). Anthrax toxin lethal factor contains a zinc metalloprotease consensus sequence which is required for lethal toxin activity. *Molecular Microbiology*, **13**, 1093–100.

Kochi, S. K., Schiavo, G., Mock, M., and Montecucco, C. (1994). Zinc content of the *Bacillus anthracis* lethal factor. *FEMS Microbiology Letters*, **124**, 343–8.

Leppla, S. H. (1991). The anthrax toxin complex. In *Sourcebook of bacterial protein toxins*, (ed. J. E. Alouf and J. H. Freer), pp. 277–302. Academic Press, New York.

Lincoln, R. E., Walker, J. S., Klein, F., Rosenwald, A. J., and Jones, W. I. (1967). Value of field data for extrapolation in anthrax. *Federation Proceedings*, **26**, 1558–62.

Lindeque, P. M. and Turnbull, P. C. B. (1994). Ecology and epidemiology of anthrax in the Etosha National Park, Namibia. *Onderstepoort Journal of Veterinary Research*, **61**, 71–83.

Little, S. F., Leppla, S. H., Burnett, J. W., and Friedlander, A. M. F. (1994). Structure–function analysis of *Bacillus anthracis* edema factor by using monoclonal antibodies. *Biochemical and Biophysical Research Communications*, **199**, 676–82.

Milne, J. C., Furlong, D., Hanna, P. C., Wall, J. S., and Collier, R. J. (1994). Anthrax protective antigen forms oligomers during intoxication of mammalian cells. *Journal of Biological Chemistry*, **269**, 20606–12.

Ness, G. B. Van (1971). Ecology of anthrax. Anthrax undergoes a propagation phase in soil before it affects livestock. *Science*, **172**, 1303–7.

Parvizpour, D. (1978). Human anthrax in Iran. An epidemiological study of 468 cases. *International Journal of Zoonoses*, **5**, 69–74.

Plotkin, S. A., Brachman, P. S., Utell, M., Bumford, F. H., and Atchison, M. M. (1960). An epidemic of inhalation anthrax, the first in the twentieth century. *American Journal of Medicine*, **29**, 992–1001.

Redmond, C., Hall, G. A., Turnbull, P. C. B., and Gillgan, J. S. Experimentally assessed public health risks associated with pigs from farms experiencing anthrax, *Veterinary Record*, **141**, 244–47.

Ross, J. M. (1955). On the histopathology of experimental anthrax in the guinea-pig. *British Journal of Experimental Pathology*, **36**, 336–9.

Ross, J. M. (1957). The pathogenesis of anthrax following the administration of spores by the respiratory route. *Journal of Pathology and Bacteriology*, **73**, 485–94.

Salmon, D. E. (1896). Anthrax. In *Special report on diseases of the horse*, pp. 526–30. Government Printing Office, Washington.

Sirard, J. C., Mock, M., and Fouet, A. (1994). The three *Bacillus anthracis* toxin genes are coordinately regulated by bicarbonate and temperature. *Journal of Bacteriology*, **176**, 5188–92.

Titball, R. W., Turnbull, P. C. B., and Hutson, R. A. (1991). The monitoring and detection of *Bacillus anthracis* in the environment. *Journal of Applied Bacteriology Symposium Supplement*, **70**, 9S–18S.

Turnbull, P. C. B. (ed.) (1990). *Proceedings of the International Workshop on Anthrax, 11–13 April 1989, Winchester, UK.* Salisbury Medical Bulletin, No. 68, Special supplement.

Turnbull, P. C. B. (1991). Anthrax vaccines: past, present and future. *Vaccine*, **9**, 533–9.

Turnbull, P. C. B., Carman, J. A., Lindeque, P. M., Joubert, F., Hübschle, O. J. B., and Snoeyenbos, G. H. (1989). Further progress in understanding anthrax in the Etosha National Park. *Madoqua*, **16**, 93–104.

Turnbull, P. C. B., Bell, R. H. V., Saigawa, K., Munyenyembe, F. E. C., Mulenga, C. K., and Makala, L. H. C. (1991). Anthrax in wildlife in the Luangwa Valley, Zambia. *Veterinary Record*, **128**, 399–403.

Turnbull, P. C. B., Doganay, M., Lindeque, P. M., Aygen, B., and McLaughlin, J. (1992a). Serology and anthrax in humans, livestock and Etosha National Park wildlife. *Epidemiology and Infection*, **108**, 299–313.

Turnbull, P. C. B. *et al.* (1992b). *Bacillus anthracis* but not always anthrax. *Journal of Applied Bacteriology*, **72**, 21–6.

Turnbull, P. C. B., Böhm, R., Chizyuka, H. G. B., Fujikura, T., Hugh-Jones, M. E., and Melling, J. (1993). *Guidelines for the surveillance and control of anthrax in humans and animals.* World Health Organization, Geneva.

Uchida, I., Hornung, J. M., Thorne, C. B., Klimpel, K. R., and Leppla, S. H. (1993). Cloning and characterization of a gene whose product is a *trans*-activator of anthrax toxin synthesis. *Journal of Applied Bacteriology*, **175**, 5329–39.

Watson, A. and Keir, D. (1994). Information on which to base assessments of risk from environments contaminated with anthrax spores. *Epidemiology and Infection*, **113**, 479–90.

Weinstein, L. (1938). The prophylaxis of experimental anthrax infection with various hormone preparations. *Yale Journal of Biology and Medicine*, **11**, 369–92.

Widdicombe, J. G., Hughes, R., and May, A. J. (1956). The role of the lymphatic system in the pathogenesis of anthrax. *British Journal of Experimental Pathology*, **37**, 343–9.

Wilson, G. S. and Miles, A. (1946). Anthrax. In *Topley and Wilson's principles of bacteriology, virology and immunity*, (3rd edn), pp. 1730–45. Edward Arnold, London.

Young, G. A., Zelle, M. R., and Lincoln, R. E. (1946). Respiratory pathogenicity of *Bacillus anthracis* spores. 1. Methods of study and observations on pathogenesis. *Journal of Infectious Diseases*, **79**, 233–45.

2 BORRELIOSIS (RELAPSING FEVER)

D. T. Dennis

SUMMARY

Louse-borne relapsing fever (LBRF) is caused by infection with *Borrelia recurrentis*. Tick-borne relapsing fever (TBRF) is caused by one of many *Borrelia* designated by the species of soft-shelled *Ornithodoros* ticks responsible for transmission in the locale of exposure. LBRF, previously distributed widely throughout Asia, Africa, and the Americas, has in recent decades been reported only from countries on the horn of Africa: Ethiopia, Somalia, and the Sudan. TBRF occurs sporadically and in small clusters throughout rural Africa, Asia, and the Americas, including the western United States. No good estimates of frequency of occurrence are available for either disease.

Tick vectors of borreliae (Argasidae, *Ornithodoros* species) become infected by feeding on spirochaetaemic rodents and transmit infection to humans via saliva and coxal fluid when they take subsequent blood meals; infection is transmitted vertically in ticks, which constitute an arthropod reservoir. Lice transmit infection when they are crushed, allowing infected body fluids to contaminate broken skin on mucous membranes. Infected lice and ticks remain contagious throughout their lives; lice are short-lived, while soft ticks may live for years.

TBRF is controlled by avoidance of exposure to tick-infested dwellings and infested natural sites, by removing rodent nests and eliminating harbourage for rodents and ticks in places of human habitation, and by selective application of acaricides to tick-infested dwellings or other circumscribed sites of transmission to humans. LBRF is controlled by eliminating body lice and by antibiotic treatment of infected persons.

HISTORY

Although Hippocrates accurately described the clinical features of relapsing fever, the distinction between borrelial fevers and other causes of similar fevers, such as typhus, was first made in outbreaks of apparent LBRF in Scotland in the nineteenth century. The causative spirochaetes were observed first by Obermeier during an outbreak in Germany in 1868; the disease was subsequently transmitted experimentally from person to person by inoculating with infective blood. Mackie, working in India, concluded that the body louse was the principal vector there. Ross, in Uganda, demonstrated that the disease known in East Africa as tick fever was likewise due to a spirochaete found in patients' blood.

Louse-borne relapsing fever was well known over the centuries as a scourge of armies and of civilians affected by war, and during the industrial revolution the disease attacked impoverished slum dwellers in Great Britain and in western Europe. In the 1840's the disease was introduced into the United States by immigrants, and outbreaks occurred in Philadelphia and other East Coast cities for a number of years. During the Second World War, LBRF spilled out of Ethiopia and spread across the Sudan to West Africa, causing hundreds of thousands of cases and a high mortality. It was an important cause of illness in China, India, and in the Near East earlier in the present century, and was reported also from the Andean regions of South America. In north-eastern Africa, LBRF has most recently been the cause of outbreaks in refugee populations fleeing war and famine, and other displaced and homeless persons. The disease has disappeared from most of the world as improvements in standards of living, sanitation, and hygiene have occurred as a result of socio-economic development. Historically, control of outbreaks has been achieved by delousing. The use of DDT and other insecticides during and shortly after the Second World War produced dramatic results.

Tick-borne relapsing fever is a zoonotic disease involving many species of rodents in widely distributed areas throughout the world. Human cases are especially frequent in sub-Saharan Africa, but also occur in countries of the Mediterranean littoral, Middle Eastern states, southern Russia, the Indian subcontinent, and in China. In the Americas, TBRF occurs in the states west of the Mississippi River, especially in the mountainous areas, where *B. hermsii* is the infectious agent. It also occurs in low frequency throughout Latin America. It occurs typically as sporadic cases or in small, often familial, clusters. Infected soft-shelled ticks can maintain infection for many years without a blood meal and can cause repeated infections among persons living or sleeping in the same dwelling. In the

United States, infectious exposures often occur in rustic mountain cabins (Boyer *et al.* 1977) and may be related to focal disappearance of rodents (e.g. as a result of epizootic plague) that serve as the usual maintenance hosts for ticks that transmit the relapsing fever borreliae. Rodent-infested caves in south-western states have been associated with small outbreaks of human infection with *B. turicatae*.

THE AGENT

Relapsing fever borreliae are helical bacteria, 0.2–0.5 × 5–20 μm, having 3–10 or more loose coils. (Schwan, Burgdorfer, and Rosa, 1995) An outer membrane, a middle peptidoglycan layer, and an inner cytoplasmic membrane enclose the cytoplasmic contents. The structures beneath the outer membrane are referred to as the protoplasmic cylinder; uniquely, periplasmic flagella, 15–20 inserted at each end of the bacteria, are situated beneath the outer membrane. *Borrelia* are Gram-stain negative, and stain well with various analine dyes. They are slow-growing and microaerophilic, and grow best at 30–35 °C. The TBRF spirochaetes grow well in a modification of Kelly's medium, Barbour–Stoenner–Kelly (BSK) medium; LBRF spirochaetes are more fastidious in the laboratory and grow poorly on artificial medium.

Table 2.1 Characteristics and distribution of louse-borne and tick-borne borreliae[a]

Borrelia spp.	Arthropod vector	Animal reservoir	Distribution	Disease
B. recurrentis (syn. *B. obermeyeri*, *B. novyi*)	*Pediculus humanus* var. *corporus*	Humans	North eastern Africa ? elsewhere	Louse-borne, epidemic relapsing fever
B. duttonii	*Ornithodoros moubata*	Humans	Central, eastern, southern Africa	East African, tick-borne, endemic relapsing fever
B. hispanica	*O. eraticus* (large variety)	Rodents	Spain, Portugal, Morocco, Algeria, Tunisia	Hispano-African tick-borne relapsing fever
B. crocidurae, *B. merionesi*, *B. microti*, *B. dipodilli*	*O. erraticus* (small variety)	Rodents	Morocco, Libya, Egypt, Iran, Turkey Senegal, Kenya	North African tick-borne relapsing fever
B. persica	*O. tholozani* (syn. *O. papillipes*, *O. crossi?*)	Rodents	From west China and Kashmir to Iraq and Egypt, former USSR, India	Asiatic-African tick-borne relapsing *fever*
B. caucasica	*O. verrucosus*	Rodents	Caucasus to Iraq	Caucasian tick-borne relapsing fever
B. latyschewii	*O. tartakovskyi*	Rodents	Iran, Central Asia	Caucasian tick-borne relapsing fever
B. hermsii	*O. hermsi*	Rodents, chipmunks, and tree squirrels	Western United States	American tick-borne relapsing fever
B. turicatae	*O. turicata*	Rodents	South-western United States	American tick-borne relapsing fever
B. parkeri	*O. parkeri*	Rodents	Western United States	American tick-borne relapsing fever
B. mazzotti	*O. talaje* (*O. dugesi?*)	Rodents	Southern United States, Mexico, Central and South America	American tick-borne relapsing fever
B. venezuelensis	*O. rudis* (syn. *O. venezuelensis*)	Rodents	Central and South America	American tick-borne relapsing fever

[a] Revised from Schwan, T. G., Burgdorfer, W., and Rosa, P. A. (1995). *Borrelia*. In *Manual of Clinical Microbiology*, (6th edn) (ed. P. R. Murray, *et al.*), pp. 626–635. American Society for Microbiology, Washington, D.C., 1995.

Spirochaetes are distinguished from other eubacteria by being placed in the order Spirochaetales. Ribosomal ribonucleic acid (RNA) typing suggests an older and more fundamental distinction. Borreliae are found within the family Spirochaetaceae. All species within the genus *Borrelia* are transmitted to vertebrates by arthropods. Table 2.1 lists the known *Borrelia* species causing relapsing fever in humans, and their associated vectors.

In lice, *B. recurrentis* is found almost exclusively in the haemolymph, while relapsing fever borreliae in ticks invade all tissues, including the salivary glands and the ovaries. In humans, relapsing fever borreliae gain entrance through the skin, multiply within the bloodstream, and circulate in enormous numbers during febrile periods. Although they probably do not multiply outside the bloodstream, the organisms may be found even in afebrile periods in the liver, spleen, CNS, bone marrow, and other tissues where they may cause congestion and petechial haemorrhage. The role of borreliae in causing the systemic disease manifestations of relapsing fever is not wholly clear; although the manifestations resemble responses to endotoxins, and the plasma of some patients with LBRF has been found to test positive for endotoxin-like materials, borreliae and other spirochaetes have not been found to contain endotoxin by *Limulus* lysate assay. However, a spirochaetal heat-stable pyrogenic factor is present that stimulates mononuclear phagocytes to express leucocyte pyrogen (Butler *et al.* 1979).

The characteristic relapsing nature of the illness is due to a remarkable ability of the borreliae to undergo spontaneous, immunity evading, antigenic changes (Barbour 1990). This variability results from DNA rearrangement within genes on linear plasmids encoding for outer surface membrane proteins.

THE HOSTS

ANIMAL HOSTS

Tick-borne relapsing fever borreliae are found in a wide range of rodent reservoir hosts (rats, mice, and squirrels) and in lagomorphs. Borreliosis in these animals is similar to that in humans, in that there may be one or more relapses of spirochaetaemia. Susceptibility differs between species of rodents and to different strains of the borreliae; immature animals are generally more susceptible than adults, and may die as a result of infection. LBRF is not a zoonosis, and humans are the only known mammalian host and reservoir of infection.

DISEASE IN HUMANS

Although there are differences in the presentation and course of illness between LBRF and TBRF, the major clinical manifestations are quite similar (Southern and Sanford 1969). The incubation period ranges between 2 and 18 days, with a mean of about 7 days, and the illness onset is sudden, with rapidly rising fever, headache, shaking chills, sweats, pains in the muscles and joints, and progressive exhaustion. Often, there is dizziness, nausea, and vomiting; sleep may be difficult and accompanied by disturbing dreams; delerium sometimes accompanies high fever. The patient is coherent but withdrawn, thirsty, but disinterested in food and other outside stimuli. Meningism may be present. The fever (usually 39–40 °C or higher) may be continuous or remitting, but is usually high and irregularly intermittent. The pulse is rapid and the patient is mildly tachypnoeic. The conjunctivae are often injected, and sometimes the sclerae are slightly icteric. The mucous membranes are often dry and the patient mildly dehydrated. Scattered petechiae on the trunk, extremities, and the mucous membranes occur in a third or more of LBRF patients and less frequently in TBRF patients. A non-productive cough is common, but chest sounds are usually normal; a pleuritic pain sometimes occurs. Heart sounds are compatible with a high output state. Mild enlargement of the spleen and liver may be present. Frequently occurring complications include thrombocytopenia, mild consumptive coagulopathy, and epistaxis (Dennis *et al.* 1976); less common complications include bleeding into the gastrointestinal tract pneumonitis, myocarditis, splenic rupture, and spontaneous abortion, stillbirth, and neonatal infection. Severe complications are uncommon in otherwise healthy persons, especially if the illness is diagnosed and treated in its early course.

Untreated, the general symptoms of relapsing fever intensify over a 4–6 day period, ending in a spontaneous and characteristic pathophysiologic crisis during which spirochaetes rapidly disappear from the circulating blood and tissues. A Jarisch-Herxheimer reaction commonly occurs within 1–4 hours of treatment with one of the rapidly acting antibiotics, such as erythromycin, tetracyclines, or chloramphenicol, and its severity is positively related to the density of spirochaetes in the blood (Warrell *et al.* 1971, 1983). In the first phase of the crisis (chill phase), rigors and rising fever are accompanied by an increase in cardiac output and increased peripheral vascular resistance. The rectal temperature commonly rises to 41 °C or higher, and the high fever is often accompanied by agitation, confusion, and sometimes delerium. The chill phase terminates after 10–30 minutes, at the time that spirochaetes rapidly disappear from the blood, giving way to a flush phase in which there is a rapid fall in body temperature, drenching sweats, and sometimes (especially in LBRF) a potentially dangerous fall in arterial pressure. Although the cardiac output is maintained at high levels, a decrease in effective circulating blood volume may occur as the peripheral vascular resistance falls. Vital signs must be monitored carefully during this period which usually lasts 8 hours or less. Clinical and electrocardiographic evidences of myocardial dysfunction include gallop rhythms, a prolonged Q-T interval, elevated central venous pressure, hypotension, and pulmonary oedema. Management of patients with myocardial dysfunction requires considerable caution in the administration of intravenous fluids and, in some cases, rapid digitalization (Parry *et al.* 1970). Digoxin should be administered by intravenous injection and oxygen given by mask if acute myocardial failure and pulmonary oedema occur. Steroids and non-steroidal anti-inflammatory agents have not been found to be useful in preventing or significantly ameliorating the crisis, although hydrocortisone and acetaminophen given at the time of antibiotic administration reduce the peak temperature of the ensuing crisis. Bleeding is not controlled by heparin, and there is little evidence of a consumptive coagulopathy. Vitamin K and other soluble vitamins are sometimes added routinely to the intravenous drip of patients with LBRF since they are often malnourished.

The crisis is followed by a period of exhaustion and a rapid and uneventful recovery to normal health. Not uncommonly, patients experience 1 or 2 days of mild fever in the first week of convalescence in the absence of detectable spirochaetaemia. In untreated cases, a relapse of spirochaetaemia and symptoms may recur after a period of several days to weeks. Only one or two relapses characterize LBRF; as many as 10 relapses may occur in persons with untreated TBRF. Usually, the illness becomes shorter and milder, and the afebrile intervals lengthen with each subsequent relapse. Because of the considerable antigenic variation between and within strains, there is no lasting immunity and repeated infections in the same individual have been recorded. Other infectious causes of fever are common in persons at risk for LBRF, especially typhus fever, typhoid, malaria, tuberculosis, and salmonellosis other than typhoid.

Diagnosis

Spirochaetes can be observed by dark-field microscopy, and in Wright-Giemsa-, or acridine orange-stained preparations of thin or dehaemoglobinized thick smears of peripheral blood, or in stained buffy-coat preparations. Organisms are most easily found in blood taken during the febrile periods. Relapsing fever spirochaetes are cultured from blood by inoculating BSK medium or by intraperitoneal inoculation of immature laboratory mice. Serum agglutinins against Proteus OX-K (Weil–Felix reaction) in convalescent serum support the diagnosis. Serum antibodies to *Borrelia* can be detected by enzyme immunoassay and immunoblotting, but the tests are unstandardized and subject to insensitivity resulting from antigenic variations between and within *Borrelia* species and strains. Serological cross-reactions occur with other spirochaetes, including *B. burgdorferi*, the causative agent of Lyme disease.

A distinction between fever of borrelial origin and other fevers may be difficult to make before a remission–relapse cycle has occurred. Relapsing fever is easily confused with malaria, typhus fevers, typhoid, leptospirosis, and arboviral causes of fever, such as dengue. In the United States, the geographical distribution of TBRF overlaps that of Colorado tick fever, a viral illness with similar symptoms in its early stages.

Treatment

Relapsing fever borreliae are exquisitely sensitive to antibiotics (Perine and Teklu 1983) (Table 2.2). Treatment with erythromycin, tetracyclines, chloramphenicol, or penicillin is highly effective in producing clearance of spirochaetes and remission of symptoms. For children less than 9 years of age and for pregnant women, erythromycin and penicillin are the preferred drugs. The use of delayed-release intramuscular penicillin may prolong or delay the clearance of spirochaetes and attenuate the accompanying Jarisch–Herxheimer reaction, but this is not entirely predictable; further, single-dose penicillin treatment sometimes results in relapse of spirochaetaemia and symptoms (Warrell *et al.*, 1983). Although single-dose treatment with erythromycin, tetracyclines, or chloramphenicol is highly effective in producing prompt remission and cure of LBRF, less is known about the efficacy of single-dose treatment of TBRF, and empirical treatment of TBRF for 7 days is recommended to reduce the risk of a persisting borreliosis, CNS infection,

Table 2.2 Antibiotic treatment of louse-borne and tick-borne relapsing fever in adults

Medication	Louse-borne relapsing fever (single adult dose)	Tick-borne relapsing fever (7-day adult doseage schedule)
Oral		
Erythromycin	500 mg	500 mg 6-hourly
Tetracycline	500 mg	500 mg 6-hourly
Doxycycline	100 mg	100 mg twice daily
Chloramphenicol	500 mg	500 mg 6-hourly
Parenteral		Until oral tolerated
Erythromycin	500 mg	500 mg 6-hourly
Tetracycline	250 mg	250 mg 6-hourly
Doxycycline	100 mg	100 mg 12-hourly
Chloramphenicol	500 mg	500 mg 6-hourly
Penicillin G	600 000 IU	600 000 IU daily

and relapsing spirochaetaemia. Because the Jarisch–Herxheimer reaction can result in transient hypotension and cardiac dysfunction, patients should be monitored closely during the first 12 hours of treatment.

Prognosis

Untreated LBRF has a considerable fatality, especially when it occurs in persons of otherwise poor health, such as famine-affected populations. The fatality rate in treated persons is usually less than 5 per cent. In general, TBRF is a milder disease than LBRF, the Jarisch–Herxheimer reaction is less pronounced following treatment of TBRF, and deaths are less frequent.

CONTROL MEASURES

Prevention of rodent access to the foundations and attics of homes or vacation cabins reduces the potential for tick exposure in these dwellings. Structures infested with soft ticks should be treated professionally with acaricides, and rodent-proofed. When in a louse-infested environment, body lice can be controlled by bathing and washing of clothing at frequent intervals, and by use of acaricides. When outbreaks occur in situations such as refugee camps, mass delousing of persons should be carried out with appropriate insecticidal dusts, such as benzene hexachloride (γ -BHC) (1 per cent dust) or malathion (1 per cent dust), and provisions made for washing and change of clothing. Impregnation of clothing with permethrin can provide long-term protection against infestation. Reporting of suspected cases of relapsing fever to health authorities is important for initiating prompt epidemiological investigation and control measures.

REFERENCES

Barbour, A. G. (1990). Antigenic variation of relapsing fever *Borrelia* species. *Annual Review of Microbiology*, **44**, 155–71.

Boyer, K. M. *et al.* (1977). Tick-borne relapsing fever: an interstate outbreak originating at Grand Canyon National Park. *American Journal of Epidemiology*, **105**, 469–79.

Butler, T., Hazen, P., Wallace, C. K., and Awoke, S., Habte-Michael, A. (1979). Infection with, *Borrelia recurrentis*: pathogenesis of fever and petechiae. *Journal of Infections Diseases*, **140**, 665–75.

Cuevas, L. E., Borgnolo, G., Hailu, B., Smith, G., Almaviva, M., and Hart C. (1995). Tumour necrosis factor, interleukin-6 and C-reactive protein in patients with louse-borne relapsing fever in Ethiopia. *Annals of Tropical Medicine and Parasitology*, **89**, 49–54.

Dennis, D. T., Awoke, S., Doberstyn, E. B., and Fresh, J. W. (1976). Bleeding in louse-borne relapsing fever in Ethiopia: clinical and laboratory features in 29 patients. *East African Medical Journal*, **53**, 220–5.

Parry, E. H., Warrell, D. A., Perine, P. L., Vukotich, D., and Bryceson, A. D. (1970). Some effects of louse-borne relapsing fever on the function of the heart. *American Journal of Medicine*, **49**, 472–9.

Perine, P. L. and Teklu, B. (1983). Antibiotic treatment of louse-borne relapsing fever in Ethiopia: A report of 377 cases. *American Journal of Tropical Medicine and Hygiene*, **32**, 1096–100.

Schwan, T. G., Burgdorfer, W., and Rosa, P. A. (1995). *Borrelia*. In *Manual of Clinical Microbiology*, (6th edn) (ed. P. R. Murray, *et al.*), pp. 626–635. American Society for Microbiology, Washington, D.C., 1995.

Southern, P. M. and Sanford J. P. (1969). Relapsing fever: a clinical and microbiological review. *Medicine*, **48**, 129–49.

Warrell, D. A., Perine, P. L., Bryceson, A. D., Parry, E. H. and Pope, H. M. (1971). Physiologic changes during the Jarisch–Herxheimer reaction in early syphilis. A comparison with louse-borne relapsing fever. *American Journal of Medicine*, **51**, 176–85.

Warrell, D. A., Perine, P. L., Krause, D. W., Bing, D. H., and MacDougal, S. J. (1983). Pathophysiology and immunology of the Jarisch–Herxheimer-like reaction in louse-borne relapsing fever: Comparison of tetracycline and slow-release penicillin. *Journal of Infectious Diseases*, **147**, 898–909.

3 BRUCELLOSIS

Michel Plommet, Ramon Diaz, and Jean-Michel Verger

SUMMARY

Brucellosis is transmitted to man from sheep and goats (*Brucella melitensis*), cattle (*Brucella abortus*), and pigs (*Brucella suis*), through direct or indirect contact with infected animals. A primary reticuloendothelial system (RES) infection with bacteraemia and fluctuating fever, brucellosis may affect various organs and tissues, resulting in granulomatous lesions. Possible complications include osteo-articular, cardiac, and neurological sequelae. Spontaneous recovery may occur after several months, sometimes followed by long-lasting, ill-defined malaise. Treatment with appropriate antibiotics is usually curative within 6 weeks. In animals, localization in the placenta may provoke abortion or result in birth of infected offspring. Localization in the udder provides also a route of excretion. Genital excretion may result in contamination of the environment, where *Brucella* can survive for several months. In the milk, the bacteria, (which are killed by pasteurization) survive in fresh dairy products made from unpasteurized milk and cheese but are progressively destroyed by acidification during ripening, depending on the processing. While brucellosis has been almost eliminated from most developed countries, it is still endemic and even increasing in Africa, the Middle East, Central and South-East Asia, South America, and in some Mediterranean countries. The predominant types, bovine, ovine-caprine, or porcine, depend on regional breeding systems. In exposed groups, such as nomads, farmers, veterinarians, laboratory and abattoir workers, prevention relies on hygiene education and medical surveillance. In animals, control (which should be applied on a whole animal community (herd) basis) relies on surveillance, vaccination, and/or elimination of infected animals or herds. Systematic vaccination can stop the spread of brucellosis rapidly but, eradication requires long-term action.

INTRODUCTION

The genus *Brucella* includes five main species (Table 3.1). Three naturally smooth (S) species cause reticuloendothelial system (RES) diseases in animals, with specific localizations in the placenta (causing abortion) and the udder. These species are responsible for a severe zoonosis with systemic and localized symptoms in man. Two naturally rough (R) species cause relatively benign infections, with genital male tract localizations and no, or only exceptional, transmission to man.

Table 3.1 *Brucella* species, their animal hosts, and their pathogenicity for humans[a]

Brucella species[b]	LPS type	Natural host	Other animal species affected	Human disease
B. melitensis	S	Goat, sheep	Wild animals, cattle, camels	Severe
B. abortus	S	Cattle	Wild ruminants, water buffalo, camels	Less severe
B. suis	S	Pig, hare (biovar 2), reindeer (biovar 4)	Various wild species	Severe (except biovar 2)
B. ovis	R	Sheep (ram)	None	None
B. canis	R	Dog	None	Benign

[a] Adapted, by permission of the World Health Organization, from Alton and Plommet (1986).
[b] A sixth species, *B. neotomae*, has been found in the American wood rat and holds little, if any, practical interest.

The three zoonoses, *B. melitensis*, (also known as Malta, Mediterranean, or undulant fever), *B. abortus*, ('enzootic abortion' in bovines), and *B. suis*, having many common features, will be considered together, while *B. ovis* ('contagious epididymitis' in rams) and *B. canis* will be mentioned briefly.

HISTORY

The most important event in the history of brucellosis happened on the island of Malta in 1887, when Bruce isolated the bacterium responsible for a human disease then called 'Malta' or 'Mediterranean' fever from the spleens of British soldiers who had died. Bruce succeeded in reproducing the disease in monkeys and in 1893 named the organism *Micrococcus melitensis*, renamed later in his honour *Brucella melitensis*. In spite of the paramount importance of this discovery, major questions remained: where and how did humans contract the disease? To answer these decisive questions the British Government, worried by the high incidence of Malta fever in army and navy personnel stationed on the island, set up the Mediterranean Fever Commission under the chairmanship of Bruce in 1904. One year later Zammit, the only Maltese member of the Commission, established the aetiology of the disease by accident. Zammit was looking for an experimental animal in which to study the disease. Goats were the only animals locally available in adequate numbers. On 14 June 1905, before attempting to infect a group of goats, he tested their blood for antibodies against Bruce's bacterium and, to his surprise, found that high dilutions of the serum of five out of six goats agglutinated the organism. This important discovery was confirmed by Horrocks who, on 21 June 1905, isolated *M. melitensis* from the milk of a naturally infected goat. The Malta fever mystery was thus solved and a new disease of animals discovered. Further investigations showed that about 40 per cent of the goats in Malta were serologically positive, and that many apparently healthy goats were excreting *M. melitensis* in their milk. Consequently, the consumption of unboiled goat's milk by all military and naval forces in Malta was forbidden. A dramatic reduction in the incidence of Malta fever resulted, which represents a classical demonstration of the importance of epidemiological findings to public health (Vassalo 1992).

At the same time in Denmark, Bang was working on contagious abortion in cattle. In 1897, he succeeded in isolating the bacterium responsible for this disease, a small bacillus, named by his contemporaries *Bacterium abortus* or Bang's bacillus. The organism was later identified in the milk of infected cows, but it took many more years before its role in human pathology was accepted unanimously.

Alice Evans in the United States was the first, in 1918, to relate Bruce's micrococcus and Bang's bacillus. She was then studying the bacterial species commonly present in fresh cow milk, and focused her attention on *Bacterium abortus* that had been suspected to be dangerous to human health. In the sample of milk bacteria she was studying, was *M. melitensis*. Alice Evans demonstrated that all strains of both species behaved similarly in all culture tests then available for differentiating bacteria and also in cross-agglutination. 'Considering the close relationship between the two organisms, and the reported frequency of virulent strains of *Bacterium abortus* in cows milk', she therefore concluded 'it would seem remarkable that we do not have a disease resembling Malta fever prevalent in this country' (Evans 1918). These results and conclusions were unfortunately greeted with scepticism by most bacteriologists and physicians. Only after a further 2 years did Meyer and Shaw confirm the work of Alice Evans and proposed the creation of the genus *Brucella* with two species *B. melitensis* and *B. abortus*. Nine years later (1929), a third species, *B. suis*, was added to the list by Huddleson, to encompass the strains of swine origin isolated in 1914 in the United States, which had long been considered as a porcine variety of Bang's bacillus. *Brucella suis* was shown to give rise to undulant fever in man (Spink 1956).

One hundred and six years after the discovery of Bruce, *B. melitensis*, *B. abortus*, and *B. suis* remain the actors of an animal disease that 'threatens millions of people' and, as such, is regarded by WHO as 'the most widespread of all zoonoses'. In spite of many scientific advances in the field of molecular biology and immunochemistry, many pages of the history of brucellosis have to be written before this zoonosis can to be eradicated globally.

THE AGENT

TAXONOMY

The current classification was devised by the Subcommittee on Taxonomy of the genus *Brucella* during the eight successive meetings held since 1962. The genus *Brucella* contains six species: *B. melitensis*, *B. abortus*, *B. suis*, *B. ovis*, *B. neotomae*, and *B. canis* (Corbel and Brinley-Morgan 1984). These species are mainly differentiated by their phage susceptibility patterns. *Brucella melitensis*, *B. abortus*, and *B. suis* are subdivided into three, seven and five biovars, respectively, on the basis of four additional tests: requirement for added carbon dioxide, production of hydrogen sulphide, growth in the presence of the dyes thionin and basic fuchsin, and agglutination by 'monospecific' anti-A and anti-M sera (Table 3.2) (Alton *et al.* 1988).

Table 3.2 Species and biovar differentiation of the three main *Brucella* spp. responsible for human brucellosis

Species	Biovar	Lysis by phages[a]			CO$_2$ requirement	H$_2$S production	Growth on dyes[b]		Agglutination in sera[c]	
		Tb	Wb	Iz			Thionin	Basic Fuchsin	A	M
B. melitensis	1	−	−	+	−	−	+	+	−	+
	2	−	−	+	−	−	+	+	+	−
	3	−	−	+	−	−	+	+	+	+
B. abortus	1	+	+	+	+[d]	+	−	+	+	−
	2	+	+	+	+[d]	+	−	−	+	−
	3	+	+	+	+[d]	+	+	+	+	−
	4	+	+	+	+[d]	+	−	+[e]	−	+
	5	+	+	+	−	−	+	+	−	+
	6	+	+	+	−	−	+	+	+	−
	9	+	+	+	+ or −	+	+	+	−	+
B. suis	1	−	+	+	−	+	+	−[f]	+	−
	2	−	+	+	−	−	+	−	+	−
	3	−	+	+	−	−	+	+	+	−
	4	−	+	+	−	−	+	−[g]	+	+
	5	−	+	+	−	−	+	−	−	+

[a] At the routine test dilution.
[b] Dye concentration, 20 μg/ml in serum dextrose medium (1 : 50 000).
[c] A, A monospecific antiserum; M, M monospecific antiserum.
[d] Usually positive on primary isolation.
[e] Some strains isolated in Canada, Great Britain, and USA do not grow on dyes.
[f] Some basic fuchsin-resistant strains have been isolated in South America and South-East Asia.
[g] Negative for most strains.

Although descriptions of atypical isolates are published periodically the current classification, when applied to pure cultures, has undoubtedly proved to be useful for practical and epidemiological purposes. Unfortunately, owing to the subjective nature of the criteria for *Brucella* species definition, i.e. mainly based on phenotypic similarities and host specificity, controversy has arisen about the classification of some taxa. It therefore appears to *Brucella* workers that there is a need for more objective and widely usable tests to better delineate taxa within the genus, and that molecular biology techniques can help give a better definition.

MOLECULAR BIOLOGY AND GENETICS

The first mention of a molecular study of *Brucella* dates back to 1960 when Belozersky and Spirin reported, for one strain of *B. abortus*, a guanine + cytosine percentage (GC%) equal to 57.9. Since then, more and more sophisticated techniques in molecular biology have been applied that undoubtedly have clarified the structure of the *Brucella* genome which, in spite of some degree of internal polymorphism, is strikingly homogeneous (Verger and Grayon 1992). All members of the genus are indeed characterized by very narrow ranges of GC content (average, 58 per cent) and of molecular weight (average, $2.61 \times 10^9 \pm 8$ per cent) of the genome DNA. Moreover, as shown by DNA–DNA hybridizations, the six species form a homogeneous DNA relatedness group that is 96 ± 5 per cent (mean ± standard deviation) related to the type strain (*B. melitensis* 16M), with ΔT_{m} below 1 °C. This is also confirmed by the high level of homology between DNA and ribosomal ribonucleic acid (rRNA), and by the similarity of both endonuclease-digested total DNA and ribosomal ribonucleic acid gene restriction patterns.

These studies clearly provide evidence that members of the six conventional species form a strikingly homogeneous DNA–DNA hybridization group that should therefore be considered as a single species, even if genome analysis by cloned oligonucleotide probes has revealed some degree of polymorphism of the *Brucella* genome.

Nevertheless, consistent differences exist in host specificity and in pathogenic properties of the six conventional species. There is thus a need for more basic information on the genetics and molecular biology of virulence factors. Some *B. abortus* genes encoding periplasmic or outer membrane proteins of potential value as protective or diagnostic antigens have been cloned recently. Genetic conjugation has also been demonstrated in the genus *Brucella* and was shown to be a convenient and effective means of introducing exogenous DNA into *Brucella* spp. These first results, and the ongoing research on genetics and molecular biology of *Brucella*, will, no doubt, lead to a better understanding of the virulence mechanisms in these bacteria.

GROWTH REQUIREMENTS

Brucella organisms are aerobic and many strains require supplementary carbon dioxide (CO_2) in the atmosphere for growth (Alton *et al.* 1988). They are considered slow growing and somewhat fastidious in comparison with other aerobic organisms. Thiamine, nicotinamide, and biotin are required for growth, but X and V factors are not required. Growth may be stimulated by the addition of 5–10 per cent normal serum. Growth is inhibited on media containing bile salts, tellurite, or selenite. Strains of *B. abortus* biovar 2 are the most sensitive to inhibitors, and in general require 5–10 per cent (v/v) serum for growth. The optimal temperature for all *Brucella* strains is 36–38 °C. Viability is generally lost at 60 °C, but higher temperatures may be required to ensure sterilization of concentrated *Brucella* suspensions. The culture media should be adequately buffered near pH 7 for optimal growth. Excessive acidity (pH at 3.5 or below), as observed during the fermentation process in some cheeses, rapidly kills *Brucella* cells.

Growth of *Brucella* is usually poor in liquid medium unless vigorous aeration is provided. In static incubation at 37 °C for 7 days, smooth strains produce moderate uniform turbidity with a light powdery deposit. Non-smooth strains may produce a granular deposit, variable turbidity, and pellicle formation. Growth in static liquid media favours dissociation from smooth to non-smooth forms.

With semisolid media, CO_2-dependent cultures of *B. abortus* produce a disc of growth a few millimetres below the surface, whereas CO_2 independent *B. melitensis* and *B. suis* strains produce a uniform turbidity from the surface down to a depth of a few millimetres.

Using reconstituted commercial dehydrated solid media suitable for *Brucella*, colonies only become visible after at least 2 days. After 4 days, they are round, 1–2 mm in diameter, with smooth margins, translucent, and of a pale honey colour. Later, they become larger and darker but remain clear. When viewed from above *Brucella* colonies are convex and pearl white. When plates after 4 days' incubation are examined by obliquely reflected light, smooth colonies appear round, glistening, and blue to blue-green in colour. Smooth *Brucella* species may undergo rough variation of colonial morphology during growth in non-optimal culture conditions. Rough colonies have a dry, granular appearance and are yellow to yellow-white in colour. Changes in colonial morphology are due to loss of LPS polysaccharide chains, and are associated with changes in infectivity and antigenicity. Smooth colonies are more pathogenic, whereas rough variants are less infective and lack the antigenic characteristics of smooth cultures. Examination of the colonial morphology of a culture is therefore an essential step in the production of live vaccines and of diagnostic antigens, and in the typing procedures of *Brucella* strains.

PATHOGENESIS AND IMMUNITY

After penetration through the mucosa or a skin abrasion, *Brucella* are taken up by phagocytic cells to the regional lymph nodes, where decisive events occur. Depending on dose, virulence, species and breed, and pre-existent humoral and cellular immunity effectors, the bacteria can be trapped and progressively destroyed as immunity develops or escape to the blood circulation and invade other RES organs, principally the liver, spleen, kidneys, bone marrow, and lymph nodes, but other organs may also be affected. Lesions develop by focal aggregation of RES cells containing numerous bacteria which form typical small granulomata and may evolve towards healing or, in more susceptible organs, towards abscess formation and necrosis (vertebrae) or other severe lesions (endocarditis). At this intracellular stage, the T-cell immune system directed against the *Brucella* cell wall proteins may be the main effector, but recruitment of granuloma cells by the hypersensitivity reaction to cytosolic proteins may also participate in immunity and pathological features.

Infection of the udder and mammary lymph nodes which frequently occurs in ruminants with only minimal symptoms, leads to long-lasting excretion of *Brucella* in the milk. Infection of the placenta and associated tissues, the main characteristic of animal brucellosis, leads to either abortion or birth of normal or infected offspring, and massive but short-term excretion (<1 month) of *Brucella*. Infection of the placenta does not result, as often stated, from a particular tropism but from entrapment by trophoblast cells of circulating bacteria, a relatively rare event, that can be almost totally eliminated by the presence of antibodies. This is followed by an unrestricted proliferation in chorio-allantoid tissues, a nutritionally rich fetal compartment in which maternal immunity is only marginally expressed (Bosseray and Plommet 1988; Samartino and Enright 1993 Tobias *et al.* 1993)

Immunity is thus complex where humoral, mainly anti-S-LPS antibodies, and cellular effectors act either separately or in concert at the successive steps of the infectious process. Pre-existent antibodies or those induced by the infection itself can restrict the infection to the RES, and T cells activate the killing mechanisms that may lead either to chronicity or cure. Basically, the immunity can be transferred in mice by administration of antibodies raised against the S-LPS and by T cells and antibodies raised against the cell wall proteins. These cell wall fraction free of S-LPS would not interfere with usual diagnostic tests in veterinary medicine and therefore are good candidates for new efficient vaccines (Plommet 1987; Winter and Rowe 1988; Smith *et al.* 1990; Winter 1990).

Live attenuated vaccines that mimic the natural immune response should survive at least 1–2 months in lymph nodes to confer good immunity, but not too long in order to avoid secondary colonization of the placenta and a durable serological response (Araya *et al.* 1989). Virulence, dose, time, and route of administration therefore should be carefully defined for optimal responses. Two vaccines, *B. abortus* S19 and *B. melitensis* Rev. 1, accepted worldwide as preventing bovine and ovine–caprine brucellosis, respectively, can be used. The vaccine may be injected subcutaneously at full or reduced dose, or by the conjunctival route. By this latter route, the strain is for the most part contained in the head lymph nodes, giving a shorter serological response and a reduced risk of generalization to the placenta if incidentally administered during pregnancy. *Brucella suis* S2 vaccine developed in China (Xie Xin 1986) is used there against ovine, bovine, and porcine brucellosis. It is administered orally in drinking water, but the immunity is lower than with Rev. 1, in relation to a shorter survival in lymph nodes (Bosseray and Plommet 1990; Verger *et al.* 1994).

Vaccines combining killed cells with adjuvant have also been largely and successfully used, notably with *B. melitensis* H38 (smooth, S-LPS), but a strong serological response made the latter incompatible with most control programmes. Vaccines using *B. abortus* 45/20 (rough, R-LPS) were not consistently protective and are therefore no longer accepted (Plommet 1990).

HUMAN BRUCELLOSIS

INCUBATION AND SYMPTOMS

The disease affects individuals of any age and is characterized by an extraordinary polymorphism in its clinical symptoms; the clinical diagnosis must always be confirmed by bacteriological and serological tests. The incubation period may extend from a few days to several weeks or months, depending on the dose and virulence of the strain and resistance of the host. The onset of the disease is, in the majority of cases, acute or subacute.

The acute form begins with fever, well tolerated and, in general, of vespertine presentation, shivering, profuse sweating, headache, constipation, cough, asthenia, and arthromyalgia. However, this 'classic'

symptomatology is observed in no more than half of the cases. On many occasions the onset is subacute or insidious, with febricule, asthenia, and flitting arthralgia. Sometimes the first symptom is a visceral or osteo-articular localization with little accompanying fever.

The most characteristic feature of the disease is the development of focal localizations, which become more numerous with time, the most common being the osteo-articular complications (sacroileitis, spondilitis with or without osifluent abscesses, arthralgias, arthritis, coxitis, bursitis, tenosinuvitis, and, on rare occasions, osteomyelitis). Among neurological, cardiovascular, cutaneous, pulmonary, genitourinary, ocular, digestive, and psychiatric complications, endocarditis is the most severe. However, the prognosis has changed thanks to surgical treatment combined with antibiotherapy (Christie 1980; Young 1989; Foz *et al.* 1992).

Nowadays the classic presentation of undulating fever and relapsing forms are less frequent because the diagnosis is carried out earlier and the treatment given sooner. Similarly, septic shock is exceptional.

In the West, it has been stated that when the disease occurs during pregnancy, the frequency of abortions is no different from that produced by any other systemic infection accompanied by bacteraemia. However, this statement is challenged by observations in countries of the Middle East (Yaprak *et al.* 1991).

It is important to point out that infantile brucellosis (Yaprak *et al.* 1991) is more frequent than usually assumed (16 per cent of brucellosis cases diagnosed in a hospital in Barcelona were children of less than 12 years of age), and can affect even newborn infants (Lubani *et al.* 1988).

Infantile brucellosis generally begins in an acute manner, with very well-tolerated fever and hardly any complications, and spontaneously cures itself. On only few occasions is it followed by sequelae. In countries where *Salmonella typhi* is endemic, infantile brucellosis is very frequently confused with typhoid fever.

Finally, it must be stated that the term 'chronic brucellosis' has been used in different ways historically and the definition of a case has been based on chronological, clinical, therapeutic response, or immunological criteria. According to the authors of the Montpellier School, chronic brucellosis is a special clinical form, 'a single manifestation', which is related to a particular hypersensitivity of tissues to the *Brucella* antigens (Jambon and Bertrand 1953).

DIAGNOSIS

All physicians treating a febrile patient who lives in an endemic area, or who has travelled to a country where the brucellosis is endemic must be aware of possible infection with *Brucella*. An epidemiological history should be elicited (profession, food ingested, and contact with animals), and a rapid agglutination test performed. The Rose Bengal (RB) test can be used as the most sensitive rapid screening test, but the results must be confirmed by other methods.

The only conclusive evidence of *Brucella* infection is the recovery of the bacterium from blood, bone marrow, spinal fluid, or other samples. Blood is the most important source and blood cultures must be performed whenever possible, preferably using the biphasic method of Castaneda with 10 per cent CO_2. It is recommended that cultures be maintained for at least 45 days before rejecting them as negative. The relative proportion of successful blood cultures reported in the literature is variable. In an extensive study carried out by Ariza *et al.* (1992*b*) the percentage of positive blood cultures in patients with high and low fever, and without fever, were 86.5, 75, and 28.5 per cent, respectively. Blood cultures must be performed always in veterinarians or other personnel who have had any possible contact with the Rev. 1 vaccine strain. The isolation of Rev. 1 from two veterinarians with brucellosis has been recently reported.

The majority of blood cultures in the biphasic medium are positive between the seventh and twenty-first day, but the new semiautomatic methods (BACTEC 9240 and Bact/Alert) improve the time of detection, and the presence of *Brucella* with these methods can be detected by the third day of incubation. We recommend, in addition to subculture on a solid media, use of the modified Ziehl–Neelsen method of Stamp, instead of the Gram stain. The *Brucella* are stained red against a blue background and can be distinguished from the artefacts present in the broth.

Recently, some authors have proposed assays based as the polymerase chain reaction (PCR) for the direct detection of *Brucella* spp. in blood. However, more experience is needed before this method replaces the traditional blood cultures (MATAR *et al.* 1996).

The main antigens of diagnostic significance are the cell surface smooth lipopolysaccharide (S-LPS) and the internal (mostly cytosolic) proteins. All serological tests with whole smooth cells detect antibodies to S-LPS, which can also be detected by a variety of tests adapted to use S-LPS-rich extracts. On the other hand, antibodies to internal proteins can only be shown using S-LPS-free cell extracts or purified proteins.

A correct serological diagnosis of human brucellosis can be made with tests that use smooth whole cells, including the RB, tube serum agglutination (SAT), 2-mercaptoethanol (2-ME), Coombs, complement fixation (CF), immunofluorescence, and enzyme immunoassays (ELISA test), but keeping in mind that different classes of immunoglobulins are found in the acute and subacute case. IgM appears early and later

IgG and IgA predominate. The results of a combination of tests such as SAT and Coombs, or ELISA with the conjugates of the proper specificity can be used to evaluate the IgM/IgG/IgA ratios, and this information is useful in the assessment of the time of evolution of the disease at the moment of the diagnosis. Although ELISA with LPS is a very promising test for estimating the Ig classes, several technical (standardization and expression of the results), and interpretation problems (results can be reported either as a titer, an optical density of a reference serum, or in units) have to be taken into account before it can be recommended to all laboratories. A correct diagnosis can be made with the less sophisticated tests (Diaz and Moriyon 1989).

The *Brucella* S-LPS cross-reacts with the corresponding antigen of species or serotypes of *Yersinia, Francisella, Salmonella, Vibrio, Escherichia coli* and others. An important point in the use of the water-soluble proteins is that serological cross-reactivity with other bacteria of clinical importance has never been found. Therefore, they can be used to discriminate infections due to *Brucella* from those due to the above bacteria. Antibodies to internal proteins have been studied by counterimmunolectrophoresis (CIEP) and ELISA. By CIEP it has been found that patients with 2-ME-resistant antibodies and high Coombs titers also had higher numbers of precipitin lines and high titers of antibodies to proteins. Obviously, the antibody response in such patients had a longer evolution than those with high 2-ME sensitive (mostly IgM) antibodies (Diaz *et al.* 1976).

Recently, it has been reported that the changes in levels of IgG antibodies to proteins correlate better with clinical recovery than do levels of IgG antibodies to lipopolysaccharide (Baldi *et al.* 1996).

In cases of neurobrucellosis it is necessary to try to isolate the *Brucella* from the spinal fluid and demonstrate the presence of antibodies against LPS and cytosolic proteins. It has also been shown that *Brucella* meningitis is characterized by an increase of IgG in the spinal fluid, and that the determination of specific IgG concentration can be of value in the diagnosis.

In nearly every case, human brucellosis can be diagnosed using epidemiological, clinical, and serological data. Although serological data are of great value, no existing serological test (including ELISA) reflects clinical progress or recovery, or predicts the risk of a relapse. The interpretation of positive serology in the absence of symptoms and previous history of brucellosis is always difficult.

TREATMENT

The treatment of human brucellosis is limited by the property of *Brucella* to remain sheltered in the monocyte–phagocyte system, which accounts for the relapses of this disease. In recent years, several randomized trials have been carried out, using different antibiotic regimes. A commonly used regime for acute septi-caemic brucellosis is:

(1) doxycycline (100 mg every 12 h) for 45 days plus streptomycin (1 g/day) for 15 days or for 3 weeks; and

(2) doxycycline (100 mg every 12 h) for 45 days plus rifampicin (15 mg/kg body weight) also for 45 days

Repeat courses are recommended in cases of relapse. In serious cases, with toxic symptoms, it is advisable to use 1 mg/kg/day of prednisone or methyl-prednisolone during the first few days (Hall 1990; Ariza 1992; Bertrand 1992).

In case of spondylitis, prolonged treatment for 8 weeks has been recommended and results of Ariza *et al.* (1992*a*) indicate that the doxycycline–strepto-mycin combination is the most effective. In endocardi-tis, besides the surgical treatment, the combination rifampicin-doxycycline–streptomycin is recommended for at least 12 weeks or more. The same treatment can be used in neurobrucellosis.

In pregnant women and infants of less than 8 years of age who cannot be treated with tetracycline, rifampicin, for at least 30 days, or alternatively trimethoprim– sulphamethoxazole, is recommended.

Nowadays the use of antigens (melitine) applied intradermally, or treatment by means of intravenous injections of dead *Brucella* cells (vaccinotherapy), have been abandoned. However, it has never been shown whether the beneficial effects indicated in the past were due to desensitization or to breaking up the equi-librium which might have been established between *Brucella* and macrophages.

PROGNOSIS

Before the antibiotic era (1946) most of the patients recovered spontaneously after several weeks or months, but many developed severe forms and/or dis-abling sequelae. Antibiotic therapy applied after early diagnosis should provide a complete cure in most patients, with a relapse rate of less than 10 per cent.

ANIMAL BRUCELLOSIS

SYMPTOMS AND INCUBATION

Brucellosis in ruminants, also known as 'enzootic abor-tion' is characterized clinically by third-term abortions, placental retentions, and endometritis, which usually evolve favourably, followed by a normal full-term preg-nancy, and only about 5 per cent have residual sterility. Other symptoms include premature delivery of new-borns with lung infection and respiratory distress, udder inflammation, articular and periarticular (hygroma) localizations. Brucellosis may also remain silent for years, with or without serological and/or bac-teriological evidence of infection. The incubation period is highly variable: a mid-term cow in close contact with an aborted one becomes seropositive in 1 week and may abort after 3 weeks. In contrast, a non-pregnant heifer may remain negative for several months, until her first calving, when serological responses will become positive in most (95 per cent of) infected females. Congenitally infected offspring (calves, lambs, and kids) usually recover, but a few (about 5 per cent in bovines) remain silently infected until first delivery.

In the male, the infection is localized in joints and genital organs (reducing fertility), and there is excre-tion in the semen which, though unimportant in bovines, is the main route of transmission of *B. ovis* and *B. canis* in rams and dogs.

In other domestic or wild animal species, the same localizations, i.e. reproductive tract, articular, and mammary, are the main features, while autopsy may discover infection of the spleen, liver, nodes, kidneys, and lungs (Alton 1985). There is a special interest in hares where brucellosis, due to *B. suis* biovar 2, is sometimes transmitted to humans and swine.

Horses in contact with infected cows often exhibit a characteristic osteo-articular lesion—fistulous withers— that is sometimes the first clinical evidence of brucel-losis in a farm. In contrast, farm dogs that may become infected by consuming placental envelops do not exhibit conspicious signs, but they should none the less, be included in test control programmes.

DIAGNOSIS

The requirements for diagnosis of animal brucellosis should be considered from three points of view:

1. Diagnosis after abortion or other suspicious signs on an individual basis requires high blood test titres, microscopic examination, and culture to give an unambiguous result.

2. In control programmes, on a herd and/or individ-ual basis, only a fraction of infected animals are positive at a time, and the tests, either collective (as the bulk milk ring test (MRT) in dairy cows), or individual, should be repeated to cover all animals at seropositive periods of infection: in test-and-slaughter programmes every 1–3 months. In periodic surveillance of a brucellosis-free herd, surveys once a year (or more in enzootic area) on a significant sample of the herd are required.

3. Diagnosis in market animals. National and inter-national organizations (Office International des

Epizooties) (OIE) have issued rules and standards for commercial exchanges to avoid transmission of brucellosis. However, individual diagnostic techniques applied on these animals (often young ones, thus in silent phase) cannot be an absolute safeguard. Only the status of the maternal herd can give this guarantee, which should be certified through a good surveillance system.

Brucellosis should be suspected in any abortion or premature delivery wherever brucellosis is enzootic. Where herd surveillance tests are applied regularly, a switch to a positive response should command prompt action, confirmation, and segregation of suspect animals to prevent propagation of the disease.

Microscopic examination of stained smears prepared from fetal membranes, stomach content, vaginal swabs, or ram semen can, when carried out by a trained technician, give a good indication of brucellosis, but confirmation by culture is necessary (Alton *et al.* 1988).

The culture of *Brucella* requires special equipment—such as a CO_2 incubator—and training, but it gives an undisputed result, and sometimes is the only proof of infection. Selective agar media, such as the Farrell's medium, are preferred for contaminated samples (colostrum and milk, fetal membranes, vaginal swabs, semen) but non-selective liquid or agar media can also be used with aseptically collected samples (milk, synovial fluid). Blood is usually not convenient in animals except in dogs. The best sample at autopsy is fetal stomach content, while at slaughter, the best, in order of preference, are supramammary, medial iliac, maxillary, parotid, retropharyngeal lymph nodes, spleen and liver.

The classic serological tests, seroagglutination (SAT) and complement fixation (CF), are based on the reaction between the cell surface antigen S-LPS (or R-LPS in *B. ovis*, and *B. canis*) and immunoglobulin (Ig) isotypes (Table 3.3). IgG1 and IgA are the more specific indicators of infection and CF, rose Bengal (RB) and milk ring test (MRT) are preferred to SAT. Other techniques and antigens, including the delayed hyper-

sensitivity brucellin skin test, may improve both specificity and sensitivity but are not yet widely accepted (e.g. ELISA). In the classic methods false positives occur in:

(1) LPS cross-reacting infections, mainly by *Yersinia*; and

(2) some long-lasting post-vaccinal responses (*c.* 2 per cent, >24 months) usually of IgM type.

Falsely negatives occur in the incubation period and in the chronic phase, as well as during pregnancy. Even after calving, when the responses are usually maximal, a few culture-positive animals (*c.*, 5 per cent) may be serologically negative.

TREATMENT

Cure rates of 50–80 per cent have been reported in cows, rams (*B. ovis*), and dogs (*B. canis*) with the classic combination of oxytetracycline-streptomycin. Such treatment (forbidden in cattle, sheep, and swine in the European Union) can be considered in valuable animals, but the risk of keeping an infected pet (*B. canis*) or an animal with residual lesions of the male genital tract (*B. ovis*) should also be considered.

PROGNOSIS

Brucellosis evolves spontaneously towards either recovery or chronic forms with eventual udder localization, a potential contaminating source, and crippling articulate lesions. The recovery rate depends on the host species, (being higher in ewes than in goats or cows,) and breed. In herds or flocks (except in small ones, <20), the disease will be maintained indefinitely by transmission to new generations (before or after birth), even if clinical episodes only occur in a cyclical manner over a period of several years

Human disease and losses in meat and milk production are the main costs for society, and are particularly high for developing countries (WHO 1986).

EPIDEMIOLOGY

OCCURRENCE

In human brucellosis, an epidemiological 'cul-de-sac' (no transmission between persons except between mother and child) reflects the nature of contact with infected animals: sporadic in tourists, endemic in professionally exposed workers, and epidemics or outbreaks in occasionally exposed groups—such as in the historical outbreak of Malta fever in the Royal Navy. In animals, because of high contagion within herds and

Table 3.3 Effectors in diagnostic tests (bovine)

	Anti S-LPS Ig				Brucellin-sensitized T cells
	G1	G2	M	A	
Seroagglutination	−	+	+	−	−
Complement fixation	+	−	(+)	−	−
Rose Bengal plate test	+	−	(+)	−	−
Milk ring test	±	±	+	+	−
Skin test	−	−	−	−	+

±, May participate; (+), variable.

the long inapparent phase of infection, the prevalence/herd/year is the only correct indicator in surveys and control programmes. Paradoxically, a decline in human cases following progress in animal control programmes, as observed in recent years in Greece, France, Spain, Italy, and Mongolia (Kolar 1987; Plommet 1992), may be concealed at the beginning of a control programme by the improvement in surveillance.

The three principal groups of people at risk are:

(1) professional: breeders, farmers, veterinarians, meat-and milk-plant workers, and technicians in diagnosis, research, or production laboratories;

(2) social: those living near infected animals, (on the farm or in nomadic groups) and those consuming raw milk, fresh cheese, or uncooked meat.

(3) Visitors to endemic regions, who eat local fresh cheese.

GEOGRAPHY

While the description of a 'Mediterranean fever' by Hippocrates in 450 BC suggests that the disease was already prevalent, as it still is around the Mediterranean Sea, the origin of the *Brucella* genus is only speculative (Spink 1956). Yet adaptation to specific hosts and genetic stability on passage in occasional hosts suggests the 'species' diverged long ago from a common ancestor and evolved independently with only minor stable modifications. The 'species' thereby followed their domestic hosts as they spread worldwide with commercial exchanges and colonization, with possibly recontamination of, and by, wild animals, as sometimes observed nowadays.

Many countries started combatting animal brucellosis in the 1950s. The following are now free (OIE 1992) or with a few residual cases (indicated by B.a or B.s for *B. abortus* or *B. suis*) with human prevalence lower than 1 per 10^5 (WHO 1992): Canada, Australia, New Caledonia, New Zealand, Japan, Korea, Taiwan, Vanuatu, Austria, Bulgaria (B.s), Cyprus, Czechoslovakia (B.s), Denmark, Estonia (B.a), Finland, Germany (B.a, B.s), Hungary, Latvia (B.s), Lithuania (B.a), The Netherlands, Norway, Romania (B.s), UK and Ireland (B.a), Sweden, Switzerland, and also Malawi and Mauritius.

A few countries are expected to be free by the year 2000: USA, France, Belgium, Malaysia; or in a few more years: Spain, Italy, Portugal, and some countries in America (Garcia-Carrillo 1987). In China, *B. melitensis* being prevalent in the northern provinces and *B. suis* in the south, great progress is now being recorded (Shen Er-Li and Lu Shiliang 1991). In most other countries, in particular in the Middle East, the prevalence is high or unknown. Human prevalence per 10^5 is higher than 10 in Tunisia, Jordan, Kuwait, Oman, and Iran; from 5 to 10 in Djibouti, Syria, Spain, and Turkey; and between 1 and 5 in Algeria, Israel, Iraq, Mexico, Italy, Greece, and the former Yugoslavia (WHO 1992).

SOURCES AND TRANSMISSION

Humans become infected by ingestion, direct contact, inhalation, or accidental inoculation by penetration through conjunctival, nasopharyngeal, pulmonary, and/or intestinal mucosae, or through skin abrasion or injury.

Milk, cream, and fresh cheese are the main sources of human brucellosis. Excretion in milk may attain 10^4/ml at the beginning of lactation and then decline to a few bacteria (*c.* 10/ml) but may persist during successive lactation periods (Plommet *et al.* 1988). During cheesemaking, the bacteria are first concentrated by about fivefold in the curd and then decline with the acidification produced by lactic bacteria. Survival depends therefore on the type of cheese and the ripening involved, which may vary from 25 days in acid-type curding (e.g. Camembert) to several months in Cheddar cheese (IDF 1980). Fortunately, *Brucella* are destroyed by pasteurization.

Excretion via the genital tract at abortion or normal birth, which continues for some weeks, is the second most important source of infection for humans; in animal herds, this is the major source. Placenta, fetus, and fluids are hugely rich in bacteria, with up to 10^{12}/g in cows (Alexander *et al.* 1981). Infection can occur by direct contact or by indirect vectors after contamination of surroundings. *Brucella* survive in the soil, water, solid, or liquid manure, depending on the material, temperature, and sun exposure—up to 8 months in liquid manure at 15 °C or below, but a shorter time at higher temperatures (Plommet 1972; Crawford *et al.* 1990). Bacteria can contaminate drinking water. Airborne dust or droplets may cause transmission especially when high pressure jets of water are used during washing of premises. Such indirect transmission is observed in villages along the transhumance routes and in abattoir workers.

Meat products, mainly spleen, liver, genital organs, lymph nodes, and meat with remnants of lymphatic tissue, constitute an important source of human and animal (pigs, dogs) infection. In developed countries, infected animals are slaughtered separately and viscera discarded. *Brucella* are destroyed by cooking.

PREVENTION AND CONTROL

IN HUMANS

Prevention in humans relies, whenever possible, upon control and eradication of the animal reservoir of infection and pasteurization of milk. People living in,

Ariza, J. (1992). Antibiotic therapy for human Brucellosis. In *Prevention of brucellosis in the Mediterranean countries*, (ed. M. Plommet), pp. 87–93. Pudoc, Wageningen.

Ariza, J. *et al.* (1992*a*). Treatment of human Brucellosis with Doxycycline plus Rifampin or Doxycycline plus Streptomycin. *Annals of Internal Medicine*, **117**, 25–30.

Ariza, J., Pellicer, T., Pallarès, R., Foz, A., and Gudiol, F. (1992*b*). Specific antibody profile in human Brucellosis. *Clinical Infectious Diseases*, **14**, 131–40.

Baldi, P. C., Miguel, S. E., Fossati, C. A., and Wallach, J. C. (1996). Serological follow-up of human brucellosis by measuring IgG antibodies to lipopolysaccharide and cytoplasmic proteins of *Brucella* species. *Clinical Infectious Diseases*, **22**, 446–55.

Belozersky, A. N. and Spirin, A. S. (1960). Chemistry of the nucleic acids in microorganisms. In *The Nucleic acids*, Vol 3 (ed. E. Chargaff and J. N. Davidson) pp. 147–85. Academic Press, New York.

Bertrand, A. (1992). *Antibiotic treatment for brucellosis*. MZCP Consultation on epidemiology and surveillance of Brucellosis involving human health care. Heraklion, Crete, 19–22 October 1992. MZCC, Athens.

Bosseray, N. and Plommet, M. (1988). Serum and cell-mediated immune protection of mouse placenta and fetus against a *Brucella abortus* challenge: expression of barrier effect of placenta. *Placenta*, **9**, 65–79.

Bosseray, N. and Plommet, M. (1990). *Brucella suis* S2, *Brucella melitensis* Rev. 1 and *Brucella abortus* S19 living vaccines: residual virulence and immunity induced against three *Brucella* species challenge strains in mice. *Vaccine*, **8**, 462–8.

Christie, A. B. (1980). *Infectious diseases. Epidemiology and clinical practice*, (3rd edn). Churchill Livingstone, Edinburgh.

Corbel, M. J. and Brinley-Morgan, W. J. (1984). Genus *Brucella* Meyer and Shaw 1920, 173 AL. In *Bergey's manual of systematic bacteriology*, Vol. 1, (1st edn), (ed. N. R. Krieg and J. G. Holt), pp. 377–88. Williams and Wilkins, Baltimore.

Crawford, R. P., Huber, J. D. and Adams, B. S. (1990). Epidemiology and surveillance. In *Animal brucellosis*, (ed. K. Nielsen and J. R. Duncan), p. 136. CRC Press, Boca Raton.

Diaz, R. and Moriyon, I. (1989). Laboratory techniques in the diagnosis of human Brucellosis. In *Brucellosis: clinical and laboratory aspects*, (ed. E. J. Young and M. J. Corbel), pp. 73–83. CRC Press, Boca Raton.

Diaz, R., Maravi-Poma, E. and Rivero, A. (1976). Comparison of counterimmuno-electrophoresis with other serological tests in the diagnosis of human Brucellosis. *Bulletin of the World Health Organization*, **53**, 417–24.

Dranovskaya, E. A. (1991). New approaches to Brucellosis vaccination of people with high risk of infection. In *Brucella and Brucellosis in man and animals*, The Turkish Microbiological Society publication No. 16, (ed. E. Tumbay, S. Hilmi, and O. Ang), pp. 87–100. Ege University Press, Izmir.

Evans, A. C. (1918). Further studies on Bacterium abortus and related bacteria; II. A comparison of Bacterium abortus with Bacterium bronchisepticus and with the organism which causes Malta Fever. *Journal of Infectious Diseases*, **22**, 140–50.

FAO (Food and Agricultural Organization) (1993). Guidelines for a regional Brucellosis control programme for the Middle East. Amman, 14–17 February 1993. FAO, Rome.

Fensterbank, R. (1986). Brucellosis in cattle, sheep and goats: diagnosis, control and vaccination. *Revue Scientifique et Technique de l'Office International des Epizooties*, **5**, 605–18.

Foz, A., Diaz, R., and Ariza, J. (1992). Brucella. In *Enfermedades Infecciosas Y Microbiologia Clinica*, (ed. E. J. Perea), pp. 682–7. Doyma, Barcelona.

Garcia-Carrillo, C. (1987). *La Brucelosis de los animales en América y su relacion con la infeccion humana*. OIE, Paris.

Hall, W. H. (1990). Modern chemotherapy for Brucellosis in humans. *Reviews of Infectious Diseases*, **12**, 1060–99.

IDF (International Dairy Federation) (1980). Behavior of pathogens in cheese. *Bulletin*, **112**, 4–23.

Jambon, J. and Bertrand, L. (1953). Le problème de la brucellose chronique. *IV Congreso Internacional de Higiene y Medicina Mediterraneas Barcelona*, pp. 143

Kolar, J. (1987). Control of *Brucella melitensis* Brucellosis in developing countries. *Annales de l'Institut Pasteur/Microbiologie*, **138**, 122–6.

Lubani, M. M. *et al.* (1988). Neonatal Brucellosis. *European Journal of Pediatrics*, **147**, 520–2.

Matar, G. M., Khnisser, I. A., and Abdelnoor, A. M. (1996). Rapid laboratory confirmation of human brucellosis by PCR analysis of a target sequence on the 31-kilodalton Brucella antigen DNA. *Journal of Clinical Microbiology*, **34**, 477–8.

OIE (Office International des Epizooties) (1992). *Santé animale mondiale*. OIE, Paris.

Plommet, M. (1972). Survie de *Brucella abortus* dans le lisier de bovins. Désinfection par le xylène. *Annales de Recherches Vétérinaires*, **3**, 621–32.

Plommet, M. (1987). Brucellosis and immunity: humoral and cellular components in mice. *Annales de l'Institut Pasteur/Microbiologie*, **138**, 105–10.

Plommet, M. (1990). Killed vaccines in cattle: current situation and prospects. In *Advances in Brucellosis research*, (ed. L. Garry Adams), pp. 215–27. Texas AM University Press, College Station.

Plommet, M. (1992). Lutte contre la Brucellose à *Brucella melitensis*: choix d'une stratégie. Résultats attendus. In *Prevention of brucellosis in the Mediterranean countries*, (ed. M. Plommet), pp. 160–5. Pudoc, Wageningen.

Plommet, M., Fensterbank, R., Vassal, L., Auclair, J., and Mocquot, G. (1988). Survival of *Brucella abortus* in ripened soft cheese made from naturally infected cow's milk. *Le Lait*, **68**, 115–20.

Samartino, L. E. and Enright, F. M. (1993). Pathogenesis of abortion of bovine Brucellosis. *Comparative Immunology, Microbiology and Infectious Diseases*, **16**, 95–101.

Shen Er-Li and Lu Shiliang (1991). The control of human Brucellosis in China. In *Strategies in diagnosis and control of Brucellosis in Asia*, FAO meeting, Beijing, 5–8 October, AGA/BRU/92/28. FAO, Rome.

Smith, R., III, Adams, L. G., Sowa, B. A., and Ficht, T. A. (1990). Induction of lymphocyte responsiveness by the outer membrane–peptidoglycan complex of rough strain of *Brucella abortus*. *Veterinary Immunology and Immunopathology*, **26**, 31–48.

Spink, W. W. (1956). *The nature of Brucellosis*. University of Minnesota Press, Minneapolis.

Sultan Al-Khalaf, S. A., Taka Mohamad, B., and Nicoletti, P. (1992). Control of Brucellosis in Kuwait by vaccination of cattle, sheep and goats with *Brucella abortus* strain 19 and *Brucella melitensis* strain Rev. 1. *Tropical Animal Health and Production*, **24**, 45–49.

Tobias, L., Cordes, D. O,. and Schurig, G. G. (1993). Placental pathology of the pregnant mouse inoculated with *Brucella abortus* strain 2308. *Veterinary Pathology*, **30**, 119–29.

Vassalo, D. J. (1992). The Corps Disease: Brucellosis and its historical association with the Royal Army Medical Corps. *Journal of the Royal Army Medical Corps*, **138**, 140–50.

Verger, J. M. and Grayon, M. (1992). Contribution de la biologie moléculaire à la taxonomie du genre *Brucella*. In *Prevention of brucellosis in Mediterranean countries*, (ed. M. Plommet), pp. 187–97. Pudoc, Wageningen.

Verger, J. M., Grayon, M., Zundel, E., Lechopier P. and Olivier-Bernardin, V. (1994). Comparison of the efficacy of *Brucella suis* strain 2 and *Brucella melitensis* Rev. 1 live vaccines against a *Brucella melitensis* experimental infection in pregnant ewes. *Vaccine*, **13**, 191–6.

WHO (World Health Organization) (1986). *Joint FAO/OMS expert committee on Brucellosis*. Technical Report No. 740. WHO, Geneva.

WHO (World Health Organization) (1992). *Animal health yearbook*, pp. 171–4. WHO, Geneva.

Winter, A. J. (1990). Mechanisms of protective immunity against *Brucella abortus* in the mouse model system of infection. In *Advances in Brucellosis research*, (ed. L. Garry Adams), pp. 137–43. Texas AM University Press, College Station.

Winter, A. J. and Rowe, G. R. E. (1988). Comparative immune responses to native cell envelope antigens and the hot sodium dodecyl sulfate insoluble fraction (PG) of *Brucella abortus* in cattle and mice. *Veterinary Immunology and Immunopathology*, **18**, 149–63.

Xie Xin (1986). Orally administrable Brucellosis vaccine: *Brucella suis* strain 2 vaccine. *Vaccine*, **4**, 212–16.

Yaprak, I., Bakiler, A. R., Kansoy, S., and Agzitemiz, M. (1991). Clinical picture in childhood Brucellosis. In *Brucella and brucellosis in man and animals*, The Turkish Microbiological Society publication No. 16, (ed. E. Tumbay, S. Hilmi, and O. Ang), pp. 109–21. Ege University Press, Izmir.

Young, E. J. (1989). Clinical manifestations of human Brucellosis. In *Brucellosis: clinical and laboratory aspects*, (ed. E. J. Young and M. J. Corbel), pp. 97–126. CRC, Boca Raton.

4 CAMPYLOBACTERIOSIS

M. B. Skirrow

SUMMARY

The only form of campylobacteriosis of major public health importance is campylobacter enteritis due to *Campylobacter jejuni* and *C. coli*. It is the most frequently identified form of infective diarrhoea in industrialized countries, with incidences in the region of 1 per cent per year. It causes economic losses amounting to many millions of pounds annually. *Campylobacter jejuni* and *C. coli* inhabit the intestinal tracts of wild birds and domestic animals. Poultry, in particular, become heavily colonized, and most broiler chickens sold in shops are contaminated. Red meats and offal are contaminated to a lesser degree. Human infection, which is mostly sporadic, may be acquired directly from animals or their products, by eating their meat raw or undercooked, or by eating foods that have become cross-contaminated from the raw product. Raw milk and contaminated water are sources that have given rise to major outbreaks of infection. Prevention depends on controlling infection in food-producing animals, especially poultry, reducing contamination during slaughter and processing, and correctly handling the raw products during food preparation. Education of the public on the basic principles of hygiene and safe food handling is an important adjunct.

HISTORY

The discovery, in the late 1970s, that campylobacters were a leading cause of acute diarrhoea can have few parallels in the history of microbiology. Bacteria formerly almost unknown in human medicine suddenly became commonplace in clinical laboratories. Although campylobacters had been known since the early 1900s as a cause of abortion in sheep and cattle, their role as enteropathogens went unnoticed, mainly because they are not detected by the methods traditionally used to culture faeces. The first indication that they might be enteropathogenic came from descriptions, dating from 1931 and 1944, that certain species could cause diarrhoea in cattle and pigs. The first instance of human infection was a milk-borne outbreak of gastroenteritis in a penitentiary in the United States in 1938 caused by a 'vibrio' that was almost certainly *Campylobacter jejuni*; all isolates were from blood. Later, also in the United States, Elizabeth King described 11 strains of a similar 'vibrio' isolated from the blood of patients with severe diarrhoea. This work was picked up in Belgium some 15 years later by Butzler, who wisely enlisted the help of veterinary colleagues to develop a method for isolating these bacteria from faeces. With this method they showed that campylobacters could be found in the faeces of 5 per cent of children with diarrhoea (Butzler *et al.* 1973). Strangely, this work was ignored until it was confirmed and extended in the United Kingdom by Skirrow (1977). It then quickly became clear that campylobacters were among the leading causes of acute diarrhoeal disease and that infection was acquired from animals and foods of animal origin.

This story acquired a nice postscript in 1985 when it was found that as long ago as 1886 Theodor Escherich described what must have been campylobacters in colonic smears of infants who had died of 'cholera infantum'. Interest in them waned because they could not be cultured. Additional historical aspects are described by Skirrow (1994).

THE AGENT

TAXONOMY

Campylobacters were first isolated by McFadyean and Stockman in 1906 during the course of an inquiry into epizootic abortion in sheep and cattle set up by the British Board of Agriculture. They thought the organism was a vibrio, and in 1919 it was named '*Vibrio fetus*' by Smith and Taylor in the United States. '*Vibrio fetus*' was the principal member of a group that became known as the microaerophilic vibrios, but work at the Institut Pasteur in 1963 showed that these bacteria were basically different from the true vibrios, so the genus *Campylobacter* was formed to accommodate them. For many years the taxonomic position of the genus was confused, but modern DNA technology has now shown that *Campylobacter*, together with *Arcobacter*, *Helicobacter*, and *Wolinella*, form a distinct group of bacteria known as rRNA Superfamily VI (Vandamme and Goossens 1992). Most of its members are adapted to living on mucosal surfaces, a feature reflected in their spiral morphology and rapid motility, which enable them to move freely in mucus.

DISEASE ASSOCIATIONS (rRNA Superfamily VI)

Although most of the 15 species of campylobacter have been isolated from human beings at some time, only a few are of public health significance. By far the most important are *C. jejuni* and *C. coli*, which account for almost all cases of campylobacter enteritis in industrialized countries and most cases in developing countries. In the former, *C. jejuni* accounts for about 90 per cent of infections and *C. coli* 10 per cent, but certain regions, notably Croatia, have a higher proportion of *C. coli* infections, probably linked with pork consumption (Popovic-Uroic 1989). A few infections are caused by *C. upsaliensis*, *C. lari*, *C. hyointestinalis*, and *Arcobacter butzleri*, but their significance is often uncertain. These species are more common in children in developing countries. *Campylobacter jejuni* subsp. *doylei* is a fastidious subspecies of *C. jejuni* also found in children living under poor social conditions (*C. jejuni* subsp. *jejuni*, the typical form, is referred to simply as *C. jejuni* elsewhere in this chapter). *Campylobacter fetus*, the type species of the genus, is an uncommon cause of systemic infection in patients with immunodeficiency or pre-existing disease. *Helicobacter cinaedi* (normally found in hamsters) and *H. fennelliae* are associated with proctocolitis in homosexual men. An account of human infection with these less common campylobacters and related bacteria is given by Mishu *et al.* (1995).

The gastric bacterium *H. pylori*, which plays a major role in the pathogenesis of peptic ulceration and gastric cancer, has no known host other than man. However, the less common gastric organism, '*H. heilmannii*', which has not yet been cultured, has a morphologically identical counterpart in dogs and cats. Time will tell whether the two are the same.

The remainder of this chapter deals only with campylobacter enteritis caused by *C. jejuni* and *C. coli*.

GROWTH AND SURVIVAL REQUIREMENTS

Campylobacter jejuni and *C. coli* are small, spiral or curved, non-sporing, Gram-negative bacteria, highly motile by means of single polar flagella. They are strictly microaerophilic and cannot normally tolerate oxygen at atmospheric tension. Thus, special gaseous conditions must be provided for their successful cultivation. Oxygen 5–10 per cent and carbon dioxide 1–10

per cent are ideal, and the addition of hydrogen improves growth. *Campylobacter jejuni* and *C. coli* (together with *C. lari* and *C. upsaliensis*) have a higher optimal growth temperature (42–43 °C) than other campylobacters and they are sometimes referred to as the 'thermophilic' group. They react to adverse conditions by rounding up into coccal forms, with intact cell walls and flagella. Lysis results if the insult persists, but otherwise these coccal forms can pass into a resting phase in which oxygen tolerance is increased. Such resting coccal forms may remain viable for several months in cold water, but they may not be culturable by ordinary methods. They may, however, still be capable of infecting susceptible hosts (Jones *et al.* 1991).

They are delicate bacteria unable to withstand heat, desiccation, or other physical and chemical agents as well as most enteric bacteria. They are destroyed by pasteurization, chlorination, and other conventional forms of disinfection (Griffiths and Park 1990), and by gamma irradiation. Survival is enhanced under cold conditions, but the process of freezing and thawing causes about a tenfold reduction in numbers. They are susceptible to a wide range of antimicrobial agents.

MOLECULAR BIOLOGY

Antigenic structure and serotyping

The cell wall of *C. jejuni* and *C. coli* contains lipopolysaccharide with a lipid-A component (endotoxin) similar to other Gram-negative bacteria. Polysaccharide components are antigenically diverse and are the heat-stable (O) antigens that form the basis of the widely used Penner serogrouping scheme. Likewise, certain flagellar and surface proteins are the heat-labile antigens on which the widely used Lior scheme is built. Some 66 O antigens have been defined in the Penner scheme and over 160 heat-labile antigens in the Lior scheme. Different combinations of these antigens go to make up many hundreds of individual serotypes. Good discrimination can be attained with a restricted set of antisera from each scheme. Serotyping is normally available only at reference laboratories, but it remains the most generally applicable method for epidemiological investigations.

Other typing methods

Biotyping is the simplest but least discriminating of typing methods. Kits that combine biotyping and resistotyping tests are available commercially and can be used in non-specialized laboratories. Phage typing has been used successfully in a few centres, but experience is limited. These methods are best used to enhance other typing methods such as serotyping. In the past

10 years a bewildering array of molecular typing methods has been described, mostly based on some form of DNA analysis. Each has its exponents and each its drawbacks. All require specially equipped laboratories, but they are theoretically capable of 'fingerprinting' all strains. There is an urgent need for an integrated approach to campylobacter typing internationally, particularly in relation to these genotyping methods. At present there is little or no standardization, so that results from different regions cannot be compared. This important subject is reviewed by Patton and Wachsmuth (1992) and Owen and Gibson 1995).

DISEASE MECHANISMS

In order to produce disease, the bacteria must be able to reach the intestinal mucosa and attach to its surface. The high degree of motility and spiral shape of campylobacters assist them in attaining this end; they are able to move along strands of mucus with extraordinary facility. The bacteria possess specific outer membrane proteins that bind to epithelial cells, but intact functioning flagella are necessary for invasion of epithelial cells. Experiments with human volunteers established that infection can be acquired from the ingestion of only 500–800 bacteria.

Tissue invasion is almost certainly a regular feature of infection. Although bacteraemia has been recorded in less than 1 per cent of infections (Skirrow *et al.* 1993), transient bacteraemia is probably more frequent; *Campylobacter jejuni* and *C. coli* do not survive for long in blood, as they are sensitive to the killing action of normal serum (unlike *C. fetus*, which is resistant), and blood cultures are seldom taken from patients with diarrhoea. There are several toxic products that might play a role in pathogenesis. First, there is the direct action of endotoxin released from the bacterial cell wall. Secondly, many strains produce a cholera-like enterotoxin, though in smaller amounts than by *V. cholerae* or enterotoxigenic *Escherichia coli*. Cytopathic toxins have also been detected in supernatant fluids of *C. jejuni* cultures. However, the significance of these various toxins is doubtful, as strains that apparently do not produce any of them have been shown to be virulent in human volunteers. Moreover, patients do not produce neutralizing antibodies to them. There is clinical and experimental evidence that hepatotoxic factors are produced.

THE HOSTS

ANIMAL HOSTS

Campylobacter enteritis is mainly a human disease, but some animals are also affected. It is difficult to assess the morbidity in animals, as the bacteria are usually found as often in healthy as in sick animals. The organisms are so widespread and common that animals become infected early in life when they may still have campylobacter antibodies acquired from their mothers. Thus infection may be mild or subclinical, yet it stimulates active immunity that persists with continuing exposure. Experimental infection in dogs, cats, cattle, sheep, and other domestic animals usually causes only mild disease, but there are clear instances of severe spontaneous campylobacter enteritis in non-human primates and dogs, sometimes linked with human infection (Skirrow 1994).

HUMAN HOSTS

Man is not a natural host of campylobacters and infection is normally transient. Man does not, therefore, constitute a significant reservoir of the bacteria. Infection is not always symptomatic, and there is considerable variation in severity of illness.

Incubation period

The average incubation period, calculated from volunteer experiments and point-source outbreaks, is 3 days (range 1–7 days).

Symptoms and signs

The illness starts either with abdominal pain and diarrhoea or with a prodromal period of fever, headache, and general influenza-like symptoms lasting from a few hours to a few days. Some patients suffer rigors, high fever, and even delirium; children may have febrile seizures. Illnesses commencing with a prodrome tend to be more severe.

The diarrhoeal illness itself is clinically indistinguishable from that due to salmonella or shigella, but when groups of patients are compared, those with campylobacter enteritis, on average, have more severe abdominal pain. The pain can be so acute that the victim is referred to hospital with suspected appendicitis. Nausea is usual, but vomiting is not a striking feature of the illness. The diarrhoea becomes watery and prostration may result in severe cases. Blood may appear in the stools on the second or third day; occasionally patients present with bloody stools and a picture of acute colitis mimicking acute ulcerative colitis.

Spontaneous resolution usually occurs after 2 or 3 days of diarrhoea, leaving the patient temporarily washed out, and lighter by several kilograms. Abdominal pain commonly persists for a few days, especially if the patient tries to eat too much too soon.

The excretion of campylobacters in the faeces after clinical recovery falls exponentially. The mean excretion period in a recent study was found to be 37.6 days, with a maximum of 69 days (Kapperud *et al.* 1992*a*). Excretion is of little consequence, as the risk of an excreter transmitting infection is extremely low. Long-term carriage has only been reported in patients with immune deficiency.

Atypical features of infection have been reported. These include skin rashes, notably urticaria, and abdominal pain without diarrhoea, particularly in schoolchildren. Children under the age of 1 year commonly have frank blood in their stools, often without much diarrhoea or fever. This picture can mimic intussusception in neonatal infants. Outbreaks of neonatal meningitis have also been reported in hospital nurseries.

Complications are rare in the acute stages of illness, but they include massive intestinal haemorrhage, toxic megacolon, and haemolytic uraemic syndrome. Reactive (aseptic) arthritis is a late complication that may arise 1–2 weeks after onset of illness; it is estimated that it affects about 1 per cent of patients. Guillain–Barré syndrome (postinfective polyneuropathy) is a less frequent, but more serious late complication (Rees *et al.* 1993). It is strongly, though not uniquely, associated with *C. jejuni* serotype O19 (Penner) infection. It has been suggested that the lipopolysaccharides of these strains possess a specific epitope that cross-reacts with peripheral nerve myelin proteins, thereby triggering an autoimmune reaction.

Diagnosis

As the clinical picture of campylobacter enteritis cannot be reliably distinguished from that of other forms of bacterial diarrhoea, diagnosis is dependent on the identification of the bacteria in the laboratory. Campylobacters can be recognized by their characteristic morphology in direct wet preparations or smears of faeces, but isolation of the bacteria in culture is the definitive method.

In order to ensure adequate sensitivity, faecal samples should be delivered to the laboratory on the day of collection, or else refrigerated overnight. If this is not possible, specimens should be placed in a transport medium recommended by the laboratory. The isolation of *C. jejuni* and *C. coli* in culture is a straightforward procedure, but the use of a special selective medium incubated in a specially gassed container is essential. Incubation is usually carried out at 42–43 °C in order to give extra selectivity and speed of growth. Growth is often visible after overnight incubation, but cultures are commonly left for 2 days before reading. Suspect campylobacter colonies can be identified by simple microscopy and reported simply as 'Campylobacter species'. This is adequate for routine clinical purposes, but there may be epidemiological reasons for identifying organisms as *C. jejuni* or *C. coli*, and to retain isolates for serotyping and further study. Species identification can be done in minutes by latex agglutination (at a cost), or by conventional biochemical tests in 1 or 2 more days; serotyping takes longer, as isolates are usually referred to a specialist laboratory.

Some laboratories use enrichment methods to increase the sensitivity of culture, but in general this is not necessary for the diagnosis of campylobacter enteritis, and it lengthens the time of final reporting to 3 or 4 days after receipt of the specimen. Enrichment culture is, however, essential for detecting campylobacters in foods and environmental samples.

The direct detection of campylobacters by DNA probing and polymerase chain reaction amplification is a promising new development. It is capable of detecting small numbers of campylobacters in water, but so far, not in faeces or foods.

Serodiagnosis is occasionally useful. It may be the only option for the diagnosis of patients with suspected late complications in whom cultures were not performed at the time of the acute illness. The appropriate test in such a case is one that detects antibody to group antigens, that is, antigens common to all strains of *C. jejuni* and *C. coli*. A complement-fixation test and enzyme-linked immunosorbent assay (ELISA) have been developed for this purpose. Another useful application of serodiagnosis is case detection in outbreaks where a particular campylobacter strain has been identified. Faecal culture may not be available, or the lapse of time might have made it unreliable. In this case agglutination, bactericidal, or immunoblotting tests are used, as they detect antibody to the specific infecting strain. Laboratory methods for the detection of campylobacter infections are described by Nachamkin (1995).

Pathology

The jejunum and upper ileum are the sites of initial infection, but infection usually spreads distally to affect the rest of the ileum and colon. The mucosa shows acute inflammatory infiltration, often with crypt abscess formation. The histological appearances are indistinguishable from those seen in salmonella and shigella infections. Mesenteric adenitis is usually seen in patients who have undergone laparotomy for suspected appendicitis. Terminal ileitis has been seen on radiography or compression ultrasonography in patients with acute abdominal pain.

Most patients show a rapid immune response to infection in the form of sharply rising titres of specific anti-campylobacter IgA, IgM, and IgG antibodies in serum. Specific IgA antibodies appear locally in intestinal secretions. These antibodies give protection against reinfection with the homologous strain and apparently against some other strains, as children in developing countries develop general immunity after only a few episodes of campylobacter infection. This immunity is reflected by a progressive rise of specific serum IgA antibody during the first few years of life (Blaser *et al.* 1986).

Treatment

Most patients with campylobacter enteritis require no more than simple supportive treatment in the form of fluid and electrolyte replacement. Antimicrobial therapy is effective if given early in the disease, but as most patients are recovering by the time a bacteriological diagnosis is made, it is seldom needed. If at that time the patient is still acutely ill, it is reasonable to give a short course (no more than 5 days) of an appropriate antimicrobial agent. Erythromycin is the agent of choice in most cases (e.g. erythromycin stearate 500 mg twice daily for adults; erythromycin ethyl succinate 40 mg/kg/day for children). Resistance to erythromycin remains generally low and is mainly confined to *C. coli*. Ciprofloxacin and other fluoroquinolones are very effective against sensitive strains, but resistance rates have risen alarmingly (up to 50 per cent) in some parts of the world, notably in Spain and The Netherlands. Such resistance has been attributed to the widespread use of enrofloxacin in poultry.

Prognosis

The prognosis in campylobacter enteritis is excellent. The disease is certainly unpleasant, but it is normally self-limiting and without sequelae, except possibly in rare cases of Guillain–Barré syndrome. Death is exceptional and almost always associated with other illness or debility.

A more detailed account of the pathological and clinical aspects of the disease is given by Skirrow and Blaser (1995).

EPIDEMIOLOGY

OCCURRENCE

Incidence

Campylobacter enteritis is the most common form of acute infective diarrhoea identified in most industrialized countries of the world. In the United Kingdom almost 50 000 laboratory confirmed infections were reported in 1994, representing an annual incidence of about 90 per 100 000. This figure has risen severalfold since reporting began in 1978, but the rise can be explained largely by increased testing, as the percentage of positive faecal specimens has remained roughly constant. Estimates of the true incidence, based on a survey of patients attending a single family practice, gave a figure of 1.1 per cent per year, i.e. about 12 times the

incidence of the laboratory confirmed infections (Kendall and Tanner 1982). A similar incidence was calculated in the United States, where the figure was derived from consultation rates in a community outbreak of campylobacter enteritis. Of the 865 persons identified as having been ill with diarrhoea, only 47 had consulted their doctor, or 1 in 18 of those ill. The application of this factor to laboratory statistics gave a national incidence of roughly 1 per cent per year (Tauxe 1992).

Although this incidence is high, it is below the level at which a population develops general immunity to campylobacter infection. As a consequence, the disease affects people of all ages, although there is a gradual lessening of incidence after about the age of 30 years. The disease has an unusual bimodal age distribution, with the highest peak in children aged 1–4 years and a secondary peak in young adults (15–24 years). This is a constant finding in industrialized countries, but the reasons for it are unknown. This pattern is partly distorted by the fact that young children tend to be sampled more intensely than adults. If the number of faecal specimens tested in each age group is taken as the denominator, and the positive ones expressed as a percentage, a different picture emerges in which the highest figure is in the 15–24-year age group (Skirrow 1987). There is a slight excess of infection in males (M : F ratio 1.3 : 1); this ratio is higher (1.7 : 1) in young adults aged 15–24 years.

Sporadic and epidemic infection

The great majority of infections are sporadic, or in the form of small family outbreaks. Family outbreaks are undoubtedly more frequent than reports suggest, for if cases are followed up diligently, other mild household cases and symptomless infections are commonly found. Community outbreaks are uncommon, but they can be of major proportions. Most are due to the consumption of raw milk or untreated water (see below).

Seasonal trends

There is a strikingly constant seasonal pattern of infection in temperate regions, with a sharp rise of incidence in late spring early summer followed by a gradual fall to base levels during late summer and autumn (Skirrow 1987). In the United States, sporadic infections show the same pattern, but outbreak-associated infections (mostly milk- and and water-borne) show sharp peaks in the spring and autumn (Tauxe 1992). What causes these seasonal patterns is unknown.

Developing countries

In developing countries infection is hyperendemic as a result of poor sanitation and close contact with animals in the home. Children are repeatedly exposed to infection from an early age, particularly during weaning. Some protection is afforded by specific antibody in breast milk, but about half of all initial infections are symptomatic. Thereafter, the ratio of symptomatic to asymptomatic infection falls as immunity is gained during the first few years of life (Calva *et al.* 1988). Older children and adults are unaffected by the disease. Although many infections are symptomless, campylobacter enteritis contributes substantially to the burden of childhood diarrhoea in developing countries (Taylor 1992).

Travellers' diarrhoea

Owing to the high prevalence of infection in the warm climates of developing countries, it is not surprising that campylobacter enteritis is a common form of travellers diarrhoea, often second only to that due to enterotoxigenic *Escherichia coli* (ETEC). About 12 per cent of campylobacter infections recorded in the United Kingdom are acquired abroad, but in Scandinavia the equivalent figure is nearer 50 per cent. Here again there is a seasonal variation. In a study of Finnish tourists visiting Morocco (Mattila *et al.* 1992), campylobacter enteritis was the leading cause of travellers diarrhoea in winter (28 per cent of cases), but not in autumn (7 per cent).

Economic costs

Campylobacter enteritis has a major economic impact in industrialized countries. A detailed study of 53 routinely diagnosed patients in the United Kingdom in 1986 showed that the direct costs of health care and investigation averaged £135 per patient, and indirect costs attributable to lost productive output averaged £130 per patient (Sockett and Pearson 1988). Intangible costs attributable to 'pain and suffering' amounted to £314 per patient. Based on these rates, the defined costs alone for laboratory-diagnosed cases gives a figure of £12 million per year. Even allowing for the fact that undiagnosed cases would be milder and cost less, the true total for all cases would be far higher, especially if the cost of 'pain and suffering' is included.

SOURCES AND TRANSMISSION

Campylobacter jejuni and *C. coli* are widely distributed in nature as inhabitants of the intestinal tract of birds and some mammals. Their essentially avian origin is reflected in their optimum growth temperature of 42–43 °C. Shedding of the bacteria by wild birds causes contamination of open waters even in remote places, and, as campylobacters can survive for several months

in water at temperatures below 15 °C, no such water is safe to drink without appropriate treatment.

Domestic animals, especially poultry, readily become colonized with *C. jejuni* and to a lesser extent *C. coli*. Pigs are unusual in that they are almost universally colonized with *C. coli* rather than *C. jejuni*. Such ubiquity among domestic food-producing animals provide many opportunities for the transmission of infection to man.

Direct transmission from animals

In general, the transmissibility of campylobacters is low, but there are definite risks associated with handling infected or colonized animals or their carcasses without taking proper hygienic precautions, which basically boil down to the frequent and thorough washing of hands. Most exposure is occupational, notably the handling of poultry, either live or during the processing and preparation of carcasses. Farmers, veterinarians, abattoir workers, butchers, and many others are at risk of occupational infection.

Direct transmission may also occur in the home through contact with infected pets. Most such instances arise through contact with a sick puppy, less often a kitten, that is itself suffering from campylobacter diarrhoea. The victim is often a young child. It is difficult to measure the proportion of infections contracted in this way, but estimates of 5 per cent in the United Kingdom and 6 per cent in the United States have been made (Saeed *et al.* 1993). Transmission from human patients is discussed below (p. 44).

Indirect transmission

Indirect transmission via milk, water, and food is believed to account for most infections. Transmission via food is a complex subject and is discussed below. First, the simpler issues of milk- and water-borne infections are examined.

Milk

The consumption of raw or inadequately heat-treated cows milk has caused major outbreaks of campylobacter enteritis, particularly in England where the largest outbreak affected over 3000 people, including about 2500 schoolchildren (Robinson and Jones 1981). In the United States, at least 26 outbreaks affecting a total of 7600 people have been reported, and case-control studies have shown consistently that the consumption of raw milk carries up to a ninefold increased risk of infection. Campylobacters have been isolated from 2.5–12.3 per cent of bulked raw milk samples in the United Kingdom, The Netherlands, and the United States (Humphrey and Hart 1988; Rohrbach *et al.* 1992).

Faecal contamination at the time of milking, which cannot be avoided even in the best-run parlours, is thought to be the main route by which the bacteria get into the milk, but they may also be excreted in milk from infected udders. Campylobacter mastitis is an uncommon condition, but as the bacteria are excreted in large numbers early in the infection before the milk has become visibly granular, it is a potentially potent source of infection. Goats' milk has also been implicated in outbreaks of campylobacter enteritis. As long as raw milk is sold to the public, milk-borne campylobacter infections will continue to occur. Campylobacters are destroyed by properly conducted pasteurization.

An unusual cause of the contamination of milk after pasteurization was identified in certain areas of the United Kingdom. Magpies (*Pica pica*) and jackdaws (*Corvus monedula*) acquired the habit of pecking through the foil tops of doorstep-delivered milk bottles, and in so doing contaminated the milk with campylobacters (Palmer and McGuirk 1995). It is thought that the bacteria are picked up from cow pats, which the birds probe for invertebrates. This activity is strongest in early summer when fledglings are being fed. Although this bizarre route of transmission accounts for a substantial part of the early summer rise of infection in certain areas, it is only a potential problem where there are home deliveries of milk. It can be prevented by the simple measure of covering the tops of milk bottles. The milk in breached bottles should be discarded or used only for cooking.

Water

As mentioned above, campylobacters can be found in any collection of open water. Sporadic infection is common in those who drink untreated water from streams or pools while engaged in trekking and other outdoor pursuits, or accidentally while swimming. More importantly, major outbreaks have been caused by the contamination of community water supplies. There have been at least 10 such outbreaks, the largest of which affected about one-fifth of the population of a town of some 16 000 inhabitants in the United States. In every case there had either been a defect in the chlorination or distribution system, or else the water was from a source considered clean enough not to need chlorination (Melby *et al.* 1991). Conventional chlorination eliminates campylobacters. Outbreaks in institutions have been caused by inadequately protected header tanks that allowed birds to contaminate the contents (Palmer *et al.* 1983).

Food

As the routes of transmission described above account for only a minority of all infections, we are left with the conclusion that most are derived from food, though precise knowledge of such foods is incomplete. There are several approaches to the problem.

1. Identification of foods most likely to be contaminated with campylobacters. Apart from milk, raw meats are the main source. Table 4.1 summarizes the results of surveys on several types of meat, from which it is seen that broiler chickens are by far the most frequently contaminated. Moreover, campylobacter counts in the region of 10^6 per carcass are commonplace in these birds, whereas much lower counts are found in red meats. This difference is accentuated after freezing, which causes at least a $\log_{10}$ fall in viable count. The fall in count between the larger abattoir carcasses and their equivalent red meat products is caused by drying of the surface of carcasses that occurs during the prolonged air chilling process.

2. Identification of foods implicated in outbreaks of infection. Food-borne outbreaks of campylobacter enteritis are uncommon and it is seldom that a particular source food can be identified with certainty. Table 4.2 summarizes the few foods that have been

Table 4.1 The prevalence of campylobacters in meats, mean percentage of samples positive (number of surveys analysed in parentheses)

	Carcass in abattoir (before chilling)	Retailed product	
		Fresh	Frozen
Broiler chickens	58 (20)	59 (17)	43 (6)
Red meats:			
beef	12 (3)	3.5 (9)	0 (1)
lamb	15 (3)	5.8 (5)	2 (1)
pork	31 (6)	3.4 (9)	1 (1)
sausages (mixed)	–	0.2 (1)	2 (1)
offal[a]	–	22 (8)	2 (3)

[a] Mostly liver, kidney, and heart from cattle, sheep, and pigs

Table 4.2 Foods (excluding milk) incriminated or suspected as the vehicle of infection in community outbreaks of campylobacter enteritis

	Number of outbreaks reported
Chicken	10
Turkey	3
Red meat	4
Shellfish (raw)	2
Egg (frozen 1; undercooked 1)	2
Cake icing	1
Specific meal (item of food undetermined)	27

Attack rates ranged from 12 to 100 per cent (mean 43.0 per cent).

Table 4.3 Foods (excluding milk) associated with risk of campylobacter infection as determined by case-control studies

Food	Number of studies	Odds ratio
Chicken (any)	8	2.0–5.7
Chicken (raw or undercooked)	3	6.3–9.0
Raw or rare fish	1	4.0
Raw or rare shellfish	1	1.5
Game hens	1	3.3
Turkey sandwiches	1	1.7
Mushrooms	1	1.5

implicated. Again, poultry head the list. Some 27 other outbreaks have been traced to the consumption of a particular meal, but with insufficient data to identify a specific food item; most of these arose in Japan where a wide variety of raw foods is commonly eaten.

3.   Search for statistical associations between infection and the consumption of various foods. Table 4.3 shows the foods associated with an increased risk of infection in case-control studies. Again chickens feature prominently. In the most comprehensive study, from the United States, it was calculated that 48 per cent of all infections were attributable to the consumption of broiler chickens (Harris *et al.* 1986). Infection from raw or rare fish, or shellfish, was probably from contaminated water rather than the fish.

4.   Measurement of the effect of interrupting transmission from a suspected source on the incidence of infection in the human population. This is a convincing tactic, but difficult to execute. The control of a particular serotype of *C. jejuni* prevalent in a broiler chicken farm in the south of England was shown to be followed by a sharp reduction of the same serotype in the associated community (Pearson *et al.* 1993). The introduction of compulsory pasteurization of milk in Scotland virtually eliminated milk-borne campylobacter enteritis.

Infection can be transmitted from raw meats, chicken carcasses and other animal products in three ways. First, when handling the product, bacteria may be transferred from the fingers to the mouth unthinkingly; this is especially likely in the case of inexperienced food handlers. Secondly, the product may be consumed raw or undercooked, either from choice or by accident. Barbecue- and fondue-cooked meats are particularly liable to be undercooked and are known to carry an increased risk of infection (Kapperud *et al.* 1992*b*). Thirdly, other 'innocent' foods may become cross-contaminated from the raw product by means of hands and utensils. This is probably the most frequent mode of infection, but it is difficult to prove. It does not require much imagination to appreciate the ease

with which a few hundred bacteria can be transferred from, say, a fresh broiler covered in a million bacteria to a nearby bit of salad or piece of bread.

At least campylobacters do not multiply in food like salmonellas (they do not grow below about 30 °C), which explains why large explosive outbreaks of campylobacter food poisoning are rarely seen. Their numbers decline on exposure to air and they cannot easily withstand drying. They are readily destroyed by normal cooking procedures.

COMMUNICABILITY

The communicability of campylobacters is low. Their survival outside the body is generally short. Point-source outbreaks of infection are usually notable for the scarcity of secondary cases. Young children are sometimes an exception: mothers may become infected from handling the soiled nappies of infected children, and toddlers may spread infection to their siblings and occasionally to other members of the family. I have never known infection to have spread from patients in hospital, even when they have had profuse campylobacter diarrhoea. Simple 'excretion precautions' are adequate for the prevention of cross-infection. Neonatal units are an exception in that five outbreaks have been recorded, one with cases of meningitis. Common factors, such as communally used rectal thermometers, have been suspected as vehicles of infection (Butzler and Goossens 1988). Newborn babies sometimes pick up infection from their mothers, usually during birth.

Healthy food handlers who are excreting campylobacters in their faeces are extremely unlikely to transmit infection through handling food, but they should not handle food if they have diarrhoea.

PREVENTION AND CONTROL

The safe disposal of sewage, the provision of safe drinking water, and the application of good hygiene in the workplace and home are fundamental measures that are already in place in most industrialized countries.

PUBLIC EDUCATION

There should be a deliberate strategy for educating adults and schoolchildren on basic hygiene, in particular the importance of washing the hands after handling sick animals and before eating or handling food. There should be instruction on good hygienic practice in the kitchen, notably the importance of handling and storing raw meats separately from cooked foods and salads. Questionnaires have revealed an extraordinary ignorance on these matters among ordinary householders in the United Kingdom. Much could be done through the intelligent use of television and other mass media. The professional caterer requires a more detailed form of instruction. Such a strategy is also applicable to the prevention of salmonellosis and other food-borne infections.

CONTROL OF INFECTION IN FOOD-PRODUCING ANIMALS AND THEIR PRODUCTS

The widespread distribution of campylobacters in wildlife makes control of the natural reservoir of infection impractical, but the control of infection in domestic food-producing animals and their products is possible. There is probably little that can be done to reduce exposure of sheep and cattle to infection, but steps can be taken to minimize the contamination of carcasses with gut contents during slaughter and processing. Milk is rendered safe by pasteurization or other heat treatment, which should be compulsory for all milk sold to the public.

The greatest impact on human infection is likely to come from the control of campylobacter colonization of poultry. As broiler chickens are grown in closed sheds and there is no evidence of vertical transmission via eggs, the bacteria must be introduced from extraneous sources, and it should be possible to prevent this. Potential sources are the boots and clothing of attendants, water supplies, and small birds, mammals, and insects that could gain access to sheds; dried feed is an unlikely source. Experimental interventions to block transmission from each of these sources have reduced colonization rates significantly (Kapperud et al. 1993). The disinfection and redesign of water supply systems, which are often from private bore holes, has been particularly effective (Pearson et al. 1993). The dosing of chicks with normal intestinal flora ('competitive exclusion') is another approach that is being explored (Schoeni and Wong 1994). The trouble is that all of these measures are uneconomic for farmers, because excluding or reducing colonization does not increase the value of the product. More research to find the most effective interventions, and the introduction of suitable incentives to help farmers implement them, are required. This will need proper research funding and co-operation between microbiologists, veterinarians, and private industry. No formal strategy or legislation exists for the control of campylobacter infection in poultry.

A subsidiary approach is to try to reduce the cross-contamination that occurs during the mass mechanized processing of broilers. Some processing plants are capable of handling 15 000 birds an hour, so the potential for the dissemination of bacteria is immense.

Birds that are free of campylobacters at the start of processing are likely to end up contaminated. Improvements in the design of machinery has helped to this end, notably the introduction of spray or forced air cooling of carcasses at the end of processing, but the essential problem remains. The subject is discussed more fully by Humphrey (1989).

A sure way to attain a bacteriologically safe product is to expose birds to terminal irradiation, which has the advantage of killing salmonellas and other pathogenic microbes. This again has cost implications and there are the problems of public acceptability.

VACCINATION

The prospect of vaccinating against campylobacter enteritis is attractive, particularly for children in developing countries where infection is hyperendemic. A vaccine consisting of inactivated campylobacter whole-cells and heat-labile ETEC enterotoxin adjuvant has shown promise in an animal model, and this is being developed for human trials at the United States Naval Medical Research Institute (Harberberger and Walker 1994). The development of a campylobacter vaccine should clearly be dovetailed into cholera and ETEC vaccine development.

SURVEILLANCE AND LABORATORY SERVICES

Surveillance is a vital part of any control programme, and as diagnosis can only be made in a laboratory, a laboratory-based monitoring service is an essential requirement. Any such service should have a reference laboratory capable of providing prompt identification and typing of field isolates (see p. 38).

REFERENCES

Blaser, M. J., Taylor, D. N., and Echeverria, P. (1986). Immune response to *Campylobacter jejuni* in a rural community in Thailand. *Journal of Infectious Diseases*, **153**, 249–54.

Butzler, J. P. and Goossens, H. (1988). *Campylobacter jejuni* infection as a hospital problem: an overview. *Journal of Hospital Infection*, **11**, (Suppl. A), 374–7.

Butzler, J. P., Dekeyser, P., Detrain, M., and Dehaen, F. (1973). Related vibrio in stools. *Journal of Pediatrics*, **82**, 493–5.

Calva, J. J., Ruiz-Palacios, G. M., Lopez-Vidal, A. B., Ramos, A., and Bojalil, R. (1988). Cohort study of intestinal infection with campylobacter in Mexican children. *Lancet*, **i**, 503–6.

Griffiths and Park (1990). Campylobacters associated with human diarrhoeal disease. *Journal of Applied Bacteriology*, **69**, 281–301.

Harberberger, R. L. and Walker, R. I. (1994). Prospects and problems for development of a vaccine against diarrhea caused by *Campylobacter*. *Vaccine Research*, **3**, 15–22.

Harris, N. V., Weiss, N. S., and Nolan, C. M. (1986). The role of poultry and meats in the etiology of *Campylobacter jejuni/coli* enteritis. *American Journal of Public Health*, **76**, 407–11.

Humphrey, T. J. (1989). Salmonella, campylobacter and poultry: possible control measures. *Abstracts on Hygiene and Communicable Diseases*, **64**, R1–R8.

Humphrey, T. J. and Hart, R. J. C. (1988). Campylobacter and salmonella contamination of unpasteurized cows' milk on sale to the public. *Journal of Applied Bacteriology*, **65**, 463–7.

Jones, D. M., Sutcliffe, E. M., and Curry, A. (1991). Recovery of viable but non-culturable *Campylobacter jejuni*. *Journal of General Microbiology*, **137**, 2477–82.

Kapperud, G., Lassen, J., Ostroff, S. M., and Aasen, S. (1992a). Clinical features of sporadic campylobacter infections in Norway. *Scandinavian Journal of Infectious Diseases*, **24**, 741–9.

Kapperud, G., Skjerve, E., Bean, N., Osroff, S. M., and Lassen, J. (1992b). Risk factors for sporadic *Campylobacter* infections: results of a case-control study in southeastern Norway. *Journal of Clinical Microbiology*, **30**, 3117–21.

Kapperud, G. *et al.* (1993). Epidemiological investigation of risk factors for campylobacter colonization in Norwegian broiler flocks. *Epidemiology and Infection*, **111**, 245–55.

Kendall, E. J. C. and Tanner, E. I. (1982). Campylobacter enteritis in general practice. *Journal of Hygiene (Cambridge)*, **88**, 155–63.

Mattila, L. *et al.* (1992). Seasonal variation in etiology of travelers' diarrhea. *Journal of Infectious Diseases*, **165**, 385–8.

Melby, K., Gondrosen, B., Gregusson, S., Ribe, H., and Dahl, O. P. (1991). Waterborne campylobacteriosis in northern Norway. *International Journal of Food Microbiology*, **12**, 151–6.

Mishu Allos, B. Lastovica, A. J., and Blaser, M. J. (1995). Atypical campylobacters and related microorganisms. In *Infections of the gastrointestinal tract*, (ed. M. J. Blaser, P. D. Smith, J. I. Ravdin, H. B. Greenberg, and R. L. Guerrant), pp. 849–65. Raven Press, New York.

Nachamkin, I. (1995). *Campylobacter* and *Arcobacter*. In *Manual of clinical microbiology*, (6th edn.), (ed. P. R. Murray, E. J. Baron, M. A. Pfaller, F. C. Tenover, and R. H. Yolken), pp. 483–91. ASM Press, Washington.

Owen, R. J. and Gibson, J. R. (1995). Update on epidemiological typing of *Campylobacter*. *PHLS Microbiology Digest*, **12**, 2–6.

Palmer, S. R. and McGuirk, S. M. (1995). Bird attacks on milk bottles and campylobacter infection. *Lancet*, **345**, 326–7.

Palmer, S. R. *et al.* (1983). Water-borne outbreak of campylobacter gastroenteritis. *Lancet*, **i**, 287–90.

Patton, C. M. and Wachsmuth, I. K. (1992). Typing schemes: are current methods useful? In Campylobacter jejuni: *current status and future trends*, (ed. I. Nachamkin, M. J. Blaser, and L. S. Tompkins), pp. 110–28. American Society for Microbiology, Washington.

Pearson, A. D. *et al.* (1993). Colonization of broiler chickens by waterborne *Campylobacter jejuni*. *Applied and Environmental Microbiology*, **59**, 987–96.

Popovic-Uroic, T. (1989). *Campylobacter jejuni* and *Campylobacter coli* diarrhoea in rural and urban populations in Yugoslavia. *Epidemiology and Infection*, **102**, 59–67.

Rees, J. H., Gregson, N. A., Griffiths, P. L., and Hughes, R. A. C. (1993). *Campylobacter jejuni* and the Guillain–Barré syndrome. *Quarterly Journal of Medicine*, **86**, 623–34.

Robinson, D. A. and Jones, D. M. (1981). Milk-borne campylobacter infection. *British Medical Journal*, **282**, 1374–6.

Rohrbach, B. W., Draughon, F. A., Davidson, P. M., and Oliver S. P. (1992). Prevalence of *Listeria monocytogenes*, *Campylobacter jejuni*, *Yersinia enterocolitica*, and *Salmonella* in bulk tank milk: risk factors and risk of human exposure. *Journal of Food Protection*, **55**, 93–7.

Saeed, A. M., Harris, N. V., and DiGiacomo, R. F. (1993). The role of exposure to animals in the etiology of *Campylobacter jejuni/coli* enteritis. *American Journal of Epidemiology*, **137**, 108–14.

Schoeni, J. L. and Wong, A. C. L. (1994). Inhibition of *Campylobacter jejuni* colonization in chicks by defined competitive exclusion bacteria. *Applied and Environmental Microbiology*, **60**, 1191–7.

Skirrow, M. B. (1977). Campylobacter enteritis: a 'new' disease. *British Medical Journal*, **2**, 9–11.

Skirrow, M. B. (1987). A demographic survey of campylobacter, salmonella and shigella infections in England. *Epidemiology and Infection*, **99**, 647–57.

Skirrow, M. B. (1994). Diseases due to *Campylobacter*, *Helicobacter* and related bacteria. *Journal of Comparative Pathology*, **111**, 113–49.

Skirrow, M. B. and Blaser, M. J. (1995). *Campylobacter jejuni*. In *Infections of the gastrointestinal tract* (ed. M. J. Blaser, P. D. Smith, J. I. Ravdin, H. B. Greenberg, and R. L. Guerrant), pp. 825–48. Raven Press, New York.

Skirrow, M. B., Jones, D. M., Sutcliffe, E., and Benjamin, J. (1993). Campylobacter bacteraemia in England and Wales, 1981–91. *Epidemiology and Infection*, **110**, 567–73.

Sockett, P. N. and Pearson, A. D. (1988). Cost implications of human campylobacter infections. In *Campylobacter IV: proceedings of the fourth international workshop on campylobacter infections*, (ed. B. Kaijser and E. Falsen), pp. 261–4. University of Göteborg, Göteborg.

Taylor, D. N. (1992). *Campylobacter* infections in developing countries. In Campylobacter jejuni: *current status and future trends*, (ed. I. Nachamkin, M. J. Blaser, and L. S. Tompkins), pp. 20–30. American Society for Microbiology, Washington.

Tauxe, R. V. (1992). Epidemiology of *Campylobacter jejuni* infections in the United States and other industrialized nations. In Campylobacter jejuni: *current status and future trends*, (ed. I. Nachamkin, M. J. Blaser, and L. S. Tompkins), pp. 9–19. American Society for Microbiology, Washington.

Vandamme, P. and Goossens, H. (1992). Taxonomy of *Campylobacter*, *Arcobacter*, and *Helicobacter*: a review. *Zentralblatt für Bakteriologie*, **276**, 447–72.

5 CAT-SCRATCH DISEASE

Michel Drancourt and Didier Raoult

SUMMARY

The aetiology of cat-scratch disease remains controversial since two bacterial species, *Afipia felis* and *Bartonella* (*Rochalimaea*) *henselae*, have been isolated from diseased lymph nodes. Most recent reports, however, demonstrated that *B. henselae* is regularly detected and isolated from such adenopathies, and that the sera of patients with a definitely diagnosed cat-scratch disease exhibit significant titres of anti- *Bartonella henselae* antibodies, but no antibodies against *Afipia felis*. Also, *B. henselae* was isolated from the reservoir (healthy domestic cats), but not *A. felis*. The precise role of the latter bacterial species remain to be clarified. Both are fastidious, facultative intracellular Gram-negative bacteria. *B. henselae*, *Bartonella quintana*, and *Bartonella elizabethae* cause endocarditis and *Bartonella bacilliformis* causes septicaemia (Oroya's fever) in non-immunocompromised hosts; *B. henselae* and *B. quintana* cause fever, bacteraemia, bacillary angiomatosis, and visceral peliosis in human immunodeficiency virus-infected patients. We also recently isolated *B. quintana* from a cat-owner with chronic adenopathy.

Clinical manifestations include a self-limited subfebrile disease with peripheral adenopathy, and Parinaud' syndrome with conjunctivitis and adenopathy. Systemic and severe forms have been reported, with granulomatous hepatitis, osseous, and splenic localizations; and neuritis, encephalitis, glomerulonephritis, thrombocytopenic purpura, and erythema nodosum have also been reported.

Current diagnosis of cat-scratch disease relies upon the history of close contacts with cats positive serology, and direct demonstration by molecular biology tools and isolation of *B. henselae* or *A. felis* in clinical samples. Experimental data and some clinical reports suggest that aminoglycosides may be useful for treating this disease. There is no effective prophylaxis, apart from avoiding contact with domestic cats.

HISTORICAL INTRODUCTION

Cat-scratch disease has been observed in France and the United States since 1931. Its initial description was published in 1950 by two French groups, Debré *et al.* 1950) and Mollaret *et al.* 1950). In the absence of a proven aetiological agent, the diagnosis of cat-scratch disease relied upon four diagnostic criteria:

(1) contact with a cat or dog and the presence of cutaneous scratch lesions or conjunctivitis;
(2) cutaneous hypersensitivity after experimental subcutaneous inoculation of filtered cat-scratch disease adenopathy;
(3) the absence of other documented aetiology; and
(4) pathological aspects, including necrotic granuloma, infiltrate with inflammatory cells and micro-abceses.

In 1983, Wear *et al.* reported the presence of bacilli in the walls of capillaries in 34/39 cat-scratch disease adenopathies after Warthin–Starry staining. They noted that these bacteria were Gram-negative after Brown–Hopps–Gram staining, and were located into vacuoles in the cytoplasm of infected macrophages and histiocytes. The same observations were made in cutaneous lesions (Margileth *et al.* 1984), and isolation of an unidentified Gram-negative bacterium on brain–heart axenic medium was reported in 1988 from 10/19 cat-scratch disease adenopathies (English *et al.* 1988). Only one of these 10 isolates was subcultured on blood–agar medium, leading to the hypothesis of a defective phase unable to grow on blood–agar, and a vegetative phase able to grow on blood–agar. The molecular identification led to the creation of a new bacterial genus, *Afipia* and the isolate was named *Afipia felis* (Brenner *et al.* 1991).

In 1988, bacilli were observed after Warthin–Starry staining in cat-scratch disease cutaneous lesions in AIDS patients (Hall *et al.* 1988; LeBoit *et al.* 1988). Also, a new clinical and pathological entity, named bacillary angiomatosis, characterized by cutaneous lesions mimicking lesions of Kaposi's sarcoma, was described in AIDS patients (Stoler *et al.* 1983; Cockerell *et al.* 1987; Berger *et al.* 1989). Some patients had contact with cats, and the lesions were characterized by capillary angiogenesis with cuboid endothelial cells, and the presence of Warthin–Starry staining bacilli in capillary walls (Berger *et al.* 1989). Kemper *et al.* proposed that bacillary angiomatosis was part of cat-scratch disease in immunocompromised patients including AIDS patients (Kemper *et al.*, 1990). Because of common Warthin–Starry tinctorial affinity, the same morphology using electron microscopy, and the occurrence of bacillary angiomatosis after contact with cats, it was hypothesis that *A. felis* was the common aetiological agent of both diseases.

In 1990, however, Relman *et al.* published the identification of a new bacterium in the cutaneous lesions of patients with bacillary angiomatosis, using the universal identification method showing 16S rRNA gene homology of 98.3 per cent with *Rochalimaea quintana*. This new bacterium, different from *A. felis* was then isolated from the blood of AIDS patients with fever and bacteraemia, visceral peliosis, and visceral bacillary angiomatosis (Perkocha *et al.* 1990). It was named *Rochalimaea henselae* (Regnery *et al.* 1992*a*). Both *R. henselae* and *R. quintana* were recently included in the genus *Bartonella* (Brenner *et al.* 1993).

At that stage, *A. felis* was regarded as the unique aetiological agent of cat-scratch disease, and *B. henselae* the unique aetiological agent of bacillary angiomatosis. However, serological study published in 1992 (Regnery *et al.* 1992*c*) found 88 per cent seropositivity for *B. henselae* and 25 per cent seropositivity for *A. felis* among 41 American patients diagnosed as cat-scratch disease. *B. henselae* was later isolated from the adenopathies of cat-scratch disease patients (Dolan *et al.* 1993), and a specific 16S rDNA sequence was obtained after PCR amplification using adenopathies (Perkins *et al.* 1992 Anderson *et al.* 1994*a*) and the material used in the past as skin test antigen (Anderson *et al.* 1993). Consequently, the concept shifted towards *B. henselae* as a unique aetiological agent for both bacillary angiomatosis and cat-scratch disease.

We recently reported the isolation of *B. quintana* from the blood of a patient with bacillary angiomatosis (Maurin *et al.* 1994), and from the chronically inflamed lymph nodes of a patient who had contact with cats (Raoult *et al.* 1994). It appears that both *B. henselae*, in the United States, and *B. quintana*, in the United States and in Europe, are the aetiological agents of bacillary angiomatosis and possibly of cat-scratch disease.

THE AGENTS

TAXONOMY AND MOLECULAR BIOLOGY

A. felis and *B. henselae* both belong to the α-subgroup of Proteobacteria. The genus *Afipia* was recently created on molecular grounds, according to current standards in the definition of genus and species in bacteriology. It encompasses six genospecies, three of them are named (*A. felis, Afijia clevelandensis,* and *Afijia broomae,*) the remaining three are unnamed. The

six species are Gram-negative bacilli, growing on axenic media, i.e. sheep-blood agar and buffered charcoal yeast extract, but not on MacConkey agar.

A. felis is a 0.2–2.5 μm long, motile Gram-negative bacillus. Tests for oxidase, catalase, indole production, H_2S production, gelatin and esculin hydrolysis, glucose, lactose, maltose and sucrose oxidation and fermentation are negative. The tests for urease production and nitrate reduction are positive. It is a facultative intracellular bacterium (Birkness *et al.* 1992).

The genus *Bartonella* encompasses six species: *B bacilliformis, B. quintana, B. henselae, B. elizabethae, B. vinsonii,* and the recently described species *B. vinsonii* subspecies *berkoffii* (Breitschwerdt *et al.* 1995). *Bartonella* species are 1–2 μm long, non-motile, Gram-negative bacteria, which share negative tests for oxidase, catalase, urease, and oxidation or fermentation of glucose. We showed that the addition of 10 per cent hemin allows for the species identification of *B. henselae, B. quintana* and *B. vinsonii* using the API-Coryne identification strip (Drancourt and Raoult 1993). One report of a 17 kb bacteriophage in *B. henselae* (Anderson *et al.* 1994*b*) has not yet been confirmed.

DISEASE MECHANISMS

The evidence that cat-scratch disease is caused by *Bartonella henselae* infection includes the following. It has been isolated from the reservoir (cat) (Regnery *et al.* 1992b) and from patients with definite cat-scratch disease (Dolan *et al.* 1993) and specific DNA fragments are demonstrated in these clinical specimens. Morever, specific immunological response is demonstrated in patients in an autologous reaction (Wear 1983) or by using a heterologous strain (Regnery *et al.* 1992c). However, because of the lack of any valid animal model for cat-scratch disease, reproducible clinical and pathological induction of the disease after *Bartonella henselae* inoculation has not been obtained.

In contrast *A. felis* although has been isolated from adenitis (Schwartzman 1992) and its DNA was detected in adenitis (Andrews *et al.* 1992) it does not induce a demonstrable immunological response in patients (Schwartzman 1992). In the initial report, 50 per cent of adenitis did not produce any isolate. However, *B. quintana* was isolated from two patients who had chronic adenitis and contact with cats, but no detectable immune response (Raoult *et al.* 1994*a*; Raoult, unpublished data).

Two possible hypotheses may explain these data; either *A. felis* and *B. henselae* are two independent aetiological agents of cat-scratch disease, they are necessary as co-infections to induce human disease, sharing the same reservoir (cat) and the same vector of inoculation. In this hypothesis, the relative contribution of each bacterial species to the disease remains to be established. It appears that *B. henselae* is able to induce an immunological response, with the production of specific antibodies and to stimulate cellular immunity (if *B. henselae* was indeed the antigen of the previously used skin test). Human macrophages may be a target cell for *A. felis* during human infection, and we demonstrated that *A. felis* is a facultative intracellular bacterium, residing within the phagosome of infected macrophage, and inhibiting the phagosome–lysosome fusion probably through to the secretion a specific inhibitory protein (Brouqui and Raoult 1993). Human vascular endothelial cells are one target of *B. henselae* during human infection, and though *Bartonella* were reported as epicellular bacteria, our observations demonstrate that at least *B. quintana* is a facultative intracellular bacterium, residing within a vacuole of the infected cell (P. Brouqui and D. Raoult, unpublished data). *B. henselae* shares with *B. bacilliformis* and *B. quintana* the unique property of inducing human endothelial cell proliferation, with a modification of the endothelial cell population (N. Teisseyre, personal communication). This property, unique among human bacterial pathogens was associated with a soluble factor, probably a protein, in *B. bacilliformis* (Garcia *et al.* 1992).

Cat-scratch disease can present as a local infection at the site of entry (scratches, lesions, or conjunctivitis), as a regional infection with an enlarged, infected lymph node associated with the site of entry, and as a systemic infection with lesions and infection demonstrated in various tissues. The relative contribution of immunodepression to the dissemination of the aetiological agent is unclear. Disseminated cat-scratch disease has been reported both in immunocompetent and immunocompromised patients with the same histological lesions. Bacteraemia and septicaemia due to *B. henselae* has been reported only in immunocompromised hosts, but *B. bacilliformis* causes a fatal septicaemic infection (Oroya's fever) in apparently immunocompetent patients. All three *Bartonella* species produce endocarditis in immunocompetent patients.

THE HOSTS

THE CAT

In most instances, cats implicated in cat-scratch disease are healthy, they do not react using skin test, and are not made ill by the injection of pus from patients with cat-scratch disease. Recently, *B. henselae* was isolated from the blood of a healthy cat (Regnery *et al.* 1992*b*). On a few occasions, however, a cat-scratch disease agent was suspected in ill cats. An argyrophilic intracellular bacterium was observed in the mandibular lymph node of a cat, but definite identification of this bacterium was never confirmed, despite the fact that slides were deposited in the collection of the Armed Forces Institute of Pathology (Kirkpatrick and Whiteley 1987).

THE HUMAN

Cat-scratch disease is a clinical and pathological entity defined as reported above. Parinaud's syndrome is a particular form of the disease, with conjunctivitis and a regional enlarged lymph node; the putative aetiological agent has been observed in the conjunctiva of such patients (Wear *et al.* 1985). Visceral localizations may be documented even in the absence of peripheral adenopathy. Hepatic localization results in granulomatous hepatitis (Malatack and Jaffe 1993), and splenic, deep lymphatic, and osseous localizations were documented (Waldvogel *et al.* 1994). Also, encephalitis was reported 1–6 weeks after cat scratches (Carithers 1985; Lewis and Tucker 1986), as well as polyneuritis (Carithers and Margileth 1991) and glomerulonephritis (D'Angati *et al.* 1990). Cat-scratch disease was reported to cause erythema nodosa (Carithers 1985) and thrombocytopenic purpura (Jim 1961). Systemic and severe forms were reported both in non-immunocompromised patients (Margileth *et al.* 1987) and in immunocompromised patients (Black *et al.* 1986), without granuloma formation.

A presumptive diagnosis can be obtained by a history of close contacts with a cat, a clinical condition as reported above, and serological tests for the detection of antibodies directed against *B. henselae*, *B. quintana* and *A. felis*. An enzyme-linked immunosorbent assay (Barka *et al.* 1993) and an immunofluorescence assay (Regnery *et al.* 1992*c*; Raoult *et al.* 1994*b*) were developed for the detection of antibodies directed against *B. henselae* and *B. quintana*, and an immunofluorescence assay for the detection of antibodies directed against *A. felis* (Drancourt *et al.* 1992). A definite diagnosis can be obtained by the excision of the enlarged lymph node or biopsy of diseased tissue for histological and, bacteriological examination, culture and direct detection of the bacterium. Characteristic histological changes include subcapsular foci of necrosis, inward spread involving germinal centres and paracortex, follicular and paracortical hyperplasia, vascular proliferation, and neutrophil fragmentation and formation of epithelioid cells, and occasionally giant cells around the necrotic zones. *Bartonella* species and *A. felis* were observed as thin, pleomorphic bacilli along the vessels after Warthin–Starry staining in cat-scratch disease adenopathies (Wear *et al.* 1983).

The isolation of *B. henselae* and *B. quintana* can be attempted by inoculation of clinical material on to sheep-blood agar, at 37 °C under a 5 per cent CO_2 atmosphere for 15–45 days, whereas buffered charcoal yeast extract agar incubated for 15–45 days at 25–30 °C should be used for the isolation of *A. felis*. Clinical material can be inoculated into human endothelial cell lines; several teams have observed that strains of *Bartonella* can be isolated using cell culture techniques. HeLa cell lines support the growth of *A. felis*. Morphological and biochemical characteristics of *A. felis* and *Bartonella* species have been described, but identification currently also relies upon immunological reactivity, the analysis of fatty acids using chromatography, and molecular identification. Whereas protein profile analysis, DNA/DNA hybridization and macrorestriction profiles obtained using pulsed-field gel electrophoresis allow the species identification (Maurin *et al.* 1994*a*), they require too much bacterial material to be useful for routine clinical identification. An alternative to 16S rRNA sequence analysis may be restriction fragment length polymorphism of the amplified citrate synthase gene. The detection of *Bartonella* in clinical specimens can be achieved by using immunofluorescence with polyclonal or monoclonal antibodies, or by molecular detection using polymerase chain reaction amplification followed by hybridization of a fragment of a heat-shock-like protein encoding gene (Anderson *et al.* 1994).

Apart from the role of *B. henselae* in the pathogenesis of cat-scratch disease, *B. henselae*, *B. quintana*, and *B. elizabethae* are agents of endocarditis (Daly *et al.* 1993; Hadfield *et al.* 1993; Spach *et al.* 1993; Drancourt *et al.* 1995). *B. bacilliformis* causes a septicaemia (Oroya's fever) in non-immunocompromised hosts. *B. henselae* and *B. quintana* cause fever, relapsing bacteraemia, bacillary angiomatosis, and visceral peliosis in immunocompromised patients (Schwartzman 1992). *B. quintana* has been isolated in alcoholic patients with bacteraemia (Spach *et al.* 1995).

EPIDEMIOLOGY

The previous criteria of definition of cat-scratch disease included contact with cats. Virtually all recorded instances of cat-scratch disease have been temporally associated with contact with domestic cats (Carithers 1985). Originally, the cat was thought to be an efficient inoculator of the agent of cat-scratch disease, which was considered to be widely distributed in the environment. However recent data indicate that the cat is in fact the reservoir of the bacterium (Kirkpatrick and Glickman 1989). Epidemiological studies indicated that owning a kitten has strongly associated with cat-scratch disease (Zangwill *et al.*

1993), and that among cat owners, patients with bacillary angiomatosis were more likely than controls to own a kitten (Tappero *et al.* 1993). (The very first young patient observed by Debré in 1931 slept with his kitten). *B. henselae* was repeatedly isolated from a cat which exhibited antibodies against the bacterium (Regnery *et al.* 1992*b*), and it was again isolated from pet cats of patients with bacillary angiomatosis and from 41 per cent of randomly screened cats in San Francisco (Koehler *et al.* 1994). Also, seroprevalence of antibodies against *B. henselae* is higher in cats linked to cat-scratch disease patients (81 per cent) than in the general cat population (38 per cent) (Zangwill *et al.* 1993). These data strongly suggest that cats, or kittens, are the reservoir of *B. henselae*, which in turn is at least one of the aetiological agents of cat-scratch disease. Whether the distribution of *A. felis* and *B. henselae* is limited to the domestic cat or extends to other animals is unknown. The route of inoculation is usually though cutaneous lesions due to cat scratches, but cat fleas may play a role in the transmission; it was shown that owning a cat with fleas was a risk factor (Zangwill *et al.* 1993), and *B. henselae* has been isolated from fleas from one infected cat (Koehler *et al.* 1994).

PREVENTION, CONTROL, AND TREATMENT

Cats are the only known reservoir of the agent of cat-scratch disease. The only prevention strategy is to avoid contact with cats; this may be particularly advisable for immunocompromised patients. There is not, currently a recommended antibiotic treatment for cat-scratch-induced wounds, and currently recommended antibiotic treatments for animal bites (amoxycillin plus clavulanate) (Goldstein 1995) have not been shown to be effective for the prevention of cat-scratch disease. Antibiotic susceptibility tests for *A. felis* indicate that this species is susceptible to imipenem, aminoglycosides, and rifampicin when tested in axenic medium, and to amikacin and tobramycin only when tested in a HeLa cells model (Maurin *et al.* 1993). *Bartonella* species, including *B. vinsonii*, *B. quintana*, and *B. henselae* were susceptible to amoxycillin, third-generation cephalosporins, aminoglycosides, tetracyclines, macrolides, rifampicin, and co-trimoxazole when tested in axenic media (Maurin and Raoult 1993). When tested using a cultured cell model, however, only the aminoglycosides were effective against *B. henselae* (Musso *et al.* 1995).

Cat-scratch disease is a self-limited disease in most cases, and there is no controlled study regarding the antibiotic treatment of this disease. Some reports mentioned the efficacy of aminoglycosides (Bogue *et al.*

1989; Lewis and Wallace 1991). The efficacy of ciprofloxacin was reported in five adult patients with a regional form of cat-scratch disease (Preston Holley 1991), and in one additional observation (Molnar 1992). Trimethoprim–sulphamethoxazole was reported to be effective in children (Collipp 1992). These scarce data and our experimental results suggest that aminoglycosides should be used in the antibiotic treatment of cat-scratch disease.

REFERENCES

Anderson, B., Kelly, C., Threlkel, R., and Edwards, K. (1993). Detection of *Rochalimae henselae* in cat-scratch disease skin test antigens. *Journal of Infectious Diseases*, **168**, 1034–6.

Anderson, B. *et al.* (1994*a*). Detection of *Rochalimaea henselae* DNA in specimens from cat scratch disease patients by PCR. *Journal of Clinical Microbiology*, **32**, 942–8.

Anderson, B., Goldsmith, C., Johnson, A., Padmalayan, I., and Baumstark, B. (1994*b*). Bacteriophage-like particle of *Rochalimaea henselae*. *Molecular Microbiology*, **13**, 67–73.

Andrews, D. M., Kurnick, J. T., and Ruoff, K. L. (1992). Case 22–1992. Pathogenesis of cat scratch disease. Reply. *New England Journal of Medicine*, **327**, 1600–1.

Barka, N. E., Hadfield, T., Patnaik, M., Schartzman, W. A., and Peter, J. B. (1993). EIA for detection of *Rochalimaea henselae*-reactive IgG, IgM, and IgA antibodies in patients with suspected cat-scratch disease. *The Journal of Infectious Diseases*, **167**, 1503–4.

Berger, T. G., Tappero, J. W., Kaymen, A., and LeBoit, P. E. (1989). Bacillary (epitheloid) angiomatosis and concurrent Kaposi's sarcoma in acquired immunodeficiency syndrome. *Archives of Dermatology*, **125**, 1543–7.

Birkness, K. A., George, V. G., White, E. H., Stephens, D. S., and Quinn, F. D. (1992). Intracellular growth of *Afipia felis*, a putative etiologic agent of cat scratch disease. *Infection and Immunity*, **60**, 2281–7.

Black, J. R., Herrington, D. A., Hadfield, T. L., Wear, D. J., Margileth, A. M., and Shigekawa, B. (1986). Life-threatening cat-scratch disease in an immunocompromised host. *Archives of Internal Medicine*, **146**, 394–6.

Bogue, C. W., Wise, J. D., Gray, G. F., and Edwards, K. M. (1989). Antibiotic therapy for cat-scratch disease? *Journal of the American Medical Association*, **262**, 813–16.

Breitschwerdt, E. B., Kordick, D. L., Malarkey, D. E., Keene, B., Hadfield, T. L., and Wilson, K. (1995). Endocarditis in a dog due to infection with a novel *Bartonella* subspecies. *Journal of Clinical Microbiology*, **33**, 154–60.

Brenner, D. J., Hollis, D. G., Mos, C. *et al.* (1991). Proposal of *Afipia* gen. nov., with *Afipia felis* sp. nov. (formerly the cat-scratch disease bacillus), *Afipia clevelandensis* sp. nov. (formerly the Cleveland clinic foundation strain), *Afipia broomae* sp. nov., and three unnamed genospecies. *Journal of Clinical Microbiology*, **29**, 2450–60.

Brenner, D. J., O'Connor, S. P., Winkler, H. H., and Steigerwalt, A. G. (1993). Proposals to unify the genera *Bartonella* and *Rochalimaea*, with description of *Bartonella quintana*, comb. nov., *Bartonella vinsonii* comb. nov., *Bartonella henselae* comb. nov., and *Bartonella elizabethae* comb. nov., and to remove the family *Bartonellaceae* from the order *Rickettsiales*. *International of Systematic Bacteriology*, **4**, 777–86.

Brouqui, P. and Raoult, D. (1993). Proteinase K-sensitive and filterable phagosome-lysosome fusion inhibiting factor in *Afipia felis*. *Microbial Pathogenesis*, **15**, 187–95.

Carithers, H. A. (1985). Cat-scratch disease. An overview based on a study of 1,200 patients. *American Journal of Diseases in Childhood*, **139**, 1124–33.

Carithers, H. A. and Margileth, A. M. (1991). Cat-scratch disease: acute encephalopathy and other neurologic manifestations. *American Journal of Diseases in Childhood*, **145**, 98–101.

Cockerell, C. J., Whitlow, M. A., Webster, G. F., and Friedman-Kien, A. E. (1987). Epitheloid angiomatosis: a distinct vascular disorder in patients with the acquired immunodeficiency syndrome or AIDS-related complex. *Lancet*, **ii**, 654–6.

Collipp, P. J. (1992). Cat-scratch disease: therapy with trimethoprim–sulfamethoxazole. *American Journal of Diseases in Childhood*, **146**, 397–9.

D'Agnati, V., McEachrane, S., Dicker, R., and Nielsen, E. (1990). Cat scratch disease and glomerulonephritis. *Nephron*, **56**, 431–5.

Daly, J. S. *et al.* (1993). *Rochalimaea elizabethae* sp. nov. isolated from a patient with endocarditis. *Journal of Clinical Microbiology*, **31**, 872–81.

Debré, R., Lamy, M., Jammet, M. L., Costil, L., and Mozziconacci, P. (1950). La maladie des griffes du chat. *Semaine des Hôpitaux de Paris*, **66**, 76–9.

Dolan, M. J. *et al.* (1993). Syndrome of *Rochalimaea henselae* adenitis suggesting cat scratch disease. *Annals of Internal Medicine*, **118**, 331–6.

Drancourt, M. and Raoult, D. (1993). Proposed tests for the routine identification of *Rochalimaea* species. *European Journal of Clinical Microbiology and Infectious Diseases*, **12**, 710–13.

Drancourt, M., Donnet, A., Pelletier, J., and Raoult, D. (1992). Acute meningoencephalitis associated with seroconversion to *Afipia felis*. *Lancet*, **340**, 558.

Drancourt, M. *et al.* (1995). *Bartonella* (*Rochalimaea*) *quintana* endocarditis in three homeless men. *New England Journal of Medicine*, **332**, 419–23.

English, C. K., Wear, D. J., Margileth, A. M., Lissner, C. R., and Walsh, G. P. (1988). Cat-scratch disease: isolation and culture of the bacterial agent. *Journal of the American Medical Association*, **259**, 1347–52.

Garcia, F. U., Wojta, J., and Hoover, R. L. (1992). Interactions between live *Bartonella bacilliformis* and endothelial cells. *Journal of Infectious Diseases*, **165**, 1138–41.

Goldstein, E. J. C. (1995). Bites. In *Mandell, Douglas and Bennett's principles and practice of infectious diseases* (ed. G. L. Mandell, J. E. Bennett, and R. Dolin), pp. 2765–9. Churchill Livingstone, New York.

Hadfield, T. L., Warren, R., Kass, M., Brun, E., and Levy, C. (1993). Endocarditis caused by *Rochalimaea henselae*. *Human Pathology*, **24**, 1140–1.

Hall, A. V., Roberts, C. M., Maurice, P. D., McLean, K. A., and Shousha S. (1988). Cat-scratch disease in patients with AIDS: atypical skin manifestation. *Lancet*, **ii**, 453–4.

Jim, R. T. S. (1961). Thrombocytopenic purpura in cat-scratch disease. *Journal of the American Medical Association*, **176**, 1036–7.

Kemper, C. A., Lombard, C. M., Deresinski, S. C., and Tompkins, L. S. (1990). Visceral bacillary epitheloid angiomatosis: possible manifestations of disseminated cat scratch disease in the immunocompromised host: a report of two cases. *American Journal of Medicine*, **89**, 216–22.

Kirkpatrick, C. E. and Glickman, L. T. (1989). Cat-scratch disease and the role of the domestic cat: vector, reservoir, and victim? *Medical Hypotheses*, **28**, 145–9.

Kirkpatrick, C. E. and Whiteley, H. E. (1987). Argyrophilic, intracellular bacteria in the lymph node of a cat: cat-scratch disease bacilli? *Journal of Infectious Diseases*, **156**, 690–1.

Koehler, J. E., Glaser, C. A., and Tappero, J. W. (1994). *Rochalimaea henselae* infection: new zoonosis with the domestic cat as reservoir. *Journal of the American Medical Association*, **271**, 531–5.

LeBoit, P. E. *et al.* (1988). Epitheloid haemangioma-like vascular proliferation in AIDS: manifestation of cat scratch disease bacillus infection? *Lancet*, **i**, 960–3.

Lewis, D. E. and Wallace, M. R. (1991). Treatment of adult systemic cat scratch disease with gentamicin sulfate. *Western Journal of Medicine*, **154**, 330–1.

Lewis, D. W. and Tucker, S. H. (1986). Central nervous system involvement in cat scratch disease. *Pediatrics*, **77**, 714–21.

Malatack, J. J. and Jaffe, R. (1993). Granulomatous hepatitis in three children due to cat-scratch disease without peripheral adenopathy. *American Journal of Diseases in Childhood*, **147**, 949–53.

Margileth, A. M., Wear D. J., Hadfield, T. L., Schlagel, C. J., Spigel, G. T., and Muhlbauer, J. E. (1984). Cat-scratch disease. Bacteria in skin at the primary inoculation site. *Journal of the American Medical Association*, **252**, 928–31.

Margileth, A. M., Wear, D. J., and English, C. K. (1987). Systemic cat scratch disease: report of 23 patients with prolonged or recurrent severe bacterial infection. *Journal of Infectious Diseases*, **155**, 390–402.

Maurin, M. and Raoult, D. (1993). Antimicrobial susceptibility of *Rochalimaea quintana*, *Rochalimaea vinsonii*, and the newly recognized *Rochalimaea henselae*. *Journal of Antimicrobial Chemotherapy*, **32**, 587–94.

Maurin, M., Lepocher, H., Mallet, D., and Raoult, D. (1993). Antibiotic susceptibilities of *Afipia felis* in axenic medium and in cells. *Antimicrobial Agents and Chemotherapy*, **37**, 1410–13.

Maurin, M., Roux, V., Stein, A., Ferrier, F., Viraben, R., and Raoult, D. (1994). Isolation and characterization by immunofluorescence, SDS-PAGE, Western-blot, RFLP-PCR, 16S rRNA sequencing and pulsed-field gel electrophoresis of *Rochalimaea quintana* from a patient with bacillary angiomatosis. *Journal of Clinical Microbiology*, **32**, 1166–71.

Mollaret, P., Reilly, J., Bastin, R., and Tournier, P. (1950). Sur une adénopathie régionale subaiguë et spontanément curable avec intradermoréaction et lésions ganglionnaires particulières. *Bulletin des Membres de la Société Médicale des Hôpitaux de Paris*, **66**, 424.

Molnar, R. R. (1992). Ciprofloxacin in cat-scratch disease. *Medical Journal of Australia*, **156**, 664.

Musso, D., Drancourt, M., and Raoult, D. (1995). Lack of bactericidal effect of antibiotics except aminoglycosides on *Bartonella* (*Rochalimaea*) *henselae* in axenic medium and associated with cells. *Journal of Antimicrobial Chemotherapy*, **36**, 101–108.

Perkins, B. A., Swaminathan, B. S., Jackson, L. A., Brenner, D. J., Wenger, J. D., and Regnery, R. L. (1992). Pathogenesis of cat-scratch disease. *New England Journal of Medicine*, **327**, 1599–600.

Perkocha, L. A. *et al.* (1990). Clinical and pathological features of bacillary peliosis hepatitis in association with human immunodeficiency virus infection. *New England Journal of Medicine*, **323**, 1581–5.

Preston Holley, H. (1991). Successful treatment of cat-scratch disease with ciprofloxacin. *Journal of the American Medical Association*, **265**, 1563–5.

Raoult, D., Drancourt, M., Carta, A., and Gastaut, J. A. (1994*a*). *Bartonella* (*Rochalimaea*) *quintana* isolation in a patient with chronic adenopathy, lymphopenia, and a cat. *Lancet*, **343**, 977.

Raoult, D., Tissot Dupont, H., and Enea-Mutilod, M. (1994*b*). Positive predictive value of *Rochalimaea henselae* antibodies in the diagnosis of cat scratch diseas (CSD). *Clinical Infectious Disease*, **19**, 355.

Regnery, R. L., Anderson, B. E., Clarridge, J. E., Rodriguez-Barradas, M. C., Jones, D. C., and Carr, J. H. (1992*a*). Characterization of a novel *Rochalimaea* species, *R. henseale* sp. nov., isolated from blood of a febrile, human immunodeficiency virus-positive patient. *Journal of Clinical Microbiology*, **30**, 265–74.

Regnery, R. L., Martin, M., and Olson, J. (1992*b*). Naturally occurring *Rochalimaea henselae* infection in domestic cat. *Lancet*, **340**, 557–8.

Regnery, R. L., Olson, J. G., Perkins, B. A., and Bibb, W. (1992*c*). Serological response to *Rochalimaea henselae* antigen in suspected cat-scratch disease. *Lancet*, **339**, 1443–5.

Relman, D. A., Loutit, J. S., Schmidt, T. M., Falkow, S., and Tompkins, L. S. (1990). The agent of bacillary angiomatosis. An approach to the identification of uncultured pathogens. *New England Journal of Medicine*, **89**, 1573–80.

Schwartzman, W. A. (1992). Infections due to *Rochalimaea*: the expending spectrum. *Clinical Infectious Diseases*, **15**, 893–902.

Spach, D. H. *et al.* (1993). Endocarditis caused by *Rochalimaea quintana* in a patient infected with human immunodeficiency virus. *Journal of Clinical Microbiology*, **31**, 692–4.

Spach, D. H. *et al.* (1995). *Bartonella* (*Rochalimaea*) *quintana* bacteremia in inner-city patients with chronic alcoholism. *New England Journal of Medicine*, **332**, 424–8.

Stoler, M. H., Bonfiglio, T. A., Steigbigel, R. T., and Pereira, M. (1983). An atypical subcutaneous infection associated with acquired immune deficiency syndrome. *American Journal of Clinical Pathology*, **80**, 714–8.

Tappero, J. W. *et al.* (1993). The epidemiology of bacillary angiomatosis and bacillary peliosis. *Journal of the American Medical Association*, **269**, 770–5.

Waldvogel, K., Regnery, R. L., Anderson, B E., Caduff, R., Caduff, J., and Nadal, D. (1994). Disseminated cat-scratch disease: detection of *Rochalimaea henselae* in affected tissue. *European Journal of Pediatry*, **153**, 23–7.

Wear, D. J., Margileth, A. M., Hadfield, T. L., Fischer, G. W., Schlagel, C. J., and King, F. M. (1983). Cat scratch disease: a bacterial infection. *Science*, **221**, 1403–5.

Wear, D. J., Malaty, R. H., Zimmerman, L. E., Hadfield, T. L., and Margileth, A. M. (1985). Cat scratch disease bacilli in the conjunctiva of patients with Parinaud's oculoglandular syndrome. *Ophthalmology*, **92**, 1282–7.

Zangwill, K. M., *et al.* (1993). Cat scratch disease in Connecticut. *New England Journal of Medicine*, **329**, 8–13.

6 CHLAMYDIOSIS

E. O. Caul and M. Sillis

SUMMARY

Chlamydiosis is a systemic, bacterial zoonotic disease associated with significant mortality if untreated. The clinical manifestations are diverse. The causative agent is *Chlamydia psittaci*, an intracytoplasmic obligate 'energy' parasite. It has a unique, complex developmental cycle involving the infectious elementary body and the vegetative, non-infectious reticulate body. Human chlamydiosis occurs worldwide, mainly affecting persons exposed to infected psittacine and other birds, especially ducks, turkeys, and pigeons, and less commonly to animals, particularly sheep. Outbreaks occur amongst aviary workers, poultry processing workers, and veterinarians. Infection is transmitted through inhalation of infected aerosols contaminated by avian droppings, nasal discharges, or products of ovine gestation or abortion. Person to person transmission is rare. Control strategies have met with variable success depending on the degree of compliance or enforcement of legislation. In the United Kingdom control is secondary, resulting from protection of national poultry flocks by preventing the importation of Newcastle disease virus using quarantine measures. Improved standards of husbandry, transport conditions, and chemoprophylaxis are useful for controlling reactivation of latent avian chlamydial infection. Vaccination has had limited effect in controlling ovine infection. Improved education of persons in occupational risk groups and the requirement for notification may encourage a more energetic approach to its control.

HISTORY

THE DISEASE

The disease, psittacosis, was first recognized by Ritter in 1879 (Harris and Williams 1985) who described several cases of unusual pneumonia or 'pneumotyphus' associated with exposure to tropical pet birds in Switzerland. Morange named the disease after the Greek word for parrot, *psittakos*, having established parrots to be the source of infection in a similar outbreak in Paris in 1894. The term 'ornithosis' was sug-gested for infection in non-psittacine birds. Currently the term 'chlamydiosis' is used to describe chlamydial infection in all avians and mammals.

THE AGENT

The original description of chlamydial elementary bodies is attributed to Halberstaedter and von Prowazek in 1907 who observed intracytoplasmic inclusions containing large numbers of minute particles in conjunctival epithelial cells from humans and apes with trachoma. They classified these 'Chlamydizoa' (Greek, meaning 'a mantle') between bacteria and protozoa incorrectly, but they rightly inferred that these inclusions were the aetiological agents of trachoma.

The causative organism of psittacosis was described initially in 1930 independently by three researchers (Coles 1930; Levinthal 1930; Lillie 1930). Each reported minute spherical bodies within reticuloendothelial cells in infected parrots. In 1930 Bedson described the agent as 'an obligate intracellular parasite with bacterial affinities' (Bedson *et al.* 1930)—a concept not generally accepted for another 30 years. Thereafter, the generic name Bedsoniae was used to describe the agent. In due course the agent was cultivated in fertile hens' eggs.

In 1932 Bedson and Bland demonstrated the complex replication cycle from initial infection to the release of progeny of *C. psittaci* (Bedson and Bland 1932). They found two cell-type populations: the small, infectious elementary body (EB) and the larger, vegetative, non-infectious reticulate body (RB), subsequently recognized to be unique and applicable, with some modifications, to all members of the *Chlamydia* genus. It is now clear that chlamydiae are small prokaryotes that have evolved to a highly parasitic existence and do not constitute the missing link between bacteria and viruses as once thought.

PATHOGENESIS

The causal relationship between elementary bodies and psittacosis was demonstrated in 1932 by Bedson and co-workers. They demonstrated pathogenicity for experimental budgerigars, viable chick embryos, and mouse tissue cultures. Burnet (1935), investigating the ecology of psittacosis, showed that fledglings acquired infection from asymptomatic parent birds. Human infections were most commonly acquired via the aerosol route from inhalation of infected avian excreta or fomites. Overt human infection with *C. psittaci* strains from lower mammals is rare, suggesting low virulence. Two human cases of conjunctivitis (Collier and Ridgway 1984) acquired from cats with pneumonitis, and a laboratory-acquired infection with the enzootic abortion of ewes (EAE) agent were described 20 years ago.

Chlamydia psittaci has considerable pneumopathogenic potential and is known to cause human disease ranging from asymptomatic infection to severe pneumonia and death. Haematogenous spread of the organism from the respiratory tract results in a systemic illness affecting multiple organ systems. The detailed clinical and pathological observations of 18 patients in a chlamydial outbreak in Louisiana (Treuting and Olson 1944) are noteworthy.

Human infection in pregnancy (Giroud *et al.* 1956) with EAE agent was recognized in 1967 as a zoonosis. Severe septicaemia and abortion, due to placentitis, with a high mortality was described.

EPIDEMIOLOGY

The disease, psittacosis, arises from human contact with psittacines, from which many of the early outbreaks were derived. As ownership of psittacines became fashionable, large-scale importation of South American birds into the United States and Europe occurred. This resulted in the 1929–30 pandemic with its associated high mortality and serious recognition of the disease. In 1935 chlamydiosis was also found to be prevalent in wild psittacines in Australia. Further sporadic cases of chlamydiosis occurred in the United States and Germany, incriminating domestically bred budgerigars. Non-psittacine birds have also been implicated in the transmission of this infection. Pneumonitis infections, due to chlamydiosis, in women in the Faroe Islands (Bedson 1940) in 1938, were probably contracted while preparing fulmar petrels for consumption. In the 1950s outbreaks occurred in turkey-processing plant employees in the United States (Irons *et al.* 1951) and later domestic ducks were implicated in outbreaks in Czechoslovakia (Strauss 1967). Poultry-associated cases were first reported in western Europe in 1975 (in Denmark). More recently outbreaks have occurred in poultry processing plants in the United Kingdom, especially among workers on eviscerating lines or who plucked birds (Newman *et al.* 1992). Serological surveys showed that asymptomatic

infections were common in persons at risk. An association between sheep contact and human abortion was noted by Giroud and co-workers, many years after the agent causing EAE was first described. Since that time a number of human *C. psittaci* infections have been ascribed to contact with lambing or aborting ewes (Palmer and Salmon 1990).

CONTROL

Recognition of the zoonotic potential of *C. psittaci* resulted in adoption of various strategies in an attempt to control the spread of chlamydial infection to humans and to protect the domestic poultry industries from the velogenic, viscerotropic Newcastle disease. National embargoes on psittacine importation were first recorded in the 1930s in the United States, United Kingdom, and Federal Republic of Germany after the pandemic in 1929–30. This resulted in an increase in bird smuggling and import bans were revoked and replaced in the 1960s with import permits, health certification, quarantine measures, and prophylactic antibiotics. In the United Kingdom, the Psittacosis or Ornithosis Order 1953 (MAFF 1953) provided statutory powers to detain and isolate affected birds and to disinfect premises. In 1976, import restrictions were reimposed through the Import of Captive Birds Order (MAFF 1976), because of an increase in human cases. These strategies met with limited success in some countries and have encouraged psittacines to be bred domestically. However, chlamydiosis still occurs globally and is more frequently associated with poultry industries. In 1983, the Foreign Quarantine Provisions of the US Federal Register (Centers for Disease Control 1983) revoked restrictions on importation of psittacines as chlamydiosis was no longer regarded a threat to public health. However, interstate quarantine of psittacines and prophylaxis with chlorotetracycline remained under USDA supervision; but there is no federal control after quarantined birds are released. Some countries made chlamydiosis a statutory notifiable disease to encourage more energetic control measures. The disease was made notifiable in 1972 in Australia and in 1978 in Norway. Chlamydiosis in humans is not notifiable in the United Kingdom, except in Cambridgeshire (Wreghitt and Taylor 1988), but in 1989 it was added to the list of prescribed industrial diseases under the Social Security Act (1975) (Industrial Injuries Advisory Council 1989). More recently the International Animal Health Code and an EEC Council Directive have stipulated animal health requirements covering international trade and importation.

Vaccination has had limited effect in controlling ovine chlamydiosis. However, in recent years a disturbing increase in incidence of this disease (Blewett *et al.* 1982) has rekindled interest and little legislation relating to infection control exists.

THE AGENT

TAXONOMY

Chlamydiae are small, coccoid, obligatory, intracellular, RNA-and DNA-containing parasites. Their life cycle is unique, involving alternation between EBs and RBs. The small (0.3 μm) spore-like infectious EB (Fig. 6.1a) binds and enters the eukaryotic host cell. It differentiates into a metabolically active RB (1.0 μm)

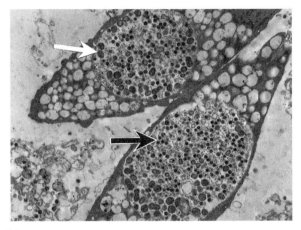

(a)

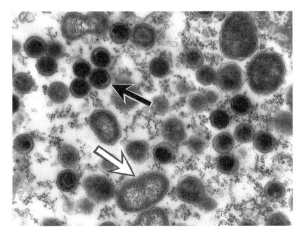

(b)

Fig. 6.1 (a) Electron micrograph of Chlamydia infected cell culture. Arrows indicate large cytoplasmic vacuole containing various stages in Chlamydia replication (× 2000). (b) Chlamydia elementrary bodies (black arrow) and reticulate bodies (white arrow) within cytoplasmic vacuoles (× 17,000).

within a cytoplasmic membrane-bound vacuole wherein division by binary fission occurs and differentiation back into EBs is followed by release from the cell to complete the cycle (Fig. 6.1b) (Treharne 1991). Their metabolic repertoire is distinct from that of free-living bacteria, relying on their hosts for ATP. The genome size is correspondingly small (1.45 megabase pairs) and, structurally, the cell wall is comprised of protein and lipopolysaccharide (LPS) and lacks peptidoglycan. Sequence analysis of the 16S ribosomal RNA has confirmed that *Chlamydia* is a single genus within the Eubacteria related to the Planctomyces (Katenboeck *et al.* 1993). The order Chlamydiales has one family, Chlamydiaceae and a single genus. Four species are recognized within the genus *Chlamydia*: *C. psittaci*, *C. trachomatis*, *C. pneumoniae*, and *C. pecorum*, which share a common LPS and overall morphology. DNA homology studies show that rationalization of chlamydial taxonomy is now appropriate (Herring 1992).

Strain differentiation within the four species is recognized where *C. trachomatis* is categorized within 15 serovars (Schachter 1978a). Antigenic diversity is also recognized within *C. psittaci* revealing at least five groups—avian, ovine abortion, ruminant non-abortion, feline, and guinea-pig. Recent evidence also suggests that antigenic diversity occurs within *C. pneumoniae*. It is likely that sequence variation within the chlamydial genome, following amplification by the polymerase chain reaction, will determine a more accurate basis for strain differentiation (Herring 1993).

MOLECULAR BIOLOGY

Molecular research of chlamydial structure has been largely focused on the outer membrane of the elementary body (EB) because of its central role in the infection process (Treharne 1991). The main constituents of the outer membrane are proteins of molecular weight 40, 57, and 12 kDa together with lipopolysaccharide (LPS).

Sixty per cent of the major outer membrane protein (MOMP), composed of the 40 kDa protein, is surface-exposed. MOMPs from different chlamydial species exhibit high sequence homology but still contain species- (biovar-) and serovar-specific epitopes. Other major protein components are the 60 kDa and 12 kDa cysteine-rich proteins. These EB-associated proteins, unlike MOMP which is also present in the RB, are developmentally regulated and probably involved in the condensation of the RB to EB process. These two proteins are responsible for the cell wall rigidity. The final major component of the membrane complex is the deeply truncated genus-specific LPS which forms the basis of laboratory diagnosis. LPS is overproduced during replication and can be incorporated into the host cell surface.

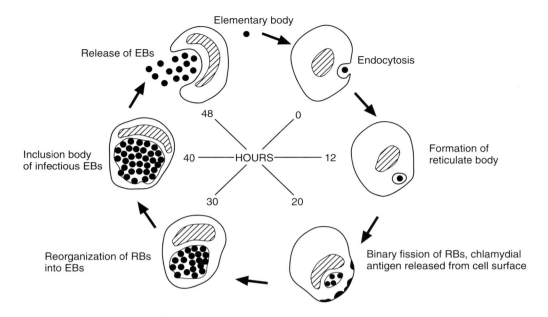

Fig. 6.2　Developmental cycle of chlamydiae.

Other chlamydial proteins of interest are the 27 kDa and 57 kDa proteins. The former is of particular interest as sequence analysis demonstrates significant homology with the surface-located macrophage infectivity potentiator protein of *Legionella pneumophila*, an important virulence factor. The heat-shock 57 kDa protein may also have an important pathogenic role. This genus-specific antigen, closely related to the groEL protein of *E. coli*, can elicit delayed conjunctival hypersensitivity in guinea-pigs (Watkins *et al.* 1986) and monkeys (Schachter 1978*b*) sensitized by prior chlamydial infection. This may explain the exacerbation of disease in some animals when whole chlamydial vaccine was used.

DISEASE MECHANISMS

Chlamydiae cause a broad spectrum of clinically distinct diseases. It is unclear whether these diverse features are mediated by differences in pathogenetic characteristics or are due to variation of the host's immune response. Disease mechanisms may, in part, involve direct activity on the host cell as shown by the dose-related immediate toxic response when injected into experimental animals. This toxicity, originally thought to be associated with the endotoxic LPS, now appears to be due to the genus-specific heat-shock protein (57 kDa). Recently, circulating chlamydial LPS immune complexes have been incriminated in the pathogenesis of some chronic disease.

Chlamydia psittaci does not exhibit host cell-type specificity and can cause productive infection in various cell types, including mononuclear phagocytes which contribute to systemic spread. It is possible that monocytes may degrade internalized immune complexes prior to acquisition by dendritic cells, which in turn are uniquely capable of eliciting primary T-cell responses (Stagg *et al.* 1992). *In vivo*, the pivotal role of dendritic cells shapes the immunological outcome, either by T-cell stimulation or by generation of non-specific killing mechanisms. This is observed in post-chlamydial reactive arthritis where dendritic cells drive inflammatory processes.

Protective immunity to chlamydial re-infection is associated with mucosal antibody, is serovar specific and short lived. Surface-exposed outer membrane constituents of the chlamydial EBs (MOMP and LPS), are immunoaccessible and are likely targets of the immune response. However, LPS neutralizing antibody is not stimulated. MOMP is antigenically complex and exhibits unique and common moieties conferring species serovariation.

Chlamydia psittaci infects primarily mucosal epithelium and resolution of infection occurs without adverse sequelae (Schachter 1992), although severe chronic inflammation may occur. Repeated exposure to chlamydial antigens may contribute to the immunopathology. Evidence from experimental animal work implies that multiple episodes of infection provoke hypersensitivity responses, causing irreversible tissue damage. Application of non-infectious detergent-extracted chlamydial antigens to the conjunctivae of immune guinea-pigs results in delayed hypersensitivity

(Watkins *et al.* 1986). The offending protein was the genus-specific heat-shock 57 kDa antigen. Clarification of the role of the host response to this protein and its invocation of autoimmunity is required.

In humans, *C. psittaci* infects via the respiratory tract and is transported to, and replicates in, the reticuloendothelial cells of the liver and spleen. Spread via the haematogenous route to the lungs produces EB-rich fibrinous exudates. This process accounts for the long incubation period (7–20 days). Man is an incidental, dead-end host.

Maternal infection with ovine *C. psittaci* results in a predilection for, and replication in, trophoblasts. EBs are released into intervillous spaces and infect other chorionic villi, inducing intense inflammation. Placental insufficiency and fetal anoxic death follow. Trophoblast destruction releases large amounts of thromboplastin, and possibly chlamydial toxins, into the circulation resulting in disseminated intravascular coagulation and shock.

Avian chlamydiosis is a generalized infection affecting all major organs (Meyer 1965). Oedema, haemorrhage, and extensive lymphocytic infiltration are common. Inapparent infection is more common than overt disease, which is precipitated by stress following capture, transport, re-housing or food shortage. EBs are shed during overt and inapparent infection. Subclinical intestinal infections are common both in abortion-affected and healthy ruminants, although their pathogeneticity remains unclear (Storz 1988).

Chlamydial adhesion consists of two factors acting in unison where specific binding to cell receptors and/or non-specific physical interactions occur. Adhesion is trypsin resistant, heat- and periodate oxidation-sensitive and inhibited by heparin and heparan sulphate. Non-specific attachment of chlamydial MOMP by electrostatic and hydrophobic interactions is also likely to be important.

Endocytosis is essential for chlamydial development, although conceivably more than one route is used. This may depend on the mode of presentation, the chlamydial strain or the host cell. Endocytosis is 'parasite determined', blocked at low temperatures (4–8 °C) involving local segmental responses of the host cell membrane similar to clathrin-dependent receptor-mediated endocytosis. Intracellular lysosomal fusion with the chlamydia-containing endocytic vesicle is probably inhibited, by undefined surface properties of the EBs, and occurs prior to replication. Reduction of the disulphide bonds, which cross-link the MOMP, causes loss of EB envelope rigidity and initiates the conversion of EBs to RBs. Increase in porin activity facilitates nutrient exchanges between the developing RB and host cell. Complete differentiation into metabolically active RBs occurs within 9 or 10 h. Macromolecular synthesis

of proteins and nucleic acids utilizes host cell ATP and nucleotides. RBs divide by binary fission and by 30 h reorganize into a new generation of EBs, stimulated probably by reduction of ATP within the endocytic vesicle. Extensive cross-linking of MOMP increases the rigidity of the outer membrane. The endocytic vacuole enlarges due to EB accumulation, followed by release into the extracelluar environment.

Non-productive and persistent infections are common in chlamydial disease but the mechanism is unknown. Chlamydiae may survive in cells for long periods in a non-replicative form or, alternatively, multiply at a low level. Tissue culture studies indicate that tryptophan concentrations are critical for persistent infection, although interferon and depletion of other cell nutrients may be involved. True latency has not been demonstrated.

Drugs inhibiting *C. psittaci* replication interfere with protein synthesis or cell wall synthesis (Collier 1984). Rifampicin has the highest antichlamydial activity, followed by tetracyclines and macrolides, e.g. erythromycin and clarithromycin. The newer quinolones, e.g. ofloxacin, also show high antichlamydial activity. Penicillins and some cephalosporins possess moderate antichlamydial activity by their action on RBs. Inhibition of binary fission and development of abnormal forms occurs and can be reversed by removal of antibiotics. Such drugs are not recommended for therapy.

EB suspensions are thermolabile, lose infectivity within hours at 35–37 °C and within days at 4 °C. Survival can be improved by buffering at pH 7.2 containing 0.4 M sucrose and can be maintained for months/years at −70 °C or in liquid nitrogen. Freeze-drying is variably successful.

Infectivity is destroyed or greatly reduced, within 1 min at room temperature, by chemical agents at concentrations routinely used for disinfection, e.g. alcohols, iodine, and hypochlorite, although 1 percent phenol was less rapid. *Chlamydia psittaci* is stable in dust, feathers, faeces, and products of abortion at ambient temperatures, an ecologically important factor in transmission. *Chlamydia psittaci* infectivity has been documented in canary feed for 2 months, in poultry litter for up to 8 months, straw and hard surfaces for 2–3 weeks, and in diseased turkey carcasses for more than 1 year.

THE HOSTS

Globally, chlamydiosis occurs throughout the animal kingdom affecting ectothermic vertebrates, avians, mammals, and man. Common reservoirs of zoonotic chlamydiae include psittacine birds, pigeons, pheasants, and seabirds. Bird species of the economically important poultry industries, for example turkeys, geese, and ducks, are also natural hosts. *Chlamydia psittaci* infections are also of economic importance in farm animals, e.g. sheep, goats, cattle, and pigs. Close domestic association between symptomatic cats and humans provides ample opportunity for zoonotic spread.

INCUBATION PERIOD

Humans: usually 4–15 days, may be as long as 1 month. Avians: unknown in natural infection but experimental infection in turkeys produced symptoms in 5–10 days. Mammals: unknown in natural infection but in experimental infection of lambs lung involvement was most severe at 5 days.

SYMPTOMS AND SIGNS

Humans

The onset of disease may be insidious or rapid, with fever, headache and generalized malaise. After a few days an irritating non-productive cough develops followed by sputum production. Chest signs are often limited to râles with little evidence of consolidation, which is at variance with the radiological findings. Epistaxis and mucocutaneous manifestations frequently occur. Complications include hepatosplenomegaly, meningitis or meningoencephalitis, myocarditis, or pericarditis (Crosse 1990). During acute illness the white cell count is often normal with leucopenia developing in about 25 per cent of cases.

Infection with ovine *C. psittaci* is particularly significant in pregnancy as several cases of abortion, critical puerperal sepsis, and shock, with significant mortality, have occurred in women in contact with sheep (Bloodworth *et al.* 1987). Uncommonly, neural involvement, flu-like illness, respiratory symptoms, and conjunctivitis have been reported in children and adults following sheep exposure.

Avians

Chlamydiosis is often asymptomatic but a generalized infection affecting all major organs may occur (Arzey *et al.* 1990). Loss of condition with yellow-green gelatinous diarrhoea, anorexia, respiratory distress and nasal discharge occurs. Conjunctivitis may be the only symptom. Ducks typically have serous or purulent nasal and ocular discharges, whereby feathers around the eyes and nostrils become encrusted.

Mammals

Feline pneumonitis manifests febrile, depressive, and anorexic illness with mucopurulent discharge from eyes and nostrils (Storz 1988). Recovery after 2–4 weeks frequently results in a subclinical carrier state which may relapse. In very young or elderly cats pneumonitis may be fatal.

In ruminants chlamydiae can cause respiratory, intestinal, placental, and arthropathogenic manifestations. Intestinal infections cause diarrhoea in young animals, initiate pathology in other parts of the body, thus representing important transmission mechanisms. Many ruminants harbour chlamydiae in the alimentary tract without clinical symptoms. Observations in dogs and pigs are similar, and intestinal chlamydial infection in mammals is comparable to acute/persistent avian infection.

Placental and fetal infections of ruminants, with ensuing abortion, are economically important causes of reproductive failure. In experimentally infected animals, clinical observations show a clear sequence of events. Fever and marked leucopenia occur 1–2 days after inoculation and continue for 3–5 days. The placental junction is breached and thereafter events *in utero* proceed independently of those in the dam. Abortion occurs approximately 40 days after infection, usually in the last trimester, but may be as early as day 100 of gestation. Ovine enzootic abortion spreads by contact at lambing, and infection acquired at this time remains latent until subsequent pregnancy when recrudescence results in abortion. Infertility problems may occur after chlamydial abortion.

Bovine mastitis (Storz 1988), caused by naturally occurring infection in milking herds, causes severe reduction, or transitory cessation, of milk production. Chlamydiae can be recovered from the milk but its epidemiological significance is unknown.

Polyarthritis of lambs (stiff lamb disease) occurs in epizootic proportions in the United States and is economically important. The age of affected lambs ranges from 4 days to several weeks. Varying degrees of mobility, anorexia, and conjunctivitis are observed and, with disease progression, lambs are reluctant to bear weight on their limbs. In Germany, chlamydiae have been isolated from synovial specimens of pigs with chronic, non-purulent synovitis.

PATHOLOGY

Humans

Infection may be generalized but major changes occur in the lungs which appear congested. Typically, areas of normal alveoli containing air, interspersed with areas of affected alveoli with an EB-rich cellular fibrinous or serous exudate are seen. Interstitial infiltration and mucosal oedema is rare. Necrotic areas and Kupffer cell vacuolation occur in the liver, and the spleen is typically congested. Cardiac muscle may be oedematous with interstitial infiltration and vegetations may occur on heart valves. Occasionally, adrenals may be haemorrhagic. When the central nervous system is affected, congestion and oedema of the brain and cord is observed, sometimes with chromatolysis of nerve cells or intracytoplasmic inclusions in meningeal cells.

Pathological features of placentitis caused by chlamydiae from ovine infection reveal a focal acute microinfarction due to patchy infiltration of inflammatory cells and fibrin deposits in the intervillous spaces (Wong *et al.* 1985). Destruction and desquamation of trophoblasts in the absence of chorio-amnionitis occurs with an associated deciduitis.

Avians

Lung and air sac congestion results from focal inflammatory cell infiltration, oedema, and haemorrhage. Histiocytic and lymphatic cells accumulate in interalveolar septa and propria of the large bronchioli. Other mucous membranes are infiltrated diffusely or focally with lymphocytes, mononuclear cells, and heterophils. Similar changes occur in other major organs. Eosinophilic necrosis occurs in the liver.

Mammals

Intestinal infection can be cytocidal, resulting in atrophied, irregularly shaped, vesiculated microvilli, and ultimately cell degeneration. Oedema and cellular infiltration of the lamina propria occurs. Diarrhoea results from loss of enterocyte function.

Placental and fetal infections are complex pathological phenomena. The major pathology is localized placentitis with necrotic cotyledons and thickened, opaque periplacentomes. Margins of placental lesions consist of zones of hyperaemia and haemorrhage. Cytoplasmic inclusions are present in chorionic cells of the intercotyledonary region and endometrial cells. Exudate is present in the inter- and peri-placentome and the chorio-allantois is oedematous.

Fetal infection occurs through haematogenous spread from the placenta to the fetal circulation. Oral, conjunctival, and respiratory lesions are reported, but fetal death is associated with terminal anoxia due to placental insufficiency.

TREATMENT

Humans

Some patients recover without specific therapy. Other severely ill patients require supportive therapy, fluid level maintenance, oxygen therapy, and measures to combat shock. Tetracyclines and macrolides, particularly erthyromycin and clarithromycin, are the drugs of choice, although some of the newer quinolones, ofloxacin and ciprofloxacin, are effective. Tetracyclines have better bioavailability in the central nervous system. They are administered either orally or parenterally, dependent on clinical severity. Early therapeutic intervention results in excellent response and is particularly important in pregnancy, but inadequate regimens may lead to relapse.

Avians

Chemotherapy is identical for treatment and prophylaxis (Grimes 1985). Treatment can be affected by feed-administered chlorotetracycline or by parenteral administration. Antibiotic concentration in feed varies according to species, e.g. 2500–5000 p.p.m. for parrots and 500 p.p.m. for budgerigars. The prescribed time for treatment is 45 days for oral administration in parrots and 30 days for budgerigars. For injection, 75 mg/kg body weight every 5 days is recommended; however, repeated injections may result in muscle damage. Blood concentrations greater than 1 μg/ml are considered adequate. Vibramycin-calcium syrup is effective and is the treatment of choice in Europe. The efficacy of some quinolones for treating avian psittacosis is being evaluated.

Mammals

Injection of a long-acting oxytetracycline preparation will maintain ovine pregnancy until nearer the expected parturition date (Aitken *et al.* 1990). It is recommended as a 'one-off' procedure to minimize the development of resistance. Tetracyclines do not eliminate placental infectivity, and it is advisable to institute treatment of the whole flock. Ewes not close to lambing may require a further dose of tetracycline after 2 weeks. Despite treatment, some ewes still abort.

PROGNOSIS

Humans

Mortality rates from avian sources were as high as 40 per cent in the pre-antibiotic era. In the Louisiana outbreak, 8 of 19 cases died and during the 1929 pandemic 20–30 per cent of infected cases died. Nowadays fatalities are rare, accounting for less than 5 per cent of affected cases, but significant morbidity is common. Ovine chlamydial infection in pregnant women may result in an 80 per cent fatality rate. Fetal or neonatal death is common.

Avians

Infection is usually inapparent with overt disease being precipitated by stress, e.g. overcrowding, inadequate nutrition, or transportation. Epizootics accompanied by high mortality rates occur among flocks of birds.

Sporadic deaths occur in older birds that escaped infection as nestlings. Unchecked, mortality in domestic poultry flocks may reach 30 per cent.

Mammals

Ovine and bovine adult infection is usually asymptomatic and rarely results in death. Infection during pregnancy can result in 25 per cent of cases aborting.

DIAGNOSIS

With minor modification, many of the laboratory tests used for chlamydial diagnosis are applicable in all

hosts. The merits of the commonly used tests are outlined in Tables 6.1 and 6.2.

Humans

The mainstay of diagnosis is the complement fixation (CF) test, but immunofluorescence tests are becoming increasingly popular. Antigen and genome detection have been evaluated recently and appear to be both reliable and rapid, although not widely used (Sillis *et al.* 1992). Culture is not routinely attempted.

Avians

Available diagnostic tests are not reliable enough to allow screening or culling programmes to be 100 per

Table 6.1   Laboratory tests in routine chlamydial diagnosis: detection of the organism

Test	Specimen type	Limitations of use	Limitations of interpretation
Histology/cytology: stain with Gimenez, Geimsa or FITC-labelled antibody	Impression smears from tissue or post-mortem tissue from avians and mammals	Easy to perform Suitable for one-off test or can be automated Does not allow for therapeutic intervention	Depends on typical morphological appearance
Direct antigen detection 1. ELISA (enzyme-linked immunosorbent assay)	Post-mortem tissue, oropharyngeal, cloacal and faecal specimens from avians Vaginal swabs, placental and fetal tissue from mammals Respiratory material from humans	ELISA: high sensitivity but may get cross-reactivity with *E. coli* or *salmonella* spp. Faecal material may cause false positive or false negative results	Positive results should be confirmed by visualization of EBs by direct IF Intermittent shedding of chlamydiae, particularly in the carrier state, may necessitate repeat testing to exclude the infective state
2. IF (immunofluorescence)	As for ELISA	DIF: subjective and requires expertise in reading the tests. Unsuitable for large numbers of specimens. Excellent sensitivity	Absence of representative cellular material in the specimen invalidates a negative result Differentiation of species depends on the antibody used, i.e. LPS, genus-specific; MOMP, species-specific
Genomic detection: Polymerase chain reaction	As for ELISA	Complex method requiring rigorous technical skill. Currently not a user-friendly method for routine laboratories. Subject to extrinsic nucleic acid contamination. Useful epidemiological tool	Possibility of contamination must be excluded. A positive result may not indicate clinical relevance. Inhibitors of PCR may be present, thus invalidating a negative result
Culture	As for ELISA	Contamination problems with faecal and post-mortem material. Technique is slow, difficult and special transport conditions are required to maintain chlamydial viability. Culture of avian strains presents a hazard to personnel and strict containment measures are required. Optimal sensitivity of cultures is necessary	The predictive value of a negative result is low unless optimal conditions for transport and culture are maintained.

Table 6.2 Laboratory tests in routine chlamydial diagnosis: detection of a serological response

Test	Limitations of use	Limitations of interpretation
Complement fixation (CF) test	Not suitable for 'one-off' testing. Technique requires optimizing for different animal species sera under test	Cannot differentiate between species, detects genus-specific antibody only. Presence of antibody indicates exposure to chlamydia at some time, not necessarily currently. CF antibody may be absent in some birds actively excreting chlamydiae
WIF test (whole cell inclusion IF)	Detects genus- and species-specific antibody and requires expertise in interpretation. Useful in diagnosis of human infection as the genus-specific response is detected early in the infection and allows timely therapeutic intervention. IgM is applicable in primary infection	Species-specific antibody peaks at approx. 4 weeks after onset of illness and detection is therefore of limited clinical value
Micro-IF (micro-immunofluorescence)	Highly dependent on selection of a correct pool of chlamydial antigens. Antigenic diversity of *C. psittaci* can be used to advantage, resulting in a highly specific epidemiological tool but with a concomitant reduction in sensitivity for diagnostic purposes	Requires considerable interpretative skill and intuitive selection of antigens for reliable result. Cross-reactivity between chlamydial species has been reported
Latex agglutination	As sensitive as CF test in avian diagnosis but detects mainly IgM antibody	Better indicator of current or recent infection in avians. Cockatiels and budgerigars do not produce IgM in chronic infection, therefore a negative result may be unreliable in these avian species

cent effective. Veterinarians only accept a positive culture result as a basis for complying with notification regulations and there is a great need for a test which is accurate, rapid and economical (Spencer 1989). Immunological and genomic techniques on ante-mortem specimens are becoming popular, whereas conventional histopathology is declining.

Mammals

Laboratory diagnosis is restricted to chlamydial detection in placentae or aborted fetal tissue using Gimenez or immunological methods.

EPIDEMIOLOGY

OCCURRENCE

Confirmation of human infection may only be sought in moderate to severe cases, resulting in many unrecognized mild and asymptomatic infections. In many countries, human disease is not notifiable whereas in Norway and Sweden notification has occurred for nearly 40 years. Incidence rates of 9.9 per 100 000 per year (range 1.1–45.8) have been reported for Norway. However, in the United States, although approx. 100 cases are reported annually this reflects only 1 per cent

of cases. In Britain (Fig. 6.3) fewer than 40 cases were reported annually before 1966 but this has now increased to more than 400 cases per year, with periodic peaks. Bird exposure was reported in only 20 per cent of cases. In Scotland, 60 per cent of cases documented bird exposure. In Japan, where pet bird keeping is very popular, the annual incidence is estimated at 250–300 cases. Most countries detected an infection peak in 1981 linked to spread by migratory geese. However, the epidemiology of chlamydial respiratory infection needs re-evaluation following the recognition of *C. pneumoniae* (Grayston *et al.* 1986). The CF test remains the most routinely used laboratory investigation for human chlamydiosis, although it cannot differentiate between the chlamydial species. Epidemics of *C. pneumoniae* occur and the contribution of this species to the reported human cases requires definition.

The incidence data of avian and ovine infections in the United Kingdom (Fig. 6.3) are also subject to similar distortions of underdiagnosis and under-reporting. Differences in ecology, surveillance and reporting over time affect this data. In the United Kingdom 84–89 per cent of reported ovine cases occur during January to March each year, hence the increased risk to pregnant women at this time.

Ovine *C. psittaci* is enzootic and large numbers of EBs are shed in fetal fluids and placentae. Ewes rarely

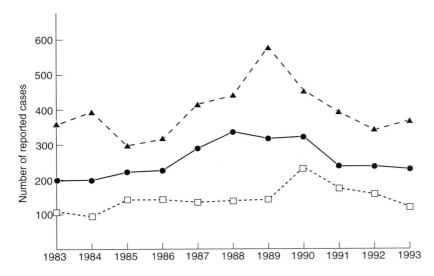

Fig. 6.3 Chlamydiosis in avians (■, reported cases), ovines (●, reported cases ×5), and humans (▲, reported cases) in the United Kingdom. (Data from VIDA Central Veterinary Laboratory, Weybridge and Public Health Laboratory Service CDSC, Colindale.)

abort twice, but chlamydial excretion occurs in the faeces and in fetal and placental products in subsequent pregnancies. Hence healthy sheep are a source of infection. Human infection with ovine *C. psittaci* is sporadic and no outbreaks have occurred. Bovine abortion is epizootic and poses minimal risk for humans as infection is relatively chronic with low-level excretion in aborted material. Serological evidence that stockmen and veterinarians face significant exposure to ruminant chlamydiae is available, although this may require further evaluation using more specific serology.

Seasonality has not been observed in most countries, but peaks are usual in July and August in Czechoslovakia and early in the year in Japan. This may provide information on the source of some infections, e.g. in the duck industry human infection relates to ducklings hatching in the spring and reaching a summer peak when birds are processed. Japanese observations may relate to continuous contact with pet birds indoors during the winter. The age groups most affected in outbreaks are 35–44 years (UK) 20–59 years (USA), and 40–60 years (Czechoslovakia). In Czechoslovakia, 80 per cent of infections occur in females, reflecting their preponderance in the duck industry workforce.

The first European chlamydiosis outbreak was related to a sick bird in a Swiss household, resulting in 50 per cent mortality. Similar outbreaks were observed worldwide until the 1930 pandemic involving at least 1000 cases with a 20 per cent mortality. The pandemic was due to large-scale importation of infected Amazon parrots to satisfy fashionable demand. Since then, over 70 types of psittacine birds have been found to harbour chlamydiae. In Britain infection among domestically bred budgerigars is uncommon.

Infection is not confined to psittacines, as exemplified by the Louisiana outbreak where egrets were implicated (Treuting and Olson 1944). Eight of 19 affected cases died, including nurses involved in caring for primary cases. Many wild game and garden birds are also known to be infected and remain an important source of infection to humans and other birds. Periodically, epizootics of infection occur in aviaries, resulting in a high avian mortality.

Feral pigeons in towns and cities worldwide are commonly infected. However, zoonotic spread of infection from asymptomatic pigeons appears to be low. Handling sick pigeons and killing or dressing wild pigeons is a major risk. Sporadic infections acquired from racing pigeons are frequent. Stress of flying long distances, housing in insanitary lofts, competing for food, and transportation are all factors which may trigger avian disease.

Since the introduction of intensive poultry rearing, several major outbreaks of chlamydiosis affecting man have been reported, mainly associated with ducks and turkeys. These were evident in Czechoslovakia when the formation of large poultry plants and increased production was associated with an increase in pneumonia. Between 1949 and 1960, 1072 cases were diagnosed, with a further 500 during the next 5 years. The mortality rate in humans was 0.7 per cent.

An outbreak of psittacosis occurred in the Minnesota turkey industry in 1986 (Hedberg *et al.* 1989). The risk of acquiring infection varied by work area, with employees in the evisceration area and those in the live hang area many more times more likely to acquire infection than employees in other areas.

Ducks have been associated with a number of outbreaks of human chlamydiosis (Table 6.3) The first

Table 6.3 Attack rates for human psittacosis in various outbreaks

Outbreak	Source of infection	Number exposed	Number infected	Attack rate % (range[a])	Reference
Israeli families	Psittacine and non-psittacine birds	37	30	83	Huminer D. *et al.* (1988). *Lancet*, **8611**, 615–18.
Denmark abattoir	Ducks	142	15	11	Mordhorst, C. (1978). *Ugerskrift for Laeger*, **140**, 2875–80.
Minnesota turkey plant	Turkeys	1233	186	15 (5–46)	Hedberg, K. *et al.* (1989). *American Journal of Epidemiology*, **130**, 569–77.
Texas/Missouri/ Nebraska Outbreak	Turkeys	645	80	12 (2–44)	Durfee P. *et al.* (1975). Journal of the American Veterinary Association, **167**, 804–8.
UK Veterinarians	Ducks	34	15	44	Palmer, S. *et al.* (1981). *Lancet*, **ii**, 798–9.
UK duck plant	Ducks	190	14	8 (3–18)	Andrews, B. *et al.* (1981). *Lancet*, **i**, 632–4.
UK duck processors	Ducks	80	13	16	Newman, P. *et al.* (1992). *Epidemiology and Infection*, **108**, 203–10.

[a] range, attack rate variation related to job assignment.

outbreak in the British duck industry occurred in 1980 when a cluster of cases led to an epidemiological survey (Andrews *et al.* 1981). Seventy-two per cent of plant workers were seropositive compared with 37 per cent of the duck farm workers. Attack rates were highest in workers on the eviscerating line. In another British duck outbreak in 1985 (Newman *et al.* 1992) new employees were three times more likely to become infected cases than established employees. An explosive outbreak of duck-associated *C. psittaci* infection among British veterinarians in 1980 (Palmer *et al.* 1981) was associated with a visit to one of the duck plants involved in the previous outbreak. The highest attack rates were associated with contact with feathers. No illness was observed in workers at the plant. The exposure of a susceptible group to a heavily contaminated environment may account for these findings.

TRANSMISSION

Transmission to man occurs by the respiratory route from healthy and sick birds through faecal droppings and conjunctival/nasal secretions. Organisms survive well on feathers or in dust. Ruminants and cats transmit *C. psittaci* to man via aerosols of infected body fluids. Outbreaks in poultry plant workers have implicated parenteral transmission via cuts and abrasions (Hedberg *et al.* 1989), although this is contentious.

In birds, exposure of nestlings to infection is the major mode of transmission. Vertical transmission may occur in some species. Wild birds are important in transmission to commercial poultry. In ruminants (Stamp *et al.* 1950), infection is spread by contact at lambing and infection remains latent until the following pregnancy when recrudescence results in abortion which contaminates pastures. The theory that birds feeding on this material may act as a vector to other flocks remains to be proved.

Lice and mites have been shown to carry chlamydiae but their role in the epidemiology of psittacosis is unknown. Survival of the agent of epizootic bovine abortion on the surface of ectoparasites has been demonstrated.

PREVENTION AND CONTROL

Regulations aimed at preventing importation of Newcastle disease virus into countries to protect the domestic poultry flocks, also prevent the importation of chlamydiae.

After the 1930 pandemic, numerous countries instituted a complete import ban of psittacine birds. However, due to inadequately controlled prohibitions, illegal smuggling became rife, resulting in the introduction in many countries of import permits with quarantine. The United States no longer imposes import restrictions as chlamydiosis is not felt to be a serious public health threat (Grimes 1985). The restriction on import permits to only a few birds per permit or to a small number of licensed premises may be more effective.

The International Animal Health Code (Office International des Epizooties) and the European Union Council Directive 92/65/EEC lay down specific trade and import conditions.

Psittacines must have appropriate health certification and birds must originate from one of the approved registered countries complying with appropriate transit legislation.

Recrudescence frequently occurs in carrier birds due to transit stress, and overt symptoms or death may occur early in quarantine, thus eliminating infective birds. Not all carriers will be identified in the quarantine period, but healthy carriers constitute less of a human or avian health hazard. Quarantine periods vary in different countries, e.g. 35 days in the United Kingdom and Europe. In the United States uninterrupted treatment of psittacines with chlortetracycline for 45 days, but only 30 days for budgerigars, is recommended by the National Association of State Public Health Veterinarians (1993); a measure designed mainly to protect the quarantine station employees. Ideally, following treatment, quarantined birds should be tested for chlamydiosis. More stringent measures apply in Germany (Gerbermann 1989).

Preventative strategies in poultry plants include the use of masks, hermetic domes over plucking machines, and installation of good ventilation to reduce spread by inhalation. Defeathering carcasses previously immersed in scalding water and heat processing of feathers/down have been used. The most effective measures focus on identifying and treating infected flocks before processing, while remembering that apparently healthy birds are infectious.

Education of exposed occupational groups is important to raise awareness and to improve husbandry. Pregnant women should avoid sheep exposure and laboratory personnel should apply good laboratory practice with strict containment measures.

Preventing domestic birds acquiring infection is difficult because of the high carriage rate in wild birds. However, poultry or pet birds kept indoors can be given prolonged antibiotic therapy. In sheep, transmission to other ewes can be reduced by isolating aborted ewes, destroying placentae, and disinfecting the area. Prophylactic tetracycline treatment of other ewes should be considered. Protective vaccines are available but they tend to give only short-lived, modest protection against disease. Formalized sheep vaccines are of questionable value, but the live, attenuated, feline vaccines have better efficacy against disease, although they do not prevent infection or shedding.

REFERENCES

Aitken, D., Clarkson, M. J., and Linklater, K. (1990). Enzootic abortion of ewes. *Veterinary Record*, **Feb.**, 136–8.

Andrews, B. E. Major, R., and Palmer, S. R. (1981). Ornithosis in poultry workers. *Lancet*, **i**, 632–4.

Arzey, K. E., Arzey, G. G., and Reece, R. L. (1990). Chlamydiosis in commercial ducks. *Australian Veterinary Journal*, **67**, 333–4.

Bedson, S. P. and Bland, J. O. W. (1932). A morphological study of psittacosis virus, with the description of a developmental cycle. *British Journal of Experimental Pathology*, **13**, 461–6.

Bedson, S. P. (1940). Virus diseases acquired from animals. *Lancet*, **ii**, 577–9.

Bedson, S. P., Western, G. T., and Simpson, S. L. (1930). Observations on the aetiology of Psittacosis. *Lancet*, **1**, 235–6.

Blewett D. A., Gisemba, F., and Miller, J. K. (1982). Ovine enzootic abortion. The acquisition of infection and consequent abortion within a single lambing season. *Veterinary Record*, **Nov.**, 499–501.

Bloodworth, D. L., Howard, A. J. Davies, A., and Mutton, K. J. (1987). Infection in pregnancy caused by *Chlamydia psittaci* of ovine origin. *Communicable Diseases Report*, **10**, 3–4.

Burnet, F. M. (1935). Enzootic psittacosis amongst wild Australian parrots. *Journal of Hygiene (London)*, **35**, 412–20.

Centers for Disease Control (1983). *Federal Register*, **48**, 143–5.

Coles, A. C. (1930). Microorganisms in psittacosis. *Lancet*, **i**, 1011–12.

Collier, L. H. (1984). Chlamydia. In *Topley and Wilson's Principles of bacteriology, virology and immunity*, (7th ed), vol. 2, (ed. M. T. Parker) Edward Arnold, London, pp. 510–25.

Collier, L. H. and Ridgway, G. L. (1984). Chlamydial diseases. In *Topley and Wilson's principles of bacteriology, virology and immunity*, (7th ed), vol. 3, (ed. G. R. Smith) Edward Arnold, London, pp. 558–73.

Crosse, B. A. (1990). Psittacosis: a clinical review. *Journal of Infection*, **21**, 251–9.

Gerbermann, H. (1989). Current situation and alternatives for diagnosis and control of chlamydiosis in the Federal Republic of Germany. *Journal of the American Veterinary Medical Association*, **195**, 1542–7.

Giroud, P., Roger, F., and Dumes, N. (1956). Certaines avortements chez la femme peuvent être dus a des agents situés a côté du groupe de la psittacose. *Comptes Rendus des Seances de L'Academie des Sciences*, **242**, 697–9.

Grayston, J. T., Kuo, C. C., Wang, S. P., and Altman, J. (1986). A new *Chlamydia psittaci* strain, TWAR, isolated from acute respiratory tract. *New England Journal of Medicine*, **315**, 161–8.

Grimes, J. E. (1985). Enigmatic psittacine chlamydiosis: Results of serotesting and isolation attempts, 1978 through 1983, and considerations for the future. *Journal of the American Veterinary Medical Association*, **186**, 1075–9.

Halberstaedter, L. and von Prowazek, S. (1907). Zur Atiologie des Trachoms. *Deutsche Medizinische Wochenschrift*, **33**, 1285–7.

Harris, R. L. and Williams, T. W. (1985). Contributions to the origin of pneumotyphus. A discussion of the original article by J. Ritter in 1980. *Reviews of the Infections Diseases*, **7**, 119–22.

Hedberg, K. *et al.* (1989). An outbreak of psittacosis in Minnesota turkey industry workers: Implications for modes of transmission and control. *American Journal of Epidemiology*, **130**, 569–77.

Herring, A. J. (1992). The molecular biology of chlamydiae—a brief overview. *Journal of Infection*, **25**, (Suppl. 1), 1–10.

Herring, A. J. (1993). Typing *Chlamydia psittaci*—a review of methods and recent findings. *British Veterinary Journal*, **149**, 455–75.

Industrial Injuries Advisory Council (1989). Social Security Act 1975. Chlamydiosis and Q fever, pp. 1–3. HMSO, London.

Irons, J. V., Mason, D. and White, R. F. (1951). Outbreaks of Psittacosis (ornithosis) from working with turkeys or chickens. *American Journal of Public Health*, **41**, 931–7.

Kaltenboeck, B., Konstantin, J., Kousoulas, G., and Storz, J. (1993). Structures of an allelic diversity and relationships among the major outer membrane protein (*omp A*) genes of the four *Chlamydial* species. *Journal of Bacteriology*, **175**, 487–502.

Levinthal, W. (1930). Die Ätiologie der Psittacosis. *Klinische Wochenschrift*, **9**, 654.

Lillie, R. D. (1930). Psittacosis: rickettsia-like inclusions in Man and in experimental animals. *Public Health Report*, **45**, 773–8.

MAFF (1953). Psittacosis or Ornithosis Order, No. 38. HMSO, London.

MAFF (1976). Import of Captive Birds Order. HMSO, London.

Märdh, P. A., La Placa, M., and Ward, M. (1992). European Society for Chlamydia Research, pp. 67–72. Uppsala University.

Meyer, K. F. (1965). *Ornithosis diseases of poultry*, (5th ed.), (ed. H. E. Biester and L. H. Schwarte), pp. 675–70. Iowa State University Press.

National Association of State Public Health Veterinarians Compendium Committee. (1993). Compendium of Chlamydiosis (psittacosis) control, 1994. *Journal of the American Veterinary Medicine Association*, **203**, 1673–80.

Newman, P. S. T. J. Palmer, S. R., Kirby, E. D. and Caul, E. O. (1992). A prolonged outbreak of ornithosis in duck processors. *Epidemiology and Infection*, **108**, 203–10.

Palmer, S. R., Andrews, B. E. and Major, R. (1981). A common source outbreak of ornithosis in veterinary surgeons. *Lancet*, **ii**, 798–9.

Palmer, S. R. and Salmon, R. L. (1990). Enzootic abortion in ewes: risks to humans. *Health and Hygiene*, **11**, 205–7.

Schachter, J. (1978*a*). Chlamydial infections. *New England Journal of Medicine*, **298**, 428–35.

Schachter, J. (1978*b*). Chlamydial infections. *New England Journal of Medicine*, **298**, 540–9.

Schachter, J. (1992). The pathogenesis of chlamydial infection. Proc Europ Soc for Chlamydia Research Ed. Märdh P-A, La Placa M, Ward M. (1992). Uppsala Univ, pp. 67–72.

Strauss, J. (1967). Microbiologic and epidemiologic aspects of duck ornithosis in Czechoslovakia. *American Journal of Ophthalmology*, **63**, 1246–59.

Sillis, M. *et al.* (1992). The differentiation of chlamydia species by antigen detection in sputum specimens from patients with community-acquired acute respiratory infections. *Journal of Infection*, **25**, (Suppl. 1), 77–86.

Spencer, L. M. (1989). Chlamydiosis research and control runs regulatory obstacle course. *Journal of the American Veterinary Medicine Association*, **195**, 853–62.

Stagg, A. J. *et al.* (1992). Dendritic cells in the initiation of immune responses to chlamydia. In *Proceedings of the European Society* for Chlamydia Research, (ed. P.- A. Märdh M. La Placa M. Ward) pp. 77–80. Uppsala University.

Stamp, J. T. *et al.* (1950). Enzootic abortion in ewes. Transmission of the disease. *Veterinary Record*, **62**, 251–4.

Storz, J. (1988). Overview of animal diseases induced by chlamydial infections. In *Microbiology of Chlamydia*, (ed. Almen L. Barron), pp. 168–91. CRC Press, Boca Raton.

Treharne, J. D. (1991). Recent developments in the biology of the Chlamydiae. *Reviews of Medical Microbiology*, **2**, 45–9.

Trenting, W. L. and Olson, B. J. (1944). An epidemic of severe pneumonitis in the Bayou region of Louisiana. *Public Health Report, Washington*, **59**, 1299–311; 1331–50.

Watkins, N. G. *et al.* (1986). Ocular delayed hypersensitivity: a pathogenetic mechanism of chlamydial conjunctivitis in guinea pigs. *Proceedings of the National Academy of Sciences USA*, **83**, 7480–4.

Wong, S. Y. *et al.* (1985). Acute placentitis and spontaneous abortion caused by *Chlamydia psittaci* of sheep origin: a histological and ultrastructural study. *Journal of Clinical Pathology*, **38**, 707–11.

Wreghitt, T. G. and Taylor, C. D. (1988). Incidence of respiratory tract chlamydial infections and importation of psittacine birds. *Lancet*, **i**, 582.

FURTHER READING

Almen L. *Barron* (ed.) (1987). *Microbiology of Chlamydia*. CRC Press, Boca Raton.

Bowie W. R. *et al.* (ed.) (1990). *Chlamydial Infections*. Proceedings of the 7th International Symposium on Human Chlamydial Infections. Cambridge University Press.

Märdh, P.-A., La Placa, M. Ward, and M. (1992). *Proceedings of the European Society* for Chlamydial Research. Uppsala University.

Storz J. (1971). *Chlamydia and chlamydia-induced diseases*. C. Thomas. Springfield, Illinois.

7 DISEASES CAUSED BY CORYNEBACTERIA AND RELATED ORGANISMS

Daniel Thomas

SUMMARY

Corynebacterial disease is caused by species of bacteria phylogentically related to, but not including, the agent of human diphtheria, *Corynebacterium diphtheriae*. Although first recognized as early as the late nineteenth century, there is still much confusion surrounding the classification and clinical significance of these bacteria. Recent reclassification of species formerly belonging to the genus *Corynebacterium*, means that for the purposes of this chapter the term 'corynebacterial disease' will be used to include not only animal and human disease caused by bacteria belonging to the genus *Corynebacterium*, but also zoonoses caused by species formerly classified in the genus *Corynebacterium*, now in the genera *Actinomyces* and *Rhodococcus*; a grouping made largely by historical rather than phylogenetic consideration.

In humans, zoonotic corynebacteria only occasionally cause clinical disease in the immunocompetent host. For this population, risk of infection appears greatest in those who drink unpasteurized milk or have contact, occupational or otherwise, with infected animals. While incidence of the non-diphtheria corynebacteria in the immunocompetent population remains low and appears to be steady over time, *R. equi* is emerging as an important pathogen of immunocompromised patients, especially those with HIV-1 infection.

Management of human infection is generally by antibacterial drugs and occasionally surgery. Control of human infection is probably best effected by avoiding the consumption of unpasteurized milk and by raising awareness in those at risk (e.g. sheep shearers, the immunosuppressed) and those clinicians involved in treating these groups. Reducing prevalence in animal populations may be achieved by improving general farm hygiene (including fly control) and husbandry practices, reducing cuts and abrasions during routine procedures, and possibly by vaccination.

HISTORY

In 1896 Lehmann and Neumann proposed that bacteria which were morphologically similar to the diphtheria bacillus should be included within the genus *Corynebacterium* (Noble and Smith 1990). Since this time, with the exception of the diphtheria bacillus *Corynebacterium diphtheriae*, the biology and clinical significance of the various species has remained poorly understood. However, it has long been recognized that a number of the corynebacteria that cause human disease are zoonoses.

Formerly called *Corynebacterium ovis*, *C pseudotuberculosis* is so named because of its ability to produce tubercle-like lesions. It is also called the Preisz–Nocard bacillus in honour of the workers who first isolated the organism from the necrotic kidney of a sheep in the 1890s. Although known to be a pathogen of sheep for a century, it was not until 1966 that a human infection was first reported (Lopez *et al.* 1966).

Corynebacterium pyogenes was first described by Lucet in 1893 (Noble and Smith 1990). Only very few cases of human disease have since been recorded.

Rhodococcus equi (formerly *Corynebacterium equi*) was first recognized as a cause of pneumonia in foals in 1923, but was not reported as a cause of human disease until 1967 (Golub *et al.* 1967). Since then almost all reports of human illness have been in patients with defective cell-mediated immunity. The first description of *R. equi* infection in a patient with AIDS was published in 1986 (Sane and Durack 1986). By reviewing published case series, Linder (1994) demonstrated the emergence of *R. equi* as an AIDS opportunist infection during the 1980s.

Corynebacterium ulcerans was first isolated in 1920 from a human patient in the United States presenting with diphtheria-like illness. In the following decade *C. ulcerans* was isolated from patients with clinical diphtheria, tonsillitis, sore throats, or no symptoms (Gilbert and Stewart 1926). In 1928 the organism was isolated from the bovine udder and since then human infection has been associated with the consumption of untreated dairy produce. It has been suggested that many historical milk-borne outbreaks of diphtheria, attributed at the time to *C. diphtheriae*, may in fact have been caused by *C. ulcerans*. Currently, human infection with *C. ulcerans* is relatively rare.

Corynebacterium bovis was first recovered from cows' milk in 1916 by Evans, who named it *Bacillus abortus* var. *lipolyticus*. Bergey renamed the organism *C. bovis* in 1925. The first case of human disease attributed to *C. bovis* was not described until 1975 (Bolton *et al.* 1975). Vale and Scott (1977) described a further six cases, confirming *C. bovis* as a cause of human disease.

Corynebacterium kutscheri a pathogen of wild and laboratory rodents, was named after Kutscher who first isolated the organism (Noble and Smith 1990).

THE AGENTS

The corynebacteriae are often referred to as diphtheroids or coryneforms. These are ubiquitous, free-living, plant-, and animal-parasitic species.

The phylogeny of bacteria causing corynebacterial disease in humans and animals has been the subject of debate. Four species classified currently in the genus *Corynebacterium* are known zoonoses, causing clinical disease to varying extents in their human and domestic animal hosts: *C. ulcerans*, *C. pseudotuberculosis*, *C. bovis*, and *C. kutscheri*. In addition to these four species, *Rhodococcus equi* and *Actinomyces pyogenes*, both formerly classified within the genus *Corynebacterium*, can cause clinical human illness, and for the purposes of this review are included in this chapter.

Although *C. diphtheriae* is not thought to have an animal reservoir, it has occasionally been isolated from cutaneous lesions on the limbs of horses, the udder and teats of cows, and from elephants; probably the result of human contamination. It has been postulated that *C. diphtheriae*, *C. pseudotuberculosis*, and *C. ulcerans* evolved from a common ancestor which parasitized ungulates in pre-human times. Evidence for this comes from the fact that these three species differ from other corynebacteria in their inability to deaminate pyrazinamide.

The taxonomic status of *C. ulcerans* is not clear. There is debate as to whether the organism should be regarded as a species, or as a strain (or a number of strains) intermediate between the species *C. diphtheriae* and *C. pseudotuberculosis*. Populations of *C. ulcerans* produce the exotoxins of both *C. diptheriae* and *C. pseudotuberculosis* to varying degrees. Carne and Onon (1982) studied the morphological and biochemical properties of 125 different strains of *C. ulcerans* isolated from man and animals and reported a high degree of intraspecific variation. The majority of

strains isolated from humans produce predominantly diphtheria toxin.

There appears to be much inter- and intraspecific variation in the virulence of zoonotic corynebacteria. Virulence of corynebacteria is determined by production of one of three toxins: (1) diphtheria toxin; (2) the dermonecrotic toxin of *C. pseudotuberculosis*, and (3) the soluble haemolysin produced by *A. pyogenes*. Diphtheria toxin production is the result of infection of the bacteria by a virus; a lysogenic bacteriophage carrying a specific 'tox' gene. Strains of *C. ulcerans* and *C. pseudotuberculosis* are known to produce this diphtheria toxin. Dermonecrotic toxin differs from diphtheria toxin in a number of biological properties and is produced by most strains of *C. pseudotuberculosis* and *C. ulcerans*. *Actinomyces pyogenes* usually produces a potent soluble haemolysin.

A full description of the biochemical and microbiological properties of the zoonotic corynebacteria and their classification can be found in the review of Lipsky *et al.* (1982). A useful review of the taxonomy and molecular biology of *R. equi* is provided by Mosser and Hondalus (1996).

THE HOSTS

ANIMAL

Corynebacteria cause disease in domestic animals worldwide. The most important as causes of economic loss are *C. pseudotuberculosis*, *A. pyogenes*, and *R. equi*.

Corynebactrium pseudotuberculosis is the aetiological agent of two specific chronic animal diseases, caseous lymphadenitis (CLA) of sheep and goats, and ulcerative lymphangitis of horses. It has also been isolated from lesions in other mammals, including cattle, deer, camels, and pigs. CLA is characterized by discrete, chronic abscesses containing a caseous pus, particularly in superficial lymph nodes but also in visceral nodes and organs. The disease occurs in most parts of the world where sheep husbandry is intensive. The major impact of the disease is economic, through condemnation of carcasses intended for meat. Australian data have demonstrated no significant difference in body weight between CLA-affected and non-affected sheep. However, in the United States workers have suggested an association with 'thin ewe syndrome'. In terms of labour for inspection and removal of lesions post-mortem, CLA is the most important disease of sheep in Australia and the leading cause of economic loss to the sheep industry. In the United States it is the third most common cause of condemnation at slaughter. Evidence suggests that *C. pseudotuberculosis* reduces wool production, costing an estimated annual loss of

A\$17 million to the Australian wool industry (Paton *et al.* 1994).

Actinomyces pyogenes is a widespread animal pathogen and a frequent cause of suppuration in cattle, sheep, pigs, and goats. It has been implicated in the aetiology of summer mastitis, a disease of economic importance affecting the non-lactating mammary gland of heifers or dry cows. Summer mastitis is caused by a mixed bacterial infection, and although there are conflicting views on the relative importance of the bacterial species making up the summer mastitis complex, *A. pyogenes* usually predominates. This bacterium may also cause secondary complication in foot-and-mouth disease, swine plague, and contagious agalactia of sheep and goats.

Rhodococcus equi causes suppurative bronchopneumonia, lymphadenitis, and enteritis in foals of less than 6 months of age. Horses over 6 months of age rarely develop clinical illness. Foals with combined immunodeficiency disease are particularly susceptible. *Rhodococcus equi* infection has also been reported in cattle, sheep, pigs, dogs, and cats. A recent report described natural co-infection in foals of *R. equi* and *Pneumocystis carinii*, a common microbial opportunist in AIDS (Ainsworth *et al.* 1993). This finding supports the case for a detailed investigation of the role of animals in the epidemiology of the opportunistic zoonoses which contribute to the clinical spectrum of AIDS.

The reservoir of *C. ulcerans* is thought to be cattle. The organism has been implicated in the aetiology of bovine mastitis, but only occasionally causes infection. The organism has been isolated from bite wounds and cervical abscesses in monkeys and from cases of gangrenous dermatitis in captured ground squirrels.

Corynebacterium bovis is present amongst the normal skin flora of domestic cattle and is a common commensal of the bovine udder. Its presence in milk causes butterfat to hydrolyse and thus turn rancid. This organism only occasionally causes mastitis and it has been proposed that subclinical infection may actually be protective.

Corynebacterium kutscheri is a pathogen of rodents and has been isolated from wild voles. Clinical disease is rare in experimental rats and mice, except in those immunosuppressed.

HUMAN

Corynebacterium ulcerans is a rare infection of humans, usually presenting as a mild sore throat (Ghose and Hutton 1988). Toxigenic strains may give rise to symptoms similar to classical diphtheria (Kisely *et al.* 1994), but in individuals previously immunized against *C. diphtheriae* symptoms may be attenuated. Other symptoms reported to be due to *C. ulcerans* have included pneumonia and ulcers on the hand or leg.

Infection by *C. pseudotuberculosis* in humans, also rare, usually presents as suppurative granulomatous lymphadenitis. Axillary lymphadenitis is not uncommon in Australian sheep shearers, suggesting that the incidence of human infection with *C. pseudotuberculosis* may be higher than currently documented. Other reports of human infection have included a case of fever and abscesses in a young butcher (Richards and Hurse 1985) and a case of eosinophilic pneumonia in a veterinary student following exposure in a microbiology laboratory.

There are seven reported human infections of *C. bovis*. Three of these involved the central nervous system (one each of meningitis, epidural abscess, and a ventriculojugular shunt infection), two cases of prosthetic valve endocarditis, one case of chronic otitis media and mastoiditis, and a case of chronic leg ulcer. Of these cases 3/7 were associated with a prosthetic device; the shunt infection was associated with shunt nephritis.

A single case of *C. kutscheri* infection has been reported in humans, a case of chorio-amnionitis in a premature infant (Fitter *et al.* 1979).

Since 1990, of 36 published cases of *R. equi* 33 have been secondary to HIV infection. Clinical presentation is generally insidious with fatigue, fever, and a non-productive cough. Significant delays have been reported between the onset of symptoms and diagnosis. Harvey and Sunstrum (1991) reviewed 30 published reports of *R. equi* infection in patients with or without HIV infection and found that the presentation of symptoms in HIV-infected patients was similar to that in non-HIV-infected patients. Pneumonia was the most common clinical presentation (77 per cent of cases). Mortality was higher for HIV-infected patients (55 per cent) than others (20 per cent), but this may have been related to the presence of simultaneous opportunistic infections in 5 of the 11 HIV-infected patients. In a recent report of an AIDS patient, the presenting lesion was a foot mycetoma which proceeded to disseminated infection, including the lung. Other unusual primary sites reported are the pelvis, bone, and eye following penetrating injury; these have occurred more often in cases without HIV infection. Multiple relapses of pulmonary infection are common, even when successful treatment is ultimately achieved. Further information on clinical presentation of *R. equi* is given by Linder (1994).

EPIDEMIOLOGY

OCCURRENCE

With the exception of recent epidemics in Russia and Eastern Europe (the Commonwealth of Independent Soviets), the incidence of *C. diphtheriae* has declined in

Western countries in recent decades and is now reported only at low levels. Conversely, zoonotic corynebacterial disease (in particular that caused by *R. equi*), whilst still relatively rare, is becoming increasingly important as an opportunistic infection of HIV-infected patients (Berger *et al.* 1994). As the size of the immunocompromised human population increases worldwide, corynebacterial disease may emerge as an important zoonosis.

C. ulcerans

Reports of human corynebacterial disease are uncommon. A study of corynebacterial disease reported to PHLS Communicable Disease Surveillance Centre by laboratories in England, Wales, Northern Ireland, Republic of Ireland, Isle of Man, and Channel Islands revealed that *C. ulcerans* was the most frequently reported zoonotic species. Between 1975 and 1993, there were 81 cases of human *C. ulcerans* infection (annual range 1–9) reported to PHLS Communicable Disease Surveillance Centre. There were more than twice as many reports for females as males, and *C. ulcerans* was most frequently isolated from the 5–14 year age group (Fig. 7.1). The highest number of reports was made by laboratories in south-west and north-west England, areas with high densities of dairy cattle. It must be noted that considerable under-reporting of human *C. ulcerans* infection probably occurs; differential diagnosis may not be considered by the clinician and people previously immunized against *C. diphtheriae* may present with only mild pharyngeal symptoms.

Despite the fact that *C. ulcerans* is not a significant veterinary problem, data are available on the prevalence of this pathogen in its animal reservoir. Meers (1979) examined 197 samples of bulk milk from herds in south-west England, and found one non-toxigenic strain. During a 2-year period, Hart (1984) isolated *C. ulcerans* from 5 of 52 dairy herds in the south-west of England, four of the five strains were toxigenic. During this period of enhanced surveillance, only one human

case of infection by *C. ulcerans* was identified as occurring in the same area; a 12-year-old boy presenting with a sore throat. Further investigation revealed that the boy drank milk from a farm on which a toxigenic strain of *C. ulcerans* had been isolated. This boy had been immunized as an infant against diphtheria and had received a pre-school booster.

C. pseudotuberculosis

In Australia, caseous lymphadenitis is the most common bacterial disease of sheep. Infection in cattle is rare but has been described in Denmark, Israel, California, and Kenya, and in buffaloes in Egypt (Shpigel *et al.* 1993). Batey (1986) examined a representative sample ($n = 8711$) from the Western Australian sheep population estimated at over 30 million and found the prevalence of caseous lymphadenitis at slaughter to be 3 per cent for lambs, 42 per cent for rams, and 54 per cent in ewes. Prevalence increased with age, as did extent of involvement and occurrence of visceral lesions, particularly in association with lesions of the body. CLA is prevalent in South America, the United States, and New Zealand. Despite control measures, CLA-infected goats were inadvertently imported into the United Kingdom in 1987.

In Australia, 10 cases of human infection by *C. pseudotuberculosis* were reported in 1966–76. This is almost certainly an underestimate. Perhaps not surprisingly, no cases of *C. pseudotuberculosis* have been reported to the Communicable Disease Surveillance Centre by laboratories in the United Kingdom. However, as CLA is a relatively recent veterinary problem in Britain it will be interesting to follow any changes in the incidence of *C. pseudotuberculosis* infection over time in both human and animal hosts.

R. equi

Between 1967 and 1989 approximately 30 cases of *R. equi* were described. From 1990 to 1993 an addi-

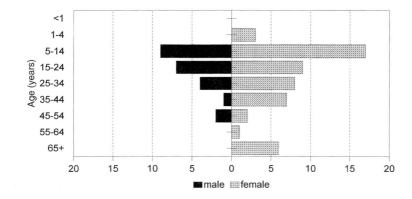

Fig. 7.1 Sex and age distribution of human *C. ulcerans* cases in the UK, 1975–93 ($n = 81$). (Source: Laboratory reports to PHLS Communicable Disease Surveillance Centre.)

tional 36 cases were published. Linder (1994) provides an excellent summary of these cases, and attributes the recent increase in the number of reports of *R. equi* infection partly to increasing awareness amongst microbiologists but also to the increasing pool of immunocompromised hosts. Laboratory reports of *R. equi* in the United Kingdom are not readily available prior to 1991. Since 1991, eight cases have been reported to PHLS Communicable Disease Surveillance Centre by laboratories in the United Kingdom.

A. pyogenes

Human infection with *A. pyogenes* is rare in the United Kingdom. However, in other countries it may be a cause of significant morbidity. A yearly outbreak of leg ulcers occurring in May to October amongst school-children in rural Thailand has been attributed to infection with *A. pyogenes*; other common pyogenic bacteria such as beta-haemolytic streptococci, mostly group A, and *Staphylococcus aureus* and *Staphylococcus epidermidis* are present as secondary infections Kotrajaras *et al.* 1982; Kotrajaras and Tagami, 1987).

In cattle, incidence of summer mastitis is highest in northern Europe, particularly amongst the black-and-white dairy breeds. However, this finding may be the result of ascertainment bias, as the disease is less economically important in beef cattle. Summer mastitis is also prevalent in Japan and parts of the United States and has been reported in Greece, Australia, Zimbabwe, and Brazil. The seasonal distribution of the disease is associated with prevalent cattle husbandry: in Eire a spring peak occurs, reflecting the predominance of spring-calving herds. By examining 8995 samples submitted to the South Dakota Animal Disease Research and Diagnostic Laboratory over a 10-year period, Kirkbride (1993) found *A. pyogenes* to be the bacterium most frequently associated (in 4.2 per cent of cases) with bovine abortions or still births. In 1992, 61 diagnoses of fetopathy and 269 diagnoses of mastitis due to *A. pyogenes*, as well as 101 diagnoses of *A. pyogenes* disease (other than mastitis or fetopathy) were made in cattle by veterinary investigation centres in England, Scotland, and Wales (CVL 1993). In the same year there were 37 diagnoses of mastitis due to corynebacterium (presumably *C. bovis*) in cattle.

SOURCES, TRANSMISSION, AND COMMUNICABILITY

Person to person spread of *C. ulcerans* has not been documented. The age and sex distribution of *C. ulcerans* reports in the United Kingdom (Figure 7.1) would indicate that infection is not primarily the result of occupational exposure.

Hart (1984) conducted an investigation of *C. ulcerans* within a religious farming community in the United Kingdom. Following the detection of a single human case, nose and throat swabs were taken from all members of the community ($n = 60$), and milk was routinely sampled from individual cows. A second clinical case and one other subclinical human case were identified and eight cows were found to be excreting toxigenic strains of *C. ulcerans*. The second clinical human case was thought to have arisen from the mechanical breakdown of the pasteurization process.

In countries where *C. pseudotuberculosis* is enzootic, its epidemiology is largely determined by its high concentration in purulent discharges (up to 5×10^7 bacteria per gram of pus) and its persistence in the environment. Bacteria may be present in the faeces of infected sheep, with environmental contamination leading to a reservoir being present in the soil, bedding, and sheep pens. Transmission in sheep is by infection of superficial skin wounds, particularly those caused by shearing (Serikawa *et al.* 1993). Contaminated sheep dip may also be important. Spread from flock to flock occurs. There is evidence that contaminated fomites may have a role in animal to animal transmission. House *et al.* (1986) suggest that the practice amongst New Zealand farmers of popping abscesses and nodes in sheep using bare hands is a risk factor for *C. pseudotuberculosis* infection.

Virtually all human clinical *R. equi* cases are in patients with predisposing immune suppression due, for example, to neoplastic disease, corticosteroid treatment, or HIV infection. Immunosuppression is a also a predisposing factor in foals. The subclinical epidemiology of *R. equi* in both animal and human populations, and consequently its communicability, is unknown.

Rhodococcus equi forms part of the normal faecal flora of horses and can persist for long periods on contaminated pasture. On horse farms clinical illness is usually sporadic but may become endemic. Outbreaks have occasionally been reported. Transmission in animals is thought to be by ingestion, but transmission by inhalation, by congenital infection, and by migrating helminth larvae has been postulated. Infection in man is thought to be acquired through the respiratory route. A history of exposure to farm animals or manure was reported by 9 of the 20 human *R. equi* cases without HIV infection reviewed by Harvey and Sunstrum (1991). Comparable exposure data for HIV-infected individuals was not available. As for other opportunistic zoonoses of HIV-infected individuals (e.g. *Pneumocystis carinii*, *Cryptosporidium parvum*), the epidemiology of *R. equi* in the immunocompromised population is poorly understood.

Transmission of *A. pyogenes* in cattle is thought to be by flies, and the sheep-head fly, *Hydrotaea irritans*, has been shown to carry *A. pyogenes*. Transmission is consequently related to the density of susceptible animals and abundance of vectors. Little is known about transmission to humans. In Thailand, infection in children is thought to occur by contamination of accidentally traumatized skin by Oriental eye flies carrying the bacteria. Lesions are then thought to become secondarily infected by other pyogenic bacteria. The attack rates in school children in two areas of Thailand were 36 per cent and 54 per cent.

TREATMENT, PREVENTION, AND CONTROL

Prevention of *C. ulcerans* is best effected by eliminating consumption of unpasteurized dairy produce. Since 1983, legislation in Scotland has required heat treatment of all cows' milk on sale to the public. This has reduced the incidence of all milk-borne infection (including *C. ulcerans* infection) as compared with previous years and compared with England and Wales, where legislation does not exist (Sharp *et al.* 1985). However, even in Scotland, raw milk continues to be drunk by dairy farmers, farmworkers and their families (where no retail sale occurs). A recent study demonstrated that this practice is also common in England: 159 of 161 dairy farmers in a representative cohort reported drinking untreated cows' milk at interview (Thomas *et al.* 1994). High standards of hygiene during pasteurization processes will reduce risk of infection, and mechanical breakdown in the pasteurization process has been implicated as a cause of *C. ulcerans* infection.

Prevention of human cases of *C. pseudotuberculosis* infection may be best effected by the covering of cuts and abrasions when handling animals or the products of animals. Health promotion may have a role in raising awareness in groups at risk, for example: sheep shearers or butchers, and in raising awareness in clinicians responsible for treatment of these groups.

Many *R. equi* cases report a history of exposure to domestic animals, but until the epidemiology of this infection is better understood it is difficult to make specific recommendations about the exposure of immunocompromised hosts to farm animals. Control of *A. pyogenes* infection in endemic areas of Thailand has been proposed by control of flies and improvement of sanitation.

Treatment of corynebacterial disease is by antibiotics and/or surgery. *Corynebacterium ulcerans* is reported to be sensitive to most antibacterial agents *in vitro* and erythromycin is favoured in practice. Whereas nearly all *R. equi* isolates from animals and soil are sensitive to penicillin, most human isolates are penicillin resistant. A study of 107 *R. equi* strains referred to Centres for Disease Control found almost all strains susceptible to co-amoxiclav, ampicillin-sulbactam, gentamicin, imipenem, rifampicin, tetracycline, trimethoprim–sulphamethoxazole, and vancomycin. Suggested treatment was an initial period of combination parenteral therapy including at least two of the drugs, followed by several months of oral combination therapy. The optimal duration of antimicrobial therapy and the role of surgery is uncertain. Preference has been expressed by some for bactericidal agents in view of the immune suppression and heavy bacterial load, not all of it intracellular. Relapses after short periods of antimicrobial therapy occur.

No vaccine against corynebacterial disease is available for use in humans but a recent trial using a whole cell vaccine provides evidence for protection against *C. pseudotuberculosis* in vaccinated sheep and goats (Menzies *et al.* 1991).

ACKNOWLEDGEMENTS

Nicola Barrett for providing UK laboratory data and Kenton Morgan for reading the manuscript.

REFERENCES

Ainsworth, D. M., Weldon, A. D., Beck, K. A., and Rowland, P. H. (1993). Recognition of *Pneumocystis carinii* in foals with respiratory distress. *Equine Veterinary Journal*, **25**, 103–8.

Batey, R. G. (1986). Frequency and consequence of caseous lymphadenitis in sheep and lambs slaughtered at a Western Australian abattoir. *American Journal of Veterinary Research*, **47**, 482–5.

Berger B. J., Hussain, F., and Roistacher, K. (1994). Bacterial Infections in HIV-infected patients. *Infectious Disease Clinics of North America*, **8**, 449–65.

Bolton, W. K., Sande, M. A., Normansell, D. E., Sturgill, B. C., and Westervelt, F. B. (1975). Ventriculojugular shunt nephritis with *Corynebacterium bovis*. Successful therapy with antibiotics. *American Journal of Medicine*, **59**, 417.

Carne, H. R. and Onon, E. O. (1982). The exotoxins of *Corynebacterium ulcerans*. *Journal of Hygiene, Cambridge*, **88**, 173–91.

CVL (1993). *Veterinary investigation diagnosis analysis III 1992 and 1985–92*. Ministry of Agriculture, Fisheries and Food, Welsh Office Agriculture Department, Scottish Office, Agriculture and Fisheries Department.

Fitter, W. F., de Sa, D. J., and Richardson, H. (1979). Chorioamnionitis and funisitis due to *Corynebacterium kutscheri*. *Archives of Diseases in Childhood*, **55**, 710–12.

Ghose, A. R. and Hutton, R. M. (1988). A case of sore throat due to *Corynebacterium ulcerans*. *Communicable Disease Report*, **88**, 16.

Gilbert, A. M. and Stewart, M. S. (1926). *Corynebacterium ulcerans*: a pathogenic microorganism resembling *C. diphtheriae*. *Journal of Laboratory and Clinical Medicine*, **12**, 756–61.

Golub, B., Falk, G., and Spink, W. W. (1967). Lung abscess due to *Corynebacterium equi*. Report of first human infection. *Annals of Internal Medicine*, **66**, 1174–7.

Hart, R. J. C. (1984). *Corynebacterium ulcerans* in humans and cattle in North Devon. *Journal of Hygiene, Cambridge*, **92**, 161–4.

Harvey, R. L. and Sunstrum, J. C. (1991). *Rhodococcus equi* infection in patients with and without Human Immuno-deficiency Virus infection. *Reviews of Infectious Disease*, **13**, 139–45.

House, R. W., Schousboe, M., Allen, J. P., and Grant, C. C. (1986). *Corynebacterium ovis* (pseudo-tuberculosis) lymphadenitis in a sheep farmer: a new occupational disease in New Zealand. *New Zealand Medical Journal*, **99**, 659–62.

Kirkbride, C. A. (1993). Bacterial agents detected in a 10-year study of bovine abortions and stillbirths. *Journal of Veterinary Diagnostic Investigation*, **5**, 64–8.

Kisely S. R., Price, S., and Ward, T. (1994). '*Corynebacterium ulcerans*': a potential cause of diphtheria. *CDR Review*, **4**, R63–R64.

Kotrajaras, R. and Tagami, H. (1987). *Corynebacterium pyogenes*: its pathogenic mechanism in epidemic leg ulcers in Thailand. *International Journal of Dermatology*, **26**, 45–50.

Kotrajaras, R., Buddhavudhikrai, P., Sukroongreung, S., and Chanthravimol, P. (1982). Epidemic leg ulcers caused by *Corynebacterium pyogenes* in Thailand. *International Journal of Dermatology*, **21**, 407–9.

Linder, R. (1994). *Rhodococcus equi:* an emerging opportunist in humans. *PHLS Microbiology Digest*, **11**, 87–91.

Lipsky, B. A., Goldberger, A. C., Tompkins, L. S., and Plorde, J. L. (1982). Infections caused by nondiphtheria coryne-bacteria. *Reviews of Infectious Diseases*, **4**, 1220–1235.

Lopez, J. F., Wong, F. M., and Quesada, M. S. (1966). *Corynebacterium pseudotuberculosis*–first case of human infection. *American Journal of Clinical Pathology*, **46**, 562.

Meers, P. D. (1979). A case of classical diphtheria and other infections due to *Corynebacterium ulcerans*. *Journal of Infection*, **1**, 139–42.

Menzies, P. I., Muckle, C. A., Brogden, K. A., and Robinson, L. (1991). A field trial to evaluate a whole cell vaccine for the prevention of caseous lymphadenitis in sheep and goat flocks. *Canadian Journal of Veterinary Research*, **55**, 362–6.

Mosser, D. M. and Hondalus, M. K. (1996). *Rhodococcus equi:* an emerging opportunistic pathogen. *Trends in Microbiology*, **4**, 29–33.

Noble, W. C. and Smith, E. R. (1990). Other Corynebacterial and coryneform infections. In Topley and Wilson's Principles of Bacteriology, Virology and Immunity, Vol. 3. (eds. G. R. Smith and C. S. F. Easman), pp. 75–79.

Paton, M. W. *et al.* (1994). New infection with *Corynebacterium pseudotuberculosis* reduces wool production. *Australian Veterinary Journal*, **71**, 47–9.

Richards, M. and Hurse, A. (1985). *Corynebacterium pseudotuberculosis* abscesses in a young butcher. *Australia and New Zealand Journal of Medicine*, **15**, 85–6.

Sane, D. C. and Durack, D. T. (1986). Infection with *Rhodococcus equi* in AIDS. *New England Journal of Medicine*, **314**, 56–7.

Serikawa, S. *et al.* (1993). Seroepidemiological evidence that shearing wounds are mainly responsible for *Corynebacterium pseudotuberculosis* infection in sheep. *Journal of Veterinary Medical Science*, **5**, 691–2.

Sharp, J. C. M., Paterson, G. M., and Barret, N. J. (1985). Pasteurisation and the control of milkborne infection in Britain. *British Medical Journal*, **291**, 463–4.

Shpigel, N. Y., Elad, D., Yeruham, I., Winkler, M., and Saran, A. (1993). An outbreak of *Corynebacterium pseudotuberculosis* infection in an Israeli dairy herd. *Veterinary Record*, **133**, 89–94.

Thomas, D. Rh. *et al.* (1994). Zoonotic illness: determining risks and measuring effects: the association between current animal exposure and a history of illness in a well characterised rural population. *Journal of Epidemiology and Community Health*, **48**, 151–5.

Vale, J. A. and Scott, G. W. (1977). *Corynebacterium bovis* as a cause of human disease. *Lancet*, **2**, 682–4.

8   EHRLICHIOSIS

S. A. Ewing

SUMMARY

Ehrlichiosis was recognized as a zoonotic disease in the Ozark Plateau of North America in the late 1980s. Earliest cases were assumed to have resulted from *Ehrlichia canis* infections, but this well-known pathogen of canine agranulocytes was later shown to cross-react with *E. chaffeensis*, a newly described organism and putative cause of what became known as human (predominantly monocytic) ehrlichiosis. Somewhat later a 'granulocytic ehrlichiosis' was recognized in human beings, first in north-central North America (Minnesota and Wisconsin) and later elsewhere; and the causative agent is thought to be identical to a long-recognized Old World ruminant pathogen, *E. phagocytophila*, which, itself, may be identical to *E. equi*, a granulocytotropic agent first described from horses in California. Evidence assembled to date suggests that ixodid ticks transmit both types of human ehrlichiosis. *Amblyomma americanum* and *Dermacentor variabilis* have been identified as likely vectors of *E. chaffeensis*, and the *Ixodes scapularis* complex has been implicated in connection with human granulocytic ehrlichiosis in several parts of North America and in Europe. White-tailed deer have been implicated as probable vertebrate hosts for *E. chaffeensis*, but the natural history of this *Ehrlichia* and its granulocytic counterpart—both only recently recognized as zoonoses in North Americans and Europeans—remains to be described. Likewise, the extent of similarities between these two zoonotic ehrlichieae and *E. sennetsu*, the first-known human ehrlichial pathogen and the cause of sennetsu fever in Japan and Malaysia, is undetermined. The natural history of *E. sennetsu* is also unknown, but 16S ribosomal DNA studies indicate that it is phylogenetically closer to *E. risticii*, an equine monocytotropic pathogen in North America with no known zoonotic significance, than to either *E. chaffeensis* or *E. phagocytophila*.

HISTORY

Human (predominantly monocytic) ehrlichiosis was first described in the United States in a patient bitten by ticks in March 1986 while visiting Arkansas (Maeda *et al.* 1987*a*). The patient returned to his home in Michigan and approximately 10 days after the bites, became febrile and suffered generalized myalgia. After several days of illness and multiple visits to medical facilities, he was finally hospitalized 16 days after ticks were removed. When preliminary diagnoses that included leptospirosis, Rocky Mountain spotted fever, and tularaemia could not be confirmed, other causes were explored. On the basis of morula-like inclusions in leucocytes and serological data, a diagnosis of ehrlichiosis was made and the causative agent reported as *Ehrlichia canis*. The conclusion that *E. canis* was the pathogen was questioned (Ewing *et al.* 1987) and attempts began to isolate an organism from a human patient. Eventually *E. chaffeensis* was discovered, also in a patient bitten by ticks in Arkansas, this time a man on temporary military duty there in 1990 (Dawson *et al.* 1991*a*).

More than 415 cases of ehrlichiosis have been recognized in several parts of North America, but they are concentrated in the Ozark Plateau and adjacent areas in south-central and south-eastern USA. One outbreak in New Jersey (Petersen *et al.* 1989) and a single case from New England (Rynkiewicz and Liu 1994*a*) suggest that there may be multiple vectors and possibly multiple ehrlichial disease conditions that must be sorted out. This is not surprising given that human ehrlichiosis has, in the past, most likely been masked by or confused with, Rocky Mountain spotted fever, murine typhus, or other rickettsial diseases.

Ehrlichia chaffeensis, like some other species in the genus, is not easily cultivated. The original isolation (Dawson *et al.* 1991*a*) was made in a canine macrophage cell line designated DH82 and has been grown subsequently in other cell lines, including that of a human endothelial cell (Dawson *et al.* 1993).

Ehrlichiosis is so recently recognized as a problem in human beings that little is known of its zoonotic origins. It seems likely that *E. chaffeensis* (and perhaps other ehrlichieae) circulates among wild hosts in nature, and human beings are more or less accidentally inserted into the cycle(s) on a sporadic basis. Substantially less is known about the even more recently discovered granulocytic ehrlichiosis (HGE) of human beings (Bakken *et al.* 1994, 1995; Chen *et al.* 1994). Presumably this disease also represents an interaction of human beings with a pathogen which is usually circulating in domestic and/or wildlife species. If preliminary indications prove true that *E. phagocytophila* and *E. equi* are more or less identical organisms (Chen *et al.* 1994) which cause this human disease, both domestic and wild herbivores will probably prove to be reservoirs, as they are in continental Europe and Great Britain. Recently, indeed, serological evidence of HGE infections has been reported from Switzerland (Brouqui *et al.* 1995) and polymerase chain reaction (PCR) evidence from dogs and horses in Sweden (Johanson *et al.* 1995) suggests that a similar or identical agent is present there. The finding of granulocytic ehrlichiosis in human beings in Minnesota and Wisconsin (and more recently in New England states, New York, Pennsylvania, Maryland, Florida, Arkansas, and California), and tentative identification of the cause as *E. phagocytophila*, raises the very important possibility of zoonotic illness in the Old World where this pathogen (often referred to as *Cytoecetes phagocytophila*) is commonly encountered in domestic herbivores and in deer. Tick-borne fever and pasture fever are spread, respectively, to sheep and cattle by *Ixodes ricinus* in continental Europe and Great Britain (Woldehiwet and Scott 1993). This tick species also feeds on human beings and presumably could play a role in zoonotic ehrlichial disease in the Old World similar to that first reported in North America in 1994.

Ehrlichia ewingii, a granulocytotropic parasite of dogs in North America, appears to be more closely related to *E. canis* and *E. chaffeensis*—both primarily associated with agranulocytes—than to other granulocytic agents (Anderson *et al.* 1992*b*). Interestingly, *Amblyomma americanum* has been shown to transmit *E. ewingii* under experimental conditions (Anziani *et al.* 1990) and preliminary evidence (Anderson *et al.* 1993; Everett *et al.* 1994) suggests that this ixodid may be a vector of *E. chaffeensis*.

Ehrlichia sennetsu, formerly *Rickettsia sennetsu*, has been studied extensively in Japan for many years. It was the first organism currently assigned to the genus *Ehrlichia* to be recognized as a human pathogen. Its apparent close phylogenetic relationship to *E. risticii*, an equine pathogen of considerable veterinary medical importance in North America, is of particular interest given that the natural means of transmission for both agents continues to elude investigators (Ristic 1990; Hahn *et al.* 1990; Rikihisa 1991).

THE AGENTS

Ehrlichia chaffeensis is closely related to two canine pathogens, *E. canis* and *E. ewingii* (Anderson *et al.* 1991, 1992*b*). It was first isolated in 1990 from a man bitten by unidentified ticks in the same general geographic region where the sentinel case was discovered (Dawson *et al.* 1991*a*). Typical of species in the genus, the organism is a tiny, Gram-negative, somewhat pleomorphic, coccus that stains blue to purple with Romanowsky-type stains.

The type species of the genus *Ehrlichia* is *E. canis*, an organism described in 1935 and originally assigned to the genus *Rickettsia*; it was reassigned in 1945 when the genus *Ehrlichia* was erected (Ewing 1969). *Ehrlichia phagocytophila* was described even earlier (1932) and was also first assigned to the genus *Rickettsia* but later reassigned by Foggie (1962) to the genus *Cytoecetes* where it resided until 1984 when it, too, was transferred (Ristic and Huxsoll 1984). The genus *Cytoecetes* was erected by Tyzzer (1938) to accommodate an organism he found in granulocytes of voles in North America; it is not known whether the agent he described is still circulating in nature nor what its relationship might be to the granulocytotropic ehrlichieae. Nevertheless, the micrographs and drawings published by Tyzzer (1938) certainly appear to represent the same organism that is currently being called human granulocytic *Ehrlichia*; and HGE has been reported from the same vicinity where Tyzzer worked (Telford *et al.* 1995). *Ehrlichia sennetsu*, originally designated *Rickettsia sennetsu*, was the first member of the genus associated with human disease, so-called sennetsu fever in Japan and Malaysia.

Ehrlichia species are obligatory intracellular parasites presently assigned to the Order Rickettsiales. Classification of the organisms mentioned in this chapter is as follows:

Order: Rickettsiales
  Family: Rickettsiaceae
    Tribe: Ehrlichieae
      Genus: *Ehrlichia*
        Species: *E. canis* (genotype species)
            E. chaffeensis
            E. ewingii
            E. phagocytophila ⎫ These two species
            E. equi ⎬ may be synonymous
            E. sennetsu ⎭
            E. risticii

In vertebrate hosts the ehrlichieae are found in membrane-lined vacuoles in the cytoplasm of leucocytes, some species having marked tropism for agranulocytes and others for granulocytes. This tropism is reflected in the names of diseases associated with the organisms. The species whose invertebrate hosts and vectors are known to be ticks have been little studied in these arthropods, and host cell preference in this phase of their life cycles is largely unknown.

According to Wells and Rikihisa (1988) vacuoles containing ehrlichieae do not fuse with lysosomes. Single organisms wrapped in a vacuolar membrane are visible by electron microscopy, but the classical morula, observed by light microscopy as an aggregate of tightly to loosely associated organisms, is diagnostic for the genus. Organisms are surrounded by thin bileaflet outer and inner membranes (Rikihisa 1991) and differ from rickettsial relatives by the absence of thickening of either leaflet of the outer membrane. The inhibition of lysosomal fusion is not a generalized process in infected cells but rather is restricted to vesicles that contain *Ehrlichia* species (Wells and Rikihisa 1988; Rikihisa 1991).

Ehrlichia species are believed to perform aerobic and asaccharolytic catabolism; those species studied can utilize glutamine and glutamate and generate ATP as do other rickettsiae, *sensu stricto*. Unlike their rickettsial relatives, ehrlichieae prefer glutamine, presumably because it penetrates phagosomes better than does glutamate (Weiss *et al.* 1988, 1990). Members of the genus *Ehrlichia* apparently cannot utilize glucose 6-phosphate or glucose, a characteristic shared with species in the genus *Rickettsia*. Metabolic activity is greatest *in vitro* at pH 7.2–8.0 and declines rapidly below pH 7 (Weiss *et al.* 1988, 1990).

Ehrlichia species that can be cultivated may be isolated in acute or chronic phase of infection. Each species seems to have a tissue tropism that affects the appearance of disease, e.g. *E. risticii* in the equine large colon wall results in watery diarrhoea (Rikihisa *et al.* 1985) whereas *E. canis*-infected cells tend to be in the microvasculature of canine lungs, kidneys, and meninges and epistaxis is a common occurrence, particularly in chronic/relapsed patients (Huxsoll *et al.* 1972; Hildebrandt *et al.* 1973; Simpson 1974).

CLINICAL DISEASE

Human ehrlichiosis appears to occur in at least three forms: sennetsu fever caused by *E. sennetsu* and recognized in Japan for decades; human (predominantly monocytic) ehrlichiosis caused by *E. chaffeensis* in the United States and first recognized in the mid- to late 1980s; and granulocytic human ehrlichiosis, thought to be caused by *E. phagocytophila* (*E. equi* synonym?) and first recognized in the Upper Midwest, United States in the early 1990s and later elsewhere in the United States and and Europe. In no instance is the host range well studied and the zoonotic aspects of this complex of diseases are largely unexplored.

SENNETSU EHRLICHIOSIS

Known variously as sennetsu fever glandular fever, infectious mononucleosis, and Hyuganetsu disease in south-western Japan since the nineteenth century, sen-netsu ehrlichiosis is characterized by acute febrile illness accompanied by lethargy, haematological abnormalities, including lymphocytosis, and by lymphadenopathy. *Ehrlichia sennetsu* was first isolated from human blood, bone marrow, and lymph node in 1953 by injection into mice (Misao and Kobayashi 1954). Mice are highly susceptible and are routinely used for cultivation of the agent; they develop lymphadenopathy in about 2 weeks and are often weakened and diarrhoeic. Non-human primates have been infected experimentally (Stephenson 1990) but horses proved refractory (Rikihisa 1991). Ristic and Holland (1993) have suggested that *E. sennetsu* may be more widespread in south-eastern Asia than previously thought, and Segreti *et al.* (1986) have reported that patients in the United States suspected to have infectious mononucleosis, but who are negative on the 'monospot' test for this disease, sometimes are positive for anti-*E. sennetsu* antibodies.

HUMAN (PREDOMINANTLY MONOCYTIC) EHRLICHIOSIS

This disease was first reported in 1987, and its aetiology was finally ascribed to the newly isolated *E. chaffeensis* in 1991 (Anderson *et al.* 1991; Dawson *et al.* 1991*a*). The sentinel case was prematurely diagnosed as a zoonosis involving *E. canis* (Maeda *et al.* 1987*a*). This initial assignment was reconsidered once the limited host range of *E. canis* and its tick vector were pointed out (Ewing *et al.* 1987; Maeda *et al.* 1987*b*). To date several hosts have been exposed experimentally to *E. chaffeensis*, and dogs (Dawson and Ewing 1992) and white-tailed deer (Ewing *et al.* 1995) have proved susceptible. Not only did some of the exposed animals seroconvert, but the organism was re-isolated via tissue culture for a considerable time. Neither dogs nor deer showed clinical evidence of disease. Serological evidence suggests that several wildlife species, especially the white-tailed deer, may be infected under natural conditions, but the vertebrate host range has not been explored extensively (Dawson *et al.* 1994). Likewise, ixodid ticks may harbour *E. chaffeensis* in nature (Anderson *et al.* 1993), but work has just begun on this aspect of the natural history of this zoonotic agent (Dawson *et al.* 1994; Ewing *et al.* 1995).

About 90 per cent of human patients have a history of tick exposure (sometimes bites) within 3 weeks of onset of illness (Eng and Giles 1989; Eng *et al.* 1990; Spach *et al.* 1993; Everett *et al.* 1994; Fishbein *et al.* 1994), which usually presents as a non-specific febrile condition somewhat resembling Rocky Mountain spotted fever (RMSF) (caused by *Rickettsia rickettsii*). In one study (Fishbein *et al.* 1994) involving almost 240 cases occurring between 1985 and 1990, more than

90 per cent had onset in the 6-month period between April and September, prime season for ticks in the northern temperate zone. In addition to fever, headache is very common. Clinicopathological features often seen about 1 week after onset include leucopenia, thrombocytopenia, and elevated serum hepatic aminotransferase levels (Spach *et al.* 1993). Other features include malaise, nausea, vomiting, myalgia, and loss of appetite (Eng *et al.* 1990). Rash is much less common in ehrlichiosis than in RMSF and palms and soles are rarely involved in ehrlichiosis (McDade 1990; Fishbein *et al.* 1994). Harkess (1989) recognized ehrlichiosis as a cause of bone marrow hypoplasia and Harkess *et al.* (1990) described a seriously ill patient with neurological abnormalities. Severe complications that are sometimes fatal include renal failure and encephalopathy. Dunn *et al.* (1992) demonstrated *E. chaffeensis* in mononuclear cells from cerebrospinal fluid. Severe illness and death may occur (Fishbein *et al.* 1994), although Petersen *et al.* (1989) have reported that symptoms are sometimes mild. Paediatric cases have been reported occasionally (Harkess *et al.* 1991; Barton *et al.* 1992).

Diagnosis depends on clinical findings, and serological results are usually relied upon for confirmation. Indirect immunofluorescent antibody (IFA) assays using *E. canis* antigen were used until *E. chaffeensis* antigen became available (Dawson *et al.* 1990, 1991*b*). Dumler *et al.* (1991, 1993*a*) described techniques to demonstrate ehrlichial organisms in human tissues. PCR techniques are now used routinely in experimental work (Anderson *et al.* 1992*a*), occasionally in diagnostic situations (Paddock *et al.* 1993; Everett *et al.* 1994), and may eventually be valuable in facilitating early diagnosis.

Lesions reported from fatal cases by Dumler *et al.* (1991) include 'esophageal ulcer; pulmonary hemorrhage; interstitial pneumonitis; focal necrosis of the liver, spleen, and lymph nodes; multisystem perivascular lymphohistiocytic infiltrates; and extensive hemophagocytosis in the spleen, liver, lymph nodes, and bone marrow'. Fatal ehrlichiosis without seroconversion has been reported in a patient with HIV infection (Paddock *et al.* 1993). Lungs of this patient had extensive alveolar haemorrhage, microvascular congestion, and haemorrhage and oedema of interlobular septa. *Ehrlichia chaffeensis* DNA was demonstrated by PCR and morulae were observed in tissues taken at autopsy.

Tetracycline (or its analogues) has been the drug of choice in treating *E. chaffeensis* infection. Chloramphenicol has also been used successfully (Eng *et al.* 1990; Fishbein *et al.* 1994). There have been no controlled experiments to establish optimal dosage or duration of therapy (Harkess 1991), but Brouqui and Raoult (1992) have conducted *in vitro* studies of antibiotic susceptibility of *E. chaffeensis*. If treatment is begun early, prognosis is good. Severe morbidity and the occasional fatal cases have most often occurred in older persons or when medical intervention was delayed. Fishbein *et al.* (1994) reported that, among hospitalized patients, median recovery time was 16 days for patients treated initially with tetracycline, 12 days for those treated initially with chloramphenicol, and 27 days for those initially treated with other antibiotics. Death or severe illness was most probable in patients aged 60 years or more and in those who did not receive tetracycline or chloramphenicol until 8 or more days after the onset of symptoms.

GRANULOCYTIC HUMAN EHRLICHIOSIS

This disease was first observed in the Upper Midwest, United States in 1990. The first report concerned six people from Minnesota and Wisconsin who contracted a febrile illness that was fatal in two cases (Chen *et al.* 1994). Morulae were found in granulocytes of all six patients. A DNA product amplified by PCR and analysed for nucleotide sequence was 99.9 and 99.8 per cent similar to *E. phagocytophila* and *E. equi*, respectively. Later, many other cases (perhaps fewer than 100 through 1995) were reported (Bakken *et al.* 1995; Telford, *et al.* 1995) and the same species were considered to be involved. Neither of these agents had been reported as a human pathogen previously; *E. phagocytophila* has been known for decades as a pathogen of ruminants in the Old World (Foggie 1951; Foggie 1962; Woldehiwet and Scott 1993) and *E. equi* since the 1960s as a cause of disease in horses in the United States, especially California (Gribble 1969; Stannard *et al.* 1969; Madigan 1993). Discovery of human granulocytic ehrlichiosis is so recent (first reported in 1994) that little can be said about likely natural host(s) of the causative agent(s) in North America. If *E. phagocytophila* (*E. equi?*) or closely related organisms proves to be the pathogen(s) involved, as now appears to be the case, wild and domestic herbivores will presumably be the logical hosts for initial studies seeking reservoirs. Likewise, if the agent described by Tyzzer (1938) is eventually proved to be closely related or identical to HGE, then rodents will be important reservoirs of infection.

EPIDEMIOLOGY

The long-known sennetsu fever or glandular fever from Japan that is now recognized as a form of ehrlichiosis remains an enigma in terms of origin and means of transmission. Though convincing evidence is lacking, ticks are assumed to be vectors (Ristic and Holland 1993); however, suggestions have been made that eating a certain kind of fish may be related to spread (Fukuda *et al.* 1973, cited by Rikihisa 1991). It is interesting that *E. sennetsu* is closely related phylogenetically to *E. risticii* (Anderson *et al.* 1992*b*), the causative agent of equine monocytic ehrlichiosis (Potomoc horse fever, PHF). In spite of numerous attempts to identify the natural mode of transmission of PHF in the United States, it is not known even if arthropod vectors are involved (Palmer 1989; Holland and Ristic 1993). Oral transmission has been demonstrated experimentally by Palmer and Benson (1988), but whether this route of infection is important epidemiologically is not known.

Human (predominantly monocytic) ehrlichiosis has been diagnosed in more than 415 patients in the United States since its discovery in 1986. A few cases have been reported from Europe (Morais *et al.* 1991; Pierard *et al.* 1995) and one from Africa (Uhaa *et al.* 1992). Collectively, that is a relatively small number of patients, of course; nevertheless, information is accumulating slowly to characterize the disease and its mode of transmission in North America. Everett *et al.* (1994) have presented convincing evidence that exposure to ticks is a highly correlated event for patients with ehrlichiosis, and Standaert *et al.* (1995) reported a cluster of cases in a community where there was high risk of exposure to *Amblyomma americanum*. Earlier, Fishbein *et al.* (1989) stated that tick exposure is commonly a part of the history for human ehrlichiosis patients, and Petersen *et al.* (1989) found that soldiers who tucked their pants into their boots to deter ticks were only half as likely as their cohorts to develop ehrlichiosis.

To date a few vertebrate species and a few ixodid ticks have been examined experimentally and from nature, but information is too meagre to provide adequate basis for firm conclusions. Anderson *et al.* (1993) found *E. chaffeensis* in wild-caught *Amblyomma americanum* via the PCR technique. Everett *et al.* (1994) found a few *A. americanum* and a few *Dermacentor variabilis* positive for *E. chaffeensis* by the indirect fluorescent antibody technique. It appears that white-tailed deer and some other wildlife species may serve as hosts under natural conditions (Dawson *et al.* 1994). Dogs can be infected experimentally (Dawson and Ewing 1992), but there is no strong evidence implicating dogs as epidemiologically important hosts. In fact, Harkess *et al.* (1989) and Rohrbach *et al.* (1990) found no increased risk among patients who had contact with dogs. Prazy *et al.* (1991) also found that contact with dogs, even animals with *E. canis* infection, did not constitute a risk for human beings, and Eng and Giles (1989) stated that ehrlichiosis was not transmitted from dogs to human beings. Ewing *et al.* (1995) have demonstrated that white-tailed deer can be infected experimentally and that *A. americanum* can transmit

the agent to naive deer, but there is no direct evidence that deer are epidemiologically important.

Ehrlichia canis is known to persist in dogs long after recovery from clinical disease (Ewing and Buckner 1965), and it is thought that this carrier state may be of veterinary medical importance. In the absence of knowledge of the natural reservoir host(s) for *E. chaffeensis*, it is premature to speculate about its carrier state. None the less, Dumler *et al.* (1993*b*) have reported persistent infection in a human patient.

Granulocytic human ehrlichiosis is so recently discovered that little is known about geographic distribution, much less reservoir host(s). Nevertheless, many cases have been recognized in the mid-1990s, especially in the Upper Midwest United States, specifically in Minnesota and Wisconsin (Bakken *et al.* 1994; Chen *et al.* 1994), in New England states (Hardalo *et al.* 1995; Telford, *et al.* 1995) and other parts of the United States where *Ixodes scapularis* complex ticks are abundant (Pancholi *et al.* 1995). Bakken *et al.* (1994) reported that 11 of 12 patients (92 per cent) had a history of arthropod bite within about 10 days of onset of illness and stated that *Ixodes scapularis* or *Dermacentor variabilis* was described as attached to eight patients (67 per cent) prior to onset of fever. Dawson (1996) has pointed to the possible importance of dual transmission of HGE and *Borrelia burgdorferi* by *I. scapularis*.

One case of human ehrlichiosis from New England is confusing because it is unclear whether it was human (predominantly monocytic) or granulocytic ehrlichiosis (Brouqui and Raoult 1994; Rynkiewicz and Liu 1994*a*, *b*). Even in the face of strong serological evidence of *E. chaffeensis* infection, the diagnosis was questioned. This confusion is understandable and not surprising given that *E. chaffeensis*, the putative cause of human (predominantly monocytic) ehrlichiosis, has also been reported to occur occasionally in granulocytes (Maeda *et al.* 1987*a*). As stated previously, granulocytic ehrlichiosis has been discovered more recently, but it appears that in at least the first 12 patients granulocytes, to the exclusion of other cells, were parasitised in every instance (Bakken *et al.* 1994; Chen *et al.* 1994). Many more cases of *E. chaffeensis* infection have been reported, but the majority are serological diagnoses. Given the small number of human beings from whom *E. chaffeensis* has been isolated, and the few in whose leucocytes the parasite has been demonstrated, one can but guess whether designating the disease anything other than simply ehrlichiosis is appropriate.

PREVENTION AND CONTROL

Although ehrlichial vaccines are becoming available for domestic animals, the zoonotic importance of the ehrlichieae is too recently recognized for any products designed for human beings to have been developed. Indeed, the extent to which the ehrlichieae are important pathogens must be determined before prevention/control will be considered seriously by the medical community. Moreover, until the natural history of *E. sennetsu* and *E. chaffeensis* is better understood there is little basis for designing prevention/control procedures. Likewise, it must be confirmed whether *E. phagocytophila* is the exclusive cause of what is now called human granulocytic ehrlichiosis; and, if so, considerable field work should be done not only in the United States but in continental Europe and Great Britain as well. There should be substantial incentive to determine the zoonotic potential for *E. phagocytophila* in areas where tick-borne fever and bovine pasture fever are important disease of domestic ruminants.

Evidence implicating ixodid ticks as vectors of *E. chaffeensis* is quite strong, and there is a growing body of evidence that *Ixodes* spp. are involved in transmitting human granulocytic ehrlichiosis. If ticks can be implicated as vectors, as they have been for Lyme disease (*Borrelia burgdorferi* infection), then tick control will be of central importance. As Korenberg (1994) stated in connection with Lyme disease, DDT was once used across vast geographic regions with considerable success in control of *Ixodes*-borne infections; he suggests that until ecologically acceptable alternatives to such pesticides can be found, personal protection from ticks seems 'to be the sole recourse'. The same can be said for human (predominantly monocytic) ehrlichiosis and probably for human granulocytic ehrlichiosis as well. If PCR or some other technique can be perfected to determine quickly whether ticks recovered from a suspected endemic area or from a person are infected with a pathogen, appropriate therapeutic intervention could be timely, even life-saving. Experience has shown that early treatment with chloramphenicol or tetracycline is important in reducing morbidity/mortality from ehrlichiosis just as from Rocky Mountain spotted fever (Fishbein *et al.* 1994). Fishbein *et al.* (1994) have even suggested that 'It is probably not necessary to distinguish ehrlichiosis from other tick-borne infections because, except for Colorado tick fever, all acute tick-borne diseases found in the United States are susceptible to tetracycline.' Indeed, some physicians make no attempt at definitive, comfirmatory diagnosis and proceed with tetracycline therapy whenever symptoms and history raise suspicion that a patient has been exposed to a tick-borne agent.

Ehrlichiosis is not a reportable disease. The numbers of cases being reported to public health authorities are likely but a small fraction of those which occur. Likewise, it is probable that many cases are misdiagnosed as Rocky Mountain spotted fever or other 'rickettsial disease' or a similarly nebulous entity. The existence in medical literature of such ill-defined terms as 'Rocky Mountain spotless fever' (Westerman 1982) and 'Oklahoma tick fever' is a clear indication that syndromes exist which beg to be defined aetiologically and delineated clinically and epidemiologically one from another. Undoubtedly, some of these patients whose disease goes essentially undiagnosed have ehrlichiosis. The good fortune that timely tetracycline therapy is curative does not obviate the need to characterize tick-borne pathogens and to solve epidemiological puzzles whose solution would provide sound basis for designing preventive measures. A great deal remains to be done to uncover the natural history of tick-borne pathogens, especially the ehrlichieae. It will not be surprising to discover additional ehrlichieae circulating in nature, and the chances are good that some among them will cause zoonotic diseases.

REFERENCES

Anderson, B. E., Dawson, J. E., and Wilson, K. H. (1991). *Ehrlichia chaffeensis*, a new species associated with human ehrlichiosis. *Journal of Clinical Microbiology*, **29**, 2838–42.

Anderson, B. E. *et al.* (1992*a*). Detection of the etiologic agent of human ehrlichiosis by polymerase chain reaction. *Journal of Clinical Microbiology*, **30**, 775–80.

Anderson, B. E., Greene, C. E., Jones, D. C., and Dawson, J. E. (1992*b*). *Ehrlichia ewingii* sp. nov., the etiologic agent of canine granulocytic ehrlichiosis. *International Journal of Systematic Bacteriology*, **42**, 299–302.

Anderson, B. E., Sims, K. G., and Olson, J. G. (1993). *Amblyomma americanum*: a potential vector of human ehrlichiosis. *American Journal of Tropical Medicine and Hygiene*, **49**, 239–44.

Anziani, O. S., Ewing, S. A., and Barker, R. W. (1990). Experimental transmission of a granulocytic form of the tribe Ehilichieae by *Dermacentor variabilis* and *Amblyomma americanum* to dogs. *American Journal of Veterinary Research*, **51**, 929–31.

Bakken, J. S., Dumler, J. S., Chen, S. -M., Eckman, M. R., Van Etta, L. L., and Walker, D. H. (1994). Human granulocytic ehrlichiosis in the Upper Midwest United States. A new species emerging? *Journal of the American Medical Association*, **272**, 212–18.

Bakken, J. S., Krueth, J., Wilson-Nordskog, C., Tilden, R. S., Asanovich, K., and Dumler, J. S. (1995). Human granulocytic ehrlichiosis (HGE): clinical and laboratory characteristics of 41 patients from Minnesota and Wisconsin. *Journal of the American Medical Association*, **275**, 199–205.

Barton, L. L., Rathore, M. H., and Dawson, J. E. (1992). Infection with *Ehrlichia* in childhood. *Journal of Pediatrics*, **120**, 998–1001.

Brouqui, P. and Raoult, D. (1992). *In vitro* antibiotic susceptibility of the newly recognized agent of ehrlichiosis in humans, *Ehrlichia chaffeensis*. *Antimicrobial Agents and Chemotherapy*, **36**, 2799–2803.

Brouqui, P. and Raoult, D. (1994). Human ehrlichiosis (letter). *New England Journal of Medicine*, **330**, 1760.

Brouqui, P., Dumler, J. S., Lienhard, R., Brossard, M., and Raoult, D. (1995). Human granulocytic ehrlichiosis in Europe. *Lancet*, **346**, 782–3.

Chen, S. -M., Dumler, J. S., Bakken, J. S., and Walker, D. H. (1994). Identification of a granulocytotropic *Ehrlichia* species as the etiologic agent of human disease. *Journal of Clinical Microbiology*, **32**, 589–95.

Dawson, J. E. (1996). Human ehrlichiosis in the United States. In *Current clinical topics in infectious diseases* (ed. J. S. Remington and M. N. Swartz), pp. 164–71. Blackwell Science, Cambridge, MA.

Dawson, J. E. and Ewing, S. A. (1992). Susceptibility of dogs to infection with *Ehrlichia chaffeensis*, causative agent of human ehrlichiosis. *American Journal of Veterinary Research*, **53**, 1322–7.

Dawson, J. E., Fishbein, D. B., Eng, T. R., Redus, M. A., and Greene, N. R. (1990). Diagnosis of human ehrlichiosis with the indirect fluorescent antibody test: kinetics and specificity. *Journal of Infectious Diseases*, **162**, 91–5.

Dawson, J. E. *et al.* (1991*a*). Isolation and characterization of an *Ehrlichia* sp. from a patient diagnosed with human ehrlichiosis. *Journal of Clinical Microbiology*, **29**, 2741–5.

Dawson, J. E., Rikihisa, Y., Ewing, S. A., and Fishbein, D. B. (1991*b*). Serologic diagnosis of human ehrlichiosis using two *Ehrlichia canis* isolates. *Journal of Infectious Diseases*, **163**, 564–7.

Dawson, J. E., Candal, F. J., George, V. G., and Ades, E. W. (1993). Human endothelial cells as an alternative to DH82 cells for isolation of *Ehrlichia chaffeensis*, *E. canis*, and *Rickettsia rickettsii*. *Pathobiology*, **61**, 293–6.

Dawson, J. E. *et al.* (1994). White-tailed deer as a potential reservoir of *Ehrlichia* spp. *Journal of Wildlife Diseases*, **30**, 162–8.

Dumler, J. S., Brouqui, P., Aronson, J., Taylor, J. P., and Walker, D. H. (1991). Identification of *Ehrlichia* in human tissue (letter). *New England Journal of Medicine*, **325**, 1109–10.

Dumler, J. S., Dawson, J. E., and Walker, D. H. (1993*a*). Human ehrlichiosis: hematopathology and immunohistologic detection of *Ehrlichia chaffeensis*. *Human Pathology*, **24**, 391–6.

Dumler, J. S., Sutker, W. L., and Walker, D. H. (1993*b*). Persistent infection with *Ehrlichia chaffeensis*. *Clinical Infectious Diseases*, **17**, 903–5.

Dunn, B. E. *et al.* (1992). Identification of *Ehrlichia chaffeensis* morulae in cerebrospinal fluid mononuclear cells. *Journal of Clinical Microbiology*, **30**, 2207–10.

Eng, T. R. and Giles, R. (1989). Zoonosis update: ehrlichiosis. *Journal of the Amercian Veterinary Medical Association*, **194**, 497–500.

Eng, T. R. *et al.* (1990). Epidemiologic, clinical, and laboratory findings of human ehrlichiosis in the United States, 1988. *Journal of the American Medical Association*, **264**, 2251–8.

Everett, E. D., Evans, K. A., Henry, R. B., and McDonald, G. (1994). Human ehrlichiosis after tick exposure. Diagnosis using polymerase chain reaction. *Annals of Internal Medicine*, **120**, 730–5.

Ewing, S. A. (1969). Canine ehrlichiosis. In *Advances in veterinary science and comparative medicine*, Vol. 13, (ed. C. A. Brandley and C. E. Cornelius), pp. 331–53. Academic Press, New York.

Ewing, S. A. and Buckner, R. G. (1965). Observations on the incubation period and persistence of *Ehrlichia* sp. in experimentally infected dogs. *Veterinary Medicine/Small Animal Clinician*, **60**, 152–5.

Ewing, S. A., Johnson, E. M., and Kocan, K. M. (1987). Human infection with *Ehrlichia canis* (letter). *New England Journal of Medicine*, **317**, 899.

Ewing, S. A. *et al.* (1995). Experimental transmission of *Ehrlichia chaffeensis* (Rickettsiales: Ehrlichieae) among white-tailed deer by *Amblyomma americanum* (Acari: Ixodidae). *Journal of Medical Entomology*, **32**, 368–74.

Fishbein, D. B., Kemp, A., Dawson, J. E., Green, N. E., Redus, M. A., and Fields, D. H. (1989). Human ehrlichiosis: prospective active surveillance in febrile hospitalized patients. *Journal of Infectious Diseases*, **160**, 803–9.

Fishbein, D. B., Dawson, J. E., and Robinson, L. E. (1994). Human ehrlichiosis in the United States, 1985 to 1990. *Annals of Internal Medicine*, **120**, 736–43.

Foggie, A. (1951). Studies on the infectious agent of tick-borne fever in sheep. *Journal of Pathology and Bacteriology*, **63**, 1–15.

Foggie, A. (1962). Studies on tick pyaemia and tick-borne fever. *Symposia of the Zoological Society of London*, **6**, 51–8.

Fukuda, T., Sasahara, T., and Kitao, T. (1973). Studies on the causative agent of Hyuganetsu disease. XI. Characteristics of rickettsia-like organism isolated from metacercaria of *Stellantchasmus falcatus* parasitic in grey mullet. *Journal of the Japanese Association of Infectious Diseases*, **47**, 474–82 [in Japanese].

Gribble, D. H. (1969). Equine ehrlichiosis. *Journal of the American Veterinary Medical Association*, **155**, 462–9.

Hahn, N. E. *et al.* (1990). Attempted transmission of *Ehrlichia risticii*, causative agent of Potomac horse fever, by the ticks, *Dermacentor variabilis*, *Rhipicephalus sanguineus*, *Ixodes scapularis* and *Amblyomma americanum*. *Experimental and Applied Acarology*, **8**, 41–50.

Hardalo, C. J., Quagliarello, V., and Dumler, J. S. (1995). Human granulocytic ehrlichiosis in Connecticut: report of a fatal case. *Clinical Infectious Diseases*, **21**, 910–14.

Harkess, J. R. (1989). Ehrlichiosis: a cause of bone marrow hypoplasia in humans. *American Journal of Hematology*, **30**, 265–6.

Harkess, J. R. (1991). Ehrlichiosis. *Infectious Disease Clinics of North America*, **5**, 37–51.

Harkess, J. R., Ewing, S. A., Crutcher, J. M., Kudlac, J., McKee, G., and Istre, G. R. (1989). Human ehrlichiosis in Oklahoma. *Journal of Infectious Diseases*, **159**, 576–9.

Harkess, J. R., Stucky, D., and Ewing, S. A. (1990). Neurological abnormalities in a patient with ehrlichiosis. *Southern Medical Journal*, **83**, 1341–3.

Harkess, J. R., Ewing, S. A., Brumit, T., and Mettry, C. R. (1991). Ehrlichiosis in children. *Pediatrics*, **87**, 199–203.

Hildebrandt, P. K., Huxsoll, D. L., Walker, J. S., Nims, R. M., Taylor, R., and Andrews, M. (1973). Pathology of canine ehrlichiosis (tropical canine pancytopenia). *American Journal of Veterinary Research*, **34**, 1309–20.

Holland, C. J. and Ristic, M. (1993). Equine monocytic ehrlichiosis (Syn., Potomac horse fever). In *Rickettsial and chlamydial diseases of domestic animals*, (ed. Z. Woldehiwet and M. Ristic), pp. 215–32. Pergamon Press, Oxford.

Huxsoll, D. L., Amyx, H. L., Hemelt, I. E., Hildebrandt, P. K., Nims, R. M., and Gochenour, W. S. (1972). Laboratory studies of tropical canine pancytopenia. *Veterinary Parasitology*, **31**, 53–9.

Johansson, K. -E., Pettersson, B., Uhlen, M., Gunnarsson, A., Malmqvist, M., and Olsson, E. (1995). Identification of the causative agent of granulocytic ehrlichiosis in Swedish dogs and horses by direct solid phase sequencing of PCR product from the 16S rRNA gene. *Research in Veterinary Science*, **58**, 109–12.

Korenberg, E. I. (1994). Comparative ecology and epidemiology of lyme disease and tick-borne encephalitis in the former Soviet Union. *Parasitology Today*, **10**, 157–60.

McDade, J. E. (1990). Ehrlichiosis – a disease of animals and humans. *Journal of Infectious Diseases*, **161**, 609–17.

Madigan, J. E. (1993). Equine ehrlichiosis. In *Rickettsial and chlamydial diseases of domestic animals*, (ed. Z. Woldehiwet and M. Ristic), pp. 209–14. Pergamon Press, Oxford.

Maeda, K., Markowitz, N., Hawley, R. C., Ristic, M., Cox, D., and McDade, J. E. (1987*a*). Human infection with *Ehrlichia canis*, a leukocytic rickettsia. *New England Journal of Medicine*, **316**, 853–6.

Maeda, K., Markowitz, N., Hawley, R. C., Ristic, M., Cox, D., and McDade, J. E. (1987*b*). Human infection with *Ehrlichia canis* (letter). *New England Journal of Medicine*, **317**, 899–900.

Misao, T. and Kobayashi, Y. (1954). Studies on infectious mononucleosis. I. Isolation of etiologic agent from blood, bone marrow, and lymph node of a patient with infectious mononucleosis by using mice. *Tokyo Iji Shinshi*, **71**, 683–6.

Morais, J. D., Dawson, J. E., Greene, C., Filipe, A. R., Galhardas, L. C., and Bacellar, F. (1991). First European case of ehrlichiosis. *Lancet*, **338**, 633–4.

Paddock, C. D. *et al.* (1993). Fatal seronegative ehrlichiosis in a patient with HIV infection (brief report). *New England Journal of Medicine*, **329**, 1164–7.

Palmer, J. E. (1989). Prevention of Potomac horse fever (Editorial). *Cornell Veterinarian*, **79**, 201–5.

Palmer, J. E. and Benson, C. E. (1988). Oral transmission of *Ehrlichia risticii* resulting in Potomac horse fever. *Veterinary Record*, **122**, 635.

Pancholi, P. *et al.* (1995). *Ixodes dammini* as a potential vector of human granulocytic ehrlichiosis. *Journal of Infectious Diseases*, **172**, 1007–12.

Petersen, L. R. *et al.* (1989). An outbreak of ehrlichiosis in members of an army reserve unit exposed to ticks. *Journal of Infectious Deseases*, **159**, 562–8.

Pierard, D., Levtchenko, E., Dawson, J. E., and Lauwers, S. (1995). Ehrlichiosis in Belgium. *Lancet*, **346**, 1233–4.

Prazy, D., Davoust, B., Bissuel, G., and Vidor, E. (1991). Human pathogenecity of *Ehrlichia canis*. *Lancet*, **337**, 1169.

Rikihisa, Y. (1991). The tribe Ehrlichieae and ehrlichial diseases. *Clinical Microbiology Reviews*, **4**, 286–308.

Rikihisa, Y., Perry, B. D., and Cordes, D. O. (1985). Ultrastructural study of rickettsial organisms in the large colon of ponies experimentally infected with Potomac horse fever. *Infection and Immunity*, **49**, 505–12.

Ristic, M. (1990). Current strategies in research on ehrlichiosis. In *Ehrlichiosis: a vector-borne disease of animals and humans*, (ed. J. C. Williams and I. Kakoma), pp. 136–53. Kluwer Academic Publishers, Boston.

Ristic, M. and Holland, C. J. (1993). Human ehrlichiosis. In *Rickettsial and chlamydial diseases of domestic animals*, (ed. Z. Woldehiwet and M. Ristic), pp. 187–94. Pergamon Press, Oxford.

Ristic, M. and Huxsoll, D. L. (1984). Ehrlichieae. In *Bergey's Manual of Systematic Bacteriology*, (ed. N. R. Krieg and J. G. Holt), pp. 704–9. Williams and Wilkins, Baltimore.

Rohrbach, B. W., Harkess, J. R., Ewing, S. A., Kudlac, J., McKee, G. L. and Istre, G. R. (1990). Epidemiological and clinical characteristics of persons with serological evidence of *Ehrlichia canis* infection. *American Journal of Public Health*, **80**, 442–5.

Rynkiewicz, D. and Liu, L. X. (1994*a*). Human ehrlichiosis in New England (letter). *New England Journal of Medicine*, **330**, 292–3.

Rynkiewicz, D. and Liu, L. X. (1994*b*). Human ehrlichiosis (letter). *New England Journal of Medicine*, **330**, 1761.

Segreti, J., Kessler, H., Cole, A. I., Holland, C., Ristic, M. and Levin, S. (1986). Seroprevalence of antibodies to *Ehrlichia sennetsu* in patients with symptoms of mononucleosis. *Clinical Research*, **34**, 533a.

Simpson, C. F. (1974). Relationship of *Ehrlichia canis*-infected mononuclear cells to blood vessels of lungs. *Infection and Immunity*, **10**, 590–6.

Spach, D. H., Liles, W. C., Campbell, G. L., Quick, R. E., Anderson, D. E., and Fritsche, T. R. (1993). Tick-borne diseases in the United States. *New England Journal of Medicine*, **329**, 936–47.

Standaert, S. M. *et al.* (1995). Ehrlichiosis in a golf-oriented retirement community. *New England Journal of Medicine*, **333**, 420–5.

Stannard, A. A., Gribble, K. H., and Smith, R. S. (1969). Equine ehrlichiosis, a disease with similarities to tick-borne fever and bovine petechial fever. *Veterinary Record*, **84**, 149–50.

Stephenson, E. H. (1990). Experimental ehrlichiosis in non-human primates. In *Ehrlichiosis: a vector-borne disease of animals and humans*, (ed. J. C. Williams and I. Kakoma), pp. 93–9. Kluwer Academic Publishers, Boston.

Telford III, S. R., Lepore, T. J., Snow, P., Warner, C. K., and Dawson, J. E. (1995). Human granulocytic ehrlichiosis in Massachusetts. *Annals of Internal Medicine*, **123**, 277–9.

Tyzzer, E. E. (1938). *Cytoecetes microti*, N. G. N. sp., a parasite developing in granulocytes and infective to small rodents. *Parasitology*, **30**, 242–57.

Uhaa, I. J., Maclean, J. D., Greene, C. R., and Fishbein, D. B. (1992). A case of human ehlichiosis acquired in Mali: clinical and laboratory findings. *American Journal of Tropical Medicine and Hygiene*, **46**, 161–4.

Weiss, E., Dasch, G. A., Kang, Y-H., and Westfall, H. N. (1988). Substrate utilization by *Ehrlichia sennetsu* and *Ehrlichia risticii* separated from host constituents by renografin gradient centrifugation. *Journal of Bacteriology*, **170**, 5012–17.

Weiss, E., Dasch, G. A., Williams, J. C., and Kang, Y.-H. (1990). Biological properties of the genus *Ehrlichia*: substrate utilization and energy metabolism. In *Ehrlichiosis: a vector-borne disease of animals and humans*, (ed. J. C. Williams and I. Kakoma), pp. 59–67. Kluwer Academic Publishers, Boston.

Wells, M. Y. and Rikihisa, Y. (1988). Lack of lysosomal fusion with phagosomes containing *Ehrlichia risticii* in P388D1 cells: abrogation of inhibition with oxytetracycline. *Infection and Immunity*, **56**, 3209–15.

Westerman, E. L. (1982). Rocky Mountain spotless fever: a dilemma for the clinician. *Archives of Internal Medicine*, **142**, 1106–7.

Woldehiwet, Z. and Scott, G. R. (1993). Tick-borne (pasture) fever. In *Rickettsial and chlamydial diseases of domestic animals*, (ed. Z. Woldehiwet and M. Ristic), pp. 233–54. Pergamon Press, Oxford.

9 ERYSIPELOID

Robert M. M. Smith

SUMMARY

Erysipelothrix rhusiopathiae, the aetiological agent of human erysipeloid, was recognized more than 100 years ago as the cause of swine erysipelas. It is a non-sporulating, Gram-positive, rod-shaped bacterium, distributed worldwide and it is found in a variety of domestic animal species, especially pigs.

There are three distinct clinical forms of human infection with *E. rhusiopathiae*, a localized cutaneous form, a diffuse cutaneous form, and a rare systemic form usually with endocarditis. Erysipelas can affect animals of all ages but is recognized more frequently in juveniles. The disease in swine exhibits similar stages to the disease in man. Management of human infection is with penicillin or, in severe cases of endocarditis, by valve replacement.

Human *E. rhusiopathiae* infections are usually associated with occupational contact with infected animals or animal products. Existing skin lesions, or intact skin, may be contaminated with the organism prior to injury.

Prevention is largely a matter of maintaining good hygiene and raising awareness in those at risk (especially butchers and farmers), and ensuring that clinicians are aware of *E. rhusiopathiae* as a possible cause of bacterial endocarditis.

HISTORY

Erysipelothrix rhusiopathiae (erysipelas; *erythros* = red, *pella* = skin), literally 'erysipelas thread of red disease') is synonymous with *Erysipelothrix insidiosa*. The human condition may also be known as erysipeloid, Rosenbach's erysipeloid, erysipelotrichosis, fish handler's disease and erythema migrans, and the animal disease as sheep joint ill, swine erysipelas, diamonds, diamond skin disease and fish rose.

Recognized for more than 100 years as the agent of swine erysipelas and as the cause of human erysipeloid, it was first isolated from mice in 1878 (Koch 1880) and subsequently from a pig with '*rouget du porc*' (Pasteur and Thuillier 1883). It was identified as the agent of swine erysipelas and as a zoonosis by Loeffler in 1886.

Pathogenicity in man was first demonstrated by a German surgeon in 1884, Friedrich Julius Rosenbach, hence 'Erysipeloid of Rosenbach'.

Fish handler's disease erysipeloid used to be common among fishermen, cleaners, porters, and those in associated occupations who were often infected through skin abrasions caused by the spines or bones of fish, especially mucilaginous species such as skate, or by splinters from the wooden boxes in which they were carried (Spencer 1959). In 1926 Klauder reported 'about a thousand' cases among commercial fisherman on the eastern seaboard of America. During the Second World War a number of outbreaks occurred in Norwegian fish-processing factories, with over 200 human cases reported from a single fish factory (Hunter 1974). A further 235 cases were reported among fish producers and trawlermen in Aberdeen (Procter and Richardson 1954). Some of these infections may have been due to the presence of *Erysipelothrix* in putrefying fish due to inadequate freezing facilities, exacerbated by delays in ships returning to port because fishing boats were required to sail to and from the fishing grounds in convoy during wartime.

In 1934, McGinnes and Spindle, investigating 210 cases of erysipeloid in a bone button factory in the USA, showed that infection was highest amongst those workers who sustained traumatic injury while working in the warm, moist environment needed to keep the bone workable. 'Seal finger' and 'whale finger' in sealers and whalers, respectively, were caused by the abrasions and other superficial injuries that were inevitable in these occupations caused mainly by wire ropes, flensing knives, and bone fragments (Hillenbrand 1953). Infection has always been considered less common in freshwater fish but in 1930 200 cases were identified in workers preparing golden perch in a processing plant in Odessa. Pork finger usually arises from contact with infected meat and game which accounts for the disease in abattoir workers, meat porters, butchers, and poultry workers.

In pigs, the disease was not considered to be economically important until 1928 when a series of epizootics was recorded in South Dakota with subsequent spread to other major pig-producing regions of the United States.

THE AGENT

Erysipelothrix is a member of the family Coryne-bacteriaceae. The genus *Erysipelothrix* has only one member, *Erysipelothrix rhusiopathiae*, widely distributed in nature and carried by a variety of animal species. It is a facultatively anaerobic, non-spore-forming, non-capsulated, and non-acid-fast bacterium.

Twenty-three serotypes of *Erysipelothrix rhusiopathiae* are recognized. Type 1 is divided into two subtypes, 1a and 1b. Serotypes 1 and 2 are the principal agents of acute swine erysipelas; this is important in the immunization of swine as only a few strains of serotype 3 produce effective bacterins against swine erysipelas (Wood and Harrington 1978).

The mechanism of pathogenicity of *E. rhusiopathiae* in animals is not clearly understood, but there is evidence of neuraminidase involvement. This enzyme is produced by all strains of *E. rhusiopathiae* so far tested, and cleaves α-glycosidic linkages in neuraminic acid, a reactive mucopolysaccharide found on the surfaces of body cells. In low or avirulent strains, neuraminidase activity is lower. Pathological activity associated with the enzyme probably results from its presence in large amounts as it is not itself a toxin; this is thought to be the case with the septicaemia characteristic of acute swine erysipelas. Neuraminidase activity can be associated with a number of aspects of the pathogenesis of the disease, such as increased permeability of cell walls, formation of excess fibrin from fibrinogen, and stimulation of erythrocyte agglutination leading to haemolysis.

There is evidence that chronic changes of erysipelatous arthritis are associated with immunological processes. The bacteria or their fragments do not entirely disappear from chronically affected joints and the lesion may progress in response to continued exposure to these antigenic components.

THE HOSTS

ANIMAL

Erysipelothrix rhusiopathiae is a cause of disease in a wide variety of animals. The bacterium is geographically widespread with a worldwide distribution and has been reported from the Americas, Europe, Asia, and Australasia.

Although the organism can cause disease in many animal species, infection with erysipeloid is a relatively serious infection of swine, presenting in one of three forms: as the relatively mild 'diamond skin' disease, with well-defined rhomboid, bluish-red lesions on the skin, the result of thrombotic vasculitis of end-arterioles; as a more severe septicaemic form, with diffuse erythema, petechiae, and tissue necrosis; or as a chronic form with polyarthritis and sometimes vegetative endocarditis. In the chronic arthritic form, swollen, joints, especially on the front legs, cause the animals to try and avoid weight-bearing by adopting a kneeling posture.

The disease in pigs is usually acquired by ingestion of infected material, often from organisms excreted by infected or colonized animals which have contaminated their environment via urine or faeces. Organisms have been isolated from the tonsils and faeces of apparently healthy pigs (Wood 1974) and are often excreted before clinical signs become apparent. Transdermal infection is also possible.

In ovines *E. rhusiopathiae* infection most commonly presents as polyarthritis, usually in lambs up to 7 months old. The serotypes responsible are usually those that occur in porcine infections. The epidemiology of infection in sheep remains poorly understood, although routes of entry are usually the umbilicus and castration or docking wounds. Cutaneous infections may also be found on the feet of sheep which have recently been dipped.

Cutaneous infections have also been described in cattle and horses with subsequent endocarditis, and in dogs, leading to arthritis, although the strains may differ from those found in pigs. A number of reports from the former USSR have described infections in free-living and captive wild mammals, including rodents, bears, deer, antelope, non-human primates, and dolphins (Wood and Schuman 1981).

Diagnosis of swine erysipelas is by microscopy of the blood or post-mortem examination of blood or viscera for the presence of the characteristic, slender, Gram-positive bacilli, or by cultivation on agar or in broth. Examination of contaminated or putrefying material may involve mouse inoculation or it can be plated on 5 per cent blood agar at pH 6.8 containing 0.1 per cent sodium azide and 0.001 per cent crystal violet (Sneath *et al.* 1951). Acute infections produce only smooth colonies and chronic infections a mixture of rough and smooth colonies of the organism. An agglutination test may be useful in animals showing evidence of joint involvement; a titre of 40 on the fifth day is considered indicative of infection.

A number of animal vaccine treatments, since the days of Pasteur, using virulent or hypervirulent bacilli, have been discontinued because they had an appreciable mortality or produced healthy carriers capable of spreading infection. A live attenuated vaccine administered by aerosol is used in Eastern Europe and Japan (Wood 1984). Elsewhere an adsorbed vaccine prepared from a serotype 2 strain grown in a complex medium containing serum is more commonly used. Most of the immunizing antigen is found in the culture filtrate. One dose is said to protect pigs for 4–6 months, and two doses for 8–12 months. Treatment of affected and in-contact pigs used to be 10–30 ml of antiserum although this has been superseded by antibiotics such as penicillin.

HUMAN

Human infection with *E. rhusiopathiae* is rare. It causes a localized cellulitis which usually develops within 2–7 days of infection around the site of inoculation, usually on the hands or arms of people handling animals or animal products. The bacteria are introduced through pre-existing skin wounds or abrasions. There are three major categories of human disease:

1. A mild cutaneous form usually localized around the hands and fingers. Most of these infections run a self-limiting course of about 3 weeks' duration, the cutaneous rash fading with central clearing. The peripheral edge of the rash advances slowly and is usually slightly elevated. These lesions are characteristically violaceous and disproportionately painful and oedematous but without suppuration.
2. A more severe generalized cutaneous infection which may develop from a localized lesion to produce lesions at remote sites. Many of these patients will have fever and a proportion will report systemic symptoms such as articular pain. The clinical course of the disease may be protracted and recurrences are not uncommon.
3. A septicaemic form, occasionally associated with endocarditis and often presenting with fever and malaise, is very rare in non-immunosuppressed patients. Approximately one-third of such cases will have the concurrent erysipeloid skin lesion and occasionally a purpuric, petechial rash accompanied by thrombocytopenia. Endocarditis may occur in patients without pre-existing valvular damage. Immunosuppressed patients, for whom the prognosis is poor, may be particularly susceptible to dissemination and endocarditis.

A fourth clinical form of infection by ingestion is rarely seen (Berg 1984).

The appearance and distribution of the skin lesions are usually diagnostic, and the absence of suppuration and pitting distinguishes erysipeloid from other pyogenic cutaneous infections such as staphylococcal or streptococcal cellulitis (Grieco and Sheldon 1970). The patient's occupation or recreational activities may also act as diagnostic indicators. There is no apparent immunity following an episode of erysipeloid.

Although the characteristic appearance of the skin lesion is often diagnostic, laboratory investigation requires a full-thickness biopsy specimen taken from the advancing edge of the violaceous area. Culture requires a 1 per cent glucose infusion broth, incubated anaerobically in 5–10 per cent CO_2 at 35–37 °C. Subcultures to blood agar plates are made at 24-hour intervals. The use of selective media is not necessary unless the specimen is heavily contaminated. Commercially available blood culture media are satisfactory for primary isolation from blood since *E. rhusiopathiae* are not particularly fastidious. In cases of chronic infection where numbers of bacteria are small, enrichment with horse, calf, or pig serum in broth followed by incubation for 10 days may be required.

Erysipelothrix rhusiopathiae may sometimes be dismissed as a skin contaminant when grown from blood culture. Although not difficult to culture, it is not always easy to identify. The best method for confirming an isolate is mouse inoculation using a suspension of biopsy material. Fluorescent antibody tests will also confirm the identification of *E. rhusiopathiae*. There are no serological tests routinely available to demonstrate antibodies to *E. rhusiopathiae*.

Erysipelothrix rhusiopathiae is very sensitive to penicillin and moderately sensitive to cephalosporins, tetracycline, chloramphenicol, clindamycin, and erythromycin. It is usually resistant to the aminoglycosides, sulphonamides, and vancomycin frequently used empirically for Gram-positive bacterial infections. Penicillin was first tested as therapy for *E. rhusiopathiae* sepsis in 1944 and remains the antibiotic of choice for both localized and systemic infections.

EPIDEMIOLOGY

Man is an accidental host of *Erysipelothrix rhusiopathiae* acquiring the infection from infected animals, their fomites, or the environment. Human erysipeloid is a largely occupational disease of slaughterhouse workers, agricultural workers, and those in the meat handling and fishing industries.

Human *Erysipelothrix* infection is rare in the United States and the United Kingdom. The Centers for Disease Control (CDC) in Atlanta receives an average of one case per year. A review of erysipeloid reported to the PHLS Communicable Disease Surveillance Centre by laboratories in England and Wales identified 12 cases of human *Erysipelothrix* infection (annual range 1–3) reported between 1975 and 1995. Reporting of infection caused by *E. rhusiopathiae* is not required by health agencies so it is unclear as to whether the incidence is increasing or decreasing (Reboli and Farrar 1989).

In the United Kingdom swine erysipelas is mainly sporadic but in some Central European countries, Asia, Canada, and Central and Southern America it

can cause epidemics with serious economic consequences. In some countries swine can only be raised
profitably where systematic vaccination is practised.
Outbreaks of disease tend to occur in valleys and low-
lying areas, especially in the summer months, although
with considerable regional variations in morbidity and
mortality. The reasons for this variability are uncertain
but it has been suggested they may be due to differences in virulence of the organism. Acute forms of the
disease tend to be rare in western Europe and in the
United States, where disease tends to occur in 4- to 5-
year cycles. In the United Kingdom the disease in
sheep occurs mainly in lowland flocks involved in fat
lamb production where replacement ewes are often
purchased annually. In such flocks this may be due to
the presence of carrier ewes or to the presence of the
organism in the soil. Some reported outbreaks
(Report, 1972, 1975, 1976, 1977) have been associated
with the spreading of pig slurry on pasture grazed by
lambs, but reliable evidence has generally proved
elusive (Jones 1979).

A seasonal pattern of the disease in warm weather
has been reported in both animals and man (King
1946; Barber 1948) but Penny and Guise (1986), in a
review of animal condemnation statistics from the
United Kingdom Ministry of Agriculture Fisheries and
Food (MAFF), demonstrated no seasonal associations
between the periods 1960–72 and 1973–84. They point
out that during this time major changes occurred in
pig husbandry and feeding practices in the United
Kingdom with fewer pigs being raised outdoors or in
yards but generally managed more intensively indoors
on partly slatted floors which make faecal spread of
disease less likely. Other factors, such as a reduction in
the number of skin parasites and the virtual elimination of the pig louse, both of which are possible vectors
of swine erysipelas, may also have contributed to a
reduction in the numbers of animal cases.

PREVENTION AND CONTROL

The disease in man is not reportable in either the
United States or Britain. Changes in manufacturing
processes have reduced occupational exposures to
animal products carrying *E. rhusiopathiae*, such as the
use of plastic rather than bone buttons, and the use of
plastic instead of wooden fish boxes. Continued
reductions in human exposures are likely to maintain
the current low levels of reported erysipeloid and of
E. rhusiopathiae endocarditis.

Control of erysipelas in swine and poultry range
from general sanitation to the use of vaccine where the
disease is enzootic. Two vaccines are generally available for veterinary use, both of which have been shown

to give satisfactory results; an adsorbed vaccine (bacterin adsorbed on aluminium hydroxide) and a live
avirulent vaccine. Immunity is provided for up to 6
months. The bacterin is given in two doses, the first
prior to weaning and the second 2–4 weeks later. The
avirulent vaccine is usually administered in drinking
water. Since the disease tends to be sporadic in birds
other than turkeys, immunization is not generally
recommended unless a recognized danger of infection
is present.

Avoidance of human infection is primarily through
implementation of good occupational practices, especially when handling diseased pigs or turkeys or for
those working in the fishing or fish-processing industries. Observation of adequate hygiene precautions,
such as hand washing with disinfectants and covering
skin wounds or abrasions, together with control of the
disease in susceptible domestic species plays an important role in preventing the disease in man. The control
of rodent populations in meat- and fish-processing
plants also form part of the control measures for this
disease.

In the United States erysipeloid was listed as a
specific occupational disease under worker's compen-
sation laws in the states of Arizona, Colorado, Iowa,
Kansas, and New Mexico (Morgis *et al.* 1967).

ACKNOWLEDGEMENT

The author would like to thank K. Halstead Smith for a
critical review of the final draft.

REFERENCES

Barber, M. (1948). Discussion on swine erysipelas infection
(*Erysipelothrix rhusiopathiae*) in man and animals. *Proceedings
of the Royal Society of Medicine*, **41**, 328–30.

Berg, R. A. (1984). *Erysipelothrix rhusiopathiae*. *Southern Medical
Journal*, **77**, (12), 1614.

Grieco, M. H. and Sheldon, C. (1970). *Erysipelothrix rhusiopathiae*. *Annals of the New York Academy of Sciences*, **174**,
523–32.

Hillenbrand, F. K. M. (1953). Whale finger and seal finger,
their relation to erysipeloid. *Lancet*, **i**, 680–1.

Hunter, D. (ed.) (1974). *The diseases of occupations*, (5th edn),
pp. 709–12. The English Universities Press, London.

Jones, T. D. (1979). Aspects of the epidemiology and control
of *Erysipelothrix insidiosa* polyarthritis in lambs. *Veterinary
Annual*, **19**, 88–96.

King, P. F. (1946). Erysipeloid. *Lancet*, **251**, 196–8.

Klauder, J. V. (1926). Erysipeloid and swine erysipelas in man.
Journal of the American Veterinary Medical Association, **86**, 536–41.

Koch, R. (1880). *Investigations into the aetiology of traumatic
infective diseases*. New Sydenham Society, London.

Loeffler, F. A. (1886). Experimentelle Untersuchungen
uber Schweinerothlauf. Arb. kais. Gesundheit. *Sante*, **1**,
46–55.

McGinnes, G. F. and Spindle, F. (1934). Erysipeloid condition among workers in a bone button factory due to the bacillus of swine erysipelas. *American Journal of Public Health*, **24**, 32–5.

Morgis, G. G., Beauregard, L. P., and Shoub, E. P. (1967). *State compensatory provisions for occupational diseases*. US Bureau of Mines Bulletin 623, Government Printing Office, Washington.

Pasteur, L. and Thuillier, L. (1883). Pathologie experimentale: la vaccination du rouget des porcs a l'aide du virus mortel attenue de cette maladie. *Compte Rendus Hebdomadaires de Seances l'Academie de Siences, Paris*, **97**, 1163–9.

Penny, R. H. C. and Guise, H. J. (1986). Swine erysipelas is a seasonal disease: fact or fiction? *Veterinary Annual*, **26**, 129–33.

Procter, D. M. and Richardson, I. M. (1954). A report on 235 cases of erysipeloid in Aberdeen. *British Journal of Industrial Medicine*, **11**, 175–9.

Reboli, A. C. and Farrar, W. E. (1989). *Erysipelothrix rhusiopathiae*: an occupational pathogen. *Clinical Microbiology Reviews*, **2**, (4), 354–9.

Report (1972). Summaries of Monthly Reports of the Veterinary Investigation Service, MAFF. *Veterinary Record*, **91**, 121.

Report (1975). Summaries of Monthly Reports of the Veterinary Investigation Service, MAFF. *Veterinary Record*, **97**, 319.

Report (1976). Summaries of Monthly Reports of the Veterinary Investigation Service, MAFF. *Veterinary Record*, **99**, 177.

Report (1977). Summaries of Monthly Reports of the Veterinary Investigation Service, MAFF. *Veterinary Record*, **100**, 521.

Rosenbach, A. J. F. (1884). *Microorganismen bei den Wundinfektionskrankheiten des Menschen*. Wiesbaden, Bergmann.

Sneath, P. H. A., Abbott, J. D., and Cunliffe, A. C. (1951). The Bacteriology of Erysipeloid. *British Medical Journal*, **2**, 1063–6.

Spencer, R. (1959). The sanitation of fish boxes. I. The quantitative and qualitative bacteriology of commercial wooden fish boxes. *Journal of Applied Bacteriology*, **22**, 73–84.

Wood, R. L. (1974). Isolation of pathogenic *Erysipelothrix rhusiopathiae* from feces of apparently healthy swine. *American Journal of Veterinary Research*, **35**, 41–3.

Wood, R. L. (1984). Swine erysipelas—a review of prevalence and research. *Journal of the American Veterinary Medical Association*, **184**, (8), 944–9.

Wood, R. L. and Harrington, R. Jr (1978). Serotypes of *Erysipelothrix rhusiopathiae* isolated from swine and from soil and from manure of swine pens in the United States. *American Journal of Veterinary Research*, **39**, 1833–40.

Wood, R. L. and Schuman, R. D. (1981). In *Infectious diseases of wild mammals*, (ed. J. W. Davis, L. H. Karstad, and D. O. Trainer), (2nd edn), p. 297. Iowa State University Press, Ames.

10 VEROCYTOTOXIN-PRODUCING *ESCHERICHIA COLI* (VTEC) INFECTIONS

S. Nelson, R. C. Clarke, and M. A. Karmali

SUMMARY

Verocytotoxin (VT)-producing *Escherichia coli* (VTEC) infection is associated with a distinct illness, the clinical spectrum of which includes non-specific diarrhoea, haemorrhagic colitis, and the haemolytic uraemic syndrome (HUS). HUS is the leading cause of acute renal failure in children.

VTEC infection has become widely recognized as a major cause of food-borne disease, particularly in industrialized societies. Infection may also be water-borne or acquired via person to person transmission. The natural reservoir of VTEC is the intestinal tracts of domestic animals, particularly cattle, and foods of bovine origin such as ground beef patties and unpasteurized milk are major sources of human disease. The significant morbidity and mortality associated with VTEC infection (largely as a result of HUS) makes it a zoonotic problem of serious public health concern.

Although over 150 different OH serotypes of VTEC have been associated with human illness, the vast majority of reported outbreaks and sporadic cases of VTEC-infection in humans have been associated with serotype O157:H7.

The incubation period of VTEC-associated illness is about 3–5 days. After ingestion of VTEC (particularly strains of serotype O157:H7) in contaminated food the organisms multiply in the bowel and colonize the mucosa of probably the large bowel in a manner similar to that seen with enteropathogenic *E. coli* serotypes. This is characterized by the destruction of microvilli and an intimate effacing adherence of the bacterium. It is likely that pathophysiological changes associated with this enterocyte pathology are responsible for the genesis of diarrhoea, but the precise mechanisms remain to be elucidated.

VTs constitute a family of related protein subunit exotoxins, the major ones implicated in human disease being VT1, VT2, and VT2c. Genes encoding these toxins have been cloned and sequenced and their mode of action elucidated at the molecular level. The specific receptor for these toxins has been determined as globotriosylceramide (Gb_3). These molecules are thought to be absorbed into the circulation during the early stages of VTEC infection and to damage specific target cells, which are probably capillary endothelial cells in the kidneys and other organs and tissues. Endothelial cell injury results in the characteristic microangiopathic disease observed in HUS.

The occurrence of large outbreaks of food-borne VTEC-associated illness has promoted close public scrutiny of this zoonosis at all levels in the chain of transmission, including the farm, abbatoir, food processing, packaging, and distribution plants, the wholesaler, the retailer, and finally the consumer. This will undoubtedly lead to new regulations and practices at these various levels in the future.

Progress in understanding the pathogenesis of VTEC infection may lead to the development of specific vaccines to prevent the disease or its severe complications.

HISTORY

The presence of a hitherto unrecognized cytotoxin, active on Vero cells, in culture filtrates of some *Escherichia coli* strains was reported by Konowalchuk and colleagues in 1977. An antiserum prepared against a partially purified Vero cytotoxin (VT) preparation from their prototype VT-producing *E. coli* (VTEC) strain H. 30 (serotype O26:H11) neutralized the activity of VT from 8 of 10 VT+ve strains but not from two others, suggesting the existence of serological heterogeneity among VTs, an observation that has since been confirmed. Seven VTEC strains were from patients with gastroenteritis, suggesting that VT was a virulence factor in enteric disease. Of the remaining three strains, one was associated with diarrhoea in a weanling pig and two were from cheese, thus providing the earliest suggestion of a food-borne, and possibly zoonotic, origin for VTEC.

In 1983 O'Brien and LaVeck purified and characterized the H.30 toxin and showed that it was a polypeptide subunit toxin that was structurally and antigenically similar to Shiga toxin produced by *Shigella dysenteriae* type 1. They thus referred to it as Shiga-like toxin (SLT).

It was not until the early 1980s that the significance of VTEC in human disease started to become appreciated.

In 1983, Riley and colleagues from the Centers for Disease Control (CDC), Atlanta, conducted epidemiological investigations on two outbreaks of a poorly understood condition referred to as 'haemorrhagic colitis' which is characterized by severe abdominal cramps, haemorrhagic diarrhoea, and a lack of significant fever. They found a close link between disease and the consumption of undercooked hamburger patties from a commercial fast-food outlet. Microbiological investigations showed an association between disease and the presence of an *E. coli* strain belonging to the 'rare' O157:H7 serotype that was later shown to be a VT producer. This organism was subsequently recovered from a preserved quality-control sample of hamburger meat from the batch that was originally implicated in the outbreaks. Many foodborne outbreaks associated with *E. coli* O157:H7 have since been reported from North America, Europe, and other regions (Griffin and Tauxe 1991).

Also in 1983, Karmali *et al.* in Toronto, established a link between infection by VTEC belonging to several serotypes, including O157:H7, and the haemolytic uraemic syndrome (HUS), a condition of unknown aetiology that was first described in 1955 (Gasser *et al.* 1955). The aetiological relationship between VTEC and the most common 'classical' form of HUS has since been confirmed in several countries. HUS consists of the triad of features: acute renal failure, thrombocytopenia, and microangiopathic haemolytic anaemia, which in the classical syndrome, occur a few days after the onset of a bloody diarrhoeal illness that resembles haemorrhagic colitis. HUS, a leading cause of acute renal failure in children, is characterized histopathologically by thrombotic microangiopathy affecting the renal glomeruli and other organs such as the gut. Karmali *et al.* suggested that VT was of direct significance in the genesis of HUS because VT was present *in vivo* (in faecal filtrates of HUS patients), it was a common denominator in strains belonging to several different serotypes, and significant antibody responses to VT were observed in the sera of several patients. They postulated that VT was responsible for the damage to capillaries in the glomeruli and other organs, probably through a direct cytotoxic action on endothelial cells (Karmali *et al.* 1989).

These initial observations by Riley *et al.* and Karmali *et al.* have now been confirmed in several centres throughout the world (Karmali 1989; Griffin and Tauxe 1991).

Significant advances have been made during the past decade in understanding the epidemiology and pathogenesis of VTEC infection, which has become widely recognized as a major zoonotic infection of humans.

THE HOSTS

HUMAN

Incubation period

The majority of reported outbreaks of VTEC infection have been associated with VTEC serotype O157:H7. Estimates of the incubation period in these outbreaks (Griffin and Tauxe 1991) have ranged from about 1 to 9 days, with an average of about 3–5 days, an incubation period that is similar to that for campylobacteriosis, but significantly longer than that for other food-borne illness such as salmonellosis (12–36 h).

Clinical features

VTEC infection is associated with a wide spectrum of clinical manifestations that include non-specific diarrhoea, haemorrhagic colitis, and HUS.

Haemorrhagic colitis

This illness (Riley *et al.* 1983), also referred to as acute 'ischaemic colitis', is characterized by the sudden onset of severe abdominal cramping, followed within hours by watery diarrhoea. Patients may experience nausea, but vomiting is not a feature. Watery diarrhoea progresses rapidly to a phase characterized by profuse bloody discharge resembling lower gastrointestinal haemorrhage. Fever is typically absent or low-grade. The white blood cell count may be elevated with a slight left shift. Barium enema examination, if performed early, shows a 'pseudotumour' or 'thumbprinting' pattern, suggesting submucosal oedema or haemorrhage, usually in the ascending or transverse colon. Colonoscopy may show erythema, haemorrhage, and oedema in the ascending and proximal transverse colon. An inflammatory exudate may also be seen. The illness is usually self-limited and resolves within about a week. Severe illness may be complicated by bowel stricture.

Haemolytic uraemic syndrome (HUS) (**Karmali *et al.* 1985b, 1989**)

HUS is defined by a triad of features: acute renal failure, thrombocytopenia, and microangiopathic haemolytic anaemia. Although there are different varieties of HUS, the most common form, by far, is 'classical', or D+ (diarrhoea associated), HUS which has its highest incidence in children; it presents, typically, a few days after the onset of an acute diarrhoeal 'prodromal' illness, which is often bloody with features indistinguishable from those of haemorrhagic colitis. The other, very uncommon, forms of HUS, also referred to as D–HUS, include the 'atypical' HUS of childhood (in which the prodrome is typically a respiratory illness), childhood forms that are inherited, and adult forms that occur in association with pregnancy, oral contraceptive usage, malignant hypertension, and various chronic illnesses.

Classical HUS is a leading cause of acute renal failure in childhood. Whereas renal and gastrointestinal features predominate in most cases, severe complications may occur as a result of microangiopathic disease in other organ systems, including the central nervous system (CNS), heart, lungs, and pancreas. 'Classical' HUS and/or VTEC-associated HUS with prominent CNS manifestations is often referred to as thrombotic thrombocytopenic purpura (TTP). This is probably unjustified because TTP, while resembling HUS, is a distinct clinical entity in which neurological signs and fever are more prominent, a diarrhoeal prodrome is uncommon, and the peak age of incidence is in the third decade.

Following the initial reports from Canada that showed an association between 'classical' HUS and VTEC infection, it is now widely recognized that VTEC is the principal cause of 'classical' HUS. However, HUS is also a major complication of Shiga dysentery associated with *Shigella dysenteriae* type 1. The factor responsible for the genesis of HUS following both VTEC infection and Shiga dysentery is probably the identical protein exotoxin, referred to as VT1 or Shiga toxin, that is elaborated by VTEC and *Sh. dysenteriae* type 1, respectively.

Treatment and prognosis

In most patients with VTEC-associated diarrhoea and haemorrhagic colitis, the illness is self-limiting and full recovery is achieved with general supportive measures.

HUS used to have a very high case-fatality rate of about 50 per cent. However improvement in the treatment of renal failure and the attendant biochemical disturbances, largely through the use of peritoneal dialysis, has substantially improved the outlook. Modern management techniques have reduced the case-fatality rate to 3–5 per cent, although up to 30 per cent of survivors may develop long-term residual disability in the form of chronic renal failure, hypertension, or a neurological deficit (Trompeter *et al.* 1983). Intravenous immune globulin therapy may be beneficial in a few children with HUS (Sheth *et al.* 1987; Siegler 1988) although the basis for this effect remains to be elucidated. The role of passive immunoprophylaxis in reducing the risk of disease in close contacts of index cases has yet to be explored.

The role of antimicrobial agents in preventing or ameliorating the symptoms of VTEC infection remains controversial. Theoretically, antimicrobial therapy might be of benefit by preventing or aborting infection in exposed individuals and/or by ameliorating the severity of disease once developed. The theoretical risks of antimicrobial administration include progression of VTEC enteritis to HUS due to an enhancement of toxin production by antimicrobials, as has been demonstrated *in vitro* using subinhibitory levels of trimethoprim (Karch *et al.* 1985), or to enhanced growth and survival of VTEC in the bowel as a result of alterations in the endogenous bowel flora. The development of HUS following Shiga dysentery in Bangladesh (Koster *et al.* 1977) has been linked to treatment with antimicrobial agents prior to the development of HUS and to the use of inappropriate antimicrobials (i.e. agents to which the infecting strain of *Sh. dysenteriae* type 1 was subsequently shown to be resistant) after admission to hospital. In contrast, Cimolai and colleagues found that 'appropriate' antibiotic use in VTEC O157 enteritis was associated with a lack of progression to HUS. On the other hand, prolonged use of antimotility agents was found to be a risk factor for progression to HUS (Cimolai *et al.* 1990)

Pathology

In fatal cases of HUS with haemorrhagic colitis, gross pathological examination shows, typically, pale swollen kidneys with petechial capsular haemorhages. Oedematous thickening and haemorrhage is seen affecting parts or all of the colon and the small intestine, and may also be evident in other organs, such as the central nervous system, lungs, heart, and pancreas. In severe cases the entire bowel may appear necrotic and gangrenous (Richardson *et al.* 1988).

The renal histopathology is characterized by glomerular thrombotic microangiopathy with endothelial cell swelling and subendothelial deposits (Habib *et al.* 1982; Richardson *et al.* 1988; Tzipori *et al.* 1988). Afferent arterioles and small-and medium-sized arteries may also be involved (Richardson *et al.* 1988; Tzipori *et al.* 1988). Similar thrombotic microangiopathy may be seen in the capillaries of the brain, gastrointestinal tract, and other organs.

Histopathological appearances in the bowel include mucosal and submucosal oedema and haemorrhage, patchy ulceration, thrombotic occlusion of vessels, and, occasionally, pseudomembrane formation (Morrison *et al.* 1986; Richardson *et al.* 1988; Hunt *et al.* 1989; Griffin *et al.* 1990). Inflammatory changes vary from mild and non-specific (Richardson *et al.* 1988) to acute inflammation resembling ischaemic colitis or infectious colitis (Kelly *et al.* 1987; Griffin *et al.* 1990). Hunt *et al.* 1989; Severe cases may exhibit severe ileal mucosal ulceration or full-thickness necrosis of the bowel wall (Richardson *et al.* 1988; Tzipori *et al.* 1988).

Colonoscopy or sigmoidoscopy in patients with haemorrhagic colitis may show a friable oedematous mucosa with evidence of inflammation, haemorrhage, ulceration, or pseudomembrane formation (Morrison *et al.* 1986). Histological examination of biopsies is often inconclusive, showing non-specific changes or variable features of both infectious colitis and ischaemic colitis. The definitive diagnosis of VTEC infection thus rests on microbiological investigations.

Diagnosis

The optimal strategy for the laboratory diagnosis of VTEC infection involves the detection and isolation of VTEC and/or the demonstration of free VT in the faeces of patients with a compatible clinical illness.

Detection of VTEC and free faecal VT in faeces

Sorbitol MacConkey agar   The method used by most laboratories for diagnosing VTEC infection involves the selective isolation of the most common VTEC serotype, O157:H7 (and also O157:H–) from faecal culture using a sorbitol-containing MacConkey (SMAC) agar. The selectivity of the SMAC medium is based on the fact that most *E. coli* O157:H7 strains, unlike 95 per cent of other *E. coli*, do not ferment sorbitol within 24 hours of incubation and thus appear colourless on this medium (March and Ratnam 1986). Non-sorbitol-fermenting colonies need to be identified as *E. coli* using biochemical tests and serotyped by antiserum to the O157 antigen (using commercially available latex agglutination reagents) and H7 antisera (usually in a reference laboratory). Some strains of the closely related *Escherichia hermanii* have been reported to cross-react with the O157 antiserum (Lior and Borczyk 1987; Rice *et al.* 1992). Isolates may be confirmed as VT producers by cytotoxicity assays using Vero or HeLa cell lines, or by genetic methods to detect specific sequences within genes encoding VT production. While easily incorporated in most diagnostic laboratories, the SMAC medium is limited because: (1) it is insensitive for detecting low inocula, and (2) it cannot diagnose infection due to non-O157 VTEC. The emergence of a clone of sorbitol-fermenting VTEC O157 in Central Europe further compromises the utility of the SMAC medium in diagnosing VTEC infections (Gunzer *et al.* 1992). The technique of

immunomagnetic separation has been found to be useful in selectively isolating *E. coli* O157 from foods and animals (Chapman *et al.* 1994).

Detection of free faecal VT and VT-producing E. coli *in primary faecal cultures*   Detection of free faecal VT is a very sensitive approach for diagnosing VTEC infection because samples may be positive for faecal VT even when VTEC are no longer detectable. It also facilitates the detection of VTEC serotypes other than O157 (Karmali *et al.* 1985*b*; Ritchie *et al.* 1992). Strategies to detect all VTEC strains in primary faecal culture require the use of methods that allow detection of VT-producing bacteria rather than individual serotypes such as O157. However, testing multiple individual colonies from primary culture is not, logistically, feasible; but Karmali *et al.* 1985*a, b*) have reported a screening method that involves testing polymyxin B extracts of colony sweeps or pools from primary agar cultures for VT production. This method was able to detect VTEC in a concentration of less than 5 per cent in mixed cultures, but was limited by the use of labour-intensive cytotoxicity assays which take up to 3 days to detect VT. The use of sensitive immunospecific methods to detect VT would make the detection of free faecal VT and the 'colony' sweep method attractive approaches for diagnosing VTEC infections in the clinical laboratory. Promising immunospecific methods have been developed to detect VT in faecal filtrates (Acheson *et al.* 1994) and in bacterial culture filtrates (Karmali *et al.* 1994*b*) (Basta *et al.* 1989). An ELISA method for rapidly detecting the O157 antigen in faeces or in meat samples is also available (Park *et al.* 1996).

Genetic methods   Successful cloning and sequencing of the genes encoding VT production has led to the development of two approaches for detecting VTEC in faecal samples. In the colony blot method, individual VTEC can be identified among isolated colonies from primary culture by DNA = DNA hybridization methods using DNA probes against regions of the toxin-encoding genes (Brown *et al.* 1989; Karch and Meyer 1989*a*) Willshaw *et al.* 1987; Newland and Neill 1988; Seriwatana *et al.* 1988). The use of non-radioactive digoxigenin-labelled probes makes this approach more convenient for the clinical lab, but the method is limited by the number of individual colonies that are isolated in a primary stool culture. The use of the polymerase chain reaction (PCR) has substantially enhanced the sensitivity of screening VTEC, both from primary stool cultures as well as directly from stools, using primers directed against sequences common to different VTs (Karch and Meyer 1989*b*; Paton *et al.* 1993) or using a multiplex assay utilizing more than one set of primer sequences to detect individual toxins (Pollard *et al.* 1990; Olsvik *et al.* 1991; Brian *et al.* 1992). As well, PCR primer sets specific for adhesive factors, such as the *eae* gene, have been developed (Gannon *et al.* 1993; Louie *et al.* 1994).

Serological methods

Patients with VTEC infection do not consistently develop serum antibodies to VTs (Karmali 1994a). Serological tests to detect such antibodies are thus of limited value in diagnosis. On the other hand, serological responses to the O157 lipopolysaccharide correlate well with recent infection by *E. coli* O157:H7, and are thus useful in diagnosing VTEC infection associated with this particular serotype (Chart *et al.* 1989; Barrett *et al.* 1991). It should be noted, however, that the O157 lipopolysaccharide (LPS) cross-reacts with the LPS of other bacteria, such as *Brucella abortus* (Corbel *et al.* 1983; Notenboom *et al.* 1987). Serological responses to LPS of serotypes other than O157 may be helpful in establishing the pathogenetic significance of these strains (Ludwig *et al.* 1996).

ANIMAL

Animals may be asymptomatic carriers of VTEC or may develop specific syndromes, depending on the host species and/or the characteristics of the infecting VTEC strains. A specific syndrome affecting weanling pigs, oedema disease, is associated with specific VTEC serotypes O138, O139, and O141, which produce a VT2-variant toxin, termed VT2e. This usually fatal illness is characterized by anorexia, oedema of the eyelids, and neurological involvement consisting of incoordination and paralysis (Shanks 1938). Histopathologically, the disease is characterized by microangiopathy of target organs (brain, stomach) (MacLeod *et al.* 1991b). Although VT2e-producing strains have occasionally been recovered from humans, their clinical significance is uncertain (Pierard *et al.* 1991). Pigs can shed other serotypes of VTEC that are VT1 and VT2 producers but their importance in human disease is unclear.

High proportions of adult cattle and calves are asymptomatic carriers of VTEC and probably constitute the main reservoir of strains implicated in human disease (Mohammad *et al.* 1986; Borczyk *et al.* 1987; Montenegro *et al.* 1990; Suthienkul *et al.* 1990; Wells *et al.* 1991; Wilson *et al.* 1992; Beutin *et al.* 1993; Renwick *et al.* 1993). Over 100 serotypes, including O157:H7, have been isolated from cattle, and a growing number of these serotypes have been isolated from humans (Butler and Clarke 1994). Calves, 2–8 weeks of age, have developed diarrhoea or dysentery associated with a number of VTEC serotypes, notably O5, O26 and O111 (Chanter *et al.* 1984; Sherwood *et al.* 1985; Moxley and

Francis 1986; Schoonderwoerd *et al.* 1988; González and Blanco 1989). VTEC strains have also been recovered from other ruminants, such as sheep and goats (Mohammad *et al.* 1986; Beutin *et al.* 1993). The full extent of the prevalence of VTEC in domestic animals and wildlife remains to be determined.

THE AGENT (VTEC)

TAXONOMY AND CLASSIFICATION

Taxonomically the genus *Escherichia*, in the family Enterobacteriaceae, is very closely related to, if not identical with, the genus *Shigella*. Thus the discovery of a toxin, VT1, in *E. coli* that is virtually identical to Shiga toxin produced by *Sh. dysenteriae* type 1 is not surprising.

The property of VT-production distinguishes VTEC from other pathogenic enteric *E. coli*, such as enterotoxigenic *E. coli*, enteroinvasive *E. coli*, enteropathogenic *E. coli* (EPEC) serotypes, and enteroaggregative *E. coli*.

Over 150 different VTEC OH serotypes have now been associated with human disease. Many others have been recovered exclusively from animals. The term enterohaemorrhagic *E. coli* (EHEC) has been applied to those VTEC serotypes that have the same clinical, epidemiological, and pathogenetic features associated with the prototype strain *E. coli* O157:H7 (Levine 1987).

Whittam and colleagues have investigated the clonal origin of VTEC O157 strains by assaying allelic variation at up to 20 different enzyme loci by multilocus enzyme electrophoresis. Strains of *E. coli* O157:H7 from a diversity of sources were found to constitute a genetically distinct clonal group that is only distantly related to VTEC of other serotypes (Whittam *et al.* 1988). On the other hand, when compared to EPEC serotype strains (with many of which *E. coli* O157:H7 shares the attaching and effacing adherence property), the O157:H7 clone was found to be most closely related to a clone of O55:H7 strains that has long been associated with worldwide outbreaks of infantile diarrhoea (Whittam *et al.* 1993).

DISEASE MECHANISMS

The specific disease mechanisms of VTEC involve their toxins and colonization factors. Host factors such as receptors and immune mechanisms form the other key components of an equation that determines the type and severity of illness.

Verocytotoxins

Structure/function

Verocytotoxins comprise a family of related subunit proteins whose prototype, VT1, is virtually identical to

Shiga toxin. The second major toxin, VT2, has a number of closely related variants including VT2c and VT2e. VTs are among the most potent biological substances known, toxic to cells at pico-to nanomolar concentrations. The use of different nomenclatures for the major toxins and toxin subtypes has led to proposals for rationalizing the nomenclature, such that the term VT is interchangeable with SLT (Shiga-like toxin) and the subtype designation is identical (O'Brien *et al.* 1994). Thus SLT IIc is interchangeable with VT2c.

With the exception of VT2e (Marques *et al.* 1987; Gyles *et al.* 1988), and a closely related variant (SLT IIva (Yee *et al.* 1993), verocytotoxins are encoded by lysogenic bacteriophage (Smith *et al.* 1983, 1984; O'Brien *et al.* 1984). The holotoxins consist of an 'A' or enzymatically 'active' chain (*c.* 32 kDa) and 'B' or cell-'binding' chains (*c.* 8 kDa). VTs are likely of the A:5B form. Isolated VT1 B subunits, when crystallized and examined by X-ray crystallography, form a pentamer with a hydrophobic pore lined by α-helices and β-sheets from subunit n and $n + 1$ interacting in an antiparallel fashion (Stein *et al.* 1992). The functional receptor for Shiga toxin, VT1, VT2, and VT2c is the mammalian cell membrane glycolipid, globotriosylceramide (Gb$_3$; galα1-4galβ1-4gluβ1-3-ceramide) (Lindberg *et al.* 1987; Lingwood *et al.* 1987; Samuel *et al.* 1990). VT2e preferentially binds to globotetraosylceramide (Gb$_4$) (Samuel *et al.* 1990), which differs from Gb$_3$ only by having an additional carbohydrate residue (galNAc) in the terminal position. Once bound to the cell, Shiga toxin/VT1 has been demonstrated to internalize by way of clathrin-coated pits (Sandvig *et al.* 1989) and target the endoplasmic reticulum via the Golgi by a process termed 'retrograde transport' (Sandvig *et al.* 1992). The A subunit, after it is proteolytically nicked to an enzymatically active A$_1$ fragment (Reisbig *et al.* 1981), cleaves the *N*-glycosidic bond at position A-4324 of the 28S rRNA of the 60S ribosomal subunit (Endo *et al.* 1988). These toxins are exquisitely potent inhibitors of translation, effective at pico- to nanomolar concentrations (Obrig *et al.* 1987; Head *et al.* 1991). The major toxin types of the VT family have been cloned and sequenced (Calderwood *et al.* 1987; DeGrandis *et al.* 1987; Jackson *et al.* 1987*a,b*; Gyles *et al.* 1988; Ito *et al.* 1990) at the transcriptional level.

Role in disease

The occurrence of widespread sterile microangiopathic lesions in various organs and tissues in HUS and pig oedema disease is consistent with systemic toxaemia. The reproduction of such lesions in experimental animals by injected toxins supports the concept that VTs have a distinct role in their genesis (MacLeod *et al.* 1991*b*; Richardson *et al.* 1992). A disease of racing greyhounds referred to as 'Alabama rot' or 'idiopathic cutaneous and renal glomerular vasculopathy' shows striking resemblance to human HUS. It has recently been shown to be associated with VTEC infection (Hertzke *et al.* 1995).

Underlying the microangiopathic lesions seen in the renal glomeruli of patients with HUS is the characteristic swelling of capillary endothelial cells accompanied by fibrin deposition and occlusion of the vessel lumen. Surrounding tissue infarction and necrosis are believed to be a result of this primary lesion. Demonstration of the direct cytotoxic effect of VT on human endothelial cells in culture (Kavi *et al.* 1987; Obrig *et al.* 1988) including human renal microvascular endothelial cells (HRVEC) (Barley-Maloney *et al.* 1990) supports the concept that endothelial cells are primary targets for VT *in vivo*. The toxin receptor, Gb$_3$, has been identified in human renal tissue (Boyd and Lingwood 1989) and toxin–endothelial cell binding has been visualized by immunofluorescent techniques in rabbits injected intravenously with toxin (Richardson *et al.* 1992) and in human renal sections (Lingwood 1994). Cytokines, such as interleukin-1β and tumour necrosis factor, have been shown to augment the cytotoxic potential of VT for cultured human umbilical vein endothelial cells, which has been correlated with an increased expression of the Gb$_3$ receptor (Louise and Obrig 1991; Kar *et al.* 1992; Kaye *et al.* 1993). However Gb$_3$ expression is maximal in HRVEC and is not further influenced by the action of cytokines.

The precise role of VT, and the possible potentiating role of cytokines, in the pathophysiology of HUS, including local intravascular coagulation, thrombocytopenia and microangiopathic haemolytic anaemia, remains to be elucidated.

The role of VT in the production of diarrhoea is not clear. There are no toxin receptors on the mucosal epithelium of the gut (Björk *et al.* 1987); however, microangiopathy, oedema, and haemorrhage have been observed in human intestinal sections of HUS patients (Richardson *et al.* 1988) which may affect the absorptive properties of the gut, resulting in diarrhoea. Rabbits injected intravenously with purified VT1 develop lesions in the gut and in the central nervous system and clinically display dose-related symptoms of diarrhoea and paralysis (Richardson *et al.* 1992). Interestingly, similar experiments with purified VT2c in rabbits demonstrated dose-related symptoms of overt haemorrhagic cecitis, with blood and mucus in the diarrhoeic stools (Head *et al.* 1988). This may thus provide a useful model for studying haemorrhagic colitis in humans.

Histopathological findings in the gut of patients with haemorrhagic colitis, characterized by microangiopathic lesions, haemorrhage, and oedema, are consistent with toxin-mediated damage of the microvasculture in the bowel wall. Experimental reproduction of the symptoms and pathology of haemorrhagic colitis in rabbits injected with VT1 and VT2c supports a direct role of systemic VT in the genesis of human haemorrhagic colitis.

The induction of fluid secretion in rabbit ileal loops by VT1 and Shiga toxin (Keusch *et al.* 1972; O'Brien and LaVeck 1983) argued for a role for these toxins in the genesis of the watery diarrhoea that precedes the symptoms of haemorrhagic colitis. The 'enterotoxic' activity of Shiga toxin in rabbit gut loops has been correlated with the presence of Gb_3 in rabbit enterocytes (Mobassaleh *et al.* 1988). However, the absence of Gb_3 in the human intestinal mucosa suggests that a local action of VT on enterocytes is not responsible for the diarrhoeal symptoms in humans. On the other hand, recent advances in knowledge about VTEC colonization of the gut mucosa suggest that the mechanisms of colonization themselves are responsible for the genesis of diarrhoeal symptoms (Donnenberg and Kaper 1992).

Colonization

The greatest insights into the nature and mechanisms of intestinal mucosal colonization by VTEC have come from studies on strains of enteropathogenic *E. coli* (EPEC) serotypes which have had a long-standing epidemiological association with outbreaks of infantile enteritis. Evidence to date suggests that certain VTEC serotypes, particularly O157:H7, have similar mechanisms.

Histological examination of intestinal biopsies from patients, or of tissues from animals with natural or experimental infection with EPEC, has shown a characteristic pattern of bacterial attachment to enterocytes which consists of the destruction of microvilli and an intimate effacing adherence of the bacterium to the epithelial membrane, which forms pedestals and partially envelopes the bacterium (Staley *et al.* 1969; Polotsky *et al.* 1977). This appearance is referred to as the attaching and effacing (AE) lesion. In the mammalian cell, high concentrations of filamentous actin and other cytoskeletal proteins are present beneath the site of bacterial attachment (Knutton *et al.* 1989).

Recent evidence (Donnenberg and Kaper 1992) indicates that the mechanisms for the AE lesion involves the interaction of various plasmid-and chromosomally mediated factors that are subject to complex genetic and environmental regulation.

Initial adherence of EPEC, prior to the AE lesion, consists of fimbrial attachment to enterocytes that is mediated by the plasmid-mediated "bundle-forming" pilus (BFP) Giron *et al.* 1991). However VTEC do not express BFP, and the occurrence of a fimbrial attachment phase has not been firmly established.

All the virulence factors necessary for the formation of the AE lesion, in both VTEC and EPEC, are encoded for by a large 35,480 bp chromosomal locus (pathogenicity island) referred to as LEE (locus for enterocyte effacement) (McDaniel *et al.* 1995). One of the LEE structural genes that is critical for AE lesion formation is eae which encodes a 94 kDa outer membrane adhesin protein "intimin" which is responsible for the bacterium's intimate attachment to the enterocyte (Jerse and Kaper 1991). Two other genes, espA and espB (Donnenberg *et al.* 1993; Jarvis *et al.* 1995; Jarvis and Kaper 1996; Kenny and Finlay 1995; Kenny *et al.* 1996) encode secreted proteins (espA and espB, respectively) that activate signal transduction pathways (Foubister *et al.* 1994; Ismaili *et al.* 1995) which lead to cytoskeletal changes in the enterocyte and to the phosphorylation of a host cell protein, Hp90 (Manjarrez-Hernandez *et al.* 1992), which binds to intimin. espA (25kDa polypeptide) and espB (37kDa polypeptide) are two of at least five different secreted proteins encoded for by LEE. The functions of secreted proteins other than EspA and EspB are not known.

Studies with VTEC have shown that strains belonging to several serotypes exhibit the AE lesion *in vitro* and in experimental animal models, and evidence to date indicates that the mechanisms of the VTEC and EPEC AE lesions are similar. However VTEC do not express BFP. An *eae* gene homologue, which has been cloned and sequenced from *E. coli* O157:H7 (Beebakhee *et al.* 1992; Yu and Kaper 1992), showed almost complete identity with the EPEC *eae* gene for the first 2200 bp (97 per cent homology), but less so (59 per cent homology) over the last 800 bp at the C terminus. It is thought (Donnenberg and Kaper 1992) that sequence heterogeneity at the C terminal end may be responsible for tissue binding and may explain the propensity of EPEC to bind to the small bowel mucosa in contrast to VTEC which tends to colonize the large bowel of animals, and probably humans, although this remains to be proven.

GROWTH AND SURVIVAL REQUIREMENTS

VTEC grow well under aerobic or facultatively anaerobic conditions. They normally inhabit the intestinal tract, where they can multiply to large numbers when host factors facilitate growth. Our understanding of the interaction between VTEC and normal gut flora is limited, but it is likely that, as with other enteric pathogens, such as *Salmonella*, the normal host flora plays an important role in inhibiting growth of VTEC in the intestinal environment. Most information on growth and survival is currently based on studies with *E. coli* serotype O157:H7. Information on environmental survival is limited (USDA:APHIS:VS 1994), but it has been demonstrated that O157 can

such contact. The extent of contamination can be magnified in the deboning and grinding operations. The current trend for concentration and rapid distribution systems in the food-processing sector have resulted in plants that produce as many as one million hamburger patties per day with distribution to large geographic areas. This can result in large outbreaks when coupled with improper cooking and handling procedures at the retail or consumer level. On the other hand, such concentration of volume can facilitate the implementation of control strategies such as HACCP (Hazard Analysis Critical Control Points) programmes which can result in the production of large volumes of high-quality, safe food.

Prevention of transmission at the food preparation level through appropriate handling and heating is critical. The higher association of VTEC infection with ground meat compared to cuts of beef is likely due to differences in processing. When cuts of beef are surface-contaminated, the organisms can be killed readliy with cooking. In ground beef patties, however, the organisms are mixed throughout the meat, and the achievement of adequate internal killing temperatures and cooking time become critical in reducing the risk of infection. Once cooked, any leftovers should be promptly refrigerated or frozen. In addition, hands and any materials coming in contact with the uncooked meat (cutting boards, utensils) should be washed thoroughly with hot, soapy water, and should not come in contact with any uncooked foods.

These basic elements of food hygiene in the home and institutional setting need to be advocated aggressively in public education campaigns, especially through the popular media.

Increasing evidence of person to person transmission of VTEC infection necessitates effective infection control procedures in hospitals, day-care centres, and other institutions. The development and implementation of rapid diagnostic techniques will lead to earlier recognition of VTEC infection and thus allow more timely implementation of public health control measures.

Research into the feasibility of vaccinating populations to prevent VTEC infection or its systemic complications is at an early stage of development. Two potential immunization options include the use of vaccines to prevent VTEC colonization of the intestinal mucosa, and toxoids or subunit components of the holotoxins to obviate the consequences of systemic VT toxaemia (Bielaszewska *et al.* 1997).

The nature of colonization factors and potential *eae* gene products such as intimin is only now becoming understood, and knowledge of the local or systemic antibody responses to these proteins is still limited.

Following infection by VTEC strains that express one or more toxins, only some individuals develop specific antibodies to VT1 (Karmali 1994a), whereas specific immune responses to VT2 and VT2c appear to be very uncommon. The reason for the inconsistent nature of the serum antitoxic response in patients with VT1-producing VTEC infection remains to be elucidated. Possible explanations (Levine *et al.* 1992) include:

(1) a low antigenic stimulus afforded by a toxin with a high biological activity;

(2) immunosuppressive effect of the toxin which is known to be cytotoxic for B lymphocytes *in vitro*;

(3) restriction of the immune response to individuals of particular major histocompatibility complex class II genotypes; or

(4) epitopes on the VT1 molecule to which immune responses occur more consistently *in vivo* may not have been adequately exposed in the assay used.

It should be noted, however, that the absence of a serological response does not necessarily preclude the ability to induce protection after toxoid immunization (Levine *et al.* 1992). Both VT1 toxoid (Richardson *et al.* 1992) and VT1 'B' subunit toxoid or components (Harari and Arnon 1990, Boyd *et al.* 1991) have been shown to induce protective immunity in laboratory animals.

In the veterinary setting, MacLeod and Gyles (1991) were able to protect pigs from a lethal challenge of purified VT2e, both by passive immunization with anti-VT2e neutralizing antibodies and by active immunization with VT2e toxoid.

METHODS/PROGRAMMES/EVALUATION

Meat inspection programmes worldwide are under review and undergoing a change from a sensory-based approach to the implementation of HACCP and other strategies with an emphasis on total quality management. The integration of the preharvest sector into food safety programmes will likely result in the HACCP approach being extended to the farm level. Internationally, food inspection systems are under increasing trade pressure to comply with international standards such as the ISO 9000 series. In many countries public health regulations dictate minimal cooking temperatures that must be achieved and good food hygiene practices to ensure that 'ready to eat' food sold at the retail level is safe.

Other proposed control methods include the use of chemical compounds or irradiation to decrease or eliminate microbial load in meat products. Detergents such as trisodium phosphate (TSP) have shown promise as treatments to decrease coliform counts on carcasses and are being licensed as a processing aid in some countries. Another means of reducing microbial load is by γ-irradiation. This process has been shown to reduce VTEC in hamburger patties effectively (Thayer and Boyd 1993) and does not appear to have an adverse effect on the product. In the past the largest problem with implementing this technique has been consumer acceptance. Recent marketing of irradiated chicken in the United States of America has shown that consumer attitudes are changing and that irradiation may be a viable approach to reduce VTEC contamination of retail foods. These developments, coupled with public education programmes promoting proper food handling and preparation techniques, will have a positive effect in reducing the exposure of the public to VTEC by contaminated food.

LEGISLATION

Currently VTEC infection in animals is not a reportable or 'named' disease in agricultural regulations worldwide. Investigations usually are the result of tracebacks from food-borne outbreaks or research prevalence surveys. This may change in some countries as farm-level control programmes for VTEC, especially serotype O157:H7, are implemented. In many countries, the sale of unpasteurized milk is illegal, thereby providing an effective measure to reduce VTEC-related milk-borne outbreaks. Also, many nations and municipalities have guidelines and regulations setting standards for internal cooking temperatures and sanitary measures at the retail level, that, when properly enforced, also serve as critically important barriers to human infection.

Public health surveillance of VTEC infection can play a major role in devising and implementing control measures. Whereas reporting of human cases of VTEC infection (or only O157:H7 infection) to public health authorities is mandatory in some countries, it is not so in others. Consistent reporting by all countries can make a vital contribution to surveillance at the international level and allow more global strategies of control to be devised.

REFERENCES

Acheson, D. W. K., De Breuker S., Donohue-Rolfe A., Kozak K., Yi A., and Keusch G. T. (1994). Development of a clinically useful diagnostic enzyme immunoassay for enterohemorrhagic *Escherichia coli*. In *Recent advances in verocytotoxin-producing* Escherichia coli *infections*, (ed. M. A. Karmali and A. Goglio), pp. 109–112. Elsevier Science, Excerpta Medica Series, Amsterdam.

Ahmed, S. and Cowden, J. (1997). An outbreak of *E. coli* 1057 in Central Scotland. 3rd International Symposium and Workshop on Shiga Toxin (Verocytotoxin)-producing *Escherichia coli* Infections, Baltimore, MD.

Barley-Maloney, L., Obrig, T., and Daniel, T. (1990). Human renal microvascular endothelial cells (HRMEC) are targets for hemolytic uremic syndrome associated verotoxin. (ABSTRACT). *Journal of the American Society of Nephrology*, **1**, 515.

Barrett, T. J., Green, J. H., Griffin, P. M., Pavia, A. T., Ostroff, S. M. and Wachsmuth, I. K. (1991). Enzyme-linked immunosorbent assays for detecting antibodies to Shiga-like toxin I, Shiga-like toxin II, and *Escherichia coli* O157:H7 lipopolysaccharide in human serum. *Current Microbiology*, **23**, 189–95.

Beebakhee, G., Louie, M., Azavedo, J. D., and Brunton, J. (1992). Cloning and nucleotide sequence of the *eae* gene homologue from enterohemorrhagic *Escherichia coli* serotype O157:H7. *FEMS Microbiology Letters*, **91**, 63–8.

Besser, R. E. *et al.* (1993). An outbreak of diarrhea and hemolytic uremic syndrome from *Escherichia coli* O157:H7 in fresh-pressed apple cider. *Journal of the American Medical Association*, **269**, 2217–20.

Beutin, L., Geier, D., Steinruck, H., Zimmermann, S., and Scheutz, F. (1993). Prevalence and some properties of verotoxin (Shiga-like toxin) producing *Escherichia coli* in seven different species of healthy domestic animals. *Journal of Clinical Microbiology*, **31**, 2483–8.

Bielasczewska, M., Clarke, I., Karmali, M. A. and Petric, M. (1997). Localisation of intravenously administered verocytotoxins (shiga-like toxins) 1 and 2 in rabbits immunized with homologous and heterologous toxoids and toxin subunits. *Infections and Immunity* **65**, 2509–16.

Björk, S., Breimer, M. E., Hansson, G. C., Karlsson, K. A., and Leffler, H. (1987). Structures of blood group glycosphingolipids of human small intestine. *Journal of Biological Chemistry*, **262**, 6758–65.

Booth, L. and Rowe, B. (1993). Possible occupational acquisition of *Escherichia coli* O157 infection. *Lancet*, **342**, 1298–9.

Borczyk, A. A., Karmali, M. A., Lior, H., and Duncan, L. M. C. (1987). Bovine reservoir for verotoxin-producing *Escherichia coli* O157:H7. *Lancet*, **i**, 98.

Boyd, B. and Lingwood, C. (1989). Verotoxin receptor glycolipid in human renal tissue. *Nephron*, **51**, 207–10.

Boyd, B., Richardson, S., and Gariépy, J. (1991). Serological responses to the B subunit of shiga-like toxin 1 and its peptide fragments indicate that the B subunit is a vaccine candidate to counter the action of the toxin. *Infection and Immunity*, **59**, 750–7.

Brian, M. J. *et al.* (1992). Polymerase chain reaction for diagnosis of enterohemorrhagic *Escherichia coli* O157 in patients with hemolytic uremic syndrome. *Journal of Clinical Microbiology*, **30**, 1801–6.

Brown, E. D., Sethabutr, O., Jackson, M. P., Lolekha, S., and Echeverria, P. (1989). Hybridization of *Escherichia coli* producing Shiga-like toxin I, Shiga-like toxin II, and a variant of Shiga-like toxin II with synthetic oligonucleotide probes. *Infection and Immunity*, **57**, 2811–14.

Butler, D. G. and Clarke, R. C. (1994). Diarrhea and dysentery in calves. In Escherichia coli in domestic animals and humans, (ed. C. L. Gyles), pp. 91–116. Commonwealth Agricultural Bureau, Wollingford, Oxford, UK.

Calderwood, S. B., Auclair, F., Donohue-Rolfe, A., Keusch, G. T., and Mekalanos, J. J. (1987). Nucleotide sequence of the Shiga-like toxin genes of *Escherichia coli*. *Proceedings of the National Academy of Sciences*, USA, **84**, 4364–8.

Caprioli, A. *et al.* (1994). Community-wide outbreak of hemolytic uremic syndrome associated with non-O157 vero-toxin-producing *E. coli. Journal of Infectious Diseases*, **169**, 208–11.

Carter, A. O. *et al.* (1987). A severe outbreak of *Escherichia coli* O157:H7-associated hemorrhagic colitis in a nursing home. *New England Journal of Medicine*, **317**, 1496–500.

CDC (Centers for Disease Control) (1993). Update: Multistate Outbreak of *Escherichia coli* O157:H7 infections from Hamburgers—Western United States, 1992–1993. *Journal of the American Medical Association*, **269**, 2194–6.

Chanter, A., Morgan, J. H., Bridger, J. C., Hall, G. A., and Reynolds, D. J. (1984). Dysentery in gnotobiotic calves caused by atypical *Escherichia coli. Veterinary Record*, **114**, 71.

Chapman, P. A., Wright D. J., and Siddons C. A. (1994). Evaluation of immunomagnetic separation for isolating verocytotoxin-producing *Escherichia coli* O157 from bovine faeces and milk. In *Recent Advances in Verocytotoxin-producing* Escherichia coli *infections*, (ed. M. A. Karmali and A. Goglio), pp. 93–6. Elsevier Science, Excerpta Medica Series, Amsterdam.

Chart, H., Scotland, S. M., and Rowe, B. (1989). Serum antibodies to *Escherichia coli* serotype O157:H7 in patients with hemolytic uremic syndrome. *Journal of Clinical Microbiology*, **27**, 285–90.

Cieslak, P. L., *et al.* (1993). *Escherichia coli* O157:H7 infection from a manured garden. *Lancet*, **342**, 367.

Cimolai, N., Carter, J. E., Morrison, B. J., and Anderson, J. D. (1990). Risk factors for the progression of *Escherichia coli* O157:H7 enteritis to hemolytic uremic syndrome. *Journal of Pediatrics* **116**, 589–92.

Clarke, R. C., McEwen, S. A., Gannon, V. P., Lior, H., and Gyles, C. L. (1989). Isolation of verocytotoxin-producing *Escherichia coli* from milk filters in south-western Ontario. *Epidemiology and Infection*, **102**, 253–60.

Corbel, M. J., Stuart, F. A., and Brewer, R. A. (1983). Observations on serological cross-reactions between smooth *Brucella* species and organisms of other genera. *Developments in Biological Standardization*, **56**, 341–8.

DeGrandis, S. A., Ginsberg, J., Toone, M., Climie, S., Friesen, J., and Brunton, J. (1987). Nucleotide sequence and promoter mapping of the *Escherichia coli* Shiga-like toxin operon of bacteriophage H-19B. *Journal of Bacteriology*, **169**, 4313–19.

Donnenberg, M. S. and Kaper, J. B. (1992). Enteropathogenic *Escherichia coli, Infection and Immunity*, **60**, 3953–61.

Donnenberg, M. S., Yu, J. and Kaper, J. B. (1993). A second chromosomal gene necessary for intimate attachment of enteropathogenic *Escherichia coli. Journal of Bacteriology* **175**, 4670–80.

Doyle, M. P. and Schoeni, J. L. (1987). Isolation of *Escherichia coli* O157:H7 from retail fresh meats and poultry. *Applied Environmental Microbiology* 53, 2394–6.

Endo, Y., Tsurugi, K., Yutsudo, T., Takeda, Y., Ogasawara, T., and Igarashi, K. (1988). Site of action of a Vero toxin (VT2) from *Escherichia coli* O157:H7 and of shiga toxin on eukaryotic ribosomes; RNA *N*-glycosidase activity of the toxins. *European Journal of Biochemistry*, **171**, 45–50.

Foubister, V., Rosenshine, I., and Finlay, B. B. (1994). A diarrheal pathogen, enteropathogenic *Escherichia coli*, triggers a flux of inositol phosphates in infected epithelial cells. *Journal of Experimental Medicine*, **179**, 993–98.

Fukushima, H., Hashizume, T., and Kitani, T. (1997). Abstract V6/VII. The massive outbreak of enterohemorrhagic *E. coli* 0157 infections by food poisoning among the elementary school children in Sakai, Japan, in 1996. 3rd International Symposium and Workshop on Shig Toxin (Verocytotoxin)-producing *Escherichia coli* infections, Baltimore, MD< June 22–26, 1997.

Gannon, V. P. J., Rashed, M., King, R. K., and Thomas, E. J. G. (1993). Detection and characterization of the *eae* gene of shiga-like toxin-producing *Escherichia coli* using polymerase chain reaction. *Journal of Clinical Microbiology*, **31**, 1268–74.

Gasser, C., Gautier, E., Steck, A., Siebenmann, R. E., and Oechslin, R. (1955). Hämolytisch-urämische syndrome: bilaterale Niereninden-Nekrosen bei akuten Erworbenen hämolytischen anämien. *Schweizerische Medizinische Wochenschrift*, **85**, 905–9.

Giron, J. A., Ho, A. S. Y., and Schoolnik, G. K. (1991). An inducible bundle-forming pilus of enteropathogenic *E. coli. Science*, **254**, 710–13.

González, E. A. and Blanco, J. (1989). Serotypes and antibiotic resistance of Verotoxigenic (VTEC) and necrotizing (NTEC) *Escherichia coli* strains isolated from calves with diarrhea. *FEMS Microbiology Letters*, **60**, 31–6.

Griffin, P. W. and Tauxe, R. V. (1991). The epidemiology of infections caused by *Escherichia coli* O157:H7, other enterohemorrhagic *E. coli*, and the associated hemolytic uremic syndrome. *Epidemiologic Reviews* **13**, 60–98.

Griffin, P. M., Olmstead, L. C., and Petras, R. E. (1990). *Escherichia coli* O157:H7-associated colitis: a clinical and histological study of 11 cases. *Gastroenterology*, **99**, 142–9.

Gunzer, F., Bohm, H., Russman, H., Bitzan, M., Aleksik, S., and Karch, H. (1992). Molecular detection of sorbitol-fermenting *Escherichia coli* O157 in patients with hemolytic uremic syndrome. *Journal of Clinical Microbiology*, **30**, 1807–10.

Gyles, C. L., Grandis, S. A. D., MacKenzie, C., and Brunton, J. L. (1988). Cloning and nucleotide sequence analysis of the genes determining verocytotoxin production in a porcine edema disease isolate of *Escherichia coli. Microbial Pathogenesis*, **5**, 419–26.

Habib, R., Levy, M., Gagnadoux, M. F., and Broyer, M. (1982). Prognosis of the hemolytic uremic syndrome in children. *Advances in Nephrology*, **11**, 99–128.

Harari, I. and Arnon, R. (1990). Carboxy-terminal peptides from the B subunit of shiga toxin induce a local and parenteral protective effect. *Molecular Immunology*, **27**, 613–21.

Head, S. C., Petric, M., Richardson, S., Roscoe, M., and Karmali, M. A. (1988). Purification and characterization of verocytotoxin 2. *FEMS Microbiology Letters*, **51**, 211–16.

Head, S. C., Karmali, M. A., and Lingwood, C. A. (1991). Preparation of VT1 and VT2 hybrid toxins from their purified dissociated subunits. *Journal of Biological Chemistry*, **266**, 3617–21.

Hertzke, D. M., Cowan, L. A., Schoning, P., and Fenwick, B. W. (1995). Glomerular ultrastructural lesions of idiopathic cutaneous and renal glomerular vasculopathy of greyhounds. *Veterinary Pathology*, **32**, 451–9.

Isaacson, M., Canter P. H., Effler P., Arntzen L., Bomans P., and Heenan R. (1993). Hemorrhagic colitis in Africa. *Lancet*, **341**, 961.

Ismaili, A., Philpott, D. J., Dytoc, M. T., and Sherman, P. M. (1995). Signal transduction responses following adhesion of verocytotoxin-producing *Escherichia coli. Infection and Immunity*, **63**, 3316–26.

Ito, H., Terai, A., Kurazono, H., Takeda, Y., and Nishibuchi, M. (1990). Cloning and nucleotide sequencing of Verotoxin 2 variant genes from *Escherichia coli* O91:H21 isolated from a patient with the hemolytic uremic syndrome. *Microbial Pathogenesis*, **8**, 47–60.

Itoh, T. *et al.* (1988). Gastroenteritis associated with verocytotoxin producing *Escherichia coli* 0145:NM. *Advances in Research on Cholera and Related Diarrheas*, **5**, 21–8.

Jackson, M. P., Neill, R. J., O'Brien, A. D., Holmes, R. K., and Newland, J. W. (1987*a*). Nucleotide sequence analysis and comparison of the structural gene for Shiga-like toxin I and Shiga-like toxin II encoded by bacteriophages from *Escherichia coli* 933J. *FEMS Microbiology Letters*, **44**, 109–14.

Jarvis, K. G., Giron, J. A., Jerse, A. E., McDaniel, T. K., Donnenberg, M. S., and Kaper, J. B. (1995). Enteropathogenic *Escherichia coli* contains a putative type III secretion system necessary for the export of proteins involved in attaching and effacing lesion formation. *Proceedings of the National Academy of Sciences (USA)* **92**, 7996–8000.

Jarvis, K. G. and Kaper, J. B. (1996). Secretion of extracellular proteins by enterohemorrhagic *Escherichia coli* via a putative type III secretion system. *Infection and Immunity* **64**, 4829–29.

Jerse, A. E. and Kaper, J. B. (1991). The *eae* gene of enteropathogenic *Escherichia coli* encodes a 94-kilodalton membrane protein, the expression of which is influenced by the EAF plasmid. *Infection and Immunity*, **59**, 4302–9.

Kar, N. C. A. J. v. d., Monnens, L. A. H., Karmali, M. A., and Hinsbergh, V. W. M. v. (1992). Tumor necrosis factor and interleukin-1 induce expression of the verocytotoxin receptor globotriaosyl ceramide on human endothelial cells: Implications for the pathogenesis of the hemolytic uremic syndrome. *Blood*, **80**, 2755–64.

Karch, H. and Meyer, T. (1989*a*). Evaluation of oligonucleotide probes for identification of Shiga-like-toxin-producing *Escherichia coli*. *Journal of Clinical Microbiology*, 1180–6.

Karch, H. and Meyer, T. (1989*b*). Single primer pair for amplifying segments of distinct Shiga-like-toxin genes by polymerase chain reaction. *Journal of Clinical Microbiology*, **27**, 2751–7.

Karch, H., Goroncy-Bermes, P., Opferkuch, W., Kroll, H. P., and O'Brien, A. (1985). Subinhibitory concentrations of antibiotics modulate amount of shiga-like toxin produced by *Escherichia coli*. In *The influence of antibiotics on the host–parasite relationship II*, (ed. D. Adam, H. Hahn, and W. Opferkuchg). Springer-Verlag, Berlin, Heidelberg.

Karmali, M. A. (1989). Infection by Verocytotoxin-producing *Escherichia coli*. *Clinical Microbiology Reviews*, **2**, 15–38.

Karmali, M. A., Petric, M., Lim, C., Cheung, R., and Arbus, G. S. (1985*a*). Sensitive method for detecting low numbers of verotoxin-producing *Escherichia coli* in mixed cultures by use of colony sweeps and polymyxin extraction of Verotoxin. *Journal of Clinical Microbiology*, **22**, 614–19.

Karmali, M. A., Petric, M., Lim, C., Fleming, P. C., Arbus, G. S., and Lior, H. (1985*b*). The association between hemolytic uremic syndrome and infection by Verotoxin-producing *Escherichia coli*. Journal of Infectious Diseases, **151**, 775–82.

Karmali, M. A. *et al.* (1994*a*). Enzyme-linked immunosorbent assay for detection of immunoglobulin G antibodies to *Escherichia coli* verocytotoxin I. *Journal of Clinical Microbiology*, **32**, 1457–63.

Karmali, M. A., Winkler M., Petric M., McDowell C., and Penn L. (1994*b*). Evaluation of a microplate latex method (Verotox F) for detecting and characterizing verocytotoxins (VTs) in *Escherichia coli*. Presented at the 95th Annual Meeting of the American Society of Microbiology, Washington, DC, 21–25 May, 1994. Abstract C-178.

Kavi, J., Chant, I., Maris, M., and Rose, P. E. (1987). Cytopathic effect of Verotoxin on endothelial cells. *Lancet*, **ii**, 1035.

Kaye, S. A., Louise, C. B., Boyd, B., Lingwood, C. A. and Obrig, T. G. (1993). Shiga toxin-associated hemolytic uremic syndrome: interleukin-1B enhancement of shiga toxin cytotoxicity toward human vascular endothelial cells in-vitro. *Infection and Immunity*, **61**, 3886–91.

Kelly, J. K., Pai, C. H., Jadusingh, I. H., Macinnis, M. L., Shaffer, E.A., and Hershfield, N. B. (1987). The histopathology of rectosigmoid biopsies from adults with bloody diarrhea due to verotoxin-producing *Escherichia coli*. *American Journal of Clinical Pathology*. **88**, 78–82.

Kenny, B. and Finlay, B. B. (1995). Protein secretion by enteropahthogenic *Escherichia coli* is essential for transducing signals to epithelial cells. *Proceedings of the National Academy of Sciences (USA)* **92**, 7991–95.

Kenny, B., Lai, L., Finlay, B. B. and Donnenberg, M. S. (1996). EspA, a protein secreted by enteropathogenic *Escherichia coli* (EPEC) is required to induce signals in epithelial cells. *Molecular Microbiology* **20**, 313–24.

Keusch, G. T., Grady, G. F., Mata, L. J., and McIver, J. (1972). The pathogenesis of *Shigella* diarrhea. 1. Enterotoxin production by *Shigella* dysenteriae 1. *Journal of Clinical Investigation*, **51**, 1212–18.

Kibel, M. A. and Barnard, P. J. (1968). The hemolytic uremic syndrome: a survey in Southern Africa. *South African Medical Journal*, **42**, 692–8.

Knutton, S., Baldwin, T., Williams, P. H., and McNeish, A. S. (1989). Actin accumulation at sites of bacterial adhesion to tissue culture cells: basis of a new diagnostic test for enteropathogenic and enterohemorrhagic *Escherichia coli*. *Infection and Immunity*, **57**, 1290–8.

Konowalchuk, J., Speirs, J. I., and Stavric, S. (1977). Vero response to a cytotoxin of *Escherichia coli*. *Infection and Immunity*, **18**, 775–9.

Koster, F. *et al.* (1977). Hemolytic uremic syndrome after shigellosis. Relation to endotoxemia and circulating immune complexes. *New England Journal of Medicine*, **298**, 927–33.

Law, D. (1994). Adhesion and its role in the virulence of enteropathogenic *Escherichia coli*. *Clinical Microbial Reviews*, **7**, 152–73.

Levine, M. M. (1987). *Escherichia coli* that cause diarrhea: enterotoxigenic, enteropathogenic, entero:invasive, enterohemorrhagic, and enteroadherent. *Journal of Infections Diseases*, **155**, 377–89.

Levine, M. M. *et al.* (1992). Antibodies to Shiga holotoxin and to two synthetic peptides of the B subunit in sera of patients with *Shigella dysenteriae* 1 dysentery. *Journal of Clinical Microbiology*, **30**, 1636–41.

Lindberg, A. A., Brown, J. E., Strömberg, N., Westling-Ryd, M., Schultz, J. E., and Karlsson, K.-A. (1987). Identification of the carbohydrate receptor for Shiga toxin produced by *Shigella dysenteriae* type 1. *Journal of Biological Chemistry*, **262**, 1779–85.

Line, J. E., Fain, A. R. Jr., and Moran, A. B. (1991). Lethality of heat to *Escherichia coli* O157:H7: D-value and Z-value determinations in ground beef. *Journal of Food Protection*, **54**, 762–6.

Lingwood, C. (1994). Verotoxin binding in human renal sections. *Nephron*, **66**, 21–8.

Lingwood, C. A. *et al.* (1987). Glycolipid binding of natural and recombinant *Escherichia coli* produced Verotoxin in-vitro. *Journal of Biological Chemistry*, **262**, 8834–9.

Lior, H. and Borczyk, A. (1987). False-positive identification of *Escherichia coli* O157. *Lancet*, **i**, 333.

Lopez, E. L. *et al.* (1989). Hemolytic uremic syndrome and diarrhea in Argentine children: the role of Shiga-like toxins. *Journal of Infectious Diseases*, **160**, 469–75.

Lopez, E. L. *et al.* (1991). Evidence of infection with organisms producing shiga-like toxins in household contacts of children with hemolytic uremic syndrome. *Pediatric infectious Disease Journal*, **10**, 20–4.

Louie, M. *et al.* (1994). Sequence heterogeneity of the *eae* gene and detection of verotoxin-producing *Escherichia coli* using serotype-specific primers. *Epidemiology and Infection*, **112**, 449–461.

Louise, C. B. and Obrig, T. G. (1991). Shiga toxin-associated hemolytic uremic syndrome: combined cytotoxic effects of shiga toxin, interleukin 1β, and tumor necrosis factor alpha on human vascular endothelial cells *in vitro*. *Infection and Immunity*, **59**, 4173–9.

Ludwig, K., Bitzan, M., Zimmerman, S., Kloth, M., Ruder, H., and Mueller-Wieffel, D. E. (1996). Immune response to non-0157 verotoxin-producing *Escherichia coli* in patients with haemolytic uraemic syndrome. *Journal of Infectious Diseases*, **174**, 1028–39.

MacLeod, D. L. and Gyles, C. L. (1991a). Immunization of pigs with a purified shiga-like toxin II variant toxoid. *Veterinary Microbiology*, **29**, 309–18.

MacLeod, D. L., Gyles, C. L., and Wilcox, B. P. (1991b). Reproduction of edema disease of swine with purified Shiga-like toxin-II variant. *Veterinary Pathology*, **28**, 66–73.

Manjarrez-Hernandez, H. A., Baldwin, T. J., Aitken, A., Knutton, S. and Williams, P. H. (1992). Intestinal epithelial cell protein phosphorylation in enteropathogenic *Escherichia coli* diarrhea. *Lancet*, **339**, 521–23.

March, S. B. and Ratnam, S. (1986). Sorbitol MacConkey medium for detection of *Escherichia coli* O157:H7 associated with hemorrhagic colitis. *Journal of Clinical Microbiology*, **23** 869–72.

Marques, L. R. M., Peiris, J. S. M., Cryz, S. J., and O'Brien, A. D. (1987). *Escherichia coli* strains isolated from pigs with edema disease produce a variant of shiga-like toxin II. *FEMS Microbiology Letters*, **44**, 33–8.

McDaniel, T. K., Jarvis, K. G., Donnenberg, M. S., and Kaper, J. B. (1995). A genetic locus of enterocyte effacement conserved among diverse enteric pathogens. *Proceedings of the National Academy of Sciences (USA)* **92**, 1664–68.

Mobassaleh, M., Donohue-Rolfe, A., Jacewicz, M., Grand, R. J., and Keusch, G. T. (1988). Pathogenesis of shigella diarrhea. Evidence for a developmentally regulated glycolipid receptor for *Shigella* toxin involved in the fluid secretory response of rabbit small intestine. *Journal of Infectious Diseases*, **157**, 1023–31.

Mohammad, A., Peiris, J. S. M., and Wijewanta, E. A. (1986). Serotypes of verocytotoxigenic *Escherichia coli* from cattle and buffalo calf diarrhea. *FEMS Microbiology Letters*, **35**, 261–5.

Montenegro, M. *et al.* (1990). Detection and characterization of fecal verotoxin-producing *Escherichia coli* from healthy cattle. *Journal of Clinical Microbiology*, **28**, 1417–21.

Morgan, D., Newman, C. P., Hutchinson, D. N., Walker, A. M., Rowe, B., and Majid, F. (1993). Verotoxin-producing *Escherichia coli* O157 infections associated with the consumption of yoghurt. *Epidemiology and Infection*, **111**, 181–7.

Morrison, D. M., Tyrell, D. L. J., and Jewell, L. D. (1986). Colonic biopsy in Verotoxin-induced hemorrhagic colitis and thrombotic thrombocytopenic purpura (TTP). *American Journal of Clinical Pathology*, **86**, 108–12.

Moxley, R. A. and Francis, D. H. (1986). Natural and experimental infection with an attaching and effacing strain of *Escherichia coli* in calves. *Infection and Immunity*, **53**, 339–46.

Newland, J. W. and Neill, R. J. (1988). DNA probes for Shiga-like toxins I and II and for toxin-converting bacteriophages. *Journal of Clinical Microbiology*, **26**, 1292–7.

Notenboom, R. H., Borczyk, A., Karmali, M. A., and Duncan, L. M. C. (1987). Clinical relevance of a serological cross-reaction between *Escherichia coli* O157 and *Brucella abortus*. *Lancet*, **ii**, 745.

O'Brien, A. D. and LaVeck, G. D. (1983). Purification an characterization of a *Shigella dysenteriae* 1-like toxin produced by *Escherichia coli*. *Infection and Immunity*, **40**, 675–83.

O'Brien, A. D., Newland, J. W., Miller, S. F., Holmes, R. K., Smith, H. W., and Formal, S. B. (1984). Shiga-like toxin converting phages from *Escherichia coli* strains that cause hemorrhagic colitis or infantile diarrhea. *Science*, **226**, 694–6.

O'Brien, A. D., Karmali, M. A., and Scotland, S. M. (1994). *A proposal for rationalizing the nomenclature of the Escherichia coli cytotoxins.* (Abstract) in the Proceedings from the 2nd International symposium and workshop on Verocytotoxin (Shiga-like toxin)-producing *Escherichia coli* infections, 27–30 June 1994. Bergamo, Italy. Elsevier, Amsterdam.

Obrig, T. G., Moran, T. P., and Brown, J. E. (1987). The mode of action of Shiga toxin on peptide elongation of eukaryotic protein synthesis. *Biochemical Journal*, **244**, 287–94.

Obrig, T. G. *et al.* (1988). Direct cytotoxic action of Shiga toxin on human vascular endothelial cells. *Infection and Immunity*, **56**, 2373–8.

Olsvik, O. *et al.* (1991). A nested PCR followed by magnetic separation of amplified fragments for detection of *Escherichia coli* shiga-like toxin genes. *Molecular and Cellular Probes*, **5**, 429–35.

Pai, C. H., Ahmed, N., Lior, H., Johnson, W. M., Sims, H. V., and Woods, D. E. (1988). Epidemiology of sporadic diarrhea due to verocytotoxin-producing *Escherichia coli*: a two-year prospective study. *Journal of Infectious Diseases*, **157**, 1054–7.

Park, C. H., Vandel, N. M., and Hixon, D. L. (1996). Rapid immunoassay for detection of *Escherichia coli* 0157 directly from stool specimens. *Journal of Clinical Microbiology*, **34**, 988–90.

Paton, A. W., Paton, J. C., Goldwater, P. N., and Manning, P. A. (1993). Direct detection of *Escherichia coli* shiga-like toxin genes in primary fecal cultures by polymerase chain reaction. *Journal of Clinical Microbiology*, **31**, 3063–7.

Pierard, D., Huyghens, L., Lauwers, S., and Lior, H. (1991). Diarrhea associated with *Escherichia coli* producing porcine oedema disease verotoxin. *Lancet*, **ii**, 762.

Pollard, D. R., Johnson, W. M., Lior, H., Tyler, S. D., and Rozee, K. R. (1990). Rapid and specific detection of Verotoxin genes in *Escherichia coli* by the polymerase chain reaction. *Journal of Clinical Microbiology*, **28**, 540–5.

Polotsky, Y. E. *et al.* (1977). Pathogenic effect of enterotoxigenic *Escherichia coli* and *Escherichia coli* causing infantile diarrhoea. *Acta Microbiological Academiae Scientiarum Hungaricae*, **24**, 221–36.

Read, S. C., Gyles, C. L., Clarke, R. C., Lior, H, and McEwen, S. (1990). Prevalence of verocytotoxigenic *Escherichia coli* in ground beef, pork, and chicken in southwestern Ontario. *Epidemiology and Infection*, **105**, 11–20.

Reisbig, R., Olsnes, S., and Eiklid, K. (1981). The cytotoxic activity of *Shigella* toxin. Evidence for catalytic inactivation of the 60S ribosomal subunit. *Journal of Biological Chemistry*, **256**, 8739–44.

Renwick, S. A. *et al.* (1993). Evidence of direct transmission of *Escherichia coli* O157:H7 infection between calves and a human. *Journal of Infectious Diseases*, **168**, 792–3.

Rice, E. W., Sowers, E. G., Johnson, C. H., Dunnigan, M. E., Strockbine, N. A., and Edberg, S. C. (1992). Serological cross-reactions between *Escherichia coli* O157 and other species of the genus *Escherichia*. *Journal of Clinical Microbiology*, **30**, 1315–16.

Richardson, S. E., Karmali, M. A., Becker, L. E., and Smith, C. R. (1988). The Histopathology of the hemolytic uremic syndrome associated with verocytotoxin-producing *Escherichia coli* infections. *Human Pathology*, **19**, 1102–8.

Richardson, S. E. *et al.* (1992). Experimental verocytotoxemia in rabbits. *Infection and Immunity*, **60**, 4154–67.

Riley, L. W. *et al.* (1983). Hemorrhagic colitis associated with a rare *Escherichia coli* serotype. *New England Journal of Medicine*, **308**, 681–5.

Ritchie, M., Partington, S., Jessop, J., and Kelly, M. T. (1992). Comparison of a direct fecal shiga-like toxin assay and sorbitol-MacConkey agriculture for laboratory diagnosis of enterohemorrhagic *Escherichia coli* infection. *Journal of Clinical Microbiology*, **30**, 461–4.

Rowe, P. C., Orrbine, E., Lior, H., Wells, G. A., and McLaine, P. N. (1993). Diarrhoea in close contacts as a risk factor for childhood haemolytic uraemic syndrome. *Epidemiology and infection*, **110**, 9–16.

Samuel, J. E., Perera, L. P., Ward, S., O'Brien, A. D., Ginsburg, V., and Krivan, H. C. (1990). Comparison of the glycolipid receptor specificities of shiga-like toxin type II and shiga-like toxin type II variants. *Infection and Immunity*, **58**, 611–18.

Sandvig, K., Olsnes, S., Brown, J. E., Peterson, O. W., and Deurs, B. v. (1989). Endocytosis from coated pits of Shiga toxin: A glycolipid-binding protein from *Shigella dysenteriae* 1. *Journal of Cell Biology*, **108**, 1331–43.

Sandvig, K., Garred, O., Prydz, K., Kozlov, J. V., Hansen, S. H., and Deurs, B. v. (1992). Retrograde transport of endocytosed Shiga toxin to the endoplasmic reticulum. *Nature*, **358**, 510–12.

Schoonderwoerd, M., Clark, R. C., Dreumel, A. A. v., and Rawluk, S. A. (1988). Colitis in calves: natural and experimental infection with a verotoxin-producing strain of *Escherichia coli* O111:NM. *Canadian Journal of Veterinary Research*, **52**, 484–7.

Sekla, L. (1990). Verotoxin-producing *Escherichia coli* in ground beef in Manitoba. *Canadian Medical Association Journal*, **143**, 519–21.

Seriwatana, J., Brown, J. E., Echeverria, P., Taylor, D. N., Suthienkul, O., and Newland, J. (1988). DNA probes to identify shiga-like toxin I- and II-producing enteric bacterial pathogens isolated from patients with diarrhea in Thailand. *Journal of Clinical Microbiology*, **26**, 1614–15.

Shanks, P. L. (1938). An unusual condition affecting the digestive organs of the pig. *Veterinary Record*, **50**, 356–8.

Sherwood, D., Snodgrass, D. R., and O'Brien, A. D. (1985). Shiga-like toxin production from *Escherichia coli* associated with calf diarrhea. *Veterinary Record*, **116**, 217.

Sheth, K. J., Gill, J. C. and Leichter, H. (1987). High dose immunoglobulin infusions in the hemolytic uremic syndrome. *Kidney International*, **31**, 217 [Abstract].

Siegler, R. L. (1988). Management of the hemolytic uremic syndrome. *Journal of Pediatrics*, **112**, 1014–20.

Smith, H. W., Green, P., and Parsell, Z. (1983). Vero cell toxins in *Escherichia coli* and related bacteria: transfer by phage and conjugation and toxic action in laboratory animals, chickens, and pigs. *Journal of General Microbiology*, **129**, 3121–37.

Staley, T. E., Jones, E. W., and Corley, L. D. (1969). Attachment and penetration of *Escherichia coli* into intestinal epithelium of the ileum in newborn pigs. *American Journal of Pathology*, **56**, 371–92.

Stein, P. E., Boodhoo, A., Tyrell, G. J., Brunton, J. L., and Read, R. J. (1992). Crystal structure of the cell-binding oligomer of verotoxin-1 from *Escherichia coli Nature (Lond.)*. **355**, 748–50.

Suthienkul, O., Brown, J. E., Seriwatana, J., Tienthongdee, S., Sastravaha, S., and Echeverria, P. (1990). Shiga-like-toxin-producing *Escherichia coli* in retail meats and cattle in Thailand. *Applied Environmental Microbiology*, **56**, 1135–9.

Tarr, P. I. and Hickman, R. O. (1987). Hemolytic uremic syndrome epidemiology: a population-based study in King County, Washington, 1971–1980. *Pediatrics*, **80**, 41–5.

Thayer, D. W. and Boyd, G. (1993). Elimination of *Escherichia coli* O157:H7 in meats by gamma irradiation. *Applied Environmental Microbiology*, **59**, 1030–4.

Trompeter, R. S. *et al.* (1983). Haemolytic uraemic syndrome: an analysis of prognostic features. *Archives of Diseases in Childhood*, **58**, 101–5.

Tzipori, S., Chow, C. W., and Powel, H. R. (1988). Cerebral involvement with *Escherichia coli* O157:H7 in humans and gnotobiotic piglets. *Journal of Clinical Pathology*, **41**, 1099–103.

USDA:APHIS:VS Report (1994). Escherichia coli O157:H7 *issues and ramifications*. Centers for Epidemiology and Animal Health, 555 South Howes, Fort Collins, Colorado, 80521, USA.

Wells, J. G. *et al.* (1991). Isolation of *Escherichia coli* serotype O157:H7 and other Shiga-like-toxin-producing *Escherichia coli* from dairy cattle. *Journal of Clinical Microbiology*, **29**, 985–9.

Whittam, T. S., Wachsmuth, I. K., and Wilson, R. A. (1988). Genetic evidence of clonal descent of *Escherichia coli* O157:H7 associated with hemorrhagic colitis and hemolytic uremic syndrome. *Journal of Infectious Diseases*, **157**, 1124–33.

Whittam, T. S. *et al.* (1993). Clonal relationships among *Escherichia coli* strains that cause hemorrhagic colitis and infantile diarrhea. *Infection and Immunity*, **61**, 1619–29.

Willshaw, G. A., Smith, H. R., Scotland, S. M., Field, A. M., and Rowe, B. (1987). Heterogeneity of *Escherichia coli* phages encoding Vero cytotoxins: comparison of cloned sequences determining VT1 and VT2 and development of specific gene probes. *Journal of General Microbiology*, **133**, 1309–17.

Wilson, J. B., McEwen, S. A., Clarke, R. C., Leslie, K. E., Waltner-Toews, D., and Gyles, C. L. (1992). A case control study of selected pathogens including verocytotoxigenic *Escherichia coli* in calf diarrhea on an Ontario veal farm. *Canadian Journal of Veterinary Research*, **56**, 184–8.

Yee, A. J., DeGrandis, S., and Gyles, C. L. (1993). Mitomycin-induced synthesis of a shiga-like toxin from enteropathogenic *Escherichia coli* H.1.8. *Infection and Immunity*, **61**, 4510–13.

Yu, J. and Kaper, J. B. (1992). Cloning and characterization of the *eae* gene of enterohemorrhagic *Escherichia coli* O157:H7. *Molecular Microbiology*, **6**, 411–17.

11 GLANDERS AND MELIOIDOSIS

Sky R. Blue, David J. Pombo, and Marion L. Woods, II

GLANDERS

SUMMARY

Glanders is a zoonotic disease which typically affects members of the soliped family (horses, asses, mules) but may also occasionally affect other animals such as camels and cats. Glanders is caused by *Burkholderia mallei*, which is Gram-negative with a bipolar staining pattern, and non-motile. The organism is probably a facultative intracellular parasite. *Burkholderia mallei* has not been identified in nature outside the animal host although the organism can survive in water for up to 4 weeks. Infection is usually acquired through contact with infected animals. Carnivores can be infected from eating glandered flesh. Historically, humans with horse exposure such as grooms, coachmen, veterinarians, and butchers were at greatest risk of acquiring disease. Glanders in humans is usually acquired from infected animals. Without appropriate antibiotic therapy, local infection typically spreads rapidly to produce septicaemia. Prior to effective antibiotic therapy, clinical disease in humans was usually fatal. With the control of the disease in equines, human glanders has become rare in the western hemisphere.

In solipeds, glanders is usually manifested as a respiratory illness (nasal discharge, cough, and pneumonia). In horses, glanders can be acute or subacute. In mules and asses the disease is usually acute and fatal. Cutaneous glanders was known as farcy and is characterized by subcutaneous abscesses and lymphadenitis. Guinea-pigs and hamsters are extremely susceptible to disease and were used for diagnostic purposes. Diagnosis is based on culture, serology, and mallein skin testing.

Treatment of human infection with sulphadiazine (100 mg/kg/day) in divided doses for 21 days has been effective. Longer courses of therapy may be advisable for an organism which can establish latency in the host. Infected animals are almost always destroyed for control measures.

HISTORY

Glanders is an ancient disease, probably encountered with early domestication of the horse. Today, the prevalence of this disease is waning because of strict animal control measures involving testing and destruction of infected animals. An overview of the history of glanders is presented in Table 11.1. A well documented report of the epidemiological and clinical features of 6 cases of human glanders acquired by laboratory personnel has been written by Howe and Miller (1947).

Table 11.1 Brief history of glanders

Third century BC	Aristotle	The first recorded description of glanders, called 'Melis', was made
1664	Jacques Labessie de Solleysel	The contagious nature of glanders and farcy was recognized
1795	Erik Viborg	Glanders and farcy were proven to be caused by the same 'heat susceptible virus'
1830	John Elliston	The zoonotic nature of glanders in man was suspected
1837	Pierre Francois Olive Rayer	The agent of human glanders was proven to be the same as the equine contagion through sound experimental methods
1882	Loeffler and Schutz	The glander's bacillus was isolated and Koch's postulates fulfilled for glanders
1891	Kalning and Helmane	The mallein test was developed
1894	Britain	The first 'Glanders and Farcy Order' was issued
1920	Britain and US	Glanders is almost completely eradicated

THE AGENT

TAXONOMY (CLASSIFICATION)

Recent work on the taxonomy of the pseudomonads has led to the creation of new genus groupings on the basis of ribosomal RNA homologies. Members of the former *Pseudomonas* homology group II (*P. pseudomallei*, *P. mallei*, *P. cepacia*, *P. gladioli*, *P. picketti*) have been the assigned to the new genus *Burkholderia*. Typical for this genus, *Burkholderia mallei* is an aerobic, or facultatively anaerobic, catalase positive, non-spore forming, Gram-negative rod, but it is the only member of the genus which lacks flagellae, and is non-motile.

MOLECULAR BIOLOGY (MICROBIOLOGY)

The biochemical characteristics of *B. mallei* have been compared with other members of the genus by Redfearn *et al.* (1966). This Gram-negative rod is an aerobic organism, or a facultative anaerobe in the presence of nitrate. All strains of *B. mallei* are able to reduce nitrate to nitrite but few strains can form gas from nitrate. Most strains are oxidase positive. *B. mallei* has limited ability to oxidize sugars as a carbohydrate source; glucose and, in some cases, mannitol can be oxidized. It is able to use a wide variety of organic compounds as its sole carbon source, but with much strain to strain variation.

Microscopically, the organism is pleomorphic but tends to form slender rods, 0.5 μm wide and 2–5 μm long in young cultures, which can appear bipolar or 'safety pin' shaped after staining because of terminal granules. Older cultures contain a variety of shapes, including branched, filamentous, and coccobacillary forms. The longer rods may appear beaded on staining. *Burkholderia mallei* grows in standard blood culture systems, but may grow slowly on solid medium unless glycerol is present. On solid medium young colonies appear shiny and translucent initially, but become mucoid with age. *Burkholderia mallei* do not produce pigment to any significant degree, and are not fluorescent (Millen *et al.* 1948).

DISEASE MECHANISMS

Knowledge of the pathogenic mechanisms of *B. mallei* is rudimentary. In experimental intraperitoneal infection in hamsters, which are extremely susceptible to *B. mallei*, the minimum lethal dose has been shown to vary from as few as 20 to over 5×10^7 organisms, for virulent and avirulent strains, respectively. In hamsters, the more virulent strains produce acute disease, while less virulent strains lead to subacute or chronic disease.

The mechanisms underlying these differences are not known. Production of proteases by *B. mallei* has been reported, but these proteases appear to be relatively weak and it is unclear whether they are the main determinants of virulence. Haemolysin is uniformly absent. The biology of other exotoxins and their role in virulence of *B. mallei* has not been reported.

GROWTH AND SURVIVAL REQUIREMENTS

The specific growth requirements of *B. mallei* in the natural state have not been well defined, in large part because it is a specialized parasitic bacterium which has not been isolated outside of the animal host. In the laboratory the glanders bacillus is relatively sensitive to extremes of heat and drying. It does not grow at 42 °C and is inactivated by direct sunlight or by drying at room temperature. It survives best in moist, dark culture conditions and is viable in tap water for up to 4 weeks, indicating the potential for transmission of disease from contaminated water sources for extended periods of time. Standard blood culture systems work well for primary isolation of the organism but growth on solid medium can be enhanced by glycerol.

HUMAN DISEASE

The clinical manifestations of *B. mallei* infection in human and equine hosts are similar. In man *B. mallei* infections occur as localized cutaneous lesions (similar to farcy), pneumonitis (similar to glanders), sepsis, or a combination of these forms. The primary focus of infection appears to relate to the route of transmission; cutaneous inoculation may lead to localized infection whereas inhalation exposure may lead to pneumonitis. Any primary site of infection may disseminate to become a septicaemic form and bacteraemia may lead to discrete localized infections. Chronic suppurative infection is occasionally seen and is characterized by relapses.

The most common sites of localized infection are the skin and the soft tissues. Primary inoculation occurs during contact with infected animals. Localized erythema, inflammatory nodules, local cellulitis, lymphangitis, regional lymphadenitis, and abscesses may develop at the site of inoculation. The incubation period for localized infection is usually 1–5 days. Systemic symptoms of fever and malaise may be present but tend to be less severe than in the septic form of the disease. Direct inoculation of mucous membranes may result in a focal infection characterized by mucopurulent discharge and ulcerating granulomatous lesions. The chronic suppurative form of glanders is characterized by multiple discrete soft tissue abscesses in which the subcutaneous and intramuscular tissues of the extremities are most often involved.

The incubation period for inhalation-acquired acute pulmonary *B. mallei* infection is approximately 2 weeks. Symptoms of chest infection may include pleuritic chest pain. Physical examination findings in the chest are related to the size of the pneumonic process. More extensive lesions may be associated with signs of consolidation. Chest radiographs characteristically show rounded circumscribed densities similar to early lung abscesses but a typical lobar or bronchopneumonia appearance can also be seen. Positive cultures from blood, sputum, or mucosal discharges will confirm the diagnosis. Serological studies are an important adjunct to diagnosis because the organism may be difficult to isolate from sputum.

Any site of infection may result in systemic dissemination and sepsis. Common symptoms seen in very toxic-appearing patients include fever, severe myalgias, malaise, headache, and pleuritic chest pain. A generalized papular-pustular rash may develop along with lacrimation, diarrhoea, lymphadenitis, and symptoms related to specific visceral involvement. In addition to the lungs and pleura, the eye, liver, spleen, skeletal system, and central nervous system may be involved. Laboratory abnormalities usually relate to the systemic septic state, but can include leucocytosis or leucopenia with a relative lymphocytosis. The acute septic form carries a very high mortality and has been fatal in 7–10 days.

DIAGNOSIS

Burkholderia mallei may be difficult to identify in sputum or body fluids. Blood cultures may be insensitive except in terminal stages. However, irregularly stained Gram-negative organisms in conjunction with a 'Pseudomonas species' on culture should alert clinicians to consider glanders in the appropriate epidemiological setting. Serological tests may be helpful in diagnosis but cannot confirm or exclude infection. Thus, the diagnosis can be substantiated with a significant or sustained rise in the agglutination titre. Complement fixation tests are less sensitive but more specific. Mallein skin tests can be used to determine whether prior infection has occurred, in a manner analogous to tuberculin skin testing.

TREATMENT

Because of the rarity of this disease, the optimum treatment regimen is not known. Experimental models and limited anecdotal human experience suggest that sulphadiazine in a dose of 100 mg/kg/day in divided doses for 21 days is an effective therapy. Since the development of more effective anti-Gram-negative aminoglycosides, cephalosporins, and carbapenems, it may be reasonable to utilize double antibiotic therapy and perform *in vitro* susceptibility studies. An *in vitro* study of antimicrobial sensitivity of *B. mallei* isolates determined that all isolates ($n = 34$) were sensitive to sulphamethizole, sulphathiazole, tetracycline, gentamicin, kanamycin, tobramycin, streptomycin, and a combination of trimethoprim and sulphamethoxazole, whereas none of the isolates were sensitive to cephalothin, colistin, ampicillin, penicillin, and nitrofurantoin (Al-Izzi and Al-Bassam 1989). Ciprofloxacin and ofloxacin were effective in models of glanders in guinea-pigs and hamsters but clinical data in humans are not available. Supportive therapy in the septic form of the disease and surgical drainage in localized infection are important adjuncts to antibiotic therapy.

ANIMAL DISEASE

Burkholderia mallei is most pathogenic for horses, mules, asses, and other members of the soliped family. Horses tend to have acute or chronic disease, whereas, mules and asses tend to have an acute fulminant disease. Camels and felines are also susceptible to acquisition of glanders. Dogs, goats, cattle, and rabbits are more resistant to infection. In Germany during the early part of the twentieth century, large circus carnivores died of glanders which was probably contracted from infected horse meat. Animals which died included polar bears, lions, tigers, leopards, and jackals. Hyenas contracted infection but recovered. Glanders was epizootic among horses on the European continent during First World War; 15 776 infected horses were destroyed in Germany and 20 585 infected horses in France were destroyed. The value of quarantine was evident in Great Britain, which had fewer than 100 cases of glanders during the same time period because of geographic isolation.

EPIDEMIOLOGY

Glanders has followed closely the movement of domesticated animals. Usually an acute infection in mules and asses, glanders can be latent or chronic in horses. Animals with acute infection are easily recognized, whereas chronically or latently infected horses may escape diagnosis and thus serve as reservoirs for the spread of glanders to healthy animals.

Burkholderia mallei can survive in moist environments for an extended period of time and can spread from animal to animal via direct contact with infected secretions or wound discharge. Contaminated fodder, water troughs, or harnesses may be involved in transmission. *Burkholderia mallei* transiently present in the soil or water may account for sporadic cases which have no known contact with infected animals.

Events which bring large numbers of horses together have been responsible for large epizootics. Over 3000 cases of glanders in horses were reported in 1885 in England. The growth of the British empire and the widespread use of horses in military campaigns around the world helped to spread glanders to Egypt, Afghanistan, India, and South Africa. The widespread use of the mallein test and infection control measures in livestock significantly lowered the rates of equine glanders in western Europe and the United States. Glanders does not have any known wild animal reservoir, hence careful control measures in domestic livestock have virtually eradicated this disease in developed countries.

Rates of human glanders parallel rates of glanders in animals. Humans contract glanders primarily from contact with infected animals. Thus, the disease is associated with occupations such as farmers, livestock and animal-processing workers, stable workers, healthcare and laboratory personnel. Transmission from person to person is also a risk, and isolation and infection control procedures should be stringent for hospitalized cases. In the developed world, laboratory exposure has become an important mode of disease acquisition.

Today equine glanders and horse to man transmission are seen only in areas of developing countries including Ethiopia, Senegal, Mauritania, Sudan, Swaziland, Central African Republic, Iraq, Iran, Lebanon, Turkey, Afghanistan, India, Pakistan, Nepal, Myanmar, Indonesia, parts of the former Soviet Union, Mongolia, and China.

PREVENTION AND CONTROL

Historically, control and prevention of glanders has been dependent upon identification and destruction of infected animals. This technique was effective in eliminating glanders in the United States and western Europe. Because no vaccine is available to prevent glanders, it would seem prudent to continue this form of control. Mallein testing (intrapalpebral, ophthalmic, or subcutaneous routes) is an effective method of identifying animals which have latent or active disease. Animals with positive mallein tests are then tested serologically to confirm the results of the mallein test. Because intrapalpebral and ophthalmic tests do not affect subsequent serological tests for glanders, they have replaced subcutaneous testing. Control of glanders in the animal host is the most important

method to reduce the incidence in humans. Appropriate laboratory safety is essential in clinical and research areas which isolate *B. mallei*.

MELIOIDOSIS

SUMMARY

Melioidosis is a tropical disease caused by the facultative intracellular parasite *Burkholderia pseudomallei* (formerly *Pseudomonas pseudomallei*), a motile, Gram-negative rod, which is oxidase positive, and usually cannot ferment lactose. Most cases of melioidosis occur between latitudes 20°N and 20°S during the monsoon or wet seasons. This seasonal occurrence is thought to be related in part to increased numbers of *B. pseudomallei* in the moist soil and increased water runoff.

Illness in humans is usually acute pneumonia. Other clinical presentations include simulated re-activation tuberculosis, genitourinary infection, soft tissue and bone infection, primary bacteraemia parotitis, focal infection of the central nervous system, as well as a distinct neurological syndrome characterized by aseptic meningitis syndrome, brain-stem encephalitis, and motor paralysis. Melioidosis may even simulate myocardial infarction (myocardial abscess). Trauma associated with inoculation with *B. pseudomallei* from soil or water in endemic areas can result in cellulitis and bacteraemia. Aspiration of organisms from water or soil may be responsible for primary pneumonia. Asymptomatic pharyngeal carriage in endemic areas is apparently infrequent and, when present, is likely to be associated with disease. Latency and relapse are important aspects of melioidosis. During the 1970s in the United States, melioidosis was referred to as 'the Vietnamese time bomb' because of its ability to recur or become manifest long after patients left endemic areas. Melioidosis is a significant disease of domestic mammals. Mortality and morbidity associated with animal disease acquisition is high and most animals are destroyed for control.

HISTORY

When Whitmore and Krishnaswami first isolated *B. pseudomallei* in 1912 from a human case they thought it was the glanders bacillus because of glanders-like pathology in the lungs of the patient. However, the lack of a history of equine exposure, coupled with the isolation of a motile organism with wrinkled colonial morphology, led these investigators to describe a new

Table 11.2   Brief history of melioidosis

1912	Whitmore and Krishnaswami discover a 'glanders-like' illness in Rangoon
1913	Whitmore publishes the pathological description of 38 cases of this 'glanders-like' disease
1913	Fletcher studied an outbreak of septicaemic disease in laboratory animals that turned out to have an aetiological agent similar to the 'Whitmore Bacillus'
1960's	The latent nature of melioidosis is recognized
1962	Seroprevalence surveys reveal the extent of endemicity and suggest that the majority of infections are subclinical
1989	Ceftazidime therapy is found to decrease mortality by 50%

organism and syndrome. In 1913, Whitmore detailed the microbiology of melioidosis, including an early animal model, and human pathology of this disease in 38 patients, most of whom were morphine addicts. Acute melioidosis was almost uniformly fatal prior to antibiotic therapy. Later, melioidosis was recognized in soldiers who were stationed in endemic areas in the Pacific during the Second World War and during the Vietnam War (Brundage *et al.* 1968). Reactivation of melioidosis following a prolonged latent period was observed as another manifestation of *B. pseudomallei* infection in returned soldiers from the Vietnam War. Seroprevalence surveys in endemic areas suggest that infection with *B. pseudomallei* is common but that most infections remain asymptomatic. (Leelarasamee and Bovornkitti 1989). Melioidosis has been recognized as a serious disease among domestic animals in endemic areas. An overview of the history of melioidosis is presented in Table 11.2.

THE AGENT

TAXONOMY

Recent work on the taxonomy of the pseudomonads has led to creation of new genus groupings on the basis of ribosomal RNA homologies (Gilligan 1995). Members of the former *Pseudomonas* homology group II (*P. pseudomallei, P. mallei, P. cepacia, P. gladioli, P. picketti*) have been the assigned to the new genus *Burkholderia*. *Burkholderia pseudomallei* and *B. mallei* are closely related on the basis of comparative DNA hybridization, high guanine–cytosine content, specificity of phage lysis, and cross-reactivity on a variety of serological assays.

MORPHOLOGY

Burkholderia pseudomallei is an aerobic, Gram-negative rod, which is catalase positive, oxidase positive, and

which can oxidize a wider range of sugars than *B. mallei* (Gilligan 1995) *Burkholderia pseudomallei* can rapidly hydrolyse gelatin, produce haemolysis, produce gas from nitrate, and grow well at 42 °C. Another major distinction is the presence of 1–4 terminal flagella.

The appearance of colonies on solid media can vary greatly. The colour is usually white or cream and opaque, but often can be orange or yellow. Colony morphology is smooth on new cultures but becomes characteristically rough and wrinkled after a few days. Wrinkling occurs more quickly on glycerol-containing agar. Similar wrinkling morphology occurs on pellicles which form on the surface of broth cultures.

DISEASE MECHANISMS

The potential virulence mechanisms of *B. pseudomallei* were recently reviewed by Kanai and Kondo (1994). One virulence factor, the lipopolysaccharide (LPS) from *B. pseudomallei* was found to be as potent as the LPS from *Salmonella abortus equi* in lethal toxicity and tumour necrosis factor (TNF) inducing capacity in mice. However, the LPS from *B. pseudomallei* was only 3 per cent as potent as LPS from *Pseudomonas aeruginosa*, in inducing cachexia in mice, a surrogate marker of TNF production.

Burkholderia pseudomallei produces exotoxins which may also contribute to the characteristic toxic presentation of acute melioidosis. The separable effects of a lethal, heat stable toxin and a dermonecrotic, heat labile protease have been demonstrated, and a 31 kDa exotoxin which was lethal for mice, with a LD_{50} of 30 μg has been purified. Other potential virulence determinants identified by Ashdown *et al.* (1979) include a protease, lipase, and lecithinase. This protease appears to both significantly enhance the ability of *B. pseudomallei* to infiltrate the lung in a rat model of pneumonia and to cleave immunoglobulins. Bacterial siderophore production, which is necessary to acquire iron in growth-limiting conditions, may also contribute to the virulence of this organism.

An additional factor which contributes to the virulence of *B. pseudomallei* is the ability to survive in phagocytic cells. *In vitro* studies demonstrate that *B. pseudomallei* can persist in rabbit macrophages and can multiply in human polymorphonuclear cells and in macrophages. These growth characteristics enable this facultative intracellular bacterial parasite to establish latency in the host.

GROWTH AND SURVIVAL REQUIREMENTS

Burkholderia pseudomallei is found in the soil and water between the latitudes 20°N and 20°S where melioidosis is endemic. Most clinical cases occur during the wet season when the organism can be more readily cultured from the environment. However, within endemic zones, the geographic distribution of melioidosis is not uniform. There are distinct 'hot spots' where melioidosis in humans and animals is known to occur with a higher frequency. Perhaps not surprisingly, *B. pseudomallei* is not uniformly distributed in the soil within a 'hot spot'. An illustration of this phenomenon was demonstrated by the investigation of a recurring annual cluster of cases of melioidosis which predictably occurred in sheep within a particular 3.3 hectare paddock located at the Oonooba Veterinary Laboratory, Townsville, Australia (Thomas *et al.* 1979). In order to determine whether soil or water harboured this pathogen, a total of 760 samples (730 soil, 30 water) from 23 different sites were cultured during an 18-month period. *Burkholderia pseudomallei* was recovered on 12 occasions from four sites located in the rhizosphere (root zone) of two trees, at a depth of 25–45 cm, in clay-containing soil. It was not isolated from seven sites which were always under water during the wet season. Isolates were only recovered during the wet season, and on 9 of the 12 occasions, isolation of the organism occurred during months when rainfall was greater than 37 mm (average, 160 mm).

One hypothesis which could explain this uneven distribution of *B. pseudomallei* in soil samples from endemic areas is that soil protozoans, such as free living amoebae, may modulate soil populations of *B. pseudomallei*. Free-living amoebae appear to be the major determinants of soil bacteria populations and may be involved in the natural life cycle of *B. pseudomallei* as they are involved in the Legionella life cycle. The distribution of *B. pseudomallei* isolates in this paddock was consistent with the expected distribution of free-living amoebae which are known to be present in particularly high numbers (10^5 amoebae/g of soil) in the rhizosphere of trees and other plants (Rodriguez-Zaragora 1994). It is conceivable that *Bulkholderia pseudomallei* a facultative intracellular bacterial parasite could live within amoebae as do *Legionella* species. We have recently isolated free living amoebae from the original soil samples collected by Dr. Thomas and are investigating this hypothesis (Woods, unpublished).

HUMAN DISEASE

High seroprevalence of antibodies to *B. pseudomallei* in melioidosis endemic areas, suggests that the majority of *B. pseudomallei* infections are asymptomatic or subclinical (Dance 1991). The primary risk factor for acquisition of infection with *B. pseudomallei* is appropriate environmental exposure. Latent infection with

B. pseudomallei is attributed to the ability of the organism to survive in phagocytes without destruction as a facultative intracellular parasite, in a fashion analogous to mycobacterial infections (Pruksachartvuthi *et al.* 1990).

Acute pulmonary melioidosis is characterized by prostration and marked toxicity. Subacute melioidosis can simulate reactivation tuberculosis. Primary bacteraemia is a common form of melioidosis in Thailand (Chaowagul *et al.* 1989). Melioidosis may even simulate myocardial infarction (myocardial abscess) or result in sudden death. Focal melioidosis can be manifested as genitourinary infections, soft tissue and bone infections, parotitis, or focal infection of the central nervous system. A neurological syndrome which may be exotoxin mediated and characterized by aseptic meningitis syndrome, brain-stem encephalitis, and motor paralysis was recognized in northern Australia (Woods *et al.* 1992). The portal of entry of this organism appears to be via the respiratory tract and breaks in integument.

Pulmonary infection is the most common clinical manifestation of *B. pseudomallei* infection (Everett and Nelson 1975). Infection may occur through direct inhalation or through haematogenous dissemination from another site. The typical acute pulmonary presentation is pneumonia with high fever, toxicity often out of proportion with the physical findings, or pulmonary involvement seen in chest radiographs. Hepatomegaly or palpable spleen may be present with disseminated disease. In Whitmore's autopsy series (1913), pneumonia with characteristic caseous consolidation was present in 34 of 38 patients and splenic involvement was present in 25 of 38 patients. Pneumonitis associated with haematogenous dissemination generally results in scattered nodular densities resembling early lung abscesses. The chest radiographs usually demonstrate consolidation early but subsequent cavitation may occur. Upper lobe cavitary disease in subacute infection can mimic the appearance of tuberculosis. Laboratory abnormalities are often non-specific, including leucocytosis, anaemia, and an elevated C-reactive protein concentration (>5 mg/dl). The differential diagnosis of acute pulmonary melioidosis includes *Staphlococcus aureus* pneumonia or bacteraemic pneumococcal pneumonia.

Focal disease may occur following trauma in which inoculation of the wound with *B. pseudomallei* occurs, e.g. bone, skin, muscle. The histological appearance of acute localized infection is abscess formation, whereas chronic disease produces granulomata. Septic arthritis, which can involve the large joints such as the elbows, knees, and ankles, may represent primary inoculation or dissemination from another primary site. Following bacteraemic dissemination, abdominal abscesses may be found in the liver and spleen. Reactivation of latent infection in the reticuloendothelial system may produce liver and spleen abscesses as well. Rupture of intra-abdominal abscesses, especially those in the hepatobiliary tree, may result in peritonitis with ascites. Urinary tract disease, including cystitis, pyelonephritis, and prostatitis, has been recognized. The epidemiology of prostatic infection is not clear, but this form of the disease could be sexually transmitted. Other focal organ involvement includes isolated pericarditis, ocular infections, and parotitis.

Focal infection of the central nervous system in melioidosis is infrequent but can present as brain abscess and meningitis. A separate neurological syndrome characterized by aseptic meningitis syndrome, brain-stem encephalitis with cranial nerve palsies, and motor paralysis mimicking Guillain–Barré syndrome occurring in the absence of demonstrable nervous system infection has been described. This syndrome may be exotoxin induced.

Acute septicaemic infections are usually remarkable for the dramatic manner in which they present. High fever, tachypnoea, myalgias, hepatosplenomegaly, and septic shock are common manifestations. Disorientation, headache, pharyngitis, diarrhoea, and pustular rash can also be seen. Signs and symptoms related to localized manifestations may predominate in some cases, e.g. pneumonitis or meningitis. Acute septic melioidosis is usually rapidly progressive with mortality approaching 90 per cent. The effect of HIV seroprevalence on expression of clinical melioidosis is unfolding. Just as pneumococcal bacteraemia rates are known to reflect HIV prevalence in a community, one may predict a similar trend for *B. pseudomallei* bacteraemia in communities with high seroprevalence of both HIV and *B. pseudomallei* infection. Primary bacteraemic melioidosis could be mistaken for malaria before culture results or malaria smears are available.

Melioidosis may be responsible for fever of unknown origin in endemic areas and in returning travellers from those areas. Melioidosis should be considered in the differential diagnosis of any febrile illness in individuals who resided in endemic areas during the monsoon season. History of potential exposure (including trauma) coupled with serology and appropriate cultures may help make the diagnosis, especially in patients who have risk factors for disease acquisition. Negative serology does not rule out the diagnosis.

LATENCY

During the 1970s in the United States melioidosis was referred to as 'the Vietnamese time bomb' because of its ability to recur or become manifest long after patients left endemic areas, a characteristic feature of

facultative intracellular parasites. Risk factors for clinical expression of melioidosis in humans include diabetes mellitus, alcohol use, other conditions in which the immune system is suppressed (AIDS, corticosteroid use, leprosy). Latency occurs because of the ability of the organism to survive in phagocytic cells, probably in the reticuloendothelial–endothelial system.

DIAGNOSIS

Diagnosis rests on isolation of *B. pseudomallei* from sites of disease (Gilligan 1995). Isolation of *B. pseudomallei* from sterile body sites is usually not difficult. However, the selective use of culture tubes containing saponin, which lyses phagocytes, may have a theoretical advantage for recovery of this facultative intracellular parasite. On solid medium, growth is enhanced by the addition of glycerol. Selective medium, such as Ashdown medium which contains crystal violet and gentamicin, is more sensitive than MacConkey's agar for the primary isolation of the organism from specimens containing mixed flora (sputum, draining wounds, abscesses).

Burkholderia pseudomallei is a small, Gram-negative bacillus which is motile in fresh culture and oxidase positive. It is aerobic, does not form spores, and exhibits bipolar staining. Colonies turn from smooth to a characteristic wrinkled appearance after a few days' incubation. Wrinkling occurs more quickly on glycerol-containing agar. Positive identification can be made by a battery of standard biochemical tests and agglutination with specific antiserum.

Serological tests include indirect haemagglutination antibody tests, complement fixation titration, indirect immunofluorescence, and enzyme-linked immunosorbent assay (ELISA). Positive results can help confirm the diagnosis, but negative results do not rule out the infection. Indirect haemagglutination antibody test is the most frequently used. More sensitive diagnostic methods are being developed to identify *B. pseudomallei*, including nucleic acid probes and polymerase chain reaction tests (PCR). Assays to detect *B. pseudomallei* antigens directly offer the possibility of rapid diagnostic efficacy.

TREATMENT

The choice of antimicrobial treatment and the route of administration will vary with the severity and form of the disease. Severe or septic melioidosis warrants aggressive intravenous treatment with two antimicrobial agents, based on susceptibility studies. The introduction of ceftazidime (6 g/day) has led to a 50 per cent reduction in the mortality of this disease, and this antibiotic can be used in conjunction with trimethoprim–

sulphamethoxazole (8–10 mg/kg/day of trimetho-prim) (White *et al.* 1989). These patients may require intensive care. The organism is consistently gentamicin resistant (Dance *et al.* 1989).

Trimethoprim–sulphamethoxazole (Tm/smx) has been the mainstay of treatment and is still used in combination regimens, but resistance is known to develop during treatment and may be present initially in a percentage of isolates from Thailand. After initial treatment with intravenous antimicrobials, a prolonged course of oral antibiotic is indicated. Total duration of therapy varies according to severity of infection and can be up to 12 months, the usual duration being 3–6 months. *In vitro* time-kill susceptibility studies suggest that newer carbapenems or semisynthetic penicillin-β-lactamase inhibitor combinations may be of use in future trials of acute disease treatment.

Less severe forms of the disease can be treated with oral antimicrobial agents. Trimethoprim–sulphamethoxazole is commonly chosen, but doxycycline or chloramphenicol are alternative choices. Antimicrobial antagonism has been observed between chloramphenicol, doxycycline, and trimethoprim–sulphamethoxazole during routine disc susceptibility testing. Antibiotic treatment is usually not given to patients with low positive serologies without other firm evidence of infection.

The overall relapse rate after treatment is reported to be about 15 per cent per year, but the rate varies with the form of the original infection (Sanford 1995). Patients with localized disease have a 10 per cent rate of relapse by the first year, compared to 38 per cent in patients with the disseminated septic form. The median time to relapse was 6 months after treatment. Other factors associated with relapse are renal failure, non-ceftazidime-containing regimens, less than 8 weeks of oral treatment, increased severity of original infection, and prior bacteraemia. Relapses may occur at the site of original disease or elsewhere and are treated according to the antimicrobial sensitivity of the isolate.

ANIMAL DISEASE

In contrast to glanders, an animal reservoir has not been identified. We have recognized melioidosis occurring in a patient following attack by an estuarine crocodile in a freshwater billabong. However, subsequent attempts to isolate *B. pseudomallei* from the teeth, oropharynx, and ventral slits of 20 yearling estuarine crocodiles (40 cultures) from a tidal river were unsuccessful (unpublished). We postulated that the crocodile bite provided the portal of entry for *B. pseudomallei* present in the local environment. A single case of

melioidosis attributed to a dog bite has been described.

Also in contrast to glanders, the susceptibility of horses and other equines to melioidosis is relatively low. In addition to equines, monkeys, sheep, goats, pigs, and even cetaceans can acquire melioidosis. Mice and rats are relatively resistant to infection and disease, whereas hamsters and guinea-pigs are very susceptible. Development of melioidosis in animals is determined by the innate immunity of the species and by the strain virulence. Dannenburg and Scott (1958*a,b*) reported on experimental respiratory infection of mice and hamsters by virulent and avirulent strains. Inhalation of large numbers of virulent organisms causes rapid development of caseous abscesses in the lung, and necrotic foci in spleen and liver. Hamsters were more susceptible than mice, but by 5 and 10 days, respectively, both species inevitably died. However, with lower doses (<6 LD_{50}) of virulent *B. pseudomallei*, mice developed chronic infections, whereas hamsters developed uniformly fatal disease. Experimental intraperitoneal inoculation of *B. pseudomallei* and *B. mallei* in male guinea-pigs produces the Strauss reaction, a swelling of the scrotum secondary to periorchitis.

EPIDEMIOLOGY

Risk factors for infection with *B. pseudomallei* are primarily related to outdoor exposure (occupations which involve working in soil or water) during the wet season, in an endemic area for melioidosis. Factors which place patients at increased risk of developing melioidosis following infection with *B. pseudomallei* include conditions which are immunosuppressive, such as AIDS and probably HIV infection, leprosy, corticosteroid use, diabetes mellitus, and alcoholism. Person to person and animal to person transmission may occur, but these modes of transmission are rare.

The majority of patients infected with *B. pseudomallei* appear to remain asymptomatic and probably harbour latent infection, analogous to infection with *Mycobacterium tuberculosis*. Serological surveys in areas of South-East Asia and Northern Australia indicate that as many as 40 per cent of indigenous people in discrete rural areas have evidence of prior infection with *B. pseudomallei* (Chaowaful *et al.* 1989, Currie *et al.* 1993).

Although the usual direction of transmission is from environment to animal (or man), environmental contamination of soil in non-endemic regions can occur from infected animals. In France during the 1970s, investigators were able to isolate *B. pseudomallei* from soil for years after an extensive epizootic. Disease transmission from animal to man almost certainly occurs, as does man to man transmission, but it is only a minor contribution to human disease. Isolation of infected patients may be prudent but has not been shown to be necessary.

Melioidosis is endemic through tropical areas of the world but appears to be concentrated in South-East Asia and northern Australia. Sporadic cases may occur outside those areas. Reactivation of latent infection stemming from travel in endemic areas may account for some of the sporadic reports.

PREVENTION AND CONTROL

Acquisition of infection usually occurs following contact with soil or water in endemic areas during the wet season when *B. pseudomallei* numbers increase and can be isolated from environmental sources. Disease prevention depends on avoidance of contact with soil or water, especially during the wet season, in melioidosis endemic areas, particularly for patients with risk factors for disease expression. If wounds occur in this setting, prompt wound cleansing should be undertaken.

REFERENCES

GLANDERS

Al-Izzi, S. A. and Al-Bassam, L. S. (1989). *In vitro* susceptibility of *Pseudomonas mallei* to antimicrobial agents. *Comparative Immunology, Microbiology and Infectious Diseases*, **12**, 5–8.

Howe, M. and Miller, W. (1947). Human glanders: report of six cases. *Annals of Internal Medicine*, **26**, 93–115.

Miller, W. *et al.* (1948). Studies on certain biological characteristics of *Malleomyces mallei* and *Malleomyces pseudomallei*. I. Morphology, cultivation, viability and isolation from contaminated specimens. *Journal of Bacteriology*, **55**, 115–26.

Redfearn, M. S., Pallerni, N. J., and Stanier, R. Y. (1966). A comparative study of *Pseudomonas pseudomallei* and *Bacillus mallei Journal of General Microbiology*, **43**, 293–313.

MELIOIDOSIS

Ashdown, L. (1979). An improved screening technique for isolation of *Pseudomonas pseudomallei* from clinical specimens. *Pathology*, **11**, 293–7.

Brundage, W. *et al.* (1968). Four fatal cases of melioidosis in U. S. soldiers in Vietnam: bacteriologic and pathologic characteristics. *American Journal of Tropical Medicine and Hygiene*, **17**, 183–91.

Chaowagul, W. *et al.* (1989). Melioidosis: a major cause of community-acquired septicemia in northeastern Thailand. *Journal of Infectious Diseases*, **159**, 890–9.

Currie, B. *et al.* (1993). The 1990–1991 outbreak of melioidosis in the Northern Territory of Australia: clinical aspects. *Southeast Asian Journal of Tropical Medicine and Public Health*, **24**, 436–43.

Dance, D. A. (1991). Melioidosis: the tip of the iceberg? *Clinical Microbiological Reviews*, **4**, 52–60.

Dance, D. A. *et al.* (1989). The antimicrobial susceptibility of *Pseudomonas pseudomallei*. Emergence of resistance *in vitro* and during treatment. *Journal of Antimicrobial Chemotherapy*, **24**, 295–309.

Dannenberg, A. and Scott, E. (1958*a*). Melioidosis; pathogenesis and immunity in mice and hamsters. I. Studies with virulent strains of *Malleomyces pseudomallei*. *Journal of Experimental Medicine*, **107**, 153–6.

Dannenberg, A. and Scott, E. (1958*b*). Melioidosis: pathogenesis and immunity in mice and hamsters. II. Studies with avirulent strains of *Malleomyces pseudomallei*. *American Journal of Pathology*, **34**, 1099–119.

Everett, E. and Nelson, R. (1975). Pulmonary melioidosis: observations in thirty-nine cases. *American Review of Respiratory Disease*, **112**, 331–40.

Gilligan, P. (1995). *Pseudomonas* and *Burkholderia*. In *Manual of clinical microbiology*, pp. 509–19. ASM Press, Washington DC.

Kanai, K. and Kondo, E. (1994). Recent advances in biomedical sciences of *Burkholderia pseudomallei* (basonym: *Pseudomonas pseudomallei*). *Japanese Journal of Medical Science and Biology*, **47**, 1–45.

Leelarasamee, A. and Bovornkitti, S. (1989). Melioidosis: review and update. *Reviews of the Infectious Diseases*, **11**, 413–25.

Pruksachartvuthi, S. *et al.* (1990). Survival of *Pseudomonas pseudomallei* in human phagocytes. *Journal of Medical Microbiology*, **31**, 109–14.

Rodriguez-Zaragoza, S. (1994). Ecology of free-living amoebae. *Critical Reviews in Microbiology*, **20**, 225–41.

Sanford, J. (1995). *Pseudomonas* species (including melioidosis and glanders). *In Principles and practice of infectious disease*, (4th edn) (ed. G. Mandell, J. Bennett, and R. Dolin), pp. 2003–9. Churchill Livingstone, New York.

Thomas, A. *et al.* (1979). Isolation of *Pseudomonas pseudomallei* from clay layers at defined depths. *American Journal of Epidemiology*, **110**, 515–21.

White, N. J. *et al.* (1989). Halving of mortality of severe melioidosis by ceftazidime. *Lancet*, **2**, 697–701.

Whitmore, A. (1913). An account of a glanders-like disease occurring in Rangoon. *Journal of Hygiene*, **13**, 1–34.

Woods, M. L. *et al.* (1992). Neurologic melioidosis: seven cases from the Northern Territory of Australia. *Clinical Infectious Diseases*, **15**, 163–9.

12 LEPTOSPIROSIS

W. A. Ellis

SUMMARY

Leptospirosis is a zoonotic disease caused by members of the genus *Leptospira*. The pathogenic leptospires are morphologically identical: they are thin, helical, motile, Gram-negative bacteria, which are often hooked at one or both ends.

Members of the genus cause major economic loss to the intensive cattle and pig industries of the developed world through their effect on reproductive performance. They also constitute an important occupational disease risk for those who work in those industries. They are important human pathogens in developing countries where poor work and living conditions maximize the opportunity for transmission from animals to man.

Leptospires persist in the kidneys and genital tracts of carrier animals and are excreted in urine and genital fluids. Survival outwith the host is favoured by warm, moist conditions. Transmission is by direct or indirect contact with a carrier animal.

Interruption of transmission from animal to man is the critical factor in the control of human leptospirosis.

HISTORY

Adolf Weil (1886) is usually attributed with the first descriptions of clinical leptospirosis and the disease is often referred to as Weil's disease. However in a comprehensive review of the literature, Faine (1994) documents much earlier descriptions. These include descriptions by Willman in 1803 of what was probably leptospirosis while working with the British Medical Mission with the Grand Visier's Army in Syria; an outbreak of 'fièvre jaune' among Napoleon's troops at Heliopolis in 1800, during the siege of Cairo; and of a similar disease in Egypt in 1851.

In nineteenth-century epidemics of jaundice, the relationships of troops, bathing, water, sewage, rats, occupations, and seasons of outbreaks of disease were noted, but a specific cause was not discovered. However, as bacteriology expanded as a discipline at the end of the nineteenth century and the first decade of the twentieth century there were a number of unsubstantiated claims which attributed the cause of Weil's disease to various bacteria.

The first demonstration of a spirochaete in a patient was recorded in 1907 when Stimson demonstrated spiral organisms with hooked ends, in kidney tissue of a fatality. The patient either died from Weil's disease, or was convalescing from Weil's disease when he contracted yellow fever and died (Faine 1994). Living leptospires were first seen in pond water examined by dark-field microscopy a few years later and reported in 1914 by Wolbach and Binger.

In 1914–15, in Japan, where Weil's disease was common among coal miners, Inada and his colleagues succeeded in transmitting the infection to guinea-pigs, from the blood of which they isolated the responsible organism; they also demonstrated that specific antiserum could confer passive protection. Independently in Europe, German workers, Hubener and Reiter, and Uhlenhuth and Fromme, transmitted the disease to guinea-pigs and demonstrated the spirochaete.

Soon after their discovery of leptospires as the cause of Weil's disease, the Japanese workers described the role of rats as carriers. This in turn opened the way for an appreciation of transmission by carrier animals and possible control methods.

Rapid progress was made in the decade following the First World War, with, for example, the recognition of further disease entities with a leptospiral origin, in particular anicturic forms; agglutination–lysis, active immunization; the serological differentiation of strains and the recognition of their association with different types of the disease (reviewed by Faine 1994).

The recognition of leptospirosis as a disease in dogs quickly followed (in 1916) its diagnosis in man. Subsequently the disease was recognized in cattle in 1935 and in pigs in 1939.

The disease in man was recognized to be of greatest importance in people living or working in warm, moist environments, where poor sanitation was prevalent, and as a consequence many of the early investigations were carried out in South-East Asia. In more temperate climates, investigations concentrated on disease associated with work in wet, rodent-infested environments, e.g. fish processing, coal mining. Associated epidemiological studies concentrated on identifying wildlife reservoirs of infection. Apart from the early recognition of the dog as a major reservoir of *canicola* infection, the recognition of domestic animals as the maintenance hosts for economically important strains of *Leptospira* did not come until much later. Pomona infection of pigs was recognized as a major cause of economic loss in pigs in most pig-producing regions—apart from the most westerly parts of Europe, including the British Isles—during the 1950s and 1960s. The cattle-maintained serovar *hardjo* was not isolated until 1960.

Developments in isolation media and improvements in immunofluorescence technology in the 1960s and early 1970s allowed further progress in the understanding of leptospirosis in domestic animals, while the movement at this time to intensive production systems provided the environmental conditions for leptospirosis to have a much greater impact on the economics of domestic food animal production. The latter half of the 1970s and the early 1980s saw major developments in the appreciation of the clinical impact, and epidemiology of *hardjo* infection in cattle, and control measures were elucidated. With this awareness of *hardjo* as a cattle pathogen of global importance came an appreciation of it as an occupational disease of those employed in the cattle industry.

The 1980s and early 1990s saw the recognition of the domestic pig as a maintenance host for *bratislava* infection. In the same time period an appreciation of the susceptibility of the horse to a spectrum of incidental leptospiral infection became apparent. The possibility of the horse being an alternative maintenance host for *bratislava* infection in many parts of the world also emerged.

For most of the recorded history of leptospirosis it was believed that long-term renal carriage was the major site of persistence in the carrier host and that consequent urinary excretion was seen as the major way in which leptospirosis could be transmitted. The 1980s saw the recognition of the male and female genital tracts as important sites of persistence in the carrier animals (cattle, pig, and dog) and reproductive disease as an the important facit of animal leptospirosis. In China, fetal disease has also been recognized as an important feature of human leptospirosis. The advent of various DNA technologies in the late 1980s and early 1990s has allowed genetic fingerprinting techniques to be applied to the typing of leptospires, allowing improvements in epidemiology and surveillance techniques.

While in the developed countries the poor environmental conditions where leptospirosis thrived have largely been removed from the workplace, the improvements in standards of living and associated increased leisure time has seen people using wet environments as a place to pursue recreation and there has been the emergence of leptospirosis as a risk associated with such activities as angling, canoeing, and raft racing. The increased opportunities for travel have also seen leptospirosis emerge as a problem for travellers to warm, wet climates, in particular to South-East Asia.

THE AGENT

Leptospires are thin, helical, motile, Gram-negative organisms, which are often hooked at one or both ends. In a suitable liquid environment, they spin constantly on their long axis. They range in length from about 10 to 20 μm, with an amplitude of approximately 0.1–0.15 μm and a wavelength of about 0.5 μm. Under adverse nutritional conditions, leptospires may be greatly elongated, while under conditions such as high salt concentrations, ageing culture, or in tissues, leptospires may form coccoid forms of about 1.5–2 μm (Faine 1994). They divide by binary fission.

The major structural components are: an outer envelope which surrounds a cell wall or peptidoglycan complex, and two polar endoflagella (one originating subterminally at each end)

TAXONOMY

The taxonomy of the leptospires is in a period of change, which can cause considerable confusion to those not intimately acquainted with the subject. Until recently a single genus *Leptospira* was recognized in the family Leptospiraceae. Two groupings were recognized within the genus—those which are found in animal species (the parasitic strains) and in water (the saprophytic strains). These two groupings, which were referred to as the *interrogans* and *biflixa* complexes, can be differentiated by their growth requirements and biochemical reactions. Only the parasitic strains are of medical and veterinary interest. For taxonomic purposes and as an aid to epidemiological studies the parasitic leptospires were divided into serogroups on the basis of antigenic relationships as determined by cross-agglutination reactions, and further subdivided into serovars by agglutination–absorption patterns. There are some 23 serogroups recognized, containing approximately 212 serovars.

The advent of genetic typing methods has provided rapid reproducible typing protocols. The current recommendations on the taxonomy of leptospires (Ellis 1995) recognized eight species of pathogenic leptospires within the family Leptospiraceae; these are *Leptospira interrogans*, *L. borgpetersenii*, *L. inadai*, *L. kirschneri*, *L. noguchii*, *L. meyer*, *L. weillii*, and *L. santarosai*.

The species definition is based on a level of DNA–DNA homology of at least 70 per cent and up to 5 per cent divergence in DNA relatedness. Taxonomy at the subspecific level continues to be based on serovars as defined by serotyping, but other valid methods which give comparable results to conventional serotyping can be used for their identification. Such methods include monoclonal antibody agglutination profiles, factor analysis, and analyses in which restriction fragment length polymorphisms or rRNA gene restriction patterns are used in pulsed field gel electrophoresis analyses. The term type is used to indicate strain differences at the subserovar level (Ellis 1995).

MOLECULAR BIOLOGY

The genus *Leptospira* is characterized by a guanine plus cytosine (G + C) ratio of 35–41 mol% in its chromosomal DNA, depending on species. The published genome size has varied between 3100 kb and 5000 kb, depending on the techniques used to measure it and reflecting differences between strains. The *Leptospira interrogans* serovars *icterohaemorrhagiae* and *pomona* have two circular chromosomes: the large (4400–4600 kb) and the small (350 kb) replicons are regarded as chromosomal because the essential *asd* gene is located on the smaller unit.

Leptospira interrogans strains contain two 23S and 16S rRNA genes, but only one 5S rRNA gene. The 5S rRNA gene is highly conserved among the pathogenic leptospires.

GROWTH REQUIREMENTS

Under laboratory conditions, the temperature range within which pathogens will grow varies, but they will not grow below 13 °C; optimum growth occurs at 28–30 °C, while some strains, particularly recent isolates, will grow at 37 °C. Heat-shock proteins are produced. Optimum growth occurs in the pH range 7.2–7.6. They are chemo-organotrophs, growing in aerobic or microaerophilic environments. For the initial isolation of some of the more fastidious strains, oxygen protective agents, such as superoxide dismutase and/or sodium pyruvate, are required. Reduced oxygen concentration aids primary isolation and growth on solid media.

The only major carbon and energy sources used by pathogenic leptospires are long-chain fatty acids. Sugars are not fermented and cannot be used as carbon sources. The essential fatty acids for nutrition and energy metabolism are also toxic so they are normally provided as polyoxyethylene sorbitan esters. In addition, bovine serum albumin is usually included as a detoxifier. Glycerol enhances the growth of some leptospires.

Ammonia is an essential nutrient, being the only recognized nitrogen source for leptospires. It may be supplied in the form of ammonium salts or by the deamination of the amino acid, asparagine, by asparaginase present in serum. Vitamins B_{12} and B_1 are required, as are phosphate, magnesium, and iron.

SURVIVAL REQUIREMENTS

Leptospires survive in water and culture media for long periods of time, but they do not survive desiccation. With the exception of Fe, most heavy metals are lethal. Very low temperatures are tolerated in a protein-containing environment: cryopreservation at −70 °C to −140 °C is used for the long-term storage of leptospire cultures. They are sensitive to acid, at a pH of 6.8 or lower, but they survive alkaline conditions of up to pH 7.8–7.9. They are very susceptible to agents which remove or damage the outer envelope, for example detergents and soaps.

Various combinations of the above factors operate together in natural environments. Leptospires can survive in soils, mud, swamps, watercourses, and the tissues of live or dead animals. Survival outwith an animal depends mainly on moisture and acidity. Serovar *pomona* has been recovered from soil with a pH 6.7–7.2 for up to 74 days. Faine (1994) has suggested that pathogenic leptospires may grow and multiply under suitable environmental conditions. Survival in experimentally infected slurry for at least 138 days has been observed, while in another study leptospires survived for up to 18 h in untreated abattoir sewage. Survival in kidneys for at least 21 days at 4 °C has been observed.

DISEASE MECHANISMS

The same range of disease processes are seen in all animals, irrespective of the animal species or the infecting serovar; however, there are significant differences in host specificity and susceptibility. There is also a relationship between age and susceptibility. Immunity to primary infection appears to be solely by humoral immune response, mainly to the outer envelope lipopolysaccharide (LPS) antigens, although cellular immunity may have a role in vaccinal induced immunity, but this is poorly understood.

Within the pathogenic leptospires, virulence ranges from non-virulent to highly virulent strains. Primary isolates from animals are often virulent but this is usually lost on subculturing. The rate at which virulence is lost on subculturing is highly variable. Virulence can be regained by some strains by animal passage. This phenomenon is based on the gradual decline of the percentage of virulent organisms in a culture. During animal inoculation the virulent organisms are selected, multiply, and can be re-isolated from the animals. When strains are subcultured for an extended period of time, all virulent organisms can be lost, and even after animal passage these strains do not regain virulence (Faine 1994)

Leptospirosis is a bacteraemic infection. Leptospires do not localize at the site of entry. They are not pyogenic, but cause inflammatory reactions through secondary tissue damage. The main lesion in all forms of leptospirosis is damage to the walls of small blood vessels, leading to leakage. Other lesions follow as secondary effects. Little is known about the properties of leptospires which are likely to be important in pathogenic mechanisms: adherence of leptospires to cells, invasion of cells, and the capability to produce cytotoxins are presumed to play a role (Faine 1994).

Adherence and invasion

Leptospires can invade the mucous membranes, abraded and water-softened skin. Virulent strains have been shown to adhere to cultured fibroblasts and epithelial cells *in vitro*, whereas avirulent strains do not adhere. Attachment is inhibited by homologous Fab fragments but enhanced by subagglutinating amounts of homologous antisera. Adherence is decreased after protease treatment but not after periodate treatment, which indicates that proteins and not LPS are involved in adherence. Detachment of tight junctions and penetration between cells by leptospires has been observed in liver and kidney. Intracellular leptospires have been observed, but it is uncertain whether *Leptospira* invade intact cells or only cells that are damaged by leptospiral toxins.

Toxicity

Cytotoxic activity has been described and has been shown to be associated with virulence. The cytotoxic component is the lipid moiety of a glycolipoprotein.

Haemolysins may play a role in the pathogenesis of leptospirosis, due to their ability to lyse erythrocytes and other cells.

Leptospiral LPS resembles Gram-negative bacterial LPS. However, although it clots *Limulus* lysate, it is relatively non-toxic to cells or animals—approximately 12 times less lethal than *E. coli* LPS for mice. Evidence indicates that it causes the haemorrhages and coagulation defects which are features of leptospirosis. It is highly immunogenic and enhances the activity of macrophages and non-specific immunity. Diphenylamine treatment of leptospires reduces their resistance against anti-leptospiral activity present in serum, indicating a role for LPS in pathogenesis.

Autoimmunity

Autoimmunity may be important in the development of renal lesions in the dog, while in horses an autoimmune uveitis can occur, particularly following *pomona* infection.

THE HOSTS

Infection of susceptible animals occurs though the mucous membranes of the eye, mouth, nose, vagina, and penis, and through abraded or water-softened skin, and is followed after a 4–10-day incubation period by a bacteraemic phase that may last from a few hours to 7 days. This phase may be subclinical but can be characterized by pyrexia, excretion of leptospires in milk and, with some serovars, by functional damage to the internal organs, especially in younger animals. During this period leptospires can be isolated from most organs of the body and also from cerebrospinal fluid. Acute clinical disease coincides with this bacteraemic phase.

This primary bacteraemic phase ends with the appearance of circulating antibodies, which are detectable usually by 10 days after infection. Peak titres and the time for which they persist vary considerably, depending on the animal species, the infecting serovar, and the route of infection. There is an initial IgM response which peaks 2–3 weeks postinfection. The IgG response is much slower.

Following the period of leptospiraemia, the leptospires localize and persist in a number of organs, especially the proximal renal tubules (all ages and species) and the genital tracts of sexually mature females and entire males of certain species (cattle, pigs, and dog). Leptospires may also persist in the central nervous system of some species (sheep).

Differences have been found in tissue tropisms exhibited by different strains of the same serovar, for example some strains of *L. borgpetersenii* serovar *hardjo* have been shown to persist primarily in the kidney, while others have a predilection for the genital tract and others persist in both organ systems.

Leptospires localized in the proximal renal tubules multiply and are voided in the urine. The duration and intensity of urinary shedding varies from species to species, animal to animal, and with the infecting serovar. In the case of incidental infections (including all human infections) the duration of excretion is usually only very short and the number of organisms excreted is low. In the case of host-maintained infections such as *L. borgpetersenii* serovar *hardjo* infection in cattle, the intensity of excretion is highest during the first 4–6 weeks of shedding. Leptospiruria is very constant during this period. A variable period of intermittent, low intensity, leptospiruria then ensues and this frequently lasts for 6–12 months in cattle but can persist for life. Similarly, brown rats infected with *icterohaemorrhagiae* may excrete for life. In contrast, in other host-maintained infections, where venereal infection is probably the more important route of infection, such as *L. interrogans* serovar *hardjo* infection in the cattle and sheep, or serovar bratislava infection in pigs, urinary shedding is of very low intensity.

The factors involved in the cessation of urinary excretion are poorly understood, but one recent study has shown that it is invariably associated with a sharp increase in urinary antileptospiral IgG and IgA antibody levels.

Localization of leptospires in the pregnant and non-pregnant uterus of domestic animals is one of the more recently recognized features of infection, particularly host-maintained infections. Serovar *hardjo*, for example, has been shown to persist in the pregnant bovine uterus for up to 142 days and in the non-pregnant uterus for 97 days postinfection. Localization in the pregnant uterus may in turn be followed by fetal infection, with subsequent chronic reproductive wastage and excretion of the leptospires in the post-calving uterine discharge. Fetal infection is most likely to occur in the second half of pregnancy. Bovine and ovine fetuses infected during the latter stages of gestation may develop detectable antibody titres.

Localization of serovars *hardjo* and *bratislava* have been reported in the testes and accessory glands of bulls and boars, respectively, while leptospires of the *pomona* and *hebdomadis* serogroups have been demonstrated in bull semen. Leptospiral antibodies have been detected in seminal plasma, suggesting local antibody production.

Persistence of serovar *hardjo* in the mammary glands of cattle and goats has also been reported (Ellis 1994).

SYMPTOMS AND SIGNS

In considering the features of clinical disease in different hosts it must be borne in mind that in man and the companion animals (dog and horse), the clinician is usually presented with an individual case, whereas in the food-producing animals cases usually present as herd problems.

Man

The disease in humans varies according to the infecting serovar of *Leptospira*, and the age, health, and nutrition of the patient. It is an acute febrile disease, the manifestations of which arise from the effects of a generalized vasculitis. There are many possible clinical presentations and courses. None of the presenting features of leptospirosis is specific for that disease,

although each serovar tends to be associated with a characteristic severity of illness.

The incubation period can vary from 2 to 30 days, but is usually in the range 5–14 days.

All forms of leptospirosis start in a similar way. The main presenting signs are sudden-onset severe headache, muscle pains, fever, conjunctival suffusion, a transient rash on the palate and skin, and photophobia. Thereafter the severity to the illness may vary from a mild form to a severe or even fatal form.

The mild form of the disease is characteristically seen with infections by serovars such as *hardjo* or *pomona*. The initial symptoms may be followed by a transient remission which may, in some instances, proceed to aseptic meningitis and renal failure. Exanthematous rashes can occur in up to 30 per cent of patients in the first week, lasting 1–2 days, sometimes localized to the trunk or shins.

At the other extreme is the severe form. This is seen in infections with serovars such as *icterohaemorrhagiae* and *copenhageni*. Illness worsens, usually rapidly, after onset so that renal failure appears within 7–10 days, sometimes accompanied by skin and mucosal haemorrhages, jaundice, haemoptysis, myocarditis, or liver failure, leading to death if untreated.

Leptospirosis of either type in pregnancy carries the risks of intrauterine infection and fetal death.

The extent to which organ systems are affected reflects the severity of disease:

1. Respiratory manifestations range from a cough and haemoptysis to pulmonary oedema and adult respiratory distress syndrome.
2. Abnormalities can be detected on urine analysis in 80–90 per cent of patients. Progressive renal dysfunction is manifested by oliguria and anuria.
3. Serous meningitis is the most common form of neurological complication. Occasionally encephalitis may occur. Convalescence from meningitis may be prolonged and involve periods of physical and muscular weakness and mental exhaustion for months. A number of patients suffer prolonged mental symptoms, ranging from mood changes, irritability, and irrationality to dementia, serious psychosis, and depression.
4. In many patients the liver is enlarged and tender. In icteric patients, jaundice usually appears on days 4–9 after onset. A raised serum bilirubin level with normal aminotransferases is highly suggestive of leptospirosis.

The mortality rate in those infected with serovars known to cause severe disease (e.g., *icterohaemorrhagiae*, *copenhageni*) can range from 5 to 40 per cent. Infections with those serovars which cause mild disease (e.g. *hardjo*) are almost never icteric or fatal.

Animals

The vast majority of animal leptospiral infections are subclinical. Two groups of animals are most likely to experience clinical infections:

(1) the young animal;
(2) sexually mature, lactating and/or pregnant females. (This feature of leptospirosis is its most important aspect in terms of effects on farm economics, and is largely, but not exclusively, caused by serovars maintained by the affected animal species.)

Where incidental leptospiral infections cause clinical disease in animals, there are close parallels with those features observed in the severe form of disease in man. Severe illness is characterized by jaundice, haematuria, haemaglobinuria, evidence of renal damage, and meningitis, and infections such as those due to *icterohaemorrhagiae* can be fatal. In addition, dogs infected with certain serovars, most notably *canicola*, can develop chronic renal disease with unthriftiness polyuria, and polydipsia (Greene 1984). Postinfection fatigue problems can have serious consequences for performance animals such as hunting dogs, greyhounds, race and competition horses.

Acute infection of adult cows gives rise to the so called 'milk drop syndrome' or 'flabby bag syndrome' in the lactating dairy cow, especially in early lactation. It is characterized by a sudden drop in milk yield. The udder appears flabby, as if the cow had already been milked—not swollen and painful as in most forms of mastitis—and all four quarters are affected. The milk is often thickened and yellow, not unlike colostrum, and may contain clots and may even be blood tinged. Cell counts are elevated and culture examination for common mastitis pathogens is negative. Affected animals may have markedly elevated rectal temperatures but appear remarkably well. They continue to eat as normal. Affected animals recover without treatment and milk yield usually returns to almost pre-infection levels over a 10–14-day period. However, cows in late lactation may dry-off prematurely and the yield of individual cows may remain depressed throughout lactation.

Dramatic outbreaks of 'milk drop' affecting up to half the cows in a herd over a short period of time (4–6 weeks) occur but are uncommon. The more usual situation is where:

(1) only one or two animals are obviously affected, usually first or second calvers;
(2) an unexplained increase in herd cell count occurs; and/or
(3) the month's milk production figures are less than the computerized predictions for that month.

An agalactia similar to that seen in cows has been observed in *hardjo*-infected sheep. Recently lambed ewes suddenly stop producing milk, giving rise to lamb deaths due to starvation. Ewes return to milk after 3–4 days without treatment.

Reproductive wastage is a chronic sequel of leptospirosis in the breeding animal. In pregnant cows, fetal infection with resulting still births, abortions, and the birth of weak offspring of reduced viability may occur. While such reproductive wastage can occur in cattle infected by many parasitic leptospires, it is particularly a feature of *pomona* and *hardjo* infections. Abortion and the other effects usually occur 1–6 weeks (*pomona* infection) and 4–12 weeks (*hardjo* infection) after the acute phase of infection; however, such animals have frequently shown no clinical evidence of acute infection.

With *pomona* infections these events usually occur in the last 3 months of gestation. Abortion has been observed in the second trimester in cases of *autumnalis* infection. With *hardjo* infection, abortion has been diagnosed at all stages from the fourth month through to term, and circumstantial evidence indicates that it may also cause early embryonic death.

The incidence of abortion can sometimes be high, particularly in first or second calvers: more than 20 per cent may be affected following the introduction of *hardjo* into a susceptible group of cattle, but most commonly, there is an insidious loss of 3 to 6 per cent of pregnancies per year, with peaks occurring every 4–7 years.

Reproductive wastage in pigs (especially serovars *pomona* and *bratislava*), and sheep (serovar *hardjo*) is also seen as late-term abortion (usually in the last 2 weeks of gestation), still birth, and the birth of weak offspring; while in the horse (various serovars), abortion has been seen from the fourth month of gestation onwards, but most commonly in the last 3 months of gestation.

Infertility has been a common field observation in *hardjo*-infected cattle herds and improvements in breeding efficiency have been noted in herds following *hardjo* vaccination. Attempts to establish herd data to support these observations and preliminary supportive findings have been reported. Infertility is an important feature of *bratislava*-infection in pigs.

DIAGNOSIS

Because of the lack of definitive clinical features, a conclusive diagnosis of leptospirosis is dependent on laboratory confirmation. A diagnosis of leptospirosis may be required not only for the clinician to confirm leptospirosis as a cause of clinical disease but also for other reasons, including:

(1) the assessment of the infection and/or the immune status of a population for the purposes of a control or eradication programme on either a local, regional, or national basis;

(2) epidemiological studies; and

(3) an assessment of the infectivity status of an individual animal to assess its suitability for international trade or for introduction into an uninfected population.

The diagnostic procedures for leptospirosis fall into two groups. The first consists of tests for the demonstration of leptospires in body fluids and in biopsy or post-mortem tissues, and the second contains tests for antibody detection. The selection of tests to be carried out depends on the stage of infection and the samples and resources available. The principles and practices in the applications of the tests are similar in animal and human leptospirosis.

Antigen detection methods in the diagnosis of acute leptospirosis

The bacteraemic phase of infection coincides with the onset of symptoms of acute leptospirosis and persists for 1–7 days. Efforts to diagnose infection during this phase should be directed towards the detection of leptospires, their DNA or antigens in blood, CSF, and tissue biopsy material. The techniques available are direct examination for leptospires, culture, and detection of specific DNA sequences following polymerase chain reaction (PCR) amplification. Should the patient survive the first week of illness, then leptospires may be demonstrated in urine. Should the patient die during the acute phase, kidney, lung, liver, aqueous humour, brain, and urine should be examined by either culture, immunochemical staining, PCR, or silver staining techniques. When interpreting the results of all antigen detection procedures the diagnostician must remember that if antibiotic therapy has already been initiated it is probable that the results will be negative. In the case of agalactia in cattle, leptospires may be cultured from milk, but this is normally impractical.

Serological diagnosis of acute leptospirosis

Antigen detection methods are often not available and in those instances the diagnostician in reliant on serology. In animals that survive infection, serology is an important diagnostic tool. In general, if a blood sample for serology is taken early in the illness and a second sample is taken a week later—and repeated at similar intervals for a further 2 weeks if feasible in human cases—it should be possible to demonstrate a diagnostic rise in leptospiral antibodies. The most useful methods used are the microscopic agglutination

test (MAT) and the enzyme-linked immunosorbent assay (ELISA) and, less frequently, the micro-capsule agglutination test (MCA). If the patient dies, or if for some other reason only one sample is available, the IgM-specific ELISA tests are very useful. The MCA test will become positive before the other two tests. CSF can be a useful fluid to test for antibodies, particularly in fatal cases.

Fetal serology can be very useful in cases of fetal disease in all species.

Antigen detection methods in the diagnosis of chronic leptospirosis

While abortion is a chronic event, it should be treated as for the microbiological diagnosis of acute fatal disease. In addition, fetal adrenal tissue and placenta should be examined.

Diagnosis of chronic leptospirosis

Serological tests have very limited applications in the diagnosis of chronic leptospirosis and in identifying renal and genital carriers. At this time antibody titres are static or declining, or may no longer be detectable, depending on the time that has elapsed since the acute phase of disease.

Identification of carrier animals

There are no reliable methods for identifying carrier animals. There is no correlation between an animal's serological status and whether it is a chronic renal or genital tract carrier. Organism detection methods are not sufficiently sensitive or reliable to detect the low numbers of organisms which may be present.

Techniques

Culture is difficult and time consuming, and to obtain reliable results it must be performed by experienced personnel, as must the identification of isolates. It is the most sensitive method of demonstrating leptospires, provided that antibiotic residues are absent, that tissue autolysis is not advanced, and that tissues for culture have been stored at a suitable temperature (4 °C) and, in the case of urine, at a suitable pH since collection.

There is no one isolation medium which will grow all leptospires, but the best general medium is semi-solid (0.1–0.2 per cent agar) EMJH medium. It can be modified by the addition of from 0.4 to 2 per cent fresh rabbit serum (Faine 1982, 1994; Ellis 1986). The E medium (Ellis 1986) is a better option when dealing with infections such *hardjo* and *bratislava*. A dilution culture method should be used. Contamination may be controlled by a variety of selective agents, e.g.

5-fluorouracil, nalidixic acid, fosfomycin, and a cocktail of rifamycin, polymyxin, neomycin, 5-fluorouracil, bacitracin, and actidione. The use of selective agents will reduce the chance of isolation where there are only small numbers of viable leptospires. Culture media, containing 5-fluorouracil at levels between 200 and 500 μg/ml, should be used as transport media for the submission of samples. Cultures should be incubated at 29–30 °C for at least 12 weeks and preferably for 26 weeks (Ellis 1986). They should be examined by dark-ground microscopy every 1–2 weeks.

The demonstration of leptospires by immunochemical staining methods is more suited to diagnostic laboratories; however, these tests depend on the number of organisms and lack the sensitivity of culture. The immunochemical methods that have been used for diagnosis include immunofluorescence, PAP, avidin–biotin, and immunogold techniques. While these methods have not proved as sensitive as culture, one of them, immunofluorescence, has been used widely, particularly in the diagnosis of fetal leptospirosis. It has the advantage of giving better contrast between the leptospires and the tissue background than the other methods. This is particularly important since leptospires are very small and filamentous, which makes them difficult to differentiate from some connective tissue elements and cilia. Immunofluorescence has the disadvantage that the production of good-quality polyclonal antisera requires long inoculation regimes in rabbits.

Dark-ground microscopy of body fluids has been widely used and can be a useful tool in the hands of an experienced diagnostician, but many tissue artefacts can be mistakenly identified as leptospires. Leptospires do not stain satisfactorily with the aniline dyes and silver staining techniques lack sensitivity and specificity.

DNA hybridization techniques are now becoming available. There have been a number of reports of blot and *in situ* hybridization, as diagnostic tools for leptospirosis, using both radioactive and non-radioactive, genomic and specific probes. Two primer sets, which between them have genus specificity, have been piloted for the rapid detection of leptospiraemia in man using PCR, by the WHO Reference Laboratory, KIT, Amsterdam. Problems due to non-specific inhibitors have reduced the sensitivity of this technology when applied to urine and tissue samples.

Serological tests

Serological testing using the microscopic agglutination test (MAT) is the most widely used laboratory procedure for the diagnosis of leptospiral abortion. The test is relatively serovar specific. The minimum antigen requirements are that the test should employ representative strains of all the serogroups known to exist in the particular country, plus those known to be maintained under investigation elsewhere.

In the diagnosis of chronic leptospirosis, the MAT is best used as a herd or flock test, rather than as a test for an individual animal. A minimum of 10 animals or 10 per cent of the herd, whichever is the greater, should be tested to obtain useful information. Increasing the sample size and sampling a number of different cohorts markedly improves disease investigation and assessments of vaccination needs. A retrospective diagnosis of leptospirosis may be made when the majority of affected animals have titres of 1:1000 or greater. The herd test approach is not very useful for the diagnosis of *hardjo*-associated abortion in endemically infected cattle herds not for *bratislava* infection in pig herds, because of the insidious and chronic nature of herd infections and the very low levels of antibody which may be found in postabortion sera.

ELISA tests and the MCA test have advantages for many human diagnostic laboratories, in that they do not require the maintenance of live leptospires for antigens and they have good cross-reactivity.

PATHOLOGY

The main pathological changes are essentially the same in all species, with the primary lesion being damage to the membranes of the endothelial cells of small blood vessels. In acute leptospirosis there are no pathognomonic gross changes. Many of the features recorded after death from leptospirosis are those which would occur in death from renal failure from other causes, accompanied by jaundice in some cases. There may be petechial or ecchymotic haemorrhages in the skin, conjunctivae, mucosal and serosal surfaces, in the subcutaneous tissues and fat, and in the endocardium. The thoracic and peritoneal cavities may contain bloodstained yellow fluid. There may be subpleural haemorrhages. Splenomegaly is occasionally a feature.

The liver may be enlarged and tense, or pale, or yellow. There may be disruption of cord and lobular structure, which is sometimes accompanied by centrilobular necrosis. The liver cells become irregular, swollen, and degenerate.

The most significant lesions are in the kidneys, which may be swollen, and yellow-green in jaundiced patients, with subsurface haemorrhages. The constant histological feature is interstitial nephritis, and tubular necrosis. Haemorrhages are apparent, particularly in the medulla.

One of the characteristic lesions of acute leptospirosis is the degeneration of striated muscle. In biopsies of the gastrocnemius muscle, individual muscle fibres can be seen to have lost their cross-striations, be swollen and vacuolated. Sarcolemmal nuclei proliferate and the area is surrounded by inflammatory cells. In cardiac muscle vacuolation and degeneration are common.

Uveitis, iritis, and iridiocyclitis are common findings in the eyes.

In chronic leptospirosis in animals, lesions are confined to the kidneys and consist of scattered small grey/white foci, often surrounded by a ring of hyperaemia. Microscopic examination shows these lesions to be a progressive focal interstitial nephritis. The interstitial leucocytic infiltrations, which consist mainly of lymphocytes, macrophages, and plasma cells, may be extensive in some areas. Focal damage may also involve glomeruli and renal tubules. Some affected glomeruli are swollen, some atrophic, and others are replaced by fibrosis. The Bowman's capsule may be thickened, containing eosinophilic granular material. Tubular changes involve atrophy, hyperplasia, and presence of necrotic debris in the lumen in some areas. Occasionally, petechial haemorrhages may be present in interstitial spaces.

TREATMENT

Man

In the mild forms of leptospirosis, management is symptomatic, as indicated by the nature and severity of the manifestations. The severe form requires intensive-care management, including the availability of peritoneal dialysis, etc (for a detailed review see Faine 1994).

Penicillin is the antibiotic of choice in human cases, while in animals it is combined with streptomycin. The efficacy of antibiotics in the treatment of human leptospirosis was for long a matter of dispute, but this has finally been put to rest by a randomized, placebo-controlled, double-blind study, involving severely ill patients with leptospirosis from Manila, which has shown that penicillin therapy will markedly shorten the duration of illness and hasten recovery of renal function (Watt *et al.* 1988). The Jarisch–Herxheimer reaction can occur as a sequel to penicillin treatment.

Animals

In dogs treatment is similar to that for man. Disease outbreaks in food-producing animals are herd rather than individual animal problems, hence it is important to put treatment in the context of the need to control infection in the herd (p. 000).

The use of antibiotic treatment in cases of *hardjo* agalactia in cattle is a matter of clinical judgement, depending on the pregnancy status of the animal and on various herd factors (p. 000). Affected animals

recover without treatment; however, if the animal is pregnant, fetal infection and subsequent fetal loss may occur, and in such circumstances antibiotics (penicillin and streptomycin) should be administered.

Streptomycin (and its dihydro-analogue), when given at a dose of 25 mg/kg, will markedly reduce the number of organisms an infected animal is excreting, but, with certain serovars, it will not give a microbiological cure. However, it is frequently used to treat carrier animals in an attempt to reduce the risk of introducing infection from them to other animals.

PROGNOSIS

Most patients with leptospirosis will recover in 2–6 weeks, if not jaundiced. The death rate in jaundiced patients depends on the facilities available to treat liver and renal failure and on the early commencement of penicillin treatment. Patients who survive the renal and myocardial failure of severe leptospirosis usually recover completely in 6–12 weeks. Convalescence may be protracted (up to 6 months) and up to 10 per cent of patients complain of recurring headaches (Faine 1994) and uveitis for some years.

In animals the prognosis is very good, provided they have not become jaundiced. Animals which abort due to leptospiral infection are extremely unlikely to abort again due to the same serovar in a later pregnancy.

EPIDEMIOLOGY

There are differences in the global distribution of some of the *Leptospira* species: *L. interrogans*, *L. borgpetersenii* and *L. kirschneriase* have a worldwide distribution, whereas *L. noguchii* and *L. santarosai* are found mainly in North and South America, while *L. weillii* is found mainly in China and eastern Asia.

The epidemiology of leptospirosis is potentially very complicated since, theoretically, any animal species can be infected by any of the pathogenic serovars. Fortunately, only a small number of serovars will be endemic in any particular region or country. Furthermore, leptospirosis is a disease which shows a natural nidality, and each serovar tends to be maintained in specific maintenance hosts. Therefore, in any region, an animal species will be infected by: (1) serovars *maintained* by that species or (2) serovars maintained by other animal species present in the area (Hathaway 1981). The relative importance of these *incidental infections* is determined by the opportunities that prevailing social, management, and environmental factors provide for contact and transmission of leptospires from other species to the target host species. *Man is always an incidental host.*

The major *Leptospira* infections of global importance and their maintenance hosts are:

(1) serovars *icterohaemorrhagiae* and *copenhageni*—maintained by the brown rat;

(2) serovar *canicola*—maintained by dogs;

(3) serovar *pomona* type kennewicki—maintained by pigs in most parts of the world but not in the United Kingdom or western Europe (with the exception of parts of Italy);

(4) serovar *hardjo*—maintained by cattle worldwide (and also possibly sheep and goats);

(5) serovar *bratislava*—this is the most recently recognized major domestic animal–leptospire association and the least understood. Its epidemiology is very complicated. There appear to be specific pig-adapted strains, strains which are maintained by pigs, dogs, horses, and hedgehogs, and strains which are found only in wildlife.

The number of *Leptospira* infections maintained by food-producing animals is very small and while regional differences occur, local geographical differences are not as important as with incidental infections. Host-maintained infections are characterized by high seroprevalences, with many animals being infected subclinically. Where disease occurs, it is primarily associated with modern intensive management systems, and limited to susceptible sexually mature females. These systems are often managed in such a way that there is a regular throughput of susceptible females, and major economic losses can occur. In contrast, in the developed regions of the world the serological prevalences of incidental infections are usually low. Clinical incidents are usually 'one-offs' and rarely pose major economic problems. The exception is the horse, which appears to be particularly susceptible to incidental infections (every serogroup known to occur in Ireland has been isolated from horse clinical/pathological material). Incidental infections of animals assume much greater significance in developing countries, where the opportunities for interspecies contact and transmission are much greater.

In the developed regions of the world, the prevalence of human leptospirosis is very low. In such regions, human leptospirosis is an occupational disease, primarily affecting those who work directly with animals, e.g. dairy farmers, slaughtermen, meat inspectors, veterinarians. Other groups particularly at risk are people who engage in water-associated recreational activity or who have jobs where there may be wet working conditions, e.g. fish farmers. Some examples are:

1. In the United Kingdom, 12 per cent of dairy farmers in Cheshire were found to have antibodies to *hardjo*.

2. In Victoria, Australia, it has been estimated that everyone who milks cows will become infected with *hardjo* over a 20-year working life.

3. Eleven per cent of railway workers in parts of northern Italy have antibodies to leptospires (mostly rodent–maintained strains).

In contrast, in the developing countries, where poor working and housing conditions prevail, and there are major water-associated occupations such as rice growing, the opportunity for contact with both rodent and domestic animal maintained leptospires is greatly increased. Prevalences can be very high: for example, an 18 per cent seroprevalence has been reported in a rural community in Nigeria; a 22 per cent seroprevalence in urban communities in Belize; a 48 per cent seroprevalence in males in rice-farming villages in the Philippines; and a 33 per cent seroprevalence in sanitation workers in Madras City.

SOURCES

The source of infection is always an infected animal. The major factors in maintaining infection in a population are:

(1) the persistently infected carrier: some animals remain carriers for life but whether they remain infective throughout that period remains uncertain;

(2) the regular supply of susceptible animals: in dairy herds, for example, the standard practice of removing replacement heifers from their dams shortly after birth and keeping them separated from the main herd until shortly before or after calving ensures such a regular supply of non-immune animals.

TRANSMISSION

Transmission may be either direct or indirect. Direct transmission is probably more important in within-host-species transmission, with indirect transmission being the important method of incidental infection. However, indirect transmission does have a role in the transmission of host-maintained infections.

Direct transmission occurs through direct contact with infected urine or the products of abortion, handling infected kidneys, by ingestion of infected milk, and by transplacental infection. Venereal infection is thought to be important in those infections where the male and female genital tracts are major sites of persistence.

Environmental conditions are important for the survival of leptospires outwith the host, and the level of environmental contamination is critical to indirect transmission. Clearly, the longer leptospires remain viable in the environment, the greater the chances of them coming in contact with and infecting a susceptible host. The optimum conditions for survival outwith the host are warm, moist conditions with a pH close to neutral.

As well as aiding survival of leptospires, water also helps in the dissemination of infection and in the actual process of infecting a host. Moving water acts as a means of mechanically spreading infection. Intact skin acts as an effective barrier to leptospiral infection; however, after skin becomes softened by immersion in water leptospires can penetrate and establish infection.

PREVENTION AND CONTROL

Preventive measures must be based on a knowledge of the location, number, and frequency of either human and/or animal cases (clinical and subclinical), the infecting serovars (and types) of leptospire, their maintenance hosts, means of transmission, and risk factors. To acquire and monitor this information requires a surveillance system which reflects the various facets of leptospirosis and its impact on different population groups (human and animal) (Faine 1994).

The main resources are: (1) case identification; (2) notification systems; (3) collating information from these two sources and linking them with seroprevalence data; and (4) culture-based data on prevalence rates in local animal populations (domestic and wild).

Case identification is particularly difficult, because of the difficulties in diagnosis, and studies (human and animal) invariably underestimate the incidence of clinical disease. In many countries human leptospirosis is a notifiable disease, but since notification statistics are dependent on case identification, these are equally flawed. Serological surveys can provide useful information about the prevalence of antibodies, and thus give a guide to infections likely to be maintained by that population and to the relative exposure levels to incidental infections. Culture surveys are very useful in both domestic and wild animal populations in that they identify those infections which particular species maintain, and when compared with serological data they can be used to discriminate between the host-maintained and the common incidental infections of that species.

MEASURES FOR CONTROL AND PREVENTION

Strategies for the control of infections in man

These must consider that man is always an incidental host for infections maintained by animals, and that the approach to control of incidental infections in man will differ in high- and low-prevalence regions.

Interruption of transmission from animal to man is the critical factor in the control of human leptospirosis. The following are key elements in achieving this, and as many as are appropriate to the situation should be included in a strategy:

1. Identify the sources of infection: where transmission is occurring and what are the host species.
2. Control infection in the host species, if that is possible. This is an important feature in controlling occupational leptospirosis resulting from contact with domestic animal hosts, e.g. *hardjo* vaccination in cattle.
3. Control of rodent carriers, e.g. rat control programmes.
4. Reduce contact with carrier animals—improved living and working conditions by, for example, introducing mechanical harvesting of rice and sugar cane.
5. Exclusion from known contaminated environments i.e., do not bathe in stagnant waterways.
6. Occupational hygiene. Provide waterproof clothing to give a barrier to infection.
7. Vaccination. This approach is adopted in parts of China.
8. Awareness/education. People at risk need to be aware of the risks and what they can do to reduce these.
9. Provision of laboratory support facilities and trained personnel to carry out control programmes.

The control of leptospirosis in people travelling from low-risk environments to high-risk environments for short periods of time

Doxycycline has been used prophylactically to protect soldiers in tropical jungles and could be used to protect others being exposed to risk for short periods of time.

Strategies for the control of incidental infections in domestic animals

These are based on the same principles outlined for man. Animal management regimes should minimize contact with carrier animals, by such means as avoiding communal watering points and ensuring separate housing. If necessary, vaccination should be carried out if vaccines are available and warranted.

Strategies for the control of host-maintained infections in domestic food-producing animals

In developing strategies for the control of leptospirosis in host-maintained infections, based on keeping a population free of infection, it is important to minimize the major risk factors involved in introducing infection to a clean herd. For example:

1. Develop a closed herd policy and thus avoid buying in carrier animals.
2. Keep only one host species on the premises, thus minimizing the risk of contact with another maintenance host, such as sheep in the case of *hardjo* infection in cattle.
3. Avoid contact with other animals of the same species; in particular:
   (a) do not share the use of a bull or boar with another enterprise;
   (b) establish secure boundaries.
4. Avoid indirect transmission, e.g. prevent access to a watercourse which has other animal hosts upstream, or a communal watering point.

In developing strategies for the control of leptospirosis in host-maintained infections based on minimizing economic loss through clinical and subclinical disease rather than keeping a population clear of infection, it is important ensure that only animals of similar immune status to a herd are brought into that herd.

Streptomycin, will significantly reduce the level of excretion by carrier animals. When used as part of a control programme it is best used either on the whole herd at the same time or on added animals which are being held in isolation. Oral tetracyclines, at levels of 600–800 g/tonne of feed will control the clinical effects of leptospirosis in pigs but will not eliminate infection from a herd.

Vaccines, though useful, will not eradicate infection from an endemically infected herd and will not stop excretion in the animal which is already leptospiruric. They will not always prevent abortion in the animal in which placental localization has already occurred prior to vaccination.

In the endemically infected herd; ideally a programme should start with treating all adult animals at a time when the cost of lost product (such as milk) can be minimized. This may mean deferring treatment until animals go dry. Vaccinate the whole herd (all females destined for breeding and all entire males) annually in the case of cattle, or prior to service in the case of pigs. Where there are doubts about vaccine efficacy, reduce cattle vaccination intervals to 6 months or less.

LEGISLATION

Legislation can provide an important incentive to carry out control measures. In the United Kingdom the Control of Substances Hazardous to Health regulations place the onus on farmers to identify whether their cattle are infected by serovar *hardjo*, to inform their employees of the situation, and to take measures to protect their employees (i.e. provide protective clothing, vaccinate their cattle). In addition, the climate of increased willingness of employees to seek redress/compensation through the courts for illness associated with negligence, has heightened awareness of many employers in the red meat and dairy industries that leptospirosis is an occupational disease of those industries, and of the need to instigate practical preventive measures.

REFERENCES

Ellis, W. A. (1986). The diagnosis of Leptospirosis in farm animals. In *The present state of leptospirosis diagnosis and control*, (ed. W. A. Ellis and T. W. A. Little), pp. 13–32. Martinus Nijhoff, Dordrecht.

Ellis, W. A. (1994). Leptospirosis as a cause of reproductive failure. *Veterinary Clinics of North America: Food Animal Practice*, **10**, 463–78.

Ellis, W. A. (1995). International Committee on Systematic Bacteriology Subcommittee on the Taxonomy of *Leptospira*. *International Journal of Systematic Bacteriology*, **45**, 872–4.

Faine, S. (1982). *Guidelines for the control of leptospirosis.* Offset Publication No. 67, World Health Organization, Geneva.

Faine, S. (1994). *Leptospira and leptospirosis.* CRC Press, Boca Raton.

Greene, C. E. (1984). Leptospirosis. In *Clinical microbiology and infectious diseases of the dog and cat*, pp. 588–98. W. B. Saunders, Philadelphia.

Hathaway, S. C. (1981). Leptospirosis in New Zealand: an ecological view. *New Zealand Veterinary Journal*, **29**: 109–12.

Watt, G. *et al.* (1988). Placebo controlled trial of intravenous penicillin for severe and late leptospirosis. *Lancet*, **1**; 433–5.

Weil, A. (1886). Uebereine eigenthümliche, mit Milztumur, Icterus and Nephritis einhergehende, acute Infectionskrankheit. *Deutsch Archive KlinMedizin*, **39**, 209.

Wolbach, S. B. and Binger, C. A. L. (1914). Notes on a filtrable speriochete from fresh water. *Spirochater fiflexa* (new species). *Journal of Medical Research*, **30**, 23.

13 LISTERIOSIS

J. McLauchlin and N. Van der Mee-Marquet

SUMMARY

Listeriosis occurs in a variety of animals, including humans, and most often affects the pregnant uterus, the central nervous system, or the bloodstream. During pregnancy, infection spreads to the fetus, which will either be born severely ill or die *in utero*. In non-pregnant individuals, listeriosis usually presents as meningitis, encephalitis, or septicaemia in the immuno-compromised and elderly. Infection can be treated successfully with antibiotics, but 20–40 per cent of human cases are fatal.

In domestic animals (especially in sheep and goats) listeriosis usually presents as encephalitis, abortion, or septicaemia, and is a cause of considerable economic loss.

The genus *Listeria* comprises six species of Gram-positive bacteria, but almost all cases of human listeriosis are due to *Listeria monocytogenes*. A similar pattern is seen in animals, except that up to 10 per cent of cases are due to *Listeria ivanovii*.

Listeriae are ubiquitous in the environment world-wide, especially in sites with decaying organic vegetable material. Many animals carry the organism in the faeces. It is generally believed that consumption of contaminated foods is the principal route of transmission for both humans and animals. Although human listeriosis is relatively rare (about 3–8 cases per million people in North America and western Europe), because of the high mortality rate it is amongst the most important causes of death from food-borne infections in industrialized countries.

Control measures should be directed at excluding *Listeria* from food or feed and inhibiting its multiplication and survival in foods. Silage which is spoiled or mouldy should not be used, and care should be taken to maintain anaerobic conditions for as long as possible.

In a number of countries (including the United Kingdom, United States, France, New Zealand, and parts of Australia) 'at-risk' individuals have been advised on food hygiene and to modify their diet, to avoid eating specific foods such as soft cheese and paté.

HISTORY

The bacterium *Listeria monocytogenes* and the disease listeriosis were first recognized, causing a spontaneous outbreak of infection amongst laboratory rabbits and guinea-pigs in Cambridge (England), by Murray and colleagues in 1924. The species name *monocytogenes* was derived from the marked mononuclear leucocytosis shown by these animals. In 1927 Pirie in South Africa isolated the same bacterium from infected gerbils, and named this *Listerella* after the surgeon and pioneer of antisepsis, Lord Lister. The generic name was changes to *Listeria* in 1940 for taxonomic reasons. Gill in New Zealand is credited with the first isolation of *L. monocytogenes* from an infected domestic animal and described an ovine encephalitis 'circling disease'.

Nyfeldt, in Denmark in 1929, isolated *L. monocytogenes* from the blood cultures of humans with a mononucleosis-like infection (a rare manifestation of the disease), and Burn 1936 in the United States, established listeriosis as a cause of infection during the perinatal period and also as meningitis in adults. Prior to 1926 there are descriptions of disease likely to have been listeriosis, indeed a 'diphtheroid' isolated from the cerebrospinal fluid of a soldier in Paris in 1919 was later identified as *L. monocytogenes*.

During the 1980s the rise in the numbers of both human and animal listeriosis in several countries (including the United Kingdom), together with a series of human food-borne outbreaks in North America and Europe (Table 13.1), led to renewed professional interest in the disease and public alarm.

THE AGENT

THE GENUS *LISTERIA*

Listeria are coccobacilli or rod-shaped, non-sporing, Gram-positive bacteria with a DNA G + C content of 36–42 mol%. The cell wall is typical for a Gram-positive organism, and contains alanine and glutamic acid cross-linked by meso-diaminopimelic acid: teichoic acids are present. The fatty acids anteiso $C_{17:0}$ and disease. Maternal infection may spread to the unborn infant, resulting in either an intrauterine death, or the birth of a neonate severely ill within the first days after delivery (early onset neonatal infection). Neonates can also develop late-onset sepsis, typically 10–12 days after delivery.

Disease presentation

Listeriosis most often affects the contents of the pregnant uterus, the central nervous system, or the bloodstream. In non-pregnant individuals, listeriosis most frequently presents as meningitis (with or without septicaemia), or septicaemia without involvement of the central nervous system. The latter form of illness is generally confined to immunocompromised individuals and rarely has identifiable foci of infection. Listeric meningoencephalitis and encephalitis occur less commonly.

In the pregnant woman, listeriosis is most often recognized as one or more self-limiting influenza-like episodes during or after the latter half of the second trimester, although infection can occur throughout gestation. Maternal listeriosis usually presents with pyrexia and other non-specific symptoms, although some individuals may be asymptomatic. Maternal listeric meningitis during pregnancy and recurrent infection in the same woman during different pregnancies is very rare.

During pregnancy infection spreads from the maternal circulatory system to the fetus, probably via the placenta, although this is not inevitable. Fetal infection developing before the third trimester usually results in intrauterine death. The fetus has severe and overwhelming multisystem infection involving internal organs, with the widespread formation of granulomatous lesions, especially in the liver and placenta (granulomatosis infantiseptica). Infection of the infant during the third trimester results in either intrauterine death, or the delivery of a severely ill neonate (early onset infection).

Early onset sepsis is characterized by non-specific signs of infection and prematurity. Cutaneous lesions may be present (sometimes with granulomas) and the neonate may be convulsive. Most early onset cases are septicaemic, some with meningitis; however, some infants appear to be infected only at superficial sites. The degree of severity may be partially dependent on the gestational age at infection. Surviving infants can exhibit long-term sequelae, especially those delivered prematurely or with involvement of the central nervous system.

Late-onset neonatal sepsis typically occurs after uncomplicated full-term pregnancies, and usually presents as meningitis about 10 days after delivery. *Listeria monocytogenes* is acquired either from maternal sites during or shortly after delivery (possibly during passage through the birth canal) or from the postnatal environment.

Focal infections caused by *L. monocytogenes* are relatively rare, and are primarily confined to immunocompromised individuals. Deep-seated infections with or without abscess formation occur in a wide variety of sites. Listeric endocarditis also occurs, and is usually confined to patients with underlying cardiac lesions or with prosthetic heart valves.

Non-systemic cutaneous and ocular listeriosis resulting from contact with infected animals or animal material has been described (McLauchlin and Low 1994). These superficial lesions may develop to serious systemic infection.

Diarrhoea or other gastrointestinal symptoms have been found as a feature of some cases of listeriosis, but may be specific to certain *L. monocytogenes* strains.

Since *L. monocytogenes* is common in the environment, individuals must be exposed to the organism through food alone on a frequent basis; it is possible that the majority of incidents of listeriosis manifest as subclinical infection, perhaps as mild influenza-like illness, or as infection of the gastrointestinal or upper respiratory tract. This is also supported by the relatively mild forms of the disease presenting as cutaneous infections or as bacteraemia in the pregnant woman.

During infection of the fetus, the pregnant woman often exhibits a series of pyrexial influenza-like episodes, resulting from the same strain of *L. monocytogenes* invading the maternal bloodstream. However, in both humans and animals it is very rare for the pregnant individual with an infected fetus to develop serious infection (such as meningitis or encephalitis), despite invasion of the bloodstream.

Diagnosis

Since the clinical symptoms of human listeriosis are not sufficiently characteristic to establish a diagnosis, it is necessary to isolate and identify *L. monocytogenes*. Special culture media and procedures are not usually required when examining samples from normally sterile sites.

Diagnosis of septicaemia or meningitis is made by culturing blood or cerebrospinal fluid. *Listeria monocytogenes* is sometimes seen in stained cerebrospinal fluid smears collected from patients with meningitis, together with a moderate leucocyte reaction (usually lymphocytic), elevated protein levels, and depressed sugar concentrations. Despite the species name '*monocytogenes*', monocytosis during septicaemia or meningitis is rarely observed.

During pregnancy, *L. monocytogenes* can be cultured from maternal blood, especially when collected during febrile episodes. Before delivery, an abnormal visual appearance of the amniotic fluid may give an early suggestion of listeriosis, especially when discoloured by meconium. At birth *L. monocytogenes* is present in high numbers both on many sites of the infected infant and in the maternal genital tract, and can be seen in stained smears. This bacterium can be cultured readily from the placenta and lochia, the infant's blood, cerebrospinal fluid, respiratory and gastric tract, skin and other surface sites, and the maternal high vagina. Amniotic fluid and meconium should be cultured when available, the former can be collected by amniocentesis prior to delivery.

Following intrauterine death and expulsion of the fetus, necropsy should be carried out. Material taken from the infant's liver, spleen, brain, and other internal organs should be examined for *L. monocytogenes*. Culturing maternal high vaginal swabs may also be useful in retrospective diagnosis of intrauterine infection within several weeks after delivery.

Methods to detect bacterial antigen and specific nucleic acid sequences have been described and are likely to become more widely used for diagnosis in the future. Procedures to detect specific antibody have also been described; however, interpretation is problematic.

Pathology

The histological changes in human listeriosis are similar to those observed in animals. Infection causes necrosis, followed by proliferative activity of cells in the reticuloendothelial system, resulting in miliary granuloma formation and focal necrosis with suppuration of the affected tissues. The bacterium is often present in the necrotic foci. The numbers and extent of the lesions vary with the sites infected as well as the resistance of the host.

Meningitis is characterized by suppurative inflammation of the meninges with granuloma and necrosis of cerebral tissue. A thick purulent exudate may be found in the subarachnoid space. During encephalitis, gross lesions may be absent, or present in the pons and medulla oblongata. In cases of encephalomyelitis, submiliary to miliary nodules are often found in the leptomeninges.

In the newborn, the disease is characterized by a massive involvement of the liver with disseminated lesions in many other organs, including the spleen, adrenal glands, lungs, oesophagus, posterior pharyngeal wall, and the tonsils. Cutaneous foci are often seen, especially on the back and lumbar region.

In the placenta, multiple white or grey necrotic areas occur within the villous parenchyma and decidua, the largest usually in the basal villi and decidua basalis. This gross appearance may allow a presumptive diagnosis of listeriosis. The necrotic foci are identical to those in the fetal organs. Gram-positive rods are usually seen within the necrotic centres of the villous and decidual abscesses, as well as within the membranes, umbilical cord, and surface of the fetus. The necrotic foci typically contain collections of polymorphonuclear leucocytes and are found between the trophoblast and stroma. Inflamed or necrotic chorionic villi are enmeshed in intervillous inflammatory material and fibrin.

Antimicrobial treatment

Various antibiotics have been recommended for treatment of listeriosis, including penicillin, ampicillin, tetracycline, erythromycin, trimethoprim–suphamethoxazole, and rifampicin. *In vitro* studies on the activities of various antimicrobial agents show that *L. monocytogenes* is almost always uniformly sensitive to ampicillin, penicillin, and erythromycin, although up to 10 per cent of cultures may be resistant to tetracycline. *Listeria monocytogenes* is uniformly highly resistant to cephalosporins, and fluoroquinolones have insufficient activity to be recommended for the treatment of listeriosis.

Studies using a number of *in vivo* animal models are difficult to interpret, although there is general agreement between these and with data from the prognosis of patients that a combination of ampicillin or penicillin plus an aminoglycoside is superior to using either drug alone.

It is recommended that central nervous system listeriosis in adults should be treated with intravenous ampicillin (200 mg/kg/day divided into six doses) plus an aminoglycoside (3–6 mg/kg/day divided into two or three doses) for 3–4 weeks.

During pregnancy, ampicillin (4–6g/day in four doses) plus an aminoglycoside (3 mg/kg/day divided into two or three doses) should be given intravenously if amnionitis is present, or amoxicillin (2–3 g orally per day in four doses) if it is not present. In both situations, treatment should continue for 2 weeks. In cases of serious allergy to ampicillin, trimethoprim (160 mg) plus sulphamethoxazole (800 mg) may be given intravenously every 12 hours.

Neonatal listeriosis should be treated with intravenous ampicillin plus an aminoglycoside. In early onset infection, ampicillin 100–150 mg/kg/day for infants with body weight respectively under or over 2 kg, plus 3–6 mg/kg of gentamicin in two doses should be given. In the second week after delivery, ampicillin 150–200 mg/kg with body weight respectively under or over 2 kg, plus gentamicin in the same doses as above should be given. Two weeks of treatment is recommended, but a longer course should be considered if a diagnosis of meningitis has been made. With late-onset neonatal listeriosis, meningitis is commonly present and ampicillin (200–400 mg/kg in 4–6 doses) plus gentamicin (3–6 mg/kg in two doses) is recommended. If the organism is present in the cerebrosinal fluid, the addition of rifampicin or trimethoprim– sulphamethoxazole may be considered. The length of treatment is variable; if prompt clinical improvement occurs and the bacterium is absent from the CSF, 2 weeks' treatment may be adequate. However, 4–6 weeks should generally be considered.

Prognosis

Fetal infection and death during early gestation is a recognized complication of maternal infection, but this is not inevitable. Once infection of the contents of the pregnant uterus has occurred, successful prepartum treatment of the mother with antimicrobial agents has resulted in the birth of apparently healthy infants. In late gestation, death of the fetus may occur, although it is more likely to result in the birth of a severely ill infant. Early onset neonatal listeriosis has a high fatality (>35 per cent), and in those that survive, sequelae such as neurodevelopmental handicaps, hydrocephalus, ptosis, and strabismus may occur. Late-onset neonatal listeriosis also has a high mortality rate, although generally not as high as early onset infection. The long-term prognosis for infants after late-onset sepsis or meningitis has not been well studied.

Mortality rates for adult and juvenile listeriosis vary from 10 to more than 50 per cent, with poor prognostic indicators including age (>50 years), pre-existing disease, early convulsions (in cases of meningitis), and the need for cardiovascular, renal, or ventilatory support. Residual disabilities may occur. Relapses of infection, some more than 2 years after the original episodes, have been described.

ANIMAL LISTERIOSIS

Disease presentation

Amongst domestic animals, sheep and goats are most susceptible, although infection also takes place in cattle (Gitter 1989; Low and Donachie 1997). Infection has been recognized in more than 40 other species of feral and domesticated animals, but this account will deal principally with sheep and cattle.

Listeriosis presents as a wide range of disorders, details of which parallel much of what has already been outlined for humans, although there are some differences. A substantial portion of the cases of abortion in sheep (but less commonly in cattle) are accounted for by *L. ivanovii*. The disease varies by species. In primates the disease is similar to that in humans.

There are six main manifestations of the disease: abortion, septicaemia, encephalitis, diarrhoea, mastitis, and ocular infections.

In sheep, goats, and cattle abortion is recognized late in pregnancy and is rarely accompanied by severe systemic disease in the dam. Aborting animals may excrete the organism in the milk without evidence of mastitis. Septicaemia in young animals occurs in the first few weeks of life; some have diarrhoea, but there is no specific symptomology. Diarrhoea and septicaemia also occur in older animals (principally ewes).

Unlike human listeriosis, the most commonly recognized form of the disease in animals is as an encephalitis (Barlow and McGorum 1985). In ruminants this takes the form of a unilateral (or, less commonly, bilateral) cranial nerve paralysis affecting the eye, eyelid, ear, and lips (with consequent dropping of cud), which is often followed by ataxia, and moving in circles—hence the name circling disease. The affected animals are dull with the head drooping to one side, sometimes with food or cud hanging from the mouth and, because of the partial paralysis of the pharynx, saliva is often drooled. Animals sometimes stand still, pressing against a fixed object, or appear recumbent. The course of the disease in bovines is quite prolonged (4–14 days), but is much more acute in sheep where death can occur within 4–48 hours. In sheep, the disease can resemble pregnancy toxaemia (ketosis). Encephalitis occurs in older animals (in sheep most often during late pregnancy or soon after lambing) as well as in the young.

Abortion, septicaemia and encephalitis are usually sporadic in cattle, but can occur as outbreaks amongst flocks of sheep where losses may be heavy. During outbreaks, septicaemia and abortion may occur together with cases of encephalitis, but this is unusual. Experimental infection indicates that the septicaemia can develop in a few days after consumption of contaminated feed, but the incubation period for encephalitis is likely to be much longer (20–30 days).

Listeria monocytogenes also causes mastitis in cows, where large numbers of the bacterium can be shed into milk. All four quarters or only one may be affected, and the disease severity can vary markedly, sometimes appearing subclinical. Excretion of the organism into milk can persist for more than 3 years.

Keratoconjunctivitis together with iritis occurs in both sheep and cattle. These conditions are usually unilateral. In cases of conjunctivitis, other bacterial or viral pathogens may also be present on the conjunctiva.

Listeric abortion, septicaemia, and encephalitis have been recognized in pigs, horses, dogs, and cats, but this is rare.

Listeriosis has been reported in more than 20 species of birds. Infection is most often recognized in chickens, turkeys, and ducks. Septicaemia and myocardial necrosis are the most common manifestations, and it has been suggested that these are often secondary to other infections.

Risk factors

Although less commonly associated with predisposing factors (as described for humans) listeriosis in animals does show characteristics of an opportunistic pathogen. The unborn and newly delivered are more susceptible to infection, and encephalitis occurs most often in the adult pregnant animal during the later stages of gestation or shortly after delivery. Outbreaks have been associated with climatic stress (sudden drops in temperature, snow falls, drought, and shortage of food), and cases most often occur in the spring when animals may be in poor condition. Increases in susceptibility of animals to experimental infection have been demonstrated by malnutrition, immunosuppression, viral infection, and other uncharacterized stress factors.

As with humans, the majority of animal listeriosis cases are assumed to be acquired via contaminated feed (a particular risk factor is the consumption of poor-quality silage). This will be outlined in the epizoology section.

Diagnosis and pathology

Diagnosis of abortion is usually achieved by the culturing of fetal organs or stomach contents. The culturing of the organism from placenta may be difficult to interpret in the absence of histological analysis, where necrosis and abscess formation will be observed. The placental lesions are pin-point, yellowish necrotic foci involving the tips of the cotyledonary villi, with a focal to diffuse intercotyledonary placentitis covered in a red/brown exudate. The fetus is usually autolytic with miliary necrotic foci scattered throughout the liver and spleen, although these are not always present. At postmortem, organs from the fetus and the newly delivered (particularly the liver and spleen) should be examined and cultured for the organism. Septicaemia is often accompanied by focal hepatic necrosis (sawdust liver).

Ante-mortem diagnosis of listeric encephalitis is problematic since there are no satisfactory diagnostic tests, and listeric encephalitis may mimic other diseases. Prior to death, L. monocytogenes may be cultured from the brain, but in some cases is absent: the organism is invariably only isolated from the brain and not from other organs. Listeria monocytogenes has been isolated from brains of apparently healthy sheep, but it is not clear how commonly this occurs. However, necropsy samples show a diagnostic pattern of histological changes and this has proved to be the only definitive means of diagnosis. It is essential that histological examination is performed to exclude the possibility of other diseases causing the condition. The typical listeric parenchymal lesions are confined to the brain-stem and medulla, and are composed of microabscesses which begin with collection of neutrophils or microglial cells. Gross pathological lesions are rarely observed. The glial nodules often persist and become infiltrated by macrophages. Adjacent to the lesions is heavy perivascular cuffing composed mainly of lymphocytes and histiocytes in addition to occasional neutrophils and eosinophils. Bacteria, either singly or in small clumps, are sometimes seen near the periphery of the lesions, but not in the perivascular cuffs. Meningitis (affecting the cerebellum and anterior cervical cord), probably developing secondarily to the parenchymal lesions, and neuritis of the trigeminal nerve may also be present. A correlation between the degree of cell-mediated immunity and brain lesion suggests that immunopathological reactions are important components of this condition.

Listeria monocytogenes is probably rare as a cause of mastitis, but should be considered during cultural procedures as part of the investigation of this condition since the organism can be misidentified as a 'diphtheroid' or a streptococcus. Clinically the condition presents with abnormal milk secretion and swelling of the affected quarter(s).

A marked monocytosis is commonly observed in infected rodents, together with focal hepatic necrosis from which the organism can be readily cultured. A diffuse myocardial necrosis is often observed in guinea-pigs.

Listeriosis in birds is characterized by conspicuous lesions of myocardial degeneration and necrosis, with necrotic foci found in the liver, spleen, and lungs from which the organism can be readily cultured. Involvement of the central nervous system also sometimes occurs.

Treatment and prognosis

Because of the disease severity and rapid onset of clinical symptoms, treatment of infected sheep or cattle is rarely attempted: infected animals may be destroyed on humanitarian grounds. During outbreaks in these animals the mortality rates are often 100 per cent, and those surviving can exhibit permanent central nervous system disorders.

As is found with humans, the pregnant dam with an intrauterine infection is rarely accompanied by severe systemic disease so it is not necessary to attempt treatment. A listeric abortion does not seem to affect the possibility of subsequent conception.

The response to antibiotic treatment in cows with listeric mastitis has been poor and the organism can be excreted for extended periods of time. Hence it is recommended that such animals should not be used for milk production and culling should be considered.

DISEASE MECHANISMS

The production of an experimental keratoconjunctivitis (Anton's eye test) performed in either guinea-pigs or rabbits by instilling a live bacterial suspension into the conjunctiva has been used to demonstrate the virulence of L. monocytogenes for the past 60 years. Mice and rabbits are now more frequently used and they suffer an acute fatal infection 1–7 days after a sufficient dose of a virulent strain (usually >10^4 bacteria) is given either intravenously or intraperitoneally. Virulence can be measured by LD_{50}, by the kinetics of growth of the bacterium in tissues, or by the extent of survival in the liver and spleen. Intraperitoneal carrageenan or mineral oil may be given to mice prior to inoculation to increase susceptibility to infection.

Ovine encephalitis accompanied by the characteristic histological features has been experimentally achieved by inoculating the organism into the dental pulp. Histological encephalitis was evident after 6 days, but the onset of clinical neurological disease varied between 20 and 40 days.

Oral inoculation of mice, rats, and guinea-pigs has been reported. Infection showed most consistency in gnotobiotic animals and interference of colonization by the microflora of the gastrointestinal tract has been suggested. Differences have been reported between both strains of *L. monocytogenes* and growth conditions used for the bacteria prior to inoculation which were not apparent when using the intravenous or intraperitoneal route. Oesophageal inoculation of 10^6 *L. monocytogenes* to juvenile rats showed about a 50 per cent infection rate in the liver or spleen. A reduction in the acidity of the stomach by cimetidine treatment reduced the infective dose.

Feeding trials in cynomologous monkeys have been reported, and only those animals receiving 10^9 cells showed fever, septicaemia, loss of appetite, irritability and occasional diarrhoea. Those animals fed up to 10^7 bacteria (some of which were completely asymptomatic) shed the organism in the faeces for up to 21 days.

In chick embryos injected by the intra-allantoic route, the LD_{50} is around 10^2 organisms. Lesions occur in the chorio-allantoic membrane, liver, and heart, and the bacterium can be readily cultured from these sites.

Chronic mastitis can be induced experimentally in cows by intramammary injection. Bacteraemia could not be detected in these animals, and typically 10^3–10^4 *L. monocytogenes*/ml were shed into milk for 9–12 months of the remaining lactation period.

Listeria monocytogenes is able to infect a range of cell types growing *in vitro*, including enterocytes, macrophages, and fibroblasts. The use of such models has contributed much to an understanding of the factors involved in intracellular invasion and growth (see below).

It is a characteristic of the natural disease in both humans and animals in that there is usually a low attack rate. The susceptibility to infection may be increased by external factors, some of which have already been mentioned. However, other factors (such as other infectious agents or products of the metabolism of other micro-organisms) may yet prove to be of importance. *Listeria monocytogenes* is a somewhat marginal pathogen. Hence experimental models reflecting the natural infection may work poorly, and relatively large numbers of animals may be needed for a small proportion of these to produce clinical symptoms of disease.

There is evidence supporting the role of antacid therapy in increasing susceptibility of some patients, and in experimental animal infection. The buffering capacity of some food types may also be of importance in facilitating the survival of the organism, which may then invade at sites further along the gastrointestinal tract, although other routes of infection may occur. Experimental septicaemia in animals can be achieved via the respiratory route, and further evidence supporting this possibility comes from one of the cases (septicaemia and aspiration pneumonia) which developed after eating contaminated coleslaw salad in the 1981 Canadian outbreak (Table 13.1).

Histopathological analysis suggests that the intestinal tract can act as the site of invasion and the M cells overlying the Peyer's patches may act as the site of penetration, although the observation that *L. monocytogenes* (as well as *L. ivanovii*) will readily invade various epithelial and fibroblast cell types growing *in vitro* suggests that there may be multiple routes by which this bacterium initially invades the host's cells. In the caecum and colon of animals following oral inoculation, the bacteria can be observed, together with an inflammatory reaction, in phagocytic cells present in the underlying lamina propria. Following this phase, invasion of the uterine contents or central nervous system (for patients with shorter incubation periods) may occur, probably via the circulatory system.

In the liver, the organism is cleared from the blood by the phagocytic Kupffer cells. In their non-activated state, some bacteria will survive, escape to the cell cytoplasm, and subsequently spread to hepatocytes. Formation of localized lesions occurs in the liver and also in the spleen.

Intrauterine infection of the fetus results from haematogenous spread from the mother. Abscess formation takes place in the placenta, and this may spread via the umbilical vein or the amniotic fluid to the fetal internal organs. The series of pyrexial episodes observed in the mother may result from re-invasion of maternal bloodstream from placental sites. *Listeria monocytogenes* is unusual in that it is able to survive and grow in amniotic fluid, and aspiration of this leads to the pathological changes in the fetal respiratory tracts. The presence of high numbers of the organism in amniotic fluid results in widespread contamination of neonatal and maternal surface sites at delivery, as well as the postnatal environment, and may results in cases of neonatal cross-infection.

Experimental and field studies suggest that encephalitis in sheep and cattle results from *L. monocytogenes* reaching the base of the brain along cranial nerves, particularly the trigeminal nerve. It is assumed that animals eat contaminated feed, particularly silage, and the organism enters the nerves after penetrating the oral mucus membrane or through pre-existing areas of trauma such as tooth root scars (which are prominent in sheep during the spring). The mechanism for travel along nerves is not understood, and it has not been established whether the polymerization of actin is involved (see below).

Listerial genes involved with invasion and intracellular movement in mammalian cells are shown in Fig. 13.1. The cell surface listerial protein internalin is involved with the initial stages of invasion and binds to the mammalian cell surface protein, E-cadherin. Subsequently, *L. monocytogenes* becomes encapsulated in a membrane bound compartment, which it dissolves by the action of the listeriolysin (and possibly also the phospholipase). The bacterium then enters into the cytoplasm where it multiplies and becomes surrounded by polymerized host cell actin. The actin is preferentially polymerized on the older pole of the bacterium by the ActA cell surface protein. This polymerization confers intracellular mobility to the bacterium and allows invasion of adjacent mammalian cells. The bacterium is then encapsulated in a double membrane bound compartment which is dissolved by the action of the lecithinase activated by the metalloprotease (although the listeriolysin and phospholipase may also be involved) and the whole process is repeated. Three further open reading frames of unknown function (ORF X, Y, and Z) are located adjacent to the p1cB gene. These genes are all regulated by the positive regulation factor (prfA gene, marked by a '+' on Fig. 13.1). The operon containing the internalin genes are locatd quite close to the other above mentioned genes on the bacterial chromosome.

It is of note that all the above-mentioned genes (or a very similar set) are present in *L. ivanovii*, which follows the same general pattern of cellular invasion and movement. Unlike *L. monocytogenes*, *L. ivanovii* does not cause plaque formation in fibroblasts growing *in vitro*, and it has been suggested that the lower virulence of the latter species may be related to lack of as yet uncharacterized cytotoxic factors. There is evidence supporting the presence of these genes in *L. seeligeri*, although it is only weakly invasive to mammalian cells. It is not clear whether *L. seeligeri* also lacks additional virulence factors or if these genes are poorly functional. An alternative explanation may be that *L. seeligeri* is adapted to survive in quite different eukaryotic environments.

Regulation of the genes involved with the virulence of *L. monocytogenes* is under the control of the positive regulation factor (prfA) gene product, and six promoters have been identified which interact with this protein (marked by '+' on Fig. 13.1), including a promoter for its own production. Listeriolysin is one of the major extracellular proteins produced by *L. monocytogenes* under conditions of heat shock, and there is evidence to suggest that some of the above-mentioned genes are also regulated by the stage of the cell cycle and temperature. Recent work has shown that the disaccharide cellobiose represses the expression of the listeriolysin and phospholipase genes by an as yet uncharacterized mechanism. It is tempting to speculate that the absence of this environmentally ubiquitous plant-derived molecule allows the induction of genes as a pathogenic response to the environment of eukaryotic cells.

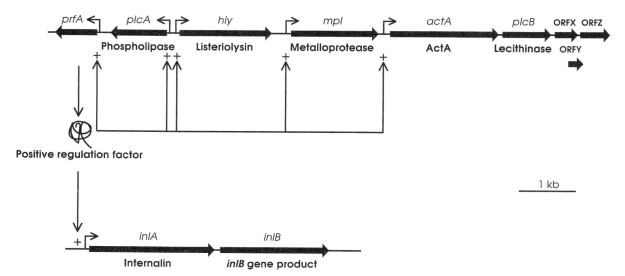

Fig. 13.1 Regulation of genes involved with the virulence of *L. monocytogenes*. The cell cycle, temperature, and cellobiose are also involved in gene regulation.

Listeria monocytogenes is an intracellular parasite, and it is in this environment that the pathogen gains protection and evades some of the host's defences. However, the host has a number of strategies to deal with such parasites. For a full account of this process, see Kaufmann (1993).

EPIDEMIOLOGY

The widespread distribution of *L. monocytogenes* provides numerous potential ways in which the disease may be transmitted to both animals and humans (Schuchat *et al.* 1991). Although there has been much current interest in infection via the oral route, this is not the only mode of transmission (Fig. 13.2).

The peak in the incidence of human listeriosis most often occurs at the end of the summer and early in the autumn. The reasons for this are not understood. Animal listeriosis principally occurs in the spring. This is probably not only because of the physiology and condition of the animals, but also because of the provision of poorly prepared food.

The reported incidence of human listeriosis varies between countries, in the range of less than 1 to more than 7 cases per million of the total population. Although these in part may reflect differences in sur-

veillance systems, they probably represent true differences in incidence. There are similar differences in the incidence of animal listeriosis in different regions: for example in the United Kingdom, listeriosis in sheep is a particular problem in Scotland and the north of England. These differences may in part be due to the ability to produce good-quality feed.

TRANSMISSION OF LISTERIOSIS IN HUMANS

Direct contact with infected animals

Listeriosis rarely may be transmitted by direct contact with infected animals or animal material. In such cases the disease occurs principally as papular or pustular cutaneous lesions, usually on the upper arms or wrists of farmers or veterinarians 1–4 days after attending bovine abortions. Since listeric infection is more common in sheep than cows, it is remarkable that such infections do not occur in association with sheep. However, the duration of manipulation and extent of skin exposure is greater when dealing with bovines abortions (McLauchlin and Low 1994).

Listeria monocytogenes is widespread in the environment and superficial infections in humans from other sources are rare. This observation, together with the likelihood that extremely high levels of *L. monocytogenes* (10^8 cfu/ml) occur in infected bovine amniotic fluid

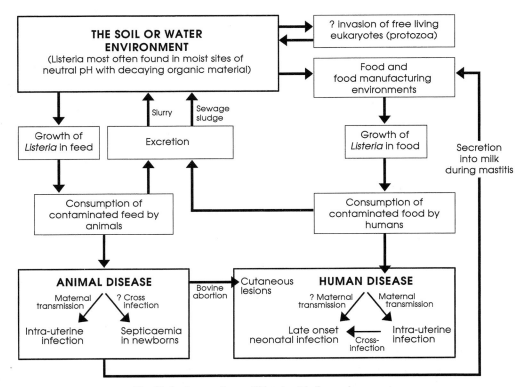

Fig. 13.2 Interactions of *Listeria* with the environment.

(as are found during intrauterine infection in humans), suggests that the infective dose for human cutaneous listeriosis is high.

Although cutaneous listeriosis in adults is invariably a mild infection with a successful resolution (even without antimicrobial therapy), systemic involvement is suggested in some cases by fever and tenderness of the axillary lymph nodes. Indeed, brucellosis has been considered as a differential cause in some cases. Furthermore, cases have also been described of acute meningitis in farmers after assisting at bovine abortions, although in these instances the route of infection is unclear.

Conjunctivitis in poultry workers has also been reported.

Cross-infection during the neonatal period

Hospital cross-infection between newborn infants occurs and these follow the pattern of congenital listeriosis (onset within 1 day of birth). In the same hospital, and within a short period of time, an apparently healthy (or more rarely more than one) neonate is born who typically develops late-onset listeriosis between the fifth and twelfth day after delivery. The same strain of *L. monocytogenes* is isolated from both infants and the mother of the late-onset case, but not from mother of the late-onset case. In most of the episodes, the cases are either delivered or nursed in the same or adjacent rooms, and consequently staff and equipment are common to both. Two larger series have been described occurring in Sweden and Costa Rica, where four and seven cases, respectively, resulted from single early onset cases (Bortolussi and Seeliger 1990). The likely source of infection involved a contaminated rectal thermometer and a mineral oil bath. In one episode, true person to person transmission occurred when, 3 days after delivery, the mother of an early onset case was nursed in an open ward and handled a neonate from an adjacent bed who subsequently developed late-onset listeriosis.

There is little evidence for cross-infection or person to person transmission outside the neonatal period.

Food-borne transmission

It is now generally agreed that the consumption of contaminated foods is the principal route of transmission for this disease: microbiological and epidemiological evidence supports an association with many food types (dairy, meat, vegetable, fish, and shellfish) in both sporadic and epidemic listeriosis (Tables 13.1 and 13.2) (WHO 1988; Miller *et al.* 1990; Schuchat *et al.* 1992). Although diverse in their constituents and manufacturing processes, foods associated with transmission often show the following common features: the capability of supporting the multiplication of *L. monocytogenes* (relatively high water activity and near-neutral

pH); relatively heavy ($>$g10^3/g) contamination with the implicated strain; processed with an extended (refrigerated) shelf-life; and consumed without further cooking. One food (alfalfa tablets), was quite disparate in that it was a dry product in which *L. monocytogenes* would not be able to grow. However, one of the ingredients (alfalfa) did show similar properties to that described above in that prior to drying and encapsulation it had been stored wet where deterioration, and presumably growth of *L. monocytogenes*, had occurred.

The incubation period from food-borne infection varies widely between individuals from 1 up to 90 days, with an average for intrauterine infection of around 30 days. It is not known whether these differences after oral ingestion are dose- or strain-dependent, or perhaps reflect unknown differences in host susceptibility. Based on data from a very small number of cases, high levels of *L. monocytogenes* (10^3–$>10^7$/g) have been found in foods consumed by patients prior to infection, suggesting that the infective dose is high. However, much caution is needed here since the infective dose is likely to vary greatly between individuals. In addition, suspect foods are generally only available for examination for relatively short periods and hence will be more likely to be collected from patients showing short incubation periods. These observations, together with the ability of *L. monocytogenes* to multiply in foods (even under ideal storage conditions) means that there are considerable difficulties in ascribing a 'safe' level of *L. monocytogenes* in food for regulatory purposes.

As has already been stated, *L. monocytogenes* is widespread in the environment, including food, although it is generally present in relatively low numbers. This feature, together with the properties and types of foods associated with transmission of infection (Tables 13.1 and 13.3), also support the likelihood of a high infective dose for infection through food.

Outbreaks of human listeriosis involving $>$100 individuals have been recognized (Table 13.1). Some outbreaks have continued over long periods of 6 months to 5 years, probably explained by long-term colonization of a single site in the food-manufacturing environment, as well as the long incubation periods shown by some patients. Sites of *L. monocytogenes* contamination within food-processing facilities involved in human infection have included wooden manufacturing equipment, wooden and metallic shelving, porous conveyor belts, cool-room condensates, and floor drains. *Listeria monocytogenes* has been shown to survive well in a variety of environments where food is manufactured, particulary those that are moist with organic material, and it is from such sites that contamination of food occurs during processing.

A comparison between the numbers of foods containing *L. monocytogenes* and the number of listeriosis

Table 13.3 Sporadic cases of food-borne human listeriosis

Country	Year	Implicated food
USA	1985	Turkey frankfurters
England	1986	Soft cheese
England	1988	Soft cheese
England	1988	Cooked chicken
England	1988	Rennet
Canada	1989	Alfalfa tablets
USA	1989	Sausage
Finland	1989	Salted mushrooms
Italy	1989	Sausage
Italy	1989	Fish
Denmark	1989	Smoked cod roe
Canada	1989	Soft cheese
Belgium	1989	Fresh cream and ice-cream
Italy	1994	Pickled olives

cases indicates that most contaminated foods (even those associated with outbreaks) have very low attack rates for infection. Some strains of *L. monocytogenes* may be of higher pathogenicity, although the basis for this is poorly understood.

Given the properties and distribution of *L. monocytogenes*, cases related by a common source may be very widely distributed both temporally and geographically. Some food-borne listeriosis outbreaks were recognized under highly unusual circumstances, and it is likely that even despite national and international surveillance systems, common source outbreaks will be unrecognized.

TRANSMISSION OF LISTERIOSIS IN ANIMALS

Abortion and septicaemia in newborn animals is clearly a result of an intrauterine infection acquired from the dam, and parallels abortion and early onset neonatal infection in humans. Septicaemia (also with meningitis in some animals) in lambs in the first few weeks of life has been attributed to umbilical infection acquired in lambing pens, possibly from contaminated soil or feed: this corresponds to late-onset neonatal infection in humans.

Iritis and keratoconjunctivitis usually occur during the winter in silage-fed sheep and cattle. These may occur by direct introduction of contaminated feed into the eye, and have been particularly associated where feed is provided in holders or racks at eye level.

As in human infection, the majority of cases of animal listeriosis are assumed to be acquired via the oral route. There is a strong association between the feeding of silage and all manifestations of listeriosis in sheep and cattle, although cases do occur where silage has not been used. However, the exact mechanism by which silage feeding leads or predisposes to listeriosis is not clear. Under normal conditions it is impossible to

produce silage free of *Listeria*: the organism has been isolated from silage with a pH of less than 4, albeit in very low numbers. However, where poor-quality silage has been produced and a low pH and anaerobic conditions are not achieved, proliferation of *Listeria* takes place and very high numbers can be found. Poor quality is often also due to insufficient herbage quality, or to contamination by soil or faeces. The recent change to production of silage in polythene bales ('big bale' silage) has seen a corresponding increase in ovine listeriosis in the United Kingdom. Although the big bale method is more economical than the traditional use of clamps, these are more prone to spoilage and growth of *Listeria*: high numbers of the organism are often associated with sites where damage to the bags has occurred or at the tied end. The peak in the numbers of animal listeriosis in the spring may reflect a decrease in the quality of silage used for feed. The observation that listeriosis is often associated with poor-quality silage where high numbers of *L. monocytogenes* occur suggests that the infective dose is high.

It has been suggested that silage may have an immunosuppressive effect, but the mechanism of this has not been characterized.

RELATIONSHIP BETWEEN ANIMAL AND HUMAN LISTERIOSIS AND INTERACTIONS OF LISTERIA WITH THE ENVIRONMENT

The possible routes of infection in both human and animal disease are represented in Fig. 13.2. For both humans and animals most infection probably results from ingestion of food or feed where excessive proliferation of *L. monocytogenes* has occurred.

It is not clear what proportion of all the strains of *L. monocytogenes* and *L. ivanovii* in the environment cause disease, and why *L. ivanovii* is such a very rare pathogen for humans. Although some non-pathogenic cultures of *L. monocytogenes* have been identified, experimental infection of animals (albeit with rather 'un-natural' models) have not indicated much variation in virulence. However, the distribution of 'types' of *L. monocytogenes* usually varies between cultures isolated from the environment and those causing disease. The proportion of *L. monocytogenes* types is significantly different between syndromes in both humans and animals. In addition, the majority of the strains responsible for the apparently unrelated large food-borne outbreaks of human listeriosis have been unexpectedly similar. The significance of these three observations is not clear; however, they may be reflecting adaptions by strains (or species) to different environmental niches which affect virulence.

Apart from human infection acquired as a direct result of attending infected animals or from food directly contaminated from an infected animal (as may be the case with milk from an animal with listerial mastitis), it is unclear what, if any, are the connections between human and animal listeriosis. Analysis of strains causing 'sporadic' human and animal listeriosis indicates a wide range of 'types' in both groups which do not generally appear to be related. The seasonal peaks in human and animal listeriosis do not coincide, also suggesting that these two groups are not causally related. This perhaps should not be unexpected of a group of marginal pathogens which are probably not host adapted and which occur widely in the environment as many different types.

Listeria monocytogenes and *L. ivanovii* are members of a group of bacteria which are adapted to saprophytic environments in soil or water and have additional adaptions to survive in eukaryotic intracellular environments. Quite how these additional factors have evolved is not clear. It may be these factors evolved for survival in mammals, or for a quite different group of eukaryotes, such as free-living protozoa.

PREVENTION AND CONTROL

Manufacturers of food and food-processing equipment should be aware of the properties of *Listeria* (Ryser and Marth 1991). The design of the factory and equipment should facilitate cleaning and sanitizing to reduce the possibility of contamination and colonization with *L. monocytogenes*. Producers, shippers, and retailers of perishable foods must utilize good refrigeration and shelf-life control, together with adequate packaging and consumer advice, including 'sell by' and 'consume by' dates and proper storage conditions. Application of a HACCP (Hazard Analysis Critical Control Point) programme or a similar comprehensive assessment and control scheme is advised for both the safety and quality of the final product. Over the past decade, the food industry in Europe and North America has been active in investigating *Listeria* in foods and the factory environment, in implementing hazard analysis, and establishing codes of practice, and there is evidence to suggest that some foods have improved in microbiological quality during this time.

Because *L. monocytogenes* is a potential pathogen, and the detection of other species of *Listeria* can indicate environmental contamination (especially in those foods which have undergone a listericidal process), the ideal should be to exclude all *Listeria* from food, and this should be pursued vigorously. The achievement of this objective is probably impractical for all foods, and is clearly unattainable for raw foods or those which have not undergone a listericidal process. The response by national regulatory authorities in various countries to the presence of *L. monocytogenes* in foods on retail sale has varied from a total exclusion in certain foods (as has been the policy in the United States and in some EU legislation), to a tolerance of some contamination (as is the policy in Britain).

Listeria monocytogenes can multiply (albeit slowly) at refrigeration temperatures, hence it is not only important to exclude the organism from foods, but also to inhibit its multiplication and survival. This problem can be addressed by improving legislation on temperature and shelf-life control. It is now possible to assess levels of *Listeria* in foods, and this provides additional valuable information on its microbiological quality, in that higher counts are more likely to reflect abuse with respect to hygiene, shelf-life, and temperature of storage.

To avoid listeriosis and other food-borne infections, the general public should be educated about the use of good food and personal hygiene practices from the time the food is purchased to consumption. This includes avoiding cross-contamination between raw and cooked foods, properly maintaining refrigerators, and not over-extending the normal shelf-life of foods. Since *Listeria* are widely distributed in the environment, total avoidance and complete elimination of *L. monocytogenes* from all food is not possible, and it is likely that all individuals will be exposed to *Listeria* at some time. However, pregnant women and immunocompromised individuals are at increased risk of contracting listeriosis. In a number of countries (including the United Kingdom, United States, France, New Zealand, and parts of Australia) 'at-risk' individuals are advised to take special precautions. Processed and ready-to-eat foods such as soft and surface-ripened cheese and pate have been identified as being particularly hazardous, and general advice has been issued in England and Wales for vulnerable individuals not to consume these. Further general advice was issued in the United States to avoid other types of soft cheese (feta and Mexican-style), to avoid delicatessen-type foods and to reheat 'cold cut' type meats. In the light of the recent outbreaks in Australasia, it might also be prudent to include advice to avoid types of cooked and ready-to-eat fish and seafood.

Susceptible individuals should avoid consuming raw or inadequately cooked meat and seafoods, wash fruits and vegetables to be consumed raw, and thoroughly re-heat all pre-cooked and 'leftover' foods before consumption, especially highly processed ready-to-eat meals.

Unexplained influenza-like illness in pregnant women and the immunocompromised should be investigated by blood cultures. In addition, those individuals attending infected animals should be aware of the possibility of cutaneous or ocular listeriosis, and should also seek medical attention if suspect lesions develop. It may also be prudent to advise the pregnant and immunosuppressed not to help with lambing, milk ewes that have recently given birth, touch the afterbirth, or come into contact with newborn lambs. This clearly represents a potential route of infection, although with the exception of the cutaneous and ocular lesions, significant associations have not been observed between listeriosis cases and rural backgrounds.

To prevent cross-infection during the neonatal period, strict infection control measures must be instigated at the time of delivery. Such measures include barrier nursing, use of heat-sterilized or single-use equipment, single use barriers and alcohol wipes for surfaces, and the wearing of gloves and aprons which are changed prior to hand washing and attending other patients.

Because human listeriosis is a rare disease, surveillance schemes and epidemiological investigations of cases are essential to identify clusters of patients related by common source and vehicles of infection. The use of case-control studies to investigate outbreaks of listeriosis has had mixed success, and common source outbreaks may only be recognized by collection of isolates from infected patients and identification of common strains. Since *L. monocytogenes* is widespread in the environment (including foods), it is important that comparisons of isolates are made using discriminatory typing schemes. Subtyping methods applied to *L. monocytogenes* have included: serotyping, bacteriocine typing, plasmid analysis, phage typing, DNA restriction fragment analysis (including pulsed field gel electrophoresis), random amplification of polymorphic DNA analysis, and multilocus enzyme electrophoresis. Traditional methods of analysis have involved serotyping and phage typing, although a combination of these with molecular methods or multilocus enzyme electrophoresis offers much higher discrimination. To utilize these systems, considerable investment in time, personnel, and equipment is required, and these are practicable only in laboratories such as national reference centres with a particular interest in *Listeria*.

To prevent listeriosis in animals, attention should be paid to feeds, especially to silage, as has already been discussed. Live attenuated vaccines have been developed for use in animals and it is claimed that this offers some protection, although results of field trails are equivocal. However, with the revolution in the understanding of the process of pathogenesis of this organism and interactions with the host's cell-mediated immunity, together with the ability to genetically manipulate *Listeria*, it seems likely that this will be an area of active investigation in the future.

ACKNOWLEDGEMENTS

The authors gratefully acknowledge the help of Dr J. C. Low (Scottish Agriculture College Veterinary Services, Edinburgh) for advice on the veterinary aspects of listeriosis.

REFERENCES

Barlow, R. M. and McGorum, B. (1985). Ovine listerial encephalitis: analysis, hypothesis and synthesis. *Veterinary Record*, **116**, 233–6.

Bortolussi, R. and Seeliger, H. P. R. (1990). Listeriosis. In *Infectious diseases of the fetus and newborn infant*, (ed. J. S. Remington and J. O. Klein), (3rd edn), pp. 812–33. Saunders, Philadelphia.

Burn, C. G. (1936). Clinical and pathological features of an infection caused by a new pathogen of the genus *Listerella*. *American Journal of Pathology*, **12**, 341–8.

Dramsi, S., Lebrun, M., and Cossart, P. (1996). Molecular and genetic determinants involved in invasion of mammalian cells by *Listeria monocytogenes*. In *Current topics in microbiology and immunology*, Vol. 209, (ed. V. L. Miller), pp. 61–71. Springer, Berlin.

Farber, J. M. and Peterkin, P. I. (1991). *Listeria monocytogenes*, a food-borne pathogen. *Microbiological Reviews*, **55**, 476–511.

Gellin, B. G. and Broome, C. V. (1989). Listeriosis. *Journal of the American Medical Association*, **261**, 1313–20.

Gill, D. A. (1933) Circling disease: A meningoencephalitis of sheep in New Zealand. *Veterinary Journal*, **89**, 258–70.

Gitter, M. (1989). Veterinary aspects of listeriosis. *PHLS Microbiology Digest*, **6**, 38–42.

Gray, M. L. and Killinger, A. H. (1966). *Listeria monocytogenes* and listeric infections. *Bacteriological Reviews*, **30**, 309–82.

Jones, D. (1990). Foodborne listeriosis. *Lancet*, **336**, 1171–4.

Kaufmann, S. H. E. (1993). Immunity to intracellular bacteria. *Annual Review of Immunology*, **11**, 129–63.

Low, J. C. and Donachie, W. (1997) A review of *Listeria monocytogenes* and listeriosis. *Veterinary Journal*, **153**, 9–29.

McLauchlin, J. and Low, J. C. (1994). Primary cutaneous listeriosis in adults: An occupational disease of veterinarians and farmers. *Veterinary Record*, **24**, 615–17.

Miller, A. L., Smith, J. L., and Somkuti, G. A. (ed.) (1990). *Foodborne listeriosis*. Elsevier, Amsterdam.

Murray, E. G. D., Webb, R. A., and Swann, M. B. R. (1926) A disease of rabbits characterised by a large mononuclear leucocytosis, caused by a hitherto undescribed bacillus *Bacterium monocytogenes* (n.sp.). *Journal of Pathology and Bacteriology*, **29**, 407–39.

Nyfeldt, A. (1929). Etiologie de la mononucleose infectieuse. *Comptes rendus des séances de la Société de Biologie*, **101**, 590–1.

Pirie, J. H. H. (1927). A New disease of veld rodents, 'Tiger River Disease'. *Publications of the South African Institute for Medical Research*, **3**, 163–86.

Portnoy, D. A., Chakraborty, T., Goebel, W., and Cossart, P. (1992). Molecular determinants of *Listeria monocytogenes* pathogenesis. *Infection and Immunity*, **60**, 1263–7.

Ryser, E. T. and Marth, E. H. (1991). *Listeria, listeriosis, and food safety*. Marcel Dekker, New York.

Schuchat, A., Swaminathan, B., and Broome, C. V. (1991). Epidemiology of Human Listeriosis. *Clinical Microbiology Reviews*, **4**, 169–83.

Schuchat, A. *et al.* (1992). Role of foods in sporadic listeriosis: 1. Case-control study of dietary risk factors. *Journal of the American Medical Association*, **267**, 2041–5.

Sheehan, B., Kocks, C., Dramsi, S., Gouin, E., Klarsfeld, A. D., and Mengaud, J. (1994). Molecular determinants of the *Listeria monocytogenes* infectious process. *Current Topics in Microbiology and Immunology*, **192**, 187–216.

WHO Working Group (1988). Foodborne listeriosis. *Bulletin of the WHO*, **66**, 421–8.

14 LYME DISEASE

Dennis J. White

SUMMARY

Lyme disease is caused by infection with the spirochete *Borrelia burgdorferi* and is transmitted to humans through the bite of an infected tick of the *Ixodes ricinus* complex, especially *Ix. scapularis*, *Ix. pacificus*, *Ix. ricinus* and *Ix. persulcatus*. *Borrelia burgdorferi* infection is acquired by immature *Ixodes ricinus* complex ticks, from infected small mammal reservoirs, a cycle responsible for the maintenance of this disease in nature. Prolonged feeding of infected nymphal, or occasionally adult, ticks on a human, can result in disease. Disease is manifested through pathological effects on any of several systems, including the skin, the nervous system, the heart, the musculoskeletal system, and the patient's state of emotional health. This spirochaetal disease is common in the United States and Europe, and is seen in increasing frequency on other continents. Although known historically by other names, Lyme disease is only now receiving a surge of research and clinical interest in many areas of the world. Until effective means of tick population control, or an effective human vaccine, become available, control of this disease relies upon education and prevention.

HISTORY

The recent characterization of the disease referred to as Lyme arthritis in the fall of 1975, following a cluster of childhood arthritis cases in Connecticut, has led to significant medical, epidemiological, ecological, and biological research (Steere *et al.* 1984). This initial cluster of cases, however, was preceded by a description of erythema chronicum migrans (ECM) in 1970 in Wisconsin. Investigation of this unusual concentration of cases with childhood arthritic symptoms in the Lyme, Old Lyme, and East Haddam areas of southern Connecticut, was prompted by expressed concerns of parents. Investigators from the Connecticut State Health Department and Yale University were asked to determine reasons for the apparent abnormal incidence of a cluster of 'juvenile rheumatoid arthritis'. Snydman, from the Connecticut State Health Department, and Steere, a Rheumatology Fellow at

Yale University, began a series of investigations (Steere *et al.* 1978.)

They developed a surveillance system to review information from a variety of resources, including parents, school nurses, physicians, and local health officers. Initial efforts were focused on identifying children with inflammatory joint disease as well as other family members who may have experienced similar disorders. Thirty-nine children and twelve adults were found to be affected with recurrent attacks of swelling and pain in the large joints, especially the knee, within this initial geographic focus. Incidence rates were far above that expected for juvenile rheumatoid arthritis and cases appeared to be clustered by space and time. Onsets of illness were predominantly during the summer and early fall. Families with more than one affected member reported onsets of illness in separate years. This information led to the suspicion that an arthropod vector was involved.

In fact, 25 per cent of the patients reported a history of an erythematous lesion they considered to be an insect bite prior to the onset of arthritic symptoms. The initial bite reaction expanded into large, red, annular lesions over a several-week period. Reviews of the medical literature led the investigators to relate these histories to descriptions of ECM reported in Europe in the early 1900s (Hellerstrom 1951). However, the European literature described the ECM reaction as a response to the bites of *Ix. ricinus* ticks with associated neurological sequelae rather than the arthritic sequelae observed in the Connecticut patients. The disease was referred to as Bannwarth syndrome or Garin–Bujadoux syndrome, and reflected the spectrum of symptoms related to infection. Afzelius reported in 1909 on the development of a red, expanding rash that persisted several weeks to months in association with the bites of sheep ticks, *Ix. ricinus*, in Switzerland. He referred to this rash as erythema chronicum migrans, yet an infectious aetiology was not established at that time (Afzelius 1910).

The disease syndrome observed in Connecticut was referred to as 'Lyme arthritis'. Within a very short time, investigations led to the further association of other disease symptoms in patients with reported 'Lyme arthritis'. In addition to the development of arthritic symptoms, some of these patients also developed neurological and cardiac symptoms. Since the syndrome now was found to affect several systems, the name of the disease was changed to 'Lyme disease' (Andriole 1989).

ORGANISM

Much of the research conducted to identify the disease agent coincided with efforts to determine the potential vector(s) as well as the natural cycle of the disease. Spielman and colleagues in Massachusetts had reviewed populations of ticks of the *Ixodes* genus and found morphological differences within populations of east coast communities of *Ixodes scapularis* ticks. These ticks were found abundantly in foci on Long Island and offshore islands of the north-eastern United States. On the basis of these structural and other behavioural differences, Spielman *et al.* renamed the northern deer tick as *Ixodes dammini* in 1979. Investigators in the north-east were reviewing the role of this tick as the vector of *Babesia microti*, the agent responsible for human babesiosis in the north-east, concurrent with the medical investigations in Connecticut on Lyme arthritis.

Epidemiological investigations in Connecticut coincided with these surveys of arthropod populations which had a potential for disease transmission in the north-east. Entomological surveys in the early 1980s provided information that deer ticks, then known as *Ixodes dammini*, were extremely prevalent in the area where Lyme disease patients lived. In fact, immature *I. dammini* as parasites on mice were found to be 13 times more prevalent, and adult *I. dammini* as parasites on deer to be 16 times more prevalent on the eastern side of the Connecticut River than on the western side. This coincided with epidemiological information that pointed to the eastern side of the Connecticut River where Lyme disease incidence rates were 30 times higher than on the western side (Steere *et al.* 1978).

During the 1970s and 1980s, investigators in New York, as well as in other states of the north-east, were investigating other tick-borne diseases, including Rocky Mountain spotted fever (RMSF) and human babesiosis. Benach, an investigator working with the New York State Department of Health on Long Island, had been collaborating with Burgdorfer at Rocky Mountain Laboratories, of the National Institutes of Health in Hamilton, Montana, on the rickettsial agent of RMSF and other potential vector species, such as the deer tick. It was during this collaborative effort studying *I. dammini* ticks, provided by Benach from Shelter Island, Long Island, New York, that Burgdorfer and A Barbour isolated a previously unrecognized spirochaete (Burgdorfer *et al.* 1982). This spirochaete was subsequently isolated from the blood and cerebro-

spinal fluids of Lyme disease patients in the laboratories of Benach and Steere, conclusively proving the etiology (Benach *et al.* 1983). Patients from which spirochaetes were isolated were also subsequently shown to have IgM and IgG serological reactivity to the spirochaete. Johnson, from the University of Minnesota named the spirochete *Borrelia burgdorferi* (Johnson *et al.* 1984).

In 1993, Oliver at the Georgia Southern University, on the basis of cross-breeding experiments between the northern and southern populations of *Ixodes scapularis* (including representatives of populations that had been renamed *Ixodes dammini*), reported that these populations were able to interbreed and produce viable progeny over several generations. This called into question whether the previous distinction of *I. dammini* as a separate species was appropriate.

In the western United States, *Ixodes pacificus*, the western black-legged tick, is responsible for Lyme disease transmission. The disease is transmitted in the eastern and upper mid-western United States by *Ixodes scapularis*. *Ixodes persulcatus* ticks are responsible for Lyme disease transmission in Asia. Each of these tick species is part of the *Ixodes ricinus* complex. *Ixodes ricinus* is responsible for Lyme disease transmission throughout Europe. *Borrelia burgdorferi* has been found in other tick genera and other biting arthropods, but the roles of these arthropods as actual vectors of the spirochaete are not understood. The syndrome now known generically as Lyme disease has been reported in several areas throughout Asia, Australia, England, Europe, Mexico, North America, Russia, and South Africa.

Heterogeneity of *B. burgdorferi* from different areas of the world could explain apparent differences seen in the clinical presentations of Lyme disease in Europe and America. *Borrelia garinii* and *Borrelia afzelii* in Europe have been identified as separate genospecies from *B. burgdorferi sensu stricto* and may be associated with other types of clinical manifestations apparently more common in Europe than in the United States. Although only *B. burgdorferi* has been identified in North America, all three genospecies have been found in Europe.

DISEASE AGENT

TAXONOMY

In 1981, the spirochaete now known to cause Lyme disease was isolated from *Ix. scapularis* ticks collected from Shelter Island, New York (Burgdorfer *et al.* 1982). The order Spirochaetales is comprised of two families (Spirochaetaceae and Leptospiraceae) and only six genera (*Serpulina*, *Cristispira*, *Spirochaeta*, *Treponema*, *Borrelia*, and *Leptospira*). The genera *Borrelia*, *Leptospira*, and *Treponema* contain species pathogenic for humans and animals. With the identification of two new *Borrelia* species in Europe in the early 1990s—*Borrelia garinii* and *Borrelia afzelii*—there are now 23 recognized species of *Borrelia*. As yet, *Borrelia burgdorferi sensu stricto* is the only genospecies found in North America, while all three genospecies have been found in Europe (Ginsberg 1993).

Spirochaetes are helically shaped bacteria with a very distinct anatomy and motility. As is true for all spirochaetes, the *Borrelia* have a protoplasmic cylinder consisting of the peptidoglycan layer, cytoplasmic membrane and cytoplasmic contents, and periplasmic flagella between the protoplasmic cylinder and a loosely associated outer envelope. The periplasmic flagella are attached subterminally at each end of the protoplasmic cylinder and extend toward the opposite end of the cell. The *Borrelia* are longer and more loosely coiled than the other spirochaetes. Basic morphological features of the Borreliae include a helical shape, roughly 0.2–0.5 μm in diameter and 3–30 μm in length, with 3–10 loose coils along the length of the cell. Of the *Borrelia* species, *Borrelia burgdorferi* is the longest and narrowest and has fewest flagella (7–11). The periplasmic flagella are responsible for the distinct flexing type of motility found in spirochaetes.

MOLECULAR BIOLOGY

The *B. burgdorferi* strain initially isolated from the Shelter Island *Ix. scapularis* deer ticks was designated B31. This strain was shown to have two dominant outer surface proteins with molecular weights of roughly 31 and 34 kDa, referred to as Outer surface protein A and B, or OspA and OspB. There is also a prominent 66 kDa polypeptide and a 41 kDa flagellar antigen. Other immunodominant antigens have been identified with further technical refinements and intensive molecular investigations. Since serological testing depends on the detection of specific antibody binding, recent molecular biology research efforts have focused on the identification of other antigenic components of *B. burgdorferi*. A number of investigators have noted prominent host antibody responses to other proteins, ranging in molecular weight from 20, 39, 60, 68, 71, 73, 83, to 93 kDa. Many of these proteins may be shared with other spirochaetes, which can result in some degree of cross-reactivity in serological analyses. In contrast, the OspA and OspB proteins are specific for *B. burgdorferi*, but a humoral response to these antigens may occur in only a small proportion of patients. Several of the genes coding for these antigens have been cloned and sequenced. This will permit a further understanding of their pathogenic and immunogenic characteristics.

Knowledge about the molecular biology of *B. burgdorferi* has grown exponentially in recent years, with new proteins identified, characterized, and sequenced. New spirochaetal strains are being identified on a regular basis, rendering any attempt to summarize such an active research field in a review text a rather difficult task. Application of this rapidly evolving information may allow for the development of new highly sensitive and highly specific diagnostic tools. The question of which spirochaetal nucleotide sequences code for the production of antigens responsible for the specific pathogenic effects on different target human systems or the sequence of symptoms may be answered in the near future. The role of non-protein antigens of *B. burgdorferi* also needs to be further elucidated.

DISEASE MECHANISMS

Pathogenesis of Lyme disease remains controversial. Early localized illness is primarily a manifestation of infection, while late disseminated and chronic manifestations may be due to a combination of infectious and autoimmune pathology or to autoimmune mechanisms alone. Tissue damage and disease manifestations may be a result of the complex interactions of cells of the immune system and humoral factors such as interleukins, circulating immune factors, prostaglandins, or collagenases. B-cell and T-cell lymphocytes proliferate in a wide variety of organ systems, and infiltrations of lymphocytes can be associated with increases of macrophages, dendritic immune cells, and tissue mast cells. Visceral damage is due to inflammation caused by an interaction of cellular and humoral factors in response to antigenic components of the spirochaetes.

GROWTH AND SURVIVAL REQUIREMENTS

The borreliae are fastidious, microaerophilic bacteria that grow best at 33 °C in a complex liquid medium referred to as modified Barbour–Stoenner–Kelly (BSK) medium. Although it is difficult to isolate *B. burgdorferi* from patients, it is relatively easy to isolate the spirochaete from ticks. Relative to other bacteria, *B. burgdorferi* grows very slowly, with binary fission occurring after a 12–24-hour period. This spirochaete will lose infectivity for laboratory animals after prolonged *in vitro* culture.

HOSTS

There is an extensive literature describing Lyme disease in domestic pets such as cats and dogs, as well as in livestock, especially in the United States. Some of the clinical work on veterinary aspects of Lyme disease has relied on serological tests demonstrating antibodies to *B. burgdorferi*. Since investigators are uncertain of the significance of such antibodies in the animal host, and clinical and exposure information are incomplete and inconsistent, the following information concentrates on human aspects of Lyme disease.

INCUBATION PERIOD

In general terms, if a patient develops symptoms in response to an infected tick bite, the dermatological signs may occur 3–30 days after the tick bite. Flu-like or virus-like illness may accompany the skin lesion or independently develop weeks to months after exposure. Generally, neurological, rheumatological or cardiac symptoms may develop months to years after exposure to the infectious tick bite, with or without earlier development of Lyme disease signs or symptoms. Onset of disease may be mediated, and apparently prevented, by the individual's immune system. Development of disease, and progression of untreated disease, may be extremely different for individual patients. Serosurveys conducted in healthy, working populations residing in endemic areas have demonstrated antibodies to *B. burgdorferi* in asymptomatic individuals without prior history of disease (Fahrer *et al.* 1991; Feder *et al.* 1995).

SIGNS AND SYMPTOMS

Lyme disease is a multisystem disorder and, if not identified and treated soon after onset, it can become a chronic, disabling infection. As is true with other spirochaetal illnesses, the clinical manifestations of Lyme disease can involve many organ systems and occur at variable intervals after exposure to the infected tick bite (Steere 1989). The progression of untreated Lyme disease may involve any of the organ systems described and is not always sequential from one system to another. What had earlier been described as Stage I disease is now referred to as 'early localized Lyme disease'. The first potential evidence of Lyme disease infection might include the detection of an attached tick or the non-specific swelling or minor inflammation that may occur from any tick bite. It is important to note that virtually all biting arthropods may produce a localized immune or allergic response in a human, whether or not the arthropod was a tick of the *Ixodes ricinus* complex, or whether or not a deer tick was infected with *B. burgdorferi*. In addition, different genospecies of this spirochaete may be responsible for different clinical outcomes. The classical initial cutaneous response to the invasion of the spirochaete has been referred to as erythema chronicum migrans (ECM), but is now more commonly referred to simply

as erythema migrans (EM). EM usually occurs within 1 month of the infectious tick bite. Recent evidence in laboratory animals points to the need for the tick to feed for at least 24 hours in order for transmission of *B. burgdorferi* to occur. Often, only about 30–50 per cent of confirmed Lyme disease patients will recall having a tick bite, so the absence of a history of a tick bite should not rule out the possibility of Lyme disease (Steere 1989).

EM begins as erythematous macules or papules, usually at the site of a tick bite, and often in the groin, thigh, axilla, or on the back of an individual. The lesion may be warm but it is usually not associated with any direct pain. Some patients report a burning or itching sensation. As opposed to the inflammation associated with an otherwise uninfected arthropod bite, a true EM will expand over time and may reach several centimetres in diameter over the course of 4–6 weeks. The median diameter of the EM is roughly 10 cm but may reach 50–60 cm in some cases. It is not unusual to see a concentric ring pattern which may otherwise be described as a bull's eye, target, or doughnut lesion. Most EM tend to be flat, or occasionally slightly raised, with red to bright red outer borders and often with central clearing. Patients infrequently present with vesiculated, indurated, or necrotic central lesions. Due to early haematogenous spread of the spirochaete, multiple secondary, or satellite, lesions may occur in some patients. If left untreated, the EM rash, including secondary lesions, will fade over a 4–6 week interval.

Early localized disease is often associated with concurrent non-specific 'flu-like' constitutional symptoms. These symptoms may include malaise, fatigue, lethargy, headache, and generalized arthralgias and myalgias.

Early disseminated Lyme disease, formerly referred to as Stage II illness, may occur within several weeks to months after the infectious tick bite. These symptoms may include neurological and cardiac manifestations. The neurological manifestations may mimic other diseases. Approximately 10–15 per cent of untreated Lyme disease patients may develop neurological manifestations associated with early disseminated Lyme disease. Appropriate antibiotic therapy instituted during early localized disease usually prevents progression to these later symptoms. In the absence of EM, the neurological symptoms may be the first expression of Lyme disease in some patients. Headache, neck pain and stiffness, memory loss, problems concentrating, and emotional problems may be present. Facial nerve palsies, either unilateral or bilateral, may occur concurrent with meningitis symptoms. Bell's palsy may occur in 50 per cent of patients with meningitis. Extreme fatigue and malaise may be present. Some patients may present with one neurological finding and subsequently develop a second distinct neurological finding. Painful radiculopathy and peripheral and central nerve damage may occur during disseminated disease. Some patients have infrequently reported psychoses, hallucinations, sleep disorders, and personality changes possibly related to Lyme disease.

A small percentage of patients (1–8 per cent) with untreated Lyme disease may develop cardiac symptoms within 4 months of the tick bite. As is true with neurological presentations, cardiac symptoms may be the first recognized signs of a Lyme disease infection. Lyme carditis can cause atrioventricular conduction defects, myopericarditis, tachyarrythmias, or mild congestive heart failure. Patients may report periods of fainting, lightheadedness, palpitations, shortness of breath, or chest pain.

Late or chronic disease signs, formerly referred to as Stage III, most prominently include musculoskeletal manifestations (Shadick *et al.* 1994). Infection with *B. burgdorferi* may cause a variety of musculoskeletal complaints, including non-inflammatory joint disease or polyarthralgia, and true inflammatory disease with hot, red, swollen joints, often affecting one or several joints and often associated with tendonitis, bursitis, or fibromyalgia. Intermittent arthritis may persist for 1–15 weeks with intervening symptom-free periods. Large joints are most often affected, especially the knee. Difficulty in walking is the primary functional disability. Erosive bone disease, bone cysts, and cartilage damage may occur.

In addition to the spectrum of musculoskeletal symptoms associated with chronic Lyme disease, tertiary neuroborreliosis, or late-stage neurological manifestations may occur (Logigian *et al.* 1990). Recently, several neurological manifestations have been associated with *B. burgdorferi* infection, including progressive encephalomyelopathy, polyneuritis, cerebral vasculitis, optic neuritis, mental and/or psychiatric disorders, and cognitive dysfunctions. These apparently may occur years after exposure to the infectious tick bite.

European Lyme borreliosis has historically been associated with a distinct spectrum of dermatological and neurological symptoms different from that seen in the United States (Weber and Pfister 1994). Certain symptoms are commonplace in early and late stage presentations in European Lyme disease which are not associated with disease seen in the United States or elsewhere. This may be due to certain *Borrelia* spp. strain differences and their associated pathogenic processes. As previously mentioned, erythema migrans following known tick bites has been observed in Europe since the early 1900s. Garin and Bujadoux described meningopolyneuritis as a response to tick bites in 1922. Research in the United States on Lyme disease since 1975 has led

to a resurgence of interest and investigation in European *Borrelia* infections. In particular, investigations have concentrated on acrodermatitis chronica atrophicans (ACA), ACA-associated polyneuritis, and spirochaetal lymphocytoma.

Unlike the mainly musculoskeletal symptoms observed in the United States, chronic European Lyme borreliosis infections appear to affect predominantly the nervous system. Progressive encephalomyelitis, sensorimotor polyneuritis associated with ACA, and other latent tertiary neuroborreliosis manifestations have been described recently. In some patients, ACA is thought to be a late manifestation of EM and/or spirochaetal lymphocytoma disease. However, many patients presenting with ACA may not have a history of either EM or spirochaetal lymphocytoma.

Clinical signs associated with cutaneous manifestations may include a tick bite lesion, erythema migrans, haematogenous dissemination and resultant secondary, or satellite lesions, lymphocytoma or acrodermatitis chronica atrophicans. Early disseminated disease may also include symptoms associated with a 'flu-like' illness such as fever, fatigue, headache, malaise, muscle and joint pains, localized or regional lymphadenopathy, or conjunctivitis. These symptoms can be intermittent in nature. At this point in the illness, laboratory findings are often negative or inconclusive. Specific *B. burgdorferi* antibodies are not usually detectable until roughly 3–4 weeks after onset of initial symptoms. Future development of more sensitive tests may improve early laboratory detection of infection.

Cardiac symptoms may occur within the first 2 months in 1–8 per cent of patients. Symptoms may include arrhythmias, myopericarditis, and various degrees of atrioventricular block, which may require the insertion of a temporary pacemaker.

Borrelia burgdorferi has shown characteristics of early neurotropism. Neurological symptoms associated with Lyme disease have been observed in roughly 15 per cent of patients with confirmed Lyme disease. Typically, neurological symptoms are present in untreated patients within the first 2–3 months of illness. Symptoms may include aseptic meningitis, encephalitis, cranial nerve palsies, peripheral radiculoneuritis, and peripheral neuropathy. Meningitis may manifest as headache or stiff neck. About 10 per cent of Lyme disease patients may have unilateral or bilateral Bell's palsy which may last for months before resolution. Radiculoneuritis may also occur in the first few months of illness. Radicular pain of the extremities with occasional loss of muscle strength may occur. Neurological sequelae in the untreated patient may progress 1–2 years after initial exposure to late-stage symptoms suggestive of nerve demyelination, cognitive dysfunction, seizures, ataxia, fibromyalgia, and chronic fatigue.

Some patients will also report encephalitic symptoms associated with difficulties in concentration, emotional problems, or lethargy.

Neuroborreliosis observed in Europe has included progressive encephalomyelitis symptoms to include multiple sclerosis-like manifestations and as multifocal encephalitis or psychosis. Acrodermatitis chronica atrophicans-associated polyneuritis has been reported. Ocular manifestations have been reported and include iritis, optic neuritis, panophthalmitis, and choroiditis.

Arthritic manifestations have been associated with Lyme disease since its discovery. This was reflected in the early diagnostic confusion with juvenile rheumatoid arthritis. Arthralgias and myalgias are common features of early disseminated disease. A variety of symptoms are reported in early disease, including migratory pain in tendons, muscles, and bones. Within months to years after initial erythema migrans presentation, a large proportion (40–60 per cent) of untreated patients may develop joint manifestations ranging from migratory, intermittent arthralgias to chronic destructive arthritis. Differences in presentation may be due to the individual host immune response and/or to genetic predisposition. Chronic Lyme arthritis is also associated with the presence of major histocompatibility genes HLA-DR4 and HLA-DR2. Presence of these genes results in chronic arthritis as well as the absence of response to antibiotic therapy. Recurrent monoarticular or asymmetric oligoarticular arthritis can occur. The knee is most commonly affected, often as a hot, intensely swollen joint. Arthritic attacks may last for weeks to months and may recur over a period of several years. Temporomandibular joint pain has also been associated with chronic illness.

DIAGNOSIS

As is true for other bacterial diseases, the definitive diagnosis of Lyme disease would be to culture *B. burgdorferi* from Lyme patients. The spirochaete has been successfully cultured from blood, CSF, synovium, and erythema migrans biopsies. However, culture of the spirochaete is extremely difficult and time consuming. Most tests available for Lyme disease confirmation rely upon the detection of the individual's immune response to *B. burgdorferi* infection.

Lyme disease remains a clinical diagnosis, with serological laboratory tests currently used as supportive evidence of infection. Serological tests should not be ordered indiscriminately or as a routine office practice, but rather to support a suspected diagnosis otherwise based on clinical and epidemiological grounds. The current serological techniques have several inherent limitations, including false-positive and false-

negative findings. Antibodies to *B. burgdorferi* develop slowly in the infected individual, making it even more difficult for the medical care provider to identify a suspect case in the presence of a vague clinical picture or early clinical symptoms. In addition, in the absence of classic clinical symptoms, a positive serological result is not definitive evidence for the diagnosis of Lyme disease.

The humoral response to *B. burgdorferi* is relatively well characterized. In the absence of antibiotic therapy, IgM antibody develops to peak levels 3–6 weeks after exposure. Antibiotic therapy provided during early illness may reduce or eliminate detectable levels of IgM antibody. Specific IgG antibody develops peak levels during the later disseminated phases of illness and may be detectable for years after exposure. The detection of stable levels of IgG antibody after antibiotic therapy does not indicate treatment failure.

To date, serological testing for Lyme disease has not been standardized. Different laboratories may use different antigens, reagents, and testing procedures, even if the same type of test is offered. In addition, laboratory results are often reported using different test units, rendering interpretation of laboratory results extremely confusing, especially if serum samples are sent to more than one laboratory. A great variability has been demonstrated among laboratories testing aliquots of the same patient and control sera. False-negative and false-positive results are still common in most available commercial Lyme disease test procedures. Indirect immunofluorescent antibody (IFA) and enzyme-linked immunosorbent assay (ELISA) tests are the predominant laboratory tests available. Other tests available now, or in the near future, include improvements in spirochaetal culture (e.g. cutaneous lavage), antigen-capture ELISA, immunoblot, urinary antigen detection, serum borreliacidal assays, and polymerase chain reaction (PCR) assays.

False-positive laboratory results may occur in the presence of polyclonal B-cell activation, syphilis, positive rheumatoid factor, positive antinuclear antibody, active infectious mononucleosis, or other reasons for cross-reactivity.

Although Western blotting remains experimental, future test improvements may increase this test's applicability. As molecular science detects specific antigenic proteins of these pathogenic spirochaetes, immunoblotting procedures may allow for the detection of patient antibodies to specific proteins earlier in illness or at levels which are lower than those detectable by current serological procedures. In addition, sequential immunoblot tests can detect temporal increases of specific antibodies to specific antigens. Depending upon the number of bands, and the intensity of patient immunological reaction to individual bands over time, immunoblot testing can allow for determination of relative duration of illness. Standardization of Western blot protocols and interpretation of the number of resultant bands and the intensity of individual band staining should be forthcoming.

The polymerase chain reaction (PCR) also appears promising with future improvement. Since *B. burgdorferi* appears to evoke an inflammatory response in the presence of very few spirochaetes, PCR of human tissues or fluids may provide the clinician with important laboratory information. The test is extremely sensitive and theoretically can detect as few as one organism in human tissues. However, the PCR's sensitivity contributes to some practical laboratory concerns. Meticulous care must be taken to avoid potential contamination of test reagents. PCR testing should not be done in a laboratory that also performs spirochaetal culture. PCR test results may indicate the current or historical presence of the disease agent in a patient, but does not necessarily indicate the presence of live organisms. *Borrelia burgdorferi* may circulate intermittently, or in extremely low numbers in patients with early disease, rendering even PCR testing of blood or serum a relatively low-yield procedure. Further research with these potentially very specific and sensitive tests is clearly indicated.

PATHOLOGY

Human Lyme disease is a complex, multisystemic infectious and inflammatory disease caused by infection with one of at least three species of *Borrelia*, including *B. burgdorferi*, *B. garinii*, and *B. afzelii*. Recent reports indicate that these *Borrelia* genotypes may have different pathogenic potentials. In general terms, the clinical syndrome is known to affect the skin, reticuloendothelial, cardiovascular, central nervous, and skeletal systems.

The primary cutaneous lesion, referred to as erythema (chronicum) migrans (ECM or EM) represents a host immunological response to the presence of spirochaetes in the dermis and is associated with a perivascular infiltration of plasma cells, lymphocytes, and macrophages. Lymphocytoma cutis, or borrelial lymphocytoma, is seen primarily in Europe and appears to be associated with a B-cell response to the presence of antigenic components of these spirochaetes.

The spirochaetes can disseminate to any organ but may demonstrate a tropism for the reticuloendothelial system, resulting in regional lymphadenopathy or splenomegaly. Frank signs of meningeal irritation signals an increase in lymphocytes, plasma cells, and total protein of the cerebrospinal fluid. Facial nerve paresis can occur, with bilateral Bell's palsy frequently

observed. Lymphocytes and plasma cells are reported to infiltrate the nerves and autonomic ganglia. Endocardial infiltration of lymphocytes and plasma cells has been reported.

Joint inflammation may be accompanied by a hyperplasia of synovial membrane and associated lymphocytic and plasma cell infiltration. Neurological involvement is accompanied by the often persistent presence of lymphocytes and plasma cells within the nerve and in the perineural area. Nerve fibres can eventually lose myelin. Cerebral parenchyma involvement may be associated with dementia or other forms of psychiatric illness.

Acrodermatitis chronica atrophicans (ACA) is associated with the infiltration of numerous lymphocytes, plasma cells, macrophages, and mast cells in the dermis between dilated blood vessels. Unique soft-tissue nodules can occur around the elbows, referred to as ulnar fibrous nodules, and are filled with collagen, macrophages, and plasma cells.

TREATMENT

Early publications demonstrated the effectiveness of penicillin and tetracycline in the treatment of early Lyme disease, although further understanding of the disease and pathogenic processes have led to refinements in selections of drug, dose, and duration of antibiotics recommended for Lyme disease therapy. Due, in part, to the lack of large, well-controlled treatment trials using different regimens on uniformly defined patients, and accompanied by long-term follow-up, optimal Lyme disease therapy protocols have yet to be fully defined (Weber and Pfister 1994).

Depending on the disease manifestations in the individual patient, appropriate antibiotic administration may be effective in curing the illness. Lyme disease symptoms can be extremely diverse among individual patients. The sooner the health-care provider includes Lyme disease within the differential diagnosis, the greater the chances for early detection and prompt institution of effective treatment. However, as alluded to earlier, there is currently no evidence to suggest that treatment of asymptomatic seropositive individuals is effective or necessary.

Early Lyme disease symptoms can usually be treated with oral antibiotics. Infrequently, patients with severe early disease can develop later disease symptoms despite proper administration of early therapy. For early disease, doxycycline (100 mg orally, twice a day) or tetracycline hydrochloride (250–500 mg orally, four times a day) for 10 days to 3 weeks has been recommended for men, non-pregnant women, and children more than 8 years old. Amoxicillin (250–500 mg orally three times a day in adults, or 20–40 mg/kg/day in three divided doses for children) for 10 days to 3 weeks has been effective and is preferred for children younger than 8 years old or in pregnant or lactating women who are not allergic to amoxicillin. Erythromycin (250 mg orally, four times a day in adults, or 30 mg/kg/day in children) has been reported but may be less effective.

Mild neurological manifestations (Bells palsy alone) may be treated with oral doxycycline, tetracycline hydrochloride, or amoxicillin as indicated above but administered for a full month. Intravenous antibiotic therapy is recommended for cranial or peripheral neuropathies, meningitis, or encephalitis due to Lyme disease infections. In adults with normal renal function, intravenous penicillin (20–24 million units/day) can be provided in divided doses every 4–6 hours (250 000–400 000 units/kg/day in children) for 10–21 days. Alternatively, intravenous ceftriaxone at 2 g once daily in adults for 14 days (50–80 mg/kg/day in children) has been reported to be effective. Similar protocols can be used in patients with later CNS symptoms.

Cardiac conduction disease can be treated similarly to early Lyme disease, with oral doxycycline, tetracycline, or amoxicillin. More serious cardiac illness requires intravenous antibiotic administration. Ceftriaxone, at 2 g/day for adults (50–80 mg/kg/day for children) or penicillin G, at 20–24 million units/day for adults (250 000–400 000 units/kg/day for children) for 10–21 days has been recommended. Conduction system abnormalities caused by *B. burgdorferi* are not permanent but, occasionally, a pacemaker may be needed on a temporary basis in certain patients.

Rheumatological abnormalities associated with Lyme disease often represent the more refractory signs and may often last for long periods of time despite the administration of what otherwise would have been effective doses of antibiotics. In adult patients with Lyme arthritis 20–24 million units/day of intravenous penicillin G for 2–3 weeks has been effective (300 000 units/kg/day for children), but the effective response may not occur until weeks or months after administration. Intravenous ceftriaxone at 2 g once daily for 2–3 weeks in adults (75–100 mg/kg/day intravenously in children) has been effective in patients who did not respond to penicillin. Doxycycline at 100 mg orally twice a day, or amoxicillin at 500 mg orally three times a day (amoxicillin in children at 50 mg/kg/day divided three times a day) given for 30 days may be effective in patients with Lyme arthritis. Effective therapy for Lyme arthritis occasionally requires repeated administration or follow-up therapy with an alternative drug. As mentioned earlier, there have been no studies to determine the optimal duration of intravenous antibiotic therapy. Most clinicians are choosing intravenous antibiotic regimens ranging from 2 to 4 weeks as opposed to the 10–14-day interval suggested in earlier publications. Most current published recommendations include the maximum duration of administration of intravenous antibiotics of 3–4 weeks.

Pregnant women with Lyme disease should be treated aggressively with a full course of antibiotics according to the stage of their illness. There are no conclusive studies that establish the need for parenteral antibiotics for early Lyme disease in pregnant women. There is also little evidence supporting the practice of treating *Ix. scapularis* tick bites prophylactically in the absence of Lyme disease symptoms.

PROGNOSIS

Clearly, the sooner Lyme disease is recognized in a patient, and appropriate therapy instituted, the better the chances for disease resolution. Early Lyme disease, in most cases, is easily and effectively treated with oral antibiotics or, in the case of early neurological disease, with intravenous antibiotics. Untreated disease, even over the course of years, has been reported to resolve on its own. On the other hand, in certain individuals it appears that certain pathological features of disease may progress despite what would be considered in other patients as adequate antibiotic therapy (Shadick *et al.* 1994). Whether the presence of individual immune response may contribute to disease complications is still open to further investigation.

Apparently, a small proportion of cases may develop symptoms similar to chronic fatigue syndrome or to certain demyelinating diseases, even in the presence of aggressive antibiotic therapy. Extensive controversy exists, and extended dialogue continues among patients, physicians, the medical insurance industry, and the public health community on this important topic. Experimental therapies have been applied in certain cases, to include extended durations of antibiotic administration, combinations of therapeutic approaches, use of unlicensed antibiotics, and the extremely questionable practice of deliberate infection with *Plasmodium falciparum*. Further research may reveal whether other disease syndromes exist which mimic the myriad symptoms associated with Lyme disease, whether *B. burgdorferi* infection causes as yet unrecognized symptoms, or whether certain individuals mount an immune response to spirochaetal infection that itself may be associated with pathogenesis.

EPIDEMIOLOGY

OCCURRENCE

In 1990, a standard Lyme disease surveillance case definition was introduced in the United States to count and confirm cases of disease reported to county, state, or federal health agencies. Prior to this it was virtually impossible to compare Lyme disease reports from different geopolitical entities.

Thousands of cases of Lyme disease are being reported every year in the United States and from most European countries, especially Germany, Austria, Switzerland, France, and Sweden (Axford and Rees 1994). Cases of Lyme disease are increasingly being reported from Russia, the Baltic Republics, China, Japan, and Australia.

In the United States, New York State has the highest cumulative case count. Epidemiological analysis of over 15 000 confirmed (Appendix A) Lyme disease case reports that had been submitted to the New York State Health Department from 1986, when the disease became officially reportable, to 1993, has provided some indication of potential 'risk groups'. Incidence rates in endemic areas vary widely and are associated with varying levels of vector tick populations and tick infection rates. Review of incidence rates in New York State has identified town-based incidence rates ranging from 0.1 to 4.7 per cent in highly endemic areas, with respective county-based incidence rates of 20–220 cases/100 000 population. Incidence rates similarly associated with focal epidemic disease activity reported in coastal Massachusetts have been as high as 35–66 per cent. Analysis by age and sex of the 15 000 case reports has identified a bimodal distribution with peak infection rates in children aged 5–9 years (17 cases/ 100 000 population) and in adults aged 40–69 years (22 cases/100 000). A distinct decrease in incidence rate occurred in the 15–29-year age group at 10 cases/ 100 000 population. In addition, significant sex differences (*T*-test, $P < 0.05$) were seen, with more cases in females in the 30–39-year age group and in males in the 60–69 and 70+ age groups. Whether these differences can be attributed to behaviour or other factors potentially associated with increased exposure risk, or with better disease symptom recognition has not yet been determined.

Rates of human infection may depend on the proximity of residence to, or participation in recreational activities near certain areas supporting populations of vector ticks and the inherent tick infection rate with *B. burgdorferi*. In certain endemic areas of eastern North America, *I. scapularis* tick infection rates may be as high as 60–80 per cent, as opposed to *Ix. pacificus* infection rates on the west coast ranging between 1 and 2 per cent. Although not fully understood, differences in the prevalence of infected ticks may result from differing local host preferences of geographically distinct populations of tick vectors. For example, subadult *Ix. pacificus* and southern populations of *Ix. scapularis* prefer to feed on reptile hosts. These hosts appear to be less competent for maintenance of the spirochaete in tick to tick transmission. In contrast, northern populations of *Ix. scapularis* have abundant populations of competent reservoir mice for their immature stages and of white-tailed deer as the preferred hosts for adult ticks. The availability of this combination of biological and ecological factors may contribute significantly to the focal establishment of high disease prevalence.

SOURCES

Several significant biological hurdles must be crossed in order for successful spirochaete transmission from a reservoir host to a susceptible and competent vector which can support a spirochaete infection itself, and become an infectious potential vector to a subsequent susceptible host. Theoretically, the potential for spirochaetal infection with *B. burgdorferi* among wild vertebrates could be extended to any species fed upon by competent tick vectors. However, even if fed upon by infected ticks, these potential hosts are not equally capable of transmitting infections to ticks which subsequently feed on them. Members of the *Ix. ricinus* complex may feed on a wide variety of mammal, reptilian, and avian hosts. Twenty to forty species of birds and mammals have been reported as hosts of these ticks. Further work is under way to determine the reservoir status of several of these hosts. In most geographic settings, the natural cycle of Lyme disease includes a competent vector tick species, healthy, large populations of rodents or other small mammals upon which immature stages of the vector tick feeds, and supportive large populations of deer which are the preferred host of the adult tick stage.

In general, the preferred habitat for vector tick species includes a deciduous forest setting with damp soil with shrubby undergrowth. Deer populations may be a significant determinant of the size of the vector population, but their role in the natural cycle of *B. burgdorferi* is still unclear. In addition, avian hosts may serve to disperse vector ticks, but they do not appear to serve as a reservoir for the spirochaete. Rather, the natural disease cycle is maintained in the small mammal reservoir hosts of the spirochaete and the immature vector ticks feeding on these competent hosts. In North America, the white-footed mouse, *Peromyscus leucopus*, fulfils this role as the competent reservoir host. Larval ticks feeding on infected *P. leucopus* during late summer and early fall months become infectious nymphs responsible for increased risks for human disease exposure the following late spring and early summer. In Europe, small rodents such as *Apodemus* and *Clethrionomys* species serve as primary reservoir hosts for immature *Ix. ricinus*.

TRANSMISSION

Transmission of human Lyme disease occurs during the prolonged feeding of infected vector tick species. Host-seeking larval ticks and nymphs are capable of acquiring the spirochaete if they feed on competent reservoir hosts for a sufficient time to ingest blood-borne spirochaetes. Upon digestion of the blood meal and moulting to the next stage, these ticks are now potentially infectious for the next host. Epidemiological analysis of human disease onset dates indicates that seasonal peaks of disease transmission most often coincide with seasonal feeding activity of nymphal ticks. Feeding success and resulting disease transmission is enhanced for the nymphal stage due in part to its small size (1–2 mm). Humans generally do not sense the presence of the nymph upon attachment to the skin or of its crawling to a feeding site. If the feeding site is on a portion of the body not regularly seen by the human host, the tick may feed for more than the 24–48 hours required to activate the infectious spirochaetes from the tick midgut tissue and transmit through the haemocoel and salivary fluid. Transovarial transmission is not common from the engorged female tick to her progeny.

COMMUNICABILITY

Although potential human to human transmission of *B. burgdorferi* may occur transplacentally or by blood transfusion, Lyme disease infection is communicable to humans primarily after the bite of a tick species of the genus *Ixodes* infected with *B. burgdorferi* in the United States or *B. burgdorferi*, *B. garinii*, and *B. afzelii* in Europe. Lyme disease has not been documented to be transmitted by sexual contact, by consumption of infected game animals, or by bites of insects. Research is being conducted to determine the potential role of biting insects, other *Ixodes* species, and other tick genera in spirochaete transmission, but results to date have been inconclusive.

PREVENTION AND CONTROL

PREVENTION

Given a basic minimum level of Lyme disease information, most individuals living, working, or playing in Lyme disease endemic areas may be able to conduct most normal activities while adhering to fairly simple Lyme disease preventive measures.

In areas where infected ticks are present, an important aspect of self-protection includes the recognition of suitable tick habitat and either avoidance or the diligent application of preventive measures when travelling through such a habitat. *Ixodes* spp. larvae can be found in woodland settings near where the gravid

female tick likely deposited her eggs. Since tick dispersal at this stage extends only as far as the territory of their dominant hosts, most larvae will be found in the woodland leaf litter. Once the larvae have attached to a host, the sibling ticks will be further dispersed throughout the range of the rodents, other mammals, or birds upon which they feed. Nymphal and adult ticks can be found in a wide variety of habitats, much removed from their original location, but tend to be located in greater numbers in wooded settings or along the edges of fields and woodlands where different habitats meet. Since ticks quest on vegetation waiting for a passing host, most ticks will attach to humans brushing against vegetation. Thus, people walking along a trail in a wooded or grassy area stand an excellent chance of avoiding contact with ticks by simply avoiding brushing against vegetation overhanging the trail. If the people in such a situation wear light-colored long trousers and shirts and frequently examine themselves and their companions, then ticks could be seen and brushed off the clothing before they had a chance to begin feeding. As a more definitive defence, individuals in tick-infested areas should also consider use of any of the several diethyltoluamide or permethrin formulations of insect repellent products. These products have been found to be effective in repelling ticks. Diethyltoluamide products, commonly referred to as 'deet', can be applied to the clothing or to skin, but may need to be reapplied every 3–4 hours especially in hot, humid weather. Controlled-release formulations may provide up to 12 hours of protection. Permethrin products are applied only to clothing and have been found to be effective in killing ticks which become attached to treated clothing.

After spending time outdoors in tick-infested areas, check clothing thoroughly. A full-body exam before going to sleep will also ensure that any ticks which may have evaded all other defences are removed before the 24–48 hours of feeding required for transmission of *Borrelia* spirochaetes.

If a tick is found attached to the skin and has begun feeding, prompt removal should be accomplished using fine-tipped forceps. Grab the tick across the mouthparts as close to the skin as possible, not across the body of the tick, and pull the tick straight out. Squeezing of the tick with fingers or forceps, or irritating the tick with chemicals, hot needles or matches, or attempting to suffocate the tick may actually cause regurgitation of gut contents into the wound, thereby increasing the chances of spirochaetal infection.

CONTROL STRATEGIES

Several strategies of vector management have been subjected to scientific review. These strategies can include measures involving any of the following:

(1) reduction of vector dispersion by targeting insecticide products directly to wild mammal hosts;
(2) reduction of local tick populations by broadscale application of insecticides in habitats supporting populations of immature or adult ticks;
(3) reduction of the tick's wildlife host populations;
(4) modification of the natural tick environment;
(5) exploitation of the host's production of anti-tick antibodies;
(6) exploitation of natural populations of parasites or predators;
(7) release of sterile male ticks; or
(8) employment of pheromonal attractants to disrupt natural mating behaviour.

While some of these potential means of control have only been hypothesized, or at best, only investigated in laboratory settings, several procedures have been fully field tested under natural conditions and found to be relatively effective. Although numerous studies have been published relating the efficacy of any of several individual strategies, what is obviously lacking in any literature review of this topic is an effort documenting the combination of any of these methods to identify the potential effect of well-designed integrated tick management procedures.

Several common insecticides have been found capable of controlling *Ixodes* populations in their natural setting in woodlands or in residential settings on lawns. Liquid or granular formulations of several common registered insecticides such as carbaryl, diazinon, chlorpyrifos, pyrethroids, and cyfluthrin have been found effective against *Ixodes* ticks in these environments. Varying degrees of success have been reported and may be related to actual formulation, dose, habitat selected for study, or season of application. Reports of population reductions range from 70 to 97 per cent. Expectation of long-term control or widescale effective population reduction depend further on the geographic area covered by such a programme. Although these procedures have been attempted on experimental plots, the literature is devoid of information derived from municipal-based programme with large tracts of land treated in such a manner. In addition, if substantial numbers of residents choose not to have their properties included in such tick control programme, a 'checkerboarding' effect could substantially reduce the potential for significant short- or long-term tick population reductions.

Another method of tick control includes the development of insecticide delivery systems that allow focusing the insecticide application directly to the tick hosts. One such approach has included the use of permethrin-treated cotton as surrogate nesting material for small mammal hosts of *Ix. scapularis*. Small mammal hosts of immature ticks will use the available cotton material as nesting material. The system is designed such that the permethrin-treated cotton used for nest material will kill immature *Ix. scapularis* parasites attached to the nesting rodents. This method has been under investigation for over 10 years and has been available commercially for homeowner purchase. Although apparently extremely effective in achieving parasite mortality on the rodent hosts, this system focuses only on one type of immature tick host. Research using this control application in several areas indicates that other immature tick hosts, such as birds and larger mammals, carry a disproportionately larger tick burden in areas where the system was used. This is a prime example of a system well designed to accomplish effective tick control in one natural component of the disease cycle that may not necessarily result in effective reduction of infestation levels on other native hosts. This system could be considered for use in an integrated tick control approach where several components of tick population reduction could be applied.

Environmental management for reduction of tick populations has been in use since the early 1900s, especially in the western United States. Ranchers and other property owners regularly burned large tracts of land to control populations of *Dermacentor andersoni*, the vector of Rocky Mountain spotted fever in that area. Recent attempts to apply this traditional technology have been somewhat difficult to achieve due, in part, to local environmental restrictions. If well timed and well monitored, especially in the early spring prior to vegetation leafing, leaf litter and low-growth grassy vegetation burning could be effective in reducing overwintering populations of *Ixodes* (and other) tick species. Decisions and legal ability to conduct such attempts at tick control must be determined by a full assessment of local conditions and regulations.

Certain investigators have conducted laboratory-based experimentation using tick colonies and have noticed a gradual decrease of tick feeding success on the same hosts. Further investigation led to the identification of host-derived anti-tick antibodies. It remains to be seen if passive immunity using such antibodies could be effective in reducing tick feeding in recipient hosts. Unlike most blood-feeding arthropods which complete their blood meal in just a few seconds or minutes, ixodid ticks most often require days to complete their blood meal. During this feeding, ticks introduce a variety of proteinaceous products into the host, including anticoagulants, haemagglutinins, and anti-inflammatory products necessary for the tick to complete its meal, and result in pathogen transmission to the host. Early observations of reduced feeding rates were noted in the 1930s with *Dermacentor variabilis* and laboratory guinea-pigs. Immunity to ticks in any given host may well depend on the host's history of specific tick infestation, unless the resulting immunity from an unrelated host species could be passively transferred to a susceptible host species.

Natural predators and parasites have been considered as potential agents for tick control for years. Several species of Hymenoptera, especially ants and parasitic wasps, have been found to predate upon, or parasitize, certain tick species. Although this may occur to some degree in nature, use of natural predators or parasites in a large-scale tick reduction programme is greatly limited by the massive numbers of such organisms that have to be released and be successfully competitive in order to achieve any significant population reduction. This particular approach, as well as sterile male releases, may be inherently limited due to the absolute numbers of organisms involved. There may exist a good potential, however, for the application of pheromones, either as aggregation or attractant compounds, in altering natural tick behaviour. Some work on *Ix. ricinus* in this field was accomplished in the 1970s. Given new technical capabilities, some of this work could have wider interest for future applications at altering *Ixodes* behaviour.

One approach which has gained a foothold in some communities is the application of methods resulting in the reduction of deer populations, since deer are the preferred host of the adult *Ix. ricinus* complex. Actual attempts at deer reduction have been accomplished in specific geographic settings, especially on off-shore islands of the north-eastern United States. In such isolated settings, especially where alternate hosts for adult tick hosts may be limited in number for any of several reasons associated with island settings, such control efforts can be effective for short- and long-term tick reductions. However, one must seriously question whether similar procedures are practical on mainland settings where deer populations are free to range over large tracts of land, and where adequate numbers of alternate medium and large mammal hosts coexist. Certain communities wishing to reduce nuisance deer populations in suburban settings may need to assess the potential alternative feeding pathways that exist for ticks that may, otherwise, be deprived of normal populations of their preferred hosts. This includes the very real possibility that human parasitism with these ticks may increase. For long-term control, it may be possible that well-designed deer reduction efforts, when combined with extensive deer and other medium and large mammal exclusion, seasonal vegetation burning, and the seasonal application of particular formulations of particular insecticides, may lead to promising results. As yet, no large-scale, municipal or experimental programme has been developed using any integrated tick management programme.

REFERENCES

Afzelius, A. (1910). Verhandlungen der Dermatologischen Gesellschaft zu Stockholm on October 28, 1909. *Arch. Dermatol. Syph.*, **101**, 404.

Andriole, V. T. (ed.) (1989). Lyme disease and other spirochetal diseases. *Reviews of the Infectious Diseases*, II, (suppl. 6), S1433–4.

Axford, J. S. and Rees D. H. E. (eds) (1994). Lyme borreliosis. *NATO Advanced Study Institute Series. Series A Life Sciences*, **260**.

Benach J. L. *et al.* (1983). Spirochetes isolated from the blood of two patients with Lyme Disease. *New England Journal of Medicine*, **308**, 740–2.

Burgdorfer, W., Barbour, A. G., Hayes, S. F., Benach, J. L., Grunwaldt E., and Davis, J. P. (1982). Lyme disease—a tick borne spirochetosis? *Science*, **216**, 1317–19.

Fahrer, H., van der Linden, S. M., Sauvain, M., Gern, L., Zhioua E., and Aeschlimann, A. (1991). The prevalence and incidence of clinical and asymptomatic Lyme borreliosis in a population at risk. *Journal of Infectious Diseases*, **163**, 305–10.

Feder, H. M., Gerber, M. A., Cartter, M. L., Sikand, V., and Krause, P. J. (1995). Prospective assessment of Lyme disease in a school-aged population in Connecticut. *Journal of Infectious Diseases*, **171**, 1371–4.

Ginsberg, H. S. (1993). Transmission risk of Lyme disease and implications for tick management. *American Journal of Epidemiology*, **138**, (1), 65–73.

Hellerstrom, S. (1951). Erythema chronicum migrans Afzelius with meningitis. *Acta Dermato- Venereologica (Stockholm)*, **310**, 227–234.

Johnson, S. E., Klein, G. C., Schmid, G. P., Gowen, G. S., Feeley, J. C., and Schulze, T. (1984). Lyme disease, a selective medium for isolation of the suspected etiological agent, a spirochete. *Journal of Clinical Microbiology*, **19**, 81–2.

Logigian, E. L., Kaplan, R. F., and Steere, A. C. (1990). Chronic neurologic manifestations of Lyme disease. *New England Journal of Medicine*, **323**, (21), 1438–44.

Shadick, N. A., *et al.* (1994). The long term clinical outcomes of Lyme disease: a population-based retrospective cohort study. *Annals of Internal Medicine*, **121**, 560–7.

Spielman, A., Clifford, C. M., Piesman, J., and Corwin, M. D. (1979). Human babesiosis on Nantucket Island, U.S.A.: Description of the vector *Ixodes (Ixodes) dammini:*, n.sp. (Acarina: Ixodidae). *Journal of Medical Entomology*, **15**, 218–34.

Steere, A. C. (1989). Medical progress–Lyme disease. *New England Journal of Medicine*, **321**, (9), 586–96.

Steere, A. C., Broderick, T. F., and Malawista, S. E. (1978). Erythema chronicim migrans and Lyme arthritis: field study of ticks. *American Journal of Epidemiology*, **108**, 322–7.

Steere, A. C., Malawista, S. E., Craft, J. E. Fischer, D. K., and Garcia-Blanco, M. (ed.) (1984). *Lyme disease: First international symposium. Yale Journal of Biology and Medicine*.

Weber, K. and Pfister, H. W. (1994). Clinical management of Lyme borreliosis. *Lancet*, **343**, 1017–19.

APPENDIX A

Lyme disease case definition used by the New York State Department of Health Lyme disease is a systemic, tick-borne disease with protean manifestations, including dermatological, rheumatic, neurological, and cardiac abnormalities. The best clinical marker for the disease is the skin lesion, erythema migrans (EM).

GENERAL DEFINITIONS INTENDED FOR
SURVEILLANCE PURPOSES:

1. Erythema migrans (EM)
    EM is a skin lesion which typically begins as a red
    macule or papule and expands over a period of
    days to weeks to form a large round lesion, often
    with partial central clearing. Secondary lesions
    may also occur. For purposes of surveillance, *a soli-
    tary lesion must reach at least 5 cm in size*. In most
    patients, the expanding EM lesion is accompanied
    by other symptoms, particularly fatigue, fever,
    headache, mild stiff neck, arthralgias, or myalgias.
    These symptoms are typically intermittent and
    changing. For purposes of surveillance, the diag-
    nosis of EM must be made by a physician.
    Laboratory confirmation is recommended for
    people with no known exposure.
2. Late manifestations
    Any of the following that occur without an alterna-
    tive explanation.
    (a) Musculoskeletal system
        Recurrent (at least two), brief attacks (weeks
        or months) of objective joint swelling in one
        or a few joints sometimes followed by chronic
        arthritis in one or a few joints. Chronic pro-
        gressive arthritis not preceded by brief
        attacks, or chronic symmetrical polyarthritis
        are not accepted as criteria for diagnosis. Of
        particular importance, arthralgias, myalgias,
        or fibromyalgia syndromes alone are not
        accepted as criteria for musculoskeletal
        involvement.
    (b) Nervous system
        Lymphocytic meningitis, cranial neuritis, par-
        ticularly facial palsy (may be bilateral),
        radiculoneuropathy and, rarely, encephalo-
        myelitis alone or in combination. Ence-
        phalomyelitis must be confirmed by showing
        antibody production against *B. burgdorferi* in
        the cerebrospinal fluid (CSF) demon-
        strated by a higher titre of antibody in CSF
        than in serum. Headache, fatigue, para-
        esthesias or mild stiff neck alone are not
        accepted as criteria for neurological
        involvement.
    (c) Cardiovascular system
        Acute onset, high grade (2° or 3°) atrioven-
        tricular conduction defects that resolve in
        days to weeks, sometimes associated with myo-
        carditis. Palpitations, bradycardia, bundle
        branch block or myocarditis alone are not
        accepted as criteria for cardiovascular
        involvement.
3. Endemic county
    An endemic country is one in which at least two
    definite cases have been previously acquired or a
    country in which a known *B. burgdorferi*-infected
    tick vector has been shown to be present.
4. Exposure
    Exposure is defined as having been in wooded,
    bushy or grassy areas (potential tick habitats) in
    an endemic county no more than 30 days prior to
    onset of EM, or travel to a recognized endemic
    area within the year before the onset of late mani-
    festations; a history of tick bite is NOT required.
5. Laboratory confirmation
    Laboratory confirmation of infection with
    B. burgdorferi is established when a laboratory iso-
    lates the spirochaete from tissue or body fluid,
    detects diagnostic levels of IgM or IgG antibodies
    to the spirochaete in serum or CSF, or detects a
    significant change in antibody levels in paired
    acute and convalescent serum samples. Syphilis
    and other known causes of biological false-positive
    serological test results, should be excluded as
    appropriate, when laboratory confirmation has
    been based on serological testing alone.

LYME DISEASE CASE DEFINITIONS

Confirmed case is defined as the following:

1. A person with EM
    or
    A person with at least one late manifestation and
    laboratory confirmation of infection.
2. Unconfirmed case is defined as a reported case
    that does not meet the above criteria.
3. Pending—investigation not complete.

Note: Summaries of surveillance data will be based
on confirmed cases unless otherwise noted.

15 MYCOBACTERIAL DISEASES

J. Gallagher and P. A. Jenkins

MYCOBACTERIUM BOVIS

SUMMARY

Tuberculosis is a chronic granulomatous disease result-ing from infection with either *Mycobacterium tuber-culosis*, *M. bovis*, or *M. avium*. Man is the natural host for *M. tuberculosis* and birds for *M. avium*. *Mycobacterium bovis* is the cause of tuberculosis in cattle but is also highly infectious for man and can pose a serious life-threatening zoonotic risk. World Health Organization data for 1990 (Anon 1993) indicated that just over 3 million people worldwide died from tuberculosis, more than all other infectious diseases combined. Over 8.5 million cases of tuberculosis were diagnosed that year. Although the very great majority of these cases were associated with infection due to *M. tuberculo-sis*, a very small, largely undetermined portion of these enormous totals resulted from *M. bovis* infections. Where data have been available, approximately 1–5 per cent of isolates from cases have proved to be *M. bovis*, implying that this zoonosis still produces a considerable toll of disease and death in man.

Tuberculosis in cattle has a global distribution. Few countries are completely free of it, although partial erad-ication has been achieved in many developed countries. Transmission of infection from cattle to man is mainly through the consumption of unpasteurized milk, which is now essentially a problem of developing countries.

Infections due to *M. bovis* are discussed in this section, whereas infections due to other mycobacteria are discussed at the end of the chapter.

HISTORY

Tuberculosis is an ancient disease with evidence of this affliction, in the form of classical spinal lesions, being seen in Egyptian mummies dating back to 2000–3000 BC, since which time it has become a scourge of most civil-izations. A variety of views were originally held as to the causation of tuberculosis. Thoughts that it was a conta-gious disease appear to have developed with the early Greek observers, Isocrates, Aristotle, and Galen, but little progress was made until Francisus Silvus defined the pathology of tuberculosis in 1671.

The infectious nature of tuberculosis was demon-strated by Villemin in 1865 in a series of experiments in which he transmitted infection to rabbits by inocula-tion of material from lesions from cattle and from man. Some years later Robert Koch identified 'bacil-lary organisms' in lesions of tuberculosis and in 1882 succeeded in cultivating these on a medium of inspis-sated bovine serum. With these cultures, Koch repro-duced tuberculosis in experimental animals, thus convincingly establishing the tubercle bacillus as the aetiological agent of this disease. Extreme views were then held with regard to the role of animals in the cau-sation of this condition in man. One of several views expounded in Germany at the time was that tuberculo-sis was contracted from cattle as a venereal infection.

Koch thought initially that the organisms respons-ible for disease in both man and cattle were the same but Theodore Smith in 1898 demonstrated a differ-ence in the rate of growth *in vitro* and the virulence of strains of tubercle bacilli recoverable from man and cattle. Ravenal in 1889 demonstrated that tuberculosis of birds was caused by a similar, yet clearly different, organism from that afflicting man or cattle. Following this work, Koch inoculated human isolates into cattle and found they produced only small, non-progressive lesions. He reasoned that cattle isolates in man would behave likewise. Announcing his conclusions at the International Tuberculosis Conference in London in 1901, Koch expounded the view that tuberculosis was virtually host-specific both in man and cattle, and stated that 'the human subject is immune against infec-tion with bovine bacilli or is so slightly susceptible that it is not necessary to take any steps to counteract risk of infection'. This assertion from so notable a figure caused great controversy in the scientific community and stimulated an enormous amount of experimental work and in-depth investigation into the nature of tuberculosis in man and animals, much of which forms the basis of our present-day knowledge. A Royal Commission was set up in Britain to carry out this work, the main persons involved being A. S. and F. Griffith and Louis Cobbett, Medical Research

Council, and John McFadyean, principal of the Royal Veterinary College, London.

The Commissioners found that the human bacillus was undoubtedly the most frequent cause of tuberculosis in man, yet 5 per cent of all deaths from this disease were due to infection with bovine strains. But the proportion of such infections was much higher in very young children, mostly under 5 years of age, being of the order of 33 per cent. Indeed, autopsy data indicated that deaths in man due to tuberculosis of bovine origin were proportionally higher in Britain than in any other of the European countries or North America. Commenting on the situation in Britain, McFadyean observed that 'Tuberculosis is immensely more frequent among cattle than in any other farm animals' and 'bovine tuberculosis is the fountain-head for the disease in these other species' (Anon 1965).

A scheme for the eradication of bovine tuberculosis was launched by the Ministry of Agriculture in 1935. At that time surveys showed that 40 per cent of dairy cows in Britain were tuberculous and that 0.5 per cent of all milk probably contained bovine tubercle bacilli. The overall prevalence rate of infection in cattle in general was thought to be between 15 and 20 per cent, based on abattoir reports and limited tuberculin testing. Pigs, which often were fed milk products (for example, whey), were estimated in one survey to show a prevalence of tuberculous lesions at slaughter of 11 per cent. Farm cats enjoying fresh raw milk in rural Cheshire, had a prevalence of 13 per cent, whereas city cats from the London area showed only a prevalence of 3.6 per cent of tuberculous lesions. Over the same period it was estimated that the human toll due to bovine tuberculosis was of the order of 2500 deaths per annum and there was a still larger amount of illness. The majority of cases were in very young children, mostly under 5 years, and cows' milk was considered the source of these infections (Anon 1965).

With the progress of the eradication scheme and the gradual introduction of pasteurization of milk at the dairies, infection of man and other species was greatly reduced The national cattle herd was declared tuberculosis-tested in 1960, when every bovine had been tuberculin tested at least once and all reactors to the test slaughtered. At that stage only 0.16 per cent of cattle tested reacted positively from 3.5 per cent of herds. By 1965 the reactor incidence fell to 0.06 per cent representing 1 per cent of herds. Thereafter progress towards eradication faltered with the finding that the herd incidence of tuberculosis, compared with other regions, was considerably higher in the south-west region of England where it was later found to be associated with an overspill of infection from populations of wild badgers. In problem areas, badgers frequently showed a prevalence of tuberculosis of 20 to 30 per cent. Many badgers were found to be severely tuberculous with 'open' lesions present in both lungs and kidneys (Muirhead *et al.* 1974). Intensive surveys indicated that the badger was indeed a primary reservoir host and destruction of infected communities in an extensive area successfully stopped further new infections of cattle (Anon 1979). This finding further confirmed the badger as the primary source but the draconian approach to control was unacceptable on a wider scale. A partial selective culling programme of infected badger communities was thus introduced and a low incidence of tuberculosis in cattle still continues in the south-west of England as well as in several smaller areas elsewhere in the country. However, in the problem areas the cattle herds are tested annually and any found with reactions are kept under restriction after the reactors have been removed to slaughter and held under restriction until testing at 60-day intervals yields no more reactors. Whereas milk from approximately 98 per cent of all cattle herds is pasteurized, where reactors occur in a herd which is retailing fresh milk, sales are immediately stopped. These measures, which have been in force throughout the eradication campaign, have successfully protected against the risk of milk-borne infections for at least three decades.

THE AGENT

The agent of tuberculosis in man, *M. tuberculosis* was at one stage considered a single species with bovine or avian variants or strains responsible for infections of cattle and birds, respectively. This opinion is still held by some workers but it is generally accepted that *M. bovis* and *M. avium* are separate species. In common with all mycobacteria they all possess a very thick, complex cell wall, comprising peptidoglycans, arabinogalactans, mycolic acids, and a range of lipids. It is mainly the mycolic acids which confer the ability to retain basic dyes such as carbol fuchsin despite acid treatment (Draper 1982). Tubercle bacilli do not produce toxins and their pathological effects result essentially from the strong antigenicity of their cell walls.

A wide range of growth media has been used to cultivate tubercle bacilli, the majority being either egg or agar based. Isolation and identification techniques have been reviewed extensively by Jenkins *et al.* (1982). Lowenstein–Jensen medium is still probably the most widely used egg-based medium in diagnostic laboratories, although in some of the larger laboratories a radiometric technique may also be used for primary isolation. One such is the BACTEC system, which utilizes radiolabelled palmitic acid in a liquid medium (Middlebrook *et al.* 1977) and has allowed more rapid detection of the presence of mycobacteria, with the average time for isolation reported as 10–14 days (Damato *et al.* 1983).

Agar-based media are used for primary isolation by some laboratories and have the benefit that a range of antibiotics can be included in the agar to make it selective, thus obviating the need for strong acid or alkali decontamination of specimens before culture, as is necessary for the egg media. Probably the most widely used of these is Middlebrook's 7H11 agar (Mitchison *et al.* 1972).

Mycobacterium tuberculosis produces a eugonic growth appearing on egg media usually in 2–3 weeks. Appearance on agar media may be slightly earlier. In contrast, *M. bovis* shows dysgonic growth and frequently will not be apparent on egg media for at least 4–5 weeks of incubation. Again, on agar media growth may be seen earlier. Growths of *M. bovis* are typically stimulated by the presence of sodium pyruvate while inhibited by glycerol. The reverse is seen with *M. tuberculosis*. Resistance to pyrazinamide is normally found with *M. bovis* isolates. Strain identification of *M. bovis* isolates by bacteriophage or biotyping has been largely unsuccessful but considerable progress has been made in DNA fingerprinting using restriction endonuclease analysis and the more discriminatory restriction fragment length polymorphism (RFLP) technique. Although not yet in routine use, these techniques are invaluable epidemiological tools (O'Reilly and Daborn 1995).

EPIDEMIOLOGY

The main reason for the considerable increase in prevalence of bovine tuberculosis in western Europe in the early twentieth century was undoubtedly the development of the dairy industry. Town dairies were set up to supply fresh milk directly to towns' people, and tuberculosis was often rife in the cramped and unsanitary conditions of these dairies. As a result of eradication measures in cattle and the introduction of pasteurization, milk no longer poses the threat of tuberculosis to man in Britain or, indeed, in the other European countries, North America, or in most of the developed countries.

The situation may be entirely different in some developing countries where a dairy industry has been encouraged but without the safeguard of pasteurization. Fortunately, although controls on infection of cattle may be lacking, the development of pasteurization plants mostly goes hand in hand with the development of the dairy sector. Local customs can have a strong effect on the likelihood of contracting infection. Traditionally, in many African countries and in much of Asia, milk is boiled before consumption. In

parts of southern Africa it is soured in calabashes, which devitalizes the tubercle bacilli (Kleeberg 1984). In areas of South America, fresh milk is rarely drunk, most of milk production being used for cheesemaking or manufacture of the more transportable products, evaporated and condensed milk.

Tubercle bacilli survive well in milk. One animal with tuberculosis of the udder amongst a herd of 100 milking cows will contaminate the whole output of the herd. Bacilli will be found in the cream layer, emulsifying with the fat globules which are readily assimilated in the gut. Some milk products also pose a risk, and yoghurt and cream cheese made from unpasteurized milk from infected cows have been found to harbour tubercle bacilli for up to 14 days after preparation. Butter made from such animals may remain contaminated for as long as 100 days after preparation (Kleeberg 1984).

Slaughterhouse inspection for evidence of tuberculosis is usually thorough, even in many developing countries Although eating meat from tuberculous cattle presents a theoretical risk, the real risk is determined by the cooking and preparation methods. Tubercle bacilli are relatively heat sensitive. However, infection of slaughterhouse workers as a result of handling infected animals and their carcasses has been recorded, and in Queensland, Australia, tuberculosis has been considered an occupational hazard of meatworkers. From 1953 to 1981 a total of 87 cases of tuberculosis due to *M. bovis* were recorded. Whereas 13 patients drank raw milk and one patient apparently contracted infection from exposure to another, a total of 57 cases had a history of work-related or domestic exposure to cattle. Of this number, 40 were meatworkers. For 16 cases no likely source of infection was apparent. Overall, 77 per cent of cases presented with pulmonary disease (Georghiou *et al.* 1989).

Direct pulmonary infection of man through aerosols from diseased cattle undoubtedly occurs, and prior to the virtual eradication of tuberculosis in cattle in Britain this was probably a significant source of infection for the farming community. Widespread contamination of walls and windows of cow sheds was noted by Jensen (1953) who commented that 'I should like to emphasise that working in highly infected cow stables has to be looked upon as being far more dangerous than working in a tuberculosis hospital'. The risk of this still remains, both in Britain and elsewhere where sporadic outbreaks of tuberculosis in cattle continue. The risks are however, now small in Britain.

The prevalence of *M. bovis* infections in man in Britain has been approximately 1 per cent of diagnosed cases of tuberculosis for many years. The great majority of these cases are considered to be the result of recrudescence of an earlier, probably childhood, infection. The majority of such patients are aged 60–70 years (Katarina 1969). A detailed study of cases of tuberculosis in south-east England from 1977 to 1979 revealed an incidence of bovine infections of 1.5 per cent but, more surprisingly, *M. bovis* was found in a similar age range of patients as was *M. tuberculosis*. While most cases occurred in 60-year-olds, many were seen in much younger age groups, with the youngest patient with the bovine strain being a 6-year-old. It was postulated that pulmonary spread of infection from man to man with bovine strains was occurring entirely independent of any bovine source (Collins *et al.* 1981).

These findings highlight the possibility that, particularly in countries where tuberculosis in cattle is well controlled, new *M. bovis* infections in man may not originate directly from a cattle source. Fortunately, it would appear that man to man spread of *M. bovis* infections occurs considerably less frequently than *M. tuberculosis* infections (O'Reilly and Daborn 1995).

Indirect transmission of tuberculosis from companion animals is now an extremely unlikely event in Britain. Curently there is now a greater risk of man infecting companion animals than the converse. There have been well-documented cases of dogs and cats developing tuberculosis on farms affected with outbreaks of tuberculosis in the cattle in North America and elsewhere, but these are exceptional. Dogs and cats are equally susceptible to human and bovine tubercle bacilli which, depending on the route of transmission, will produce progressive disease with widespread lesions (Lepper and Corner 1983). Parrots are notable amongst birds in being susceptible to infection with *M. tuberculosis*, and there is some evidence that *M. bovis* may also be pathogenic for them (Francis 1958). Recently, a rare chronic arthritic condition of cats has been found in Britain to be associated with a mycobacterial infection. The isolate recovered from the joints, but not from elsewhere, appears to be an atypical variant of *M. tuberculosis*. The infections seen so far have been 'closed' and would appear to offer little risk to man (Gunn-Moore and Jenkins 1994). These infections are discussed further in the latter section of this chapter.

Tuberculosis due to *M. bovis* in farmed deer is a problem found in a small number of herds in Britain over the past decade or so. Tuberculosis in this species, as in cattle, is a notifiable disease and strict controls are placed on affected herds. Red and roe deer (*Cervus elaphus* and *Capreolus capreolus*) are mainly involved, but the meat inspection procedures should result in a negligable risk to man through consumption of venison. Sporadic localized infection of feral deer has been recorded in Britain (Gunning 1985) but subsequent surveys have shown this to be a very rare occurrence. However, infection of farmed red deer in New

Zealand has become a serious problem requiring rigorous control measures. In Canada, farmed elk (*Cervus elaphus* var. *canadensis*), with some herds showing a prevalence of infection of almost 40 per cent, were considered the source of infection of a veterinarian and several farm workers through handling the animals and their carcasses (Fanning and Edwards 1991).

Eradication of tuberculosis from cattle in a number of countries has faltered as reservoirs of infection have been disclosed in other species sharing the same habitat. In Britain and in Ireland progress has been impaired by the finding of well-established reservoirs of infection in badgers (*Meles meles*). Although the problem in Britain is essentially regional, that in Ireland is widespread (O'Connor and O'Malley 1989). When disease is occurring at a high prevalence in cattle the effects of a wildlife source are not evident, and it is typically only when controls have reduced the incidence to very low levels that they may become apparent, as was the case in Britain. The significance of the reservoir infection is determined by its manifestation in the reservoir species, or more particularly whether 'open' lesions capable of discharging infection are present and whether there is sufficient opportunity for that infection to be spread to the host. Cattle and badgers do share the same habitat, and with lung, kidney, and discharging bite-wound lesions in badgers there is ample opportunity for spread (Gallagher *et al.* 1976).

Badgers may also share habitat with man and will raid domestic gardens, gorging on carrots, strawberries, raspberries, and blackberries, etc. and there is a theoretical risk that eating unwashed produce from the garden may pose a risk of infection to man, should the invading badger be severely tuberculous. However, no such cases have been recorded in man so far.

In New Zealand a considerable reservoir of infection has been found in brush-tail possums (*Trichosurus vulpecula*) and the problem now affects large areas of North and South Islands (Julian 1981). Additionally, feral red deer have become infected, mainly from the possums, and have introduced infection to farmed deer herds. Several cases of cutaneous tuberculosis have been recorded in trappers following the removal of pelts from infected possums. Affected possums show a suppurative lymphadenitis of the superficial nodes, frequently with discharging fistulas, and well-developed suppurative lung lesions may also be present.

In Australia infected feral water buffaloes (*Bubalus bubalus*) caused problems in eradication in the Northern Territories (McCool and Newton-Tabrett 1979); whereas wild pigs (*Sus scrofa*) were also found infected, they were not considered a risk to cattle. The prevalence in the pigs was quite high, but opportunities for spread to stock were lacking (Corner *et al.* 1981).

The risk of man presenting as a source of infection for cattle has also become considerably more apparent with the progress of eradication programmes. Instances of this, although uncommon, have been reported from Britain, Holland, Germany, Canada, and New Zealand (Lesslie 1960, Huitema 1969; Black 1972; Wigle *et al.* 1972; Werner 1981. Infection of cattle by man mostly derives from patients with pulmonary disease, although a number of outbreaks have been due to farm workers affected with renal tuberculosis. Urination in cattle sheds or sometimes on bales of hay and straw used for the animals has been reported in different instances. Most of such cases have involved *M. bovis* with its greater propensity to cause extrapulmonary lesions. Cattle infections have been recorded due to both human and bovine tubercle bacilli. *Mycobacterium tuberculosis* does not cause progressive disease in cattle, but will cause tuberculin sensitization. Post-mortem examination of reacting animals often shows caseous lesions restricted to the primary complex (Lesslie 1968). However, in one outbreak lesions of tuberculous mastitis were found in a cow with a history of mastitis, which had been treated by the cowman, who 2 months earlier had died from generalized tuberculosis (Lesslie 1968). In all herds with this infection, stopping contact with the human source halted further cases in the cattle (Lesslie 1968). But it has been shown, both in experimental and natural infections, that cattle infected with *M. tuberculosis* may excrete organisms in the milk in the absence of clinical mastitis (Lepper and Corner 1983). There is thus a potential risk of milk becoming infected as a result of tuberculous persons working with dairy cows, as well as the more obvious one of their directly contaminating the milk.

THE HOSTS

HUMAN

Mycobacterium bovis is equally as virulent as *M. tuberculosis* for man (Jensen *et al.* 1940). The pathogenesis of infection by either is much the same and is essentially dependent on the route of infection. Direct pulmonary infection with bovine tubercle bacilli will result in the development of phthisis or pulmonary tuberculosis and shows the same pattern of clinical progression as occurs with the human bacilli. However, a greater tendency for the development of extrapulmonary lesions has been noted with bovine infections, most particularly in the development of renal tuberculosis (Collins *et al.* 1981). In pulmonary infections the initial lesion which develops in the lung, the Ghon focus, usually a small caseous abscess, is frequently discernible. This lesion, together with lesions in the drainage lymph nodes, the hilar nodes, represents the primary focus. Tuberculin hypersensitivity develops from 3 to 8 weeks postinfection, and the onset may be heralded by fever. Primary lesions frequently heal and may resolve completely or fibrose and calcify. Non-healing lesions often liquefy and discharge infection into bronchi, producing bronchopneumonia or empyema. Cavity formations can develop and often result in a high level of infectiousness. These processes may not occur for several years after initial infection, when they would then be termed postprimary disease (Grange 1980).

In Britain, most cases of bovine tuberculosis in man have been acquired through ingestion of infected milk, either during the 1950s or earlier. Frequently infection gained entry via the tonsils, producing tonsillar swelling, sore throat, and enlargement of the cervical nodes, later developing to scrofula or purulent cervical adenitis. Such lesions can also develop following generalization from cases of phthisis or tuberculous pneumonia, but these lesions have been seen as the most frequent manifestation of bovine infection, being the characteristic manifestation of infection acquired through drinking tuberculous milk. Tuberculosis of the gut is also generally associated with milk-borne infection and may result in the development of mesenteric lymph node masses causing abdominal cramps and later with peritonitis and tuberculous hepatitis. Genitourinary, bone, joint and meningeal lesions, as well as kidney lesions, may arise from haematogenous spread from either pulmonary or non-pulmonary acquired infection (Grange 1980).

Savage (1929) reviewed the manifestations of bovine strain infections in man at a time when milk infection was prevalent and noted that in his series of cases pulmonary lesions were present in only 1 per cent, the remainder being non pulmonary infections. In these a full range of lesions was seen, with 45 per cent exhibiting classical cervical lymphatic lesions of scrofula, 32 per cent scrofuloderma, and 51 per cent showing skin lesions of lupus vulgaris. Genitourinary lesions were present in 17 per cent bone and joint lesions in 18 per cent, and meningitis in 27 per cent. Cutaneous tuberculosis, lupus vulgaris, was frequently associated with bovine strain infection amongst the rural community from occupational contact with cattle. Historically, facial lesions were not uncommon in milkers as a result of close contact with cattle.

ANIMAL

Tuberculosis in cattle in most instances presents as an infection of pulmonary origin. Whether infection occurs by direct inhalation of infected aerosols or from ingestion, the pattern of lesion development is much the same. Ingested organisms deposit in the rumen or first stomach, which contains liquor with a variety of bacteria and protozoan organisms and functions as a digestive fermentor. During fermentation large quantities of methane and carbon dioxide are generated from the food base. These gases must be cleared frequently by eructation and in so doing aerosols of organisms are drawn into the lungs to be first inhaled before expulsion. Pulmonary and upper respiratory tract lymph nodes thus represent the main drainage nodes affected following deposition of tubercle bacilli in the lungs. The Ghon focus in the lung may be very difficult to locate, but lymph node lesions of caseation and calcification are evident in the bronchomediastinal or retropharyngeal nodes. Following the establishment of pulmonary lesions in cattle, disease is generally progressive, in contrast to man where lengthy containment or sometimes resolution often occurs. When visceral lesions develop in cattle, Klimmer (1946) observed that the lungs showed lesions in 75 per cent of cases slaughtered as tuberculous. The liver was affected in 28 per cent, the spleen in 19 per cent, the uterus in 10 per cent, and the udder, intestines and ovary each in 1 per cent, whereas the kidneys were only seen to show lesions in 0.7 per cent of cases.

This pattern of lesions was seen at a time when tuberculosis was widespread in Europe. Outbreaks of tuberculosis in cattle in Britain are now of a more sporadic nature, approximately 90 per cent of them appearing to be associated directly with infection from badgers by contamination of pasture. The annual testing of the eradication programme in the problem areas effectively detects early disease, so that rarely are advanced, generalized cases found. Infected cattle now encountered are likely to show lesions of the retropharyngeal and bronchomediastinal lymph nodes in from 70 to 80 per cent of cases, whereas gross lung lesions are only found in approximately 2 per cent, the remaining cases showing lymph node lesions of the mesenteric, prescapular, and small numbers of infections in other nodes. Tuberculosis of the udder is now extremely rare.

Most cattle show no clinical signs until disease is advanced, when gradual loss of condition and eventually emaciation occur. A capricious appetite and fluctuating temperature may be noted. Superficial lymph nodes may be enlarged. Occasionally retropharyngeal node enlargement can result in dysphagia, and noisy breathing or even snoring can be heard, particularly after exertion. Where pulmonary disease is present, a chronic, soft cough may be heard and as it advances hyperpnoea and eventually dyspnoea develop. Evidence of tuberculous mastitis will often produce palpable induration of the upper part of the udder and supramammary nodes. A variety of other signs may more rarely be seen with involvement of other systems.

PREVENTION AND CONTROL

There has been a commonly held opinion that milk from infected cattle generally provided a low dose of organisms which effectively acted for many as an immunogen, conferring a protective immunity (Collins and Grange 1983). This opinion was indeed confirmed by Sjogren and Sutherland (1975), who confirmed that there was a protective effect of childhood bovine infection and showed an inverse relationship between the incidence of tuberculosis in cattle populations and that in man. However, the protection of populations in this manner results in an unacceptable risk of disease to the minority. A campaign of BCG vaccination with removal of the risks posed by infected cattle by pasteurization of milk and eradication of tuberculosis from cattle is the ideal approach to the problem.

National cattle tuberculosis eradication schemes have greatly reduced or minimized the risk of bovine tuberculosis for man in most of Europe, North America, and other developed countries. However, the cost of national eradication, together with requirement for the veterinary infrastructure necessary to operate it, means that in developing countries this may not always be feasible. However, in such countries, where large dairy concerns are established, usually involving European breeds which may be more susceptible to general disease problems and also tuberculosis, pasteurization of the milk and a policy of test and slaughter of stock should be required (Kleeberg 1984).

In situations of sporadic infection of cattle, as is currently the case in Britain, a risk assessment will be required to determine the appropriate action necessary. For this close medical veterinary liaison is desirable. Whether the cattle failing the tuberculin test were found to show gross lung lesions causing them to be 'open cases' needs to be considered in making a judgement as to the likely risks to the cowman or handlers. If udder lesions were found, which is now very rarely so in Britain, these will pose a far wider risk. If the farm is retailing raw milk, this will be stopped forthwith under the public health regulations, but even if the farm milk is sent for pasteurization it is likely that fresh raw milk will be drunk by the farmer's and farm workers' families. Initial action should be to determine the Heaf test status of those at risk. Where strong reactions are found, clinical examination and X-ray may be considered. Further action with regard to chemotherapy would be dependent on the findings.

Routine prophylactic chemotherapy is not justified as no evidence of acquisition of infection from such outbreaks over the past two decades has been recorded in Britain.

Vaccination of cattle with BCG has been examined by trials on a number of occasions, but the immunity conferred has been found to be variable, often poor, and vaccination has not proved to be an effective means of control in cattle (Lepper and Corner 1983).

Surveillance for *M. bovis* infection of man requires that all isolates from man be typed, which is an aspect of tuberculosis bacteriology that has been lacking in many countries (Collins and Grange 1983). Without this information the contribution made by animals to the human problem remains a matter of speculation. *Mycobacterium bovis* is usually resistant to pyrazinamide and often isoniazid and thus, where it is found, it may be necessary to change the regimen.

OTHER ZOONOTIC MYCOBACTERIA

The majority of the other mycobacteria that infect patients are widespread in the environment and have no particular relationship with animals. They have been variously called atypical, anonymous, non-tuberculous, or mycobacteria other than tubercle bacilli (MOTT). A more accurate collective name for them is 'opportunist mycobacteria' as they usually require some defect such as pre-existing lung disease or immunosuppression before they can establish infection (Marks 1964). Of the 13 species of opportunist mycobacteria that are well documented as capable of causing human disease, only two are truly zoonotic—*M. avium* and *M. marinum*. Recently a tuberculosis-like organism has been isolated from cats. The public health significance of this is at present unknown (see below).

MYCOBACTERIUM AVIUM (CHESTER 1901)

Mycobacterium avium is the cause of tuberculosis in a wide range of bird species and has also been isolated from other animals including pigs, cattle, and deer. In humans it causes pulmonary disease in adults, cervical lymphadenopathy in children, and disseminated disease in immunosuppressed individuals. Taxonomically it is closely related to *M. intracellulare* and to a lesser extent to *M. scrofulaceum* and is thus often referred to as a member of the *Avium–intracellulare* (MAI) complex or the *Avium–intracellulare–scrofulaceum* (MAIS) complex. A majority now regard *M. scrofulaceum* to be sufficiently different for it to be a separate species. Within the MAI complex over 20 different serotypes are recognized (Schaefer 1967) and, of

these, types 1–6 and 8–11 are considered to be truly *M. avium*.

In birds *M. avium* infection is acquired via the alimentary tract. This gives rise to granulomatous lesions in the intestines, liver, spleen, and bone marrow. The lesions in the gastric mucosa can become necrotic tuberculous foci which ultimately destroy the mucosa and form ulcers through which the contents escape into the intestinal canal. The material that is discharged contains large numbers of acid-fast bacilli (AFB). The isolation of *M. avium* from other animals such as pigs and cattle is unlikely to be of importance clinically as carcasses are routinely inspected. Deer for human consumption are not inspected so closely but then it is difficult to imagine how *M. avium* could be transmitted to humans.

PULMONARY DISEASE

This is predominantly a disease of middle-aged to elderly males with chronic bronchitis and emphysema or some other form of lung damage. The signs, symptoms, and radiographic appearances are indistinguishable from those due to *M. tuberculosis* and it is not until the laboratory has isolated and identified the organism that the clinician is aware that he or she is dealing with disease caused by *M. avium*. Symptoms develop gradually and the picture is one of a subacute or chronic illness rather than an acute one.

Sputum may be positive for AFB on direct microscopy but there is no evidence of patient to patient transmission, unlike classical tuberculosis which is transmitted via infectious aerosols produced by coughing or sneezing. Exactly how *M. avium* infection is acquired is not known. There is little evidence of infection being directly acquired from birds and it is assumed that the organisms are excreted and remain viable in the environment. Suwankrugharn and Leat (1977) showed that *M. avium* artificially inoculated into soil survived for up to 6 months, and there are references in Francis (1958) which claim that avian bacilli can remain viable in the 'barnyard' for up to 4 years.

The incidence of disease due to *M. avium* is difficult to determine as there is no statutory requirement for cases to be notified as there is with infection due to *M. tuberculosis*. Prior to the advent of AIDS there were between 30 and 40 new cases of pulmonary disease due to *M. avium* each year in England and Wales. *Mycobacterium avium* infections in patients with AIDS have increased these figures dramatically (Campbell and Jenkins 1990).

The treatment of pulmonary disease due to *M. avium* is difficult as strains are resistant *in vitro* to the commonly used antituberculosis drugs. However, the correlation between this resistance and an *in vivo* response is unclear. Hunter *et al.* (1981) showed that a significant number of patients infected with strains of the

MAI complex responded satisfactorily to a regimen containing rifampicin and ethambutol despite *in vitro* resistance. However, it was necessary to give the drugs for 2 years rather than the standard 6–9 months. Studies are in progress by the British Thoracic Society to investigate further standard regimens and the newer drugs such as clarithromycin and the quinolones.

MYCOBACTERIUM AVIUM AND AIDS

As stated above, the advent of AIDS has had a significant effect on the incidence of *M. avium* infections. The species occurs as a late complication of HIV disease and may be localized or disseminated. Other opportunist mycobacteria can infect AIDS patients, but by far the most common opportunist mycobacterial pathogen is *M. avium*. Why this should be is not known.

These cases can be difficult to diagnose and it is important that bacteriological confirmation of the diagnosis be obtained. Specimens which are not normally examined in tuberculosis bacteriology, such as faeces, can be very rewarding from a clinical point of view. They are often highly positive on direct microscopy but cultures can be difficult to obtain because of the concomitant contamination with other bacteria.

CERVICAL LYMPHADENOPATHY

Opportunist mycobacteria, particularly the MAI complex and *M. malmoense* can cause superficial cervical lymphadenopathy, mainly in children. As with pulmonary disease there is little evidence of infection being directly acquired from infected animals and the most likely source is environmental. Bacilli are thought to enter via the tonsils or following minor trauma to the gums after, for example dental treatment. The nodes are unilateral and there is no systemic upset. The treatment of choice is total excision of the affected nodes but if this is not possible they will resolve spontaneously in time. Antituberculosis chemotherapy is not indicated (White *et al.* 1986).

The incidence of this problem is difficult to determine as some cases are diagnosed by histopathology without bacteriological confirmation. In England and Wales between 1981 and 1994 there were over 200 cases due to the MAI complex but an unknown number of these would have been caused by *M. intracellulare* rather than *M. avium*.

MYCOBACTERIUM MARINUM
(ARONSON 1926)

Mycobacterium marinum is a pathogen of fish and causes discrete self-limiting granulomatous lesions in humans. These have been acquired from swimming pools

(Linnel and Norden 1954) or more frequently from aquaria, hence the term 'fish-tank granuloma'. (Gray *et al.* 1990). The fish themselves develop a disseminated granulomatous disease which ultimately leads to wasting and death.

In humans the granulomas appear as tender, erythematous, small papules. These later coalesce to form a nodule which may become pustular. When acquired from swimming pools the lesions tends to occur on the elbows, knees, or feet which have been abraded by contact with the sides of the pool. In fish-tank granuloma the lesions occur on the hands and wrists, often following cuts. Occasionally there may be a sporotrichoid type spread up the forearm.

In the laboratory AFB are sometimes seen by microscopy of a biopsy but culture is still needed to confirm the diagnosis. This can take several weeks and slopes need to be incubated at 30 °C as *M. marinum* is unlikely to grow at 37 °C on primary isolation. The species is photochromogenic and identification is relatively simple.

The lesions will resolve spontaneously but this can take several months. Many regimens have been used, often with success, but it is not clear if this is due to the drugs or spontaneous healing. A combination of co-trimoxazole and minocycline appears to be the most efficacious (Gray *et al.* 1990).

'M. TUBERCULOSIS' IN CATS

It has long been recognized that cats can develop skin lesions in which it was possible to demonstrate AFB by direct microscopy but cultures were rarely if ever positive. This was thought to be cat leprosy or possibly caused by *M. leprae-murium*. In recent years tissues from cats have been cultured in the Bactec 460 radiometric system (Becton Dickinson, Oxford) and after 6–8 weeks incubation have given a positive growth. On subculture to solid media these strains have grown very slowly but appear to have the cultural characters of *M. tuberculosis*. More importantly, they have given a positive result with a DNA probe specific for the tuberculosis complex. This probe detects the insertion sequence IS 6110 which is specific for the complex (Gen-probe, San Diego, USA). The exact significance of these findings from a public health point of view is not clear. So far similar strains have not been isolated from human material (Gunn-Moore and Jenkins 1994).

CONCLUSIONS

Mycobacterium bovis and *M. marinum* are clearly transmitted from the animal host to humans. Fortunately, in developed countries the reservoir of *M. bovis* disease in cattle has been greatly reduced and as a result most cases are now re-activation of disease acquired many years earlier. However, the discovery of foci of infection in other species such as badgers means that surveillance of the disease in cattle must be maintained. In developing countries, eradication schemes, if they exist at all, are erratic and inconsistent and there is a dearth of accurate information on the incidence of the disease.

Mycobacterium marinum is relatively unimportant as a zoonosis. The disease is self-limiting and can easily be avoided by taking sensible precautions such as wearing gloves when cleaning fish tanks etc.

The position of *M. avium* as a zoonosis is more difficult to determine. The vast majority of infections are not contracted directly from infected animals and must therefore be a result of organisms persisting in the environment. This being the case, exposure is impossible to avoid.

REFERENCES

Anon (1965). Bovine tuberculosis. In *A Centenary of Animal Health 1865–1965*. HMSO, London.

Anon (1979). *Bovine tuberculosis in badgers*, Report from Ministry of Agriculture, Fisheries and Food. HMSO, London.

Anon (1993). *A global emergency*. WHO Report: TB. World Health Organization, Geneva.

Aronson J. D. (1926). Spontaneous tuberculosis in salt-water fish. *Journal of Infectious Diseases*, **39**, 314.

Black, H. (1972). The association of tuberculosis in man with a recurrent infection in a dairy herd. *New Zealand Veterinary Journal*, **20**, 14–15.

Campbell, I. A. and Jenkins, P. A. (1990). *Opportunist mycobacterial infections. In Respiratory Medicine* (ed. R. A. L. Brewis, G. J. Gibson, and D. M. Geddes). Baillière, Tyndall and Cox, London.

Chester, F. D. (1901). *A manual of determinative bacteriology*. MacMillan, New York.

Collins, C. H. and Grange, J. M. (1983). The bovine tubercle bacillus. *Journal of Applied Bacteriology*, **55**, 13–29.

Collins, C. H. Yates, M. D., and Grange, J. M. (1981). A study of bovine strains of *Mycobacterium tuberculosis* isolated from humans in south east England 1977–1979. *Tubercle*, **62**, 113–16.

Corner, L. A., Barrett, R. H., Lepper, A. W. D., Lewis, V., and Pearson, C. W. (1981). A survey of mycobacterioses in feral pigs in northern territory. *Australian Veterinary Journal*, **57**, 537–42.

Damato, J. J., Collins, M. T., Rothlauf, M. V., and McClatchy, J. K. (1983). Detection of mycobacteria by radiometric and standard plate procedures. *Journal of Clinical Microbiology*, **17**, 1066–73.

Draper, P. (1982). The anatomy of *Mycobacteria*. In *The biology of Mycobacteria*, Vol. 1, (ed. C. Ratledge and J. L. Stanford). Academic Press, London.

Fanning, A. and Edwards, S. (1991). *Mycobacterium bovis* infection in human beings in contact with elk (*Cervus canadensis*) in Alberta, Canada. *Lancet*, **338**, (8777), 1253–5.

Francis, J. (1958). *Tuberculosis in animals and man*. Cassell, London.

Gallagher, J., Muirhead, R. H., and Byrne, K. J. (1976). Tuberculosis in wild badgers (*Meles meles*) in Gloucestershire: Pathology. *Record*, **98**, 9–14.

Georghiou, P. Patel, A. M. and Konstantinos, A. (1989). *Mycobacterium bovis* as an occupational hazard in abattoir workers. *Australian and New Zealand Journal of Medicine*, **19**, 409–10.

Grange, J. (1980). *Tuberculosis. In Mycobacterial Diseases*, Current Topics in Infection, Series 1. Arnold, London

Gray, S. F., Stanwell-Smith R., Reynolds, N. J. and Williams, E. W. (1990). Fish tank granuloma. *British Medical Journal*, **300**, 1069.

Gunning, R. F. (1985). Bovine tuberculosis in the roe deer. *Veterinary Record*, **116**, 300.

Gunn-Moore, D. A. and Jenkins, P. A. (1994). Tuberculosis in cats. *Veterinary Record*, **134**, 395.

Huitema, H. (1969). The eradication of bovine tuberculosis in cattle in the Netherlands and the significance of man as a source of infection for cattle. *Selected papers of the Royal Netherlands Tuberculosis Association*, **12**, 62.

Hunter, A. M., Campbell, I. A., Jenkins, P. A., and Smith, A. P. (1981). Treatment of pulmonary infections caused by mycobacteria of the *Mycobacterium avium–intracellulare* complex. *Thorax*, **36**, 326.

Jenkins, P. A., Pattyn S. R., and Portaels, F. (1982). Diagnostic bacteriology. In *The Biology of the Mycobacteria*, Vol. 1, (ed. C. Ratledge and J. Stanford). pp. 411–70. Academic Press, London.

Jensen, K. A. (1953). Bovine tuberculosis in man and cattle. In *Advances in the control of zoonoses*. WHO/FAO seminar on zoonoses, Vienna, 1952. WHO monograph series 19. pp. 11–24. World Health Organization, Geneva.

Jensen, K. A., Lester, V. and Toderlund, K. (1940). The frequency of of bovine infection among tuberculous patients in Denmark, *Acta Tuberculosea Scandinavica*, **14**, 125–57.

Julian, A. F. (1981). Tuberculosis in the possum (*Trichosurus vulpecula*). In *Proceedings of the first symposium on marsupials in New Zealand* (ed. B. D. Bell) pp. 163–74. Zoological Publications from Victoria, University of Wellington.

Katarina Y. P. (1969). Observations on human infection with *Mycobacterium bovis*. *Tubercle*, **50**, 14–21.

Kleeberg, H. H. (1984). Human tuberculosis of bovine origin in relation to public health. *Revue Scientifique et Technique, Office Internationale des Epizooties*, **3**, 11–32.

Klimmer, J. (1946). Tuberculosis. In *Special pathology and theraputics of the diseases of domestic animals*, (5th edn, Hutya, F. Marek, J., Manninger, R., Greig, J. R., Mohler, J. R., and Eichorn, A.) Vol. 1, pp. 555–659. Baillière Tindall and Cox, London.

Lepper A. W. D. and Corner, L. A. (1983). Naturally occuring mycobacterioses of animals. In *The biology of the mycobacteria*, Vol. 2, (ed. C. Ratledge and J. Stanford), pp. 418–521. Academic Press, London.

Lesslie, I. W. (1960). Tuberculosis in attested herds caused by the human type tubercle bacillus. *Veterinary Record*, **72**, pp. 218–24.

Lesslie, I. W. (1968). Cross infections with mycobacteria between animals and man. *Bulletin of the International Union against Tuberculosis*, **41**, 285–8.

Linnel, F. and Norden, A. (1954) *Mycobacterium balnei*. A new acid-fast bacillus occurring in swimming pools and capable of producing skin lesions in humans. *Acta Tuberculosea Scandinavia, Suppl.*, **33**, 1.

McCool C, J. and Newton-Tabrett, D. A. (1979). The route of infection in tuberculosis in feral buffalo. *Australian Veterinary Journal*, **55**, 401–2.

Marks, J. (1964). Nomenclature of mycobacteria. *American Review of Respiratory Disease* **90**, 278.

Middlebrook, G., Reggiardo, Z., and Tigertt, W. D. (1977). Automatable radiometric detection of growth of *Mycobacterium tuberculosis* in selective media. *American Review of Respiratory Disease*, **115**, 1067–9.

Mitchison, D. A., Allen, B. W., Carrol, L. Dickinson J. M., and Aber, V. R. (1972). A selective oleic albumin agar medium for tubercle baccilli. *Journal of Medical Microbiology*, **5**, 165–75.

Muirhead, R. H., Gallagher J., and Birn K. J. (1974). Tuberculosis in wild badgers in Gloucestershire: Epidemiology. *Veterinary Record*, **95**, 522–55.

O'Connor, R. and O'Malley, E. (1989). *Badgers and bovine tuberculosis in Ireland*. Report prepared by The Economic and Social Research Institute for the Eradication of Animal Disease Board, Department of Agriculture and Food, Dublin.

O'Reilly, L. M. and Daborn, C. J. (1995). The epidemiology of *Mycobacterium bovis* infections in animals and man: a review. *Tubercle and Lung Disease*, **76**, 1–46.

Savage, W. G. (1929). *The prevention of human tuberculosis of bovine origin*. Macmillan, London.

Schaefer, W. B. (1967). Type-specificity of atypical mycobacteria in agglutination and antibody absorption tests. *American Review of Respiratory Disease*, **96**, 1165.

Sjögren, I. and Sutherland J. (1975). Studies of tuberculosis in man in relation to tuberculosis in cattle. *Tubercle*, **56**, 113–27.

Suwankrugharn, N. and Leat, J. (1977). Artificial colonisation as a method for studying the normal habitat of mycobacteria. *Tubercle*, **58**, 25.

Werner, V. E. (1981). Transmission of tuberculosis to a cattle herd from a livestock attendant with renal tuberculosis. *Monatsheft für Veterinarmedizin*, **36**, 819–20.

White, M. P., Bangash, H., Goel K. M., and Jenkins, P. A. (1986). Non tuberculous mycobacterial lymphadenitis. *Archives of Diseases in Childhood*, **61**, 368.

Wigle, W. D., Ashley, M. J., Killough, E. M., and Cosens, M. (1972). Bovine tuberculosis in humans in Ontario: the epidemiological features of 31 active cases occurring between 1964 and 1970. *American Review of Respiratory Diseases*, **106**, 528–34.

Wilkins, E. G. L., Griffiths, R. J., and Roberts, C. (1986). Bovine tuberculosis of the skin. *Journal of Infection*, **12**, 280–1.

16 PASTEURELLOSIS

Nicola J. Barrett

SUMMARY

'Pasteurellosis' (also known in animals as shipping fever or pneumonia, transport or transit fever, stock-yard pneumonia, bovine pneumonic pasteurellosis, haemorrhagic septicaemia, or avian, bird or fowl cholera), embraces a multitude of diseases caused by different *Pasteurella* species in animals and humans. Disease in animals usually occurs as a consequence of stress such as overcrowding, chilling, transportation, or as a result of a concurrent infection. Human infections occur after bites, scratches, or licks from infected animals. Infection may be prevented through the avoidance of animal bites and the prompt hygienic care of wounds.

HISTORY

There is some dispute in the literature as to whether Troussaint was the first to isolate *P. multocida* in 1879 in France (Rimler and Rhoades 1989), or whether it was Pasteur in 1880 and 1881 who also successfully isolated a bacterium from blood and organs of birds infected with fowl cholera (Mutters *et al.* 1989). The first name that was given to this organism was *Micrococcus gallicidus* by Burrill in 1883; Zopf called it *M. cholerae gallinarum* in 1885, and Trevisan changed the name to *Bacterium cholerae-gallinarum* (Frederiksen 1989*a*). The generic name *Pasteurella* was subsequently suggested by Trevisan in 1887 who wanted to commemorate Pasteur's work on the earlier elucidation of the type species (Mutters *et al.* 1989). The first published case of human pasteurellosis appears to have been that described by Debre in 1919, although some authors believe that it was Brugnatelli in 1913 (Frederiksen 1989*b*).

THE AGENT

TAXONOMY AND MOLECULAR BIOLOGY

The genus *Pasteurella*, family Pasteurellaceae, are classically aerobic and facultatively anaerobic, fermentative, Gram-negative, small non-motile coccoid, ovoid, or rod-shaped organisms that do not produce spores (Mutters *et al.* 1989). The taxonomy of Pasteurella is still debated (MacInnes and Borr 1990; Bisgaard 1993)

Pasteurella sensu stricto

According to (Mutters *et al.* 1989) this group of 11 species, based on common biochemical features as well as phenotypic criteria, now comprises: *P. multocida*, *septica*, and *gallicida*. The first two have been described in mammals, man, and birds, and the third from birds alone. The other recognized species include *P. gallinarum*, the avian respiratory pathogen, found particularly in chickens; *P. dagmatis* (previously *P. pneumotropica* biotype Henriksen, *Pasteurella* 'gas' or *Pasteurella* new species 1), found in both animals, particularly dogs and cats, and humans; *P. canis* biotype 1 (formerly biotype 6 of *P. multocida*), found in dogs and humans following bites or scratches from these animals; and *P. canis* biotype 2 (formerly Bisgaard's taxon 13) found in calves; *P. stomatis*, usually found in dogs, cats, and human injuries caused by these animals' bites; *P. anatis* (identical to Bisgaard's taxon 1) that colonizes the intestinal tract of ducks, and *P. langaa* (identical to Bisgaard's taxon 4) in the respiratory tracts of chickens; *P. avium* (NAD requiring), *P. volantium*, and the provisional *Pasteurella* species A (most of which were formerly attributed to *Haemophilus avium*, in part now re-classified as *P. avium*) are principally found in fowl (*P. avium* also comprises an NAD-independent type found in calves); and finally the provisional *Pasteurella* species B (previously a biotype of *P. multocida*) reported in dogs, cats, and man. Further to this there are other taxa, some of which are zoonotic such as the *Actinobacillus/Pasteurella*-like organisms (previously Bisgaard's taxon 16) which have been isolated from dogs and occasionally humans, that exhibit common features of *Pasteurella sensu stricto* but for which no genetic affiliation has been observed. Similarly *P. 'bettii'* (or *P. bettyae*), a designation given by some to a group of organisms mainly found in the human genitourinary tract, remains as *species incertae sedis*, as does the SP-group, identified in guinea-pigs and a human stool specimen, and the SP-like (Bisgaard's taxon 6) also found in guinea-pigs. The existence of such 'strains' may indicate the occurrence of more, but as yet unrecognized, species in this genus. Even more recently other species of *Pasteurella* have been reported, including *P. granulomatis* found in cattle in Brazil, and *P. caballi* found in horses in the USA and Sweden, and from an infected wound of a Danish veterinary surgeon. The ongoing identification of new species and the reclassification of previously described strains means that the interpretation of any published data is difficult (Bisgaard 1993).

Other *Pasteurella*

The species and taxa that have been excluded from *Pasteurella sensu stricto* in the recent reclassification include: *P. haemolytica* (reported from cattle, sheep, goats, and man), *P. aerogenes* (isolated from pigs and man), *P. pneumotropica* biotypes Heyl and Jawetz, and *P. multocida* biotype 1 (both found in laboratory mammals), and *P. testudinis* (identified in tortoises). However, while these species have currently maintained their generic name, others have been both removed and renamed, such as *P. ureae* which is strictly adapted to the human host and now redesignated as *Actinobacillus ureae*.

P. multocida

Several serological classification systems have been devised to correlate specific strains of *P. multocida* with host specificity, virulence, or disease. Carter's classification in the 1950s and 1960s grouped *P. multocida* into five serotypes based on polysaccharide antigens determined by a passive or indirect haemagglutination test; A, B, D and E are all capsular types, whereas C, a component of the normal flora of the respiratory tract of dogs and cats, is a non-capsulated strain.

P. haemolytica

Two general approaches to the typing of the *P. haemolytica* complex have been adopted (Mutters *et al.* 1989): biotyping and serological typing.

DISEASE MECHANISMS

The virulence and multifunctional pathogenicity of members of the Pasteurellaceae has been reviewed by Nicolet (1990).

GROWTH AND SURVIVAL REQUIREMENTS

Pasteurella grow between 30 and 40 °C. They may show bipolar staining, particularly as fresh isolates stained with Romanowsky stains such as Wright or Geimsa. *Pasteurella multocida* and *P. haemolytica* are glucose positive, sucrose positive, urease negative, and H_2S nega-

tive. Certain strains produce capsules of varying size and are believed by some to be more virulent than the non-capsulated strains.

Initial isolation from clinical specimens is usually made on enriched agar media supplemented with 5 per cent inactivated serum or bovine, horse, or sheep blood in air or air plus five per cent carbon dioxide. Cultures can be maintained and colonial variants selected on BBL-trypticase soy, Difco-tryptose, Gibco-dextrose starch or other comparable agars, with or without serum supplement. Several selective media have been developed to recover *Pasteurella* from specimens that are grossly contaminated (Rimler and Rhoades 1989). Alternatively, virulent strains of *P. multocida* can be recovered by subcutaneous inoculation of mice and cultures subsequently made from liver, spleen, and heart, but such methods are not appropriate for large numbers of specimens. The growth requirements for *P. multocida* have been the subject of numerous studies (Rimler and Rhoades 1989).

Much less work has been carried out on the other zoonotic agents of pasteurellosis, namely *P. pneumotropica*, *P. dagmatis*, *P. stomatis*, *P. canis*, and *P. aerogenes*, with regard to their molecular biology, disease mechanisms, growth and survival requirements. Mutters *et al.* (1985) describe the characteristics of the genus *Pasteurella* and the species now included in *Pasteurella sensu stricto*.

THE HOSTS

ANIMAL

The range of susceptible mammals and birds is now known to be very wide and the organism has been frequently isolated from the nasopharyngeal region of healthy animals. *Pasteurella multocida* in particular is so widespread amongst terrestrial and aquatic mammals and birds (well over 100 different species have been identified) that it would probably be unwise to exclude any of these species as possible hosts (Biberstein 1981; Rimler and Rhoades 1989).

Pasteurella multocida is associated with several different clinical entities, such as haemorrhgic septicaemia (HS) and bronchopneumonia of cattle, and more rarely meningitis, localized infections, abortions, mastitis, and arthritis; septicaemia in birds; HS, pneumonia, and atrophic rhinitis in pigs; rhinitis, pneumonia, and septicaemia in rabbits; pneumonia and HS in sheep; less frequently mastitis, localized infections, abortions, and meningitis or meningoencephalitis in cattle; and possibly atrophic rhinitis and pneumonia in goats. *Pasteurella multocida* also occurs as wound infections in dogs and cats and the subspecies *septica* has been associated with infections of the central nervous system

(CNS) in cats. It has often been identified as a secondary invader in animals, rather than the sole cause of the above symptoms and signs. Disease may result from invasion of commensal organisms during periods of stress or following infections with viruses, mycoplasmas, or rickettsias. *Pasteurella multocida* are normal oral and pharyngeal flora of dogs, cats, wild and domestic ruminants, horses, swine, rabbits, opossums, rodents, birds, and reptiles. Carriage rates are variable and may range from 3.5 per cent in buffalo to 90 per cent in cats (Jones and Lockton 1987).

Pasteurella haemolytica is found commonly in ruminants and has been identified as the causative agent of: enzootic pneumonia of and systemic infections in sheep, septicaemia of lambs; pneumonia or bovine respiratory disease complex (*BRDC*) in cattle, in association with *P. multocida*; and less frequently meningitis and arthritis in lambs; atypical pneumonia in sheep and pneumonia in goats; mastitis in ewes and cows; and rarely septicaemia of newborn calves. Infections may also occur in pigs. *Pasteurella haemolytica* is commonly found in the nasal cavity of healthy cattle, sheep, and goats.

Pasteurella pneumotropica is a major cause of pasteurellosis in laboratory rodents, including rats, mice, hamsters, and guinea-pigs. Mice and rabbits suffer enzootic pneumonia; septicaemia, genital infections, abscesses, and mastitis have all been reported in rodents. Laboratory rodents may carry the organism on the oropharyngeal mucous membranes.

Pasteurella dagmatis and *P. stomatis* are mainly found in the nasopharynx of dogs and cats, *P. canis* biotype 1 is found in dogs, and biotype 2 has been isolated from the lungs of calves with pneumonia and from sheep, and *P. aerogenes* in the respiratory and gastrointestinal tract of pigs.

HUMAN

Pasteurella multocida is the most commonly reported zoonotic infection in this group, resulting usually from infected dog and cat bites. *Pasteurella haemolytica* has also been associated with dog-bite wounds. *Pasteurella pneumotropica* (possibly *P. dagmatis*) has been reported as causing wound infections and very rarely septicaemia, meningitis, respiratory tract, and bone and joint infections. *Pasteurella dagmatis*, *P. stomatis*, and *P. canis* biotype 1 infections have all been associated with dog bites and other animal wounds; sometimes more than one species may be isolated from a single wound. *Pasteurella dagmatis* and *P. canis* may also be found in patients with chronic respiratory tract disease, but infrequently. *Pasteurella dagmatis* may also result in systemic infections following animal bites. *Pasteurella aerogenes* wound infections usually associated with pig bites are rarely seen in man.

Pasteurella multocida, *P. haemolytica*, and *P. pneumotropica* (possibly *P. dagmatis*) have been found in the respiratory tract of healthy people.

Incubation period
Usually within 24 to 48 hours from the bite.

Symptoms and signs, and pathology
Infections may range from trivial sepsis to severe abscesses that may be accompanied by septicaemia. A typical infection results in a diffuse cellulitis at the site of the lesion, accompanied by pain and swelling. Lymphangitis occurs in about 20 per cent of cases and regional lymphadenitis in 10 per cent. Local complications such as osteomyelitis, tenosynositis and arthritis may cause prolonged disability. Septic arthritis particularly affects the knee joint. Other organisms such as *Staphylococcus aureus* and *Pseudomonas aeruginosa* may also be isolated from the infected sites. Conjunctivitis or endophthalmitis may occur following animal scratches or bites to the cornea.

Diagnosis
Early diagnosis is important, especially in the young and elderly, as well as in immunosuppressed patients including pregnant women. Clinical features are varied and mostly non-specific. A history of animal contact must be sought. A possible pitfall in the subsequent identification of the causative *Pasteurella* spp. with the (API) system has recently been highlighted. *Haemophilus influenzae* and *H. parainfluenzae* may be misidentified as *P. pneumotropica*, or less frequently as *P. multocida* or *P. haemolytica*. Hamilton-Miller (1993) suggests that isolates identified as one of these species using the API system should be tested for X and V dependency. *Pasteurella* spp. should grow well on the nutrient agar required for this test whereas *Haemophilus* spp. grow only around the appropriate supplements.

Treatment
The majority of wound infections will heal following local treatment with or without systemic antibiotics. *Pasteurella* are highly susceptible to penicillin and ampicillin.

The role of antibiotics in the prophylaxis of infections in bite or scratch wounds is controversial. *Pasteurella multocida* and other *Pasteurella* spp. account for only some of the resulting infections, and other micro-organisms especially *S. aureus* should also be considered. Most infections will heal on local treatment only, but those with lowered resistance (on steroids for example), those with wounds involving the hands or face, immunocompromised, or diabetic patients may require prophylactic antibiotics.

The evaluation, management, and treatment of animal bites has been reviewed by (Weber and Hansen 1991).

Prognosis

The disease is effectively self-limiting but septicaemia and other serious symptoms may occur.

EPIDEMIOLOGY

Infected animal wounds have been identified as a major public health problem in developed countries. In Denmark in the 1970s there were an estimated 10 000 dog bites annually. In the United States it was assumed that over 1 million animal bites occurred annually, of which only one-sixth to one-half were reported (Frederiksen 1989*b*; Weber and Hansen 1991). In England and Wales in the 1980s there were an estimated 209 000 dog bites of man that resulted in presentation at hospital each year (Young 1988). In France there were an estimated 17 million cats and dogs with 500 000 animal bites each year. Cat bites may occur less frequently, although some believe that they more often result in infection which may be due either to the nature of cat bites in that their sharp teeth penetrate more deeply, or due to the pathogenicity or virulence of the responsible organism (Weber and Hansen 1991). Although most bite wounds are trivial and most victims do not seek medical attention, they result in significant medical costs. In the United States dog bites account for 70–93 per cent of animal bites, cat bites 3–15 per cent, and 'wild' animals less than 1 per cent. The risk of acquiring infection from a penetrating dog bite is between 2 and 29 per cent.

Occupational groups at risk from animal bites or other injuries, and infections arising from indirect contact with animals, include veterinary surgeons, laboratory workers, farmers and, in general, any individuals working with wild or domesticated animals.

In Sweden an analysis of *Pasteurella* strains identified between 1989 and 1992 revealed that of the 159 isolates 95 were *P. multocida* subspecies *multocida*, 21 subspecies *septica*, 28 *P. canis* biotype 1, 10 *P. stomatis*, and five *P. dagmatis* (Holst *et al.* 1992). Ninety-four per cent of infections were wounds; there were five cases of septicaemia, and three of meningitis. In a 12-year study of *Pasteurella* infections in England, Wales, and Ireland reported by laboratories from 1975 to 1986, 3699 cases were identified (Young 1988) of which 93 per cent were *P. multocida*. Skin infections were identified in 3185 cases (86 per cent); 9 per cent were respiratory tract infections, 2.4 per cent septicaemias, and less than

1 per cent each were abdominal infections, meningitis, bone and joint, eye, and urinary tract infections.

PREGNANCY-ASSOCIATED CASES

Recent reviews and case reports of infections in pregnancy include that by Roll of *et al.* (1992) who reported on two cases of severe infections that occurred in the second trimester of pregnancy in previously healthy women, one of whom suffered meningitis and the other had cellulitis and deep abscess formation. The fetuses were not apparently affected. Both women had contact with cats and dogs; neither had been bitten, but they had been licked by their pets from which *P. multocida* and *P. stomatis* were subsequently isolated. Waldor *et al.* (1992) reported a case of *in utero* infection in the first trimester of pregnancy. Following treatment the 31-year-old mother from the United States recovered rapidly from the bacteraemia but the 12-week-old fetus was spontaneously aborted. *Pasteurella multocida* was isolated from the woman's blood and vagina, and also from her two cats and dog. The authors cited five previous cases of suspected or proven pasteurella bacteraemia during pregnancy recorded in the literature. All occurred in the third trimester; three fetuses died, as did one mother due to disseminated intravascular coagulation. Three of the women had been bitten/scratched by cats and one other had been in contact with pets. Wong *et al.* (1992) also reported on a case of *P. multocida* infection in a 21-year-old female in Scandinavia with a twin pregnancy. The woman developed chorio-amnionitis at 27 weeks' gestation after prolonged rupture of membranes. One twin in a separate sac suffered infection and died shortly after birth; the other twin was not infected. Infection is believed to have been caused by ascending infection from asymptomatic colonization of the vaginal tract. In Finland a 37-year-old pregnant woman gave birth normally at 37 weeks following ruptured membranes but the infant died the next day of fulminant bacterial pneumonia (Andersson *et al.* 1994). The mother became feverous postpartum but recovered after antibiotic treatment. *Pasteurella multocida* subspecies *septica* was isolated from her cervix and the infants nasopharynx, and lung post-mortem. Swabs from the tonsils of the family's cat were also positive for the same organism although the mother did not recall any bites or scratches in the weeks preceding delivery. The mode of transmission to the child was uncertain; it may have occurred *in utero* through subclinical chorio-amnionitis, or in the vagina during delivery from an ascending infection of the mother. In 1994 Thorsen *et al.* described a case of *P. aerogenes* infection in a stillborn baby and its mother at 31 weeks' gestation in Denmark. During an uncomplicated pregnancy the mother had worked on a pig farm but the organism was not subsequently isolated from some of the sows housed there. The authors suggested a relationship between the isolation of the bacterium and sudden fetal death, and that transmission may have occurred haematogenously or from the lower genital tract to the uterus and fetus.

TRANSMISSION

Transmission is primarily via bites or scratches from dogs and cats, and less frequently from other animals. Other routes of transmission have also been described; *P. multocida* infections may be acquired from animals by their licking on mucosal surfaces or on injured skin (Rollof *et al.* 1992). Cases of *P. multocida* meningitis and ear infections have been associated with dog and cat licks to the faces and ears, and of endocarditis via the licking of leg ulcers by a dog (Hombal and Dincsoy 1992). Man may also become infected from the respiratory aerosol of infected cattle, sheep, pigs, poultry, and cats. Non-zoonotic transmission may also occur. Transmission of *Pasteurella multocida* direct from man to man has not been reported but might occur amongst patients with respiratory tract disease.

PREVENTION AND CONTROL

Vaccination for some forms of pasteurellosis in livestock are available worldwide (Donachie 1992).

Elimination of stray dogs and cats can reduce the chances of bites and therefore prevent some cases. Guidelines covering education of children and information for pet owners on how to avoid animal bites has been produced in the United States but their effectiveness has not been evaluated. Wounds, particularly bites, should be thoroughly cleansed. Those working with animals should have a high index of suspicion, particularly if immunocompromised or pregnant.

REFERENCES

Andersson, S. *et al.* (1994). Fatal congenital pneumonia caused by cat-derived *Pasteurella multocida*. *Paediatric Infectious Disease Journal*, **13**, 74–5.

Biberstein, E. L. (1981). *Haemophilus–Pasteurella–Actinobacillus:* their significance in veterinary medicine. In Haemophilus, Pasteurella *and* Actinobacillus, (ed. M. Kilian, W. Frederiksen and E. L. Biberstein), pp. 61–73. Academic Press, London.

Bisgaard, M. (1993). Ecology and significance of Pasteurellaceae in animals. *Zentralblatt fur Bakteriologie. International Journal of Medical Microbiology, Virology, Parasitology and Infectious Diseases*, **279**, 7–26.

Donachie, W. (1992). Prevention of pasteurellosis. *British Veterinary Journal*, **148**, 93–5.

Frederiksen, W. (1989*a*). A note on the name *Pasteurella multocida*. In Pasteurella *and pasteurellosis*, (ed. C. Adlam and J. M. Rutter), pp. 35–6. Academic Press, London.

Frederiksen, W. (1989*b*). Pasteurellosis of man. In Pasteurella *and pasteurellosis*, (ed. C. Adlam and J. M. Rutter), pp. 303–20. Academic Press, London.

Hamilton-Miller, J. M. T. (1993). A possible pitfall in the identification of *Pasteurella* spp. with the API system. *Journal of Medical Microbiology* **39**, 78–9.

Holst, E., Rollof, J., Larsson, L., and Nielsen, J. P. (1992). Characterization and distribution of *Pasteurella* species recovered from infected humans. *Journal of Clinical Microbiology*, **30**, 2984–7.

Hombal, S. M. and Dincsoy, H. P. (1992). *Pasteurella multocida* endocarditis. *Clinical Microbiology and Infectious Diseases*, **98**, 565–8.

Jones, A. G. H. and Lockton, J. A. (1987). Fatal *Pasteurella multocida* septicaemia following a cat bite in a man without liver disease. *Journal of Infection*, **15**, 229–35.

MacInnes, J. I. and Borr, J. D. (1990). The family Pasteurellaceae: modern approaches to taxonomy. *Canadian Journal of Veterinary Research*, **54**, S6–11.

Mutters, R., Ihm, P., Pohl, S., Frederiksen, W., and Mannheim, W. (1985). Reclassification of the genus *Pasteurella* Trevisan 1887 on the basis of deoxyribonucleic acid homology, with proposals for the new species *Pasteurella dagmatis*, *Pasteurella canis*, *Pasteurella stomatis*, *Pasteurella anatis*, and *Pasteurella langaa*. *International Journal of Systematic Bacteriology*, **35**, 309–22.

Mutters, R., Mannheim, W., and Bisgaard, M. (1989). Taxonomy of the group. In Pasteurella *and pasteurellosis*, (ed. C. Adlam and J. M. Rutter), pp. 3–34. Academic Press, London.

Nicolet, J. (1990). Overview of the virulence attributes of the HAP-group of bacteria. *Canadian Journal of Veterinary Research*, **54**, S12–15.

Rimler, R. B. and Rhoades, K. R. (1989). *Pasteurella multocida*. In Pasteurella *and pasteurellosis*, (ed. C. Adlam and J. M. Rutter), pp. 37–73. Academic Press, London.

Rollof, J., Johansson, H., and Holst, E. (1992). Severe *Pasteurella multocida* infections in pregnant women. *Scandinavian Journal of Infectious Diseases*, **24**, 453–6.

Thorsen, P., Moller, B. R., Arpi, M., Bremmelgaard, A., and Frederiksen, W. (1994). *Pasteurella aerogenes* isolated from stillbirth and mother. *Lancet*, **343**, 485–6.

Waldor, M., Roberts, D., and Kazanjian, P. (1992). *In utero* infection due to *Pasteurella multocida* in the first trimester of pregnancy: case report and review. *Clinical Infectious Diseases*, **14**, 497–500.

Weber, D. J. and Hansen, A. R. (1991). Infections resulting from animal bites. *Infectious Disease Clinics of North America*, **5**, 663–80.

Wong, G. P., Cimolai, N., Dimmick, J. E., and Martin, T. R. (1992). *Pasteurella multocida* chorioamnionitis from vaginal transmission. *Acta Obstetricia et Gynecologica Scandinavica*, **71**, 384–7.

Young, S. E. J. (1988). Pasteurella infections 1975–86. *PHLS Microbiology Digest*, **5**, 4–5.

17 Q FEVER

Thomas J. Marrie

SUMMARY

Q fever is a wide spread illness affecting wild and domestic animals and man. The etiological agent, *Coxiella burnetii*, has both a wild life and domestic animal cycle. In mammals infection localizes to the endometrium and the mammary glands. The organism is reactivated during pregnancy reaching high concentrations in the placenta. At the time of parturition the organism is aerosolized. Inhalation of *Coxiella burnetii* by susceptible animal results in Q fever. In man Q fever may be acute (self limited febrile illness, pneumonia, hepatitis) or chronic (mostly endocarditis). Abortion and stillbirth are manifestations of Q fever in domestic animals and in animal models of disease (such as Q fever in pregnancy in a mouse model). A vaccine is available for abattoir workers and veterinarians and others in high risk occupations for acquiring Q fever.

HISTORY

In August 1935, E. H. Derrick, the Director of the Laboratory of Microbiology and Pathology at the Queensland Health Department at Brisbane, Australia was asked to investigate an outbreak of undiagnosed febrile illness among abattoir workers in Brisbane (Derrick 1937). This illness he named Q for 'query fever'. Burnet and Freeman inoculated guinea-pigs, mice, monkeys, and embryonated eggs with materials that they received from Derrick. In a haematoxylin–eosin-stained section from a mouse spleen they found areas filled with lightly stained material of faint, uniformly granular texture. Smears stained by Castaneda's method and with Gimesa stain revealed bodies which appeared to be of rickettsial nature (Burnet and Freeman, 1937). The organisms they saw were in the forms of tiny rods less than 1 μm in length and about 0.3 μm across—the shape varied from well-formed rods to coccoid. At about the same time Cox and G. Davis at the Rocky Mountain Laboratory in Montana, working on possible vectors of Rocky Mountain spotted fever and tularaemia, identified rickettsias (the Nine Mile agent) from ticks. In April 1938 Burnet sent Dyer spleen specimens from mice infected with the Q fever agent, Dyer showed that the Q fever agent was identical to the Nine Mile agent (McDade 1990). Derrick (1939) proposed the name *Rickettsia burnetii* for the Q fever agent; however, in 1948 Philip proposed that *Rickettsia burnetii* be considered as a single species of a distinct genus, *Coxiella* since it was now apparent that this organism was unique among the rickettsia. The Q fever agent is now known as *Coxiella burnetii*.

Early in the course of work with *C. burnetii* it was evident that it was highly infectious and, indeed, there were several reports of laboratory-acquired outbreaks of Q fever among employees at the National Institutes of Health from 1940 to 1946 (Hornibrook 1940; Huebner 1947; Spicknall *et al.* 1947)

In 1944 outbreaks of Q fever occurred among British troops stationed in Italy, Greece, and Corsica during the second World War. Outbreaks were also reported among American troops returning to the United States from duty in the Mediterranean area (Robbins and Regan 1946; Robbins *et al.* 1946).

Outbreaks of Q fever were observed at meat-packing houses in Amarillo, Texas (Topping *et al.* 1947) and Chicago, Illinois (Shepard 1947). As part of these studies Sheppard implicated aerosols as the route of transmission of Q fever in Chicago.

In a series of studies from southern California, Lennette and co-workers found that Q fever was associated with exposure to sheep and goats and that *Coxiella burnetii* could be isolated from the air of premises housing infected animals (Lennette *et al.* 1949; Lennette and Welsh 1951). In 1948 Huebner and Aleagnes isolated *Rickettsia burnetii* from raw milk obtained from cows in southern California. In 1950 Luoto and Huebner were able to isolate *C. burnetii* from placentas of naturally infected parturient dairy cows.

In 1956 Stoker and Fiset described phase variation in *Rickettsia burnetii*. This observation has proven to be a sentinel one in the history of *Coxiella burnetii*. As will be discussed later, phase variation is important in the pathogenesis of Q fever. By 1959 Q fever had been found in man and animals from 16 countries in Africa, nine in America, 23 in Europe, Asia, Australia, and Oceania (Babudieri 1959) and *C. burnetii* had been isolated from a wide variety of arthropods, wild, and domestic animals.

The discovery of phase variation was instrumental in vaccine studies of *C. burnetii*. In 1957 Abinanti and Marmion found that antibody against phase I antigen had a protective effect against infection in mice and guinea-pigs. Work during the 1960s examined the antibody response to inactivated whole-cell phase I vaccine in human volunteers (Bell *et al.* 1964), and in 1984 Marmion and co-workers reported the results of a clinical trial of a low-dose (30 μg), formalin-inactivated *C. burnetii* phase I vaccine, Henzerling strain, that they had used in Australian abattoir workers.

THE AGENT

Coxiella burnetii is a highly pleomorphic coccobacillus with a Gram-negative cell wall (Figs 17.1, 17.2). It measures 0.2×0.7 μm. It has a developmental cycle— this term applies to parasites that in addition to pleomorphism have developed forms with different functions to withstand physiological and biochemical variations in their habitats and immunological challenges (McCaul 1991). There are two cell types, distinguished on the basis of size, sensitivity to osmotic lysis, ability to metabolize exogenously supplied substrates, and peptidoglycan content. The development cycle of *C. burnetii* begins with attachment and ingestion of the small cell variant (SCV) by a host cell. Fusion of the primary lysosome with the phagosome containing the small cell variant occurs. (Figs 17.1, 17.2) After this there is metabolic activation of the SCV starting vegetative growth, leading to differences in morphological appearance. The acid pH of the phagolysosome activates the metabolic enzymes of

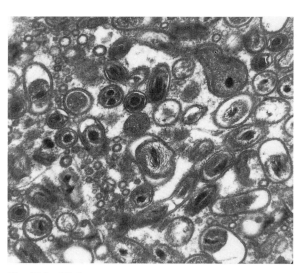

Fig. 17.2 Higher power view of the *C. burnetii* cells shown in Fig. 17.1. The electron-dense material is condensed DNA. Note the characteristic Gram-negative cell wall. (Magnification ×21 632.)

C. burnetii. During the early stage of bacterial growth the intermediate cell maintains the small cell variant morphology but loses its resistant property. Further bacterial growth leads to the development of a large cell variant and *C. burnetii* begins to undergo sporogenesis. Upon release from the mother cell the endogenous cell undergoes further development to achieve the full resistant capability of the small resting cell.

Following lysis from the cell *C. burnetii* is released into the external environment. Spores are also released. Both the small and large cell variants have Gram-negative cell walls. The formation of spores explains the ability of *C. burnetii* to withstand harsh environmental conditions. It survives for 7–10 months on surfaces at 15–20 °C, for more than 1-month on fresh meat in cold storage, and for more than 40 months in skimmed milk at room temperature (Christie 1974). *Coxiella burnetii* can be destroyed by 2 per cent formaldehyde but the organism has been isolated from infected tissues stored in formaldehyde for up to 4–5 months. It has also been isolated from fixed paraffinized tissues. Lysol 1 per cent and 5 per cent hydrogen peroxide will kill *C. burnetii*.

Coxiella burnetii undergoes phase variation (Stoker and Fiset 1956). In nature and laboratory animals it exists in the phase I state in which organisms react with late (45 day) convalescent guinea-pig sera and only slightly with early (21-day) sera. Repeated passage of phase I organisms in embryonated chicken eggs leads to gradual conversion to phase II avirulent forms. There are no morphological differences between the two phases although they differ in the sugar composition of their lipopolysaccharides (Schramek and Mayer 1982), and

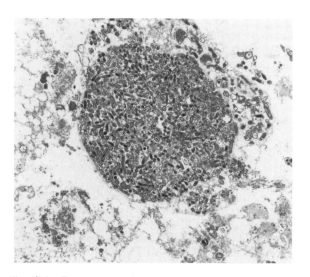

Fig. 17.1 Transmission electron micrograph of a vegetation from a patient with Q fever endocarditis. Note the many *C. burnetii* cells in a phagolysosome. (Magnification ×3865.)

their buoyant density in caesium chloride and in their affinity for basic fuchsin dyes. *Coxiella burnetii* lipopolysaccharide (LPS) is non-toxic to chicken embryos at doses of over 80 μg per embryo, in contrast to *Salmonella typhimurium* smooth and rough-type LPS, which is toxic in nanogram amounts (Hacksteadt *et al.* 1985).

Plasmids have been found in both phase I and phase II cells (Samuel *et al.* 1985). Three different plasmids varying from 36 to 45 kb have been described (Sawyer *et al.* 1987). The first plasmid, named Q_pH_1 was found in a Nine Mile phase I isolate. It is 36 kb and is present at about three copies per cell. The second plasmid, designated Q_pRS was obtained from an isolate named Priscilla which was recovered from the placenta of a goat that had aborted. This plasmid has been found in four isolates obtained from patients with Q fever endocarditis (Michael *et al.* 1990; Mallavia *et al.* 1991). Q_pRS has considerable homology with Q_pH_1 and is 39 kb in size. The third, a 51 kb plasmid, was obtained from feral rodent isolates near Dugway, Utah and has been designated Dugway (Stoennes and Lachman 1960). Isolates with no plasmids have plasmid DNA integrated into the genome. Stein and Raoult (1992b) examined eight new *C. burnetii* isolates from patients with chronic Q fever and found that seven of the eight had plasmids which were about 40 kb in size.

There is no correlation between plasmid type and disease caused by *C. burnetii*. The Q_pH_1 plasmid has been found in isolates from cases of acute Q fever while the Q_pRS plasmid and chromosomally integrated sequences with homology to this plasmid are found in isolates of patients with Q fever endocarditis (Minnier *et al.* 1991).

It has been suggested by some workers that there are at least six strains of *C. burnetii*. These are Hamilton, Bacca, Rasche, Biotzere, Corazon, and Dod. The first three strains contain the Q_pH_1 plasmid and have been associated with acute Q fever. Biotzere has plasmid Q_pRS and Corazon has no plasmid but plasmid-related sequences are present in the genome. These two strains are associated with chronic Q fever. The Dod strain, which contains the Q_pDG plasmid, is avirulent.

More recently Thiele *et al.* (1993) have used pulsed field gel electrophoresis to examine isolates of *C. burnetii* and have shown that there is considerable heterogeneity among isolates. It is very likely that there are more strains of *C. burnetii* than have been recognized to date.

The ability of *C. burnetii* to survive in the phagolysosome has been linked to its ability to produce superoxide dismutase which protects it from host cell generated superoxide anion and hydrogen peroxide (Akporiaye 1983). *Coxiella burnetii* inhibits the respiratory burst of phagocytosing human neutrophils, a property similar to that possessed by *Legionella* and *Leishmania* (Baca *et al.* 1993). Acid phosphatase is a possible virulence factor for *C. burnetii*.

Only a few of the *C. burnetii* genes are known; two of these comprise the heat-shock inducible *htp*AB operon (*htp*A and *htp*B genes) which encode the heat-shock protein that is homologous to similar proteins in mycobacteria and *E. coli* (Vodkin and Williams 1988). The *C. burnetii* genes for the two heat-shock proteins and for citrate synthase have been cloned and expressed in *Escherichia coli*. Hendrix *et al.* (1993) have cloned and-sequenced the gene *com*1 which codes for an outer membrane protein.

TAXONOMY

Coxiella burnetii is the sole species of its genus (Weiss *et al.* 1991). On the basis of 16S RNA sequence similarities, it has been placed in the gamma subdivision of proteobacteria with a specific but rather distant relationship to *Legionella*. Only *Wolbachia persica* belongs in the gamma subdivision with minor relatedness to the *Coxiella–Legionella* cluster.

PATHOGENICITY

When guinea-pigs are inoculated intraperitoneally with *C. burnetii* granulomas develop in the liver, bone marrow, and spleen. Guinea-pigs exposed to aerosols containing *C. burnetii* develop pneumonia within the first 5 days. The pneumonia begins to resolve by day 15 following exposure and is complete by day 29. Hepatic and splenic granulomas develop. Mice inoculated with *C. burnetii* either intranasally or intraperitoneally also develop pneumonia, hepatic, and splenic granulomas, bone marrow, and liver involvement (Baca 1991).

In studies with persistently infected L929 mouse fibroblasts or macrophage cell lines such as J774 and P3881, different isolates of *C. burnetii* produce different effects. Cells infected with Q_pRS isolates exhibit multivacuolation and do not proliferate in suspension cultures or infect J774 cells. Proteins of *C. burnetii* are inserted into the cell membrane of these cells and this leads to the antibody-dependent cell cytotoxicity found in Q fever (Marecki *et al.* 1978). Isolates implicated in short-term acute disease caused the insertion of more antigen into the host cell membrane than did isolates associated with chronic disease (Baca 1991). These observations may be a partial explanation as to why some patients develop acute Q fever and others develop chronic Q fever.

THE HOSTS

ANIMALS

Coxiella burnetii can infect a large number of animal species including livestock, but infection is usually asymptomatic. In his 1959 review Babudieri describes bronchopneumonia in goats due to Q fever and continuous fever lasting several days in infected cattle. Catarrhal mastitis in cows and bronchopneumonia in a dog have been reported. Studies from the United States suggested that there was no morbidity in cattle and sheep naturally infected with *C. burnetii* and no reports of effects on milk yields. Endocarditis, the major form of chronic Q fever in man, does not seem to occur in other animals.

Coxiella burnetii localizes to the uterus and mammary glands of infected animals. Cattle have been resistant to experimental infection by intranasal, intravenous, intravaginal inoculation, and by the feeding of contaminated bran. Intranasal infection of a pregnant cow by means by an atomizer did lead to infection. *Coxiella burnetii* has been isolated from the placentas of naturally infected cows and naturally infected and experimentally infected sheep (Long 1990). It has been transmitted transplacentally in a guinea-pig model of infection.

Once infected, cows have shed *C. burnetii* in milk for up to 32 months. Grist (1959) in his 4-year longitudinal study of a diary herd found that no more than 15 per cent of the milk cows showed evidence of infection at any one time. He suggested that infection is maintained within a herd largely by infection of younger non-immune animals. Sheep have shed the organism in faeces for 11–18 days postpartum (Welsh *et al.* 1958).

Outbreaks of abortion due to *C. burnetii* have been reported in goats, in cattle, and sheep. Inflammation of the placenta has been demonstrated in sheep and goats in instances where *C. burnetii* has caused abortion (Palmer *et al.* 1983). Stresses such as overcrowding and pregnancy are associated with multiplication of *C. burnetii* in the placenta. The placentas of infected sheep can contain 10^9 guinea-pig infective doses per gram of tissue.

In addition to cattle, sheep, and goats, which are the traditional reservoirs of *C. burnetii*, the following domestic animal species have been found to be infected with this organism in some areas:-pigs, horses, dogs, cats, camels, buffaloes, pigeons, geese, and fowl (Babudieri 1959; Marrie *et al.* 1985, 1993)

Coxiella burnetii has been found in many species of ticks and in lice and flies. Under experimental conditions it has been possible to infect fleas and cockroaches. Infection with *C. burnetii* is widespread throughout the wild animal population and the rate of this infection varies from country to country. Where Q fever is endemic there may very well be a differential infection rate among the wildlife; hares and rabbits are more commonly infected than other animals (Marrie *et al.* 1993).

Table 17.1 summarizes our studies of a variety of animals in Nova Scotia, carried out using a micro-immunofluorescence test. Our experience in Nova Scotia illustrates that the data regarding infected

Table 17.1 Rate of *Coxiella burnetii* infection of various animals in Nova Scotia as measured by antibodies to *C. burnetii* phase I and phase II antigens. Data are from (George and Marrie 1987; Marrie *et al.* 1985).

Animal	Number Tested	Percent positive IFA[a] test	
		Phase I	Phase II
Domestic			
Sheep	329	0	6.7
Cattle	214	24.2	23.8
Goats	29	3.5	7.0
Cats	216	6.0	24.1
Dogs	447	0	0
Wild			
Snowshoe hare (*Lepus americanus*)	730	49	12
Moose (*Alces alces americana Clinton*)	243	16.5	11.5
White-tailed deer *Odocoileus virginianus*)	68	1.5	4.4
Raccoon (*Procyon lotor*)	42	7.1	9.5

[a] IFA, indirect fluorescence antibody.

animals has to be correlated carefully with the epidemiology of this infection in man. We have studied several outbreaks of Q fever following exposure to infected parturient cats (Marrie *et al.* 1988a,b). We also have observed cases of Q fever following exposure to wild rabbits and to deer. We have been able to associate only three of our cases (out of >300) of Q fever with exposure to infected cattle. Yet Table 17.1 shows that a considerable percentage of the cattle are infected. In a seroepidemiological survey of a random sample of the Nova Scotia population we found that there was a statistically significant association between residence in four counties and seropositivity for *C. burnetii*. These four counties account for 75 per cent of the cattle, sheep, and goats in our province. However, exposure to cattle, sheep, and goats as reported by questionnaire data was not a risk factor for seropositivity. It is likely that indirect exposure resulted in subclinical Q fever in this population.

THE HUMAN HOST

Clinical features

Humans are the only animals known to develop illness regularly as a result of *C. burnetii* infection. There are several distinct syndromes of *C. burnetii* infection in man, and while such infections are usually divided into acute and chronic Q fever, the entities listed below are convenient and clinically important ways of dividing *C. burnetii* infection for purposes of discussion:

1. A self-limited febrile illness of 2–14 days' duration.
2. Pneumonia.
3. Endocarditis.
4. Hepatitis.
5. Osteomyelitis.
6. Q fever in the immunocompromised host.
7. Q fever in infancy.
8. Q fever in pregnancy.
9. Neurological manifestations.

Table 17.2 shows the symptoms of acute Q fever in patients from six different countries from 1948 to 1989. Fever and fatigue are the predominant manifestations in almost all of the patients in all series. Headache is also a prominent symptom, although its frequency ranges from a low of 65 per cent in the California series to a high of 98 per cent in the patients reported from Uruguay. Cough was reported in only 24 per cent of the patients in the Northern California series but in 90 per cent of the patients from Uruguay. Rash is infrequently reported. Neurological manifestations are generally uncommon but in the series from the West Midlands, UK, 23 per cent of the patients had neurological symptoms.

Self-limited febrile illness

Where Q fever is endemic a significant percentage of the general population, often of the order of 11–12 per cent, have been found to have antibodies to *C. burnetii*. Most of these individuals do not recall pneumonia or any other illness that could readily be attributable to this infection. The extent to which

Q fever contributes to undifferentiated febrile illnesses in the population may be very high, as suggested by a study from the south of Spain where 21 per cent of 505 adults who had fever of more than 1 week's and less than 3 weeks' duration had Q fever (Viciana 1992). All of these individuals had normal chest radiographs.

Pneumonia

Pneumonia is one of the predominant manifestations of acute Q fever in man, but there is tremendous variation in its reported frequency. It is the predominant manifestation of acute Q fever in Nova Scotia, but in France where hepatitis is the major manifestation of acute Q fever, and pneumonia is rarely seen (Dupont 1992).

Cough may not be present even though pneumonia is evident radiographically. In most instances the pneumonia is of mild to moderate severity, but it can be rapidly progressive, resulting in respiratory failure.

Physical examination of the chest is often normal. About 5 per cent of patients with pneumonia have splenomegaly. The rapidly progressive form of Q fever pneumonia mimics Legionnaires' disease, the pneumonic form of tularaemia, severe *Chlamydia pneumoniae* pneumonia, and in even pyogenic bacterial pneumonia.

The radiographic picture of Q fever pneumonia is variable (Fig 17.3–17.5). Segmental and subsegmental pleural opaced opacities are common (Gordan *et al.* 1984) Multiple rounded opacities are seen, and in Nova Scotia this is very suggestive of Q fever that follows exposure to infected parturient cats. Pleural effusions are found in up to one-third of cases.

Table 17.2 Symptoms of acute Q fever in patients from six different countries

	Percentage with indicated symptom					
	Northern California 1948–49; 180 patients (Clark *et al.* 1951)	Australia 1962–81; 111 patients (Spelman 1981)	Switzerland 1983; 191 patients (Dupuis *et al.* 1985)	Uruguay 1975–1985; 1358 patients[a] Somma–Moveirn *et al.* 1987)	Nova Scotia 1983–1986; 51 patients (Marrie *et al.* 1988a)	West Midlands UK March–April 1989; 102 patients (Smith *et al.* 1993)
Fever	100	100	88	98	94	99
Fatigue	100	NS[b]	97	98	98	NS
Chills	74	68	NS	NS	88	NS
Headache	65	86	77	98	73	68
Myalgia	47	60	64	NS	69	54
Sweats	31	NS	NS	98	84	NS
Cough	24	32	70	90	28	51
Nausea	22	25	25	NS	49	NS
Vomiting	13	42	25	NS	25	
Chest pain	10	NS	34	NS	28	45
Diarrhoea	5	7	NS	NS	22	NS
Sore throat	5	NS	27	NS	14	NS
Rash	4	8	5	NS	18	NS
Neurological	NS	NS	NS	NS	NS	23

[a] All cases occurred in workers at meat-processing plants.
[b] NS, not stated.

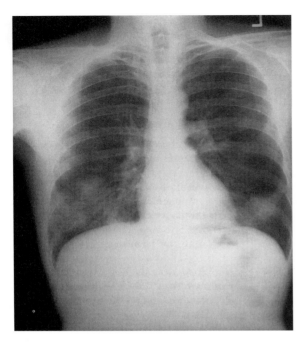

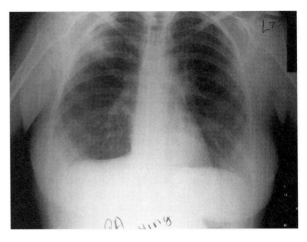

Fig. 17.4   Chest radiograph of a 20-year-old female with right upper lobe pneumonia due to *C. burnetii*.

The rare fatalities from *C. burnetii* pneumonia usually occur in patients with severe co-morbid illnesses. Information regarding the histology of Q fever in pneumonia in man is extremely limited. In one of

Fig. 17.3   Chest radiograph of a young man with Q fever pneumonia. Note the multiple rounded opacities.

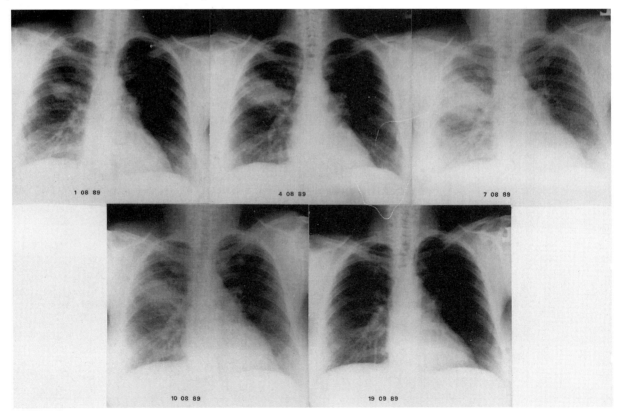

Fig. 17.5   Serial chest radiographs of a patient with Q fever pneumonia. Note the rapidity with which the opacity increases in size and the speed with which it resolves.

our patients with severe pneumonia the bronchial epithelial lining was denuded in part due to necrosis. The interstitium showed oedema and infiltration by lymphocytes and macrophages. Alveolar spaces were filled with macrophages and other cells resembling detached epithelium (Figs 17.6, 17.7). In another patient there was a lung mass composed of mixtures of macrophages, giant cells, plasma cells, and lymphocytes (Janigan and Marrie 1983)

White blood cell count is usually normal but one-third of patients have an increased count. A slight elevation occurs in the hepatic transaminase levels in almost all patients. Rarely, the syndrome of inappropriate secretion of antidiuretic hormone complicates the pneumonia (Biggs *et al.* 1984).

Diagnosis

The diagnosis of *C. burnetii* pneumonia is usually confirmed by demonstration of a fourfold rise in anti-

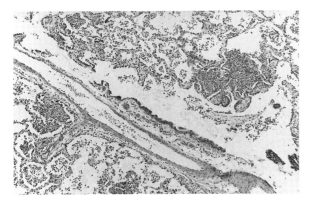

Fig. 17.6   Photomicrograph of an open lung biopsy from a patient with *C. burnetii* pneumonia. Note the extensive inflammatory response which is both alveolar and interstitial. (Magnification ×175.)

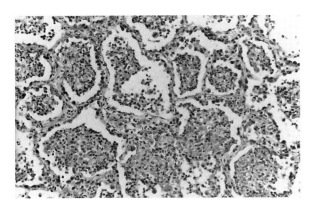

Fig. 17.7   Photomicrograph of an open lung biopsy from a patient with *C. burnetii* pneumonia. The alveoli are filled with an inflammatory exudate. There is hyperplasia of the pneumocytes lining the alveoli. (Magnification ×175.)

body titre between acute and convalescent sera, since most laboratories do not have the facilities required to isolate this micro-organism. Recently Stein and Raoult (1992a) were able to detect *C. burnetii* DNA by amplification using a polymerase chain reaction. They developed primers derived from the *C. burnetii* superoxide dismutase gene. This should allow the detection of *C. burnetii* in a variety of clinical specimens although the sensitivity of this test in *C. burnetii* pneumonia is still unknown. Since *C. burnetii* is an intracellular pathogen, there may be very little in the way of *C. burnetii* DNA in respiratory secretions.

A variety of laboratory tests have been used to detect antibodies to *C. burnetii*, including microagglutination, complement fixation, microimmunofluorescence, and enzyme-linked immunoabsorbent assay. The complement fixation and microimmunofluorescence tests are most commonly used. Antibodies should be determined to both phase I and phase II antigens. In acute Q fever, antibodies to phase II predominate while in chronic Q fever antibodies to phase I predominate.

Some authors have advocated using the indirect immunofluorescence test to detect antibodies to IgM so that a single serum sample may be used in the diagnosis of acute Q fever (Hunt *et al.* 1983). However, IgM antibodies may persist for up to 678 days following acute infection and in one study 3 per cent of 162 patients still had significant IgM antibody levels 1 year after infection (Dupius *et al.* 1985).

Treatment

The treatment of choice for *C. burnetii* pneumonia is tetracycline or doxycycline. Tetracycline is given in a dose of 500 mg every 6 hours for 7–10 days. Doxycycline is given in a dosage of 100 mg twice daily for 7–10 days. *In vitro* studies performed by Yeaman *et al.* (1987) suggest that several quinolones, including difloxacin, ciprofloxacin, and oxolinic acid, should also be effective in the treatment of Q fever. Rifampin is the most active antibiotic *in vitro* against *C. burnetii*.

Chronic Q fever

Clinical features

The major manifestation of chronic Q fever is endocarditis, but infection of vascular prostheses, aneurysms, osteomyelitis, hepatitis, prolonged fever and purpuric eruptions are reported (Brouqui *et al.* 1993).

As with other forms of endocarditis, infection usually develops on abnormal or prosthetic cardiac valves (Raoult *et al.* 1987). The incidence of Q fever endocarditis seems to be increasing, although this may reflect increased recognition of this entity. Turck *et al.* (1976) drew attention to this form of Q fever when they reported 16 cases of chronic Q fever that they diagnosed between 1968 and 1973. Their review of the literature yielded only 55 other cases of chronic Q fever. This contrasts with 79 cases of chronic Q fever reported from the Public Health Laboratory Service's Communicable Disease Surveillance Centre in England from 1975 to 1980 (Palmer and Young 1982). From 1975 to 1981 *C. burnetii* accounted for 3 per cent of all cases for endocarditis reported in England and Wales. In the small province of Nova Scotia, Canada with a population 900 000, 11 cases of Q fever endocarditis have been diagnosed between 1979 and 1993.

The clinical presentation is that of culture-negative endocarditis. Prolonged fever and negative blood cultures in a patient with an abnormal prosthetic valve should suggest this diagnosis. If these findings are combined with marked clubbing of the fingers and hyperglobulinaemia one should be even more suspicious of this diagnosis. Splenomegaly and hepatomegaly are found in about half the patients, and a purpuric rash due to leucocytoclastic vasculitis occurs in about 20 per cent of patients. The sedimentation rate is usually quite high (often >100 mm/h); anaemia and microscopic haematuria are present. Arterial emboli complicate the course of one-third of patients.

The vegetations in chronic Q fever are different for those found in pyogenic bacterial endocarditis. In chronic Q fever the vegetation is usually smooth and may form nodules on the valve (Fig. 17.8). Microscopically there is a subacute and chronic inflammatory infiltrate and many large, foamy macrophages (Fig. 17.9) full of the characteristic micro-organisms are readily seen with electron microscopy (Figs. 17.1 and 17.2).

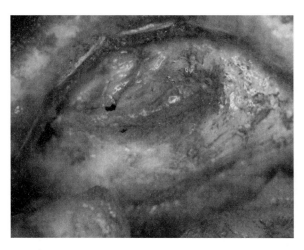

Fig. 17.8 *Coxiella burnetii* vegetation on a prosthetic valve. The 'ridge' is the vegetation (reproduced with permission from Raoult, D., Raza, A., and Marrie, T. J. (1991). Q fever endocarditis and other forms of chronic Q fever. In *Q fever.* Volume 1: *The disease*, (ed. T. J. Marrie pp. 179–99. CRC Press, Boca Raton, FLA.).

Diagnosis

Confirmation of the diagnosis of Q fever endocarditis is usually made serologically. A complement fixation titre of ≥1:200 to phase I antigen is said to be diagnostic of chronic Q fever, although not all patients in the series reported by Turck *et al.* (1976) had this titre. *Coxiella burnetii* can be isolated from the blood of patients with Q fever endocarditis by using a shell vial technique.

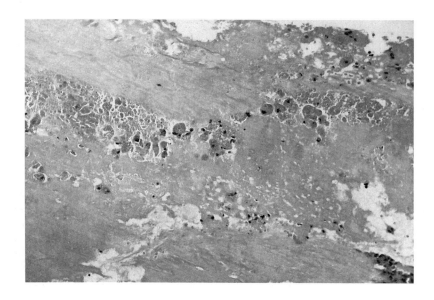

Fig. 17.9 Photomicrograph of vegetation of a patient with Q fever endocarditis. The large round cells are foamy macrophages. (Magnification ×114.)

Treatment

There have been no controlled clinical trials of the treatment of Q fever endocarditis. A variety of antibiotics have been used and some authorities recommend that treatment be continued indefinitely. However, a consensus is emerging that combination antibiotic therapy is necessary to treat this severe illness successfully (Levy *et al.* 1991). We have used doxycycline in combination with trimethoprim–sulphamethoxazole or rifampin for a total of 2 years. Others have used doxycycline in combination with either ofloxacin or ciprofloxacin. A recent finding that the bactericidal effect of doxycycline is enhanced when alkalinization of the phagolysosome is accomplished with chloroquine or amantadine may have major implications for the future treatment of endocarditis (Maurin *et al.* 1992) Raoult and co-workers are now routinely using this doxycycline and hydroxychloroquin with great success (D. Raoult, personal communication).

Antibody titres to *C. burnetii* should be determined every 6 months during the therapy of chronic Q fever and every 3 months for the first 2 years after cessation of therapy. Successful treatment is accompanied by a falling erythrocyte sedimentation rate, correction of anemia and hyperglobulinaemia, and a steady decline in the phase I antibody titre. In our experience there have been no relapses after 2 years of combination, for example doxycycline and rifampin, therapy. Valve replacement is often necessary for haemodynamic reasons.

Hepatitis

There are three main manifestations of Q fever hepatitis (Hofmann and Heaton 1982):

1. Infectious hepatitis-like picture.
2. Hepatitis as an incidental finding in a patient with acute Q fever.
3. Fever of unknown origin with characteristic granulomas on liver biopsy.

The hepatic granuloma in Q fever hepatitis, the so-called doughnut granuloma, consists of a dense fibrin ring surrounded by a central lipid vacuole. These granulomas are not specific for Q fever since they have also been seen in Hodgkin's disease and infectious mononucleosis. Two weeks of antibiotic therapy with a tetracycline compound is usually sufficient. Most cases of hepatitis represent the acute form of the disease, although an occasional patient with hepatitis can have the serological profile of chronic Q fever—these patients should be treated for longer than 2 weeks.

Neurological manifestations

Severe headache is the most common neurological manifestation of Q fever. Aseptic meningitis and/or encephalitis is rare (Marrie and Raoult 1992).

Two recent studies from the United Kingdom report a very high incidence of neurological manifestations of Q fever infection. In a study from Plymouth, Riley *et al.* (1990) reported an incidence of neurological complications in 22 per cent of 103 patients with Q fever. Forty-six of the patients had acute Q fever, five had chronic Q fever, and 52 had remote infections. Six of the 45 patients with acute Q fever had residual neurological impairment, including weakness, recurrent meningismus, blurred vision, residual paraesthesis, and sensory loss involving the left leg. In the study from the West Midlands (Smith *et al.* 1993), 23 of 101 patients reported neurological symptoms. Eight complained of hallucinations—in six these were visual, in one auditory, and in one olfactory. Six patients described symptoms compatible with an expressive dysphasia. Three had hemifacial pain suggestive of trigeminal neuralgia. Diplopia and dysarthria were described by one patient each, and one patient had a visual-field disturbance. These deficits lasted for only a few days. The rate of neurological involvement in these two studies is so much higher than that reported from any other country in the world that it raises the possibility that a neurotrophic strain of *C. burnetii* was circulating in the United Kingdom.

Rarely, Q fever meningoencephalitis may be accompanied by seizures and coma. Other neurological manifestations of Q fever include behavioural disturbances, cerebellar signs and symptoms, cranial nerve palsies, extrapyramidal disease, and the MillerFisher syndrome.

Q fever in the immunocompromised host

Raoult and co-workers (1993) found that 10 per cent of 500 HIV-positive individuals had IgG antibodies at a titre of $\geq 1:25$ to *C. burnetii*, twice the rate in healthy blood donors. They also found that 5 of 68 (7.3 per cent) of patients hospitalized with Q fever from 1987 to 1989 in Marseilles were HIV positive. They went on to estimate that in HIV-positive individuals the number of cases of Q fever was 13 times higher than that in the general population. The same investigators reviewed all cases of chronic Q fever in France from 1982 to 1990 (Brouqui *et al.* 1993) and they found that 20 per cent of these 84 patients were immunocompromised.

Q fever in pregnancy

Coxiella burnetii was isolated from the placenta of a woman who became pregnant 2 years after an episode of acute Q fever. This suggests that re-activation of Q fever occurs during human pregnancy as it does in other animals (Syrucek *et al.* 1958). In this same study three women who had Q fever during pregnancy had normal children and *C. burnetii* was isolated from the placenta of two of them. The third had her pregnancy interrupted because of rubella and *C. burnetii* was isolated from her placenta. The fifth woman's child had hypospadias—*C. burnetii* was isolated from her placenta.

A 21-year-old Israeli woman had Q fever at 21 weeks of pregnancy (Reichmann *et al*. 1988). Her course was complicated by thrombocytopenia and labour was induced at 28 weeks—the baby was normal.

We recently reported two cases of Q fever in pregnancy (Marrie 1993). One of these cases was subclinical —her husband developed Q fever pneumonia following exposure to parturient cats. At this point she was 36 weeks into her pregnancy but she had never had never had any symptoms of infection. However, serological testing demonstrated a fourfold rise in antibody titre and *C. burnetii* was isolated from her placenta. The second patient had Q fever pneumonia at 12 weeks of gestation. She was treated with antibiotics and recovered from her pneumonia; however, she went on to deliver at 31 weeks' gestation. Her infant weighed 1550 g and required 1 month in the neonatal intensive care unit. When examined at 1 year of age his head circumference was in the tenth percentile, weight was between the tenth and twenty-fifth percentile and developmental milestones and physical examination was normal. *Coxiella burnetii* was isolated from her placenta.

Other manifestations of Q fever

Q fever may occur in infancy where it has caused pneumonia, febrile seizures, pyrexia of unknown origin, malaise, and meningeal irritation. Haematological manifestations of Q fever include bone marrow necrosis haemophagocytosis, haemolytic anaemia, lymphadenopathy mimicking lymphoma, transient hypoplastic anaemia, reactive thrombocytosis, thrombocytopenia, and splenic rupture. Optic neuritis and erythema nodosum have also been reported in association with Q fever.

EPIDEMIOLOGY

Coxiella burnetii has been a remarkably successful pathogen. It has spread to most countries in the world. When Kaplan and Beartagna reviewed the literature up to 1955 they found that Q fever was present in 51 countries on 5 continents. At that time they noted that Ireland, The Netherlands, New Zealand, and Poland did not have Q fever. In the interim, Q fever has been demonstrated in Ireland, The Netherlands, and Poland. New Zealand still remains free of Q fever.

TRANSMISSION

Aerosols are the most important means of transmission to man. A dose-response effect is evident. For example, guinea-pigs exposed to 10^4 infectious dose units had an incubation period of 6 days whereas those exposed to 10 units had an incubation of 10 days (Tiggert and Benenon 1956). Human volunteers who inhaled 1 infectious unit had an incubation period of 16 days, whereas those who were exposed to 1500 infectious units had an incubation period of 10 days. We have observed that individuals who cleaned up the products of conception of their infected parturient cats had the shortest incubation period for Q fever and the most severe illness. In this group the incubation period ranged from 7 to 30 days, according to the intensity of the exposure.

Indirect exposure to contaminated aerosols was also important as British residents who lived along a road over which farm vehicles travelled developed Q fever as a result of exposure to contaminated straw, manure, or dust from the farm vehicles (Salmon *et al*. 1981). Four hundred and fifteen residents of a Swiss valley who lived along a road over which sheep travelled to and from mountain pastures developed Q fever (Dupuis 1987)

A number of recent outbreaks indicate the importance of indirect exposure to *C. burnetii*. In an outbreak of Q fever in a truck-repair plant, 16 of 32 employees were infected (Marrie *et al*. 1989). One of the employees had a cat which had given birth to kittens 2 weeks prior to the outbreak. The cat refused to let the kittens suckle and the employee, after donning his work clothes, fed the kittens from a bottle and then went to work. The attack rate for the employees who worked upstairs where the cat owner worked was 67 per cent, compared with 25 per cent for those who worked downstairs. The cat and the kittens had antibodies to *C. burnetii*. The contaminated clothing of the cat's owner may have served as a vehicle whereby *C. burnetii* was introduced into the truck-repair plant. An outbreak described by Marmion and Stoker (1956) involved 10 of 30 people who performed a play in a village church. The only source of Q fever was indirect contact with sheep through a shepherd who had a role in the play and who came to the rehearsals in his working clothes, accompanied by his sheep-dog. Twenty four samples of dust from the shepherd's clothing and others who came into contact with the two known infected flocks of sheep were obtained with a suction device. *Coxiella burnetii* was isolated from one specimen of dust collected from the shepherd's clothing. Contaminated clothing from the Rocky Mountain Laboratory in Montana, a Q fever research facility, led to cases of Q fever among laundry workers (Oliphant *et al*. 1949).

In Baddeck, Nova Scotia a parturient cat with vaginal bleeding for 3 weeks after delivery led to an outbreak of Q fever affecting 2.8 per cent of the population of the town (Marrie *et al*. 1988b). Sixteen people who attended a birthday party became ill with Q fever. At

3 p.m. on the day of the party the hostess' cat gave birth to kittens in the bedroom closet. The hostess closed the closet and bedroom doors and prepared for the party which began at 6 p.m. None of the guests entered the bedroom; however, all spent time in the kitchen which adjoined the bedroom. *Coxiella burnetii* was isolated from the cat's uterus (Marrie *et al.* 1988a). Even activity as tame as playing poker can be a risk factor for Q fever if an infected parturient cat gives birth during the course of the poker game (Langley *et al.* 1988).

Outbreaks of Q fever that have occurred in institutions, illustrate how infectious are the aerosols of *C. burnetii*. Prior to the recognition that sheep were infected with *C. burnetii* they were often transported to a research institute that, in many instances, was part of a hospital. Several large outbreaks of Q fever have occurred as a result of the use of infected pregnant sheep in research (Hall *et al.* 1982). In these outbreaks most of the people who became ill (63–70 per cent) did not have direct contact with the sheep but worked along the route along which the sheep were transported to the laboratory.

Several authors have suggested that ingestion of raw (presumably contaminated milk) is a risk factor for acquisition of Q fever. *Coxiella burnetii* was not killed by pasteurization techniques used in the 1940s and 1950's (Went worth 1955); however, current pastenization techniques are effective. A study carried out at the Idaho State Penitentiary showed that seroconversion to *C. burnetii* could occur after ingestion of raw contaminated milk, but clinical disease did not (Benson *et al.* 1963). This observation correlates with findings from a study in which cats experimentally infected via the oral route did not become ill, whereas cats infected via the subcutaneous route became ill and lethargic (Gillespie and Baker 1952). In one study 11 Portuguese volunteers ingested food contaminated with *C. burnetii* but only two developed complement fixing antibodies (anonymous 1950). In another study reported from Milwaukee, 34 human volunteers consumed unpasteurized raw milk naturally infected with *C. burnetii*. None became ill and none developed antibodies that could be detected by the complement fixation test, the capillary agglutination, or the radioisotope precipitation test (Krumbiegel and Wisniewski 1970).

Percutaneous transmission has been demonstrated experimentally; 29 Portuguese volunteers who were infected intradermally developed signs of disease (anonymous 1950). A 24-year-old male who crushed ticks between his fingers while hiking in the mountains in Montana became ill with Q fever 16 days later (Eklund *et al.* 1947). There is one report of transmission of Q fever via a blood transfusion (anonymous 1977).

Coxiella burnetii has been isolated from human placenta and one study, at least, demonstrated immunological evidence of human fetal infection with *C. burnetii* (Fiset *et al.* 1975). However, it is unlikely that vertical transmission has much of a role in the epidemiology of Q fever in man.

Person to person transmission is very uncommon, although there have been instances where the evidence is suggestive (Mann *et al.* 1986). There are two reports of the transmission of *C. burnetii* to attendants during autopsies (Harman 1949; Genth *et al.* 1982), but while these cases are cited as instances of person to person transmission, it is possible that aerosols generated during the autopsy could have resulted in the infection. Because of the rarity of person to person transmission of Q fever there is no need to isolate patients hospitalized with this illness, but precautions should be taken during autopsy of patients with presumed or documented Q fever infection.

EPIZOOLOGY

There is an extensive wildlife reservoir of *C. burnetii*, as reviewed above. Since many species of ticks are known to be infected with *C. burnetii*, it was assumed that ticks infected wild and domestic animals. Other possible routes of infection from wild animals to domestic animals are by contamination of the environment by infected products of conception (aerosols from these products could infect domestic animals and man.), ingestion of contaminated grass, or ingestion of contaminated animals, such as mice, by cats. A seasonal variation in the prevalence of antibodies among deer was evident in one study—antibody prevalence peaked in mid-winter (January), was lowest in late spring just prior to parturition in May, and increased thereafter (Enright *et al.* 1971).

PREVENTION AND CONTROL

Outbreaks of Q fever in laboratory workers in the 1940s led to the production of a formalin-inactivated whole-cell vaccine. This vaccine seemed to be protective, although no formal trials were carried out. A formalin-killed, ether-extracted 10 per cent suspension of *C. burnetii*-infected yolk sac had a complement fixation antigen titre of 1:8 and seemed to be effective. (Ormsbee and Marmion 1991)

Early vaccines were accompanied by occasional severe reactions in the form of an indolent, indurated mass at the vaccination site or the formation of a sterile abscess which pointed and discharged and sometimes formed a chronic draining sinus requiring excision. Reactions were associated with frequent vaccination and the possession of antibody before inoculation. This led to a pre-vaccination screening programme to detect pre-existing cellular immunity or hypersensitivity. A small dose of diluted Q fever vaccine was inoculated intradermally and those who reacted in 5–7 days with erythema at the inoculation site were excluded from vaccination.

After Stoker and Fiset described phase variation in *C. burnetii*, it was recognized that antibody against phase I antigen had protective effects in immunized mice and guinea-pigs. The next development was the observation that phase I antigen, like bacterial lipopolysaccharide, could be extracted from *C. burnetii* with phenol–water mixtures, dimethylsulphoxide, formamide or trichloroacetic acid; the extracts had haptenic, antigenic and, in some instances, immunogenic activity. Following this, methods were devised to purify *Coxiella* cells from yolk sac protein and lipid.

The use of formalin-inactivated, low-dose phase I highly purified *C. burnetii* suspensions together with pre-vaccination serotesting and skin testing facilitated the prophylactic use of the vaccine in laboratory workers and eventually in industrial groups. Between 1966 and 1968 vaccine trials with a purified Henzerling phase I vaccine were carried out by Hornick. Doses ranging from 1 to 30 μg were given subcutaneously. Three to ten months later subjects were challenged with a *C. burnetii* aerosol. Protection ranged from 71 per cent for the 1 μg dose to 89–100 per cent for the 30 μg dose.

In Australia, Marmion and co-workers, in response to an increase in the prevalence of Q fever in abattoirs following the introduction of feral goats into the slaughtering programme, produced a formalin-inactivated Henzerling strain of *C. burnetii* vaccine from infected yolk sac by low–high salt extraction. They went on to perform a trial involving abattoir workers in South Australia. The vaccine was effective. While the yearly rates of Q fever among the unvaccinated workers fluctuated, a typical result in the trial was three cases of Q fever among 2716 vaccinated workers compared with 52 cases among 2012 unvaccinated workers. Common reactions included fever, headache, and local tenderness.

Measurement of antibody by traditional serological tests (such as the complement fixation test) after vaccination does not accurately reflect protection. Only 56–64 per cent of vaccine recipients in the South Australia trials had measurable antibody by these tests at 20–60 months after vaccination. Eighty-four per cent had measurable antibody 0.6–3 months post-vaccination. The implication is that cell-mediated immunity is important in providing protection from infection and that a positive cell-mediated immune response can be produced by vaccination even though a humoral immune response cannot be detected. The finding that a single microgram dose of whole-cell *C. burnetii* vaccine induces a lymphoproliferative response in 80–90 per cent of vaccines tends to substantiate this.

Fries *et al.* (1993) recently reported their results of an evaluation of the safety and immunogenicity of a chloroform–methanol residue (CMR) vaccine for Q fever. They immunized 35 healthy adults with a single CMR subcutaneous dose of 30, 60, 120, or 240 μg. No adverse reactions were seen at the 30 or 60 μg doses. However, 7 of the 10, 240 μg recipients reported erythema and/or induration at the inoculation site. Two subjects reported malaise and one had low-grade fever. Serum IgM responses, best detected with phase II antigen, developed in 30, 60, 73, and 90 per cent of recipients with the 30, 60, 120, and 240 μg doses, respectively. results were encourag enough to proceed with field trials.

A *C. burnetii* vaccine suitable for easy mass inoculation of those at risk is not yet available. Presently, vaccination should be limited to individuals, such as veterinarians and abattoir workers, who are at high risk of acquiring Q fever.

VACCINATION OF ANIMALS

A phase I formalin-inactivated vaccine was administered to 1400 Holstein–Friesian dairy calves and heifers. Only 1 per cent of vaccinated cows shed *C. burnetii*, whereas 39 of 164 (24 per cent) of non-vaccinated cows shed *C. burnetii* (Biberstein *et al.* 1977). Four immunized cows were challenged with 4×10^8 infected guinea-pig doses via the subcutaneous route. These cows had normal full-term calves, whereas two non-vaccinated cows aborted late in pregnancy and *C. burnetii* was isolated from the tissue of the fetuses. While organisms were recovered from the milk, colostrum, and placenta of both vaccinated and unvaccinated cows, the number of organisms recovered from unvaccinated cows was 1000 times greater than that from vaccinated cows (Behymer *et al.* 1976). Similar results were obtained when a whole-cell, phase I Henzerling strain vaccine or a chloroform method residue vaccine was used in ewes (Brooks *et al.* 1986).

OTHER PREVENTATIVE MEASURES

Use of only seronegative sheep in research facilities should prevent outbreaks of Q fever in most institutions. Pregnant sheep should not be transported through hospitals. Research facilities should be designed so that outside access to the animal quarters is direct, with contact confined to the animal quarters. The care of animals in such facilities should conform to nationally accepted standards.

Consumption of pasteurized milk only will serve to eliminate the few cases that may be transmitted in this manner.

In Cyprus the incidence of *C. burnetii* infection among goats and sheep was reduced by a programme in which aborted material was destroyed, affected dams isolated, and the premises disinfected (Polydorou 1985). Control of ectoparasites on cattle, sheep, and goats may also be important in the control of Q fever.

REFERENCES

Abinanti, F. R. and Marmion, B. P. (1957). Protective or neutralizing antibody in Q fever. *American Journal of Hygiene*, **66**, 173–95.

Akporiaye, E. T. and Baca, O. G. (1983). Superoxide anion production and superoxide dismutase and catalase activities in *Coxiella burnetii*. *Journal of Bacteriology*, **154**, 520–3.

Anonymous (1950). Experimental Q fever in man. *British Medical Journal*, **1**, 1000.

Anonymous (1977). Comment on Q fever transmitted by blood transfusion—United States. *Canadian Disease Weakly Report*, **3**, 210.

Babudieri, B. (1959). Q fever: A zoonosis. *Advances in Veterinary Science*, **5**, 81–182.

Baca, O. G. (1991). Pathogenesis of rickettsial infection: emphasis on Q fever. *European Journal of Epidemiology*, **7**, 222–8.

Baca, O. G., Roman M. J., Glew, R. H., Christner, R. F., Buhler, J. E., and Aragon, A. S. (1993). Acid phosphatase activity in *Coxiella burnetii*: a possible virulence factor. *Infection and Immunity*, **61**, 4232–9.

Behymer, D. E. *et al.* (1976). Q fever (*Coxiella burnetii*) investigations in dairy cattle: challenge of immunity after vaccination. *American Journal of Veterinary Research*, **37**, 631–4.

Bell, J. F., Luoto, L., Casey, M., and Lackmand, D. B. (1964). Serologic and skin test response after Q fever vaccination by the intracutaneous route. *Journal of Immunology*, **93**, 403–8.

Benson, W. W., Brock, D. W., and Mather, J. (1963). Serologic analysis of a penitentiary group using raw milk from a Q fever infected herd. *Public Health Reports*, **78**, 707–10.

Biberstein, E. L. *et al.* (1977). Vaccination of diary cattle against Q fever (*Coxiella burnetii*): results of field trials. *American Journal of Veterinary Research*, **38**, 189–93.

Biggs, B. A. *et al.* (1984). Prolonged Q fever associated with inappropriate secretion of anti-diuretic hormone. *Journal of Infection*, **8**, 61–3.

Brooks, L. *et al.* (1986). Q fever vaccination of sheep. Challenge of immunity in ewes. *Journal of Veterinary Research*, **47**, 1235–8.

Brouqui, P. *et al.* (1993). Chronic Q fever: Ninety-two cases from France; including 27 cases without endocarditis. *Archives of Internal Medicine*, **153**, 642–9.

Burnet F. M. and Freeman, M. (1937). Experimental studies on the virus of Q fever. *Medical Journal of Australia*, **2**, 299–305.

Christie, A. B. (1974). *Infectious diseases, epidemiology and clinical practice*, pp. 876–91. Churchill Livingston, Edinburgh.

Clark, W. H., Lennette, E. H., Railsback, O. C., and Romer, M. S. (1951). Q fever in California. VII. Clinical features in one hundred and eighty cases. *Archives of Internal Medicine*, **88**, 155–67.

Derrick, E. H. (1937). 'Q' fever, new fever entity: clinical features, diagnosis and laboratory investigation. *Medical Journal of Australia*, **2**, 281–99.

Derrick, E. H. (1939). Rickettsia burnetii: the cause of 'Q' fever. *Medical Journal of Australia*, **1**, 14.

Dupont, H. T. *et al.* (1992). Epidemiologic features and clinical presentation of acute Q fever in hospitalized patients: 323 French cases. *American Journal of Medicine*, **93**, 427–34.

Dupuis, G., Peter, O., Pedroni, D., and Petite, J. (1985). Aspects cliniques observeés lors d'une épidémie de 415 cas de fiévre Q. *Schweizerische Medizinische Wochenschrift*, **115**, 814–18.

Dupuis, G., Petite, J., Peter, O., and Vouilloz, M. (1987). An important outbreak of human Q fever in Swiss Alpine Valley. *International Journal of Epidemiology*, **16**, 282–7.

Eklund, C. M., Parker, R. R., and Lackman, D. B., (1947). Case of Q fever probably contracted by exposure to ticks in nature. *Public Health Reports*, **62**, 1413–16.

Enright, J. B., Franti, C. E., Behymer, D. E., Longhurst, W. M., Dutson, V. J., and Wright, M. E. (1971). *Coxiella burnetii* in a wildlife-livestock environment. Distribution of Q fever in wild mammals. *American Journal of Epidemiology*, **94**, 79–90.

Fiset, P., Wisseman, C. L. Jr, and El-Bataine, Y. (1975). Immunologic evidence of human fetal infection with *Coxiella burnetii*. *American Journal of Epidemiology*, **101**, 65.

Fries, L. F., Waag, D. M., and Williams, J. C. (1993). Safety and immunogenicity in human volunteers of a chloroform–methanol residue vaccine for Q fever. *Infection and Immunity*, **61**, 1251–8.

George, J. and Marrie, T. J. (1987). Serological evidence of *Coxiella burnetii* infection in horses in Atlantic Canada. *Canadian Veterinary Journal*, **28**, 425–6.

Gerth, H.-J. and Leidig, U. (1982). Reimenschneider Th. Q-fieber-epidemie in einem Institute fur Humanpathologie. *Deutsche Medizinische Wochenschrift*, **107**, 1391–5.

Gillespie, J. H. and Baker, J. A. (1952). Experimental Q fever in cats. *American Journal of Veterinary Research*, **13**, 91–4.

Gordon, J. D. *et al.* (1984). The radiographic features of epidemic and sporadic Q fever pneumonia. *Journal of the Canadian Associatia of Radiography*, **35**, 293–6.

Grist, N. R. (1959). The persistence of Q fever infection in a dairy herd. *Veterinary Record*, **71**, 839–41.

Hacksteadt, T., Peacock, N. G., Hitchcock, P. J., and Cole, R. L. (1985). Lipopolysaccharide variation in *Coxiella burnetii*; intrastrain heterogenicity in structure and antigenicicty. *Infection and Immunity*, **48**, 359–65.

Hall, C. J., Richmond, S. J., Caul, E. O., Pearce, N. H., and Silver, I. A. (1982). Laboratory outbreak of Q fever acquired from sheep. *Lancet*, **1**, 1004–6.

Harman, J. B. (1949). Q fever in Great Britain; clinical account of eight cases. *Lancet*, **2**, 1028.

Hendrix, L. R., Mallavia, L. P., and Samuel, J. E. (1993). Cloning and sequencing of *Coxiella burnetii* outer membrane protein gene *com*1. *Infection and Immunity*, **61**, 470–7.

Hofmann, C. E. R. and Heaton, J. W. (1982). Q fever hepatitis. Clinical manifestations and pathological findings. *Gastroenterology*, **83**, 474–9.

Hornibrook, J. W. (1940). An institutional outbreak of pneumonitis. 1. Epidemiologic and clinical studies. *Public Health Reports*, **55**, 1936–44.

Huebner, R. J. (1947). Report of an outbreak of Q fever at the National Institute of Health. II. Epidemiological features. *American Journal of Public Health*, **37**, 431–40.

Huebner, R. J., Jellison, W. L., Beck, M. D., Parker, R. R., and Shepard, C. C. (1948). Q fever studies in Southern California. I. Recovery of *Rickettsia burnetii* from raw milk. *Public Health Reports*, **63**, 214–22.

Hunt, J. G., Field, P. R., and Murphy, A. M. (1983). Immunoglobulin responses to *Coxiella burnetii* (Q fever): Single-serum diagnosis of acute infection using an immunofluorescence technique. *Infection and Immunity*, **39**, 977–81.

Janigan, D. T. and Marrie, T. J. (1983). An inflammatory pseudotumor of the lung in Q fever pneumonia. *New England Journal of Medicine*, **30**, 86–8.

Kaplan, M. M. and Bertagna, P. (1955). The geographical distribution of Q fever. *Bulletiu of the WHO*, **13**, 829–60.

Krumbiegel, E. R. and Wisniewski, H. J. (1970). Q fever in Milwaukee. II. Consumption of infected raw milk by human volunteers. *Archives of Environmental Health*, **21**, 63–5.

Lang, G. H. (1990). Coxiellosis in animals. In *Q fever—the disease*, (ed. T. J. Marrie), pp. 23–48. CRC Press, Boca Raton, FLA.

Langley, J. M., Marrie, T. J., Covert, A. A., Waag, D. M., and Williams, J. C. (1988). Poker players pneumonia—an urban outbreak of Q fever following exposure to a parturient cat. *New England Journal of Medicine*, **319**, 354–6.

Laughlin, T., Waag, D., Williams, J., and Marrie, T. J. (1991). Q fever: from deer to dog to man. *Lancet*, **337**, 676–7.

Lennette, E. H. and Welsh, H. H. (1951). Q fever in California. X. Recovery of *Coxiella burnetii* from the air of premises harbouring infected goats. *American Journal of Hygiene*, **54**, 44.

Lennette, E. H., Clark, W. H., and Dean, B. H., (1949). Sheep and goats and the epidemiology of Q fever in Northern California. *American Journal of Tropical Medicine*, **29**, 527–41.

Levy P. Y. *et al.* (1991). Comparison of different antibiotic regimens for therapy of 32 cases of Q fever endocarditis. *Antimicrobial Agents and Chemotherapy*, **35** 533–7.

Luoto, L. and Huebner, R. J. (1950). Q fever studies in Southern California. IX. Isolation of Q fever organisms from parturient placentas of naturally infected cows. *Public Health Reports* **65**, 541–4.

McCaul, T. F. (1991). The developmental cycle of *Coxiella burnetii*. In Q fever: (ed. J. C. Williams and H. A. Thompson), pp. 224–58. CRC Press, Boca Raton, FLA.

McDade, J. E. (1990). Historical aspects of Q fever. In *Q fever: the disease*, (ed. T. J. Marrie), Vol. 1, pp. 5–21. CRC Press, Boca Raton, FLA.

Mallavia, L. P., Samuel, J. E., and Frazier, M. E. (1991). The genetics of *Coxiella burnetii*: Etiological agent of Q fever and chronic endocarditis. In *Q fever: The biology of Coxiella burnetii*, (ed. J. C. Williams and H. A. Thompson), pp. 259–85. CRC Press, Boca Raton, FLA.

Mann, J. S., Douglas, J. S., Inglis, J. M., and Leitch, A. G. (1986). Q fever: person to person transmission within a family. *Thorax*, **41**, 974–5.

Marecki, N., Becker, F., Baca, O. G., and Paretsky, D. (1978). Changes in liver and L-cell plasma membranes during infection with *Coxiella burnetii*. *Infection and Immunity*, **19**, 272–80.

Marmion, B. P. and Stoker, M. G. P. (1956). The varying epidemiology of Q fever in the South East region of Great Britain. II. In two rural areas. *Journal of Hygiene*, **54**, 547–61.

Marmion, B. P. *et al.* (1984). Vaccine prophylaxis of abattoir-associated Q fever. *Lancet*, **2**, 1411–14.

Marrie, T. J. (1993). Q fever in pregnancy: Report of two cases. *Infectious Diseases in Clinical Practice*, **2**, 207–9.

Marrie, T. J. and Raoult, D. (1992). Rickettsial infections of the central nervous system. *Seminars in Neurology*, **12**, 213–24.

Marrie, T. J. *et al.* (1985). Seroepidemiology of Q fever among domestic animals in Nova Scotia. *American Journal of Public Health* **75**, 763–6.

Marrie, T. J., Durant, H., Williams, J. C., Mintz, E., and Waag, D. M. (1988*a*). Exposure to parturient cats is a risk factor for acquisition of Q fever in Maritime Canada. *Journal of Infections Diseases*, **158**, 101–8.

Marrie, T. J., MacDonald, A., Durant, H., Yates, L., and McCormick, L. (1988*b*). An outbreak of Q fever probably due to contact with a parturient cat. *Chest*, **93**, 98–103.

Marrie, T. J., Langille, D., Papukna, V., and Yates, L. (1989). An outbreak of Q fever in a truck repair plant. *Epidemiology and Infection*, **102**, 119–27.

Marrie, T. J., Embil, J., and Yates, L. (1993). Seroepidemiology of *Coxiella burnetii* among wildlife in Nova Scotia. *American Journal of Tropical Medicine and Hygiene*, **49**, 613–15.

Maurin, M., Benoliel, A. M., Bongrand, P., and Raoult, D. (1992). Phagolysomal alkalinization and the bactericidal effect of antibiotics: The *Coxiella burnetii* paradigm. *Journal of Infectious Diseases*, **166**, 1097–102.

Michael, F., Minnick, R., Heinzen, A., Dowthrait, R., Mallavia, L. P., and Frazier, M. E. (1990). Analysis of QpRS specific sequences from *Coxiella burnetii*. *Annals of the New York Academy of Sciences*, **5990**, 514–23.

Minnick, M. F., Heinzen, R. A., Reschke, D. K., Frazier, M. E., and Mallavia, L. P. (1991). A plasmid-encoded surface protein found in chronic disease isolates of *Coxiella burnetii*. *Infection and Immunity*, **59**, 4735–9.

Oliphant, J. W., Gordon, D. A., Meis, A., and Parker, R. R. (1949). Q fever in laundry workers, presumably transmitted from contaminated clothing. *American Journal of Hygiene*, **49**, 76–82.

Ormsbee, R. A. and Marmion, B. P. (1991). Prevention of *Coxiella burnetii* infection: vaccines and guidelines for those at risk. In *Q fever*. Volume 1: *The disease*, (ed. T. J. Marrie), pp. 225–40. CRC Press, Boca Raton, FLA.

Palmer, S. R. and Young, S. E. J. (1982). Q fever endocarditis in England and Wales, 1975–81. *Lancet*, **ii**, 1148–9.

Palmer, N. C., Kierstead, M., Key, D. W., Williams, J. C., Peacock, M. G., and Vellend, H. (1983). Placentitis and abortion in sheep and goats in Ontario caused by *Coxiella burnetii*. *Canadian Veterinary Journal* **24**, 60–1.

Philip, C. B. (1948). Comments on the nature of the Q fever organism. *Public Health Reports*, **63**, 58.

Polydorou, K. (1985). Q fever in Cyprus—recent progress. *British Veterinary Journal*, **141**, 427–30.

Raoult, D. *et al.* (1987). Q fever endocarditis in the south of France. *Journal of Infections Diseases*, **155**, 570–3.

Raoult, D. *et al.* (1993). Q fever and HIV infection. *AIDS*, **7**, 81–6.

Reichmann, N., Raz, R., Keysary, A., Goldwasser, R., and Faltau, E. (1988). Chronic Q fever and severe thrombocytopenia in a pregnant woman. *American Journal of Medicine*, **85**, 253–4.

Reilly, S., Northwood, J. L., and Caul, E. O. (1990). Q fever in Plymouth, 1972–88. A review with particular reference to neurological manifestations. *Epidemiology and Infection*, **105**, 91–408.

Robbins, F. C. and Regan, C. A. (1946). Q fever in the Mediterranean area: report of its occurrence in allied troops. I. Clinical features of the disease. *American Journal of Hygiene*, **44**, 6–22.

Robbins, F. C., Gauld, R. L., and Warner, F. B., (1946). Q fever in the Mediterranean area: reported of its occurrence in allied troops. II. Epidemiology. *American Journal of Hygiene*, **44**, 23–50.

Salmon, M. M., Howells, B., Glencross, E. J. G., Evans, A. D., and Palmer, S. R. (1981). Q fever in an urban area. *Lancet*, **1**, 1004.

Samuel, J. E., Frazier, M. E., and Mallavia, L. P. (1985). Correlation of plasmid type and disease caused by *Coxiella burnetii*. *Infection and Immunity*, **49**, 775–7.

Sawyer, L. A., Fishbein, D. B., and McDade, J. E. (1987). Q fever: current concepts. *Reviews of the Infections Diseases*, **9**, 935–46.

Schramek, S. and Mayer, H. (1982). Different sugar compositions of lipopolysaccharides isolated from phase I and pure phase II cells of *Coxiella burnetii*. *Infection and Immunity*, **38**, 53–7.

Shepard, C. C. (1947). An outbreak of Q fever in a Chicago packing house. *American Journal of Hygiene*, **46**, 185–92.

Smith, D. L. *et al.* (1993). A large Q fever outbreak in the West Midlands: clinical aspects. *Respiratory Medicine*, **87**, 509–16.

Somma-Moreira, R. E., Caffarena, R. M., Somma, S., Pérez, G., and Monteiro, M. (1987). Analysis of Q fever in Uruguay. *Reviews of the Infections Diseases*, **9**, 386–7.

Spelman, D. W. (1981). Q fever: a study of 111 consecutive cases. *Medical Journal of Australia*, **1**, 547–53.

Spicknall, C. G., Huebner, R. J., Finger, J. A., and Blocker, W. P. (1947). Report of an outbreak of Q fever at the National Institute of Health. I. Clinical features. *Annals of Internal Medicine*, **27**, 28–40.

Stein, A. and Raoult, D. (1992*a*). Detection of *Coxiella burnetii* by DNA amplification using polymerase chain reaction. *Journal of Clinical Microbiology*, **30**, 2462–6.

Stein, A. and Raoult, D. (1992*b*). Phenotypic and genotypic heterogenicity of eight new human *Coxiella burnetii* isolates. *Acta Virologia*, **36**, 7–12.

Stoenner, H. G. and Lachman, D. E. (1960). The biological properties of *Coxiella burnetii* isolated from rodents collected in Utah. *American Journal of Hygiene*, **71**, 775–9.

Stoker, M. G. P. and Fiset, P. (1956). Phase variation of the nine mile and other strains of *Rickettsia burnetii*. *Canadian Journal of Microbiology*, **2**, 310–21.

Syrucek, L., Sobeslavsky, O., and Gutvirth, L. (1958). Isolation of *Coxiella burnetii* from human placentas. J Hyg Epidemiol *Journal of Hyglene, Epidemiology, Microbiology and Immunology*, **2**, 29–35.

Thiele, D., Willems, H., Kopf, G., and Krauss, H. (1993). Polymorphism in DNA restriction patterns of *Coxiella burnetii* isolates investigated by pulsed field gel electrophoresis and image analysis. *European Journal of Epidemiology*, **9**, 419–25.

Tiggert, W. D. and Beneson, A. S. (1956). Studies on Q fever in man. *Transactions of the Association of American Physicians*, **69**, 98–104.

Topping, N. H., Shepard, C. C., and Irons, J. V. (1947). Q fever in the United States. I. Epidemiologic studies of an outbreak of among stock handlers and slaughterhouse workers. *Journal of the American Medical Association*, **33**, 813–15.

Turck, W. P. G. *et al.* (1976). Chronic Q fever. *Quarterly Journal of Medicine*, **45**, 193–217.

Viciana, P., Pachon, J., Cuello, J. A., Palomino, J., Jimenez-Mejias, M. E., and Cisneros, J. M. (1992). *Fever of indeterminate duration in the community. A seven year study in the South of Spain.* Abstract no 683. 32nd Interscience Conference on Antimicrobial Agents and Chemotherapy, 11–14 October 1992. *American Society for Microbiology*, Washington, DC.

Vodkin, M. H. and Williams, J. C. (1988). A heat shock operon in *Coxiella burnetii* produces a major antigen homolgous to a protein in both mycobacteria and *Escherichia coli*. *Journal of Bacteriology*, **170**, 1227–34.

Weiss, E., Williams, J. C., and Thompson, H. A. (1991). The place of *Coxiella burnetii* in the microbial world. In *Q fever: The biology of Coxiella burnetii*, (ed. J. C. Williams and H. A. Thompson), pp. 2–19. CRC Press, Boca Raton, FLA.

Welsh, H. H., Lennette, E. H., Abinanti, R. F., and Winn, J. F. (1958). Air-borne transmission of Q fever: The role of the parturition in the generation of infective aerosols. *Annals of the New York Academy of Sciences*, **70**, 528–40.

Wentworth, B. B. (1955). Historical review of the literature on Q fever. *Bacteriological Reviews*, **19**, 129–49.

Yeaman, M. R., Mitscher, L. A., and Baca, O. G. (1987). *In vitro* susceptibility of *Coxiella burnetii* for antibiotics, including several quinolones. *Antimicrobial Agents and Chemotherapy* **31**, 1079–84.

18   RAT-BITE FEVERS

R. L. Salmon and M. B. McEvoy

*STREPTOBACILLARY FEVER—R. L. SALMON
AND M. B. MCEVOY*

SUMMARY

Infection with *Streptobacillus moniliformis*, known as streptobacillary fever, rat-bite fever, epidemic arthritic erythema (Haverhill fever) occurs worldwide. Only three outbreaks have been described. It is caused by the bite of a rat or other infected rodent, or by ingestion of water or milk contaminated by rats. Control is by prevention of rat infestation.

HISTORY

Streptobacillus moniliformis was first isolated in 1925 from the blood of a laboratory worker and became recognized as one of the two causes of rat-bite fever (the other is *Spirillum minis*). At the same time, an epidemic form of the disease, Haverhill fever, was recognized during an outbreak in the United States (Parker and Hudson 1926) which was ascribed to milk. Accounts of cases have been rare in the world literature but in 1983 the largest outbreak ever described occurred among pupils at a boarding school in England following the probable contamination by rat urine of a private water supply from a spring (McEvoy *et al.* 1987).

THE AGENT

Streptobacillus moniliformis is a pleomorphic Gram-negative bacterium which may occur as short coccobacillary forms as well as chains and intertwining wavy filaments. Previously believed to be related to the actinobacilli, it is now thought to have more in common with the mycoplasmates (Costas and Owen 1987). It is a facultative anaerobe and slow growing on blood, serum, or other bodily fluid. The optimal growth temperature is 35–37 °C and optimal pH 7.4–7.6. L-Forms may arise spontaneously. It is inhibited by Liquoid (sodium polyanethol sulphonate) and killed at 55 °C in 30 min or less. Except for the L-form, *S. moniliformis* is penicillin sensitive. The L-form is sensitive to tetracycline and presumably to erythromycin.

THE HOSTS

ANIMAL

Streptobacillus moniliformis is carried in the nasopharynx or excreted in the urine of healthy rats (Strangeways 1933). It may be carried in other rodents where, as in the case of mice, it may also give rise to disease, notably septicaemia or arthropathy, which may be fatal.

HUMAN

Incubation period

The incubation in the original outbreak described was 1–4 days (Parker and Hudson 1926) and is rarely longer than 10 days.

Symptoms and signs

Fever followed after a median of 2 days by a symmetrical erythematous, usually maculopapular, rash affecting the palms of the hands, the feet, shins and ankles and, in about half the cases, the face. Asymmetrical arthralgia, and also arthritis, affecting usually more than one joint, occurs in most cases ('epidemic arthritic erythema').

Diagnosis

By culture of blood, synovial fluid, or lymph nodes. Strains may be distinguished by the electrophoretic profiles of cellular proteins (Costas and Owen 1987).

Treatment

Penicillin, erythromycin, and tetracycline have all been used with evidence of success (Shanson *et al.* 1983). Penicillin may encourage the development of L-forms and prolong the course of the illness (Roughgarden 1965).

Prognosis

The duration of illness ranges from 2 to 32 days (median 16 days). At least one relapse occurs in about half the cases and more than one relapse in 17 per cent. Mortality is low but severe complications, including endocarditis, pneumonia, metastatic abscesses, and anaemia have been described, largely before the advent of antibiotic treatment (Roughgarden 1965; Taber and Feigen 1979).

EPIDEMIOLOGY

OCCURRENCE

Sporadic cases occur worldwide. Three outbreaks have been described (Parker and Hudson 1926; Place and Sutton 1934; McEvoy *et al.* 1987). These include the first to be described which was at Haverhill, Massachusetts, which gave the epidemic form of the disease its name of 'Haverhill fever' (Parker and Hudson 1926).

In the most recent and largest outbreak which was at a boarding school (McEvoy *et al.* 1987), the school was situated on a 100 acre site in a rural area near a market town in England. Within the grounds are extensive gardens, stables, and a farm which, at the time, provided the school with unpasteurized milk. There were about 700 people on the site, including 500 schoolgirls, aged 8–19 years, of which 370 were boarders and 130 attended daily.

The first case of fever was reported on 11 February, 1983, and a further 24 cases presented the next day. Cases continued to occur in children and staff members, with a peak on 14 February, when 86 people became ill. The onset of the last known cases was 21 February, by which time a total of 304 cases had occurred.

Analysis of these 304 cases by day of onset of symptoms suggested a common source for the outbreak, with exposure probably continuing over several days in early February. It is likely that the earliest cases, which were recognized retrospectively, had occurred on 6–8 February. All cases had lived on or visited the site of the school, and there were no reported cases of secondary transmission.

A random sample of 230 pupils was interviewed in greater detail. There were significant associations between the development of illness and the consumption of cold milk (relative risk = 3.3, P = 0.02) and cold water (relative risk = 10, P = 6×10^{-5}) at the school. No other exposures were associated with illness.

Milk and water consumption were examined further, with data collected from the whole at-risk population. Although both milk and water drinking remained significantly associated with the development of illness, water was associated independently of milk, but milk was not associated independently of water.

The major source of supply to the school was mains chlorinated water. However, water was also supplied by a spring. In addition, the sewage system had been transferred from the old filter-bed method to the mains system 2 weeks before the onset of the outbreak. The filter-bed and cesspit were situated on high ground above the spring. Inspection of this area revealed the presence of rats. Moreover, water could have filtered back into the spring pond, where rats were also seen. The spring water fed a well in an old courtyard. The well water passed through a chlorine-dosing unit and calorifiers to a pressurized storage unit in the school basement, where it was then used to feed the hot-water system. Inspection revealed no domestic hot water return to the calorifiers. It was reported to be impossible to raise the water temperature above 50 °C. Despite the presence of the chorine-dosing unit there was no evidence of chlorine in the water feeding the calorifiers. An inspection of the raw milk supplied from the school farm showed no evidence that the milk could have been contaminated with rat urine.

Streptobacillus moniliformis was isolated from the blood cultures of four boarders who had returned home and were subsequently admitted to hospital (Shanson *et al.* 1983). The organism was not cultured from the samples of milk or water or from rats trapped in the school grounds after 16 February.

The attack rate was 49 per cent (304/700). The duration of illness ranged from 2 to 32 days (median 16 days). All cases had fever and 95 per cent had a rash. The distribution of the rash, unlike the joint involvement (which affected 97 per cent), tended to be symmetrical.

Over half had two or more joints involved and a third three or more joints. Altogether, 56 per cent of patients experienced one recurrence, 11 per cent two recurrences, and 6 per cent had three.

The conclusion that water was the vehicle of infection was strongly supported by epidemiological evidence and by circumstantial evidence that opportunity existed for the consumption of water from a spring infected with rats.

The hot-water supply was probably contaminated intermittently between 5 February and 12 February. During the first 2 weeks of February, operations on the building site involved digging around the foundations and the weather was exceptionally stormy. These factors may have disturbed the local rat population, causing it to contaminate the spring pond. The mains water supply was shut off for frequent short spells during this period, and drinking water could have been drawn from the hot taps. There was evidence that the 'hot' water was cool, and heavy demands on the supply would have caused the temperature to fall further. A higher attack rate which was observed among the boarders (54 per cent v. 20 per cent in day pupils) can be explained by their greater exposure to contaminated water. The total absence of cases outside the school suggests that the mains water was not contaminated.

SOURCES AND TRANSMISSION

Up to 50 per cent of rats carry the organism, as do, rarely, other rodents (Strangeways 1933). Sporadic cases usually occur following rat bites ('rat-bite fever') but may occur following living or working in a rat-infested building. Outbreaks may result from the contamination by rats of milk (Parker and Hudson 1926) or water (McEvoy *et al.* 1987).

COMMUNICABILITY

Person to person transmission does not occur.

PREVENTION AND CONTROL

Preventing the infestation by rats of human dwellings and workplaces is the key to control and would plausibly explain the apparent absence of cases in North America and Europe. Disease clusters must prompt the systematic search for a common source.

REFERENCES

Costas, M. and Owen, R. J. (1987). Numerical analysis of electrophoretic protein patterns of *Streptobacillus moniliformis* strains from human, murine and avaian infections. *Journal of Medical Microbiology*, **23**, 303–11.

McEvoy, M. B., Noah, N. D., and Pilsworth, R. (1987). Outbreak of fever caused by *Streptobacillus moniliformis*. *Lancet*, **II**, 1361–3.

Parker, F. and Hudson N. P. (1926). The etiology of Haverhill fever. *American Journal of Pathology*, **II**, 357–9.

Place, E. H. and Sutton L. E. (1934). Erythema arthriticum epidemicum (Haverhill fever). *Archives of internal Medicine*, **54**, (5), 659–84.

Roughgarden, J. W. (1965). Antimicrobial therapy of rat-bite fever. *Archives of Internal Medicine*, **39**, 116.

Shanson D. C. *et al.* (1983). *Streptobacillus moniliformis* isolated from blood in four cases of Haverhill fever; first outbreak in Britain. *Lancet*, **II**, 92–4.

Strangeways, W. I. (1933). Rats as carriers of *Streptobacillus moniliformis*. *Journal of Pathological Bacteriology*, **37**, 45–51.

Taber, L. H. and Feigen R. D. (1979). Spirochetal infections. *Pediatric clinics of North America*, **26**, 337.

SPIRILLARY FEVER—R. L. SALMON

HISTORY

Spirillary fever was first described in a Bombay rat by Henry Van Dyke Carter, a distinguished physician and pathologist who was the original illustrator of *Gray's Anatomy*, in 1888 (Hiatt and Hiatt 1995). *Spirillum minus* became recognized as one of the two causes of rat-bite fever (the other is *Streptobacillus moniliformis*). Accounts of cases have been rare but occur worldwide (Pritchard 1990).

THE AGENT

Spirillum minus is a minute (0.2 μm wide by 2–5 μm in length) spirillar bacterium, which has 2–3 rigid spirals of 0.8–1.0 μm wavelength and one or more flagella attached at each pole. It may be stained with methylene blue and with Giemsa. Its true taxonomic place is unknown (Skirrow 1990). It is aerobic and can be cultured only *in vivo* in mice and guinea-pigs (Pritchard 1990).

THE HOSTS

ANIMAL

Spirillum minus is found in rats, mice, and guinea-pigs and does not seem to be pathogenic in animals.

HUMAN

Incubation period

The incubation period is generally 7–21 days but may extend to months (Pritchard 1990).

Symptoms and signs

These can be differentiated clinically from strepto-bacillary fever (Holmgren and Tunevall 1970). Redness and swelling are visible at the wound site initially but may be healed before the onset of systemic disease, which is heralded by paroxysmal fever accompanied by lymphadenopathy and an extensive dark-red exanthema. Myalgia and arthralgia, more pronounced on the side of the body affected by the bite, occur. Arthritis seldom occurs.

Diagnosis

The organism is present in the local lesion or lymph nodes but may occasionally be demonstrated, with difficulty, by dark-field microscopy. Subcutaneous inoculation of fluid or lymph nodes in guinea-pigs is followed by a chancre and enlargement of regional lymph nodes. In both of these sites *Spirillum minus* may be demonstrated (Pritchard 1990). Unlike strepto-bacillary fever, leucocytosis is usually absent in spirillo-sis (Holmgren and Tunevall 1970).

Treatment

Parenteral penicillin is the drug of choice, although may cause a Jarisch–Herxheimer reaction. Erythromycin or chloramphenicol may be used in patients allergic to penicillin. Sulphonamides are ineffective.

Prognosis

Attacks last 3–4 days but, in the absence of treatment, can recur, usually at a regular interval, for months or even years. Case fatality rate is 2–10 per cent (Pritchard 1990).

EPIDEMIOLOGY

Sporadic cases occur worldwide. Outbreaks are not described. Wild rats, living in close proximity to man, were examined in Vancouver in 1950 and 14 per cent carried *Spirillum minus* (Pritchard 1990). Carriage by laboratory rats, mice, and guinea-pigs is also described. Disease is exclusively transmitted to humans by the bite of an infected animal, in contrast to *Streptobacillus moniliformis* where transmission by the contamination of milk or water by the urine of infected animals is described.

Person to person transmission does not occur.

PREVENTION AND CONTROL

Preventing the infestation by rats of human dwellings and workplaces is the key to control. Also of importance is the taking of general precautions to avoid being bitten when handling laboratory animals. Meticulous local wound care of any bites that do occur is also necessary.

REFERENCES

Hiatt J. R. and Hiatt N. (1995). The forgotten first career of Doctor Henry Van Dyke Carter. *Journal of the American College of Surgeons*, **181**, (5), 464–6.

Holmgren E. B. and Tunevall, G. (1970). Case report—rat bite fever. *Scandinavian Journal of Infections Disease*, **2**, 71–4.

Pritchard, D. G. (1990). In *Topley and Wilson's Principles of bacteriology, virology and immunity*, (8th edn), (ed). M. T. Parker and L. H. Collier), Vol. III, pp. 618–19 Edward Arnold, London.

Skirrow, M. B. (1990). In *Topley and Wilson's Principles of bacteriology, virology and immunity*, (8th edn), (ed. M. T. Parker and B. I. Duerden), Vol. II, pp. 545–7. Edward Arnold, London.

19 SALMONELLOSIS

T. J. Humphrey, E. J. Threlfall, and J. G. Cruickshank

SUMMARY

Over 2000 food poisoning serotypes of salmonella (bacterium) exist and the prevalence of individual serotypes constantly changes. Host-adapted strains may cause serious illness (e.g. *S. dublin* in cattle, *S. pulorum* in chickens), but most human food poisoning salmonellas do not cause clinical signs in animals. The main reservoirs for human infection are poultry, cattle, sheep, and pigs. Infection in animals is maintained by recycling slaughterhouse waste as animal feed, faecal–oral spread, and faecal contamination of hatching eggs. Transmission occurs when organisms, introduced into the kitchen in, for example, poultry carcasses, meat, or unpasteurized milk, multiply in food due to inadequate cooking, cross-contamination of cooked foods, and inadequate storage. Person to person spread is common in institutions such as hospitals.

In human the presence and severity of symptoms depends on the infecting dose. Typically there is watery diarrhoea for a few days, possibly leading to dehydration, with abdominal pain and low-grade fever. Septicaemia and abscess formation are rare.

In animals subclinical infection is common and many animals may be intermittent or persistent carriers. However, cows may suffer with fever, diarrhoea, and abortion. Calves undergo epizootic outbreaks of diarrhoea with high mortality. In pigs, fever and diarrhoea are less common than in cattle. Infected sheep, goats, and poultry usually show no signs of infection.

Prevention and control of food poisoning include educating food handlers in good kitchen hygiene, ensuring thorough cooking of meat, refrigerating cooked foods and preventing cross-contamination, pasteurizing all milk and ensuring personal hygiene, and reducing contamination of poultry carcasses at abattoirs. Finally, irradiation of meat and other foods before purchase will reduce contamination.

INTRODUCTION

Human salmonellosis may manifest as one of two clinical entities. The most severe is enteric fever and is caused by *Salmonella typhi* or *S. paratyphi A, B,* or *C.* With few exceptions, in the case of paratyphoid B infection transmission is from person to person without animal involvement. All other salmonellas are primarily of animals and some can be transmitted to man causing 'non-typhoid salmonellosis'. These latter infections are zoonotic and are discussed in this chapter.

THE AGENT

Gaertner (1888) is credited with the first isolation of a salmonella, probably *S. enteritidis* from both victims and suspect food in an outbreak of food poisoning. The term salmonella was only adopted many years later in honour of an American veterinary surgeon, Daniel E. Salmon, who was involved in early studies.

Salmonella serotypes are distributed into seven subspecies. Almost all those which infect warm-blooded animals (including man) belong to group 1. The other groups affect cold-blooded animals and rarely infect man. Salmonellas are Gram-negative, usually flagellate rods, and grow readily on simple culture media and in a wide range of foods in either aerobic or anaerobic conditions at temperatures from about 7 °C to 46 °C. Individual salmonellas showed considerable antigenic diversity and White (1929) developed a scheme which was modified by Kauffmann, based on antigenic structure, whereby individual strains could be identified by serotyping, thus paving the way for studies of outbreaks, sources, and other facets of epidemiological analysis.

Up to the early 1940s comparatively few salmonellas were recognized and about 14 serotypes were responsible for the majority of cases. Thereafter, with increasing interest in food poisoning and the development of improved isolation and typing techniques, many more salmonellas were characterized. Over 2000 serotypes have now been identified but comparatively few are of major importance in human disease.

Salmonellas can share antigens with other enteric bacteria, which can create diagnostic difficulties. Further discrimination amongst serotypes can be achieved by other techniques, for example phage typing, plasmid analysis, and pulsed field gel electrophoresis (see below). Such precision has proved invaluable in epidemiological studies, particularly those involving common serotypes.

TYPING AND FINGERPRINTING OF SALMONELLA

For the most common salmonella serotypes, and for serotypes of particular clinical significance such as *S. typhi*, subdivision within serotype is often an essential prerequisite for meaningful epidemiological investigations. Traditionally a variety of phenotypic characteristics have been used for this purpose. However, in recent years such techniques have been supplemented by a range of DNA-based methods which can provide a molecular 'fingerprint' of the organism, which often cannot be detected by phenotypic methods. The phenotypic characteristics which have been most used for subdivision within serotype are bacteriophage typing (phage typing), biotyping, and antibiogram typing (R-typing), and these have occasionally been supplemented by analysis of lipopolysaccharide content (LPS) or outer membrane-proteins (OMPs) for specific investigations. DNA-based methods involve the analysis of plasmid DNA and, more recently, the analysis of chromosomal DNA.

The underlying principle of phage typing is the host specificity of bacteriophages and, on the basis of their susceptibility to lysis by different phages or races of phages, a number of salmonella serotypes have been subdivided. Published phage typing schemes are in existence for *S. typhi*, *S. paratyphi* A and B, *S. enteritidis*, *S. typhimurium*, *S. virchow*, and *S. hadar* reviewed by Threlfall and Frost 1990). Using such schemes, over 30 phage types of *S. enteritidis* (Ward *et al.* 1987) and over 200 phage types of *S. typhimurium* (Anderson *et al.* 1977) have been designated.

Biotyping, based on the fermentation of various substrates and on other tests such as motility and the presence of haemagglutinating fimbriae, has been used to subdivide several salmonella serotypes. However, in contrast to phage typing, biotyping is laborious and probably less discriminatory, and for these reasons the method is not used extensively for epidemiological investigations.

Because of the fluidity of resistance plasmids and transposons, and because antibiotic resistance is relatively uncommon in many serotypes, antibiogram typing (R-typing) cannot be regarded as a satisfactory primary method for subdivision within serotype. Nevertheless, for some serotypes and phage types, for example *S. typhimurium*, antibiotic resistance patterns can provide a useful epidemiological marker. This method has been used extensively for the subdivision of certain zoonotic phage types of *S. typhimurium*, such

as definitive phage types (DTs) 204c and 104 (Threlfall *et al.* 1986, 1994*c*).

Analysis of lipopolysaccharide (LPS) content, although not a useful tool for subdivision within serotype, has proved useful for investigating interactions within certain phage types. For example, irreversible loss of the ability to synthesize LPS has been shown to be responsible for the conversion of *S. enteritidis* phage type 4 to *S. enteritidis* phage type 7 (Chart *et al.* 1989). In contrast, analysis of outer membrane protein patterns has been shown to be of little value for differentiation within serotype (Helmuth *et al.* 1985).

Methods based on the characterization of plasmid DNA include plasmid profile typing, plasmid fingerprinting, and the identification of plasmid-mediated virulence genes. These methods are based on the numbers and molecular weights (MWs) of carried plasmids in different strains. In particular, plasmid profile typing has been used extensively in support of epidemiological investigations for differentiation both within serotype and phage type (reviewed by Threlfall *et al.* 1994*e*). Of necessity, plasmid profile typing is restricted to those serotypes which possess plasmids and is of limited use in serotypes in which the majority of isolates contain only one plasmid. However, if required, further discrimination may be achieved by cleaving plasmid DNA with restriction endonucleases and the resultant plasmid 'fingerprint' may be used to subdivide plasmids of similar M_r. However, as with plasmid profile typing, plasmid fingerprinting is restricted to plasmid-carrying strains. The presence or absence of serotype-specific plasmids (SSPs) (see below) may also be a useful epidemiological marker and a large number of strains can be rapidly screened using a DNA probe specific for the *spv* genes.

The methods described above are applicable only to plasmid-carrying strains. More recent methods have sought to identify small regions of heterogeneity within the bacterial chromosome. Four such methods which have been used for the differentiation of salmonellas are ribotyping, random cloned chromosomal sequence (RCCS) typing, insertion sequence (IS) *200* typing and pulsed field gel electrophoresis (PFGE). The first three methods use DNA–DNA hybridization to identify restriction fragment length polymorphisms (RFLPs) by detection of single or multicopy gene sequences across the bacterial genome; the fourth method (PFGE) permits analysis of the whole bacterial genome on a single gel.

Ribotyping, which was originally used primarily as a taxonomic tool, can provide a molecular fingerprint based on the distribution of conserved 16S *rrn* genes across the bacterial genome. RCCS typing, which utilizes randomly cloned sequences of chromosomal DNA as single-stranded gene probes, can provide a method of observing heterogeneity in chromosomal restriction enzyme-generated fragment patterns. This method of typing has provided a means of subdividing *S. typhimurium* (Tompkins *et al.* 1986) and may be useful in laboratories which do not have access to phage typing. The salmonella-specific insertion sequence (IS*200*) has been shown to be distributed on conserved loci on the chromosome of many salmonella serotypes with copy numbers ranging from one to 25 and, in some serotypes, identification of the number and distribution of IS*200* elements in the genome has provided a method of discrimination suitable for epidemiological investigations. For example, in *S. typhi*, 15 IS*200* types (clonal lineages) were identified in 49 Vi-phage types (Threlfall *et al.* 1994*d*). Similarly, IS*200* fingerprinting has been used for discrimination within *S. heidelberg* (Stanley *et al.* 1992), *S. brandenburg* (Baquar *et al.* 1994), *S. infantis* (Pelkonen *et al.* 1994) and *S. paratyphi B/java* (Ezquerra *et al.* 1993). For *S. paratyphi B*, this method of typing was used recently in combination with phage typing for the typing of strains from a large outbreak of *S. enterica* serotype *paratyphi B* infection in France caused by a contaminated goats' milk cheese (Desenclos *et al.* 1996).

In contrast to the DNA-based methods described above, which are based on the identification of specific gene sequences across the bacterial genome, pulsed field gel electrophoresis (PFGE) provides a macro fingerprint of the whole genome. This method is becoming increasingly used for the fingerprinting of salmonella, and has been used for subdivision both within serotype and phage type. For example, PFGE has provided a method of discrimination within *S. enteritidis* PT4 (Powell *et al.* 1994) and in 1995 the method provided a means of defining a strain of *S. agona* PT15 associated with a contaminated snack food (Threlfall *et al.* 1996), which caused outbreaks in at least four widely separated countries (Anonymous 1995*a*). Similarly, when used in conjunction with ribotyping and IS*200* fingerprinting, PFGE has provided a method for subdividing strains of *S. panama* isolated in several countries (Stanley *et al.* 1995).

For the meaningful typing of salmonella, it is important that a structured approach is adopted and the use of phenotypic methods such as phage typing and antibiogram analysis for the primary subdivision of strains be supplemented, when appropriate, by epidemiologically validated molecular techniques such as those described above.

PATHOGENESIS

A few serotypes are host adapted; for example, *S. typhi* infects only man and *S. pullorum* and *S. gallinarum* only fowls. Most salmonellas, however, enjoy a wide host range in exotic as well as domestic animals. Mechan-

isms of toxicity are not fully understood. Claims that exotoxins are demonstrable remain controversial and unconfirmed. While many salmonella types may occasionally cause invasive disease, some are especially prone to do so in man, for example *S. dublin*, *S. typhimurium* (some), and *S. cholerae-suis*. Several factors likely to be associated with or responsible for increased virulence have been identified in such strains.

INTERACTIONS OF NON-TYPHOIDAL SALMONELLA ORGANISMS WITH MAMMALIAN EPITHELIAL CELLS

The ability of salmonellas to invade, survive, and replicate within eukaryotic cells is essential for successful infection. Salmonellas posses several virulence-promoting factors which contribute to the disease process. These factors are generally conserved between species, as are the mechanisms by which these bacteria interact with the host cell. These factors facilitate invasion into nonphagocytic cells, survival in the intracellular environment, and replication within host cells (reviewed by Finlay *et al.* 1992).

Following ingestion of the organism the next stage in the disease process is penetration of the intestinal epithelium. Transmission electron microscopy has revealed that invasive salmonellas interact with the well-defined apical microvilli of epithelial cells, thereby disrupting the brush border. Once these cells have been penetrated, the bacteria are enclosed in membrane-bound vacuoles within the host cytoplasm. Virulent salmonellas survive and multiply within these vacuoles after a lag period of about four hours, eventually lysing their host cells and disseminating to other parts of the body. It has been demonstrated for *S. typhimurium* that such intracellular replication is essential for pathogenicity. The salmonellas remain within membrane-bound inclusions and their survival involves blockage of phagosome–lysosome fusion. Salmonellas also depolarize epithelial barriers by affecting the integrity of tight junctions between cells, which has the result of promoting significant cytotoxic damage to epithelial cells.

In contrast to other invasive enteric bacteria, such as *Yersinia* spp. and enteropathogenic *Escherichia coli*, salmonellas require neither motility nor fimbriae to adhere to and invade eukaryotic cells. The induction of *de novo* protein synthesis is necessary for invasion and is regulated by the microenvironment (low oxygen), growth phase, or the epithelial cell surface. Only viable, metabolically active salmonellas can adhere to host cell surfaces. Adherence is followed almost immediately by internalization into the host cells. The bacterial genes necessary for salmonellas to enter eukaryotic cells have yet to be fully characterized but at least six different genetic loci appear to be involved and an additional hyperinvading locus has recently been identified (Finlay *et al.* 1992).

SEROTYPE-SPECIFIC 'VIRULENCE' PLASMIDS

Analysis of the plasmid content of salmonella strains belonging to a range of serotypes has demonstrated that some (but not all) serotypes possess plasmids of high relative molecular mass (M_r) which can be regarded as 'serotype-specific'. Serotypes which harbour such plasmids include *S. enteritidis*, *S. typhimurium*, *S. dublin*, *S. cholerae-suis*, *S. pullorum*, and *S. gallinarum*. In contrast, SSPs have not been identified in other important zoonotic serotypes, such as *S. virchow* or *S. hadar*. Such plasmids range in M_r from about 30 MDa in *S. cholerae-suis* to 62 MDa in *S. typhimurium* (Helmuth *et al.* 1985). In general, SSPs are non-conjugative and do not carry easily identifiable phenotypic markers like drug resistance, although in epidemic strains of *S. typhimurium* DT 193, a conjugative SSP of approximately 80 MDa coding for multiple drug resistance has recently been identified (Threlfall *et al.*, 1994*a*).

The results of animal challenge experiments have indicated that SSPs are involved in the virulence of their host strains for certain strains of inbred mice, like BALB/c. In particular, studies by Pardon *et al.* (1986) and Gulig and Curtis (1987) have demonstrated that for *S. typhimurium*, the 60 MDa SSP genetically determined the spread of the organism beyond the small intestine to the deeper tissues such as the mesenteric lymph nodes or the spleen. They also observed the attenuation of virulence of plasmid-cured strains in parenterally inoculated mice.

SSPs from different serotypes all posses a highly conserved common DNA region which carries genes—*s*almonella *p*lasmid *v*irulence (*spv*) genes—responsible for virulence for mice (Williamson *et al.* 1988*a*). In *S. dublin* such *spv* genes have been shown to be clustered within an 8 kb *Sal*I–*Xho*I restriction endonuclease fragment (Williamson *et al.* 1988*b*) and a homologous region has been identified in the SSPs of *S. typhimurium*, *S. enteritidis*, *S. cholerae-suis*, and several other serotypes (Williamson *et al.* 1988*a*). Within this region, a highly conserved 3.5 kb *Hind* III fragment has been shown to have homology with the virulence regions of the SSPs of *S. dublin* and *S. enteritidis* (Woodward *et al.* 1989).

Six *spv* genes within the common 8 kb *Sal* I–*Xho*I fragment R, A, B, C, D and have now been sequenced. The *spv* E gene encodes a 13 kDa protein, the *spv* D gene a 25 kDa protein, and the *spv* C gene, a 28 kDa protein, which is located both in the outer membrane and the cytoplasm. The latter protein has a demonstrable role in virulence as transposon insertion mutants in the *spv* C gene resulted in a significant drop in the

number of *S. typhimurium* isolated from the spleen of orally infected mice. Moreover, only one-fifth of such mice died following infection with a SSP transposon-attenuated strain as compared to those infected with wild-type bacteria (Norel *et al.* 1989). The *spv* B gene encodes a 65 kDa protein of unknown function which is located both in the outer membrane and the cytoplasm, and the *spv* A gene a 28 kDa protein also of unknown function.

Although essential for the virulence in certain strains of mice, the role of SSP virulence plasmids in the pathogenesis of disease in humans and other animal species is not clear. Results with cattle have suggested that such plasmids are required for bacteraemia (Pardon *et al.* 1986) but not necessarily for gastroenteritis. SSP-like plasmids have been shown to be necessary for intracellular survival of salmonellas in mouse phagocytes (Buchmeier and Heffron 1991) and it has been suggested that such plasmids may enhance the survival of their host organism in extraintestinal infections in humans (Fierer *et al.* 1992). However, recent studies have demonstrated that for *S. enteritidis*, the possession of a SSP is not necessary for the induction of enteritis in humans (Threlfall *et al.* 1994*b*). Likewise, similar SSPs have not been identified in certain phage types of *S. typhimurium* isolated from cases of diarrhoea in humans (Brown *et al.* 1986).

NON-TYPHOID SALMONELLOSIS IN MAN

CLINICAL MANIFESTATIONS

Salmonella infection most commonly results in a gastroenteritic illness with diarrhoea and, from time to time, a number of other symptoms (Table 19.1). The infective dose is often quoted as being high, greater than 10^5 cells, for example (Anonymous 1993). Although this may still be broadly correct for most salmonella serotypes in most vehicles, there is increasing evidence from the analysis of outbreaks and the implicated foods that in foodstuffs where the bacteria

Table 19.1   Symptoms of salmonella infection

Symptom	Percentage of cases[a]
Diarrhoea	87
Abdominal pain	84
Feeling feverish	75
Nausea	65
Muscle pain	64
Vomiting	24
Headache	21
Blood in stools	6

[a] From an egg-associated outbreak of *S. enteritidis* (Stevens *et al.*, 1989).

are protected from gastric acidity lower numbers can initiate infection. In a Cheddar cheese-associated outbreak in Canada (D'Aoust 1985) the infective dose of *S. typhimurium* for previously healthy adults was calculated to be less than 10 cells. Analysis of a large number of outbreaks demonstrated that, for non-typhoid salmonellosis, there was a relationship between infecting dose and the severity of illness (Glynn and Bradley 1992; Mintz *et al.* 1994).

The mean attack rate in salmonella outbreaks where poultry meat was the vehicle was estimated to be 20 per cent (Hobbs 1971). More recent work (Glynn and Bradley 1992), where analysis was applied to 47 outbreaks in the United States with a range of vehicles and caused by either *S. enteritidis*, *S. infantis*, *S. thompson*, or *S. typhimurium*, calculated the mean attack rate to be 56 per cent with a range of 3–100 per cent of exposed persons.

The incubation period is usually within the range of 12–72 hours, but occasionally may extend up to a week. In some outbreaks, where large numbers of organisms are believed to have been consumed, incubation periods as short as 2.5 hours have been reported (Stevens *et al.* 1989). Stools do not usually contain blood and in the majority of cases the acute gastrointestinal symptoms will clear with supportive therapy only within 4–5 days. Malaise, lassitude, and weakness may continue for substantially longer. In severe infections dehydration and prostration may develop rapidly and patients may require hospitalization. The very young, the elderly, the immunosuppressed and those with underlying chronic diseases are more susceptible to infection and are particularly liable to develop complications. For most serotypes, including *S. enteritidis* and *S. typhimurium*, the two most common in humans, only a small proportion of patients (1–2 per cent), especially those with high susceptibility or those infected with invasive strains, may become bacteraemic with fever and other manifestations of Gram-negative sepsis. With certain, less common serotypes, such as *S. dublin* and *S. cholerae-suis* and also for some strains of *S.virchow*, the incidence of extraintestinal infections is higher. In up to 25 per cent of cases of *S. dublin*, 75 per cent of *S. cholerae-suis*, and 4 per cent of *S. virchow* infections the organisms can be isolated from blood cultures (Threlfall *et al.* 1992). Such cases carry an appreciable mortality, though most will recover with antibiotic therapy.

Sequelae of disseminated infection may include metastatic abscesses in organs such as bone, particularly vertebrae, the wall of the aorta, and kidney. Other complications are non-specific and include reactive arthritis and ankylosing spondylitis, the pathogenesis of which is not understood.

Asymptomatic infections are thought to be common, although the proportion of patients who do not manifest disease is not known. It is not unusual in the investigation of outbreaks to find up to 50 per cent of contacts of cases excreting the organisms but remaining free of symptoms.

The clinical outcome of most salmonella infections is complete resolution of all symptoms. About half of the patients with uncomplicated infections will continue to excrete the organism in the faeces 5 weeks after recovery, 10 per cent at 9 weeks and less than 1 per cent after a year (Buchwald and Blazir 1984). This prolonged carrier state is unique amongst food-borne infections and is the cause of much testing and exclusion of victims from various food-handling activities. Its practical significance will be discussed later.

Septicaemic illness will require antibiotic treatment. While most infecting strains are susceptible to a wide variety of antibiotics, the quinolone ciprofloxacin is currently the preferred choice when treatment is indicated on the grounds that, as well as being effective in control of the disease, it will also reduce the duration of subsequent carriage (Willcox and Spencer 1992). However, relapses of carriage are common and repeated courses may be necessary. Antibiotic resistance in salmonellas is becoming more common and is no longer confined to a relatively small number of phage types of *S. typhimurium*. For example, recent surveys in the United Kingdom have demonstrated that since 1990 the incidence of multiple resistance has increased in *S. typhimurium*, and the incidence of resistance to ciprofloxacin has increased in *S. hadar* and *S.virchow* (Frost, *et al.* 1995).

EPIDEMIOLOGY

RECENT TRENDS IN INCIDENCE

Human salmonellosis continues to be a major international problem both in terms of morbidity (Anonymous 1989) and economic cost (Barnass *et al.* 1989). While a variety of vehicles from, for example, potato crisps (Hobbs and Roberts 1993) to bean sprouts (O'Mahony *et al.* 1990) have been implicated in outbreaks, salmonellosis is primarily associated with products of animal origin. The number of reported cases of non-typhoid salmonellosis has increased substantially in many countries over the past 10 years. This is associated largely with *S. enteritidis*, with phage type (PT) 4 predominating in western Europe, PT1 in eastern Europe, and PTs 8 and 13a in the United States. Given the ubiquity of *S. enteritidis* and other salmonellas, it is surprising that infection rates can be so different in neighbouring countries. This is illustrated in Fig. 19.1 which shows data from England and Wales,

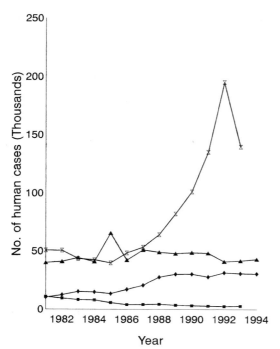

Fig. 19.1   Recent trends in salmonella infections. ▲, USA; ◆, England and Wales; ■, The Netherlands; ⊠ Germany.

the United States, The Netherlands, and Germany (Stöhr, personal communication). The increase in reported cases in England and Wales occurred in the second half of the 1980s (Fig. 19.1) and this trend is typical of much of western Europe. As in North America, however, there were exceptions to this. Thus, while cases increased markedly in Germany from 50 633 in 1981 to 195 378 in 1992, cases in The Netherlands fell from 10 783 to 2590 in the same period (Fig.19.1; Stöhr, personal communication). Infection rates are falling in many countries although they remain much higher than those in the early to mid-1980s.

TRANSMISSION

Salmonellosis is acquired either by ingestion of organisms in raw, undercooked, or cross-contaminated food or water, or by the passing of the organisms from person to person via the faecal–oral route by either direct contact with infected excreta or indirectly through the handling of objects such as bedding, toys, and clothing which have been contaminated with excreta. Outbreaks of human salmonellosis are not uncommon (see Table 19.2) but most infections are sporadic. Identification of the source(s) of infection in sporadic cases is rarely possible because of the nearly universal distribution of common potential vehicles of

transmission in households, catering establishments, and the environment, for example eggs, poultry, red meats, dairy products. Only when there are numbers of related cases (i.e. outbreaks) in which common factors can be sought and identified is there a real likelihood of successful source tracing.

OUTBREAKS

In any outbreak, primary cases occur through the consumption of contaminated food and subsequent and secondary cases may arise through person to person contact with primary cases. This tendency for person to person transmission to follow earlier cases is characteristic of salmonella infections and is rare with other food poisoning bacteria.

Food-borne outbreaks tend to be of the 'point source' type, with most of the victims or primary cases becoming ill over a period from 12 to 72 hours after the common consumption of contaminated food. Cases with later onset (secondary cases) have probably become infected from direct or indirect contact with one of the primary cases. Outbreaks of this kind occur in circumstances where a single catering establishment is serving groups of people; for example, hospitals, schools, nursing homes, receptions, and other recreational facilities.

Less common are 'continuing or extended common source' outbreaks where a contaminated food or medicament is widely distributed and cases are related through organism type but not obviously in time or place. Such outbreaks can be confused with sporadic cases, particularly when cases are distributed nationally or even extended to other countries. Recent vehicles in outbreaks of this type included salami sticks (Cowden *et al.* 1989*a*) and mung bean sprouts (O'Mahony *et al.* 1990) in the United Kingdom and undercooked eggs and chicken in a great many countries (St. Louis *et al.* 1988; Cowden *et al.* 1989*b*). Paradoxically, the rarer the serotype the more likely widely disseminated outbreak is to be recognized.

Person to person outbreaks are most often seen in institutions where there may be difficulties in maintaining good hygiene, for example psychogeriatric wards. The organism may be introduced by an unrecognized case or by a convalescent excreter and over a period of time other patients on the ward acquire the infection by faecal–oral transfer. Such outbreaks may extend over weeks or months.

Some outbreaks seem to have features of all three of those defined above and may defy explanation. One such occurred in a children's hospital with an unusual, and hence easily identifiable and readily traceable, salmonella serotype. The infection invaded many wards in an apparently haphazard way and was never traced to any source. Only temporary closure of the hospital brought the outbreak under control.

SALMONELLOSIS IN ANIMALS

When infected, domestic animals, particularly poultry and pigs, frequently become asymptomatic carriers for variable periods, although some serotypes, in some animals, can give rise to severe infections. Disease may manifest as septicaemia and/or enteritis, although the severity of the illness can be governed by the age of the animal. For example, in young calves, septicaemia with a high mortality is common in infections caused by *S. dublin* and phage types of *S. typhimurium*, while in older animals the pattern is more usually of asymptomatic infection or of an enteritis followed by asymptomatic carriage which is frequently long term. Enteritis in cows infected with *S. dublin*, a cattle-adapted serotype, is frequently precipitated by calving, and diarrhoea, rapidly progressing to dysentery, may occur with weight loss, emaciation, and death. Similar clinical manifestations can be seen in sheep after lambing.

The above events are relatively uncommon and in discussions on the zoonotic transmission of salmonellas it is necessary to differentiate between short-term problems, which may result from a chance infection which leads to the contamination of a particular product or foodstuff, and the underlying background of human salmonellosis brought about by sustained infection or carriage in some food animals. Thus, the occasional colonization or infection of dairy cows (Gay *et al.* 1994) may result in salmonella outbreaks associated with either raw (Maguire *et al.* 1992), improperly pasteurized (Ryan *et al.* 1987), or improperly heat-treated (Rowe *et al.* 1987) milk products. A similar relationship exists between salmonella infection in pigs and contamination of pork products (Maguire *et al.* 1993; Cowden *et al.* 1989*a*). A more recent, and more serious, example in the United Kingdom concerns the very rapid rise in *S. typhimurium* DT 104 infections.

Since 1991 this particular phage type has become increasingly common in cattle and humans, and also in poultry and pigs. This national outbreak is causing particular concern as the epidemic strain is resistant to a number of antibiotics (Threlfall *et al.*, 1994*c*), including chloramphenicol, ampicillin, and tetracyclines, and, more recently, to trimethoprim and ciprofloxacin (Threlfall *et al.* 1996).

Outbreaks of the type outlined above are clearly important to those afflicted, the producers/suppliers involved, and may have significant sociological and economic consequences. Their control can be helped by improvements in production and catering hygiene, and this will be discussed later. It is clear, however, that a substantial proportion of human salmonellosis, in a great many countries, is a consequence of asymptomatic salmonella infection of poultry. A variety of sero- and phage types have been involved (Humphrey *et al.* 1988). In most cases a particular salmonella becomes important for a short while and then declines. Two examples of this are nationwide outbreaks, in England and Wales, involving *S. agona*, in 1975 and *S. hadar* between 1977 and 1981 (Anonymous 1989). They both were associated with chicken and turkeys infected from contaminated imported feed. As discussed earlier, the recent pattern of human infections internationally has been dominated by *S. enteritidis* since the middle 1980s (Rodrigue *et al.* 1990). This bacterium is strongly associated with poultry, principally chickens, and continues to be the dominant salmonella serotype in a great many countries, although the number of cases would appear to be on the decline.

Table 19.2 shows data from general salmonella outbreaks in England and Wales between 1988–91. The information illustrates the importance of poultry meat and eggs. For example, of the 429 outbreaks during that period where it was possible to implicate a vehicle, 177 (41 per cent) involved eggs and egg products and 110 (25 per cent) poultry meat. *Salmonella enteritidis* PT4 was the pathogen implicated in 233 outbreaks (54 per cent). Of these, 135 (58 per cent) involved eggs

Table 19.2 Foodstuffs and salmonella serotypes implicated in general outbreaks of human salmonellosis in England and Wales 1988–91[a]

Serotype	Number of outbreaks where following foods were implicated				
	Eggs	Poultry meat	Red meat	Other foods[b]	Not known
Salmonella enteritidis					
all phage types	160	62	12	54	1621
PT4	135	45	8	45	1250
Other *Salmonella* serotypes	17	48	29	48	1034

[a] Taken from data given in PHLS/SVS reports 1989–92.
[b] Other foods includes meals or food containing poultry meat and/or eggs.

and 45 (19 per cent) poultry meat. (In 1987 there were six egg-associated outbreaks identified in England and Wales. *Salmonella enteritidis* was implicated in none of these). The outbreak patterns identified in England and Wales show many similarities with those in the rest of western Europe, North America, and elsewhere (Rodrigue *et al.* 1990). Measures to either limit or prevent the infection of chickens with *S. enteritidis* have clear public health benefits.

SOURCES OF SALMONELLA INFECTION IN FOOD ANIMALS

The three principal sources of salmonellas which infect food animals are: infected breeding stock, contaminated foodstuffs, and the environment. The importance of individual routes of infection are dependant, in part, on the salmonella serotype and food animal involved. The overall cycle of salmonella transmission is complex (Baird-Parker 1991) but in practice, with individual incidents or with particular serotypes, routes of transmission may be easier to unravel.

The role of infected breeding stock

With certain salmonellas, usually those that show either partial or total host adaptation, vertical transmission from infected breeding stock is the principal route of infection. Examples of this are *S. dublin* in cattle and *S. enteritidis* PT4 in chickens, particularly in broiler chicken production.

Contaminated foodstuffs in the transmission of salmonellas to food animals

The presence of salmonellas in feedstuffs can often result in the infection/colonization of food animals and contamination of products derived from them. This would seem to be particularly important in poultry (Williams 1981). A relationship is apparent between contaminated feed, the incidence of particular serotypes in poultry, and the appearance of these organisms in outbreaks of human salmonellosis.

Heat processing in feed production should be sufficient to destroy salmonellas or to reduce levels below those required to infect animals, but may fail to do so, especially when conditions of treatment are inadequate or opportunities exist for recontamination of the finished product.

The contaminated farm environment and salmonella infection in food animals

The use of animal excreta on farmland presents potential health hazards to domestic animals and man (Wray 1975). Salmonellas are capable of prolonged survival in either faecal material, slurry, or on pasture (Wray 1975). There can also be difficulties in the cleaning and disinfection of farm premises, and salmonellas were isolated from 8 per cent of floor-swab samples taken from calf-rearing units after cleaning and disinfection (Wray *et al.* 1990). In further studies, these authors (Wray *et al.* 1991) also demonstrated that salmonellas could be isolated, on at least one occasion, from 50 per cent of samples taken from calf markets and 21 and 7 per cent of samples taken from transport vehicles before and after cleaning, respectively. A variety of salmonellas have also been isolated, in a number of studies, from water courses and farm-associated wild animals (Davies and Wray 1994). Gulls, in particular, are believed to be important in the dissemination of salmonellas. Those sampled at or around refuse tips or slaughterhouses show a raised incidence of salmonella carriage (Fenlon 1983). Infection of grazing animals following the contamination of pasture with gull faeces has also been demonstrated (Coulson *et al.* 1983), although the importance of gulls as salmonella vectors has been questioned (Girdwood *et al.* 1985).

Mice may be important in the dissemination of *S. enteritidis* to laying hens (Eckroade *et al.* 1991) and the artificial infection of wild mice with a strain of *S. enteritidis* PT4 resulted in the excretion of the bacterium for over 6 months (Davies and Wray 1994).

CONTAMINATION OF FOODS

MEAT

Raw meats, whether as cuts or processed, must be regarded as potentially contaminated with salmonellas. Sausages, minced meat, and offal obtained from retail shops can have high rates of contamination, though there is considerable variation between surveys.

CONTAMINATION OF CARCASSES

Salmonellas can contaminate carcass meat by a variety of routes, but faecal contamination is the most important. The extent to which this happens is governed by the degree of carriage in the live animal and the hygiene of the slaughter process. There are wide variations in reported isolation rates of salmonellas from red meat animals. For example, salmonellas are rarely isolated from adult sheep and cattle in the United Kingdom (Mackey 1989). In parts of Australia and the United States, however, high levels of intestinal carriage have been demonstrated (Samual *et al.* 1980). There is rather more general agreement on poultry, and surveys, in a variety of countries, have shown that carriage rates in live birds and contamination rates in carcasses can be high. The prevalence of salmonella-positive red-meat animals will increase as a result of mixing at markets (Wray *et al.* 1991) and the stress of transportation of all animals can lead to the recrudescence of latent infections (Williams and Spencer 1973). Salmonellas can also spread rapidly during transportation or in the lairage prior to slaughter. Grau and Smith (1974) demonstrated that the prevalence of salmonella-positive lamb carcases was related to the length of time the animals were held before they were killed.

Carcass contamination can occur at almost any stage of the slaughter process but is more likely, in red-meat animals, where the intestines and hide are removed. Much work has been carried out on salmonella contamination of poultry carcasses. Studies have shown that the incidence of carcass contamination often exceeds that of infection in the live bird (McBride *et al.* 1980). This is the result of cross-contamination which can occur during transport to the factory and at many points on the slaughter line, but immersion scalding, to loosen the feathers prior to mechanical plucking, is of particular importance. Scalding can result in contamination of carcass surfaces and deep tissues with pathogenic micro-organisms (Lillard 1973; Mulder *et al.* 1978). It is also inefficient in killing or removing organisms attached to chicken skin (Notermans and Kampelmacher 1975), and those that survive scalding are more difficult to remove during the later stages of processing.

Contamination of carcasses of any food animal is most usually confined to the surfaces, and the examination of deep muscle tissues from beef carcasses, for example, did not yield any potential human pathogens (Gill 1979). As mentioned above, this is not the case with chicken, and two independent investigations in the United Kingdom (Humphrey 1991a; Rampling, personal communication) isolated *S. enteritidis* PT4 from aseptically collected muscle samples from chickens purchased at retail outlets. The public health implications of such isolations have yet to be fully assessed but a case-control study in the UK found that PT4 infection was associated with the consumption of hot, cooked, take-away chicken (Cowden *et al.* 1989b). The bacterium was probably present in tissues either as a result of invasive disease (Lister 1988) or the ingress of contaminated scald tank water (Lillard 1973).

CONTAMINATION OF EGGS

Infection of laying hens with *S. enteritidis* and the resultant contamination of eggs is believed to have been important in the increase in human salmonellosis seen in many countries since the mid-to-late 1980s (Rodrigue *et al.* 1990).

Salmonellas can be isolated from either egg shells or contents. Their presence on egg shells is usually the result of faecal carriage, although, with *S. enteritidis* in particular, infection of the lower reproductive tract may also be important (Humphrey *et al.* 1991*a*). Salmonellas on egg shells can contaminate egg contents either by passage through the shell (Sparks and Board 1985) or at breaking. With the intact hens' egg the former is a rare event and it is accepted scientific opinion that contents contamination with *S. enteritidis*, in particular, is more usually the result of infection of reproductive tissue, principally the oviduct (Hoop and Pospischil 1993).

Surveillance in the United Kingdom and United States has demonstrated that the prevalence of contents-positive eggs on sale to the general public is low (<0.1 per cent). However, given the large number of eggs consumed, even such apparently low contamination rates may be significant. Although fresh eggs contain only a few cells of *S. enteritidis* (Humphrey *et al.* 1989, 1991*b*; Mawer *et al.* 1989) the bacterium is capable of growth in contaminated eggs, particularly where storage conditions have weakened the yolk membrane and permitted salmonellas access to yolk contents (Humphrey and Whitehead 1993 Humphrey 1994).

MILK AND MILK PRODUCTS

Milk-producing animals, including cattle, can be infected with salmonellas. While market surveys have shown a low overall prevalence of infected cows (Gay *et al.* 1994) carriage can be prolonged. Giles *et al.* (1989) found that *S. typhimurium* DT 49a persisted in a dairy herd for $3\frac{1}{2}$ years. The principal vehicle in milk-associated human salmonellosis is unpasteurized milk and many outbreaks have been reported. Prohibition of the sale of unpasteurized milk imposed in Scotland in 1983 has all but eliminated milk-borne outbreaks in that country.

In general, raw milk will become salmonella-positive as a result of faecal contamination, although some studies have shown no relationship between farm hygiene scores, the levels of indicator bacteria, and the presence of salmonellas in milk (McEwen *et al.* 1988).

All salmonellas so far examined, are sufficiently heat sensitive to be destroyed by pasteurization, and pasteurized milk has an enviable safety record, although some outbreaks have been associated with this product. This may be due to faults in the pasteurization process but contamination after heat treatment is more likely. Pasteurized milk was the vehicle of infection in an outbreak in 1956, but bottle tops were found contaminated with mouse faeces (Galbraith and Pusey 1984). It is more usual for outbreaks to arise as a result of contamination of the heat-treated product with raw milk. An example of this was a large, multi-state outbreak of salmonellosis in the United States (Ryan *et al.* 1987).

Salmonellas can survive in certain cheeses, and such products have been implicated in some large outbreaks. In Canada, 1500 people were infected after consuming contaminated Cheddar-type cheese (D'Aoust 1985). More recently, in the United Kingdom, an outbreak of infection with *S. dublin* was associated with soft unpasteurized cows' milk cheese (Maguire *et al.* 1992). Similarly, a large outbreak of *S. enterica* serotype *paratyphi B* infection in France in 1993, in which over 273 cases were identified, was caused by a contaminated goats' milk cheese (Desenclos *et al.* 1996). It should, however, be noted that the most common symptomology in this outbreak was that of gastroenteritis, which suggests that the strain involved was that normally designated as *S. paratyphi B* var *java*, or *S. java*. It is clear that acid production alone cannot be regarded as a control measure against salmonellas in cheese.

FOOD HANDLERS

Food handlers found to be excreters are often accused of being the source of the outbreak. Evidence, albeit indirect, suggests that any person, including excreters, who has a formed stool and practises reasonable hygiene are rarely responsible for either initiating or extending an outbreak (Cruickshank and Humphrey 1987). Salmonellas are readily removed by hand washing (Pether and Gilbert 1971). Catering staff are often found to have eaten the food that has caused an outbreak and are victims rather than perpetrators. Food handlers with diarrhoea do, however, constitute a significant risk and should be excluded from work for 48 hours following recovery (Anonymous 1990).

While the direct involvement of carrier food handlers as disseminators of salmonellas is doubtful, their potential role in food cross-contamination is beyond dispute. Salmonella-contaminated raw products, principally meat and poultry, have been shown to bring about extensive contamination of the kitchen environment (de Wit *et al.* 1979; de Boer and Hahne 1990). The homogenization of contaminated egg contents resulted in the production of contaminated droplets which distributed *S. enteritidis* widely in the environment around the mixing bowl (Humphrey *et al.* 1994). Survival at 20 °C was prolonged (>24 hours) in small egg droplets or smears.

Many salmonella outbreaks have been caused by poor kitchen practice, and Roberts (1986) estimated that, in approximately 14 per cent, cross-contamination was an important contributory factor. Salmonellas are also able to grow well on a variety of

cooked or raw foods (Ingham *et al.* 1990; Golden *et al.*, 1993) and storage at non-refrigeration temperatures has been shown to be important in many outbreaks (Roberts 1986). For example, Luby *et al.* (1993) reported a large outbreak in which customers became infected with either *S. agona* or *S. hadar* because cooked turkey was held unrefrigerated in a small restaurant kitchen for several hours, rinsed with water to remove offensive odour, and incompletely reheated before serving.

CONTROL

It may be possible to intervene at a number of points on the feed–food chain to either reduce or eliminate the risk of human salmonellosis. The practicality of intervention and its cost effectiveness may depend on the salmonella serotype involved and the degree of its spread. Thus, infections in the United Kingdom with *S. typhimurium* DT 124 resulting from the contamination of salami sticks (Cowden *et al.* 1989*a*) were prevented by a temporary withdrawal of the product and improvements in production hygiene. Milk-borne salmonellosis can be prevented by the simple expedient of proper pasteurization of milk and milk products. Where infection is widespread, such as the multinational pandemic caused by *S. enteritidis* (Rodrigue *et al.* 1990) control may be more difficult to achieve, particularly if the vehicles of infection are foods such as eggs or chicken which are consumed in large numbers. The successful control of this type of problem may require intervention at many points on the food chain (Anonymous 1994*a*).

CONTROL MEASURES DURING ANIMAL PRODUCTION

The control of zoonotic salmonellosis can present a variety of practical difficulties and, as a consequence, may require long-term strategies and, possibly, legislation. For example, the importance of vertical transmission of certain salmonellas in poultry production has been recognized by the European Union which has put in place legislation to deal with this problem (Anonymous 1992*b*). This requires the regular monitoring of poultry breeding flocks. Those where the presence of either *S. enteritidis* or *S. typhimurium* is confirmed are slaughtered. Such a policy, while having laudable aims, can prove to be an economic burden on the industry involved, particularly where, as with *S. enteritidis* in poultry, infection is widespread and often at a high prevalence. As a consequence of the economic concerns, alternative strategies are being explored. Competitive exclusion, where cultures of intestinal micro-organisms from infection-free mature hens are administered to day-old chicks, has been shown to limit salmonella infection (Nurmi and Rantala 1973) and is being used increasingly.

In the United Kingdom legislation has been introduced to control the contamination of animal feedstuffs with salmonellas. Relevant legislation includes the Zoonoses Order (1989), the Processed Animal Protein Order (1989) and the Importation of Processed Animal Protein Order (1981). Animal feeds can only be tested in laboratories authorized under the Processed Animal Protein Order (1989).

The above Orders have been remarkably successful and the contamination rates in processed animal protein and fishmeal produced in the United Kingdom has declined from 10 per cent in 1986 to 2 per cent in 1993 (Anonymous 1994*b*). There is, however, the possibility of recontamination of animal feed on the farm. To guard against this it is possible to incorporate antimicrobial compounds such as organic acids. Humphrey and Lanning (1988) found that such treatment of feed given to breeding hens reduced the vertical transmission of salmonellas. Acid feed treatment has also been shown to limit the horizontal spread of *S. enteritidis* PT4 in some broiler flocks (Humphrey 1991*b*). Rodent control programmes must also be seen as an important control measure, particularly in poultry production.

Antibiotics are used to treat clinical salmonella infections in livestock. Such treatments, while successful in controlling clinical signs, often do not produce a bacteriological cure. Indeed, some antimicrobials have been shown to prolong the salmonella carrier-state in poultry by disturbing the ecological balance of the gut and inhibiting key organisms responsible for limiting intestinal populations of salmonellas. Various antimicrobial feed additives, especially those permitted for animal growth promotion, were examined by Smith and Tucker (1978) and some, including nitrovin, flavomycin, lincomycin, or tylosin, increased the numbers of salmonellas being shed and often prolonged the period of excretion to the point of slaughter.

Cattle are the main farmed species in which salmonellosis frequently causes clinical problems and the great majority of these arise from either *S. dublin* or *S. typhimurium* infections. A wide range of 'exotic' serotypes cause sporadic outbreaks of disease in cattle and, to a far lesser extent, in sheep, whereas clinical salmonellosis is very rare in pigs. Thus, developments in vaccination have generally been restricted to cattle, and commercial vaccines against *S. dublin* and *S. typhimurium* are widely in use. Unlike other salmonella serotypes in poultry, *S. enteritidis* can cause clinical problems, especially in broilers and this, as well as the associated epidemic in man, stimulated considerable and very promising work on vaccine development in this species. Field and pilot studies on a vaccine against *S. enteritidis* in chickens have demonstrated a good protection, although generally only a reduction in carriage/infection is seen (Barrow *et al.* 1990). A recent vaccine using a strain of *S. enteritidis* grown under conditions of iron limitations reduced mortality, clinical illness, faecal shedding, and egg contents contamination rates in birds infected artificially (Schofield, personal communication).

The control of environmental contamination can be difficult, although the storage of slurry and faeces before they are spread on to pasture will do much to reduce the salmonella load. Potential hazard can also be reduced by allowing the maximum delay between the manuring of grazing land and its use by food animals. However, spread of infection by wild birds, especially gulls from extensive rubbish tips, adds a further significant means of environmental contamination. Protection of housed animals, such as pigs and poultry, may present fewer problems but the intensive nature of much of this type of production will facilitate the spread of salmonellas. Nevertheless, salmonellosis in animals is not ubiquitous, with, in general, only a very small proportion of slaughter animals being infected. The chances of producing salmonella-free animals is increased by proper biosecurity, rodent control programmes, and efficient cleaning and disinfection.

It is often necessary to identify salmonella-positive animals, particularly in control programmes. The samples taken should taken account of the epidemiology and behaviour of the salmonella serotype under investigation, if this is known, and the techniques used during examination should be sensitive and as rapid as practically possible. The current international pandemic of *S. enteritidis* infection (Rodrigue *et al.*, 1990) has led to extensive monitoring of poultry flocks. This bacterium is invasive in poultry and can be isolated from tissues, including reproductive tissues, in the absence of intestinal carriage (Hoop and Pospischil 1993). Thus techniques which rely on the examination of gut contents only may either underestimate or miss infection. A better approach is to carry out environmental or serological screening with confirmation of positive results by more detailed examination of birds. Measurement of yolk antibodies against *S. enteritidis* is effective in the detection of positive breeder or layer flocks (Van de Giessen *et al.* 1992) and provides a cost-effective, non-invasive technique which is worthy of wider use. Very few salmonellas are invasive in red-meat animals, under normal commercial conditions, and the testing of faecal samples is much less likely to lead to false negative results.

CONTROL IN FOOD PRODUCTION

There is increasing agreement that salmonella control may be most successfully applied on the farm, and a prime example of this is in poultry production in the United Kingdom where, as a result of government- and industry-inspired intervention, the prevalence of salmonella-positive chicken carcasses has been markedly reduced from *c.* 70 per cent to *c.* 35 per cent (Anonymous, 1995*b*). However, in milk production, particularly where dairy animals may be colonized with salmonellas which do not cause infection, control is better applied during food production, and the pasteurization of milk is a good example of successful, cost-effective intervention. Control is clearly more difficult during slaughter but a great variety of studies, in many countries, have explored the possibility of reducing the prevalence of salmonella- contaminated carcasses.

CONTROL OF CARCASS CONTAMINATION

The public health importance of salmonella-contaminated poultry carcasses has generated many investigations into possible decontamination measures. In general, in poultry processing, experimental methods which have been shown to be successful in pilot scale are either too expensive in a commercial situation or bring about unacceptable changes in carcass quality. One of the more effective end-product treatments is γ-irradiation and Dempster (1985) demonstrated that this process can destroy salmonellas on chicken carcasses. There is, however, considerable consumer resistance to this procedure, and it is unlikely to be adopted in the short term. With red meat, spraying with either hot water (80 °C) or lactic acid have been shown to have applications as carcass decontaminants (Smulders 1987, Davey and Smith 1989).

The degree of cross-contamination is influenced by both the number of colonized/infected animals and slaughter hygiene. In addition to the on-farm measures outlined above, the prevalence of salmonella-positive animals entering the slaughterhouse can be reduced by a reduction in transport times and a limitation on the time spent by animals in the lairage. Measures, such as tying of the anus, to prevent the contamination of carcases with faeces will also reduce the extent and degree of carcase contamination.

CONTROL IN RETAIL OUTLETS, FOOD CATERING ESTABLISHMENTS, AND IN THE HOME

Control is based upon the practice of meticulous hygiene in all aspects of the handling of food. Staff educational programmes should be established and should emphasize the importance of hand washing, proper storage and refrigeration of food, kitchen sanitation, and prevention of cross-contamination. The risks when certain foods are undercooked should also

be emphasized. Staff with gastroenteric symptoms must be excluded until recovery. Outbreak control is based upon the isolation and treatment of patients (in institutions); identification and surveillance of contacts and others exposed to the same source; the blocking of further transmissions; and the tracing and elimination of the original of the outbreak. Investigations are frequently extensive and may involve several bodies and organizations; for example laboratory and epidemiological services, environmental health departments, government agencies, food manufacturers, and retail and catering establishments.

The great majority of salmonellas so far studied are unable to grow on food stored below 7 °C and will only grow slowly at temperatures below 10 °C. Thus the refrigeration of perishable foods will not only extend shelf-life but will also prevent the growth of salmonellas. There has been much recent discussion in Europe over the refrigerated storage of eggs as a means of limiting the risk of infection with *S. enteritidis*. The ability of this bacterium to grow in egg contents is largely controlled by the integrity of the yolk membrane. The rate of yolk membrane breakdown is accelerated by storage at high and/or fluctuating temperatures and high humidities. In the United Kingdom, consumers have been advised to store eggs under refrigeration following purchase (Anonymous, 1992*a*). This has the advantages of suppressing or inhibiting the growth of salmonellas, rendering them more heat sensitive (Humphrey 1990) and preserving the integrity of the yolk membrane (Williams 1992). In the United States eggs are held under refrigeration in shops. In most of Europe control in retail outlets is confined to limitations on shelf-life and a suggestion that storage temperatures should not exceed 20 °C.

The successful control of salmonellosis requires intervention at all points on the food chain. Consumers and caterers can do much with regard to kitchen hygiene and the proper cooking of 'at risk' foods to limit risk. The ease with which cross-contamination can occur in the kitchen (de Wit *et al.* 1979), coupled with an increasing desire amongst consumers to eat foods that are only lightly cooked, mean that control may be best applied during food and animal production.

REFERENCES

Anderson, E. S., Ward, L. R., de Saxe, M. J., and de Sa, J. D. H. (1977). Bacteriophage-typing designations of *Salmonella typhimurium. Journal of Hygiene* (Cambridge), **78**, 297–300.

Anonymous (1989). *Salmonella in eggs*, Vol. II. House of Commons Agriculture Committee. HMSO, London.

Anonymous (1990). Notes on the control of human sources of gastrointestinal infections, infestations and bacterial intoxications in the United Kingdom. Communicable Disease Report, Public Health Laboratory Service, Supplement I, 1–13.

Anonymous (1992*a*). *Eggs and salmonella—the facts.* British Egg Industry Council, London, UK.

Anonymous (1992*b*). Council of the European Communities Directive 92/117/EEC. 17 December 1992.

Anonymous (1993). *Interim report on campylobacter.* Advisory Committee on the Microbiological Safety of Food. HMSO, London.

Anonymous (1994*a*). *Annual report (1993) of Steering Group on the Microbiological Safety of Food.* HMSO, London.

Anonymous (1994*b*). *Salmonella in animal feeding stuffs and ingredients.* MAFF Animal Health (Zoonosis) Division, Tolworth, UK.

Anonymous (1995*a*). An outbreak of *Salmonella agona* due to contaminated snacks. *CDR Weekly*, **5**, 29–32.

Anonymous (1995*b*). Salmonella contamination. Survey of UK-produced raw chicken. *Food Safety Information Bulletin*, No. 576–9.

Baird-Parker, A. C. (1991). Foodborne salmonellosis. In *Foodborne illness*, pp. 53–61. Edward Arnold, London.

Baquar, N., Burnens, A., and Stanley, J. (1994). Comparative evaluation of molecular typing of strains from a national epidemic due to *Salmonella brandenburg* by rRNA gene and IS*200* probes and pulsed-field gel electrophoresis. *Journal of clinical Microbiology*, **32**, 1876–80.

Barnass, S., O'Mahony, M., Sockett, P. N., Garner, J., Franklin, J., and Tabaqchali, S. (1989). The tangible cost implications of a hospital outbreak of multiple-resistant salmonella. *Epidemiology and Infection*, **103**, 227–34.

Barrow, P. A., Lovell, M. A., and Berchieri, A. (1990). Immunisation of laying hens against *Salmonella enteritidis* with live attenuated vaccines. *Veterinary Record*, **126**, 241–2.

Brown, D. J., Munro, D. S., and Platt, D. J. (1986). Recognition of the cryptic plasmid, pSLT, by restriction fingerprinting and a study of incidence in Scottish salmonella isolates. *Journal of Hygiene* (Cambridge), **97**, 193–7.

Buchmeier, N. A. and Heffron, F. (1991). Inhibition of macrophage phagosome–lysosome fusion by *Salmonella typhimurium. Infection and Immunity*, **59**, 2232–8.

Buchwald, D. S. and Blazer, M. J. (1984). A review of human salmonellosis: II. Duration of excretion following infection with non-typhoid salmonella. *Reviews of Infectious Diseases*, **6**, 345–56.

Chart, H., Rowe, B., Threlfall, E. J., and Ward, L. R. (1989). Conversion of *S. enteritidis* phage type 4 to *S. enteritidis* phage type 7 involves loss of lipopolysaccharide with concomitant loss of virulence. *FEMS Microbiology Letters*, **58**, 299–304.

Coulson, J. C., Butterfield, J., and Thomas, C. (1983). The Herring Gull, *Larvis argentatus*, as a likely transmitting agent of *Salmonella montevideo* to sheep and cattle. *Journal of Hygiene*, **91**, 437–43.

Cowden, J. M. *et al.* (1989*a*). A national outbreak of *Salmonella typhimurium* DT124 caused by contaminated salami sticks. *Epidemiology and Infection*, **103**, 219–25.

Cowden, J. M., Lynch, D., and Joseph, C. A. (1989*b*). Report of a national case control study of *Salmonella enteritidis* phage type 4 infection. *British Medical Journal*, **299**, 771–3.

Cruickshank, J. G. and Humphrey, T. J. (1987). The carrier food handler and non-typhoid salmonellosis. *Epidemiology and Infection*, **98**, 223–30.

D'Aoust, J. Y. (1985). Infective dose of *Salmonella typhimurium* in cheese. *American Journal of Epidemiology*, **122**, 717–20.

Davey, K. R. and Smith, M. G. (1989). A laboratory evaluation of a novel hot water cabinet for the decontamination of sides of beef. *International Journal of Food Science and Technology*, **24**, 305–16.

Davies, R. H. and Wray, C. (1994). Salmonella pollution in poultry units and associated enterprises. In *Pollution in livestock production systems.* (ed. I. Ap Dewi, R. F. E. Axford, I. Fayez, M. Marai, and H. Omed), pp. 137–65. CAB International.

de Boer, E. and Hahne, M. (1990). Cross-contamination with *Campylobacter jejuni* and *Salmonella* spp. from raw chicken products during food preparation. *Journal of Food Protection*, **53**, 1067–8.

Dempster, J. F. (1985). Radiation preservation of meat and meat products: a review. *Meat Science* **12**, 61–89.

Desenclos, J. C. *et al.* (1996). Large outbreak of *Salmonella enterica* serotype *paratyphi B* infection caused by a goats' milk cheese, France, 1993: a case finding and epidemiological study. *British Medical Journal*, **312**, 91–3.

de Wit, J. C., Broekhuizen, G., and Kampelmacher, E. H. (1979). Cross-contamination during the preparation of frozen chickens in the kitchen. *Journal of Hygiene*, **83**, 27–32.

Eckroade, R. J., Davison, S., and Benson, C. E. (1991). Environmental contamination of pullet and layer houses with *Salmonella enteritidis*. In *Proceedings of the symposium on Diagnosis and Control of Salmonella*, San Diego, California, USA, 29 October 1991, pp. 14–17.

Ezquerra, E., Burnens, A., Jones, C., and Stanley, J. (1993). Genotypic typing and phylogenetic analysis of *Salmonella paratyphi B* and *S. java* with IS*200*. *Journal of General Microbiology*, **139**, 2409–14.

Fenlon, D. R. (1983). A comparison of salmonella serotypes found in the faeces of gulls feeding at a sewage works with serotypes present in the sewage. *Journal of Hygiene*, **91**, 47–52.

Fierer, J., Krause, M., Tauxe, R., and Guiney, D. (1992). *Salmonella typhimurium* bacteraemia: association with the virulence plasmid. *Journal of Infectious Diseases*, **166**, 639–42.

Finlay, B. B., Leung, K. Y., Rosenshine, I., and Garcia-del Portillo, F. (1992). Salmonella interactions with the epithelial cell. *ASM News*, **58**, 487–9.

Frost, J. A., Threlfall, E. J., and Rowe, B. (1995). Antibiotic resistance in non-typhoidal salmonellas isolated from humans in England and Wales, 1994. *PHLS Microbiology Digest*, 131–3.

Galbraith, N. S. and Pusey, J. J. (1984). Milkborne infectious disease in England and Wales 1939–1982. In *Health hazards of milk*, (ed. D. L. J. Freed), pp. 27–59. Bailliere and Tindall, London.

Gay, J. M., Rice, D. H., and Steiger, J. H. (1994). Prevalence of faecal salmonella shedding by cull dairy cattle marketed in Washington State. *Journal of Food Protection*, **57**, 195–7.

Giles, N., Hopper, S. A., and Wray, C. (1989). Persistence of *Salmonella typhimurium* in a large dairy herd. *Epidemiology and Infection*, **103**, 235–41.

Gill, C. O. (1979). A review: intrinsic bacteria in meat. *Journal of Applied Bacteriology*, **47**, 367–78.

Girdwood, R. W. A., Fricker, C. R., Munro, D., Shedden, C. B., and Monaghan, P. (1985). Incidence and significance of salmonella carriage by gulls (*Larus* spp.) in Scotland. *Journal of Hygiene*, **95**, 229–41.

Glynn, J. R. and Bradley, D. J. (1992). The relationship between dose and severity of disease in reported outbreaks of salmonella infection. *Epidemiology and Infection*, **109**, 371–88.

Golden, D. A., Rhodehamel, E. J., and Kautter, D. A. (1993). Growth of *Salmonella* spp. in Cantaloupe, Watermelon and Honeydew melons. *Journal of Food Protection*, **56**, 194–6.

Grau, F. H. and Smith, M. G. (1974). Salmonella contamination of sheep and mutton carcases related to pre-slaughter holding conditions. *Journal of Applied Bacteriology*, **37**, 111–16.

Gulig, P. A. and Curtis, R. III. (1987). Plasmid-associated virulence of *Salmonella typhimurium*. *Infection and Immunity*, **55**, 2891–901.

Helmuth, R., Stephan, R., Bunge, C., Hoog, B., Steinbeck, A., and Bulling, E. (1985). Epidemiology of virulence-associated plasmids and outer membrane protein patterns within seven common salmonella serovars. *Infection and Immunity*, **48**, 175–82.

Hobbs, B. C. (1971). In *Poultry disease and world economy* (ed. R. F. Gordon and B. M. Freeman p. 65.

Hobbs, B. C. and Roberts, D. (1993). Food Poisoning and Food Hygiene. 6th Edition London. Edward Arnold. p. 96

Hoop, R. K. and Pospischil, A. (1993). Bacteriological, serological, histological and immuno-histochemical findings in laying hens with naturally acquired *Salmonella enteritidis* phage type 4 infection. *Veterinary Record*, **133**, 391–3.

Humphrey, T. J. (1990). Heat resistance in *Salmonella enteritidis* phage type 4: the influence of storage temperatures before heating. *Journal of applied Bacteriology*, **69**, 493–7.

Humphrey, T. J. (1991*a*). Food poisoning–a change in patterns? *Veterinary Annual*,. **31**, 32–7.

Humphrey, T. J. (1991*b*). The influence of feed treatment with organic acids on the colonisation of broiler chickens with Salmonella enteritidis PT4. In *Quality Poultry Products III. Safety Marketing Aspects*, Proceedings of the combined sessions of the 10th Symposium on the quality of Poultry Meat and the 4th Symposium on the Quality of Eggs and Egg Products. Doorweth, Holland, 12–17 May 1991, (ed. R. W. A. W. Mulder and A. W. de Vries), pp. 39–47.

Humphrey, T. J. (1994). Contamination of egg shell and contents with *Salmonella enteritidis*: a review. *International Journal of Food Microbiology*, **21**, 31–40.

Humphrey, T. J. and Lanning, D. G. (1988). The vertical transmission of salmonellas and formic acid treatment of chicken feed: a possible strategy for control. *Epidemiology and Infection*, **100**, 43–9.

Humphrey, T. J. and Whitehead, A. (1993). Egg age and the growth of *Salmonella enteritidis* PT4 in egg contents. *Epidemiology and Infection*, **111**, 209–19.

Humphrey, T. J., Mead, G. C., and Rowe, B. (1988). Poultry meat as a source of human salmonellosis in England and Wales. *Epidemiology and Infection*, **100**, 175–84.

Humphrey, T. J., Cruickshank, J. G., and Rowe, B. (1989). *Salmonella enteritidis* phage type 4 and hens' eggs. *Lancet*, **i**, 281.

Humphrey, T. J., Chart, H., Baskerville, A., and Rowe, B. (1991*a*). The influence of age on the response of SPF hens to infection with *Salmonella enteritidis* PT4. *Epidemiology and Infection*, **106**, 33–43.

Humphrey, T. J., Whitehead, A., Gawler, A. H. L., Henley, A., and Rowe, B. (1991*b*). Numbers of *Salmonella enteritidis* in the contents of naturally contaminated hens' eggs. *Epidemiology and Infection*, **106**, 489–96.

Humphrey, T. J., Martin, K., and Whitehead, A. (1994). Contamination of hands and work surfaces with *Salmonella*

enteritidis PT4 during the preparation of egg dishes. *Epidemiology and Infection*, **113**, 403–9.

Ingham, S. C., Alford, R., A., and McCown, A. P. (1990). Comparative growth rates of *Salmonella typhimurium* and *Pseudomonas fragii* on cooked crab meat stored under air and modified atmosphere. *Journal of Food Protection*, **53**, 566–7.

Lillard, H. S. (1973). Contamination of blood system and edible parts of poultry with *Clostridium perfringens* during water scalding. *Journal of Food Science*, **38**, 151–4.

Lister, S. A. (1988). *Salmonella enteritidis* infection in broilers and broiler breeders. *Veterinary Record*, **123**, 50.

Luby, S. P., Jones, J. L., and Horan, J. M. (1993). A large salmonellosis outbreak associated with a frequently penalised restaurant. *Epidemiology and Infection*, **110**, 31–9.

McBride, G. B., Skura, B. J., Yada, R. Y., and Bowmer, E. J. (1980). Relationship between incidence of salmonella contamination among pre-scalded, eviscerated and post-chilled chickens in poultry processing plant. *Journal of Food Protection*, **43**, 538–42.

McEwen, S. A., McClure, L. H., and Martin, S. W. (1988). Farm inspection scores and milk quality criteria and indices of salmonella in bulk milk. *Journal of Food Protection*, **51**, 958–62.

Mackey, B. M. (1989). The incidence of food poisoning bacteria on red meat and poultry in the United Kingdom. *Food Science and Technology Today*, **3**, 246–9.

Maguire, H. *et al.* (1992). An outbreak of *Salmonella dublin* infection in England and Wales associated with a soft unpasteurised cows' milk cheese. *Epidemiology and Infection*, **109**, 389–96.

Maguire, H. C. F., Codd, A. A., Mackay, V. E., Rowe, B., and Mitchell, E. (1993). A large outbreak of human salmonellosis traced to a local pig farm. *Epidemiology and Infection*, **110**, 239–46.

Mawer, S. L., Spain, G. E., and Rowe, B. (1989). *Salmonella enteritidis* phage type 4 and hens' eggs. *Lancet*, **i**, 280–1.

Mintz, E. D., Carter, M. L., Hadler, J. L., Wassell, J. T., Zingeser, J. A., and Tauxe, R. V. (1994). Dose-response effects in an outbreak of *Salmonella enteritidis*. *Epidemiology and Infection*, **112**, 13–23.

Mulder, R. W. A. W., Dorresteijn, L. W. J., and Van Der Broek, J. (1978). Cross-contamination during the scalding and plucking of broilers. *British Poultry Science*, **19**, 61–70.

Norel, F., Coynault, C., Miras, I., Hernant, D., and Popoff, M. (1989). Cloning and expression of plasmid DNA sequences involved in salmonella serotype *typhimurium* virulence. *Molecular Microbiology*, **3**, 733–43.

Notermans, S. and Kampelmacher, E. H. (1975). Heat destruction of some bacterial strains attached to broiler skin. *British Poultry Science*, **16**, 351–61.

Nurmi, E. and Rantala, M. (1973). New aspects of salmonella infection in broiler production. *Nature*, **241**, 210–11.

O'Mahony, M. *et al.* (1990). An outbreak of *Salmonella saint paul* infection associated with bean sprouts. *Epidemiology and Infection*, **104**, 229–35.

Pardon, P., Popoff, M. Y., Coynault, C., Marly, J., and Miras, I. (1986). Virulence-associated plasmids of salmonella serotype *typhimurium* in experimental murine infection. *Annales de Microbiologie de l'Institut Pasteur*, **137B**, 395–405.

Pelkonen, S., Rompanen, E-L., Siltonen, A., and Pelkonen, J. (1994). Differentiation of *Salmonella* serovar *infantis* from human and animal sources by fingerprinting IS*200* and 16S *rrn* loci. *Journal of Clinical Microbiology*, **32**, 2128–33.

Pether, J. V. S. and Gilbert, R. J. (1971). The survival of salmonellas on finger-tips and transfer of the organisms to food. *Journal of Hygiene*, **69**, 673–81.

Powell, N. G., Threlfall, E. J., Chart, H., and Rowe, B. (1994). Subdivision of *Salmonella enteritidis* PT4 by pulsed-field gel electrophoresis: potential for epidemiological surveillance. *FEMS Microbiology Letters*, **119**, 193–8.

Roberts, D. (1986). Factors contributing to outbreaks of foodborne infection and intoxication in England and Wales 1970–1982. In *2nd World Congress Foodborne Infections and Intoxication, Berlin*, Vol. 1, pp. 157–9.

Rodrigue, D. C., Tauxe, R. V., and Rowe, B. (1990). International increase in *Salmonella enteritidis*: a new pandemic. *Epidemiology and Infection*, **105**, 21–7.

Rowe, B. *et al.* (1987). *Salmonella ealing* infections associated with consumption of infant dried milk. *Lancet*, **ii**, 900–3.

Ryan, C. A. *et al.* (1987). Massive outbreak of antimicrobial-resistant salmonellosis traced to pasteurised milk. *Journal of the American Medical Association*, **258**, 3269–274.

St. Louis, M. E. *et al.* (1988). The emergence of grade A eggs as a major source of *Salmonella enteritidis* infections: new implications for the control of salmonellosis. *Journal of the American Medical Association*, **259**, 2103–7.

Samual, J. L., O'Boyle, P. A., Mathers, W. J., and Frost, A. J. (1980). Distribution of salmonella in the carcases of normal cattle at slaughter. *Research in Veterinary Science*, **28**, 368–72.

Smith, H. W. and Tucker, J. F. (1978). The effect of feed additives on the colonisation of the alimentary tract of chickens by *Salmonella typhimurium*. *Journal of Hygiene*, **80**, 217–31.

Smulders, F. J. M. (1987). Prospectives for microbial decontamination of meat and poultry by organic acids with special reference to lactic acids. In *Elimination of pathogenic organisms from meat and poultry*, Proceedings of an International Symposium: Prevention of Contamination, and Decontamination in the Meat Industry, Zeist, The Netherlands, 2–4 June 1986, (ed. F. J. M. Smulders), pp. 319–44. Elsevier, Amsterdam.

Sparks, N. H. C. and Board, R. G. (1985). Bacterial penetration of the recently oviposited shell of hens' eggs. *Australian Veterinary Journal*, **62**, 169–70.

Stanley, J., Burnens, N., Powell, N., Chowdrey, N., and Jones, C. (1992). The insertion sequence IS*200* fingerprints chromosomal genotypes and epidemiological relationships in *Salmonella heidelberg*. *Journal of General Microbiology*, **138**, 2329–2336.

Stanley, J., Baquar, N., and Burnens, A. (1995). Molecular subtyping for *Salmonella panama*. *Journal of Clinical Microbiology*, **33**, 1206–11.

Stevens, A., *et al.* (1989). A large outbreak of *Salmonella enteritidis* phage type 4 associated with eggs from overseas. *Epidemiology and Infection*, **103**, 425–33.

Threlfall, E. J. and Frost, J. A. (1990). The identification, typing and fingerprinting of salmonella: laboratory aspects and clinical applications. *Journal of Applied Bacteriology*, **68**, 5–16.

Threlfall, E. J., Rowe, B., Ferguson, J. L., and Ward, L. R. (1986). Characterisation of plasmids conferring resistance to gentamicin and apramycin in strains of *Salmonella typhimurium* phage type 204c isolated in Britain. *Journal of Hygiene* (Cambridge), **97**, 419–26.

Threlfall, E. J., Hall, M. L. M., and Rowe, B. (1992). Salmonella bacteraemia in England and Wales, 1981–1990. *Journal of Clinical Pathology*, **45**, 34–6.

Threlfall, E. J., Hampton, M. D., Chart, H., and Rowe, B. (1994a). Identification of a conjugative plasmid carrying antibiotic resistance and salmonella plasmid virulence (*spv*) genes in epidemic strains of *Salmonella typhimurium*. *Letters in Applied Microbiology*, **18**, 82–5.

Threlfall, E. J., Hampton, M. D., Chart, H., and Rowe B. (1994b). Use of plasmid profile typing for surveillance of *Salmonella enteritidis* phage type 4 from humans, poultry and eggs. *Epidemiology and Infection*, **112**, 25–32.

Threlfall, E. J., Frost, J. A., Ward, L. R., and Rowe B. (1994c). Epidemic in cattle and humans of *Salmonella typhimurium* DT 104 with chromosomally integrated multiple drug resistance. *Veterinary Record*, **134**, 577.

Threlfall, E. J., Torre, E., Ward, L. R., Dávalos-Pérez, A., Rowe, B., and Gibert, I. (1994d). Insertion sequence IS*200* fingerprinting of *Salmonella typhi*: an assessment of epidemiological applicability. *Epidemiology and Infection*, **112**, 253–61.

Threlfall, E. J., Powell, N. G., and Rowe, B. (1994e). Differentiation of salmonellas by molecular methods. *PHLS Microbiology Digest*, **11**, 199–202.

Threlfall, E. J., Frost, J. A., Ward, L. R., and Rowe, B. (1996). Increasing spectrum of resistance in multiresistant *Salmonella typhimurium* DT104 epidemic in humans in England and Wales. *Lancet*, 1053–4.

Tompkins, L. S., Troup, N., Labaigne-Roussel, A., and Cohen, M. L. (1986). Cloned, random chromosomal sequences as probes to identify salmonella species. *Journal of Infectious Diseases*, **152**, 156–62.

Van de Giessen, A. W., Dufrenne, J. B., Ritmeester, W. S., Berkers, P. A. T. A., Van Leeuwen, W. J., and Notermans, S. H. W. (1992). The identification of *Salmonella enteritidis*-infected poultry flocks associated with an outbreak of human salmonellosis. *Epidemiology and Infection*, **109**, 405–11.

Ward, L. R., de Sa, J. D. H., and Rowe, B. (1987). A phage-typing scheme for *Salmonella enteritidis*. *Epidemiology and Infection*, **99**, 291–4.

White, P. B. (1929). Notes on intestinal bacilli with special reference to smooth and rough races. *Journal of Pathology and Bacteriology*, **32**, 85–94.

Willcox, M. H. and Spencer, R. C. (1992). Quinolones and salmonella gastroenteritis. *Journal of Antimicrobial Chemotherapy*, **30**, 221–8.

Williams, E. F. and Spencer, R. (1973). Abattoir practices and their effect on the incidence of salmonellae in meat. In *The microbiological safety of food*, (ed. B. C. Hobbs, and J. H. B. Christian), pp. 41–6. Academic Press, London.

Williams, J. E. (1981). Salmonellas in poultry feeds—a worldwide review. Part I. *World's Poultry Science Journal*, **37**, 6–19.

Williams, K. C. (1992). Some factors affecting albumen quality with particular reference to Haugh unit score. *World's Poultry Science Journal*, **48**, 5–16.

Williamson, C. M., Baird, D., and Manning, E. J. (1988a). A common virulence region on plasmids from eleven serotypes of salmonella. *Journal of General Microbiology*, **134**, 975–82.

Williamson, C. M., Pullinger, G. D., and Lax, A. J. (1988b). Identification of an essential virulence region on salmonella plasmids. *Microbial Pathogenesis*, **5**, 469–73.

Woodward, M. J., McLaren, I., and Wray, C. (1989). Distribution of virulence plasmids within salmonellae. *Journal of General Microbiology*, **135**, 503–11.

Wray, C. (1975). Survival and spread of pathogenic bacteria of veterinary importance within the environment. *Veterinary Bulletin*, **45**, 543–50.

Wray, C., Todd, N., McLaren, I. M., Beedell, Y. E., and Rowe, B. (1990). The epidemiology of salmonella infection of calves: the role of dealers. *Epidemiology and Infection*, **105**, 295–305.

Wray, C., Todd, N., McLaren, I. M., and Beedell, Y. E. (1991). The epidemiology of salmonella in calves: the role of markets and vehicles. *Epidemiology and Infection*, **107**, 521–5.

20 ROCKY MOUNTAIN SPOTTED FEVER

Daniel J. Sexton and Edward B. Breitschwerdt

SUMMARY

Rocky Mountain spotted fever carried by infection with *Rickettsia rickettsii*, is an acute tick-borne disease which, in its classic form, is characterized by a cutaneous rash, fever, and widespread organ dysfunction. Illness is related to direct endothelial injury caused by *R. rickettsii*. The name Rocky Mountain spotted fever is a misnomer as the disease occurs through the continental United States, southern Canada, Mexico, Central America, and even in parts of South America. Synonyms for Rocky Mountain spotted fever include tick typhus, Tobia fever (Columbia), Sao Paulo fever, and fiebre maculosa (Brazil) and fiebre marchada (Mexico). The severity of clinical illness is highly variable, ranging from a mild viral-like malady to a fulminant fatal disease.

Rickettsia rickettsii is maintained in nature in a complex cycle involving a variety of hard-shelled (Ixodid) ticks and both small and large mammals; man is only a accidental host.

HISTORY

The earliest reports of rickettsial disease in the New World described early settlers to the Bitterroot Valley in western Montana and the Snake River Valley in eastern Idaho who were stricken with a exanthematous illness known as 'black measles'. This mysterious disease which became known as 'Rocky Mountain spotted fever' caused substantial medical and economic problems by the time a brilliant young physician-investigator, Howard T. Ricketts, arrived in the Bitterroot Valley in April, 1906 to investigate its cause. By careful observation, deduction, canny scientific reasoning, and well-designed but simple experiments, Ricketts discovered the cause of the illness by inoculating blood from ill patients into guinea-pigs. In addition, he simultaneously discovered the vector (*Dermacenter andersonii*) and accurately characterized the basic epidemiological cycle of the disease (Ricketts 1907). Soon after Ricketts published the results of his classic experiments, European investigators such as Nicolle realized the potential applications of his observations and laboratory methods for the study of epidemic typhus. Using Ricketts' methods, Nicolle isolated the causative organism of epidemic typhus and confirmed his earlier epidemiological observations that the vector was the body louse. These discoveries, coupled with the classic studies of von Prowazek and da Rocha-Lima, led to the widespread use of simple but effective preventative measures centred around control of body louse infestation. Following his brilliant experiments in Montana, Ricketts travelled to Mexico City in December 1909 to study epidemic typhus. Unfortunately he contracted the disease he was studying and died in May 1910. Thereafter, a succession of other American investigators expanded Ricketts' observations. S. Burt Wolbach first described the pathological features of Rocky Mountain spotted fever, and successfully visualized *R. rickettsii* organisms in human tissue. Wolbach's pathological observations, along with those of early clinicians, led to a basic understanding of the pathophysiology of *R. rickettsii* infection. It is fitting and appropriate that the genus name *Rickettsia* was chosen by da Rocha Lima to honour Ricketts for his important contributions to microbiology.

In 1931 Brazilian and American investigators demonstrated that the cause of Sao Paulo exanthematic typhus was *R. rickettsii* (Dias and Martins 1939), That same year Badger and Dyer recognized that Rocky Mountain spotted fever was an endemic zoonosis east of the Mississippi River. In fact, Rocky Mountain spotted fever is now recognized as a relatively common tick-borne illness in the north-eastern, mid-Atlantic, south-eastern, and south-western states. During the past 40 years, the incidence of Rocky Mountain spotted fever in Montana and Idaho has inexplicably declined, while much higher incidence rates of disease persist in Oklahoma, North Carolina, and Virginia.

THE AETIOLOGICAL AGENT

TAXONOMY

Like other Gram-negative bacteria, spotted-fever group (SFG) rickettsiae (Table 20.1) belong to the α-group of purple bacteria. Along with the families Bartonellaceae and Anaplasmataceae they are members of the order Rickettsiales. The order Rickettsiales is in turn divided into three tribes: Rickettsieae, Ehrlichieae and Wolbachieae. Until recently the tribe Rickettsieae was further divided into three genera: *Rickettsia, Rochalimeae,* and *Coxiella.* On the basis of recent phenotypic and genotypic studies, including the use of polymerase chain reaction and sequencing of the DNA encoding the 16S rRNA gene, *Rochalimeae* have been reclassified into the family Bartonellaceae and *Coxiella* have been moved to the α-subgroups of the Protobacteria. The sole remaining genus, *Rickettsia,* is divided into three groups or biotypes: typhus, scrub typhus, and spotted fever. *Rickettsia rickettsii* is the prototypic organism in the spotted fever group which now contains at least 17 separate species. Phylogenetic studies utilizing polymerase chain reaction technology and sequencing the DNA encoding the 16S rRNA gene ribosome have shown that *R. rickettsii* is closely related to other members of the spotted fever group such as *R. conorii* and *R. sibirica,* whereas its phylogenetic relationship to other spotted fever members such as *R. akari, R. australis,* and *R. belli* is substantially more distant.

MICROBIOLOGY AND ULTRASTRUCTURE

SFG rickettsiae are weakly Gram-negative, non-motile, coccobacilli, measuring 0.3–0.7 μm by 0.8–2.0 μm. Like other rickettsiae, they are difficult to see in tissue sections without special stains but can be visualized using Giemsa, Machiavello, and Giménez staining and by the use of fluorescent antibody staining techniques. Ultrastructurally, *R. rickettsii* has ribosomes and indistinct strands of DNA in an amorphous cytosol surrounded by a plasma membrane. In addition, there is an indistinct microcapsular layer on the outer surface of the rickettsial cell. An electron-lucent zone separates this layer from the host cytosol. This zone, which is thought to represent a slime layer, can be stained with ruthenium red and methenamine silver (Walker 1989) Although its role in virulence is uncertain, the slime layer may be important in pathogenicity.

GROWTH AND SURVIVAL CHARACTERISTICS

Like all other members of the genus *Rickettsia,* SFG rickettsiae are obligate intracellular bacteria that cannot be propagated on cell-free media. *Rickettsia rick-* *ettsii* can be propagated *in vitro* in the yolk sac of developing chick embryos, but it is more conveniently grown on primary or established cell culture monolayers such as chick embryo fibroblasts, monkey kidney cells (Vero), mouse L cells, and golden hamster cells. Unlike typhus group rickettsiae, which grow only in the cytoplasm of host cells, members of the spotted fever group grow both in the nucleus and cytoplasm.

Rickettsial entry into host cells is mediated by induced phagocytosis, as drugs that block phagocytosis also block cellular entry of rickettsiae in experimental studies. Host cell entry requires metabolically active rickettsiae and is directly or indirectly related to phospholipase activity. When inside host cells, rickettsiae rapidly escape from their phagocytic vacuole and reside directly in the cytosol or nucleus.

Rickettsia rickettsii has the curious ability to spread from cell to cell by traversing cell membranes without causing obvious membrane damage. Individual rickettsial organisms exit from infected cells via host cell filopodia and rarely accumulate in large numbers within individual cells. The precise mechanisms by which SFG rickettsiae damage host cells are still poorly understood, but cell death does not appear to be due to production of extracellular toxins or due to mechanical lysis (Walker 1989).

Rickettsia rickettsii derives energy from the metabolism of glutamate via the citric acid cycle, but it does not utilize glucose or have the ability to synthesize or degrade nucleoside monophosphates. Numerous specialized adaptations allow *R. rickettsii* to exist as an intracellular organism. These special mechanisms include the ability to acquire host ATP using a rickettsia-derived ATP translocator protein, and the ability to utilize host-derived glutamine as an energy source. In addition *R. rickettsii* thrives in the presence of high concentrations of potassium and proteins (Walker 1989).

ANTIGENIC STRUCTURE

Studies of the antigenic structure of rickettsiae led to the current classification of multiple rickettsial species. A still poorly understood cross-reacting surface antigen is responsible for the Weil–Felix reaction, in which sera from patients with a primary rickettsial infection cross-react with somatic antigens of three strains of *Proteus* (OX-19, OX-2, and OX-K). Because of poor specificity, this test is no longer used clinically and is now only of historical and laboratory research interest. Antigens have been developed for complement fixation, agglutination, indirect haemagglutination, indirect fluorescent antibody, and enzyme-linked immunoabsorbent assay (ELISA) tests. The use of monoclonal antibody techniques has, for the first time, allowed practical serological separation of the various members of the spotted fever group. Instead of rickettsial isolation, which lacks clinical utility, the use of a defined epitope blocking modification of the ELISA technique provides a highly specific and practical way to separate infections caused by different SFG members. (Radulovic *et al.* 1993).

The cell surface of SFG rickettsiae contains several outer membrane proteins (rOmps) and lipopolysaccharides. The best characterized and most important rOmps residing on the surface of *R. rickettsii* have molecular masses of 190 and 120 kDa. Although their exact function is unknown, these two dominant outer membrane proteins and a minor 17 kDa lipoprotein antigen have been cloned *in vitro* and their DNA sequence have been determined. The abundance of similar outer membrane proteins in other rickettsiae and the regularly arrayed surface structure of both rOmps suggests that they have a structural function. In addition, both the 190 and the 120 kDa rOmps are major immunogens capable of eliciting protective immune responses in experimental animals.

BASIS FOR VIRULENCE

Virulence of members of the spotted fever group vary in severity. Some species (e.g. *R. parkeri* and *R. rhipicephali*) are non-virulent for animals and humans; other species (e.g. *R. australis*) typically produce a mild disease in both humans and laboratory animals. No satisfactory hypothesis has been proposed to explain the striking variations in virulence among different species of the spotted fever group or between individual strains of the same species (e.g. *R. rickettsii*). For example, it was noted almost 100 years ago that the mortality rate for cases of Rocky Mountain spotted fever was over 80 per cent in the Bitterroot Valley of Montana, yet the mortality rate for the same disease in the adjacent Snake River Valley was approximately 3 per cent Subsequently these geographic differences in virulence have disappeared without explanation (Walker 1989).

Individual strains of *R. rickettsii* isolated from ticks have been shown to vary in virulence, but isolates made from humans with fulminant and mild disease appear to be identical when injected into laboratory animals. Furthermore, results of animal infectivity studies vary widely when different species of animals are studied. Various investigators have attempted to correlate laboratory virulence markers (such as plaque morphology in various cell lines) with pathogenicity in animal models of infection. Such attempts have largely been unsuccessful or inconclusive (McDade 1990).

Results of *in vitro* studies have demonstrated that individual strains of *R. rickettsii* can mutate from highly virulent to relatively avirulent organisms. For instance,

Cox found that the Iowa strain of *R. rickettsii* lost its virulence for guinea-pigs between the 50th and 125th egg passage. Animals infected with relatively avirulent *R. rickettsii* strains develop immunity and are refractory to challenge with large doses of highly virulent *R. rickettsii* strains (McDade 1990). In addition, the virulence of the same strain of *R. rickettsii* varies in individual ticks, depending on their feeding status. The virulence of *R. rickettsii* in overwintered or starved ticks is restored only after the ingestion of a blood meal or after incubation at 37 °C for 1–2 days (Spencer and Parker 1930). The mechanism for this 're-activation phenomenon' is uncertain, but it may be related to the thickness of extracellular slime layer (which is much thicker around rickettsiae within the cells of fed ticks than in starved ticks) (Hayes and Burgdofer 1982; Winkler 1990).

One strain of *R. rickettsii*, the HLP strain, is so phenotypically and ecologically distinct from other strains that it appears to be a unique subspecies. This strain was originally found in the rabbit tick (*Haemaphysalis leporispalustris*). The HLP strain, has only been isolated from ticks that do not feed on humans. It is weakly virulent in laboratory animals such as guinea-pigs and has never been shown to cause human disease. Unique heat-labile epitopes on each of the major surface proteins (120 and 155 kDa) distinguish HLP strains from other strains of *R. rickettsii*.

Dose of inoculum appears to be an important determinant of virulence in dogs and humans. Humans inoculated with 10 median guinea-pig infectious doses ($GPID_{50}$) of *R. rickettsii* have shorter incubation periods, longer duration of fever after institution of antirickettsial treatment, and higher attack rates than subjects inoculated with one $GPID_{50}$ (Dupont *et al.* 1973). A similar dose response has also been demonstrated in dogs experimentally infected with *R. rickettsii* (Keenan *et al.* 1977).

A number of host factors appear to affect the severity of human infection due to *R. rickettsii*. For example, increasing age is accompanied by a higher fatality to case ratio. This phenomenon of increasing severity of illness associated with increasing age was observed in the pre-antibiotic era and has persisted during the era in which effective antirickettsial drugs are widely available for treatment of Rocky Mountain spotted fever. Male gender appears to be an additional risk factor for severe disease. Males with Rocky Mountain spotted fever have a higher risk of dying than females within all age groups (Hattwick *et al.* 1976). Finally, the presence of glucose 6-phosphate dehydrogenase deficiency, more commonly identified in Black individuals, appears to be risk factor for severe and/or fatal disease due to both *R. rickettsii* and *R. conorii* (Walker *et al.* 1983). Black race and heavy alcohol consumption have also been associated with increased risk of severe disease and a fatal outcome, but these factors are difficult to separate from other risk factors for severe or fatal outcome, such as delay in seeking or receiving appropriate antimicrobial therapy (Kirkland and Sexton 1995).

DISEASE MECHANISMS

After inoculation into the body via the saliva of an infected tick or via mucous membrane or cutaneous contact with infectious tick tissue, rickettsiae proliferate intracellulary and then subsequently spread throughout the body via the bloodstream and lymphatics. Like other SFG organisms, *R. rickettsii* appears to have tropism for endothelial cells.

The mechanism by which *R. rickettsii* produces characteristic damage to small blood vessels is unknown. Endothelial cell death is not due to a rickettsial-derived toxin or unchecked rickettsial proliferation leading to mechanical cell lysis. Rather, cell death appears to occur as a direct rickettsial effect by, as yet, uncertain mechanisms. Cell injury by SFG rickettsiae has been associated with phospholipase A activity, protease activity, and free-radical-induced lipid peroxidation (Walker 1989). Whether these disease-causing factors contribute in a minor or major way to the pathophysiology of rickettsial infection and phagocytic cellular responses, the net effect is endothelial cell injury followed by host cell-mediated humoral antibody responses. Widespread rickettsia-induced vasculitis characteristically leads to increased vascular permeability, oedema, and the activation of humoral inflammatory and coagulation mechanisms. In severe cases vascular thrombosis and haemorrhage may result in body-wide organ dysfunction, often associated with hypovolaemia or shock.

VECTORS

The epidemiology of the various SFG rickettsial diseases is directly or indirectly related to the geographic distribution and life cycle of the vector. The natural history of Rocky Mountain spotted fever is intimately associated with the life cycle of various species of Ixodid ticks that are both vectors for transmission and reservoirs of the organism in nature. In the United States and Canada the two most important vectors are the wood tick (*Dermacentor andersonii*) and the American dog tick (*Dermacentor variabilis*). In addition, the lone star tick (*Amblyomma americanum*) is an unproven but potential vector in some regions. The rabbit tick

(*H. leporispalustris*) is involved in transmission of *R. rickettsii* to small mammals, but it is not believed to be a vector for man. The brown dog tick (*Rhipicephalus sanguineus*) is an important vector in Mexico. *Amblyomma cajennense* is the main vector in Central and South America. In the United States *D. andersonii* is the principal vector west of the Mississippi River; *D. variabilis* is the predominant vector east of the Mississippi River, Texas, Oklahoma and the mid-western states. Neither *Dermacentor* species is host specific. Larval and nymphal forms of both ticks feed on a variety of rodents and small mammals. Adult forms feed on larger wild and domestic animals and occasionally bite humans.

Following a blood meal from a rickettsaemic animal, rickettsiae proliferate in the gut wall of the host tick and soon thereafter penetrate gut epithelium and infect the tick haemocytes. Within a few days all tick tissues are infected. This generalized rickettsial infection persists throughout the tick's life span, including subsequent developmental stages (trans-stadial transmission). Furthermore, rickettsial proliferation in the tick oogonia and oocytes leads to transovarian transmission (Burgdorfer 1992). Tick to tick venereal transmission occurs as well: rickettsiae can be transferred either in spermatozoa or in fluids from infected males during the process of mating.

Although ticks infected with *R. rickettsii* are able to develop normally and reproduce, continuous maintenance of such strains by transovarian passage eventually has adverse effects on the biological processes of the tick. Beginning with the fifth generation, infected females often die within 2 weeks following a blood meal; those females that survive produce small numbers of eggs that fail to develop (Burgdorfer 1992). Thus, although trans-stadial and transovarian transmission are important in the maintenance of *R. rickettsii* in nature, continuing transmission between ticks and their natural mammalian hosts is required for the persistence of *R. rickettsii*-infected ticks. Limited information exists on the percentage of *R. rickettsii*-infected ticks in specific endemic regions. Studies to determine the prevalence of infected ticks have been hampered by the fact that ticks often contain nonpathogenic members of the spotted fever group which are difficult to distinguish from *R. rickettsii* unless cumbersome animal inoculation studies are undertaken. Despite these difficulties, it appears that only a small fraction (less than 1 per cent) of tick populations contain *R. rickettsii* in most endemic regions. However, the phenomenon of clustering of cases of Rocky Mountain spotted fever in dogs, or people from the same households or community during short time spans suggests that 'hyperendemic foci' of infected ticks may periodically exist in small geographic areas.

HOSTS

ANIMALS

Maintenance of *R. rickettsiae* in nature occurs via transmission between ticks and their mammalian hosts. Man and dogs are infected incidentally when an infected arthropod takes a blood meal. The complexity of these arthropod–mammal cycles of infection is remarkable. Not all vertebrate hosts for the tick vectors of *R. rickettsii* function as reservoirs of rickettsial infection (i.e. experience a transient or sustained rickettsaemia following a blood meal by an infected tick). Many small mammals, including field mice (*Microtus pennsylvanicus* and *Peromyscus leucopus*), pine voles (*Pitymys pinetorum*), cotton rats (*Sigmodon hispidus*), rabbits and hares (*Silvagus floridanus* and *Lepus americanus*), opossums (*Didelphis marsupialis virginia*), chipmunks and squirrels (*Eutamius amoenus* and *Spermaophilus lateralis tescorum*), develop transient or sustained rickettsemia following exposure to infected ticks. These animals are the primary reservoir for Rocky Mountain spotted fever in the North America. Other animals, such as the cavy (*Cavia apecea*) and the capybara (*Hydrochoerus capybara*), probably function as wild vertebrate hosts and reservoirs for *R. rickettsii* in South America. The role of larger vertebrates as reservoirs of Rocky Mountain spotted fever is less certain. Even though adult *Dermacenter* species have a host preference for medium and large mammals such as dogs, domestic animals, deer, raccoons, foxes, and coyotes, a role for these animals as reservoirs is unlikely (Marchette 1982).

Following experimental inoculation with *R. rickettsii*, canines develop a transient rickettsaemia associated with illness varying in severity from subclinical to fatal (Green and Breitschwerdt 1993). Experimentally, severity of illness correlates with the infectious dose of *R. rickettsii*. Dogs in endemic regions frequently develop clinical illness after natural infection with *R. rickettsii* including fever, anaemia, neutropenia followed by neutrophilia, thrombocytopenia, and occasionally gangrenous necrosis of the nose, ears, or extremities. Furthermore, dogs from endemic areas and households with known cases of Rocky Mountain spotted fever frequently have anti-rickettsial antibodies, reflecting prior exposure to either non-pathogenic or (less frequently) pathogenic spotted fever group antigens (Breitschwerdt *et al.* 1987). Despite these observations, and despite the fact that dogs are a primary host for adult *Dermacenter variabilis* ticks, it is unlikely that dogs serve a significant natural vertebrate reservoir for *R. rickettsii*. Dogs inoculated with *R. rickettsii* are rickettsaemic for approximately 7 days (Breitschwerdt *et al.* 1988). Yet only 1 per cent of *R. sanguineous* ticks feeding on rickettsaemic dogs became infected (Norment and Burgdorfer 1984).

Dogs may occasionally contribute to the human epidemiology of Rocky Mountain spotted fever by serving as a vehicle for transport of infected ticks into the household or back yards of humans.

HUMANS

Rocky Mountain spotted fever is often a severe disease and, unlike after spotted fever group rickettsiae, eschars are rare. Clinical illness due to *R. rickettsii* varies from a mild viral-like febrile ailment to fulminating and devastating fatal disease characterized by dysfunction of major organ systems and shock. The incubation period ranges from 2 to 12 days, but as many patients cannot recall a recent tick bite, this time interval is of limited clinical use. Virtually all patients have fever which is often an initial symptom of illness. Most patients have a skin rash that in its typical form begins as a macular or macular-papular non-pruritic exanthem on the ankles and wrists that later spreads to the remainder of the extremities and the trunk. Later the rash often becomes petechial. In severe cases skin rash may coalesce into large areas of haemorrhagic skin necrosis; rarely gangrene of the digits, genitals, and or ears may occur (Kirkland *et al.* 1993) In approximately 10 per cent of reported cases a skin rash is not observed. Some cases of so-called 'Rocky Mountain spotless fever' may be severe and end fatally due to delayed initiation of antirickettsial treatment (Helmick *et al.* 1984, Sexton and Corey 1992). In a small percentage of cases, onset of rash may be delayed until the end of the first week of illness or even later. Rarely, skin rash is fleeting or localized to a small segment of the body. In addition to rash, most patients experience a severe headache and generalized myalgias. Nonspecific gastrointestinal symptoms such as nausea, vomiting, and even diarrhoea are common (>50 per cent of patients), particularly in the early phases of illness. In fact, these gastrointestinal symptoms may be so severe or prominent that they overshadow other more typical symptoms of illness, leading to misdiagnosis or delay in initiation of appropriate therapy. Rarely, patients with Rocky Mountain spotted fever have symptoms that lead to erroneous diagnoses such as cholecystitis or appendicitis. As the pathophysiology of Rocky Mountain spotted fever is directly related to a generalized rickettsial-induced small vessel vasculitis, a wide variety of neurological, cardiopulmonary, and musculoskeletal symptoms may occur in the early or late phases of illness. Encephalopathy, seizures, symptoms of focal neurological dysfunction, arthralgias, arthritis, chest pain, arrhythmias, cough, and dyspnoea may occur during the course of Rocky Mountain spotted fever, leading to both misdiagnosis and a wide array of complications.

The course of individual illness is highly variable. Many patients initially become ill with non-specific symptoms and most initially lack a skin rash; in most cases these individuals quickly become sicker unless specific antirickettsial therapy is given. A typical skin rash usually appears during the second to the fifth day of illness (Helmick *et al.* 1984). Rarely, illness is fulminant leading to death as early as the fourth or fifth day of illness. Some patients are initially mildly ill and then suddenly deteriorate. Some patients who receive no effective antirickettsial therapy have a mild illness with no early or late complications.

Thrombocytopenia, renal insufficiency, and unremitting high fevers and severe headache are usual manifestations of Rocky Mountain spotted fever. Laboratory tests indicating disturbances of coagulation, acute renal failure, jaundice, and elevated liver function tests are common, as are the presence of pulmonary infiltrates. Disseminated intravascular coagulation, when present, is often a terminal event. Cardiac dysfunction ranging from arrhythmias to congestive heart failure is occasionally seen in severe cases. In addition, most patients with severe Rocky Mountain spotted fever have alterations in mentation ranging from confusion to coma. Seizures, stroke, and hallucinations may occur as well. Most patients with neurological dysfunction have normal cerebrospinal fluid; however, there may be a mild pleocytosis with moderate elevations of the protein concentration. Cerebrospinal fluid pleocytosis can lead to an erroneous diagnosis of encephalitis if neurological features dominate the clinical presentation.

Untreated, patients with Rocky Mountain spotted fever typically experience illness that lasts 2–3 weeks ending with either death in approximately one quarter of cases or recovery. Most patients who receive antirickettsial therapy begin to improve within 72–96 hours of the onset of therapy, but in severe cases improvement may take substantially longer. Defervescence occurs in experimentally infected dogs within 24 hours of initiation of oral antibiotics. Lack of clinical improvement within 72 hours after the onset of treatment indicates that a rickettsial cause is less likely. Some patients who recover from severe illness due to Rocky Mountain spotted fever are left with long-term sequelae such as deafness, neurogenic bladders, or other permanent neurological deficits.

Diagnosis

It is axiomatic that the diagnosis of Rocky Mountain spotted fever and all other spotted fever group rickettsioses must be made on clinical and epidemiological grounds. There is no definitive laboratory test that is sufficiently reliable for diagnosis in the early phases of illness. Only a minority of patients with Rocky

Mountain spotted fever have the classic triad of headache, skin rash, and fever when they first seek medical care (Kirkland and Sexton 1995). Of necessity, initial therapy is virtually always empiric. A diagnosis can be confirmed by demonstrating a significant rise in antibody titre between acute and convalescent serum samples, by skin biopsy stained with direct immunofluorescent conjugates, and by culture (Walker *et al.* 1978). Skin biopsy is a useful test in Rocky Mountain spotted fever when it is positive, but a negative result does not exclude the diagnosis. In addition, early initiation of antirickettsial therapy can produce false-negative results. Skin biopsy is not a practical technique for most out-patients and it is obviously not useful in patients lacking a skin rash. Rickettsial cultures are available only in specialized laboratories found in a few large medical centres. Techniques utilizing polymerase chain reaction technology have been employed successfully to diagnose Rocky Mountain spotted fever during the early phase of illness, but such methods lack sensitivity, and unless arduous quality control measures are employed, specificity is difficult to maintain consistently (Sexton *et al.* 1994) Rocky Mountain spotted fever may masquerade as one of a diverse array of other diseases, including meningococcaemia, staphylococcal or Gram-negative sepsis, erhlichiosis, a drug reaction, infectious mononucleosis, measles, and a non-specific viral illness. Misdiagnosis is common. For instance in one series including 100 patients seen at Duke Medical Center over half of the patients with Rocky Mountain spotted fever were misdiagnosed at the time of their first physician visit (Kirkland *et al.* 1993).

Pathology

The pathological hallmark of Rocky Mountain spotted fever is a lymphohistiocytic vasculitis (Fig. 20.1). Endothelial damage occurs early in infection. As infection proceeds, progressive damage to blood vessels occurs. Lymphocytes and macrophages accumulate in these sites of injury leading to the characteristic pathological features of the disease. Rickettsial-induced vascular injury often results in innumerable minute foci of endothelial damage accompanied by haemorrhage, a generalized increase in permeability, and movement of plasma and plasma proteins into the interstitium (Fig. 20.2). As a result, rapid and substantial loss of intravascular volume may occur. Although thrombocytopenia, a reduced fibrinogen concentration, and elevated fibrin split products may be found in some patients with severe Rocky Mountain spotted fever, disseminated intravascular coagulation is rare. However, thrombocytopenia, probably due to platelet utilization

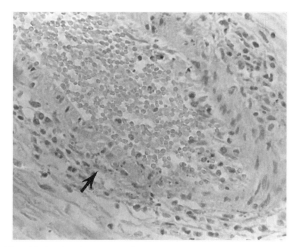

Fig. 20.1 Focal segmental necrosis (arrow) in a pulmonary artery from a dog with Rocky Mountain spotted fever (Hematoxylin and Eosin, × 462.5). The dog died acutely due to natural infection with *Rickettsia rickettsii*. There were similar lesions in arteries in the testes, skin, and brain. (Courtesy of Dr Don Meuten, North Carolina State University, Raleigh, NC.)

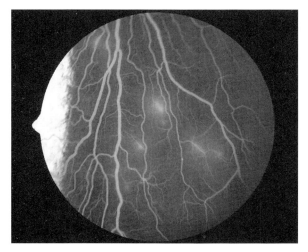

Fig. 20.2 Late-stage (day 13 following inoculation) fluorescein angiogram of the non-tapetal fundus of a dog experimentally infected with *Rickettsia rickettsii*. There are multiple areas of fluorescein dye leakage (hyperfluorescence) along retinal blood vessels, reflecting focal rickettsial-induced vascular leakage. Ocular abnormalities are frequently encountered in association with Rocky Mountain spotted fever in dogs and people. (Courtesy of Dr Michael Davidson, North Carolina State University, Raleigh, NC.)

at sites of rickettsia-mediated vascular injury, though often absent in the early phases of illness, is present in most patients who are hospitalized with Rocky Mountain spotted fever.

Treatment

Only two drugs are of proven benefit in spotted fever group rickettsioses: tetracycline and chloramphenicol. Experimentally, chloramphenicol enrofloxacin (which is converted to ciprofloxacin) and tetracycline are equally efficacious for treating *R. rickettsii* infection in dogs (Breitschwerdt *et al.* 1991). Chloramphenicol is usually reserved for human cases in which alternate diagnoses such as meningococcaemia are being entertained or for the treatment of pregnant women. Tetracycline therapy, which is as effective as chloramphenicol, is substantially safer. Although repeated doses of tetracycline can cause dental staining in children, a short course of therapy has little chance of dental damage. Thus tetracycline is usually considered to be the drug of choice even in children. Some quinolones have been shown to have antirickettsial activity *in vitro*, but, despite a limited amount of *in vivo* data from experimental studies, the efficacy of quinolones as therapy for spotted fever group rickettsioses in people has not been adequately demonstrated.

Prognosis

In addition to the presence of the virulence factors mentioned previously, prognosis in Rocky Mountain spotted fever is related to the time interval from onset of illness to time of initiation of treatment. Patients who are treated within the first 5 days of illness have a lower mortality and less morbidity than cases treated later (Hattwick *et al.* 1978; Kirkland and Sexton 1995). In addition, patients with normal levels of glucose 6-phosphate dehydrogenase have better outcomes than patients who have this hereditary enzyme deficiency (Raoult *et al.* 1986). Long-term sequelae may occur in patients with severe Rocky Mountain spotted fever; rarely sequelae such as persistent mononeuropathy may occur even in patients with mild illness (Archibald and Sexton 1995).

EPIDEMIOLOGY

TRANSMISSION AND COMMUNICABILITY

Transmission of *R. rickettsii* occur via a tick bite. Experimental transmission of *R. rickettsii* can occur via aerosols of infectious tick tissues or faeces and via contact with mucous membranes or even via contact with intact skin. Thus it is possible that transmission may occur via transfer of infectious tick tissue or faeces to conjunctivae, via minor skin abrasions, or via inhalation of aerosols generated when engorged tissues are crushed. Approximately 40 per cent of people with documented Rocky Mountain spotted fever cannot recall having a recent tick bite; thus the absence of a history of a tick bite should not influence the clinician's decision to begin empirical therapy (Walker 1995). Even though human to human transmission of *R. rickettsii* does not occur, occasionally cases of Rocky Mountain spotted fever occur in clusters in single households or neighbourhoods, (Schaffner *et al.* 1965) and a kennel epizootic has been reported in dogs (Breitschwerdt *et al.* 1985). In such instances it is likely that hyperendemic foci of infected ticks are responsible. All rickettsiae, including *R. rickettsii*, are notorious causes of illness in laboratory workers who are involved in the processing of rickettsial cultures and clinical specimens. Transmission in such instances may occur via accidental inoculation with needles or sharp objects or via infectious aerosols generated during centrifugation or via laboratory accidents.

DISTRIBUTION AND INCIDENCE

Rocky Mountain spotted fever occurs in south-western Canada, in virtually all the states in the continental United States, Mexico, Central American, Columbia, and Brazil. In the United States the disease is most common in the mid-Atlantic and south-eastern states and Oklahoma (although foci of endemic disease occur in other locations such as Long Island, Cape Cod, and central Ohio). Yet even in endemic areas the annual risk of disease is low. For reasons that remain unclear the annual incidence of disease in North Carolina varies by region from 1–2 to 15 cases/ 100 000. The annual incidence of Rocky Mountain spotted fever fluctuates widely in the United States. Furthermore, the regional incidence of disease in the United States has fluctuated even more remarkably

during the past 50–60 years. For example, the incidence of Rocky Mountain spotted fever in the Rocky Mountain region was more than 50 cases per 100 000 population during the 1920s and 1930s but the incidence of disease is currently only a small fraction of this number (Walker 1989). No one has been able to fully explain these annual and regional fluctuations in incidence, although lifestyle changes (e.g. increasing suburbanization in the eastern United States) and fluctuations in the annual survival of ticks are possibly important (Fig. 20.3).

PREVENTION AND CONTROL

Measures such as the use of tick repellents by those exposed to areas of high tick density and prompt removal of attached ticks, using measures to protect the fingers and mucous membranes from exposure to infectious tick tissues, are generally recommended hygienic control measures. But there is no realistic way to prevent the human acquisition of *R. rickettsii* as the number of ticks per hectare may number in the millions, and the number of human tick bites in areas such as the United States undoubtedly numbers in millions each year.

During the past 70 years a variety of killed rickettsial vaccines derived from ticks, embryonated eggs, and cell cultures have been developed. None of these vaccines has provided adequate immunity in human volunteers and/or in large field trials. At present no vaccine is commercially available to prevent Rocky Mountain spotted fever or any other SFG rickettsioses. Furthermore, the prospects are dim for widespread use

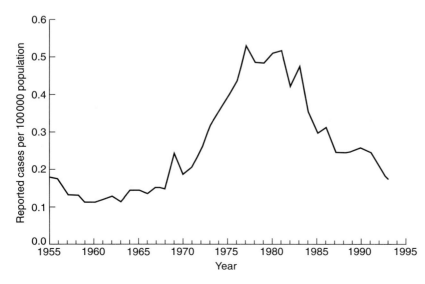

Fig. 20.3 Incidence of Rocky Mountain spotted fever in the United States, 1955–93.

even if a vaccine becomes available. Prompt recognition and treatment of illness remain the only viable ways to prevent morbidity and mortality. As the early clinical phases of Rocky Mountain spotted fever are non-specific and mimic so many common benign illnesses, a high index of suspicion coupled with a knowledge of the local and regional epidemiology should result in the early empirical use of antirickettsial therapy. This approach remains the cornerstone of any strategy to prevent disability and death. In many cases illness can be aborted or significantly lessened by the early use of safe and inexpensive therapy such as oral tetracycline.

REFERENCES

Archibald, I. K. and Sexton, D. J. (1995). Long term sequelae in Rocky Mountain spotted fever. *Clinical infectious Diseases*, **12**, 1122–5.

Breitschwerdt, E. B. *et al.* (1985). Canine Rocky Mountain spotted fever—a kennel epizootic. *American Journal of Veterinary Research*, **46**, 2124–8.

Breitschwerdt, E. B. *et al.* (1987). Antibodies to spotted fever-group rickettsiae in dogs in North Carolina. *American Journal of Veterinary Research*, **48**, 1436–40.

Breitschwerdt, E. B. *et al.* (1988). Clinical, hemotologic, and humoral response in female dogs inoculated with *Rickettsia rickettsii* and *Rickettsia montana*. *American Journal of Veterinary Research*, **49**, 70–6.

Breitschwerdt, E. B. and *et al.* (1991). Efficacy of chloramphenicol, enrofloxacin and tetracycline for treatment of experimental Rocky Mountain spotted fever in dogs. Antimicrobial Agents and Chemotherapy, **35**, 2375–81.

Burgdorfer, W. (1992). Ecological and epidemiological considerations of Rocky Mountain spotted fever and scrub typhus. In Walker D. H., ed. *Biology of rickettsial diseases*, CRC Press, Boca Raton, Florida. (ed. D. H. Walker), Vol. 1, pp. 33–51.

Dias, E. and Martins, A. V. (1939). Spotted fever in Brazil a summary. *American Journal of Tropical Medicine and Hygiene*, **19**, 103–8.

DuPont, H. L. *et al.* (1973). Rocky Mountain spotted fever: a comparative study of the active immunity induced by inactivated and viable pathogenic *Rickettsia rickettsii*. *Journal of Infectious Diseases*, **128**, 340–4.

Greene, C. E. and Breitschwerdt, E. B. (1993). Rocky Mountain spotted fever in dogs. In Rickettsial and chlamydial diseases of domestic animals, (ed. Z. Woldenhiwet and M. Ristic), pp. 153–67. Pergamon Press, Oxford.

Hattwick, M., O'Brien, R. J. , and Hanson, B. F. (1976). Rocky Mountain spotted fever: epidemiology of an increasing problem. *Annals of Internal Medicine*, **84**, 732–9.

Hattwick, M. *et al.* (1978). Fatal Rocky Mountain spotted fever. *Journal of the American Medical Association*, **240**, 499–503.

Hayes, S. K. and Burgdorfer, W. (1982). Reactivation of *Rickettsia rickettsii* in *Dermacenter andersonii* ticks: an ultrastructural analysis. *Infection and Immunity*, **37**, 779–85.

Helmick, C. G., Bernard, K. W., and D'Angelo, L. J. (1984). Rocky Mountain spotted fever: clinical labortory and epidemiological features of 262 cases. *Journal of Infectious Diseases*, **150**, 480–8.

Keenan, K. P. *et al.* (1977). Pathogenesis of infection with *Rickettsia rickettsii* in the dog: a disease model for Rocky Mountain spotted fever. *Journal of Infectious Diseases*, **135**, 911–17.

Kirkland, K. K. and Sexton, D. J. (1995). Therapeutic delay in Rocky Mountain spotted fever. *Clinical Infectious Diseases*, **12**, 1118–21.

Kirkland, K. B. *et al.* (1993). Rocky Mountain spotted fever complicated by gangrene: report of six cases and review. *Clinical Infectious Diseases*, **16**, 629–34.

McDade, J. E. (1990). Evidence supporting the hypothesis that rickettsial virulence factors determine the severity of spotted fever and typhus group infectious. *Annals of the New York Academy of Sciences*, **590**, 20–6.

Marchette N. (1982). The tick-borne rickettsiae of the spotted fever or tick typhus group. In *Ecological relationships and evolution of the rickettsiae*, CRC Press, Boca Raton, Florida. (ed. N. J. Marchette and D. Stiller), pp. 75–112.

Norment, B. R. and Burgdorfer, W. (1984). Susceptibility and reservoir potential of the dog to spotted fever-group rickettsiae. *American Journal of Veterinary Research*, **45**, 1706–10.

Radulovic, S. *et al.* (1993). EIA with species-specific monoclonal antibodies: A novel seroepidemiologic tool for determination of the etiologic agent of spotted fever group rickettsiosis. *Journal of Infectious Diseases* **168**, 1292–5.

Raoult, D. *et al.* (1986). Haemolysis with Mediterranean spotted fever and glucose-6-phosphate dehydrogenase deficiency. *Transactions of the Royal Society of Tropical Medicine and Hygiene*, **80**, 961–2.

Ricketts, H. T. (1907). Recent studies of Rocky Mountain spotted fever. *Medical Sentinel*, **15**, 68–71.

Schaffner, W., McLeod, A. C., Koenig, M. G. (1965). Thrombocytopenic Rocky Mountain spotted fever—a case study of a husband and wife. *Achives of Internal Medicine*, **116**, 857–65.

Sexton, D. J. and Corey, G. R. (1992). Rocky Mountain 'spotless' and 'almost spotless' fever—a wolf in sheeps clothing. *Clinical in Infectious Diseases*, **15**, 439–48.

Sexton, D. J. *et al.* (1994). The use of polymerase chain reaction as a diagnostic test for Rocky Mountain spotted fever. *American Journal of Tropical Medicine and Hygiene*, **50**, 59–63.

Spencer, R. R. and Parker, R. R. (1930). *Studies on Rocky Mountain spotted fever infection by means other than tick bite*. Hygienic Laboratory Bulletin No. 154, pp. 60–3. US Public Health Service, Washington, DC.

Walker, D. H. (1989). Rocky Mountain spotted fever: A disease in need of microbiological concern. *Clinical Microbiological Reviews*, **2**, 227–40.

Walker, D. H. (1995). Rocky Mountain spotted fever. a seasonal alert. *Clinical Infectious Diseases*, **12**, 1111–17.

Walker, D. H., Cain, B. G., and Olmstead P. M. (1978). Specific diagnosis of Rocky Mountain spotted fever by immunofluorescent demonstration of *Rickettsia rickettsii* in cutaneous lesions. *American Journal of Clinical Pathology*, **69**, 619–23.

Walker, D. H., Radisch, D. L., and Kirkman, H. N. Haemolysis with rickettsiosis and glucose-6-phosphate dehydrogenase deficiency. *Lancet*, **2**, 217.

Winkler, H. H. (1990). Rickettsia species (as organisms). *Annual Review of Microbiology*, **44**, 131–53.

different names (Indian tick typhus, Kenyan tick typhus, South African tick bite fever).

In southern Africa, in 1912, a Mozambican physician described a disease of unknown aetiology associated with bites of tick larvae, which were identified as *Amblyomma hebraeum* and *Rhipicephalus simus*. Itching, sometimes accompanied by 'vesicular' or papular lesions at the bite site, was followed by myalgia, headache, regional lymphadenopathy associated with the tick bite, fever, and a slight maculopapular eruption (Sant' Anna 1912). Two decades later, studies undertaken in South Africa showed that there were two distinct clinical features in patients presenting with African tick-bite fever. An urban form was found in patients in contact with dogs and dog ticks *Rhipicephalus* spp and *Haemaphysalis leachi*) and had clinical features similar to those of Mediterranean spotted fever. The second form was found in patients with a history of recent trips into rural areas and contact with cattle and their ticks (*Amblyomma hebraeum*). This form of the disease was characterized by an almost total lack of cutaneous rash (Pijper 1936). Although cross-protection assays in guinea-pigs showed that the causative agents of the two forms were probably different, these findings could not be demonstrated in subsequent experiments and Mediterranean spotted fever, or African tick-bite fever, was considered to be the single pathogenic tick-transmitted rickettsiosis in this African area (Gear 1954). However studies undertaken in Zimbabwe have recently determined that there are in fact two pathogenic spotted fever group rickettsiae coexisting in the southern part of Africa, mainly *R. conorii* and *R. africae* (Kelly and Mason 1990).

A further rickettsial disease of the Old World, called Siberian tick typhus or North Asian tick typhus, was described in the early 1930s in the Krasnoyarsk region of the USSR (Rehacek and Tarasevich 1988). In the subsequent decade, the main vector was shown to be *Dermacentor nuttalli*, and isolates of the rickettsial agent were obtained from blood and necrotic cutaneous tissues of patients.

Other similar diseases have subsequently been described from all over the world (Queensland tick typhus, Israeli spotted fever, Japanese spotted fever) (Table 21.1).

Rickettsialpox was first described in the 1940s in New York and in other areas of the United States. Once isolated from the blood of patients, although it did not cross-react with *Proteus* OX-19 strain, *R. akari* was classified as a spotted fever group rickettsia because it grows in both the cytoplasm and the nucleus of infected cells. Antigenic cross-reactions with spotted fever group rickettsiae supported this classification. Other isolates have been obtained from the former Soviet Union Woodward and Jackson 1965 (Rehacek and Tarasevich 1988).

The routine application of molecular biology techniques has led, in the past 5 years, to the detection and description of several new spotted fever group rickettsiae, which have been isolated in Africa, Europe, the former USSR, Australia, and the United States.

SPOTTED FEVER GROUP RICKETTSIAE: THE ORGANISMS

PHYLOGENY AND CLASSIFICATION

Since the first reports on rickettsioses, the classification of their causative agents has been a subject of much debate. After initially having been considered as protozoa or viruses, rickettsiae have been classified into the order Rickettsiales which included a wide group of organisms all with the unique common feature of being dependent upon eukaryotic cells for their growth and replication. Chlamydiae and Rickettsiae were classified in the same order. The initial difficulty in studying rickettsiae and other related organisms was the fact that they could not be grown on artificial media. Although the clinical, ecological, and epidemiological features of rickettsial diseases could be readily established, rickettsiologists had to discover that rickettsiae could be grown in yolk sacs of embryonated eggs, and cell cultures, before the study of the biology of the organisms could begin.

After 1984, according to the eight edition of *Bergey's manual of determinative bacteriology*, three families were classified in the order Rickettsiales: the Bartonellaceae, Anaplasmataceae, and Rickettsiaceae. Organisms as different as Rickettsiae, Rochalimaea, Wolbachiae, Ehrlichiae, and *Coxiella* were included into the family Rickettsiaceae because they were all 'intimately associated with arthropod tissues, usually in an intracellular position' (Weiss and Moulder 1984). Rickettsiae were classified into three main groups: the typhus group rickettsiae (*R. prowazekii*, *R. typhi* and *R. canada*), the scrub typhus rickettsia with its unique representative, (*R. tsutsugamushi*, and the spotted fever group rickettsiae represented by eight different recognized strains (*R. rickettsii*, *R. conorii*, *R. sibirica*, *R. australis*, *R. rhipicephali*, *R. montana*, *R. parkeri*, and *R. akari*). The classification of rickettsiae into these three groups was based on ecological characteristics (association with different vectors), geographical origin, clinical features or biological criteria (growth conditions, ability to invade cell nuclei), and on serological cross-reactions. G+C percentage composition of typhus (29–30 per cent) and spotted fever group rickettsiae (32–33 per cent) was the first information available on rickettsial genomes (Wyatt and Cohen 1952; Tyeryar *et al.* 1973). More recently, molecular biology has provided new

Table 21.1 Spotted fever group rickettsiae and their vectors around the world

	Organism	Human disease	Geographical distribution	Source of isolates
Europe	R. conorii	Mediterranean spotted fever or Boutonneuse fever	Mediterranean coast Black Sea basin	R. sanguineus ticks, humans
	R. sibirica	Sibirian tick typhus or North Asian tick typhus	Former USSR (European part)	D. nuttalli, D. marginatus D. silvarum, H. concinna, humans
	R. slovaca	Meningoencephalitis	Czechoslovakia, Switzerland, France, Portugal	D. marginatus
	R. helvetica		Switzerland	I. ricinus
	R. rhipicephali		France	R. sanguineus
	R. massiliae		France, Greece, Portugal	R. sanguineus, R. turanicus
	'Mtu 5, Bar 29, PoTiR 1 strains'		France, Spain, Portugal	R. snaguineus, R. turanicus
	'Po TiR8 strain' (= MC16, Hmr strains*)		Portugal	Hy. marginatum marginatum
	'Astrakhan SFG rickettsia'	Astrakhan spotted fever	Astrakhan	R. sanguineus, R. pumilio
	R. akari	Rickettsialpox	Former USSR	A. (or L.) sanguineus, humans
Asia	R. sibirica	Siberian tick typhus or North Asian tick typhus	Former USSR (Asian part) China	D. nuttalli, D. marginatus, D. silvarum, D. sinicus, H. concinna, humans
	R. japonica	Japanese spotted fever or Oriental spotted fever	Japan	Unknown vector, humans
	R. conorii (Indian tick typhus)	Mediterranean spotted fever	India	R. sanguineus
	'Israeli spotted fever rickettsia'	Israeli spotted fever	Israel	R. sanguineus
	'Thai tick typhus rickettsia'		Thailand	R. sanguineus and Ixodes spp. pooled
	'HA-91'		Inner Mongolia	Hy. asiaticum
Australia	R. australis	Queensland tick typhus	Australia (north-east)	I. holocyclus, humans
	'R. honei'	Flinders Island spotted fever	Tasmania	Unknown vector, humans
Africa	R. conorii (Moroccan strain)	Mediterranean spotted fever or boutonneuse fever	Mediterranean area	R. sanguineus, humans
	R. conorii (Kenyan strain, Simko strain, Malish 7 strain)	Kenyan tick typhus, South African tick-bite fever	Eastern, Central and Souther Africa (Kenya, Ethiopia, Zimbabwe, South Africa, Central African Republic)	R. simus, H. leachi, R. mushamae (*)
	'R. africae'	African tick-bite fever	Zimbabwe, Ethiopia, Central African Republic	A. hebraeum, A. variegatum
	'Hmr strain * (= MC16, = PoTiR8)'		Zimbabwe	Hy. marginatum rufipes
	'MC 16 strain'		Morocco	Hy. marginatum marginatum
	R. rhipicephali (*)		Central African Republic	R. of the compositus group, R. lunulatus
	R. massiliae (*)		Central African Republic	R. lunulatus, R. sulcatus, R. mushamae
	'Mtu5 strain' (*)		Central African Republic	R. mushamae, R. senegalensis, H. paraleachi
America	R. rickettsii	Rocky Mountain spotted fever	United States	D. andersoni, D. variabilis
	R. bellii		United States	D. variabilis
	R. montana		United States	D. variabilis, D. andersoni
	R. rhipicephali		United States	R. sanguineus, Dermacentor spp.
	R. parkeri		United States	A. maculatum
	'R. amblyommii'		United States	A. americanum
	R. akari	Rickettsialpox	United States	A. (or L.) sanguineus

(*) detected only by PCR.

tools for the statistical analysis of relatedness between organisms, by the study of DNA–DNA homology, restriction profiles of genomic fragments or of whole genomes, or by sequencing the 16S rRNA gene. According to 16S rRNA gene sequencing, the genus *Rickettsia* belongs to the phylum α.2 of the *Proteobacteria* (Fig. 21.2), and it is likely that the order Rickettsiales will be completely revised in the next edition of *Bergey's manual* (Weisburg 1989; Weisburg *et al.* 1989). It is

interesting to point out that rickettsiae, inside the phylum alpha, are phylogenetically related to a wide range of bacteria, which are associated in a symbiotic or parasitic way with eukaryotic host cells (Weisburg 1989). Among them are the plant pathogens *Agrobacterium* and *Rhizobium* species (Weisburg *et al.* 1985), as well as the plant mitochondria themselves (Weisburg 1986). They also share a common ancestor with arthropod symbionts, the *Wolbachia pipientis* group

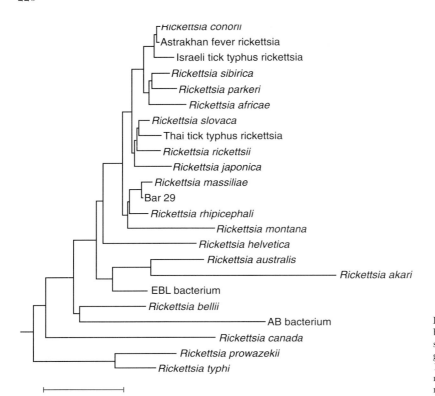

Rickettsia conorii
Astrakhan fever rickettsia
Israeli tick typhus rickettsia
Rickettsia sibirica
Rickettsia parkeri
Rickettsia africae
Rickettsia slovaca
Thai tick typhus rickettsia
Rickettsia rickettsii
Rickettsia japonica
Rickettsia massiliae
Bar 29
Rickettsia rhipicephali
Rickettsia montana
Rickettsia helvetica
Rickettsia australis
Rickettsia akari
EBL bacterium
Rickettsia bellii
AB bacterium
Rickettsia canada
Rickettsia prowazekii
Rickettsia typhi

Fig. 21.2 Phylogenetic tree for members of the order Rickettsiales and other species representing the α- and γ-subgroups of the Proteobacteria obtained by 16S rRNA gene sequencing (scale bar represents 5 per cent differences in nucleotide sequences).

of organisms, which are responsible for distortions of sex ratios in the offspring of infected individuals by inducing cytoplasmic incompatibility (Turelli and Hoffmann 1991; O'Neill *et al.* 1992) or parthenogenesis (Stouthamer and Werren 1993), and with a bacterial strain which provokes male killing in the ladybird beetle (Werren *et al.* 1994). Rickettsiae are characterized by a relatively short genome (1.1–1.3 Mb), when compared to extracellular bacteria (Roux *et al.* 1992; Roux and Raoult 1993). These bacteria, by invading a new ecological niche, the eukaryotic cytoplasm, and by learning how to exploit the metabolic resources of the host cell, could have 'lost' the fragments of their genome necessary for their extracellular life and those genomic fragments, function of which has been replaced by the metabolic processes of host cell.

The spotted fever group rickettsiae were first grouped together because they were associated with ticks, had common antigenic features (Weiss and Moulder 1984), and because they all stimulated the formation of agglutinins to *Proteus* OX-19 strain in the Weil–Felix test (Weil and Felix 1916).

Although the antigenic determinants of their immunological reactions were unknown, the distinctive immunogenic properties of rickettsial antigens were used in the first half of the century to distinguish among spotted fever rickettsiae. Cross-immunity and vaccine protection tests (Pijper 1936) in guinea-pigs, complement fixation (Plotz *et al.* 1944), or toxin neutralization tests (Bell and Stoenner 1960) were successfully applied to the differentiation of *R. rickettsii*, *R. sibirica*, and *R. conorii*. Similarly, the indirect microimmunofluorescence serological typing with mouse sera was developed in 1978 and it is still the current reference method for the identification of new spotted fever group rickettsiae (Philip *et al.* 1978). Accordingly, the classically recognized spotted fever group rickettsial species, are in fact serotypes. Purification methods enabling the separation of rickettsiae from host cell components, have opened the way to the study of rickettsial proteins and the understanding of the mechanisms on which all previously applied serological identification techniques have been based.

Genomic DNA–DNA relatedness studies on the spotted fever group are still fragmentary, but it has been demonstrated that some members are so closely related that, according to the criteria accepted by the International Committee for Systematic Bacteriology, they should be considered to be a single species (Wayne *et al.* 1987; Walker 1989*b*). Since there is not, and there will probably never be, a total agreement in the scientific community about what can be considered

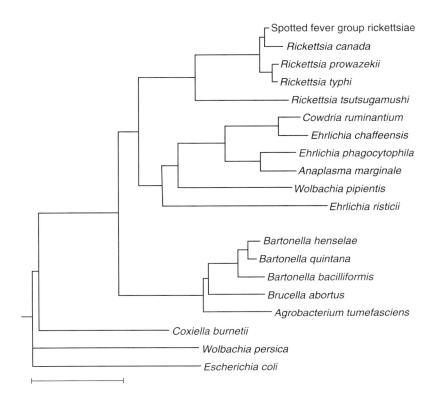

Fig. 21.3 Phylogenetic tree of the spotted fever group rickettsiae obtained by 16S rRNA sequencing (scale bar represents 0.5 per cent differences in nucleotide sequences).

to be a distinct rickettsial 'species', for our purposes a species will be defined as a group of isolates which are genotypically differentiable from all other rickettsiae—genotypes having been determined by 16S rRNA gene sequencing (Fig. 21.3) (V. Roux, unpublished data), pulsed field gel electrophoresis (Roux *et al.* 1992; Roux and Raoult 1993) and PCR/RFLP (Regnery *et al.* 1991). For practical reasons, it is obviously useful to give different names to rickettsial serotypes causing clinically different spotted fevers.

MORPHOLOGY

Spotted fever group rickettsiae are obligate intracellular organisms growing free into the cytoplasm of their eukaryotic host cell. These bacteria can be stained by Giemsa or Giménez staining methods. They can occasionally invade the nucleus of the cells they are infecting. *Rickettsia rickettsii*, by electron microscopy, shows a typical Gram-negative bacterial cell surface made up of a cellular membrane, the inner and outer leaflets of the cell wall, a microcapsular layer, and a further polysaccharide slime layer (Silverman *et al.* 1978). A similar structure characterizes all spotted and typhus group rickettsiae (Popov *et al.* 1986; Silverman 1991). Although it was accepted that rickettsiae enter the cytoplasm of the host cell by a phagocytosis process,

the presence of a transient phagocytic vacuole has only been demonstrated recently by electron microscopy (N. Teyssire, unpublished data). The escape from the phagosome could be due to activation of a phospholipase acting on the membrane of the phagosome. The mechanisms of invasion of cells by spotted fever group rickettsiae differs greatly from that of typhus group rickettsiae. When compared to cells infected with *R. prowazekii*, cells infected with *R. rickettsii* have fewer organisms but much greater cytopathological changes (Wisseman 1985; Silverman 1991). Dilatation of the rough endoplasmic reticulum is detected 48 hours after the beginning of the infection (Silverman *et al.* 1981; Iwamasa *et al.* 1992). It has also been observed that spotted fever group rickettsiae have the capacity of bi-directional movements into and out of the cell (Ito and Rikihisa 1981; Silverman *et al.* 1981). Recent experiments showed that the progression of *R. conorii* into human endothelial cells (Teysseire *et al.* 1992) and that of R. rickettsii into Vero cells is associated with actin polymerization (Heinzen *et al.* 1993) (Fig. 21.4). The actin filamentous structures extend from the pole of each bacteria and could be at the basis, as has been shown for other bacteria (*S. flexneri* or *L. monocytogenes*), of the motility of the organisms inside the infected cells and of the ability of one organism to leave one cell for another through cytoplasmic

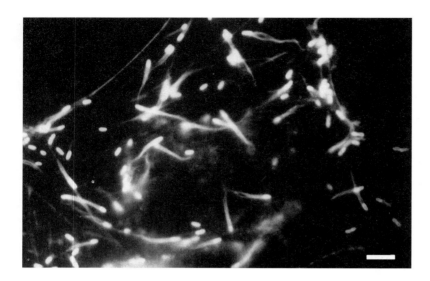

Fig. 21.4 Vero cells infected with *Rickettsia conorii* and labelled with NBD-phallacidin for polymerized actin. Each organism presents an actin tail 0.3–15 μm in length. Bar = 3 μm. (Teysseire *et al.* 1992.)

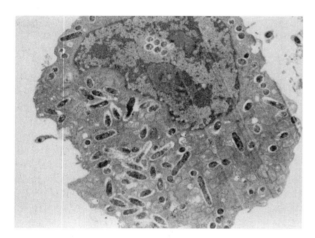

Fig. 21.5 Electron micrograph of a Vero cell infected with *Rickettsia conorii*. Rickettsiae are scattered in the cytoplasm, while they are organized in 'colonies' into the nucleus.

extrusions. In the nucleus, where rickettsiae are not connected to actin tails, the bacteria produce 'colonies' similar to those produced by typhus group rickettsiae in the cytoplasm (Fig. 21.5).

ANTIGENIC PROPERTIES

Antigenic properties of spotted fever group rickettsiae have been investigated for two main reasons. The first purpose was mainly taxonomic; to establish biochemical or serological methods to differentiate these closely related organisms. The second was to detect rickettsial

antigens which induce protective immune response in inoculated animals, in other words antigens for candidate vaccines.

Spotted fever group rickettsiae may be differentiated on the basis of their distinct migration patterns after polyacrylamide gel electrophoresis (Tzianabos *et al.* 1974; Pedersen and Walters 1978; Anacker *et al.* 1980; Williams *et al.* 1986). Protein profiles of rickettsiae are characterized by different components: the high molecular weight species-specific proteins (SPAs) and the lipopolysaccharide-like fragments (LPS) (Osterman and Eisemann 1978; Anacker *et al.* 1987; Raoult and Dasch 1989). The electrophoretic mobilities of the SPAs are different from one strain to another, whereas the LPS have rather common features in all spotted fever group rickettsiae. Immunological reactions of laboratory animals and humans are mainly directed against the LPS fractions (Philip *et al.* 1976; Ormsbee *et al.* 1978; Ancker *et al.* 1983), which explains the predominance of cross-reacting antibodies in their sera. Cross-reactions with high molecular weight epitopes are, however, frequently observed in human sera (Feng *et al.* 1986; Beati *et al.* 1994). In mice, the reaction is directed mainly against the SPAs, so that in indirect immunofluorescence antibody (IFA) testing, homologous titres are higher than heterologous titres (Philip *et al.* 1976, 1978). This has led to mice being used for differentiating rickettsiae in comparative IFA testing (Yu *et al.* 1990; Beati *et al.* 1994). In spite of the fact that powerful molecular biology techniques are now available for the classification of rickettsiae, recently isolated organisms have to be tested by the indirect microimmunofluorescence serotyping method, which is still the reference technique for characterizing spotted fever group rickettsiae, before they can be considered to be novel species (Uchida *et al.* 1989; Beati and Raoult 1993; Beati *et al.* 1992; Kelly *et al.* 1994). However, it is likely that this laborious technique, often subjective, will be replaced by more sensitive and specific methods. The analysis of restriction profiles of rickettsial DNA after amplification by polymerase chain reaction has already been used successfully for identification of rickettsiae in cell culture (Regnery *et al.* 1991; Beati *et al.* 1992; Eremeeva *et al.* 1994a and ticks (Beati *et al.* 1993*b*) Gage *et al.* 1994). This method enables one to identify organisms without isolating or growing them in cell cultures.

Protection against rickettsial infections is a complex mechanism involving humoral and cellular immune responses. Observations in laboratory animals have suggested that the SPAs, especially their heat-labile epitopes, were involved in producing immune protection against rickettsiae (Anacker *et al.* 1985; Feng *et al.* 1987; Li *et al.* 1988; Gage and Jerrells 1992). Monoclonal antibodies reactive with some of these epitopes protected laboratory animals from a challenge with rickettsiae belonging to the same or to a different serotype (Vishwanath *et al.* 1990). These properties made the SPAs, now called rOmpA and rOmpB, suitable candidates for subunit vaccine production. The rOmpA outer membrane protein of *R. rickettsii* corresponds to the previously named 190 kDa protein, the solubilized products of which appeared as the 150 kDa protein on sodium dodecyl sulphate–polyacrylamide gel electrophoresis (SDS-PAGE), while the rOmpB protein is the former 120 kDa protein. Due to the growth conditions of rickettsiae, these proteins can not be obtained and purified in sufficient amounts for vaccine purposes. For these reasons, recent studies devoted to the production of recombinant forms of rickettsial antigens (Vishwanath *et al.* 1990) have led to the description of the sequence and structure of the genes encoding for the immunogenic high molecular weight proteins of *R. rickettsii* and *R. conorii* (McDonald *et al.* 1987; Gilmore *et al.* 1989, 1991; Gilmore 1990; Gilmore and Hackstadt 1991; Hackstadt *et al.* 1992; Crocquet-Valdes *et al.* 1994; Schuenke and Walker 1994).

THE EPIDEMIOLOGY

GEOGRAPHICAL DISTRIBUTION

Classically, six spotted fever group rickettsiae were recognized as human pathogens and were characterized by distinct geographical distribution areas: *R. rickettsii, R. conorii, R. sibirica, R. australis, R. japonica,* and *R. akari* (Walker 1989*a*). Over the past 5 years, several other rickettsiae have been described following the dramatic evolution of new detection and identification techniques provided by molecular biology. Some of the newly described rickettsiae are now recognized pathogens.

Rickettsia rickettsii was, and still is, the pathogenic strain in the New World. Spotted fever diseases in South America have been attributed to infections with *R. rickettsii or R. sibirica* on the basis of serological cross-reactions in human sera in the 1930s and 1940s (Bustamante and Varela 1947; Hoogstraal 1967; Sexton *et al.* 1993). Other rickettsiae, *R. rhipicephali, R. montana, R. parkeri,* and *R. bellii,* and a new strain isolated from *Amblyomma americanum,* and provisionally named *Rickettsia amblyommii* (Pretzman *et al.* 1994), are American serotypes of unknown pathogenicity.

In the Mediterranean area, in the Middle East and the Far East, *R. conorii* is the main spotted fever agent and is classically transmitted through the bite of the brown dog tick, *Rhipicephalus sanguineus.* A review published in 1957 reported all data dealing with the geographical distribution of boutonneuse fever (or Mediterranean spotted fever) in the Mediterranean area and southern Europe, with cases reported from Italy, Spain, Portugal, Greece, Turkey, Cyprus, Palestine, Romania, Bulgaria, Tunisia, Algeria, Morocco, Libya, and Egypt (Olmer and Olmer 1957*a*). Another rickettsia, the agent of the Israeli spotted fever is transmitted by the same tick species in Israel (Goldwasser *et al.* 1974*b*). Rickettsiae have not been characterized in other countries around Israel, so that it is not possible to establish if the distribution areas of *R. conorii* and the Israeli spotted fever are clearly distinct, contiguous, or overlapping. In the past few years novel rickettsial sero-and genotypes of unknown pathogenicity have been described in the Mediterranean area, for example *R. massiliae, R. rhipicephali,* and the Mtu5 strain (Beati *et al.* 1992; Drancourt *et al.* 1992).

Two main serotypes seemed to occupy distinct geographical regions in the centre of Europe. *Rickettsia helvetica,* isolated from *I. ricinus* ticks in Switzerland, is widely distributed in that country on both sides of the Alpine range (Beati *et al.* 1993*b*; *R. slovaca,* isolated from *D. marginatus* ticks in the former Czechoslovakia (Rehacek 1984), has been subsequently found in several other European countries (Switzerland, France, Portugal, and the former Soviet Union) (Beati *et al.* 1993*ab*; Bacellar *et al.* 1995). A further pathogenic rickettsia of the Old World is *R. sibirica,* the agent of North Asian tick typhus (or Siberian tick typhus). This serotype has been isolated from different tick species belonging to the genus *Dermacentor.* Its geographical distribution spreads from the European through the Asian part of the former USSR and crosses the Chinese border (Yu *et al.* 1993). A pathogen, isolated from *R. sanguineus* and *R. pumilio* ticks in the Astrakhan region, is the newly recognized agent of Astrakhan spotted fever (Eremeeva *et al.* 1994*b*). Other strains of unknown pathogenicity, isolated in China and the former USSR, have been characterized (Eremeeva *et al.* 1993; Yu *et al.* 1993). It has been shown that at least four rickettsial genotypes, *R. sibirica, R. slovaca; R. conorii* and a strain called 'S' are present in the Black Sea and the Caspian Sea regions (Balayeva *et al.* 1993; Eremeeva *et al.* 1993). In Asia, other rickettsiae have been described several decades ago, the Indian tick typhus rickettsia and the Thai tick typhus rickettsia (TT-118 strain) (Robertson and Wissemann 1973). Although the latter is included in the usual reference spotted fever group rickettsial panel, its pathogenicity has not been investigated. *Rickettsia japonica* is a human pathogen so far confined to the southern islands of Japan (Uchida 1993). The vector of this disease has yet to be described (Uchida *et al.* 1992). The presence of spotted fever group rickettsioses has been serologically determined in other Asian countries (Wilde *et al.* 1991; Sirisanthana *et al.* 1994). Their aetiological agents still need to be identified.

Rickettsia conorii was thought to be the only agent of spotted fever all over Africa, but the isolation of *Rickettsia africae*, a new rickettsia from patients in Zimbabwe and from European travellers coming back from this country, has shown that there are at least two pathogenic rickettsiae on the African continent (Kelly *et al.* 1994). The primary isolation of *R. africae* from an *Amblyomma variegatum* tick from Ethiopia (Philip *et al.* 1966; Burgdorfer *et al.* 1973) suggests that this strain has a wide distribution area. The immature stages of *Amblyomma hebraeum* and *variegatum* are very 'anthropophilic' when compared with other African spotted fever group rickettsial vectors, which could explain the fact that high serological prevalence of tick-borne rickettsioses is associated with the presence of *Amblyomma* ticks. The detection of spotted fever group rickettsiae in ticks of the Central African Republic (Tissot Dupont *et al.* 1994) and Egypt (El Dessouky *et al.* 1991), the characterization of new strains isolated from *Hyalomma marginatum marginatum* ticks from Morocco and from *Hyalomma marginatum rufipes* from Zimbabwe (L. Beati, unpublished data) seem to suggest that our knowledge of tick-related rickettsiae on the African continent is still fragmentary. Moreover, there is serological evidence that spotted fever group rickettsioses are present in all other African countries where seroepidemiological surveys have been undertaken (H. Tissot Dupont, unpublished data).

In Australia, *R. australis* is the agent of Queensland tick typhus and is transmitted by the bite of *Ixodes holocyclus* ticks. More recently a new pathogenic rickettsia, provisionally called *Rickettsia honei*, has been isolated from patients in the Flinder Islands, Tasmania (Stewart

1991; Baird *et al.* 1992). The vectors of the disease need to be identified. The geographical distribution of pathogenic spotted fever group rickettsiae on the Australian continent seems to extend along the entire eastern coast (Sexton *et al.* 1991*b*).

Cases of rickettsialpox have been reported from the United States and the former USSR, where the disease is transmitted by the bite of different mite vectors.

All these data are summarized on geographical maps (Figs 21.6–21.10). We are nevertheless aware that these will be modified over and over in the next few years, following the rapid spread of new identification techniques.

VECTORS AND INFECTIOUS CYCLES

From the beginning of the century, rickettsia-like organisms and spotted fever vectors have been described from all over the world. It is now sometimes difficult to interpret these findings, because the identification techniques used in early reports were often not specific when compared to the reference identification method (serotyping) and especially to modern techniques of molecular characterization. For example, *R. conorii* was supposed to be transmitted by a large number of tick genera in Africa (Charters 1946; Hoogstraal 1956; Camicas 1975). Because *R. conorii* was considered to be the only African rickettsia belonging to the spotted fever group, all ticks infected by rickettsia-like organisms were regarded as new vectors of *R. conorii*. We now know, that rickettsiae transmitted by at least some *Amblyomma* and *Hyalomma* species are different from the Mediterranean spotted fever agent in the southern part of Africa and Morocco, and that further genotypes, different from *R. conorii*, have been detected by PCR/RFLP in Central African ticks (Tissot Dupont *et al.* 1994). Similarly, it was thought that *R. sibirica* was present in sylvatic cycles in regions where there were no reported cases of Siberian tick typhus. Recent analysis of the strains originally isolated in those regions, showed that some of the *R. sibirica* strains were in fact *R. slovaca* (Eremeeva *et al.* 1993). Consequently, we should be cautious in describing tick vectors, vertebrate reservoirs, or sylvatic cycles of spotted fever group rickettsiae, with all attempts being made to meet the recognized criteria for rickettsial identification

In the typical zoonotic cycle (Fig. 21.11) rickettsiae of the spotted fever group are tick-borne organisms which infect and multiply in almost all the organs of their invertebrate hosts. When the ovarias and oocytes of an adult female are infected, rickettsiae may be transmitted transovarially to at least some of its offspring. The percentage of infected eggs obtained from females of the same tick species, infected with the

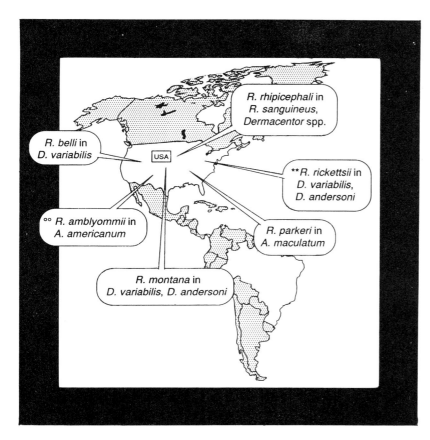

R. rhipicephali in
R. sanguineus,
Dermacentor spp.

R. belli in
D. variabilis

USA

**R. rickettsii in
D. variabilis,
D. andersoni

°° **R. amblyommii** in
A. americanum

R. parkeri in
A. maculatum

R. montana in
D. variabilis, D. andersoni

Fig. 21.6 American spotted fever group rickettsiae. In this map only major vectors are mentioned. **, Pathogenic rickettsiae;°°, strains which have yet to be officially recognized. Although countries where the presence of spotted fever group rickettsiae has been serologically confirmed in animals or humans are in white, it does not mean that rickettsiae are present over the whole area of the country.

same rickettsial strain, may vary, depending on factors that have yet to be elucidated (Burgdorfer and Varma 1967; Burgdorfer and Brinton 1975). Once an egg is infected, all the following life stages of the tick will be infected. Therefore, the rate of trans-stadial transmission is usually 100 per cent. Ixodid ticks are bloodsucking arthropods in all their development stages, apart from some of the adult male ticks in some *Ixodes* species. Rickettsiae infecting the ticks salivary glands can be transmitted to vertebrate hosts during feeding. Therefore, since larvae, nymphs, and adults may all be infective for susceptible vertebrate hosts, the tick must be regarded as the main reservoir host of rickettsiae. Moreover, although sexual transmission from male to female ticks has been described in *I. ricinus* ticks (Hayes *et al.* 1980), rickettsiae are transmitted cytoplasmically (or maternally inherited) through successive female generations of ticks. This kind of transmission pattern suggests that the present tick–rickettsiae associations could be the result of a long co-evolution process.

While there is a wide consensus on this part of the rickettsial cycle, the role of vertebrate reservoirs in maintaining zoonotic foci has yet to be agreed upon. For vertebrates to be efficient reservoirs of rickettsiae

they should be normal hosts of the vector, they should be susceptible to the rickettsia, and they should develop a relatively long-duration rickettsiaemia. Otherwise, ticks would not be able to recover rickettsiae from the bloodstream of their hosts. Man, therefore, is obviously not a good reservoir for rickettsiae, since he is seldom infested with large numbers of ticks for a long period and rickettsiaemia is of short duration, especially after antibiotic treatments.

Although yet to be demonstrated, there is another potential way that rickettsiae may be transmitted from infected to uninfected ticks. The 'social' behaviour of ticks is mainly determined by the effects of different pheromones (Hamilton 1992; Pavis and Barré 1993), some of which are responsible for aggregation of ticks on the host. This enables feeding and copulation to occur at the same time and results in mouthparts of several different ticks being in the skin of the host in very close proximity. It is therefore possible that under such feeding conditions direct spread of rickettsiae to uninfected ticks might be possible at the actual feeding sites without rickettsiaemia being present.

Rickettsialpox (*R. akari*) is an urban disease which involves mites of the genus *Allodermanyssus*, the house

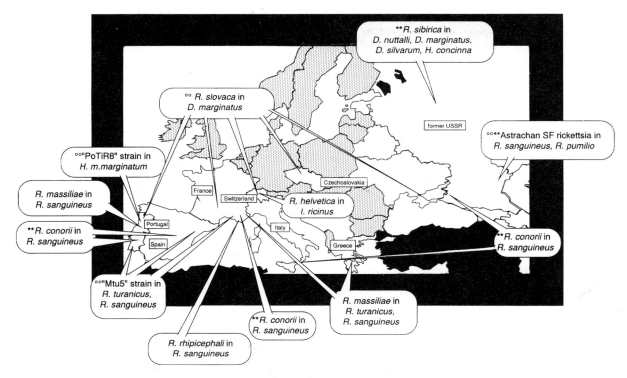

Fig. 21.7 European spotted fever group rickettsiae. In this map only major vectors are mentioned, **, Pathogenic rickettsiae,°°, strains which have yet to be officially recognized. Although countries where the presence of spotted fever group rickettsiae has been serologically confirmed in animals or humans are in white, it does not mean that rickettsiae are present over the whole area of the country.

mouse *Mus musculus* and, accidentally, man. The two nymphal stages and both the female and the male adult stage of the mite mainly feed on mice, which are highly susceptible to infection with *R. akari*. Although mice can be considered to be natural reservoirs of *R. akari*, since this organism can be transmitted transovarially, the mite may cta not only as vector but also as reservoir of rickettsialpox. Humans are classically attacked by mites after mice extermination campaigns. In the former Soviet Union, rickettsialpox is also known as an urban illness, but in rural areas, wild mice are also involved in the cycle and humans get infected when they invade the ecological niche of mites/rodents (Woodward and Jackson 1965). Suspected cases of rickettsialpox have been reported from South Africa, but there is no information about the natural cycle of the disease in this part of the world.

Europe, Mediterranean Sea, former USSR (including the Asian part)

In the Mediterranean area, *Rhipicephalus sanguineus*, the brown dog tick, is the usual vector of *R. conorii* (Fig. 21.12). It has been recognized as the vector of

this organism in northern Africa, in the former USSR, and India. Larvae and nymphs of this *Rhipicephlus* tick have been found feeding on other vertebrates, but the dog seems to be the main host of each developmental stage *R. sanguineus* along the Mediterranean coast (Gilot 1984). For this reason, the dog has been considered as a potential reservoir of the agent of boutonneuse fever. Although dogs seroconvert after having been bitten by infected ticks, the immunofluorescence titres decrease progressively during the winter months, when ticks are undergoing their diapausal life stage (Espejo *et al.* 1993). Moreover, it seems that dogs do not develop a disease when bitten by infected ticks, and there are no reports of rickettsial strains isolated from dogs in southern Europe. Based on these observations, the role of dogs in maintaining *R. conorii* does not appear to be important. Other pathogenic strains (Israeli spotted fever and Astrakhan spotted fever rickettsiae), as well as strains of unknown pathogenicity (*R. massiliae*, *R. rhipicephali* and the Mtu5 strain) have also been isolated from *R. sanguineus*. Moreover, the Mtu5 strain and *R. massiliae* have been isolated from the haemolymph of *Rhipicephalus turanicus* ticks (Beati *et al.* 1992), which are included into the *Rhipicephalus*

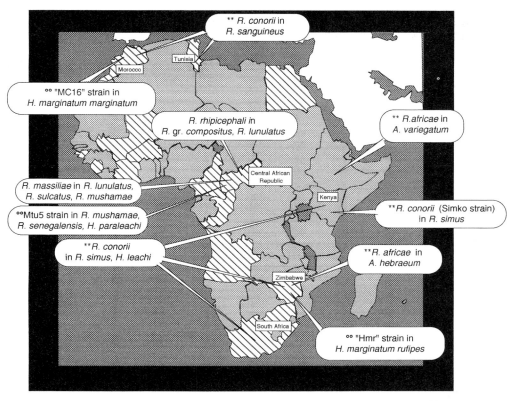

Fig. 21.8 African spotted fever group rickettsiae. In this map only major vectors are mentioned.[**], Pathogenic rickettsiae;[oo], strains which have yet to be officially recognized. Although countries where the presence of spotted fever group rickettsiae has been serologically confirmed with animals or humans are in white, it does not mean that rickettsiae are present over the whole area of the country.

sanguineus complex. *Rhipicephalus pumilio*, a further vector of the Astrakhan spotted fever, is also included into the *R. sanguineus* complex of ticks (Eremeeva *et al.* 1994*b*). From a phylogenetical point of view, the three pathogenic rickettsiae are closely related, and the three other 'non virulent' strains are also closely related, but according to the 16S rRNA gene analysis, the two groups of rickettsiae constitute two clearly distinct clusters (Fig. 21.3). The natural cycle of these organisms, their relationships, the effects they have on dogs, still need to be thoroughly investigated. However, it is evident that, especially in the South of France, where four different rickettsiae have been found in the same area in *R. sanguineus*, it is not yet possible to determine which rickettsial strain (or strains) are responsible for humoral immune response in man and animals. Nevertheless, the predominance of one of these rickettsiae in distinct regions may explain the different seroprevalence data recorded in different areas of the Mediterranean basin.

Rickettsia helvetica, has been isolated from *I. ricinus* ticks in different regions of Switzerland where this tick species predominates. It has a wide range of hosts including domestic and wild animals, birds, reptiles, and man. *I. ricinus* has been found to be infected with rickettsia-like organisms in other countries (Czechoslovakia, France), and it seems likely that the distribution area of *R. helvetica* may be wide (Rehacek and Tarasevich 1988). In Switzerland, antibodies against spotted fever group rickettsiae were found in several wild and domestic animals at rates varying from 10 to 30 per cent depending on the geographical area and the host (Péter 1985). This could indicate that this rickettsia is often inoculated by ticks into their hosts, but there is no information about potential natural reservoirs. In a preliminary study, the seroprevalence of antibodies against rickettsiae in a sample of sera, obtained from people reported to have been bitten by ticks, was compared to the seroprevalence in a population living outside the distribution area of *I. ricinus*. In the latter, the seroprevalence was significantly lower. Consequently, *R. helvetica* appears to be inoculated into humans often enough to elicit antibody production, even though clinical signs suggesting rickettsial infection have never been reported.

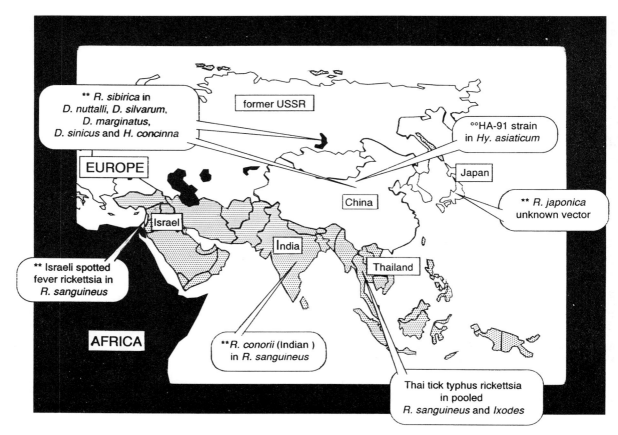

Fig. 21.9   Asian spotted fever group rickettsiae. In this map only major vectors are mentioned,[**], Pathogenic rickettsiae; [oo], strains which have yet to be officially recognized. Although countries where the presence of spotted fever group rickettsiae has been sero-logically confirmed in animals or humans are in white, it does not mean that rickettsiae are present over the whole area of the country.

Rickettsia slovaca was first isolated from *Dermacentor marginatus* ticks in the former Czechoslovakia, where this strain has been incriminated as the aetiological agent of a single case of acute meningoencephalitis. Its pathogenic role for humans has never subsequently been confirmed (Rehacek and Tarasevich 1988). Seroprevalence data have been collected from a wide range of domestic and wild animals in this area, showing that birds, insectivores, bats, lagomorphs, rodents, carnivores, artiodactyla, and reptiles are sometimes infected with rickettsiae. Moreover, lago-morphs and rodents showed rickettsiaemic phases after inoculation with *R. slovaca*. Even though all rick-ettsiae detected in Czechoslovakian ticks (*Dermacentor, Ixodes,* or *Haemaphysalis*) have been considered to be *R. slovaca*, it seems likely that other rickettsiae (*R. helvetica*) may be widespread in *Ixodes* ticks. With non-specific tests, it is difficult to determine seropreva-lences, potential pathogenicity, or the ecological cycles of different rickettsial strains coexisting in the same area. As previously mentioned, several other isolates of rickettsiae genotypically identical to the 'B' strain of *R. slovaca* have been reported from Portugal (Bacellar *et al.* 1995), France (Beati *et al.* 1993*a*), Switzerland (Beati *et al.* 1993*b*), Armenia, and Crimea (Eremeeva *et al.* 1993), showing that this is probably the most widely distributed rickettsia in Europe.

Epidemiological data on spotted fever group rick-ettsioses in the former USSR, have already been sum-marized in detail (Rehacek and Tarasevich 1988). Rickettsia-like organisms have been detected in *Dermacentor, Haemaphysalis, Rhipicephalus, Hyalomma* and *Ixodes* ticks. Seroprevalences have been reported in birds and wild and domestic animals, indicating that these are often exposed to rickettsiae. An increase in titres in rodents appears to follow the activity periods of juvenile stages of ticks, and rickettsial strains have been successfully isolated from them. *Rickettsia sibirica* was thought to be transmitted through the bite of a very wide range of tick genera. It has recently been

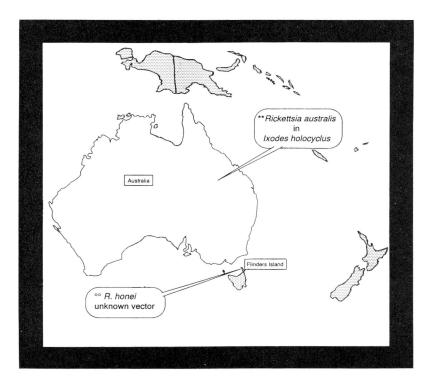

Fig. 21.10 Australian spotted fever group rickettsiae. In this map only major vectors are mentioned.**, Pathogenic rickettsiae;°°, strains which have yet to be officially recognized. Although countries where the presence of spotted fever group rickettsiae has been serologically confirmed in animals or humans are in white, it does not mean that rickettsiae are present over the whole area of the country.

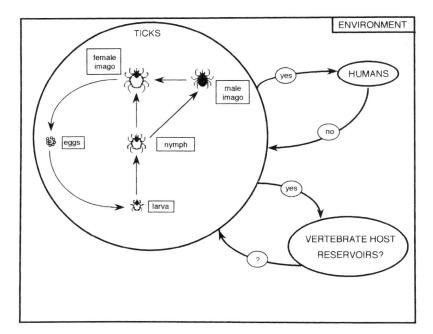

Fig. 21.11 Infectious cycle of spotted fever group rickettsiae in their Ixodid vectors.

shown that at least some of the USSR isolates are in fact different from *R. sibirica*. Of these, the Barbash strain has been found to be identical to *R. conorii* (Wang *et al.* 1987), and several 'mild' strains (Tarasevich 1978) of *R. sibirica* isolated from *D. marginatus* have been found to be identical to *R. slovaca* (Eremeeva *et al.* 1993). However it has been confirmed that the main vector of *R. sibirica* is *Dermacentor nuttalli*,

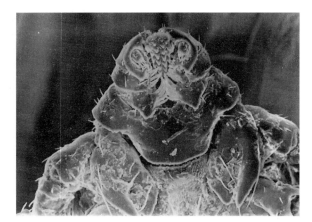

Fig. 21.12 Ventral view of the mouthparts of an adult *Rhipicephalus sanguineus*, the vector of Mediterranean spotted fever.

which can be replaced by *Haemaphysalis concinna*, D. marginatus and D. silvarum, depending on the geographic areas (Eremeeva *et al.* 1993).

Africa

Three main ecological cycles of spotted fever group rickettsioses have been so far identified on the African continent. In northern Africa, the cycle and transmission patterns of rickettsia are identical to those given for *R. conorii* in the Mediterranean area. *Rickettsia conorii* has, however, been isolated from throughout the continent including South Africa. Under a line which could be drawn under the Sahel region, and which includes Ethiopia (Philip *et al.* 1966), Kenya (Heisch *et al.* 1957, 1962), Zimbabwe (Kelly and Mason 1990), and South Africa (Gear and Douthwaite 1938), *R. conorii* appears to be transmitted by two other dog ticks, *Rhipicephalus simus* and *Haemaphysalis leachi*. While *R. sanguineus* is distributed all over the African continent and it has sometimes been incriminated as a vector of *R. conorii*, no isolates have been made from this tick in the South (Heisch *et al.* 1957, 1962). In a sample containing 600 *R. sanguineus* ticks collected in Zimbabwe, none were found to be infected with rickettsia-like organisms, although they were collected from dogs which were infested with *H. leachi* and *R. simus* ticks, from which *R. conorii* could be isolated. Since rickettsiaemia follows experimental infection of dogs with a Zimbabwean strain of *R. conorii* (Kelly *et al.* 1992*b*), the transmission of rickettsiae from one tick to another does not appear to only depend on rickettsiaemia in the host. Also aggregation on the host does not appear to play a role as *R.simus* and *R. sanguineus* are often found feeding together in the ears of

infested dogs. The lack of infection in *R. sanguineus* ticks may therefore be a result of other properties of the tick, probably of a genetic nature, which have yet to be determined. Genetic properties of rickettsiae could also play a role, as it appears that the Kenyan strain and the Zimbabwean strains of *R. conorii* are slightly different from the Mediterranean strains. Although they are identical by PCR/RFLP or 16S rDNA sequencing, they show distinct migration patterns on SDS-PAGE and the sequences of the gene encoding for the 190 kDa protein are clearly different (V.Roux, unpublished data).

Another cycle in Africa is maintained by *Amblyomma* ticks. Although *A. hebraeum* (Fig. 21.13) and *A. variegatum* ticks usually infest cattle and large wild ungulates, their juvenile stages are highly anthropophilic when compared to the above mentioned dog ticks. These arthropods are responsible for the transmission of a newly identified pathogenic spotted fever rickettsia, *R. africae* (Kelly *et al.* 1994). The transmission of this rickettsia trans-stadially and transovarially by *A. hebraeum* ticks has been confirmed under laboratory conditions (Kelly and Mason 1991), and rickettsiaemia can be demonstrated in the blood of goat and cattle experimentally or naturally infected with *R. africae* (Kelly *et al.* 1991*a,b*).

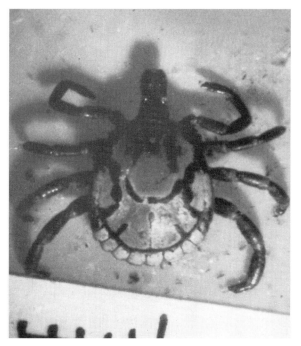

Fig. 21.13 Dorsal view of a male, adult *Amblyomma hebraeum*, the newly recognized vector of *Rickettsiae africae*.

Australia

The ecology of Queensland tick typhus was reviewed in 1991, just before the isolation and characterization of a new pathogenic rickettsia, *R. honei*, the Flinder Island spotted fever agent. Therefore, cases reported from this archipelago, have been considered to be caused by *R. australis*, and the distinctive ecological features of the two organisms are yet to be described. The infection rates of the ticks, seroprevalences in wild animals, and the presence of vertebrate reservoirs have not been thoroughly investigated in Australia. It is clearly established though, that the main vector of *R. australis* is *Ixodes holocyclus*. Complement fixation seroprevalence data showed that 6 to 15 per cent of wild vertebrates in the foci of Queensland tick typhus have been exposed to rickettsiae (Sexton *et al.* 1991*b*). By indirect immunofluorescence assays, it has recently been demonstrated that 11 per cent of the dog population of south-eastern Australia has antibodies reactive with spotted fever group rickettsiae. These results supported the hypothesis that the distribution area of spotted fevers, previously thought to be only in the north-east, extends to other regions of Australia (Sexton *et al.* 1991*a*). Vertebrates inoculated with *R. australis* have failed to develop detectable rickettsiaemia and therefore the role of dogs and other mammals as reservoirs of infection has not been determined. The relative high anthropophilic nature of *I. holocyclus* incriminates it as the main vector of human rickettsioses, though *I. tasmani*, the most widely distributed *Ixodes* tick in the country, has also been found to be infected with rickettsiae. These ticks have overlapping distribution areas (Sexton *et al.* 1991*b*), a very wide range of vertebrate hosts, and both may feed on humans. Since *I. tasmani* seems to be less 'apparent' when biting man than *I-holocyclus*, the former has been suspected to be a potential vector of Flinder Island spotted fever and in this form of disease tick bites are less often reported than in Queensland tick typhus.

Asia

Japan

While information about rickettsial isolates, their geographical distribution, their identification and classification are numerous (Okada *et al.* 1990; Uchiyama *et al.* 1990), the ecology of Japanese spotted fever seems to be poorly understood. Although tick bites have been reported by patients (Uchida *et al.* 1985), the vector of the disease has yet to be identified. Since a high percentage of rodents belonging to the *Apodemus* and *Rattus* genera have detectable antibody titres against spotted fever group rickettsiae, it is likely that the vector may be a common parasite of these animals (Uchida 1993). Electron microscopy studies of *Dermacentor taiwanensis* showed that this tick contains rickettsia-like organisms, probably belonging to the spotted fever group (Yano *et al.* 1993). However, these encouraging results must be followed by isolation of the organisms to establish if this tick species is the vector of *R. japonica*, or if it is infected by another rickettsia-like organism.

China

A recent comprehensive review of the Chinese literature, which was previously inaccessible to Western researchers, has provided information about spotted fever group rickettsioses in China (Fan *et al.* 1987*b*). Although using serological data, it was possible to establish (Fan *et al.* 1987*a*) that spotted fever group rickettsioses were widespread in China, the lack of human and tick isolates made it difficult to determine the causative agents of illness. Further studies led to the isolation of rickettsial strains from patients, from six species of ticks, and from rodents in the northern regions of China (Fan *et al.* 1987*a*). Two previously undescribed serotypes, provisionally named *R. sinkiangensis* and *R. heilongjiangi*, have been isolated from ticks, and human isolates were serotypically identical to *R. sibirica*. Spotted fever group rickettsiae have been found in *D. nuttalli*, *D. marginatus*, *Dermacentor silvarum*, *Haemaphysalis concinna*, and *Haemaphysalis japonica* (Fan *et al.* 1987*b*). By immunoblotting, human isolates, as well as the provisionally named *R. sinkiangensis*, were identical to *R. sibirica* (Fan *et al.* 1988). These data were later confirmed by PCR/RFLP analysis. Further tick isolates from *Dermacentor sinicus* collected in the Beijing area were genotypically closely related to *R. sibirica*. However, rickettsiae (strain HA-91) from a *Hyalomma asiaticum* tick showed unique migration patterns by immunoblotting and PCR/RFLP (Yu *et al.* 1993). Accordingly it would appear that *R. sibirica* is the main pathogenic spotted fever group rickettsia in China, and its southern distribution is much wider than previously supposed, reaching the latitude 40°N (Yu *et al.* 1993).

INCIDENCE

The geographic distribution of spotted fever group rickettsiae is very wide, although reliable data on the incidence or prevalence of the diseases they cause are very fragmentary, especially in developing countries. Such diseases are often undiagnosed, because their clinical signs are usually non-specific. In countries where tick-borne rickettsioses are well known and easily recognized, physicians often treat their patients without reporting the cases. Moreover, the distinct epidemiological features of each spotted fever group rickettsiosis result in totally different prevalences being reported from almost each endemic area. Data are often collected in one endemic focus, or even in a small part of an endemic area, and it is difficult, therefore, to compare such information (WHO 1993). It is also important to note that serological studies do not automatically indicate the presence of pathogenic rickettsiae, as there is extensive serological cross-reactivity between these organisms and the non-pathogenic species (Hechemy *et al.* 1989). However, in the 1980s, a widespread and increased incidence of spotted fever cases was been reported from different Mediterranean countries (Otero *et al.* 1982; Raoult *et al.* 1984; Mansueto *et al.* 1986).

SPOTTED FEVERS: THE DISEASES

PATHOGENESIS

Like other rickettsiae, the main cellular targets of spotted fever group organisms are endothelial and smooth muscle cells of peripheral vessels. Following tick bite, the vascular walls are infected following haematogenous and lymphogenous spread of the organism. The entry of rickettsiae into the endothelial cells seems to be due to a receptor-mediated mechanism. If the *in vitro* model of rickettsial infection reflects what happens *in vivo*, it is likely that the organisms spread from one infected cell to the other, without inducing the rupture of target cells, like typhus group rickettsiae. Vascular damage leads to an increased vascular permeability, oedema, hypotension, and hypovolaemia. In severe forms of the disease, renal failure and non-cardiogenic pulmonary oedema are observed. Digestive and neurological signs may also be present. Due to the same pathology, but more easy to see, the cutaneous rash and the eschar at the bite site are distinctive signs of spotted fever group rickettsioses (Walker *et al.* 1987).

CLINICAL FEATURES

Nine species of spotted fever group rickettsiae are now recognized as human pathogens. Until recently, the endemic areas of the diseases were distinct and no overlap had been observed. We now know that at least in the south and the east of the African continent, there are two different spotted fever group rickettsiae coexisting in the same areas and causing different clinical signs of disease in man. Since more and more tourist activity is bringing people into contact with the ecological niches of foreign rickettsioses (safari, trekking, camping) it is useful to mention the main clinical features accompanying the infection induced by each of these different pathogens.

Common features for spotted fever group rickettsioses are fever, headache, cutaneous maculopapular rash, the distribution of which includes palms and soles, an inoculation eschar at the tick-bite site, associated with local lymphadenopathy. Depending on the aetiological rickettsial strain, some of these clinical signs may be absent. Therefore, the diagnosis may be delayed or incorrect, resulting in inappropriate treatments and in severe forms of the disease. Severe forms of both Mediterranean and Rocky Mountain spotted fever have been observed in patients with glucose 6-phosphate dehydrogenase deficiency. Old age, cardiac insufficiency, diabetes, alcoholism, heavy smoking, and respiratory insufficiency have also been mentioned as predisposing factors for the development of severe forms of spotted fever (Walker and Kirkman 1981; Raoult *et al.* 1986*a,b*)

Mediterranean spotted fever

Although *R. conorii* has always been considered to produce a less severe disease than *R. rickettsii*, severe forms are reported in 6 per cent of patients, and the mortality rate may reach 2.5 per cent. For this reason we can not consider it to be a mild form of spotted fever. Because of the frequent lack of several classical clinical features, a diagnosis score has been proposed to facilitate the diagnosis of this disease (Table 21.2) (Raoult *et al.* 1993). The onset of signs is generally

Table 21.2 Diagnostic score for Mediterranean spotted fever (according to Raoult *et al.* 1993)

	Points
Epidemiological criteria	
Life or recent travel in endemic area	2
Onset between May and September	2
Contact with dog ticks	2
Clinical criteria	
Fever higher than 39 °C	5
Eschar ('*tache noire*')	5
Maculopapular or purpuric eruption	5
Two of the three clinical criteria	3
The three clinical criteria together	5
Unspecific biological criteria	
Platelet count < $150 \times 10^9/1$	1
Liver enzymes > 50 IU/1	1
Bacteriological criteria	
Isolation of *Rickettsia conorii* from blood	25
Detection of *Rickettsia conorii* in skin biopsy using IFA	25
Serological criteria	
Sole serum with total Ig ≥ 1:128	5
Sole serum with IgG ≥ 1:128 and IgM ≥ 1:64	10
2 sera with fourfold titre elevation within 2 weeks	20

A total score > 25 is consistent with a presumptive diagnosis of Mediterranean spotted fever.
IFA, indirect immunofluorescence assay.

abrupt and typical cases have fever (>39 °C), rash, and eschar. Headache, myalgia, and arthralgia are characteristic accompanying symptoms of boutonneuse fever. Malignant forms have a petechial rash, neurological, renal, or cardiac problems, especially in elderly people (Raoult *et al.* 1986*a*). Thrombosis of the deep venous vessels and acute pericarditis have also been mentioned as complications of boutonneuse fever Drancourt *et al.* 1991; Landau *et al.* 1992)

Siberian tick typhus

This disease has been well described in the former USSR, where literature relating to spotted fever and typhus group rickettsioses is abundant. Its incubation period is usually 4–7 days after the tick bite. Thereafter, an ulcerated necrotic lesion appears at the inoculation site, often accompanied by regional lymphadenophaty. Fever (38–39 °C), headache, myalgia, and digestive disturbances are concomitant symptoms and can last for 6–10 days without treatment. The rash, which may be purpuric, usually occurs 2–4 days after the onset of clinical symptoms. The central nervous system is often affected during infection. This disease is considered to be a mild form of spotted fever and it is seldom associated with complications (Rehacek and Tarasevich 1988).

African tick bite fever

The first case that could reliably be attributed to infection with *R. africae*, was reported from Zimbabwe in 1992 (Kelly *et al.* 1992*a*). Although only one case has been described so far, the clinical features of the patient correspond to those described at the beginning of the century in Mozambique (Sant'Anna 1912)

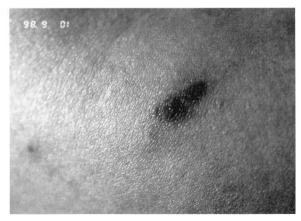

Fig. 21.14   Inoculation eschars in a case of African tick-bite fever, due to multiple bites of larvae of *A. hebraeum* (kindly supplied by Dr. Harle)

and South Africa, in people living in rural rather than urban areas. At that time it was called the 'forme fruste' of Mediterranean spotted fever (Pijper 1936). In this disease, headache, fever, eschar (Fig. 21.14) at the tick bite site, and regional lymphadenopathy are the usual clinical findings. Since these signs could also be attributed to Mediterranean spotted fever, it is understandable that the two diseases have long been confused. However, a cutaneous rash is lacking or very transient in African tick bite fever cases (Kelly *et al.* 1994).

Queensland tick typhus and Flinder Island spotted fever

Even though Queensland tick typhus has been recognized as a disease since 1946 when the first cases were observed amongst Australian troops training in the bush of Northern Queensland, only 21 cases were reported subsequently until 1989. More recently, the number of reported cases has increased to 62, showing that rickettsioses are widespread all along the eastern Australian coast (Sexton *et al.* 1991*a,b*). However, the causative agents are not the same. *Rickettsia australis*, which is the aetiologic agent of Queensland tick typhus, is clearly prevalent in the north, while *R. honei* has been isolated from patients in the Flinder Islands, which are localized in an archipelago near Tasmania in the far south of the country. The distribution areas of the two organisms have yet to be established. Although *R. australis* and *R. honei* show clear biological and genotypical differences (Baird *et al.* 1992), the clinical features of the diseases they cause are quite similar. After an abrupt onset, characterized by fever, headache, and myalgia, patients usually develop a rash (maculopapular or vesicular) within the first 10 days. An eschar seems to be more prevalent in cases from the north (65 per cent) than in Flinder Island spotted fever patients (28 per cent). Bites clearly associated with ticks are reported more often in the north than in the south, where lesions attributed to 'insect' bites are, however, frequently mentioned. Lymphadenopathy is a common features in both diseases, even though its prevalence is slightly higher in the classical Queensland tick typhus. The two diseases are regarded as mild forms of spotted fever group rickettsioses, with 30 per cent of patients recovering despite inappropriate treatment. Fifty per cent of patients were hospitalized, however, and a severe form of Flinders Island spotted fever developed in one elderly patient. A single fatal case of Queensland tick typhus has been reported to date.

Japanese spotted fever or Oriental spotted fever

The first reports of spotted fever group rickettsiosis in Japan date back to 1984 (Uchida 1993; Uchida *et al.*

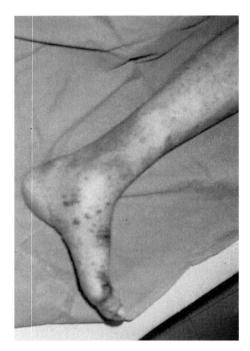

Fig. 21.15 Rash due to an infection with *Rickettsia japonica* (kindly supplied by Dr Mahara).

1985). During the following years several isolates were obtained from patients, mainly in the south-eastern areas of Japan. The disease has an abrupt onset, with headache and high fever (39–40 °C), followed by the occurrence of a macular rash, sometimes petechial and haemorrhagic. The rash is found all over the body, including palms and soles. Eschars at the bite site (Fig. 21.15) are often reported and tick bites recalled, but the vector of the disease has yet to be determined (Uchida *et al.* 1986). Severe forms have not been reported and the defervescence seems to occur about 10 days after the onset of the disease even after inappropriate treatment.

Israeli spotted fever

The first cases of rickettsial spotted fever in Israel were reported in the late 1940s, and were diagnosed as Rocky Mountain spotted fever. The number of cases increased following the progression of new settlements in the rural areas of Israel. Although the disease shares the main clinical features of Mediterranean spotted fever, the typical eschar at the inoculation site is usually lacking. Several fatal cases and severe forms have been described, and the prevalence of the disease seems to be increasing (Gross and Yagupsky 1987; Goldwasser *et al.* 1974*a*). An epidemiological survey showed that amongst infected children, 74 per cent of

patients were male and 74 per cent less than 9 years old. The incubation period was estimated at about 7–8 days after tick bite. Symptoms observed in 100 per cent of the cases were fever and rash, which usually started on hands and feets and extended centripetally. The prevalence of arthralgia, headache, vomiting, and myalgia varied from 13 to 33 per cent. A primary lesion, resembling a small pinkish papule rather than a real eschar, was found less often (7 per cent) than spleno- or hepatomegaly (35, and 30 per cent, respectively) (Gross and Yagupsky 1987).

Astrakhan spotted fever

This disease has clinical features similar to those of Israeli spotted fever and Mediterranean spotted fever. It is more frequently diagnosed in males (61 per cent) than in females. The first signs are high fever (38–39 °C) and rash (Fig. 21.16) which seldom develops into a petechial form (14 per cent). An eschar is present in only 23 per cent of patients, while severe headache and myalgia are reported frequently (>80 per cent). Severe or lethal forms have not been described to date (Tarasevich *et al.* 1991*a,b*).

Rickettsialpox

The onset of this mild disease usually occurs 7–10 days after a mite bite. At the inoculation site a painless red

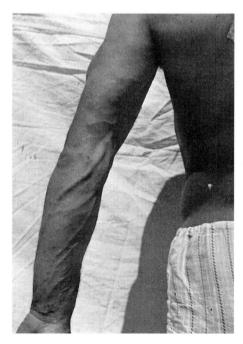

Fig. 21.16 Cutaneous eruption in a case of Astrakhan spotted fever (kindly supplied by Dr Tarasevich).

papule appears and becomes vesicular over the following days. The scab that usually appears when the vesicular lesion bursts persists for about 3 weeks. Regional lymph nodes may be slightly enlarged. Fever appears suddenly, accompanied by chills, headache, myalgia, anorexia, and photophobia. The rash sometimes develops simultaneously with these signs, but may also develop several days later. Cutaneous lesions are maculopapular and develop into a vesicular form. When the vesicles dry out, they are usually replaced by crusts, which do not produce scars. Even if not treated, patients recover spontaneously in 1–3 weeks. Varicella and, in the early stage of rickettsialpox, other rickettsioses have to be considered in the differential diagnosis of this disease (Saah and Hornick 1985, Christie 1987).

DIAGNOSIS

Rickettsial infection is sugested when, fever, headache, and rash occur during the tick season. The presently recognized diagnostic method is based on indirect immunofluorescence. IgG titres of 1/128 and greater and IgM of 1/64 or or more, or seroconversion with a twofold increase in titres over a 2-week period are regarded as sufficient for diagnosis (Raoult et al. 1993). Although this method and Western immunoblotting (Raoult and Dasch 1989) can be used to confirm a suspected case of spotted fever, they can not determine the causative agent of the rickettsiosis. Furthermore, serological seroconversions usually do not occur in the early phases of the disease; an appropriate treatment must therefore be instituted on a clinical basis. Direct isolation of rickettsiae from patient material is necessary for definitive diagnosis. However, this procedure is lengthy and can only be used for confirming a previous diagnosis of rickettsiosis. Indirect immunofluorescence assays performed on skin biopsies of the cutaneous rash is a further technique enabling rapid diagnosis, it is, however, useless in spotless forms of the disease (Woodward and Hornick 1985). ELISA tests based on the specific properties of monoclonal antibodies have recently been developed for the direct determination of causative agents of spotted fevers (Radulovic et al. 1993). Since the practical use of such technique requires a complete panel of monoclonal antibodies directed specifically against all 22 recognized strains, it does not seem to be applicable in the near future. PCR/RFLP techniques, once adapted to the detection of rickettsiae in blood samples, could greatly facilitate the identification of the causative agent.

TREATMENT AND PROPHYLAXIS

In vitro antibiotic susceptibility tests have been performed using the two main representatives of the spotted fever group rickettsiae, *R. conorii* and *R. rickettsii*. The assays were first carried out using embryonated eggs, and later on cell culture monolayers. In these models, tetracycline and doxycycline have been shown to be highly effective, although rifampin and chloramphenicol may also be effective. The quinolone antibiotics (ciprofloxacin, ofloxacin and pefloxacin) have recently proved to be effective in treating adults with Mediterranean spotted fever. Studies are now under way to establish whether josamicin, which could become the treatment of choice for children and pregnant women, is effective (Raoult 1989; Drancourt and Raoult 1993).

Initial vaccination studies were made by Ricketts, who established that blood and sera collected from laboratory animals which had recovered from Rocky Mountain spotted fever were protective when inoculated into other animals (Ricketts and Gomez 1908). In other early studies, laboratory animals were vaccinated with phenolized emulsions of infected ticks (Spencer and Parker 1925) and later these trials were carried out on monkeys (Kenyon et al. 1975; Sammons et al. 1976), guinea-pigs, and human volunteers (Clements et al. 1983). Although these vaccines induced protection in laboratory animals, they were never applied on a large scale in medical practice (Ascher et al. 1978; Kenyon et al. 1979), because their effectiveness in protecting man could not be clearly established. As a result of antibiotic therapy being shown to be very effective, vaccination trials have been suspended (Woodward 1986).

Prophylactic antibiotic treatment of people reporting recent tick bites has been proposed (Kenyon et al. 1978). Since the antibiotics of choice are bacteriostatic, rather than bactericidal, prophylactic treatment, by reducing the immune reaction of the infected individuals, induces a delayed disease instead of preventing it.

The best prophylactic measures are those aimed at avoiding tick bites. In rural areas infested by ticks, repellents can be applied to the clothing and the skin. Insecticides are usually commercially available for the control of ticks on domestic animals. This may not be sufficient in the case of dog ticks, such as *Rhipicephalus sanguineus*, which can survive for long periods in the protected environment of human dwellings. Apartments infested by this tick species have been found in the centre of France and in Switzerland, regions far removed from the ticks' natural distribution area. Micro-outbreaks of boutonneuse fever have occurred in Switzerland 6 years after the introduction of ticks on a pet dog into an apartment (Péter et al. 1984). Ticks were found not only on the dog, but also in cupboards, drawers, and behind furniture against the wall. The presence of infected ticks outside the endemic area may be responsible for a spotted fever infection which become hard to diagnose, especially if the patient does not remember travel to endemic areas years previously. Once the tick has attached it is necessary to remove it as soon as possible, as the transmission of infectious organisms appears to occur only 20 hours after tick attachment, but detection of feeding ticks is often difficult, as larvae may be less than 1 mm in length, even after engorging.

ACKNOWLEDGEMENTS

Special thanks to Professor Patrick J. Kelly for reviewing the English manuscript.

REFERENCES

Anacker, R. L., McCaul, T. F., Burgdorfer, W., and Gerloff, R. K. (1980). Properties of selected rickettsiae of the spotted fever group. *Infection and Immunity*, **27**, 468–74.

Anacker, R. L., *et al.* (1983). Biological properties of rabbit antibodies to a surface antigen of *Rickettsia rickettsii*. *Infection and Immunity*, **40**, 292–8.

Anacker, R. L., List, R. H., Mann, R. E., Hayes, S. F., and Thomas, L. A. (1985). Characterization of monoclonal antibodies protecting mice against *Rickettsia rickettsii*. *Journal of Infectious Diseases*, **151**, 1052–60.

Anacker, R. L., Mann, R. E., and Gonzales, C. (1987). Reactivity of monoclonal antibodies to *Rickettsia rickettsii* with spotted fever and typhus group rickettsiae. *Journal of Clinical Microbiology*, **25**, 167–71.

Ascher, M. S., Oster, C. N., Harber, P. I., Kenyon, R. H., and Pedersen, C. E. (1978). Initial clinical evaluation of a new Rocky Mountain spotted fever vaccine of tissue culture origin. *Journal of Infectious Diseases*, **138**, 217–21.

Bacellar, F., Regnery, R. L., Núncio, M. S., and Filipe A. R. (1995). Genotypic evaluation of rickettsial isolates recovered from various species of ticks in Portugal. *Epidemiology and Infection*, **114**, 169–78.

Baird, R. W., Lloyd, M., Stenos, J., Ross, B. C., Stewart, R. S., and Dwyer, B. (1992). Characterization and comparison of Australian human spotted fever group rickettsiae. *Journal of Clinical Microbiology*, **30**, 2896–902.

Balayeva, N. M. *et al.* (1993). Genotypic and biological characterisics of non-identified strain of spotted fever group rickettsiae isolated in Crimea *Acta Virologica*, **37**, 475–83.

Beati, L. and Raoult, D. (1993). *Rickettsia massiliae* sp.nov., a new spotted fever group rickettsia. *International Journal of Systematic Bacteriology*, **43**, 839–40.

Beati, L., Finidori, J. -P., Gilot, B., and Raoult, D. (1992). Comparison of microimmunofluorescence serologic typing, sodium dodecyl sulfate-polyacrylamide gel electrophoresis, and polymerase chain reaction followed by restriction fragment length polymorphism analysis for identification of rickettsiae: characterization of two new rickettsial strains. *Journal of Clinical Microbiology*, **30**, 1922–30.

Beati, L., Finidori, J. -P., and Raoult, D. (1993*a*). First isolation of *Rickettsia slovaca* from *Dermacentor marginatus* in France. *American Journal of Tropical Medicine and Hygiene*, **48**, 257–68.

Beati, L., Humair, P. -F., Aeschlimann, A., and Raoult, D. (1993*b*). Identification of spotted fever group rickettsiae isolated from *Dermacentor marginatus* and *Ixodes ricinus* ticks collected in Switzerland. *American Journal of Tropical Medicine and Hygiene*, **5**, 138–48.

Beati, L., Péter, O., Burgdorfer, W., Aeschlimann, A., and Raoult, D. (1993*c*). Confirmation that *Rickettsia helvetica* sp. nov., is a distinct species of the spotted fever group of rickettsiae. *International Journal of Systematic Bacteriology*, **43**, 521–6.

Beati, L., Kelly, P. J., Mason, P. R., and Raoult, D. (1994). Species-specific Balb/c mouse antibodies to rickettsiae studied by western blotting. *FEMS Microbiology Letters*, **119**, 339–44.

Bell, E. J. and Stoenner, H. G. (1960). Immunologic relationships among the spotted fever group of rickettsias determined by toxin neutralization tests in mice with convalescent animal serums. *Journal of Immunology*, **84**, 171–82.

Boinet, J. and Piéri, J. (1927). Epidémies d'exanthème infectieux. *La Presse Medicale*, **89**, 3–15.

Burgdorfer, W., and Brinton, L. P. (1975). Mechanisms of transovarial infection of spotted fever rickettsiae in ticks. *Annals New York Academy of Sciences*, **266**, 61–72.

Burgdorfer, W. and Varma, M. G. R. (1967). Trans-stadial and transovarial development of disease agents in arthropods. In *Annual Review of Entomology*, (ed. R. F. Smith and T. E. Mittler), pp. 347–76. Annual Reviews, Palo Alto.

Burgdorfer, W., Ormsbee, R. A., Schmidt, M. L., and Hoogstraal, H. (1973). A search for the epidemic typhus agent in Ethiopian ticks. *Bulletin of the World Health Organization*, **48**, 563–9.

Bustamante, M. E. and Varela, G. (1947). Distribucion de las rickettsiasis en Mexico. *Revista del Instituto de salubridady enfermedades tropicales*, **8**, 3–14.

Camicas, J. -L. (1975). Conceptions actuelles sur l'épidémiologie de la fièvre boutonneuse dans la région éthiopienne et la sous-région européenne méditerranéenne. *Cahiers de l' ORSTOM, ser Ent. med. Parsitol.*, **13**, 229–32.

Charters, A. D. (1946). Tick-typhus in Abyssinia. *Transactions of the Royal Society of Tropical Medicine and Hygiene*, **39**, 335–42.

Christie, A. B. (1987). Rickettsial disease: typhus. In *Infectious diseases: epidemiology and clinical practice*, pp. 1070–97. Churchill Livingstone, Edinburgh.

Clements, M. L. *et al.* (1983). Reactogenicity, immunogenicity, and efficacy of a chick embryo cell-derived vaccine for Rocky Mountain spotted fever. *Journal of Infectious Diseases*, **148**, 922–30.

Conor, A. and Bruch, A. (1910). Une fièvre éruptive observée en Tunisie. *Bulletin de la Société de Pathologie exotique*, **8**, 492–6.

Crocquet-Valdes, P. A., Weiss, K, and Walker, D. H. (1994). Sequence analysis of the 190-kDa antigen-encoding gene of *Rickettsia conorii* (Malish 7 strain). *Gene*, **140**, 115–19.

Drancourt, M. and Raoult, D. (1993). Antimicrobial therapy of rickettsial spotted fever. In *Antimicrobial agents and intracellular pathogens*, (ed. D. Raoult), pp. 139–53. CRC Press, Boca Raton.

Drancourt, M., Brouqui, P., Chiche, G., and Raoult, D. (1991). Acute pericarditis in Mediterranean spotted fever. *Transactions of the Royal Society of Tropical Medicine and Hygiene*, **85**, 799.

Drancourt, M., Kelly, P. J., Regnery, R. L., and Raoult, D. (1992). Identification of spotted fever group rickettsiae using polymerase chain reaction and restriction endonuclease length polymorphism analysis. *Acta Virologica*, **36**, 1–6.

Durand, P. (1932). Rôle du chien comme réservoir de virus dans la fièvre boutonneuse. *Archives de l'Institut Pasteur de Tunis*, **21**, 239–50.

El Dessouky, A., Manor, E. A., Lange, J. V., and Azad, A. F. (1991). Detection of spotted fever group rickettsiae in ticks from the North Sinai, Egypt. In *Rickettsiae and rickettsial diseases*, (ed. J. Kazar and D. Raoult), pp. 383–7. Publishing House of the Slovak Academy of Sciences, Bratislava.

Eremeeva, M. E., Balayeva, N. M., Ignatovich, V. F., and Raoult, D. (1993). Proteinic and genomic identification of spotted fever group rickettsiae isolated in the former USSR. *Journal of Clinical Microbiology*, **31**, 2625–33.

Eremeeva, M., Yu, X. J., and Raoult, D. (1994*a*). Differentiation among spotted fever group rickettsiae species by analysis of restriction fragment length polymorphism of PCR-amplified DNA. *Journal of Clinical Microbiology*, **32**, 803–810.

Eremeeva, M. E. *et al.* (1994*b*). Astrakhan fever rickettsiae: antigenic and genotypic analysis of isolates obtained from human and *Rhipicephalus pumilio* ticks. *American Journal of Tropical Medicine and Hygiene*, **51**, 697–706.

Espejo, E., Alegre M. D., Font, B., Font, A., Segura, F., and Bella, F. (1993). Antibodies to *Rickettsia conorii* in dogs: seasonal differences. *European Journal of Epidemiology*, **9**, 344–6.

Fan, M. Y. *et al.* (1987*a*). Rickettsial and serologic evidence for prevalent spotted fever rickettsiosis in inner mongolia. *American Journal of Tropical Medicine and Hygiene*, **36**, 615–20.

Fan, M. Y., Walker, D. H., Yu, S. R., and Liu, Q. H. (1987*b*). Epidemiology and ecology of rickettsial diseases in the People's Republic of China. *Reviews of Infectious diseases*, **9**, 823–40.

Fan, M. Y., Yu, X. J., and Walker, D. H. (1988). Antigenic analysis of Chinese strains of spotted fever group rickettsiae by protein immunoblotting. *American Journal of Tropical Medicine and Hygiene*, **39**, 497–501.

Feng, H. M., Kirkman, C. and Walker, D. H. (1986). Radioimmunoprecipitation of [^{35}S] methionine-radiolabeled proteins of *Rickettsia conorii* and *Rickettsia rickettsii*. *Journal of Infectious Diseases*, **154**, 717–21.

Feng, H. M., Walker, D. H., and Wang, J. G. (1987). Analysis of T-dependent and -independent antigens of *Rickettsia conorii* with monoclonal antibodies. *Infection and Immunity*, **55**, 7–15.

Gage, K. L. and Jerrells, T. R. (1992). Demonstration and partial characterization of antigens of *Rickettsia rhipicephali* that induce cross-reactive cellular and humoral immune responses to *Rickettsia rickettsii*. *Infection and Immunity*, **60**, 5099–106.

Gage, K. L., Schrumpf, M. E., Karstens, R. H., Burgdorfer, W., and Schwan, T. G. (1994). DNA typing of rickettsiae in naturally infected ticks using a polymerase chain reaction/ restriction fragment length polymorphism system. *American Journal of Tropical Medicine and Hygiene*, **50**, 247–60.

Gear, J. H. S. (1954). The rickettsial diseases of southern Africa. *South African Journal of Clinical Science*, **5**, 158–75.

Gear, J. H. S. and Douthwaite, M. (1938). The dog tick *Haemaphysalis leachi* as a vector of tick typhus. *South African Medical Journal*, **12**, 53–5.

Gilmore, R. D. (1990) Characterization of the 120-kDa surface protein gene of *Rickettsia rickettsii* (R strain). In *Rickettsiology: current issues and perspectives*, (ed. K. E. Hechemy, D. Paretsky, D. H. Walker, and L. P. Mallavia), pp. 459–67. Annals of the New York Academy of Sciences, New York.

Gilmore, R. D. and Hackstadt, T. (1991). DNA polymorphism in the conserved 190 kDa antigen gene repeat region among spotted fever group rickettsiae. *Biochimica et Biophysica Acta*, **1097**, 77–80.

Gilmore, R. D., Joste, N., and McDonald, G. A. (1989). Cloning, expression and sequence analysis of the gene encoding the 120 kD surface-exposed protein of *Rickettsia rickettsii*. *Molecular Microbiology*, **3**, 1579–86.

Gilmore, R. D., Cieplak, W., Policastro, P. F., and Hackstadt, T. (1991). The 120 kilodalton outer membrane protein (rOmp B) of *Rickettsia rickettsii* is encoded by an unusually long open reading frame: evidence for protein processing from a large precursor. *Molecular Microbiology*, **5**, 2361–70.

Gilot, B. (1984). Biologie et écologie de *Rhipicephalus sanguineus* (Latreille, 1806) (Acariens: Ixodoidea) dans le sud-est de la France. *Sciences Vétérinaires et Médicales Comparées*, **86**, 25–33.

Goldwasser, R. A., Klingberg, M. A., Klingberg, W., Steinman, Y., and Swartz, T. A. (1974*a*). Laboratory and epidemiologic studies of rickettsial spotted fever in Israel. *Frontiers of Internal Medicine, 12th Int. Congr. Internal Med., Tel Aviv*, pp. 270–5 270–5.

Goldwasser, R. A., Steinman, Y., Klingberg, W., Swrtz, T. A., and Klingberg, M. A. (1974*b*). The isolation of strains of rickettsiae of the spotted fever group in Israel and their differentiation from other members of the group by immunofluorescence methods. *Scandinavian Journal of Infectious Diseases*, **6**, 53–62.

Gross, E. M. and Yagupsky, P. (1987). Israeli rickettsial spotted fever in children. *Acta Tropica*, **44**, 91–6.

Hackstadt, T., Messer, R., Cieplak, W., and Peacock, M. G. (1992). Evidence for proteolytic cleavage of the 120-kilodalton outer membrane protein of rickettsiae: identification of an avirulent mutant deficient in processing. *Infection and Immunity*, **60**, 159–65.

Hamilton, J. G. C. (1992). The role of pheromones in tick biology. *Parasitology Today*, **8**, 130–3.

Hayes, S. F., Burgdorfer, W., and Aeschlimann, A. (1980). Sexual transmission of spotted fever group rickettsiae by infected male ticks: detection of rickettsiae in immature spermatozoa of *Ixodes ricinus*. *Infection and Immunity*, **27**, 638–42.

Hechemy, K. E., Raoult, D., Fox, J., Han, Y., Elliott, L. B., and Rawlings, J. (1989). Cross-reactions of immune sera from patients with rickettsial diseases. *Journal of Medicine and Microbiology*, **29**, 199–202.

Heinzen, R. A., Hayes, S. F., Peacock, M. G., and Hackstadt, T. (1993). Directional actin polymerization associated with spotted fever group rickettsia infection of Vero cells. *Infection and Immunity*, **61**, 1926–35.

Heisch, R. B., McPhee, R., and Rickman, L. R. (1957). The epidemiology of tick-typhus in Nairobi. *East African Medical Journal*, **34**, 459–77.

Heisch, R. B., Grainger, W. E., Harwey, A. E., and Lister, G. (1962). Feral aspects of rickettsial infections in Kenya. *Transactions of the Royal Society of Tropical Medicine and Hygiene*, **56**, 272–86.

Hoogstraal, H. (1956). *African Ixodoidea. I. Ticks of the Sudan (with special reference to Equatoria Province and with preliminary reviews of the genera* Boophilus. Margaropus, and Hyalomma). Dep. US Navy, Bur. Med. Surg., Washington, DC.

Hoogstraal, H. (1967). Ticks in relation to human diseases caused by rickettsia species. *Annual Review of Entomology*, **12**, 377–420.

Ito, S. and Rikihisa, Y. (1981). Techniques for electron microscopy of rickettsiae. In *Rickettsiae and rickettsial diseases*, (ed. W. Burgdorfer and R. L. Anacker), pp. 213–27. Academic Press, New York.

Iwamasa, K., Okada, T., Tange, Y., and Kobayashi, Y. (1992). Ultrastructural study of the response of cells infected *in vitro* with causative agent of spotted fever group rickettsiosis in Japan. *APMIS*, **100**, 535–42.

Kelly, P. J. and Mason, P. R. (1990). Serological typing of spotted fever group rickettsia isolates from Zimbabwe. *Journal of Clinical Microbiology*, **28**, 2302–4.

Kelly, P. J. and Mason, P. R. (1991). Transmission of a spotted fever group rickettsia by *Amblyomma hebraeum* (Acari: Ixodidae). *Medical Entomology*, **28**, 598–600.

Kelly, P. J., Mason, P. R., Manning, T., and Slater, S. (1991a). Role of cattle in the epidemiology of tick-bite fever in Zimbabwe. *Journal of Clinical Microbiology*, **29**, 256–9.

Kelly, P. J., Mason, P. R., Rhode, C., Dziva, F., and Matthewman, L. A. (1991b). Transient infections of goats with a novel spotted fever group rickettsia from Zimbabwe. *Research in Veterinary Science*, **51**, 268–71.

Kelly, P. J. et al. (1992a). African tick-bite fever: a new spotted fever group rickettsiosis under an old name. *Lancet*, **340**, 982–3.

Kelly, P. J., Matthewman, L. A., Mason, P. R., Courtney, S., Katsanda, C., and Ruhwaka, J. (1992b). Experimental infection of dogs with a Zimbabwean strain of *Rickettsia conorii*. *Journal of Tropical Medicine and Hygiene*, **95**, 322–6.

Kelly, P. J., Beati, L., Matthewman, L. A., Mason, P. R., and Raoult, D. (1994). A new pathogenic spotted fever group rickettsia from Africa. *Journal of Tropical Medicine and Hygiene*, **97**, 129–37.

Kenyon, R. H., Sammons, L. S., and Pedersen, C. E. (1975). Comparison of three Rocky Mountain spotted fever vaccine. *Journal of Clinical Microbiology*, **2**, 300–4.

Kenyon, R. H., Williams, R. G., Oster, C. N., and Pedersen, C. E. (1978). Prophylactic treatment of Rocky Mountain spotted fever. *Journal of Clinical Microbiology*, **8**, 102–4.

Kenyon, R. H., Kishimoto, R. A., and Hall, W. C. (1979). Exposure of guinea pigs to *Rickettsia rickettsii* by aerosol, nasal, conjunctival, gastric, and subcutaneous routes and protection afforded by an experimental vaccine. *Infection and Immunity*, **25**, 580–2.

Landau, Z., Feld, S., Kunichezky, S., Grinspan, M., and Gorbacz, M. (1992). Thrombosis of the mesenteric vein as a complication of Mediterranean spotted fever. *Clinical Infectious Diseases*, **15**, 1070–1.

Li, H., Lenz, B., and Walker, D. H. (1988). Protective monoclonal antibodies recognize heat-labile epitopes on surface proteins of spotted fever group rickettsiae. *Infection and Immunity*, **56**, 2587–93.

McDonald, G. A., Anacker, R. L., and Garjian, K. (1987). Cloned gene of *Rickettsia rickettsii* surface antigen: candidate vaccine for Rocky mountain spotted fever. *Science*, **235**, 83–4.

Mansueto, S., Tringali, G., and Walker, D. H. (1986). Widespread, simultaneous increase in the incidence of spotted fever group rickettsioses. *Journal of Infectious Diseases*, **154**, 539–40.

Okada, T., Tange, Y., and Kobayashi, Y. (1990). Causative agent of spotted fever group rickettsiosis in Japan. *Infection and Immunity*, **58**, 887–92.

Olmer, D. and Olmer, J. (1957a). Epidémie des rickettsioses sur le littoral méditerranéen. La fièvre boutonneuse. *Revue de Pathologie Générale et Comparée*, 80–92.

Olmer, D. and Olmer, J. (1957b). Répartition géographique actuelle de la fièvre boutonneuse. *Marseille Médical*, **94**, 525–36.

O'Neill, S. L., Giordano, R., Colbert, A. M. E., Karr, T. L., and Robertson, H. M. (1992). 16S rRNA phylogenetic analysis of the bacterial endosymbionts associated with cytoplasmic incompatibility in insects. *Proceedings of the National Academy of Sciences USA*, **89**, 2699– 702.

Ormsbee, R. A. et al. (1978). Antigenic relationships between the typhus and spotted fever groups of rickettsiae. *American Journal of Epidemiology*, **108**, 53–9.

Osterman, J. V. and Eisemann, C. S. (1978). Surface proteins of typhus and spotted fever group rickettsiae. *Infection and Immunity*, **21**, 866–73.

Otero, R., Fenoll, A., and Casal, J. (1982). Resurgence of Mediterranean spotted fever. *Lancet*, ii, 1107.

Pavis, C. and Barré, N. (1993). Kinetics of male pheromone production by *Amblyomma variegatum* (Acari: Ixodidae). *Journal of Medical Entomology*, **30**, 961–5.

Pedersen, C. E. and Walters, V. D. (1978). Comparative electrophoresis of spotted fever group rickettsial proteins. *Life Science*, **22**, 583–8.

Péter, O. (1985). Présence d'anticorps contre la 'Rickettsie suisse' chez les mammifères sauvages et domestiques du Canton de Neuchâtel. *Schweizerische Archive für Tierheilkunde*, **127**, 461–8.

Péter, O., Burgdorfer, W., Aeschlimann, A., and Chatelanat, P. (1984). *Rickettsia conorii* isolated from *Rhipicephalus sanguineus* introduced into Switzerland on a pet dog. *Zeitschrift für Parasitenkunde*, **70**, 265–70.

Philip, C. B., Hoogstraal, H., Reiss-Gutfreund, R., and Clifford, C. M. (1966). Evidence of rickettsial disease agents in ticks from Ethiopian cattle. *Bulletin of the World Health Organization*, **35**, 127–31.

Philip, R. N., Casper, E. A., Ormsbee, R. A., Peacock, M. G., and Burgdorfer, W. (1976). Microimmunofluorescence test for the serological study of Rocky Mountain spotted fever and typhus. *Journal of Clinical Microbiology*, **3**, 51–61.

Philip, R. N., Casper, E. A., Burgdorfer, W., Gerloff, R. K., Hughes, L. E., and Bell, E. J. (1978). Serologic typing of rickettsiae of the spotted fever group by indirect microimmunofluorescence. *Journal of Immunology*, **121**, 1961–8.

Pijper, A. (1936). Etude expérimentale comparée de la fièvre boutonneuse et de la tick-bite-fever. *Archives de l'Institut Pasteur de Tunis*, **25**, 388–401.

Plotz, H., Reagan, R. L., and Wertman, K. (1944). Differentiation between Fièvre boutonneuse and Rocky Mountain spotted fever by means of complement fixation. *Proceedings of the Society of Experimental Biology and Medicine*, **55**, 173–6.

Popov, V. L., Dyuisalieva, R. G., Smirnova, N. S., Tarasevich, I. V., and Rybkina, N. N. (1986). Ultrastructure of *Rickettsia sibirica* during interaction with the host cell. *Acta Virologica*, **30**, 494–8.

Pretzman, C., Stothard, D. R., Ralph, D., and Fuerst, P. A. (1994). A new species of rickettsia, isolated from the lone star tick, *Amblyomma americanum* (Ixodidae). *11th Sesqui-Annual Meeting, American Society for Rickettsiology and Rickettsial Diseases, St. Simons Island, Georgia, USA*, 24 (Abstract).

Radulovic, S., Speed, R., Feng, H. M., Taylor, C., and Walker, D. H. (1993). EIA with species-specific monoclonal antibodies: a novel seroepidemiologic tool for determination of the ethiologic agent of spotted fever rickettsiosis. *Journal of Infectious Diseases*, **168**, 1292–5.

Raoult, D. (1988). Rickettsioses en dehors de la fièvre Q. *Encyclopédie Medico-Chirurgicale (Paris–France), Maladies Infectieuses 8077 G10*, **3**, 1–18.

Raoult, D. (1989). Antibiotic susceptibility of rickettsia and treatment of rickettsioses. *European Journal of Epidemiology*, **5**, 432–5.

Raoult, D. and Dasch, G. A. (1989). Line blot and Western blot immunoassays for diagnosis of Mediterranean spotted fever. *Journal of Clinical Microbiology*, **27**, 2073–9.

Raoult, D. *et al.* (1984). Recrudescence de la fièvre boutonneuse méditerranéenne dans le Sud de la France. *Méditerranée Médicale*, **3**, 47–8.

Raoult, D., Weiller, P. J., Chagnon, A., Chaudet, H., Gallais, H., and Casanova, P. (1986*a*). Mediterranean spotted fever: clinical, laboratory and epidemiological features of 199 cases. *American Journal of Tropical Medicine and Hygiene*, **35**, 845–50.

Raoult, D *et al.* (1986*b*). Incidence, clinical observations and risk factors in the severe form of Mediterranean spotted fever among patients admitted to hospital in Marseilles 1983–1984. *Journal of Infection*, **12**, 111–16.

Raoult, D., Tissot Dupont, H., Chicheportiche, C., Péter, O., Gilot, B., and Drancourt, M. (1993). Mediterranean spotted fever in Marseille, France: correlation between prevalence of hospitalized patients, seroepidemiology, and prevalence of infected ticks in three different areas. *American Journal of Tropical Medicine and Hygiene*, **48**, 249–56.

Regnery, R. L., Spruill, C. L., and Plikaytis, B. D. (1991). Genotypic identification of rickettsiae and estimation of intraspecies sequence divergence for portions of two rickettsial genes. *Journal of Bacteriology*, **173**, 1576–89.

Rehacek, J. (1984). Rickettsia slovaca, *the organism and its ecology.* Acta Scientarum Natularium Acadamiae Scientarum Bohemoslovarae Brno.

Rehacek, J. and Tarasevich, I. V. (1988). *Acari-borne rickettsiae and rickettsioses in Eurasia*, Veda publishing house of the Slovac Academy of Sciences, Bratislava.

Ricketts, H. T. and Gomez, L. (1908). Studies on immunity in Rocky Mountain spotted fever. First communication. *Journal of Infectious Diseases*, v, 221–44.

Robertson, R. G. and Wissemann, C. L. (1973). Tick-borne rickettsiae of the spotted fever group in West Pakistan. *American Journal of Epidemiology*, **97**, 55–64.

Roux, V. and Raoult, D. (1993). Genotypic identification and phylogenetic analysis of the spotted fever group rickettsiae by pulsed-field gel electrophoresis. *Journal of Bacteriology*, **175**, 4895–904.

Roux, V., Drancourt, M., and Raoult, D. (1992). Determination of genome sizes of *Rickettsia* spp. within the spotted fever group, using pulsed-field gel electrophoresis. *Journal of Bacteriology*, **174**, 7455–7.

Saah, A. J. and Hornick, R. B. (1985). Rickettsiosis. *Rickettsia akari* (Rickettsialpox). In *Principles and practice of infectious diseases*, (ed. G. L. Mandell, R. G. Douglas, and J. E. Bennett), pp. 1087–8. Wiley, New York.

Sammons, L. S., Kenyon, R. H., and Pedersen, C. E. (1976). Effect of vaccination schedule on immune response of *Macaca mulatta* to cell culture-grown Rocky Mountain spotted fever vaccine. *Journal of Clinical Microbiology*, **4**, 253–7.

Sant'Anna, J. F. (1912). On a disease in man following tick-bites and occurring in Lourenco-Marques. *Parasitology*, **9**, 87–8.

Schuenke, K. W. and Walker, D. H. (1994). Cloning, sequencing, and expression of the gene encoding for an antigenic 120-kilodalton protein of *Rickettsia conorii. Infection and Immunity*, **62**, 904–9.

Sexton, D. J., Banks, J., Graves, S., Hughes, K. and Dwyer, B. (1991*a*). Prevalence of antibodies to spotted fever group rickettsiae in dogs from southeastern Australia. *American Journal of Tropical Medicine and Hygiene*, **45**, 243–8.

Sexton, D. J., Dwyer, B., Kemp, R., and Graves, S. (1991*b*). Spotted fever group rickettsial infections in Australia. *Review of Infectious Diseases*, **13**, 876–86.

Sexton, D. J. *et al.* (1993). Brazilian spotted fever in Espirito Santo, Brazil: description of a focus of infection in a new endemic region. *American Journal of Tropical Medicine and Hygiene*, **49**, 222–6.

Silverman, D. J. (1991). Some contributions of electron microscopy to the study of the rickettsiae. *European Journal of Epidemiology*, **7**, 200–6.

Silverman, D. J., Wisseman, A. D., Waddell, A. D., and Jones, M. (1978). External layers of *Rickettsia prowazekii* and *Rickettsia rickettsii*: occurence of a slime layer. *Infection and Immunity*, **22**, 233–46.

Silverman, D. J., Wisseman, C. L., and Waddell, A. (1981). Envelopment and escape of *Rickettsia rickettsii* from host membranes. In *Rickettsiae and rickettsial diseases*, (ed. W. Burgdorfer and R. L. Anacker), pp. 241–55. Academic Press, New York.

Sirisanthana, T., Pinyopornpanit, V., Sirisanthana, V., Strickman, D., Kelly, D. J., and Dash, G. A. (1994). First cases of spotted fever group rickettsiosis in Thailand. *American Journal of Tropical Medicine and Hygiene*, **50**, 682–6.

Spencer, R. R. and Parker, R. R. (1925). Rocky Mountain spotted fever: vaccination of monkeys and man. *Public Health Reports*, **40**, 2159–78.

Stewart, R. S. (1991). Flinders Island spotted fever: a newly recognised endemic focus of tick typhus in Bass Strait. Clinical and epidemiological features. *Medical Journal of Australia*, **154**, 94–9.

Stouthamer, R. and Werren, J. H. (1993). Microbes associated with parthenogenesis in wasps of the genus *Trichogramma. Journal of Invertebrate Pathology*, **61**, 6–9.

Tarasevich, I. V. (1978). Ecology of rickettsiae and epidemiology of rickettsial diseases. In *Proceedings of the 2nd International Symposium on Rickettsiae and rickettsial diseases*, (ed. J. Kazar, R. A. Ormsbee, and I. V. Tarsevich), pp. 330–49. Veda publishing house of the Slovac Academy of Sciences, Bratislava.

Tarasevich, I. V. (1991*a*). Astrakhan fever, a spotted fever rickettsiosis. *Lancet*, **337**, (8734) 172–3.

Tarasevich, I. V., Makarova, V. A., Fetisova, N. F., Stepanov, A. V., Miskarova, E. D., and Raoult, D. (1991*b*). Studies of a 'new' rickettsiosis 'Astrakan' spotted fever. *European Journal of Epidemiology*, **7**, 294–8.

Teysseire, N., Chiche-Portiche, C., and Raoult, D. (1992). Intracellular movements of *Rickettsia conorii* and *Rickettsia typhi* based on actin polymerization. *Research in Microbiology*, **143**, 821–9.

Tissot Dupont, H., Cornet, J. -P., and Raoult, D. (1994). Identification of rickettsiae from ticks collected in the Central African Republic using the polymerase chain reaction. *American Journal of Tropical Medicine and Hygiene*, **50**, 373–80.

Turelli, M. and Hofmann, A. A. (1991). Rapid spread of an inherited incompatibility factor in California *Drosophila. Nature*, **353**, 440–2.

Tyeryar, F. J., Weiss, E., Millar, D. B., Bozeman, F. M., and Ormsbee, R. A. (1973). DNA base composition of Rickettsiae. *Science*, **180**, 415–17.

Tzianabos, T., Palmer, E. L., Obijeski, J. F., and Martin, M. L. (1974). Origin and structure of the group-specific, complement-fixing antigen of *Rickettsia rickettsii*. *Applied Microbiology*, **28**, 481–8.

Uchida, T. (1993). *Rickettsia japonica*, the etiologic agent of Oriental spotted fever. *Microbiology and Immunology*, **37**, 91–102.

Uchida, T., Mahara, F., Tsuboi, Y., and Oya, A. (1985). Spotted fever group rickettsiosis in Japan. *Japanese Journal of Medical Science and Biology*, **38**, 151–3.

Uchida, T., Tashiro, F., Funato, T., and Kitamura, Y. (1986). Isolation of a spotted fever group rickettsia from a patient with febrile exanthematous illness in Shikoku, Japan. *Microbiology and Immunology*, **30**, 1323–6.

Uchida, T., Yu, X. J., Uchiyama, T., and Walker, D. H. (1989). Identification of a unique spotted fever group rickettsia from humans in Japan. *Journal of Infectious Diseases*, **159**, 1122–6.

Uchida, T., Uchiyama, T., Kumano, K., and Walker, D. H. (1992). *Rickettsia japonica* sp. nov., the etiological agent of spotted fever group rickettsiosis in Japan. *International Journal of Systematic Bacteriology*, **42**, 303–5.

Uchiyama, T., Uchida, T., and Walker, D. H. (1990). Species-specific monoclonal antibodies to *Rickettsia japonica*, a newly identified spotted fever group rickettsia. *Journal of Clinical Microbiology*, **28**, 1177–80.

Vishwanath, S., McDonald, G. A., and Watkins, N. G. (1990). A recombinant *Rickettsia conorii* vaccine protects guinea pigs from experimental boutonneuse fever and Rocky mountain spotted fever. *Infection and Immunity*, **58**, 646–53.

Walker, D. H. (1989*a*). Rickettsioses of the spotted fever group around the world. *Journal of Dermatology*, **16**, 169–77.

Walker, D. H. (1989*b*). Rocky Mountain spotted fever: a disease in need of microbiological concern. *Clinical Microbiological Review*, **2**, 227–40.

Walker, D. H. (1991). *Biology of rickettsial diseases*. CRC Press, Boca Raton, Florida.

Walker, D. H. and Kirkman, H. N. (1981). Genetic states possibly associated with enhanced severity of Rocky Mountain spotted fever. In *Rickettsiae and rickettsial diseases*, (ed. W. Burgdorfer and R. L. Anacker), pp. 621–9. Academic Press, New York.

Walker, D. H., Herrero-Herrero, J. I., Ruiz-Beltràn, R., Bullon-Sopelana, A., and Ramos-Hidalgo, A. (1987). The pathology of fatal mediterranean spotted fever. *American Journal of Clinical Pathology*, **37**, 669–72.

Wang, J. G., Walker, D. H., Li, H., Lenz, B., and Jerrels, T. R. (1987). Barbash strain spotted fever group rickettsia is a strain of *Rickettsia conorii* and differs from *Rickettsia sibirica Acta Virologica*, **31**, 489–98.

Wayne, L. G. *et al.* (1987). Report of the ad hoc committee on reconciliation of approaches to bacterial systematics. *International Journal of Systematic Bacteriology*, **37**, 463–4.

Weil, E. and Felix, A. (1916). Zur serologischen Diagnose des Fleckfiebers. *Wiener Klinische Wochenschrift*, **29**, 33–5.

Weisburg, W. G. (1986). Molecular approach to the study of rickettsial phylogeny. *Clinical Microbiology*, **198**, 191–3.

Weisburg, W. G. (1989). Polyphyletic origin of bacterial parasites. In *Intracellular parasitism*, (ed. J. W. Moulder) pp. 1–15. CRC Press, Boca Raton, Florida.

Weisburg, W. G., Woese, C. R., Dobson, M. E., and Weiss, E. (1985). A common origin of rickettsiae and certain plant pathogens. *Science*, **230**, 556–8.

Weisburg, W. G. *et al.* (1989). Phylogenetic diversity of the rickettsiae. *Journal of Bacteriology*, **171**, 4202–6.

Weiss, E. and Moulder, J. W. (1984). Order I. Rickettsiales Gieszczkiewicz 1939, 25AL. In *Bergey's manual of systematic bacteriology*, (ed. N. R. Kreig and J. G. Holt), pp. 687–704. Williams and Wilkins, Baltimore.

Werren, J. H., Hurst, G. D. D., Zhang, W., Breeuwer, J. A. J., Stouthamer, R., and Majerus, M. E. N. (1994). Rickettsial relative associated with male killing in the ladybird beetle (*Adalia bipunctata*). *Journal of Bacteriology*, **176**, 388–94.

WHO (World Health Organization) (1993). Global surveillance of rickettsial diseases: memorandum from a WHO meeting. *Bulletin of the World Health Organization*, **71**, 293–6.

Wilde, H., Pornsilapatip, J., Sokly, T., and Thee, S. (1991). Murine and scrub typhus at Thai-Kampuchean border displaced persons camp. *Tropical and Geographical Medicine*, **43**, 363–9.

Williams, J. C., Walker, D. H., Peacock, M. G., and Stewart, S. T. (1986). Humoral immune response to Rocky Mountain Spotted Fever in experimentally infected guinea pigs: immunoprecipitation of lactoperoxidase ^{125}I-labeled proteins and detection of soluble antigens of *Rickettsia rickettsii*. *Infection and Immunity*, **52**, 120–7.

Wisseman, C. L. (1985). Selected observations on rickettsiae and their host cells. In *Rickettsiae and rickettsial diseases*, (ed. J. Kazar), pp. 167–84. Publishing House of the Slovak Academy of Sciences, Bratislava.

Woodward, T. E. (1986). Rickettsial vaccines with emphasis on epidemic typhus. *South African Medical Journal*, October Supplement 73–6.

Woodward, T. E. and Jackson, E. B. (1965). Spotted fever rickettsiae. In *Viral and rickettsial infections of man*, (ed. F. L. Horsfall and I. Tamm), pp. 1095–129 Lippincott, Philadelphia.

Woodward, W. E. and Hornick, R. B. (1985). Rickettsiosis. *Rickettsia rickettsii* (Rocky Mountain spotted fever). In *Principles and practice of infectious diseases*, (ed. G. L. Mandell, R. G. Douglas, and J. E. Bennett), pp. 1082–7. Wiley, New York.

Wyatt, G. R. and Cohen, S. S. (1952). Nucleic acids of rickettsiae. *Nature*, **170**, 846–7.

Yano, Y., Ta kada, N., and Fujita, H. (1993). Ultrastructure of spotted fever rickettsialike microorganisms observed in tissues of *Dermacentor taiwanensis* (Acari: Ixodidae). *Journal of Medical Entomology*, **30**, 579–85.

Yu, X., Walker, D. H., and Jerrells, T. R. (1990). Polypeptides constituting the antigenic basis for identification of *Rickettsia sibirica* species by the standard serotyping method for spotted fever group rickettsiae. *Acta Virologica*, **34**, 71–9.

Yu, X., Jin, Y., Fan, M., Xu, G., Liu, Q., and Raoult, D. (1993). Genotypic and antigenic identification of two new strains of spotted fever group rickettsiae isolated from China. *Journal of Clinical Microbiology*, **31**, 83–8.

22   STREPTOCOCCOSIS

R. T. Mayon-White

SUMMARY

Two species of streptococci are of zoonotic interest: *Streptococcus suis* and *S. zooepidemicus*. Pigs are the primary hosts of *S. suis*, and human disease is concentrated in people who have contact with pigs or pork. The main human disease from *S. suis* is meningitis. *Streptococcus zooepidemicus* causes pharyngitis in humans, complicated rarely by glomerulonephritis. In these cases, the source is unpasteurized milk. Cattle and horses are natural hosts, but other species may also have pyogenic infections. All the pyogenic (beta-haemolytic) streptococci of clinical significance have animal connections, sometimes by disease and often by sharing group antigens. Penicillin is the mainstay of treatment and the prevention of human disease is by milk pasteurization and hygiene in the meat industry.

INTRODUCTION

The genus *Streptococcus* consists of non-motile, non-sporing, Gram-positive bacteria that grow in chains. Most streptococci live as part of the normal flora of animals, and some have single species as their natural hosts. The earliest subdivision of the genus was by the haemolysis of mammalian blood used to enrich culture media. All the streptococci of zoonotic interest are beta-haemolytic and so are broadly classified as pyogenic streptococci. In the 1930s, Lancefield developed a grouping system based on antigens that could be extracted from the cell walls by hot acids. This became the most practical and commonly used classification of streptococci, with the group-specific antigens denoted by letters. Within the groups are one or more species, and a few species have more than one group antigen. Several streptococcal species cause zoonoses, with different illnesses. This chapter considers the different species separately within their groups. Before beginning on the zoonotic streptococcoses, it may be helpful to mention that group A and group B streptococci, *S. pyogenes* and *S. agalactiae*, can give a false appearance of being zoonotic infections. So there are short accounts of these two species at the end of this chapter.

Biochemically, streptococci are catalase-negative and ferment sugars, producing lactic acid. They are aerobic and faculatively anaerobic. The pyogenic streptococci grow best on enriched laboratory media. The production of acid tends to limit growth, so the highest yields of bacteria are obtained in buffered media such as Todd–Hewitt broth. The features that are common to all zoonotic streptococci are the production of exotoxins that destroy tissue: haemolysins, hyaluronidases, and proteinases. These properties are used in laboratory diagnosis. The beta-haemolysis that is visible when cultured on blood agar is a well-known feature, by which a clear, colourless zone surrounds the colonies on agar plates. The antibodies formed against some of these toxins are used in serological tests of infection by group A streptococci and may in time prove useful in the investigation of other streptococcal disease. The streptococci described here are killed by most disinfectants and heat above 60 °C. They are sensitive to penicillin. Other microbiological features are described under the individual groups or species.

GROUP C STREPTOCOCCI

There are four species of streptococci which possess the group C antigen. *Streptococcus dysgalactiae*, *Streptococcus equi*, *Streptococcus equisimilis*, and *Streptococcus zooepidemicus*. Hitherto human microbiology laboratories have not distinguished these species. Indeed, many clinical microbiologists have taken little interest in streptococci that were not group A or B. The detection of outbreaks of glomerulonephritis associated with *S. zooepidemicus* show that there is interest to be found in this pathogen that occurs in horses, cattle, and rodents. Of the four species, *S. zooepidemicus* has the most definite zoonotic potential.

STREPTOCOCCUS ZOOEPIDEMICUS

THE AGENT

This group C streptococcus is capsulated and is more widely distributed across mammalian species than other pyogenic streptococci. It has at least 15 serotypes that have been identified from cultures taken from horses. Type 2 is one of the most common and infects a number of species, including humans. Some strains of *S. zooepidemicus* have been found to have M protein antigens which are similar, if not identical, to those of *S. pyogenes*, a finding that may explain the occasional occurrence of diseases normally associated with *S. pyogenes*.

DISEASE IN ANIMALS

Streptococcus zooepidemicus has been associated with outbreaks of respiratory tract infection in horses, manifest by catarrh. In these circumstances, it may be a secondary invader in pathological lesions started by viral infections. It can cause septic lesions in a range of mammals, from cattle and horses to guinea-pigs and rabbits. It has been isolated from the umbilical infections in newborn horses and from the lungs of sheep with pneumonia. It can cause mastitis in cattle and this may be the main route of transmitting infection in humans.

DISEASE IN MAN

Streptococcus zooepidemicus infection in man occurs in the respiratory tract, both as a cause of acute pharyngitis, and as a commensal organism. The infection may be complicated by spread into the lungs, or via the bloodstream to cause meningitis, endocarditis, and septic arthritis. The more severe human infections have been associated with drinking unpasteurized milk, often when the cows have had mastitis (Barrett 1986).

An unusual complication has been seen in two outbreaks of acute glomerulonephritis, both linked to drinking unpasteurized milk. The first outbreak affected 85 people in Romania (Duca *et al.* 1969). The account of the second of these outbreaks in a farming family provides a good review of this zoonotic streptococcus (Barnham *et al.* 1983). This outbreak began with mild upper respiratory tract infections in five of the six people in the family living on a small dairy farm in Yorkshire. The farmer and two of his children developed malaise, oedema, abdominal pain, haematuria, and hypertension—the signs and symptoms of acute glomerulonephritis. The two children recovered within a few weeks, but the farmer suffered weakness and tiredness for 6 months. The youngest child in the family and a second family living on the farm were not affected. All five who were ill had *S. zooepidemicus* isolated from their throats (two cases) or serological evidence of streptococcal infection (high antibody titres to streptococcal exotoxins). The people living on the farm had consumed unpasteurized milk for many years. The herd had had mastitis in the spring when the illness started, but *S. zooepidemicus* was not found in milk samples, which were not tested until 2 months later.

Infections are treatable with penicillin. Prevention is by pasteurization of milk.

OTHER GROUP C STREPTOCOCCI

Streptococcus equisimilis is a group C streptococcus chiefly associated with human throat and skin infections. Some strains resemble *S. pyogenes* (group A streptococci) in possessing T antigens (cell wall proteins which are useful in classifying group A streptococci for epidemiological purposes). The human infections probably originate from person to person spread and are not zoonoses, although this streptococcus has also been reported to cause septic arthritis in piglets.

Streptococcus equi is associated with strangles in horses and has not been linked to human disease. *Streptococcus dysgalactiae* is less haemolytic and is a cause of mastitis in cattle and arthritis in sheep. It is not a recognized cause of human disease.

GROUP G STREPTOCOCCI

This group of streptococci has no species name. It is a cause of pharyngitis in humans, and, like *S. equisimilis*, sometimes possesses T-type antigens identified with *S. pyogenes*. Although organisms of the same group can infect dogs, there is no established link between human and canine strains.

GROUP L STREPTOCOCCI

Group L Streptococci are beta-haemolytic organisms known to cause infection in dogs, cattle, pigs, and sheep. In studies of skin infections in meat workers, group L streptococci have been found by Barnham and co-workers in Yorkshire, England (Barnham and Neilson 1987). The skin lesions were impetigo, wounds and paronychia in 15 people. In half of the cases, the lesions were also infected with *Staphylococcus aureus*. As the latter is a well-known pathogen, it is not certain whether the group L streptococci were secondary pathogens or colonizers. Human group L streptococcal infections are too rare, or too infrequently recognized, to have been studied systematically as the object of prevention and control. Skin hygiene, including protecting the skin to reduce injury, hand washing and the covering of open cuts, may help to prevent human infections from this and other streptococcal infections in meat workers.

GROUP R STREPTOCOCCUS, STREPTOCOCCUS SUIS Type 2

Streptococcus suis type 2 is a cause of meningitis in piglets and human beings. Most of the human infections have occurred in people who have contact with pigs or pork (Zanen and Engel 1975; Arends and Zanen 1988). The route of infection from pigs to humans is uncertain, but may be through inhaled droplets, either from the respiratory tract of pigs or from pork during the processing of meat.

HISTORY

Streptococcus suis was first identified as a species of streptococci by de Moor in 1959, having isolated these bacteria from septicaemic lesions in pigs. The species can be divided into two groups by the polysaccharide group antigens R and S. Both groups cause disease in pigs, but only *Streptococcus suis* type 2 (group R) has an established place as zoonotic human pathogens. The first reports of human disease came from Denmark between 1960 and 1966. More cases followed in The Netherlands, France, and Britain, so by 1983 there had been 50 reported cases in Europe. The disease has been reported as the most common cause of adult meningitis in Hong Kong, on the basis of eight definite cases and another 12 possible cases in a 3-year period, 1978–80 (Chau *et al.* 1983). In the Hong Kong series, it was noted that more cases occurred in the summer.

THE AGENT

Streptococcus suis is a haemolytic diplococcus which grows on enriched laboratory culture media. It has a group D antigen made of teichoic acid and a polysaccharide capsule which contains the type-specific antigen. There are two types. Type 1 causes outbreaks of infection in newborn piglets, and does not cause human infection. Type 2 causes disease in weaned pigs and is the topic of this section.

THE ANIMAL HOST

The natural habitat of *Streptococcus suis* is the tonsils of pigs. Infection in piglets may occur at an early age of 3–20 weeks, and cause outbreaks of meningitis in litters. It may be important that the human cases occur in countries where pigs are reared in close confinement.

THE HUMAN HOST

The incubation period of *Streptococcus suis* infection in human beings has not been determined. The sporadic and rare occurrence of the human infections and the lack of any direct evidence on the portal of entry combine to make a mystery of the incubation period of this disease in human beings. By extrapolating from other streptococcal infections, from the general pattern of bacterial meningitis, and from the disease in pigs, it is possible that the incubation is about 2 or 3 days.

Bacterial meningitis is the main clinical condition in the majority of reported cases. The features of this condition are headache, fever, confusion leading to coma, photophobia, and vomiting. Deafness can occur as a result of cranial nerve damage, and remain as a sequel of infection. Septicaemia is less common as a clinical condition, but it is likely that bacteraemia is the route by which *S. suis* type 2 reaches the meninges. Septic arthritis is a rare presentation but one that also occurs with *S. suis* infections in pigs and with other species of streptococci infecting human beings. In a review of 60 cases (Arends and Zanen 1988), 10 cases had medical factors that may predispose to meningitis and septicaemia: head injuries, neurosurgery, asplenia, abdominal carcinomas, liver disease, and Zollinger–Ellison syndrome.

The treatment of this infection is by penicillin. Like other streptococci, it is resistant to aminoglycoside antibiotics, but there is synergy with penicillin and aminoglycosides given together.

EPIDEMIOLOGY

The illnesses caused by *S. suis* type 2 are the same as those due to several capsulated bacteria. Almost all human cases of *S. suis* type 2 infection have been associated with contact with pigs or pork. The weakest association has been in housewives who have been preparing meals using pork. Much stronger associations occur in cases of veterinary surgeons attending pigs, slaughtermen, and butchers. The route of infection is not clear. Infection from pig tissues (flesh or lymphoid tissue, including tonsils) through broken skin seems the most likely, but few of the people who have this disease give a history of an inflamed skin lesion. This suggests that systemic disease does not depend on a focal skin lesion, but rather on dissemination through the bloodstream from a small inoculum. Although there have been studies aimed at isolating streptococci from cuts and abrasions on the skin of meat workers, *S. suis* type 2 has not been found, in contrast to the frequent finding of group A streptococci.

23 EPIDEMIC AND MURINE TYPHUS

D. J. Sexton, E. B. Breitschwerdt, I. Beati, and D. Raoult

SUMMARY

Typhus group rickettsiae produce three distinct clinical illnesses: epidemic typhus, a louse-borne disease caused by *Rickettsia prowazekii*; scrub typhus, a chigger-borne disease caused by *Orientia tsutsugamushi*; and murine typhus, a flea-borne disease caused by *Rickettsia typhi*. All three pathogens typically cause an acute illness with skin rash, headache, myalgias, fever, and chills. Epidemic typhus may relapse after apparent recovery, even 30 years or more after primary infection, resulting in an illness known as Brill–Zinsser disease.

Epidemic typhus is now a rare disease, but previously it was worldwide in distribution. Typically epidemic typhus occurred during instances in which humans were forced to live in crowded, cold, and unhygienic conditions (e.g. aboard ships, in jails, and during military operations). Until recently, man was considered to be the only reservoir for *R. prowazekii*, but in 1975 a new sylvatic cycle involving the flying squirrel and its ectoparasites was discovered in the eastern United States.

Murine typhus occurs throughout the world. Its epidemiology is primarily linked to the distribution of rats and the rat flea, *Xenopsylla cheopis*. However, recently both a new reservoir (opossums in southern California) and a new potential vector (the cat flea) have been discovered.

Control or avoidance of the vectors are the cornerstones of strategies to prevent morbidity and mortality.

HISTORY

The history of the typhus fevers is closely linked with the history of men in battle. Epidemic typhus has been credited with deciding the outcome of more battles than any general's best-laid strategy.

Early Greeks such as Thucydides and Hippocrates described patients who probably had louse-borne typhus. Physicians during the Middle Ages described the clinical features of epidemic typhus accurately in reports describing vast and devastating epidemics that killed tens of thousands. For example, during the conquest of Granada by the army of Ferdinand and Isabella of Spain in 1492, an estimated 17 000 Spanish soldiers died of a severe exanthematous illness that probably was epidemic typhus. In 1552, Emperor Charles V was forced to abandon his campaign at Metz when over 10 000 soldiers died of an illness that was probably epidemic typhus. Additional outbreaks of typhus affected armies of virtually every nationality during the next three centuries. In many cases infected soldiers then spread disease throughout the civilian population when armies disbanded in disarray or defeat. Devastating losses were experienced by the Russian army when over 60 000 men died of epidemic typhus during a 2-month period in the winter of 1912. Thereafter lice infested French and Russian soldiers and prisoners of war spread typhus throughout central Europe, resulting in infection of nearly 2 million people.

Typhus continued to cause massive suffering into the twentieth century. For example, during the 8-year period from 1917 to 1925 an estimated 25 million cases of epidemic typhus occurred in Russia, causing approximately 3 million deaths (Weiss 1988). During the Second World War epidemic typhus occurred in numerous German concentration camps. Since the end of this war there have been no major outbreaks of epidemic typhus but WHO recently identified epidemic typhus as a lingering public health problem in Africa (Groupe de travail OMS 1982; WHO 1993).

The mode of transmission of epidemic typhus was not established until 1909 when Nicolle discovered the causative organism in the human body louse, *Pediculus humanus corporis* (Nicolle *et al.* 1900). Later the causative organism was isolated from the blood of infected patients and named *R. prowazekii* to honor both Howard Taylor Ricketts, who discovered *R. rickettsii*, and Stanislaus von Prowazek, a pioneering European rickettsiologist.

In 1910 Nathan Brill described a mild typhus-like illness in New York immigrants from eastern Europe. This illness came to be known as Brill's disease (Brill 1910). After Brill's report appeared, most sporadic or (endemic) typhus-like infections occurring in patients in the south-eastern coastal region of United States were usually (erroneously) called Brill's disease. In 1933 Zinsser and Castaneda isolated *R. prowazekii* from several cases of Brill's disease. Their careful analysis of epidemiological data and deductive reasoning led them to conclude accurately that recrudescent typhus infection may occur decades after primary infection with *R. prowazekii*. This recrudescent form of typhus is now known as Brill–Zinsser disease.

Murine typhus was not recognized as a separate form of typhus until the beginning of twentieth century. Early investigators in the western hemisphere (including Howard Ricketts) realized that there were two forms of typhus fever: a European form which was severe and often fatal, and a Mexican form which was milder and rarely caused death. Mooser and others subsequently found that typhus patients with the mild form of typhus were usually free of body lice. Thereafter, Maxcy used clinical and epidemiological criteria to separate murine typhus (also called endemic typhus or Brill's disease) from both epidemic typhus and recrudescent epidemic typhus (Brill–Zinsser disease) (Maxcy 1926). Subsequent investigators demonstrated that the rat was the reservoir and the cat flea was the principal vector of murine typhus (Dyer *et al* 1931; Mooser *et al* 1931).

AETIOLOGICAL AGENTS

TAXONOMY

Like other Gram-negative bacteria, typhus rickettsiae are members of the α-group of the purple bacteria. Along with the families Bartonellaceae and Anaplasmataceae, they are members of the order Rickettsiales and the family Rickettsiaceae. The family Rickettsiaceae in turn is divided into three tribes: Ehrlichieae, Wolbachieae and Rickettsieae. Until recently the tribe Rickettsieae was divided into three genera: *Rochalimaea*, *Coxiella*, and *Rickettsia*. But studies associating polymerase chain reaction technology with sequencing the DNA encoding the 16S rRNA have resulted in findings that suggest *Coxiella* should be reclassified to the γ-subgroup of the *Proteobacteria* and *Rochalimaea* should be united with the genus *Bartonella*. The tribe *Rickettsieae* now has two genera, *Rickettsia* and *Orientia*: the sole species of *Orientia* is *O. tsutsugamushi*. The genus *Rickettsia* is divided into spotted fever and typhus groups. The typhus group consists of *R. prowazekii*, *R. typhi*, *R. canada*, and *R. felis*.

The mol G+C content of typhus group rickettsiae (29 per cent) is lower than that of the spotted fever group (33 per cent) and similar to that of scrub typhus group rickettsiae (28 to 30.5 per cent, depending on the strain). The sizes of the genome of typhus group rickettsiae previously established by DNA renaturation

and sedimentation rate methods (Tyeryar *et al.* 1973; Myers and Wisseman 1980), have been revised on the basis of data using pulsed field gel electrophoresis techniques (Eremeeva *et al.* 1993). The genome of *R. prowazekii* possesses 1106 kb (±54 kb); the genome of *R. typhi* has 1133 kb (±44 kb). Restriction patterns of different strains of typhus group rickettsiae showed that there are slight differences between the Breinl and the Evir strains of *R. orowazekii*.

Recently a rickettsial-like organism initially called the ELB agent and subsequently named *R. felis* has been observed in the midgut of cat fleas (*Ctenocephalides felis*) and has been isolated from a single human in Texas with an illness clinically indistinguishable from murine typhus (Schriefer *et al.* 1994). Selective serological and gene sequence studies indicate that this micro-organism has genetic and antigenic characteristics of both typhus and spotted fever group rickettsiae. Results of studies utilizing polymerase chain reaction technology and restriction fragment length polymorphism suggest that *R. felis* belongs in a cluster or 'clade' with the agent of rickettsialpox (*R. akari*) and Queensland tick typhus (*R. australis*) (Higgins *et al.* 1996). *Rickettsia felis* cannot be distinguished from *R. typhi* using currently available serological tests but it can be detected using polymerase chain reaction technology. Sequencing of the 16S ribosomal DNA gene of *R. felis* indicates 98.5 per cent hamology with *R. typhi* (Schriefer *et al.* 1994*b*).

MICROBIOLOGY AND ULTRASTRUCTURE

Typhus rickettsiae, like other rickettsiae, are non-motile coccobacilli measuring 0.3–0.7 μm by 0.8–2.0 μm. All typhus rickettsiae are weakly Gram-negative and are difficult to visualize in tissue sections unless special stains such as Geimsa, Machiovello, or Gimenez are used, or unless fluorescent antibody-based staining techniques are employed.

The envelope of *R. typhi* and *R. prowazekii* is similar to those of spotted fever group rickettsiae in that it consists of a bilayer inner membrane, a peptidoglycan layer, and a bilayer outer membrane. In the typhus group and spotted fever group rickettsiae the inner leaflet of the two-unit outer membrane is the thickest.

Typhus rickettsiae have a slime layer which can be stained with ruthenium and silver methenamine if special care is taken in cell preparation. The influence of the slime layer in determining virulence and pathogenicity of individual species is uncertain.

GROWTH AND SURVIVAL CHARACTERISTICS

Like all rickettsiae, the typhus group rickettsiae are obligate intracellular pathogens that cannot be propa-

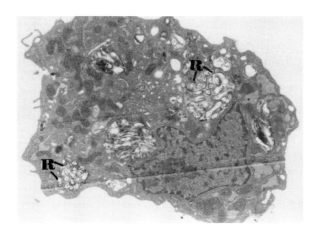

Fig. 23.1 A Vero cell infected with *Rickettsia typhi*. Rickettsiae are clustered together in different 'colonies' which are not surrounded by any membrane (R, *Rickettsia*).

gated on cell-free media. All typhus rickettsiae can be propagated *in vitro* in the yolk sac of the developing chicken embryo or on primary or established cell culture monolayers such as chick embryo fibroblasts, mouse L cells, and golden hamster cells. Typhus group rickettsiae produce plaques on primary chick embryo fibroblast monolayers 10–12 days after inoculation, but only certain virulent strains of *R. prowazekii* and *R. typhi* form plaques on Vero cell monolayers. Typhus group rickettsiae characteristically grow only in the cytoplasm of host cells where they reside directly in the cytosol free of host cell membranes (Fig. 23.1).

Typhus rickettsiae gain access to host cell cytoplasm by stimulating their own phagocytosis (induced phagocytosis) (Weiss 1982). *In vitro*, prior to cell entry, typhus rickettsiae absorb to host cell membranes. This absorption requires metabolically active rickettsiae and is essentially irreversible (Austin and Winkler 1988). Once inside cells, rickettsiae escape almost immediately from the phagosome and begin to proliferate.

Rickettsia prowazekii grows in conformity to a one-step growth curve. Typically the intracellular rickettsial burden becomes high 36–48 hours' after infection, at which time the host cell ruptures releasing rickettsiae into the extracellular space. *Rickettsia prowazekii* does not produce important cytopathogenic changes in infected cells. High bacterial density may be detected in infected cells, without observing any important signs of cell injury (Wisseman 1985; Silverman 1991). (Fig. 23.1). The death of the host cell seems to be due to physical breakdown caused by the overwhelming number of organisms in the cytoplasm.

Intracellular rickettsial growth occurs independently of host protein synthesis. Members of the typhus group biotype require a CO_2-enriched atmosphere to grow in

chick embryos. Neither typhus or scrub typhus group rickettsiae metabolize glucose. In fact, *R. prowazekii* lacks transport systems for glucose and glucose 6-phosphate (Austin and Winkler 1988) Unlike most bacteria, all rickettsiae, including the scrub typhus and typhus group rickettsiae have an additional energy source in the form of a carrier-mediated transport system for di-and triphosphates. Growing rickettsiae use an ADP–ATP transport system to acquire host ATP and have the ability to utilize host-derived glutamine as an energy source (Austin and Winkler 1988). Several genes of *R. prowazekii* have been cloned and expressed in *E. coli* and the gene for citrate synthase ATP/ADP translocase (the 17 kDa protein) has been elucidated. Some or all of the cloned genes may play a role in virulence or in eliciting protective immunity (Mallavia 1991).

ANTIGENIC STRUCTURE

Animal studies done 50 years ago demonstrated that cell wall extracts from *R. prowazekii* and *R. typhi* conferred specific homologous protection. The nature of these host-sensitive soluble antigens has been studied extensively and related to serotype-specific polypeptide antigens (SPA). These antigens in turn have been used to develop subunit vaccines that provoke dose-dependent antibody and cell-mediated immune responses in guinea-pigs (Walker 1988*b*) Dasch has proposed that the SPA of both *R. prowazekii* and *R. typhi* are actually heat sensitive epitopes of a protein that can be released from the surface of rickettsial cell walls by various *in vitro* manoeuvres. Once released, SPA may exist as a disulphide-linked polymer (Dasch *et al.* 1985).

Antigens of typhus group rickettsiae are composed mainly of high and low molecular weight proteins, and lipopolysaccharide (LPS)-like antigens of low molecular weight. High molecular weight proteins have mobility patterns that differ among strains. Essential immunogens such as a 120 kDa SPA are able to induce protection when inoculated into guinea-pigs, mice, and monkeys. Furthermore these 120 kDa proteins are also species–species epitopes (Black *et al.* 1983) which can be used to differentiate between typhus group rickettsiae.

BASIS FOR VIRULENCE

Although *R. prowazekii* infection typically occurs in distressed populations with underlying health problems such as poor nutrition, it is frequently fatal to otherwise healthy individuals. In contrast, *R. typhi* virtually always produces a mild illness in which fatalities are extremely rare. The basis for differences in virulence between or among species is poorly understood, but there is evidence that differences in virulence relate to factors involving both the host and the organism.

Studies examining the differences in virulence between individual human isolates of typhus rickettsiae have shown no direct correlation between fatality rates in humans and those in guinea-pigs or mice (McDade 1991). For example, isolates of *R. prowazekii* recovered from fatal human cases of epidemic typhus are unable to produce fatal illness in experimentally infected guinea-pigs, whereas isolates of *R. typhi* made from humans with mild illness typically produce mild-illness in guinea-pigs yet invariably cause fatal infection in mice. Dogs infected with *R. prowazekii* seroconvert but do not develop clinical or haemostatic abnormalities. These observations illustrate the fact that typhus group rickettsiae vary in their virulence for different animal species, that results of studies in experimental animals cannot be extrapolated to disease in humans, and that the results of animal infectivity studies vary considerably depending upon the species of animal that is studied (McDade 1991).

Nearly 60 years ago Clavero and Perez Gallardo observed that a highly virulent strain of *R. prowazekii* (Madrid-1) suddenly became avirulent for guinea-pigs after a few passages in embryonated eggs (Clavero and Perez Gallardo 1943). This E (for Espana) strain was subsequently shown by the same investigators to be non-pathogenic when injected into human volunteers. In studies using the E strain as an attenuated vaccine 32 of 36 human vaccinees remained afebrile after challenge with a virulent strain of *R. prowazekii*, whereas 17 of 18 unvaccinated controls developed classic symptoms and signs of louse-borne typhus (McDade 1991). The nature of the E strain mutation remains a mystery despite intensive laboratory studies and subsequent experiments in which passages of the original Madrid-1 strain failed to result in similar changes in virulence.

Strain differences in *R. prowazekii* may explain the differences virulence of infection when louse-borne typhus is compared to sylvatic (flying squirrel-associated) typhus. However, comparative analysis of *R. prowazekii* strains from flying squirrels and isolates from outbreaks of epidemic typhus have shown only minimal differences in DNA sequences or protein profiles (Walker 1991).

Our understanding of host-related virulence factors following rickettsial infection is primarily based on epidemiological studies. Such studies have usually shown that increasing age, male, sex, African origins, and glucose 6-phosphate dehydrogenase-deficiency are all associated with increased disease severity and a fatal outcome (Walker 1991). For example, severe murine typhus occurring in glucose 6 phosphate dehydrogenase-deficient US soldiers during the Vietnam war appeared to be a more virulent and severe infection (Whelton *et al.* 1968).

DISEASE MECHANISMS

After inoculation into the body via the bite of a flea (murine typhus), or after transcutaneous entry of infectious louse or flea faeces (epidemic and murine typhus), rickettsiae spread throughout the body via the bloodstream or lymphatics. Once inside their human host, rickettsiae enter enthothelial cells and proliferate intracellularly by binary fission. Unlike spotted fever group rickettsiae, which are released early from endothelial cells and spread rapidly to contiguous endothelial cells, *R. prowazekii* proliferates intracellularly until the cell bursts and releases rickettsiae into the extracellular space.

The precise mechanisms by which typhus group and scrub typhus group rickettsiae produce cellular injury is still uncertain, but experimental studies suggest that a complex and multifactorial sequence of events culminates in endothelial injury (both swelling and necrosis) and secondary immune and phagocytic host responses (lymphocytes and macrophages) (Walker 1988*a*). Typhus rickettsiae have the ability to injure cells directly in the absence of immune and inflammatory responses. Attachment of *R. prowazekii* to cell membranes is followed by increased phospholipase activity and secondary injury to host cell membranes (Winkler and Miller 1981). *Rickettsia prowazekii*-infected cells appear normal in ultrastructural studies, even while vast numbers of rickettsial organism accumulate intracellularly. Subsequent 'burst release' of rickettsiae appears to cause death of the host cell.

Typhus group rickettsia-induced cellular injury results in the pathological hallmarks of all rickettsial infections: widespread vasculitis with increased vascular permeability, oedema, and activation of humoral inflammatory and coagulation mechanisms.

EPIDEMIOLOGY: GEOGRAPHICAL DISTRIBUTION

Only a few foci of epidemic typhus were still active over the past two decades: they were in Burundi, Rwanda, and Ethiopia (Brouqui *et al.* 1992). In South America, cases are still found on the Andes Mountains. In these foci, epidemic typhus has evolved into an epidemic-endemic form, due to the fact that people are immunized continuously from a young age.

Murine typhus is a worldwide disease. This disease has often been associated with ports were rats and men live in close contact. This disease has, however, been recognized in almost all countries where surveys to detect it have been undertaken (Gear 1941; Retel-Laurentin *et al.* 1974, Traub *et al.* 1978; Kennou and Edlinger 1984; Williams *et al.* 1992; WHO 1993). In the United States, endemic typhus occurs in suburban areas of Los Angeles, California, and in Texas

(Williams *et al.* 1992). Recent reports have documented murine typhus in Israel, Egypt, Thailand, Kampuchea, and eastern African countries Redus *et al.* 1986; Shaked *et al.* 1988; Boros *et al.* 1989; Samra *et al.* 1989; Wilde *et al.* 1991). The epidemiology of epidemic, murine typhus is directly or indirectly related to the geographic distribution or the life cycles of their louse or flea vectors.

The principal vector of epidemic typhus is the human louse *P. humanus*. Two subspecies, *P. humanus humanus* (human body louse) and *P. humanus capitus* (human head louse) feed naturally on man. Although *R. prowazekii* can be acquired and maintained by the head louse, the body louse is the major and most important vector for man. Until recently, *P. humanus* was thought to be the sole vector of epidemic typhus. However, in 1975 *R. prowazekii* infection was found in flying squirrels in Florida and Virginia (Bozeman *et al.* 1975). Subsequent studies disclosed that both the squirrel flea (*Orchospea howardii*) and the squirrel louse (*Neohaematopinus sciuropteri*) are important vector for transmission of *R. prowazekii* among flying squirrels. Unlike *N. sciuropteri*, which is host-specific and does not feed on man, *O. howardii*, the vector for human sylvatic typhus infection, will bite man when its principal host is unavailable (Sonenshine *et al.* 1978).

Lice feeding on rickettsiaemic patients may quickly become infective. Human body lice may take new blood meals as often as every 5 hours. After ingestion, rickettsiae multiply in gut epithelial cells of the louse. As infected gut cells progressively rupture, the rickettsiae are excreted in the faeces of the louse. Louse faeces may remain infectious for as long as 100 days.

The body louse spends its life on the skin or clothes of man. Eggs are laid on clothes and hatch in about 8 days. Larvae (also called nymphs) moult three times before they become adults. Lice require a blood meal during each of their life cycles. Following a blood meal by the louse, faeces are deposited at the site of each bite. Rickettsiae in faeces or in lice tissue may be introduced into the skin by scratching or minor trauma due to the irritation. Contamination of the conjunctiva or inhalation via aerosols may also result in disease transmission. In fact, when the human host has high fever (or dies), the louse will try to move to another host. This characteristic behaviour is the basic mechanism allowing epidemic typhus to spread rapidly from one man to another, especially when humans have to live in overcrowded conditions.

The principal vector of murine typhus is the rat flea, *Xenopsylla cheopis*. In addition, the cat flea, *C. felis*, and the mouse flea (*Leptopsylla segnis*) may also serve as occasional vectors (Irons *et al.* 1944). Natural infection with *R. typhi* has been reported for six additional species of fleas, three species of lice, three species of mites, and one tick genus (*Hyalomma*) but it is unclear and if these ectoparasites actually transmit *R. typhi*. Their role in the epidemiology of disease, if any, is certainly minor (Farhang-Azad 1988). Once infected with *R. typhi*, fleas remain infected for their entire life span (which is not shortened by the presence of rickettsiae). Infected fleas pass viable rickettsiae in their faeces during the course of their lifetime. *Rickettsia typhi* may remain infective in flea faeces for several years, thus aerosols from rat or mice nests may result in human infection without direct contact with fleas or rats (Silverman *et al.* 1974). The mechanism by which rickettsiae remain viable in dried faeces has not been explained.

HOSTS

The principle vector of *R. felis* is thought to be the cat flea (Schriefer *et al,* 1994*b*) *Rickettsia typhi* is normally maintained in a cycle between fleas and rodents such as rats. Other vertebrate hosts, such as house mice, cats, shrews, opossums and skunks, may occasionally substitute for rodents in this cycle. However, the vast majority of cases of murine typhus are associated with sites where rats such as *Rattus novegicus* and *R. rattus* accumulate in large numbers. These rats serve both as hosts for the vectors of murine typhus and as 'amplifiers' for rickettsial infection by becoming rickettsaemic after contact with an infected flea, and in turn act as a source for infection for simultaneously feeding ectoparasites. Indeed, uninfected fleas readily become infected while feeding on a rickettsaemic rodent under experimental conditions.

A similar cycle of infection between the flea *Ctenocephalides felis* and the opossum probably occurs for *R. felis*.

In most parts of the world *R. prowazekii* circulates in a man–louse–man cycle. Man is the principal reservoir of infection as the human body louse is extremely host-specific. *Pediculus humanus* typically spends its entire life on the same host and does not leave unless manually removed or unless poor sanitary conditions, overcrowding, and close contact allow transfer to a second human host. The louse acquires *R. prowazekii* after feeding on a rickettsaemic human, but does not become infective until 5–7 days later. Transmission of *R. prowazekii* from louse to human occurs by contamination of the bite site with faeces containing rickettsiae, or by contamination of conjunctivae or mucous membranes with the crushed bodies or faeces of infected ticks. Individuals with Brill–Zinsser disease provide a mechanism for the interepidemic survival of *R. prowazekii*. If individuals with recurrent *R. prowazekii* infection are simultaneously infested with lice, an epidemic focus of *R. prowazekii* can become established.

As mentioned previously, *R. prowazekii* also exists in a sylvatic cycle of infection between flying squirrels and their lice or flea ectoparasites. However, to date other squirrels and native mammals have not been found to be naturally infected.

CLINICAL FEATURES

The clinical features of epidemic typhus and murine typhus are similar although the severity of illness and complications of infection vary considerably. Both diseases typically begin abruptly. Headache, myalgias, and non-specific constitutional symptoms such as malaise, anorexia, chills, and fever are common. After an incubation period of 10–14 days, the majority of patients with epidemic typhus develop malaise and vague symptoms before the onset of fever and severe headache (Perrine *et al.* 1992). Most patients complain of fever, chills, myalgias, arthralgias, and anorexia early in the course of their illness. Non-specific complaints such as cough, nausea, abdominal pain, diarrhoea, photophobia, and dizziness occur in less than one-half of patients, but when present, such symptoms may lead to diagnostic confusion and misdiagnosis. Although a localized eschar does not occur in epidemic typhus, most patients develop a skin rash that classically begins on the trunk and spreads to the periphery. The rash may be macular, maculopapular, or petechial and it may be difficult to detect in dark-coloured individuals. Rarely, severe cases may develop gangrene of the distal extremities necessitating amputation. The majority of patients with epidemic typhus manifest one or more abnormalities of central nervous system function, such as signs of meningeal irritation or signs of focal or generalized cortical dysfunction ranging from seizures to confusion, drowsiness, and coma. Thrombocytopenia, jaundice, and abnormal liver function tests may occur in severe cases. Clinical and electrocardiographic evidence of myocarditis may occur in a small percentage of patients. Pulmonary involvement may manifest as interstitial pneumonitis, bronchitis, or bronchiolitis.

In contrast to epidemic typhus, murine typhus is typically a mild illness and fatalities are extremely rare. Similar to other forms of typhus, the incubation period ranges from 8 to 16 days (mean 11) (Woodward 1988). Onset of illness is usually relatively abrupt. Fever, headache, chills, myalgia, and gastrointestinal symptoms such as nausea, vomiting, abdominal pain, and diarrhoea are usually prominent early in illness. *The only known case* of human infection with Rickettsia felis involved a patient from southern Texas who had an illness indistinguishable from murine typhus (Schriefer 1994*a*).

In murine typhus, skin rash occurs in most but not all patients near the end of the first week of illness. Like the rash of other forms of typhus this rash classically begins on the trunk and spreads peripherally, but unlike other rickettsial infections it rarely involves the palms and the soles (Fig. 23.2). Often the rash is faint, thus it is easily overlooked in dark-skinned individuals. Rarely the skin rash may become petechial; even more rarely, it becomes necrotic. As in other forms of typhus, severe cases may occasionally manifest signs of central nervous system, cardiac, renal, and hepatic dysfunction. Untreated, murine typhus lasts 9–18 days. Most patients, even those who do not receive antirickettsial therapy, recover without complications or sequelae.

Recrudescent typhus or Brill–Zinsser disease can appear in patients who totally recovered from epidemic typhus, years after the onset of the first infection (Reilly and Kalinske 1980). The late relapse of R.prowazekii infection is often associated with the

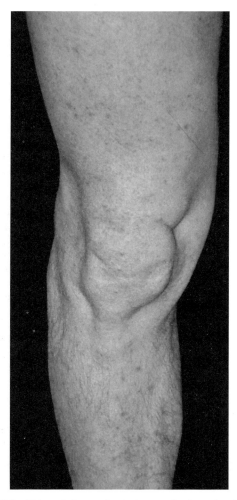

Fig. 23.2   Skin rash in a patient who acquired murine typhus while visiting New Delhi, India (reproduced from *Clinical Infectious Diseases* (1995 with permission of Murray Abramson).

breakdown of immunity. The mechanism by which rickettsiae survive in the body for decades is not understood. Patients with Brill–Zinsser disease typically develop a mild form of epidemic typhus. If body lice are present when the recrudescent attack occurs, these lice may be the vectors of a new epidemic focus, the classic form of epidemic typhus. The typical clinical features of patients with Brill–Zinsser disease include rash and fever. However, skin rash may be absent in some cases, thus diagnosis may be difficult unless historical data can be elicited about previous typhus infection or contracted residence in a place and time when epidemic typhus was common.

DIAGNOSIS

No laboratory test is diagnostic in the early phase of any rickettsial disease. Diagnosis of the various forms typhus is usually suspected by the presence of typical clinical findings such as fever, headache, and skin rash in a patients residing in a typical epidemiological setting. For instance, epidemic typhus is usually suspected when fever and skin rash occur in lice-infested persons who are living in crowded, cold, and unhygienic circumstances. Illness often occurs in clusters, but it may also occur as isolated illness in the winter months in areas where flying squirrels make their nests in proximity to man. The initial clinical features of murine typhus are often non-specific, thus misdiagnosis as a viral illness, malaria, or a large array of bacterial diseases is not uncommon.

Differentiation between increases in IgG and IgM antibody titres may help to distinguish between a primary infection and a Brill–Zinsser disease. Epidemic and endemic typhus cannot be differentiated by serology, unless previous cross-adsorptions of sera are done (Dasch and Bourgeois 1981; Saah and Hornick 1985).

As with other rickettsial diseases, the diagnosis of murine typhus or epidemic typhus can be confirmed by four methods: culture, serology, biopsy, and polymerase chain reaction technology. Cultures are available only in specialized laboratories found in a few large medical or research centres. Biopsy of either an eschar or the generalized skin rash can lead to a definitive diagnosis by demonstrating the characteristic changes of rickettsial vasculitis and the presence of rickettsia in tissue using fluorescent antibody conjugates. A diagnosis of recent epidemic or murine typhus rickettsial infection can be established by demonstrating a fourfold or greater rise in antibody titre in properly collected acute and convalescent serum samples. Antibody against all three pathogens can be detected using indirect immunoflourescent, micro-agglutination, complement fixation, and enzyme-linked immunoassay methods.

The immunofluorscent antibody test can distinguish between IgM and IgG antibody responses which is particularly useful in the diagnosis of recrudescent *R. prowazekii* infection (Brill–Zinsser disease). Such individuals manifest an IgG but not an IgM response to the convalescent stage of illness.

For decades the Weil–Felix reaction, which was based on fortuitously discovered cross-reaction between anti-rickettsial antibodies and *Proteus* antigens, was used to diagnose the various forms of typhus fever. For example, patients convalescent from murine and epidemic typhus and Rocky Mountain spotted fever often have antibody against OX-2 and OX-19 antigens. The Weil–Felix test is now only of historical interest, as it has been supplanted by more sensitive and more specific serological tests using specific rickettsial antigens. If the Weil–Felix test is used as the primary method for diagnosis, both false-positive results (due to a coincidental recent or remote *Proteus* infection) and false-negative results are important problems.

Techniques using polymerase chain reaction (PCR) technology have been used to diagnose scrub typhus and murine typhus and to detect these organisms in their respective vectors. The limited availability of PCR technology and the difficulties in insuring rigorous quality control of the laboratory methods for PCR testing make these diagnostic methods impractical and largely limited to research centres.

PATHOLOGY

The pathological hallmark of all typhus infections is a lymphohistiocytic vasculitis. Damage to endothelial cells occurs early in infection. As illness advances, progressive endothelial damage leads to widespread vascular dysfunction. In addition, rickettsia-induced cell damage leads to the accumulation of lymphocytes and macrophages around small blood vessels. In severe infection endothelial damage results in permeability changes and the egress of plasma and plasma proteins from the intravascular compartment to the interstitium. In addition, endothelial injury leads to disruption of vessel integrity manifesting as microscopic and macroscopic foci of haemorrhage.

Thombocytopenia, probably due to platelet utilization at the sites of rickettsia-induced vascular injury, often occurs in patients with advanced and severe illness, but disseminated intravascular coagulation is uncommon. The vasculitis of epidemic typhus infection may be accompanied by mural and intimal thrombi in small vessels surrounded by inflammatory infiltrates consisting of macrophages, lymphocytes, and plasma cells. These lesions may occur focally throughout the central nervous system, where they are called typhus nodules. These nodular inflammatory lesions may be associated with secondary changes induced by minute foci of haemorrhage. Typically the grey matter, which contains more blood vessels, is more affected than white matter. As the vasculitis of *R. prowazekii* infection is generalized, virtually any organ may be involved. Lesions are usually prominent in the spleen, heart, liver, lungs, kidney, and skeletal muscle (Walker 1991).

Murine typhus is almost always a mild illness, thus its pathology of infection has been studied to a lesser extent. In the few cases of fatal murine typhus examined at autopsy, pathological changes nearly identical to those seen in epidemic typhus were identified (Walker 1991).

TREATMENT

Tetracycline and chloramphenicol are the only effective treatments for epidemic and murine typhus. In areas of the world where diagnostic facilities are unavailable or inaccessible, chloramphenicol is widely used as empirical treatment since its broad spectrum includes coverage for other serious illness, such as meningococcaemia and typhoid fever, that can initially mimic epidemic typhus. However, many clinicians prefer to use tetracycline for all typhus infections as it is cheap and safer than chloramphenicol. In addition, in the opinion of many clinicians, tetracycline appears to produce a faster clinical response than chloramphenicol. But most patients treated with either antibiotic improve markedly within 48 hours following the initiation of therapy. In fact, failure to respond within 48–72 hours of starting empirical treatment is often considered to be clinical evidence that a rickettsial disease is not present.

PROGNOSIS

At present, the typhus fevers have excellent prognosis if tetracycline or chloramphenicol is begun early in the course of illness. In general, the earlier such therapy is begun, the milder and less complicated is the infection. However, if antirickettsial therapy is not used, serious complications and even a fatal outcome may occur in patients with epidemic typhus. Although rare fatalities have been reported in patients with murine typhus, most patients recover spontaneously even if therapy is not given.

As with Rocky Mountain spotted fever, the presence of glucose 6-phosphate dehydrogenase deficiency may be associated with severe illness in patients infected with *R. typhi* or *R. prowazekii*. Also, as in Rocky Mountain spotted fever, illness due to typhus fever appears to have a poorer prognosis in elderly patients.

That untreated epidemic typhus can end fatally has been noted since the Middle Ages when vast epidemics resulted in the deaths of tens of even hundreds of thousands of patients. Indeed, the deaths of Howard Ricketts and Stanislaus von Prowazek were both directly related to infection with *R. prowazekii*. In the pre-antibiotic era, it was estimated that 10–40 per cent of infected patients succumbed (McDade 1991). But in a recent report from Ethiopia describing 60 patients with epidemic typhus, no patients died although transient neurological deficits, hypotension, and jaundice occurred in a minority (Perrine *et al.* 1992).

EPIDEMIOLOGY

TRANSMISSION AND COMMUNICABILITY

Transmission of *R. prowazekii* does not occur directly by the bite of the human body louse. Rather, the louse deposits rickettsia-laden faeces at the feeding site. The host in turn inoculates these faeces into the site of the louse bite by scratching or by inadvertent contamination of the conjunctivae or mucous membranes. Massive numbers of viable rickettsiae may be present in lice faeces which, incredibly, may remain infective for up to 100 days (Farhang-Azad 1988).

As mentioned earlier, transmission of sylvatic typhus is quite complicated and because of the limited number of cases reported thus far, the importance of various factors influencing transmission remain speculative. Because the flying squirrel louse. (*N. sciuropteri*) is highly host specific and is not known to feed on humans, it is presumed that the flying squirrel flea (*O .howardii*) is the probable vector for human infection. *Orchospea howardii* has been known to parasitize man when its preferred host, the flying squirrel (Fig. 23.3)

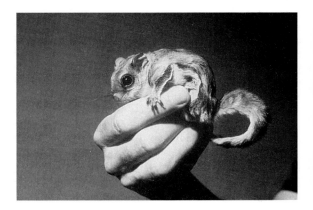

Fig. 23.3 Flying squirrel (*Glaucomys volans*), an intermediate host for *R. prowazekii* in the eastern and central United States (reproduced from *Parasitology Today* (1967), **3**; 85–7, with permission of Joseph E. McDade).

has become unavailable (e.g. when squirrel nests in the attics of homes are discovered and destroyed).

The principal vector of murine typhus, the rat flea (*X. cheopis*), does not normally parasitize man, but when their normal hosts are unavailable (e.g. because of mass efforts at rodent control), *X. cheopis* may bite man. Similar to the transmission of *R. prowazekii* by louse fleas, *R. typhi* is excreted in large amounts in the faeces of feeding fleas. Transmission to humans may occur when the bite, a skin abrasion, conjunctivae, or other mucous membranes are contaminated by the infected flea faeces. In addition, fleas may transmit *R. typhi* orally during the process of feeding by regurgitating rickettsiae from their gut into the bite wound. As aerosol transmission of infection can occur in laboratory conditions, it is possible that air-borne transmission can also occur when humans breathe dust that is heavily contaminated with infective flea faeces.

DISTRIBUTION AND INCIDENCE

Formerly worldwide in distribution, epidemic typhus has become an uncommon disease in the developed nations of the world during the past 40 years. During the period 1981–90 the World Health Organization received reports of 20 454 cases of epidemic typhus. These figures were probably an underestimate of the true incidence of disease in less developed nations, but several trends are notable. Almost 70 per cent of the total cases reported occurred in Ethiopia, and an additional 25 per cent were from Nigeria. In addition, scattered cases were reported from several countries in Central and South American (Perrine *et al.* 1992). Since 1963 a small number of sylvatic typhus cases have been reported from the eastern United States. All of these cases occurred in the autumn or winter when squirrels tend to nest in the attics of homes in the south-eastern United States. A small number of cases of Brill–Zinsser disease occur annually in the United States, South America, and Europe. In most instances these patients are individuals from eastern Europe who previously had epidemic typhus during the First or Second World Wars.

Murine typhus has been reported from every continent except Antarctica. Cases tend to occur in port cities and in areas where rats and man coexist in the same living spaces. Sporadic cases continue to be reported from Africa, South America, Australia, Asia, and Europe, but reliable figures on the incidence and prevalence of infection do not exist. Travellers to areas with poor sanitation and inadequate rat control occasionally acquire infection and then return home during the incubation period. In the United States most cases of murine typhus are recognized and reported from Texas, but it is likely that numerous additional cases are misdiagnosed as viral illnesses or other benign self-limiting infections. Recently a cluster of murine typhus cases reported from Los Angeles led to the discovery that animals such as the opossum may play a role in the propagation of *R. typhi* in nature (Williams *et al.* 1992).

Rickettsia felis has thus far only been recognized in commercial flea colonies and in opossums from southern California and Texas and in a single human from Texas. As further studies are undertaken, it is likely that its distribution will be wider than has currently been reported.

PREVENTION

Measures that prevent the acquisition of body lice will effectively prevent the transmission of epidemic typhus. In areas where human lice infestation is common, the use of long-acting insecticides and regular washing of clothes are the mainstays of typhus prevention. Although strains of lice that are resistant to insecticides such as DDT, malathion, and lindane have been reported, the synthetic pyrethroid permethrin remains an effective and long-lasting agent when applied as a dust or spray on clothing or bedding (Irons *et al.* 1944). Fabric treated with permethrin can retain toxicity to body lice after as many as 20 washings. Although the use of tetracycline or chloramphenicol can help to interrupt a typhus outbreak, such measures are generally of lesser importance than control and prevention of infestation by lice. Since doxycycline is effective as a single-dose treatment for epidemic typhus, it is likely that it would also be effective given once-weekly as prophylaxis even though such a regimen has never been tested in field studies.

Both inactivated and live vaccines against *R. prowazekii* have been developed. Inactivated vaccines provide moderate protection as manifested by reduced severity of disease in vaccinated persons after exposure. Live attentuated vaccines using the E strain of *R. prowazekii* have been developed and field tested. Mild local and systemic side-effects were common; approximately 15 per cent of patients develop mild illnesses 1–2 weeks after vaccination (Perrine *et al.* 1992). Because of the concerns that the E strain could spontaneously revert back to wild-type *R. prowazekii*, inactivated vaccines against epidemic typhus are not currently available.

Prevention of murine typhus is best accomplished by the control of rodent populations. Since *R. typhi* is maintained in nature by rats and fleas, efforts to control fleas on household pets such as cats will secondarily reduce the chance of human infection.

REFERENCES

Abramson, M., Sexton, D. J. (1995). Murine Typhus. Clinical Infectious Diseases, **21**, 991.

Austin, F. E. and Winkler, H. H. (1988). Relationship of rickettsial physiology and composition to the rickettsia-host cell interaction. In *Biology of rickettsial disease*, (ed. D. H. Walker), CRC Press, Boca Raton, Florida. Vol. II, pp. 29–51.

Azad, A. F., Sacci, J. B., Nelson, W. M., Dasch, G. A., Schmidtmann, E. T. and Carl, M. (1992). Genetic characterisation and transovarial transmission of a tyhpus-like rickettsia found in cat fleas. *Proceedings of the National Academy of Sciences USA,*, **89**, 43–6.

Black, C. M., Tzianabos, T., Rowmillat, L. F., Redus, M. A., McDade, J. E. and Reimer, C. B. (1983). Detection and characterization of mouse monoclonal antibodies to epidemic typhus rickettsiae. *Journal of Clinical Microbiology*, **18**, 561–8.

Botros, B. A. M., Soliman, A. K., Darwish, M., El Said, S., Morrill, J. C. and Ksiazek, T. G. (1989). Seroprevalence of murine typhus and fievre boutonneus in certain human populations in Egypt. *Journal of Tropical Medicine and Hygiene*, **92**, 373–8.

Bozeman, F. M. *et al.* (1975). Epidemic typhus rickettsiae isolated from flying squirrels. *Nature*, **255**; 545–7.

Brill, N. (1910). An acute infectious disease of unknown origin. A clinical study based on 221 cases. *American Journal of Medical Science*, **139**, 482–502.

Brouqui, P., Delmont, J., Raoult, D. and Bourgeade, A. (1992). Etat actuel des connaissances sur 1 epidemiologie des rickettsioses en Afrique. *Bulletin de la Société de Pathologies exotique*, **85**, 1–6.

Clavero, G. and Perez Gallardo, F. (1943). Estudio experimental da una cepa apatogenicay immunizante de Rickettsia prowazekii. *Rev Sanidad Hlg Pub*, **17**, 1–27.

Dasch, G. A. and Bourgeois, A. L. (1981). Antigens of the typhus group of rickettsiae: importance of the species-specific protein antigens in eliciting immunity. In *Rickettsiae and rickettsial diseases*, (ed. W. Burgdorfer, and R. L. Anacker), pp. 61–70. Academic Press, New York.

Dasch, G. A. *et al.* (1985). Distinctive properties of components of the cell envelopes of typhus group rickettsiae. In *Rickettsiae and Rickettsial diseases*, (ed. J. Kazar), pp. 55–61. Public House of the Slovak Academy of Sciences, Bratislava, Czechoslovak.

Dyer, R. E., Rumreich, A. and Badger, L. F. (1931). Typhus fever. A virus of the typhus type derived from fleas collected from wild rats. *Public Health Reports*, **46**, 334–8.

Eremeeva, M. E., Roux, V. and Raoult, D. (1993). Determination of genome size and restriction pattern polymorphism of *Rickettsia prowazekii* and *R. typhi* by pulsed field gel electrophoresis. *FEMS Microbiology Letters*; **112**, 105–12.

Farhang-Azad, A. (1988). Relationship of vector biology and epidemiology of louse-and flea-borne rickettsioses. In *Biology of rickettsial diseases*, CRC Press (ed. D. H. Walker), Vol. I, pp. 51–63. Boca Raton, Florida.

Gear, J. (1941). The typhus group of fevers. *The Leech*, **1941**, 7–15.

Groupe de travail OMS, (1982). Rickettsioses: un problème de morbidité persistant. *Bulletin of the World Health Organisation* **60**, 693–701.

Higgins, J. A., Radulovic, S., Schriefer, M. E. and Azad, A. F. (1996). *Rickettsia felis*: a new species of pathogenic rickettsia isolated from cat fleas. *Journal of Clinical Microbiology*, **34**, 671–4.

Irons, J. V. (1944). *et al.* Probable role of the cat flea, *Ctenocephalides felis*, in transmission of murine typhus. *American Journal of Tropical Medicine and Hygiene*, **24**, 359–62.

Kennou, M. F. and Edlinger, E. (1984). Donnees actuelles sur les rickettsioses en Tunisie. *Archives de l'Institut Pasteur de Tunis*, **61**, 427–33.

McDade, J. E. (1991). Evidence supporting the hypothesis that rickettsial virulence factors determine the severity of spotted fever and typhus group infections. *Annals of the New York Academy of Sciences*, **540**, 20–6.

Mallavia, L. P. (1991). Genetics of rickettsiae. *European Journal of Epidemiology*, **7**, 213–21.

Maxcy, K. L. (1926). An epidemiological study of endemic typhus (Brill's disease) in the southeastern United States with special reference to its mode of transmission. *Public Health Reports*, **41**, 12967–90.

Mooser, H., Castenda, M. R., and Zinsser, H. (1931). Rats as carriers of Mexican typhus fever. *Journal of the American Medical Association*, **97**, 231–2.

Myers, W. F. and Wisseman, C. L. (1980). Genetics relatedness among the typhus group of rickettsiae. *International Journal of Systematic Bacteriology*, **30**, 143–50.

Nicolle, C., Compote, C., and Conseil, E. (1900). Transmission experimetale du typhus exanthematique par le pou du corps. *Comples Rendus: de l'Academic des Sciences*, **149**, 486–9.

Penire, P. L. *et al.* (1992). A clinico-epidemiological study of epidemic typhus in Africa. *Clinical Infectious Diseases*, **19**, 1149–58.

Redus, M. A., Parker, R. A., and McDade, J. E. (1986). Prevalence and distribution of spotted fever and typhus infections in Sierra Leone and Ivory Coast. *International Journal of Zoonoses*, **13**, 104–11.

Reilly, P. J. and Kalinske, R. W. (1980). Brill–Zinsser disease in North America. *Western Journal of Medicine*, **133**, 338–40.

Retel-Laurentin, A., Capponi, M., and Gidel, R. (1974). Enquete sur les rickettsioses dans la region Bobo (rive droite de la Volta-Noire). *Bulletin de la Société Medicale d' Afrique Noire de Langue Francaise*, **19**, 411–20.

Saah, A. J. and Hornick, R. B. (1985). Rickettsiosis. *Rickettsia prowazekii* (epidemic or louseborne typhus). In *Principles and practice of infectious diseases*, (ed. G. L. Mandell, R. G. Douglas, and J. E. Bennett), pp. 1092–4. Wiley & Sons, New York.

Samra, Y., Shaked, Y., and Maier, M. K. (1989). Delayed neurologic display in murine typhus. Report of two cases. *Archives of Internal Medicine*, **149**, 949–51.

Schriefer, M. E., Sacci, J. B. J., Dumler, J. S., Bullen, M. G., and Azad, A. F. (1994*a*). Identification of a novel rickettsial infection in a patient diagnosed with murine typhus. *Journal of Clinical Microbiology*, **32**, 949–54.

Schriefer, M. E., Sacci, J. B. J., Taylor, J. P., Higgens, J. A., and Azad, A. F. (1994*b*). Murine typhus: updated roles of multiple urban components and a second typhus like rickettsia. *Journal of Medical Entomology*, **31**, 681–5.

Shaked, Y., Samra, Y., Maeir, M. K., and Rubinstein, E. (1988). Murine typhus and spotted fever in in the eighties: retrospective analysis. *Infection*. **16**, 283–7.

Silverman, D. J. (1991). Some contributions of electron microscopy to the study of the rickettsiae. *European Journal of Epidemiology*, **7**, 200–6.

Silverman, D. J., Boese, J. L., Wisseman, C. L. (1974). Ultrastructural studies of *Rickettsia prowazekii* from louse midgut cells to faeces: search for 'dormant forms'. *Infection and Immunity*, **10**, 257–63.

Sonenshine, D. E. *et al.* (1978). Epizootiology of epidemic typhus (*Rickettsia prowazekii*) in flying squirrels. *American Journal of Tropical Medicine and Hygiene*, **27**, 339–49.

Traub, R., Wisseman, C. L., and Azad, F. A. (1978). The ecology of murine typhus—a critical review. *Tropical Diseases Bulletin*, **75**, 237–317.

Tyeryar, F. J., Weiss, E., Millar, D. B., Bozeman, F. M., and Ormsbee, R. A. (1973). DNA base composition of *Rickettsiae. Science*, **180**, 415–17.

Walker, D. H. (1988*a*). Pathology and pathogenesis of the vasculotropic rickettsioses. In *Biology of rickettsial diseases*, (ed. D. H. Walker), CRC Press, Boca Raton, Florida. Vol. I, pp. 115–39.

Walker, D. H. (1988*b*). Role of composition of rickettsiae in rickettsial immunity: typhus and spotted fever groups. In Walker D. H. ed *Biology of rickettsial diseases*, CRC Press, (ed. D. H. Walker), Vol. II, pp. 101–11. Boc Raton, Florida.

Walker, D. H. (1991). The role of host factors in severity of spotted fever and typhus rickettsioses. *Annals of the New York Academy of Sciences*, **540**, 10–19.

Weiss, E. (1982). The biology of rickettsiae. *Annual Review of Microbiology*, **36**, 345–70.

Weiss, K. (1988). The role of rickettsioses in history. In *Biology of rickettisal diseases*, (ed. D. H. Walker), Vol. I, pp. 1–15. CRC Press Boca Raton, Florida.

Whelton, A., Donadio, J. V., Jr. and Elisberg, B. (1968). Acute renal failure complicating rickettsial infections in glucose-6-phosphate dehydrogenase deficient individuals. *Annals of Internal Medicine*, **69**, 323–8.

WHO (1993). Global surveillance of rickettsial diseases: memorandum from a WHO meeting: *Bulletin of the World Health Organisation*, **71**, 293–6.

Wilde, H., Pornsilapatip, J., Sokly, T., and Thee, S. (1991). Murine and scrub typhus at Thai—Kampuchean border displaced persons camp. *Tropical and Geographical Medicine*, **43**, 363–9.

Williams, S. G. *et al.* (1992). Typhus and typhus-like rickettsiae associated with opossums and their fleas in Los Angeles County, California. *Journal of Clinical Microbiology*, **30**, 1758–62.

Winkler, H. H. and Miller, E. T. (1981). Immediate cytotoxicity and phospholipase A: the role of phospholipase A in the interaction of *R. prowazekii* and L cells. In *Rickettsiae and rickettsial diseases*, (ed. W. Burgdorfer and R. L. Anacker), pp. 327–8. Academic Press, New York.

Wisseman, C. L. (1985). Selected observations on rickettsiae and their host cells. In *Rickettsiae and rickettsial disease*, (ed. J. Kazar), pp. 167–84. Publishing House of the Slovak Academy of Sciencies, Bratislava.

Woodward, T. E. (1988). Murine typhus fever: its clinical and biologic similarity to epidemic typhus. In *Biology of rickettsial diseases*, (ed. D. H. Walker) Vol. I, pp. 79–93. CRC Press, Boca Raton, Florida.

Zinsser, H. and Castenada, M. R. (1933). On the isolation from a case of Brill's disease of a typhus state resembling the European type. *New England Journal of Medicine*, **209**, 815–19.

24   SCRUB TYPHUS

Lorenza Beati, Didier Raoult, Daniel J. Sexton, and Edward Breitschwerdt

SUMMARY

Scrub typhus, also called chigger-borne typhus or tsut-sugamushi disease, is a febrile illness widely distributed in the eastern hemisphere, especially in south-eastern Asia. Its causative agent is *Orientia tsutsugamushi*, previously named *Rickettsia orientalis* and *Rickettsia tsutsugamushi*, which is transmitted to humans through the bite of the larval stage of trombiculid mites, acarians belonging to the genus *Leptotrombidium*. The geographical distribution of scrub typhus overlaps the distribution of these arthropods.

HISTORY

The presence of tsutsugamushi disease and its association with chigger bites has been recognized by some of the native populations of Japan and China for centuries. The term 'akamushi', the origin of the Japanese name for this rickettsiosis, means 'red chigger'. Rural residents of these countries often knew that the best way to avoid being infected was to avoid areas infested by these arthropods (Weiss 1981; Walker 1991). Early Chinese and Japanese investigators suspected that the illness was related to small mites. In 1920 Hayashi isolated an agent from mites that he called '*Theileria tsutsugamushi*'. In retrospect, this agent was not the cause of scrub typhus, but the term '*tsutsugamushi*' (for 'noxious mite') has persisted. In retrospect, the first identification of the causative agent of scrub typhus was by Nagayo and co-workers in 1930 (Nagayo *et al.* 1930). They called this organism *Rickettsia orientalis* but the name was changed to *R. tsutsugamushi* in 1948 (Bengston 1948) and then to *Orientia tsutsugamushi* in 1996. Prior to Nagayo's isolation of *O. tsutsugamushi*, investigators working what is now Malaysia used epidemiological data to classify locally occurring disease into urban (or 'shop') typhus or rural typhus. Rural typhus, which occurred predominately in grass or shrub land, later came to be called shrub typhus by British and Americans during Second World War. The term scrub typhus is now used throughout the world except in Japan where the name 'tsutsugamushi disease' is preferred. However, other synonyms have

also been used, including chigger-borne rickettsioses, Kedani (hairy mite) fever, akamushi (red mite) fever, flood fever, Japanese river fever, and tropical typhus.

The interest of physicians and scientists in this disease increased during the Second World War, when more than 15 000 cases of infection were diagnosed among the allied forces, with a mortality rate varying from 1 to 35 per cent (Weiss 1981). However, the disease cannot be associated with war conditions or natural disasters as is the case with epidemic typhus. The high incidence of scrub typhus during the Second World War and, to a lesser extent during the Vietnam War, can be ascribed to the fact that, during military field operations, large numbers of non-immune individuals were introduced into ecological niches inhabited by trombiculid mites. Therefore, scrub typhus should not be directly associated to the lack of hygiene and health care, which are characteristic features of war conditions. The term 'scrub' typhus was adopted because it was thought that the vectors were mainly found on scrub vegetation.

Although the high incidence of scrub typhus among the allied troops may be partly due to false-positive serological results, its occurrence led to a better description of the epidemiology and clinical features of the disease, and to the introduction of appropriate treatments. The disease shares common features with epidemic typhus, for example fever, headache, and rash, but the presence of an eschar and generalized lymphadenopathies is distinctive of scrub typhus.

In 1982, the WHO pointed out that, based on specific serological tests, a high proportion of fevers of unknown origin in endemic areas were probably undiagnosed scrub typhus cases and that the characteristic clinical signs, fever, eschar, and adenopathies, are often lacking (Groupe de travail OMS 1982). In 1993, a WHO meeting on global surveillance of rickettsial disease reported that, if the amount of epidemiological data collected on rickettsioses was considered rather inadequate in developing countries, then the information on scrub typhus was downright non-existent (WHO 1993). Emergence of scrub typhus has recently been observed in Australia and Japan, proving that endemic foci of the disease persist and that the disease should not be underestimated (Yamshita *et al.* 1988, 1994; Currie *et al.* 1993).

ORIENTIA TSUTSUGAMUSHI: THE ORGANISM

PHYLOGENY AND CLASSIFICATION

According to the last edition of *Bergey's manual of systematic bacteriology* (1984), *O. tsutsugamushi* belongs to the order Rickettsiales, family Rickettsiaceae, tribe Rickettsiae, and genus *Rickettsia*. This classification was based mainly on phenotypical data, geographical origin, relationships to vectors, or serological cross-reactions (Weiss and Moulder 1984). The classification of the organisms in the order Rickettsiales is currently under revision, as a result of the application of modern techniques of molecular biology, that have provided new insights into rickettsial phylogeny. As a result, the genus name *Orientia* was recently designated to include the agent of scrub typhus.

Sequencing of the 16S rRNA gene of these bacteria has recently shown that the genus *Rickettsia* belongs to a single phylum in the α-subdivision of the Proteobacteria (Weisburg 1989). The spotted fever group, typhus group and the AB bacterium are clustered together (at least 97 per cent homology). *Orientia tsutsugamushi* seems to have diverged earlier from the other rickettsiae (90 per cent homology), but it still remains more related to rickettsiae than to other bacteria of the same phylum (V. Roux, unpublished data). This last observation seems to contradict the conclusions drawn from the analysis of the structure and immunology of stress proteins (HSP60) of different organisms, which suggested that *O. tsutsugamushi* should be excluded from the genus *Rickettsia* (Dasch *et al.* 1990). The G+C content of *O. tsutsugamushi* (28.1–30.5 per cent), which has only recently been evaluated (Kumura *et al.* 1991), is different from that of *R. rickettsii*, but similar to that of the typhus group rickettsiae.

MORPHOLOGY

Orientia tsutsugamushi is an obligatory intracellular organism, which multiplies free in the cytoplasm of the host cell. Like other rickettsiae, it may be stained with the Giménez staining method. However, the Giemsa stain, preceded by a Carnoy's fixation, the method of choice for the staining of *O. tsutsugamushi*. It is a Gram-negative organism, with bilayer inner and outer membranes. By electron microscopy (Ito and Rikihisa 1981), the thickness of the leaflet of the outer membrane of *O. tsutsugamushi* enables one to differentiate it from the other rickettsiae, which usually show thinner outer membrane leaflets (Silverman 1991; Weiss 1982). Furthermore, there are some doubts about the presence of a peptidoglycan layer in *O. tsutsugamushi*, which is atypical for Gram-negative bacteria (Silverman 1991). The outer membrane is coated with a micro-capsular layer which is surrounded by a large translucent area called the slime layer (thinner than in other rickettsiae).

The organism can be cultured in embryonated eggs or in cell culture monolayers, where it produces small plaques (1 mm diameter) after 17 days of infection. The escape of *O. tsutsugamushi* from infected cells occurs through cell projections (Walker 1989) and does not seem to be related to cell damage. In mesothelial cells, the organisms are extruded from the cell in a vesicle of cell membrane and are phagocytosed by another cell while still coated with the cell membrane (Wisseman 1985). *Orientia tsutsugamushi* in L929 cells is a 1.2–1.6 μm long rod, with a diameter of 0.5–0.6 μm.

In arthropod cells *O. tsutgamushi* may be longer (up to 4 μm), containing characteristic cytoplasmic microtubular structures connected by a plate to the cytoplasmic membrane (Wright *et al.* 1984). The function of these microtubules has still to be determined. In the ovaries of infected mites, rickettsiae have been observed 'budding' out from the cell membrane or surrounded by a membrane in the cytosol.

ANTIGENIC PROPERTIES

Various strains of *O. tsutsugamushi* isolated from humans, chigger, or animals all belong to one of several different serotypes of the same species. These serotypes are not specifically associated with a vector species, a geographical area, or host species (Weiss 1981; Yamamoto *et al.* 1986; Ohashi *et al.* 1990). Studies, undertaken in the Japanese Gifu Prefecture, showed that it is not possible to find a single vector for each rickettsial serotype, and that rodents and humans can be infected by different strains (Yamashita *et al.* 1994). Karp, Gilliam, Kawasaki, and Kato are the best known serotypes. All three strains are used together as antigens in reagents used for the detection of antibodies reactive with *O. tsutsugamushi* (Eisemann and Osterman 1985; Yamamoto *et al.* 1986; Yamashita *et al.* 1994). Serotypes other than the preceding four strains have been described (Yamashita *et al.* 1988; Ohashi *et al.* 1990). Although these strains share common antigens, they can be differentiated from one another on the basis of their protein composition in different tests (fluorescence, cross-neutralization in guinea-pigs, toxin neutralization, cross- vaccination, or complement fixation) (Bell *et al.* 1946; Smadel *et al.* 1946; Rights *et al.* 1948; Iida *et al.* 1964; Shishido 1964). Occasionally the occurrence of cross-reactive antibodies in mouse sera can make classification of certain strains difficult, or impossible (Chang *et al.* 1990). In such instances, specific monoclonal antibodies are useful for the identification of newly isolated organisms (Weiss and Moulder 1984; Eisemann and Osterman 1985; Chang *et al.* 1990; Yamashita *et al.* 1994).

Studies using electrophoresis have shown that some of the major surface exposed antigens of *O. tsutsugamushi* do not react with heterologous sera. Outer membrane polypeptides with a molecular weight of 54–56 kDa are considered to be strain-specific, while the 43 and 70 kDa polypeptides are group-specific (Tamura *et al.* 1985; Urakami *et al.* 1986; Ohashi *et al.* 1988, 1990). The variability of the 54–56 kDa protein is at the basis of the phenotypic variations which characterize the different *O. tsutsugamushi* serotypes. These proteins seem to be involved in absorption to the host cell surface (Ohashi *et al.* 1992; Urakami *et al.* 1983). In laboratory animals and in humans, cross-immunity produced by one serotype may protect from a subsequent infection with another serotype, but this protection, when present, is transient (Oaks *et al.* 1987).

Humans infected with *O. tsutsugamushi* produce antibodies reactive with several surface antigens of the organism. These immunogenic antigens include rickettsial proteins in with a molecular weight of 110, 58, 56, and 47 kDa. The 58 kDa protein, called Sta58, is one the most conserved proteins among scrub typhus strains. Cloning of the gene encoding this protein has demonstrated that the amino acid sequence of Sta58 has a high homology with that of the heat-shock protein of *E. coli* (Hsp60, stress protein). Infection with one strain of *O. tsutsugamushi* does not preclude reinfection with another strain. This antigenic heterogeneity among strains complicates immunodiagnosis; as a result a battery of antigens must be utilized to detect infection with *O. tsutsugamushi* serologically.

EPIDEMIOLOGY

GEOGRAPHICAL DISTRIBUTION

Cases of tsutsugamushi disease have been reported from South-East Asia, Japan, Malaysia, Kampuchea, Thailand, Vietnam, southern China, Taiwan, Papua New Guinea, South-eastern Siberia, Sri Lanka, Indonesia, the Philippines, Korea, western Pacific Islands, Pakistan, Astrakhan, India, and northern Australia (Fig. 24.1) (Williams *et al.* 1994; Berman and Kundin 1973; Shirai and Wisseman 1975; Shirai *et al.* 1979; Weiss 1981; Groupe de travail OMS 1982 Weiss 1981; Groupe de travail OMS 1982; Weiss and Moulder 1984; Christie 1987; Currie *et al.* 1993; Yamashita *et al.* 1994) Depending on the region, scrub typhus may be either seasonal or endemic throughout the year.

VECTORS AND INFECTIOUS CYCLE

The main hosts of *O. tsutsugamushi* are different species of *Leptotrombidium* mites. *Leptotrombidium deliense* is the major vector in forest and scrub areas through tro-

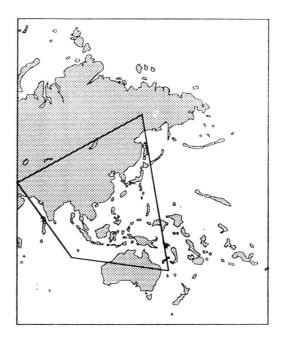

Fig. 24.1   The approximate distribution area of scrub typhus is delimited with a black line.

pical and subtropical Asia; *L. fletcheri* transmits scrub typhus in Indonesia, Malaysia, New Guinea and the Philippines; *L. arenicol* is a vector in Malaysia, and *L. imphatum* is a vector in Thailand. Other species of *Leptotrombidium* such as *L. pavlovskyi*, *L. papale*, *L. pallidum*, and *L. scutellare* are vectors of scrub typhus in cooler regions such as Japan, Korea, China, and parts of Siberia. In Japan two forms of scrub typhus occur: classical tsutsugamushi disease occurs primarily in the summer months and is transmitted by *L. akamushi*, whereas a milder form of disease, transmitted by *L. palliaum* and *L. scutellare*, occurs in winter. The occurrence of both forms of disease are closely related to the prevalence and distribution of these vectors. For instance, when the temperature rise above 20 °C in early summer, *L. akamushi* becomes especially prevalent along river banks. When temperatures fall below 18–20 °C, *L. pallidum* and *L. scutellare* increase in prevalence in woodlands and along hedgerows between tilled fields (Rapmund 1984).

Within 48 hours after emerging from eggs, chiggers attach to a host and feed for the next 2–12 days. After feeding they enter a pupa-like stage from which they emerge as a eight-legged nymph. Approximately 2 weeks later the nymphs pass through a second pupa-like stage and emerge as adults. Both nymphs and adults are scavengers and predators that feed on arthropods and their eggs in the soil and on debris on the surface of the soil. After mating, female adults may lay as many as 400 eggs which eventually hatch into six-legged chiggers. Trombiculid mites feed on mammals only during the chigger stage.

Although the results of several experimental studies have shown that several chiggers can simultaneously acquire *O. tsutsugamushi* while feeding on a rickettsaemic animal, such chiggers do not develop a generalized infection nor do they pass their rickettsial infection to the F_1 generation.

The precise sequence of events by which *O. tsutsugamushi* survives in mites is poorly understood. The efficiency of transovarial transmission varies from 100 per cent to as low as 22 per cent. The factors responsible for these variations are not understood. After hatching, chiggers aggregate in clusters on grass stems or on leaves in areas of secondary forestation and wait for potential hosts to come into contact with them. This clustering of progeny of an infected female in small geographic areas results in the formation of 'mite islands' ranging in size from a few inches to several metres (Currie *et al.* 1993).

Trombiculid mites have a patchy distribution, depending on the strict ecological demands characterizing each species. Chiggers are sedentary animals that wait for potential hosts to come into contact with them. They do not actively search for hosts. These factors explain the occurrence of hyperendemic foci, which overlap areas usually defined as 'mite islands'. In these restricted areas, ideal climatic and vegetation conditions as well as suitable hosts must all be present.

Following the first descriptions of endemic areas of scrub typhus, it was thought that chiggers were associated strictly with scrub vegetation and rivers. However, more recently, different species of *Leptotrombidium* infected with *O. tsutsugamushi* have been collected in ecologically heterogeneous areas, such as semi-deserts, sandy beaches, rain forests, or alpine mountains (Weiss 1981).

Rickettsiae multiply in cells of different arthropod organs. *Orientia tsutsugamushi* can be transmitted transovarially from an infected female to its progeny. Sexual transmission from infected males to uninfected males does not occur, since rickettsiae totally disappear from the cytoplasm of germ cells during spermatogenesis (Urakami *et al.* 1994). The infection rate of the progeny from infected female mites may vary from 20 to 100 per cent (Roberts and Robinson 1977).

The infection of *L. arenicola* and *L. fletcheri* with *R. tsutsugamushi* produces sex-ratio variations in the offspring of infected females. While progenies of non-infected strains have sex ratios (female: male) of 2:1 and 2:3 respectively, in the infected colonies there are only female offspring (Roberts *et al.* 1977). Whether this fact is due to the occurrence of thelytochus parthenogenesis, or to chromosomal alterations in the male gametes has yet to be clarified. The number of eggs laid by infected female mites is usually normal, so that a male killing process does not seem to be the cause of this phenomenon.

Rodents, particularly rats, are the principal hosts of the trombiculid mites that transmit *O. tsutsugamushi*. However, rodents play an insignificant role as sources for infecting chiggers with *O. tsutsugamushi*. In Japan and the Himalayas and other parts of north Asia, microtines such as voles are important hosts for chiggers. As chiggers are not host specific, any species of domestic animal or birds that enter their habitat may acquire infection with *O. tsutsugamushi*. In addition to man, *O. tsutsugamushi* has been recovered from pigs, rabbits, shrews, and birds (Burgdorfer 1988).

Rickettsaemia in naturally infected mice or rats is long lasting, and organisms can be recovered several months after infection. Since mites do not feed on blood, but tissue juices, it is rather unlikely that rodents are a source of infection for chiggers. Some authors reported infections of mite larvae fed on rickettsaemic mice; a continuous infection cycle into the mite could, however, not been established by this method. Therefore the maintenance of endemic foci seems to depend on transovarial transmission rather than on the presence of vertebrate reservoirs (Weiss 1981).

INCIDENCE

The precise incidence of tsutsugamushi disease is difficult to determine. Infection commonly occurs in rural areas with poor health surveillance and many cases either fail to seek medical case or are misdiagnosed as having another illness, such as malaria. However, an increased incidence of the disease and the emergence of new endemic foci have been reported in the past 15 years in Japan and Australia Yamashita *et al.* 1988; Currie *et al.* 1993). A recent study of patients with febrile illnesses in refugee camps at the border between Kampuchea and Thailand revealed that many cases of scrub and murine typhus were lumped together with many other illnesses collectively categorized as fever of unknown origin (Wilde *et al.* 1991).

SCRUB TYPHUS: THE DISEASE

PATHOGENESIS

Experimental studies of mice with *O. tsutsugamushi* have revealed that both the route of inoculation and the infecting strain affect pathogenicity. For example, intraperitoneal inoculation of *O. tsutsugamushi* is highly lethal for mice; mice can survive injection with 100 000 times more organisms administered subcutaneously (Groves and Kelly 1989). In addition, individual strains of *O. tsutsugamushi* vary widely in their virulence for mice and humans. The molecular or genetic basis for intra-or inter-strain variations in virulence is unknown.

DISEASE MECHANISMS

After inoculation into the body via the bite of a mite, rickettsiae spread throughout the body via the bloodstream or lymphatics. Once inside their human host, rickettsiae enter enthothelial cells and proliferate intracellularly by binary fission.

The precise mechanisms by which scrub typhus group rickettsiae produce cellular injury is still uncertain, but experimental studies suggest that a complex and multifactorial sequence of events occurs, culminating in endothelial injury (both swelling and necrosis) and secondary immune and phagocytic host responses (lymphocytes and macrophages) (Walker 1988). Typhus rickettsiae have the ability to injure cells directly in the absence of immune and inflammatory responses. *Orientia tsutsugamushi* is released from infected host cells by long filopodia into which rickettsiae pass during their cellular exit. Cellular release of typhus rickettsiae likely injuries host cell membranes in a manner similar to that which occurs in infection with *R. rickettsii* (Whelton *et al.* 1968).

CLINICAL FEATURES

Scrub typhus typically begins 7–10 days after a chigger bite (range 6–19). Some patients develop a localized eschar at the site of the chigger bite (Fig. 24.2). In many cases the eschar develops before the onset of systemic symptoms. Approximately one-half of all patients with scrub typhus develop a skin rash. In typical cases

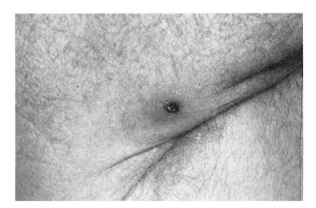

Fig. 24.2 Scrub typhus: eschar developed at the site of the chigger bite (kindly supplied by L. Watt).

the rash begins on the abdomen and spreads to the extremities. The face is often involved. The rash is usually macular or maculopapular; only rarely does it become petechial. In severe cases, some or all of the following complications may occurs: interstitial pneumonia, pulmonary oedema, arhythmias, nausea and vomiting, and a wide array of signs and symptoms of central nervous system dysfunction, including delirium, seizures, and confusion. Without treatment, scrub typhus usually lasts for 2–3 weeks. The risk of fatal outcome varies widely in different geographic regions. In fatal cases, death usually occurs late in the second week of illness due to one or more of the following: pneumonia, circulatory collapse, pulmonary oedema, or seizures. Most patients with severe disease are thrombocytopenic. Laboratory abnormalities indicative of renal and hepatic dysfunction are also common.

The pathological changes associated with scrub typhus are also similar to changes seen in epidemic typhus. The histological changes observed in biopsies of eschars depend upon the duration of the illness. The site of an infected chigger bite typically begins as a papule that sequentially evolves into a vesicopaule, an eschar, an ulcer and, in some cases, later becomes a scar. *Orientia tsutsugamushi* can be visualized in endothelial cells in a typical eschar which often consists of a focal area of cutaneous necrosis surrounded by a zone with intense vasculitis manifesting the classic changes of all rickettsial infection: perivascular infiltration of blood vessels with lymphocytes and macrophages. Thrombosis of small vessels is also present in some eschars. As in epidemic typhus, involvement of the central nervous system by *O. tsutsugamushi* may result in a mononuclear cell meningitis and the formation of typhus nodules. Some patients with scrub typhus develop interstitial pneumonitis as a direct effect of their rickettsial vasculitis. Lymphadenopathy accompanied by inflammation within the lymphatic sinuses may occur in the region of an eschar or be generalized. In addition, many patients have splenomegaly and some have portal triaditis.

Diagnosis

As recently reported from Australia, scrub typhus cases may be difficult to diagnose in regions not known as endemic areas. In these foci, some cases have been misdiagnosed in their early phases (Currie *et al.* 1993). The presence of fever and lymphadenopathy in a patient who has been in endemic areas should suggest a diagnosis of scrub typhus. Non-specific signs are neutropenia and a mononucleosis-like syndrome.

Diagnosis was originally obtained by inoculation of the blood of suspected cases into mice. The first indirect test used for the diagnosis of scrub typhus was the

Weil–Felix test, based on cross-reactions between antibodies to *O. tsutsugamushi* and the strain OX-K of *Proteus mirabilis*. However, positive reactions were found in cases of louse-borne relapsing fever, leptospirosis, or *Proteus* urinary tract infections. Although this test could detect fewer than 20 per cent of scrub typhus cases, it has been used since the Second World War (Dasch *et al.* 1979).

Specific diagnosis is now based on indirect immunofluorescence tests (Bozeman and Elisberg 1963), with a cut-off titre of 1 : 128 (IgG and IgM). Since human sera often do not cross-react with all protype strains of *O. tsutsugamushi*, it is necessary to use antigens from at least four different strains (Karp, Kato, Kawasaki, and Gilliam) for specific immunofluorescence diagnosis (Chang *et al.* 1990). Seroconversions are often delayed and antibodies may appear 10 days after the onset of the disease.

More recently, new techniques have been adapted to the diagnosis of scrub typhus. A passive haemagglutination test using a recombinant 56 kDa polypeptide gives specific reactions with sera collected from scrub typhus patients (Kim *et al.* 1993). PCR with primers derived from the 56 kDa gene of Karp (Kelly *et al.* 1990) have been developed and applied to *R.tsutsugamushi* detection in blood samples. This method is of higher sensitivity when compared to the serological tests (Sugita *et al.* 1993) but is usually not available in areas where the disease is common. Furthermore, PCR testing requires great technical expertise to avoid false-positive and false-negative results.

Treatment and prophylaxis

As for spotted fever and typhus group rickettsioses, tetracycline is the treatment of choice for scrub typhus. The recommended treatment is two 100 mg doses of doxycycline for 3–10 days. Defervescence is usually observed 24 hours after the first dose. In fact, failure to respond within 72 hours of starting empirical treatment is often considered to be clinical evidence that a rickettsial disease such as scrub typhus is not present.

Since there is no vaccine available against rickettsial diseases, in endemic areas the application of DEET-containing repellents to the skin or permethrin-containing repellents to cloth is recommended (Currie *et al.* 1993). The meal of mites lasts several days, but it seems that infectious organisms are not transmitted during the first 6–8 hours after attachment. Thus rapid removal of attached chiggers may be helpful in avoiding infections. Tetracycline, given as a weekly dose of doxycyline, is also effective as prophylaxis for individuals living or working in areas where scrub typhus is highly endemic. As this therapy may produce unwanted side-effects such as gastrointestinal distress, diarrhoea, or photosensitivity, prophylaxis is generally reserved for special circumstances, such as military operations in endemic regions.

Prognosis

The prognosis for humans infected with scrub typhus varies in different regions and even for different individuals within the same region. This variability may be due to variations in the virulence of different strains of *O. tsutsugamushi* or may be due to variability in the immunological responses of the host. Results of serological surveys in endemic regions indicate that asymptomatic, subclinical, or unrecognized infection with *O. tsutsugamushi* is common.

ACKNOWLEDGEMENTS

Special thanks to Professor Patrick J. Kelly for his patience in reviewing the English manuscript.

REFERENCES

Bell, E. J., Bennett, B. L., and Whitman, L. (1946). Antigenic differences between strains of scrub typhus as demonstrated by cross-neutralisation tests. *Proceedings of the Society of Experimental Biology and Medicine*, **62**, 134–7.

Bengston, I. A. (1948). Rickettsiales Gieszcyzkiewicz (6th edn). In *Bergey's mannual of definitive bacteriology*, (ed. R. S. Breed, E. G. P. Murray and A. P. Hitchens), Baltimore, Maryland. Williams and Wilkins, Baltimore, Maryland.

Berman, S. J. and Kundin, W. D. (1973). Scrub typhus in South Vietnam: a study of 87 cases. *Annals of Internal Medicine*, **79**, 26–30.

Bozeman, F. M. and Elisberg, B. L. (1963). Serological diagnosis of scrub typhus by indirect immunofluorescence. *Proceedings of the Society of Experimental Biology and Medicine*, **112**, 568–73.

Burgdorfer, W. (1988). Ecological and epidemiological considerations of Rocky Mountain Spotted fever and scrub typhus. In *Biology of rickettsial diseases*, (ed. D. H. Walker), Vol. 1, pp. 33–51. CRC Press, Boca Raton, Florida.

Chang, W. H., Kang, J. S., Lee, W. K., Choi, M. S., and Lee, J. H. (1990). Serological classification by monoclonal antibodies of *Rickettsia tsutsugamushi* isolated in Korea. *Journal of Clinical Microbiology*, **28**, 685–8. Christie (1987)

Currie, B., O'Connor, L., and Dwyer, B. (1993). A new focus of scrub typhus in tropical Australia. *American Journal of Tropical Medicine and Hygiene*, **49**, 425–9.

Dasch, G. A., Halle, S., and Bourgeois, L. (1979). Sensitive microplate enzyme-linked immunosorbent assay for detection of antibodies against the scrub typhus rickettsia, *Rickettsia tsutsugamushi. Journal of Clinical Microbiology*, **9**, 38–48.

Dasch, G. A., Ching, W. M., and Kim, P. Y. (1990). A structural and immunological comparison of rickettsial HSP60 antigens with those of other species. In *Rickettsiology: current issues and perspectives*, (ed. K. E. Hechemy, D. Paretsky, D. H. Walker, and I. P. Mallavia), pp. 352–69. Annals of the New York Academy of Sciences, New York.

Eisemann, C. S. and Osterman, J. V. (1983). Identification of strain-specific and group-reactive antigenic determinants on the Karp, Gilliam and Kato strains of *Rickettsia tsutsugamushi*. *American Journal of Tropical Medicine and Hygiene*, **34**, 1173–8.

Groupe de travail O. M. S. (1982). Rickettsioses: un probleme de morbidité persistant. *Bulletin of the World Health Organisation*, **60**, 693–71.

Groves, M. G. and Kelly, D. J. (1989). Characterization of factors determining. *Orientia tsutsugamushi* pathogenicity for mice. *Infection and Immunity*, **57**, 1476–82.

Iida, T., Kawshima, H., and Kawamura, A. (1964). Direct immunofluorescence for typing of tsutsugamushi disease rickettsia. *Journal of Immunology*, **95**, 1120–33.

Ito, S. and Rikihisa, Y. (1981). Techniques for electron microscopy of rickettsiae. In *Rickettsiae and rickettsial diseases*, (ed. W. Burgdorfer and R. L. Anacker), pp. 213–27. Academic Press, New York.

Kelly, D. J., Marana, D. P., Stover, C. K., Oaks, E. V., and Carl, M. (1990). Detection of *Rickettsia tsutsugamushi* by gene amplification using polymerase chain reaction techniques. In *Reickettsiology: current issues and perspectives*, (ed. K. E. Hechemy, D. Paretsky, D. H. Walker, and L. P. Mallavia); pp. 564–71. Annals of the New York Academy of Sciences, New York.

Kim, I. S., Seong, S. Y., Woo, S. G., Choi, M. S., Kang, J. S., and Chang W. H. (1993). Rapid diagnosis of scrub typhus by a passive hemagglutination assay using recombinant 56-kilodalton polypeptides. *Journal of Clinical Microbiology*, **31**, 2057–60.

Kumura, K., Minamishima, Y., Yamamoto, S., Ohashi, N., and Tamura, A. (1991). DNA base composition of *Rickettsiae tsutsugamushi* determined by reversed-phase high-performance liquid chromatography. *International Journal of Systematic Bacteriology*, **41**, 247–8.

Nagayo, M., Tamiya, T., Mitamura, T. *et al.* (1930). On the virus of tsutsugamushi disease and its demonstration by a new method. *Japanese Journal of Experimental Medicine*, **8**, 309–18.

Oaks, E. V., Stover, C. K., and Rice, R. M. (1987). Molecular cloning and expression of *Rickettsia tsutsugamushi* genes for two major protein antigens in *Escherichia coli*. *Infection and Immunity*, **55**, 1156–62.

Ohashi, N., Tamura, A., and Suto, T. (1988). Immunoblotting analysis of anti-rickettsial antibodies produced in patients of tsutsugamushi disease. *Microbiology and Immunology*, **32**, 1085–92.

Ohashi, N., Tamura, A., Sakurai, H., and Yamamoto, S. (1990). Characterisation of a new antigenic type, Kuroki, of *Rickettsia tsutsugamushi* isolated from a patient in Japan. *Journal of Clinical Microbiology*, **28**, 2111–13.

Ohashi, N., Nashimoto, H., Ikeda, H., and Tamura, A. (1992). Diversity of immunodominant 56-kDa type-specific antigen (TSA) of *Rickettsia tsutsugamushi*. *Journal of Biological Chemistry*, **267**, 12728–35.

Rapmund, G. (1984). Rickettsial diseases of the far east, new perspectives. *Journal of Infectious Diseases*, **149**, 330–7.

Rights, F., Smadel, J. E., and Jackson, E. B. (1948). Studies on scrub typhus (tsutsugamushi disease). III. Heterogeneity of strains of *R. tsutsugamushi* as demonstrated by cross-vaccination studies. *Journal of Experimental Medicine*, **87**, 339–51.

Roberts, L. W. and Robinson, D. M. (1977). Efficiency of transovarial transmission of *Rickettsia tsutsugamushi* in *Leptotrombidium arenicola* (Acari: Trombiculidae). *Journal of Medical Entomology*, **13**, 493–6.

Roberts, L. W., Rapmund, G., and Cadigan, F. C. (1977). Sex ratios in *Rickettsia tsutsugamushi*-infected and noninfected colonies of *Leptotrombidium*. *Journal of Medical Entomology*, **14**, 89–92.

Shirai, A. and Wisseman, C. L. (1975). Serologic classification of scrub typhus isolates from Pakistan. *American Journal of Tropical Medicine and Hygiene*, **1**, 87–99.

Shirai, A., Robinson, D. M., Brown, G. W., Gan, E., and Huxsoll, D. L. (1979). Antigenic analysis by direct immunofluorescence of 114 isolates of *Rickettsia tsutsugamushi* recovered from febrile patients in rural Malaysia. *Japanese Journal of Medical Science and Biology*, **32**, 337–44.

Shirai, A., Coolbaugh, J. C., Gan, E., Chan T. C., Huxsoll, D. L., and Groves, M. G. (1982). Serologic analysis of scrub typhus isolates from the Pescadores and Philippine islands. *Japanese Journal of Medical Science and Biology*, **35**, 225–9.

Shishido, A. (1964). Strain variation of *Rickettsia orientalis* in the complement fixation test. *Japanese Journal of Medical Science and Biology*, **17**, 59–72.

Silverman, D. J. (1991). Some contributions of electron microscopy to the study of the rickettsiae. *European Journal of Epidemiology*, **7**, 200–6.

Smadel, J. E., Jackson, E. B., Bennett, B. L., and Rights, E. L. (1946). A toxic substance associated with the Gilliam strain of *R.tsutsugamushi*. *Proceedings of the Society of Experimental Medicine*, **62**, 138–40.

Sugita, Y., Yamakawa, Y., Takahashi, K., Nagatani, T., Okuda, K., and Nakajima, H. (1993). A polymerase chain reaction system for rapid diagnosis of scrub typhus within six hours. *American Journal of Tropical Medicine and Hygiene*, **49**, 636–40.

Tamura, A., Ohashi, N., Urakami, H., Takahashi, K., and Oyanagi, M. (1985). Analysis of polypeptide composition and antigenic components of *Rickettsia tsutsugamushi* by polyacrylamide gel electrophoresis and immunoblotting. *Infection and Immunity*, **48**, 671–5.

Urakami, H., Tsuruhara, T., and Tamura, A. (1983). Penetration of *Rickettsia tsutsugamushi* into cultured mouse fibroblast (L cells): an electron microscopic observation. *Microbiology and Immunology*, **27**, 251–63.

Urakami, H., Ohashi, N., Tsuruhara, T., and Tamura, A. (1986). Characterisation of polypeptides in *Rickettsia tsutsugamushi*: effect of preparative conditions on migration of polypeptides in polyacrylamide gel electrophoresis. *Infection and Immunity*, **51**, 948–52.

Urakami, H., Takahashi, M., Hori, E., and Tamura, A. (1994). An ultrastructural study of vertical transmission of *Rickettsia tsutsugamushi* during oogenesis and spermatogenesis in *Leptotrombidium pallidum*. *American Journal of Tropical Medicine and Hygiene*, **50**, 219–28.

Walker, D. H. (1988). Pathology and pathogenesis of the vasculotropic rickettsioses. In Walker DH, ed. *Biology of rickettsial disease*, (ed. D. H. Walker), Vol. I, pp. 115–39. CRC Press, Boca Raton, Florida.

Walker, D. H. (1989). The rickettsia–host interaction. In *Intracellular parasitism*, (ed. J. W. Moulder), pp. 79–91. CRC Press, Boca Raton, Florida.

Walker, D. H. (1991). *Biology of rickettsial diseases*. Vol. I. CRC Press, Boca Raton, Florida.

Weisburg, W. G. (1989). Polyphyletic origin of bacterial parasites. In *Intracellular parasitism*, (ed. J. W. Moulder), pp. 1–15. CRC Press, Boca Raton, Florida.

Weiss, E. (1981). The family Rickettsiaceae: human pathogens. In *The prokaryotes. A handbook on habitats, isolation, and identification of bacteria*, (ed. M. P. Starr, H. Stolp, H. G. Truper, A. Balows, and H. G. Schlegel), pp. 2138–60. Springer-Verlag, Berlin-Heidelberg.

Weiss, E. (1982). The biology of rickettsiae. *Annual Reviews of Microbiology*, **36**, 345–70.

Weiss, E. and Moulder, J. W. (1984). Order I. Rickettsiales Gieszcakiewicz. 1939, 25AL. In *Bergeys' manual of systematic bacteriology* (ed. N. R. Kreig, and J. G. Holt), pp. 687–704. Williams and Wilkins, Baltimore.

Whelton, A., Donadio, J. V., Jr and Elisberg, B. L. (1968). Acute renal failure complicating rickettsial infections in glucose-6-phosphate dehydrogenase deficient individuals. *Annals of Internal Medicine*, **69**, 323–8.

WHO (1993). Global surveillance of rickettsial diseases: memorandum from a WHO meeting. *Bulletin of the World Health Organisation*, **71**, 293–6.

Wilde, H., Pornsilapatip, J., Sokly, T., and Thee, S. (1991). Murine and scrub typhus at Thai–Kampuchean border displaced persons camp. *Tropical and Geographical Medicine* **43**, 363–9.

Williams, S. W., Sinclair, A. J. M., and Jackson, A. V. (1944). Mite-borne (scrub) typhus in Papua and the mandated Territory of New Guinea: report of 626 cases. *Medical Journal of Australia*, **ii**, 525–39.

Wisseman, C. L. (1985). Selected observations on rickettsiae and their host cells. In *Rickettsia and rickettsial diseases*, (ed. J. Kazar), pp. 167–84. Publishing House of the Slovak Academy of Sciences, Bratislava.

Wright, J. D., Hastriter, M. W., and Robinson, D. M. (1984). Observations on the ultrastructure and distribution of *Rickettsia tsutsugamushi* in naturally infected *Leptotrombidium arenicola* (Acari: Trombiculidae). *Journal of Medical Entomology*, **21**, 17–27.

Yamamoto, S. *et al.* (1986). Immunological properties of *Rickettsia tsutsugamushi*, Kawasaki strain, isolated from a patient in Kysushu. *Microbiology and Immunology*, **30**, 611–20.

Yamshita, T, Kasuya, S., Noda, S., Nagano, I., Ohtsuka, S., and Ohtomo, H. (1988). Newly isolated strains of *Rickettsia tsutsugamushi* in Japan identified by using monoclonal antibodies to Karp, Gilliam, and Kato strains. *Journal of Clinical Microbiology*, **26**, 1859–60.

Yamashita, T., Kasuya, S., Noda, N., Nagano, I., and Kang, J. S. (1994). Transmission of *Rickettsia tsutsugamushi* strains among humans, wild rodents, and trombiculid mites in an area of Japan in which tsutsugamushi disease is newly endemic. *Journal of Clinical Microbiology*, **32**, 2780–5.

25 TULARAEMIA

Andrew Pearson

SUMMARY

Tularaemia is a plague-like disease of animals and man caused by *Francisella* species. Sporadic human infection occurs in residents and travellers to endemic areas and may cause epidemics at times of rodent increase. Transmission is from bites of ticks and mosquitoes; water-borne outbreaks occur from drinking water in rural areas. Airborne outbreaks arise from moving rodent-contaminated hay, when threshing corn, or from laboratory accidents.

Francisella tularensis subspecies *tularensis* only occurs naturally in North America; but cultures are held in laboratories around the world; this highly virulent agent has been considered to have potential for biological warfare.

Francisella tularensis subspecies *holarctica* biogroup I occurs throughout the northern hemisphere but predominates in western and northern Europe, eastern Siberia, the Far East, and Kazakhstan; cases are only rarely reported from North America. *Francisella tularensis* subspecies *holarctica* biogroup II is distributed only in Eurasia, central and eastern Europe, the Caucasus, and it is predominant in western Siberia and Kazakhstan. *Francisella tularensis* subspecies *holarctica* biovar *japonica* is distributed on the Japanese islands; *F. tularensis* subspecies *mediasiatica* occurs in central Asian parts of the former USSR.

Francisella tularensis subspecies *tularensis* principally causes ulceroglandular tularaemia, both by contact with infected lagomorphs and rabbits and from tick bites. Rarely, eating undercooked rabbit or hare meat causes a typhoidal-like illness; cleaning contaminated carcasses may lead to an oculoglandular presentation. Any form of the disease may be complicated by pneumonia which is one of the two presenting conditions in laboratory-acquired infections, the other being the typhoidal or the abdominal form. European and Asian forms of disease are far more diverse, reflecting the less virulent nature of the agent, the widespread distribution and type of ecological foci, and the greater diversity of hosts and vectors.

HISTORY

European and Russian doctors have long recognized the existence of human disease outbreaks in association with times of rodent abundance (highs). In 1532 Jacob Ziegler described how lemmings crowded together and died of epidemic disease and then caused disease among human beings '*ex quarum corruptione aer fir pestilens et ad ficit Norduegos uertigire et icteri*'. In 1653, Olaus Wormius wrote of the Norwegians' fear of lemming invasions and he described a disease which included swelling of the glands. From the early times the clergy used to read a Latin prayer of exorcisement against lemmings, 'I exorcise you, pestiferous worms mice, birds or locusts, or other animals, by God the Father, … that you department immediately from these fields, or vineyards, or waters, and dwell in them no longer, but go away to those places in which you can harm no person'. This statement represents the first written public health intervention for a tularaemia-like disease!

By the end of the nineteenth century 'lemming fever' was a well-recognized clinical entity. In 1895, Collett wrote:

It is obvious that great masses of individuals which perish incessantly during a migratory year, must have an influence on sanitary conditions, especially during the warm season of the year. Everyone who has visited a mountain plateau during a prolific year will have noticed their oblong pellets of dung which are to be found strewed about everywhere and in such great quantities that it is often difficult to place one's foot on a spot that is entirely clear of them. It follows of itself that all running water will be contaminated by this decaying excrement. To this may be added the dead animals, which will be found lying scattered about in great numbers, and which, during hot summers, become quickly decomposed. The rain carried the putrid matter onto the nearest water course, when it makes its way to wells, and becomes mixed with drinking water of the inhabitants. During some great prolific years definite forms of sickness have appeared in certain of the over-run districts, and the people have given these the name of 'Lemming Fever' as they presumed that they were connected with the appearance of these animals. Many of the doctors practising in the country have turned their attention to the disease and diagnosed it in their case reports.

The discovery of tularaemia is attributed to McCoy (1911) who reported a plague-like illness in Californian ground squirrels (*Citellus beecheyi*, Richardson) and who, with Chapin, isolated an apparently new agent (McCoy and Chapin 1912). Pure cultures of this organism, which they called *Bacterium tularensis* after the Californian county Tulare, were used to reproduce the disease in guinea-pigs. A similar agent had been observed in Europe by Horne (1912), who saw tiny plague-like, bipolar-staining coccobacilli in Scandinavian lemmings (*Lemmus lemmus*), and transferred the agent to guinea-pigs in which it produced an epizootic in the animal colony at the Veterinary Institute in Oslo.

The first case in North America for which the diagnosis was established by isolation of the organism was described by Wherry and Lamb in 1914, but the possible extent of human infection in America was not realized until an investigation of 'deerfly fever' by Francis in the Pahvant valley of Utah. The investigation of these early cases and outbreaks caused a significant morbidity and a mortality amongst the investigators and laboratory workers. In the USA between 1924 and 1950 there were 23 309 recorded cases with a 9.5 per cent case fatality ratio before the introduction of streptomycin in 1949, between 1960 and 1968 there are reports of 2594 cases with only 23 deaths.

In western Europe the first established cases of *F. tularensis holarctica* (type B) were diagnosed in Norway and Sweden by Thjotta (1931*a,b*). Tularaemia has been reported from both the European and Asiatic parts of the USSR (Tiggertt 1962); and most

other countries of northern, central and eastern Europe (Jusatz 1962); and in Japan (O'Hara *et al.* 1971). Indigenous tularaemia has not been recorded in the United Kingdom but cases are occasionally imported (Blomley and Pearson 1972; Wood *et al.* 1976).

THE AGENT

TAXONOMY

The taxonomic designation of the seven bacterial agents causing tularaemia-like disease is given in Table 25.1. In the past, strains of *tularensis* have been assigned variously to the *Pasturella* group (on the basis of various characters, including its bipolar staining and its solubility in 1 in 800 sodium ricinoleate) and to the *Brucella* group (on the basis of such characters as its weak fermentative ability and its sensitivity to methylene blue). A separate genus, *Francisella*, was proposed after it was appreciated that its DNA base composition, fatty acid profile, and biochemical reactivity are quite different from those of bacteria in the genera *Pasteurella*, *Yersinia*, and *Brucella*. The G + C content of

Table 25.1   Designation of Genus *Francisella*

Subspecies and synonyms	Reference strains and first isolation
F. tularensis subsp. *tularensis*[a] (synonyms: type A; *F. tularensis* subsp. *nearctica*) Virulent typical strain is GIEM Schu Type strain is avirulent ATCC 6223	Avirulent type strain is ATCC 6223 Virulent typical strain is GIEM strain Schu which was first isolated in 1941 from humans in the United States
F. tularensis subsp. *holarctica*[a] biogroup I (erythromycin susceptible) (synonyms: type B; *F. tularensis* subsp. *palaearctica*) Reference strains GIEM c/a 7 (Reference strains HN 63) (Reference strains TN 52)	Reference strain GIEM c/a7 isolated from humans in 1976 in the Moscow region of USSR. First isolated Norway 1896. (Horne 1912)
F. tularensis subsp. *holarctica*[a] biogroup II (erythromycin resistant) (synonyms: type B; *F. tularensis* subsp. *palaearctica*) Reference strain is GIEM 503 ATCC 29684	Reference strain GIEM 503 is the type strain of this subspecies
F. tularensis subsp. *holarctica*[a] biogroup japonica (synonym: *F. tularensis* var. *palaearctica japonica*) Reference strain is GIEM Miura	Reference strain GIEM Miura was isolated from humans in 1975. Originally isolated in Japan in 1926 from a human lymph node
F. tularensis subsp. *mediasiatica*[a] Reference strain is GIEM 543	Isolated in the middle Asian region of the USSR (Alma-Ata) in 1965 from a gerbil. Maintained only by ticks and strains of *Lepus* and *Gerbillinae*
F. novicida[b] Reference strain is ATCC 15482	First isolated from a water sample in Utah USA in 1951 and later from human cases in USA
F. philomiragia[b] (synonym: *Yersinia philomiragia*) Type strain is ATCC 25015	First isolated in 1959 from a dying muskrat in Utah USA, other strains isolated from water and human cases

[a] Validly described by Olsufjev and Meshcheryakova in 1983 who revised their previous nomenclature of these subspecies.
[b] Validly described by Hollis *et al.* in 1989.

Francisella DNA is 33–36 mol %, as compared with 40–45 mol % for *Pasteurella*, 46–50 for *Yersinia*, and 55–58 for *Brucella*.

MOLECULAR BIOLOGY

Francisella tularensis has a high lipid content (21 per cent by dry weight) and contains two major phospholipids, phosphatidylethanolamine and phosphatidylglycerol. There are several unusual fatty acids, for example long-chain (C_{20}–C_{26}) acids and 2-hydroxyhexadecanoate and 3-hydroxyoctadecanoate—which could be of diagnostic value; the non-hydroxy fatty acid composition is considered to represent a valuable taxonomic characteristic (Nichols *et al.* 1985). The antigens of *F. tularensis*, including the lipopolysaccharides, and their immuno-genicity have been studied to assess their potential importance as components of vaccines (Nutter 1971). There is an extensive literature on the molecular aspects of the host–bacterial interactions of *F. tularensis* in man and animals (Lofgren *et al.* 1980, 1983).

MORPHOLOGY, GROWTH, AND SURVIVAL REQUIREMENTS

Morphology

The different subspecies and biogroups of *F. tularensis* are morphologically indistinguishable. *In vivo*, the organism occurs as tiny coccobacilli (0.2–0.7 μm) surrounded by a clear area which corresponds to the capsule. It is frequently pleomorphic; ovoid, bacillary, bean-shaped, dumb-bell, and filamentous forms may occur (Eigelsbach *et al.* 1946). The organism is Gram-negative and non-motile and does not form spores. The capsule may be demonstrated by negative staining. Loss of the capsule may occur with repeated subculture on laboratory media, but the bacteria remain viable and infective. *Francisella tularensis* stains most readily with hot carbol fuchsin or aniline gentian violet.

Isolation and cultural characters (Table 25.2)

Cysteine is required for growth. Primary isolation from animals, birds, and man requires the use of either enriched media, inoculation into the chick embryo or preliminary animal passage: the last appears to be essential for the isolation of *F. tularensis* from water. Media used for primary isolation include coagulated egg-yolk, glucose–cysteine blood agar (GCBA), peptone–cysteine agar, glucose serum agar, and Brain Veal infusion agar. During the 1967 Swedish outbreak, Ringertz and Dhalstrand (1968) used successfully a medium containing tryptose broth, cysteine, sodium thioglycollate, glucose, and rabbit blood. The use of antibiotics in selective media has been recommended for the isolation of *F. tularensis* from contaminated

Table 25.2 Detection and typing methods for *Francisella* species

Method	Source
Bacterial culture	
Blood agar (GCBA)	Lake and Francis (1922)
Peptone cysteine agar	Eigelsbach and McGann (1984)
Tryptose broth medium	Ringertz and Dahlstrand (1968)
Animal inoculation	
Infant white mice	
Guinea-pigs	Anthony *et al.* (1991)
Adult white mice	Ito *et al.* (1985)
Chick embryo	
Non-cultural and genomic method	
Enumeration of viable non-culturable bacteria	
16s RNA hybridization	Forsman *et al.* (1990)
Immunological methods	
Fluorescent antibody detection of antigen	Zuerlein and Smith (1985)
Rapid slide microagglutination	Haug and Pearson (1972)
Microagglutination test (MAT)	Behan and Klein (1982)
Tube agglutination	Francis and Evans (1926)
Microtitre plate agglutination	Massey and Mangiafico (1974)
Haemagglutination inhibition	Saslaw and Carlisle (1961)
Gel diffusion	Ohara *et al.* (1974)
ELISA using lipopolysaccharide	Carlsson *et al.* (1979)
Elisa using sonicated extract	Viljanen *et al.* (1983)
Radiometric assay	Canonico *et al.* (1975)
Monoclonal antibody	Fulop *et al.* (1991)
Intradermal skin test	Buchanan *et al.* (1971)
Lymphocyte stimulation	Syrjälä *et al.* (1984)
Interleukin-2 production	Karttunen *et al.* (1985)

material; penicillin, polymyxin B, and cycloheximide have been used.

Francisella tularensis colonies on GCBA are 1–3 mm in diameter after 48–72 h, greyish, and usually viscous with a greenish discolouration of the surrounding medium, but colonial characters may differ markedly on other media. The optimum temperature for growth is 37 °C. The organism will not grow under full anaerobic conditions; CO_2 is beneficial for growth. *Francisella tularensis* is cytotrophic. It grows well in the developing chick embryo in which it causes death of the embryo in 3–4 days when inoculated onto the chorio-allantoic membrane. Animal passage is the optimal method for isolation of wild strains. Subcutaneous inoculation into the guinea-pig of *F. tularensis* subspecies *tularensis* (type A) leads to death in 5–8 days. Subscapular injection into white mice is the preferred method for the isolation of the subspecies *holarctica* (type B).

Biochemical and biological properties

Francisella tularensis gives a weak catalase reaction and, under optimal conditions, forms acid but no gas in glucose and usually in maltose, mannose, and laevulose, but not in sucrose. Its oxidase reaction is negative but it forms H_2S. Differentiation between *tularensis* and the *holarctica* subspecies relies on the ability of the former to ferment glycerol and on its possession of a citrulline urease system (Fleming and Foshay 1955).

THE HOSTS

Francisella species are intracellular pathogens producing fulminant acute infection in the susceptible animal hosts, chronic granulomatous infection in moderately susceptible species, or long-term immunity in resistant species. The severity and type of infection and incubation period (range 1–14 days) in man depends on the subspecies or biogroup, the route of infection (Table 25.3), and the dose. The LD50 for man of the laboratory-prepared schu strain can be as little as one organism by the airborne route as compared to several hundred bacteria when ingesting holarctic strains from contaminated water. Infection in man may be localized or generalized (Table 25.4). Localized infection results from an insect or tick bite or a scratch from an infected carcass or animal; the lesion may vary from a local indurated ulcer to no visible lesion, but there is usually swelling of the local lymph nodes which may, if the infection is not treated, enlarge or rupture. The histology of the lymph node is a non-caseating granuloma in which *Francisella tularensis* may be detected by culture, immunological, or genomic methods. Bacteraemic spread and immunological reactions may complicate the disease process in man.

Published work on animal susceptibility in the past often failed to characterize fully the type of laboratory strain used in experimental work, or to distinguish whether the isolate from wild animals was of subspecies *tularensis* or *holarctica*. The classical plague-like illness described in ground squirrels and reproduced in laboratory guinea-pigs is caused by organisms of the *tularensis* subspecies. The LD_{50} is between one and ten

Table 25.3 Comparison of contact and airborne outbreaks

Symptoms and signs	Contact No. cases[a]	Outbreak %	Airborne No. cases[b]	Outbreak %
Fever	38	97	343	85
Chills	23	59	285	70
Myalgia	22	56	–	–
Malaise	20	51	179	44
Diaphoresis	11	28	–	–
Headache	9	23	230	57
Nausea and/or vomitting	3	8	73	18
Lymphadenitis	31	79	65	16
Fatigue	–	–	350	86
Exanthem	–	–	142	35
Sore throat	–	–	129	32
Chest pain (pleuritic)	2	5	–	–
Cough (non-productive)	2	5	–	–
Ulceration (cutaneous)	29	74	–	–
Infected ulcers/oral ulcers	–	–	81	20
Conjunctivitis	–	–	107	26
Muscle/joint pains	–	–	136	34
Symptoms of pneumonia	–	–	46	11

[a] Young *et al.* (1969). Vermont epidemic in 1968 of 39 symptomatic cases.
[b] Dahlstrand *et al.* (1971). Jantland epidemic between 1966 and 1967 of 405 serologically verified cases.

Table 25.4 Clinical presentations of human tularaemia

Caused by *F. tularensis tularensis*
  American type
    Ulceroglandular
    Typhoidal (abdominal)
    Oculoglandular
    Pulmonary
Caused by *F. tularensis holarctica, japonica, novicida*, and *philomiragia*
  Primary localized infection (PLI)
    Ulceroglandular
    Oculoglandular
    Oral–tonsillar–glandular
  Primary generalized infection (PGI)
    Influenzal
    Pulmonary
    Abdominal
  Secondary generalized disease (SGD)
    Generalized glandular swelling
    Multiple lung infiltrations
    Abdominal (typhoidal) illness
    Central nervous system involvement
    Immune reaction
      erythema nodosum
      multiple papular lesions
    Complications
    Relapsing disease

organisms. After subcutaneous injection the guinea-pig dies between 5 and 8 days later. At necropsy there are caseous granules in the regional lymph nodes, spleen, and liver. Infections with virulent strains may be induced by oral, intranasal, or conjunctival inoculation as well as by the intraperitoneal route. Strains of subspecies *holarctica* produce a more varied host response that depends on the route of infection, animal species, size of inoculum, age, and degree of passage of the laboratory culture.

Francisella philomiragia

The organism has been isolated from the blood of nine patients, from the lung or pleura of three more, and from the peritoneum and the meninges, each in a single case. All 13 of the patients for whom records are available had suffered from a pyrexial illness; in five there was evidence of pneumonia. Only one of the patients was previously healthy; five of them had chronic granulomatous disease, two had myeloproliferative disorders, and one recurrent pleural effusions. Five other patients had recently suffered from a near-drowning incident in sea or estuarine water (*F. philomiragia* is a halophile).

DIAGNOSIS

In endemic regions a provisional diagnosis often can be made on clinical evidence supported by informa-

tion about the patient's occupation and recent movements, particularly when a primary lesion is present. When there is no local ulcer, and if the patient has left the area in which the infection was acquired, the illness presents simply as a persistent and debilitating case of 'fever', pneumonitis, or tonsillitis in which laboratory investigations are essential for diagnosis.

Detecting the causative organism

Attempts should be made to isolate *F. tularensis* on an appropriate medium from swabs of the local lesion or aspirate from a lymph gland. Strains of the *holarctica* subspecies grow slowly on primary culture and are best isolated by subcutaneous injection of material into white mice. *Attempts to isolate* tularensis *(type A) strains should be made only when suitable containment facilities are available and laboratory staff are aware of the hazards of handling the organism.* These risks may be reduced by using an immunofluorescence method to identify organisms in tissue smears. Antigen may also be detected in tissues from dead animals by means of a thermoprecipitation method rather like that used for the diagnosis of anthrax.

Serodiagnosis

A Widal-type tube-agglutination test usually gives a positive result—a fourfold rise in titre, or a titre of 320 in a single sample—by the end of the second week of illness, but the specificity of the test is questioned; strong cross-reactions occur in brucellosis. Antibody *F. tularensis* persists for years after infection. An enzyme-linked immunosorbent assay (ELISA) has been introduced (Viljanen *et al.* 1983). This has the advantage that class-specific immunoglobulins can be detected separately.

Other immunological methods

Delayed hypersensitivity to products of *F. tularensis* develops early in infection and can be detected by means of an intradermal test (Buchanan *et al.* 1971). This is a sensitive method of diagnosis but has the disadvantage of interfering with subsequent *in vitro* tests. Cell-mediated immunity may also be detected by means of lymphocyte-stimulation tests (Syrjälä *et al.* 1984). These have been recommended as means of diagnosis but, as with antibody tests, they may give positive results for years after infection.

PATHOLOGY AND PATHOGENESIS

The incubation period of tularaemia varies inversely with the dose of organisms: ulceroglandular presentations have an incubation of 2–6 days. In volunteers, injection of a large inoculum into the skin results in 48 h in a macular erythematous lesion. The patient becomes febrile as the lesion becomes papular, pruritic, and as it slowly enlarges; the overlying skin becomes taut, thin, and shiny; rarely is the papule fluctuant. Around 96 h, ulceration occurs, giving a lesion which has sharply demarcated edges, frequently with a black and dry base. In untreated patients infected with *F. tularensis* subspecies *tularensis* type A organisms, the draining lymph nodes enlarge and become caseous. Infection with *F. tularensis* subspecies *holarctica* is accompanied by a less severe systemic reaction, but a similar ulceroglandular response. If untreated, the lesion and lymph nodes may persist for months. After inoculation, an immune individual will not develop an ulcer, but rather will demonstrate a small indurated papule similar to a positive tularaemia skintest. Biopsy of skin lesions induced by killed *F. tularensis* or by live attenuated vaccine (LVS) strains reveals mononuclear perivascular infiltrates. Minute defects in the epidermis, especially of the hands, due to trivial trauma are common. Entrance into the dermis and lymphatics through such openings could, in retrospect, be conceived as penetration through intact skin. The nail fold is an apparent portal of entry; the mantle area commonly has small tears in the region adjacent to the nail. Presumably, this is a common access route, since ulcers occur frequently in this area. The tick deposits the organisms on the skin adjacent to its bite wound, and rubbing this area could lead to contamination of that wound. Patients have been described in whom rubbing of an eye following apparent contamination of the fingers has led to oculoglandular manifestations of tularaemia. It is not known how long the organisms remain viable in human skin, but it is probably only for a relatively short time after antibiotic therapy is started.

Ingesting a large inoculum of tularaemia usually results in few or no signs of gastrointestinal disease. Aerogenic infection accounts for primary pneumonic tularaemia, the most serious form of disease. The respiratory tract is readily infected by small-particle aerosols containing as few as 1–50 bacteria. Aerosols are created as an animal is skinned or eviscerated, since there are many organisms in liver ($>10^7$/g tissue) and spleen, and the usual rough extraction of these organs during field-dressing could easily cause aerosolization of an infectious dose of *F. tularensis* as well as contaminate the uncovered skin. Pneumonia is probably initiated by terminal bronchial and/or alveolar localization of the inhaled small particles (<5 μm diameter) containing *F. tularensis*. The inflammatory reaction is acute and progressive in the animals infected with the virulent strain of tularaemia. This results in necrosis of alveolar walls which evolves into small areas of pneumonitis. Virulent organisms multiply rapidly in the lung. Microscopic findings are apparent at 24 and 48 h, with organisms demonstrated by fluorescent staining inside macrophages by 20 min after inhalation. These macrophages were in the lumina of the numerous anatomical openings, for example hair follicles, through which the organism can gain entrance to the dermis.

TREATMENT AND PROGNOSIS

Chemotherapy

Aminoglycosides are bactericidal for *F. tularensis*, and should be used for the treatment of *tularensis* and severe *holarctica* infections. Intramuscular streptomycin, if given early, may produce a dramatic clinical response; other aminoglycosides may be used. Because the organism survives intracellularly and often gives rise to a protracted and relapsing illness, aminoglycoside administration for 7–14 days may be needed. Tetracyclines are only bateriostatic; nevertheless 2 g/day by mouth, given without intermission for 2 weeks, will eliminate mild infections (Sawyer and Dangerfield 1966) and could also be used as a prophylactic regimen in areas where only *holarctica* strains occur.

Francisella philomiragia infections of the organisms tested formed a β-lactamase and were ampicillin resistant; all were sensitive to quinolones and aminoglycosides, and to chloramphenicol and cefoxitin (Hollis *et al.* 1989).

EPIDEMIOLOGY

The epidemiology of human tularaemia is exceedingly complex and varies with subspecies and virulence, ecosystem, and geographical region. The subspecies of *F. tularensis* differ in host specificity. Natural infections have been demonstrated in at least 14 species of ticks, six species of fleas, several mosquito species, over 100 wild mammal species, including 39 species of rodent and eight carnivores, nine domestic animals including cattle, sheep, cats, and dogs, and 25 species of birds.

The distribution of known foci, where animal epizootics, endemic and epidemic human tularaemia have been described are depicted in Figs 25.1–25.3. Human infection occurs in most countries of the northern hemisphere between latitudes 30° and 71°N. The incidence of the disease is poorly documented because of highly variable ascertainment. Rates have fallen since a peak between the two World Wars after recognition of occupational hazards, the introduction of streptomycin, and vaccination campaigns in the

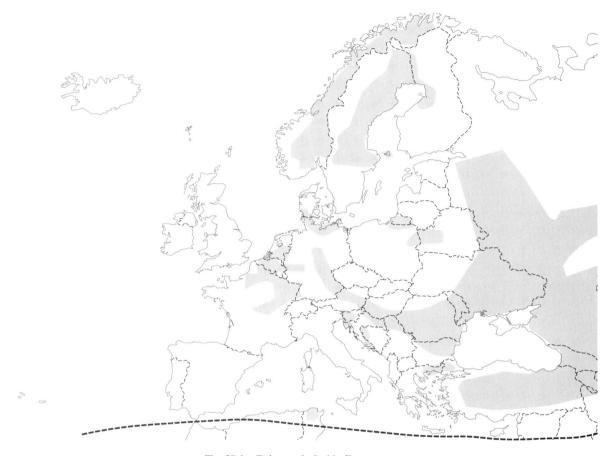

Fig. 25.1   Tularaemia foci in Europe.

former USSR reduced the number of reported cases from a period of 100 000 cases of *F. tularensis holarctica* per year in the former USSR between 1926 and 1942 to a few hundred per year at the present time.

Laboratory-acquired infections have been a significant problem (Overholt *et al.* 1961).

THE UNITED STATES OF AMERICA

Francisella tularensis subspecies *tularensis* is the main cause of serious tularaemia in the United States. The highest annual incidence reported was over 2000 cases in 1939. It is harboured by ground squirrels, cotton-tail rabbits, hares, and jack-rabbits, and it can be found from time to time in other wild and domestic animals. Human infections are in the main sporadic and occur in two seasonal peaks, one in the summer, associated with tick bites, and the other in the winter attributed to hunting, mainly of rabbits (Taylor *et al.* 1991). Various ticks of the genera *Dermacentor*, *Amblyomma*, *Haemaphysalis*, and *Ixodes* transmit the organism. Infections have been attributed to dog ticks and

contact with sick dogs. Assal *et al.* (1967), studied 536 cases in the United States and traced the origin of 26 per cent to tick bites, 13 per cent to direct contact with rabbits, and 2.6 per cent to other sources. However, according to Klock *et al.* (1973) in Utah, 72 per cent of 39 cases were associated with the bite of deer-flies (*Chrysops* sp.), though *F. tularensis* subspecies *tularensis* was transmitted among the local jack-rabbits by ticks.

Human infection with *Francisella tularensis* subsp. *holarctica* (type B) organisms have been much less frequently described in the United States. Strains of this description have been isolated from muskrats in whom they cause water-borne epizootics. Such a strain was responsible for an outbreak of mild infections in Vermont among trappers who had come into contact with infected muskrats (Young *et al.* 1969).

EUROPE AND ASIA

In the former republics of the USSR, *holarctica* (type B) strains are harboured in a wide variety of different ecological situations in meadow, steppe, forest, swamp,

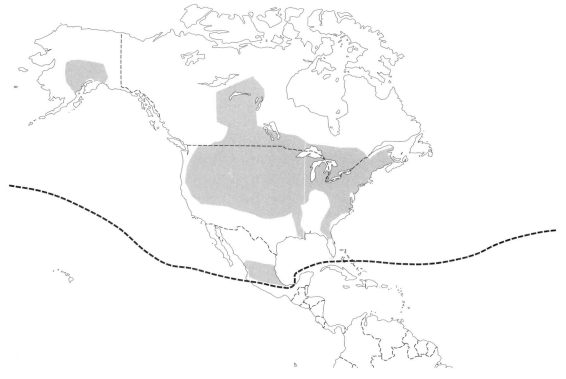

Fig. 25.2   Tularaemia foci in North America.

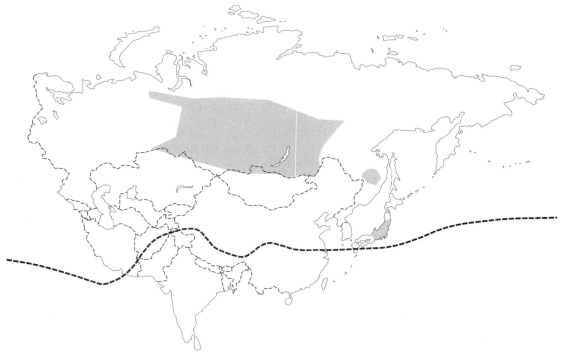

Fig. 25.3   Tularaemia foci in Asia.

Table 25.5 Classification of tularaemia foci in the former USSR (from Olsufjev and Rudnev 1960)

Kind of foci	Main reservoir	Tick involved	Season of outbreaks
Meadow-field type	*Microtus arvalis*	*Dermacentor pictus*	Winter
Steppe (ravine) type	Voles, mice, hamsters, hares, etc.	Mainly *Dermacentor marginatus*	Autumn and winter
Forest type	Red vole (*Clethyrionymous glareolus*), forest mice, hares	*Ixodes ricinus, I. frianguliceps*	Tick season
Floodland-swamp type	Water rats	*Dermacentor, Rhipicephalus, Ixodes* sp.	Season of water-rat hunting
Foothill type	Water rats (voles, etc.)	*Ixodes apronophorus*	Summer
'Tungai' type	Hares, gerbils, mice, and muskrats	*Rhipicephalus pumilio*	Season of hare hunting

foothills, and tungai, by a variety of mammals, mainly rodents, including mice, voles, water rats, muskrats, and gerbils, as well as hares. The main tick vectors are of the genera *Dermacentor*, *Ixodes*, and *Rhipicephalus*.

The epidemiological conditions have been classified according to the ecosystem in which the foci occurred (Table 25.5). For example, field voles were the dominant reservoir in field and steppe areas; *Arvicola terrestris* in the river valleys, banks, and forest; and mice, hares, and squirrels in the forests and heathland. Three epidemic types have predominated: water-borne outbreaks, where 60–80 per cent of the cases were of the oropharyngeal type (angino-bubonic) and which have been associated with contamination by the carcasses or excreta of infected animals (*F. tularensis* subspecies *holarctica* can survive in water at 4 °C for at least 5 months); vector-borne epidemics associated with mosquitoes and other arthropods; and airborne epidemics from inhalation of contaminated dust from rodent-infected hay. In addition, there have been outbreaks resulting from hunting, skinning, and preparing hides and carcasses of rabbits, water rats, and other wild game and fur-bearing animals, and agricultural or mouse outbreaks amongst farmers from direct contact with mice during epizootics.

In Norway, infections have been attributed to lemmings and hares (Haug and Pearson 1972), in Sweden to hares and voles, and in Germany and south-eastern Europe to field mice. Mosquito bites were the commonest means of acquiring tularaemia in central Sweden and an airborne outbreak was described by Dahlstrand *et al.* (1971) in Sweden. Table 25.6 gives the epidemiology classifications of cases in two areas of Sweden between 1966 and 1973.

PREVENTION AND CONTROL

The first objective is to reduce as far as possible human contact with potentially infected animal species and to avoid ticks and mosquito bites in known infected areas. This requires knowledge of the local epidemiology of tularaemia foci. When contact with potentially infected material is inevitable, specific immunization becomes necessary. Since the Second World War, preventive measures in endemic areas have been based on the dual process of education and vaccination in selected high-risk groups. Table 25.7 summarizes the approach of epidemiologists in the former USSR to prevent and control the four epidemic types of tularaemia.

Live attenuated strains of *holarctica* biotype have been used extensively as vaccines since the 1940s and have been shown to be effective (Tiggert 1962). The preferred method of vaccination was by the inhalation of dried viable vaccine. Subsequently an attenuated Russian strain (LVS) was selected for study in the United State. It was shown to be superior to a killed vaccine in immunizing activity in human subjects (Saslaw *et al.* 1961) and in experimental animals. Hornick and Eigelsbach (1966) exposed human volunteers to LVS vaccine by inhalation; this led at most to a mild self-limiting illness. They were subsequently challenged by the aerial route with a virulent strain of *F. tularensis* and were shown to have substantial, though

Table 25.6 Epidemiological classification of type of tularemia cases in Sweden: Probable routes of transmission relating to clinical presentations in Jamtland 1966–67 and Norrbotten 1966–1973

	Type I contact epidemic	Type II vector-borne	Type III water/food-borne	Type IV airborne	Unknown	Total number of cases
Jamtland	216	358	68	366	29	679
Norrbotten	333 (13%)	455 (18%)	82 (3.2%)	373 (15%)	1286 (51%)	2529

Table 25.7 Epidemic types of tularaemia: prevention and control of *Francisella tularensis* subspecies *holarctica*

Origin of epidemic	Groups of the population exposed to the infection	Mode of infection	Predominant form of the disease and location of the buboes	Time of origin of the outbreak	Source of infection	The principal methods of prophylaxis and eradication of the epidemic
Type 1 Epidemic resulting from wounds or mucous membrane infection—contact epidemic						
The water vole fur trade. Trapping of hares and other animals susceptible to tularaemia in flood-plain foci	Persons engaged in hunting and handling the carcasses	Contact with the carcass or dead body of an infected animal	The bubonic form. Buboes localized mainly in the axillary and cubital regional nodes	At the time of the spring floods and the hunting season	Water voles, hares and other animals	Prophylactic vaccination of vulnerable groups
Meat-processing factories handling sheep and hare carcasses	Workers in the carcass dressing and cutting departments	As above	As above	Any time of the year	Hares, sheep	In the event of an outbreak work should be stopped for the duration of the incubation period and until vaccination has been carried out
Rodent control work or epizootic disease surveys	Persons engaged in work of this type	As above	As above	The time of year at which the work is carried out	Murine rodents	Attention to personal prophylaxis
Hay-cutting in marshy meadows	Persons engaged in this work. The incidence is normally low	Contact with contaminated water and other substrates	The bubonic form with buboes mainly in the inguinal region	Spring and summer (i.e. the hay cutting season)	Murine rodents	
Type II Epidemic in which the infection is transmitted by an arthropod vector (vector-borne)						
The presence of human beings in the characteristic biotopes of arthropod vectors	Random members of groups working near water, marshy ground, or bushes and trees	The bite of mosquitoes, horse flies, and other arthropod vectors	The ulcerous bubonic form. The ulcers are located mainly on exposed parts of the body if dipteran insects are responsible for the bites	From July to September. The period when arthropods are most active	The water vole and murine rodents	Protection from bites by the use of repellents and other means; prophylactic vaccination of the inhabitants of natural foci of tularaemia
Type III Epidemic in which infection is contracted orally (water and food-borne epidemic)						
Contamination of water by the discharges or corpses of diseased rodents	The disease is restricted to people using water from a contaminated source. Usually a large proportion of those drawing water from one particular source contract the disease within a short space of time	The use of contaminated water in its raw state for drinking purposes	The anginous-bubonic and the intestinal forms. An intermediate form is probably the most common, however	Summer and autumn usually. Winter outbreaks have also been recorded	Murine rodents and more rarely water voles	Sterilization of water and purification and disinfection of wells. The chlorination of piped water supplies, rodent control, and prophylactic vaccination of the inhabitants of natural foci

Table 25.7 (Continued)

Origin of epidemic	Groups of the population exposed to the infection	Mode of infection disease and location of	Predominant form of the outbreak epidemic the buboes	Time of origin of the eradication of the	Source of infection	The principal methods of prophylaxis and
Contamination of foodstuffs by the discharges of diseased rodents	People consuming contaminated food stuffs which have not been adequately cooked. In contrast to water-borne epidemics the incidence is low	Consumption of contaminated foodstuffs	The intestinal form is the most common but the anginous-bubonic form may also be observed	Autumn and winter	Murine rodents	Protection of foodstuffs from the activities of rodents, extermination of rodents, and prophylactic vaccination of the inhabitants of natural foci

Type IV Epidemic where infection is the result of inhalation of contaminated air (aspiration epidemic)

The threshing of stacked corn, the carting of straw and the handling of threshed grain and rodent-contaminated vegetables	The disease is confined to persons engaged in this type of work or sleeping on contaminated straw. A high incidence of disease is normally associated with epidemics of this type	Inhalation of droplets or dust contaminated by the discharges of diseased rodents	Tularaemia of the respiratory tracts and occasionally of the intestinal canal	Winter (early) spring and sometimes autumn	Murine rodents	The use of respirators during work, the use of fir branches instead of straw for bedding, prophylactic vaccination of the inhabitants of natural foci of tularaemia and the extermination of rodents

not total, immunity. Burke (1977) reported that the routine use of LVS vaccine in laboratory workers who were regularly handling *F. tularensis* led to a reduction in the number of attacks of tularaemia infection, but cases still occurred.

REFERENCES

Anthony, L. S. D., Burke, R. D., and Nano, F. E. (1991). Growth of *Francisella* spp. in rodent macrophages. *Infection and Immunity*, **59**, 3291–6.

Assal, N., Blenden, D. C., and Price, E. R. (1967). Epidemiologic study of human tularaemia reported in Missouri *Public Health Reports*, **82**, 627. Washington DC.

Behan, K. A. Klein, and G. C. (1982). Reduction of *Burcella* species and *Francisella tularensis* cross-reacting agglutinins by dithiothreitol. *Journal of Clinical Microbiology*, **16**, 756–7.

Blomley, D. J. and Pearson, A. D. (1972). A case of tularaemia in England *British Medical Journal*, **4**, 235.

Buchanan, T. M., Brooks, G. F., and Brachman, P. S. (1971). The tularemia skin test. 325 skin tests in 210 persons: serologic correlation and review of the literature. *Annals of Internal Medicine*, **74**, 336–43.

Burke, D. S. (1977). Immunization against Tularaemia: analysis of the effectiveness of live *Francisella tularensis* vaccine in prevention of laboratory-acquired Tularaemia. *Journal of Infectious Diseases*, **135**,(1), 55–60.

Canonico, P. G., McManus, A. T., Mangiafico, J. A., Sammons, L. S., McGann, V. G., and Dangerfield, H. G. (1975). Temporal appearance of opsonizing antibody to *Francisella tularensis*: detection by a radiometabolic assay. *Infection and Immunity*, **11**, 466–9.

Carlsson, H. E. *et al.* (1979). Enzyme-linked Immunosorbant assay for Immunological diagnosis of tularaemia *Journal of Clinical Microbiology*, **10**, 615.

Dahlstrand, S. Ringertz, O., and Zetterberg, B. (1971). Airborne tularaemia in Sweden. *Scandinavian Journal of Infectious Diseases*, **3**, 7–16.

Eigelsbach, H. T. and McGann, V. G. (1984). Genus *Francisella* Dorofr'ev 1947, 176^AL. In *Bergey's manual of systematic bacteriology*, (ed. N. R. Krieg and J. G. Holt Vol. 1, pp. 394–9. Williams and Wilkins, Baltimore.

Eigelsbach, H. T., Chambers, L. A., and Coriell, L. L. (1946). Electron microscopy of *B. tularense. Journal of Bacteriology*, **52**, 179–85.

Fleming, D. E. and Foshay, L. (1955). Studies on the physiology of virulence of *Pasteurella tularensis*. I citrulline urease and deamidase activity. *Journal of Bacteriology*, **70**, 345–9.

Forsman, M., Juoppa, K., Sjostedt, A., and Tarnvik, A. (1990). Use of RNA hybridization in the diagnosis of a case of ulceroglandular tularaemia. *European Journal of Clinical Microbiology and Infectious Diseases*, **9**, 784–5.

Francis, E. and Evans, A. C. (1926). Agglutination, cross agglutination and agglutinin absorption in tularaemia. *U S Public Health Report*, Reprint No. 1089, **41**, 1273–95.

Fulop, M. J., Webber, T., Manchee, R. J., and Kelly, D. C. (1991). Production and characterization of monoclonal antibodies directed against the lipopolysaccharde of *Francisella tularensis. Journal of Clinical Microbiology*, **29**, 1407–12.

Haug R. J. and Pearson, A. D. (1972). Human infections with *F. tularensis* in Norway. *Acta Pathologica Microbiologica Scandinavica Section B*, **80**, 273–80.

Hollis, D. G., Weaver, R. E., Steigerwalt, A. G., Wenger, J. D., Moss, C., and Brenner, D. J. (1989). *Francisella philomiragia* comb. nov (formerly *Yersinia philomiragia*) and *Francisella tularensis* biogroup *novicida* (formerly *Francisella novicida*) associated with human disease. *Journal of Clinical Microbiology*, **27**, (7), 1601–8.

Horne, H. (1912). A lemming pest and a guinea pig epizootic; a contribution intended to elucidate the reasons for the mortality among lemmigns during the 'lemming years', so-called. *Zentralblatt für Bakteriologie, Parasitenkunde, Infektionskrankheiten und Hygiene*, I Abt. Orig. **66**, (2/4), 169.

Hornick, R. B. and Eigelsbach, H. T. (1966). Aerogenic immunization of man with live tularaemia vaccine *Bacteriological Review*, **30**, 532.

Ito, M., Nishiyama, K., Hyodo, S., Shigeta, S., and Io, T. (1985). Weight reduction of thymus and depletino of lymphocytes of T-dependent areas in peripheral lymphoid tissues of mice infected with *Francisella tularensis. Infection and Immunity*, **49**, 812–18.

Jusatz, H. G. (1962). Tularemia in Central Europe 1933–1953 II/37. in *World Atlas of Infectious Disease*, Pt III (ed. E Roderwaldt), pp. 1–8.

Karttunen, R., Ilonen, J., and Herva, E. (1985). Interleukin 2 production in whole blood culture: a rapid test of immunity to *F. tularensis. Journal of Clinical Microbiology*, **22**, 318–319.

Klock, L. E., Olsen, P. F., and Fukushima, T. (1973). Tularaemia Epidemic associated with the Deerfly *Journal of the American Medical Association*, **226**, 149.

Lake, G. C. and Francis, E. (1922). *Six cases of tularemia occuring in laboratory workers*. Bull. 130, p. 81 *Hyg. Lab. U. S. P. H. S.*

Lofgren, S., Tarnvik, A., and Carlsson, J. (1980). Demonstration of opsonizing antibodies to *Francisella tularensis* by leukocyte chemiluminescence. *Infection and Immunity*, **29**, (2), 329–44.

Lofgren, S., Tarnvik, A., Bloom, G. D., and Sjoberg, W. (1983). Phagocytosis and killing of *Francisella tularensis* by human polymorphonuclear leukocytes. *Infection and Immunity*, **39**, (2), 715–20.

McCoy, G. W. (1911). A plague-like disease of rodents. *Public Health Bulletin, Washington*, **43**, 53–71.

McCoy, G. W. and Chapin, C. W. (1912). Further observations on a plague-like disease of rodents with a preliminary note of the causative agent *P. tularense. Journal of Infectious Diseases*, **10**, 61–72.

Massey, E. D. and Mangiafico, J. A. (1974). Microagglutination test for detecting and measuring serum agglutinins of *Francisella tularensis. Applied Microbiology*, **27**, 25–7.

Nichols, P. D., Mayberry, W. R., Antworth, C. P., and White, D. C. (1985). Determination of monounsaturated doublebond position and geometry in the cellular fatty acids of the pathogenci bacterium *Francisella tularensis. Journal of Clinical Microbiology*, **21**, (5), 728–40.

Nutter, J. E. (1971). Antigens of *B. tularensis*; preparative procedures. *Applied Microbiology*, **22**(1), 44–8.

O'Hara, S., Sato, T., and Homma, M. (1971). Serological studies on *Francisella tularensis, Francisella movicida, Yersinia philmiragia*, and *Brucella abortus. International Journal of Systematic Bacteriology*, **2**, 336–43.

Olsufjev, N. G. and Rudne G. P. (1960). *Tularaema. Publishing House for Medical literature*, Moscow.

Overholt, E. L. *et al.* (1961). Analysis of 42 cases of laboratory acquired tularemia. Treatment with broad spectrum antibiotics. *American Journal of Medicine*, **30**, 785–806.

Ringertz, O. and Dahlstrand, S. (1968). Culture of *P. tularensis* in the 1966–67 outbreaks of tularemia in Sweden. Laboratory methods and precautions against laboratory infections. *Acta Pathologica et Microbiologica Scandinavica*, **72**, 464.

Saslaw, S. and Carlisle, H. N. (1961). Studies with tularemia vaccines in volunteers. VI. Brucella agglutinins in vaccinated and non-vaccinated volunteers challenged with tularensis. *American Journal of Medical Science*, **242**, 166–72.

Saslaw, S. Eigelsbach, H. T., Wilson, H. R., Prior, J. A., and Carhart, S. (1961). Tularemica vaccine study. II. Respiratory challenge. *Archieves of Internal Medicine*, **107**, 702–14.

Sawyer, W. D. and Dangerfield, H. G. (1966). Antibiotic prophylaxis and therapy of airborne tularemia. *Bacteriological Reviews*, **30**, 542–50.

Syrjälä, H., Herva, E. Ilonen, J., Saukkonen, K., and Salminen, A. (1984). A whole-blood lymphocyte stimulation test for the diagnosis of human Tularemia. *Journal of Infectious Diseases*, **150**, 912–15.

Taylor, J. P. *et al.* (1991). Epidemiologic characteristics of human tularemia in the southwest central states, 1981–1987. *American Journal of Epidemiology*, **133**, 1032–8.

Thjotta, T. (1930). Three cases of tularaemia disease hitherto not diagnosed in Norway. *Norsk Mag of Laegevidensk*, **92**, 32–40.

Thjotta, T. (1931*a*). Continued investigations into occurrence of tularaemia in Norway; cases originating from the infectious carriers than the hare *Norsk mag of Laegevidensk*, **92**, 32–40.

Thjotta, T. (1931*b*). Tularaemia in Norway *Journal of Infectious Diseases*, **49**, 99.

Tiggert, W. D. (1962). Soviet viable *Pasteurella tularensis* vaccines. A review of selected articles. *Bacteriological Reviews*, **26**, 354–73.

Viljanen, M. K., Nurmi, T., and Salminen, A. (1983). Enzyme-linked immunosorbent Assay (ELISA) with bacterial sonicate antigen for IgM, and IgG antibodiesto *Francisella tularensis*: comparison with bacterial agglutination test and ELISA with lipopolysaccharide antigen. *Journal of Infectious Diseases*, **148**, 715–20.

Wood, J. B. Valteris, K., Hardy, R. H., and Pearson, A. D. (1976). Imported tularaemia *British Medical Journal*, I, 811.

Young, L. S. *et al.* (1969). Tularemia epidemic: Vermont 1968, 47 cases linked to contact with muskrats. *New England Journal of Medicine*, **280**, 1253–60.

Zuerlin, T. J. Smith, P. W. (1985). The diagnostic utility of the febrile agglutinin test. *Journal of the American Medical Association*, **254**, 1211–14.

26   YERSINIOSIS AND PLAGUE

Thomas Butler

INTRODUCTION

The genus *Yersinia* consists of three principal pathogenic species *Y. enterocolitica*, *Y. pseudotuberculosis*, and *Y. pestis. Yersinia enterocolitica* and *Y. pseudotuberculosis* are the two principal pathogens of human non-plague yersiniosis. *Yersinia pestis* is the sole pathogen of human plague. Other species that are rarely identified and have less pathogenic potential are *Y. intermedia*, *Y. frederickseni*, and *Y. kristensenii. Yersinia ruckeri* is a pathogen in fish. DNA hybridization studies indicated such close relatedness between *Y. pestis* and *Y. pseudotuberculosis* that the plague bacillus was renamed *Y. pseudotuberculosis* subspecies *pestis*. However, the older name *Y. pestis* remains in use and will be employed in the following chapter.

The division of *Yersinia* infections into the two groups of non-plague yersiniosis and plague is practical because the two groups differ fundamentally in regard to human disease, epidemiology, animal reservoirs, and control strategies. Accordingly, the following chapter will deal separately with non-plague *Yersinia* infections, referred to simply as 'yersiniosis,' and *Y. pestis* infection referred to as 'plague'.

YERSINIOSIS

SUMMARY

Disease in humans is caused mostly by *Y. enterocolitica* belonging to serotypes 03, 05,27, 08, and 09 and by *Y. pseudotuberculosis*. The clinical presentations include fever, diarrhoea, abdominal pain that may mimic appendicitis, and chronic arthritis. There are typically lesions of enteritis and mesenteric lymphadenitis. Yersiniosis occurs in all European countries, with highest prevalence in northern countries and Scandinavia, as well as Canada, the United States, Australia, and Japan. Transmission is mainly from contaminated animal products such as pork and milk, sometimes from blood transfusion, and rarely from person to person spread by the faecal–oral route. Control of yersiniosis can be achieved by careful handling and cooking of meats and by pasteurization of milk and other dairy products.

The interested reader should look at publications of the International Symposia on Yersinia (Carter *et al.*

1979; Prpic and Davey 1987; Une *et al.* 1991) and monographs and reviews (Butler 1983; Cornelis *et al.* 1987; Cover and Aber, 1989; Carniel and Mollaret 1990; Andersen *et al.* 1991).

HISTORY

The discoveries of *Y. enterocolitica* and *Y. pseudotuberculosis* were not attended by the same excitement and drama as the discovery of *Y. pestis*, and Alexandre Yersin certainly had nothing to do with characterizing these species. Human infection by *Y. enterocolitica* was first reported in 1939 by Schleifstein and Coleman. It was then called *Bacterium enterocoliticum* but was renamed *Pasteurella X* by Daniels and Goudzwaard in 1963 and finally was grouped in the genus *Yersinia* by Frederiksen in 1964.

Pfeiffer in 1889 first described *Bacillus pseudotuberculosis*, which he renamed *Pasteurella pseudotuberculosis* in 1929. Additionally, it was called *Shigella pseudotuberculosis* in 1935 until Smith and Thal placed it into the genus *Yersinia* in 1965.

Before 1970, there was little attention given to yersinioses in the medical literature or in public health. In 1975, there were only 84 cases of *Y. enterocolitica* infection reported in the United States and about 6000 cases in the world literature. However, during the 1980s there occurred an increased interest and recognition of this organism as an important cause of diarrhoea and the appendicitis-like syndrome. Most of the reported cases were in Scandinavia, other European countries, Canada, and the United States.

Efforts to control yersinioses are still in their infancy. Only in the past decade have public health officials recognized the roles of contaminated pork, recontamination of pasteurized milk, and contaminated blood in blood banks as sources of *Yersinia* infection. Effective applications of control measures remain to be shown.

THE AGENTS

Yersinia enterocolitica and *Y. pseudotuberculosis* are Gram-negative, non-lactose-fermenting, urease-positive bacilli that are motile when grown at 25 °C but not at 37 °C. Both organisms grow on blood, heart infusion, MacConkey, and SS agars at room temperature and at 37 °C, and in buffered saline at 4 °C. Colonies are often very small after incubation for 24 hours but are readily apparent at 48 hours. More than 50 serotypes and five biotypes of *Y. enterocolitica* have been described (Wauters 1981). Most strains from patients belong to serotypes 03, 08, and 09 and to biotypes 2, 3, and 4. Six serotypes (I–VI) and four subtypes of *Y. pseudotuberculosis* have been identified, with O-group I accounting for approximately 80 per cent of human cases.

The virulence of the yersiniae depends on V and W antigens, which confer dependency on calcium for growth at 37 °C. Pathogenic strains are resistant to serum complement, penetrate human epithelial cells (HeLa cells) or guinea-pig conjunctivae, are lethal to mice, and demonstrate cytotoxicity (Goguen *et al.* 1986; Cornelis *et al.* 1987). Some of these characteristics are mediated by plasmids with weights of 41–82 MDa (Portnoy *et al.* 1981; Kay *et al.* 1982). The 70 kb plasmid encodes for virulence determinants that include a secreted protein kinase (Galyov *et al.* 1993) and an outer membrane protein with protein tyrosine phosphatase activity (Guan and Dixon 1990), and *Yersinia* outer membrane proteins (YOPs) that inhibit phagocytosis (Straley *et al.* 1993). The organisms penetrate eukaryotic cells using a surface protein called invasin, which is encoded by a chromosomal gene (Simonet *et al.* 1996). *Yersinia enterocolitica* does not produce a siderophore for iron transport and thus grows better in the presence of other bacteria that produce siderophores and allow the bacteria to transport iron for its growth (Cantinieaux *et al.* 1988). Many isolates produce a heat-stable enterotoxin that is similar to the heat-stable enterotoxin produced by *Escherichia coli* (Boyce *et al.* 1979). This enterotoxin, which is produced at 22 °C but not at 37 °C, is probably not important in causing diarrhoea during *Yersinia* infection. The organisms produce lipopolysaccharide endotoxin, which has biological properties similar to that of other Gram-negative bacteria.

THE HOSTS

ANIMALS

The natural reservoirs of *Y. enterocolitica* include a variety of domestic and wild species. The prominent hosts are pigs, rodents, rabbits, sheep, goats, cattle, horses, dogs, and cats. *Yersinia pseudotuberculosis* resides in many of the same animals, including rodents, rabbits, deer, and farm animals, but has also been found extensively in birds, including turkeys, ducks, geese, pigeons, pheasants, and canaries.

The organisms are localized in the oropharyngeal cavities and lumens of the gastrointestinal tract of these animals. They are excreted into the faeces to allow faecal–oral transmission among animals. Studies of pigs in slaughterhouses suggested that the tonsils and tongues contained *Y. enterocolitica* more frequently than other tissues. In experimental infections of pigs, organisms persisted longer on tonsils than in faeces (Wauters 1979). Raw intestines of pigs (chitterlings) are also implicated as a source of human infection. The presence of *Y. enterocolitica* in unpasteurized milk suggests that bacteria reach the bloodstream from the intestine and are secreted into milk by mammary glands. Alternatively, milk could be contaminated through faecal contact or through localized mastitis due to this infection.

Generally, infections of animals by *Yersinia* are asymptomatic carriages that do not produce clinical illness. On the other hand, illness in household dogs has been associated with transmission of infection to humans. Sheep in Australia were shown to develop intestinal microabscesses but did not appear to be clinically ill in one study (Slee and Skilbeck 1992). On the other hand, Philbey *et al.* (1991) found *Yersinia* infection in 4 per cent of Australian sheep with diarrhoea, ill thrift, or mortality. Intestinal lesions included acute segmental suppurative erosive enterocolitis and haemorrhagic enterocolitis. One animal had a perforation of the intestine. Lesions were less frequent and less severe in sheep with *Y. enterocolitica* than in animals with *Y. pseudotuberculosis*. *Yersinia* infection was associated with recent changes in husbandry of affected flocks, including changes in diet, shearing, and weaning; this suggested that environmental stress could have interacted with infection to result in clinical disease. In experimental infections of sheep with *Y. enterocolitica*, dexamethasone treatment resulted in a higher incidence of intestinal abscesses, suggesting that stress and/or immunosuppression could promote disease (Slee and Button 1990). Another factor contributing to expression of disease in *Yersinia* infection of sheep could be concomitant infection with nematodes and *Coccidia*, which are common in infected flocks.

Treatment of infected animals has rarely been attempted. Tetracyclines have been reported as effective against *Y. pseudotuberculosis* infection in cattle and against *Y. enterocolitica* infection in sheep.

HUMANS

Humans are accidental hosts for *Yersinia* bacteria, after they ingest contaminated animal products, and they play no important role in maintaining the organisms in nature and transmitting it to other humans. The alimentary tract is the portal of entry in most cases. An inoculum of 10^9 organisms may be required to cause infection. After an incubation period of 4–7 days, this infection causes mucosal ulcerations in the terminal ileum (rarely ascending colon), necrotic lesions in Peyer's patches, and enlargement of mesenteric lymph nodes (Bradford *et al.* 1974). In most cases, the appendix is histologically normal or shows mild inflammation. If septicaemia develops, suppurative lesions may occur in various organ systems (e.g. lung, liver, meninges). A reactive polyarthritis develops in some patients and is more common among patients with histocompatibility antigen HLA-B27. Molecular mimicry between HLA-B27 antigen and *Yersinia* antigen has been postulated as a mechanism for reactive arthritis. Superantigenic activity has been found in cultures of *Y. enterocolitica* and could be a mechanism for reactive arthritis (Stuart and Woodward 1992).

Enterocolitis accounts for two-thirds of all reported cases and is characterized by fever, diarrhoea, and abdominal pain lasting 1–3 weeks (Marks *et al.* 1980). In serious cases, rectal bleeding and perforation of the ileum may occur (Rabinovitz *et al.* 1987). Faecal excretion of the organism may continue for weeks after symptoms have subsided. Leucocytes, and less commonly blood or mucus, may be present in the stool. Most patients with this syndrome are less than 5-years of age. Patients with mesenteric adenitis and/or terminal ileitis have fever, right lower quadrant pain, and leucocytosis. The syndrome is most common in older children and adolescents and may be clinically indistinguishable from acute appendicitis.

A reactive polyarthritis, seen in 10–30 per cent of adults with *Y. enterocolitica* infection in Scandinavia, begins a few days to a month after onset of acute diarrhoea and may involve the knees, ankles, toes, fingers, and wrists. In most cases, two to four joints become inflamed in rapid succession over a period of 2–14 days. Symptoms persist for more than 1 month in two-thirds of cases and for more than 4 months in one-third. After 12 months, most patients are symptom less, but a few will have persisting low back pain, including sacroileitis, which has been specifically related to the presence of HLA-B27 (Leirisalo-Repo 1987). Ankylosing spondylitis rarely occurs. Synovial fluid examination reveals fewer than 25 000 white blood cells/mm^3, with 60–95 per cent polymorphonuclear leucocytes. Synovial fluid cultures are usually negative. Reiter syndrome with arthritis, urethritis, and conjunctivitis has also been reported. Like arthritis, this complication is much more likely to develop in individuals with the HLA-B27 antigen (Aho *et al.* 1973; Borg *et al.* 1992).

Erythema nodosum occurs in up to 30 per cent of the Scandinavian cases. Skin lesions appear on the patient's legs and trunk 2–20 days after onset of fever

and abdominal pain and resolve spontaneously within a month in most cases. Women outnumber men by 2 to 1.

Recently, exudative pharyngitis has been documented as part of the spectrum of illnesses caused by *Y. enterocolitica*. In one large outbreak in the United States, 8 per cent of patients presented with acute pharyngitis and fever, without accompanying diarrhoea (Rose *et al.* 1987). Cases of pneumonia, empyema, and lung abscess have been reported (Greene *et al.* 1993).

Yersinia enterocolitica septicaemia is less common and is most often reported in patients with diabetes mellitus, severe anaemia, haemochromatosis, cirrhosis, malignancy, and in elderly patients. Patients with iron overload, such as thalassaemic patients who receive frequent transfusions, are at risk for septicaemia. The treatment of iron-overloaded patients with desferrioxamine has been particularly associated with *Yersinia* sepsis because this iron chelator enhances the growth of the organism and also appears to inhibit polymorphonuclear leucocyte defence against the infection (Chiu *et al.* 1986; Cantinieaux *et al.* 1988). Septicaemic patients may develop hepatic or splenic abscesses, osteomyelitis, wound infections, or meningitis. Endocarditis and mycotic aneurysms due to *Y. enterocolitica* have been reported (Applebaum *et al.* 1983). Septicaemia caused by transfusion of contaminated blood has been reported (Pietersz *et al.* 1992).

By far the most common manifestation of *Y. pseudotuberculosis* infection in humans is mesenteric adenitis, which causes an acute appendicitis-like syndrome with fever and right lower quadrant abdominal pain (Weber *et al.* 1970). At laparotomy, there is usually a normal appendix and enlarged mesenteric lymph nodes that may be accompanied by inflammation of the terminal ileum. The infection is usually self-limited, and patients who have undergone surgery generally begin to improve promptly after laparotomy. Erythema nodosum and polyarthritis have also been described in patients with *Y. pseudotuberculosis* infection. Less than 30 cases of *Y. pseudotuberculosis*-induced septicaemia have been reported in the world literature (Yamashiro *et al.* 1971). About 50 per cent of septicaemic patients have underlying disease such as cirrhosis, haemochromatosis, or diabetes mellitus.

For diagnosis, culture of stool, mesenteric lymph node, pharyngeal exudate, peritoneal fluid, or blood may yield *Yersinia*, depending on the clinical syndrome. Recovery of organisms from otherwise uncontaminated material such as blood, cerebrospinal fluid, or mesenteric lymph node tissue is not difficult, but isolation of yersiniae from faeces is hampered by their slow growth and by overgrowth of normal faecal flora. Yield of positive stool cultures can be increased by using cold enrichment, alkali treatment, or selective CIN agar, but these methods are not cost-effective in routine diagnosis because usual enteric culturing methods can detect most clinically significant infections (Kachoris *et al.* 1988).

Serological tests are useful in diagnosing *Yersinia* infections provided sera are absorbed appropriately (Wauters 1981). *Yersinia enterocolitica* and *Y. pseudotuberculosis* cross-react with each other and with other organisms such as *Brucella, Vibrio*, and *E. coli. Yersinia pseudotuberculosis* types II and IV cross-react with *Salmonella* groups B and D. Agglutinating antibodies appear soon after onset of illness but generally disappear within 2–6 months.

For therapy, *Yersinia enterocolitica* is usually susceptible *in vitro* to aminoglycosides, chloramphenicol, tetracycline, trimethoprim–sulphamethoxazole, piperacillin, and the third-generation cephalosporins (Hoogkamp-Korstanje 1987). Isolates are usually resistant to penicillin, and resistance to ampicillin, carbenicillin, and first-generation cephalosporins occurs frequently. The value of antimicrobial therapy in cases of enterocolitis and mesenteric adenitis is unclear, since these infections are usually self-limited. Treatment of enterocolitis with antibiotics shortened the persistence of IgG anti-*Yersinia* antibodies to about 3 months (Kihlstrom *et al.* 1992). Patients with *Y. enterocolitica*-induced septicaemia, which has a mortality of 50 per cent despite treatment, should receive antibiotic therapy. The drug of choice has not yet been identified, but gentamicin, 5 mg/kg/day intravenously in divided doses, or chloramphenicol, 50 mg/kg/day orally or intravenously in divided doses, are suggested. Good responses have been reported with trimethoprim–sulphamethoxazole, doxycycline, and ciprofloxacin, whereas failures have occurred with cefuroxime, ceftazidime, cefoperazone, and gentamicin (Hoogkamp-Korstanje 1987). Laparotomy for suspected appendicitis should be avoided when *Yersinia* infection is a likely diagnosis.

Yersinia pseudotuberculosis is usually sensitive *in vitro* to ampicillin, tetracycline, chloramphenicol, cephalosporins, and aminoglycosides. Although antibiotic therapy is probably not warranted in most patients with mesenteric adenitis, patients with septicaemia should receive ampicillin, 100–200 mg/kg/day intravenously, or streptomycin, 20–30 mg/kg/day intramuscularly, or tetracycline, 20–30 mg/kg/day orally or intravenously in divided doses. The reported mortality in *Y. pseudotuberculosis* septicaemia is 75 per cent despite antibiotic therapy.

EPIDEMIOLOGY

Yersinia enterocolitica is a relatively infrequent cause of diarrhoea and abdominal pain in the United States but is more common in northern Europe. Infections have been documented in other parts of the world including South America, Africa, and Asia, but *Y. enterocolitica* is rarely a cause of tropical diarrhoea (Carniel *et al.* 1986). Most isolates from Europe are serotypes 03 and 09, while a majority of the isolates from Canada and the United States are serotypes 03 and 08, respectively. Recently serotype 03 isolates have been recovered from patients in the New York City area (Bottone 1983), and serious infections due to serotype 08 have been reported from The Netherlands (Hoogkamp-Korstanje *et al.* 1986).

Children and adults and both sexes are susceptible, but children are more often infected than are adults. Transmission of infection occurs by ingestion of contaminated food or water and, less commonly, by direct contact with infected animals or patients (Fig. 26.1). Butchers in Finland are at increased risk of infection (Merilahti-Palo *et al.* 1991).

Transmission of infection from animals to humans has been suggested through household dogs. In northern European countries, *Y. enterocolitica* is frequently acquired by ingestion of incompletely cooked pork (Tauxe *et al.* 1987). The ability of this organism to grow at 4 °C means that refrigerated meats can be sources of infection. The organisms have been isolated from lakes, streams, and drinking water, but only a few cases have been linked to infection of water. Epidemics of food-borne disease have occurred in the United States, including one due to contaminated chocolate milk in New York (Black *et al.* 1978), one associated with pasteurized milk in Tennessee, one due to bean sprouts in Pennsylvania, and others in Atlanta and Baltimore associated with consumption of raw pork intestine (chitterlings) during holiday festivities (Lee *et al.* 1991). A large outbreak occurred at a Japanese school in 1972 causing 198 pupils to develop fever and abdominal pain. The majority of cases occur in the winter.

Person to person spread of yersiniosis rarely occurs. Marks *et al.* (1980) reported intrafamilial spread of yersiniosis in Canada, and Toivanen *et al.* (1973) reported nosocomial spread of infection in a Finnish hospital. Contaminated blood in blood banks has been a source of *Y. enterocolitica* infection, resulting in shock and death in several cases (Anonymous 1991). The donors of the contaminated blood were presumably bacteraemic at the time of donation, but they were not noticeably ill. Multiplication of bacteria in the refrigerators of the blood banks probably played a role in causing severe disease in the recipients of the transfusions.

Infection due to *Y. pseudotuberculosis* is the rarest of the yersinioses. Although this infection has a world-wide distribution, more cases have been reported from Europe than from other continents. The majority of

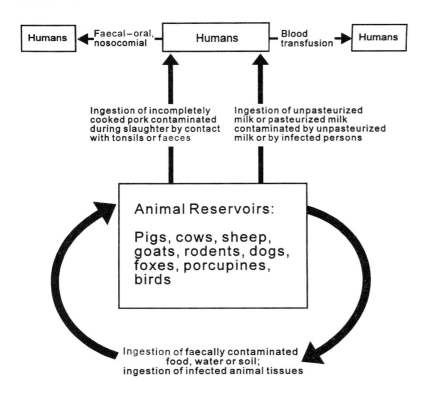

Fig. 26.1 Transmission of yersinioses among animal reservoirs and from animals to humans and from humans to animals. Wide arrows indicate common transmission, medium arrows indicate occasional transmission, and thin arrows indicate rare transmission.

patients have been children aged 5–15 years. Males are affected three times more often than females. Most patients developed their illnesses in the winter. Transmission of this infection is presumed to occur by ingestion of organisms from contact with an infected animal, or common source contamination within a family, such as food or water.

The epizoology of yersiniosis is based on faecal–oral transmission among individual animals in a flock or to members of distant species that ingest faecally contaminated food, water, or soil. *Yersinia enterocolitica* of serotypes 03 and 09 were cultured from more than 50 per cent of pork tongue in butcher shops in Belgium during all seasons of the year, indicating widespread infection of pigs in Belgium year-round (Wauters 1979). Pigs also constitute the major reservoir in other countries, such as Denmark (Christiansen 1987), The Netherlands (de Boer and Nouws 1991), and Japan (Shiozawa *et al.* 1991), but not in Australia (Slee and Skilbeck 1992). The pigs are healthy carriers. In Australia, sheep and goats are the most commonly infected animals. Both *Y. enterocolitica* and *Y. pseudo-tuberculosis* are transmitted among sheep in the cool, damp weather of the winter and spring, under experimental conditions (Slee and Skilbeck 1992). Under natural field conditions, *Y. enterocolitica* was excreted year-round. Infection occurred mostly in young lambs, with older sheep showing immune protection. No

cross-immunity was shown between *Y. enterocolitica* and *Y. pseudotuberculosis* because animals previously infected by one species could be infected by the other.

In the United States, *Yersinia enterocolitica* 08 that has caused large food-borne outbreaks was not found in a survey of domestic animals (Shayegani and Parsons 1987). However, the pathogenic serotype was found in some wild animals, including a fox and porcupine.

PREVENTION AND CONTROL

Public health measures to control *Yersinia* infection should focus on the animal reservoirs in any particular location. No successful attempts have been made to interrupt transmission by the faecal–oral route among host animals, and no animal vaccines are currently available.

Complete cooking of meats and proper pasteurization of dairy products should render potentially contaminated foods safe for consumption. Nevertheless, other approaches to reducing the frequency of contamination of uncooked foods deserve consideration. The methods of slaughtering pigs could be modified to reduce contamination of meat. For example, Christiansen (1987) proposed that abbatoir workers might prevent contact of meat with the contents of the oral cavity and intestinal tract during slaughter. He suggested removal of pigs' heads so that the contaminated tonsils would not have contact with other body parts. Kapperud (1991) advises excision of the tongue and tonsils as a separate operation after removal of the lungs, heart, diaphragm, and liver. Tongues and head meat could be scalded before removal from the slaughterhouse. Faecal contamination of meat should be avoided. Kapperud (1991) suggests a method of circumanal incision followed by removal of intestines, or enclosing the anus and rectum in a plastic bag after use of a bung cutter. In Danish pigs, use of a mechanical bung cutter (Jarvis, Middleton, Connecticut, USA) resulted in a lower incidence of contamination of meat by *Yersinia* than a normal technique of gut removal (Andersen *et al.* 1991). Christiansen (1987) also advised that meat should not be refrigerated for prolonged periods before consumption because of the unique ability of *Yersinia* to multiply at 4 °C. Consumption of uncooked meats, like chitterlings, should, of course, be avoided.

In dairies, care must be taken to prevent contamination of milk after pasteurization. Milk-associated outbreaks in the United States revealed that pasteurization methods were adequate, but that after pasteurization workers probably recontaminated the milk. Therefore, it would be prudent to design dairy plants to ensure that unpasteurized milk and workers handling unpasteurized milk have no opportunity to make contact with pasteurized milk. This could be accomplished by physically separating areas that receive unpasteurized milk from those that handle milk after it is pasteurized.

Transfusion-associated yersiniosis could be reduced by screening donors for histories of recent diarrhoea or fever. However, some of the donors involved in these contaminated transfusions were reported to be asymptomatic. It is not practical in blood banks to culture all donated blood before it is transfused. Incubation of donated blood overnight before separation of packed red cells has been proposed to reduce the incidence of contaminated transfusions (Pietersz *et al.* 1992), but it is not known whether this method will be effective or feasible.

PLAGUE

SUMMARY

Plague is a disease of animals and humans caused by one bacterial species, *Y. pestis*. The most common clinical form in humans is acute febrile lymphadenitis, called bubonic plague. Less common forms include septicaemic, pneumonic, and meningeal plague. Mortality is high in untreated plague, but early antibiotic treatment reduces mortality significantly. The major animal reservoirs are rodents, principally urban and domestic rats as well as squirrels and prairie dogs and field mice, and less commonly rabbits, cats, and other carnivores. Transmission among animals and from animals to man occurs mainly by flea bites and less commonly by ingestion, by inhalation of infected respiratory tract secretions, and by handling infected animal tissues. Plague is endemic in several countries of Africa, Asia, and South America and in the southwestern United States, but is absent from Europe, Canada, Australia, and Japan. Control of plague requires avoidance of human contact with infected animals, use of plague vaccine in high-risk situations, selectively trapping and killing animals, and applying insecticide dusts.

HISTORY

Plague is a disease of antiquity that has persisted to modern times. Epidemic bubonic plague was vividly described in biblical and medieval times. This disease was estimated to have killed one-quarter of Europe's population in the Middle Ages. The present pandemic of plague began in China in the 1860s and spread to Hong Kong in the 1890s. The genus is called *Yersinia* because Alexandre Yersin (1863–1943) went to Hong Kong in 1894 and successfully isolated the causative organism in pure culture. This pandemic was subsequently spread by rats transported on ships to California and port cities of South America, Africa, and Asia. Transmission by flea bites was suggested by Ogata in 1897. Efficiency of *Xenopsylla cheopis* fleas for transmission of plague by blockage of swallowing was shown by Bacot and Martin in 1914. Urban plague transmitted by rats was brought under control in most affected cities, but the infection was transferred to sylvatic rodents, which allowed it to become entrenched in rural areas of these countries. In the first half of this century, India was severely affected by plague epidemics and suffered more than 10 million deaths. In 1948, streptomycin was shown to reduce sharply the case fatality rate in humans. In the 1960s and 1970s, Vietnam became the leading country for plague; during the war it reported more than 10 000 cases a year (Butler 1983). Before 1970, *Y. pestis* was called by its earlier name, *Pasteurella pestis*.

Vaccines, using either attenuated strains or killed cultures of *Y. pestis*, were developed by Haffkine in India, the United States Army, and the Pasteur Institute. Vaccines were used widely in the Second World War. During the Vietnam war, more than 10 million Vietnamese people were vaccinated with the attenuated EV76 strain of *Y. pestis*.

THE AGENT

Yersinia pestis is a Gram-negative bipolar-staining bacillus that belongs to the bacterial family Enterobacteriaceae. It grows aerobically on most culture media, including blood agar and MacConkey agar. It does not ferment lactose and forms small colonies on MacConkey agar after 24-hour incubation at 35 °C. On triple-sugar-iron agar, *Y. pestis* produces an alkaline slant and acid butt. It is non-motile and negative for citrate utilization, urease, and indole.

Like the other yersiniae, the plague bacillus produces V and W antigens and *Yersinia* outer membrane proteins (Straley *et al.* 1993), which confer a calcium requirement for growth at 37 °C (Ferber and Brubaker 1981). This property, mediated by a 45 MDa plasmid (70 kb), is essential for virulence and plays a role in adapting the organism for intracellular survival and growth. Monoclonal antibody against V antigen given to animals protected them against experimental plague (Brubaker 1991). Other important virulence factors include the production of lipopolysaccharide endotoxin, a capsular envelope containing the antiphagocytic principle fraction I antigen, the ability to absorb organic iron into the form of haemin, and the presence of the temperature-dependent enzymes coagulase and fibrinolysin.

THE HOSTS

ANIMALS

Throughout the world, the urban and domestic rats *Rattus rattus* and *R. norvegicus* are the most important reservoirs of the plague bacillus. In sylvatic foci of plague, such as occurs in the United States, the important reservoirs are the ground squirrel, rock squirrel, and prairie dog. Rabbits and domestic cats are occasionally infected and can bring disease to man. Each endemic area has its own prominent host species. For example, in Brazil, the most numerous infected animal is the field mouse, *Zygodontomys pixuna*.

The organism is transmitted among the natural animal reservoirs by flea bites, or by ingestion of contaminated animal tissues. The most efficient vector for transmission is the oriental rat flea, *Xenopsylla cheopis*. When a flea ingests a blood meal from a bacteraemic animal infected with *Y. pestis*, the coagulase of the organism causes the blood to clot in the foregut, leading to blockage of the flea's swallowing. *Yersinia pestis* multiplies in the clotted blood. During attempts to ingest a blood meal, a blocked flea may regurgitate thousands of organisms into an animal's skin. The inoculated bacteria migrate by cutaneous lymphatics to the regional lymph nodes. The flea-borne bacilli possess a small amount of envelope antigen (fraction I) and are readily phagocytosed by the host's polymorphonuclear leucocytes and mononuclear phagocytes. *Yersinia pestis* resists destruction within mononuclear phagocytes and may multiply intracellularly with elaboration of envelope antigen. If lysis of the mononuclear cell occurs, the bacilli released are relatively resistant to further phagocytosis. The involved lymph nodes show polymorphonuclear leucocytes, destruction of normal architecture, haemorrhagic necrosis, and dense concentrations of extracellular plague bacilli.

Disease in animals varies from subclinical bacteraemia to illness with lymphadenitis and abscess formation in many organs, to sudden death with overwhelming sepsis. Large die-offs of rodents occur periodically, and plague is one of the major determinants of rodent population size in certain endemic areas. Generally, the enzootic hosts of plague tolerate infection well and recover, enabling a species to be an effective and durable reservoir of infection.

HUMANS

The most common presentation is bubonic plague, which presents a distinctive clinical picture. During an incubation period of 2–8 days following the bite of an infected flea, bacteria proliferate in the regional lymph nodes. Patients are typically affected by the sudden onset of fever, chills, weakness, and headache. Usually at the same time, after a few hours or on the next day, patients notice the bubo, which is signalled by intense pain in one anatomic region of lymph nodes, usually the groin, axilla, or neck. A swelling evolves in this area, which is so tender that the patients typically avoid any motion that would provoke discomfort.

The buboes of patients with plague are oval swellings that vary from 1 to 10 cm in length and elevate the overlying skin, which may appear stretched or erythematous. They may appear either as smooth, uniform, egg-shaped masses or as an irregular cluster of several nodes with intervening and surrounding oedema. There is warmth of the overlying skin and an underlying, firm, non-fluctuant mass. Around the lymph nodes there is usually considerable oedema, which can be either gelatinous or pitting in nature. Although infections other than plague can produce acute lymphadenitis, plague is virtually unique for the suddenness of onset of the fever and bubo, the rapid development of intense inflammation in the bubo, and the fulminant clinical course that can produce death as quickly as 2–4 days after the onset of symptoms.

The groin is the most common site of the buboes in plague. Other common sites are the axillae and cervical region. The reason for a given distribution of buboes is presumed to be the distribution of flea bites.

Body temperature is elevated, in the range of 38.5–40.0 °C, and pulse rates are increased to 110–140 per minute. Blood pressures are characteristically low, in the range of 100/60 mmHg, due to extreme vasodilation. Lower pressures that are unobtainable may occur if shock ensues. The liver and spleen are often palpable and tender (Crook and Tempest 1992).

The majority of patients with bubonic plague do not have skin lesions; however, about one-quarter of the patients in Vietnam did show varied skin findings. The most common were pustules, vesicles, eschars, or papules near the bubo or in the anatomic region of skin that is lymphatically drained by the affected lymph nodes, presumably representing sites of the flea bites. Rarely, these skin lesions progress to extensive cellulitis or abscesses. Ulceration, however, may lead to a large plague carbuncle.

Another kind of skin lesion in plague is purpura, which is a result of the systemic disease. The purpuric lesions may become necrotic, resulting in gangrene of distal extremities, the probable basis of the epithet 'Black Death' attributed to plague through the ages. These purpuric lesions contain blood vessels affected by vasculitis and occlusion by fibrin thrombi, resulting in haemorrhage and necrosis.

A distinctive feature of plague, in addition to the bubo, is the propensity of the disease to overwhelm patients with a massive growth of bacteria in the blood. In the early acute states of bubonic plague, all patients probably have intermittent bacteraemia. Single blood cultures obtained at the time of hospital admission in Vietnamese patients were positive in 27 per cent of cases. A hallmark of moribund patients with plague is high-density bacteraemia, so that a blood smear revealing characteristic bacilli has been used as a prognostic indicator in this disease. Occasionally in the pathogenesis of plague infection, bacteria are inoculated and proliferate in the body without producing a bubo. Patients may become ill with fever and actually die with bacteraemia but without detectable lymphadenitis (Hull *et al.* 1987). This syndrome has been termed 'septicaemic plague' to denote plague without a bubo.

One of the feared complications of bubonic plague is secondary pneumonia. The infection reaches the lungs by haematogenous spread of bacteria from the bubo. In addition to the high mortality, plague pneumonia is highly contagious by airborne transmission. It presents in the setting of fever and lymphadenopathy as cough, chest pain, and often haemoptysis. Radiographically there is patchy bronchopneumonia, cavities, or confluent consolidation (Centers for Disease Control 1992). The sputum is usually purulent and contains plague bacilli.

Primary inhalation pneumonia is rare now but is a potential threat following exposure to a patient with plague who has a cough. Recent cases in the United states were exposed to sick domestic cats that had pneumonia or submandibular abscesses (Centers for Disease Control 1992). Plague pneumonia is invariably fatal when antibiotic therapy is delayed more than 1 day after the onset of illness.

Plague meningitis is a rarer complication and typically occurs more than 1 week following inadequately treated bubonic plague. It results from haematogenous spread from a bubo and carries a high mortality rate compared with that of uncomplicated bubonic plague. There appears to be an association between buboes located in the axilla and the development of meningitis. Less commonly, plague meningitis presents as a primary infection of the meninges without antecedent lymphadenitis. Plague meningitis is characterized by fever, headache, meningismus, and pleocytosis with a predominance of polymorphonuclear leucocytes. Bacteria are frequently demonstrable with a Gram stain of spinal fluid sediment, and endotoxin has been demonstrated in spinal fluid with the limulus test.

Plague can produce pharyngitis that may resemble acute tonsillitis. The anterior cervical lymph nodes are usually inflamed, and *Y. pestis* may be recovered from a throat culture or by aspiration of a cervical bubo. This is a rare clinical form of plague that is presumed to follow the inhalation or ingestion of plague bacilli.

Plague presents sometimes with prominent gastrointestinal symptoms of nausea, vomiting, diarrhoea, and abdominal pain. These symptoms may precede the bubo or, in septicaemic plague, occur without a bubo and commonly result in diagnostic delay (Hull *et al.* 1986).

A bacteriological diagnosis is readily made in most patients by smear and culture of a bubo aspirate. The aspirate is obtained by inserting a 20 gauge needle on a 10 ml syringe containing 1 ml of sterile saline into the bubo and withdrawing it several times until the saline becomes blood-tinged. Because the bubo does not contain liquid pus, it may be necessary to inject some of the saline and immediately reaspirate it. Drops of the aspirate should be placed on to microscopic slides and air-dried for both Gram and Wayson stains. The Gram stain will reveal polymorphonuclear leucocytes and Gram-negative coccobacilli and bacilli ranging from 1 to 2 μm in length. Wayson stain is prepared by mixing 0.2 g of basic fuchsin (90 per cent dye content) with 0.75 g of methylene blue (90 per cent dye content) in 20 ml of 95 per cent ethyl alcohol. This mixture is then poured slowly into 200 ml of 5 per cent phenol. A smear, after being fixed for 2 minutes in absolute methanol, is stained for 10–20 seconds in Wayson's stain, washed with water, and dried. *Yersinia pestis* appears as light-blue bacilli with dark-blue polar bodies, and the remainder of the slide has a contrasting pink counterstain. Smears of blood, sputum, or spinal fluid can be handled similarly (Butler *et al.* 1976).

The aspirate, blood, and other appropriate fluid should be inoculated on to blood and MacConkey agar plates and into infusion broth. For definitive identification, cultures can be mailed in double containers to the Centers for Disease Control, Plague Branch, PO Box 2087, Fort Collins, Colorado 80522, USA (telephone: 303-221-6450). At this same laboratory, a serological test, the passive haemagglutination test utilizing fraction I of *Y. pestis*, can be performed on acute-and convalescent-phase serum. In patients with negative cultures, a fourfold or greater increase in titre, or a single titre of $\geq 1:16$ is presumptive evidence for plague infection.

Early treatment of patients with antibiotics is life-saving. Untreated plague has an estimated mortality rate of greater than 50 per cent. Streptomycin is the drug of choice because it reduces the case fatality rate to less than 5 per cent. No other drug has been demonstrated to be more efficacious or less toxic. Streptomycin should be administered intramuscularly in two divided doses daily totalling 30 mg/kg of body weight/day for 10 days. Most patients improve rapidly and become afebrile in about 3 days. The 10-day course of streptomycin is recommended to prevent relapses because viable bacteria have been isolated from buboes of patients with plague during convalescence.

For patients allergic to streptomycin, or in whom an oral drug is strongly preferred, tetracycline is a satisfactory alternative. It is administered orally in a dose of 2–4 g/day in four divided doses for 10 days. For patients with meningitis who require a drug with good penetration into the cerebrospinal fluid and for patients with profound hypotension in whom an intramuscular infection may be poorly absorbed, chloramphenicol should be administered intravenously. This is given as a loading dose of 25 mg/kg of body weight, followed by 60 mg/kg/day in four divided doses. After clinical improvement, chloramphenicol should be continued orally to complete a total course of 10 days.

Other antimicrobial drugs have been used in plague, with varying success. These include sulphonamides, trimethoprim–sulphamethoxazole, kanamycin, and ampicillin. These drugs all appear to be either less effective or more toxic than streptomycin and therefore should not be chosen.

Antibiotic resistance in human isolates of *Y. pestis* has never been reported, nor has resistance emerged during antibiotic therapy. The antibiotics streptomycin, tetracycline, and chloramphenicol given alone are clinically very effective and relapses are exceedingly rare. Therefore, there is no rationale for using multiple antibiotics to treat plague (Welty *et al.* 1985).

The buboes usually recede without need of local therapy. Occasionally, however, they may enlarge or become fluctuant during the first week of treatment, requiring incision and drainage. The aspirated fluid should be cultured for evidence of superinfection with other bacteria, but this material is usually sterile.

EPIDEMIOLOGY

Plague occurs worldwide, with most of the human cases reported from developing countries of Asia and Africa. During 1980–89, 8554 cases of human plague were reported to the World Health Organization from 17 countries. Of these cases, 981 died. The countries that reported more than 100 cases during 1980–89, from greatest to least, were Tanzania, Vietnam, Zaire, Brazil, Madagascar, Peru, Uganda, Burma, Bolivia, United States, and Botswana. In the United States, all the plague cases occurred in the south-western states of New Mexico, Arizona, Colorado, Utah, and California. Most of these occur during the months of May to October, when people are outdoors and come into contact with rodents and their fleas.

Plague is primarily a zoonotic infection. Humans become accidental hosts in the natural cycle of plague when bitten by infected rodent fleas; humans appear to play no role in the maintenance of plague in nature. Only rarely, during epidemics of pneumonic plague, is the infection passed directly from person to person. Humans also rarely develop infection by the direct handling or inhalation of contaminated animal tissues and fluids (Fig. 26.2).

In the United States, males and females have been equally affected. Sixty per cent of cases occurs in persons less than 20 years old. Although a majority of cases occur in Caucasians, the attack rate among American Indians living in endemic areas such as Arizona, New Mexico, and Utah is ten times the rate among non-Indians living in the same states (1.4 cases/100 000 population and 0.1/100 000 populations, respectively) (Kaufmann *et al.* 1980). Within endemic areas, risk factors associated with acquiring plague include direct contact with rodents or carnivores, the presence of harbourage and food sources for wild rodents in the immediate vicinity of the home, and possible failure to control fleas on pet dogs and cats (Mann *et al.* 1979).

In the epizoology of urban plague, the domestic black rat *R.rattus* has probably been the most important host historically. It climbs well, inhabits ships as well as houses, and is a good host for the efficient plague flea vector *X. cheopis*. Plague in other than the urban setting, however, has taken on many complex variations. The classic theory of plague reservoirs

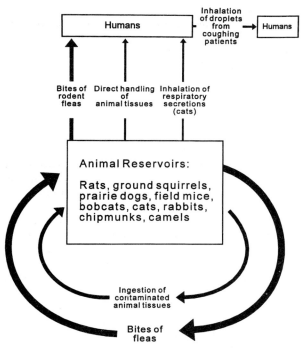

Fig. 26.2 Transmission of plague among animal reservoirs and from animals to humans and from humans to humans. Wide arrows indicate common transmission, medium arrows indicate occasional transmission, and thin arrows indicate rare transmission.

requires one or more relatively resistant small mammal species, which serve as the enzootic reservoir species, and one or more relatively susceptible species, which serve as the epizootic hosts and may be involved in the so-called rat die-offs or ratfalls. In urban plague, the same species of rats can be both the enzootic and epizootic species, whereas in rural or sylvatic plague, there are usually two or more separate species. For example in India, Baltazard and Bahmanyar (1960*a*) found that the field gerbil *Tatera indica* was resistant to plague and served as the enzootic reservoir. The domestic rats were 'liaison rodents', carrying plague from gerbils to man. In Java, the resistant field species was *R. exulans* and, again, the domestic rats were merely liaisons to man (Baltazard and Bahmanyar 1960*b*). In the sylvatic plague that occurs in the United States, the ecology of plague does not neatly fit this pattern. Although the colonizing rodents, ground squirrels, and prairie dogs have frequently brought plague to man, the resistant enzootic species has been difficult to define. Kartman *et al.* (1958) suggested that the meadow vole was responsible for enzooticity in California. More recently in New Mexico and Arizona, the carnivorous coyotes and bobcats, as well as rabbits, were shown to be

infected with plague, but the modes of transmission among these animals remain to be delineated.

In Vietnam, the brown street rat *R. norvegicus* was an important plague reservoir, in addition to *R. rattus*. The house shrew *S. murinus* also carried plague and appeared to be an important host for carrying infection to man (Cavanaugh *et al.* 1968, 1969).

In Africa, the wild rodent complex *Mastomys natalensis* has been demonstrated to be an important reservoir for the maintenance of both plague and the virus of Lassa fever by Green *et al.* (1978). Issacson *et al.* (1981) in South Africa examined the susceptibility of *Mastomys* to experimental plague infection and found that *M. natalensis* was relatively resistant to fatal infection, as shown by a 50 per cent death rate after a dose of 19×10^5 bacteria given subcutaneously. By contrast, another species, called *Mastomys coucha*, which differs from other species by having diploid chromosomes of numbers 32 and 36, was susceptible to death when inoculated with only 1.9×10^2 bacteria. This suggests that genetically determined differences among species of rodents could allow the same genus to provide a relatively resistant enzootic reservoir and a more susceptible epizootic reservoir for plague infection. In Tanzania, a serousurvey of rodents in the active focus of Lushoto District in the 1980s revealed that several species were infected (Kilonzo *et al.* 1992). The most numerous seropositive species were *R. rattus* and *M. natalensis*.

Some of the fluctuations in plague occurrence have been related to changing populations of the rodent reservoirs. In Indian cities, Seal (1960) described replacement of *R. rattus* by *B. bengalensis* at the same time that human plague diminished. Although both rodents were good hosts for *Y. pestis*, *R. rattus* was more heavily parasitized with the efficient flea vector *X. cheopis* than were the bandicoot rats. The virtual elimination of plague infection from India after 1950 was an astonishing event and could have other explanations. One possibility is that insecticide spraying to control mosquitoes as vectors of malaria also had a controlling effect on the fleas that transmitted plague.

Another part of the epizoology of plague is the relationship of the potential flea vectors to their mammalian hosts. Generally, the flea species that are narrowly adapted to a particular host are so poorly adapted to man that they have only transient existences on man, but this can, of course, be long enough for a few bites and the transmission of plague. The human flea *Pulex irritans* is not an efficient plague vector and rarely, if ever, has transmitted plague from man to man.

The proliferation of fleas on rodents is believed to be crucial for the propagation of plague epizootics. Much has been made of the flea index (the average number of fleas per rodent). When the flea index is high, that is, exceeding one, the chances for an epizootic among rodents are greater. The multiplication of fleas on rodents is highly seasonal, being greatest in the warm and dry times when epidemics are most likely to occur. In Vietnam, the rainy season curtailed sharply the transmission of plague and concomitantly reduced flea indices (Olson 1969).

Although rodent fleas are specific for their host species and, thus, are rarely exchanged, the intermingling of different rodent species and their fleas has been observed in the field and might explain the migration of plague from an urban focus to a sylvatic focus, and vice versa. The wild rodent flea *M. telchinum* was found on the urban rat *R. norvegicus* in San Francisco in 1938 (Kartman *et al.* 1958). Furthermore, rodent fleas have been found on dogs. Fleas of domestic dogs and cats have been implicated in the transmission of plague to man in the United States (von Reyn *et al.* 1977), but infection of these fleas with *Y. pestis* has only rarely been identified. Dogs in Tanzania were frequently seropositive for plague and carried approximately eight fleas per dog (Kilonzo *et al.* 1993). However, it is not known whether dogs played any role in the transmission of infection or they were simply a 'dead-end' transmission following the ingestion of infected rodents.

PREVENTION AND CONTROL

All patients with suspected plague should be reported to the Public Health Department and to the World Health Organization. Patients with uncomplicated infections who are promptly treated present no health hazards to other persons. Those with cough or other signs of pneumonia must be placed in strict respiratory isolation for at least 48 hours after the institution of antibiotic therapy or until the sputum culture is negative. The bubo aspirate and blood must be handled with gloves and with care to avoid the formation of aerosois of these infected fluids. Laboratory workers who process the cultures should be alerted to exercise precautions; however, standard bacteriological techniques that safeguard against skin contact with, and aerosolization of, cultures should be adequate.

A formalin-killed vaccine, Plague Vaccine USP (Greer Laboratories, PO Box 800, Lenoir, North Carolina 28645, USA) is available for travellers to epidemic or hyperendemic areas, for individuals who must live and work in close contact with rodents, and for laboratory workers who must handle live *Y. pestis* cultures. A primary series of two injections is recommended with a 1–3 month interval between them. Booster injections are given every 6 months for as long

as exposure continues. The vaccine is not currently in use for the protection of the inhabitants of endemic localities. The last large-scale use of plague vaccines was in American military personnel in Vietnam in 1965–75 and in Vietnamese civilians during the same years. Persons living in endemic areas should provide themselves with as much personal protection against rodents and fleas as possible, including living in rat-proof houses, wearing shoes and garments to cover the legs, and applying insecticide dusts to houses when plague is anticipated.

Once an epidemic of plague has been identified by confirming the infection in several human cases in one locality, the explosive epidemic potential of plague requires emergency action on the part of public health authorities. The first step is to ensure that medical facilities, personnel, and antibiotics are available in the locality for treating human cases. This medical treatment will save lives but will have no significant impact on prevention because nearly all human cases result from bites of infected rodent fleas.

The next step is to prevent further human cases by interrupting transmission of infection from the animal reservoirs caused by flea bites. Before embarking on any strategic plan, local health authorities should report the epidemic to the central health authorities. Eventually the World Health Organization should be notified and would likely respond by offering advice and help. The interested reader should consult publications from Geneva regarding plague control (Bahmanyar and Cavanaugh 1976; World Health Organization 1990).

First priority is given to insecticide dusting because infected fleas are the most immediate threat to humans. The choice of insecticide will depend on whether local fleas might be resistant to any insecticide on account of recent applications of insecticide in a previous control effort against malaria. Testing of fleas for insecticide susceptibility using WHO kits is advised. The commonly used insecticides in plague control are DDT, BHC, carbaryl, diazinon, and malathion. It is essential that experienced personnel apply insecticides appropriately in places that will reach the animals that carry fleas.

The second priority is rodent control. This should be undertaken with caution only after insecticide application has been started because infected fleas on poisoned rodents may depart dying animals and infect humans. Nevertheless, reducing the numbers of rodents, both infected and susceptible animals, can be highly effective in curtailing an epizootic. The strategy will depend on the rodent species involved in the epizootic and the geographic location. The usual methods of rodent control are trapping and application of rodenticides. Experienced personnel to apply rodenticide are desirable because of the dangers of accidentally poisoning humans and other unintended animals. Rodenticides that have been used in plague epidemics include sodium fluoroacetate, thallium sulphate, and zinc phosphide.

REFERENCES

Aho, K. *et al.* (1973). HL-A antigen and reactive arthritis. *Lancet*, **2**, 157.

Andersen, J. K., Sorensen, R., and Glensbjerg, M. (1991). Aspects of the epidemiology of *Yersinia enterocolitica*: a review. *International Journal of Food Microbiology*, **13**, 231–8.

Anonymous (1991). Update: *Yersinia enterocolitica* bacteremia and endotoxin shock associated with red blood cell transfusions—United States, 1991. *Morbidity Mortality Reports*, **40**, 176–8.

Applebaum, J. S., Wilding, G., and Morse, L. J. (1983). *Yersinia enterocolitica* endocarditis. *Archives of Internal Medicine*, **143**, 2150–1.

Bahmanyar, M. and Cavanaugh, D. C. (1976). *Plague manual.* World Health Organization, Geneva.

Baltazard, M. and Bahmanyar, M. (1960*a*). Recherches sur la peste en Inde. *Bulletin of World Health Organization*, **23**, 169–215.

Baltazard, M. and Bahmanyar, M. (1960*b*). Recherches sur la peste a Java. *Bulletin of World Health Organization*, **23**, 217–46.

Black, R. E. *et al.* (1978). Epidemic *Yersinia enterocolitica* infection due to contaminated chocolate milk. *New England Journal of Medicine*, **298**, 76–9.

Borg, A. A., Gray, J., and Dawes, P. T. (1992). Yersinia-related arthritis in the United Kingdom. A report of 12 cases and review of the literature. *Quarterly Journal of Medicine New Series 84*, **304**, 575–82.

Bottone, E. J. (1983). Current trends of *Yersinia enterocolitica* isolates in the New York City area. *Journal of Clinical Microbiology*, **17**, 63–7.

Boyce, J. M., Evans, D. J., Evans, D. G. *et al.* (1979). Production of heat-stable, methanol-soluble enterotoxin by *Yersinia enterocolitica*. *Infection Immunity*, **25**, 532–7.

Bradford, W. D., Noce, P. S., and Gutman, L. T. (1974). Pathologic features of enteric infection with *Yersinia enterocolitica*. *Archives of Pathology*, **98**, 17–22.

Brubaker, R. R. (1991). The V antigen of Yersiniae: an overview. *Contributions to Microbiology and Immunology*, **12**, 127–33.

Butler, T. (1983). *Plague and other* Yersinia *infections*. Plenum, New York.

Butler, T. *et al.* (1976). *Yersinia pestis* in Vietnam. II. Quantitative blood cultures and detection of endotoxin in the cerebrospinal fluid of patients with meningitis. *Journal of Infectious Disease*, **133**, 493–9.

Cantinieaux, B. *et al.* (1988). Impaired neutrophil defense against *Yersinia enterocolitica* in patients with iron overload who are undergoing dialysis. *Journal of Laboratory and Clinical Medicine*, **111**, 524–8.

Carniel, E. and Mollaret, M. M. (1990). Yersiniosis. *Comparative Immunology Microbiology Infectious Diseases*, **13**, 51–8.

Carniel, E. *et al.* (1986). Infrequent detection of *Yersinia enterocolitica* in childhood diarrhea in Bangladesh. *American Journal of Tropical Medicine and Hygiene*, **35**, 370–1.

Carter, P. B., Lafleur, L., and Toma, S. (ed.) (1979). Yersinia enterocolitica. *Biology, epidemiology, and pathology*. S. Karger, Basel.

Cavanaugh, D. C. *et al.* (1968). Some observations on the current plague outbreak in the Republic of Vietnam. *American Journal of Public Health*, **58**, 742–52.

Cavanaugh, D. C., Ryan, P. F., and Marshall, J. D. (1969). The role of commensal rodents and their ectoparasites in the ecology and transmission of plague in Southeast Asia. *Bulletin of Wildlife Disease Association*, **5**, 187–94.

Centers for Disease Control (1992). Pneumonic plague—Arizona, 1992. *Journal of the American Medical Association*, **268**, 2146–7.

Chiu, H. Y. *et al.* (1986). Infection with *Yersinia enterocolitica* in patients with iron overload. *British Medical Journal*, **292**, 97.

Christiansen, S. G. (1987). The *Yersinia enterocolitica* situation in Denmark. *Contributions to Microbiology and Immunology*, **9**, 93–7.

Cornelis, G. *et al.* (1987). *Yersinia enterocolitica*, a primary model for bacterial invasiveness. *Reviews of Infectious Diseases*, **9**, 64–87.

Cover, T. L. and Aber, R. C. (1989). *Yersinia enterocolitica*. *New England Journal of Medicine*, **321**, 16–24.

Crook, L. D. and Tempest, B. (1992). Plague. A clinical review of 27 cases. *Archives of Internal Medicine*, **152**, 1253–6.

de Boer, E. and Nouws, J. F. M. (1991). Slaughter pigs and pork as a source of human pathogenic *Yersinia enterocolitica*. *International Journal of Food Microbiology*, **12**, 375–8.

Ferber, D. M. and Brubaker, R. R. (1981). Plasmid in *Yersinia pestis*. *Infection Immunity*, **31**, 839–41.

Galyov, E. E. *et al.* (1993). A secreted protein kinase of *Yersinia pseudotuberculosis* is an indispensable virulence determinant. *Nature*, **361**, 703–2.

Goguen, J. D. *et al.* (1986). Plasmid-determined cytotoxicity in *Yersinia pestis* and *Yersinia enterocolitica*. *Infection Immunity*, **51**, 788–94.

Green, C. A., Gordon, D. H., and Lyons, N. F. (1978). Biological species in *Praomys* (*Mastomys*) *natalensis* (Smith), a rodent carrier of Lassa virus and bubonic plague in Africa. *American Journal of Tropical Medicine and Hygiene*, **27**, 627–9.

Greene, J. N. *et al.* (1993). Case report: Yersinia enterocolitica necrotizing pneumonia in an immunocompromised patient. *American Journal of Medical Sciences*, **305**, 171–3.

Guan, K. and Dixon, J. E. (1990). Protein tyrosine phosphatase activity of an essential virulence determinant in *Yersinia*. *Science*, **249**, 553–6.

Hoogkamp-Korstanje, J. A. A. (1987). Antibiotics in *Yersinia enterocolitica* infections. *Journal of Antimicrobial Chemotherapy*, **20**, 123–31.

Hoogkamp-Korstanje, J. A. A., de Koning, J., and Samson, J. P. (1986). Incidence of human infection with *Yersinia enterocolitica* serotypes 03, 08, and 09 and the use of indirect immunofluorescence in diagnosis. *Journal of Infectious Diseases*, **153**, 138–41.

Hull, H. F., Montes, J. M., and Mann, J. M. (1986). Plague masquerading as gastrointestinal illness. *Western Journal of Medicine*, **145**, 485–7.

Hull, H. F., Montes, J. M., and Mann, J. M. (1987). Septicemic plague in New Mexico. *Journal of Infectious Diseases*, **155**, 113–18.

Isaacson, M., Arntzen, L., and Taylor, P. (1981). Susceptibility of members of the *Mastomys natalensis* species complex to experimental infection with *Yersinia pestis*. *Journal of Infectious Disease*, **144**, 80.

Kachoris, M. *et al.* (1988). Routine culture of stool specimens for *Yersinia enterocolitica* is not a cost-effective procedure. *Journal of Clinical Microbiology*, **26**, 582–3.

Kapperud, G. (1991). *Yersinia enterocolitica* in food hygiene. *International Journal of Food Microbiology*, **12**, 53–66.

Kartman, L., Prince, F. M., Quan, S. F., and Stark, H. E. (1958). New knowledge on the ecology of sylvatic plague. *Annals of New York Academy of Sciences*, **70**, 668–711.

Kaufmann, A. F., Boyce, J. M., and Martone, W. J. (1980). Trends in human plague in the United States. *Journal of Infectious Diseases*, **141**, 522–4.

Kay, B. A., Wachsmuth, K., and Gemski, P. (1982). New virulence-associated plasmid in *Yersinia enterocolitica*. *Journal of Clinical Microbiology*, **15**, 1161–3.

Kihlstrom, E. *et al.* (1992). Intestinal symptoms and serological response in patients with complicated and uncomplicated *Yersinia enterocolitica* infections. *Scandinavian Journal of Infectious Diseases*, **24**, 57–63.

Kilonzo, B. S., Mbise, T. J., and Makundi, R. H. (1992). Plague in Lushoto district, Tanzania, 1980–1988. *Transactions of the Royal Society of Tropical Medicine and Hygiene*, **86**, 444–5.

Kilonzo, B. S., Gisakanyi, N. D., and Sabuni, C. A. (1993). Involvement of dogs in plague epidemiology in Tanzania. Serological observations in domestic animals in Lushoto district. *Scandinavian Journal of Infections Disease*, **25**, 503–6.

Lee, L. A. *et al.* (1991). *Yersinia enterocolitica* 0:3: an emerging cause of pediatric gastroenteritis in the United States. *Journal of Infectious Diseases*, **163**, 660–3.

Leirisalo-Repo, M. (1987). *Yersinia* arthritis. *Contributions to Microbiology and Immunology*, **9**, 145–54.

Mann, J. M. *et al.* (1979). Endemic human plague in New Mexico: risk factors associated with infection. *Journal of Infectious Diseases*, **140**, 397–401.

Marks, M. T. *et al.* (1980). *Yersinia enterocolitica* gastroenteritis: a prospective study of clinical, bacteriologic, and epidemiologic features. *Journal of Pediatrics*, **96**, 26–31.

Merlahti-Palo, R. *et al.* (1991). Risk of *Yersinia* infection among butchers. *Scandinavian Journal of Infectious Diseases*, **23**, 55–61.

Olson, W. P. (1969). Rat-flea indices, rainfall, and plague outbreaks in Vietnam, with emphasis on the Pleiku area. *American Journal of Tropical Medicine and Hygiene*, **18**, 621–8.

Philbey, A. W., Glastonbury, J. R. W., Links, I. J., and Matthews, L. M. (1991). *Yersinia* species isolated from sheep with enterocolitis. *Australian Veterinary Journal*, **68**, 108–10.

Pietersz, R. N. I. *et al.* (1992). Prevention of *Yersinia enterocolitica* growth in red-blood-cell concentrates. *Lancet*, **340**, 755–6.

Portnoy, D. A., Moseley, S. L., and Falkow, S. (1981). Characterization of plasmids and plasmid-associated determinants of *Yersinia enterocolitica* pathogenesis. *Infection and Immunity*, **31**, 775–82.

Prpic, J. K. and Davey, R. D. (ed.) (1987). *The genus* Yersinia: *epidemiology, molecular biology and pathogenesis*. Karger, Basel.

Rabinovitz, M. *et al.* (1987). *Yersinia enterocolitica* infection complicated by intestinal perforation. *Archives of Internal Medicine*, **147**, 1662–3.

Rose, F. B., Camp, C. J., and Antes, E. F. (1987). Family outbreak of fatal *Yersinia enterocolitica* pharyngitis. *American Journal of Medicine*, **82**, 636–7.

Seal, S. C. (1960). Epidemiological studies of plague in India. 2. The changing pattern of rodents and fleas in Calcutta and other cities. *Bulletin of World Health Organization*, **23**, 293–300.

Shayegani, M. and Parsons, L. M. (1987). Epidemiology and pathogenicity of *Yersinia enterocolitica* in New York State. *Contributions to Microbiology and Immunology*, **9**, 41–7.

Shiozawa, K., Nishina, T., Miwa, Y., Mori, T., Akahane, S., and Ito, K., (1991). Colonization in the tonsils of swine by *Yersinia enterocolitica*. *Contributions to Microbiology and Immunology*, **12**, 63–7.

Simonet, M., Riot, B., Fortineau, N., and Berche, P. (1996). Invasin production by *Yersinia pestis* is abolished by insertion of an IS200-like element within the *inv* gene. *Infection and Immunity*, **64**, 375–9.

Slee, K. J. and Button, C. (1990). Enteritis in sheep and goats due to *Yersinia enterocolitica* infection. *Australian Veterinary Journal*, **67**, 396–8.

Slee, K. J. and Skilbeck, N. W. (1992). Epidemiology of *Yersinia pseudotuberculosis* and *Y. enterocolitica* infections in sheep in Australia. *Journal of Clinical Microbiology*, **30**, 712–15.

Straley, S. C., Skrzypek, E., Plano, G. V., and Bliska, J. B. (1993). Yops of *Yersinia* spp. pathogenic for humans. *Infection and Immunity*, **61**, 3105–10.

Stuart, P. M., and Woodward, J. G. (1992). *Yersinia enterocolitica* produces superantigenic activity. *Journal of Immunology*, **148**, 225–33.

Tauxe, R. V. *et al.* (1987). *Yersinia enterocolitica* infections and pork: the missing link. *Lancet*, **1**, 1129–32.

Toivanen, P., Toivanen, A., Olkkonen, L., and Aantaa, S. (1973). Hospital outbreak of *Yersinia enterocolitica* infection. *Lancet*, **1**, 801–3.

Une, T., Tsutomu, M., and Tsubokura, M. (ed.) (1991). Current investigations of the microbiology of *Yersiniae*. S. Karger, Basel.

von Reyn, C. F. *et al.* (1977). Epidemiologic and clinical features of an outbreak of bubonic plague in New Mexico. *Journal of Infectious Diseases*, **136**, 489–94.

Wauters, G. (1979). Carriage of *Yersinia enterocolitica* serotype 3 by pigs as a source of human infection. *Contributions to Microbiology and Immunology*, **5**, 249–52.

Wauters, G. (1981). Antigens of *Yersinia enterocolitica*. In Yersinia enterocolitica, CRC Press, Boca Raton, Florida. (ed. E. J. Buttone), pp. 41–53.

Weber, J., Finlayson, N. B., and Mark, J. B. D. (1970). Mesenteric lymphadenitis and terminal ileitis due to *Yersinia pseudotuberculosis*. *New England Journal of Medicine*, **283**, 172–4.

Welty, T. K. *et al.* (1985). Nineteen cases of plague in Arizona. A spectrum including ecthyma gangrenosum due to plague and plague in pregnancy. *Western Journal of Medicine*, **142**, 641–6.

World Health Organization Consultation on Plague (1990). World Health Organization, Geneva.

Yamashiro, K. M. *et al.* (1971). *Pasteurella pseudotuberculosis*. Acute sepsis with survival. *Archives of Internal Medicine*, **128**, 605–8.

PART 2   VIRAL ZOONOSES

27   ARENAVIRUSES

Colin R. Howard

SUMMARY

The arenaviruses, which take their name from the sand-sprinkled appearance under the electron microscope, are single-stranded RNA viruses which can cause severe haemorrhagic disease (e.g. Lassa fever, Argentinian, Bolivian and Venezuelan haemorrhagic fevers).

Haemorrhagic fevers have an incubation period usually of 7–16 days, with insidious onset of fever, malaise, rigors, fatigue, headache, vomiting, constipation or diarrhoea, conjunctival congestion, epistaxis, and petechial haemorrhages beneath skin, palate, and gums. In severe cases there is haematemesis and encephalopathy. The fatality rate is 5–30 per cent in outbreaks.

Argentinian haemorrhagic fever, caused by Junín virus, affects mainly farm workers in the wet pampas areas used for cereal cultivation. The reservoir is principally *Calomys* field voles and virus is excreted in the urine and saliva. Transmission is possibly airborne from dust, contaminated food, or by direct contact with skin abrasions. Incidence coincides with peak rodent populations during the maize harvest from April to July. Bolivian haemorrhagic fever, caused by Machupo virus, has affected farm workers in northeastern Bolivia exposed to voles. Lassa fever occurs in western and central Africa. The reservoir is the multimammate rat *Mastomys natalensis*. Person to person transmission occurs in rural hospital settings from contact with body fluids. Venezuelan haemorrhagic fever, caused by Guanarito virus was first described in 1989 in the mid west of Venezuela. Virus has been isolated from the cotton rat *Sigmodon alstoin*. Unlike the other arenaviruses, lymphocytic choiromeningitis virus infection is usually asymptomatic or causes mild flu-like symptoms, but occasionally aspectic meningitis or meningo-encephalomyelitis. The reservoir is domestic mice, and reports of human infection are mainly from laboratory workers.

INTRODUCTION

There are few groups of viral zoonoses that have attracted such widespread publicity as the arenaviruses, particularly during the 1960s and 1970s when Lassa emerged as a major cause of haemorrhagic disease in West Africa. Unlike other zoonoses, members of the group are used routinely for the study of virus–host relationships and several members remain endemic within restricted geographical localities. Thus the study of this unique group of enveloped, single-stranded RNA viruses has been pursued for two quite separate reasons. First, lymphocytic choriomeningitis virus (LCM) has been used as a model of persistent virus infections for over half a century; its study has contributed, and continues to contribute, a number of cardinal concepts to our present understanding of interactions between viruses and the host immune system. Although LCM infections of humans are rare, this virus remains the prototype of the Arenaviridae and is a common infection of laboratory mice, rats, and hamsters. Secondly, certain arenaviruses cause severe haemorrhagic diseases in man, notably Lassa fever in Africa, Argentinian haemorrhagic fever in South America, and more recently Guaranito infection in Venezuela. The latter is a prime example for the need of ever-continuing vigilance for the emergence of new viral diseases; more recently a further arenavirus (Sabia) has been isolated from Brazil.

In common with LCM, the natural reservoir of these infections is a limited number of rodent species (Howard 1986). Although the initial isolates from South America were at first erroneously designated as newly defined arboviruses, there is no evidence to implicate arthropod transmission for any arenavirus. However, similar methods of isolation and the necessity of trapping small animals have meant that the majority of arenaviruses have been isolated by workers in the arbovirus field. A good example of this is the recently identified Guanarito virus that emerged during investigation of a dengue virus outbreak in Venezuela (Salas *et al.* 1991).

There is an interesting spectrum of pathological processes among these viruses. All the evidence so far available suggests that the morbidity of Lassa fever and South American haemorrhagic fevers due to arenavirus infection results from the direct cytopathic action of these agents. This is in sharp contrast to the immunopathological basis of 'classic' lymphocytic choriomeningitis disease seen in adult mice infected with LCM virus. (For a general overview of the arenaviruses, see Salvato 1993).

PROPERTIES OF THE VIRUS

NOMENCLATURE AND NATURAL HISTORY

The morphological, physicochemical, and serological properties of the arenaviruses were first summarized by Pfau (1974). The grouping was first recognized on the basis of a serological cross-reaction observed between LCM and Machupo viruses. The Arenaviridae take their name from their sand-sprinkled appearance when viewed in the electron microscope (Latin: *arena* = sand). The members of the family are listed in Table 27.1. The various strains and isolates of LCM are now considered to be a genus within the Arenaviridae. A close serological relationship exists between LCM, Lassa virus, and other arenaviruses from Africa. For this reason, they are loosely referred to as the 'Old World' arenaviruses, in contrast to those from the Americas, although now LCM can be found worldwide except in Australia (Howard and Simpson 1980). The 'New World' arenaviruses show varying degrees of serological relationships with Tacaribe virus, first isolated in Trinidad. For this reason, viruses from the Americas are frequently regarded as members of the Tacaribe complex.

With the exception of LCM, all are referred to by names that reflect the geographical area in which they were isolated. Various strain designations are also commonly used, in particular for LCM and arenaviruses isolated from man. Multiple isolations of non-pathogenic viruses that infect New World rodents are made less frequently, with the exception of Pichinde virus where a large number of field isolates from Columbia have been characterized.

All but one of the 16 members of the Arenaviridae so far described have rodents as their natural reservoir hosts. The exception is the Tacaribe virus, which was originally isolated from the fruit-bat, *Artibeus literatus*. Although rodents are divided into over 30 families distributed worldwide, arenaviruses are predominantly found within two major families, the Muridae (e.g. mice and rats) and Cricetidae (e.g. voles, lemmings, gerbils). The nature of the original reservoir for LCM virus remains obscure, but it appears to be mainly in species of the Muridae which evolved in the Old World and subsequently spread to most parts of the globe. There is a wide range of tropism and virulence among laboratory strains of LCM virus originally isolated from laboratory mouse colonies.

The natural reservoir of Lassa virus, *Mastomys natalensis*, is also a member of Muridae and, in common with the host of LCM, frequents human dwellings and food stores. In contrast, nearly all arenaviruses isolated from the South American continent are associated

Table 27.1   Arenaviridae: host and geographic distribution

Virus	Vertebrate host	Geographic distribution
New World		
Amapari	*Oryzomys goeldi*	Brazil
	Neocomys guinae	Brazil
Flexal	*Neocomys* spp.	Brazil
Guanarito	*Sigmodon alstoni*	Venezuela
Junín	*Calomys laucha*	Argentina
	Calomys musculinus	Argentina
	Akadon azarae	Argentina
Latino	*Calomys callosus*	Bolivia
Machupo	*Calomys callosus*	Bolivia
Parana	*Oryzomys buccinatus*	Paraguay
Pichinde	*Oryzomys albigularia*	Colombia
Tacaribe	*Artibeus literatus*	Trinidad
	Artibeus jamaicensis	Trinidad
Tamiami	*Sigmodon hispidus*	USA
Old World		
Ippy	*Mastomys natalensis*	Central African Republic
LCM	*Mus musculus*	Worldwide
Lassa	*Mastomys natalensis*	West Africa
Mobala	*Praomys jacksoni*	Central African Republic
Mopeia	*Mastomys natalensis*	Mozambique
		Zimbabwe

Members causing human infections underlined; severe human infections with LCM occur on passage through hamsters and gerbils.

with cricetid rodents whose members frequent open grasslands and forest.

In recent years, several new arenaviruses have come to our attention. In the instance of Guanarito virus, this new form of haemorrhagic fever from Venezuela was originally mistaken as dengue (Gonzalez *et al.* 1995). A virus from Brazil dubbed Sabia virus has recently caused a laboratory-associated infection during investigations of a new outbreak of hitherto unrecorded febrile illness in the southern provinces. Both instances bring into sharp relief once again the need for continuing vigilance of these zoonoses.

ULTRASTRUCTURE OF ARENAVIRUSES AND INFECTED CELLS

Negative-staining electron microscopy of extracellular virus shows pleomorphic particles ranging in diameter from 80 to 150 nm.

The virus envelope is formed from the plasma membrane of infected cells. A significant thickening of both bilayers of the membrane together with an increase in the width of the electron-translucent intermediate layer is characteristic of arenavirus development. Little is known about the internal structure of the arenavirus particle, although thin sections of mature and budding viruses clearly show the ordered, and often circular, arrangements of host ribosomes that are typical of this virus group and confer the 'sandy' appearance from which its name is derived. Distinct, well-dispersed filaments, 5–10 nm in diameter, are released from detergent-treated virus. Two predominant size classes are present, with average lengths of 649 nm and 1300 nm, respectively; these lengths do not show a close relationship with the two virus-specific L and S RNA species. Each is circular and beaded in appearance. Convoluted filamentous strands up to 15 nm in diameter can be seen in preparations of spontaneously disrupted Pichinde virus. These appear to represent globular condensations which arise from an association between neighbouring turns of the underlying helix. The basic configuration of the filaments shows a linear array of globular units up to 5 nm in diameter, probably representing single molecules of the viral polypeptide. These filaments progressively fold through a number of intermediate helical structures to produce the stable 15 nm diameter forms (Young 1987).

Arenaviruses replicate in experimental animals in the absence of any gross pathological effect. However, cellular necrosis may accompany virus production, not unlike that seen in virus-infected cell cultures. The variable pathological changes associated with arenavirus infections are further complicated by the occasional appearance of particles in tissue sections that react strongly with fluorescein-conjugated antisera. Granular fluorescence with convalescent serum in the perinuclear region of acutely infected Vero cells is often seen. In addition, intracytoplasmic inclusion bodies are a prominent feature in virus-infected cells both *in vitro* and *in vivo*. These usually appear early in the replication cycle and consist largely of single ribosomes which later become condensed in an electron-dense matrix, sometimes together with fine filaments (Murphy and Whitefield 1975).

CHEMICAL COMPOSITION

Nucleic acid

The genome of arenaviruses consists of two single-stranded RNA segments of different sizes, designated L and S. Analysis of RNA is complicated by the presence of ribosomal 18S and 28S RNA although these cellular RNA species are not essential for virus replication. The total ribosomal RNA content may, in turn, be influenced by the varying proportions of infectious to non-infectious particles present in virus stocks. A role for these host RNA molecules in the establishment and maintenance of persistent infections is now emerging (see below).

Extracted virion RNA is not infectious and the detection of a viral DNA polymerase led to the belief that arenaviruses adopt a negative-strand coding strategy with respect to viral protein synthesis. Complete molecular sequence data confirm that each species is unique with an established total protein coding capacity of between 250 and 300 kDa from the L strand and 125–150 kDa from the S RNA.

Genetic studies have shown that the S strand codes for the nucleoprotein (N) and the envelope glycoprotein precursor (GPC) in two main open reading frames located on RNA molecules of opposite polarity. The 3′ half of the S RNA codes for the N protein by production of an mRNA with a nucleotide sequence complementary to the viral genome. In contrast, the GPC is expressed by the 5′ half of the S RNA strand, which is required to undergo replication before the production of a mRNA with a viral-sense sequence specific for the GPC protein. Thus expression of the genome is by synthesis of subgenomic RNA from full-length templates of opposite polarities. This strategy of 'ambisense' coding for viral protein has so far been described only for the arenaviruses and some bunyaviruses. The reading frames for the two major gene products are separated by a hairpin structure of approximately 20 paired nucleotides. This intergenic region may act as a control mechanism for genome expression but there is as yet no experimental evidence to support this possibility.

The L RNA strand represents about 70 per cent of the viral genome, but less is known of its genetic organization. Reassortment studies with virulent and avirulent strains of LCM virus have shown that lethal disease in guinea-pigs is associated with the L RNA strand. The L protein is encoded by a large open reading frame covering 70 per cent of the L RNA strand: it is expressed via a mRNA complementary in sense to the viral genome.

Proteins

The arenavirus genome codes for at least five proteins; an RNA-dependent RNA polymerase and a zinc-binding (Z) protein from the L strand, and three structural proteins from the smaller, S strand. Extracellular particles contain a major nucleocapsid-associated protein of molecular weight 54–68 kDa with two glycoproteins in the outer viral envelope. These envelope glycoproteins are not primary gene products but arise by proteolytic cleavage of a larger, 75 kDa glycoprotein precursor polypeptide (GPC). Maturation and release of virus does not seem to be markedly inhibited in the presence of tunicamycin, an inhibitor of glycosylation; glycoprotein processing appears to be essential for infectivity, however.

The major glycoprotein species (GP2) in the molecular weight range of 34–42 kDa represents the C-terminal cleavage product of the GPC envelope glycoprotein precursor. A major antigenic site has been located between amino acids 390 and 405, and cross-reactive monoclonal antibodies bind to epitopes in this region. The corresponding N-terminal product of GPC cleavage (GP1) is probably highly glycosylated with at least four antigenic domains. Neutralizing monoclonal antibodies to LCM virus map to two of these regions and there is less sequence homology between the GP1 than between the GP2 molecules of different arenaviruses. Polyclonal neutralizing antibody appears to react predominantly with conformation-dependent structures within one of these domains. Until recently, a puzzling feature of arenavirus structure was the finding of a single glycoprotein in the envelopes of Tacaribe and Tamiami viruses. This is despite the close relationship known to exist between Tacaribe and Junín virus, the latter possessing the more typical duplex of envelope glycoproteins, and sequence analysis predicting the existence of a GP1 glycoprotein. This issue has now been resolved, however, with the identification of a second, similarly sized glycoprotein in the outer envelope of Tacaribe virus (M. J. Buchmeier, personal communication).

The internal nucleocapsid-associated (N) protein accounts for much of the virus-specific protein present in purified virus and infected cells, and remains bound to the virus genome after solubilization of the virus with non-ionic detergents. Molecular cloning studies have shown a surprisingly high degree of homology between the N proteins of Old and New World arenaviruses, and this would account for the serological cross-reactions seen using certain monoclonal antibodies to the N protein. A high degree of conservation between such epidemiologically distinct viruses may indicate precise functional roles for certain areas of the N polypeptide in virus replication. Cleavage is not noticeable in Vero cells; yields of arenaviruses are lower in these cells, perhaps due to reduced availability of N for packaging. A fragment of the N protein is often seen in the nucleus of these cells although the exact function of this is not clear.

A minor component with a molecular weight in excess of 150 kDa is often observed in infected cells. This L protein is coded by the larger RNA genome segment, as shown by the study of reassortant viruses. This large protein is considered to be the virus-specific RNA polymerase (Fuller-Pace and Southern 1989). Amino acid sequences common to the viral polymerase are present along the open reading frame coding for the L protein, which suggests the conservation of certain functional domains. A small, 12 kDa viral polypeptide, the so-called Z, or zinc-binding protein, is considered to play a role in controlling the replication and expression of the genome, although this has not been confirmed.

REPLICATION

Arenaviruses replicate in a wide variety of mammalian cells although either BHK-21 cells or monkey kidney cell lines are used for biochemical studies (Howard 1986). Most arenaviruses also grow well in mouse L cells but the simultaneous production of C-type retroviruses restricts their usefulness. Maximal virus adsorption to cell surfaces is at 2 hours at 37 °C. At low multiplicities of infection (i.e. below 0.1) the latent period is approximately 6–8 hours, after which cell-associated virus increases exponentially. The titre of extracellular virus reaches a maximum 36–48 hours after infection. The passage history of any particular virus stock is probably one of the most critical factors determining the kinetics of arenavirus replication.

Infected cells undergo only limited cytopathic changes in the cell lines commonly employed, with little or no change in the total level of host cell protein synthesis; virus yields vary in different susceptible cell types. Cell metabolism is only minimally affected and in some cells only a reduction in differentiated, or 'luxury' cell functions can be observed. Cultures of persistently infected cells are readily established, the morphology and growth kinetics of which are similar to those of uninfected cells.

Only limited information is available concerning the replication and expression of viral RNA within infected cells, although possible replication events can be predicted from the nucleotide sequences of L and S genome segments. The major feature of an ambisense coding strategy is that it allows for independent expression and regulation of the N and GPC genes from the S RNA segment. The N protein is independently expressed late in acute infection and in persistently infected cells in the absence of low levels of glycoprotein production. This is explained by the production of subgenomic mRNA from a negative polarity, virus-sense template.

A control mechanism must therefore exist which determines the fate of nascent RNA of negative polarity, destined either for encapsidation or as a template for N protein-specific mRNA. In contrast, the template for glycoprotein-specific mRNA is of complementary sense to viral RNA and as such would not be required for nascent virus production. The lack of glycoprotein late in the replicative cycle or in persistently infected cells would therefore imply selective transcriptional or translational control of this gene product.

Both viral RNA and its complementary strand contain hairpin sequences which may provide recognition points for termination of transcription by viral RNA polymerase. The nucleotide sequence in the hairpin region is of coding sense and may be transcribed, either as a discrete mRNA species or as a result of extended transcription of N or GPC messengers through this region. The postulated reading frames for viral gene products transcribed from LCM and Pichinde viral genomes would fit this hypothesis. In addition, a sequence for ribosomal 18S subunit binding is present on both mRNA molecules, although the significance of this is not clear.

DIAGNOSIS AND ANTIGENIC RELATIONSHIPS

The diagnosis of arenavirus infections may be made by demonstration of a fourfold rise in specific antibody titre, the presence of IgM viral antibodies, or isolation of the virus. Although arenaviruses can easily be grown in a variety of mammalian cell cultures, it must be remembered that clinical specimens from patients presenting with a clinical picture of viral haemorrhagic fever should always be handled in containment facilities. For this reason, tests for antibody are more useful, and inactivated viral antigens for serology can be easily prepared. For routine isolation, the E6 clone of Vero cells is the cell line of choice, although all arenaviruses grow well in primate-and rodent-derived fibroblast cell lines. However, a cytopathic effect is often difficult to see, and inoculated cultures often require examination by immunofluorescence (IF) or enzyme-linked immunosorbent assay (ELISA) in order to detect the presence of viral antigens.

IF is now the preferred method for the diagnosis of human arenavirus infections. In the case of Lassa fever, infected cell substrates are used that have been treated by ultraviolet (UV) light, acetone, and cobalt irradiation to ensure safety. Drops of cell cultures dried on to glass slides can be prepared in a central laboratory and these preparations remain stable for many months. Most of the antigen detected within acetone-fixed infected cells represents cytoplasmic nucleocapsid protein. In the case of the New World arenaviruses, serological cross-reactions in the IF test (e.g. with sera from patients with Bolivian (Machupo) and Argentinian (Junín) haemorrhagic fevers) are found with fixed cultures. Substrates prepared from other members of the Tacaribe complex, which includes Junín and Machupo viruses also react with sera taken from these patients during the acute phase and early convalescence. Greatest cross-reactivity can be seen between the closely related Junín and Machupo antigens, closely followed by Tacaribe virus-infected cells. ELISA has been used as an alternative to IF for early and rapid diagnosis, although its use is restricted by the small amounts of antigen available for coating the solid-phase.

Each member of the Arenaviridae is antigenically related to other members of the group, although the degree of cross-reactivity depends on the assay system used. The complement fixation (CF) test reveals the broadest relationships (Casals 1975). A particularly strong relationship between Tacaribe, Junín, and Machupo viruses can be readily demonstrated by CF, with more distant cross-reactivity being discernible between these viruses and other members of the Tacaribe complex, although Pichinde and Tamiami are not so closely related to each other nor to other New World arenaviruses (Casals *et al.* 1975). With the CF test, LCM and Lassa viruses show some relationship to each other. All the available evidence suggests that the complement-fixing antigen is associated with the internal nucleoprotein.

Monoclonal antibodies are increasingly used to distinguish between virus strains because they can be prepared against epitopes which go unrecognized when polyclonal antisera are used. Buchmeier *et al.* (1981) summarized the patterns of reactivity with a panel of monoclonal antibodies directed against laboratory strains of the homologous virus, and Lassa and Mopeia viruses. Reagents directed against the smaller, GP2 envelope glycoprotein cross-reacted by immunofluorescence with all substrates examined, whereas antibodies directed against the larger GP1 glycoprotein were either strain-specific or reacted with a subset only of the strains examined, presumably by binding to previously unrecognized epitopes. The observations that certain of these broadly cross-reactive antibodies also reacted with Pichinde virus suggests that epitopes on surface envelope structures among Old World and New World arenaviruses are conserved. A similar comparison has also been undertaken with monoclonal antibodies to Lassa tested against the Mopeia and Mobala viruses from Africa. Again, various degrees of cross-reactivity were observed with reagents specific for the GP2 external glycoprotein. Mobala virus from the Central African Republic, however, appears to be distinct, as several cross-reactive monoclonal antibodies originally prepared against LCM virus failed to recognize Mobala-infected substrates. Clegg and Lloyd (1984) analysed an extensive range of different Lassa and Mopeia strains, and found antigenic determinants common to all strains of both viruses on the internal nucleocapsid and on at least one of the two glycoproteins.

The neutralization test is highly specific for all members of the Arenaviridae; it is notable that the few examples of cross-reactivity were obtained with high-titre animal antisera raised against Junín, Tacaribe, and Machupo viruses. However, the ease with which neutralizing antibodies can be quantified varies greatly. No cross-reactions have been observed between Junín and Machupo viruses in plaque-reduction tests with human convalescent sera despite the close relationship demonstrable by CF. A similar marked specificity of neutralization has been demonstrated with LCM and Lassa sera, and both viruses are readily distinguishable from one another by this technique. The sensitivity of the neutralization test for LCM virus can be increased by incorporating either complement or anti-gammaglobulin into the test system. However, neutralizing antibodies to Lassa virus can be detected only with great difficulty.

RESPONSES IN THE RODENT HOST

IMMUNE RESPONSE

The classic example of virus-induced immunopathological disease is LCM virus infection of adult mice (Casals 1975), in which intracerebral inoculation causes severe disease and death. In contrast, if mice are infected before or shortly after birth they develop a non-pathogenic life-long carrier state. The newborn mouse is immunologically immature and the virus does not stimulate an immune response; in these circumstances the virus causes no illness. The immunologically mature mouse mounts an immune response following LCM virus infection and a fatal choriomenin-

gitis results, but without evidence of neuronal damage (Lehmann-Grube 1971). Immunosuppression, either by neonatal thymectomy or by use of antilymphocytic serum, protects adult mice against fatal LCM infection; the pathological damage thus appears to be cell-mediated.

The immune responses are best understood in acute infection of mice. Intraperitoneal injection of adults gives rise to an asymptomatic acute infection of 2–3 weeks' duration. Studies of such infections have resulted in a number of findings with implications beyond the field of arenavirus research. First, the description by Rowe (1954) of the immune-mediated pathology of acute LCM infection was the first demonstration that the pathogenicity of the viruses may not be solely related to their cytolytic effects. The observation that LCM virus-infected cells were lysed by cytotoxic T cells led to the concept that recognition of a target cell requires the presence of both viral antigen and class T antigen of the host's major histocompatibility complex (Zinkernagel and Doherty 1979). Secondly, the persistence of virus in mice infected shortly after birth has provided a model for both host and viral factors involved in the establishment and maintenance of chronic infection. The finding of virus antigen–antibody complexes in persistently infected animals shows that B-cell tolerance is not involved. Finally, activation of natural killer cell activity early in acute infection, which coincides with the production of interferon, has helped increase our knowledge of innate immunity against virus infection.

The direct demonstration of virus replication in lymphocytes is of substantial importance for understanding arenavirus pathogenesis, as these cells provide a continued source of virus that enters the circulation and plays a key role in the temporal and quantitative control of the immune response (Murphy and Whitfield 1975). Viral antigen is present in the cells of the lymphatic system in mice persistently infected with LCM virus. Most of the virus in the blood of carrier mice is associated with approximately 2 per cent of the total circulating lymphocyte population. Precursor or immature lymphocytes may support the replication *in vitro* of LCM virus when they are stimulated to proliferate by phytohaemagglutinin, in agreement with the general finding that arenaviruses grow best in actively dividing cells. Such clonal expansion may be triggered *in vivo* by viral antigen binding to appropriate lymphocyte receptors.

Arenaviruses can replicate in peritoneal and tissue macrophages. Virus can be recovered from mononuclear cells and macrophages of adult mice infected with LCM virus when these cells become activated as a result of the uptake of heterologous antigens.

This does not occur in athymic mice, suggesting that infection of macrophages may require T-cell activity.

Interferon

Interferon is induced early in acute LCM virus infection of mice, and its appearance correlates with the appearance of infectious virus in the blood. There have been few studies of the levels of γ-interferon in acute arenavirus infection of man. Elevated levels can be detected in the early stages of Argentinian haemorrhagic fever, and these coincide with the onset of fever and backache. Although there is no correlation between the titres of interferon and circulating virus, Levis and colleagues (1984) have suggested that at least some of the clinical signs may be directly attributable to interferon, particularly the depression of platelet and lymphocytic numbers that result from Junín virus infection of leucocytes and macrophages.

The role of natural killer cells in controlling arenavirus infection is not clear, although many are found in the blood and spleen of LCM virus-infected mice as early as 1 day after infection. This response declines rapidly, however, until by the fourth day almost all the cytolytic immune activity is H-2 restricted.

Antibodies

Antibody against the nucleocapsid can be detected by CF and immunofluorescence early in the acute phase of most arenavirus infections. Infectious virus–antibody complexes can be detected 4 days after LCM virus infection of mice, but there is no evidence that B-cell responses play a role in the pathology of the acute infection. Immunity to arenaviruses appears in general to be type-specific; an infection with one member of the family does not necessarily confer protective humoral or cellular immunity against arenaviruses that can be distinguished by neutralization tests *in vitro*. However, cross-reactive antibodies may confer some degree of protection in some instances. For example, immunization of experimental animals with Tacaribe virus protects against subsequent challenge with the normally virulent Junín virus. These responses are clearly different from the anamnestic responses that may be induced as a result of antigenic similarities between nucleocapsid proteins of the two viruses concerned.

Cell-mediated immunity

The role of cell-mediated immunity during acute LCM infection is manifested by a cytotoxic T-cell response associated with the clearing of virus; e.g. T cells cultured and cloned *in vitro* and injected intravenously reduce the amount of virus 100-fold in the spleens of acutely infected mice. The restriction of the cytotoxic T-cell responses by the need to recognize both viral antigen and host cell proteins encoded by the H-2 region has altered our concept of the mechanisms by which the infected host clears virus from infected tissue; it has since been reported in every virus system examined. The generation of specific cellular toxicity is related to the replication of the virus in target organs; inoculation with live virus appears necessary, as a primary cytotoxic T-cell response is not seen if the virus is inactivated. This has implications for the development of inactivated arenavirus vaccines, should the stimulation of cellular immunity prove essential for protection. T-cell clones from mice infected with the Armstrong strain of LCM virus lyse a wide range of LCM virus strains. This finding demonstrates that cytotoxic responses to arenaviruses are haplotype-restricted but show a broad cross-reactivity for conserved viral determinants. Some of these determinants have now been mapped to an immunodominant domain of GP2 between amino acids 278 and 286 (Whitton *et al.* 1988). Such T-cell clones can discriminate between cells infected with a given strain of virus and others infected with the same virus containing only a single amino acid substitution in this region; this implies that mutations in this region of the genome may lead to selection of a virus variant with altered pathogenicity.

In contrast to LCM virus, the role of cell-mediated immunity in Lassa infection seems to play only a minor role. The human host is clearly restricted in its ability to clear the virus and prevent its replication in tissues, possibly because of impairment of cytotoxic T-cell reactions. The poor neutralizing antibody response and the high degree of viraemia contrast sharply with those in patients with South American haemorrhagic fevers, in whom there is little viraemia and neutralizing antibodies develop rapidly during acute infection. The prospects of immunotherapy thus seem poor and greater emphasis is, therefore, placed on the use of antiviral agents.

PERSISTENT INFECTION

Antibodies

Mice persistently infected with LCM virus produce antibodies to all the major structural proteins. This finding was contrary to the view previously held that viral persistence is established or maintained *in vivo* as a result of an absence of specific B-cell responses to some or all viral antigens. As viral proteins continue to be produced in the tissues of such animals, circulating antigen–antibody complexes are formed which can be detected by binding Clq. It is worth nothing that, despite the existence of antibody to all LCM virus structural polypeptides, sera from persistently infected mice are negative by CF tests; this was the original basis for the belief that carrier animals do not produce a humoral response to the virus. Antibody in the sera of such animals binds to the surface of virus-infected cells, but is unable to mediate complement-dependent cytolysis, suggesting that viral antigens at the plasma membrane may be either masked, thereby preventing further immune reactions, or removed by antigenic modulation. This notion would imply that persistently infected mice are deficient in viral antibody of the complement-fixing subclass of IgG, but this has not been proven.

Cell-mediated immunity

Mice persistently infected with LCM virus should mount a normal T-cell response to unrelated immunogens, indicating a state of tolerance only to specific antigens. However, it has been difficult to distinguish T-cell suppression from an absence of virus-specific T-cell clones. Here it is pertinent to mention that persistence of LCM virus in mice infected at birth or *in utero* was one of the important observations made by Burnet and Fenner to support the concept of tolerance to 'self' antigens. The time of infection is critical, as LCM infection induced 24 hours after birth results in a cytotoxic T-cell response typical of acute disease. The failure of mice infected before this time to mount an adequate cytotoxic response is presumably related to maturation of T-cell function; it appears to be virus-specific because adult carrier mice challenged with other unrelated arenaviruses mount normal cytotoxic T-cell responses. Thus the block appears to be either in recognition of infected cells, or in their expression of type-specific antigenic determinants.

PATHOLOGY OF ARENAVIRUS INFECTIONS

The mechanisms by which arenaviruses cause disease in man are not fully understood. There is no evidence that either immunopathological or allergenic processes play any part in causing disease; it appears to be more likely that disease is caused by direct damage of cells by the virus. Post-mortem studies on patients who died from Junín virus infection have shown generalized lymphadenopathy, endothelial swelling in the capillaries and arterioles of almost every organ, and depletion of lymphocytes in the spleen. Virus first replicates in lymphoid tissue from whence it invades

the reticuloendothelial system and those cells concerned in the immune and cellular immune responses; the host's defence mechanisms are thus impaired. Fatal illness is invariably associated with capillary damage leading to capillary fragility, haemorrhages, and irreversible shock (Johnson *et al.* 1973).

Disseminated intravascular coagulation is not a typical feature. Although Lassa fever is often regarded as being hepatotropic, the extent of hepatic damage is insufficient to account for the severity of the clinical disease. Studies of Lassa virus-infected rhesus monkeys have shown that changes in vascular function may play a much greater role in pathogenesis, as a result either of viral replication in the vascular epithelium or of secondary effects of virus activity in different organs. Platelet and epithelial cell functions fail immediately before death and are accompanied by a drop in the level of prostacyclin; these functions rapidly return to normal in animals surviving infection (Fisher-Hoch *et al.* 1987). Impairment of the functions of vascular epithelium in the absence of histological changes appears to be a common feature of the final stages of viral haemorrhagic diseases in general and suggests that hypovolaemic shock may be amenable to treatment with prostacyclin.

The pathogenesis of Argentinian haemorrhagic fever has been studied in guinea-pigs infected with Junín virus, this being a suitable model of human disease. There is a pronounced thrombocytopenia and leucopenia characteristic of human infections, and animals die of severe haemorrhagic lesions. Bone marrow cells are destroyed with release of proteases and acid and alkaline phosphatases into the blood; this leads to consumption of the C4 component of complement. These effects may lead in turn to progressive alterations in vascular permeability and platelet function (Rimoldi and de Bracco 1980).

The most extensive histopathological studies have been made on tissues from patients with Lassa fever (Walker and Murphy 1987). However, there are many similarities in the pathological lesions found in man following Junín and Machupo virus infections. Focal non-zonal necrosis in the liver has been described in all three conditions, with hyperplasia of Kupffer cells, erythrophagocytosis, and acidophilic necrosis of hepatocytes. Councilman-like bodies can be observed together with cytoplasmic vacuolations and nuclear pyknosis or lysis. As with other organs, there is little evidence of cellular inflammation. Lesions in other organs have been described, including interstitial pneumonitis, tubular necrosis in the kidney, lymphocytic infiltration of the spleen, and minimal inflammation of the central nervous system and myocardium (Walker and Murphy 1987). The hepatic changes may be grouped into three categories:

(1) mild to moderate infection with evidence of focal necrosis in less than 20 per cent of hepatocytes;

(2) hepatic regeneration but extensive damage probably centred on other organs; and

(3) severe damage with multifocal necrosis involving up to 50 per cent of hepatocytes.

These changes are consistent with a direct cytolytic action of the virus; nevertheless, the simultaneous presence of Lassa virus and specific antibodies during the later stages of the acute disease suggest that antibody-dependent cellular immune reactions may also occur. Microscopic changes in the kidneys are minimal; however, it is not clear whether the functional impairment is due to the deposition of antigen–antibody complexes.

LYMPHOCYTIC CHORIOMENINGITIS

Clinical and pathological features

Infection is often inapparent but may present as an influenza-like febrile illness, as aseptic meningitis, or as severe meningoencephalomyelitis. The great majority of LCM infections are, however, benign.

The incubation period is 6–13 days. In the influenza-like illness there is fever, malaise, coryza, muscular pains, and bronchitis. The meningeal form is more common; the same symptoms may remain mild and be of short duration and patients recover within a few days, but there can be more pronounced illness with severe prostration lasting 2 weeks or more. Chronic sequelae have been reported on occasion. They include headache, paralysis, and personality changes. The few deaths have followed severe meningoencephalomyelitis. In one case there was mild pharyngitis and a diffuse erythematous rash followed by haemorrhages and death.

An early leucopenia followed by lymphocytosis is a constant finding. In central nervous system disease, the cerebrospinal fluid (CSF) is at increased pressure, with a slight rise in protein concentration, normal or slightly reduced sugar concentration, and a moderate number of cells, mainly lymphocytes (150–$400/mm^3$). These changes are not, of course, restricted to LCM infections. Virus can be isolated from blood, CSF and, in fatal cases, from brain tissue.

Epidemiology

Man is usually infected through contact with rodents. Many infections have been acquired in laboratories, where LCM may be a contaminant in laboratory colonies of mice and hamsters. Hamsters kept as pet animals have also played a role in human infection. The mechanism of transmission of the virus is not fully understood but is likely to involve dust contaminated by urine, the contamination of food and drink, or via skin abrasions.

LASSA FEVER

History

Lassa virus made a dramatic appearance in Nigeria in 1969 as a lethal, highly transmissible disease. The first victim was an American nurse who was infected in a small mission station in the Lassa township in north-eastern Nigeria, whence the virus and the disease derive their names. The origin of the infection was never determined, although it is thought to have been acquired through direct contact with an infected patient in Lassa. When the nurse's condition steadily deteriorated she was flown to the Evangel Hospital in Jos, where she died the following day.

While she was in hospital she was cared for by two other American nurses, one of whom also became infected by direct contact, probably through a skin abrasion. This nurse became unwell after an 8-day incubation period and died following an illness lasting 11 days. The head nurse of the hospital, who had assisted at the post-mortem of the first patient, fell ill 7 days after the death of the second patient from who she had cared, and from whom she probably acquired the infection.

This third case was evacuated to the USA by air in the first-class cabin of a commercial airliner with two attendants and screened from economy-class passengers only by a curtain. After a severe illness under intensive care she slowly recovered. A virus, subsequently named Lassa, was isolated from her blood by workers at the Yale Arbovirus Unit. One of these virologists became ill but improved after an immune plasma transfusion donated by the third case. Five months after this infection, a laboratory technician in the Yale laboratories, who had not been working with Lassa virus, fell ill and died. The manner in which this infection was acquired has never been determined.

This trail of events not unnaturally earned for Lassa virus a formidable notoriety, which was sharply enhanced by two more devastating hospital outbreaks—one in Nigeria, the other in Liberia. The fourth epidemic was seen in Sierra Leone in October 1972. In sharp contrast to the previous outbreaks, this one was not confined to hospitals, although hospital staff were at considerable risk and several became infected. Most of the patients acquired their illness in the community and there were several intrafamilial transmissions. This led to a revision of the initial view—formed from experience of nosocomial infections—that Lassa fever has a high mortality.

Lassa fever has since continued in West Africa, usually as sporadic cases (Monath 1987). Between 1969 and 1978 there were 17 reported outbreaks affecting 386 patients in whom the mortality was 27 per cent. which Eleven of the episodes were in hospitals, where the case fatality rate reached 44 per cent; two were laboratory infections, two were community-acquired outbreaks, and two were prolonged community outbreaks. Eight patients were flown to Europe or North America. One of them was evacuated with full isolation precautions and the remainder, of whom five were infections, travelled on scheduled commercial flights as fare-paying passengers. Fortunately, no contact cases resulted.

Clinical features

Lassa virus causes a spectrum of disease ranging from subclinical to fulminating fatal infection. The incubation period ranges from 3 to 16 days and the illness usually begins insidiously. The disease is difficult to distinguish in the early stages from other systemic febrile illnesses, the most reliable clinical signs being a sore throat and vomiting. Between the third and sixth day of illness the symptoms suddenly worsen and there is high fever, severe prostration, chest and abdominal pains, conjunctival injection, diarrhoea, dysphagia, and vomiting. Chest pain, located substernally and along the costal margins, is often associated with tenderness on pressure and is exacerbated by coughing and deep inspiration. One important physical finding is a distinct pharyngitis; yellow-white exudative spots may been seen on the tonsillar pillars together with small vesicles and ulcers. The patients appears toxic, lethargic, and dehydrated; the blood pressure is low and there is sometimes a bradycardia relative to the body temperature. There may be cervical lymphadenopathy, coated tongue, puffiness of the face and neck, and blurred vision. Occasionally a faint maculopapular rash may be seen during the second week of illness, on the face, neck, trunk, and arms. In severe cases, haemorrhages also occur. Cough is a common symptom, and light-headedness, vertigo, and tinnitus appear in a few patients. Deafness has also been noted in about 20 per cent of patients and, although it may be reversible, is more often permanent.

The fever generally lasts for 7–17 days and is variable. Convalescence begins in the second to fourth weeks, when the temperature returns to normal and the symptoms improve. Most patients complain of extreme fatigue for several weeks. Loss of hair and deafness are often observed, and there may be brief bouts of fever.

Patients in whom the disease is fatal not uncommonly have a high sustained fever. Acutely ill patients suddenly deteriorate between days 7 and 14 with a sudden drop in blood pressure, peripheral vasoconstriction, hypovolaemia, and anuria; there may be pleural effusions and ascites. In addition, coma, stupor, tremors, and myoclonic twitching may occur. Death is due to shock, anoxia, respiratory insufficiency, and cardiac arrest.

Epidemiology

Lassa virus has been repeatedly isolated from the multimammate rat *Mastomys natalensis* in Sierra Leone and Nigeria. This rodent is a common domestic and peridomestic species, and large populations are widely distributed in Africa south of the Sahara. During the rainy season it may leave the open fields and seek shelter indoors. Some genetic variation has been shown in *Mastomys* populations inhabiting different ecological niches; however, there appears to be no difference in the prevalence of antibody and virus in at least two of the karyotypes found in West Africa. The animals are infected at birth or during the perinatal period. Like other arenaviruses, Lassa virus produces a persistent, tolerated infection in its rodent reservoir host with no ill effects and without any detectable immune response. The animals remain infective during their lifetime, freely excreting Lassa virus in urine and other body fluids. The correlation between the prevalence of antibody in a community and the degree of infestation by infected rodents, however, is poor.

Studies of the ratio of clinical illness to infections have recently confirmed that Lassa fever is endemic in several regions of West Africa. It has been estimated that only 1–2 per cent of infections are fatal, substantially less than the figures of 30–50 per cent originally associated with the early nosocomial outbreaks. However, there may still be up to 300 000 infections year with as many as 5000 deaths (McCormick *et al.* 1986). The seroconversion rates among villagers in Sierra Leone vary from 4 to 22 per 100 susceptible individuals per year; up to 14 per cent of febrile illness in such population groups is due to Lassa virus infection. These data confirm the relatively high rate of asymptomatic and mild infections in endemic areas. One reason for this may be the frequency of reinfections; although about 6 per cent of the population lose antibody annually, rises in antibody titre are also often observed. It is not clear if reinfection results in clinical disease. A frequent finding of incomplete immunity after infection would have profound implications for the use of a vaccine.

There may be secondary spread from person to person in conditions of overcrowded housing, and this is particularly important in rural hospitals.

Table 27.2 Differential diagnosis of Lassa fever

Malaria
Bacterial septicaemia
Enteric fevers (typhoid, paratyphoid)
Typhus
Trypanosomiasis
Streptococcal pharyngitis
Leptospirosis
Other viral haemorrhagic fevers

Medical attendants or relatives who provide direct personal care are most likely to contract the infection; as noted above, accidental inoculation with a sharp instrument and contact with blood have caused infection in few cases. Airborne spread may take place, as well as mechanical transmission. Although in Sierra Leone there has been no evidence of airborne spread in hospital outbreaks, one of the 1970 outbreaks in Nigeria is believed to have been caused by airborne transmission from a woman with severe pulmonary infection.

Diagnosis

The diagnosis of Lassa fever is confirmed by isolation of the virus or demonstration of a specific serological response. Infection in the early stages can be confused clinically with a number of other infectious disease, particularly malignant malaria (Table 27.2; Woodruff 1978).

Lassa virus grows readily in Vero cell culture and virus can usually be isolated within 4 days. Virus can be cultured from serum, throat washings, pleural fluid, and urine; it is excreted from the pharynx for up to 14 days after the onset of illness and in urine for up to 67 days after onset. Lassa infection can be diagnosed early by detection of virus-specific antigens in conjunctival cells using indirect immunofluorescence. It is important to note that virus isolation should be attempted only in laboratories equipped (level P4) to provide maximum containment to protect the investigator. Suspected cases should be reported immediately to local and national public health authorities.

The most sensitive serological test for the detection of Lassa antibodies is indirect immunofluorescence; antibodies can be dectected by this method in the second week of illness. Complement-fixing antibodies develop more slowly and are rarely detectable before the third week after onset. On occasion, complement-fixing antibodies failed to develop in patients from whom Lassa virus has been isolated. Neutralizing antibodies are difficult to measure *in vitro*, in sharp contrast to infections by the South American arenaviruses, for reasons that are unclear.

The two most reliable prognostic markers of fatal infections are the titres of circulating virus and of aspartate aminotransferase (AST). Patients in whom the titre of virus exceeds 10^4 $TCID_{50}$/ml and with AST levels above 150 IU have a poor prognosis, and fatality rates approach 80 per cent. In contrast, patients with virus and enzyme levels below these values have a greater than 85 per cent chance of survival (Johnson *et al.* 1987). This demonstration of an association between the degree of viraemia and mortality is unique for virus infections and contrasts with the difficulty in predicting the outcome in patients with Argentinian and Bolivian haemorrhagic fevers. Although Lassa fever can be diagnosed accurately from the presence of IgM antibodies on admission, there is no correlation between the time of appearance and the titre of specific antibodies and clinical outcome. Lassa fever is particularly severe in pregnant women. A study of 75 women in Sierra Leone showed that 11 of 14 deaths were the result of infection during the third trimester; a further 23 patients suffered abortion in the first and second trimesters.

Therapy

Although the passive administration of Lassa immune plasma may suppress viraemia and favourably alter the clinical outcome, it does not always do so, particularly if the patient has a high virus burden (McCormick *et al.* 1986). Failure may be due to the difficulty in assessing accurately the titre of viral neutralizing antibodies in the plasma, the late and non-uniform nature of this response in convalescence, and antigenic variation. The widespread occurrence of human immunodeficiency virus (HIV) infections in West Africa precludes at present the use of immune plasma from convalescent individuals in this region. Conversely, immune plasma may be of benefit in the treatment of Junín infections (Maiztegui *et al.* 1979; Enria *et al.* 1986). This may be due to the high titre of neutralizing antibodies that develops soon after the acute phase.

Greater success has been achieved with antivirals. In one study, patients with a poor prognosis treated for 10 days with intravenous ribavirin (60–70 mg/kg/day), begun within 6 days after the onset of fever, show a reduced case fatality of 5 per cent (McCormick *et al.* 1986). In contrast, patients who began treatment 7 or more days after the onset of fever had a case fatality rate of 26 per cent. In the Sierra Leone study, viraemia of greater than $10^{3.6}$ $TCID_{50}$/ml on admission was associated with a case fatality rate of 76 per cent. Patients with this risk factor who were treated with intravenous ribavirin within 6 days of the onset of fever had a case fatality rate of 9 per cent compared with 47 per cent in those treated 7 days or more after the onset of illness. Further studies are now in progress to determine the effectiveness of orally administered ribavirin.

ARGENTINIAN HAEMORRHAGIC FEVER

ARGENTINIAN HAEMORRHAGIC FEVER
(JUNÍN VIRUS)

Clinical and pathological features

Argentinian haemorrhagic fever has been known since 1943 and Junín virus, the causative agent, was first isolated in 1958. The virus causes annual outbreaks of severe illness—with between 100 and 3500 cases—in an area of intensive agriculture known as the wet pampas in Argentina. Mortality in some outbreaks has ranged from 10 to 20 per cent, although the overall mortality is generally 3–15 per cent.

After an incubation period of 7–16 days, the onset of illness is insidious, with chills, headache, malaise, myalgia, retro-orbital pain, and nausea; these are followed by fever, conjunctival injection and suffusion, and an anthem, exanthema, and oedema of the face, neck, and upper thorax. A few petechiae may be seen, mostly in the axilla. There is hypervascularity and occasional ulceration of the soft palate. Generalized lymphadenopathy is common. Tongue tremor is an early sign, and some patients present with pneumonitis. In the more severe cases the patient's condition becomes appreciably worse after a few days, with the development of hypotension, oliguria, hemorrhages from the nose and gums, haematemesis, haematuria, and melaena. Oliguria may progress to anuria and pronounced neurological manifestations may develop. Laboratory findings have included leucopenia with a decrease in the number of CD4-positive cells, thrombocytopenia, and urinary casts containing viral antigen. Patients recover when the fever falls, followed by diuresis and rapid improvement. Death may result from hypovolaemic shock. Subclinical infections also occur. Person to person transmission has not been observed.

Epidemiology

Argentinian haemorrhagic fever has a marked seasonal incidence, coinciding with the maize harvest between April and July, when rodent populations reach their peak. Agricultural workers, particularly those harvesting maize, are, not surprisingly, the most commonly affected.

The main reservoir hosts of Junín virus are *Calomys* field voles that live and breed in burrows under the maize fields and in the surrounding grass banks. Other rodent species may also be infected. *Calomys* spp. have a persistent viraemia and viruria, and virus is also present in considerable quantities in the saliva.

The mode of transmission of Junín virus to man has not been conclusively established. The virus may be carried in the air from dust contaminated by rodent excreta, or may enter by ingestion of contaminated foodstuffs.

Therapy

In contrast to Lassa fever, antibodies play a major role in recovery from Junín infection. Controlled trial of immune plasma collected from patients at least 6 months into convalescence have shown a dramatic reduction in mortality if plasma was given within the first 8 days of illness (Maiztegui *et al.* 1979). The efficacy of this therapy is directly related to the titre of neutralizing antibody in the plasma; as a result, a dose of no less than 3000 'therapeutic units'/kg body weight has been recommended (Enria *et al.* 1984).

The late development of a neurological syndrome is seen in up to 10 per cent of patients treated with immune plasma; it is often benign and self-limiting, but points to the possible persistence of viral antigens on cells of the CNS well into convalescence. Treatment with immune plasma also restores the response of peripheral blood lymphocytes to antigenic stimuli, suggesting that the administration of plasma also results in the modulation of cellular immunity.

Prophylaxis

There have been attempts to produce a vaccine against Argentinian haemorrhagic fever. The XJ-CI$_3$ strain of virus grown in the brains of suckling mice is relatively non-pathogenic and was administered to 636 volunteers between 1968 and 1970. However, the vaccine often induced a mild febrile reaction or a subclinical infection, and its use was discontinued despite the fact that over 90 per cent of vaccines maintained neutralizing antibody for up to 9 years. There have been renewed attempts during recent years to develop a new strain sufficiently attenuated for human use, and clinical trials of this candidate 1 vaccine are under way in Argentina.

BOLIVIAN HAEMORRHAGIC FEVER
(MACHUPO VIRUS)

Clinical features

Bolivian haemorrhagic fever was first recognized in 1959 in the Beni region in north-eastern Bolivia. The disease continued in that region more or less annually for a number of years in the form of sharply localized epidemics. Its incidence has decreased considerably since the late 1970s and human infections are now rarely reported. The mortality in individual outbreaks varied from 5 to 30 per cent. The most notable outbreak affected 700 people in the San Joaquin township between late 1962 and the middle of 1964. The mortality was 18 per cent. It is worth noting that the discovery of a common morphology and serological cross-reaction between Machupo and LCM virus led to the concept of the arenavirus family.

The clinical disease is similar to Argentinian haemorrhagic fever. The incubation period ranges from 7 to 14 days and the onset is insidious. About one-third of patients show a tendency to bleed, with petechiae on the trunk and palate, and bleeding from the gastrointestinal tract, nose, gums, and uterus. Almost half the patients develop a fine tremor of the tongue and hands, and some may have more pronounced neurological symptoms. The acute disease may last 2–3 weeks and convalescence may be protracted, generalized weakness being the most common complaint. Clinically inapparent infections are rare.

Machupo virus, the responsible agent, is readily isolated from lymph nodes and spleen taken at necropsy. However, isolation of the virus from acutely ill patients has proved difficult, the best results being obtained from specimens taken 7–12 days after the onset of illness.

Epidemiology

The rodent reservoir of Machupo virus is *Calomys callosus*; over 60 per cent of this species of vole caught during the San Joaquin epidemic were found to be infected. The distribution of cases in the township was associated with certain houses, and *C. callosus* was trapped in all households where cases occurred. Transmission to humans is probably by contamination of food and water or by infection through skin abrasions. Transmission from person to person is unusual, but a small episode took place in 1971, well outside the endemic zone. The index case, infected in Beni, carried the infection to Cochabamba and, by direct transmission, caused five secondary cases, of which four were fatal. Abnormally low rainfall, combined with an increase in the use of insecticide, led to a rapid decline in the numbers of cats, with the result that the population of Machupo-infected rodents increased dramatically, thus increasing the opportunity for human contact with contaminated soil and foodstuffs. This balance has since been restored and largely accounts from the reduction in the number of reported cases over the past two decades.

VENEZUELAN HAEMORRHAGIC FEVER (GUANARITO VIRUS)

This agent was first described in 1989, with 26 deaths being recorded among 105 cases originally suspected as being dengue infections (Salas *et al.* 1991). Most of the cases have been adults and all from the state of Portuguesa in the mid-western part of Venezuela. Lasting from 3 to 12 days, the infection is typified by fever, sore throat, nausea with vomiting, and other symptoms associated with arenavirus infections in the New World. Up to 90 per cent of the patients showed a marked thrombocytopenia and leucopenia. Post-mortem examination of the fatal cases revealed extensive hemorrhage in the lungs and liver, accompanied by cardiomegaly, splenic enlargement, and congestion of the lungs. Oedema of the kidneys was also observed, together with blood in the intestines and bladder.

The virus has since been isolated repeatedly from the cotton rat, *Sigmodon alstoni*, although there have been no significant recorded cases since the original outbreak. The route of transmission remains unclear, with person to person spread being rare. However, the infections are likely to have been acquired peridomestically, as in the study of Sales *et al.* (1991) virus was recovered from a rodent trapped in the house of one case. Little further information has become available, but continuing surveillance is now being undertaken. The relatively high mortality of the infection parallels that seen in the early reported cases of Machupo and Junín infections; in the event of further outbreaks this level should be reduced as diagnosis improves and appropriate treatment instigated earlier in the course of the disease.

FUTURE DIRECTIONS

Unique among the viral zoonoses, the arenaviruses show a host–parasite relationship which has received intensive study. In the case of LCM virus, this has resulted in the discovery of fundamental concepts in viral immunopathogenesis and clearance. Yet much remains to be learnt, particularly from the standpoint of public health. The recent emergence of Venezuelan haemorrhagic fever illustrates well the need for public health microbiologists to be ever vigilant for hitherto unknown agents to cause sudden outbreaks. The epidemiology of almost all arenaviruses remains poorly understood; for example, Lassa is clearly widespread among the rural areas of West Africa, but there is an inexact correlation between the distribution of infected rodents and human infections. There is also much to be learnt in terms of the susceptibility of the natural hosts to infection; a rodent of the *Calomys* family wild-caught in Venezuela, for example, may be refractory to infection, whereas its cousin from elsewhere in South America can be readily infected. It is tempting to speculate that arenaviruses are instrumental in controlling rodent population numbers and that only when man radically alters the rodent habitat do zoonotic infections result. Thus there is ample scope for further studies of the natural history, epidemiology, and pathology of this unique and fascinating group of viruses. By such work, we may better understand the host–parasite relationship of these agents and thus be better prepared for preventing further outbreaks of severe and debilitating human infections.

REFERENCES

Buchmeier, M. J., Lewick, H. A., Tomori, O., and Oldstone, M. B. A. (1981). Monoclonal antibodies to lymphocytic choriomeningitis virus and Pichinde viruses: generation, characterization and cross-reactivity with other arenaviruses. *Virology*, **113**, 73–85.

Casals, J. (1975). Arenaviruses. *Yale Journal of Biology and Medicine*, **48**, 115–40.

Casals, J., Buckley, S. M., and Cedenoe, R. (1975). Antigenic properties of the arenaviruses. *Bulletin of the World Health Organization*, **52**; 421–7.

Clegg, J. C. S. and Lloyd, G. (1984). The African arenaviruses Lass and Mopeia: Biological and immunochemical comparisons. In *Segmented negative strand viruses*, (ed. R. W. Compans and D. H. L. Bishop), pp. 341–7. Academic Press, Orlando.

Enria, D. A. *et al.* (1984). Importance of dose of neutralizing antibodies in treatment of Argentine haemorrhagic fever with immune plasma. *Lancet*, **2**, 255–6.

Enria D. A. *et al.* (1986). Sindrome neurologico tardo en enfermos de fiebre hemorragica Argentina tratados con plasma immune. *Medicina (Buenos Aires)*, **45**, 615–17.

Fisher-Hoch, S. P., Mitchell, S. W., Sasso, D. R., Lang, J. V., Ramsey, R., and McCormick, J. B. (1987). Physiologic and immunologic disturbances associated with shock in Lassa fever in a primate model. *Journal of Infectious Diseases*, **155**, 465–74.

Fuller-Pace, F. and Southern, P. (1989). Detection of virus-specific RNA-dependent RNA polymerase activity in extracts from cells infected with lymphocytic choriomeningitis virus: *In vitro* synthesis of full-length viral RNA species. *Journal of Virology*, **63**, 1938–44.

Gonzalez, J.-P., Sanchez, A., and Rico-Hesse, R. (1995). Molecular phylogeny of Guanarito virus, an emerging arenavirus affecting humans. *American Journal of Tropical Medicine and Hygiene*, **53**, 1–6.

Howard, C. R. (1986). Arenaviruses. In *Perspectives in medical virology*, Vol. 2, (ed. A. J. Zuckerman). Elsevier, Amsterdam.

Howard, C. R. and Simpson, D. H. L. (1980). The biology of arenaviruses. *Journal of General Virology*, **51**, 1–14.

Johnson, K. M., Webb, P. A., and Justines, G. (1973). Biology of Tacaribe-complex virus. In *Lymphocytic chorimoeningitis virus and other arenaviruses*, (ed. F. Lehmann–Grube), pp. 241–58. Springer Verlag, Vienna.

Johnson, K. M., McCormick, J. B., Webb, P. A., Smith, E., Elliott, L. H., and King, I. J. (1987). Lassa fever in Sierra Leone: clinical virology in hospitalized patients. *Journal of Infectious Diseases*, **155**, 456–63.

Lehmann-Grube, F. (1971). Lymphocytic choriomengitis virus. *Virology Monographs*, **10**, 1.

Levis, S. C. *et al.* (1984). Endogenous interferon in Argentine haemorrhagic fever. *Journal of Infectious Diseases*, **149**, 28–33.

McCormick, J. B. *et al.* (1986). Lassa fever: effective therapy with ribavirin. *New England Journal of Medicine*, **314**, 20–6.

Maiztegui, J. I., Fernandez, N. J., and de Damilano, A. J. (1979). Efficacy of immune plasma in treatment of Argentine haemorrhagic fever and association between treatment and a late neurological syndrome. *Lancet*, **2**, 216–17.

Monath, T. P. (1987). Lassa fever—new issues raised by field studies in West Africa. *Journal of Infectious Diseases*, **155**, 433–36.

Murphy, F. A. and Whitfield, S. G. (1975). Morphology and morphogenesis of arenaviruses. *Bulletin of the World Health Organization*, **52**, 409–19.

Pfau, C. J. (1974). Biochemical and biophysical properties of the arenaviruses. *Progress in Medical Virology*, **18**, 64–80.

Rimoldi, M. T. and de Bracco, M. M. (1980). *In vitro* inactivation of complement by a serum factor present in Junin virus-infected guinea pigs. *Immunology*, **39**, 159–64.

Rowe, W. P. (1954). *Studies on pathogenesis and immunity in lymphocytic choriomeningitis virus of the mouse.* US Naval Medical Research Institute, Research Report. NM 005.048.14.01. Department of Defense, Washington, DC.

Salas, R. *et al.* (1991). Venezuela haemorrhagic fever. *Lancet*, **338**, 1033–6.

Salvato, M. S. (ed.) (1993). *The Arenaviridae*. Plenum Press, New York.

Walker, D. H. and Murphy, F. A. (1987). Pathology and pathogenesis of arenavirus infections. *Current Topics in Microbiology and Immunology*, **133**, 89–113.

Whitton, J. L. *et al.* (1988). Molecular definition of a major cytotoxic T-lymphocytic in the glycoprotein of the lymphocytic choriomeningitis virus. *Journal of Virology*, **62**, 687–95.

Woodruff, A. W. (1978). In *Modern topics in infection*, (ed. J. D. Williams), p. 240. Heinemann Medical, London.

Young, P. R. (1987). Arenaviridae. In *Animal virus structures*, (ed. M. V. Nermut and A. C. Steven), pp. 185–98. Elsevier, Amsterdam.

Zinkernagel, R. M. and Doherty, P. C. (1979). MHC-restricted cytotoxic T-cells: studies on the biological role of polymorphic major transplantation antigens determining T-cell-restriction-specificity, function and responsiveness. *Advances in Immunology*, **27**, 51–77.

28 CRIMEAN–CONGO HAEMORRHAGIC FEVER

R. Swanepoel

SUMMARY

Crimean–Congo haemorrhagic fever (CCHF) is an acute disease of humans, caused by a tick-borne virus which is widely distributed in eastern Europe, Asia, and Africa. Cattle, sheep, and small mammals such as hares undergo inapparent or mild infection with transient viraemia, and serve as hosts from which the tick vectors of the virus can acquire infection. Despite serological evidence that there is widespread infection of livestock in nature, infection of humans is relatively uncommon. Humans acquire infection from tick bite, or from contact with infected blood or other tissues of livestock or human patients, and the disease is characterized by febrile illness with headache, malaise, myalgia, and a petechial rash, frequently followed by a haemorrhagic state with necrotic hepatitis. The mortality rate is approximately 30 per cent. Inactivated vaccine prepared from infected mouse brain has been used for the protection of humans in eastern Europe and the former Soviet Union in the past, but the development of a modern vaccine is inhibited by limited potential demand. The voluminous literature on the disease has been the subject of several reviews from which the information presented here is drawn, except where indicated otherwise (Chumakov 1974; Hoogstraal 1979, 1981; Watts *et al.* 1989; Swanepoel 1994*a,b*).

HISTORY

Descriptions of a disease in eastern Europe and Asia resembling CCHF can be traced back to antiquity, but a condition given the name Crimean haemorrhagic fever was first recognized in an outbreak affecting about 200 soldiers and peasants who were exposed to ticks while harvesting crops and sleeping outdoors on the Crimean Peninsula in 1944. In the following year it was demonstrated through the inoculation of human subjects with filtered suspensions of ticks and tissues of patients, that the disease was caused by a tick-transmitted virus. However, the virus itself was only isolated in laboratory hosts, namely mice, in 1967. In

1969, it was shown that the agent of Crimean haemorrhagic fever was identical to a virus named Congo which had been isolated in 1956 from the blood of a febrile child in Stanleyville (now Kisangani) in what was then the Belgian Congo (now Democratic Republic of the Congo), and since that time the two names have been used in combination.

During the three decades which followed the initial description of the disease in the Crimea, the presence of the virus came to be recognized in many east European and Asian countries, in some instances as a result of the conducting of deliberate surveys, but often as a consequence of the occurrence of nosocomial outbreaks or large epidemics, many of which were precipitated by circumstances which involved the exposure of large numbers of humans to ticks, such as the implementation of major and reclamation or resettlement schemes in Bulgaria and the Soviet Asian republics. In contrast, only 15 cases of the disease had been reported in Africa prior to 1981, eight of them laboratory infections, and only one patient had developed haemorrhagic manifestations and died. Since then, sporadic cases of haemorrhagic disease and deaths have been diagnosed regularly each year in southern Africa, probably as a result of increased awareness among clinicians, and a few cases of severe disease have also been recorded West Africa. Contrary to earlier speculation, therefore, it is now clear that the disease which occurs in Africa is no less severe than that in Eurasia.

Epidemics of the type formerly observed in Eurasia are now infrequent, although an outbreak involving 90 cases of the disease occurred in Khazakstan in 1989 (Lvov 1994). Over the past decade CCHF has been diagnosed most regularly in Bulgaria and South Africa, with an annual incidence varying from 5 to 25 cases in each of the two countries. In parts of the former Soviet Union, the decrease in the occurrence of the disease has been ascribed to more intensive agricultural utilization of land, with cattle largely being confined to feedlots, and with populations of the wild hosts of the tick vectors being reduced by hunting. Nevertheless, it is clear from surveys conducted in Africa and Eurasia that there is extensive circulation of the virus in livestock and wild vertebrates, with very high antibody prevalence rates occurring in adult livestock in some areas. In contrast, the prevalence of antibody in rural human populations is generally low, in the range of less than 0.1–2 per cent, but there are notable exceptions, as in northern Senegal where up to 20.6 per cent of people had antibody in locations where nomadic shepherds had regular contact with sheep, and slept outdoors where they were exposed to ticks. The evidence suggests that the disease of humans is probably underdiagnosed in many countries due to lack of awareness and/or non-availability of appropriate medical and laboratory services, but also that there is generally a low rate of transmission of infection to humans, as discussed below.

THE VIRUS

TAXONOMY AND MOLECULAR BIOLOGY

The causative agent of CCHF is a member of the *Nairovirus* genus of the family Bunyaviridae, which at present contains 32 viruses arranged in seven serogroups on the basis of antigenic affinities, with CCHF virus, Hazara from Pakistan, and Khasan from the former USSR constituting one of the serogroups. All members of the genus are believed to be transmitted by either ixodid or argasid ticks, and only three are known to be pathogens of humans, namely, CCHF, Dugbe, and Nairobi sheep disease viruses. Dugbe commonly cause mild infection of sheep and cattle in West Africa and is infrequently associated with benign febrile illness of humans. Nairobi sheep disease virus, which is believed to be identical to Ganjam virus of India, is a pathogen of sheep and goats in East Africa and India which occasionally causes benign illness in humans.

Nairoviruses are spherical, 90–120 nm in diameter, and have a bilipid-layer envelope from which glycoprotein spikes project. The virions contain three major structural proteins: two envelope glycoproteins, G1 and G2, with molecular weights 72–84 and 30–40 kDa, respectively; a nucleocapsid protein, N (48–54 kDa); and minor quantities of a large protein, L (>200 kDa), believed to be the viral transcriptase. Hazara virus is unique in having three glycoproteins. The viruses have a three-segmented, single-stranded RNA genome which is in the negative sense (complementary to mRNA). Each RNA segment, L (large), M (medium), and S (small), is contained in a separate nucleocapsid within the virion. The L RNA segment (molecular weight $4.1–4.9 \times 10^6$ Da) codes for the viral transcriptase, the M segment ($1.5–2.3 \times 10^6$ Da) for the G proteins, and the S segment ($0.6–0.7 \times 10^6$ Da) for the N protein. Precursors of the glycoproteins have been found in infected cells, but non-structural proteins found during the replication of viruses of other genera of the Bunyaviridae have not as yet been demonstrated in association with nairoviruses.

Nairoviruses attach to receptors on susceptible cells, are internalized by endocytosis, and replicate in the cytoplasm. The virions mature by budding through endoplasmic reticulum into cytoplasmic vesicles in the Golgi region, which are presumed to fuse with the plasma membrane to release virus.

PATHOGENESIS

The mechanisms of pathogenesis by CCHF virus are incompletely understood, but by analogy with other arthropod-borne viruses it can be surmised that there may be some replication in tissues at the the site of inoculation, with haematogenous and lymph-borne spread of infection to regional lymph nodes and certain target organs, such as the liver which is a major site of replication of the virus. Capillary fragility is a feature of the disease, and although it has not been demonstrated conclusively that endothelial cells are infected, there is evidence of the formation of circulating immune complexes with activation of complement, and this would contribute to damage of the capillary bed and hence to the genesis of the skin rash and renal and pulmonary failure. Endothelial damage would lead to platelet aggregation and degranulation, with activation of the intrinsic coagulation cascade. Tissue damage in organs such as the liver would result in further release of procoagulants into the bloodstream, and the impairment of the circulation through the occurrence of disseminated intravascular coagulopathy would, in turn, contribute to further tissue damage. Damage to the liver would limit clearance of fibrin degradation products and impair synthesis of coagulation factors to replace those consumed. Abnormalities in clinical pathology values observed in patients indicate that the occurrence of disseminated intravascular coagulopathy is probably an early and central event in the pathogenesis of the disease.

CULTURE OF THE VIRUS

In the past, CCHF virus has been propagated and titrated most commonly by intracerebral inoculation of suckling mice. The virus is non-pathogenic for other laboratory animals, including rabbits, guinea-pigs, and monkeys. It can be grown in a wide variety of primary and line cell cultures, including Vero, CER, BHK-21, and SW13 cells, but it is poorly cytopathic and hence infectivity is titrated by plaque production or demonstration of immunofluorescence in infected cells.

Little information is available on the stability of CCHF virus, but infectivity is destroyed by low concentrations of formalin or β-propriolactone. Being enveloped, the virus is sensitive to lipid solvents. It is labile in infected tissues after death, presumably due to a fall in pH, but infectivity is retained for a few days at ambient temperature in separated serum, and for up to 3 weeks at 4 °C. Infectivity is stable at temperatures below –60 °C, but is rapidly destroyed by boiling or autoclaving.

INFECTION OF DOMESTIC AND WILD ANIMALS

Experimentally inoculated domestic ruminants and small mammals, such as little susliks, hedgehogs, hares, and myomorph rodents, were found to undergo inapparent infection or mild fever and viraemia, with maximum recorded titres of infectivity ranging from $10^{2.7}$ to $10^{4.2}$ mouse intracerebral 50 per cent lethal doses/ml ($MICLD_{50}$/ml), and with a demonstrable immune response. The virus was not abortigenic in heifers and ewes inoculated late in pregnancy (Swanepoel and Shepherd 1983–88, unpublished observations). However, when ticks of a laboratory strain of *Hyalomma truncatum* capable of causing sweating sickness, a toxicosis, were inadvertently placed on CCHF-infected sheep and cattle in the course of tick infection experiments, some of the animals became severely ill (Shepherd *et al.* 1991). Thus, animals which undergo simultaneous infection with CCHF virus and specific tick-borne pathogens of livestock in nature, constitute a source of infection for humans who treat or butcher sick animals; an observation which would explain the circumstances under which some patients have been observed to acquire infection in the former USSR and in South Africa, as discussed below.

In limited experiments, birds have been found to be refractory to the virus, but recent evidence suggests that certain non-passerines may be capable of infecting ticks despite failing to circulate detectable levels of virus, as discussed below.

INFECTION OF HUMANS

The incubation period is generally short, ranging from 1 to 3 days (maximum 9 days) following infection by tick bite, and is usually 5 or 6 days (maximum 13) in persons exposed to infected blood or other tissues of livestock or human patients. There is usually a very sudden onset of illness with fever, rigors, chills, severe headache, dizziness, neck pain and stiffness, sore eyes, photophobia, malaise, and myalgia with intense backache or leg pains. Nausea, sore throat, and vomiting are common manifestations early in the disease and some patients experience non-localized abdominal pain and diarrhoea at this stage. Fever may be intermittent and patients may undergo sharp changes of mood over the first 2 days, with feelings of confusion and aggression. By the second to fourth day of illness they may exhibit lassitude, depression, and somnolence, and have a flushed appearance with injected conjunctivae or chemosis. Tenderness of the abdomen localizes in the right upper quadrant, and hepatomegaly may be discernible. Tachycardia is common and patients may be slightly hypotensive. There may be lymphadenopathy, and enanthem and petechiae of the throat, tonsils, and buccal mucosa.

Patients develop a petechial rash on the trunk and limbs on the third to sixth day of illness, and this may be followed rapidly by the appearance of large bruises and ecchymoses, especially in the anticubital fossae, upper arms, axillae, and groin. Development of a haemorrhagic tendency may be evident only from the oozing of blood from injection or venipuncture sites, but epistaxis, haematemesis, haematuria, melaena, gingival bleeding, and bleeding from the vagina or other orifices may commence on day 4–5 of illness, or even earlier. There may also be internal bleeding, including retroperitoneal and intracranial haemorrhage. Severely ill patients enter a state of hepatorenal and pulmonary failure from about day 5 onwards and progressively become drowsy, stuporous, and comatose. Jaundice becomes apparent during the second week of illness. Deaths generally occur on days 5–14 of illness. Patients who recover usually begin to improve subjectively on day 9 or 10 of illness, but asthenia, conjunctivitis, slight confusion, and amnesia may continue for a month or longer.

Viraemia has been detected from the time of onset up to day 13 of illness, with highest titres occurring during the first 5 days. The viraemia is of greater intensity and longer duration in humans than in lower animals, with a maximum recorded titre of $10^{6.2}$ $MICLD_{50}$/ml, but is less intense than the viraemias commonly recorded in the other so-called formidable viral haemorrhagic fevers, such as Marburg disease, and Ebola and Lassa fevers.

Changes in clinical pathology values are more marked in fatal than in non-fatal infections, and abnormalities recorded during the first few days of illness include leucocytosis or leucopenia, elevated serum aspartate transaminase (AST), alanine transaminase (ALT), γ-glutamyl transferase, lactic dehydrogenase, alkaline phosphatase and creatine kinase levels, thrombocytopenia, prolonged activated partial thromboplastin (APTT) and thrombin times, elevated prothrombin ratio and fibrin degradation product levels, and depression of fibrinogen and haemoglobin values. Bilirubin, creatinine, and urea levels increase and serum protein levels decline during the second week of illness.

DIAGNOSIS

Specimens to be submitted for laboratory confirmation of a diagnosis of CCHF include blood from live patients and, in order to avoid performing full autopsies, heart blood and liver samples taken with a biopsy needle from deceased patients. On account of the propensity of the virus to cause laboratory infections, and the severity of the human disease, investigation of CCHF is generally undertaken in maximum security laboratories in countries which have appropriate biosafety regulations and facilities.

Virus can be isolated from blood and organ suspensions in a wide variety of primary and line cell cultures, including Vero, CER and BHK-21 cells, and identified by immunofluorescence. Isolation and identification of virus can be achieved in 1–5 days, but cell cultures lack sensitivity and usually only detect high concentrations of virus present in the blood of severely ill patients during the first 5 days or so of illness. Suckling mice inoculated intracerebrally are more sensitive than cell cultures for the isolation of virus present in blood in low concentrations for up to 13 days after the onset of illness, but they take 6–9 days to succumb to the infection. Virus antigen can sometimes be demonstrated in the blood of severely ill patients with intense viraemia, or in liver suspensions, by enzyme-linked immunoassay. Viral nucleic acid can be demonstrated in serum and liver homogenates of patients by the reverse transcription–polymerase chain reaction technique (Burt and Swanepoel 1993). Observation of necrotic lesions compatible with CCHF infection in sections of liver provides presumptive evidence in support of the diagnosis.

Antibodies, both IgG and IgM, become demonstrable by indirect immunofluorescence in a few patients from day 4 of illness, but most commonly become detectable from day 7 onwards, and are present in the sera of all survivors of the disease by day 9 at the latest. The IgM antibody activity declines to undetectable levels by the fourth month after infection, and IgG titres may begin to decline gradually at this stage, but remain demonstrable for at least 5 years. Recent or current infection is confirmed by demonstrating seroconversion, or a fourfold or greater increase in antibody titre in paired serum samples, or IgM antibody activity in a single sample. The antibody responses may also be demonstrated by enzyme-linked immunoassay. Patients who succumb rarely develop a demonstrable antibody response and the diagnosis is confirmed by isolation of virus from serum, or from liver specimens (Burt *et al.* 1994).

The disease must be distinguished from the other viral haemorrhagic fevers which partially overlap in distribution with CCHF: Lassa fever, Marburg disease, Ebola fever, Omsk haemorrhagic fever, Kyasanur Forest disease, and the haemorrhagic fever with renal syndrome (HFRS) group of diseases associated with hantavirus infections. Other febrile illnesses which can be acquired from contact with animal tissues within the same geographic range as CCHF include Rift Valley fever, Q fever, brucellosis and systemic anthrax, while diseases which can be acquired from ticks include Q fever and tick-borne typhus (*Rickettsia conorii* infection, commonly known as tick-bite fever). However, severe forms of many other common infections may resemble CCHF, including the various types of viral hepatitis, malaria, and bacterial septicaemias.

PATHOLOGY

Macroscopic and microscopic lesions seen in CCHF are suggestive, but not pathognomonic, of the disease. Lesions in the liver vary from disseminated foci of coagulative necrosis, mainly mid-zonal in distribution, to massive necrosis involving over 75 per cent of hepatocytes, and a variable degree of haemorrhage, with little or no inflammatory cell response. Lesions in other organs include congestion, haemorrhage, and focal necrosis in the central nervous system, kidneys and adrenals, and general depletion of lymphoid tissues. Fibrin deposits may be seen in small blood vessels in parenchymatous organs including the liver.

TREATMENT

Patients should be treated under conditions of barrier-nursing for the protection of medical personnel. Theoretically, therapy appropriate for disseminated intravascular coagulopathy, such as the use of heparin, could be applied early in the course of the disease, but patients rarely come to medical attention at a sufficiently early stage, and the procedure is considered to be risky so that it should only be contemplated by clinicians well versed in the treatment of haemostatic failure. Standard treatment consists of replacement of red blood cells, platelets, other coagulation factors, protein (albumin) and intravenous feeding as indicated by clinical pathology findings. Immune plasma from recovered patients has been used in therapy, but there has been no controlled trial with a uniform product of proven virus-neutralizing ability. Moreover, treatments have been initiated at various stages of illness up to and including terminal coma, so that no firm conclusions can be drawn on the efficacy of the treatment. Ribavirin inhibits virus replication in cell cultures and suckling mice, and promising results were obtained in a trial on human patients in South Africa, but discontinuation of the production of the intravenous formulation has prevented treatment of adequate numbers of patients for proper evaluation of the drug (the rapid course and gastrointestinal complications of the disease render oral treatment less effective).

PROGNOSIS

The mortality rate is approximately 30 per cent (range 20–50 per cent), but this can be reduced considerably by careful monitoring of patients and the application of appropriate blood product replacement therapy. The occurrence during the first 5 days of illness of any of the following clinical pathology values is highly predictive of fatal outcome: leucocyte counts $\geq 10 \times 10^9/l$; platelet counts $\leq 20 \times 10^9/l$; AST ≥ 200 U/l; ALT ≥ 150 U/l; APTT ≥ 60 seconds; and fibrinogen ≤ 110 mg/dl. Curiously, leucopenia early in the disease does not have the same poor prognostic connotation as leucocytosis, and all clinical pathology values may be grossly abnormal after day 5 of illness without necessarily being indicative of a poor prognosis. Since an antibody response is rarely demonstrable in fatal illness, the occurrence of a detectable immune response is generally a favourable sign (Burt *et al.* 1994).

EPIDEMIOLOGY

CIRCULATION OF THE VIRUS IN NATURE

The causative agent of CCHF is widely distributed in eastern Europe, Asia, and Africa: the presence of the virus or antibody to it has been demonstrated in the former USSR, Bulgaria, Greece, Turkey, Hungary, Yugoslavia, France, Portugal, Kuwait, Dubai, Sharjah, Iraq, Iran, Afghanistan, Pakistan, India, China, Egypt, Ethiopia, Mauritania, Senegal, Burkina Faso, Benin, Nigeria, Central African Republic, Democratic Republic of the Congo, Kenya, Uganda, Tanzania, Zimbabwe, Namibia, South Africa, and Madagascar. However, the evidence for France and Portugal is based on limited serological observations and needs to be confirmed.

Although CCHF virus has been isolated from at least 30 species of ticks, including two argasids and 28 ixodids, there is no definitive evidence for most species

that they are capable of serving as vectors, and in many instances virus recovered from engorged ticks may merely have been present in the blood meal imbibed from a viraemic host. Argasid ticks are unlikely to be vectors since the virus failed to replicate in three species inoculated intracoelomically. Members of three genera of ixodid ticks, *Hyalomma*, *Dermacentor*, and *Rhipicephalus*, have been shown to be capable of transmitting infection trans-stadially and transovarially, but the bulk of the evidence suggests that *Hyalommas* are the principal vectors in nature, and in broad terms the known distribution of CCHF virus coincides with the world distribution of members of this genus of ticks. The prevalence of antibody to CCHF virus in the sera of wild vertebrates in southern Africa was found to be highest in large herbivores (the size of kudu antelope and greater), which are known to be the preferred hosts of adult *Hyalomma* ticks, and in small mammals up to the size of hares which are the preferred hosts of immature *Hyalommas*; wild mammals of intermediate size, which are parasitized by other genera of ticks, generally lacked evidence of infection. Virus or antibody has also been demonstrated elsewhere in the sera of small mammals of Eurasia and Africa, such as little susliks, hedgehogs, hares, and certain myomorph rodents, and in some instances it has been shown that these hosts develop viraemia of sufficient intensity to infect ticks. Furthermore, it has been demonstrated that CCHF virus can be passed from infected to non-infected ticks which feed together on non-inoculated or immune mammals which fail to develope demonstrable viraemia. The phenomenon of 'non-viraemic' transmission of infection between ticks, which had been demonstrated earlier with other viruses, is believed to be mediated by factors present in tick saliva. Transovarial transmission of virus in ticks occurs with low frequency, but appears to be facilitated when virus is transmitted venereally from infected males to females.

Certain passerine birds and domestic chickens were found to be refractory to CCHF virus, while guinea fowl developed transient viraemia of low intensity following experimental inoculation, and an antibody response which was demonstrable for a few weeks only. The relatively high prevalences and titres of antibody found in farmed ostriches (hosts to adult *Hyalomma* ticks) in South Africa, suggest that these birds are more susceptible to CCHF virus infection than are passerines. Most recently, antibody to CCHF virus was detected in the sera of certain ground-frequenting birds in Senegal, notably the red-billed hornbill (*Tockus erythrorhyncus*), and this species was found to be capable of infecting immature *Hyalomma* ticks following experimental inoculation, despite the fact that the birds did not manifest demonstrable viraemia; they nevertheless developed a more marked antibody response than did starlings or chickens (Zeller *et al.* 1994*a,b*). Immature ticks of some species of *Hyalomma*, notably *H. marginatum rufipes* in Africa, utilize ground-frequenting birds as hosts, and it has long been accepted that the millions of birds which migrate annually on a north–south axis between Africa and Eurasia can serve to disseminate CCHF virus through the carriage of transovarially infected immature ticks. The implication of the recent findings in Senegal is that certain non-passerines may well play a significant role in infecting ticks, and that even birds with a limited flight range, such as hornbills, can disseminate infected ticks locally.

High prevalences of antibody occur in domestic ruminants in areas infested by *Hyalomma* and the virus causes inapparent infection or mild fever in cattle, sheep, and goats, with viraemia of sufficient intensity to infect adult ticks. However, since transovarial transmission of infection in ticks occurs with low frequency, the role of livestock in the circulation of the virus is theoretically limited: it is mathematically improbable that the infection of adult ticks followed by transovarial transmission would ensure indefinite perpetuation of the virus. Hence, it is believed that the infection of immature ticks on small mammals and possibly ground-frequenting birds, constitutes an important amplifying mechanism.

TRANSMISSION OF INFECTION TO HUMANS

Sheep, goats, and cattle generally acquire natural infection with CCHF virus early in life in areas with high challenge rates, and are viraemic for about a week. Hence, it is found that humans become infected when they come into contact with the viraemic blood of overtly healthy young animals in the course of performing procedures such as castrations, vaccinations, inserting ear tags, or slaughtering the animals. Young ruminants are innately resistant to specific tick-borne diseases of livestock, such as anaplasmosis, babesiosis, and cowdriosis, but animals which are raised under tick-free conditions and moved to infested locations later in life may acquire the tick-borne diseases at the same time that they become infected with CCHF virus; consequently humans also become infected from contact with viraemic blood in the course of treating sick animals or butchering those that die. Common-source outbreaks involving more than one case of the disease can occur when several people are exposed to infected tissues. The available evidence suggests that the infection in humans is acquired through contact of viraemic blood with broken skin, and this accords with the fact that nosocomial infection in medical personnel usually results from accidental pricks with

needles contaminated with the blood of patients, or similar mishaps. Infection appears to be limited to those who have contact with fresh blood or other tissues, probably because infectivity is destroyed by the fall in pH which occurs in tissues after death, and there has been no indication that CCHF virus constitutes a public health hazard in meat processed and matured according to normal health regulations. Many human infections result directly from tick bite, and it has been observed that people can also become infected from merely squashing ticks between the fingers. Some patients are unable to recall contact with blood or other tissues of livestock, or having been bitten by ticks, but live in or have visited a rural environment where such exposure to infection is possible. Town dwellers sometimes acquire infection from contact with animal tissues or tick bite while on hunting or hiking trips.

The majority of patients tend to be adult males engaged in the livestock industry, such as farmers, herdsmen, slaughtermen, and veterinarians. The observation that infection of humans is relatively uncommon despite serological evidence of widespread infection occurring in livestock, may be explained by the facts that viraemia in livestock is short lived, and of low intensity compared to that in other zoonotic diseases such as Rift Valley fever, and that humans are not the preferred hosts of *Hyalomma* ticks. The low prevalences of antibody generally found in populations at risk, and the relative paucity of evidence of inapparent infection encountered among the cohorts of cases of the disease, suggests that infection is frequently symptomatic.

PREVENTION AND CONTROL

The control of the vectors of CCHF virus through the use of acaricides is impractical, particularly under the extensive or nomadic farming conditions which prevail in the arid areas where the disease is most prevalent. Stockmen, veterinarians, slaughtermen, and others involved with the livestock industry should be made aware of the disease and take practical steps to limit or evade exposure of naked skin to fresh blood and other tissues of animals, and to avoid handling and being bitten by ticks. Precautions should include the use of gloves and other protective clothing in slaughtering and treating animals, or in performing autopsies. Pyrethroid acaricides, such as permethrin, can be used at low concentration (0.05 per cent) to kill ticks which come into contact with human clothing (Screck *et al.* 1980), and in some countries liquid or aerosol formulations are commercially available for this purpose: clothing is either dipped in the liquid and dried, or sprayed with the aerosol. Inactivated mouse brain vaccine for the prevention of human infection has been used on a limited scale in eastern Europe and the former USSR, but the sporadic and unpredictable occurrence of the disease renders it difficult to identify target populations. A corollary to this problem is that the development of a safe and effective modern vaccine is inhibited by limited potential demand.

REFERENCES

Burt, F. and Swanepoel, R. (1993). *Evaluation of the polymerase chain reaction for the detection of Crimean–Congo haemorrhagic fever virus RNA.* Abstracts of the IXth International Congress of Virology, Glasgow, 8–13 August, 1993.

Burt, F. J., Leman, P. A., Abbott, J. A., and Swanepoel, R. (1994). Serodiagnosis of Crimean–Congo haemorrhagic fever. *Epidemiology and Infection*, **113**, 551–62.

Chumakov, M. P. (1974). [On 30 years of investigation of Crimean hemorrhagic fever.] *Trudy Instituta Poliomielita i Virusnykh Entsefalitov, Akademii Meditsinskikh Nauk SSSR*, **22**, 5–18. [In Russian; English translation NAMRU3-T950.]

Hoogstraal, H. (1979). The epidemiology of tick-borne Crimean–Congo haemorrhagic fever in Asia, Europe and Africa. *Journal of Medical Entomology*, **15**, 307–417.

Hoogstraal, H. (1981). Changing patterns of tick-borne diseases in modern society. *Annual Review of Entomology*, **26**, 75–99.

Lvov, D. K. (1994). Arboviral zoonoses of northern Eurasia (Eastern Europe and the Commonwealth of Independent States). In *Handbook of zoonoses, Section B: Viral*, (2nd edn), (ed. G. W. Beran), pp. 237–60. CRC Press, Boca Rotan, Florida.

Screck, C. E., Snoddy, E. L., and Mount, G. A. (1980). Permethrin and repellants as clothing impregnants for protection from the lone star tick *Amblyomma americanum*. *Journal of Economic Entomology*, **73**, 436–9.

Shepherd, A. J., Swanepoel, R., Shepherd, S. P., Leman, P. A., and Mathee, O. (1991). Viraemic transmission of Crimean–Congo haemorrhagic fever virus to ticks. *Epidemiology and Infection*, **106**, 373–82.

Swanepoel, R. (1994a). Crimean–Congo haemorrhagic fever. In *Infectious diseases of livestock with special reference to Southern Africa*, (ed. J. A. W. Coetzer, G. R. Thomson, and R. C. Tustin), pp. 723–9. Oxford University Press Southern Africa, Cape Town.

Swanepoel, R. (1994b). Crimean–Congo haemorrhagic fever. In *Handbook of zoonoses, Section B: Viral*, (2nd edn), (ed. G. W. Beran), pp. 157–70. CRC Press, Boca Rotan, Florida.

Watts, D. M., Ksiazek, T. G., Linthicum, K. J., and Hoogstraal, H. (1989). Crimean–Congo hemorrhagic fever. In *The arboviruses: epidemiology and ecology*, Vol. II, (ed. T. P. Monath), pp. 177–222. CRC Press, Boca Raton, Florida.

Zeller, H. G., Cornet, J. P., and Camicas, J. L. (1994a). Crimean–Congo haemorrhagic fever virus infection in birds: field investigations in Senegal. *Research in Virology*, **145**, 105–9.

Zeller, H. G., Cornet, J. P., and Camicas, J. L. (1994b). Experimental transmission of Crimean–Congo haemorrhagic fever virus by West African ground-feeding birds to *Hyalomma marginatum rufipes* ticks. *American Journal of Tropical Medicine and Hygiene*, **50**, 676–81.

FURTHER READING

Peters, C. J. and Shelokov, A. (1990). Viral hemorrhagic fever. *Current Therapy in Infectious Disease*, **3**, 355–60.

Swanepoel, R. (1995). Bunyaviridae. In *Principles and practice of clinical virology*, (3rd edn), (ed. A. J. Zuckerman, J. R. Pattison, and J. E. Banatvala), 517–44. John Wiley and Sons, Chichester.

Swanepoel, R. (1995). Nairoviruses. In *Handbook of infectious diseases*, Vol. 3, *Viruses*, (ed. J. S. Porterfield), 285–93. Chapman & Hall, London.

Swanepoel, R. and Shepherd, A. J. (1983–8). National Institute for Virology, Private Bag X4, Sandringham 2131, South Africa. Unpublished observations.

Swanepoel, R. *et al.* (1987). Epidemiologic and clinical features of Crimean–Congo hemorrhagic fever in southern Africa. *American Journal of Tropical Medicine and Hygiene*, **36**, 120–32.

Swanepoel, R., Gill, D. E., Shepherd, A. J., and Leman, P. A. (1989). The clinical pathology of Crimean–Congo hemorrhagic fever. *Reviews of Infectious Diseases*, **11**, 5794–800.

29 FOOT-AND-MOUTH DISEASE, VESICULAR STOMATITIS, NEWCASTLE DISEASE, AND SWINE VESICULAR DISEASE

P. Morgan-Capner and A. S. Bryden

The four infections described below are of major veterinary importance, but zoonotic infection is rare, or associated only with minor illness. Readers should refer to the veterinary literature for a more complete description of their manifestations in animals, and their epidemiology and control (e.g. Fenner *et al.* 1993; Radostits *et al.* 1994).

FOOT-AND-MOUTH DISEASE

SUMMARY

Foot-and-mouth disease (FMD) is still of major economic importance in many parts of the world, despite its successful control, and indeed eradication, in many others. Although the virus (FMDV) can infect a wide range of hooved animals, it is primarily in cattle and pigs that severe problems ensue. The virus is in the genus *Aphthovirus* of the family Picornaviridae and symptomatic infection usually presents as vesicles of the mouth and hooves. Human infection has been reported, but appears to be rare and of no health significance. There are a number of modes of transmission, but aerosol spread is the most important, with very high titres of virus being excreted by infected animals and infectious droplets capable of being carried over long distance by prevailing winds. The availability of a killed vaccine for almost 50 years, and quarantine and slaughter policies, enable control if used aggressively.

HISTORY

It was in the late nineteenth century that improved animal husbandry led to the recognition of FMD as a problem of major economic importance. FMD was the first animal virus identified, in 1898, and killed vaccines became available in the late 1940s.

AGENT

FMDV strains are the sole members of the *Aphthovirus* (from the Greek for 'vesicles in the mouth') genus of the Picornaviridae. They are small, 30 nm, non-enveloped single-strand RNA viruses of icosahedral symmetry. Seven serotypes are recognized: A (Allemagne), O (Oise), C, SAT 1, SAT 2, SAT 3 (South African territories), Asia 1. Within each of these serotypes there are subtypes which show antigenic drift similar to that seen with influenza A. The serotypes and subtypes differ significantly enough that cross-protection, whether following natural infection or vaccination, does not occur. FMDV differs in a number of respects from other members of the Picornaviridae. The major antigenic site is seen in FMDV as protrusions at the surface, possibly reflecting the ability of synthetic peptides to induce protective antibody, and the absence of pits on the surface may be of importance in cell attachment (Acharya *et al.* 1990). Further insight into transmission and source of FMDV is being gathered from nucleotide sequencing of the viral genome. Wild virus can be distinguished from vaccine strains and the evolution of strains can be followed (Kitching 1992). For instance, characterization of the virus imported into Italy in 1993 suggested it was a new introduction, possibly from Asia or Africa (Robson and Dalsgaard 1994). It is also being used to address the origin of outbreaks in domestic cattle in Africa; the strains are very similar to those found in buffalo, supporting asymptomatic carrier buffalo as the source (Kitching 1992).

FMDV has a very narrow range of pH at which infectivity is maintained, with the virus becoming unstable below pH 5–6. It is also susceptible to drying but can survive up to 6 months in slurry in the cold.

ANIMAL INFECTION

A wide range of domestic and wild animals may be infected naturally, some 70 species within 20 families. Birds have also occasionally been shown to be infected, as have a range of experimental laboratory animals such as guinea-pigs. Ungulates are the main hosts, however, and cattle and pigs are those most severely affected. In sheep and goats infection is often subclinical, and the horse appears resistant to infection. In wild animals FMD ranges from the inapparent to the severe. The incubation period can vary from 1 to 14 days, 3–4 days being most frequent. In cattle the infection presents as pyrexia, dullness, anorexia, nasal discharge, and a vesicular eruption in the mouth and on the hooves. The vesicles affect the tongue, hard palate, lips, muzzle and dental pad of the mouth, and the coronary band and interdigital space of the hooves, leading to lameness. In dairy cattle the udder may also be affected, and an early sign is often decline in milk yield. Pregnant cattle may abort. The vesicles soon rupture to leave ulcerated areas prone to bacterial superinfection. Although morbidity is high, mortality is low and largely confined to calves less than 6 months old and is due to a myocarditis. Although the acute infection may resolve in 1–2 weeks, the major economic importance is due to the residual effects. In beef cattle poor growth persists, and in dairy cattle there may be loss of milk for a considerable time. With bacterial superinfection of the feet and nasal cavities, lameness and nasal discharge may become chronic.

In pigs, the vesicles on the feet are the main clinical problem, becoming superinfected and leading to persistent lameness. Vesicles may develop on the snout, but those in the mouth are usually minor. In sheep and goats, infection, if apparent, is usually limited to the feet, leading to lameness.

Infection is usually acquired by inhalation of droplets, with local replication in the pharynx leading to viraemia and disseminated infection. Large amounts of virus are present in many tissues, and may be excreted for 24 hours or more prior to the onset of clinical disease, and may be disseminated in droplets for 5–10 days. Pigs can produce aerosol concentrations many thousands of times higher than those of cattle.

In some animals virus may persist in the pharynx for long periods; over a month in more than half of those infected, and more than 2 years in some cattle, and up to 6 months to a year in sheep and goats, although such persistence does not occur in pigs. Persistence occurs despite high concentrations of specific antibody. Similar persistence can occur in some wild animals, and is considered particularly important in buffalos in the epidemiology of FMD in sub-Saharan Africa where they are thought to be the natural host

and possibly infected for life. Long-term carriage can occur after subclinical infection as well as from acute clinical infection.

Infection may also result from ingestion of contaminated foodstuffs, inoculation or contamination of abrasions from various fomites such as clothes and veterinary instruments, or use of inadequately processed vaccines still containing live virus.

DIAGNOSIS

Achieving a rapid diagnosis is of critical importance for control. Other vesicular diseases can easily be confused, particularly swine vesicular disease, vesicular stomatitis (VS) and vesicular exanthema of swine in pigs, and VS in cattle and sheep. Antigen detection in vesicular epithelium or fluid by enzyme-linked immunosorbent (ELISA) is now the preferred approach, and can give a result in a few hours. Virus culture can be performed on vesicular fluid and epithelium, blood, milk, pharyngeal scrapings, and other tissues if the animal has died. Virus can be isolated in a range of cell culture types, including primary bovine thyroid and BHK-21 cells, and isolated virus typed by ELISA or neutralization. Maintaining viability during transport is essential due to the pH lability of the virus, and samples should be transported frozen or in glycerol/phosphate buffer at pH 7.6. Serum antibody can also be detected by ELISA.

HUMAN INFECTION

FMDV can be detected readily in the noses of personnel exposed to infected animals, or even after laboratory exposure (Sellers *et al.* 1970). In the study of Sellers *et al.* (1970) there was no evidence of replication, although virus could be detected for over 24 hours, and was transmitted on one occasion to a close contact. There were no clinical consequences or serological evidence of infection in this study, however. Similarly, those regularly exposed to animals with FMD in a research institute have not shown clinical signs of infection (Sellers *et al.* 1970). Reports of human infection are rare (e.g. Armstrong *et al.* 1967), but have resulted from drinking infected milk, and either inoculation or contamination of breaches in the skin. The case reported by Armstrong *et al.* (1967) had vesicles on his hands and feet, and lesions on the tongue. FMDV type O was isolated from the hand, and specific antibody detected. Of the 37 cases reviewed by Sellers *et al.* (1970), 23 were type O, 13 type C, and 1 type A. Low titres of antibody, particularly to type O, were found in serological surveys of exposed workers (Suhr Rasmussen 1968; Wisniewski and Jankowska 1968).

EPIDEMIOLOGY

Few countries have escaped FMD in the past century, but the infection is now eradicated in western Europe, North and Central America, the Caribbean, Japan, Australia, and New Zealand. Infection continues to be endemic in many parts of Asia, Africa, and South America, and still occurs in eastern Europe and the states of the former USSR. Infection can spread readily because of the high titres of virus excreted by infected animals, commencing prior to the onset of clinical disease, infection persisting in some cases for years, and the ability for the virus to spread by aerosol. Infection spreads rapidly by aerosol between closely confined animals, and the very high titres of virus produced by pigs can lead to dissemination up to 250 km on the wind, as happened in 1981 when FMD spread from Brittany to the Isle of Wight. Over land, however, virus is unlikely to spread more than 10 km. Infection can also be spread by animal products, fomites such as clothing, and many outbreaks have resulted from inadequately killed vaccines. In some parts of the world infection can be maintained in wild animals, such as the buffalo in Africa. There is no cross-protection after infection with one serotype, and even serotype-specific immunity can wane and become non-protective as the antigenic profile of the virus drifts.

PREVENTION AND CONTROL

Prevention has centred on the use of killed vaccines, control of animal movement, and slaughter and ring-fencing foci of infection. Killed vaccines have been used successfully to reduce the prevalence of disease, but experience has shown their use alone cannot achieve eradication, and that immunized cattle can still carry the virus. Vaccines are cell culture grown virus, inactivated with *N*-acetylethyleneimine, bromoethylamine hydrobromide (BEA), or similar, and administered with an adjuvant such as aluminium hydroxide (Barteling and Vreeswijk 1991). Protection is induced against the immunizing serotype only, so there has to be careful matching with the prevalent local strains. The immunity may also not be sufficient to protect against virus of the same serotype, but exhibiting antigenic drift. There has been hope for some years that recombinant or peptide vaccines could replace the killed vaccines. Recombinant protein vaccines have shown only low immunogenic capacity, when compared to killed whole virus vaccines. FMD seemed to be an ideal candidate for a peptide vaccine when it was shown that peptides of 20 and 14 amino acids could induce neutralizing antibody in guinea-pigs when polymerized or after other chemical or presentational modification. However, the response in cattle and pigs was disappointing (Brown 1992).

The requirement to prevent the introduction of FMD has led to major constraints to free trade of animals and meat products. In many countries FMD is a notifiable disease and control is by the slaughter of infected animals and their contacts, quarantine, and prevention of animal movement, and thorough disinfection of premises and possible carrier fomites by alkali or acid solutions combined with detergents.

The UK has been free of FMD since 1981, and the success of control policies in Europe led to the phasing out of vaccination in 1991–92. That reintroduction could still occur was shown by two outbreaks, in Italy in 1993, possibly via Croatia (Robson and Dalsgaard 1994), and in Greece in 1994.

VESICULAR STOMATITIS

SUMMARY

Vesicular stomatitis (VS) is largely confined to the western hemisphere, and is enzootic in tropical/subtropical parts of the Americas, and epizootics occur at regular intervals in the temperate zones. The causative agents are in the genus *Vesiculovirus* of the family Rhabdoviridae. Many types exist but vesiculovirus (VSV)-New Jersey (VSV-NJ) and VSV-Indiana (VSV-I) predominate in the Americas. Types found in other parts of the world rarely cause disease. Although a wide range of domestic and wild animals can be infected, it is horses, cattle and pigs which suffer most from vesicular disease of the mouth and hooves. Mortality is low, and recovery usually complete. Insect vectors such as sandflies are strongly implicated in transmission. Human infection can be common in those having a close working relationship with infected animals, but is often inapparent or giving a mild flu-like illness only. Although vaccines have been produced, they are little used and control is not vigorously pursued.

HISTORY

An illness compatible with VS in horses was first noted in the early eighteenth century, with a virus aetiology being suggested in 1927. Although presumed human infections had been noted in the first half of the century, confirmed human infections were first recorded in the early 1950s. The past 30 years have seen an increasing number of vesiculoviruses identified from various parts of the world.

AGENT

VSVs belong to the genus *Vesiculovirus* of the family Rhabdoviridae. They are bullet-shaped enveloped paticles of some 170 nm long and 70 nm diameter, containing a nucleoprotein of 50 nm diameter and having helical symmetry. They contain single-stranded negative-sense RNA and the nucleoprotein contains an RNA-dependent RNA polymerase to enable a complementary RNA strand to be synthesized after cell penetration. There are some 29 members of the genus (Francki *et al.* 1991), but the majority have been isolated from invertebrates only, or have not yet been proved to be relevant to humans or animals. The types of major importance and responsible for animal and human disease in the Americas are VSV-NJ and VSV-I. Other types of veterinary or human importance are: VSV-Alagoas, associated with vesicular disease of horses, mules, and cattle in Brazil (Tesh *et al.* 1987); Isfahan isolated from sandflies in Iran (Tesh *et al.* 1977); Chandipura from humans in India (Bhatt and Rodrigues 1967); Calchaqui from humans and horses in Argentina (Calisher *et al.* 1987); and Piry from humans in Brazil and laboratory workers (Anonymous 1975). Vesiculoviruses have been isolated from a wide variety of insects, including sandflies, mosquitoes, midges, and some flies.

Vesiculoviruses have a common group antigen localized in the nucleoproteins and serotype-specific antigens in the envelope. Genomic RNA fingerprinting using T1 RNase has shown homogeneity of isolates during epizootics, but great heterogeneity of strains isolated from enzootic areas in South America. The virus is stable between pH 5 and 10, but rapidly inactivated at 56 °C.

ANIMAL INFECTION

In the Americas VSV-NJ and VS-I are the predominant cause of animal infection, with the former being more common and tending to give more severe illness. Clinically apparent infection is associated particularly with horses, cattle, and pigs. Sheep and a wide range of wild animals can also be infected, but with the exception of deer are asymptomatic. After an incubation of 1–5 days, cattle develop fever and salivation. Vesicles develop in the mouth, on the tongue and oral mucosa, on the teats, and on the coronary bands of the hooves. The vesicles soon break and those on the hooves may become superinfected. The result is lameness, cessation of lactation, and loss of weight due to difficulty feeding. Full recovery with no sequelae usually follows in 7–10 days. In the horse the oral manifestations are usually paramount, whereas in the pig it is the snout and coronary bands that are primarily affected. The infection is rarely fatal except in the pig. When infection occurs in a herd of cattle 5–75 per cent may be overtly affected, but asymptomatic infections also occur.

Infection is usually acquired through abrasions in the mouth, or on the teats or coronary bands, although transmission by insect bites or mechanically is a possibility. Infection remains localized, and if viraemia does occur it is transient and low level. Virus is not excreted in urine, faeces, or milk. Immunity develops, but may decline leaving the animal susceptible to reinfection.

DIAGNOSIS

Specific antigen can be detected in vesicular fluid or scrapings taken from the vesicle base by complement fixation testing (CFT) or ELISA. Virus can be readily isolated from such specimens by culture in a wide range of cells, for example BHK-21 and Vero cells, with cytopathic effect developing rapidly. The virus is identified and typed by neutralization or CFT. Antibody can be detected by CFT, neutralization, and ELISA.

HUMAN INFECTION

Subclinical infection, or clinical features too minor to recall, are common as judged by seroprevalence studies. For instance during an epizootic of VSV-NJ in Colorado, 17 of 133 (13 per cent) veterinarians and other workers highly exposed to the virus had antibody, compared to only 3 of 52 (6 per cent) not highly exposed. Forty-eight of the 133 gave a history of compatible illness, including 11 of the 17 who were antibody positive, while only one of the 52 non-exposed persons did so (Reif *et al.* 1987). This study also confirmed the low infectivity of VSV for humans. However, where VSV is enzootic infection can be more common. For example up to 95 per cent of adults in some localities had antibodies to VSV-I (Tesh *et al.* 1974).

Clinically apparent infection with VSV-NJ or VSV-I usually presents 1–6 days after exposure (Patterson *et al.* 1958). The illness is usually flu-like, with acute fever, myalgia, headache, retro-orbital pain, malaise, pharyngitis, nausea, vomiting, and diarrhoea. In up to a quarter of cases, herpes-like vesicles occur in the mouth or gums, tongue, buccal cavity and pharynx, or on the lips or nose. Resolution occurs within 8 days. Two severe infections have been reported, both in children and one fatal, where encephalitis occurred. Infection has also been reported commonly in exposed laboratory workers (Patterson *et al.* 1958).

Transmission to humans in the community is usually associated with close contact with infected animals, such as being exposed to sneezing, examining the oral cavity of infected animals, or getting infected saliva on broken skin or in an eye (Reif *et al.* 1987). Transmission by blood-sucking insects such as sandflies cannot be excluded, however. In laboratory acquired infection, transmission has arisen by aerosol, eye splash, and contamination of skin abrasion, so confirming the advisability of wearing protective gloves and goggles.

Chandipura virus has been associated with flu-like illness (Bhatt and Rodrigues 1967) and an acute fatal encephalopathy syndrome (Rodrigues *et al.* 1983) in India. Human infection with Calchaqui (Calisher *et al.* 1987), Isfahan (Tesh *et al.* 1977), VSV-Alagoas (Tesh *et al.* 1987), and Piry (Anonymous 1975), has also been demonstrated, but only with the last has clinical illness resulted.

Diagnosis is serological, but virus isolation can be attempted although it has been unsuccessful to date.

EPIDEMIOLOGY

VSV-NJ, VSV-I, and VSV-Alagoas are restricted to the Americas, with the last probably being enzootic within parts of South America (Hanson and McMillan 1990). The former two are enzootic within the subtropical and tropical parts of the Americas. In tropical/subtropical areas epizootics occur annually or every 2–3 years, but every 5–10 years epizootics occur in the temperate zones. The geographical areas affected are sharply limited to favourable habitats, although there would appear to be potential for wider spread. VSV-NJ is the predominant strain implicated.

An epidemiological feature of epizootics which is difficult to explain is the simultaneous appearance of very closely related strains in disparate foci. A possible explanation would be transmission by insects. Supportive features are that infection occurs in the summer and declines markedly with the first frost, and that virus has been readily isolated from a range of insects including sandflies, horse flies, and mosquitoes. However, some epizootics have continued over the winter period, and viraemia is transient. Insects could act as simple mechanical vectors carrying virus from mucosal lesions. Transovarial transmission in sandflies has also been shown (Tesh *et al.* 1987), suggesting a possible mechanism for maintenance of the virus and the capability of acting as a reservoir.

PREVENTION AND CONTROL

The clinical similarity of VS to FMD gives added importance to correct diagnosis and control. Although attenuated vaccines are available, and infection in dairy cattle can have major economic consequence, they are little used in North America. Vaccination does have some success in Venezuela, however (Hanson and McMillan 1990).

NEWCASTLE DISEASE

SUMMARY

Newcastle disease (ND) is caused by a paramyxovirus (NDV), and potentially all species of birds may be infected. Clinical illness depends largely on an avian species susceptibility and infecting strain. NDV strains may be classified as high (velogenic), medium (mesogenic), and low (lentogenic) pathogenicity. The disease is of major importance in chickens as the death rate in an outbreak may be high, especially if a velogenic strain is involved, and there may be a marked reduction or cessation of egg-laying. Racing and show pigeons are also highly susceptible to infection. Virus is spread by aerosols, dust, and fomites.

Signs of infection include enteric, respiratory, and neurological manifestations. Some infections by lentogenic strains may be asymptomatic. The predominant symptom of human NDV infection is a self-limiting conjuctivitis but 'flu-like' symptoms have also been reported. Persons in close contact with poultry, or laboratory staff handling NDV in high concentration are those most liable to infection.

Control of NDV depends on local circumstances but includes limitation of access to flocks by outside personnel, culling of infected birds, and vaccination, for example of racing pigeons.

HISTORY

Newcastle disease was first described in 1926 following major outbreaks in domestic fowl on a farm near Newcastle-upon-Tyne, UK (hence the name) and in Java in the Far East (Cross 1991). The virus had almost certainly existed previously, probably in many avian species, but apparently without causing any major problems. Its emergence as a major pathogen probably reflects changes in husbandry, with the development of larger commercial flocks and increasing trade between establishments being major factors. Previously flocks had been small or chickens were kept in small numbers to supply individual families. It was thought initially that ND was classical fowl plague, caused by avian influenza virus A, and it was not until 1949 that the two viruses were differentiated.

Domestic fowl are the birds usually associated with ND but since 1983 ND has been a problem of panzootic proportions in racing pigeons.

AGENT

NDV is the type species of the paramyxoviruses and is classified as avian paramyxovirus type 1 (PMV 1); nine avian types have been described (Alexander 1988). Like all paramyxoviruses, NDV is usually present in circular form, measuring 150–200 nm in diameter, but pleomorphic filamentous forms are not uncommon. The genome is single-stranded helical RNA, 18 nm in diameter. This is contained within a lipid bilayer membrane on which are the haemagglutinin-neuraminidase and fusion spikes. Unlike myxoviruses, the haemagglutinin and neuraminidase are contained at separate sites in a single molecule. The virus attaches to cells via the haemagglutinin but it is the fusion (F) protein that effects infection by lysing the host cell membranes, leading in turn to fusion of virus and host cell membrane and release of virus nucleo-capsid into the cell cytoplasm. An important aspect of this process is cleavage of the F protein by host cell proteases as the F protein is incapable of initiating infection on its own. This has a bearing on the pathogenic potential and tissue tropism of individual strains of NDV and indicates that the disease process is dependent on both cell type and virus strain. F protein cleavage of virulent NDV strains occurs in a wider range of cell types, including some cells of non-avian origin, whereas the types of cells producing such cleavage of an avirulent strain are limited. This pantropism of virulent NDV strains presumably allows dissemination throughout the avian host, producing extensive disease (Chanock *et al.* 1990).

Like all paramyxoviruses, NDV is sensitive to a wide range of lipid solvents, disinfectants, and high or low pH. It is, however, comparatively heat stable and may remain infectious in tissues from infected birds, notably chickens, for 6 months or more at −20 °C or up to 4 months at 4 °C. In eggs from infected hens it may survive for several months at room temperature, or over 12 months at 4 °C. Under field conditions, long-term survival in infected premises and on feathers has also been noted. NDV survives well in sea and fresh water.

Following infection of a susceptible host, replication occurs in the mucosa of the upper respiratory and intestinal tracks. A primary viraemia takes place with spread to the spleen and bone marrow. In turn, a secondary viraemia occurs, permitting dissemination to other important organs such as the central nervous system and lungs. Respiratory symptoms may result from congestion of the lungs and neurological damage. Pathological changes may be widespread, with haemorrhages occurring in the respiratory and intestinal tracks. Necrotic foci may be found in the intestinal mucosa and lymphatic tissue and most organs may show hyperaemic changes.

As virus is excreted from both respiratory and alimentary tracts for 4 months or more, spread, which may show some strain variation, is by aerosol or faecal–orally, albeit via fomites and food. Viable virus may also persist in tissues of infected birds, so carcasses, if not properly disposed of, may also be a source of infection.

The immune response to infection is rapid, and antibodies, detectable by haemagglutination inhibition, may be present 4–6 days postinfection. Passive antibodies are transferred from hen to chick via egg yolk and afford some protection for 1 month after hatching.

All strains of NDV are serologically indistinguishable but may vary greatly in pathogenicity. They may be grouped into pathotypes: 'velogenic' which causes high mortality and morbidity, 'mesogenic' causing high morbidity and low to moderate mortality, and 'lentogenic' causing low morbidity, neglible mortality, and frequently asymptomatic infection (Alexander 1994). Pathotype may be related to tissue tropism (described above).

INFECTION IN BIRDS

NDV is widespread in the avian kingdom but the species giving greatest concern are chickens and racing pigeons.

The severity of ND in chickens is very variable and dependent not only on infecting pathotype but also on other factors such as age of host, co-infection with other organisms, stress, immune status, etc. Consequently, presentation may be extremely variable. Furthermore the clinical signs of ND are not pathognomonic and other pathogens may give a similar presentation (Alexander 1994).

Infection with velogenic strains may present as viscerotropic or neurotropic. Both result in high mortality and death may be very rapid with few, if any, clinical signs. Viscerotropic velogenic ND (VVND) has a sudden onset with rapid progression. Affected birds become listless, stop eating, and have ruffled feathers. Combs become cyanotic and oedematous and conjunctivitis with a mucopurulent discharge is present. Respiratory signs such as sneezing, coughing, and nasal discharge are common, as is diarrhoea which may be greenish yellow. Egg production usually ceases.

In neurotropic velogenic ND (NVND) respiratory signs are also present but the condition is characterized by neurological signs such as tremors, loss of limb co-ordination, and torticollis. NVND tends to affect older birds. With both VVND and NVND mortality may approach 100 per cent.

Infection with mesogenic NDV strains, although causing high morbidity especially in younger birds, is associated with low to moderate mortality which on occasions may be as high as 50 per cent.

By contrast, lentogenic strains have low morbidity and neglible mortality. Some mild respiratory signs may be present but many such infections, both respiratory and enteric, are totally subclinical.

A varient of NDV (PPMV-1) (Alexander 1988) has been responsible for a major panzootic in racing pigeons since about 1980. The incubation period may vary from a few days to several weeks. The first sign is excessive thirst followed by watery or haemorrhagic diarrhoea; nervous signs such as paralysis, tremor, torticollis, etc. develop subsequently. Respiratory signs are never present. Recovery may be protracted, lasting up to 6 months, and a chronic enteritis may occur, taking several months to resolve. PPMV-1 virus may also affect domestic fowl, exhibiting similar signs as in pigeons.

Susceptibility to NDV amongst other species of birds varies greatly (Cross 1991). Waterfowl and others living in the aquatic environment are usually very resistant to disease although when infected they may become long-term carriers. NDV strains affecting water-birds would seem to be generally avirulent. Conversely, psittacine species and some game species such as pheasant and partridge would appear to be highly susceptible to infection, often with VVND strains. International trade (and smuggling) of infected birds has been a major factor in the dissemination of NDV to domestic poultry. The clinical manisfestations of ND in pet and susceptible non-aquatic birds are the same as in poultry.

DIAGNOSIS

Because of the similarity of clinical features, it is impossible to differentiate NDV infection from other agents, such as avian influenzavirus, on this basis. Consequently, laboratory diagnosis is essential (Beard 1992). Isolation of virus by allantoic inoculation of 10-day-old embryonated hens' eggs with clinical samples is the method of choice. Suitable specimens are tracheal swabs, faeces, and post-mortem material such as brain, spleen, and tissue from the respiratory and alimentary tracts. Inoculation of cell cultures of avian origin such as chick embryo monolayer may also be attempted, but would not seem to be as sensitive as isolation in eggs. Any isolate has to be characterized by pathotype, i.e. velogenic, mesogenic, or lentogenic. There are several assays for this, such as the mean death time in 9–11-day-old chick embryos, the intracerebral pathogenicity index using day-old chickens, and the intravenous pathogenicity index in 6-week-old chickens. None is entirely satisfactory and there may be problems with passively acquired antibody. There is consequently a need for non-animal tests for such purposes. Tests using monclonal antibodies or oligonucleotide fingerprinting may be of value in the future.

Serological diagnosis, especially of chronic ND, may be undertaken by haemagglutination inhibition.

HUMAN INFECTION

Human NDV infection was first described in a laboratory worker who developed conjunctivitis following accidental inoculation of an eye with allantoic fluid from an infected egg (Burnet 1943). Thereafter further cases were described, including one in a salesman who had assisted with inoculation of chickens with live vaccine (Lippmann 1952). Following a splash of vaccine in one eye, conjunctivitis developed and resolved within a few days. About 2 months later the patient received a splash of vaccine in his other eye, again developing conjunctivitis, albeit of a milder nature.

Conjunctivitis is regarded as the principal manifestation of NDV infection in humans. It is similar to that caused by adenoviruses and normally resolves in 3 or 4 days, although occasionally this may take up to 3 weeks. The infection is acquired by direct inoculation of the eye or by aerosol, and the incubation period is 1–2 days. Usually only one eye is affected. No treatment is available or necessary but care should be taken to avoid secondary bacterial infection as this may result in permanent damage.

Other signs of illness are uncommon but varying claims of influenza-like illness after inhalation have been reported. However, very mild respiratory symptoms may not be noticed or considered insignificant by those infected. Following infection, low-level neutralizing antibody is produced, but this does not protect against reinfection.

Almost without exception, clinical cases have been reported only in patients with close contact with poultry and in laboratory workers handling NDV in high concentration. The pathotype, i.e. velogenic, mesogenic or lentogenic, appears to have no effect on the severity of human infection.

Antibody prevalence studies are limited but tend to support the relationship of exposure to poultry. An Indian study (Charan et al. 1981) showed that 38 per cent of those in contact with poultry were antibody positive, compared with only 4 per cent of the general population, while another study, although not stating the overall proportion possessing antibody, demonstrated greater antibody titres in poultry workers than in those without such exposure (Pedersden et al. 1990). It has also been shown that 4 per cent of US blood donors were anti-NDV positive but in patients with a range of clinical conditions it was 20–30 per cent, while in patients with infectious mononucleosis it was over 50 per cent (Powell 1984). The significance of this is unknown and may reflect non-specific factors.

EPIDEMIOLOGY AND CONTROL

Although susceptibility to disease may vary, it would seem that virtually all avian species may be infected with NDV (Cross 1991). As many birds migrate seasonally, covering vast distances, they may therefore disseminate NDV in their travels to both wild and domestic species. It is also evident that total exclusion of NDV from a country or region is likely to be impossible.

Trade may also be a direct or indirect route for spreading NDV. The past 70–80 years have witnessed a vast increase in the poultry industry, with fowl being transported not only between areas in a particular country but also between countries. Personnel such as veterinary practitioners, delivery or egg collection drivers, etc., or anyone who may travel between farms or large poultry establishments, may act as mechanical vectors carrying virus on clothing, vehicles, or equipment.

Trade, legal and illegal, in exotic species, some of which, such as psittacines, are highly susceptible to NDV, is another route of potential spread, as are racing pigeons, some of which participate in international races.

Since NDV was first recognized in 1926, three panzootics seem to have occurred. The first one lasted from the mid-1920s to about 1950. It has been suggested that the virus circulated in South-East Asia and was introduced by chance into other countries, such as England in 1926. NDV in England seemed to have died out by 1928 and other countries may have experienced a similar elimination of virus.

The second panzootic apparently centred on the Middle East in the late 1960s but spread much more quickly than the first panzootic via international trade in psittacine species.

The third and current panzootic is related to the PPMV-1 strain in racing pigeons with spread to domestic fowl occurring sporadically, often via foodstuff contaminated by feral birds. Outbreaks of this nature occurred in Great Britain in 1984 but there has been none since then. However, sporadic incidents have been reported in Ireland (both Northern Ireland and the Republic of Ireland). In Europe isolated outbreaks increased during the early 1990s, causing concern in veterinary circles. Principally affected were Germany, Italy, Belgium, and The Netherlands, although most other countries in the European Community have reported an occasional incident. Many of those incidents were reported in hobby or 'backyard' flocks over which there is little control.

Control measures include good husbandry, restriction of movement when an outbreak occurs, and in certain circumstances vaccination. Commercial establishments should ensure restricted access to the flocks, especially by persons and vehicles which may travel between farms. If any such person, such as a veterinary practitioner, does require access then appropriate hygienic measures, such as change of clothing, should be observed.

Live and killed vaccines may also be used but are of limited value as they may not prevent subsequent infection with wild NDV although markedly reducing the severity of any illness. Consequently, a vaccinated bird may be virtually disease free but could be excreting, at a lower level, highly pathogenic velogenic NDV. Vaccination of chickens is therefore most useful in areas where NDV is endemic.

Control of PPMV-1 in pigeons has met with varying success. In Great Britain a voluntary vaccination policy has been encouraged but outbreaks in pigeon lofts continue. Consequently, legislation was passed in 1994 in accordance with a European Community Directive that all racing pigeons should be vaccinated (Alexander 1994).

SWINE VESICULAR DISEASE

SUMMARY

Swine vesicular disease virus (SVDV) was identified in 1966 and is a member of the family Picornaviridae. It is closely related antigenically to coxsackievirus B5. The primary veterinary importance of SVDV is that it causes disease in swine that can be clinically indistinguishable from FMD. Control is by notification and slaughter. Human infection has been reported rarely, but illnesses similar to those seen with enteroviruses have occurred.

HISTORY

Swine vesicular disease (SVD) is a relatively recently recognized infection of pigs, having first been recognized in Italy in 1966 (Nardelli *et al.* 1968). In the following years infection was described across Europe and in the Far East, but the infection is now largely controlled in developed countries. Description of the causative organism as an enterovirus-like member of the Picornaviridae was part of the original report (Nardelli *et al.* 1968). Although primarily a vesicular disease, early transmission experiments demonstrated that it was a systemic infection, but of low mortality.

Transmission to man was shown to occur both in the laboratory and by contact with infected pigs on the farm. A number of routes of transmission were shown to occur, but infection of pigs probably occurred by contamination of skin abrasions with virus in the local environment. The impetus for control came from the difficulty in distinguishing clinically SVD from FMD, and led to control primarily by slaughter and banning the movement of infected animals.

AGENT

Swine vesicular disease virus is a member of the Picornaviridae, characterized by having a single-stranded RNA genome enclosed in a capsid of icoso-hedral symmetry. It is non-enveloped and 30 nm in diameter. Major interest has focused on SVDV because of its similarity to coxsackievirus B5 (CVB5), an established human pathogen (Graves 1973). Indeed it has been suggested that SVDV resulted from transmission of CVB5 from man to the pig. Pigs can be infected experimentally with CVB5, remaining asymptomatic, although microscopic lesions can be shown in the central nervous system and anti-CVB5 antibody develops. There is a very close antigenic similarity between CVB5 and SVDV, as shown by two-way cross-neutralization with polyclonal sera. The two viruses can be distinguished, however, by immunodiffusion. RNA–RNA hybridization also showed a close similarity. Both viruses have now been nucleotide sequenced and their protein structure deduced (Zhang *et al.* 1993). The outer capsid proteins of the two viruses show a remarkable similarity, suggesting antigenic variants of a single serotype. The non-structural polypeptides of CVB5, however, are more closely related to the other coxsackievirus B serotypes than to SVDV. Three possibilities have been suggested for the origin of SVDV and its close relationship with CVB5 (Zhang *et al.* 1993). First, that they have a common ancestor; secondly, that they have separate ancestors which have shown a convergent evolution of the part of the genome defining the capsid proteins; and, thirdly that both viruses arose by recombination. Genetic recombination is well-established between enteroviruses, and it is possible that either or both viruses have resulted from recombination events involving the coming together of different regions of genome. Defining the base sequence of a wider range of strains of CVB5 and SVDV may enable firmer conclusions to be drawn.

The virus is stable over a wide range of pH, can withstand drying, and has been shown to be capable of surviving in the environment or frozen for many months.

ANIMAL INFECTION

After an incubation period of 48–72 hours, infection in the pig is characterized by fever and vesicular lesions, primarily affecting the junction of the heel and coronary band. This results in lameness, which can persist for some while after the lesions have resolved, usually in 2–3 weeks. In 10 per cent or so of infections, vesicles appear on the snout and in the buccal cavity. Vesicular lesions occasionally spread a short way up the limbs, and even present on the thorax or abdomen. Although the infection is usually manifest only as superficial lesions, the systemic nature of the infection has been shown in experimental studies (Burrows *et al.* 1974), and rare cases have shown signs of an encephalomyelitis such as ataxia and convulsions. Asymptomatic and mild infection also occur, but less commonly after natural infection than after experimental infection by the oral or nasal route. Although morbidity is high, mortality is very low in adult pigs, although it may reach 10 per cent in piglets. No persistent infections have been identified, and all infected pigs develop protective antibody on recovery.

Infection commonly occurs through breaks in the skin or the mucosa of the gastrointestinal tract after ingestion, although infection by oral and nasal routes can occur. Infected pigs produced high titres of virus in skin lesions, nose, mouth, pharynx, gut, and genital tract for the first week, with titres markedly declining in the second week, but virus may persist for up to 3 weeks in the faeces (Burrows *et al.* 1974).

DIAGNOSIS

Laboratory diagnosis is essential due to the clinical similarity to FMD. Specific antigen can be detected in vesicle fluid by enzyme immunoassay (ELISA) to give a rapid result, but virus isolation in porcine kidney cells may also produce results within 24–48 hours. Antibody can be detected using a range of assays such as ELISA, neutralization, and immunodiffusion.

HUMAN INFECTION

Reports of human infection are few (Garland and Mann 1974; Brown *et al.* 1976; Minor and Bell 1990), but under-reporting may be substantial due to the non-specific manifestations of human infection and the potential for confusion with CVB5 if a virus is isolated. The manifestations are those associated with non-poliovirus enterovirus infection.

In one report, however, a number of laboratory workers were said to have been infected, although human infection was said to have a low incidence, both in those naturally exposed to pigs and those exposed to the virus in the laboratory (Garland and Mann 1974). Symptoms have ranged from non-specific febrile illnesses to viral meningitis, with no deaths having been recorded. Asymptomatic infection also occurs. Convalescent sera had high-titre neutralizing antibody to both CVB5 and SVDV, but immunodiffusion confirmed SVDV infection. Specific diagnosis is likely to be serological, but virus isolation should be attempted from throat, faeces, and CSF. Two routes of transmission seem feasible for human infection: inhalation of aerosols from infected pigs or contamination of abrasions.

EPIDEMIOLOGY

After its description in Italy in 1966, SVD was soon reported from many countries in Europe, including the United Kingdom where the epidemic started in December 1972 (Dawe *et al.* 1973). Epidemics also occurred in Hong Kong and Japan. The virus can be transmitted by a number of routes. Airborne spread seems highly unlikely (Sellars and Herniman 1974), and certainly did not seem to occur over any distance. The contamination of the environment by an infected pig is a ready source for infecting further generations of pigs in the pig pen or transport lorry, especially as SVDV retains infectivity for many months. Infected pig swill is a further possible means of dissemination, as is the persistence of viable virus in frozen meat products.

PREVENTION AND CONTROL

Although there have been putative killed vaccines, control has relied on slaughter of infected pigs, restricting movement, and banning swill feed from infected areas. Because of the inability to distinguish SVD from FMD clinically, SVD is a notifiable disease in the United Kingdom. Sporadic outbreaks of infection continue throughout the European Community, recent outbreaks having occurred in Italy, Belgium, Spain, and The Netherlands, although the disease has not been seen in the United Kingdom since 1982.

REFERENCES

Acharya, R., Fry, E., Stuart, D., Fox, G., Rowlands, D., and Brown, F. (1990). The structure of foot-and-mouth disease virus: implications for its physical and biological properties. *Veterinary Microbiology*, **23**, 21–34.

Alexander, D. J. (1988) Newcastle disease viruse—an avian paramyxovirus. In *Newcastle disease*, (ed. D. J. Alexander), pp. 11–22. Kluwer Academic Publishers, Norwell, MA.

Alexander, D. J. (1994). Newcastle disease. *State Veterinary Journal*, **4**, 7–10.

Anonymous (1975). *International catalogue of arboviruses including certain other viruses of vertebrates*. US Department of Health, Education and Welfare, Washington, DC.

Armstrong, R., Davie, J., and Hedger, R. S. (1967). Foot-and-mouth disease in man. *British Medical Journal*, **4**, 529–30.

Barteling, S. J. and Vreeswijk, J. (1991). Developments in foot-and-mouth disease vaccines. *Vaccine*, **9**, 75–88.

Beard, C. W. (1992). Newcastle disease. In *Veterinary diagnostic virology*, (ed. A. E. Castro and W. P. Hevschele), pp. 54–6. Mosby Year Book, St Louis.

Bhatt, P. N. and Rodrigues, F. M. (1967). Chandipura: a new arbovirus isolated in India from patients with febrile illness. *Indian Journal of Medical Research*, **55**, 1295–305.

Brown, F. (1992). New approaches to vaccination against foot-and-mouth disease. *Vaccine*, **10**, 1022–6.

Brown, F., Goodridge, D., and Burrows, R. (1976). Infection of man by swine vesicular disease virus. *Journal of Comparative Pathology*, **86**, 409–14.

Burnet, F. M. (1943). Human infection with the virus of Newcastle disease in fowls. *Medical Journal of Australia*, **2**, 313–14.

Burrows, R., Mann, J. A., and Goodridge, D. (1974). Swine vesicular disease: virological studies of experimental infections produced by the England/72 virus. *Journal of Hygiene*, **72**, 135–43.

Calisher, C. H. *et al.* (1987). A newly recognized Vesiculovirus, Calchaqui virus, and subtypes of Melao and Maguari viruses from Argentina, with serological evidence for infections of humans and horses. *American Journal of Tropical Medicine and Hygiene*, **36**, 114–19.

Chanock, R. M. and McIntosh, K. (1990). Parainfluenza viruses. *Fields virology*, (2nd edn), Vol. 1, (ed. B. N. Fields and D. M. Knipe), pp. 963–88. Raven Press, New York.

Charan, S., Mahajan, V. M., and Agarwal, L. P. (1981). Newcastle disease antibodies in human sera. *Indian Journal of Medical Research*, **73**, 303–7.

Cross, G. M. (1991). Newcastle disease. *Veterinary Clinics of North America: Small Animal Practice*, **21**, 1231–9.

Dawe, P. S., Forman, A. J., and Smale, C. J. (1973). A preliminary investigation of the swine vesicular disease epidemic in Britain. *Nature*, **241**, 540–2.

Fenner, F. J., Gibbs, E. P. J., Murphy, F. A., Rott, R., Studdert, M. J., and White, D. O. (1993). *Veterinary virology*, (2nd edn). Academic Press, San Diego.

Francki, R. I. B. Fauquet, C. M., Knudson, D. L., and Brown, F. (ed.) (1991). Classification and nomenclature of viruses. *Fifth Report of the International Committee on Taxonomy of Viruses*, pp. 252–4. Springer-Verlag, Vienna.

Garland, A. J. M. and Mann, J. A. (1974). Attempts to infect pigs with Coxsackie virus type B5. *Journal of Hygiene*, **73**, 85–96.

Graves, J. H. (1973). Serological relationship of swine vesicular disease virus and Coxsackie B5 virus. *Nature*, **245**, 314–15.

Hanson, R. P. and McMillan, B. (1990). Vesicular stomatitis virus. In *Virus infection of ruminants*, (ed. Z. Dinter and B. Morein, pp. 381–91. Elsevier, Amsterdam.

Kitching, R. P. (1992). The application of biotechnology to the control of foot-and-mouth disease virus. *British Veterinary Journal*, **148**, 375–88.

Lippmann, D. (1952). Human conjunctivitis due to Newcastle disease virus of fowls. *American Journal of Ophthalmology*, **35**, 1021–8.

Minor, P. D. and Bell, E. J. Picornaviridae. In *Topley & Wilson's principles of bacteriology, virology and immunity*, (8th edn), Vol. 4,. *Virology*, (ed. L. H. Collier and H. L. Timbury), p. 340. Edward Arnold, London.

Nardelli, L. *et al.* (1968). A foot-and-mouth disease syndrome in pigs caused by an enterovirus. *Nature*, **219**, 1275–6.

Patterson, W. C., Mott, L. O., and Jenney, E. W. (1958). A study of vesicular stomatitis in man. *Journal of the American Veterinary Medicine Association*, **133**, 57–62.

Pedersden, K. A., Sadasiv, E. C., Chang P. W., and Yates, V. J. (1990). Detection of antibody to avian viruses in human populations. *Epidemiology and Infection*, **104**, 519–25.

Powell, J. A. (1984). Studies on human antibodies to Newcastle disease virus. *Dissertation Abstract International*, **44**, 3662B.

Radostits, O. M., Blood, D. C., and Gray, C. C. (1994). *Veterinary medicine*, (8th edn). Baillière Tindall, London.

Reif, J. S. *et al.* (1987). Epizootic vesicular stomatitis in Colorado, 1982: infection in occupational risk groups. *American Journal of Tropical Medicine and Hygiene*, **36**, 177–82.

Robson, J. and Dalsgaard, H. (1994). Foot and mouth disease in the European Community. *State Veterinary Journal*, **4**, 1–3.

Rodrigues, J. J. *et al.* (1983). Isolation of Chandipura virus from the blood in acute encephalopathy syndrome. *Indian Journal of Medical Research*, **77**, 303–7.

Sellers, R. F. and Herniman, K. A. J. (1974). The airborne excretion by pigs of swine vesicular disease virus. *Journal of Hygiene*, **72**, 61–5.

Sellers, R. F., Donaldson, A. I., and Herniman, K. A. J. (1970). Inhalation, persistence and dispersal of foot-and-mouth disease virus by man. *Journal of Hygiene*, **68**, 565–73.

Suhr Rasmussen, E. (1968). Mund-og klovsyge hos mennesket. *Ugeskrift for Laeger*, **130**, 1619.

Tesh, R. B., Chaniotis, B. N., Peralta, P. H., and Johnson, K. M. (1974). Ecology of viruses isolated from Panamian phlebotomine sandflies. *American Journal of Tropical Medicine and Hygiene*, **23**, 258–69.

Tesh, R., Saidi, S., Javadian, E., Loh, P., and Nadim, A. (1977). Isfahan virus, a new *Vesiculovirus* infecting humans, gerbils and sandflies in Iran. *American Journal of Tropical Medicine and Hygiene*, **26**, 299–306.

Tesh, R. B. *et al.* (1987). Natural infection of humans, animals, and phlebotomine sandflies with the Alagoas serotype of vesicular stomatitis virus in Colombia. *American Journal of Tropical Medicine and Hygiene*, **36**, 653–61.

Wisniewski, J. and Jankowska, J. (1968). Symptomless infection of men with foot-and-mouth disease virus. *Bulletin of the Veterinary Institute in Pulawy*, **12**, 15–18.

Zhang, G., Wilsden, G., Knowles, N. J., and McCauley, J. W. (1993). Complete nucleotide sequence of coxsackie B5 virus and its relationship to swine vesicular disease virus. *Journal of General Virology*, **74**, 845–53.

30 HANTAVIRUSES

J. Clement, P. Mc Kenna, G. van der Groen, A. Vaheri, and C. J. Peters

SUMMARY

Hantavirus (HTV) is one of the recently discovered (1977) aetiological agents of acute viral haemorrhagic fever, and belongs as such to the group of 'emerging viruses' such as Ebola (1977), Guanarito (1991), and Sabia viruses (1994). HTV is the newest described genus in the Bunyaviridae family, and the only genus in that family that is *not* arthropod-borne, but transmitted by murid rodents.

At least 10 distinct serotypes have now been isolated, and seven more have been genetically characterized (Table 30.1). Of these 17 types of hantaviruses at least eight have been shown to have a clinical significance: Hantaan (HTN) (1977), Seoul (SEO) (1982), Puumala (PUU) (1984), Dobrava (DOB) (1992), Sin Nombre virus (or Four Corners) (SNV) (1993), New York (NYV) (1994), Black Canal Creek (BCC) (1994) and Bayou (BAY) (1995). Each 'serotype' has its own principal rodent vector, its own geographic distribution and its own more or less specific clinical expression. Several other hantaviruses are being evaluated for their public health significance. The majority of HTV serotypes have the kidney as the chief target organ, hence the commonly used official WHO denomination 'haemorrhagic fever with renal syndrome' (HFRS). Thus, acute renal failure in the context of a 'flu-like' illness, particularly when accompanied by thrombocytopenia and/or eye symptoms, should evoke the diagnosis. However, Sin Nombre virus (SNV), isolated after a 1993 epidemic in the United States, seems to affect primarily the lungs, where it causes an often lethal form of adult respiratory distress syndrome, now called hantavirus pulmonary syndrome (HPS). The three other 'SNV-like' viruses NYV, BCC, and BAY, seem also to target primarily the human lung, whereas the newly discovered (1994) European strain Tula (TUL), has no known pathogenicity so far.

Infected rodents remain apparently healthy, but have a probably life-long capacity to shed infectious HTV in their excreta. Recent data point to the growing importance of the wild rat as a vector for hitherto unrecognized forms of hantavirus disease (HTVD) on a worldwide scale. Man is the only known disease end-point of infection, and transmission occurs mainly via inhalation of aerosolized viral particles in open field or in laboratory conditions. Diagnosis can be secured through serological demonstration of specific HTV antibodies. Newer techniques for viral nucleic acid or antigen detection in human and rodent tissues by PCR genotyping or immunohistochemistry have recently been introduced.

Except for intravenous ribavirin in some forms, there is no virus-specific therapy for these diseases, but acute dialysis and/or mechanical ventilation may be indicated in severe cases. Vaccines based on inactivated virus or vectored recombinant viral genes are in development or in field trial phases.

INTRODUCTION

Until 1993, hantavirus disease (HTVD) could be considered as the prototype of a 'new' viral affliction: unknown by many physicians, ill-known even by many virologists, HTVD was considered a rare, somewhat arcane zoonosis with an exotic flavour, being primarily of interest to nephrologists and rodent specialists. However, explosive fresh evidence in 1993 of epidemics in Europe and particularly in the United States has focused worldwide attention on these viruses. It became clear that we were dealing with a rapidly expanding viral zoonosis of global concern.

During these recent epidemics, it also became apparent that physicians were confronted not with a 'new' virus, altered by point mutations and/or genetic reassortment (as can be seen in influenza or in rotaviruses), but rather with an agent having an already archaic presence in its rodent vectors, which had surfaced due to ecological disturbances in the local rodent population (Kilbourne 1990; Childs *et al.* 1994; Hjelle *et al.* 1994a, 1995d; Spiropoulou *et al.* 1994). Strictly speaking, it is better to refer to the recent hantaviral outbreaks not as a 'new' disease, but rather as a 'newly emerging disease', or as a 'newly recognized disease' (Clement *et al.* 1997).

Table 30.1 Major hantavirus serotypes[a] in chronological order of isolation

Hantavirus serotype (year + reference)	Main rodent vector (geographical spread)	Human illness (type of spread)
1. Thottapalayam (TPM)[b] (1971; Carey *et al.* 1971)	*Suncus murinus* (shrew) (?) (India)	Not recorded
2. Hantaan 76–118 (HTN) (1977; H. W. Lee *et al.* 1978), (1994; Avsic-Zupanc *et al.* 1994)	*Apodemus agrarius* (field mouse) (Asia, eastern Russia and southern Europe) (Slovenia)	Severe: KHF, EHF, HFRS (rural)
3. Prospect Hill (PH) (1982; P. W. Lee *et al.* 1982)	*Microtus pennsylvanicus* (meadow vole) (USA) and *Microtus* sp. (Russia)	Not recorded
4. Seoul (SEO) (1982; H. W. Lee *et al.* 1982; G. Song 1982*b*)	*Rattus norvegicus* (brown rat) (worldwide)	Intermediate HFRS (urban and rural)
5. Puumala (PUU) and *et al.* (POZ-M1) (1984; Niklasson and LeDuc 1984) (1990; Diglisic *et al.* 1994) (Chumakov *et al.* 1981) (Kariwa *et al.* 1995)	*Clethrionomys glareolus* (red bank vole) (Eurasian continent) *Mus musculus* (house mouse) (Serbia) *C. rutilus* (western Russia)[c] *C. rufocanus* (northern Japan)[c]	Mild: NE, HTVD (rural) Severe HFRS NE Not recorded
6. Thailand (THAI) (1985; Elsell *et al.* 1985)	*Bandicota indica* (bandicoot) (Thailand)	Not recorded
7. Dobrava (DOB) (1992; Avsic-Zupanc *et al.* 1992) (1992; Gligic *et al.* 1992)	*Apodemus flavicollis* (yellow necked field mouse) (ex-Yugoslavia)	Very severe HFRS (rural?)
8. Sin Nombre virus (SNV) (1993; Elliott *et al.* 1994) (1993; Schmaljohn *et al.* 1995*a*)	*Peromyscus maniculatus* (deer mouse) (south-western USA)	Often lethal HPS
9. Tula (TUL)[c] (Plyusnin *et al.* 1994)	*Microtus arvalis* (common vole) *Microtus rossiameridionalis* (Russia, Czechia, and Slovakia)	Not recorded
10. New York (NYV) (1994; J. W. Song *et al.* 1994)	*Peromyscus leucopus* (white-footed mouse) (eastern USA, Canada)	HPS
11. El Moro Canyon (ELMC)[c] (Hjelle *et al.* 1994*d*)	*Reithrodontomys megalotis* (western harvest mouse) (USA, Mexico, Canada)	Not recorded
12. Black Creek Canal (BCC) (1994; Rollin *et al.* 1995)	*Sigmodon hispidus* (cotton rat) (eastern and southern USA to Venezuela, Peru)	HPS
13. Rio Segundo (RIOS)[c] (Hjelle *et al.* 1995*a*)	*Reithrodontomys mexicanus* (?) (Mexican harvest mouse) (South America, Costa Rica, Mexico)	Not recorded
14. Bayou (BAY)[c] (Morzunov *et al.* 1995) (Torrez-Martinez and Hjelle 1995)	*Oryzomys palustris* (rice rat) (Louisiana)	HPS
15. Isla Vista (ILV)[c] (W. Song *et al.* 1995*a*)	*Microtus californicus* (California meadow vole) (California, Oregon, Baja Cal., Mexico)	Not recorded
16. Bloodland Lake (BLLL)[c] (W. Song *et al.* 1995*b*)	*Microtus ochrogaster* (prairie vole) (Mid-West USA, southern Canada)	Not recorded
17. Rio Mamore (RMV)[c] (Hjelle *et al.* 1996)	*Oligoryzomys microtis* (small-eared rice rat) (Bolivia)	Not recorded

EHF, Epidemic haemorrhagic fever; HFRS, haemorrhagic fever with renal syndrome (current WHO denomination); HPS, hantavirus pulmonary syndrome; HTVD, hantavirus disease (proposed new common denomination); KHF, Korean haemorrhagic fever; NE, nephropathia epidemica.

[a] A strain of a 'serotype' is neutralized to more than 50 per cent in plaque reduction neutralization tests (PRNT) by homologous antisera. A 'serotype' is thus defined as having no cross-reactions in PRNT with other serotypes or having a homologous to heterologous titre ratio of >1/16 in both directions.

[b] TPM was first considered a novel arbovirus and only recently genetically confirmed as a distinct hantavirus (Xiao *et al.* 1994). For the serotypes 1 through 8 listed here, a perfectly similar division in eight distinct lineages was found by polymerase chain reaction (PCR) genotyping (see text and Fig. 30.1).

[c] To date, these viruses have not been isolated, but most often only characterized by molecular genetic analysis.

(?) = uncertainty about this species being the primary host (see text).

HISTORY

HTV epidemics have been described under various (mostly geographic) denominations, resulting in up to 60 synonyms (Gajdusek 1962). HTVD has an impressive military past, going back probably as far as the American Civil War and the First World War (Brown 1916; Bradford 1916), throughout the Second World War (Stuhlfauth 1943) and other armed conflicts (Fischer-Hoch and McCormick, 1985; Clement 1987*a*).

Paradoxically, Western medicine first 'discovered' HTVD under its severe Far-Eastern form, later called 'Korean haemorrhagic fever' (KHF), during yet another armed conflict in the early 1950s, the Korean War. US Army physicians were suddenly confronted with an up to then unknown acute febrile illness with multiorgan dysfunction (mainly shock, acute renal failure, and haemorrhage), with a mortality rate between 10 and 15 per cent, and affecting over 3000 United Nations troops (Earle 1954). Despite an enormous investigative effort by a special Hemorrhagic Fever Commission of the US Army, it was not until 1976 that H. W. Lee, P. W. Lee, and K. Johnson discovered a virus-specific antigen in the lungs of a Korean striped field mouse (*Apodemus agrarius coreae*), which subsequently led to the isolation and characterization of the responsible agent in 1977, the same year as Ebola virus was first identified (H. W. Lee *et al.* 1978). This first prototype agent was called Hantaan (HTN), after the river which runs near to the famous 38th parallel between North and South Korea, where most of the battles were fought, but also where most of the KHF cases were recorded, and where the HTN-infected rodents were trapped. Thanks to the diligent efforts of the Hemorrhagic Fever Commission, however, an unique collection of more than 600 sera from 245 soldiers admitted with KHF between December 1951 and August 1954, was preserved for posterity, lyophilized in glass ampoules, and labelled with the patient's name, date of onset of disease, and of sampling. This epidemiological treasury, neatly packed in cardboard boxes in three metal trunks, was reopened in 1990, rehydrated and tested for IgM- and IgG-specific antibodies to Hantaan (HTN) and other hantaviral serotypes. Of these patients, 94 per cent (230/245) possessed HTN antibodies, and most sera contained high titred IgM on admission (LeDuc *et al.* 1990). Thus the clinical diagnosis of KHF in hundreds of patients was confirmed by modern and reliable serological techniques more than 40 years after samples were taken, a unique accomplishment in serology.

A further important contribution in recognition in the early 1960s of HTVD as a worldwide problem was the extensive bibliographic and comparative research of D. C. Gajdusek (1962), relating disease in one part of the world with that in another. With the isolation of new serotypes from the early 1980s onward (Table 30.1), allowing serological comparison between proven human cases with Scandinavian so-called 'nephropathia epidemica' (NE) or with Asian KHF, it finally became evident that both infections were caused by an antigenically similar, but not identical HTV (H. W. Lee *et al.* 1979; Svedmyr *et al.* 1980). In a disease bedevilled by a multiple terminology, the revised bibliography of Gajdusek *et al.* (1987) was all the more valuable. A general denomination such as 'hantavirus disease' (HTVD) (Desmyter *et al.* 1984) could now end the confusion. Indeed the hitherto official WHO denomination of 'haemorrhagic fever with renal syndrome' (HFRS) is more and more confusing to the clinician, since 'haemorrhagic' complications are rare or absent in the European and the current American forms of HTVD, whereas a 'renal syndrome' is rather the exception than the rule in the American forms.

THE AGENT

MORPHOLOGY, MOLECULAR BIOLOGY, AND TAXONOMY

Hantaviruses exhibit somewhat greater polymorphism than the other members of the Bunyaviridae family. Round and oval forms are most frequently visualized in electron microscopy, having a mean diameter of 122 nm, but with large variations in size from 78 to 210 nm (Tao *et al.* 1985, 1987). The virus is lipid-enveloped, with regular hollow surface projections. Like other lipid-enveloped viruses, HTVs are susceptible to most disinfectants, e.g. phenolics, dilute hypochlorite solutions, detergents, 70 per cent alcohol, and most general-purpose household disinfectants.

HTVs possess a tripartite, single-stranded, negative-sense RNA genome. These three segments are designated as small (S), medium (M), and large (L), and encode respectively the nucleocapsid (N) protein of 50–53 kDa, the two envelope proteins (G1 and G2) of 65–74 kDa and 55–60 kDa respectively, and a virion-associated polymerase of ± 200 kDa (Schmaljohn *et al.* 1985, 1986, 1987). G1 and G2 are highly glycosylated and have an important role in inducing neutralizing antibodies, used in the plaque reduction neutralization test (PRNT), which is the most sensitive serological technique for differentiating HTVs. Based on PRNT and other serological relationships, at least five distinct groups had been proposed until recently, each carried by a specific main rodent vector, and each having its own geographical distribution: Hantaan (HTN), Seoul (SEO), Thailand (THAI), Puumala

(PUU), and Prospect Hill (PH) (Chu *et al.* 1994) (Table 30.1).

Recent advances in genetic molecular biology have confirmed this classification: by comparing partial nucleotide sequences of a 333 base pair (bp) region which was amplified from the medium (M) genome segment by reverse transcriptase polymerase chain reaction, (RT–PCR), a consensus phylogenetic tree for 30 hantaviruses could be constructed (Xiao *et al.* 1994), which showed the same five lineages (HTN, SEO, THAI, PUU, and PH) as the serotypes already known before (Fig. 30.1). Moreover, a sixth distinct lineage was found (Xiao *et al.* 1994), close to, but not identical with HTN, represented by Dobrava (DOB) virus, isolated from an *Apodemus flavicollis* in Slovenia (Avsic-Zupanc *et al.* 1992) and isolated also from patients in Serbia under the name Belgrade (Gligic *et al.* 1992).

Molecular genetic analysis has proved to be a valuable tool, complementing and extending serology for classification of new hantaviruses. It is also striking to see the utility of this analysis in demonstrating the similar topology of the virus phylogenetic dendrogram to that of the rodent hosts. This provides strong evidence of the close and ancient relationship of the virus to the rodent, and confirms again the important role of the rodent–man link in HTV disease.

By amplifying in RT–PCR a 241 bp region of the small (S) segment of Thottapalayam (TPH) virus, a dis-

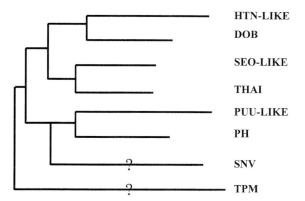

HTN-LIKE

DOB

SEO-LIKE

THAI

PUU-LIKE

PH

? SNV

? TPM

Fig. 30.1 Phylogram summarizing in a very schematic way the data of 32 different HTV isolates. This is a consensus tree based mainly on 100 bootstrap replications of the 333 bp M segment nucleotide sequences (from Xiao *et al.* 1994, with permission from the author). For the sake of completion, TPM and the recently isolated SNV have been added. Since different techniques have been used for their genotyping (see text), comparative branch lengths of TPM and SNV cannot be used, hence the question marks. Vertical distances are for visual clarity only. The 32 isolates have been grouped into eight different serotypes (HTN, DOB, SEO, THAI, PUU, PH, SNV, TPM). For the explanation of abbreviations, see Table 30.1).

tantly related HTV isolated in 1971 from a shrew captured in India (Carey *et al.* 1971), a seventh lineage was found, different from 13 other HTV isolates examined by the same technique (Xiao *et al.* 1994). It is interesting to note that TPH is not only genetically distinct from all other known HTVs, but that also its geographic origin (India) and its host (an insectivore rather than a murid rodent) are totally different from other known hantaviruses (Table 30.1, Fig. 30.1).

The most spectacular demonstration of the possibilities of genetic molecular biology, however, was given during the outbreak of the mysterious epidemic of acute respiratory failure in south-western USA, later to be called 'hantavirus pulmonary syndrome' (HPS). A mere 3 months after the discovery of the first fatal HPS cases, Nichol *et al.* (1993) submitted to *Science* a report, describing part of the G2-encoding M genome of viral RNA extracted from human *and* rodent tissues, and amplified by RT–PCR. Thus, almost from the start a genetic link was made to the responsible rodent vector, the deer mouse *Peromyscus maniculatus*. Nucleotide sequences established for 278 bp differed from that of any of the known HTVs by at least 30 per cent and indicated that the 'HPS agent' was a novel HTV, representing a new eighth lineage, first called four Corners virus (FCV) or Muerto Canyon virus (MCV), and later coined Sin Nombre virus (SNV) (Table 30.1, Fig. 30.1). Subsequent complete sequencing of all three RNA segments has shown that each segment of the new virus is independent of previously known hantaviruses and occupies the same evolutionary topology in relation to the other known viruses, demonstrating that SNV is not a re-assortant virus (Hjelle *et al.* 1994a; Spiropoulou *et al.* 1994) Further PCR-typing confirmed this genetic diversity of SNV, with geographic clines of distinct genotypes all across the United States, suggesting that HPS and associated viruses had existed in North America for many years (Childs *et al.* 1994; Hjelle *et al.* 1994a,b,c 1995d; Spiropoulou *et al.* 1994).

The surprising finding of a new North American HTV was strengthened very quickly by the description of almost identical M-genome nucleotide sequences in samples from *Peromyscus maniculatus*, collected in 1983 (Nerurkar *et al.* 1993) and the retrospective diagnosis from autopsy tissues of a HPS case who died from respiratory failure in 1983 (Zaki *et al.* 1994). All this was achieved before even the responsible agent was actually isolated in November 1993 (Elliott *et al.* 1994; Schmaljohn *et al.* 1995a): a genetic molecular *tour de force*, that was aptly described as 'virology without a virus' (Marshall and Stone 1993). This outbreak of highly lethal adult respiratory distress syndrome (ARDS) in relatively young, previously healthy persons thus launched in the United States one of the most intensive, medical sleuth programmes in recent history.

As of August 1997, a total of 172 cases of HPS have been reported in United States, with an overall mortality of ±45.3 per cent (ProMED-mail on 4 Sept'97 12.00 pm).

Four other new human pathogenic HTVs have been identified in the Americas, distinct from SNV. Three were inferred from genetic sequences detected by RT–PCR in lung tissue from deceased HPS patients. One of these cases succumbed to HPS after a probable exposure on Shelter Island, New York, i.e. outside the normal habitation range of the suspected rodent vector *P. maniculatus*. M genomic RT–PCR analysis of necropsy lung tissue differed by only 1.1 per cent from the amplicon obtained from white-footed mice (*P. leucopus*), trapped on Shelter Island, but both amplicons differed by 23 per cent from 'classical' SNV (Hjelle *et al.* 1995*b,c*). Indeed, a distinctive non-SNV HTV could later be isolated from white-footed mice, and is now called New York virus (NYV) (J. W. Song *et al.* 1994).

Another patient died in shock, ARDS, and acute renal failure (ARF) in Louisiana, again a region where *P. maniculatus* is not present (Khan *et al.* 1995). Although this virus has not been isolated so far, sequence analysis and expression of the N protein reveal it to be a new hantavirus, now referred to as Bayou (BAY), and related to, but distinct from SNV (Morzunov *et al.* 1995). Genotypic comparison with RT–PCR products obtained from rice rats (*Oryzomys palustris*), formerly trapped in southern Louisiana,

pointed to these rodents as the most likely natural reservoir (Torrez-Martinez and Hjelle 1995).

A third case died in Brazil with classic HPS, and limited sequence analysis of RNA extracted from the lung and amplified by RT–PCR showed the presence of a distinct virus (Khabbaz, 1994).

A fourth patient recovered from hypotension, ARDS, and ARF in Florida, again a region outside the normal biosphere of *P. maniculatus*. This last patient remained serologically inconclusive when tested against SNV antigen, but 12 (13 per cent) of 90 cotton rats (*Sigmodon hispidus*), trapped in his living area, were HTV seropositive. PCR genotyping from their lungs resulted in nucleotide sequences related to, but distinct from, SNV and BAY virus (MMWR 1994*a*). Once the virus, called Black Creek Canal virus (BCC), was isolated and used as antigen, IgM serology of this patient became positive (Rollin *et al.* 1995). Interestingly, a slight cross-reactivity was also noted in recombinant Western blot format between the G1 antigen of BCC and SNV (Hjelle *et al.* 1994*b*). Extensive sequence analysis has confirmed it as a new species of HTV with no evidence of re-assortment with SNV or BAY (Ravkov *et al.* 1995). Thus, rapidly accumulating evidence points to different HTV agents and different New World murid rodent vectors inducing HPS (Fig. 30.2).

Finally, several not previously described HTV were discovered by PCR cloning in the European common voles *Microtus arvalis* and *M. rossiameridionalis*, first trapped in the Tula region, south of Moscow (Plyusnin

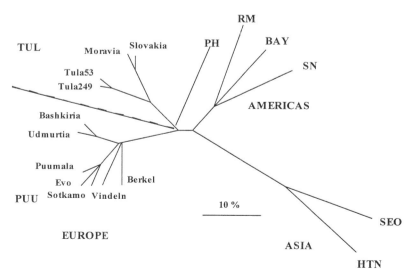

Fig. 30.2 Phylogenetic tree of hantaviruses based on S segment nucleotides, with their geographic distribution. PUU, Puumala virus; TUL, Tula; PH, Prospect Hill; RM, hantavirus carried by *Reithrodontomys megalotis* (western harvest mouse) now called El Moro Canyon virus (ELMC); BAY, Bayou; SN, Sin Nombre; SEO, Seoul; HTN, Hantaan. Tula53 and Tula249 are examples of two strains derived from the same location. Other names refer to other European PUU and TUL hantavirus strains. The bar length indicates the approximate length of a 10 per cent difference in the S segment nucleotide sequences.

et al. 1994), later also in Moravia, Czech Republic (Plyusnin *et al.* 1995) and in Slovakia (Sibold *et al.* 1995). All these central European HTV appeared related to, but distinct from PUU, and were designated as Tula virus (TUL) (Table 30.1, Fig. 30.2). So far, TUL has no known human pathogenecity, but a high degree of serological cross-reaction has been observed between TUL and PUU nucleocapsid antigen, both for IgM and for IgG, so that human TUL infections could have been incorrectly diagnosed as PUU in the past (Niklasson *et al.* unpublished observation). Moreover, it is of great interest that TUL maps on the phylogenetic tree close to (non-pathogenic) Prospect Hill (PH) and the other (very pathogenic) American HTVs (Fig. 30.2) (Clement *et al.* 1997).

GROWTH

HTVs are notoriously difficult to isolate and to grow in culture; several blind passages are frequently necessary, and the results are difficult to judge since a cytopathogenic effect (CPE) is most often lacking. This is even more true for PUU isolations where supernatants are often of low titres. Moreover, the viraemic phase seems to be very short, particularly in PUU infections, explaining perhaps the frequently negative isolation attempts in PUU infections, even when PCR products clearly indicate the presence of a PUU-like RNA (Pilaski *et al.* 1995). Thus, diagnosis has to rely on serology or on newer techniques (see p. 343–4) (Clement *et al.* 1995). The prototype Korean isolate Hantaan (HTN) was first adapted to tissue culture by French *et al.* (1981) using the A-549 cell line, derived from a human lung carcinoma. Growth in Vero E6 culture, a continuous kidney cell line from the African green monkey, resulted in development of a satisfactory plaque-reduction neutralization test (PRNT) and sufficiently high titred virus growth for further characterization (McCormick *et al.* 1982).

TRANSMISSION

HTV is carried to man by excretions and aerosols, consisting of infected respiratory and urinary droplets from apparently healthy rodent carriers, who excrete the virus in saliva, in urine, in faeces, and from their lungs. The survival time of HTVs in the environment in liquids or aerosols or in a dried state is not known.

Whereas most of proven HTVD patients actually can recall sighting of rodents, both in Europe (Clement *et al.* 1994*d*, 1996) and in the United States (Zeitz *et al.* 1995), a physical contact with rodents is almost never mentioned (Dournon *et al.* 1984), except in laboratory conditions (Desmyter *et al.* 1983). Epidemiological studies in farm workers in China (Xu *et al.* 1985) and

in shepherds and woodcutters in Greece (Antoniadis *et al.* 1987*b*) revealed a high infection rate among individuals sleeping on the ground, a finding that was confirmed in a case-control study among US military in the region of Ulm (Southern Germany), after an 1990 outbreak nephropathia epidemica during a winter field exercise (Clement *et al.* 1996). In the United States most cases are rural in origin and often have a history of agricultural activities or cleaning outbuildings; there is a correlation with increased rodent populations locally (Zeitz *et al.* 1995). Infections may well be acquired indoors in many cases because of the propensity of the major reservoir, *Peromyscus maniculatus*, to enter houses (Childs *et al.* 1994). On a worldwide scale, the same may be true for the wild rat (*Rattus norvegicus*), an often underestimated source of indoor HTV infections (G. Song *et al.* 1982*b*; Clement *et al.* 1994*d*; McKenna *et al.* 1994).

Intercage airborne transmission of HTN virus between laboratory cages of *Apodemus* sp., housed 1–4 m apart, was demonstrated by H. W. Lee *et al.* (1981), whereas Gavrilovskaya *et al.* (1990) showed airborne transmission of a PUU-like virus between cages of bank voles 1.5 m apart. In a laboratory setting, 12–16 week old Wistar rats appeared susceptible to aerosol exposure of extremely small amounts of HTN, SEO, and PUU viruses (Nuzum *et al.* 1988). The high aerosol infectivity of hantaviruses requires special precautions in the virology laboratory, particularly if viral concentrates or infected animals are involved. The substantial mortality of SNV infections has led to the recommendation that the latter be performed only at biosafety level 4 (MMWR 1994*b*). In addition, laboratory manipulations involving the introduction of rat-derived immunocytomas or hybridomas originating from HTV-infected rat colonies into HTV-free colonies has also been shown to represent an efficient means of HTV transmission among laboratory animals (McKenna *et al.* 1992).

Contamination of food (particularly by wild rats) and direct contact with rodent excreta through skin abrasions may be another occasional route of infection (Kopela and Lähdevirta 1978, Xu *et al.* 1985). Person to person transmission, or infection of personnel nursing HTVD cases, including HPS, has never been documented so far. The fact that outbreaks of HTVD can be extremely localized in circumscribed foci or even microfoci (Clement *et al.* 1996) has prompted the concept of a 'place disease' (Smadel 1953), although it must be recognized that 90 per cent of cases are solitary. There is an important need to understand the dynamics of rodents and viral infection in rodents that leads to these findings.

Interestingly, HTV isolates were also obtained from mites and/or fleas parasitizing *Apodemus* and *Clethrio-*

nomys species in China (Chen and Qiu, 1993). However, the role of these arthropods in the transmission of HTVD is not clear, and to our knowledge this finding has not been reported so far from the West.

PATHOPHYSIOLOGY

Remarkably little is known of the ways by which HTVs can cause multisystem illness and—at least in some severe cases—a multiple organ dysfunction syndrome (MODS) or even a multiorgan failure. It is clear, however, that HTVD is mainly a *microvascular* disease, and that the endothelium is the most extensively involved cell type, somehow leading to vascular hyper-permeability or 'capillary leakage' as the principal pathophysiological finding (Zaki *et al.* 1995). Endothelial susceptibility was showed in laboratory conditions in infant mice infected with HTN (Kurata *et al.* 1983; McKee *et al.* 1985), in bank voles experimentally infected with PUU (Yanagihara *et al.* 1985), and in human umbilical vein endothelial cell cultures inoculated with several HTV strains (Yanagihara and Silverman 1990). Endothelin, a potent vasoconstrictor produced by endothelial cells, may contribute to the transient forms of acute renal failure seen in patients with NE, in whom elevated plasma levels were reported (Forslund *et al.* 1993). Moreover, in the highly lethal hantavirus pulmonary syndrome (HPS), immuno-histochemical (IHC) staining showed the presence of hantaviral antigen mainly in the endothelium of lung capillaries, providing another important pathogenetic link (Nichol *et al.* 1993; Zaki *et al.* 1995).

The disease process itself is probably immunological, with a high level of cellular immune reaction, leading to a so-called state of systemic inflammatory response syndrome (SIRS), recently identified by critical care specialists as an early, but often life-threatening reaction to a variety of severe clinical insults (Anonymous 1992). Lymphocytes play a key role, and a decrease (Guang *et al.* 1994) as well as an increase (Nolte *et al.* 1995) of T lymphocytes in the acute phase has been described. The CD4 : CD8 ratio is generally decreased, however, and the presence in the circulation of atypical cells with the aspect of immunoblasts has been considered typical for the recent HPS cases (Hjelle *et al.* 1995*d*; Nolte *et al.* 1995; Zaki *et al.* 1995). There are abundant CD4+ and CD8+ lymphocytes present in the lung interstitium, but there are few polymorphonuclear cells, and there is relatively little necrosis of pneumocytes or other cells as often seen in 'conventional' ARDS (Zaki *et al.* 1995). The lymphocytes may induce migration of macrophages and other inflammatory cells, resulting in the production of cytokines such as tumour necrosis factor-α, (TNF-α), IL-1, IL-2, and γ-interferon, which may in their turn increase vascular permeability. Soluble interleukin-2 receptor (sIL-2 R) levels in sera or plasma of Chinese HTVD patients were in concordance with the degree of illness, i.e. highest during the oliguric phase (Huang *et al.* 1994). Increased levels of pro-inflammatory cytokines have recently been reported in NE cases (Linderholm *et al.* 1995).

We have recently documented very high serum nitrate levels, a measure of nitric oxide (NO), in PUU infected NE patients, showing a high and significant correlation with the Acute Physiological And Chronic Health Evaluation (APACHE II) score and with serum creatinine levels, and an inverse correlation with platelet counts (Groeneveld *et al.* 1995). NO is a highly reactive vasodilatory agent, mainly produced in endothelial cells after stimulation with (amongst other) pro-inflammatory cytokines, and has been implicated in vasodilatation of septic shock (Gomez-Jimenez *et al.* 1995). The highest nitrate levels were found in the two most severe cases, both complicated with ARDS, suggesting a possible role of NO in the, as yet ill-understood, pathogenesis of HPS.

THE HOSTS

THE RODENT VECTOR

In the literature, HTVD is often exclusively mentioned as a rodent-borne disease with strong geographical delineations. In fact, HTVs infect many different animals in nature and have a worldwide distribution. However, it is unknown whether any of the animals other than the natural rodent hosts (Table 30.1) are epidemiologically significant. The correspondence of viral phylogeny and rodent phylogeny argue that the relationship is a close one, and the finding that SNV RNA is less often detectable in antibody-positive animals other than the natural rodent reservoir suggests that persistence may not occur in many of these other infections (Childs *et al.* 1994). In a recent review of available data on this topic, we listed evidence of HTV infection in two different classes of animals (mammals and birds), eight different orders, 24 different families, and a total of 164 different species (Clement *et al.* 1994*c*).

Birds have been described in Russia and Korea (Baek and Lee 1993) as HTV seropositive, and a positive isolation of HTV from a yellow-throated bunting (*Emberizia elegans*) has even been obtained (Slonova *et al.* 1992). Bats (Kim *et al.* 1994) and particularly cats have also been named recently as potential HTV vectors: in 200 feline serum samples from Austria, an IFA seroprevalence for PUU and/or for HTN antibodies of 5 per cent was found (Nowotny 1994). The significance of these findings for human HTVD is still unclear: to our knowledge, excretion of infectious virus has not been documented yet in these animals. In a recent epidemiological study in The Netherlands, no evidence of PUU antibodies was found in a total of 2025 domestic animals, including 385 dogs and 200 cats (Groen *et al.* 1995). Nevertheless, cat ownership has been described as an epidemiological risk factor for developing HTVD in China (Xu *et al.* 1987). Insectivores such as shrews (Carey *et al.* 1971) and moles (Verhagen *et al.* 1986; Clement *et al.* 1994*c*) can also be infected with HTV, and we registered serologically proven NE cases in Belgium of patients who allegedly became ill after catching a *Neomys fodiens* (water shrew) near a fish pond, or after killing a mole in the garden (unpublished observations).

It is clear, however, that rodents are by far the most important vector for HTV transmission to man (see p. 345). HTVs do not cause apparent illness in these reservoir hosts, which remain infected carriers for life. After experimental PUU infection in bank voles, viruses were detected in the blood, kidneys, liver, urinary bladder, salivary glands, thymus, brown fat, brain, spinal cord, and particularly in the lungs (Gavrilovskaya *et al.* 1990; Yanagihara 1990). The abundance of viral antigen in virtually all organs is found despite an apparently life-long presence of humoral antibodies, also including neutralizing antibodies, as evidenced by the results of plaque reduction neutralization tests (PRNT) (LeDuc *et al.* 1986). This immunological paradox is the hallmark of HTV infection in most, if not all rodent species, and explains the capacity to transmit virus horizontally to other rodents and to man. However, the duration of virus shedding and the period of maximum infectivity remain largely unknown.

HUMANS: ENDPOINT OF AN OTHERWISE INAPPARENT INFECTION

Incubation time is difficult to estimate, since physical contact with rodents is rather an exception than the rule (see p. 338), but is mostly between 4 and 42 days (Zeitz *et al.* 1995). The clinical symptomatology derived from Korean, Russian, and Chinese war literature on HFRS has traditionally been divided in five phases: (1) febrile, (2) hypotensive, (3) oliguric, (4) diuretic, and (5) convalescent (Smadel 1953; Earle 1954). This description is less relevant to the milder European NE forms, and even less so to the severe American HPS forms, but the time framing remains valid for most if not all symptoms:

Febrile phase

Onset is often abrupt and without any prodrome; many patients can situate the exact day and even the

moment of the day when symptoms started. Chills, high fever ($\geq$ 39.5 °C), and weakness are often followed by headache, myalgia, and gastrointestinal disturbances (vomiting and/or diarrhoea). Ophthalmological signs are very specific (e.g. not present in flu) but often 'overlooked': acute myopia, blurred vision, photophobia, eye pain, conjunctival injection, and periorbital oedema. Impaired vision in the initial phase can be present in up to 38 per cent of NE cases (Penalba *et al.* 1994) but has never been mentioned so far in American HPS cases. Acute glaucoma can occur, and we encountered two cases of acute bilateral glaucoma presenting in the early phase of NE (unpublished observations). Severe uni- or bilateral lumbar pain due to swelling of the kidney develops 1 or 2 days later. The triad headache + eye pain + lumbar pain is very suggestive and is poorly, or not at all, relieved by analgesics or NSAIDs. The most important laboratory anomaly found in this early phase—and often a clue to diagnosis—is thrombocytopenia (Van Ypersele and Méry 1989; Duchin *et al.* 1994; Penalba *et al.* 1994; Colson *et al.* 1995), the severity of which is often a prognostic sign of complications to come. Conversely, in milder NE forms thrombocytopenia can be so transient as to normalize within 7 days, and can thus be missed (Colson *et al.* 1995).

Hypotensive phase

Hypotension is exceptional in European NE, occasional in severe HTN-induced Asian cases, and usual in American HPS. There is often a rapid progression to marked proteinuria, which can reach levels of 30 g/l (unpublished observations), but is as a rule transitory after a few days. This transient but heavy proteinuria is, together with the cited ophthalmological signs, important in the differential diagnosis with leptospirosis, which can otherwise perfectly mimic HTVD. Episodes of sinus bradycardia despite the feverish condition (Colson *et al.* 1995), and signs of haemoconcentration due to capillary leakage can also be seen in this period.

Oliguric phase

Renal involvement, with a temporary rise in serum creatinine from scarcely pathological levels (90 μmol/l) up to peak levels as high as 1500 μmol/l, can be seen in most Asian series, but seems less frequent in NE, particularly now that more atypical and/or milder cases are recognized by an increased awareness of the physicians. During the 1993 epidemic in the Ardennes, levels of serum creatinine $\geq$ 150 μmol/l were observed in 75 per cent (40/53) of the Belgian patients (Colson *et al.* 1995), and in only 55 per cent (42/76) of the French patients (Penalba *et al.* 1994). Remission occurs mostly within 2–3 weeks, and is often heralded by the resolution of thrombocytopenia. Except for a prolonged (several months) loss of urinary concentrating ability, a restoration to normal without sequelae is the rule. Slightly impaired kidney function has sporadically been mentioned as a sequel after severe HTN-like cases in the Balkans (Papadimitriou and Antoniadis 1994) but to our knowledge, irrefutable proof of progression to endstage renal failure has never been documented, i.e. with serial kidney biopsies.

In this stage severe haemorrhagic complications can occur in the Asian HTN-induced forms, but are rare (except for petechiae and/or epistaxis) in NE and uncommon in HPS: 'haemorrhagic' fever without haemorrhages.

Diuretic phase

Diuresis heralds renal, and often general, improvement. Important urinary volumes, however, (up to 12 l/day) can further complicate fluid balance and electrolyte disturbances.

Convalescent phase

This can be prolonged with severe postviral asthenia lasting months. We observed long-standing normocytic anaemia in some NE cases, apparently due to deficient erythropoietin synthesis, which is a product of peritubular tissue in the kidney. Since inflammatory interstital nephritis is the main lesion in NE, this may affect primarily the peritubular region (Clement *et al.* 1993).

Specific features of the hantavirus pulmonary syndrome (HPS)

HPS is characterized by a brief prodromal illness consisting of fever, myalgia, and headache which typically last 3–5 days. Gastrointestinal symptoms are common and, like in PUU virus infections, may simulate a surgical condition. Rapidly progressive, non-cardiogenic pulmonary oedema and severe hypotension (systolic BP $\leq$ 85 mmHg) then follow. With current management, about 40 per cent of patients will die within the first 48 hours of hospitalization from uncorrected hypoxia and/or from intractable shock (Duchin *et al.* 1994; Zaki *et al.* 1995). The syndrome differs clinically from that seen with most ARDS patients, although the distinctive findings may not be present at the time of hospitalization in all cases (Butler and Peters 1994; Ketai *et al.* 1994; Hjelle *et al.* 1995d). Clinical haematology values consisting of absolute leucocytosis, relative increase in polymorphonuclear leucocytes, left shift, presence of immunoblasts on smear, and thrombocytopenia are helpful (Hjelle *et al.* 1995d; Nolte *et al.* 1995). Pathological findings consist of minimal or moderate interstitial infiltrates of immunoblasts in the

lung, congestion and interalveolar oedema (Nolte *et al.* 1995; Zaki *et al.* 1995). SNV antigen is abundant in the endothelium of the lung capillaries, but there is no evidence of a viral cytopathic effect nor viral inclusions (Zaki *et al.* 1995), nor is there a genetic explanation as to why this novel virus seems to attack primarily the lungs (Spiropoulou *et al.* 1994). Where the median value of serum creatinine in the first 17 cases described by Duchin *et al.* (1994) was only of 97.2 μmol/l (range 53.4–221), single cases of HPS in Louisiana and Florida, respectively due to Bayou and BCC viruses, also had acute renal failure (ARF), may be due to the fact that a genetically different (non-SNV) HTV was implicated (see p. 337).

HPS appears to differ consistently from 'classical' HFRS due to PUU and HTN viruses, however. The early period of flushing and conjunctival injection is absent, and the permeability changes are virtually confined to the thoracic cavity in HPS. Mild nonoliguric renal failure is commonly seen in SNV infections, but tubular necrosis and oliguria are not usual. Notably, the first indications of severe disease in HPS are manifest by dyspnoea, hypoxia, and pulmonary infiltrates (Duchin *et al.* 1994; Ketai *et al.* 1994) rather than the renal failure seen in HFRS. However, noncardiogenic pulmonary oedema and/or full-blown ARDS is not unique to the American forms of HTVD. During the 1993 outbreak of PUU-induced nephropathia epidemica (NE) in the Belgian Ardennes (Clement *et al.* 1994a), we described seven patients with varying degrees of non-cardiogenic acute respiratory insufficiency and tachypnoea, indistinguishable from ARDS or its less severe form, now called 'acute lung injury' (ALI) (Clement *et al.* 1994b). Heart failure and/or volume expansion could be excluded in all these cases. A similar ALI case during the same NE epidemic was reported from France (Bouly *et al.* 1993). In 1996, two German female patients, both working in the same wool-knitting mill, were described with pulmonary symptoms without kidney involvement. At least one of these presented with all the clinical features suggestive for ALI. In both, nested RT–PCR in serum detected sequences closely related to PUU (Schreiber *et al.* 1996). During the war in Bosnia, a British soldier had to be repatriated after (presumably) a SEO infection. He developed both ARF and severe ALI without signs of fluid overload, prompting intensive ventilation therapy (Stuart *et al.* 1996).

Pulmonary oedema may, of course, be a consequence of volume expansion together with generalized increased capillary permeability, without having the proper (haemodynamic) characteristics of HPS. A majority of the following cases had pulmonary oedema at a time of renal failure, but cardiac and haemodynamic data are often lacking to exclude heart failure:

1. Among severe Chinese forms of HTVD, death in some series has been attributed more frequently to pulmonary oedema (10 fatal cases out of 48) than to haemorrhage (7/48) (Guang *et al.* 1989).

2. The Greek HTN-like isolate *Porogia* virus was obtained from a severely ill soldier with both ARF and ARDS, who had to be ventilated and dialyzed (Antoniadis *et al.* 1987*a*).

3. A German case with PCR products from the urine typical for PUU, was published as a severe non-fatal NE case with lung complications (Pilaski *et al.* 1995). However, the general clinical picture, including generalized oedema, was strongly suggestive for fluid overload, and neither cardiac nor haemodynamic data were given.

DIAGNOSIS

Since most of the clinical signs are atypical, diagnosis should rely on a strong index of suspicion with serological confirmation (Clement *et al.* 1995).

Immunofluorescent assay (IFA) remains for many laboratories the 'gold standard' diagnostic assay for the detection of HTV-specific antibodies. By comparing the titres obtained upon screening with several HTV antigens, IFA can give an indication of the HTV serotype involved in an infection. To obviate the need for P3 biosafety containment, hantaviral antigens can be inactivated by heat (Saluzzo *et al.* 1988), by gamma irradiation (van der Groen *et al.* 1983) or by treatment with β-propionolactone (van der Groen and Elliott 1982). The presence of the HTV-specific antibodies in serum is detected indirectly using a suitable conjugate labelled with fluorescein isothiocyanate (FITC). The assay may be adapted to measure the avidity (functional affinity) of the IgG class of HTV-specific antibodies. It has been reported that this so-called IgG avidity test is up to four times more sensitive than the conventional IgG serology (Hedman *et al.* 1991). Moreover, this test enables an estimation of the moment of infection (whether in humans or rodents) to be made with one single sample. This is possible as low-avidity antibody is generally restricted to the acute or early convalescent phase of illness.

We could also estimate the time of infection with one single serum sample, using enzyme-linked immunosorbent assay (ELISA) for quantification of serum antibodies against group-specific epitopes of HTV glycoproteins and nucleoproteins (Groen *et al.* 1992) and the different classes and subclasses of Ig antibodies formed after infection (Groen *et al.* 1994).

The WHO has recommended that the prototype Hantaan (HTN) virus (isolated from *Apodemus agrarius coreae*, the striped field mouse) and the Puumala (PUU) virus (isolated from *Clethrionomys glareolus*, the

bank vole) should be used as routine screening antigens (WHO report, 1991). However, it has been found that the sensitivity of the IFA assay can still be improved upon if a rat-derived Seoul (SEO) HTV strain is included in the battery of IFA screening antigens (Hinrichsen *et al.* 1993; Clement *et al.* 1994*d*; McKenna *et al.* 1994; Stuart *et al.* 1996). In the Americas, a combination of SEO and SNV would be desirable (Feldmann *et al.* 1993; Ksiazek *et al.* 1995).

Since in man (as in rodents) IgG antibodies seem to persist for life, IFA-seropositivity for IgG may not always reflect a recent infection. Moreover, a diagnostic rise in IgG titres has not always been observed in recent clinical cases. Screening for IgM in IFA being less sensitive (Ivanov *et al.* 1988), IgM enzyme immunoassay (EIA) is now generally accepted as the serologic prerequisite for confirming suspected clinical cases. The newer version of this assay, μ-capture EIA, is so sensitive and specific that, when properly performed, it provides an excellent and inexpensive early diagnostic tool (LeDuc *et al.* 1990; Niklasson *et al.* 1990; Ksiazek *et al.* 1995). Similar techniques have been reported to be reliable such as complex-trapping blocking EIA (CTB-EIA) (Groen *et al.* 1989), and μ-capture EIA with recombinant nucleoproteins expressed in *E. coli* (Zöller *et al.* 1991). In the United States, autopsy tissue RNA was reverse-transcribed, amplified by PCR, and ligated to use for expression in *E. coli* to synthesize a recombinant nucleocapsid protein (N) screening antigen for the Western blot and EIA diagnosis of HPS cases, even before the responsible Sin Nombre virus was actually isolated, another major achievement of genetic molecular biology (Feldmann *et al.* 1993; Jenison *et al.* 1994).

The use of recombinant-antigen Western blots with IgG and IgM formats has made rapid clinical diagnosis of HPS possible in the United States and Canada (Hjelle *et al.* 1994*b*, 1995*d*; Jenison *et al.* 1994). In addition to the broadly cross-reactive N protein, the envelope glycoprotein G1 of SNV is recognized by patients with acute SNV-HPS, but G1 exhibits minimal or no cross-reactivity with closely related hantaviruses. Using a series of deletion clones expressing the G1 and N antigens, Jenison and colleagues determined that the predominant linear epitopes of these proteins were localized to 31-amino acid and 59-amino acid domains near the amino-terminus, respectively (Hjelle *et al.* 1994*b*; Jenison *et al.* 1994; Yamada *et al.* 1995). This advance enabled the development of diagnostic tests with higher specificity than available with whole-virus or full-length recombinant N protein diagnostic assays. One especially promising outcome has been the development of a prototype hantavirus recombinant immunoblot assay RIBA™, to be commercialized under the form of a strip, which utilizes both recom-

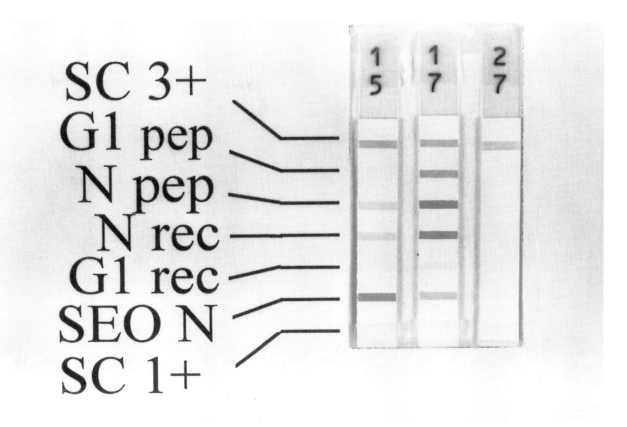

Fig. 30.3 Prototype (for research use only) (Chiron®) RIBA™ hantavirus SIA. Antigens immobilized in bands on the strips are, from top to bottom: (1) a 'serum control' (SC) band in which non-specific IgG antibodies are detected, and arbitrarily rated at 3+ visual intensity; (2) SNV G1 synthetic peptide; (3) SNV N synthetic peptide; (4) SNV N recombinant protein; (5) SNV G1 recombinant protein; (6) SEOV N recombinant protein; (7) a weak serum control (1 + intensity). To be considered positive, a band must be at least as dark as the 1+ serum control band. Strip 15 was probed with serum from a Japanese patient with SEO infection (generously provided by Dr H. W. Lee). Strip 17 was probed with serum from an Arizona patient with acute SNV infection and HPS. Strip 27 was probed with a negative control serum. A 1:50 dilution was used in this 5 hour assay. SNV, Sin Nombre virus; SEOV, Seoul virus; G1, glycoprotein 1; N, nucleocapsid protein; HPS, hantavirus pulmonary syndrome.

binant SNV N and G1 proteins, as well as synthetic peptides that constitute the minimal N and G1 epitopes themselves. This SIA (strip immuno assay) also incorporates recombinant SEO-N protein, to ensure that the assay is sensitive to SEO antibodies as well (Fig. 30.3).

Although the RIBA™ assay is an IgG assay, it has shown considerable promise in the detection of early SNV infection, including the detection of three infections in patients in the prodromal phase of HPS, i.e. before development of lung disease (B. Hjelle, personal communication). As a membrane-based assay that is interpreted visually, it can be used as a rapid (5 hour) diagnostic format in field environments, including settings in which ELISA readers are not available. The high specificity of the G1 antigen for SNV infection in the RIBA™ format has been utilized in the diagnosis of non-SNV HPS cases such as Bayou virus (BAY)

in the south-eastern United States (B. Hjelle, personal communication).

The relatively high specificity of G1 antibodies has been confirmed by studies using the radioimmunoprecipitation format (Ravkov *et al.* 1995), which may serve as a reference method for serological typing among related hantaviruses.

The enormous possibilities of PCR genotyping have been discussed already on p. 336. With appropriate primers, this technique allows detection and even genetic classification of viral RNA present in rodent and/or human tissues. However, PCR genotyping still has to prove its value for routine screening of serum or plasma, perhaps due to low HTV titres and/or very transient viraemic phases. RT–PCR performed on freshly frozen tissue is quite sensitive for SNV diagnosis if sera are not available and also provides genetic information concerning the virus (Nichol *et al.* 1993; Ksiazek *et al.* 1995). Acute blood (mononuclear cells) may also yield a PCR product, although IgM capture serology is more than adequate for routine diagnosis. Because of the low concentrations of RNA in most clinical samples, the sensitivity of the PCR reaction must be enhanced, leading to serious danger of cross-contamination and the need for extreme precautions and verification of the independence of PCR products by sequencing.

Using monoclonal and polyclonal antisera that cross-react with conserved HTV nucleoprotein epitopes, *immunohistochemistry (IHC)*-staining of HTV antigen was possible in formalin-fixed autopsy tissues (Nichol *et al.* 1993; Zaki *et al.* 1995). This technique allows even retrospective diagnosis on stored blocks of cases that died years ago (Zaki *et al.* 1994). Immunostaining with gold particles seems also to be an interesting alternative for the future (Yang *et al.* 1994). The application of RT–PCR to formalin-fixed tissues has been successful but requires careful individualization for a routine procedure and probably offers no advantage in sensitivity (Schwarz *et al.* 1995).

EPIDEMIOLOGY

Until recently, HTVD has been considered a rare disease, with the majority of cases on the Eurasian landmass, and no or only a few case reports from the American and the African continents. On both of these continents, however, evidence existed since many years of HTV infections both in man and in rodents (LeDuc *et al.* 1982, 1984, 1985, 1986; Gonzalez *et al.* 1984; Clement 1987; Yanagihara 1990). However, it is unlikely that the more typical forms of HFRS, particularly when presenting in outbreaks, would have been missed by American and African physicians. It is also possible that many of the HTV infections on these two continents could be subclinical, mild, or atypical (Yanagihara 1990), with the evident exception of the recent American HPS outbreak. Subclinical NE infections are probably the rule in Europe: in a study comparing NE incidence (recorded over 14 years) with IgG IFA PUU antibody prevalence in a highly endemic area of Sweden, it was found that the antibody prevalence rate in the oldest age groups (>60 years) was 14 to 20 times higher than the accumulated life-risk of being hospitalized with NE for men and women, respectively (Niklasson *et al.* 1987). Thus, admissions to hospital are only the top of the iceberg, whereas all other cases are possibly considered as a flu-like viral illness (Kulzer *et al.* 1992) or a viral hepatitis (Yanagihara 1990). This rather reassuring picture was confirmed during sero-epidemiological studies in normal population cohorts in Belgium (Clement and van der Groen

1987) and in The Netherlands (Groen *et al.* 1995), where we found overall positive IgG PUU seroprevalence of 257/21059 (1.3 per cent), and 83/8892 (0.9 per cent), respectively, each time without clinical implications, i.e. the vast majority of IgG seropositives had no suggestive history of renal or other clinical symptoms whatsoever.

The impact of HTVD on public health is best illustrated in two other countries, where the disease has been recognized since the early thirties:

1. In the People's Republic of China, HTVD (or epidemic haemorrhagic fever (EHF) under its local denomination), has been recognized since 1931. The first isolations of *Apodemus*-spread HTN and *Rattus*-spread SEO virus were reported in 1982 (Song *et al.* 1982*a,b*). The accumulated number of officially registered cases in the whole country from 1950 to 1990 reached 904995 with an average morbidity of 2.69 per 100000 inhabitants and an average case fatality rate of 4.3 per cent (range 14.2 per cent in 1969 to 2.1 per cent in 1990). The peak year was 1986, during which 115985 serologically confirmed cases were recorded, with a total of 2561 deaths (fatality rate 2.2 per cent) and a morbidity of 11.08/100000 (Chen and Qiu 1993). From 1988 on, a mean of 40 000 to 50000 annual cases were registered officially (G. Song, personal communication). Although specific serological diagnosis is not routinely practised, it is believed that *Rattus*-spread SEO infections have increased during recent years, even in rural settings, so that nowadays most epidemic areas in the People's Republic of China are of the mixed *Apodemus* and *Rattus* type, i.e. HTN and SEO (WHO Report 1991; Chen and Qui 1993). The age distribution ranges from newborn to 80 years old, but the disease occurs mainly in adolescents and young adults, with a net predominance in males, reflecting probably the agricultural professional exposure, at least for the *Apodemus*-spread infections.

2. In the former USSR, HTVD has been recognized since 1934 and officially registered since 1978. Seroprevalence studies carried out in IFA or direct blocking RIA on a total of 115765 subjects resulted in an overall seropositivity of 3.3 per cent, ranging from 3.5 per cent in the European part to 0.9 per cent in the Far-Eastern part (WHO Report 1991). A total of 68612 cases were registered between 1988 and 1992 (65906 from the European part and 2706 from the Far-Eastern part), with morbidity rates ranging between 1.2 (1982) and 8.0 (1985) per 100000 habitants. The peak year was 1985 with 11413 registered cases. Most patients were in the 20–45-year age group, and males outnumbered females by a ratio of 6:1. Children under the age of 14 years were underrepresented, comprising approximately 5 per cent of the cases. Cases which occurred in the Asian part were

usually caused by viruses similar or identical to HTN virus, and patients frequently experienced severe clinical disease, with case fatality rates of 10–15 per cent.

In the European part, most cases were due to milder infection with PUU-related viruses, with case fatality rates of 1–2 per cent (WHO Weekly Epidemiological Record 1993). The interesting observation that isolates of PUU-like viruses were obtained from two patients of the Asian part of Russia (WHO Weekly Epidemiological Record 1993) were confirmed in Korea (WHO Report 1991), where clinical involvement was noted with a HTV similar to, but not identical with, PUU viruses (H. W. Lee, personal communication). Moreover, PUU-like viruses were recently described in voles (*Cl. rufocanus*) in Hokkaido, Japan (Kariwa *et al.* 1995). So, PUU or PUU-like viruses seem to be present not only in Europe, but in the Far-East as well. Moreover, human infection with the rat-transmitted SEO strain was confirmed serologically among Far-Eastern Russian patients, and by serology and SEO virus isolation in an outbreak of about 50 cases in the European part of Russia (WHO Weekly Epidemiological Record 1993).

It is of interest to compare with the situation in North America. Most diagnosed HTV infections there have been due to SNV or SNV-like viruses and have manifested as HPS. This may be due in part to the severity of HPS and the increased cognisance of the clinical entity. Mild or subclinical SNV infections have been sought and have not been common. Unlike the Eurasian disease, HPS affects both men and women equally, perhaps reflecting the house and surroundings as the principal site of infection (Butler and Peters 1994; Zeitz *et al.* 1995) (Clement *et al.* 1997).

In summary, the picture gets increasingly confused, with different HTV serotypes existing in parallel in the same geographical areas. Moreover, in at least seven recent Belgian cases of ARF, presenting with all the now classical features of nephropathia epidemica (NE) (three patients even presenting with a typical renal biopsy) we were unable to detect at any moment IgG or IgM antibodies against all major HTV serotypes (unpublished data). If confirmed, this leaves the fascinating possibility that we might be confronted with still other related or unrelated viruses, apparently inducing the same clinical picture. Alternatively, PCR signals typical for PUU have been described in two cases which remained seronegative in EIA and in ELISA assays with HTN and PUU antigens (Schreiber *et al.* 1996).

EPIZOOTIOLOGY

HTVD is a zoonosis with a highly specific relationship between each viral serotype and its reservoir species (Table 30.1, Fig. 30.1). In fact, this rodent species,

rather than the geographic location, is the most important determinant of the antigenic and genetic profile of a given HTV isolate: e.g. Seoul serotypes from brown rats (*Rattus norvegicus*) all over the world are more closely related to each other than isolates from other rodent species from the same country (Xiao *et al.* 1994; LeDuc *et al.* 1984, 1985; 1986; Schmaljohn *et al.* 1985). This holds true even for the newer isolates such as Dobrava (DOB) (Fig. 30.1). That is, DOB, isolated in Slovenia from *Apodemus flavicollis*, subfamily Murinae of the Muridae family, is genetically close to the other *Apodemus* isolates from Asia, such as HTN. THAI, isolated from a *Bandicota* related to *Rattus*, falls in the same clade as other viruses carried by murid rodents, subfamily Murinae, but is particularly similar to *Rattus*-isolates i.e. SEO-like viruses (Xiao *et al.* 1994) (Fig. 30.1).

However, this strict host–virus relationship was put into question by a report of isolation of a PUU-like virus called POZ-M1, from house mice (*Mus musculus*) captured in and around habitats of patients with a severe form of HTVD in Serbia (Diglisic *et al.* 1994). Moreover, another PUU-like virus without relation to human disease, had already been isolated in Leakey, Texas, USA from *Mus musculus* (Baek *et al.* 1988). There is growing suspicion that this Leaky isolate was not independent (Xiao *et al.* 1994). Additional confirmation is needed to demonstrate that *Mus* sp., including laboratory mice, might harbour pathogenic HTV. Regardless, there is a hazard for laboratory personnel in handling laboratory rats that have not been properly screened and maintained free of hantaviruses (Mc Kenna *et al.* 1992).

Despite this possible exception, it can be maintained that the four clinically most important HTV strains are Hantaan (HTN), Seoul (SEO), Puumala (PUU), and Sin Nombre virus (SNV), respectively spread by *Apodemus agrarius*, *Rattus norvegicus*, *Clethrionomys glareolus*, and *Peromyscus maniculatus* (Table 30.1). So far, HTVs carried by other murid rodent species of the same subfamily always appeared to be closely related to each other. SEO is the only serotype with a worldwide distribution and an ever growing importance, perhaps due to the fact that *Rattus* sp. and their associated viruses have been transported for many years throughout the world on cargo ships (LeDuc *et al.* 1984, 1986) (Clement *et al.* 1997).

In the People's Republic of China, HTV isolates and/or HTV antigen were detected in 55 species of Vertebrata including 37 species of Rodentia; the field mouse (*Apodemus agrarius*) and the Norway rat (*Rattus norvegicus*) being the most important vectors, with 5.3 per cent (3497/65824) and 4.9 per cent (3789/77295) positivity, respectively. *Apodemus agrarius* was confirmed as most frequently present in rural areas (53.7 per cent of all captured rodents), versus *Rattus norvegicus* in residential areas (52.1 per cent) (Chen and Qiu 1993).

In the former USSR, a total of 300000 small mammals belonging to 63 species were collected from all ecological zones, and 45 species were found to be antigen positive (WHO, Weekly Epidemiological Record 1993). HTN in the Far-Eastern part was mainly found in *Apodemus agrarius*, whereas PUU in European and Siberian areas was mainly spread by *Clethrionomys glareolus*.

In Europe, the red bank vole (*Clethrionomys glareolus*) was shown by several authors to be the most important rodent vector for NE (Niklasson and LeDuc 1984; Groen *et al.* 1995; Verhagen *et al.* 1986). We confirmed these findings during a zoosurvey set up in Belgium, The Netherlands, and Germany between 1986 and 1990, during which 5038 wild small mammals were captured. Of a total of 2225 animals examined, 153 (6.88 per cent) showed (by IFA or ELISA) the presence of a PUU-like antigen in the lungs, whereas 194 (5.22 per cent) of a total of 3718 examined showed the presence of IFA IgG hantaviral antibodies in the serum. *Clethrionomys glareolus* was the second most abundant (total number captured, 2012), and in each country by far the most infected rodent species, showing antigen in 14.5 per cent and antibody in 13.3 per cent of the examined animals. However, significantly higher PUU-like antigen presence was found in the lungs of *Cl. glareolus* in Chimay (Belgium, 1986) with 35.5 per cent (11/31), in Enschede (The Netherlands, 1989) with 40 per cent (4/10), and in Ulm (Germany, 1990) with 22.9 per cent (8/35). In all these localities, a cluster of human NE had been noted shortly before (Clement *et al.* 1992, 1996).

A much more complex picture is seen in the Balkans (Table 30.1), where at least four clinically important HTV strains have been reported, each with their respective rodent vector: PUU spread by *Clethrionomys*, and possibly also by *Mus* (Diglisic *et al.* 1994), HTN or HTN-like spread by *Apodemus* (Antionadis *et al.* 1987*b*; Gligic *et al.* 1989; Avsic-Zupanc *et al.* 1994) and DOB by *Apodemus* (Avsic-Zupanc *et al.* 1992). Moreover, we have reported SEO-induced acute human disease in a Canadian UN soldier in 1992 in Sarajevo (Bosnia) after a clear history of rat exposure (Clement *et al.* 1994*d*). This was the first PRNT-proven evidence of SEO-infection in Europe, followed by another SEO-suspected case from the same region in a British soldier (Stuart *et al.* 1996). With these, the rat can be confirmed as an underestimated vector for spreading less benign forms of HTVD, not only in the laboratory (Desmyter *et al.* 1983; Mc Kenna *et al.* 1992), but also in urban and rural settings. We have described the first 16 acute cases of HTVD in Northern Ireland, a region where *Cl. glareolus* is not present, all reacting in IFA to R22, a rat-borne SEO serotype (McKenna *et al.* 1994).

Since 1982, wild rats have been described as HTV reservoirs (SEO-serotype) in ports and other cities in the United States, showing IgG IFA prevalences as high as 74 per cent in some alleys of Baltimore (LeDuc *et al.* 1982; Yanagihara 1990). However, only recently have mild SEO-induced human cases of HTVD been described in the United States (Glass *et al.* 1994). Moreover, in a study conducted in 8080 Baltimore city residents, an intriguing epidemiological association was found between seropositivity for a local SEO-strain called 'Baltimore rat virus', and hypertensive chronic renal disease, apparently unrelated to other renal disease (Glass *et al.* 1993).

Rats in South America have also been described as heavily infected with a SEO serotype, with prevalence rates up to 56 per cent in Belem (Brazil) (LeDuc *et al.* 1985). Already in 1990 we found in 8 (5.1 per cent) out of 156 Brazilian patients, first suspected of having leptospirosis, serological evidence of a SEO infection (Hinrichsen *et al.* 1993). In retrospect, these appeared to be the first reported cases of serologically proven HTV infection on the American continent.

Another important rodent vector in North America is the meadow vole (*Microtus pennsylvanicus*) carrying the Prospect Hill (PH) serotype (Table 30.1). No human disease has been ascribed to PH so far, despite the fact that PH-seropositive mammalogists were found, some of them with a history of non-A non-B hepatitis (Yanagihara 1990).

A major breakthrough in the understanding of the role of rodents in HTV transmission came after the May 1993 outbreak of hantavirus pulmonary syndrome (HPS) in the south-western United States. Probably due to a disturbance of the local ecological balance (heavy rains and snow during the previous spring, after a long drought), an abundance of rodent food, including piñon nuts and grasshoppers, suddenly appeared. The increased forage, and perhaps other factors, resulted in a marked population increase in the deer mouse (*Peromyscus maniculatus*), a sigmodontine rodent of the Muridae family and one of the most common mammals in North America. Between May 1992 and May 1993, deer mouse numbers were estimated as tenfold above usual (Stone, 1993), particularly in the semiarid regions of the states New Mexico, Arizona, and Colorado. Thirty per cent of the *P. maniculatus* trapped in or around habitats of proven HPS cases appeared to be seropositive to (cross-reacting) Prospect Hill (PH) (Childs *et al.* 1994; Ksiazek *et al.* 1995). Interestingly, all newer non-SNV viruses inducing HPS, such as NYV, BCC, and BAY, are also harboured in New World species of the subfamily Sigmodontinae, family Muridae, whereas all Old World HTV are hardboured by species of the subfamily Arvicolinae (*Clethrionomys* sp., *Microtus* sp.) or subfamily Murinae

(*Rattus* sp., *Apodemous* sp), suggesting again that HTV and their predominant rodent hosts have co-evolved for a very long time (Butler and Peters 1994) (Hjelle *et al.* 1995*d*).

TREATMENT, PREVENTION, AND CONTROL

THERAPY

As in so many other viral diseases, therapeutic possibilities are limited. Supportive medicine may be sufficient in the majority of cases, since self-remittance is the rule, at least in the milder European NE cases. For the flu-like symptoms, a safe analgesic such as paracetamol should be preferred over the more potent non-steroidal anti-inflammatory drugs (NSAID), in view of the potentially deleterious effect of the latter on kidney function. A further advantage of prescribing paracetamol is the fact that this drug does not enhance the risk of haemorrhagic complications. In severe HTV cases, acute dialysis for one or several sessions may be indicated, often for regulating fluid overload after prolonged oliguria. In our Belgian NE series (Colson *et al.* 1995), as in most other European series (Lähdevirta *et al.* 1984; Settergren *et al.* 1988; Van Ypersele and Méry 1989), artificial kidney treatment was necessary in 1–5 per cent of the cases. In Greece, however, the clinical picture due to a HTN-like virus Porogia virus was more severe, prompting dialysis in 30 per cent (41/138) of the patients (Papadimitriou and Antoniadis 1994).

Mechanical ventilation was often indicated as supportive treatment for the respiratory insufficiency characteristic or the American HPS cases (Duchin *et al.* 1994;) (Hjelle *et al.* 1995*d*), but appeared also to be necessary in severe European cases complicated with pulmonary oedema, induced by HTN-like serotypes (Antoniadis *et al.* 1987*a*), SEO cases (Stuart *et al.* 1996), and even by the 'benign' PUU serotype (Clement *et al.* 1994*a,b* Pilaski *et al.* 1995). Since in the latter cases, both lungs and kidneys may be affected, and haemorrhagic complications are often present, we are confronted with extremely ill patients needing the full array of intensive care medicine. The same might also apply to patients infected with the recently isolated Dobrava strain, having a reported fatal outcome of 20 per cent (Gligic *et al.* 1992).

DRUG TREATMENT

The antiviral drug ribavirin (a nucleoside analogue), when given in early treatment, has proven beneficial for the therapy of severe Far-Eastern cases (Huggins *et al.* 1991). Ribavirin therapy of HPS in an open-label trial gave inconclusive results, resulting in the organ-ization of a randomized, controlled trial. The drug seems less suited for the mostly mild PUU-induced cases.

VACCINES

As for most other viral diseases, the final answer to HTVD will be prevention by means of a safe, cheap, and generally applicable (i.e. worldwide) vaccine, a goal that has not yet been reached. However, the possibilities for priming for immunopathology exist (Yao *et al.* 1992). Target populations, in which attack rates and disease severity are sufficiently high to justify vaccination, have not been clearly defined, although areas of Asia with high HTN virus transmission and no likelihood of effective rodent control, would certainly be candidates. In the Republic of Korea a vaccine, based on a formalin-inactivated HTN virus (ROK 84–105), derived from infected suckling mouse brains, was issued (WHO Report 1991), but is awaiting further field trials. In China, field trials are under way with inactivated vaccines from golden hamster (*Mesocricetus auratis*) kidney cell cultures (GHKC), suckling mouse brains (MB), and Mongolian gerbil (*Meriones unguiculatus*) kidney cell (MGK) cultures (WHO Report 1991). Encouraging preliminary results with up to 93.2 per cent seroconversion rates have been reported (G. Song *et al.* 1991). Finally, C. Schmaljohn and co-workers, in the United States, developed a vaccinia-vectored recombinant vaccine against HTN, giving excellent humoral and cell-mediated immune responses in preclinical and phase I clinical trials (Schmaljohn *et al.* 1995*b*). However, all these vaccines are based upon only one serotype (HTN), or at best on both HTN and SEO (G. Song *et al.* 1991), which may be a problem for a full protection in view of the (ever-growing) list of clinically important hantaviral strains (Table 30.1, Fig. 30.1). It may be necessary to prepare vaccines against multiple strains, although cross-protection may be useful among more closely related viruses. The situation is best exemplified in Bosnia, where soldiers living under war conditions would have been the first to benefit from a plurivalent vaccine (Clement *et al.* 1994*d*, 1996; Stuart *et al.* 1996). To broaden the efficacy of the vaccine, and to increase safety, the use of alternate pox-viruses as recombinant vaccine vectors for both HTN and PUU viruses are now under investigation (Schmaljohn *et al.* 1995*b*).

RODENT CONTROL MEASURES

So far, China seems to be the only country where control measures and particularly large-scale rat extermination programmes may have curved the epidemiological figures of HTVD cases downwards, at least those induced by the rat-transmitted SEO serotype (WHO Report, 1991). For recently proven highly endemic areas (i.e. foci with proven recent human cases and a proven recent high infection rate in the local rodent population), it may be indicated to discourage intensive outdoor activities such as camping, caravaning, digging, and particularly low-crawl training (e.g. during military manoeuvres), at least in areas with numerous rodent burrows (Clement *et al.* 1996). For the 1993 HPS epidemic in the United States, nation-wide guidelines on leaflets, TV and even on video cassettes were distributed and focused on the removal of rodent shelters and food sources in and around houses, eliminating rodents inside houses, and limiting access of rodents to human habitats (MMWR 1993*a*). These recommendations were based on data showing increased numbers of infected rodents in case homes and other indications suggesting that infection occurred in or around households (Zeitz *et al.* 1995). Studies are now under way to evaluate the impact of these measures.

In a recent case-control study of HPS integrating rodent trapping data, not only agricultural activities such as hand-plowing appeared to be risks, but also entering and cleaning closed buildings such as food storage areas and animal sheds (Kopela and Lähdevirta 1978; Zeitz *et al.* 1995). Even exercising in a rat-infested building can be a risky activity (Clement *et al.* 1994*d*). Disturbing rodents results in the shedding of urine, and cleaning activities may produce secondary aerosols from recent excreta.

Probably such structures should be opened for a period and rodents eliminated, before cleaning using appropriate wetting and disinfection, e.g. with a dilute hypochlorite solution (MMWR 1993*a*; Zeitz *et al.* 1995).

It has proved feasible to eradicate HTVs from infected laboratory rat colonies by applying Caesarean section and foster mother techniques. This approach enables the transmission of the virus to be curbed, even under laboratory breeding and maintenance conditions (McKenna *et al.* 1992).

ACKNOWLEDGEMENTS

We wish to thank Professor Brian Hjelle of the University of New Mexico, Albuquerque, USA for the gracious remittance of the SIA strips as depicted in Fig. 30.3, and his useful comments on the possibilities of this new Chizon® assay.

We are further indebted to Mr Paul Heyman for his assistance in laboratory techniques and his skilful preparation of this manuscript.

REFERENCES

Anonymous (1992). American College of Chest Physicians/Society of Critical Care Medicine Consensus Conference: definitions for sepsis and organ failure and guidelines for the use of innovative therapies in sepsis. *Critical Care Medicine*, **20**, 864–74.

Antoniadis, A., Grekas, D., Rossi, C. A., and LeDuc, J. W. (1987*a*). Isolation of a Hantavirus from a severely ill patient with hemorrhagic fever with renal syndrome in Greece. *Journal of Infectious Diseases*, **156**, 1010–12.

Antoniadis, A., LeDuc, J., and Daniel-Alexiou, S. (1987*b*). Clinical and epidemiological aspects of haemorrhagic fever with renal syndrome (HFRS) in Greece. *European Journal of Epidemiology*, **3** (3), 295–301.

Avsic-Zupanc, T., Xiao, S. Y., Stojanovic, R., Gligic, A., van der Groen, G., and LeDuc, J. W. (1992). Characterization of Dobrava virus: a hantavirus from Slovenia, Yugoslavia. *Journal of Medical Virology*, **38**, 132–7.

Avsic-Zupanc, T., Poljak, M., Furlan, P., Kaps, R., Xiao, S. Y., and Leduc, J. W. (1994). Isolation of a strain of a Hantaan virus from a fatal case of hemorrhagic fever with renal syndrome in Slovenia. *American Journal of Tropical Medicine and Hygiene*, **51**, 393–400.

Baek, L. J. and Lee, H. W. (1993). Hantavirus infection in wild birds and bats in Korea. In: *Proceedings of the IXth International Congress of Virology, Glasgow, Scotland, 8–13 August*, W52–2, p. 84.

Baek, L. J., Yanagihara, R., Gibbs, C. J., Miyazaki, M., and Gajdusek, D. C. (1988). Leaky virus: a new hantavirus isolated from *Mus musculus* in the United States. *Journal of General Virology*, **69**, 3129–32.

Bouly, S., Hoen, B., Ciureanu, A., and Canton, Ph. (1993). Pneumonie atypique au cours de la fièvre hémorrhagique avec syndrome rénal. *Presse Médicale*, **22**, 1929.

Bradford, J. R. (1916). Nephritis in the British troops in Flanders. A preliminary note. *Quarterly Journal of Medicine*, **9**, 125–37.

Butler, J. C. and Peters, C. J. (1994). Hantaviruses and hantavirus pulmonary syndrome. *Clinics in Infections Diseases*, **19**, 387–95.

Brown, W. L. (1916). Trench nephritis. *Lancet*, **1**, 391–9.

Carey, D. E., Reuben, R., Panicker, K. N., Shope, R. E., and Myers, R. M. (1971). Thottapalayam virus: a presumptive arbovirus isolated from a shrew in India. *Indian Journal of Medical Research*, **59**, 1758–60.

Chen, H. X. and Qiu, F. X. (1993). Epidemiological survey: epidemiologic surveillance on the hemorrhagic fever with renal syndrome in China. *Chinese Medical Journal*, **106**, 857–63.

Childs, J. E. *et al.* (1994). Serologic and genetic identification of *Peromyscus maniculatus* as the primary rodent reservoir for a new hantavirus in the southwestern United States. *Journal of Infectious Diseases*, **169**, 1271–80.

Chu, Y. K., Rossi, C., LeDuc, J. Lee, H. W., Schmaljohn, C. S., and Dalrymple, J. M. (1994). Serological relationships among viruses in the hantavirus genus, family Bunyaviridae. *Virology*, **198**, 196–204.

Chumakov, M. P. *et al.* (1981). Detection of hemorrhagic fever with renal syndrome (HFRS) virus in the lung of bank voles (*Clethrionomys glareolus*) and redbacked voles (*C. rutilus*) trapped in HFRS foci in the European part of U.S.S.R. and serodiagnosis of this infection in man. *Archives of Virology*, **69**, 295–300.

Clement, J. (1987*a*). Trench nephritis: past and present. In *Hantaviruses*, Proceedings of the 29th International Colloquium of the Institute of Tropical Medicine, Antwerp (Belgium), 10–11 December, pp. 1–20.

Clement, J. and van der Groen, G. (1987*b*). Acute hantavirus nephropathy in Belgium: preliminary results of a sero-epidemiological study. Advances in experimental medicine and biology. In: Amerio A, ed. *Acute renal failure: clinical and experimental*, (ed. A. Amerio), pp. 251–64. Plenum Press, New York.

Clement, J. *et al.* (1992). Epizootiological aspects of nephropathia epidemica (NE) in Belgium, the Netherlands and Germany. *Nephrology, Dialysis, and Transplantation*, **2**, 970–1.

Clement, J., De Bock, R., and Beguin, Y. (1993). Pathophysiology of anaemia in nephropathia epidemica. *Nephrology, Dialysis, and Transplantation*, **8**, 1162–5.

Clement, J. *et al.* (1994*a*). Hantavirus epidemic in Europe, 1993. *Lancet*, **343**, 114.

Clement, J., Colson, P., and McKenna, P. (1994*b*). Hantavirus pulmonary syndrome in New England and Europe. *New England Journal of Medicine*, **331**, 45–6.

Clement, J. *et al.* (1994*c*). Hantavirus infections in rodents. In Vol. 5, (ed. Horzinek) *Virus infections of rodents*, Elsevier Amsterdam Science B. V., pp. 295–316.

Clement, J., McKenna, P., Avsic-Zupanc, T., and Skinner, C. R. (1994*d*). Rat-transmitted hantaviruses disease in Sarajevo. *Lancet*, **344**, 131.

Clement, J. *et al.* (1995). Epidemiology and laboratory diagnosis of Hantavirus (HTV) infections. *Acta Clinica Belgica*, **50**, 9–19.

Clement, J., Underwood, P., Ward, D., Pilaski, J., and LeDuc, J. (1996). Hantavirus (HTV) outbreak during military manoeuvres in Germany. *Lancet*, **347**, 336.

Clement, J., Heyman, P., Mc Kenna, P., Colson, P., Avsic-Zupanc, T. (1997). The Hantaviruses of Europe: from the bedside to the bench. *Emerging Infectious Diseases*, **3**, 205–11.

Colson, P. *et al.* (1995). Hantavirose dans l'Entre-Sambre-et-Meuse. Année 1992–1993. *Acta Clinica Belgica*, **50**, 197–205.

Desmyter, J., Johnson, K. M., Deckers, C., LeDuc, J. W., Brasseur, F., and van Ypersele de Strihou, C. (1983). Laboratory rat associated outbreak of haemorrhagic fever with renal syndrome due to Hantaan-like virus in Belgium. *Lancet*, **2**, 1445–8.

Desmyter, J., van Ypersele de Strihou, C., and van der Groen, G. (1984). Hantavirus disease or haemorrhagic fever with renal syndrome. *Lancet*, **ii**, 158.

Diglisic, G. *et al.* (1994). Isolation of a Puumala-like virus from *Mus musculus* captured in Yugoslavia and its association with severe hemorrhagic fever with renal syndrome. *Journal of Infectious Diseases*, **169**, 204–7.

Dournon, E. *et al.* (1984). HFRS after a wild rodent bite in the Haute-Savoie and risk of exposure to Hantaan-like virus in a Paris laboratory. *Lancet*, **1**, 676–7.

Duchin, J. S. *et al.* (1994). Hantavirus pulmonary syndrome a clinical description of 17 patients with a newly recognized disease. *New England Journal of Medicine*, **330**, 949–55.

Earle, D. P. (1954). Symposium on epidemic hemorrhagic fever. *American Journal of Medicine*, **16**, 617–793.

Elliott, L. H. *et al.* (1994). Isolation of the causative agent of hantavirus pulmonary syndrome. *American Journal of Tropical Medicine and Hygiene*, **51**, 102–8.

Elwell, M. R., Ward, G. S., Tingpalapong, M., and Leduc, J. W. (1985). Serologic evidence of Hantaan-like virus in rodents and man in Thailand. *Southeast Asian Journal of Tropical Medicine and Public Health*, **16**, 349–54.

Feldmann, H. (1993). Utilization of autopsy RNA for the synthesis of the nucleocapsid antigen of a newly recognized virus associated with hantaviral pulmonary syndrome. *Virus Research*, **30**, 351–67.

Fisher-Hoch, S. and McCormick, J. B. (1985). Haemorrhagic fever with renal syndrome: a Review. *Abstracts on Hygiene and Communicable Diseases*, **60**, R1–R20.

Forslund, T., Liisanantti, R., Saijonmaa, O., and Fyhrquist, F. (1993). Raised plasma endothelin-1 concentration in patients with nephropathia epidemica. *Clinical Nephrology*, **40**, 69–73.

French, G. R., Foulke, R. S., Brand, O. A., Eddy, G. A., and Lee, H. W. (1981). Korean hemorrhagic fever: propagation of the etiologic agent in a cell line of human origin. *Science*, **211**, 1046–8.

Gajdusek, D. C. (1962). Virus hemorrhagic fevers with special reference to hemorrhagic fever with renal syndrome. *Journal of Pediatrics*, **60**, 841–57.

Gajdusek, D. C., Goldfarb, L. G., and Goldgaber, D. (1987). *Bibliography of hemorrhagic fever with renal syndrome*, (2nd edn.). NIH Publication No. 88–2603. US Department of Health and Human Services, Public Health Service, National Institutes of Health, Bethesda, Maryland, USA.

Gavrilovskaya, I. N. *et al.* (1990). Pathogenesis of hemorrhagic fever with renal syndrome virus infection and mode of horizontal transmission of Hantavirus in bank voles. *Archives of Virology*, **1**, 57–62.

Glass, G. E., Watson, A. J., LeDuc, J. W., Kelen, G. D., Quinn, T. C., and Childs, J. E. (1993). Infection with a ratborne hantavirus in US residents is consistently associated with hypertensive renal disease. *Journal of Infectious Diseases*, **167**, 614–20.

Glass, G. E., Watson, A. J., LeDuc, J. W., and Childs J. E. (1994). Domestic cases of hemorrhagic fever with renal syndrome in the United States. *Nephron*, **68**, 48–51.

Gligic, A. *et al.* (1989). Hemorrhagic fever with renal syndrome in Yugoslavia: antigenic characterization of Hantaviruses isolated from *Apodemus flavicollis* and *Clethrionomys glareolus*. *American Journal of Tropical Medicine and Hygiene*, **41**, 109–15.

Gligic, A. *et al.* (1992). Belgrade virus: A new hantavirus causing severe hemorrhagic fever with renal syndrome in Yugoslavia. *Journal of Infectious Diseases*, **166**, 113–20.

Gomez-Jimenez, J. *et al.* (1995). Arginine: nitric oxide pathway in endotoxemia and human septic shock. *Critical Care Medicine*, **23**, 253–8.

Gonzalez, J. P. *et al.* (1984). Serological evidence for Hantaan-related virus in Africa. *Lancet*, **ii**, 1036–7.

Groen, J., van der Groen, G., Hoofd, G., and Osterhaus, A. (1989). Comparison of immunofluorescence and enzyme linked immunosorbent assays for the serology of Hantaan virus infections. *Journal of Virological Methods*, **23**, 195–203.

Groen, J., Dalrymple, J., Fisher-Hoch, S., Jordans, J. G. M., Clement, J. P., and Osterhaus, A. D. M. E. (1992). Serum antibodies to structural proteins of hantavirus arise at different times after infection. *Journal of Medical Virology*, **37**, 283–7.

Groen, J., Jordans, J. G. M., Gerding, M., Clement, J. P., and Osterhaus, A. D. M. E. (1994). Class and subclass distribution of Hantavirus-specific serum antibodies arise at different times after the onset of Nephropathia epidemica. *Journal of Medical Virology*, **43**, 39–43.

Groen, J., Gerding, M., Jordans, J. G. M., Clement, J. P., Nieuwenhuijs, H. M., and Osterhaus, A. D. M. E. (1995). Hantavirus infections in The Netherlands: epidemiology and disease. *Epidemiology and Infection*, **114**, 373–83.

Groeneveld, P. H. P., Colson, P., Kwappenberg, K. M. C., and Clement, J. (1995). Increased production of nitric oxide in patients infected with the European variant of Hantavirus. *Scandinavian Journal of Infectious Diseases*, **27**, 453–6.

Guang, M., Liu, G. Z., and Cosgriff, T. (1989). Hemorrhage in hemorrhagic fever with renal syndrome in China. *Reviews of Infectious Diseases*, **2**, S884–S889.

Hedman, K., Vaheri, A., and Brummer-Korvenkontio, M. (1991). Rapid diagnosis of hantavirus disease with an IgG avidity assay. *Lancet*, **338**, 1353–6.

Hinrichsen, S. *et al.* (1993). Evidence of Hantavirus infection in Brazilian patients from Recife with suspected Leptospirosis. *Lancet*, **341**, 50.

Hjelle, B. *et al.* (1994*a*). A novel Hantavirus associated with an outbreak of fatal respiratory disease in the Southwestern United States: Evolutionary relationships to known Hantaviruses. *Journal of Virology*, **68**, 592–6.

Hjelle, B. *et al.* (1994*b*). Dominant glycoprotein of four corners hantavirus is conserved across a wide geographical area. *Journal of General Virology*, **75**, 2881–8.

Hjelle, B., Spiropoulou, C. F., Torrez-Martinez, N. Morzunov, S., Peters, C. J., and Nichol, S. T. (1994*c*). Detection of Muerto Canyon virus RNA in peripheral blood mononuclear cells from patients with hantavirus pulmonary syndrome. *Journal of Infectious Diseases*, **170**, 1013–17.

Hjelle, B. *et al.* (1994*d*). Genetic identification of a novel Hantavirus of the Harvest mouse *Reithrodontomys megalotis*. *Journal of Virology*, **68**, 6751–4.

Hjelle, B., Anderson, B., Torrez-Martinez, N., Song, W., Gannon, W. L., and Yates, T. L. (1995*a*). Prevalence and geographic genetic variation of hantaviruses of New World harvest mice (*Reithrodontomys*): identification of a divergent genotype from a Costa Rican *Reithrodontomys mexicanus*. *Virology*, **207**, 452–9.

Hjelle, B., Krolikowski, J., Torrez-Martinez, N., Chavez-Giles, F., Vanner, C., and Laposata E. (1995*b*). Phylogenetically distinct hantavirus implicated in a case of hantavirus pulmonary syndrome in the northeastern United States. *Journal of Medical Virology*, **46**, 21–7.

Hjelle, B. *et al.* (1995*c*). Molecular linkage of hantavirus pulmonary syndrome to the white-footed mouse, *Peromyscus leucopus*: genetic characterization of the M genome of New York virus. *Journal of Virology*, **69**, 137–41.

Hjelle, B., Jenison, S. A., Goade, D. E., Green, W. B., Feddersen, R. M., and Scott, A. A. (1995*d*). Hantaviruses: clinical, microbiologic, and epidemiologic aspects. *Critical Reviews in Clinical Laboratory Sciences*, **32**, 469–508.

Hjelle, B., Torrez-Martinez, N., and Koster, F. T. (1996). Hantavirus pulmonary syndrome-related virus from Bolivia. *Lancet*, **347**, 57.

Huang, C., Jin, B., Wang, M., Li, E., and Sun, C. (1994). Hemorrhagic fever with renal syndrome: Relationship between pathogenesis and cellular immunity. *Journal of Infectious Diseases*, **169**, 868–70.

Huggins, J. W. *et al.* (1991). Prospective, double-blind concurrent, placebo-controlled, clinical trial of intravenous ribavirin therapy of hemorrhagic fever with renal syndrome (HFRS). *Journal of Infectious Diseases*, **164**, 1119–27.

Ivanov, A. P. *et al.* (1988). Enzyme immunoassay for the detection of virus specific IgG and IgM antibody in patients with HFRS. *Archives of Virology*, **100**, 1–7.

Jenison, S. *et al.* (1994). Characterization of human antibody responses to four corners hantavirus infections among patients with hantavirus pulmonary syndrome. *Journal of Virology*, **68**, 3000–6.

Kariwa, H. *et al.* (1995). Evidence for the existence of Puumala-related virus among *Clethrionomys rufocanus* in Hokkaido, Japan. *American Journal of Tropical Medicine and Hygiene*, **53**, 222–7.

Ketai, L. H. *et al.* (1994). Hantavirus pulmonary syndrome: radiographic findings in 16 patients. *Radiology*, **191**, 665–8.

Khabbaz, R. F. (1994). Epidemiology of hantavirus pulmonary syndrome. In *Proceedings of 34th Interscience Symposium on Antimicrobial Agents and Chemotherapy, 4–7 October*, p. 285.

Khan, A. S. *et al.* (1995). A fatal illness associated with a new hantavirus in Louisiana. *Journal of Medical Virology*, **46**, 281–6.

Kilbourne, E. D. (1990). New viral diseases. A real and potential problem without boundaries. *Journal of the American Medical Association*, **264**, 68–70.

Kim, G. R., Lee, Y. T., and Park, C. H. (1994). A new natural reservoir of Hantavirus: isolation of Hantaviruses from lung tissues of bats. *Archives of Virology*, **134**, 85–95.

Kopela, H. and Lähdevirta, J. (1978). The role of small rodents and patterns of living in the epidemiology of nephropathia epidemica. *Scandinavian Journal of Infectious Diseases*, **10**, 303–5.

Ksiazek, T. *et al.* (1995). Identification of a new North American Hantavirus that causes acute pulmonary insufficiency. *American Journal of Tropical Medicine and Hygiene*, **52**, 117–23.

Kulzer, P., Schaefer, R. M., Heidbreider, E., and Heidland, A. (1992). Retrospective diagnosis of small epidemic of haemorrhagic fever with renal syndrome. *Lancet*, **339**, 940–1.

Kurata, T., Tsai, T. F., Bauer, S. P., and McCormick, J. B. (1983). Immunofluorescence studies of disseminated Hantaan virus infection of suckling mice. *Infection and Immunity*, **41**, 391–8.

Lähdevirta, J., Savola, J., Brummer-Korvenkontio, M., Berndt, R., Illikainen, R., and Vaheri, A. (1984). Clinical and serological diagnosis of nephropathia epidemica, the mild type of a haemorrhagic fever with renal syndrome. *Journal of Infectious Diseases*, **9**, 230–8.

LeDuc, J. W., Smith, G. A., Bagley, L. R., Hasty, S. E., and Johnson, K. M. (1982). Preliminary evidence that Hantaan or a closely related virus is enzootic in domestic rodents. *New England Journal of Medicine*, **307**, 624.

LeDuc, J., Smith, G., and Johnson, K. (1984). Hantaan-like viruses from domestic rats captured in the United States. *American Journal of Tropical Medicine and Hygiene*, **33**, 992–8.

LeDuc, J., Smith, G., Pinheiro, F., Vasconcelos, P., Rosa, E., and Maiztegui, J. (1985). Isolation of a Hantaan-related virus from Brazilian rats and serologic evidence of its widespread distribution in South-America. *American Journal of Tropical Medicine and Hygiene*, **34**, 810–15.

LeDuc, J. *et al.* (1986). Global survey of antibody to Hantaan-related viruses among peridomestic rodents. *Bulletin of the World Health Organization*, **64**, 139–44.

LeDuc, J. W., Ksiazek, T. G., Rossi, C. A., and Dalrymple, J. M. (1990). A retrospective analysis of sera collected by the Hemorrhagic fever commission during the Korean conflict. *Journal of Infectious Diseases*, **162**, 1182–4.

Lee, H. W., Lee, P. W., and Johnson, K. M. (1978). Isolation of the etiologic agent of Korean Hemorrhagic fever. *Journal of Infectious Diseases*, **137**, 298–308.

Lee, H. W., Lee, P. W., Lähdevirta, J., and Brummer-Korvenkontio, M. (1979). Aetiological relation between Korean hemorrhagic fever and nephropathia epidemica. *Lancet*, **1**, 186–7.

Lee, H. W., Lee, P. W., and Baek, L. J. (1981). Intraspecific transmission of Hantaan virus, etiologic agent of Korean haemorrhagic fever, in the rodent *Apodemus agrarius*. *American Journal of Tropical Medicine and Hygiene*, **30**, 1106–12.

Lee, H. W., Baek, L. J., and Johnson, K. M. (1982). Isolation of Hantaan virus, the etiologic agent of Korean hemorrhagic fever from wild urban rats. *Journal of Infectious Diseases*, **146**, 638–44.

Lee, P. W., Amysc, H. L., Gajadnsek, D. C., Yanagihara, R. T. *et al.* (1982). New haemorrhagic fever with renal syndrome-related virus in indigenous wild rodents in United States. *Lancet*, **2**, 1405.

Linderholm, M., Ahlm, C., Settergren, B., and Tärnvik, A. (1995). Elevated plasma levels of tumor necrosis factor-α, Interleukine-6 and Interleukine-10 in patients with Nephropathia epidemica. *Proceedings of the 3rd International Conference on HFRS and Hantaviruses. 31 May-3 June, Helsinki, Finland*, p. 40.

McCormick, J. B., Sasso, D. R., Palmer, E. L., and Kiley, M. P. (1982). Morphological identification of the agent of Korean Haemorrhagic Fever (Hantaan virus) as a member of the Bunyaviridae. *Lancet*, i, 765–8.

McKee, K. T., Kim, G. R., Green, D. E., and Peters, C. J. (1985). Hantaan virus infection in suckling mice: Virologic and pathologic correlates. *Journal of Medical Virology*, **17**, 107–17.

McKenna, P. *et al.* (1992). Eradication of hantavirus infection among laboratory rats by application of caesarian section and foster mother technique. *Journal of Infection*, **25**, 181–90.

McKenna, P., Clement, J., Matthys, P., Coyle, P., and McCaughey, C. (1994). Serological evidence of Hantavirus disease in Northern Ireland. *Journal of Medical Virology*, **43**, 33–8.

Marshall, E. and Stone, R. (1993). Hantavirus outbreak yields to PCR. *Science*, **262**, 832–6.

MMWR (1993*a*) *Centers for disease control and prevention. Hantavirus infection—southwestern United States: interim recommendations for risk reduction. MMWR*, **42** (RR-11), 1–13.

MMWR (1993*b*) *Centers for disease control and prevention. Update: Hantavirus disease. MMWR* 42: 612–614.

MMWR (1994*a*) *Newly identified Hantavirus—Florida, 1994. MMWR*, **43**, 99–105.

MMWR (1994*b*) *Laboratory management of agents associated with Hantavirus pulmonary syndrome: Interim biosafety guidelines. MMWR*, **43**(RR-7), 1–7.

Morzunov, S. P. *et al.* (1995). A newly recognized virus associated with a fatal case of hantavirus pulmonary syndrome in Louisiana. *Journal of Virology*, **69**, 1980–3.

Nerurkar, V. R., Song, K. J., Gajdusek, D. C., and Yanagihara, R (1993). Genetically distinct hantavirus in deer mice. *Lancet*, **342**, 1058–9.

Nichol, S. *et al.* (1993). Genetic identification of a Hantavirus associated with an outbreak of acute respiratory illness. *Science*, **262**, 914–17.

Niklasson, B. and LeDuc, J. W. (1984). Isolation of the Nephropathia epidemica agent in Sweden. *Lancet*, **1**, 1012–13.

Niklasson, B. LeDuc, J., and Nyström, K. (1987). Nephropathia epidemica: incidence of clinical cases and antibody prevalence in an endemic area of Sweden. *Epidemiology and Infection*, **99**, 559–62.

Niklasson, B. *et al.* (1990). Haemorrhagic fever with renal syndrome: evaluation of ELISA for detection of Puumala-virus-specific IgG and IgM. *Research in Virology*, **141**, 637–48.

Nolte, K. B. *et al.* (1995). Hantavirus pulmonary syndrome in the United States: a pathological description of a disease caused by a new agent. *Human Pathology*, **26**, 110–20.

Nowotny, N. (1994). The domestic cat: a possible transmittor of viruses from rodents to man. *Lancet*, **343**, 921.

Nuzum, E. O., Rossi, C. A., Stephenson, E. H., and LeDuc, J. W. (1988). Aerosol transmission of Hantaan and related viruses to laboratory rats. *American Journal of Tropical Medicine and Hygiene*, **38**, 636–40.

Papadimitriou, M. and Antoniadis, A. (1994). Hantavirus nephropathy in Greece. *Lancet*, **343**, 1038.

Papadmitrion, M. (1995). Nephrology Forum: Hantavirus rephiopalty. *Kidney Int*, **48**, 887–902.

Penalba, C., Halin, P., Lanoux, P., Reveil, J. C., Le Guenno, B., and Camprasse, A. M. (1994). Fièvre hémorrhagique avec syndrome rénal (FHSR). Aspects épidémiologique et clinique dans le département des Ardennes (76 observations). *Médecine et Maladies Infectievses*, **24**, 506–11.

Pilaski, J. *et al.* (1995). Genetic identification of a new Puumala vrius strain causing severe hemorrhagic fever with renal syndrome in Germany. *Journal of Infectious Diseases*, **170**, 1456–62.

Plyusnin, A. *et al.* (1994). Tula virus: a newly detected hantavirus carried by European common voles. *Journal of Virology*, **68**, 7833–9.

Plyusnin, A. *et al.* (1995). Genetic variation in Tula hantaviruses: sequence analysis of the S and M segments of strains from Central Europe, *Virus Research*, **39**, 237–50.

Ravkov, E. V., Rollin, P. E., Ksiazek, T. G., Peters, C. J., and Nichol, S. T. (1995). Genetic and serologic analysis of Black Creek Canal virus and its association with human disease and *Sigmodon hispidus* infection. *Virology*, **210**, 482–9.

Rollin, P. E. *et al.* (1995). Isolation of Black Creek Canal virus, a new hantavirus from *Sigmodon hispidus* in Florida. *Journal of Medical Virology*, **46**, 35–9.

Saluzzo, J. F., Leguenno, B., and van der Groen, G. (1988). Use of heat inactivated viral hemorrhagic fever antigens in serological assays. *Journal of Virological Methods*, **22**, 165–72.

Schmaljohn, O. *et al.* (1985). Antigenic and genetic properties of viruses linked to Hemorrhagic fever with renal syndrome. *Science*, **227**, 1041–4.

Schmaljohn, C. S., Hasty, S. E., Rasmussen, L., and Dalrymple, J. M. (1986). Hantaan virus replication: effects of monensin, tunicamycin and endoglycosidases on the structural glycoproteins. *Journal of General Virology*, **67**, 707–17.

Schmaljohn, C. S., Schmaljohn, A. L., and Dalrymple, J. M. (1987). Hantaan virus M RNA: coding strategy, nucleotide sequence, and gene order. *Virology*, **157**, 31–9.

Schmaljohn, A. L. *et al.* (1995*a*). Isolation and initial characterization of a newfound hantavirus from California. *Virology*, **206**, 963–72.

Schmaljohn, C. S., Chu, Y. K., Jennings, G. B., Summers, P., Schmaljohn, A. L., and McClain, D. J. (1995*b*). Prospects for immunization to Hantaviruses. *Proceedings of the 3rd International Conference on HFRS and Hantaviruses. Helsinki, Finland. 31 May-3 June*, p. 52.

Schreiber, M., Laue, T., and Wolff, C. (1996). Hantavirus pulmonary syndrome in Germany. *Lancet*, **347**, 336–7.

Schwarz, T. F., Zaki, S. R., Morzunov, S., Peters, C. J., and Nichol, S. T. (1995). Detection and sequence confirmation of Sin Nombre virus RNA in paraffin-embedded human lung tissues using one-step RT-PCR. *Journal of Virological Methods*, **51**, 349–56.

Settergren, B., Juto, P., Trollfors, B., Wadell, G., and Norrby, R. S. (1988). Hemorrhagic complications and other clinical findings in Nephropathia epidemica in Sweden: A study of 385 serologically verified cases. *Journal of Infectious Diseases*, **157**, 380–2.

Sibold, C. *et al.* (1995). Genetic characterization of Malacky virus: a new hantavirus detected in Microtus arvalis from Slovakia. *Virus Genes*, **10**, 277–81.

Slonova, R. A., Tkachenko, E. A., Kushmarev, E. L., Dzagurova, T. K., and Astakova, T. I. (1992). Hantavirus isolation from birds. *Acta Virologica*, **36**, 493.

Smadel, J. E. Epidemic hemorrhagic fever. *American Journal of Public Health*, **43**, 1327–30.

Song, G., Qiu, X., Ni, D., Zhao, J., and Kong, B. (1982a). Etiological studies of epidemic hemorrhagic fever. Virus isolation in *Apodemus agrarius* from the non-endemic area and its antigenic characterization. *Acta Academiae Medica Sinica*, **4**, 73–7.

Song, G. *et al.* (1982b). Isolation of EHF-related agent from *Rattus norvegicus* captured in patients' homes in endemic area of the mild type of hemorrhagic fever. *Acta Microbiologica Sinica*, **22**, 373–7.

Song, G., Hang, C. S., Huang, Y. C., and Hou, F. Y. (1991). Preliminary trials of inactivated vaccine against haemorrhagic fever with renal syndrome. *Lancet*, **337**, 801.

Song, J. W. *et al.* (1994). Isolation of pathogenic hantavirus from white-footed mouse (*Peromyscus leucopus*). *Lancet*, **344**, 1637.

Song, W. *et al.* (1995a). Isla Vista virus: a genetically novel hantavirus of the California vole *Microtus californicus*. *Journal of General Virology*, **76**, 3195–9.

Song, W., Quintana, M., Torrez-Martinez, N., Ascher, M., Jay, M., and Hjelle, B. (1995b). High genetic complexity of hantavirus radiation of New World microtine voles (Rodentia: *Microtus*). *Congress book 3rd International Conference on HFRS and Hantaviruses. Helsinki, Finland, 31 May–3 June*, p. 18.

Spiropoulou, C., Morzunov, S., Feldman, H., Sanchez, A., Peters, C. J., and Nichol, S. T. (1994). Genome structure and variability of a virus causing hantavirus pulmonary syndrome. *Virology*, **200**, 715–23.

Stone, R. (1993). The Mouse-Pinon nut connection. (Report) *Science*, **262**, 833.

Stuart, L. M., Rice, P. S., Lloyd, G., and Beale R. J. (1996). A soldier in respiratory distress. *Lancet*, **347**, 30.

Stuhlfauth, K. (1943). Nachtrag zu dem 'Bericht über ein neues schlammfieberähnliches Krankheitsbild bei Deutschen Truppen in Lappland.' *Deutsche Medizinische Wochenschrift*, **69**, 439–43.

Svedmyr, A., Lee, P. W., Gajdusek, D. C., Gibbs, C. J. Jr, and Nyström, K. (1980). Antigenic differentiation of the viruses causing Korean hemorrhagic fever and epidemic (endemic) nephropathy of Scandinavia. *Lancet*, **2**, 315–16.

Tao, H., Zin Yi, C., Tung Xin, Z., Se Mao, X., and Chang Shou, H. (1985). Morphology and morphogenesis of viruses of hemorrhagic fever with renal syndrome (HFRS). I. Some peculiar aspects of the morphogenesis of various strains of HFRS virus. *Intervirology*, **23**, 97–108.

Tao, H., Xia, S. M., Chan, Z. Y., Song, G., and Yanagihara, R. (1987). Morphology and morphogenesis of viruses of hemorrhagic fever with renal syndrome. II. Inclusion bodies—ultrastructural markers of hantavirus-infected cells. *Intervirology*, **27**, 45–52.

Torrez-Martinez, N. and Hjelle, B. (1995). Enzootic of Bayou hantavirus in rice rats (*Oryzomys palustris*) in 1983. *Lancet*, **346**, 780–1.

van der Groen, G. and Elliott., L. H. (1982). Use of β-propionolactone inactivated Ebola, Marburg and Lassa intracellular antigens in immunofluorescent antibody assay. *Annales de la Société Belge de Médicine Tropicale*, **62**, 49–54.

van der Groen, G., Kurata, T., and Mets, C. (1983). Modification to indirect immunofluorescence tests on Lassa, Marburg and Ebola material. *Lancet*, **1**, 654–5.

Van Ypersele de Strihou, C. and Méry, J. P. (1989). Hantavirus-related acute interstitial nephritis in Western Europe: expansion of a world-wide zoonosis. *Quarterly Journal of Medicine*, **73**, 941–50.

Verhagen, R., van der Groen, G., Ivanov, A., Van Rompaey, J., Leirs, H., and Verheyen, R. (1986). Occurrence and distribution of Hantavirus in wild living mammals in Belgium. *Archives of Virology*, **31**, 43–52.

WHO Report (1991). Working group on the development of a rapid diagnostic method and vaccine for Haemorrhagic Fever with Renal Syndrome. Seoul, Republic of Korea, 26–28 September. *WHO Report* RS/91/GE/19 (Kor) p. 9.

WHO Weekly Epidemiological Record (1993). Haemorrhagic fever with renal syndrome. *WHO Weekly Epidemiological Record*, **68**, 189–92.

Xiao, S. Y., LeDuc, J., Yong, K. C., and Schmaljohn, C. (1994). Phylogenetic analyses of virus isolates in the genus Hantavirus, Family Bunyaviridae. *Virology*, **198**, 205–17.

Xu, Z. Y., Guo, C. S., Wu, Y. L., Zhang, X. W., and Liu, K. (1985). Epidemiological studies of hemorrhagic fever with renal syndrome: analysis of risk factors and mode of transmission. *Journal of Infectious Diseases*, **152**; 137–44.

Xu, Z. Y., Tang, Y. W., Kan, L. Y., and Tsai, T. F. (1987). Cats-source of protection or infection? A case-control study of hemorrhagic fever with renal syndrome. *American Journal of Epidemiology*, **126**, 942–8.

Yamada, T., Hjelle, B., Lanzi, R., Morris, C., Anderson, B., and Jenison, S. (1995). Antibody response to Four Corners hantavirus infections in the deer mouse (*Peromyscus maniculatus*): identification of an immunodominant region of the viral nucleocapsid protein. *Journal of Virology*, **69**, 1939–43.

Yanagihara, R. (1990). Hantavirus infection in the United States: Epizootiology and epidemiology. *Reviews of Infectious Diseases*, **12**, 449–57.

Yanagihara, R. and Silverman, D. J. (1990). Experimental infection of human vascular endothelial cells by pathogenic and nonpathogenic hantaviruses. *Archives of Virology*, **111**, 281–6.

Yanagihara, R., Amyx, H. L., and Gajdusek, D. C. (1985). Experimental infection with Puumala virus, the etiologic agent of Nephropathia epidemica in bank voles (*Clethrionomys glareolus*). *Journal of Virology*, **55**, 34–8.

Yang Shoujing, Liu Yanfang, Liu Yingying, Li Yuanzhi, and Xu Zhikai (1994). Tracing of the viral antigens by gold-labelled antibodies In the experimentally infected suckling mice with Chen strain hemorrhagic fever with renal syndrome virus and ultrastructural observation. *Journal of the Medical College of the People's Liberation Army*, **9**, 155–60.

Yao, J. S., Arikawa, J., Kariwa, H., Yoshimatsu, K., Takashima, I., and Hashimoto, N. (1992). Effect of neutralizing monoclonal antibodies on Hantaan virus infection of the macrophage P388D1 cell line. *Japanese Journal of Veterinary Research*, **40**, 87–97.

Zaki, S. R. *et al.* (1994). Retrospective diagnosis of a 1983 case of fatal hantavirus pulmonary syndrome. *Lancet*, **343**, 1037.

Zaki, S. R. *et al.* (1995). Hantavirus pulmonary syndrome: pathologenesis of an emerging infectious disease. *American Journal of Pathology*, **146**, 552–79.

Zeitz, P. S. *et al.* (1995). A case-control study of hantavirus pulmonary syndrome during an outbreak in the southwestern United States. *Journal of Infectious Diseases*, **171**, 864–70.

Zöller, L., Yang, S., and Zeyer, M. (1991). Rapid diagnosis of hemorrhagic fever with renal syndrome due to Hantavirus. *Lancet*, **338**, 183.

31   HERPES B VIRUS

D. W. G. Brown

SUMMARY

B virus or herpes simiae is a skin infection of monkeys mainly of the *Macaca* genus, which is transmitted by close contact and possibly sexually. Laboratory workers exposed to infected monkeys have been infected by bites and scratches, and through abraded skin, leading, 4–59 days later to an ascending encephalo-myelitis, and death. Prevention of infection requires quarantine of imported monkeys and stringent laboratory safety precautions. Treatment with acyclovir has been successful.

HISTORY

B virus was first isolated in 1932 from Dr W.B. who developed a fatal acute ascending myelitis following a bite on the dorsum of the left ring and little fingers by an apparently normal rhesus monkey (*Macaca mulatta*). Three days after the bite pain and swelling were noticed at the bite site, and he was admitted to hospital after 6 days with a fever, superficial redness at the bite site and lymphangitis. Subsequently vesicles developed at the bite site followed by generalized abdominal cramps, nausea and vomiting. Thirteen days after the bite hyperaesthesia of the lower limbs developed and neurological examination revealed generalized hyperalgesia below the umbilicus, and a flaccid paralysis with absent reflexes. The paraesthesia progressed rapidly and the patient died of respiratory paralysis 16 days after the bite.

Clinical samples from this case were investigated separately by two groups: Gay and Holden (1933) reported the isolation of a herpesvirus from post-mortem material. They proposed the name W virus and suggested the virus was a variant of herpes simplex. In 1934 Sabin and Wright isolated a filterable agent from brain, medulla, spinal cord and spleen by intracranial and intradermal inoculation of rabbits. They named the agent B virus and suggested it was distinct from herpes simplex. This name was universally adopted and is often used together with the descriptive term herpesvirus simiae in the literature.

A second case was reported by Sabin 1949 in which an investigator contracted a fatal neurological illness following contamination of a minor cut by monkey saliva. At the same time sera from macaques were shown to contain neutralizing antibodies to B virus. This, together with the exposure history of the two human cases, led to the recognition that B virus was a monkey virus. However, it was not until 1954 that Melnick and Banker isolated B virus from its natural host, when virus was cultured from the brain of a rhesus monkey in the course of studies of polio virus. Subsequent serological studies showed that B virus infection was widespread in a range of macaque species. B virus infection was first linked to disease in its natural hosts species when Keeble and colleagues in 1958 reported herpes-like ulcers on the lips and tongues of recently imported rhesus monkeys, from which B virus was subsequently isolated. Subsequently B virus infection was shown to be widespread in many macaque species. Less than 40 human cases have been reported since the original report and these all occurred following contact with macaques species or their tissues in the course of biomedical research.

THE AGENT

Herpes B virus, or herpes simiae as it is sometimes called is now formally classified as Cercopithecine herpes virus type 1 (Murphy *et al.* 1995). It is a herpesvirus, a member of the genus simplex virus which is part of the alphaherpes subfamily (Murphy *et al.* 1995).

Alphaherpesviruses have been isolated from several primates species, and Table 31.1 lists the primate species from which alphaherpesviruses have been isolated. B virus is closely related antigenically and genomically to other primate simplexviruses, such as human herpes simplex viruses (HSV) and simian agent 8 (SA8) in African green monkeys (Malherbe and Strickland 1970). The close relationship between the viruses in different species (HSV, SA8, B virus) reflects a common evolutionary origin. Thus the diversity of the primate simplexviruses is likely to have evolved with the individual host species following the

Table 31.1 Recognized primate alphaherpesvirus species by host species

Primate family	Primate species (common name)	Indigenous alphaherpesvirus
1. Catarrhini	Macaque	B virus Medical Lake virus
Old World monkeys	Baboon African green monkey	Simian agent 8
		Simian agent 8 LVMV
	Colobines	pH Delta
	Orang-utan Gorilla Chimpanzee	
Apes	Humans	Herpes simplex 1 and 2 Varicella-Zoster virus
	Gibbons	
2. Platyrrhini	Marmoset Capuchin Squirrel	Herpes virus Tamarinus
New World monkeys	Aotus	
	Howler Woolly	
	Spider	Spider monkey herpesvirus

introduction of a common progenitor herpesvirus into a common ancestor in the primate evolutionary line.

The antigenic, genomic and biological characteristics of B virus have received only limited investigation (Hull 1973; Weigler 1992; Whitley 1993). These properties are very similar to the better known HSV (Roizman 1982). Electron microscopy of B virus infected tissue culture demonstrated that B virus has typical herpesvirus morphology. Virions range between 100 and 200 nm in diameter and consist of an electron-dense core with iscohedral structure of 100–110 nm surrounded by the viral tegument and envelope (Reubner et al. 1975).

B virus is a double-stranded DNA virus, its genome has a molecular weight of 107×10^6 Da which corresponds to a genome size of 162 kbp. B virus DNA has a very high G + C content of 75 per cent (Whitley 1993). The genomic structure of B virus has not been fully determined, but from restriction endonuclease cleavage patterns it is known that the B virus genome, like that of HSV, forms four isomers, which differ with respect of the orientation of large and small unique regions (Harrington et al. 1992). Limited sequence data are available for B virus in the unique small (US) region (Bennett et al. 1992; Killeen et al. 1992; Slomka

et al. 1995). The genome organization in the US region shows co-linearity with equivalent HSV genes. Glycoprotein D (US6) and glycoprotein J (US5) homologues in B virus have been fully sequenced and show 69 per cent and 57 per cent amino acid identity with HSV-1, respectively (Bennett et al. 1992). Recently the glycoprotein G equivalent has been characterized and shown to be similar in size to HSV-2 (593 amino acids) but shares little amino acid similarity with HSV-1 and HSV-2 (Slomka et al. 1995).

B virus, SA8, and HSV show extensive antigenic cross-reactivity, in many test systems (Cabasso et al. 1967; Pauli and Ludwig 1977; Hutt et al. 1981; Ludwig et al. 1983; Hilliard et al. 1989). More than 50 B virus polypeptide bands have been identified by electrophoresis and immune precipitation of tissue-culture-grown virus. At least nine glycoprotein bands have been identified and the gD and gB shown to share antigenic determinants with HSV-1. Multiple other infected cell polypeptides (ICPs) produced in tissue culture infected with B virus have been shown by Western blot and immune precipitation to share antigenic determinants with HSV (Hilliard et al. 1989).

REPLICATION

B virus grows to high titre in a range of cell lines derived from several species, including primary monkey kidney, chick embryo cell lines and vero E6 cells, which are all suitable for diagnostic isolation. In these cell lines typically B virus produces a characteristic syncytial cytopathic effect. B virus can be propagated on the chorio-allantoic membrane of embryonated eggs (Burnett et al. 1939). B virus will produce a clinical illness in mice, rabbits and New World monkeys following intradermal inoculation (Sabin and Wright 1934; Gosztonyi et al. 1992).

The reproductive cycle of B virus is short: host-cell DNA synthesis is inhibited within 4 hours after infection and infectious virus is detectable within 6 hours. Peak virus levels are found between 24 and 35 hours after infection. B virus, like other herpesviruses, causes intranuclear inclusions in cell culture.

NON-HUMAN PRIMATE INFECTION

EPIZOOLOGY

B virus has been most extensively studied in rhesus and cynomolgus monkeys, because these two species are most widely used for biomedical research. B virus probably occurs in all 16 macaque species and it has been isolated from naturally infected rhesus (M. mulatta), cynomolgus (M. fascicularis), bonnet (M. radiata) monkeys and M. cyclopis (Endo et al. 1960; Hartley

Table 31.2 B virus antibody prevalence of sera collected from wild-caught Old World monkeys submitted to the Virus Reference Division, Central Public Health Laboratory, Colindale, for screening in 1989

Origin	Species	Number of sera tested	Prevalence of B virus Ab (neutralization) (%)
China	Rhesus	25	32
Philippines	Cynomolgus[a]	80	7.5
Philippines	Cynomolgus	372	4
Mauritius	Cynomolgus	263	–
Indonesia	Cynomolgus	366	42.6
Ethiopia	Baboon	87	13.7
Africa	Vervets	15	86
Total tested		1208	

[a] Colony bred.

1964; Espana 1973). B virus antibodies have been detected in most macaque species (Shah and Morrison, 1969; DiGiacano and Shah 1972; Palmer 1987) (Table 31.2). B virus antibodies have also been detected in sera from a range of African primates and humans (Van Hoosier and Melnick 1961; Cabasso 1967), but these represent antibodies against the closely related SA8 and HSV viruses, since B virus specific antibody tests have only recently been developed (Katz *et al.* 1986; Norcott and Brown 1993).

Several studies have investigated the age of acquisition of B virus antibodies in macaques (Palmer 1987). Interpretation of the published studies is complicated because some refer to wild-caught and others to colony-held monkeys, and several factors can affect the acquisition of antibody. However, a few general points can be made: newborn monkeys are generally uninfected with B virus even if born to a seropositive mother. Antibody prevalence remains low in young animals and the peaks in sexually mature adults. Zwartouw and Boulter 1984 first suggested that this picture, together with the isolation of B virus from the sacral ganglia of seropositive animals, fits best with a sexual route of transmission (Boulter 1975; McCarthy and Tosolini 1975; Vizoso 1975). However, particularly amongst captive animals, the importance of oral transmission through close contact has been highlighted as an alternative explanation (Weigler *et al.* 1990, 1993). Since B virus can be isolated from oral and genital lesions, both routes may play a part in monkey to monkey transmission and the relative importance may vary in wild and colony-bred animals.

Infection is endemic in local groups or colony-raised monkeys, but epidemics have been reported following the introduction of an infected animal into a B virus free colony (Zwartouw *et al.* 1984). The communicability of B virus to humans is low. There are only 40 reported human cases despite the high numbers of primates used for biomedical research. Communicability is raised following re-activation due to stressing of the animals and high seroconversion rates have been

reported in groups of newly imported animals associated with stress-induced re-activation (Keeble 1960). The rate of re-activation of B virus in well-managed animals may be one factor affecting this apparent low communicability. Zwartouw and Boulter 1984 were unable to demonstrate shedding of B virus from seropositive animals except following immunosuppression therapy. However, a more extensive recent study has suggested that re-activation does occur at a similar rate to that observed for HSV in seropositive humans (Weigler *et al.* 1993).

TRANSMISSION

Surveys of colony-held monkeys reveal that B virus antibody acquisition is rapid after capture and caging of the animals together (Keeble 1960). Keeping monkeys together in gang cages can result in overcrowding and stress, which can induce re-activation and may lead to more opportunity for spread through direct salivary contact or via salivary contamination of shared objectives. If monkeys are singly caged after capture, then transmission by the sexual route or close contact can be prevented or at least greatly controlled. Respiratory transmission of B virus has been shown to be possible (Chappell 1960) and one respiratory-associated outbreak has been reported in a colony of bonnet monkeys (Espana 1973). However, the observation that individually caging animals effectively prevents virus spread argues against the aerosol route being a significant route of transmission of B virus in normal circumstances.

INFECTION IN MACAQUES

B virus infection in macaques resembles human HSV infection, with primary genital or oral infection followed by latency in nerve ganglia, with periodic recurrence (Boulter 1975; Palmer 1987). Most infections are very mild or subclinical. Clinical disease in macaques has been described in rhesus but not cynomolgus monkeys (Lees *et al.* 1991). The incubation period is short and virus excretion can be detected within 2 days of infection. Keeble *et al.* (1958) first described natural B virus infection in a group of rhesus monkeys newly imported into the United Kingdom from India. Cases first developed vesicles on the tongue and oral cavity which later became ulcers and these took up to 14 days to heal. No neurological symptoms were observed in these animals, although possible lesions were identified in the medulla and pons of several animals which were thought to be related to B virus (Keeble *et al.* 1958). The frequency of clinical illness in macaques is not known, but Keeble (1960) reported similar lesions in 2.3 per cent of a larger series of 1400 monkeys. Neurological disease can be induced in the macaques by intracerebral inoculation of B virus (Sabin and Wright 1934) but it appears to be an unusual outcome of natural infection. Rare, more generalized infection has been identified, particularly in association with immunosuppression (Simon *et al.* 1993). No specific treatment is indicated for macaque B virus infection.

PATHOGENESIS OF INFECTION IN ANIMALS

The primary lesion of B virus infection is very similar to that of HSV in humans (Keeble 1960). The histological appearance of the primary lesions was of a necrotic epithelium overlying an ulcer, which extended into the papillary layer. A polymorph nuclear infiltrate was observed and ballooning degeneration noted at the edge of the lesions where cells contained intranuclear inclusions typical of herpes virus infection. In addition, the African green monkey (*Cercopithecus aethiops*), the patas monkey (*Erythrocebuspatas*), and the cynomolgus monkey can be infected experimentally with B virus but show no evidence of disease (Lees *et al.* 1991). Experimental infection of New World monkeys with B virus can lead to a devastating neurological illness similar to that seen in untreated human cases (Zwartouw *et al.* 1989).

A number of small laboratory animals have been experimentally infected with B virus, and both rabbit (Gay and Holden 1933; Sabin and Wright 1934) and mice (Gosztonyi *et al.* 1992) infected with B virus develop neurological lesions similar to those seen in human infection and have been the most widely used models to study infection.

HUMAN INFECTION

Human B virus infection has most frequently presented clinically as an ascending encephalomyelitis similar to that of the first reported case (Sabin and Wright 1934). The incubation period of human B virus infection is not well defined and between 4 and 59 days have been reported. The two fatal cases identified in the Pensacola incident (Centers for Disease Control 1987*a*; Holmes *et al.* 1990) developed local vesicular lesions within a week of a documented exposure and signs indicating severe central nervous system disease were apparent 7–14 days later. A few cases have presented early with a history of a bite and vesicular lesions at the site, but most cases have presented later in the course of illness when signs of neurological involvement are apparent. The local lesions can present with severe itching and pain at the bite site, but the local lesions are not consistently present. Local infection is followed by regional lymphadenopathy within a few days and the development of fever and involvement of central nervous system, early signs reported are persistent headache, limb stiffness, nausea and vomiting. Later in the infection a range of other neurological signs reflecting widespread brainstem damage have been reported, such as diplopia, dysarthria, dysphagia, dizziness, and ataxia. Other signs of CNS impairment such as hemiparesis, hemiplegia, convulsions or altered mental states have also been described.

The majority of B virus cases have developed severe neurological disease following an exposure to primates. However, one reported case occurred in a virologist who presented with a syndrome resembling ophthalmic zoster and claimed to have had no direct contact with non-human primates for some years (Fierer *et al.* 1973). This, together with the two mild cases reported (Bryan *et al.* 1975; Benson *et al.* 1989), suggests that B virus has the potential to cause mild or subclinical human infection illness. The recent development of B virus specific antibody tests (Hilliard *et al.* 1986; Heberling and Kalter 1987; Norcott and Brown 1993) has led to study of the scale of human B virus infection. The one study reported (Freifeld *et al.* 1995) so far suggests that the prevalence of unrecognized infection in monkey handlers is low.

LABORATORY DIAGNOSIS

Laboratory confirmation of B virus infection in humans is complicated by the extensive antigenic cross-reactivity between HSV-1 and HSV-2, common human viruses, and B virus. Definitive confirmation of human infection is by the isolation of B virus from human samples in tissue culture. B virus grows successfully in a number of primary cell lines and a continuous cell line; Vero cells are convenient for diagnostic laboratories. B virus produces a cytopathic effect in cell culture. B virus isolates are characterized serologically using immunoflorescence or neutralization with specific polyclonal sera. Identification often proved difficult because of the cross-reactivity with HSV seen with these polyclonal sera. The development of mono-clonal antibodies to B virus (Cropper *et al.* 1992) has resolved serological typing difficulties and both restric-tion enzyme digestion (Hilliard *et al.* 1986; Wall *et al.* 1989) and virion polypeptide patterns (Hilliard *et al.* 1987) have also been useful for confirming the identity of an infecting B virus strain.

As an enveloped virus, B virus is relatively heat labile, and clinical specimens for isolation require to be kept cool and transported quickly to the laboratory. Isolation of B virus strains has been most successful from CSF, conjunctival or vesicular specimens. Recom-mendations for appropriate investigations have been published (Holmes *et al.* 1995). Once in tissue culture the virus is relatively stable and can be stored for short periods at 4 °C or at −70 °C for longer periods.

The recent availability of sequence information has enabled polymerase chain reaction (PCR) tests to be developed for B virus (Scinicariello *et al.* 1993*a*; Slomka *et al.* 1993). These have been shown to be more sensi-tive than culture for detecting B virus in clinical samples and they are likely to play an important role in diagnostic testing for B virus, in a similar manner to that established for the HSV PCR test in cases of herpes simplex encephalitis (Scinicariello *et al.* 1993*b*).

Specific serological diagnosis for B virus has not been possible until recently because of the extensive antigenic cross-reactions between B virus and herpes simplex, which meant that it was very difficult to dis-tinguish an immune response to B virus from pre-existing antibody to herpes simplex virus. However, three antibody test formats have recently been described which are able to discriminate B virus anti-bodies from HSV antibodies. Katz *et al.* (1986) described an ELISA test in which sera were tested against B virus, HSV and SA8 before and after absorption with homologus and heterologous virus. Heberling and Kalter (1987) described an immuno-blot assay and Norcott and Brown (1993) used a B virus specific monoclonal antibody as the basis of a B virus specific epitope blocking assay. The sensitivity and specificity of these assays has not been fully evalu-ated for human cases because of the small numbers of samples available. In the small number of case investi-gated, antibody detection has not always proved reliable for diagnosis because B virus antibody may take some weeks to develop following infection, and individual cases have been reported to lose antibody after proven infection (Holmes *et al.* 1990; Norcott and Brown 1993; Davenport *et al.* 1994). Early treatment with acyclovir may compromise the development of a detectable immune response.

The detection of virus and antibodies for confirm-ation of infection in non-human primates can be undertaken using the same techniques. Serological screening of macaque sera to establish their B virus status is widely practised before they are used for research.

PATHOGENESIS OF HUMAN INFECTION

Disease in humans usually follows a bite by a macaque, although disease that is the consequence of re-activa-tion (Fierer *et al.* 1973) has been reported. Following the bite, local replication of virus at the inoculation site takes place. Often local vesicular lesions develop and there is evidence of local inflammation with mono-nuclear cell infiltrate, followed by evidence of lym-phangitis and subsequent lymph node involvement.

The most striking characteristic of human B virus infection is the neurological involvement. As in the first reported case, transverse myelitis is a prominent neurological finding, with ultimate progression of infection to the brain. All regions of the brain can be infected with no evidence of localization to a particular region or to a specific neuronal cell. This is different from HSV infection of the CNS in adults, which tends to localize in the temporal lobe. Histopathological findings of the brain include haemorrhagic foci, necrosis, and inflammatory changes with perivascular cuffing with mononuclear infiltrates. Degeneration of the motor neurones and gliosis and astrocytosis are late histopathological findings. Myelitis, encephalo-myelitis, or encephalitis, or different combinations of each of these conditions, have all been reported in human B virus infection.

The primary mode of virus spread is through nerve tracts (Gosztonyi *et al.* 1992). Other organs of the body are often involved, either through lymphatic spread or as a consequence of transient viraemia, although this has not been demonstrated in humans. The involved organs are usually the viscera, particularly the liver and lungs. Under such circumstances, focal haemorrhagic necrosis is common.

TREATMENT

Prior to 1980 no specific treatment was available for human B virus infection and the mortality rate was more than 70 per cent, which is very similar to that of untreated herpes simplex encephalitis. In addition to the high mortality rate, a number of the survivors were left with neurological sequelae (Table 31.3).

The development of the antiviral drug acyclovir has dramatically altered the outcome of infection. Tissue-culture studies showed that B virus was sensitive to acy-clovir although B virus is less sensitive than HSV

Table 31.3 Documented human B virus infections

Number	Year	Exposure	Outcome of infection	Reference
1	1932	Bite to the hand Rhesus monkey	Fatal infection Survived 17 days	Sabin and Wright (1934)
2	1949	Saliva contamination of wound on hand Rhesus monkey	Fatal infection	Sabin (1949)
3	1956	Scratch Monkey species not known	Recovered with moderate neurological sequelae	Davidson and Hummeler (1960)
4	1957	Bite on hand Monkey species not known	Fatal infection Survived for 30 days	Hummeler (1959)
5	1957	Suspected aerosol Rhesus monkeys	Fatal infection Survived for 7 days	Davidson and Hummeler (1960)
6	1957	Cleaned monkey skull Rhesus monkey	Fatal infection	Davidson and Hummeler (1960)
7	1957	Bite on finger Rhesus monkey	Fatal infection Survived 8 days	Davidson and Hummeler (1960)
8	1957	Bite on finger Rhesus or cynomolgus monkey	Recovered with mild neurological impairment	Breen *et al.* (1958)
9	1957	No details	Fatal infection	Davidson and Hummeler (1960)
10	1958	Cut on hand while working with primary monkey tissue culture	Fatal infection Survived 15 days	Hummeler (1959)
11	1958	Needle-stick injury to hand	Fatal infection Survived 17 days	Davidson and Hummeler (1960)
12	1958	Needle-stick and biting injuries	Fatal infection	Davidson and Hummeler (1960)
13	1960	Scratch on forearm Rhesus monkey	Fatal infection Survived 38 days	Love (1962)
14	1963	Suspected aerosol Contact with Rhesus and African green monkeys	Survived for 4 years with severe neurological sequelae	Hull (1973)
15	1965	Bite from African green monkey	Fatal infection Survived 20 days	Palmer (1987)
16	1970	Suspected recurrence No monkey contacts for several years	Survived for 12 years with severe neurological sequelae	Fierer *et al.* (1973)
17	1973	Bite from rhesus monkey	Recovered with minimal neurological sequelae	Bryan *et al.* (1975)
18	1987	Bite on thumb by rhesus monkey	Fatal infection Survived 6 months	Holmes *et al.* (1990)
19	1987	Bite to forearm by rhesus monkey	Fatal infection Survived 30 days	Holmes *et al.* (1990)
20	1987	Scratch from cage	No clinical illness[a]	Holmes *et al.* (1990)
21	1987	From husband	No clinical illness[a]	Holmes *et al.* (1990)
22	1989	Needle-stick injury. Rhesus monkey	No clinical illness[a]	Artenstein *et al.* (1991)
23	1989	Bite to chest Contact with rhesus and cynomolgus monkeys	Fatal infection Survived 8 days	Davenport *et al.* (1994)
24	1989	Bite on thumb Rhesus and cynomolgus monkeys	Full recovery from encephalomyelitis	Davenport *et al.* (1994)
25	1989	Multiple scratches	Full recovery from aseptic meningitis	Davenport *et al.* (1994)

[a] Treated with acyclovir before the onset of neurological symptoms.

(Boulter *et al.* 1980). Further studies in rabbits demonstrated that acyclovir treatment was effective in preventing disease (Boulter and Grant 1977; Zwartouw *et al.* 1989) and suggested that early treatment might be effective in preventing infection.

B virus is also sensitive to ganciclovir, which has been used in recent severe clinical cases (Zwartouw *et al.* 1989). There have been nine virologically confirmed human B virus cases diagnosed since acyclovir became available, and all cases treated early have recovered from clinical illness. The impact of treatment with acyclovir is apparent since only four of the nine cases since 1987 have been fatal (44 per cent). In the Pensacola cluster of four cases (Holmes *et al.* 1990; Centers for Disease Control 1987*a*), two patients had developed severe neurological disease before treatment and subsequently died. Two cases who were treated after the development of local lesions at the bite site, but before the onset of neurological disease recovered without clinical sequelae. Two subsequent cases (Davenport *et al.* 1994) treated with acyclovir and ganciclovir after the onset of neurological illness also recovered. In one case B virus re-excretion was detected after acyclovir treatment was discontinued following clinical recovery (Holmes *et al.* 1990). Consequently, all of the cases who have recovered since 1987 continue on maintenance acyclovir therapy, since the likely effect of discontinuing treatment is unknown.

The role of early treatment of clinical B virus infection is well established, intravenous doses of 10 mg/kg given 8 hourly intravenously are recommended, followed by oral therapy with 800 mg acyclovir given five times per day.

The role of oral acyclovir prophylactic treatment is more contentious. Three weeks of prophylactic acyclovir treatment (800 mg five times daily) has been recommended, starting immediately following a potential exposure (Wansbrough-Jones *et al.* 1989). However, because human B virus infection is rare and early treatment is effective, this has led to more emphasis being placed on careful monitoring of individuals following a potential exposure and early treatment if indicated by the clinical course (Holmes *et al.* 1995).

It has been suggested that immunoglobulin may have a role in the early treatment of B virus infection (Boulter *et al.* 1982). However, this approach has now been superseded by antiviral treatment.

EPIDEMIOLOGY

Human B virus infection is rare, indeed less than 40 cases have been recorded in the world literature since the first case in 1932 (Palmer 1987; Holmes *et al.* 1990; Artenstein *et al.* 1991; Davenport *et al.* 1994). Table 31.3 lists the twenty-five cases documented in the literature. A significant proportion of these cases occurred during the 1950s, when 12 cases were identified. This has been linked to the large numbers of macaques used for poliovirus vaccine safety testing during that time. Between 1973 and 1987 there were no recorded cases, but nine further cases have subsequently been reported in the United States. No cases have been reported in local populations in South-East Asia, where exposure to macaques might be expected to be common.

All but two of the cases have been linked to direct handling of macaques. The majority of infections were associated with a direct bite, but in a number of cases no obvious exposure was documented (Table 31.3). Two recent cases in which infection was linked to a needle-stick injury (Artenstein *et al.* 1991) and to touching a contaminated cage (Centers for Disease Control 1989; Davenport *et al.* 1994) illustrate this point. Only two cases have not been linked to direct handling of monkeys:

CASE 1

A 21-year-old laboratory technician engaged in polio vaccine production in January 1958 (Davidson and Hummeler 1960). His accident record revealed that on two occasions he had minor lacerations on his hands from broken glass containing tissue cultures of primary monkey kidney. This was a fatal infection and B virus was isolated from the CNS. B virus has been isolated from batches of primary monkey kidney which are widely used for isolating influenza virus in diagnostic virus laboratories and the importance of considering this route of exposure was recently highlighted (Wells *et al.* 1989).

CASE 2

In 1987 four human cases of B virus infection were admitted to hospitals in Pensacola, Florida (Holmes *et al.* 1990). One patient was a 29-year-old woman, the wife of a biology technician who died from B virus infection. This woman had no direct contact with monkeys, but she did apply hydrocortisone cream to her husband's skin lesions and also applied the cream to an area of contact dermatitis under a ring on her finger. B virus was isolated from this lesion, she was treated with acyclovir and the disease did not progress further. This is the only reported case of a human to human spread of B virus and no further cases were identified in this incident despite careful surveillance of more than 150 contacts.

No human infections have been reported due to SA8 virus, the alphaherpes virus of baboons and

African green monkeys, which is closely related to B virus. One death attributed to B virus (Table 31.3, case number 15) resulted from a bite by an African green monkey (*Cercopithecus aethiops*), but no virus isolate was made from the case. Despite this, it is a reasonable presumption that SA8 was responsible. There has also been one presumptive human infection with herpesvirus tamarinus, a similar virus of New World monkeys. The worker involved was in contact with New World primates, he recovered from encephalitis and developed antibodies to herpesvirus tamarinus (Medical Research Council 1985).

B virus infection is widespread in macaque species that have been used for research. Despite this and the large scale use of cynomolgus monkeys, in particular for biomedical work, human B virus cases have been linked almost exclusively to contact with rhesus monkeys. It remains to be established if the rhesus monkey B virus strain is more pathogenic that B virus strains from other macaques, or if this apparent difference reflects different rates of re-activation or behaviour differences between the different species, since the cynomolgus B virus strains and SA8 strains isolated from baboons and vervet monkeys can cause neurological illness in rabbits. It is probably wise to treat exposure to African monkeys as a potential hazard and monitor individuals potentially exposed to these and other primate herpes viruses.

PREVENTION AND CONTROL

Human B virus infection is preventable, by control of the contacts between humans and macaques. B virus infection is likely to be an uncommon outcome of macaque-related injury since thousands of monkey-related exposures occur each year. There are three main areas in which control strategies can be employed: the selection of macaques for use in biomedical research, the development of screening and safe primate handling polices (Medical Research Council 1985), and the dissemination of guidelines for the management of potential B virus exposure in staff working with primates (Wansbrough-Jones *et al.* 1988; Brown *et al.* 1988; Holmes *et al.* 1995).

The simplest way to prevent B virus infection is to allow only B virus free animals to be used for biomedical research. This has proved difficult because B virus infection is widespread in wild-caught macaques from many countries. All primates used for biomedical work are now required to be purpose bred, and breeding colonies have been set up in Europe, Asia, and America. At present one B virus free colony has been set up successfully in the United Kingdom, using a policy of serological screening followed by exclusion of infected

macaques (Zwartouw *et al.* 1984). Other colonies should be encouraged to adopt a similar approach; however, it is likely to take some years before only B virus free animals are available in the required numbers. A policy of screening sera from all Old World monkeys for B virus so that their status is known has been practised in the United Kingdom for 10 years. B virus infected animals can then be used for less hazardous work and not used for work involving immunosuppression or neuroinvasive procedures. At present the most effective method of controlling B virus infection is the monkey handling practice used within colonies. Guidelines have been published (Medical Research Council 1985; Centers for Disease Control 1987*b*) and the United States guidelines were recently updated following the importation of Ebola–Reston virus into the USA in batches of cynomolgus monkeys. These give detailed recommendations of how to handle monkeys, which are outside the scope of this review. The important issues are in restricting exposures by controlling monkey handling procedures with the use of crush cages, ketamine anaesthetic, protective gauntlets, and face protection, which all contribute to preventing penetrating injuries.

Detailed recommendations about how to manage potential exposures have been published in the United Kingdom (Brown *et al.* 1988; Wansbrough-Jones *et al.* 1989) and very recently in the United States (Holmes *et al.* 1995). These policies are broadly similar and recommend five major actions in the event of an exposure: (1) immediate cleaning of the wound site; (2) risk assessment of the incident; (3) investigation of the monkey and worker involved; (4) monitor health of the at-risk workers for several weeks; and (5) consider prophylactic treatment with oral acyclovir. There is broad agreement about the approaches to be used except for the role of immediate prophylactic acyclovir treatment. It is established that early treatment with acyclovir may prevent symptomatic B virus infection, and initiation within minutes of exposure may even prevent latent B virus infection. Against prophylactic treatment is the rarity of B virus infection, which means that therapy is unnecessary in most incidents, and the success of early treatment. The ability of immediate therapy to prevent latent infection is not yet established and prophylactic acyclovir therapy may compromise attempts to make a diagnosis.

Evaluation of the effectiveness of these control methods is difficult because of the rarity of infection, but it is likely that the use of crush cages and ketamine anaesthetic during the 1970s led to the reduction in case numbers. Accidents leading to bites by macaques require to be entered into an accident book and be reported to the relevant authorities (Health and Safety Executive in the United Kingdom). Suspected human cases are not legally notifiable but should be reported to the relevant public health authorities so that appropriate surveillance measures can be introduced.

The production of recombinant proteins from B virus may lead to the development of a B virus vaccine using the same approach as for HSV (Slomka *et al.* 1995). This might have a role in developing B virus free colonies. However, the early studies of a B virus vaccine have not been followed up (Hull 1971).

CONCLUSIONS

Fortunately, symptomatic B virus infection in humans is uncommon. However, because of its rarity, much remains to be learned about the most effective means of preventing B virus infection in exposed persons, the value of prophylactic therapy and the optimal long-term management of B virus infected patients. The rarity of these cases means that it is important that veterinary and medical personnel involved in primate work carefully document and report information on the circumstances of exposure, initial evaluation, clinical course, laboratory studies, medical management, and follow-up so that our knowledge of this virus infection is enhanced.

REFERENCES

Artenstein, A. W., Hicks, C. B., Goodwin, B. S., and Hilliard, J. K. (1991). Human infection with B virus following a needlestick injury. *Reviews of the Infectious Diseases*, **13**, 288–91.

Bennett, A. M., Harrington, L., and Kelly, D. C. (1992). Nucleotide sequence analysis of genes encoding glycoproteins D and J in simian herpes B virus. *Journal of General Virology*, **73**, 2963–7.

Benson, P. M., Malane, S. L., Banks, R., Hicks, C. B., and Hilliard, J. (1989). B virus (Herpesvirus simiae) and human infection. *Archives of Dermatology*, **125**, 1247–8.

Boulter, E. A. (1975). The isolation of monkey B virus (Herpesvirus simiae) from the trigeminal ganglia of a healthy seropositive rhesus monkey. *Journal of Biological Standards*, **3**, 279–80.

Boulter, E. A. and Grant, D. P. (1977). Latent infection of monkeys with B virus and prophylactic studies in a rabbit model of this disease. *Journal of Antimicrobial Chemotherapy*, **3**, 107.

Boulter, E. A., Thornton, B., Bauer, D. J., and Bye, A. (1980). A successful treatment of experimental B virus (Herpesvirus simiae) infection with acyclovir. *British Medical Journal*, **280**, 681–3.

Boulter, E. A., Zwartouw, H. T., and Thornton, B. (1982). Postexposure immunoprophylaxes against B virus infection. *British Medical Journal*, **284**, 746.

Breen, G. E., Lamb, S. G., and Otaki, A. T. (1958). Monkey bite encephalomyelitis: report of a case with recovery. *British Medical Journal*, **2**, 22–3.

Brown, D., Cropper, I., Lees, D., and Gardner, S. (1988). Prophylaxis against B virus infection? *British Medical Journal*, **297**, 1332.

Bryan, B. L., Espana, C. D., Emmons, R. W., Vijayan, N., and Hoeprich, P. D. (1975). Recovery from encephalomyel caused by Herpesvirus simiae, report of a case. *Archives of Internal Medicine*, **135**, 868–70.

Burnett, F. M., Lush, D., and Jackson, A. V. (1939). The propagation of herpes B and pseudorabies viruses on the chorioallantois. *Australian Journal of Experimental Biology and Medical Sciences*, **17**, 35–40.

Cabasso, V. J., Chappell, W. A., Avampato, J. E., and Brittle, I. L. (1967). Correlation of B virus and herpes simplex virus antibodies in human sera. *Journal of Laboratory and Clinical Medicine*, **70**, 170–6.

Centers for Disease Control (1987a). B virus infection in humans—Pensacola, Florida. *MMWR*, **36**, 289–90, 295–6.

Centers for Disease Control (1987b). Guidelines for prevention of Herpes simiae (B virus) infection in monkey handlers. *MMWR*, **36**, 680–2, 687–9.

Centers for Disease Control (1989). B virus infections in humans—Michigan. *MMWR*, **38**, 453–4.

Chappell, W. A. (1960). Animal infectivity of aerosols of monkey B virus. *Annals of the New York Academy of Sciences*, **851**, 931–4.

Cropper, L. M., Lees, D. N., Patt, R., Sharp, I. R., and Brown, D. (1992). Monoclonal antibodies for the identification of herpesvirus simiae (B virus) *Archives of Virology*, **123**, 267–77.

Davenport, D. S. *et al.* (1994). Diagnosis and management of human B virus (Herpesvirus simiae) infections in Michigan. *Clinics in Infectious Diseases*, **19**, 33–41.

Davidson, W. L. and Hummeler, K. (1960). B virus infection in man. *Annals of the New York Academy of Sciences*, **85**, 970–9.

DiGiacano, R. F. and Shah, K. V. (1972). Virtual absence of infection with Herpesvirus simiae in colony-reared rhesus monkeys (*macaca mulatta*) with a literature review on antibody prevalence in natural and laboratory rhesus populations. *Laboratory Animal Science*, **22**, 61–7.

Endo, M. *et al.* (1960). Etude du virus B au Japan II le premier isolement du virus B au Japan. *Japanese Journal of Experimental Medicine*, **30**, 385–92.

Espana, C. (1973). Herpesvirus simiae infection in *Macaca radiata*. *American Journal of Physical Anthropology*, **38**, 447–454.

Fierer, J., Bazeley, P., and Braud, A. I. (1973). Herpes B virus encephalomyelitis presenting as ophthalmic zoster. *Annals of Internal Medicine*, **79**, 225–8.

Freifeld, A. *et al.* (1995). A controlled seroprevalence survey of primate handlers for evidence of asymptomatic herpes B virus infection. *Journal of Infectious Diseases*, **171**, 1031–34.

Gay, F. P. and Holden, M. (1933). The herpes encephalitis problem II. *Journal of Infectious Diseases*, **53**, 287–303.

Gosztonyi, G., Falke, D., and Ludwig, H. (1992). Axonal and transynaptic (transneuronal) spread of Herpes vi simiae (B virus) in experimentally infected mice. *Histology and Histopathology*, **7**, 63–74.

Harrington, L., Wall, L. V. M., and Kelly, D. C. (1992). Molecular cloning and physical mapping of the genome of simian herpes B virus and comparison of genome organisation with that of herpes simplex type 1. *Journal of General Virology*, **73**, 1217–26.

Hartley, E. G. (1964). Naturally occurring 'B' virus infection in cynomolgus monkey. *Veterinary Record*, **76**, 555–557.

Heberling, R. L. and Kalter, S. S. (1987). A dot-immunobinding assay on nitrocellulose with psoralen inactivated Herpes virus simiae (B virus) *Laboratory Animal Science*, **37**, 304–8.

Hilliard, J. K., Munoz, R. M., Lipper, S. L., and Eberle, R. (1986). Rapid identification of herpesvirus simiae (B virus) DNA from clinical isolates in nonhuman primate colonies. *Journal of Virological Methods*, **13**, 55–62.

Hilliard, J. K., Eberle, R., Lipper, S. L., Munoz, R. M., and Weiss, S. A. (1987). Herpes virus simiae (B virus): replication of the virus and identification of viral polypeptides in infected cells. *Archives of Virology*, **93**, 185–198.

Hilliard, J. K., Black, D., and Eberle, R. (1989). Simian alphaviruses and their relation to the human herpes simplex viruses. *Archives of Virology*, **109**, 83–102.

Holmes, G. P. *et al.* (1990). B virus (herpesvirus simiae) infection in humans: epidemiological investigation of a cluster. *Annals of Internal Medicine*, **112**, 833–9.

Holmes, G. P., Chapman, L. E., Stewart, J. A., Straus, S., Hilliard, J. K., and Davenport, D. S. (1995). Guidelines the prevention and treatment of B virus infections in exposed persons. *Clinics in Infectious Diseases*, **20**, 421–39.

Hull, R. N. (1971). B virus vaccines. *Laboratory Animal Science*, **21**, 1068–71.

Hull, R. N. (1973). The simian herpesviruses. In *The herpesviruses*, (ed. A. S. Kaplan), pp. 389–425. Academic Press, New York.

Hummeler, K. Davidson, W. L., Henlew, LaBouetta, A. C., Rush, H. (1959). Encephalomyelitis due to infection with Herpes virus simiae (herpes B virus): a report of two fatal, laboratory acquired cases. *New England Journal of Medical*, **281**, 64–8.

Hutt, R., Guajardo, J. E., and Kalter, S. S. (1981). Detection of antibodies to Herpesvirus simiae and Herpesvirus hominis in non-human primates. *Laboratory Animal Science*, **31**, 184–9.

Katz, D., Hilliard, J. K., Eberle, R., and Lipper, S. L. (1986). ELISA for detection of group-specific and virus-specific antibodies in human and simian sera induced by herpes simplex and related simian viruses. *Journal of Virological Methods*, **14**, 99–109.

Keeble, S. A. (1960). B virus infection in monkeys. *Annals of the New York Academy of Sciences*, **85**, 960–9.

Keeble, S. A., Christofinis, G. J., and Wood, W. (1958). Natural virus B infection in rhesus monkeys. *Journal of Pathological Bacteriology*, **76**, 189–99.

Killeen, A. M., Harrington, K., Wall, L. V. M., and Kelly, D. C. (1992). Nucleotide sequence analysis of a homologue of herpes simplex virus type 1 gene US9 found in the genome of simian herpes B virus. *Journal of General Virology*, **73**, 195–9.

Lees, D. N., Baskerville, A., Cropper, L. M., and Brown, D. W. (1991). Herpesvirus simiae (B virus) antibody response and virus shedding in experimental primary infection of cynomolgus monkeys. *Laboratory Animal Science*, **41**, 360–4.

Love, F. M. and Jungherr, E. (1962). Occupational infection with virus B of monkeys. *Journal of the American Medical Association*, **179**, 160–2.

Ludwig, H., Pauli, G., Gelderblom, H., Darai, G., Korh, H. G., Hugel, R. M., Norrild, B, Daniel, M. D. (1983). B virus (Herpes virus simiae), In, Herpes virus Volume 2 (ed. B. Roizman) *New York and London Plenum Press*, 385–428.

McCarthy, K. and Tosolini, F. A. (1975). Hazards from simian Herpes Viruses: reactivation of skin lesions with virus shedding. *Lancet*, **I**, 649–50.

Malherbe, H., and Strickland, C. M. (1970). The viruses of vervet monkeys and baboons in South Africa. *Journal of the South African Veterinary and Medical Association*, **41**, 177–89.

Medical Research Council (1985). *The management of simians in relation to infectious hazards to staff.* MRC, London.

Melnick, J. L. and Banker, D. D. (1954). Isolation of B virus (herpes group) from the central nervous system of a rhesus monkey. *Journal of Experimental Medicine*, **100**, 181–94.

Murphy, F. A. *et al.* (ed.) (1995). Virus taxonomy classification and nomenclature of viruses. *Archives of Virology*, Suppl. 10, 114–27.

Norcott, J. P. and Brown, D. W. (1993). Competitive radioimmunoassay to detect antibodies to herpes B virus and SA8 virus. *Journal of Clinical Microbiology*, **31**, 931–5.

Palmer, A. E. (1987). B virus, herpes simiae: historical perspective. *Journal of Medical Primatology*, **16**, 99–130.

Pauli, G. and Ludwig, H. (1977). Immunoprecipitation of herpes simplex virus type 1 antigen with different antisera and human cerebrospinal fluids. *Archives of Virology*, **53**, 139.

Roizman, B. (1982). The family herpesviridae: general description, taxonomy and classification. In *The Herpesviruses*, Vol. 1, (ed. B. Roizman), pp. 1–23. Plenum Press, New York.

Ruebner, B. H., Debereux, D., Rorvik, M., Espana, C., and Brown, J. F. (1975). Ultrastructure of Herpesvirus simiae (herpes B virus). *Experimental Molecular Pathology*, **22**, 317.

Sabin, A. B. (1949). Fatal B virus encephalomyelitis in a physician working with monkeys. *Journal of Clinical Investigation*, **28**, 808.

Sabin, A. B. and Wright, A. M. (1934). Acute ascending myelitis following a monkey bite, with the isolation of a virus capable of reproducing the disease. *Journal of Experimental Medicine*, **59**, 115–36.

Scinicariello, F., Eberle, R., and Hilliard, J. (1993*a*). Rapid detection of B virus (herpesvirus simiae) DNA by polymerase chain reaction. *Journal of Infectious Diseases*, **168**, 747–50.

Scinicariello, F., English, W. J., and Hilliard, J. (1993*b*). Identification by PCR of meningitis caused by herpes B virus. *Lancet*, **341**, 1660–1.

Shah, K. V. and Morrison, J. A. (1969). Comparison of three rhesus groups for antibody patterns to some viruses: absence of active simian virus 40 transmission in the free-ranging rhesus of Cayo Santiago. *American Journal of Epidemiology*, **89**, 308–15.

Simon, M. A., Daniel, M. D., Lee-Parritz, D., King, N. W., and Ringler, D. J. (1993). Disseminated B virus infection in a cynomologus monkey. *Laboratory Animal Science*, **43**, 545–50.

Slomka, M. J., Brown, D. W. G., Clewley, J. P., Bennett, A. M., Harrington, L., and Kelly, D. C. (1993). Polymerase chain reaction for detection of herpesvirus simiae (B virus) in clinical specimens. *Archives of Virology*, **131**, 89–99.

Slomka, M. J., Harrington, L., Arnold, C., Norcott, J. P. N., and Brown, D. W. G. (1995). Complete nucleotide sequence of the Herpesvirus simiae glycoprotein G gene and its expression as an immunogenic fusion protein in bacteria. *Journal of General Virology*, **76**, 2161–68.

Van Hoosier, G. L. and Melnick, J. L. (1961). Neutralizing antibodies in human sera to Herpesvirus simiae (B virus). *Texas Report of Biological Medicine*, **19**, 376–80.

Vizoso, A. D. (1975). Recovery of Herpes simiae (B virus) from both primary and latent infections in rhesus monkeys. *British Journal of Experimental Pathology*, **56**, 485–8.

Wall, L. V. M., Zwartouw, H. T., and Kelly, D. C. (1989). Discrimination between twenty isolates of herpesvirus simiae (B virus) by restriction enzyme analysis of the viral genome. *Virus Research*, **12**, 283–96.

Wansbrough-Jones, M. H., Jones, M. H., Cooper, B., and Sarantis, N. (1989). Prophylaxis against B virus infection. *British Medical Journal*, **297**, 909.

Weigler, B. J. (1992). Biology of B virus in macaque and human hosts: A review. *Clinics in Infectious Diseases*, **14**, 555–67.

Weigler, B. J., Roberts, J. A., Hird, D. W., Lerche, N. W., and Hilliard, J. K. (1990). A cross sectional survey for B virus antibody in a colony of group housed rhesus macaques. *Laboratory Animal Science*, **40**, 257–61.

Weigler, B. J., Hird, D. W., Hilliard, J. K., Lerche, N. W., Roberts, J. A., and Scott, L. M. (1993). Epidemiology of cercopithecine herpesvirus 1 (B virus) infection and shedding in a large breeding cohort of rhesus macaques. *Journal of Infectious Diseases*, **167**, 257–63.

Wells, D. L. *et al.* (1989). Herpesvirus simiae contamination of primary rhesus monkey kidney cell cultures: CDC recommendations to minimize risks to laboratory personnel. *Diagnostic Microbiology and Infectious Disease*, **12**, 333–5.

Whitley, R. J. (1993). The biology of B virus (Cercopithecine virus 1). In *The human herpesviruses*, (ed. B. Roizman and R. J. Whitley), pp. 317–28. Raven Press, New York.

Zwartouw, H. T. and Boulter, E. A. (1984). Excretion of B virus in monkeys and evidence of genital infection. *Laboratory Animal Science*, **18**, 65–70.

Zwartouw, H. T., Macarthur, J. A., Boulter, E. A., Seamer, J. H., Marston, J. H., and Chamore, A. S. (1984). Transmission of B virus infection between monkeys especially in relation to breeding colonies. *Laboratory Animals*, **18**, 125–130.

Zwartouw, H. T., Humphreys, C. R., and Collins, P. (1989). Oral chemotherapy of fatal B virus (herpesvirus simiae) infection. *Antiviral Research*, **11**, 275–83.

32 INFLUENZA

I. H. Brown and D. J. Alexander

SUMMARY

Influenza is a highly contagious, acute illness which has afflicted humans and animals since ancient times. Influenza viruses form the Orthomyxoviridae family and are grouped into types A, B, and C on the basis of the antigenic nature of the internal nucleocapsid or the matrix protein. Influenza A viruses infect a large variety of animal species, including humans, pigs, horses, sea mammals, and birds, occasionally producing devastating pandemics in humans, such as in 1918 when over 20 million deaths occurred worldwide. The two surface glycoproteins of the virus, haemagglutinin (HA) and neuraminidase (NA), are the most important antigens for inducing protective immunity in the host and therefore show the greatest variation. For influenza A viruses 15 antigenically distinct HA and nine NA subtypes are recognized at present; a virus possesses one HA and one NA subtype, apparently in any combination. Although viruses of relatively few subtype combinations have been isolated from mammalian species, all subtypes, in most combinations, have been isolated from birds.

In the twentieth century the sudden emergence of antigenically different strains in humans, termed antigenic shift, has occurred on four occasions, 1918 (H1N1), 1957 (H2N2), 1968 (H3N2), and 1977 (H1N1), resulting in pandemics; while frequent epidemics have occurred between the pandemics as a result of gradual antigenic change in the prevalent virus, termed antigenic drift. Currently, epidemics throughout the world occur in the human population due to infection with influenza A viruses of H1N1 and H3N2 subtype or with influenza B virus. Phylogenetic studies have led to the suggestion that aquatic birds could be the source of all influenza A viruses in other species. Some pandemic strains are thought to have emerged by genetic reassortment (occurring as a result of the segmented genome of the virus) of avian and human influenza A viruses infecting the same host. Influenza viruses do not pass readily between humans and birds but transmission between humans and other animals has been demonstrated. This has led to the suggestion that the proposed reassortment of human and avian viruses takes place in an intermediate animal with subsequent transference to the human population. Pigs have been considered the leading contender for the role of intermediary because they may serve as hosts for productive infections of both avian and human viruses, and there is good evidence that they have been involved in interspecies transmission of influenza viruses; particularly the spread of H1N1 viruses to humans.

The main control measure for influenza in human populations is immunoprophylaxis aimed at the epidemics occurring between pandemics.

HISTORY

The highly contagious, acute respiratory illness now known as influenza appears to have afflicted human beings since ancient times. The individual symptoms and epidemiological characteristics of the disease are sufficiently distinct that it is possible to identify a number of major epidemics in the distant past. One such epidemic was recorded by Hippocrates in 412 BC, and numerous episodes were described in the Middle Ages.

The name influenza has its origins in early fifteenth century Italy and was adopted in Europe to explain the sudden and unexpected appearance of an epidemic disease thought to be under the influence of the stars (Kaplan and Webster 1977).

The first well-recorded pandemic in humans, in which mortality was frequently high, particularly in areas of dense population, occurred in 1580 and was believed to have originated in Asia before spreading to Africa and Europe. During the following three centuries, although record keeping was irregular and reporting was often inaccurate, there were recognizable clinical accounts of a number of serious influenza pandemics. The first pandemic for which there is more than descriptive reports was that of 1889, as retrospective research in recent years has partially identified the virus responsible by testing for influenza antibodies in serum of people who were alive at that time (Tumova 1980). Possibly the most devastating influenza pandemic recorded occurred in 1918. It has been estimated that during this pandemic between 20 and 40 million deaths occurred throughout the world and that in a developed country, such as the United States, about 0.5 per cent of the population died. In some parts of Alaska and the Pacific islands more than half the population was lost. There was an enormous impact on society in terms of mortality, morbidity, and economic factors. At the height of the epidemic community life in many cities was brought almost to a standstill. The repercussions of the pandemic were felt by armed forces engaged in the First World War, with some 43 000 deaths in the US forces alone, representing about 80 per cent of the total number of US battle deaths in the war. It is still uncertain why the pandemic was so lethal. Secondary bacterial infections causing pneumonia and other serious conditions may have accounted for some of the deaths. Today, such exacerbative infections can be treated effectively with antibiotics. Another factor may have been unusually high virulence of the virus, but attempts to recover the causative agent from frozen specimens have so far failed.

For centuries there had been wild speculation on the cause of influenza, but by the end of nineteenth century the microbiological concept of infectious disease had become accepted. Following on from this was the discovery of a bacillus in the throats of many influenza patients. This bacillus, *Haemophilus influenzae*, was for many years the leading suspect for the causative agent of influenza. The first evidence of the true viral cause came in the late 1920s when a virus was found in pigs showing disease similar to influenza in humans and successfully transmitted between pigs using filtered material. A related strain was finally isolated from a human patient in 1933 by inoculating a filtrate of throat washings into the noses of ferrets. Rapid progress followed the demonstration that influenza virus could be transmitted to ferrets and mice. A second type of influenza virus from man was transmitted experimentally to ferrets in 1940. This virus was designated influenza B to distinguish it from the first type found, which became known as influenza A. In 1933 it was found that influenza viruses would multiply in cells lining the allantoic cavity of the developing chicken embryo. This was followed by the observation that infective allantoic fluid caused agglutination of chicken red blood cells. These developments laid the foundations for early work on influenza viruses and today these techniques are still fundamental to work with influenza virus. The agglutination or haemagglutination (as it became known) reaction could be inhibited by specific serum antibodies to influenza viruses, thereby a simple assay could facilitate strain differentiation and the detection of an individual's immunological response to influenza virus infection.

The history of influenza in animals is equally confused, not least because influenza may be used as a general term for respiratory illness in animals, as it is in humans, and the wide range of microbial agents that can infect the upper respiratory tract causing influenza-like signs. However, there are many historical reports of influenza occurring simultaneously or sequentially in humans and domestic animals (Beveridge 1977) suggesting an early understanding of a possible link between the disease in animals and humans. Close correlation between human and animal influenza was made during the 1918 pandemic, and the term swine influenza was applied to a 'new' disease of pigs described at that time which produced clinical signs similar to those in humans (Dorset *et al.* 1922). Following the first isolation of influenza virus it was known that H1N1 (Hsw1N1) virus remained endemic in pig populations, particularly in the United States.

Little consideration was given to the possibility of influenza infections of other animals until 1955. In that year it was demonstrated that the causative virus of a highly pathogenic disease of chickens known as 'fowl plague', which had been isolated and described as a filterable agent as early as 1901 (Centanni and Savonuzzi, cited by Stubbs 1965), was a type A influenza virus (Schafer 1955). Several, less virulent, viruses that had been isolated from domestic poultry up to that time were also shown to be influenza A viruses. In 1956 evidence was obtained of influenza A virus infections in horses (Sovinova *et al.* 1958) and in the next 2 years respiratory disease in horses caused by this virus became widespread in Europe. These findings aroused the interest of many scientists working on influenza in humans, which was further concentrated by the H2N2 'Asian flu' pandemic of 1957. Since that time the World Health Organization has endeavoured to encourage and co-ordinate work on the epidemiology of animal viruses, particularly in relation to human influenza (Kaplan 1980). However, it was not until the late 1970s that the true picture of vast reservoirs of influenza viruses that exist in animals, particularly birds, had been formed.

THE AGENT

TAXONOMY

The influenza viruses from the Orthomyxoviridae family of which there are three genera, one consisting of type A and B viruses, a second containing type C viruses, and a third containing 'Thogoto-like-viruses' (International Committee on Taxonomy of Viruses 1995). Influenza virus types A, B, and C infect humans, but, except for occasional reports, infections of other animals are restricted to type A influenza viruses. Only influenza A viruses have been isolated from birds. Types A and B viruses both cause similar clinical disease in humans and both may be responsible for epidemics in humans. However, only influenza A viruses have produced the devastating pandemics that have made such an impact on the human population throughout recorded history.

Influenza A virus particles appear roughly spherical or filamentous, 80–120 nm in diameter. The nucleocapsid shows helical symmetry and is enclosed within a protein matrix. External to the matrix is a lipid membrane, the surface of which is covered by two types of glycoprotein projections, or spikes, with which haemagglutinin and neuraminidase activities are associated. These two surface glycopeptides, particularly the haemagglutinin, appear to be the most important antigens in terms of stimulation of protective immunity in the host. Consequently, considerable antigenic variation is seen in these polypeptides while other polypeptides are antigenically more stable.

The classification and nomenclature of influenza viruses take account of the antigenic variation that exists (World Health Organization Expert Committee 1980). Influenza viruses are grouped into types A, B, and C on the basis of the antigenic nature of the internal nucleocapsid or the matrix protein. Both these antigens are common to all viruses of the same type. Viruses of influenza A type are further divided into subtypes on the basis of the haemagglutinin (HA) and neuraminidase (NA) antigens. There are, at present, 15 HA and nine NA subtypes; a virus possesses one HA and one NA subtype, apparently in any combination.

MOLECULAR BIOLOGY

The genomes of influenza A and B viruses consist of eight unique segments of single-stranded RNA which are of negative polarity. Influenza C viruses possess seven segments of RNA. The viral RNA is transcribed to complementary messenger RNA by a virus-associated polymerase complex (designated PB1, PB2, and PA). To be infectious, a single virus particle must contain each of the eight unique RNA segments. It is likely that the incorporation of RNAs into the virion is at least partly random. The random incorporation of RNA segments allows the generation of progeny viruses containing novel combinations of genes when cells are dual infected with two different parent viruses. This phenomenon is referred to as genetic reassortment.

The eight influenza A viral RNA segments encode 10 recognized gene products. These are PB1, PB2, and PA polymerases, HA, nucleoprotein (NP), NA, matrix proteins (M1 and M2), and non-structural proteins (NS1 and NS2).

The three largest proteins (PB1, PB2 and PA) and one intermediate size protein (NP) are found in the RNA polymerase complex, which has transcriptase and endonuclease activities. This complex is involved in the synthesis of the three classes of virus-specific RNA molecules detected in infected cells, mRNA, virion RNA (vRNA), and complementary RNA (cRNA). PB2 functions during the initiation of viral mRNA transcription, recognizing the 5′ terminal caps of host cell mRNAs for use as viral mRNA transcription primers and is involved in the endonucleolytic cleavage of these primers. PB1 is responsible for the elongation of the primed nascent viral mRNA, template RNA and vRNA. The precise role of PA is unknown. NP is transported into the infected cell nucleus, where it binds to and encapsidates viral RNA. In addition to its structural role, it is believed to function in the switching of viral RNA polymerase activity from mRNA synthesis to cRNA and vRNA synthesis. NP is phosphorylated, the pattern of which is host cell dependent and may be related to viral host range restriction.

The HA protein is an integral membrane protein and the major surface antigen of the influenza virus virion. It is responsible for binding of virions to host cell receptors and for fusion between the virion envelope and the host cell. Newly synthesized HA is cleaved to remove the amino-terminal hydrophobic sequence which is the signal sequence for transport to the cell membrane. Carbohydrate side-chains are added, the number and position of which vary with the virus strain. Palmitic acid is added to cysteine residues near the HA carboxy terminus. Fusion activity requires post-translational cleavage of HA by cellular proteases into the disulphide-linked fragments HA1 and HA2. This cleavage of the HA does not affect its antigenic or receptor-binding properties, but is essential for the virus to be infectious and is an important determinant in pathogenicity. HA molecules form homotrimers during maturation. The three-dimensional structure of the complete trimer has been determined, consisting of a globular head (HA1) on a stalk (HA1/2). The head contains the receptor-binding cavity as well as most of the antigenic sites of the molecule. The carboxy terminus of HA2 anchors the glycoprotein in the cell or virion membrane. The HA is subject to a high rate of mutation due to error-prone viral RNA polymerase activity. Selection for amino acid substitutions is driven at least in part by immune pressure, as the HA is the major target of the host immune response. The amino acids making up the receptor binding site are highly conserved but the remainder of the HA molecule is highly mutable. The 15 subtypes of HA recognized currently differ by at least 30 per cent in the amino acid sequence of HA1 and are not cross-reactive serologically. Subtypes may include several variant strains which are only partially cross-reactive in serological assay.

The NA is the second major surface antigen of the virus which, like HA, is an integral membrane glycoprotein. It functions to free virus particles from host cell receptors, to enable progeny virions to escape from the cell in which they arose, and so facilitate virus spread. This activity destroys the HA receptor on the host cell preventing progeny virions reabsorbing to the host cell. Like HA, the NA is highly mutable, with variant selection driven by host immune pressure. The nine subtypes so far identified in nature are not cross-reactive serologically, although variants within subtypes are partially cross-reactive serologically.

Two matrix proteins, M1 and M2, are encoded by a bicistronic gene. The co-linear transcript of the matrix gene is translated to form M1 and M2. M1 protein forms a shell surrounding the nucleocapsids underneath the virion envelope. M2 is an integral membrane protein which functions in virus uncoating, and in the later stages of replication it allows transport of the HA to the cell surface.

The non-structural proteins NS1 and NS2 are encoded by the same gene. NS1 mRNA is co-linear with the vRNA, whereas NS2 mRNA is derived by splicing. Both proteins appear to have a role in virus replication, although information is not complete.

DISEASE MECHANISMS

In the twentieth century there have been three major pandemics, caused by viruses antigenically 'new' to the host population (antigenic shift), interspersed with both minor and major epidemics. Pandemic strains generally appear through genetic reassortment. Because vRNA is segmented, genetic reassortment can readily occur in mixed infections with different strains of influenza A viruses. This means that when two viruses infect the same cell, progeny viruses may inherit sets of RNA segments made up of combinations of segments identical to those of either of the parent viruses. This gives a theoretical possible number of 2^8 (=256) different combinations that can form a complete set of RNA segments from a concurrent infection, although in practice only a few progeny virions possess the correct gene constellation required for viability. The new subtypes of influenza viruses which appeared in humans in 1957 (Asian influenza), 1968 (Hong Kong influenza), and 1977 (Russian influenza) had several features in common. Their appearance was sudden, they were antigenically distinct from the influenza viruses then circulating in humans, they were confined to H1, H2, and H3 subtypes and the first outbreaks occurred in South-East Asia. Phylogenetic evidence suggests that these pandemic strains were derived from avian influenza viruses either after reassortment or by direct transfer. There is evidence for genetic reassortment between human and animal influenza A viruses *in vivo* (Brown *et al.* 1994) and between human influenza viruses (Guo *et al.* 1992*a*). The appearance of the H2N2 and H3N2 subtypes was paralleled by the disappearance from the human population of the previously circulating subtypes, H1N1 and H2N2, respectively. This phenomenon probably occurred in 1918 when emerging H1N1 viruses replaced H3-like viruses. The reasons for the sudden disappearance of previously circulating human strains are unknown, but it is possible that the earlier strain is disadvantaged compared with the new strain because it has already elicited widespread immunity in the human population. This may explain the failure of the H1N1 virus to replace H3N2 on its re-emergence in 1977, as a large proportion of the population would have been infected with H1N1 prior to 1957 and retained some immunity.

It appears that at frequent but irregular intervals between the major pandemics, variants of pandemic viruses arise which are sufficiently different antigenically to be capable of passing the immunological barriers of a proportion of the population and thus cause an epidemic. In general, each new 'epidemic' variant appears to wane gradually in its ability to find new susceptible hosts and dies out, it is then replaced by the next epidemic variant. These variants arise due to gradual change, i.e. by mutation and selection of the original pandemic virus, and this is termed antigenic drift. Occasionally, the epidemics occurring between pandemics may be sufficiently severe and widespread to mimic a true pandemic. In 1946 an influenza A virus produced worldwide infections that were considered by some to represent a pandemic. However, epidemiological patterns were unlike those of true pandemics, and subsequent antigenic and genetic analyses revealed that the virus was a variant of the H1N1 subtype rather than a representative of antigenic shift.

The phenomenon of antigenic variation by shift and drift in influenza A viruses contrasts with influenza B viruses which show antigenic drift but not antigenic shift, resulting in regular epidemics but not explosive pandemics. Influenza C viruses do not show antigenic drift or shift, apparently only producing sporadic infections.

Two hypotheses have been proposed for the rhythm of occurrence of human influenza A viruses: an influenza circle or cycle or an influenza spiral (Shortridge 1992). The circle or cycle theory suggests there is simply a recycling of H1, H2, and H3 subtypes. If this is so, the HA subtypes of the next pandemic virus would be expected to be H2. The spiral theory presupposes that humans are capable of being infected with all known HA subtypes of influenza A viruses; these presently number 15. There are serological grounds for this in that rural dwellers in the influenza epicentre (see pp. 000–00) have been found to possess antibodies to the avian subtypes H4 to H13 examined (Shortridge 1992). It is possible that the hypotheses are not mutually exclusive, as there is no reason that recycling should not occur within the spiral.

GROWTH AND SURVIVAL REQUIREMENTS

Mammalian influenza A viruses replicate primarily in the epithelial cells of the respiratory tract, whereas avian influenza viruses replicate in both the respiratory and the intestinal tracts of birds and shedding of virus in the faeces provides the major mechanism for virus transmission from and between birds. It would appear that the ability of influenza A viruses to replicate in the lungs is determined by temperature, while replication in the intestinal tract is dependent on pH. Replication of mammalian influenza A viruses is optimal at 33–35 °C, reflecting the superficial temperature in the respiratory tract which is lower than 37 °C. Avian influenza viruses replicate efficiently at 40–42 °C, whereas human influenza viruses do not. In contrast, some swine and equine strains possess the ability to replicate at 42 °C, showing intermediate characteristics between avian and human influenza viruses. Furthermore, avian influenza viruses replicate to high titres in the respiratory tract of pigs and can be transmitted readily to other pigs. Similarly, avian influenza viruses appear to have crossed the species barrier into horses and have been maintained independently of the avian population (Guo *et al.* 1992*b*). The enterotropic avian influenza A viruses are more resistant to low pH, which enables them to pass through the low pH values in the upper digestive tract of the host. However, a number of influenza A viruses have the potential to replicate in the intestinal tissues of some mammals such as ferrets.

The receptor specificity of the HA differs among influenza viruses and corresponds to the cell receptors in the replication site of the host from which the virus was isolated. Avian influenza viruses preferentially bind the sialic acid-α-2,3-galactose linkage, while human influenza viruses preferentially bind the sialic acid-α-2,6-galactose linkage on cell surface receptors, whereas both linkages are found in the epithelial cells (the site of virus replication) lining the pig trachea, in contrast to both birds and humans. The ability of an influenza virus to replicate in avian or mammalian tissues may be genetically linked to the PB2 gene. Studies suggest that the amino acid at residue 627 of the PB2 gene is a determinant of host range, whereas glycosylation of the HA gene appears to control the host range of H1 viruses. It would appear therefore that both viral and host genetic factors determine the tissue tropism of influenza viruses in mammals.

In vitro growth of influenza viruses is usually done in 9- to 11-day-old embryonated fowls' eggs following inoculation of infective material into the allantoic or amniotic cavities. Incubation is carried out according to the virus host's requirements for 2 to 4 days, prior to the collection of allantoic/amniotic fluids. In addition, various cell systems have been used for growth, including canine kidney cells, calf kidney cells, human embryonic lung cells, chicken embryo fibroblasts, and conjunctival cells. Organ cultures from fetal and adult trachea have also been used. Whereas embryonated fowls' eggs are widely used for primary isolation and growth of influenza viruses due to their sensitivity, caution must be exercised in their wholesale application since, with human influenza viruses, genetically distinct variants are selected on passage in the allantoic cavity when compared to those of tissue culture cells, and the egg-adapted variant is not always representative of virus circulating in the human population.

Large amounts of virus are produced by influenza A infections of bird populations. For example, the huge numbers of ducks congregating on lakes in Canada prior to their migration south and the intestinal site of multiplication of influenza virus in these animals result in large doses of virus being excreted into the lake water (Webster *et al.* 1978). Not only has it been shown that infections may be present at such levels to allow virus isolation from untreated samples of lake water (Hinshaw *et al.* 1979), but also that infectious virus may persist for up to 207 days at 17 °C and for even longer periods at 4 °C. The infectivity of influenza viruses in water is dependent on the strain of virus, salinity, pH, and temperature of the water. Pigs infected with H1N1 influenza A virus of low virulence may retain live virus in their frozen tissues for up to 3 weeks after slaughter (Romijn *et al.* 1989). It has been postulated that the reappearance of an H1N1 influenza virus in humans in 1977 (following its disappearance in 1950), was due to reintroduction from a frozen source (Webster *et al.* 1992).

THE HOSTS

Influenza viruses are found in a wide variety of mammalian and avian species. Pathogenicity differences among influenza viruses result in the production of a spectrum of clinical diseases that range in severity from fatal systemic disease to mild, sometimes inapparent, respiratory disease. Severity of the disease is also determined by the host species infected and in part by factors such as age, sex, virus dose, environment, and concurrent infections with other pathogens.

INCUBATION PERIOD AND CLINICAL SIGNS

In humans, the incubation period will vary between 1 and 3 days, depending on the virus strain and dose. Typically, the onset of clinical signs is rapid, characterized by malaise, fever, nasal symptoms, an unproductive cough, myalgia, and headache. The illness leads rapidly to prostration which usually lasts from 3 to 5 days, being most severe in children and the elderly. Complications include primary viral or secondary bacterial pneumonia.

The disease in pigs and horses is similar to that in humans. After an incubation period of 1–3 days, disease signs appear suddenly in all or a large number of animals of all ages within a unit. An acute febrile, respiratory disease is characterized by fever, apathy, anorexia, coughing, sneezing, nasal discharge, conjunctivitis, a low mortality rate and a rapid recovery. Secondary bacterial infections in both pigs and horses can often increase the severity of the illness and may result in complications such as pneumonia.

In birds the disease signs can vary considerably. Typical clinical signs of highly pathogenic avian influenza in chickens or turkeys include decreased egg production, respiratory signs, rales, excessive lacrimation, sinusitis, cyanosis of unfeathered skin especially combs and wattles, oedema of head and face, ruffled feathers, diarrhoea, nervous disorders, and high mortality. Nonpathogenic avian influenza viruses may replicate in the epithelial cells of the respiratory tract and the intestine of birds without inducing signs of disease, but virus may be shed at high concentrations in the faeces. Exacerbative conditions, including infection with other organisms, may result in avian influenza viruses which are normally not pathogenic causing severe disease in infected birds.

Generally, influenza virus infections of other animals such as ruminants and sea mammals result in subclinical disease. However, H7N7, H4N5, and H3N3 influenza A viruses were associated with a high mortality in harbour seals at Cape Cod, USA in 1979 (Lang *et al.* 1981), 1982 (Stuart-Harris *et al.* 1985) and 1991 (Callan *et al.* 1995), virus being isolated from lung and brain of dead animals. Mustelids may be more susceptible to influenza infections; in addition to the historical laboratory infections of ferrets, outbreaks of severe respiratory disease with 100 per cent morbidity and 3 per cent mortality in commercial mink in Sweden were considered due to infections with influenza virus of H10N4 subtype. Isolates made from the mink showed close genomic homology with H10N4 viruses circulating concomitantly in avian species (Berg *et al.* 1990). In all these cases the epidemics tended to be self-limiting, and the newly introduced viruses did not appear to be maintained in sea mammals or mink.

PATHOLOGY

The respiratory pathology following infection with influenza virus is difficult to define precisely, since it is frequently complicated by the effects of infection with secondary bacteria. Severe damage to the epithelium of the respiratory tract is the main feature in infections of mammals with influenza virus. The resulting damage to the epithelium facilitates secondary infection by bacterial respiratory pathogens.

In humans there is typically a rhinitis followed by tracheobronchitis and, infrequently, an interstitial pneumonitis. The disease process usually damages the respiratory tract from the nose to the small bronchi, but rarely damages alveolar cells. However, in some cases influenza A virus infection results in gross lung lesions which are patchy and randomly distributed throughout the lobes. The altered lung areas are depressed and consolidated, dark red or purple red in colour, contrasting sharply with normal lung tissue.

In typical infections of pigs the bronchi and bronchioli are dilated and filled with exudate. Bronchial and mediastinal lymph nodes are usually hyperaemic and enlarged. Histologically, there is widespread degeneration and necrosis of the epithelium in the bronchi and bronchioli. The lumen of bronchi, bronchioli, and alveoli are filled with exudate containing desquamated cells and neutrophils progressing to mainly monocytes. Furthermore, dilatation of the capillaries and infiltration of the alveolar septae with lymphocytes, histiocytes, and plasma cells occurs. Widespread interstitial pneumonia and emphysema accompany these lesions, although the severity of the former is dependent on the infecting strain (Brown *et al.* 1993*a*). In North America a proliferative necrotizing pneumonia of pigs is characterized by widespread hyperplasia of type II epithelial cells.

Significant pathological changes in other organs have not been consistently observed among infected mammals. Infections of birds with highly virulent avian viruses is characterized by haemorrhagic, necrotic, congestive, and transudative changes. Haemorrhagic changes are frequently severe in the oviducts and intestines. Encephalitis may develop in the cerebrum and cerebellum, especially in broilers. Alterations to myocardial tissues have been observed following infection with highly pathogenic strains.

DIAGNOSIS

Clinical diagnosis of infection with influenza virus is only presumptive since there are no pathognomonic signs. In addition to acute disease there may be subclinical infection or atypical courses of infection such as in a partially immune population. A definite diagnosis is only possible in the laboratory, either through isolation of virus or by demonstration of specific antibodies.

Generally, the best material for virus isolation is nasal mucus from mammals and faecal samples from birds. These are obtained using sterile swabs, which are immediately suspended in transport medium, i.e. 40 per cent glycerol, 60 per cent saline, to prevent them drying out. Samples should be collected at the acute phase of the disease. In addition, tissues from the respiratory tract of mammals and from respiratory, intestinal, and systemic organs of birds are suitable for virus isolation. Tissues are homogenized in saline containing antibiotics and antimycotics and clarified to obtain a clear supernatant. The most suitable, easily available and reliable host system for the isolation of influenza viruses is 9- to 11-day-old embryonated fowl's eggs. The swab media or supernatants of tissue homogenates are inoculated into the allantoic or amniotic cavity.

Various cell cultures may also be used for the isolation of influenza viruses, but Madin Darby canine kidney cell line is most frequently used for influenza isolation from humans and other mammals. Usually it is necessary to add trypsin to the growth medium, as a conditioning factor for the cleavage of the HA and the production of infectious virus.

After incubation at 35 °C (mammalian influenza) or 37 °C (avian influenza) for 2–4 days, the allantoic/amniotic or cell culture fluids are collected and tested for the presence of HA in the haemagglutination test using chicken red blood cells. Positive haemagglutination is presumptive for the presence of an influenza virus for mammals, but avian species are commonly infected with Newcastle disease and other paramyxoviruses. Initial identification of a virus is performed by immunodiffusion test with specific antisera to nucleoprotein or matrix protein of the three types of influenza virus. This confirms the isolate as an influenza virus of type A, B, or C, and distinguishes it from all other agents that exhibit haemagglutination. Further characterization of influenza A viruses is done to identify the antigenic nature of the surface antigens, HA and NA, in haemagglutination inhibition (HI) and neuraminidase inhibition (NI) tests, respectively, using a panel of monospecific antisera for each of the 15 HA and nine NA types. The specific inhibition of HA and NA permits subtype identification of the influenza A virus.

Influenza virus antigens can be detected using enzyme immunoassay. These tests are generally type specific, using an anti-NP antibody to either capture viral antigen or detect antigen bound to a solid phase.

The application of modern molecular technology for the detection of influenza virus RNA can be particularly useful if a rapid result is required or if it is possible that the clinical sample may not contain infectious virus. The polymerase chain reaction has been widely investigated as an alternative to more traditional methods, particularly in laboratories handling large numbers of clinical specimens, and has comparable sensitivity and specificity (Claas *et al.* 1993).

The use of serology for diagnosis is particularly useful when virus shedding is brief and is of low titre, as is often the case with respiratory viruses, in addition to the unavailability of materials for virus isolation, or when an animal or individual is no longer in the acute phase of the disease.

The HI test (Palmer *et al.* 1975), is most widely used in the diagnosis of influenza and offers the advantages of being relatively simple to perform, sensitive, easily adaptable, and inexpensive. The single radial immunodiffusion test is an alternative assay which is also inexpensive and simple to perform. Paired sera taken in the acute stage of illness and approximately 2–3 weeks later during convalescence are required for diagnosis, in order to demonstrate an increase in specific antibodies. In epidemic situations when influenza is suspected and paired sera are unavailable, a rapid diagnosis can often be made by examining single serum specimens from selected individuals for elevated levels of influenza antibody.

The serum of many species, particularly mammals, contains inhibitory substances that may interfere with the specificity of HI and other tests. Various treatments of sera have been suggested to remove these inhibitors, possibly the best and most widely used being incubation with receptor destroying enzyme. In addition to non-specific inhibitors of the HA, some sera contain non-viral substances that may agglutinate certain species of red blood cells used in the HI test. These substances may be removed by pre-treating the serum with erythrocytes to be used in the HI test. Large-scale serological surveillance of influenza has used the single radial haemolysis test, which gives comparable results to the HI test. Apart from heating at 56 °C for 30 minutes, in this test sera do not require treatment to remove non-specific inhibitors before use.

TREATMENT

There is no specific therapy for influenza, treatment being essentially palliative. Antibiotics and other antibacterial agents do not affect the viral infection, but may sometimes be used to prevent complications such as co-infection with bacteria. Specific control measures include the use of antiviral drugs and vaccination. General prophylactic measures in mammals and birds are based mainly on preventing the introduction of influenza viruses of wild aquatic birds into domestic pig herds and poultry flocks. Infected herds or flocks are kept warm and free from stress for a more rapid recovery.

Although many workers have claimed success with antiviral substances against infection with influenza viruses, very few have proved effective *in vivo*. Amantadine hydrochloride and its analogue rimantadine have antiviral properties against all subtypes of influenza A virus (Lang *et al.* 1970) but not against influenza B or C viruses (Hayden *et al.* 1980). Under certain conditions simulating natural transmission of virus, amantadine-and rimantadine-resistant viruses can arise and be transmitted to in-contact animals (Lang *et al.* 1970). Amantadine inhibits influenza A virus replication by blocking the action of M2, which functions in virus uncoating and in the later stages of virus replication. However, the effect of amantadine may be dose dependent. Amantadine may have a therapeutic effect by increasing the rate of improvement of pulmonary function in the terminal airways, where the most serious pathological changes occur following infection with influenza virus (Jackson 1976).

Two computer-designed, sialic acid-based, inhibitors of influenza virus neuraminidase have shown high potency *in vitro* and *in vivo* against both influenza A and B viruses and may be useful leads for the development of novel anti-influenza drugs.

PROGNOSIS

In humans the effects of infection with influenza viruses in a population are most easily measured by comparing excess overall mortality with 'pneumonia–influenza' death rates, and are used to indicate the extent of an epidemic rather than the lethality of the virus. It is estimated that the 1918 pandemic resulted in 20 to 40 million deaths worldwide in all age groups. Subsequent pandemics in 1957 and 1968 showed dramatically increased excess mortality, but the effects compared to the 1918 pandemic were much reduced, possibly reflecting the availability of antibiotics in preventing deaths as a result of secondary bacterial infections. The combined pandemics of 1957 and 1968, in the United States, accounted for approximately 98 000 excess deaths; however, the epidemics from 1957 to 1975, excluding the pandemic years, accounted for over twice that number of excess deaths (Dowdle 1976), indicating that epidemic influenza occurring as a result of antigenic drift is a significant 'killer' disease in humans.

In most age groups influenza infections produce high morbidity, but recovery is usually rapid and uneventful. Mortality is highest in the elderly, frequently accounting for 90 per cent of all mortality associated with influenza virus. If a vaccine provided 100 per cent protection, about 80 per cent of influenza-related deaths could be prevented by vaccinating all people above 70 years of age (Sprenger *et al.* 1993).

In other mammals the disease usually produces a short illness, characterized by low mortality, high morbidity, and rapid recovery, but varies with the infecting strain of virus and the affected species. An H7N7 influenza A virus was associated with a high mortality in harbour seals in the United States in 1980, but was apathogenic for chickens and turkeys. A novel strain of equine influenza virus (H3N8) which emerged in horses in China in 1989 was associated with a high morbidity and relatively high mortality (up to 20 per cent). The virus appeared to originate from birds (Guo *et al.* 1992*b*). The introduction of an avian-like H1N1 virus into an immunologically naive pig population resulted in a large number of disease outbreaks characterized by high morbidity but low mortality (Brown *et al.* 1993*b*).

Most influenza viruses infecting birds produce asymptomatic disease. Outbreaks in poultry due to highly pathogenic avian influenza viruses are rare, but when the disease does occur it may result in up to 100 per cent mortality, often with few clinical signs preceding sudden death.

EPIDEMIOLOGY

Influenza A viruses infect a large variety of animal species (reviewed by Kaplan and Webster 1977; Hinshaw *et al.* 1981; Alexander 1982) including humans, pigs, horses, sea mammals, and birds (Tables 32.1 and 32.2). Recent phylogenetic studies of influenza A viruses have revealed species-specific lineages of viral genes and have demonstrated that the prevalence of interspecies transmission depends on the animal species. In the early 1970s the World Health Organization initiated long-term global studies on the influenza viruses of mammals and birds to determine the diversity of influenza A viruses in nature and whether it was possible to isolate a future pandemic strain of virus from them in advance of its appearance in humans. To the present day a vast number of viruses have been isolated from a wide variety of birds and a range of terrestrial and sea mammals. As a result there have been 15 HA subtypes and nine NA subtypes recognized among the isolates, suggesting there may be a limited range of antigenic subtypes in nature. Virus subtype combinations recognized previously predominated, e.g. H3N8, H4N6, and H1N1; new or novel ones, e.g. H12N5 and H13N2, were relatively few, implying host range and viable reassortment restrictions. Although an enormous diversity of animal species has been shown to be susceptible to influenza A virus infections, three groups of animals appear to be far more important in

Table 32.1   Haemagglutinin (H) subtypes of influenza A viruses isolated from humans, pigs, horses, and birds

Subtype	Examples[a] of viruses of the subtype isolated from the specified host group			
	Humans	Pigs	Horses	Birds
H1	PR/8/34 (H1N1)	Swine/Iowa/15/30 (H1N1)	–[b]	Duck/Alberta/35/76 (H1N1)
H2	Singapore 1/57 (H2N2)	–	–	Duck/Germany/1215/73 (H2N3)
H3	Hong Kong 1/68 (H3N2)	Swine/Taiwan/70 (H3N2)	Equine/Miami /1/63 (H3N8)	Duck/Ukraine/1/63 (H3N8)
H4	–	–	–	Duck/Czechoslovakia/56 (H4N6)
H5	–	–	–	Tern/S. Africa/61 (H5N3)
H6	–	–	–	Turkey/Massachusetts/3740/65 (H6N2)
H7	–	–	Equine/Prague/ 1/56 (H7N7)	FPV/Dutch/27 (H7N7)
H8	–	–	–	Turkey/Ontario/6118/68 (H8N4)
H9	–	–	–	Turkey/Wisconsin/1/66 (H9N2)
H10	–	–	–	Chicken/Germany/N/49 (H10N7)
H11	–	–	–	Duck/England/56 (H11N6)
H12	–	–	–	Duck/Alberta/60/76 (H12N5)
H13	–	–	–	Gull/Maryland/704/77 (H13N6)
H14	–	–	–	Duck/Gurjev/263/82 (H14N5)
H15	–	–	–	Duck/Australia/341/83 (H15N8)

[a] The reference strains of influenza viruses, or the first isolates of the subtype from the host group.
[b] Not found in this species.

Table 32.2   Neuraminidase (N) subtypes of influenza A viruses isolated from humans, pigs, horses, and birds

Subtype	Examples[a] of viruses of the subtype isolated from the specified host group			
	Humans	Pigs	Horses	Birds
N1	PR/8/34 (H1N1)	Swine/Iowa/15/30 (H1N1)	–[b]	Chicken/Scotland/59 (H5N1)
N2	Singapore/1/57 (H2N2)	Swine/Taiwan/70 (H3N2)	–	Turkey/Massachusetts/3740/65 (H6N2)
N3	–	–	–	Tern/S. Africa/61 (H5N3)
N4	–	–	–	Turkey/Ontario/6118/68 (H8N4)
N5	–	–	–	Shearwater/Australia/1/72 (H6N5)
N6	–	–	–	Duck/Czechoslovakia/56 (H4N6)
N7	–	Swine/England/92 (H1N7)	Equine/Prague/ 1/56 (H7N7)	FPV/Dutch/27 (H7N7)
N8	–	–	Equine/Miami/ 1/63 (H3N8)	Duck/Ukraine/1/63 (H3N8)
N9	–	–	–	Duck/Memphis/546/74 (H11N9)

[a] The reference strains of influenza viruses, or the first isolates of the subtype from the host group.
[b] Not found in this host group.

terms of numbers and the epidemic/endemic nature of the disease than other animals: these are birds, pigs, and horses.

OCCURRENCE IN BIRDS

Influenza viruses have been shown to infect naturally a great variety of birds (reviewed by Lvov 1978; Hinshaw *et al.* 1981; Alexander 1993), including wild birds, captive caged birds, domestic ducks, chickens, turkeys, and other domestic poultry. Viruses have been isolated from species of wild bird covering all the major families of birds. This has led to the findings that non-pathogenic avian influenza viruses are ubiquitous,

particularly in aquatic birds, and that all of the different subtypes of influenza A viruses (H1 to H15 and N1 to N9) are perpetuated in aquatic birds, particularly migrating waterfowl. Furthermore, phylogenetic studies have revealed that aquatic birds are probably the source of all influenza viruses in other species.

The frequency at which viruses have been isolated from samples taken from feral waterfowl has varied considerably. Hinshaw *et al.* (1980) contrasted the frequent isolation of virus from ducks congregated on lakes in Alberta, Canada with the much lower isolation rates obtained from birds on migration. Some of the factors that govern whether or not waterfowl are likely to be infected and excrete virus are the age of the bird, the geographical location relative to migration, the time of year, the species, and the characteristics of a particular virus. Each year waterfowl congregate in extremely large flocks, usually on lakes, before migratory flights are under taken. At this stage, viruses may spread easily to susceptible birds on the crowded lakes. Isolation rates from juvenile ducks may exceed 60 per cent. The importance of waterfowl is not only in the antigenic diversity and size of virus pools they harbour, but also the rapid dissemination of these viruses around the world due to the migratory nature of these birds. In wild ducks influenza viruses replicate mainly in the intestinal tract and are excreted in high concentrations in the faeces. Many birds, particularly juveniles, are infected by the virus shed into the lake water; however, viral genetic information does not persist in the individual after clearance of infectious virus, which is usually 5–7 days after infection. Certain subtypes of influenza virus predominate in wild ducks along a particular flyway, but the predominant virus differs from one flyway to another from year to year. Studies of ducks and swans from Siberia wintering in Japan have shown an influenza isolation rate during the winter months which varied from year to year (0.5–9 per cent).

Influenza viruses of a variety of HA and NA subtypes have also been isolated from wild waterfowl in other parts of the world, including Russia, southern China, western Europe, and Australia demonstrating the worldwide distribution of avian influenza virus gene pools in nature. Phylogenetic studies have indicated that influenza viruses from Eurasia and Australia are genetically distinct from those in North America. These studies indicated that the incidence and prevalence of influenza subtypes will vary due to physical barriers which prevent intermixing of their hosts.

Recent studies by Sharp *et al.* (1993), suggest that whereas wild ducks perpetuate some influenza A viruses, they do not act as a reservoir for all such viruses. It has been suggested that the remainder of the influenza gene pool is maintained in shorebirds and gulls, from which the predominant number of isolated influenza viruses are of a different subtype to those isolated from ducks.

Circumstantial evidence suggests that initial outbreaks in domestic poultry most often occur as the result of spread from wild birds, although there have been several reports of influenza viruses being transmitted from pigs to turkeys. As a consequence, considerable antigenic variation is seen in disease outbreaks in domestic poultry. These viruses can be divided into two groups dependent on their pathogenicity. The first group of viruses are highly virulent for chickens, causing close to and including 100 per cent mortality experimentally. These viruses are all of H5 and H7 subtypes, although not all the viruses of these subtypes are highly virulent. The disease caused by the highly virulent viruses was termed fowl plague, but is now more correctly termed highly pathogenic avian influenza. In recent years outbreaks caused by infection of viruses of this group have been rare. The second group, which represents the vast majority of infections of poultry (and all other birds), have a variety of HA subtypes and cause little or no mortality in chickens infected experimentally.

Influenza viruses have been isolated less frequently from feral passerine birds than from waterfowl. Studies following a highly pathogenic H7N7 outbreak in chickens in Australia concluded that there had not been significant spread to feral birds, although virulent virus was isolated from a starling found on the affected farm (Morgan and Kelly 1990). Captive, caged, and pet birds may also have a role to play in the propagation and dissemination of influenza viruses. Monitoring of such birds throughout the world has resulted in the isolation of many viruses.

It may be concluded that enormous pools of both genetically and antigenically diverse influenza viruses exist within the bird population, and provide the source of virus for the mammalian population.

OCCURRENCE IN PIGS

Influenza A viruses of subtypes H1N1 and H3N2 have been widely reported in pigs, frequently associated with clinical disease. These include classical swine H1N1, avian-like H1N1, and human and avian-like H3N2 viruses (Table 32.3). The available evidence suggests that classical swine H1N1 virus is antigenically and genetically similar to the type A virus responsible for the human pandemic of 1918. Since that time swine influenza has remained in the pig population and has been responsible for one of the most prevalent respiratory diseases in pigs.

Table 32.3   Strains of influenza A viruses endemic in pigs

Subtype	Location	Comments
H1N1	North America, Europe, Asia, and South America	'Classical' virus [SIV], first isolated in 1930 in USA
H1N1	Europe and Asia	'Avian-like' virus, first isolated in 1979 in Europe
H3N2	Asia, Europe, North America, South America	'Human-like' virus, first isolated in 1970 in Asia
H3N2	Asia	'Avian-like' virus, first isolated in 1978

'Human-like' H1N1 viruses often infect pigs, but do not appear to be readily transmitted from pig to pig.

Swine influenza is related to the movement of animals from infected to susceptible herds, clinical disease generally appears with the introduction of new pigs into a herd. Once a herd is infected the virus is likely to persist through the production of young susceptible pigs and the introduction of new stock. Outbreaks of disease occur throughout the year but usually peak in the colder months. Infection with classical swine H1N1 influenza virus is frequently subclinical, and typical symptoms are seen often in only 25–30 per cent of a herd. Blaskovic *et al.* (1970) showed that classical swine H1N1 influenza virus was excreted from one infected pig for over 4 months, although 7–10 days is more usual. Continuous circulation of swine influenza viruses within a herd without the apparent need for an intermediate host has been shown by the isolation of virus from a herd all the year round.

Serological studies of pigs in the United States have shown that classical swine H1N1 influenza virus was prevalent throughout the pig population, with approximately 25 per cent of animals having evidence of infection. Marked regional variation in prevalence has been demonstrated and in north-central United States an average incidence of 51 per cent has been reported. Classical swine H1N1 influenza virus isolates in the United States have remained conserved both genetically and antigenically, but viruses antigenically distinguishable, although closely related, have been reported by Olsen *et al.* (1993) and Wentworth *et al.* (1994). In Canada, an H1N1 virus was associated with a new and distinctive pathology in pigs which appeared in 1990; however, the virus was most closely related to classical swine influenza viruses. Subtype H3 viruses antigenically similar to human H3 viruses circulate at a low frequency in the United States and virus is isolated rarely.

Influenza A viruses causing clinical disease reappeared in European pigs in 1976, with the introduction of classical swine H1N1 influenza virus to Italy from North America. This virus is now endemic throughout Europe with a seroprevalence of 20–25 per cent (Brown *et al.* 1995b). However, since 1979 the dominant H1N1 viruses in European pigs have been avian-like H1N1 viruses which are antigenically and genetically distinguishable from North American classical swine H1N1 influenza viruses. The 'European' swine influenza viruses appear to be most closely related to H1N1 viruses isolated from ducks.

Although usually regarded as an endemic disease, influenza infections of pigs may result in epidemics when introduction of virus to an immunologically naive population occurs. Great Britain had remained free of avian-like H1N1 virus until 1992 when respiratory disease was seen spreading rapidly throughout the country as a result of infections with an H1N1 virus

related to, but antigenically distinguishable from, the prototype strains of avian-like H1N1 viruses (Brown *et al.* 1993b).

H1N1 viruses of swine and avian origin are now co-circulating in European pigs (Donatelli *et al.* 1991) and present a potential for the emergence of new strains by genetic reassortment. Human H1N1 viruses can also infect pigs, but although pig to pig transmission has been demonstrated under experimental conditions, most strains are not readily transmitted among pigs in the field. Serological surveillance studies in Great Britain suggest that the prevailing human H1N1 strains are readily transmitted to pigs but are not maintained independently of the human population (Brown *et al.* 1995b).

Human H3N2 influenza A viruses related to a human strain from 1973, continue to circulate in European pig populations long after their disappearance from the human population. These viruses now produce clinical signs in pigs which are typical of swine influenza. Seroprevalence is usually in the range 30–50 per cent, but can be as high as 75 per cent. This apparently high level of H3N2 infections in Europe is in sharp contrast to the low prevalence in pigs in North America.

Infections of pigs with H1N1 and H3N2 viruses have been widely reported in other countries, particularly Asia, where the first isolation of a human H3N2 virus from a pig was made by Kundin (1970) shortly after the appearance of the virus in humans. However, some H3N2 viruses isolated from pigs in Asian countries appear to be entirely avian-like.

There is good evidence that genetic reassortment can occur in nature between influenza A viruses in pigs, but this has not resulted in new epidemics in the pig population in which it has occurred. Influenza A H1N2 viruses, derived from swine H1N1 and H3N2 viruses, have been isolated in Japan (Sugimura *et al.* 1980) and France (Gourreau *et al.* 1994) but, apparently, neither virus spread. Phylogenetic analyses of human H3N2 viruses circulating in Italian pigs revealed that genetic reassortment had been occurring between avian and human-like viruses since 1983. The unique co-circulation of influenza A viruses within European swine may lead to pigs serving as a mixing vessel for reassortment between influenza viruses from mammalian and avian hosts, with unknown implications for both humans and pigs. Further evidence for influenza virus reassortment in the pig is provided by the isolation of an H1N7 virus from pigs in England, apparently derived from human and equine viruses, and the isolation of an H1N2 virus from pigs in Great Britain, apparently derived from human and swine viruses (Brown *et al.* 1995a). Unlike H1N2 viruses detected elsewhere, this H1N2 appeared to spread widely within pigs in Great Britain.

Pigs serve as major reservoirs of H1N1 and H3N2 influenza viruses and are often involved in interspecies transmission of influenza viruses. The maintenance of these viruses in pigs and the frequent introduction of new viruses from other species could be important in the generation of pandemic strains of human influenza.

OCCURRENCE IN HORSES

Influenza is a common disease of horses throughout the world. Apart from rare reports of isolations or serological evidence of infection with other subtypes, only two subtypes of influenza A virus, H7N7 and H3N8, have been identified as infecting and causing disease in horses. It is possible that H7N7 viruses have disappeared largely from the horse population, as there are no substantiated reports of virus isolated from horses since 1980. However, recent worldwide serological surveillance has suggested that H7N7 may be circulating in eastern Europe (Madic *et al.* 1996) and Central Asia (Webster *et al.* 1992). Recently, equine influenza outbreaks due to infection with H3N8 virus were observed in South Africa, India, China, Hong Kong, and Nigeria, where equine influenza viruses were not known to be circulating. Recent outbreaks in China have been due to both conventional strains of H3N8 virus, and viruses which, although they contained the same surface antigens as the other equine viruses of this subtype, had genetic features that were avian-like, indicating that the virus had been introduced from birds. In North America and Europe two distinct groups of H3N8 (equine-2) virus are circulating, centred largely on geographical origin. Sporadic outbreaks typically occur and may in part be due to antigenic drift, which may compromise the efficacy of the available vaccines.

OCCURRENCE IN OTHER SPECIES

Influenza A viruses of HA subtypes H1, H3, H4, H7, and H13 have been isolated from dead and dying seals and whales (Hinshaw *et al.* 1986). These sea mammals were probably infected from the faeces of birds, shed into the water at communal gathering sites (Shortridge 1992), as it is known that these viruses were of avian origin (Callan *et al.* 1995). Influenza viruses have been isolated from mink raised on farms. These viruses (H10N4) which were of avian origin (Berg *et al.* 1990), caused systemic infection and disease in the mink and spread to contacts. In all these cases the epidemics tended to be self-limiting, and the newly introduced viruses did not appear to be maintained in sea mammals or mink.

OCCURRENCE IN HUMANS

Influenza epidemics in humans can occur following infection with influenza A or B viruses, but pandemics result only from infection with influenza A virus. Only influenza A viruses of H1, H2, and H3 subtypes have been associated with infection in humans since the mid-nineteenth century. Pandemics occur following antigenic shift, whereas epidemics result from antigenic drift (see pp. 000–00). Antigenic shifts have resulted in new subtypes of human influenza A viruses appearing in 1918 (H1N1); in 1957, when the H2N2 subtype replaced the H1N1 subtype; in 1968, when the H3N2 virus appeared, replacing the H2N2 subtype; and in 1977 when the H1N1 virus reappeared. In the last case the reappearance of H1N1 did not result in the replacement of H3N2 viruses and both continue to circulate. Pandemic strains appear to arise at one focus and spread rapidly worldwide. Each of the new subtypes since 1957 first appeared in China and spread across all continents as a result of the available, fully susceptible world population. For example, the current H1N1 virus reappeared in May 1977 in humans in northern China, by November it had spread to much of South-East Asia, and by February 1978 it was already present in Europe and the United States. Within 9 months, this virus had been distributed almost worldwide (Kendal 1987).

Every few years a new antigenic variant of the prevailing subtype appears that is capable of spreading in the population and causing a significant epidemic. In temperate climates, epidemics nearly always start at the beginning of winter. They are of varying severity dependent on the infecting strain but are characterized by rapid spread, often infecting between 30 and 40 per cent of the population of the affected area. Epidemic strains usually arise at one focus and spread rapidly worldwide. After their rapid start, the epidemics tend to end no less abruptly, often within several weeks at the local level, or within 3 months nationwide. The sudden cessation of epidemics, often when susceptible individuals are still plentiful in the population, has not been explained.

Currently, epidemics occur worldwide in the human population due to infection with influenza A viruses of H1N1 or H3N2 subtype or with influenza B virus. Rarely, infections can occur with reassorted influenza A viruses such as H1N2 and H3N1 although spread of such viruses appears to have been very limited.

Occurrence rates for influenza virus infection are highest in children. This is partly attributable to the increased immunity in older individuals that results from prior infections with related viruses. Children and young adults play an important role in the dissemination of virus into the community. When older adults (particularly >65 years of age) are exposed to influenza virus in a setting such as a nursing home, the infection rate can be as high as in younger persons, but with the potential for more severe consequences. Deaths from influenza during an epidemic are invariably high enough to affect the overall death rate and it is chiefly in the aged that such deaths occur. Other groups at risk include people with chronic disorders of the pulmonary or cardiovascular systems, children with asthma, immunosuppressed patients or those with metabolic disorders, persons infected with human immunodeficiency virus, pregnant women, regular foreign travellers and those involved in the health care of some of the aforementioned groups.

SOURCES

The detection of vast pools of influenza viruses of many different subtypes among animals, particularly aquatic birds gave considerable impetus to research aimed at determining where new subtypes, particularly those that cause pandemics, emerge. A number of theories has been suggested, of which the most widely accepted is that by adaptation, involving genetic reassortment, transference of virus from other animals to humans occurs which results in an antigenically novel virus with the ability to infect and spread in humans. Following genetic reassortment, viruses may arise that possess the necessary genes to enable infection of humans but may have surface antigens new to the host immune system.

Genetic and biochemical studies have shown that the 1957 and 1968 pandemic viruses arose by genetic reassortment. The 1957 Asian H2N2 strain obtained its HA, NA and PB1 genes from an avian virus and the remaining five genes from the preceding human H1N1 strain (Kawaoka et al. 1989). The 1968 Hong Kong H3N2 strain contained HA and PB1 genes from an avian donor and the NA and other five genes from the Asian H2N2 strain. A diagrammatic representation of the theoretical origin of influenza A viruses in humans is shown in Fig. 32.1.

The pig has been the leading contender for the role of intermediate host for reassortment of influenza A viruses. Pigs are the only mammalian species which are domesticated, reared in abundance and are susceptible to, and allow productive replication of, avian and human influenza viruses. This susceptibility is due to the presence of both $\alpha2,3$- and $\alpha2,6$-galactose sialic acid linkages in cells lining the pig trachea (see pp. 000-00), which can result in modification of the receptor binding specificities of avian influenza viruses from $\alpha2,3$ to $\alpha2,6$ linkage; thereby providing a potential link from birds to humans. Furthermore, it has been shown that humans occasionally contract influenza viruses from pigs (see p. 000). The internal protein genes of human influenza viruses share a common ancestor with the genes of most swine influenza viruses. Also, the pig has a broader host range concerning the compatibility of the NP gene of viruses derived from other species (Scholtissek et al. 1985). Recent studies by Kida

et al. (1994), investigating experimentally the growth potential of a wide diversity of avian influenza viruses in pigs, indicate that these viruses (including representatives of all subtypes H1 to H13), with or without HA types known to infect humans, can be transmitted to pigs. Therefore the possibility for the introduction of avian influenza virus genes to humans via pigs could occur. Furthermore, these studies showed that avian viruses which do not replicate in pigs can contribute genes in the generation of reassortants when co-infecting pigs with a swine influenza virus. Evidence for the pig as a mixing vessel of influenza viruses of non-swine origin has been demonstrated in Europe by Castrucci et al. (1993), who detected reassortment of human and avian viruses in Italian pigs. In addition, reassortant viruses derived from human and equine viruses (Brown et al. 1994) or from human and swine viruses (Brown et al. 1995a) have been isolated from pigs in Great Britain. Other studies of influenza viruses isolated from pigs in North America and southern China failed to detect any reassortant viruses containing internal protein gene segments of non-swine origin, although genetic heterogeneity of the HA of swine H3 influenza viruses occurs in nature in China.

Alternatively, new pandemic viruses could occur in the human population if an avian strain or a strain from another mammal became infectious for humans. Phylogenetic evidence supports this mechanism for the appearance of the Spanish influenza virus (H1N1) in 1918. Analyses of the NP gene (which is associated with host specificity) of human, swine, and avian H1N1 viruses reveals that the classical swine viruses and the contemporary human viruses probably evolved from a common avian ancestor prior to the appearance of the 1918 human pandemic strain (Gorman et al. 1991). Furthermore, avian-like H1N1 viruses circulating in European pigs since 1979 have been implicated as the precursors of the next human pandemic virus (Ludwig et al. 1995). In addition, avian H1N1 viruses antigenically and genetically related to, but distinct from European avian-like swine viruses have been detected in pigs in South-East Asia since 1993 (Webster et al. 1996).

Finally, the appearance of pandemic virus may be in fact be the re-emergence of a virus which may have caused an epidemic many years earlier. The appearance of Russian influenza (H1N1) provides support for this concept. The virus that reappeared in China in 1977 and spread subsequently to all parts of the world, was identical in all of its genes to the virus which caused a human influenza epidemic in 1950 (Nakajima et al. 1978). Webster et al. (1992) suggested that this virus was most likely reintroduced to humans from a frozen source and Shoham (1993) has proposed a biotic mechanism for the preservation of influenza viruses. Influenza viruses of the H3N2 subtype persist

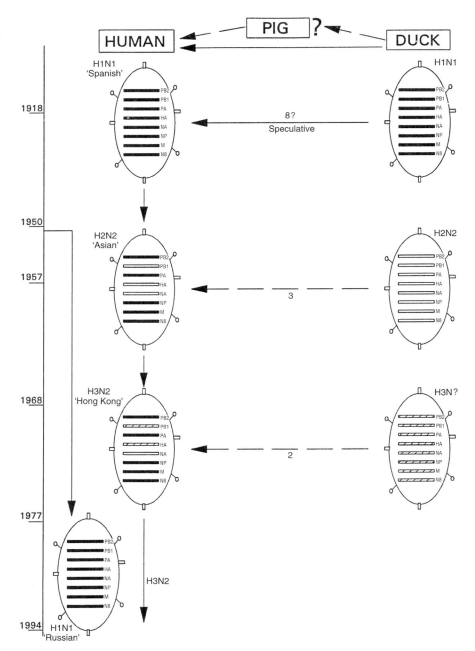

Fig. 32.1 Theoretical origin of influenza A viruses circulating in humans since 1918. Phylogenetic evidence suggests that an influenza A virus possessing eight gene segments from avian influenza reservoirs may have been transmitted to humans and pigs before 1918. This virus is believed to have caused the severe Spanish influenza pandemic of 1918. In 1957 the Asian pandemic virus H2N2, appears to have acquired three genes (PB1, HA, and NA) from the avian influenza gene pool in wild ducks by genetic reassortment with the circulating human strain from which it retained five other genes. Following the appearance of this virus, the H1N1 strain disappeared from humans. In 1968 the Hong Kong pandemic virus, H3N2, appears to have acquired two genes (PB1 and HA) from the duck reservoir by reassortment, and retained six genes from the virus circulating in humans. The appearance of H3N2 virus in humans coincided with the disappearance of the previous pandemic strain, H2N2. It has been suggested that the reassortment event leading to the production of Asian and Hong Kong pandemic viruses may have occurred in the pig, since it is receptive to, and allows productive replication of, both human and avian influenza viruses. In 1977 the Russian influenza virus H1N1, that had circulated in humans prior to 1950 reappeared and has continued to co-circulate with H3N2 viruses in the human population.

in pigs many years after their antigenic counterparts have disappeared from humans and therefore present a reservoir of virus which may in the future infect a susceptible human population. Pandemic strains may also be antigenically conserved in the avian reservoir, since counterparts of the Asian pandemic strain of 1957 continue to circulate with increased prevalence in wild ducks, domestic fowl, and live bird markets, and are coming into closer proximity to susceptible human populations.

The majority of pandemic strains have originated in China, raising the possibility that this region is an influenza epicentre (Shortridge and Stuart-Harris 1982; Shortridge 1992). In the tropical and subtropical regions of China, influenza occurs all year round. In China, influenza viruses of all subtypes are prevalent in ducks and in water frequented by ducks. The agricultural practices provide that there is close contact between domestic ducks, pigs, and humans, thereby presenting the opportunity for interspecies transmission and genetic exchange among influenza viruses, with the pig acting as an intermediary between domestic ducks and humans, as the transmission of mammalian virus strains directly to domestic poultry is unlikely to be a factor in the generation of new pandemic strains. Aquatic birds migrating or overwintering in the region might provide a source of virus for domestic ducks. Yasuda *et al.* (1991) have shown that domestic ducks harbour H3 influenza viruses antigenically and genetically similar to those in pigs, suggesting they may play a role in the transfer of avian influenza viruses from feral ducks to pigs.

TRANSMISSION

Influenza viruses infect a large variety of animals, and species barriers are less important in their ecology than they were thought to be. Given the worldwide interaction between humans, pigs, birds, and other mammalian species there is a high potential for cross-species transmission of influenza viruses in nature. A proposed model of the animal reservoir of influenza A viruses is shown in Fig. 32.2.

The ability of an influenza virus to cross between species is controlled by the viral genes, and the prevalence of transmission will depend on the animal species. The theory that pandemic influenza viruses arise as a result of adaptation and/or genetic reassortment requires that viruses pass either from other animals to humans or vice versa, and that genetic reassortment then occurs by dual infection which results in progeny virus with the ability to infect and cause disease in humans, but with antigenic determinants different from recent viruses affecting the human population. It would seem reasonable to suppose that such

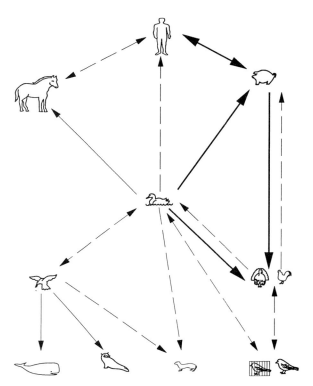

Fig. 32.2 Reservoirs and transmission of influenza A viruses. It is postulated that wild aquatic birds are the reservoir of all influenza viruses for avian and mammalian species. There is overwhelming biological, biochemical, and epidemiological evidence (———) for transmission between some species, such as pigs and humans. There is strong evidence (———) for transmission between other species, such as seabirds and sea mammals, and some evidence (— —) for other transmissions, such as between horses and humans.

transference between species would occur many more times than when the conditions are optimal for the emergence of pandemic viruses. While viruses do not pass to and from humans and animals with complete freedom, under some conditions such transmission does occur.

Transmission between humans and pigs

Early theories suggesting that the transmission of virus from pigs to humans resulted in the 1918 pandemic were speculative, although recent studies have shown that H1 influenza viruses in pigs and humans at the time of the 1918 pandemic were likely to have been very closely related. This belief explains the extraordinary events that occurred in the United States following what has become known as the Fort Dix incident. In January 1976 a virus of H1N1 subtype, identical to viruses isolated from pigs in the United States, was isolated from a soldier who had died of influenza at Fort

Dix, New Jersey, USA. At least five other servicemen were shown by virus isolation to be infected, and serological evidence suggested that some 500 personnel at Fort Dix were, or had been, infected with the same virus (Hodder *et al.* 1977; Top and Russell 1977). With the 1918 pandemic in mind this stimulated a universal vaccination programme in the USA, that was eventually abandoned when it became clear that the virus had not spread any further.

The Fort Dix incident cannot be regarded as evidence of zoonosis, since pigs as the source of the virus, although likely, was never established. However, there is considerable evidence that transmission from pigs to humans does occur. Kluzka *et al.* (1961) reported that humans working with pigs in Czechoslovakia had antibodies to the H1 subtype from pigs, and Schnurrenberger *et al.* (1970) reported that people in the United States who had close contact with pigs were more likely to have antibodies to classical swine H1N1 influenza virus than those who did not. Final confirmation of the zoonotic nature of H1N1 influenza viruses from pigs came in 1976, when clinical influenza appeared in a herd of pigs on a farm in Wisconsin 2–3 days before a caretaker also became ill with influenza. Viruses isolated from the pigs and the man were shown to be both antigenically and genetically identical swine H1N1 influenza viruses (Easterday 1980). Subsequently there have been several reports from North America of swine virus being isolated from humans with respiratory illness, occasionally with fatal consequences (Wentworth *et al.* 1994). All cases examined followed contact with sick pigs and were due to viruses most closely related to classical swine H1N1 influenza virus. In Europe, De Jong *et al.* (1986) reported the isolation of classical swine H1N1 influenza virus from three unrelated human cases of respiratory illness, one of which involved a 3-year-old child who had apparently not been in contact with pigs, although there had been recent epizootics in pigs in the region in which she was living. Perhaps of greater significance for humans is a report of two distinct cases of infection of children in the Netherlands during 1993 with H3N2 viruses, whose genes encoding internal proteins were of avian origin (Claas *et al.* 1994). Genetically and antigenically related viruses had been detected in European pigs, (Castrucci *et al.* 1993), raising the possibility of potential transmission of avian influenza virus genes to humans following genetic reassortment in pigs.

Influenza viruses of subtype H3N2 are ubiquitous in animals and endemic in most pig populations worldwide, resulting in many isolations of virus. There is no apparent evidence of pigs being infected with this subtype prior to the pandemic in humans in 1968. Indeed, the appearance of a H3N2 subtype variant strain in the pig population of a country appears to coincide with the epidemic strain infecting the human population at that time (Brown *et al.* 1995*b*).

Further evidence of the spread of influenza viruses from humans to pigs was the appearance in pigs of H1N1 viruses (or antibodies to H1N1) related to those circulating in the human population since 1977. (Nerome *et al.* 1982; Brown *et al.* 1995*b*). Genetic analysis of two strains of H1N1 virus isolated from pigs in Japan revealed that the HA and NA genes were most closely related to those of human H1N1 viruses circulating in the human population at that time. In addition, reassortant viruses with some characteristics of human H1 viruses have been isolated from pigs in England (Brown *et al.* 1995*a*).

Transmission between humans and horses

In historical accounts of pandemics in humans, frequent reference is made to similar disease in horses occurring either simultaneously or preceding that in humans. Beveridge (1977) noted such references in the accounts of 12 pandemics occurring during the eighteenth and nineteenth centuries.

Serological studies have revealed the presence of antibodies to equine H3 (equine-2) viruses in the sera of people born in the nineteenth century, and this has been considered as possible evidence that virus of this subtype was responsible for the pandemic of 1889–90. Experimental infection of human volunteers with H3 (equine-2) viruses has produced an influenza-like illness with virus-shedding and seroconversion. There is no evidence of infection of humans with the other subtype of influenza, H7 (equine-1), which has caused widespread epizootics in horses.

There have been several isolated reports of infection of horses with subtypes H1N1, H2N2, and H3N2, usually associated with human infections. Experimental infections of horses with human-derived H3N2 virus has confirmed their susceptibility to this virus (Blaskovic *et al.* 1969).

Transmission between avian and mammalian species

Although there is convincing evidence that all 15 subtypes of influenza A viruses are perpetuated in the aquatic bird populations of the world, only a few of the numerous subtypes have been observed in non-avian hosts. Phylogenetic analyses have revealed that some human pandemic strains most probably emerge following reassortment between avian and human influenza viruses, with the pig being favoured as the possible intermediate host. The H3 HA gene of the progenitor virus of the 1968 human pandemic strain was derived from an avian virus. Avian H3N2 viruses are readily transmitted to pigs in South-East Asia.

There is no evidence of direct transmission of influenza virus from avian species to humans. Experimental infection of volunteers with various avian subtypes resulted in mild clinical symptoms and no detectable antibody response (Beare and Webster 1991). There is one report of the isolation of a virus of H7N1 subtype from a man who was suffering from hepatitis, but no antibodies to that subtype were detected in the patient's serum.

Outbreaks of influenza in pigs in Europe since 1980 have been associated with influenza A viruses which are antigenically and genetically distinguishable from classical swine H1N1 viruses but closely related to H1N1 viruses isolated from ducks. All of the gene segments of the prototype viruses were considered to be typical of viruses of avian origin, indicating that transmission of a whole avian virus into pigs had occurred. These viruses continue to circulate in European pigs; they have been reintroduced to turkeys causing economic losses.

In 1979, around the Cape Cod peninsula in North America, high mortality in the population of harbour seals was attributed to an H7N7 influenza virus which was isolated from the lungs and brains of dead seals. Antigenic and genetic analyses revealed that the virus was most closely related to viruses from avian species. During the initial studies, four people involved in post-mortem examinations of the seals had developed purulent conjunctivitis within 2 days of known contamination with seal material. Although no virological studies were done on these cases, in subsequent laboratory studies an infected seal, known to be shedding virus, sneezed directly into the eye of one of the investigators who developed conjunctivitis within 2 days. Virus identical to the seal virus was isolated from the affected eye for 4 days after this incident (Webster *et al.* 1981).

In March 1989 a severe outbreak of respiratory disease in horses occurred in China. An influenza virus of subtype H3N8 was isolated and was antigenically and genetically distinguishable from equine-2 (H3N8) viruses, being most closely related to avian H3N8 influenza viruses. Genetic evidence suggests that this virus was transmitted to horses without reassortment.

Transmission of avian influenza viruses to other species of mammal (see p. 000) such as whales and mink have been reported. Genetic analysis of the viruses from whales confirmed that they had probably been introduced from birds. The potential susceptibility of mink to avian influenza viruses had been demonstrated following experimental infections.

Viruses antigenically identical to human variants of H3N2, H2N2, and H1N1 subtypes have been isolated from wild birds and domestic poultry, some have been reported to cause disease outbreaks in chickens that have shown a temporal relationship to influenza epidemics in humans.

Classical swine influenza viruses have also been isolated from ducks (Butterfield *et al.* 1978; Hinshaw *et al.* 1978), providing further supportive evidence for the natural transmission of influenza A viruses between avian and mammalian species.

COMMUNICABILITY

The ability of an influenza virus to spread is related to both the virus and the host involved. The age, population density, and air space may all affect transmissibility. Host-specific or host-adapted viruses have higher affinity for spread within a given host, than after transmission to a 'foreign' host. For example, the human viruses which cause epidemics and pandemics have a high capacity for spread amongst susceptible individuals. In contrast, the transfer of non-reassorted influenza viruses derived from birds or pigs, produce only mild or inapparent infection in humans and rarely result in secondary transmission. The majority of infections of humans in the United States with classical swine H1N1 viruses have not resulted in transmission from infected to in-contact individuals (Dasco *et al.* 1984; Patriarca *et al.* 1984).

The success of interspecies transmission of influenza viruses depends on the viral gene constellation. Successful transmission between species can follow genetic reassortment, with a progeny virus containing a specific gene constellation having the ability to replicate in the new host. Reassorted viruses with other gene constellations may have a relatively low fitness, and will not be able to perpetuate in the new host. A number of authors have proposed the NP gene as a determinant of host range (Scholtissek *et al.* 1985; Tian *et al.* 1985; Snyder *et al.* 1987) controlling the successful transmission of virus to a 'new' host. These observations support the potential role of the pig as a mixing vessel of influenza viruses from avian and human sources. The pig appears to have a broader host range in the compatibility of the NP gene in reassortant viruses than both humans and birds. Furthermore, cell receptors for both avian and human viruses are present in the pig trachea and the intermediate temperature of pigs compared to humans and birds may be important since virus synthesis is influenced by temperature control.

PREVENTION/CONTROL

PREVENTION

At present two control measures are available for influenza in humans: immunoprophylaxis with vaccines, and chemoprophylaxis or therapy with the antiviral drug amantadine hydrochloride.

Since the late 1940s, the principal preventive measures against influenza have been inactivated virus vaccines. The efficacy of vaccines has varied between 60 and 90 per cent and has been dependent on the closeness of the 'antigenic match' between the vaccine virus and the epidemic virus. However, even for those not completely protected, vaccination reduces the severity of the disease, thereby reducing costs and mortality. Two basic approaches for immunization have been pursued: the use of inactivated virus preparations and the use of live, attenuated viruses. At present only vaccines prepared with inactivated or killed virus particles are licensed for use in the European Community and the United States.

Influenza vaccine is prepared from purified, embryonated egg-grown viruses that have been rendered non-infectious. Numerous refinements have been introduced into the process over the years, and present-day inactivated vaccines are quite different from their predecessors. Four major innovations have been incorporated: the use of zonal centrifugation, the use of ether or other lipid solvents to disrupt the virus, the introduction of high-yield reassortants to improve yields in the chick embryo, and the development of better methods to quantitate the amount of viral antigens present in the vaccines. All of these efforts have led to inactivated vaccines that are better purified and more predictable in their reactogenicity and immunogenicity (Wright *et al.* 1976).

Each year the influenza vaccine is redefined to reflect changes in the antigenicity of circulating virus strains and contains virus strains representing influenza viruses believed likely to circulate in the forthcoming 'influenza season'. At present this involves two type A viruses, H1N1 and H3N2, and one type B virus. The exact strains of these viruses to be used are identified by an international network of laboratories that maintain surveillance for new influenza virus variants throughout the world. These laboratories are coordinated through the World Health Organization.

The composition of the vaccine rarely causes systemic or febrile reactions. Whole virus, subvirion, and purified surface antigens are available. To minimize febrile reactions, only subvirion or purified surface antigen preparations are used for children. Depending on the age group, the response to inactivated vaccines is either a primary or booster type of immune response. Children who have not been exposed to influenza mount a primary antibody response, and titres after the first dose of vaccine are low. After a second dose of vaccine, which provides a boost, antibody titres rise in these children. Most adults, unless they are being exposed to an entirely new antigen, will mount a booster antibody response, even to strains whose antigens are marginally different. Antibodies to influenza

vaccines are generally of the IgG subclass, and they react against the HA and NA of the vaccine strains. Antibody titres usually peak at 10–14 days after vaccine boost, then decline in the ensuing months. Serum antibodies appear to be very important in protecting against infection with influenza viruses. Extensive data show that the serum HI antibody titre correlates inversely with the occurrence of established infection with influenza viruses.

Most vaccinated children and young adults develop high post-vaccination HI antibody titres. These titres are protective against infection by strains similar to those in the vaccine or the related variants that emerge during outbreak periods. Elderly people and those with certain chronic diseases may develop lower post-vaccination antibody titres than healthy young adults and thus remain susceptible to influenza upper respiratory tract infection. Nevertheless, even if such people develop influenza illness, the vaccine has been shown to be effective in preventing lower respiratory tract involvement or other complications, thereby reducing the risk of hospitalization and death.

The effectiveness of influenza vaccine in preventing or attenuating illness varies, depending primarily on the age and immunocompetence of the vaccine recipient and the degree of antigenic similarity between the virus strains included in the vaccine and those circulating during the influenza season. When there is a good match between vaccine and circulating viruses, influenza vaccine has been shown to prevent illness in approximately 70 per cent of healthy children and young adults, while preventing hospitalization for pneumonia and influenza among elderly people living in the community.

Adverse reactions to vaccination can occur locally at the vaccination site, including pain and erythema, dependent on the age group, vaccine type, and route of inoculation. Fever and systemic signs occur less frequently, in the range of 5–30 per cent, and allergic reactions have been noted rarely, presumably to a vaccine component such as egg protein.

In some countries, notably the former Soviet Union, live attenuated vaccines have been used, but problems in ensuring attenuated safe usage has prevented widespread use. The most promising research effort has been the development of a live attenuated, cold-adapted (ca) reassortant influenza virus vaccine. This vaccine relies on the use of an attenuated donor virus to confer the property of attenuation to contemporary wild-type strains by genetic reassortment. This vaccine is very stable, owing partly to the multigenic requirement for the attenuated phenotype, and is at least as good as the inactivated vaccine in a population previously exposed to influenza virus (Heilman and La Montagne 1990). The ca vaccine is claimed to be extremely safe and efficacious in young children and it has been considered that mass vaccination of this age group with ca vaccine may control influenza epidemics.

Deoxyribonucleic acid (DNA) vaccines represent a new and potentially powerful approach to the development of subunit vaccines (Robinson *et al.* 1993; Ulmer *et al.* 1993). Vaccination by DNA inoculation is achieved by the uptake and expression of the inoculated DNA. The protein that is expressed by host cells raises the immune response including stimulation of T-cell responses and presentation by class I major histocompatibility antigens. Initial studies suggest it may be possible to afford broader protection against antigenic drift than that provided by natural infection.

Amantadine hydrochloride (see p. 000) is effective against all type A influenza viruses. If employed at the beginning of an outbreak, it can prevent disease and spread of the virus. Of those receiving amantadine within 24–48 hours of the onset of the disease, 70–90 per cent have greatly reduced symptoms. An advantage of amantadine prophylaxis is that it does not interfere with antibody production since the drug probably does not completely prevent infection. The widespread use of amantadine has been limited by side-effects (Stoof *et al.* 1992) and the rapid emergence of resistant viral strains (Hayden *et al.* 1989).

CONTROL STRATEGIES

Vaccination of people at high risk before each annual influenza season is currently the most effective measure for reducing the impact of human influenza. When vaccine and epidemic strains of virus are well matched, achieving high vaccination rates among closed populations can reduce the risk of outbreaks by inducing 'herd' immunity. This occurs when the overall number of susceptible people in a population becomes too low for virus to spread and infect a significant number of the susceptible individuals.

To maximize protection of persons at high risk, they and their close contacts should be targeted for organized vaccination programmes. Influenza vaccination is strongly recommended for any person above 6 months of age who, because of age or an underlying medical condition, is at increased risk for complications of influenza. The high-risk group consists of: persons above 65 years of age, residents of nursing homes and other chronic-care facilities, people with chronic disorders of the pulmonary or cardiovascular systems, and people who have suffered chronic metabolic diseases or immunosuppression (including as a result of medication) within the past year. In addition, people who may transmit influenza to those at high risk, i.e. hospital and nursing home personnel and household members of people in high-risk groups, should also be vaccinated.

Other groups may be included on individual merit, such as pregnant women, people infected with human immunodeficiency virus, and foreign travellers.

Currently, in the United Kingdom and the United States, fewer than 30 per cent of people among high-risk groups are vaccinated each year and more effective strategies are required for delivering vaccine to members of high-risk groups. In general, successful vaccination programmes have combined education for healthcare workers, publicity and education targeted towards potential recipients, and a plan for identifying people at high risk.

METHODS AND PROGRAMMES

Although an influenza vaccine may contain one or more of the antigens administered in previous years, annual vaccination using the current vaccine is necessary because immunity declines within the year following vaccination. Old batches of vaccine should not be administered as the constituent virus strains are updated annually to reflect the predicted epidemic strains for the coming year.

Beginning each September, when vaccine becomes available for the forthcoming influenza season, people at high risk should be offered vaccine. Because influenza activity usually peaks between late December and early March in the northern hemisphere, people in this part of the world should be vaccinated by mid November. However, it is important to avoid administering the vaccine too far in advance of the influenza season in such places as nursing homes because antibody levels may begin to decline within a few months of vaccination. Earlier vaccination is warranted, however, in particular situations, such as the early onset of an epidemic. Unvaccinated children need two doses of vaccine, at least a month apart, and, under normal circumstances, the second dose should be given before December.

EVALUATION

Each year influenza viruses isolated from epidemics are characterized antigenically in WHO influenza reference laboratories, and this information is used to evaluate the antigenic similarity with the virus strains incorporated into the current vaccine. This will provide some information on the potential efficacy of the vaccine, since the strains included in the vaccine had been selected ahead of the new 'influenza season'.

REFERENCES

Alexander, D. J. (1982). Ecological aspects of influenza A viruses in animals and their relationship to human influenza: a review. *Journal of the Royal Society of Medicine*, **75**, 799–811.

Alexander, D. J. (1993). Orthomyxovirus infections. In *Viral Infections of Vertebrates, Vol. 3, Viral Infections of Birds*, (ed. J. B. McFerran and M. S. McNulty), pp. 287–316. Elsevier, Amsterdam.

Beare, A. S. and Webster, R. G. (1991). Replication of avian influenza viruses in humans. *Archives of Virology*, **119**, 37–42.

Berg, M., Englund, L., Abusugra, I. A., Klingeborn, A., and Linne, T. (1990). Close relationship between mink influenza (H10N4) and concommitantly circulating avian influenza viruses. *Archives of Virology*, **113**, 61–71.

Beveridge, W. I. B. (ed.) (1977). *Influenza—the last great plague*. Heinemann, London.

Blaskovic, D., Kapitancik, B., Sabo, A., Styk, B., Vrtiak, O., and Kaplan, M. (1969). Experimental infection of horses with A/equi2/Miami/1/63 and human A2/Hong Kong/1/68 influenza viruses. The course of infection and virus recovery. *Acta Virologica*, **13**, 499–506.

Blaskovic, D., Jamrichova, O., Rathova, V., Skoda, R., Kociskova, D., and Kaplan, M. M. (1970). Experimental infection of weanling pigs with A/swine influenza virus. 2. The shedding of virus by infected animals. *Bulletin of the World Health Organisation*, **42**, 767–70.

Brown, I. H., Done, S. H., Spencer, Y. I., Cooley, W. A., Harris, P. A., and Alexander, D. J. (1993*a*). Pathogenicity of a swine influenza H1N1 virus antigenically distinguishable from classical and European strains. *Veterinary Record*, **132**, 598–602.

Brown, I. H., Manvell, R. J., Alexander, D. J., Chakraverty, P., Hinshaw, V. S., and Webster, R. G. (1993*b*). Swine influenza outbreaks in England due to a new H1N1 virus. *Veterinary Record*, **132**, 461–2.

Brown, I. H., Alexander, D. J., Chakraverty, P., Harris, P. A., and Manvell, R. J. (1994). Isolation of an influenza A virus of unusual subtype (H1N7) from pigs in England, and the subsequent transmission from pig to pig. *Veterinary Microbiology*, **39**, 125–34.

Brown, I. H., Chakraverty, P., Harris, P. A., and Alexander, D. J. (1995*a*). Disease outbreaks in pigs in Great Britain due to an influenza A virus of H1N2 subtype. *Veterinary Record*, **136**, 328–9.

Brown, I. H., Harris, P. A., and Alexander, D. J. (1995*b*). Serological studies of influenza viruses in pigs in Great-Britain 1991–2. *Epidemiology and Infection*, **114**, 511–20.

Butterfield, W. K., Campbell, C. H., Webster, R. G., and Shortridge, K. F. (1978). Identification of swine influenza virus (Hsw1N1) isolated from a duck in Hong Kong. *Journal of Infectious Diseases*, **138**, 686–9.

Callan, R. J., Early, G., Kida, H., and Hinshaw, V. S. (1995). The appearance of H3 influenza viruses in seals. *Journal of General Virology*, **76**, 199–203.

Castrucci, M. R., Donatelli, I., Sidoli, L., Barigazzi, G., Kawaoka, Y., and Webster, R. G. (1993). Genetic reassortment between avian and human influenza A viruses in Italian pigs. *Virology*, **193**, 503–6.

Claas, E. C. *et al.* (1993). Prospective application of reverse transcriptase polymerase chain reaction for diagnosing influenza infections in respiratory samples from a children's hospital. *Journal Clinical Microbiology*, **31**, 2218–21.

Claas, E. C. J., Kawaoka, Y., De, Jong J. C., Masurel, N., Webster, R. G., and De Jong J. C. (1994). Infection of children with avian human reassortment influenza virus from pigs in Europe. *Virology*, **204**, 453–7.

Dasco, C. C., Couch, R. B., Six, H. R., Young, J. F., Quarles, J. M., and Kasel, J. A. (1984). Sporadic occurrence of zoonotic swine influenza virus infections. *Journal of Clinical Microbiology*, **20**, 833–5.

De Jong, J. C. *et al.* (1986). Isolation of swine influenza-like A (H1N1) viruses from man in Europe, 1986. *Lancet*, **2**, (8519), 1329–30.

Donatelli, I., Campitelli, L., Castrucci, M. R., Ruggieri, A., Sidoli, L., and Oxford, J. S. (1991). Detection of two antigenic subpopulations of A (H1N1) influenza viruses from pigs. *Journal of Medical Virology*, **34**, 248–57.

Dorset, M., McBryde, C. N., and Niles, W. B. (1922). Remarks on 'Hog Flu'. *Journal of the American Veterinary Medical Association*, **62**, 162–71.

Dowdle, W. R. (1976). Influenza: epidemic patterns and antigenic variation. In *Influenza: Virus, Vaccines, and Strategy*, (ed. P. Selby), pp. 17–21. Academic Press, London.

Easterday, B. C. (1980). The epidemiology and ecology of swine influenza as a zoonotic disease. *Comparative Immunology, Microbiology and Infectious Diseases*, **3**, 105–9.

Gorman, O. T., Bean, W. J., Kawaoka, Y., Donatelli, I., Guo, Y., and Webster, R. G. (1991). Evolution of influenza A virus nucleoprotein genes: implications for the origin of H1N1 human and classical swine viruses. *Journal of Virology*, **65**, 3704–14.

Gourrean, J. M., Raiser, C., Valette, M., Donglao, A, R., Labie, J., Aymard, M. (1994). Isolation of two H1N2 influence viruses from Swine in France. *Archives of Virology*, **135**, 365–82.

Guo, Y., Xu, X., and Cox, N. J. (1992*a*). Human influenza A (H1N2) viruses isolated from China. *Journal of General Virology*, **73**, 383–8.

Guo, Y. *et al.* (1992*b*). Characterisation of a new avian-like influenza A virus from horses in China. *Virology*, **188**, 245–55.

Hayden, F. G., Cote, K. M., and Douglas, R. G. (1980). Plaque inhibition assay for drug susceptibility testing of influenza viruses. *Antimicrobial Agents Chemotherapy*, **17**, 865–70.

Hayden, F. G., Belshe, R. B., Clover, R. D., Hay, A. J., Oakes, M. G., and Soo, W. (1989). Emergence and apparent transmission of rimantadine-resistant influenza A virus in families. *New England Journal of Medicine*, **321**, 1696–702.

Heilman, C. and La Montagne, J. R. (1990). Influenza: status and prospects for its prevention, therapy and control. *Pediatric Clinics of North America*, **37**, 669–88.

Hinshaw, V. S., Webster, R. G., and Turner, B. (1978). Novel influenza A viruses isolated from Canadian feral ducks: including strains antigenically related to swine influenza (Hsw1N1) viruses. *Journal of General Virology*, **41**, 115–27.

Hinshaw, V. S., Webster, R. G., and Turner, B. (1979). Waterborne transmission of influenza A viruses. *Intervirology*, **11**, 65–8.

Hinshaw, V. S., Webster, R. G., and Turner, B. (1980). The perpetuation of orthomyxoviruses and paramyxoviruses in Canadian waterfowl. *Canadian Journal of Microbiology*, **26**, 622–9.

Hinshaw, V. S., Webster, R. G., and Rodriguez, J. (1981). Influenza A viruses: Combinations of haemagglutinin and neuraminidase subtypes isolated from animals and other sources. *Archives of Virology*, **67**, 191–206.

Hinshaw, V. S., Bean, W. J., Geraci, J. R., Fiorelli, P., Early, G., and Webster, R. G. (1986). Characterisation of two influenza A viruses from a pilot whale. *Journal of Virology*, **58**, 655–6.

Hodder, R. A., Gaydos, J. C., Allen, R. G., Top, F. H., Nowosiwsky, T., and Russell, P. K. (1977). Swine influenza A at Fort Dix, New Jersey. Extent of spread and duration of the outbreak. *Journal of Infectious Diseases*, **136**, 369–75.

International Committee on Taxonomy of Viruses (1995). Classification and nomenclature of viruses. In *Sixth report of the International Committee on Taxonomy of Viruses*, (ed. F. A. Murphy *et al.*) pp. 293–9. Springer Verlag, Vienna.

Jackson, G. G. (1976). Chemoprophylaxis and chemotherapy. In *Influenza: virus, vaccines and strategy*, (ed. P. Selby), pp. 123–33. Academic Press, London.

Kaplan, M. M. (1980). The role of the World Health Organisation in the study of influenza. *Philosophical Transactions of the Royal Society of London*, **B288**, 417–21.

Kaplan, M. M. and Webster, R. G. (1977). The epidemiology of influenza. *Scientific American*, **237**, 88–106.

Kawaoka, Y., Krauss, S., and Webster, R. G. (1989). Avian to human transmission of the PB1 gene of influenza A virus in the 1957 and 1968 pandemics. *Journal of Virology*, **63**, 4603–8.

Kendal, A. P. (1987). Epidemiologic implications of changes in the influenza virus genome. *American Journal of Medicine*, **82**, 4–14.

Kida, H. *et al.* (1994). Potential for transmission of avian influenza viruses to pigs. *Journal of General Virology*, **75**, 2183–8.

Kluzka, V., Macku, M., and Mensik, J. (1961). Evidence for pig influenza virus antibodies in humans. *Ceskoslovenska Pediatrie*, **16**, 408–11.

Kundin, W. D. (1970). Hong Kong A-2 influenza virus infection among swine during a human epidemic in Taiwan. *Nature*, **228**, 857.

Lang, G., Narayan, O., and Rouse, B. T. (1970). Prevention of malignant avian influenza by 1-amantadine hydrochloride. *Archiv für die Gesamte Virusforschung*, **32**, 171–84.

Lang, G., Gagnon, A., Gerani, J. R. (1981). Isolation of an influenza. A virus from Seals. *Archives of Virology*, **68**, 189–95.

Ludwig, S., Stitz, L., Planz, O., Van, H., Fitch, W. M., and Scholtissek, C. (1995). European swine virus as a possible source for the next influenza pandemic? *Virology*, **212**, 555–61.

Lvov, D. K. (1978). Circulation of influenza viruses in natural biocoenosis. In *Viruses and environment*, (ed. E. Kurstak and K. Maramovosch), pp. 351–80. Academic Press, New York.

Madic, J., Martinovic, S., Naglic, T., Hajsig, D., and Cvetnic, S. (1996). Serological evidence for the presence of A/equine-1 influenza virus in unvaccinated horses in Croatia. *Veterinary Record*, **138**, 68.

Morgan, I. R. and Kelly, A. P. (1990). Epidemiology of an avian influenza outbreak in Victoria in 1985. *Australian Veterinary Journal*, **67**, 125–8.

Nakajima, K., Desselburger, U., and Palese, P. (1978). Recent human influenza A (H1N1) viruses are closely related genetically to strains isolated in 1950. *Nature*, **274**, 334–9.

Nerome, K., Ishida, M., Oya, A., Kanai, C., Suwicha, K. (1982). Isolation of an influenza HIN1 virus from a pig. *Virology*, **117**, 485–9.

Olsen, C. W., McGregor, M. W., Cooley, J., Schantz, B., Hotze, B., and Hinshaw, V. S. (1993). Antigenic and genetic analysis of a recently isolated H1N1 swine influenza virus. *American Journal of Veterinary Research*, **54**, 1630–5.

Palmer, D. F., Coleman, M. T., Dowdle, W. R., and Schild, G. C. (1975). *Advanced laboratory techniques for influenza diagnosis*. Immunology Series No. 6, US Department of Health, Education and Welfare.

Patriarca, P. A. *et al.* (1984). Lack of significant person to person spread of swine influenza-like virus following fatal infection in an immunocompromised child. *American Journal of Epidemiology*, **119**, 152–8.

Robinson, H. L., Hunt, L. A., and Webster, R. G. (1993). Protection against a lethal influenza virus challenge by immunisation with a haemagglutinin-expressing plasmid DNA. *Vaccine*, **11**, 957–60.

Romijn, P. C., Swallow, C., and Edwards, S. (1989). Survival of influenza virus in pig tissues after slaughter. *Veterinary Record*, **124**, 224.

Schafer, W. (1955). Sero-immunologic studies on incomplete forms of the virus of classical fowl plague. *Archives of Experimental Veterinary Medicine*, **9**, 218–30 [In German].

Schnurrenburger, P. R., Woods, G. T., and Martin, R. J. (1970). Serologic evidence of human infection with swine influenza virus. *American Review of Respiratory Disease*, **102**, 356–61.

Scholtissek, C., Burger, H., Kistner, O., and Shortridge, K. F. (1985). The nucleoprotein as a possible major factor in determining host specificity of influenza H3N2 viruses. *Virology*, **147**, 287–94.

Sharp, G. B., Kawaoka, Y., Wright, S. M., Turner, B., Hinshaw, V. S., and Webster, R. G. (1993). Wild ducks are the reservoir for only a limited number of influenza A subtypes. *Epidemiology and Infection*, **110**, 161–76.

Shoham, D. (1993). Biotic abiotic mechanisms for long term preservation and reemergence of influenza type A virus genes. *Progress in Medical Virology*, **40**, 178–92.

Shortridge, K. F. (1992). Pandemic influenza: a zoonosis? *Seminars in Respiratory Infections*, **7**, 11–25.

Shortridge, K. F. and Stuart-Harris, C. H. (1982). An influenza epicenter? *Lancet*, **2**, 812–13.

Snyder, M. H., Buckler-White, A. J., London, W. T., Tierney, E. L., and Murphy, B. R. (1987). The avian influenza virus nucleoprotein gene and a specific constellation of avian and human virus polymerase genes each specify attentuation of avian/human influenza A/Pintail/79 reassortant viruses from monkeys. *Journal of Virology*, **61**, 2857–63.

Sovinova, O., Tumova, B., Poutska, F., and Nemec, J. (1958). Isolation of a virus causing respiratory disease in horses. *Acta Virologica*, **2**, 52–61.

Sprenger, M. W. J., Beyer, W. E. P., Kempen, B. M., Mulder, P. G. H., and Masurel, N. (1993). Risk factors for influenza mortality? In *Options for the Control of Influenza II*, (ed. C. Hannoun, A. P. Kendal, H. D. Klenk, and F. L. Ruben), pp. 15–23. Elsevier, Amsterdam.

Stoof, J. C., Booij, J., Drukarch, B., and Wolters, E. C. (1992). The anti-Parkinsonian drug amantadine inhibits the N-methyl-D-aspartic acid-evoked release of acetylcholine from rat neostriatum in a non-competitive way. *European Journal of Pharmacology*, **213**, 439–43.

Stuart-Harris, C. H., Schild, G. C., Oxford, J. S. (Eds) (1985). Influenza: is animals and birds. *In Influenza: The Viruses and the Disease* (2nd Edn). Edward Arnold Baltimore, Maryland, 83–102.

Stubbs, E. L. (1965). Fowl plague. In *Diseases of poultry*, (5th edn), (ed. H. E. Biester and L. H. Schwarte), pp. 813–22. Iowa State University Press, Ames.

Sugimura, T., Yonemochi, H., Ogawa, T., Tanaka, Y., and Kumagai, T. (1980). Isolation of a recombinant influenza virus (Hsw1N2) from swine in Japan. *Archives of Virology*, **66**, 271–4.

Tian, S. F., Buckler-White, A. J., London, W. J., Recle, L. J., Channock, R. M., and Murphy, B. R. (1985). Nucleoprotein and membrane protein genes are associated with restriction of influenza A/mallard/NY/78 virus and its reassortants in squirrel monkey respiratory tract. *Journal of Virology*, **53**, 771–5.

Top, F. H. and Russell, P. K. (1977). Swine influenza A at Fort Dix, New Jersey (January–February 1976). IV. Summary and speculation. *Journal of Infectious Diseases*, **136**, (Suppl.), S376–80.

Tumova, B. (1980). Equine influenza—a segment in influenza virus ecology. *Comparative Immunology, Microbiology and Infectious Diseases*, **3**, 45–59.

Ulmer, J. B., Donnelly, J. J., Parker, S. E., Rhodes, G. H., Feigner, P. L., and Dwarki, V. J. (1993). Heterologous protection against influenza by injection of DNA encoding a viral protein. *Science*, **259**, 1745–49.

Webster, R. G., Yakhno, M. A., Hinshaw, V. S., Bean, W. J., and Murti, K. G. (1978). Intestinal influenza: replication characterisation of influenza viruses in ducks. *Virology*, **84**, 268–78.

Webster, R. G., Geraci, J. R., Petursson, G., and Skirnisson, K. (1981). Conjunctivitis in human beings caused by influenza A virus of seals. *New England Journal of Medicine*, **304**, 911.

Webster, R. G., Bean, W. J., Gorman, O. T., Chambers, T. M., and Kawaoka, Y. (1992). Evolution and ecology of influenza A viruses. *Microbiological Reviews*, **56**, 152–79.

Webster, R. G., Guan, Y., Shortridge, K. F., Rohm, C., and Kawaoka, Y. (1996). The emergence of influenza A viruses in mammalian and avian species. In *Proceedings of Options for the Control of Influenza, 4–9 May, Cairns, Australia*, p. 40.

Wentworth, D. E. *et al.* (1994). An influenza A (H1N1) virus, closely related to swine influenza virus, responsible for a fatal case of human influenza. *Journal of Virology*, **68**, 2051–8.

World Health Organisation. Committee (1980). A revision of the system of nomenclature for influenza viruses: a W.H.O. memorandum. *Bulletin of the World Health Organisation*, **58**, 585–91.

Wright, P. F., Dolin, R., and La Montagne, J. R. (1976). Summary of clinical trials of influenza vaccines II. *Journal of Infectious Diseases*, **134**, 633–8.

Yasuda, J., Shortridge, K. F., Shimizu, Y., and Kida, H. (1991). Molecular evidence for a role of domestic ducks in the introduction of avian H3 influenza viruses to pigs in Southern China, where the A/Hong Kong/68 (H3N2) strain emerged. *Journal of General Virology*, **72**, 2007–10.

33 MARBURG AND EBOLA VIRUSES

G. Lloyd

SUMMARY

Marburg and Ebola viruses cause severe and often fatal haemorrhagic disease in humans and non-human primates. They are the two established members of the family Filoviridae and have a distinctive filamentous and irregular morphology with a genome consisting of a very large (about 19 kb) single-stranded RNA of negative polarity. Features of their organization and structure at the molecular level have led to their inclusion in the taxonomic order Mononegavirales, together with the paramyxoviruses and the rhabdoviruses.

From its original description (in 1967) to 1987 there have been six reported outbreaks of human Marburg virus infection. The first being three simultaneous outbreaks that occurred in Europe at Marburg, Frankfurt, and Belgrade, following the importation of infected African green monkeys (*Ceropithecus aethiops*) from Uganda. The remaining outbreaks occurred in South Africa 1975 and Kenya 1980 and 1987. These six episodes involved a total of 36 cases with 10 deaths, an overall fatality rate of 25 per cent. All the deaths to date have occurred in the primary cases.

Between 1976 and 1995 outbreaks of human Ebola haemorrhagic fever have been identified in Zaire (1976, 1977, 1995); Sudan (1976, 1979); Kenya (1980); Côte d'Ivoire (1994, 1995) and He Gabon (1996). All age groups and sexes were affected. In addition, a laboratory-derived infection occurred during the studies of the 1976 Zaire and Sudan epidemic. There is no known endemic incidence of the disease and the mortality rates are based on the limited numbers of epidemics identified. This has involved a total of 1008 cases with 719 deaths, an overall case fatality rate of 71 per cent.

A new Ebola virus named Reston was unexpectedly isolated from an epizootic of dying cynomolgus monkeys that had been shipped to the United States (1989, 1990) and Italy (1992) from the Philippines. The virus has been shown to be antigenically and genetically distinct from the African Ebola viruses. Human infections documented during the United States epizootic proved asymptomatic. No epidemiological link with Africa could be identified.

In Africa, the transmission of haemorrhagic fever caused by Ebola and Marburg has been associated with the reuse of unsterile needles and syringes and with the provision of patient care without appropriate barrier precautions preventing exposure to virus-containing blood and other body fluids. Epidemiological studies in humans indicate that infection is not readily transmitted from person to person by the airborne route. By contrast, studies of Ebola and Marburg virus infections in non-human primates has suggested possible airborne spread among these species. The risk of person to person transmission is highest during the latter stages of illness. Infection has not been reported in persons whose contact with an infected patient occurred during the incubation period.

As the natural history and reservoir of the filoviruses are still unknown, no specific precautions can be identified which would avoid infection from the natural environment. Although monkeys are known to have introduced Marburg virus into Europe and Ebola viruses into the United States and Italy, they are not regarded as the natural reservoir of the viruses. However, primates imported from Africa and Asia should be regarded as infectious and placed in quarantine for a minimum of 6 weeks. Since there are no antiviral drugs or effective vaccines, early identification of patients or infected animals is essential. Prevention of transmission in endemic and non-endemic areas has been based on the strict isolation of febrile patients and rigorous use of barrier precautions.

HISTORY

Filovirus infections were unknown until 1967, when 31 human cases of an acute haemorrhagic fever occurred simultaneously in Marburg and Frankfurt, Federal Republic of Germany, and Belgrade, former Yugoslavia (Martini 1969). Laboratory workers, medical personnel, animal care personnel and their relatives were infected, seven of whom died. The primary cases were infected through contact with kidney tissue, blood, and cell cultures derived from vervet or African green monkeys (*Ceropithecus aethiops*) imported from Uganda. The virus isolated from patient's blood and tissue was found by electron microscopy to be morphologically unique (see Fig. 33.2a) and antigenically unrelated to

Table 33.1 Summary of human filovirus infections during identified outbreaks

Year	Virus	Place of infection	All cases deaths/total	Overall mortality rate (%)	Source	Origin
1967	Marburg	Germany, Marburg Germany, Frankfurt Yugoslavia, Belgrade	5/23 2/6 0/2	23	Vervet monkeys	Imported from Uganda
1975	Marburg	Zimbabwe	1/2	33	Unknown	Index case infected in Zimbabwe. Secondary cases:–travelling companion and nurse
1976	Ebola (Zaire)	Northern Zaire	280/318	88	Unknown	Index case introduced virus into hospital
1976	Ebola (Sudan)	Maridi, Sudan Nazara, Sudan Tembura, Sudan Juba, Sudan	116/213 31/67 3/3 1/1	53	unknown	Disease amplified by transmission in large active hospital Outbreak in Nazara originated in cotton factory
1976	Ebola	United Kingdom	0/1	0	Laboratory infection	Needle-stick
1977	Ebola (Zaire)	Tandala, Zaire	1/1	100	Unknown	Tandala
1979	Ebola (Sudan)	Yambo-Nazar District, southern Sudan	22/34	65	Unknown	Nazara
1980	Marburg	Mount Elgon, Kenya	1/2	50	Unknown	Nzoia
1987	Marburg	Mount Elgon, Kenya	1/1	100	Unknown	Expatraite travelling in western Kenya (Kisumu)
1989	Ebola (Reston)	Richmond, Virginia	0/4	0	Monkeys	Imported monkeys from export facility in Philippines
1990	Ebola (Reston)	Manila, Philippines	0/12	0	Monkeys	Export facility
1992	Ebola (Reston)	Siena, Ilay	0	0	Monkeys	Imported from same export facility in Philippines as in 1989
1994	Ebola	Tai forest, Côte d'Ivoire	0/1	0	Chimpanzees	Contracted in during post-mortem of chimpanzee— repatriated to Switzerland
1995	Ebola	Kikwit, Zaire	244/315	77	Unknown	Confined to Bandundo region around Kikwit
1995	Ebola	Côte d'Ivoire	1	0	Unknown	Refugee from Liberia, four possible cases in home village
1996	Ebola	Gabon	21/37	57	Chimpanzees	Contact with dead primates

any known mammalian pathogen. This pathogen was named Marburg virus (MBG) after the city of Marburg, where most of the cases occurred and where much of the initial work on the virus was performed. There have only been three primary human Marburg infections and only three secondary cases located in Africa (Table 33.1). One was an Australian tourist in Zimbabwe and the others residents from the Mount Elgon region of western Kenya (Gear *et al.* 1975; Smith

et al. 1982; Teepe *et al.* 1983) (Fig. 33.1). Epidemiological investigations of both areas revealed no information on the origin of these infections.

A decade later in 1976, a severe and often fatal viral haemorrhagic fever occurred in nearly simultaneous outbreaks in the equatorial provinces of southern Sudan and northern Zaire (Fig. 33.1). Several hundred cases of infection were identified, with fatality rates of about 90 and 60 per cent, respectively, and several gen-

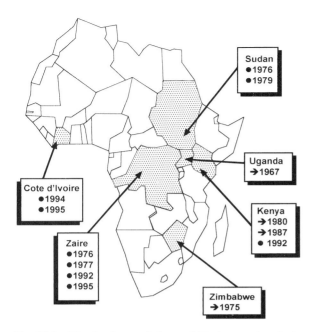

Fig. 33.1 Distribution and dates of filovirus outbreaks in Africa. ➜, Marburg virus disease; ●, Ebola virus disease.

close personnel contact with infectious body fluids. This was aggravated by the lack of modern medical facilities and supplies that could protect medical personnel from those patients initially affected. Unlike previous Ebola outbreaks, concern centred on the potential for community-wide spread from Kikwit, a large and densely populated area, to the larger cites of Kinshasa and Brazzaville close by. Control of the outbreak coincided with the introduction of protective equipment and barrier nursing techniques. The recognition of Ebola has recently extended to a confirmed case in the Côte d'Ivoire of a refugee from neighbouring Liberia in late 1995, other cases were reported to exist in his home village in Liberia (WHO 1995c). An outbreak of Ebola also identified in Gabon (WHO 1996).

Unexpectantly, Ebola virus has also appeared outside Africa in imported cynomologus monkeys (*Macaca fasicularis*) in the United States in 1989 (Jahrling *et al.* 1990) and Siena, Italy in 1992. Shipments of wild-caught cynomolgus monkeys originated from the same handling facility in the Philippines, where the presence of the virus was also documented. Although a truly Asian origin for these virus strains cannot be discounted, preliminary serological and sequencing studies suggest a close similarity with isolates from the 1976 African outbreaks.

THE AGENT

TAXONOMY

Ebola and Marburg are members of the family Filoviridae (Kiley *et al.* 1982; Pringle 1991), named for their filamentous appearance under the electron microscope (Fig. 33.2a). Similarities of genome structure and comparable mechanisms of gene expression suggest that the filoviruses have an evolutionary origin in common with the families Paramyxoviridae (which include measles and mumps) and Rabdoviridae (which includes rabies) (Sanchez *et al.* 1992). These three virus families have been grouped into a taxonomic order (Fig. 33.3), the Mononegavirales (Bishop and Pringle 1995).

MOLECULAR BIOLOGY

The genome consists of a single molecule of non-segmented negative-stranded RNA about 19 kilobases in length. It is organized into a linear arrangement of genes following a sequence beginning with a 3′ non-coding untranslated region, the core protein genes, envelope genes, and the polymerase gene attached to the untranslated region at the 5′ end (Feldmann *et al.* 1993; Sanchez *et al.* 1993). Non-structural proteins have not been detected.

erations of human to human spread. The two virus strains isolated from patients in Sudan and Zaire where found to be morphologically identical to Marburg but antigenically and biologically distinct (Bowen *et al.* 1977; WHO 1978a,b). The virus was named Ebola after a river in Zaire.

Numerous ecological studies failed to discover the reservoir. During studies of the above epidemic a non-fatal Ebola infection occurred within the United Kingdom in 1977 after a laboratory accident (Emond *et al.* 1977). Just over 6 months after the original outbreaks in Zaire, a 9-year-old girl died of acute haemorrhagic fever in Tandala, northern Zaire (Heymann *et al.* 1980). A further small epidemic occurred in the same region of Sudan in 1979 when 22 (65 per cent) of 34 infections were fatal, with transmissibility being associated with person to person spread (Baron *et al.* 1983). The latest instances of Ebola virus infection have been the severe illness of a Swiss zoologist working with infected chimpanzees in western Côte d'Ivoire in late 1994 (LeGuenno *et al.* 1995) and a larger-scale outbreak in Kikwit, Bandundu Province, Zaire 1995 which demonstrated to a worldwide audience a severe haemorrhagic illness involving some 316 cases, of which 244 died, a mortality rate of 77 per cent (WHO 1995a). A third of the cases were identified as healthcare workers. The Kikwit outbreak was similar to the original episode that occurred in 1976, 1000 km to the north. As in previous outbreaks, secondary cases occurred through

The genetic sequence of Marburg virus (MBG) and the available partial sequence of Ebola virus (EBO) indicate that in both cases seven structural proteins are encoded, which are expressed through transcription of monocistronic mRNA species. The structural proteins include an L protein that is an RNA transcriptase–polymerase (M_r 267 000); a single surface glycoprotein (GP; M_r 170 000) a major nucleoprotein (NP; M_r 94 000) and a minor nucleoprotein (VP30; M_r 32 000); a matrix or membrane-associated VP40 protein (M_r 32 000); a second matrix or membrane-assciated VP24 protein (M_r 24 000), and a VP35 protein thought to be a transcriptase–polymerase component that is considered to be the P(NS) protein equivalent of paramyxo-and rhabdoviruses. The nucleocapsid is composed of RNA, L, NP, VP35, and VP30. Analysis of the NP gene shows a short putative leader sequence at the extreme 3 end followed by the complete nucleoprotein gene. The transcriptional start (3′…UUCUUCUUAUAAUU…) and termination (3′ …UAAUUCUUUUU) signals of the MBG NP gene are very similar to those seen with EBO virus.

In comparison to other non-structural non-segmented negative-strand (NNS) RNA viruses, filovirus transcriptional signals are very similar to those of members of the paramyxovirus and morbillivirus genera. Nucleotide sequence analysis of the 3′ end, including the entire NP and L protein encoding genes of the MBG and EBO genome, has shown similar structure and organization with other NNS RNA viruses. The similarity of the filovirus NP genes and gene products to those of the paramyxoviruses imply a closer biological and phylogenetic relationship to these agents than to rhabdoviruses.

GROWTH AND SURVIVAL

Filoviruses undergo rapid, lytic replication in the cytoplasm of a wide range of host cells. The mode of entry of filoviruses into cells remains unknown, although some ultrastructural studies have suggested that virions are associated with entry by endocytosis. Uncoating occurs in a way similar to that of other negative-strand viruses. Messenger RNA is abundant in infected cells, but virion RNA is not detectable, indicating that there is a rapid packaging of genomic RNA and a rapid release of virions. Nucleocapsids also accumulate in the cytoplasm, forming prominent inclusion bodies. Virion assembly involves the preformed nucleocapsids acquiring the envelope with its surface projections by budding from the cell membranes. Laboratory infection of tissue cells shows intracytoplasmic vesiculation and mitochondrial swelling followed by a breakdown of organelles and terminal rarification and condensation. These cytoplasmic changes occur simultaneously with the accumulation of viral nucleocapsid material in intracytoplasmic inclusion bodies and the large numbers of virions extracellularly (Fig. 33.2b).

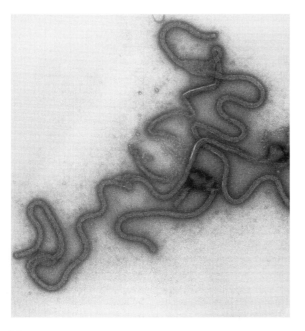

(a)

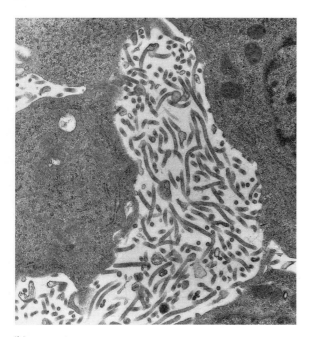

(b)

Fig. 33.2 (a) Electron micrograph, showing filamentous forms of Ebola (Reston) virus (×18 360). (b) Ebola (Sudan) virus thin section, showing virions extruding from cells into extracellular spaces (×14 040). (Courtesy of B. Dowsett.)

Family	Genus	Virus
Filoviridae	*Filovirus*	Marburg Ebola
Rhabdoviridae	*Vesiculovirus*	Vesicular stomatitis virus Chandipura virus
	Lyssavirus	Rabies
Paramyxoviridae	*Morbillivirus*	Measles
	Paramyxovirus	Newcastle disease virus Mumps Parainfluenza type 3
	Pneumovirus	Respiratory syncytial virus Pneumonia virus of mice

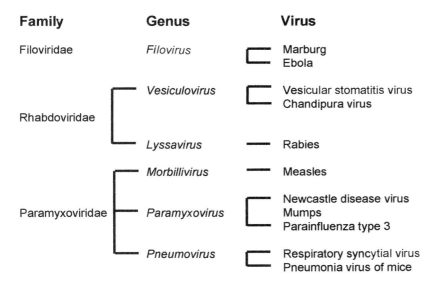

Fig. 33.3   The order Mononegavirales.

The filovirus virion is bacilliform in structure and is composed of a helical nucleocapsid, consisting of a central axis (20–30 nm in diameter), surrounded by a helical capsid (40–50 nm in diameter). A host cell membrane derived lipid outer envelope, with regular 10 nm projections surrounds the nucleocapsid and completes the striking and characteristic appearance under the electron microscope (Fig. 33.2a). Although there are often structures of varying length, with loops, branches, and other irregularities, evidence exists that infectious particles consist mainly of simple linear forms about 1 μm in length.

Marburg and Ebola virus infectivity are stabilized at ambient temperature (18–20 °C) but inactivated within 30 min at 60 °C. Ultraviolet and gamma irradiation, lipids, solvents, β-propiolactone, hypochlorite, and phenolic disinfectants all destroy infectivity.

DISEASE MECHANISMS

The exact mechanism by which filoviruses cause such a serious illness is unknown, but there is extensive viral involvement of liver, lymphoid organs, and kidneys. Extensive visceral effusions, pulmonary interstitial oedema, and renal tubular dysfunction occurring after endothelial damage leading to hypovolaemic shock are all observations contributing to death. Severe, acute fluid loss accompanied by bleeding into the tissue and gastrointestinal tract is characteristic and leads to dehydration, electrolyte and acid–base imbalance. In primates and clinical cases studied early, lymphopenia is followed by a marked neutropenia (Fisher-Hoch *et al.* 1983). In the later stages of the infection, and in association with the thrombocytopenia, the remaining platelets are unable to aggregate in response to ADP

or collagen. It has been suggested that the dysfunction of platelets and endothelia extends to other elements of the endothelial system, such as macrophages (Fisher-Hoch *et al.* 1985). In experimental monkey Ebola infections, virus has been identified in vascular endothelial cells. Humans convalescent from Marburg and Ebola infections have had virus isolated up to 3–4 months later in semen or, in a patient with uveitis, anterior chamber fluid. There is no evidence of long-term persistence, latency or late degenerative disease in the small number of patients observed or in monkeys recovering from the disease (Fisher-Hoch *et al.* 1992*a*).

THE HOSTS

HUMAN

Incubation period

The incubation period for Marburg virus disease is 3–9 days (Martini 1971) and for Ebola virus about 10 days; 5–7 days for needle transmission (Emond 1978) and 6–12 days for person to person spread.

Symptoms and signs

The illnesses caused by Marburg and Ebola viruses are virtually indistinguishable. Following exposure and incubation period both infections have an abrupt onset of illness with initial non-specific symptoms such as fever, severe frontal headache, malaise, and myalgia. Early signs include tachy cardia and conjunctivitis, and there is a maculopapular rash (5–7 days) with prior desquamation in survivors. Within a week to 10 days those destined for recovery begin to improve, even though recovery from the severe debilitating effects of the disease often takes weeks. A large number of patients in both Marburg and Ebola outbreaks develop severe bleeding between the fifth and seventh days. Patients with severe infections often experience pharyngitis, severe nausea, and vomiting, progressing to haematemesis and melena. Petechiae, ecchymoses, uncontrolled bleeding from venepuncture sites, and post-mortem evidence of visceral haemorrhagic effusions are characteristic of severe illness (Smith *et al.* 1978). Death usually occurs between the 7–10 days (range 1–21 days) after onset of clinical disease and is usually preceded by severe blood loss and shock. Convalescence is slow and marked by prostration, weight loss, and amnesia for a considerable period after the acute illness.

Clinical laboratory findings include early lymphopenia, followed by neutrophilia, marked thrombocytopenia, and abnormal platelet aggregation. Serum aspartate aminotransferase (AST)/alanine aminotransferase (ALT) enzyme levels are raised and characterized by a high AST/ALT ratio (10–3 : 1).

As the differential diagnosis in the early acute phase is difficult, other causes must be considered. The most common causes of imported infections showing a severe, acute febrile disease are malaria and typhoid fever. Therefore, differential diagnosis and treatment should not be delayed. Alternative causes include: bacterial diseases such as meningococcal septicaemia, *Yersinia pestis* infection, leptospirosis, anthrax; rickettsial diseases such as typhus and murine typhus; and viral diseases such as sandfly fever, yellow fever, chikungunya fever, Rift Valley fever, hantavirus, Congo Crimean haemorrhagic fever

Diagnosis

The diagnosis of Ebola or Marburg should be considered in patients showing acute, febrile illness having travelled in known epidemic or suspected endemic areas of rural sub-Saharan Africa and Asia, particularly when haemorrhagic signs are present. All tissues, blood, and serum collected in the acute stages of illness contain large amounts of infectious virus. Extreme care should be taken when drawing or handling blood specimens as the virus is stable for long periods at room temperature (Elliott *et al.* 1982). All needles and syringes should be discarded in punctureresistant containers with lids, and incinerated. Specimens of blood should be taken without anticoagulant. Blood or serum should be transferred to a leakproof plastic container and double wrapped in leakproof containers for transportation to a high containment laboratory. Transportation should be under appropriate biocontainment within dry or wet ice

according to international transportation or national regulations (Department of Health and Social Security and Welsh Office 1986; Centers for Disease Control 1995*c*) after consultation with any of the maximum containment reference laboratories. Sera may be safely handled for immunoassay tests by inactivating with irradiation or heating at 60 °C for 30 min. Although morphologically similar, Marburg and Ebola are immunologically distinct. The immunofluorescence assay (IFA) has been the basic diagnostic test for filovirus infection and the only one that has widespread acceptance for the diagnosis of human Ebola disease (Wulff and Johnson 1979; Rollin *et al.* 1990). A rising antibody in paired serum or a high IgG titre (>64) and presence of IgM antibody, together with clinical symptoms compatible with a haemorrhagic fever, are consistent with a diagnosis. Marburg antibody is considered specific but Ebola virus low-titre, non-specific, false-positive serological reactions do occur. When using IFA the problem of low-titre false positives makes interpretation difficult when nonhuman primate and human seroepidemiological surveys are being undertaken. For the IFA, the antigen substrate consists of virus-infected Vero cells dried on to spot slides. Recent advances in molecular biology have expressed the nucleoprotein gene of Ebola virus in a baculovirus expression system. Thus large amounts of non-infectious protein can be produced and used as antigen in many serological tests (IFA, ELISA). Currently their value is being evaluated with the aim of improving the detection capability in seroepidemiological field studies and in the screening of imported primates.

Filoviruses can be easily isolated from inoculation of fresh or stored (−70 °C) specimens of blood or serum collected during the acute phase of illness into Vero monkey kidney tissue cultures cells using laboratory containment level 4 facilities. Vero cells (particularly clone E6) and MA-104 have proved to be the most sensitive and useful cells for the propagation and assay of fresh isolates and laboratory passage filovirus strains. Primary isolation using tissue culture rarely produces a specific cytoplasmic effect, thus evidence of infection is based on the appearance of cytoplasmic inclusion bodies demonstrated 2–5 days after inoculation, by immunofluoresence staining, using antipolyclonal antisera or virus subtype or strain-specific monoclonal antibodies. Some filovirus strains such as Ebola Sudan are difficult to grow in primary cultures and success is improved through the intraperitoneal inoculation of young guinea-pigs. A monitored febrile response coincides with high levels of virus in the blood which can be recovered by tissue culture or examined directly by the electron microscope. In each of the Filoviridae outbreaks electron microscopy has proven useful in the identification of Marburg or Ebola in body fluids and tissue, and cell culture supernatants. During the Reston epizootic, immunoelectron microscopy, when used in conjunction with standard transmission microscopy (TEM) of infected cells, provided consistent results (Geisbert and Jahrling 1990). However, the technique will not distinguish between the Filoviridae strains. Specimens, including throat washings, semen and anterior eye fluid, may also be a source of virus. The presence, of Ebola and Marburg in tissues of monkeys, both experimentally and during primate outbreaks, has been demonstrated by electron microscopy (Baskerville *et al.* 1985; Geisbert and Jahrling 1990); and detection of high titres in the blood of infected patients and monkeys indicated the usefulness of an antigen capture ELISA system (Ksiazek *et al.* 1992). Such a system has been described and found to be of considerable use in the recent Kikwit epidemic. Immunobilized mouse monoclonal antibodies on a solid plastic surface capture Ebola antigen contained in tissue or blood specimens. Rabbit polyclonal anti-filovirus serum detects the antigen. The antigen immunoabsorbent detection assay has proved a rapid and reliable procedure for the early detection of filovirus infections and would prove useful as a method for the routine screening of imported primates.

The use of cross-reacting and strain-specific probes for the reverse transcriptase polymerase chain reaction (RT-PCR) has shown considerable promise as a valuable early diagnostic tool in the detection of filovirus infections.

PRIMATES

African green monkeys imported from Uganda were shown to be the source of the Marburg outbreak (Henderson *et al.* 1971), and cynomolgus monkeys the source of the newly discovered Asian filovirus. Both species were imported and closely associated with medical research.

The general characteristics of primate filovirus infections amongst experimentally and naturally infected primates suggest that the incubation period varies between 4 and 20 days, during which time the virus replicates to high titre in the liver, spleen, lymph nodes, and lungs. The clinicopathological features noted include high fever, severe weight loss, anorexia, haemorrhages, and a distinctive skin rash in association with splenomegaly, marked elevation of lactate dehydrogenase, alanine aminotransferase and aspartate aminotransferase. The AST levels are constantly 2–10 times higher than that of ALT. Evidence of thrombocytopenia is a pronounced feature but anaemia is not. Both lymphocytopenia and leucocytosis are evident and dependent on the stage of the

infection (Fisher-Hoch *et al.* 1983). Severe prostration with diarrhoea and bleeding leads to rapid death in almost all animals. The severity of the disease in primates depends on the filovirus infection and host involved. African green monkeys are far less susceptible to severe or fatal disease due to Ebola virus (Sudan) or Ebola (Reston) than cynomolgus monkeys. However African green monkeys experimentally infected with Marburg virus after the 1967 outbreak all died irrespective of route of infection (Hass and Mass 1971). Marburg virus infection of rhesus monkeys is less severe or fatal, similar to Ebola (Sudan) infection. Infection by Ebola virus (Zaire) is reported as being uniformly fatal in all species so far challenged, regardless of inoculum.

Histopathological findings include severe hepatocellular necrosis, necrosis of the zona glomerulosa of the adrenal cortex, and interstitial pneumonia, all associated with the presence of intracytoplasmic amphophilic inclusion bodies. The necrotic lesions result from direct virus infection of the parenchymal cells. Little inflammatory response occurs at the site of the lesions.

Experimental pathophysiological studies have demonstrated endothelial cell and platelet dysfunction accompanied by oedema, multiple effusions, haemorrhage, and hypovolaemic shock (Fisher-Hoch *et al.* 1985). Recent studies in *Macaca fascicularis* and *Cercopithecus aethiops* suggest that the recently isolated Asian filoviruses are less pathogenic for primates than the African filoviruses (Fisher-Hoch *et al.* 1992*b*).

TREATMENT AND PROGNOSIS

Therapy for Marburg and Ebola virus infection is limited to the provision of supportive measures and general nursing care, as there is no available vaccine and no effective antiviral drugs. Intensive supportive care is currently considered most important: prevention of shock, cerebral oedema, renal failure, bacterial superinfection, hypoxia, and hypotension may be lifesaving. Patient care is complicated by the need for isolation and protection of medical and nursing personnel. The use of plastic patient isolators is a requirement in many countries, including the United Kingdom and Europe, despite the return to the strict barrier nursing techniques now favoured in the United States and in the recent African outbreaks in Zaire, Côte d'Ivoire and Gabon.

Although used in early cases, the efficacy of human convalescent immunoplasma and interferon is doubtful since, when used experimentally, they did not protect animals from lethal infection.

EPIDEMIOLOGY

Marburg virus disease

A fulminating haemorrhagic fever caused by the Marburg virus was first recognized in August 1967 when it affected laboratory workers in three simultaneous outbreaks in Marburg and Frankfurt, Germany, and Belgrade, former Yugoslavia (Martini 1969). Altogether there were 31 human infections, of whom 25 had primary infections acquired through contact of blood and tissues from shipments of African green monkeys (*Cercopithecus aethiops*) imported from Uganda, via London. The largest number of primary infections (20) occurred among workers of a Marburg pharmaceutical firm who prepared kidney cells for vaccine production. Among those infected, exposure was attributed to autopsies (13), cleaning of contaminated glassware (5), dissection of kidneys (1), and laboratory accident involving contaminated broken glassware (1). Personnel not in direct contact with contaminated material or who wore protective gloves or masks for work with monkeys was not infected. In Frankfurt four further primary infections occurred in workers exposed to tissue culture. A veterinary officer carrying out routine post-mortems was the single recorded primary case in Belgrade. Four of the secondary infections occurred in hospital personnel who came into close contact with patients. The fifth was the wife of the veterinary surgeon, who fell ill 10 days after nursing her husband at home. The sixth case involved the wife of a patient who had transmitted the disease through sexual intercourse 83 days after the illness. Seven of the primary cases were fatal, but no fatalities occurred amongst the six secondary cases.

Around 600 animals originating from four shipments reached Europe from Uganda over a 3-week period. Frankfurt received 50–60 animals from two shipments, Belgrade approximately 300 animals from three shipments, and the remainder went to Marburg. All spent between 60 and 87 days in a holding facility in Uganda before being shipped to London, Heathrow where they spent 6–36 hours in the animal hostel before being forwarded to Germany. Details on the Belgrade enzootic indicated that 46 of 99 animals imported from the first shipment died, and 20 and 30 from the second and third shipments, respectively. This epizootic was characterized by daily deaths of one or more animals throughout the 6-week quarantine period, suggesting ongoing transmission between animals. Epidemiological evidence of the outbreak suggested that transmission between monkeys in quarantine facilities was through direct contact with contaminated equipment. Direct contact with infected blood and tissue was recorded for all human cases, and

there was evidence of aerosol transmission. No epizootics were found in Uganda although uncorroborated information had suggested a large number of monkey deaths in colonies on the island near Lake Kyoga, north of Lake Victoria, to the east of Mount Elgon in Kenya. The Ugandan monkeys were captured in this area, transported to Entebbe, where they were held for 3 days prior to shipment.

The first recognized outbreak of Marburg virus disease in Africa, and the first since the 1967 outbreak, occurred in South Africa in February 1975 (Gear *et al.* 1975). The index case involved a young Australian tourist who had hitchhiked through Zimbabwe and died after admission to a Johannesburg hospital. Shortly afterwards two non-fatal secondary cases occurred, one his female travelling companion and a nurse (Table 33.1). Again there was evidence that the virus persisted in the body; the virus was recovered from fluid aspirated from the anterior chamber of the nurse's right eye 80 days after onset of illness. In January 1980 Marburg re-appeared in Kenya (Smith *et al.* 1982). The index patient was an electrical engineer who acquired the fatal infection in western Kenya. A non-fatal secondary infection occurred 9 days later. This involved a doctor who attended the patient and had attempted mouth to mouth resuscitation. Epidemiological studies in Zimbabwe and on Mount Elgon revealed no information concerning the sources of the infections. Presently it is thought that the habitat of the natural host of Marburg virus is within, but not limited to, the Mount Elgon area and possibly overlaps the distribution of Ebola.

Ebola virus disease (Africa)

Two large simultaneous outbreaks of an acute haemorrhagic fever (subsequently named Ebola haemorrhagic fever) occurred in southern Sudan (WHO 1978*a*) and northern Zaire in 1976 (WHO 1978*b*). The first outbreak was identified in southern Sudan in June, continuing through to November 1976. There was a total of 284 cases; 67 in Nazara, 213 in Maridi, 3 in Tembura, and 1 in Juba. The focus of the epidemic was Nazara, a small town with clusters of houses scattered in dense woodland bordering the African rain-forest zone. The outbreak in Nazara originated in three employees of a cotton factory situated near the town centre. Detailed factory records for the previous 2 years did not show any fatal haemorrhagic disease in Nazara until June 1976. At that time one or two workers started dying each week. By September, six factory workers and 25 of their contacts had developed the same illness, of which 21 died. Before the outbreak died out spontaneously cases were reported in two neighbouring areas. The first was in Tembura, a small town 160 km north of Nazara, where an ill woman went to be nursed by her family. Before she died, three women who cared for her also died of the same haemorrhagic disease. No other cases were discovered. Secondly, the epidemic was dramatically amplified by the larger hospital-associated outbreak (213 cases) in Maridi, following the introduction of a patient from Nazara. Maridi, a town east of Nazara, had an estimated population of 10 000 people. Ninety-three cases (46 per cent) acquired their disease in hospital, and 105 (52 per cent) in the community. Of the 230 staff at Maridi hospital, 72 became infected while at work and 41 died. The highest rate of infection was associated with nursing haemorrhagic patients who, at the height of the epidemic, occupied most wards. After Maridi, further cases (one from Nazara and three from Maridi) were transferred to the regional hospital in Juba. A further three patients were flown to Khartoum (1200 km north), where two died. A nurse from Juba was the only secondary case identified as a result of these patient transfers.

Overall there were 151 deaths (mortality rate, 53 per cent) out of a total of 284 cases. The outbreak in Nazara continued until October, infecting a total of 67 people of whom 31 (46 per cent) died, compared to 116 (54 per cent) in Maridi. Studies on 36 families who nursed 38 primary cases indicated that of 232 contacts 30 (14 per cent) developed disease. Similar rates of transmission were observed in subsequent generations, giving an overall secondary attack rate of 12 per cent. Between July and October 1979, 34 cases of Ebola haemorrhagic fever recurred in the Yambio-Nazara District. Five family groups and two individuals were affected. The index case, a cotton-factory worker, transmitted the virus to several members of his family. The outbreak was amplified to other families through nosocomal transmission during his hospitalization and the hospitalization of subsequent cases. Mortality in this outbreak was 65 per cent (22 deaths). It was unclear whether the cotton factory was the source of the index case of infection.

Also during September to October 1976, a large outbreak of Ebola haemorrhagic fever took place in the equatorial rain forest of northern Zaire (WHO 1978b). The index case had been touring and presented himself to the out-patient clinic at Yamkuka Mission Hospital (YMH) for treatment of acute malaria, and received an injection of chloroquine. He was admitted to hospital 10 days later with gastrointestinal bleeding and died. During the following week nine other patients who had received treatment at the out-patient clinic of the YMH were admitted with Ebola haemorrhagic fever. Almost all subsequent cases had received injections or had been in close contact with other patients. The highest incidence was amongst women of 15–29 years, who had attended antenatal and out-patient clinics at this hospital and returned to their villages. After 13 of 17 staff had acquired the disease and

11 patients died, the hospital was closed. The major risk factor proved to be the re-use of non-sterilized needles which were found to be in short supply. Between 1 September and 24 October, there were 318 known cases of Ebola haemorrhagic fever with 280 deaths, a case fatality of 88 per cent. There were over 55 villages in the endemic area (Bumba zone), containing some 550 recorded cases. The overall secondary attack rate was calculated to be 5 per cent, but nearer 20 per cent in close relatives of a case. A further single fatal case was identified in Tandala Hospital in north-western Zaire in 1977 (Heymann et al. 1980). Studies in the Tandala region revealed two possible Ebola cases dating back to 1972, and a 7 per cent Ebola seroprevalence rate in the local population.

In January 1995, a charcoal-maker near Kikwit, a town in Bandudu Province, 550 km east of Kinshasa, was the first fatal case of Ebola (WHO 1995a). By early March 12 members of his family had died. Simultaneously, a Shigella I dysentery epidemic was taking place and masked the early stages of the Ebola outbreak. Hospitals may have been infected during February when an Ebola patient was seen at the Kikwit health centre and was later transferred to the general hospital. During April a resuscitating team became infected after handling a patient misdiagnosed as having typhoid. Rapid transmission of unprotected health workers and other patients occurred, many carrying the disease back into the community. Between January and June a total of 315 cases had occurred, of which 244 died (77 per cent). The female : male ratio was 166 : 149, which 74 per cent (123) females and 81 per cent (121) males died. Provisional data identified 75 (26 per cent) nurses or students and 61 (21 per cent) housewives who contracted the disease. Two hundred and sixty-six (84 per cent) of the cases resided within the Kikwit North and South Zones de Santé. No cases were identified outside the Bandundu region.

The geographic distribution of Ebola virus widened in November 1994 when a non-fatal Ebola haemorrhagic fever case emerged for the first time in West Africa (LeGuenno et al. 1995). In the Tai National Park, Côte d'Ivoire, a 34-year-old ethnologist infected herself while carrying out a post-mortem on a wild chimpanzee found dead with signs of haemorrhages. Eight days later she was admitted to hospital in Abidjan and treated for suspected malaria. As there was no improvement in her condition she was repatriated by Swiss Air Ambulance and admitted to the University Hospital of Basel. As haemorrhagic fever was considered unlikely, she was treated with ciprofloxacin and deoxycyclin for suspected Gram-negative sepsis (typhoid fever), leptospirosis, or rickettsial disease. Retrospective studies isolated the Ebola virus. No clinical illness nor seroconversions were detected among 22 contact persons in the Côte d'Ivoire or 52 hospital and air-ambulance staff based in Switzerland, despite the lack of an early Ebola diagnosis. Late in 1995 a 25-year-old refugee from neighbouring Liberia was admitted to the health facility of Gozon, Côte d'Ivoire, confirming the presence of Ebola virus in West Africa (Centers for Disease Control 1995*c*). Patient isolation and barrier nursing prevented further spread of infection within and from the health facility. Preliminary investigation of his household contacts in the village of Plibo, Maryland County, Liberia found that two male contacts showed the signs and symptoms of early Ebola infection.

The mechanism of transmission of infection in the Ebola virus outbreaks is mainly by direct contact with infected blood or tissue, by very close and prolonged contact with acutely ill patients, or by inoculation with contaminated syringes and needles. Transmission through the airborne route does not seem to be a factor in the maintenance of any of the epidemics.

EPIZOOTICS

Ebola virus

Several filoviruses closely related to Ebola were isolated in 1989 and early 1990 from sick or dying cynomolgus macaques in quarantine facilities located in Reston, Virginia, in Texas, and in Pennsylvania (Centers for Disease Control 1990*a*; Jahrling *et al.* 1990). Shipments to a quarantine facility in Siena, Italy in 1992 also contained animals that died with laboratory-confirmed Ebola-like virus infections (WHO 1992). The monkeys involved in each epizootic had been imported from the Philippines and traced to the same major export facilities. The identification of an Ebola-like virus in each facility led to the termination of all stocks, to reduce the risk of community spread. In the absence of any established link with Africa or African animals, the episode must represent evidence of Asian filoviruses. The first reported epizootic in the United States was complicated by the animals being co-infected with simian haemorrhagic fever; however, 223 of 1050 exposed animals died. The natural host and geographic distribution is unknown.

Active transmission was documented at one Philippine export facility (Hayes *et al.* 1992). Antigen capture ELISA using liver homogenates revealed that 85 out of 161 (53.2 per cent) monkeys that died within a 3-month period proved positive for filovirus antigen. The incidence was calculated to be 24.4 per 100 animals. Here captive monkeys were held in gang cages, increasing the opportunity for monkey to monkey transmission of virus by close contact with virus-laden blood or body secretions. The source of the infection remains unknown. Laboratory experimentation also shows the presence of high concentrations of viral antigen in pulmonary secretions, raising the possibility that this Ebola-like virus may be spread by the airborne route (Jaax *et al.* 1995). Parenteral inoculation with virus-contaminated blood is another possible route during the epizootics as all monkeys were tuberculin tested and given antibiotics. The common practice was to inoculate many monkeys with the same syringe and needle.

ASIA: EBOLA-LIKE VIRUS (RESTON)

Serological evidence of filovirus exposure was found in 12 (6 per cent) of 186 people who lived in wildlife collection areas or worked in primate facilities in Manila (Miranda *et al.* 1991). Within the export facility experiencing the epizootic, 22 per cent of employees tested were found positive. No illness was documented in any of the positives. In the Reston facility, five animal handlers had been identified as having a high level of daily exposure to sick and dying animals. Four were found by IFA to have had serological evidence of recent infection, three seroconverting during the period of the epizootic. No filovirus illness developed. None of the 16 contacts of monkeys with Ebola-like virus imported into Italy showed any clinical or serological signs of infection.

The origin in nature and the natural history of Marburg and Ebola viruses remain unknown. It would seem that the viruses are zoonotic and transmission to humans occurs from ongoing life cycles in animals. Studies attempting to discover the source of the Marburg outbreaks in Europe or Africa, or the recent Ebola outbreak in the United States and Italy, have failed to uncover the reservoir. Whatever their source, person to person transmission is a means by which outbreaks and epidemics progress. This involves close contact; secondary cases have rarely exceeded 10 per cent, indicating that transmission is not efficient. Nosocomial infection is a special case; extreme care should be taken when dealing with infected blood, secretions, tissues, and hospital waste.

PREVENTION AND CONTROL

PREVENTION

Without an understanding of the natural history of the viruses, ecological controls capable of preventing the sporadic human cases that have started outbreaks and epidemics in the past are impossible. The exception would be the containment of monkeys which might have the infections. While there is a strong suspicion that Ebola and Marburg diseases are zoonoses, the search continues for the origin and reservoir host(s) of the virus.

CONTROL STRATEGIES

Although both Marburg and Ebola infections are rare events, they represent a dangerous nosocomial hazard. Prompt identification of active cases is essential and is dependent upon an accurate and detailed history (Department of Health and Social Security and Welsh Office 1986; Centers for Disease Control 1995 WHO 1995*b*). It is clear from the filovirus epidemics encountered to date that hospitals have acted as the main amplifier of the disease to the community. Therefore it is important that physicians working in the areas where haemorrhagic fevers occur should be aware that these diseases exist and that nosocomial spread is a high possibility if not recognized early and patients placed in complete isolation under barrier nursing conditions. In non-endemic areas it is important to maintain awareness of the current viral epidemiological developments and the threat of importation. Prevention of person to person spread of the virus is essential to control. Three weeks prior to illness patients at highest risk have either travelled into areas where viral haemorrhagic fever (VHF) has recently occurred; had direct contact with blood, body fluids, secretions, or excretions of a person or animal with VHF; or worked in a laboratory or facility that handles the viruses. It must be emphasized that the likelihood of acquiring Ebola or Marburg is extremely low if patients do not meet any of the criteria. Contacts of such patients must be placed under surveillance and not allowed to travel. High-risk contact is associated with direct contact with blood or body fluids from acutely ill humans or animals; sexual contact with a convalescent case; or through laboratory accidents. Thus effective surveillance of high-risk contacts and isolation of further cases ensures rapid control of an outbreak. The cause of fever in patients returning from Marburg and Ebola endemic areas is more likely to be other infectious diseases (malaria or typhoid), therefore evaluation and treatment of such infections should not be delayed.

PATIENT CONTAINMENT

Control of outbreaks in endemic and non-endemic areas has been associated with the introduction of good hospital and laboratory infection control practices, with the isolation of febrile patients, careful handling of laboratory specimens and rigorous use of gloves and disinfectants. The containment of patients in plastic-film patient isolators (Trexlar) is favoured in the United Kingdom (Department of Health and Social Security and Welsh Office, 1986). These are located within a room having filtered negative air pressure gradients, a separate effluent treatment plant for waste, an in-suite autoclave for solid waste, a shower, and a staff changing room. Many consider that the

patient isolator reduces manual dexterity, introduces fatigue, inhibits the effectiveness of intensive care procedures, and hinders communication. Of most concern is that these isolators do not reduce the risk of injury by any sharp instruments and have no provision for resuscitation. This system is not used in endemic areas or recommended in the United States (Centers for Disease Control 1995) since the main risks are associated with direct inoculation of virus in blood or other material and the aerosol hazard is considered a low risk. Thus it is considered acceptable to confine patients to isolation in a single room with or without controlled filtered air. The most important consideration is staff training and supervision, the use of gloves and masks, and the mandatory use of a disinfection policy. The recommendations issued concerning the management of AIDS patients are also considered adequate for containment of filoviruses.

The repatriation to Switzerland of an acutely ill Ebola case originating in the Côte d'Ivoire demonstrates the need for vigilance, since filovirus infection was not considered or diagnosed until the patient had recovered. Had the normal barrier precautions not been undertaken, the potential for spread could have been devastating. Filovirus-infected patients should be isolated and barrier-nursed to prevent secondary infections. Handling, transportation, and testing of clinical material containing a high concentration of viruses should follow international and national guidelines.

PRIMATE GUIDELINES

As non-human primates are known to have introduced Marburg to Europe, and Ebola to the United States and Italy, the management of transportation and quarantine facilities should ensure that personnel understand the hazards associated with handling non-human primates. Although the risk of infection is low, guidelines have been issued to minimize such risks in persons exposed to non-human primates during transport and quarantine (Centers for Disease Control 1990*b*; WHO 1990). Those at risk of infection include persons working in temporary or long-term holding facilities and persons who transport animals to these facilities (cargo handlers and inspectors). Monkeys, particularly those imported from Africa and Asia, are potential sources of a range of diseases, and severe illness or deaths in recently imported primates should be reported to health and veterinary authorities and investigated for a variety of infectious agents, including Ebola.

Captive monkeys frequently held in gang cages increase the opportunity for monkey to monkey transmission by virus-laden blood or body secretions. Studies of the epizootic in the United States and experimental infection studies have found high concentrations of viral antigen in pulmonary secretions, raising the possibility that filoviruses spread through the aerosol route.

Although the newly recognized Ebola virus from Asia apparently causes a fatal disease in cynomolgus macaques, initial evidence indicates that its ability to produce infection in humans may be less than that of the Ebola and Marburg viruses from Africa. However, because of the known severity of disease caused by other members of the Filoviridae, it would be premature to ignore the possibility of a possible public health threat posed by the Asian filoviruses. Four independent accounts concerning the importation of Filoviridae-infected primates into the United States and Europe from two areas of the world, Asia and Africa, increase the importance of introducing an infrastructure for the recognition, identification, and elimination polices to remove the possibility of spread.

The high degree of transmissibility among monkeys housed in confined conditions indicates the need for early identification of infected animals, both to protect the monkeys and to minimize the risk of human infection. The early detection of filovirus antigenaemia or nucleic acid would allow identification of infected animals before they become ill. Whether their elimination would prevent any outbreak has yet to be proven. At present the potential threat from filovirus antibody-positive animals remains unclear, although there is no evidence that latent or constant infection has played any role in monkey-associated outbreaks. Improved quarantine and animal handling procedures need to be universally implemented to ensure no future outbreaks associated with wild-caught monkeys. Therefore, contact between monkeys and man should be limited and animal husbandry tightly controlled. Personnel handling animals should wear protective clothing, including rubber gloves and face respirator. All animal waste, cages, and other potentially contaminated items should be treated with appropriate disinfectants.

Finally, the increased concern for wildlife conservation and licensing of exporters/importers will further decrease the risk of filovirus spread to man.

REFERENCES

Baron, R., McCormick, J., and Zubeir, O. (1983). Ebola virus disease in southern Sudan: hospital dissemination in intrafamilial spread. *Bulletin World Health Organisation*, **61**, 997–1003.

Baskerville, A., Fisher-Hoch, S. P., Neilds, G. H., and Dowsett, A. B. (1985). Ultrastructure pathology of experimental Ebola haemorrhagic fever virus infection. *Journal of Pathology*, **147**, 199–209.

Bishop, D. H. L. and Pringle C. R. (1995). Order Mononegavirales. In *Virus Taxonomy, Sixth Report of the International Committee on Taxonomy of Viruses*, (ed. F. A. Murphy *et al.*), pp. 265–267. Springer-Verlag, Vienna.

Bowen, E. T. W., Platt, G. S., Lloyd, G., Baskerville, A., Harris, W. J., and Vella, E. C. (1977). Viral haemorrhagic fever in southern Sudan and northern Zaire: preliminary studies on the aetiologic agent. *Lancet*, **1**, 571–3.

Centers for Disease Control (1990*a*). Ebola virus infection in imported primates—Virginia, 1989. *Morbidity and Mortality Weekly Record*, **38**, 831–8.

Centers for Disease Control (1990*b*). Ebola related filovirus infection in non-human primates and interim guidelines for handling non-human primates during transit and quarantine. *Morbidity and Mortality Weekly Report*, **39**, 22–30.

Centers for Disease Control (1995*c*). Management of patients with suspected viral haemorrhagic fever—US. *Morbidity and Mortality Weekly Record*, **44**, 475–9.

Department of Health and Social Security and Welsh Office (1986). The control of viral haemorrhagic fevers. HMSO, London.

Elliot, L. H., McCormick, J. B., and Johnson, K. M. (1982). Inactivation of Lassa, Marburg, and Ebola viruses by Gamma irradiation. *Journal of Clinical Microbiology*, **16**, (4), 704–8.

Emond, R. T. D. (1978). Isolation, monitoring, and treatment of a case of Ebola infection. In *Ebola virus infection*, (ed. S. R. Pattyn), pp. 27–32. Elsevier/North Holland Biomedical Press, Amsterdam.

Emond, R. T. D., Evans, E., Bowen, E., and Lloyd, G. (1977). A case of Ebola virus infection. *British Medical Journal*, **2**, 541–4.

Feldman, H., Klenk, H. D., and Sanchez, A. (1993). Molecular biology and evolution of filoviruses. *Archives of Virology Supplement*, **7**, 87–100.

Fisher-Hoch, S. P., Platt, G. S., Lloyd, G., Simpson, D. I., Neils, G. H., and Barett, A. J. (1983). Haematological and biochemical monitoring of Ebola infection in rhesus monkeys: implications for patient management. *Lancet*, **2**, 1055–8.

Fisher-Hoch, S. P. *et al.* (1985). Pathophysiology of shock and haemorrhage in a fulminating viral infection (Ebola). *Journal of Infectious Diseases*, **152**, 887–94.

Fisher-Hoch, S. P., Perez-Oronoz, G. I., Jackson, E. L., Hermann, L. M., and Brown, B. G. (1992*a*). Filovirus clearance in non-human primates. *Lancet*, **340**, 451–3.

Fisher-Hoch, S. P. et al. (1992*b*). Pathogenic role of geographic origin of primate host and virus strain. *Journal of Infectious Diseases*, **166**, (4), 753–63.

Gear, J. S. S. *et al.* (1975). Outbreak of Marburg virus disease in Johannesburg. *British Medical Journal*, **4**, 489–93.

Geisbert, T. W. and Jahrling P. B. (1990). Use of immunoelectron microscopy to show Ebola virus during the 1989 United States epizootic. *Journal of Clinical Pathology*, **43**, 813–16.

Haas, R. and Mass, G. (1971). Experimental infection of monkeys with the Marburg virus. In *Marburg virus disease*, (ed. G. A. Martini and R. Siegert), pp. 136–43. Springer-Verlag, Berlin.

Hayes, C. G. *et al.* (1992). Outbreak of fatal illness among captive macaques in the Philippines caused by an Ebola-related filovirus. *American Journal of Tropical Medicine and Hygiene*, **46**, 664–71.

Henderson, B. E., Kissling, R. E., Williams, M. C., Kafuko, G. W., and Martin, M. (1971). Epidemiological studies in Uganda relating to 'Marburg agent'. In *Marburg virus disease*, (ed. G. A. Martini and R. Siegert), pp. 19–23. Springer-Verlag, Berlin.

Heymann, D. L., Weisfeld, J. S., Webb, P. A., Johnson, K. M., Cairns, T., and Berquist, H. (1980). Ebola haemorrhagic fever: Tandala, Zaire, 1977–1978. *Journal of Infectious Disease*, **56**, 247–70.

Jaax, M. *et al.* (1996). Transmission of Ebola virus (Zaire strain) to uninfected monkeys in a biocontainment laboratory. *Lancet*, **343**, 1669–71.

Jahrling, P. B. *et al.* (1990). Preliminary report: isolation of Ebola virus from monkeys imported to USA. *Lancet*, **335**, 502–5.

Kiley, M. P. *et al.* (1982). Filoviridae: a taxonomic home for Marburg and Ebola viruses? *Intervirology*, **18**, 24–32.

Ksiazek, T. G., Rollin, P. E., Jahrling, P. B., Johnson, E., Dalgard, D. W., and Peters, C. J. (1992). Enzyme immunosorbent assay for Ebola virus antigens in tissues of infected primates. *Journal of Clinical Microbiology*, **30**, (4), 947–50.

Le Guenno, B., Formentry, P., Wyers, M., Gounon, P., Walker, F., and Christopher, B. (1995). Isolation and partial characterisation of a new strain of Ebola. *Lancet*, **345**, 1271–4.

Martini, G. A. (1969). Marburg agent disease in man. *Transactions of the Royal Society of Tropical Medicine and Hygiene*, **63**, 295–302.

Martini, G. A. (1971). Marburg virus disease, clinical syndrome. In *Marburg virus disease* (ed. G. A. Martini and R. Siegert), pp. 1–9. Springer Verlag, Berlin.

Miranda, M. E. G., White, M. E., Dayrit, M. M., Hayes, C. G., Ksiazek. T. G., and Burns, J. P. (1991). Seroepidemiology study of filovirus related to Ebola in the Philippines [letter]. *Lancet*, **337**, 425–6.

Pringle, C. R. (1991). Order Mononegavirales. *Archives of Virology*, **117**, 137–40.

Rollin, P. E., Ksiazek, T. G., Jahrling, P. E., Haines, M., and Peters, C. J. (1990). Detection of Ebola-like viruses by immunofluorescence. *Lancet*, **336**, 1591.

Sanchez, A., Kiley M. P., Klenk, H. D., and Feldman, H. (1992). Sequence analysis of the Marburg virus nucleoprotein gene: comparison to Ebola virus and other non-segmented negative stand RNA viruses. *Journal of General Virology*, **73**, 347–57.

Sanchez, A., Kiley, M. P., Holloway, B. P., and Asuperin, D. D. (1993). Sequence analysis of the Ebola virus genome: organisation, genetic elements, and comparison with the genome of Marburg virus. *Virus Research*, **29**, 215–40.

Smith, D. G., Francis, F., and Simpson, D. I. H. (1978). African haemorrhgic fever in the southern Sudan, 1976: the clinical manifestations. In *Ebola virus haemorrhagic fever*, (ed. S. R. Pattyn), pp. 1–6. Elsevier, Amsterdam.

Smith, D. H. *et al.* (1982). Marburg-virus disease in Kenya, *Lancet*, **1**, 816–20.

Teepe, R. G. *et al.* (1983). A probable case of Ebola virus haemorrhagic fever in Kenya. *East African Medical Journal*, **60**, 718–22.

World Health Organisation/International Commission to Sudan. (1978*a*). Ebola haemorrhagic fever in Sudan; 1976. *Bulletin World Health Organisation*, **56**, 247–70.

World Health Organisation/International Commission to Zaire (1978*b*). Ebola haemorrhagic fever in Zaire; 1976. *Bulletin World Health Organisation*, **56**, 271–93.

World Health Organisation (1990). Interim guidelines for handling nonhuman primates during transit and quarantine. *Weekly Epidemiological Record*, **65**, 45–52.

World Health Organisation (1992). Viral haemorrhagic fever in imported monkeys. *Weekly Epidemiological Record*, **67**, 142–3.

World Health Organisation (1995*a*). Ebola haemorrhagic fever, Zaire. *Weekly Epidemiological Record*, **70**, 241–2.

World Health Organisation (1995*b*). Viral haemorrhagic fevers—management of suspected cases. *Weekly Epidemiological Record*, **35**, 249–52.

World Health Organisation (1995*c*). Ebola haemorrhagic fever—confirmed case in Côte d'Ivoire and suspected cases in Liberia. *Weekly Epidemiological Record*, **70**, 359.

World Health Organisation (1996). Ebola haemorrhagic fever. *Weekly Epidemiological Record*, **71**, 320.

Wulff, H. and Johnson, K. M. (1979). Immunoglobulin M and G responses measured by immunofluorescence in patients with Lassa or Marburg virus infections. *Bulletin World Health Organisation*, **57**, 631–5.

34 MOSQUITO-BORNE ARBOVIRUSES

Colin J. Leake

SUMMARY

Human infections caused by mosquito-borne arboviruses range from numerous inapparent infections, through non-fatal but debilitating fevers, to life-threatening severe haemorrhagic complications and shock, or acute encephalitis with high mortality and serious neurological after-effects in survivors. Similarly, frequent inapparent infections occur in animals, with overt disease ranging to the severe end of the scale, with haemorrhage, encephalitis, abortion, and birth defects as principal symptoms. These arboviruses are all relatively simple single-stranded RNA viruses, although they belong to several taxonomic families. Natural transmission is in the saliva injected during the biting of female mosquitoes previously infected during blood-feeding on a viraemic animal host. Transmission is highly seasonal, dictated principally by environmental temperature, the availability of water-filled breeding sites for the aquatic life stages of the mosquitoes, and the population dynamics and host-biting preferences of the adults. These arboviruses are mainly tropical in distribution and can occupy considerable geographic ranges; although some are more temperate. Many of the viruses are sporadic or persistent endemic problems of rural agricultural communities with occasional, but potentially explosive, epidemic risk to urban populations. Hereditary transovarial transmission by infected female mosquitoes to their offspring is probably important in natural maintenance, particularly with certain temperate bunyaviruses. Control methods depend on the epidemiology of the particular virus. Control of the sylvatic animal reservoir is often impossible, although several veterinary vaccines have been used successfully in domestic animals. Epidemic vector control has largely been dependent on insecticide spraying, although this may have only temporary impact on adult vector populations. Clinically, care is supportive only and, with a couple of important exceptions, vaccines are not generally available for widespread human use.

HISTORY

Because of their severe symptoms, most of these virus diseases have been known for many years, but it is only comparatively recently that these arboviruses have been isolated and characterized in the laboratory. Tables 34.1–34.3 summarize the dates of the first reliable reports of these diseases, the dates of primary isolation of the agents, and other key information regarding the epidemiology and disease symptoms of the major mosquito-associated arboviruses.

The discovery of the natural cycle of these viruses between vectors and vertebrate hosts has lead to the arthropod-borne viruses, or arboviruses, being defined as 'Viruses maintained in nature principally, or to an important extent, through biological transmission between susceptible vertebrate hosts by haematophagous arthropods, or through transovarian and possible venereal transmission in arthropods; the viruses multiply to produce viraemia in the vertebrates, multiply in the tissues of arthropods and are passed on to new vertebrates by the bites of arthropods after a period of extrinsic incubation' (WHO 1985).

Currently, 535 viruses are catalogued (Karabatsos 1985) and, of these, over 100 have been implicated in producing human illness. However, the majority of these viruses are unimportant in human disease, causing either subclinical or relatively mild influenza-like infections. A number cause debilitating fevers variously presenting with rash, polyarthritis, arthralgia, and myalgia from which recovery is usually complete, although, at times, may be prolonged. Only a minority cause serious life-threatening symptoms of haemorrhage/shock or encephalitis. In animals the most obvious signs of disease are at the severe end of the scale, manifesting as haemorrhage, encephalitis, abortion, and neonatal birth defects.

These arboviruses are primarily rural problems maintained in animal–mosquito cycles associated with agricultural practices. Principal at-risk groups are therefore agricultural communities, or development workers breaking into previously unknown or epidemi-

Table 34.1 Principal mosquito-borne members of Alphavirus genus

Virus name	ABBR.	Initial report-isolate	Geographic region						Naturally infected mosquitoes isolate +	Principal human vector	Naturally infected vertebrates isolate +	Human disease	Animal disease
			Afr.	Asia	Aust	Eur	N Am	S Am					
Chikungunya	CHIK	1779–1953	+	+	–	–	–	–	*Aedes aegypti,* forest *Aedes* species	*Aedes aegypti*	Primates, bird, bat, squirrel	Fever + rash, severe arthralgia	None recorded
Eastern equine encephalitis	EEE	1831–1933	–	(+)	(+)	(+)	+	+	23 species, 6 genera	*Coquilletidia perturbans, Culiseta melanura,* many others	Many wild birds, equines, rodents, bats, reptiles, amphibians	Encephalitis	Death: CNS involvement or inapparent
O'Nyong-nyong	ONN	1959–1959	+	–	–	–	–	–	*Anopheles gamblae, Anopheles funestus*	*Anopheles gamblae, Anopheles funestus*	None	Fever, severe joint pain	None recorded
Ross River	RR	1928–1963	–	–	+	+	+	+	22 species, 5 genera	*Culex annulirostris Aedes vigilax* several others possible	Large mammals, marsupials	Fever + rash, polyarthritis	Inapparent infection
Venezuelan equine encephalomyelitis	VEE	1925–1936	–	–	–	–	+	+	41 species (enzootic strains)	*Aedes aegypti* + 34 species in epidemics	Rodents, bats, birds marsupials, equines	Encephalitis	Encephalitis in horses
Western equine encephalitis	WEE	1930–1930	–	–	–	–	+	+	28 species	*Culex tarsalis*	Rodents, birds, equines	Encephalitis	Some deaths birds, rodent; encephalitis in horses

Compiled from Karabatsos (1985) and Monath (1988).
(+), Only a single isolate recorded in these areas.

403

Table 34.2 Principal mosquito-borne members of *Flavivirus* genus

Virus name	ABBR.	Initial report–isolate	Afr.	Asia	Aust	Eur	N Am	S Am	Naturally infected mosquitoes isolate +	Principal human vector	Naturally infected vertebrates isolate +	Human disease	Animal disease
Japanese encephalitis	JE	1870–1935	–	+	–	–	–	–	> 25 species	*Culex tritaeniorhynchus*, other ricefield *Culex*	Birds, swine, many others + antibody	Encephalitis	Encephalitis, abortion
Murray Valley encephalitis	MVE	1917–1951	–	+	+	–	–	–	*Culex annulirostris*, several others	*Culex annulirostis*	Birds	Encephalitis	No major disease recorded
Rocio	ROC	1975–1975	–	–	–	–	–	+	*Psorophora ferox*	? *Psorophora ferox*, ? *Aedes scapularis*	Sparrow	Encephalitis	None reported
St Louis encephalitis	SLE	1933–1933	–	–	–	–	+	+	Many *Culex* species	*Cx tarsalis, nigripalpus, quinquefasciatus, pipiens*	Principally birds, many mammals	Encephalitis	Asymptomatic
Wesselsbron	WSL	1955–1955	+	–	–	–	–	–	> 30 species, *Aedes caballus, Aedes circumluteolus, Aedes lineatopennis*	? mosquito transmission, infected carcass handling, laboratory infection	Cattle, sheep, rodents	Febrile illness some rash, arthralgia	Abortion teratological effects in newborn
West Nile	WN	1937–1937	+	+	–	+	–	–	24 species	*Culex univittatus*	Birds, bats, horses, large mammals.	Fever + rash neurotropic hepatitis,	Some bird deaths
Yellow Fever	YF	1648–1927	+	–	–	–	+	+	Several *Aedes, Haemagogus* and Sabethine species	*Aedes aegypti, Aedes bromeliae*	Principally primates, marsupials	Hepatotropic haemorrhagic fever	Hepatotropic primate death

Compiled from Karabatsos (1985) and Monath (1988).

Table 34.3 Principal mosquito-borne members of *Bunyavirus*, *Phlebovirus*, and *Vesiculovirus* genera

Virus name	ABBR.	Initial report–isolate	Geographic region						Naturally infected mosquitoes isolate +	Principal human vector	Naturally infected vertebrates isolate +	Human disease	Animal disease
			Afr.	Asia	Aust	Eur	N Am	S Am					
Bunyavirus													
California encephalitis	CE	1943–1943	–	–	–	–	+	–	*Aedes melanimon*, *Culex tarsalis*	*Aedes melanimon*, *Aedes dorsalis*	Ground squirrel, rabbits	Mild to encephalitis, few cases ever	None recorded
Jamestown Canyon	JC	1961–1962	–	–	–	–	+	–	*Culiseta inornata*	*Culisetas inornata*, many other *Aedes*	White tail deer, large mammals	Mild to encephalitis	None recorded
La Crosse	LAC	1943–1964	–	–	–	–	+	–	*Aedes triseriatus*, other *Aedes* spp.	*Aedes triseriatus*	Chipmunk, squirrel, fox, rabbit	Mild to encephalitis	None recorded
Tahyna	TAH	1958–1958	–	–	–	+	–	–	*Aedes caspius*, *Aedes cinereus*	*Aedes vexans*	Hares, rabbit	Febrile illness, CNS signs	None recorded
Phlebovirus													
Rift Valley Fever	RVF	1912–1930	+	–	–	–	–	–	23 species	Floodwater *Aedes* (sub-Sahara), *Culex pipiens* (Egypt) carcass handling	Ruminants, sheep, cattle + others	Fever, encephalitis, ocular signs, haemorrhage	Hepatotropic haemorrhage, abortion, death
Vesiculovirus													
Vesicular stomatitis	VS	1901–1925	–	–	–	–	+	+	*Aedes dosalis*, *Culex nigripalpus*, *Mansonia indubitans*	Not confirmed (direct contact with infected animals is risk factor)	Cattle, horse, swine, many others involved	Febrile illness vesicular lesions	Inapparent to severe resembles foot-and mouth disease

Compiled from Karabatsos (1985) and Monath (1988).

ologically silent foci, for example during clearing of forest or land for road and new town development. Although zoonotic transmission may be intense, these cycles may be largely silent in terms of disease in the animal host. Periodically, these viruses have the potential to expand explosively into major epizootic disease activity and to extend into serious human epidemic involvement. Also due to the ever-increasing development of transport of man, animals and vectors there is an increasing risk of the introduction of these viruses into completely new geographic areas, potentially resulting in major new outbreaks in immunologically naive animal and human populations (Johnson and Chanas 1981).

Animals with relatively short life spans are essential in the maintenance of these viruses. Their high annual population turnover results in the introduction of large numbers of new susceptible individuals into the population. With several viruses, birds are important hosts (Tables 34.1–34.3). Similarly large-scale turnover of domestic animals such as pigs (e.g. JE virus, Table 34.2) may be significant in the transmission cycle. The relatively long-lived animals such as horses and cattle which develop long-lasting immunity may act as epidemiological dampers by absorbing substantial numbers of potentially infectious mosquito bites without acting as amplifying hosts.

The biology and population dynamics of the individual vector mosquitoes concerned are also critical components in virus epidemiology. Vector mosquitoes require water-filled breeding sites to lay their eggs and for the larval stages to develop. The availability of seasonal rains and the development of major irrigation schemes allied to agricultural development therefore have a major impact on vector productivity. For example, a major source of vector breeding around the world is in rice-field environments (Leake 1988). A second major environmental influence is the impact of temperature which affects vector productivity and also virus replication. As summer-time temperatures reach high levels the seasonal increase in vector numbers plus the more rapid completion of the virus development cycle in the vectors combine to produce intense epizootic transmission extending into epidemic outbreaks, often focused over a very short period each year. The final important component is the host preference of the vector mosquitoes. In many situations it is known that the important vector species are primarily zoophilic in habit but during the peak of transmission a small proportion of these host-seeking mosquitoes may opportunistically bite humans. For example, with JE virus, the principal vector mosquito *Culex tritaeniorhynchus* preferentially bites cattle, with less than 1 per cent of blood-fed female mosquitoes being shown to take human blood (Burke and Leake 1988). More complex situations are known as well. There may be situations where mosquito hosts apparently switch their blood-feeding behaviour. *Culex tarsalis*, a major vector of SLE virus (Table 34.2), bites nestling birds early in the season, moving to vertebrates and humans later in the summer when the fledglings have left the nest (Tsai and Mitchell 1988). Link vectors may be involved, such as *Aedes bromeliae* (*Aedes simpsoni*), an African mosquito, that bites both primates and humans in forest-edge plantation environments. This species ensures the connection of the purely zoonotic jungle transmission cycle of YF virus between monkeys and forest-dwelling *Aedes* mosquitoes to the potential epidemic cycle. These epidemic vectors may be highly anthropophilic in biting preference and highly restricted to the locale of human habitation (Strode 1951). The best example of this is undoubtedly the yellow fever mosquito, *Aedes aegypti*, which is far more important today as a vector of the dengue viruses, the world's most prevalent flaviviruses. Detailed consideration of the dengue viruses has been largely excluded from this chapter because the majority of dengue transmission is now directly between humans by urbanized *Aedes* species. However, it is worth pointing out that there is a tree-top jungle cycle of dengue viruses between sylvatic mosquitoes and primates (Gubler 1988) and there is every probability that the dengue viruses represent an example of an originally zoonotically transmitted virus that has successfully exploited the expanding ecological niches provided by human urbanization to become a hyper-endemic/epidemically maintained virus.

Control of these arboviruses has always been difficult and is dealt with more fully below.

THE AGENTS

TAXONOMY

These arboviruses are relatively simple in structure, being composed of an outer glycoprotein envelope which encloses a nucleocapsid core containing protein and a single-stranded RNA molecule. The viruses have been classified into a number of taxonomic groups based on details of their morphology, structure, and replication strategy. The principal families considered here (Tables 34.1–34.3) are the family Togaviridae/genus *Alphavirus* (old Group A arboviruses), the family Flaviviridae/genus *Flavivirus* (old Group B arboviruses), the family Bunyaviridae/genus *Bunyavirus*, genus *Phlebovirus*, and the family Rhabdoviridae/genus *Vesiculovirus* (Karabatsos 1985).

MOLECULAR BIOLOGY

Alphaviruses

In total 27 viruses have been assigned to the *Alphavirus* genus, all but one being isolated from mosquitoes.

Several viruses, namely Mayaro, Ockelbo, Sindbis, and Semliki Forest, cause generally mild fevers in man and are not considered further here. Those alphaviruses causing more serious human disease are shown in Table 34.1. Structurally, alphaviruses are enveloped icosahedral particles, 60–70 nm in diameter, with surface spikes 6–10 nm in length overlying a nucleocapsid core with a diameter of 35–39 nm. The nucleocapsid ribonucleoprotein contains a single core or capsid C protein, and one segment of single-stranded positive-sense (infectious) RNA with a molecular weight of 4×10^6 Da. There are typically three structural proteins. Two of these are envelope proteins E1 and E2 and one is a non-glycosylated capsid protein with a molecular weight of $30–34 \times 10^3$ Da. The surface spikes are important in the initial adsorption and fusion of the virion with the host cell, followed by rapid internalization of virions into host cells in vesicles called endosomes by a process of receptor-mediated endocytosis. Within the cell there is the primary endocytotic pathway leading into the cell, several recycling pathways, and an exocytotic pathway transporting newly formed proteins from the endoplasmic reticulum into lysosomes, into secretory vesicles (a signal-mediated regulatory pathway), or directly to the outside world (constitutive or signal-independent default pathway). All parts of the assembly line are constantly being repaired by housekeeping proteins (Koblet 1990).

Within the endosome the viral membranes fuse with the endosomal membranes, thereby releasing nucleocapsids into the cytoplasm for transport to ribosomes where the genomic RNA is liberated and transcribed. The infecting genomic positive-sense strand is first transcribed into a minus-strand 49S RNA which, in turn, forms the template for progeny positive-strand 49S RNA, template for non-structural proteins comprising the RNA-dependent RNA polymerase which transcribes and replicates the viral RNAs, and for the 26S mRNA that serves as the subgenomic message producing all the structural proteins. The complete nucleotide sequence is known for several alphaviruses. The genes coding for the structural proteins are located at the 3′ one-third of the genome immediately following a non-translated section of 150–450 bases in the order 5′, nsP1, nsP2, nsP3, nsP4, C, E3, E2, 6K, E1–3′. The 6K peptide functions as a signal. Membrane proteins are produced on membrane-bound polysomes on the luminal side of the rough endoplasmic reticulum (RER) and the newly synthesized envelope proteins are transported to and inserted into the cell's plasma membrane. Newly synthesized core C protein is bound to the large ribosomal subunit and, together with progeny genomic RNA, forms new nucleocapsids in the cytoplasm, which are then transported to the cell membrane. They attach below the membrane in areas where newly formed envelope protein precursors have been inserted and the nucleocapsids bud out through the membrane by a process of reverse endocytosis, aquiring envelope protein in the process (Koblet 1990).

Flaviviruses

33 flaviviruses are known to be associated with mosquitoes and the most important in human disease are shown in Table 34.2. The dengue viruses have been excluded for reasons described above. Flaviviruses are spherical particles approximately 40 nm in diameter with surface projections of 5–10 nm. The virions contain a nucleocapsid 25–30 nm in diameter surrounded by a lipid bilayer derived from host membranes containing the envelope proteins E and M (or preM). Flaviviruses probably enter cells by receptor-mediated endocytosis, or by direct fusion with the cell membrane, in prelysosomal vesicles which are acidified within the cytoplasm to release the nucleocapsid via fusion with the liposomal membrane. Early events in uncoating, translation of the infecting RNA, and initiation of RNA replication, have not been extensively studied, but is thought to occur in association with the cellular RER. The incoming positive-sense genomic RNA is replicated to form complimentary minus strands and then genome-length plus-strand molecules are produced by a semiconservative mechanism involving replicative intermediates and replicative forms. The plus strands are then used for translation of structural and non-structural polypeptides, minus-strand synthesis, or are incorporated into new virions. The non-structural proteins NS3 and NS5 are presumed to be replicase components as they are conserved among flaviviruses and are homologous with helicases and polymerases (Chambers *et al.* 1990).

The virion RNA comprises one segment of single-stranded positive-sense RNA of molecular weight 4×10^6 Da (approx. 11 kb) in size, and three structural proteins; an envelope glycoprotein (E) with a molecular weight of $51–59 \times 10^3$ Da, a second core protein C with a molecular weight of $13–16 \times 10^3$ Da which encloses the RNA, and a third membrane-like protein (M) with a molecular weight of $7–9 \times 10^3$ Da. The RNA codes for three structural and five non-structural proteins. The flavivirus genome is organized similarly to that of the picornaviruses, code for the structural proteins being located at the 5′ one-third of the genome. There is no subgenomic message, and there is one single long open reading frame. 5′-non-coding region; C, pM/M, E, NS1, NS2A, NS2B, NS3, NS4A, NS4B, NS5-3′.

Translation initiates near the 5′ end of the molecule and individual proteins are produced by proteolytic cleavage at signalase sites by virus and host origin proteases. The non-structural proteins NS3 and NS5 are presumed to be enzymatic components of the viral replicase and the hydrophobic NS2A, NS2B, NS4A and NS4B proteins may be membrane associated. After translation of the anchored C hydrophobic sequence, the flavivirus polysome presumably becomes associated with the host cell RER and translation of the viral proteins is therefore likely to be membrane associated. Particle assembly takes place at these sites when the highly basic domain of newly synthesized core C protein interacts with viral genomic RNA to form new nucleocapsids. The prM and E proteins are translocated to these membrane sites and anchored by their hydrophobic termini in the lipid bilayer with their free ends in the lumen of the endoplasmic reticulum, suggesting that the nucleocapsid acquires its envelope by budding into the lumen (Chambers *et al.* 1990).

Morphogenesis occurs in association with intracellular membranes. Virions accumulate within disorderly arrays of membrane-bound vesicles and mature virions accumulate in the lumen of the endoplasmic reticulum. Dramatic alteration of the intracellular membranes is typical of flaviviruses. Nascent virions are transported from the endoplasmic reticulum to the cell surface where exocytosis occurs, and is believed to involve vesicles that may arise from the endoplasmic reticulum or other components of the host secretory system. Alternatively, there may be complete cytolysis; budding of flaviviruses does not seem to be a major release mechanism (Chambers *et al.* 1990).

Bunyaviruses

This large collection of over 300 viruses was originally grouped together as the Bunyamwera supergroup, but more recently the family Bunyaviridae has been divided into five genera. Only two genera, the genus *Bunyavirus* and the genus *Phlebovirus*, have members associated with mosquitoes. Several of these viruses have been associated with mild fevers in man namely Bunyamwera, Bwamba, Germiston, Group C (10 viruses), Ilesha, and Tataguine, but only those viruses associated with more severe human illness are reviewed here (Table 34.3).

Members of the Bunyaviridae are typically spherical enveloped particles, 75–115 nm in diameter with 10 nm surface spikes and a 4 nm thick bilayer structure. They contain three circular ribonucleoprotein complexes, each composed of many copies of the nucleoprotein N, a small number of the L protein transcriptase, and a single negative-sense RNA strand in L (large), M (medium), and S (small) segments, with the M segment containing determinants of neurovirulence. The remaining G1 and G2 structural proteins form the surface spikes. Bunyaviruses and phleboviruses express two non-structural proteins NS_m and NS_s. Unlike other enveloped viruses, the Bunyaviridae do not contain an internal matrix protein, suggesting that the ribonucleoproteins interact directly with the envelope. The G1 and G2 proteins are synthesized on the rough endoplasmic reticulum and transported and localized in the Golgi apparatus, where maturation occurs by budding at smooth membrane vesicles with only occasional budding having been observed at the plasma membrane. (Bouloy 1991).

Genus bunyavirus

This genus contains 138 viruses in 15 groups, of which 110 have been isolated from mosquitoes. However, only the California group are important human pathogens particularly LAC, JC, and TAH viruses. Members of this group have a negative-sense RNA replication and two of the four structural proteins are glycosylated (G1 and G2) with molecular weights of 100–125 and $29–40 \times 10^3$ Da, respectively. The nucleocapsid protein (N) has a molecular weight of $19–27 \times 10^3$ Da, and a minor large protein (L) has a molecular weight of $180–200 \times 10^3$ Da (Bouloy 1991).

Genus phlebovirus

There are 37 viruses in the *Phlebovirus* genus, mainly sandfly-associated, and the only important mosquito-associated virus is RVF (Table 34.3). Phleboviruses have what is termed an ambisense RNA replication strategy where the N and NS_s proteins are coded by two subgenomic mRNAs of opposite polarity. Two of the four structural proteins are glycosylated (G1 and G2) with molecular weights of 55–70 and $50–60 \times 10^3$ Da, respectively. The nucleocapsid protein (N) has a molecular weight of 28×10^3 Da and a minor large protein (L) has a molecular weight of $180–200 \times 10^3$ Da (Bouloy 1991).

Rhabdoviruses
Genus vesiculovirus

The genus *Vesiculovirus* contains the bullet-shaped vesicular stomatitis serogroup viruses. Virions are 170 nm × 70 nm in size with one segment of single-stranded negative-sense RNA and four structural proteins (L, G, N, M). Vesicular stomatitis group viruses are transmitted by culicine mosquitoes or phebotomine sandflies and the most important here is VS virus (Table 34.3). Features of replication are thought to be similar to other enveloped viruses. The single 42S RNA molecule is transcribed into five mRNAs coding for four structural proteins: a glycoprotein G, a matrix phosphoprotein M which underlies the envelope, a nucleocapsid protein N, and a large L protein, and a single non-structural NS protein (Fraenkal-Conrat *et al.* 1988).

VIRUS VARIATION AND EVOLUTION

Variation in viral RNA is a common theme for all these viruses (Steinhauer and Holland 1987). Variation occurs as a result of intramolecular events or segment reassortment at high frequency compared to DNA, presumably because of the fidelity of viral replication enzymes and the lack of proof-reading enzymes. It is likely that a single progeny RNA of 12 kb differs from its parent by at least 1 base. Well over half the nucleotide positions can be substituted without loss of virus viability, but the fact that these viruses show highly conserved regions suggests that the majority of these point mutations are lethal to the virus. In the non-segmented genomes in alphaviruses, flaviviruses and rhabdoviruses, genomic changes are a result of nucleotide sequence deletions, inversions or substitutions, whereas in the bunyaviruses segment reassortment is also possible (Steinhauer and Holland 1987).

A major selection pressure on the virus is the presence of host neutralizing antibody. It is known from many experimental studies that escape mutants can be generated that can evade the host response. Also it is known that at low dilutions antibody can fail to neutralize but can play a significant role in antibody-mediated enhancement of infection. This may be particularly important with the pathogenesis of the dengue viruses (Gubler 1988) and the flaviviruses in particular are known to produce cross-reactive antibody that can enhance infection with other members of the group.

DISEASE MECHANISMS

The pathogenesis of these viruses depends on their sites of replication and the nature of the host reponse, forming two major groups: viruses that are somatotropic, replicating in various organs, and viruses that are neurotropic, replicating in the brain. During the initial stages of infection it is assumed that all these viruses generate a viraemia, with disease onset characteristically of an undifferentiated fever. The somatotropic viruses primarily cause haemorhagic complications (Walker 1988). With YF virus, necrotic damage results in characteristic coagulative cell death, producing Councilman bodies in the liver and a deficit in the synthesis of coagulation factors. Damage in organs and other tissues cannot then be controlled and results in widespread haemorrhaging in many mucous membranes. Haemorrhages in the gastric and duodenal mucosa produce large amounts of partially digested blood in the digestive tract, resulting in black

vomit. Myocardial injury and acute renal failure have also been observed. Similar damage has been reported with RVF virus (Walker 1988).

In contrast, the neurotropic arboviruses develop only transient, or undetectable, viraemia, but are capable of traversing the blood–brain barrier, targeting their replication in neuronal cells. Many encephalitis viruses are pan-tropic in the brain, but the brain-stem may be particularly affected. This area plays a key role in motor functions and therefore many acute patients die rapidly from their infection. It is known that a normal cellular defence is mounted with activation of B and T lymphocytes which migrate from blood capillaries into the neuronal matrix and begin to attack infected cells by phagocytosis and by the production of intrathecal virus-specific antibody (Johnson *et al.* 1985). The resulting loss of neurones means that surviving patients may express varying levels of mental/physical sequelae.

GROWTH AND SURVIVAL REQUIREMENTS

All these arboviruses are obligate intracellular parasites and must invade living susceptible cells to replicate. Unlike viruses such as polio, which are extremely stable, these enveloped viruses cannot survive adverse conditions outside the host cell for any length of time. Temperature, pH and desiccation results in rapid loss of viability. These viruses are thus totally dependant on vertebrate and vector biology for own their survival.

THE HOSTS

INCUBATION PERIODS

Incubation periods in animals and man have been recorded from as short as 20–30 hours after infection with VS virus (Webb and Holbrook 1988) (Table 34.3) but are generally in the range 3–14 days between receiving an infectious bite and developing overt symptoms of infection, depending on the virus.

SYMPTOMS AND SIGNS IN ANIMALS

Symptoms in animals are varied, depending on the virus. A series of examples are illustrative here. (Tables 34.1–34.3). With RR virus (Kay and Aaskov 1988), MVE (Marshall 1988), ROC (Iverrson 1988) and WN viruses (Hayes 1988) and the California group bunyaviruses (Grimstad 1988), animal infections are asymptomatic, although viraemia is present. JE virus infections in ardeid birds, pigs, bats, cattle and reptiles are typically asymptomatic, although birds and pigs do develop high viraemias, and the only adverse effects of JE virus infection in animals are abortion in pregnant sows and encephalitis in horses (Burke and Leake 1988). Similarly, with EEE (Morris 1988), WEE (Reisen and Monath 1988) and VEE (Walton and Grayson 1988) viruses, birds and various other animals develop viraemia with only a few deaths being recorded, whereas in horses the animal initially becomes less responsive to stimuli and may demonstrate unusual behaviour, walking slowly in small circles. Subsequently symptoms of encephalitis develop rapidly with severe motor effects, resulting finally in prostration associated with violent uncoordinated limb, head, mouth, and eye movements preceding death.

YF (Strode 1951) and RVF (Meegan and Bailey 1988) viruses are primarily hepatotrophic, causing haemorrhage and death. RVF and WSL viruses (Swanepol 1988) cause abortion, and WSL can also cross the placenta in pregnant animals causing teratological changes resulting in abortion or neonatal death. VS virus (Webb and Holbrook 1988) causes vesicular lesions in the mucous membranes of infected animals, indistinguishable from those of foot-and-mouth virus disease.

SYMPTOMS AND SIGNS IN MAN

Human disease ranges from undifferentiated fevers to haemorrhagic symptoms and encephalitis. Undifferentiated fever symptoms are typically of a systemic febrile illness with numerous subclinical infections, or a simple fever of 1–3 days' duration, with a headache, some degree of arthralgia and myalgia, and an occasional rash. More severe fevers have an abrupt onset, headache, photophobia, retro-orbital and lower back pain, rapidly followed by general malaise, crippling myalgias and arthralgias, and prostration. There may be a transient improvement on day 3–4 followed by a relapse (saddleback fever), during which lymphadenopathy (swollen lymph nodes) and rash may appear. There are no fatalities. Convalescence may be marked by prolonged asthenia (lack of strength). Differential dignosis is extremely difficult and readily confused with malaria, influenza, or fever of unknown origin. Viruses showing these symptoms are CHIK, ONN, and RR (Table 34.1), WSL and WN (Table 34.2), TAH and usually RVF (Table 34.3). In addition, some signs of neurotropism and hepatitis has been noted with WN virus, and TAH (Table 34.3), and haemorrhagic symptoms and neurotropism with RVF. The possibility that RR virus (Table 34.1) can cross the human placenta has been pointed out (Kay and Aaskov 1988). VS virus (Table 34.3) infection causes a fever with lesions similar to that described for animals.

In the development of haemorrhagic fever there is a prodromal phase of about 3 days when it is uncertain whether the symptoms may progress beyond either an undifferentiated fever (as with dengue viruses) or a more abrupt onset of high fever. At the end of this period there may be a short period of remission for a few hours before haemorrhagic features appear. These features are: petechiae (small extravasations of blood), haemorrhage echymoses (larger extravasations of blood) such as bleeding from nose and gums, haematemesis (vomiting blood), melaena (black stools due to gastrointestinal bleeding), metrorrhagia (uterine bleeding), abortion, proteinuria (excessive protein in urine), azotaemia (abnormal urea in blood), sudden cardiovascular collapse, and rapidly terminal shock. Viruses showing these features are YF and RVF. RVF can also cause retinal lesions in the eye in a small proportion of patients, or late onset encephalitis.

The prodromal phase in encephalitis patients is similar to an undifferentiated fever marked by some systemic symptoms. A sudden rise in fever marks the start of the full-blown syndrome, with vomiting, stiff neck, dizziness, drowsiness, disorientation, confusion and rapid progression to stupor, coma, and death. Viruses showing encephalitis symptoms are the EEE, VEE and WEE viruses (Table 34.1), JE, MVE, ROC, SLE, and, to a minor extent, WN viruses (Table 34.2) and the California group bunyaviruses CE, JC, LAC and to a minor extent TAH (Table 34.3).

DIAGNOSIS

With skill, presumptive clinical diagnosis can frequently be quite accurate, but definitive diagnosis is frequently retrospective as it requires detailed virological studies to either isolate and identify the virus or to carry out specific antibody tests against reference viruses. There are several regional WHO designated reference laboratories that can support such work. Some rapid ELISA tests have now been developed, i.e. MACELISA for diagnosis of JE virus infection (Burke and Leake 1988), but these are generally not commercially available.

PATHOLOGY

General pathological changes have been described above under disease mechanisms. Further details on individual viruses are given in Monath (1988).

TREATMENT

Treatment is generally supportive only. Fevers may be treated with bed rest, plenty of fluids, and symptomatic relief of headache and pain with paracetamol. Aspirin is contra-indicated due to the haemorrhagic potential of some of these viruses. Patients suffering long-term arthralgia have, on occasion, received corticosteroid treatment. For the clinical treatment of haemorrhagic fever and associated hypovolaemic shock, provision of blood-volume expanders and platelets may be appropriate. In the case of clinical encephalitis, mechanical ventilation during the acute illness may be of help. In animal models the use of interferon has been helpful.

PROGNOSIS

Recovery from acute fevers is usually uncomplicated, although some individuals may suffer prolonged attacks of joint pain, i.e. RR virus, or prolonged exhaustion. Haemorrhagic illness is serious and may result in significant mortality. Clinical encephalitis is a very serious condition, and mortality can be very high, depending on the virus (e.g. typically 30 per cent with JE virus). The ability to isolate virus from cerebrospinal fluid and the depth of coma are ominous prognostic signs. There may be a high frequency of neurological and motor deficits in survivors, for example only 10–15 per cent of JE patients make a full recovery.

EPIDEMIOLOGY

The geographic distribution of the major viruses are shown in Tables 34.1–34.3. Incidence is highly seasonally governed by environmental factors, with prevalence often at low or undetectable levels during winter periods and very high during epidemic peaks in late summer-time, and the beginning of the rainy period in tropical areas. For example, during the acutely focused epidemics of JE virus in Thailand, seroconversion occurs in virtually all sentinel pigs over a very narrow time frame and seroconversion rates in man can approach 5–10 per cent annually (Burke and Leake 1988). Many studies have indicated substantial levels of transmission with many of these viruses. Principal risk groups are immunologically naive individuals. Periodic explosive large-scale epizootics and epidemics may occur after a protracted inter-epidemic period during which there has been progressive loss of herd immunity in the field populations, or due to the emergence of virulent variants. Such outbreaks are particularly worrying due to their unpredictablity. For example, the VEE epizootic in Colombia in 1967–68, which spread throughout the region, killed 27 000 donkeys and 40 000 horses and mules, and some 250–500 000 people were infected (Walton and Grayson 1988.). Outbreaks may also occur as a result of a major change in epidemiology. RVF virus is such an example, being introduced into the Nile delta region of Egypt in 1977, and causing a large epizootic in animals and a serious

human outbreak. A common foul-water breeding urban mosquito *Culex quinquefasciatus*, previously unimportant in RVF transmission, was unexpectedly implicated as the competent anthropophilic vector (Meegan and Bailey 1988). At the other end of the scale, epidemic transmission can occur with great regularity, particularly linked to agricultural practices. Although JE virus, the world's most serious encephalitis virus, may not seem to be particularly important, causing some 45 000 cases and 11 000 deaths annually in an Asian population exceeding 2 billion people, the regular epidemic activity has focused incidence into the younger, previously unexposed age groups. This is because, fortunately, a high proportion of infections are subclinical, with only 1 : 300 infections resulting in clinical encephalitis, with a slight preponderance in males. Nevertheless, during the few weeks of the intense annual epidemic healthcare facilities are still swamped with distressingly large numbers of seriously ill children. The impact this has on the local community is substantial not only in terms of personal loss or the burden of having to care for severely handicapped survivors, but also in pure economic terms, such as the cost of clinical care, losses to livestock, or the cost of control operations (Burke and Leake 1988).

TRANSMISSION

Transmission of the virus to man or animals is by the bite of infected female mosquitoes. Female mosquitoes require the protein in a blood meal to develop their egg batches. Perhaps a day or two after emergence from her larval development site and mating, an uninfected female will acquire the virus from a viraemic host in her first blood meal. The blood is then digested and the mature eggs laid 2–3 days later, with the female mosquito continuing to take blood meals perhaps every 3–5 days to develop further egg batches. In the meantime, the virus is on a different time schedule. In competent vectors there are a number of complete cycles of virus replication involving different vector tissues. The initial site of replication is in the single layer of midgut cells, followed by release of newly formed virions into the haemocoel of the mosquito, followed by many other tissues. It is now known that there are a number of intrinsic factors that may influence the susceptibility and vector competence of mosquitoes (Leake 1992), but in competent mosquitoes the virus finally replicates to substantial levels in the salivary glands and perhaps 10–14 days after the initial infectious meal she becomes capable of transmitting the virus by bite. The newly formed virus particles present in the anticoagulant saliva are then injected into the wound site by the female mosquito as she ingests a subsequent blood meal. Competent female vectors are thus usually quite old in terms of a total field population.

Apart from the salivary glands, infection of the ovarian tissue can lead to hereditary transovarial transmission where the next generation are infected by maternal inheritance. It is important to realize that the earlier egg batches laid by a female are unlikely to be infected as the virus will not have reached the ovary (Leake 1984). A marked difference has been seen experimentally in the frequency of transovarial transmission, with high rates being recorded for some of the bunyaviruses, very low rates for some of the flaviviruses and a paucity of data supporting alphavirus transovarial transmission. (Leake 1984). Transovarial transmission may be very important in natural maintenance of these viruses, as the next generation of transovarially infected insects does not need to acquire and replicate the virus in a blood meal, and is thus capable of transmitting the virus much earlier in their lifetime. The virus is not dependent on the vector achieving a long life, or needing to acquire multiple, potentially risky, blood meals. Finally, it is known that mosquitoes can develop stabilized infections of the ovarian tissue resulting, potentially, in long-term maintenance of the virus by transovarial transmission over many generations without the requirement for horizontal amplification (Leake 1984). Currently there is little evidence that male mosquitoes play any significant role in arbovirus maintenance, although there is experimental evidence that male mosquitoes can transmit virus venereally to females (Leake, 1984).

It is interesting that the principal arbovirus vectors are usually culicine mosquitoes and surprising that the highly anthropophilic anopheline mosquitoes have only infrequently been incriminated as virus vectors (Leake 1992). The best example of anopheline transmission is that of the alphavirus O'nyong-nyong which caused a major human epidemic of crippling fever involving up to 90 per cent of the population (Table 34.1). The source of the virus was never established or any potential animal reservoir identified (Johnson 1988). Culicine vectors fall into two groups. First, mainly tropical species such as *Culex* species that lay egg rafts that cannot withstand desiccation and must therefore breed continually throughout the year, and secondly, often temperate floodwater *Aedes* species mosquitoes that lay drought-resistant eggs that can survive adverse conditions for long periods. Hereditary virus transmission through maternal transovarial transmission has been clearly demonstrated in these mosquitoes. In sub-Saharan Africa, mosquitoes such as *Aedes callabus*, *Aedes circumluteolus*, and *Aedes lineatopennis* lay their eggs in the surrounds of moist, vegetated depressions called *dambos* which may not refill with rain water for several seasons. When rains do occur

there is rapid mosquito emergence and subsequent virus transmission. Epizootics of transovarially maintained RVF virus (Table 34.3) have clearly been associated with wet years in this region (Meegan and Bailey 1988). In temperate North. America, tree-hole breeding *Aedes triseriatus* mosquitoes are important in the maintenance of the bunyavirus LAC (Table 34.3) by horizontal transmission during the summer, surviving the cold winter by vertical transmission secure within the mosquito egg. Further examples of these transovarially maintained bunyaviruses are CE, JC, and TAH viruses (Table 34.3), and there is an extensive literature on the other extensively studied members of this group that are not covered here (Grimstad 1988). Transovarial transmission provides a secure survival mechanism for the virus under adverse climatic conditions or through inter epidemic/epizootic periods, and this has important implications for disease control, as eradication of the maintenance vectors becomes the only feasible control strategy (Leake 1984).

COMMUNICABILITY

Aside from mosquito bite there is only limited evidence for occupational acquisition of infection through handling infected carcasses (RVF virus, Table 34.3). In the clinical setting, aerosol transmission is rare, but is more common in the research laboratory, and infections can readily be acquired via accidents involving accidental injection of viable material into clinical or technical personnel.

PREVENTION AND CONTROL

Prevention of human infections, and particularly animal disease, has focused on the prophylactic use of vaccines. The following summary is taken from various authors cited by Monath (1988). No vaccines have yet been developed for use against the alphaviruses ONN and RR, the flaviviruses MVE and WN, or the California group viruses CE, LAC, JC, or TAH. Experimental CHIK and ROC virus vaccines have been produced, and although a peptide vaccine against SLE is promising, it is considered a requirement that it must be highly immunogenic as there can be substantial intervals between human outbreaks. Live attenuated and killed vaccines against VS viruses have been developed for veterinary use, but success with these vaccines has been rather mixed. Inactivated bivalent vaccines against EEE/WEE viruses have proved effective in horses, but annual boosters are required and the vaccines are not suitable for human use. A live attenuated VEE vaccine was used extensively in animals in 1969–72 and was very effective. Exceptionally, this vaccine was also used in at-risk humans at that time, although formalin-inactivated vaccine is now recommended for human use in groups such as laboratory workers. In animals, 26 million doses of a live attenuated WSL virus vaccine have been used, but no human use is thought to be warranted. A live attenuated RVF virus veterinary vaccine is effective with a single dose, but can cause some abortion in sheep, whereas the inactivated vaccine requires multiple boosting, which is expensive. A formalin-inactivated vaccine has shown good responses in humans.

Widely used vaccines for human use against JE (inactivated) and YF (live attenuated) viruses have been very successful. Incidence of clinical cases of JE in Japan is now extremely low, focusing in the very old and the very young that have not been previously vaccinated. However, routine sentinel animal and entomological surveillance still continues to detect an active zoonotic transmission cycle in birds, swine, and certain rice-field *Culex* mosquitoes, emphasizing the continued requirement for a national vaccination programme. Similarly, YF vaccination has reduced reported incidence of YF to relatively small numbers annually, although the zoonotic transmission cycle continues with the potential for large-scale outbreaks. (WHO 1986).

Vector control also poses major problems. As the maintenance vectors of these viruses are primarily zoophilic in their biting preferences, they may be distributed substantial distances from human habitation making control unrealistic. Personal protection measures against the biting of those few hungry zoophilic mosquitoes that may feed opportunistically on man, and the principal anthropophilic epidemic vectors, can be very effective if used correctly. The use of skin repellents, and impregnated bed nets are strongly recommended in relatively poorer areas of the world, and in more affluent regions house screening is effective. The role of health education through the primary healthcare system and the use of media such as radio and TV are increasingly important measures.

Organized vector control approaches have focused on control of epidemic vectors such as *Aedes aegypti*, usually by large-scale usage of insecticides aimed at a rapid reduction in vector numbers (Gratz 1991). Problems with this strategy are the potential emergence of insecticide resistance in the vectors and a reluctance of communities to use chemicals in the environment. As an alternative, considerable interest is being shown in the development of cost-effective appropriate control approaches (Curtis 1991). Unfortunately, the recent trend by many governments has been to respond to epidemic outbreaks in a cheaper short-term response, rather than investing in the expertise required to develop a long-term pro-active surveillance and control strategy.

Existing structured control programmes depend locally on surveillance, immunization, if necessary, and vector control, with manpower and financial implications for the public health services. Frequently the primary commitment of the vector control programme is to malaria vector control, a secondary commitment to pest control, and lastly to respond to sporadic explosive arbovirus outbreaks where necessary. Although many countries have some vector control capability, the effectiveness of these programmes have rarely been rigorously evaluated. It is only in well-resourced programmes, such as the mosquito abatement programmes in North America and notably in the dengue control programmes in Singapore and Cuba, that targeting mosquito vectors has been evaluated and proven to be effective.

LEGISLATION

In terms of international measures, YF is currently the only mosquito-borne arbovirus subject to International Health Regulations by WHO member states. In outline, legislation provides for a number of primary obligations in the event of epidemic activity. First, to notify WHO without delay. WHO then informs member states and publishes details in the *Weekly Epidemiological Record* Secondly, in endemic areas airports must be maintained as mosquito-free areas and facilities must exist for diagnosis, isolation, and treatment of patients. Thirdly, before entry to a country which has *Aedes aegypti*, persons who have travelled within 6 days in an YF-infected area must present a valid vaccination certificate or risk being isolated for 6 days. Finally, aircraft, ships, and vehicles arriving from infected areas must be disinfected (for full details see WHO 1986)

Epizootic information on animal diseases is centralized by the Food and Agriculture Organization (FAO) of the UN and the Office International des Epizooties (OIE). Member countries are informed via the *Monthly Epizootic Circular* of the OIE.

REFERENCES

Bouloy, M. (1991). Bunyaviridae: Genome organisation and replication strategies. *Advances in Virus Research*, **40**, 235–75.

Burke, D. S. and Leake C. J. (1988). Japanese encephalitis. In *The arboviruses: epidemiology and ecology*, Vol. 2, (ed T. P. Monath), pp 63–92. CRC Press, Boca Raton, FL.

Chambers, T. J., Hahn, C. S., Galler, R., and Rice, C. M. (1990). Flavivirus genome organization, expression and replication. *Annual Review of Microbiology*, **44**, 649–88.

Curtis, C. F. (1991). *Control of disease vectors in the community.* Wolfe, London.

Fraenkal-Conrat, H., Kimball, P. C., and Levy, J. A. (1988). Minus strand RNA viruses. In *Virology*, (2nd edn). Prentice Hall, Englewood Cliffs, N. J.

Gratz, N. (1991). Emergency control of *Aedes aegypti* as a disease vector in urban areas. *Journal of American Mosquito Control Association*, **7**, 353–65.

Grimstad, P. R. (1988). California Group Virus Disease. In *The arboviruses: epidemiology and ecology*, Vol. 3, (ed. T. P. Monath), pp. 99–136. CRC Press, Boca Raton, FL.

Gubler, D. (1988). Dengue. In *The arboviruses: epidemiology and ecology*, Vol. 2, (ed. T. P. Monath), pp. 223–60. CRC Press, Boca Ratan, FL.

Hayes, C. (1988). West Nile Fever. In *The arboviruses: epidemiology and ecology*, Vol. 5, (ed. T. P. Monath), pp. 60–88. CRC Press, Boca Ratan, FL.

Iverrson, L. B. (1988). Rocio encephalitis. In *The arboviruses: epidemiology and ecology*, Vol. 4, (ed. T. P. Monath), pp. 77–92. CRC Press, Boca Raton, FL.

Johnson, B. K. (1988). O'nyong-nyong virus disease. In *The arboviruses: epidemiology and ecology*, Vol. 3, (ed. T. P. Monath), pp. 218–23. CRC Press, Boca Raton, FL.

Johnson B. K. and Chanas A. C. (1981). The potential for the spread of arboviruses into new areas and for their subsequent persistence: A Review. *Abstracts of Hygiene and Tropical Disease*, **56**, 165–80.

Johnson, R. T. *et al.* (1985). Japanese encephalitis: immunocytochemical studies of viral antigen and inflammatory cells in seven fatal cases. *Annals of Neurology*, **18**, 567–73.

Jupp, P. G. and MCIntosh, B. M. (1988). Chikungunya virus disease. In *The arboviruses: epidemiology and ecology*, Vol. 2, (ed. T. P. Monath), pp. 138–57. CRC Press, Boca Raton, FL.

Karabatsos, N. (ed.) (1985) *International Catalogue of Arboviruses 1985, including certain other viruses of vertebrates*, (3rd edn and supplements). American Society of Tropical Medicine and Hygiene.

Kay, B. H. and Aaskov, J. G. (1988). Ross river virus (epidemic polyarthritis). In *The arboviruses: epidemiology and ecology*, Vol. 4, (ed. T. P. Monath), pp. 93–112. CRC Press, Boca Raton, FL.

Koblet, H. (1990). The 'merry-go-round': Alphaviruseses between vertebrate and invertebrate cells. *Advances in Virus Research*, **38**, 343–402.

Leake, C. J. (1984). Transovarial transmission of arboviruses by mosquitoes. In *Vectors in virus biology*, (ed. M. A. Mayo and K. A. Harrap), pp. 63–91. Academic Press, New York.

Leake, C. J. (1988). Strategies for vector-borne disease control in rice production systems in developing countries: Arboviruses other than Japanese encephalitis. In *Vector-borne disease control in humans through rice agroecosystem management*, pp. 161–73. International Rice Research Institute, PO Box 933, Manila, Philippines.

Leake, C. J. (1992). Arbovirus—mosquito interactions and vector specificity. *Parasitology Today*, **8**, 123–8.

Marshall, I. D. (1988). Murray Valley and Kunjin Encephalitis. In *The arboviruses: epidemiology and ecology*, Vol. 3, (ed. T. P. Monath), pp. 151–89. CRC Press, Boca Raton, FL.

Meegan, J. M. and Bailey, C. L. (1988). Rift Valley Fever. In *The arboviruses: epidemiology and ecology*, Vol. 4, (ed. T. P. Monath), pp. 51–76. CRC Press, Boca Raton, FL.

Monath, T. P. ed. (1988). *The arboviruses: epidemiology and ecology*, Vols 1–5. CRC Press, Boca Raton, FL.

Morris, C. D. (1988). Eastern equine encephalitis. In *The arboviruses: epidemiology and ecology*, Vol. 2 (ed. T. P. Monath), pp. 2–20. CRC Press, Boca Raton, FL.

Reisen, W. K. and Monath, T. P. (1988). Western equine encephalitis. In *The arboviruses: epidemiology and ecology*, Vol. 5, (ed. T. P. Monath), pp. 90–137. CRC Press, Boca Raton, FL.

Steinhauer, D. A. and Holland, J. J. (1987). Rapid evolution of RNA viruses. *Annual Review of Microbiology*, **41**, 409–33.

Strode, G. K. (ed.) (1951). *Yellow Fever*. McGraw-Hill, New York.

Swanepol, R. (1988). Wesselsbron virus disease. In *The arboviruses: epidemiology and ecology*, Vol. 5, (ed. T. P. Monath), pp. 31–57. CRC Press, Boca Raton, FL.

Tsai, T. F. and Mitchell, C. J. (1988). St Louis Encephjaltis. In *The arboviruses: epidemiology and ecology*, Vol. 4, (ed. T. P. Monath), pp. 113–43. CRC Press, Boca Raton, FL.

Walker, D. H. (1988). The pathogenesis and pathology of the hemorrhagic state in viral and rickettsial infections. In *CRC Handbook of Viral and Ricketsial Hemorrhagic Fevers*, (ed. J. H. S. Gear), pp. 9–45. CRC Press, Boca Raton, FL.

Walton, T. E. and Grayson, M. A. (1988). Venezuelan equine encephalomyelitis. In *The arboviruses: epidemiology and ecology*, Vol. 3, (ed. T. P. Monath), pp. 204–31. CRC Press, Boca Raton, FL.

Webb, P. A. and Holbrook, F. R. (1988). Vesicular stomatitis. In *The arboviruses: epidemiology and ecology*, Vol. 5, (ed T. P. Monath), pp. 2–29. CRC Press, Boca Raton, FL.

World Health Organization (1985). Arthopod-borne and rodent-borne viral diseases. *Technical Report Series*, Number 719, pp. 1–116. WHO, Geneva.

World Health Organization (1986). *Prevention and Control of Yellow Fever in Africa*, pp. 1–94. WHO, Geneva.

35 POXVIRUSES

Hugh W. Reid

SUMMARY

The poxviruses are a large family of complex viruses infecting many species of vertebrates as well as arthropods, and members of the three genera *Orthopoxvirus, Yatapoxvirus* and *Parapoxvirus* are the cause of sporadic zoonotic infections originating from both wildlife and domestic livestock. Infections of man are generally associated with localized lesions, regarded as inconvenient rather than life-threatening, although severe reactions have occurred, particularly in immunologically compromised individuals. The most celebrated of the orthopoxvirus infections is cowpox—a zoonotic infection which has been exploited to the enormous benefit of man as it had a pivotal role in the initiation of vaccinal strategies that eventually led to the worldwide eradication of smallpox. Cowpox occurs only in Europe and in recent years it has become evident that infection of cattle is fortuitous and the reservoir of infection is probably a wild rodent. Monkeypox is another orthopoxvirus causing zoonotic infections in Central and West Africa resembling smallpox and is the most serious of diseases in this category. While monkeypox does not readily spread between people, the potential of the virus to adapt to man is of concern and necessitates sustained surveillance in enzootic areas. The other orthopoxvirus of concern is buffalopox in the Indian subcontinent, which is probably a strain of vaccinia that has been maintained in buffalo for at least 10 years following the cessation of vaccination of the human population.

Orf virus, the most common of the parapoxviruses to cause zoonotic infection, is largely restricted to those in direct contact with domestic sheep. Generally, infection is associated with a single localized macule affecting the hand which resolves without complications. Infection would appear to be prevalent in all sheep and goat populations and human orf is a relatively common occupational hazard. Sporadic parapoxvirus infections of man also occur following contact with cattle infected with pseudocowpoxvirus, and wildlife, in particular seals.

Transmission of all the poxvirus infections requires contact with infected animals or contaminated fomites and generally results following introduction through an abrasion in the skin. The handling or eating of meat from certain wild animals appears to be a risk factor in acquiring monkeypox, while tanapox, another zoonotic poxvirus infection of Africa, is probably transmitted by mosquitoes from an unidentified reservoir.

Good hygienic practices and the wearing of protective gloves when handling infected animals does achieve a substantial degree of protection in most cases.

THE POXVIRUSES

The poxviruses of vertebrates are classified into eight genera within the subfamily Chordopoxviridae, three of which are associated with zoonotic infections (Table 35.1). In general, such infections in man are benign, though in immunologically compromised individuals the reaction can be severe. It is also recognized that this group of viruses is genomically labile, which permits adaptation and recombination to occur, and thus they have the potential to emerge in novel disease associations (Moss 1990).

Table 35.1 Chordopoxviridae which are associated with zoonoses

Genera	Name	Natural host
Orthopoxvirus	Buffalopox virus	Water buffalo in India
	Cowpox virus	Probably a rodent in Europe
	Monkeypox virus	Probably squirrels in Central and West Africa
Parapoxvirus	Orf virus	Domestic sheep/goats, worldwide
	Pseudocowpox virus	Cattle, worldwide
	Papular stomatitis virus	Cattle, worldwide
	Sealpox virus	Various species of seals, Europe/America
Yatapoxvirus	Tanapox virus	Unknown in Africa
	Yaba monkey disease virus	Monkeys in Africa

PROPERTIES

The morphology of poxviruses is complex. They are characteristically brick-shaped, 200–400 nm in length by 150–300 nm across. The external surface of the orthopoxviruses is ridged with tubules 10–20 nm in diameter, arranged in parallel rows, while the parapoxviruses have a single continuous helix appearing as the characteristic basketweave when examined by electron microscopy. The protein composition of poxviruses is also complex and more than 100 polypeptides have been identified in the most extensively studied representative, vaccinia virus. Within the outer membrane is an electron-dense core which, in the case of the orthopoxviruses, is biconcave with two structures known as lateral bodies present on either side. The core consists of a twisted and folded nucleoprotein fibre interconnected by DNA fibres which consist of a single double-stranded molecule. Replication occurs in the cytoplasm of infected cells and is characterized by ballooning of the cells and formation of intracytoplasmic inclusions. Virus is released either by budding or when the cell lyses; some particles acquire an outer membrane during this process.

The poxviruses have many common antigens and cross-reactivity between members of the orthopoxvirus and parapoxvirus genera can be shown by a variety of serological techniques. Within the orthopox genera there is also generally a high degree of cross-protection, but this provides no protection from members of the parapox genera. In general, the orthopoxviruses have a wide host range and induce good immunity in recovered animals, while the parapoxviruses have a narrow host range and produce short-lived and often incomplete immunity.

Characteristically, poxviruses cause acute infection associated with productive viral replication and shedding of virus. In the case of the orthopoxviruses this is followed by solid immunity to subsequent challenge for at least a number of years. With orthopoxviruses there is no carrier state, no latent infection occurs and hence they require a substantial population of available hosts for their survival. In contrast, infection with the parapoxviruses tends to result in incomplete protection from subsequent challenge and chronic infections also do occur. Such viruses can thus survive in much more restricted populations than the orthopoxviruses.

ORTHOPOXVIRUSES

Of the diseases to have affected mankind, smallpox caused by the orthopoxvirus variola was probably the greatest scourge. Periodic pandemics occurred throughout Asia and Europe and invaded the Americas coincidentally with the arrival of Europeans. Infection was associated with a 20–30 per cent mortality and those that recovered were often scarred for life. Such was the threat that up to the end of the eighteenth century variolation, in which fully virulent scab material was applied by scarification as a form of immunization, was widely practised despite causing 1–2 per cent mortality. The observation that milkmaids often escaped the ravages of the disease and the confirmation by Jenner that cowpox could protect against subsequent challenge with smallpox virus was therefore possibly the greatest single advance in medical history. The benefit that this zoonosis has been to mankind is thus enormous, as the rapid and widespread acceptance of vaccination led to the control of smallpox in the West and ultimately to its worldwide eradication.

COWPOXVIRUS

It is now realized that this virus is inappropriately named as infection in cattle is relatively uncommon and there is an alternative natural reservoir which has still to be identified. Infection occurs only in Europe, suggesting a similar distribution for the reservoir host.

Infection of man is characterized generally as a single lesion which commences as a papule followed by the development of vesicles, then crusting, and the lesion will usually resolve in 4–5 weeks. In the initial phase of infection patients experience malaise, pyrexia and lymphadenopathy of the draining nodes. Recovery is normally complete and uncomplicated but the reaction may be severe, and in one case of infection of a patient with severe endogenous eczema the reaction became generalized and had a fatal outcome.

Primary lesions are normally on the hand or lower arm, but facial lesion are also quite common. Person to person spread does not occur. Contact with animals is generally established in reported cases and in recent years the most frequent established source of infection has been the domestic cat.

In cattle, infection is considered to be rare and is characterized by pox-like lesions appearing on the teats of milking cows. Infection occurs erratically and good dairy hygiene normally ensures that only a few cases occur in an outbreak. In domestic cats the infection can be very much more severe and it is noteworthy that in the UK it is reported from only a few veterinary practices, suggesting that it may be under-reported. However, serological surveys do not suggest that infection is common in cats and it is not considered that they could represent the natural host.

Almost all diagnosed cases in cats occur in animals known to be rodent hunters and most cases are reported in the autumn (Bennett *et al.* 1986).

In cats, visible signs of infection generally appear first as a single small bite-like lesion which frequently develops into a large abscess which may give rise to cellulitis. After 10–14 days disseminated lesions appear as erythematous macules which develop into ulcerating papules, but vesicles are only rarely observed. Scabs form over these lesions which then fall off during the next 2–3 weeks. Cats are pyrexic, inappetent and depressed during the acute phase of the disease but normally will recover unless there are secondary bacterial complications (Bennett *et al.* 1990).

Although a rodent is suspected, the natural host of cowpox in most of Europe has not been identified. The detection of antibody to orthopoxvirus in sera from wild-caught bank voles (*Clethrionomys glareolus*) and short-tailed voles (*Microtus agrestis*) cannot be regarded as evidence of cowpoxvirus infection as it is equally possible that the antibody reflects infection with ectromelia virus, an orthopox virus infection of mice (Kaplan *et al.* 1980). Virus very similar to cowpox has been isolated from a gerbil (*Rhombomys opimus*) in Turkmenia but such rodents have a restricted range and can not be the natural host elsewhere.

Infection has also occurred in a number of species, mainly Felidae, held in zoological collections, but only in the Moscow Zoo outbreak was the source of infection identified. Infection had apparently been transmitted from rats fed to the carnivores, as infection was shown to be prevalent on the breeding farm from which the rats were obtained.

Clinical appearance and history of contact with infected animals can allow a presumptive diagnosis. Scab scrapings removed and processed for electron microscopic examination following negative staining can be used to identify characteristic viral particles. Although embryonated eggs traditionally have been used to isolate virus, the use of conventional tissue culture is more convenient in most laboratories. A variety of serological tests can also be used to provide retrospective confirmation of orthopoxvirus infection.

BUFFALOPOX

Buffalopox is a disease of buffalo (*Bubalus bubalis*) which has been reported from Indonesia, Russia, Egypt, Italy, Pakistan, Bangladesh, and India, where it is of economic importance in the milking buffalo. Clinically the disease resembles cowpox, although lesions may be more extensive affecting the whole udder, inner thighs, head, and mouth. Mastitis is a frequent sequela. However, the biological characteristics of isolates and analysis of the DNA establish that buffalopox virus is sufficiently distinct to justify classification as a separate subspecies of vaccinia (Dumbell and Richardson 1993).

Human infection is generally restricted to the hand, wrist, and thumbs of those milking affected buffalo

and consists of 1–5 pocks. Fever and swelling of the regional lymph nodes frequently occur also, and when the scabs detach scars are usually left.

The disease in India has persisted for over 10 years following the cessation of vaccination, thus it is assumed that infection can be sustained in the buffalo population. Infection tends to occur in local epizootics affecting only a proportion of the animals at risk. Infected human milkers would appear to be responsible for spreading infection between herds. Cattle also sometimes become infected, but the disease is mild, and sheep also are susceptible to infection.

Diagnosis is generally made on clinical evaluation and history. But virus can either be identified directly by electron microscopy or following isolation in embryonated eggs or tissue culture.

MONKEYPOX

This is the most serious zoonotic poxvirus infection and is regularly associated with significant mortality. It is also of greatest concern because of the possible emergence of a human-adapted form. Though normally person to person transmission is inefficient, it is possible that in an immunocompromised population it could occur more readily and permit the selection of human-adapted mutants (Douglass *et al.* 1994). Selection pressure on orthopoxviruses is known to allow the emergence of variants of enhanced or diminished pathogenicity, as exemplified by myxomatosis virus in rabbit populations. It is thus essential that surveillance for monkeypox infection is man is sustained to ensure that any such development is detected at an early stage.

Monkeypox was identified originally as an infection in a primate colony in Copenhagen in 1958 and later in other centres in Europe and the United States. Subsequently, in 1970, outbreaks of smallpox-like disease in people inhabiting the tropical rainforest regions in western and Central African were reported. As this was considered to potentially to jeopardize the global smallpox eradication campaign, which had commenced in 1967, there followed intense investigations to establish the risk posed (Khodakewich *et al.* 1988).

The original outbreak affected primates from Asia. They suffered a severe generalized disease with papules, vesicles, and pustules, which formed scabs after 7–10 days affecting the whole body, particularly on the soles of the feet and palms of the hands, with orang-utans proving particularly susceptible. Subsequent investigation failed to identify any antibodies in over 1000 sera collected from Asian primates. In contrast, in sera collected in Africa from 10 species of primate and four species of squirrel, antibody could be detected consistently.

Monkeypox virus is antigenically closely related to variola but can be distinguished by tests with adsorbed sera. Comparison of the DNA of strains derived from different regions of Africa confirmed that monkeypox was a distinct viral species and that isolates from different geographical locations were distinct strains. Analysis of the DNA of so-called whitepox virus isolates established that it was genetically not possible for them to have arisen through mutation from monkeypox and that these 'isolates' represented laboratory contamination with variola virus.

Human cases of monkeypox have occurred only in tropical rainforest regions of Central and West Africa and have been restricted to those living in small villages where hunting is an integral activity. From the time of recognition in 1970 there appeared to have been a real increase in incidence through to 1984 and thereafter there was a decline. The reason for this decline is unclear because it has occurred during a period when the human population has become increasingly susceptible through the cessation of vaccination against smallpox (Cook 1988).

The clinical features of monkeypox cannot be differentiated from smallpox, except for the lymph node enlargement that is pronounced in monkeypox and may be generalized or confined to the nodes of the neck and inguinal region. Patients become fevered prior to developing typical pox virus lesions of papule, vesicle, peduncles, scab and desquamation, which can involve the entire body. The disease is more severe in individuals not vaccinated against smallpox, in which case the fatality rate is over 10 per cent.

In contrast to smallpox, monkeypox usually occurs singly or as a small cluster with little evidence of person to person transmission. Most cases occur in children, particularly boys over 5 years of age, suggesting that their activities result in greater exposure. The source of infection for 70 per cent of cases would appear to be wild animals and it is thought that several species may be involved. Examination of sera collected from wild animals in West and Central Africa have identified 10 species of monkeys as being infected in addition to four species of squirrel.

Epidemiological evidence would suggest that squirrels are the most likely source of infection for man as they tend to inhabit the secondary forest surrounding the agricultural zone where most cases appear to originate. Person to person transmission probably accounts for 30 per cent of cases, generally following close contact, and even in a population unprotected by vaccination it has been calculated that the theoretical maximum number of transmissions from an index case would be 11 generations. The model used for these calculations assumed individuals were immunologically competent and it is possible that in a population in which a significant number were immunologically compromised further spread and human adaptation could occur. Thus, despite the relative rarity of this infection in man and its restricted geographical distribution, monkeypox has the potential to adapt under appropriate selection pressures to give rise to variants with increased virulence and the capability to disseminate in the human population, which would have serious global repercussions.

In Africa, presumptive diagnosis will generally be reached on the basis of clinical presentation and history. However, virus can readily be demonstrated in scab material and can be recovered in tissue culture or by egg inoculation. Recovered virus can be characterized by restriction enzyme fragment analysis to confirm its identity. Serological tests have also been used in retrospective diagnosis and to identify inapparent infections.

YATAPOXVIRUS

TANAPOXVIRUS

First isolated in 1962, tanapox virus infection is associated with a mild disease in man characterized by a febrile response associated with the development of one or two nodular lesions. It first appeared in the Tana River basin in Kenya, causing epidemics in 1957 and 1962. Subsequently, infection was recognized on many occasions in Zaire and it is probably enzootic in several countries in equatorial Africa (Jezer *et al.* 1985). It has also occurred in primate centres in the United States where animal handlers have become infected.

The disease in man characteristically is biphasic with a pre-eruptive phase when the patient is febrile for 2–4 days, which is sometimes accompanied by severe headache. Thereafter, one or more intensely itchy macules develop, which enlarge to about 1 cm, surrounded by a large erythematous zone and ringed by swollen oedematous skin. Regional lymph nodes become enlarged. The macules contain necrotic tissue which may slough, resulting in ulceration which may increase to 2 cm in diameter. Healing, which is often slow, is associated with a permanent scar. Lesions generally appear on areas of the body which would normally be uncovered by clothing and there is no evidence of disseminated spread from human infection in any case examined.

The epidemiology of tanapox is obscure. Tanapox does spread rapidly amongst captive monkeys but it is unclear if they act as the natural reservoir. Almost all cases occur in people with close access to rivers. There is a seasonal increase in incidence coincidental with increased mosquito activity and it has been suggested that culicine mosquitoes transmit the virus mechanically. In animal handlers infection is transmitted through skin abrasions. Previous vaccination against smallpox provides no protection from infection with tanapox virus.

Diagnosis is made on the basis of history and clinical appearance. Skin scrapings or necrotic tissue from lesions contain virus particles readily detected by electron microscopy. Morphologically, the particles differ from other orthopoxviruses in that many particles are enveloped and the surface tubular arrays are much more pronounced.

YABAPOX

In 1957, rhesus monkeys held at Yaba in Nigeria developed subcutaneous growths which were shown to be caused by a distinct poxvirus. These 'tumours' could be transmitted experimentally and caused the development of histiocytomas which spontaneously regressed by 6–12 weeks. Similar subcutaneous growths developed at the site of inoculation in a man who was accidentlly infected and in six volunteers. Antibody to yabapox virus has been detected in sera from a variety of African monkeys as well as cynomolgus monkeys from Malaysia. The natural host of this virus is assumed to be primates, probably restricted to Africa, and there may be a related virus in primates of South-East Asia.

PARAPOXVIRUS

Human parapoxvirus infections are relatively common and generally produce local lesions which are an inconvenience and subsequently resolve leaving little or no residual scar. The most frequent infection is with orf virus from sheep and goats, but pseudocowpox, sealpox and unidentified sources, presumed to be transmitted from wildlife, can also be responsible for human infections. Infections are generally restricted to those who are occupationally at risk, and because infection is normally uncomplicated, often recognized by those who become infected, and benefits little from treatment, parapoxvirus infections are probably markedly under-reported. There is no cross-protection between the orthopoxviruses and parapoxviruses despite considerable antigenic and genomic cross-reactivity.

ORF

Orf would appear to be prevalent in all domestic sheep and goat populations and has a worldwide distribution.

Infection in sheep

Orf is associated with proliferative skin lesions, particularly around the lips of neonatal lambs, but all ages and categories of animal may be affected. Infection occurs in areas of exposed skin subjected to traumatic insult as virus will establish only in newly regenerated epithelium. Lesions tend to be most frequent around the lips of lambs, teats of ewes, and legs and mouths of those grazing rough pasture. Lesions are characteristic of poxvirus infection—macule, vesicle, pustule, and scab—but in a proportion, extensive epithelial proliferations occur and lesions may persist. Virus is shed in the scabs of lesions, and infectivity can be retained for long periods provided they remain dry. Dried scabs in buildings would appear to be the principal means by which infection survives between years. However, infection would often appear to be mild or inapparent, and it is considered that such subclinical infections may also be important in the epidemiology. Immunity following infection is incomplete and re-infection can occur readily, although secondary infections are, in general, less severe.

Human infection

Orf in man is most frequently diagnosed in those directly handling sheep, in particular those bottle-feeding lambs in the spring and those involved in shearing and slaughtering sheep at other times (Robinson and Peterson 1983). However, infection also can be transmitted by fomites and sometimes contact with sheep or goats is difficult to establish.

Virus infection will establish following introduction through the epidermis, thus the fingers of those feeding lambs are particularly at risk. Infection occurs only at the site of traumatized epidermis. Following an incubation period of 3–7 days the maculopustular reaction establishes, surrounded by an erythematous rim. This tends to increase in size with a weeping surface and central vesiculation and pustulation. The lesion then crusts overlying a papillomatous surface which is liable to be haemorrhagic if the crust is detached at this stage. The crust then dries and will detach after 6–8 weeks leaving no scar. Normally only a single lesion is present and spread to other areas does not usually occur (Groves et al. 1991).

Secondary bacterial infection of orf lesions can cause complications but can normally be controlled through antibiotic application. Lymphangitis and lymphadenitis of the draining lymphatics is a frequent complication and may be associated with flu-like symptoms. Less frequently, infection is associated with a generalized reaction including widespread maculopapular eruption and erythema multiforme. Extensive lesions have been described also in those with burns received at the time of infection and in immuno-suppressed patients, which have resulted in the development of 'giant orf' resembling pyogenic granuloma and requiring amputation of the affected digit. Patients with atopic dermatitis may also be more vulnerable to infection. Diagnosis is often made on the basis of clinical presentation and history. Virus isolation is not generally successful but characteristic parapoxvirus particles can be observed in scab or vesicular fluid collected early in the course of infection. Histological examination of biopsy material will differentiate orf infection from other proliferative skin disorders. Recovered patients will have antibody to orf virus which is most readily detected by ELISA.

It should be noted that any immunity is only of short duration and re-infection occurs readily.

Infection can normally be avoided through good hygienic practices and the wearing of protective gloves when handling infected animals or raw sheep products. Individuals who may be more vulnerable to infection due to immunosuppression or other factors should avoid contact with sheep or goats. It should also be recognized that the vaccine used for sheep is in fact fully virulent virus and operators must take great care not to autoinoculate while vaccinating.

PSEUDOCOWPOX

This is a virus disease of the teats of milking cattle which establishes as a chronic herd infection appearing periodically some 2 weeks after calving. Lesions are generally single and control can be achieved through good hygiene with the milking machine teat clusters and in the preparation of teats prior to milking. Preventing damage to the teats is also essential.

The cause is a parapoxvirus of cattle which has a worldwide distribution. Though closely related to the virus of papular stomatitis, its exact relationship is not clear, although some authors do consider them the same entity.

The clinical course of infection in man is essentially similar to orf although contact with affected cattle is the source of infection.

BOVINE PAPULAR STOMATITIS

This is generally a mild, often inapparent infection, mainly of young cattle. Lesions appear as reddened foci developing into hyperaemic papules with central necrosis. Lesions may be present on the muzzle, nostrils, lips, tongue, buccal papillae, and hard and soft palate, persisting for a few days or weeks. Infection is highly contagious and most animals in a group will become infected. When infection occurs shortly after transportation and mixing, lesions may be more severe and there may also be loss of appetite and excessive salivation. The causal virus is considered by some authors to be the same as the parapoxvirus of pseudocowpox.

Human infection follows contact with clinically affected animals and the lesions are similar to those caused by other parapoxviruses of ruminants.

SEALPOX

Skin lesions in a variety of species of seals have been described associated with both orthopoxvirus and parapoxvirus infection. However, those infections caused by parapoxvirus are more commonly reported and have been associated with transmission to man. Lesions have generally been observed in captive animals, most frequently in pups reared in sanctuaries, and consist of raised cutaneous swellings 1.5–2 cm in diameter which may appear proliferative, most often affecting the ventral surface and flippers as well as around the nose and lips. The lesions may be relatively few or multiple and may become eroded and susceptible to secondary bacterial infection.

Originally, reports of affected animals involved American seals: California sealion (*Zalophus californianus*), South American sealion (*Otaria byronia*), harbour seal (*Phoca vitulina*) and northern fur seals (*Callorhinus ursinus*), but more recently it has been observed to be widespread in European populations of grey seals (*Halichoerus grypus*).

People exposed to such infected animals have become infected through abrasions in the skin. The course of infection in man is very similar to that of other parapoxvirus infections. Protective clothing and gloves should always be worn when handling seals due to risk of this and other infections that they can carry.

PARAPOXVIRUS OF REINDEER AND MUSK OX

Outbreaks of parapoxvirus infection affecting reindeer and musk ox have occurred in which the disease has severely affected animals and been associated with considerable mortality. The virus has been shown morphologically to be a parapoxvirus and the lesions in man were reported to resemble tumours and, on initial infections, fever, enlarged lymph nodes, and nausea occurred. Surgical removal was considered necessary, and in the one case that was not operated on, a 2-cm diameter proliferative growth persisted for 6 months. Infection occurred in herdsmen, and in those who handled potentially contaminated clothing or were in contact with affected patients (Falk 1978). The authors of the report believe that the severity of the disease in man indicates that the virus is distinct from orf virus. However, it has been reported that infection can be transmitted from musk oxen to sheep, which may indicate that they are the same virus.

PARAPOXVIRUS INFECTIONS OF WILDLIFE

Parapoxvirus infections have been identified in squirrels in Europe and the United States, and in kangaroos, and parapoxvirus-induced disease has been described in free-living deer in the United States, while quite severe disease has occurred in farmed red deer in New Zealand. Infection of man does not appear to occur readily from these sources, although there is a report of two cases of parapoxvirus infection in which a wildlife source was implicated. In both cases the lesions were discrete epidermal nodules which enlarged progressively over several months. Parapoxvirus infection was confirmed by ultrastructural examination of biopsy material. Infection was considered distinct from orf and does raise the possibility that wildlife may harbour a variety of, as yet uncharacterized, parapoxviruses with zoonotic potential.

REFERENCES

Bennett, M., Gaskell, C. J., Gaskell, R. M., Baxby, D., and Gruffydd-Jones, T. J. (1986). Poxvirus infection in the domestic cat: some clinical and epidemiological observations. *Veterinary Record*, **118**, 387–90.

Bennett, M., Gaskell, C. J., Baxby, D., Gaske, R. M., Kelly, D. F., and Naidoo, J. (1990). Feline cowpox virus infection. *Journal of Small Animal Practice*, **31**, 167–73.

Cook, G. C. (1988). Human monkeypox: a viral disease with an uncertain future in Africa. *Tropical Diseases Bulletin*, **85**, (2).

Douglass, N. J., Richardson, M., and Dumbell, K. R. (1994). Evidence for recent genetic variation in monkeypox viruses. *Journal of General Virology*, **75**, 1303–9.

Dumbell, K. and Richardson M. (1993). Virological investigations of specimens from buffaloes affected by buffalopox in Maharashtra State, India between 1985 and 1987. *Archives of Virology*, **128**, 257–67.

Falk, E. S. (1978). Parapoxvirus infections of reindeer and musk ox associated with unusual human infections. *British Journal of Dermatology*, **99**, 647–54.

Groves, R. W., Wilson-Jones, E., and MacDonald, D. M. (1991). Human orf and milkers' nodule: A clinicopathologic study. *Journal of American Academy of Dermatology*, **25**, 706–11.

Jezek, Z., Arita, I., Szczeniowski, M., Paluko, K. M., Ruti, K., and Nakano, J. H. (1985). Human tanapox in Zaire: clinical and epidemiological observation on cases confirmed by laboratory studies. *Bulletin of the World Health Organisation*, **63**, 1027–35.

Kaplan, C., Healing, T. D., Evans, N., Healing, L., and Prior, A. (1980). Evidence of infection by viruses in small British field rodents. *Journal of Hygiene*, **84**, 285–94.

Khodakevich, L., Jezek, Z., and Messinger, D. (1988). Monkeypox virus: ecology and public health significance. *Bulletin of the World Health Organisation*, **66**, 747–52.

Moss, B. (1990). Poxviridae and their replication. In *Virology*, (2nd edn), (ed. B. N. Fields *et al.*), pp. 2079–111. Raven Press, New York.

Robinson, A. J. and Petersen, G. V. (1983). Orf virus infection of workers in the meat industry. *New Zealand Medical Journal*, **96**, 81–5.

36 PRION PROTEIN-RELATED DISEASES OF MAN AND ANIMALS

James Hope

SUMMARY

Scrapie, Creutzfeldt–Jakob disease (CJD), Gerstmann–Straussler–Sheinker (GSS) syndrome and related diseases of mink (transmissible mink encephalopathy), mule deer, and elk (chronic wasting disease) are the founder members of a group of diseases called the transmissible degenerative (or spongiform) encephalopathies (TSE); the range of species affected by these disorders has grown in recent years to include cattle (bovine spongiform encephalopathy), cats (feline spongiform encephalopathy), and a variety of captive zoo antelope, such as the kudu and African oryx. These diseases can be transmitted from affected to healthy animals by inoculation or by feeding diseased tissues. Iatrogenic transmission of CJD in man has occurred. The transmissible factor or prion has yet to be fully characterized but transmission to laboratory rodents provides a way of measuring the amount of infectivity in tissues and body fluids by quantal titration. This chapter outlines our current understanding of scrapie, bovine spongiform encephalopathy (BSE) and other TSEs. It highlights recent progress in defining the molecular components of the TSE agents, the role of the prion protein, PrP, and its cell and molecular biology.

INTRODUCTION

SCRAPIE

Scrapie of sheep has been known in Europe for centuries and has spread to most parts of the world with the migrations of man and his livestock. Australia, New Zealand and Argentina are about the only countries with a major sheep population which appear to be free of this disease. Its synonyms, goggles, staggers, *traberkrankheit* or trotting disease, *la tremblante*, conjure up pictures of a range of clinical conditions—altered behaviour, hypersensitivity to sound or touch, loss of condition, pruritus and associated fleece loss and skin abrasions, incoordination of the hind limbs—which are diagnostic to the experienced shepherd but usually require confirmation by examination of brain tissue for a triad of histopathological signs: vacuolation, loss of neurones and gliosis (Hadlow 1995)

Onset of the natural clinical disease peaks in flock animals at 3.5 years, with most cases occurring in the age range of 2.5–4.5 years (Hunter *et al.* 1992). In the incubation period, the infected animal is clinically normal and indistinguishable from its uninfected flockmates. Whether it sheds pathogen and acts as a reservoir for infection during the long, preclinical phase is not known, and the lack of an *in vivo* diagnostic test for the infectious particle means that the true prevalence of infection and of the carrier status of unaffected animals within a flock is also unknown.

Scrapie has been reported in most breeds of sheep and, within a flock, it appears to occur in related animals. The within-flock incidence is usually 1–2 cases/100 sheep/year but there have been several instances of 40–50 per cent of animals of a flock succumbing to the disease within a year. The scrapie status of the dam is a major risk factor for the development of disease in progeny, and introduction of a new sire into a previously clear flock has been noted (anecdotely) to provoke outbreaks of clinical disease. A number of genetic markers have recently been identified as risk factors and the introduction of gene typing has greatly facilitated interpretation of field studies on the incidence of natural and experimental disease (Hunter *et al.* 1993; Goldmann *et al.* 1994).

The prognosis on observation of clinical signs is invariably death within a few days, weeks, or months, hence in veterinary work this usually results in a recommendation to cull the affected animal from the flock, and similarly to slaughter its dam and other maternally related sheep.

KURU AND CREUTZFELDT–JAKOB DISEASE

Kuru is a chronic, degenerative disease of the central nervous system discovered in the Fore and related tribes of the eastern highlands of Papua New Guinea in the early 1950s. It takes its name from the native word for shivering. Affecting adults and children (above 4 years of age) alike, it accounted for 1 in 100 deaths per year in this small group of people. First clinical signs were falling over and difficulty in co-ordination, which progressed rapidly over a few months to severe cerebellar dysfunction, immobilization, and death. Incubation period may vary from 5 years to 50 years. Histopathological analysis of brain tissue revealed hyperplasia and hypertrophy of astrocytes and microglia, neuronal vacuolation, and status spongiosis. Amyloid plaques, particularly in the cerebellum, were seen in most cases but little demyelination or inflam-mation was observed. These characteristics so resem-bled scrapie in sheep that Hadlow suggested they were related and, that kuru might be a transmissible disease; in 1966, this transmissibility was confirmed by the production of a clinical disease with similar brain pathology in chimpanzees. The time lag between intracerebral inoculation and clinical disease in these animals was extremely long and ranged from 18 to 21 months. Kuru was the first human degenerative con-dition of the CNS to be transmitted to an artificial host and immediately focused attention on other obscure conditions which might have a similar aetiology (Brown and Gajdusek 1991). One of these was Creutzfeldt–Jakob disease, which had earlier been noted to have brain pathology reminiscent of kuru.

Creutzfeldt–Jakob disease was first described by Creutzfeldt (1920) and Jakob (1921) as a progressive dementia with clinical signs suggesting dysfunction of the cerebellum, basal ganglia, and lower motor neu-rones. Paradoxically, the initial case report may have included a condition which in retrospect would not now be regarded as CJD—a situation in parallel to the current re-appraisal of the definition of prion dis-eases—and certainly this disease has been described under various names (reviewed by Kirschbaum 1968). The clinical signs are more variable than kuru but most commonly the disease is associated with gradual mental deterioration leading to dementia and confu-sion, and a progressive impairment of motor function, including myoclonus. CJD occurs mainly in the fifth and sixth decades of life. Most patients die within 6 months of onset of clinical signs and there are no verified cases of recovery. Pathologically the lesions of the brain included variable vacuolation of the neu-ropil, astrocytosis and, in about 10 per cent of CJD cases, kuru and other types of amyloid plaques. By 1968, recognition of its similarity to kuru and scrapie had stimulated its transmission to a chimpanzee by intracerebral inoculation of biopsy tissue and confirmed its classification with these diseases. Gerstmann–Straussler syndrome, a progressive dementia with cere-bellar amyloid plaques, is a familial variant of CJD with an extended clinical time course (Brown and Gajdusek 1991).

Epidemiologically, these human forms of prion disease can be classified as familial, sporadic, and iatro-genic. The incidence of CJD-related disease in man is remarkably constant at 0.5–1 cases per million of popu-lation per year throughout the world and is not linked to the incidence of any of the animal disease. This low incidence casts doubt on the role of infection in its propagation within the population. Some 13–14 per cent of cases are familial and linked to mutations in the open reading frame (ORF) of the *PrP* gene. There have been many clinical and pathological studies on human cases of neurological disease which seem to be associated with these rare mutations of the *PrP* gene, including Jakob's original family (Brown *et al.* 1994) and the first GSS case (Kretzschmar *et al.* 1991) (reviewed by Goldfarb *et al.* 1994). In some families, there is complete penetrance of the phenotype and so the mutation is regarded as the cause of the disease. Apart from iatrogenic cases induced by transplantation of infected tissues or inoculation of contaminated pharmaceuticals of human origin, there is no epidemi-ological evidence for horizontal transmission of the disease. A stochastic event involving conversion of the PrP protein to its disease-associated isoform or the chance mutation of a benign, ubiquitous viral-like agent are two mechanisms which have been suggested to explain the incidence of sporadic cases (see p. 000). There is no cure for the clinical condition although genetic counselling, where applicable, may effectively prevent transmission of disease from one generation to the next.

There is considerable clinical and pathological hete-rogeneity in the human prion diseases and although genetic typing and nucleotide sequencing of the *PrP* ORF has provided some unifying concepts, mutation in the PrP protein does not appear to be the whole story. Other genetic factors including linkage to the E4 allele of *ApoE* gene have been implicated as risk factors for the occurrence of CJD (Amouyel *et al.* 1994) (but see also Salvatore *et al.* 1995).

In April 1996 Will *et al.* (1996) reported a new variant of CJD (NVCJD) possibly linked to bovine spongiform encephalopathy. Ten cases, all in young adults or teenagers presented with behavioural and psychiatric disturbances and early ataxia. The duration of illness was prolonged (up to 2 years) and typical EEG changes of CJD were absent. There was extensive kuru-type amyloid plaque formation surrounded by vacuoles. Spongiform changes were most evident in the basal ganglia and thalamus with high-density prion protein accumulation on immunocytochemical analy-sis, especially in the cerebellum.

FATAL FAMILIAL INSOMNIA

Fatal familial insomnia (FFI) is the newest member of the human transmissible encephalopathies. It is characterized by a dysfunction of the autonomic nervous system, usually presenting with insomnia and problems of appetite, temperature, and blood pressure regulation. At post-mortem, the pathology of the brain is mostly neuronal loss and degeneration of the thalamus with little or no vacuolation of the neuropil. Its classification as a prion disease was originally based on its association with an asparagine (N) to aspartic acid (D) mutation at codon 178 of the *PrP* gene, a mutation which is also linked to a classical form of CJD. Which of the two phenotypes prevails appears to depend on the amino acid encoded by codon 129 of the same *PrP* allele: in FFI, codon 129 encodes methionine while in CJD, codon 129 encodes valine (Goldfarb *et al.* 1992). Homozygosity at codon 129 also appears to be risk factor in the development of sporadic CJD, but each polymorphism at this codon is fairly common and not thought to be pathogenic *per se* (Palmer *et al.* 1991). The classification of FFI has recently been confirmed by transmission of disease to laboratory mice (Tateishi *et al.* 1995)

MYOPATHIES

Both Alzheimer's precursor protein (beta-APP) and PrP and their mRNAs are located in human muscle macrophages unrelated to their localization within muscle tissue or pathology. These proteins may play a role in the biology of muscle macrophages (Askanas *et al.* 1995) and in muscle development and regeneration. Overexpression *PrP* mRNA and protein in transgenic mice can lead to severe degeneration of skeletal muscle (Westaway *et al.* 1994) and has recently focused attention on a new group of prion protein-related, neurodegenerative diseases. Sporadic inclusion-body myositis is a common progressive muscle disease involving mononuclear cell inflammation and vacuolated muscle fibres, and a similar non-inflammatory, inclusion-body myopathy is familial. In both muscle diseases, PrP (as well as beta-APP, phosphorylated tau and apolipoprotein E) abnormally accumulate in vacuolated muscle fibres. In contrast to the brain PrP disorders, the accummulation of PrP protein in muscle fibres is associated with increased levels of *PrP* mRNA (Sarkozi *et al.* 1994). There is no evidence for the transmissibility of these muscle disorders.

BOVINE SPONGIFORM ENCEPHALOPATHY

Bovine spongiform encephalopathy (BSE) has devastated the UK cattle industry for the past decade (Bradley and Wilesmith 1993). From isolated cases first reported in 1986 and some retrospectively identified in May 1985, a major epidemic was under way by 1988 which has to date claimed over 160 000 cattle within the British Isles. Some other countries have also confirmed cases: Switzerland (205), Ireland (120), Portugal (30), France, and Germany, with one or two cases in Italy, Denmark, Canada, Oman, and the Falkland Islands.

The disease produces a progressive degeneration of the central nervous system and was named because of the sponge-like appearance of BSE brain tissue when seen under the light microscope (Wells *et al.* 1987). Warning signs of the illness include changes in the behaviour and temperament of the cattle. The affected animal becomes increasingly apprehensive and has problems of movement and posture, especially of its hind limbs. The cow (or bull) has increased sensitivity to touch and sound, loss of weight and, as the disease takes hold of its nervous system, a creeping paralysis sets in. This clinical phase of BSE lasts from a fortnight to over 6 months. Although the majority of animals affected have been dairy cows, this neurological disease can occur in either sex with a modal age of onset of 4–4.5 years (range 1.8–18 years). Most cases of BSE have occurred in cattle between the ages of 3 and 5 years and for most of its development time the disease gives no telltale sign of its presence (Wilesmith *et al.* 1988). This inability to detect the asymptomatic carrier of BSE or scrapie limits the measures which can be taken to prevent infected bovine or ovine tissues from use in feed and pharmaceutical products.

The neurological lesions in BSE-affected cow brains are virtually identical to those found in scrapie-affected sheep and include the spongiform change which gives BSE its name. From its clinical and neuropathological signs, BSE was immediately suspected to belong to the scrapie family of transmissible spongiform encephalopathies. This has been confirmed by biochemical studies (Hope *et al.* 1988*a*) and by experimental transmission of BSE to mice (Fraser *et al.* 1988), cattle (Dawson *et al.* 1990*a*), mink (Robinson *et al.* 1994), marmoset (Baker *et al.* 1993), cynomolgus macaques (Lasmezas *et al.* 1996), sheep and goats (Foster *et al.* 1993) and a pig (Dawson *et al.* 1990*b*).

The origins and control of BSE and its current status

Epidemiological analyses of BSE-affected herds identified a protein feed supplement to be the most likely source of infection (Wilesmith *et al.* 1988). During the late 1970s changes in the rendering process which salvages compounds of nutritional and commercial value from abbatoir waste are thought to have led to a less efficient system for inactivating scrapie-affected sheep offal and, in turn, to a contaminated protein supplement. Subsequent recycling of BSE-infected cattle waste in this process may have contributed to the persistence of the disease.

Ruminant feed legislation aimed at removing the source of infection from cattle born after 1988 was introduced in 1989–90 and the epidemic is now showing signs of rapid decline; by April, 1996, the number of confirmed BSE cases had dropped to below 1200 a month following a peak incidence of over 1000 cases a week in 1993. There have been over 26 000 cases of BSE in cattle born after the feed ban but the very low within-herd incidence (about 2 per cent) of the disease makes vertical or horizontal transmission within herds unlikely. Illegal or unknowing feeding of contaminated protein to calves is suspected as the reason for these 'born after the ban' (BAB) cases. A comprehensive report on the epidemiology of BSE has recently been published (Anderson *et al.* 1996).

In parallel with the BSE epidemic, natural cases of transmissible spongiform encephalopathies have been also been reported for the first time in cattle-related species—greater kudu, eland, nyala and gemsbok, Arabian and scimitar-horned oryx (Kirkwood and Cunningham 1994), and in the cat family—puma, cheetahs (Kirkwood and Cunningham 1994), and domestic cats (Pearson *et al.* 1992). Apart from some cases in the greater kudu, contaminated feed is suspected but difficult to prove because of the absence of detailed feeding records.

ARE TSES ZOONOSES?

Creutzfeldt–Jakob disease and the other human TSEs are incurable but very rare, affecting just over 1 person in 2 million every year (see above). However, the BSE epidemic gave rise to worries that BSE or other animal TSEs would cause human disease if introduced into man via food or by a product of the biotechnology industry. Although there is no epidemiological link of scrapie and the other animal TSEs with CJD, there have been several cases of human to human transmission via cadaver-derived therapeutics or tissues—as, for example, an unfortunate consequence of corneal transplantation (Hogan and Cavanagh 1995), pituitary growth hormone injection (Devillemeur *et al.* 1992), or dura mater grafting (Esmonde *et al.* 1993). Several studies of risk factors from classical CJD have been carried out, but there are no consistently observed associations with occupation or foods (SEAC 1994). However, zoonotic hypotheses have been proposed (Davanipour *et al.* 1986; Diringer 1995).

The new variant CJD infection is clearly a candidate zoonosis, and UK government policy has been to accept the possibility in order to introduce control measures. At present evidence that NVCJD was acquired from BSE-infected cattle is accumulating (see p. 429). Recent work by Collinge *et al.* (1996) suggests that new variant CJD has biochemical characteristics distinct from other types of CJD but which resemble those of BSE transmitted to mice, domestic cat, and macaque.

WHAT IS THE SCRAPIE/BSE AGENT?

TAXONOMY

Modern virus classification uses the morphology and biochemistry of virions and their mode of replication as the basis for taxonomy; for example, the nature of the virion nucleic acid—DNA or RNA—its size, symmetry, the presence or absence of a lipid envelope, genome integration, mechanism of cell entry, use of vectors, etc. The scrapie and related agents remain undefined in this sort of detail and so their classification has not been easy, although many structures have been described as specific for scrapie-infected fractions (Cho 1976; Cho *et al.* 1977): 'nemaviruses' (Narang 1990), scrapie-associated fibrils (Merz *et al.* 1981, 1984) or prion rods (McKinley *et al.* 1986) and small, pentangular structures of 10 nm diameter (Ozel and Diringer 1994), or in tissue sections as spheres and tubes (Baringer *et al.* 1981) or tubulo-vesicular vesicular structures (TSVs) (Liberski *et al.* 1988).

STRAINS OF AGENT

Viruses, bacteria, bacteriophages, and all other conventional forms of life show phenotypic or strain variation which is encoded by their nucleic acid genomes. Strain variation is also a common feature of various scrapie isolates in mice, hamsters, sheep, and goats, but while selection and mutation of murine scrapie strains is documented, a coding molecule has yet to be defined. The two main criteria used to distinguish strains of mouse-passaged scrapie are (1) the ranking of the incubation periods they produce in mice of the three *Sinc* genotypes—s7s7, s7p7; and p7p7; and (2) the severity and location of vacuolar degeneration induced in the brains of terminal cases of disease (Fraser 1976). The occurrence of different strain of pathogen has implications for much of the epidemiology and genetics of these diseases (see below). For example, passage of BSE from seven unrelated cattle sources into a panel of *Sinc* s7s7, s7p7, and p7p7 mice have given a remarkably uniform pathology and ranking of incubation period, differing from over 20 other transmissions of sheep and goat scrapie. Transmissions to mice of spongiform encephalopathy from six species (including sheep and goats, kudu, and oryx) which have been experimentally or naturally infected with BSE have given similar results to direct BSE transmissions from cattle (Bruce *et al.* 1994). Although the molecular basis of this uniformity is uncertain, similar transmissions from the 'suspect-BSE' CJD cases recently described in the UK (Will *et al.* 1996) and France (Chazot *et al.* 1996) may distinguish between a cattle or some other source of disease. Interim results of transmissions of sporadic CJD and NVCJD to mice provide strong evidence that the same agent strain is involved in both BSE and NVCJD (Bruce *et al.*, 1997).

BIOCHEMISTRY OF INFECTIVITY: FIBRILS, RODS, AND THE PRION PROTEIN

High titres of infectivity are recovered in preparations of membranes purified from TSE-affected brain and other tissues; this infectivity is not significantly reduced by disruption of membranes using deoxycholate (DOC), sarcosinate (Sarkosyl), and other mild detergents, and can be concentrated and pelleted by differential centrifugation. This infectious material is heterogeneous in size and physical properties and has yet to be isolated as a band by density gradient centrifugation. This has hindered its biophysical characterization. Viewed by electron microscopy, these highly enriched fractions of infectivity contain fibrils of various shapes and sizes as well as ferritin particles and amorphous material. Surprisingly, these fractions are homogeneous biochemically. One isolate of hamster scrapie (263K) survives prolonged treatment with high concentrations of proteinase K and contains little else but a 27–30 000 M_r protein. This is the prion protein (PrP27–30) and, although different isolates from mouse and other species are more susceptible to proteases than the 263K-protein and so are sometimes harder to detect, PK-resistant PrP (PrP-res or PrP^{Sc}) is found in all TSE isolates and has become a biochemical marker for disease and the infectious agent (Hope *et al.* 1986, 1988 *a,b*).

Several groups have reported a stoichiometry of 100 000 molecules of PrP^{Sc} per infectious particle using rodent models of these diseases (Scott *et al.* 1991). The fibrils (scrapie-associated fibrils or rods) are aggregates of PrP^{Sc} and provide a morphological marker of infection/disease; in some models, they can be visualized in tissue by thin-section electron microscopy and shown to be composed of PrP by immunogold staining (Jeffrey *et al.* 1992, 1996). In retrospect, these sparingly soluble fibrils of a normal cellular protein (PrP^c) had been seen as plaque-like deposits of amyloid in human (kuru) and mouse (experimental scrapie) brain several years before their biochemical characterization.

PrP^c is a phosphoinositol-glycolipid-anchored membrane glycoprotein found in brain and, to a lesser extent, other tissues. The primary structure of the PrP is virtually constant in mammalian species (Schatzl *et al.* 1995), including man, mouse, and cow (Goldmann 1993) and there is an avian homologue (Harris *et al.* 1991). It is a glycoprotein of 33–35 000 Da which is anchored to the cell plasma membrane by a phosphatidyl-inositol glycolipid attached to its carboxy-terminal amino acid (Stahl *et al.* 1987). The hamster protein (PrP^c and PrP^{Sc}) has 208 amino acids (PrP$^{23-231}$) and the normal isoform is completely degraded by proteases under conditions which leave a 27–30 000 Da, protease-resistant core of the PrP^{Sc} isoform intact (PrP$^{27-30}$) (Bolton *et al.* 1982, 1985; Hope *et al.* 1986; McKinley *et al.* 1983). PrP$^{81-230}$ is equivalent to the proteinase-K-resistant core of mouse PrP^{Sc} (Hope *et al.* 1988*a*) and its expression in transgenic mice has been shown to be sufficient to support replication of infectivity and the development of disease (Fischer *et al.* 1996).

In vitro formation of PrP^{Sc} from PrP^C has been shown in infected cell cultures (see below) and in a cell-free system where the conversion is driven by addition of PrP^{Sc} template (Kocisko *et al.* 1994). The cell-free system mimics several aspects of the *in vivo* disease, including species and strain specificities (Bessen *et al.* 1995; Kocisko *et al.* 1995; Raymond *et al.*, 1997). From these test-tube studies, two distinct models for the formation of PrP^{Sc} have evolved: in both, exogenous PrP^{Sc} forms catalytic heterodimers with PrP^C which results in the formation of more PrP^{Sc}; in one, these 'heterodimers' are real (Kaneko *et al.* 1995) while in the other they actually represent the growing face of a PrP^{Sc} fibril or aggregate (Caughey *et al.* 1995). This latter, 'seeded' polymerization model fits better with the kinetics of *in vitro* conversion PrP^C to protease-resistant PrP, although *de novo* 'PrP^{Sc}' made in a test-tube has yet to be shown to be infectious. This mechanism of conversion resembles a crystallization process in that it is rate-limited by nucleus formation and accelerated by seeding (Caughey *et al.* 1995).

Although the structures and pathway of conversion between PrP^C and PrP^{Sc} have yet to be worked out, the atomic coordinates of a soluble, independent folding domain of the protein (residues 121–230) have recently been defined by nuclear magnetic resonance spectroscopy (Riek *et al.* 1996). Knowledge of the full structure of PrP^C and PrP^{Sc} may help the design of chemicals engineered to prevent the conversion process and so help predict transmission between species and limit the effects of these diseases. To date, simple comparison of the primary sequences of PrP from different species has failed to aid the prediction of whether or not a particular source or new strain of TSE will transmit from one species to another (Goldmann *et al.* 1996; Krakauer *et al.* 1996). Old conundrums such as why the mouse-passaged ME7 strain transmits to rats but not guinea-pigs or rabbits following intracerebral inoculation have not yet been solved by molecular biology (Barlow and Rennie 1976).

THE STABILITY OF INFECTIVITY AND ITS MEASUREMENT

The physical heterogeneity of infectious particles has been one of the major drawbacks preventing their molecular characterization. During fractionation of tissue homogenates of scrapie-infected brain by rate-zonal density gradient centrifugation, infectivity ranges in size from 40S to >500S (Prusiner *et al.* 1977). This behaviour is probably due to its association with the PrP protein. The range in size observed may be due to the interaction of this protein with various membrane fragments and cell debris. The use of filters, ultracentrifugation, gel filtration, and other sizing techniques to define the minimum size of the pathogen have been hindered by this problem. Irradiation techniques using high-energy ionizing particles are unaffected by the purity of the infectious particles and have consistently given estimates of less than 200 kDa for the target size of the replicating particle (reviewed by Alper 1993), although these estimates continue to be disputed (Rowher 1991). Most recently, detergent lysis, membrane filtration and mouse titration using a mouse-passaged isolate of CJD have been used to define a maximum size of this agent at less than 25 nm (Tateishi *et al.* 1993).

Physical and chemical treatments of infectious fractions can alter the pathogenesis of infection in the animals used in the quantal titration of infectivity, and these complex effects are often neglected when fractionation/titre data is analysed. For example, boiling reduces the titre of inocula as measured by an intracerebral route but not by peripheral inoculation (Dickinson and Fraser 1969; Taylor and Diprose 1996). The cellular and molecular basis of these effects on titre are poorly understood and hence much of our knowledge on inactivation is anecdotal and difficult to interpret in terms of molecular structure. To complicate the situation still further, it appears that different strains of scrapie and other TSEs may have different relative resistance to thermal (and possibly other forms of) inactivation. However, rules of thumb developed from work on the model of murine scrapie may also apply to the sterilization of CJD- and BSE-infected materials (Taylor *et al.* 1994). For example, scrapie infectivity is inactivated by oxidizing agents (2 per cent available chlorine, bleach), high alkalinity (1–2 M sodium hydroxide), extremes of temperature (138 °C for 20 min) and other conditions which destroy proteins and their biological activities (Taylor 1993). Current UK Department of Health guidelines recommend steam autoclaving at 136–138 °C for 18 min for the sterilization of possible CJD-exposed instruments and materials.

SINC, THE PRION PROTEIN GENE AND PRP-LESS MICE

Genetic linkage studies in various species have implicated PrP as a product of the *Sinc* (or homologous locus), and further evidence for this congruency has recently been provided using mice genetically engineered to lack one or both copies of their *PrP* gene (Weissmann *et al.* 1994). Mice lacking a *PrP* gene appear normal and these PrP^{null} mice neither replicate infectivity nor develop disease when challenged with doses of infectivity that would be lethal to their $PrP^{+/+}$ littermates. Levels of PrP^C appear to be crucial in determining the timing and duration of clinical disease; hemizygous $PrP^{+/-}$ mice which express roughly half the normal ($PrP^{+/+}$) amount of PrP^C in the brain, have a significantly longer clinical phase and incubation period of disease compared with the survival characteristics of their $PrP^{0/0}$ littermates (Manson *et al.* 1994*a*). These experiments have confirmed a key role for PrP^C as either substrate for a pathogenic isoform (PrP^{Sc}) or as a receptor molecule for a more conventional pathogen. Transgenic mice with human or bovine *PrP* genes in place of their own may be more susceptible than their wild-type littermates to inoculation with human (Collinge *et al.* 1995; Hope 1995; Telling *et al.* 1995) or bovine infectious particles.

PRION, VIRINO OR VIRUS?

There are three structures commonly proposed for the BSE/scrapie pathogen: the virus, a conventional structure of host-independent protein protecting and encapsidating a replication template of nucleic acid; the virino, a composite structure of host protein and host-independent molecule (possibly a small nucleic acid) which determines the strain of scrapie; or the Prion, where one version of a prion structure has some form of the PrP protein as the sole component of the pathogen. It is the Prion which is currently most widely accepted.

NATURAL TRANSMISSION

The life cycle of an infectious agent can be defined at three levels, its mechanism of transmission within and between populations; at the level of the organism, where one needs to understand route of entry, spread, replication and shedding from an individual; this also includes its pathogenesis; and, thirdly, for intracellular parasites such as viruses it is beneficial to understand how the agent hijacks the cell and uses its biosynthetic machinery to reproduce. Hence, as far as it is understood, the three cycles of a typical TSE-like infection are documented below.

TRANSMISSION AND MAINTENANCE WITHIN A POPULATION

One of the main problems of understanding the epidemiology of human TSE disease is to explain its low incidence, an incidence which appears incompatible with a sustainable infection within the population. There are two main views on this dichotomy: that the disease is not infectious but arises *de novo* in each individual as the result of a somatic or germline mutation in the prion protein gene; the other stresses our lack of knowledge of the prevalence of infection rather than the incidence of clinical disease and proposes that there is a widespread inapparent infection of the population by a benign agent and only in certain genetically susceptible individuals or by its mutation to a pathogenic form will this ubiquitous agent produce disease. In either case, the predominant form of natural transmission is predicted to be vertical in accordance with field observation in man.

In scrapie of sheep, the other common natural TSE, there is evidence for both vertical and horizontal transmission of disease. Maternal transmission of the infection from ewe to offspring either *in utero* or immediately after birth is thought to be the major route of propogation of the disease within a flock, but lateral transmission is also documented (Dickinson *et al.* 1974). Factors associated with the horizontal spread of infections, such as host susceptibility, source, and route of infection have been investigated for many years in sheep and rodent models of disease. The low incidence of clinical disease in affected flocks is usually interpreted to mean the agent is not highly contagious and this is supported by the low or zero infectivity in body fluids or secretions. Recently, hay mites cohabiting the pasture of flocks of sheep in Iceland have been implicated as an insect vector of disease (Wisniewski *et al.* 1996).

Medium levels of infectivity in placentae and amniotic fluids may contaminate pasture or pens and surrounds where lambing occurs and persist for long periods (Pattison *et al.* 1974). Desemination of agent by other routes—in faeces, urine, milk—is less likely as little or no infectivity has ever been detected in these excretions. Of the common routes of entry (or re-entry) into the body—ingestion, inhalation, contact, and coitus—the natural route is probably via the mouth or skin abrasions. Both are well-documented portals of entry for experimental transmission of scrapie and other spongiform encephalopathies to rodents and ruminants. Infectivity has been detected in the eyes and lungs of natural cases of disease and conjunctival instillation of scrapie in mice can produce disease (Scott *et al.* 1993) but there have been no accounts of experimental aerosol transmission, and infectivity in lungs may be due to secondary transport and infection; however, this emphasizes the need for adequate protection when handling tissues infected with TSE and recommended safety precautions for laboratory workers include the use of face masks, avoidance of aerosols, and eye protection. Sexual intercourse does not seem to be a risk factor in the transmission of these diseases in man or animal.

SPREAD OF PATHOGEN WITHIN THE NATURAL HOST

Apart from the recognized familial incidence, the oral route of transmission of natural scrapie and the pathogenesis of disease is based on painstaking work by many workers, notably Hadlow and colleagues. They measured infectivity by rodent bioassay in various neonatal and maternal sheep tissues and body fluids in flocks of sheep with a high incidence of natural scrapie or in experimentally infected animals. The early appearance of infectivity in tonsil, retropharyngeal and mesenteric-portal lymph nodes, and intestine suggested that primary infection was occurring by way of the alimentary tract, either prenatally from pathogen in amniotic fluid or postnatally from a contaminated environment (Hadlow *et al.* 1982). Exactly where in the alimentary tract the pathogen gains access to sites of replication and transport is a point of debate at the moment. Uptake by the oropharyngeal tract may circumvent normal protective processes against oral infection and this route into the central nervous system has been implicated for scrapie and BSE. The acidic pH of the stomach is an effective barrier against this mode of transmission for a wide variety of organisms, but not for scrapie-like agents which are highly stable at low pH; similarly, other physicochemical inactivators such as cholate in bile salts which protect against enteric, enveloped viruses may simply disperse prions, enhancing their uptake and transport across the gut epithelium. For some viruses, there is uptake of non-replicating particles by cells overlying Peyer's patches (in the ileum) and intact virus particles in smooth-surfaced cytoplasmic vesicles in these cells have been seen by EM. These cells appear to hand over virus particles to adjacent mononuclear cells for antigen-processing and replication, and some of the particles then enter the local lymphatic system (Mimms and White 1984). This paradigm matches the kinetics of infectivity levels in various tissues following oral infection of rodents with scrapie but it is difficult to show it in the natural disease. After oral infection of mice, neural spread of pathogen occurs from the gastrointestinal tract, perhaps via the enteric and sympathetic nervous systems to spinal cord. Neuroinvasion may be initiated either via infection of Peyer's patches or directly by infection of nerve endings in the gut wall, and the lymphoreticular system may be by-passed completely (Kimberlin and Walker 1989a). However, with alternative routes of infection (intraperitoneal, subcutaneous), the spleen and other lymphatic tissues are important sites where the pathogen appears to replicate to a threshold level before breakthrough into the peripheral nervous system and transport to the lower spinal cord (Fraser and Dickinson 1978; Kimberlin and Walker 1989b; Lasmezas et al. 1996). It is the PrP-producing follicular dendritic cell which appears important for replication in the spleen (Kitamoto et al. 1991). Retrograde axonal transport to the CNS then precedes its devastating effects on brain and brain-stem.

Since the physiology and living conditions of man, sheep, cattle, and laboratory rodent differ widely, it would be surprising if this model for the entry and spread of agent through the body were generally applicable, and much still needs to be done to understand pathogenesis in man and ruminant. In their early kuru studies, Asher and colleagues found epidemiological evidence that agent may enter the body through breaks in the skin and mucous membranes; this agreed with contemporary data that following subcutaneous injection, scrapie in rodents showed early replication in lymphoid tissue and later in other organs. Taylor and colleagues have recently shown that scrapie infection can be established readily through skin abrasions in immunocompetent but not immunodifficient (SCID) mice (Taylor et al. 1996b). However, in kuru and CJD studies (from clinically ill patients), brain was regularly found to be infected but only occasionally was infectivity detected in other organs such as spleen and lymphoid tissue. Paradoxically, as the titre increased in the CNS it decreased or disappeared from lymphoid tissue (Asher et al. 1976). Current failure to detect infectivity (and PrP^{Sc}) in peripheral tissues of CJD/GSS patients and BSE-affected cattle cautions against making too many general statements about pathogenesis based on sheep and rodent studies.

There is no evidence of maternal transmission of human or rodent spongiform encephalopathies (Anderson et al. 1996), although this has often been noted in field studies of natural scrapie in sheep and some evidence of a 'maternal effect' in the transmission of BSE has been reported (Cumow et al., 1997). Attempts to circumvent maternal transmission in sheep, by embryo transfer techniques have had mixed success, not least because of the 'carrier status' problem, and the lack of information on the range of

natural strains of scrapie and their interaction with the host genome (Foster et al. 1992, 1996; Foote et al. 1993)

Obviously the vertical and horizontal methods of transmission are not mutually exclusive and may change in relative importance with time. For example, the mini-epidemic of spongiform encephalopathy in African Kudu may have had a common source with BSE—feeding of contaminated protein—but in subsequent cases lateral transmission is implicated (Kirkwood et al. 1993, 1994). This emphasizes that the initial wave of disease may be started by one mechanism but continued by another with maintenance at a low level by lateral or maternal transmission.

CELL BIOLOGY OF SCRAPIE REPLICATION

The presence of PrP^c in a cell or organism appears to be a necessary, if not sufficient condition for it to be able to replicate the TSE pathogen. Although the *PrP* gene is expressed in many embryonic and adult mouse tissues (Manson et al. 1992), its deletion from the mouse genome does not appear to affect normal development, behaviour, and fertility (see above). Animals homozygous (0/0) and heterozygous (0/+) for this mutation can be inbred to produce stable lines of mice and appear normal (Bueler et al. 1992; Manson et al. 1994a). Some workers (Collinge et al. 1994; Manson et al. 1995; Colling et al. 1996) but not others (Herms et al. 1995; Lledo et al. 1996) have observed a subtle deficit in synaptic transmission in tissue slices, while altered circadian rhythms and sleep pattern have also recently been described (Tobler et al. 1996) in these *PrP*-less (0/0) mice. Gross abnormalities, such as loss of Purkinje cells and cerebellar ataxia, are an inconsistent observation (Sakaguchi et al. 1996) and need to be further substantiated as specific deficits of *PrP* gene deletion. However, 0/0 mice survive intracerebral inoculation of doses of scrapie agent lethal to wild-type mice, and 0/+ animals, which have decreased levels of PrP protein in the brain, have significantly extended survival times compared to +/+ mice (Bueler et al. 1993; Manson et al. 1994b). Titration of infectivity in brain and spleen of 0/0 mice following challenge with prions has failed to detect replication although infectivity persists in these animals long after infection (Sailer et al. 1994): these experiments show that expression of the *PrP* gene is a prerequisite for replication and development of disease in the mouse.

In vitro replication also appears dependent on the expression in cells of PrP protein and, in the absence of other markers for infectivity, the site of conversion of PrP^C to PrP^{Sc} has been studied to elucidate where in the cell replication is taking place. Time-course studies in infected neuroblastoma cells indicate that the conversion takes place following transit of PrP^c to the cell surface, either at the surface or on endocytosis in the endosomal-lysosome system (Caughey and Raymond 1991; Harris *et al.* 1996; Borchelt *et al.* 1992; Laszlo *et al.* 1992; Caughey 1994; *in vivo* PrP (either PrP^c or PrP^{Sc}) can be observed accummulating at the plasma membrane and in the intercellular space well before neuronal loss, vacuolation, and gliosis (Jeffrey *et al.* 1992, 1996) and may have a direct toxic or mitogenic effect on neighbouring cells. Some of these effects can be mimicked *in vitro* on cultured cells by PrP^{Sc} (Muller *et al.* 1993) or PrP fragments (Forloni *et al.* 1993; Hope *et al.* 1996) and can be ameliorated by NMDA receptor antagonists (Perovic *et al.* 1995); *in vivo* uptake and processing of PrP by microglia and their subsequent cytokine response may also play a role in the neuro-degenerative process (Brown *et al.* 1996)—a process which is clearly dependent on neuronal expression of PrP^c (Brandner *et al.* 1996; Brown *et al.* 1996).

Much further work needs to be done to understand these cellular interactions in the brain and peripheral tissues, not least because their understanding should guide the development of therapeutics. Interestingly, polyanions such as dextran sulphate, Congo Red and pentosan sulphate, which can inhibit PrP^c to PrP^{Sc} formation *in vitro* (Caughey and Raymond 1993), may also extend the survival time of hamsters or mice co-infected with some strains of scrapie (Ehlers and Diringer 1984; Farquhar and Dickinson 1986; Kimberlin and Walker 1986; Ladogana *et al.* 1992; Ingrosso *et al.* 1995); the large doses and extended therapy needed in these cases may preclude their use in practice. To date, no conventional antiviral agent or antibiotic has been effective in delaying the time course of scrapie or other natural TSE.

CONTROL

The UK control policy for preventing BSE transmission to humans is, first, to eradicate BSE from the UK beef herds. It was made illegal to feed ruminant-derived protein to ruminants in July 1988, to prevent possibly infected bovine and ovine material from entering the food chain, particularly brain and spinal cord. To avoid human exposure to BSE, a ban on the use of specific cattle tissues for human consumption was introduced in November 1989–January 1990 in the UK, and, in September 1990, this ban was extended to their use as feed to any animal or bird. These specified bovine offals (SBOs) were brain, spinal cord, tonsil, thymus, spleen, and the lower intestine (duodenum to rectum) from cattle over the age of 6 months. This high-risk category of tissues was based on the levels of infectivity detected by mouse bioassay in natural cases of sheep scrapie. New data on the direct assay of infectivity by mouse bioassay in these cattle tissues indicates

that the levels of agent may not be as high or as widespread in cattle as they are in sheep (Fraser and Foster 1993; Wells *et al.* 1994; Taylor *et al.* 1995 1996a). However, cattle to cattle transmission appears much more efficient than the equivalent cattle to mouse experiment and there is no estimate of the relative efficiency of cattle to human transmission.

Guidance has been issued for minimizing risks for laboratory (SEAC, 1994; Department of Health, 1996) and occupational (ACDP 1996) exposures. Strict measures for slaughtering, processing, and rendering cattle have been implemented.

REFERENCES

ACDP (Advisory Committee on Dangerous Pathogens) (1996). *BSE (Bovine spongiform encephalopathy) Background and general occupational guidance.* ACDP, HMSO, London.

Alper, T. (1993). The scrapie enigma: insights from radiation experiments. *Radiation Research*, **135**, 283–92.

Amouyel, P., Vidal, O., Launay, J. M., and Laplanche, J. L. (1994). The apolipoprotein-E alleles as major susceptibility factors for Creutzfeldt-Jakob-disease. *Lancet*, **344**, 1315–18.

Anderson, R. M. *et al.* (1996). Transmission dynamics and epidemiology of bovine spongiform encephalopathy (BSE) in cattle in Great Britain: past, present, and future. *Nature*, **382**, 779–88.

Asher, D. M., Gibbs, C. J. Jr, and Gajdusek, D. C. (1976). Pathogenesis of subacute spongiform encephalopathies. *Annals of Clinical and Laboratory Science*, **6**, 84–103.

Askanas, V., Sarkozi, E., Bilak, M., Alvarez, R. B., and Engel, W. K. (1995). Human muscle macrophages express beta-amyloid precursor and prion proteins and their messenger-RNAs. *Neuroreport*, **6**, 1045–9.

Baker, H. F., Ridley, R. M., and Wells, G. A. (1993). Experimental transmission of BSE and scrapie to the common marmoset. *Veterinary Record*, **132**, 403–6.

Baringer, J. R., Prusiner, S. B., and Wong, J. S. (1981). Scrapie-associated particles in postsynaptic processes. Further ultra-structural studies. *Journal of Neuropathology and Experimental Neurology*, **40**, 281–8.

Barlow, R. M. and Rennie, J. C. (1976). The fate of ME7 scrapie infection in rats, guinea-pigs and rabbits. *Research in Veterinary Science*, **21**, 110–11.

Bessen, R. A., Kocisko, D. A., Raymond, G. J., Nandan, S., Lansbury, P. T., and Caughey, B. (1995). Non-genetic propagation of strain-specific properties of scrapie prion protein. *Nature*, **375**, 698–700.

Bolton, D. C., McKinley, M. P., and Prusiner, S. B. (1982). Identification of a protein that purifies with the scrapie prion. *Science*, **218**, 1309–11.

Bolton, D. C., Meyer, R. K., and Prusiner, S. B. (1985). Scrapie PrP 27–30 is a sialoglycoprotein. *Journal of Virology*, **53**, 596–606.

Borchelt, D. R., Taraboulos, A., and Prusiner, S. B. (1992). Evidence for synthesis of scrapie prion proteins in the endocytic pathway. *Journal of Biological Chemistry*, **267**, 16188–99.

Bradley, R. and Wilesmith, J. W. (1993). Epidemiology and control of bovine spongiform encephalopathy (BSE). *British Medical Bulletin*, **49**, 932–59.

Brandner, S. *et al.* (1996). Normal host prion protein necessary for scrapie-induced neurotoxicity. *Nature*, **379**, 339–43.

Brown, D. R., Schmidt, B., and Kretzschmar, H. A. (1996). Role of microglia and host prion protein in neurotoxicity of a prion protein-fragment. *Nature*, **380**, 345–7.

Brown, P. and Gajdusek, D. C. (1991). The human spongiform encephalopathies: kuru, Creutzfeldt–Jakob disease, and the Gerstmann–Straussler–Scheinker syndrome. *Current Topics in Microbiology and Immunology*, **172**, 1–20.

Brown, P., Cervenakova, L., Boellaard, J. W., Stavrou, D., Goldfarb, L. G., and Gajdusek, D. C. (1994). Identification of a prnp gene mutation in Jakob's original Creutzfeldt–Jakob-disease family. *Lancet*, **344**, 130–1.

Bruce, M., Chree, A., McConnell, I., Foster, J., Pearson, G., and Fraser, H. (1994). Transmission of bovine spongiform encephalopathy and scrapie to mice—strain variation and the species barrier. *Philosophical Transactions of the Royal Society of London Series B-Biological Sciences*, **343**, 405–11.

Bruce, M. E. *et al.* (1997). Transmissions to mice indicate that 'new variant' CJD is caused by the BSE agent. *Nature*, **389**, 498–501.

Bueler, H. *et al.* (1992). Normal development and behaviour of mice lacking the neuronal cell-surface prp protein. *Nature*, **356**, 577–82.

Bueler, H. *et al.* (1993). Mice devoid of PrP are resistant to scrapie. *Cell*, **73**, 1339–47.

Caughey, B. (1994). Scrapie-associated prp accumulation and agent replication–effects of sulfated glycosaminoglycan analogs. *Philosophical Transactions of the Royal Society of London Series B-Biological Sciences*, **343**, 399–404.

Caughey, B. and Raymond, G. J. (1991). The scrapie-associated form of PrP is made from a cell-surface precursor that is both protease-sensitive and phospholipase-sensitive. *Journal of Biological Chemistry*, **266**, 18217–23.

Caughey, B. and Raymond, G. J. (1993). Sulfated polyanion inhibition of scrapie-associated PrP accumulation in cultured cells. *Journal of Virology*, **67**, 643–50.

Caughey, B., Kocisko, D. A., Raymond, G. J., and Lansbury, P. T. (1995). Aggregates of scrapie-associated prion protein induce the cell-free conversion of protease-sensitive prion protein to the protease-resistant state. *Chemistry and Biology*, **2**, 807–17.

Chazot, G., Broussolle, E., Lapras, C., Blattler, T., Aguzzi, A., and Kopp, N. (1996). New variant of Creutzfeldt–Jakob-disease in a 26-year-old French man. *Lancet*, **347**, 1181.

Cho, H. J. (1976). Is the scrapie agent a virus? *Nature*, **262**, 411–12.

Cho, H. J., Greig, A. S., Corp, C. R., Kimberlin, R. H., Chandler, R. L., and Millson, G. C. (1977). Virus-like particles from both control and scrapie-affected mouse brain. *Nature*, **267**, 459–60.

Colling, S. B., Collinge, J., and Jefferys, J. G. R. (1996). Hippocampal slices from prion protein null mice–disrupted Ca^{2+}-activated K^+ currents. *Neuroscience Letters*, **209**, 49–52.

Collinge, J. *et al.* (1994). Prion protein is necessary for normal synaptic function. *Nature*, **370**, 295–7.

Collinge, J. *et al.* (1995). Unaltered susceptibility to BSE in transgenic mice expressing human prion protein. *Nature*, **378**, 779–83.

Collinge, J., Sidle, D. C. L., Meads, J., Ironside, J., and Hill, A. F. (1996). Molecular analysis of prion strain variation and the aetiology of 'new variant' CJD. *Nature*, **383**, 685–90.

Curnow, R. N., Hodge, A., and Wilesmith, J. W. (1997). Analysis of the bovine spongiform encephalopathy maternal cohort study: the discordant case-control pairs. *Applied Statistics-Journal of the Royal Statistical Scoiety Series C*, **46**, 345–9.

Davanipour, Z., Alter, M., Sobel, E., Asher, D. M., and Carleton Gadjdusek, D. (1986). Transmissible virus dementia: evaluation of a zoonotic hypothesis. *Neuroepidemiology*, **5**, 194–206.

Dawson, M., Wells, G. A. H., and Parker, B. N. J. (1990*a*). Preliminary evidence of the experimental transmissibility of bovine spongiform encephalopathy to cattle. *Veterinary Record* **126**, 112–13.

Dawson, M., Wells, G. A. H., Parker, B. N. J., and Scott, A. C. (1990*b*). Primary parenteral transmission of bovine spongiform encephalopathy to the pig. *Veterinary Record*, **127**, 338–9.

Department of Health (1996). *New Variant of Creutzfeldt–Jakob disease (CJD)*. PL CMO (96) 5. HMSO, London.

Devillemeur, T. B. *et al.* (1992). Creutzfeldt–Jakob disease in 4 children treated with growth-hormone. *Revue Neurologique*, **148**, 328–34.

Dickinson, A. G. and Fraser, H. (1969). Modification of the pathogenesis of scrapie in mice by treatment of the agent. *Nature*, **222**, 892–3.

Dickinson, A. G., Stamp, J. T., and Renwick, C. C. (1974). Maternal and lateral transmission of scrapie in sheep. *Journal of Comparative Pathology*, **84**, 19–25.

Diringer, H. (1995). Proposed link between transmissible spongiform encephalopathies of man and animals. *Lancet*, **346**, 1208–10.

Ehlers, B. and Diringer, H. (1984). Dextran sulphate 500 delays and prevents mouse scrapie by impairment of agent replication in spleen. *Journal of General Virology*, **65**, 1325–30.

Esmonde, T., Lueck, C. J., Symon, L., Duchen, L. W., and Will, R. G. (1993). Creutzfeldt–Jakob disease and lyophilised dura mater grafts: report of two cases. *Journal of Neurology Neurosurgery and Psychiatry*, **56**, 999–1000, [Review].

Farquhar, C. F. and Dickinson, A. G. (1986). Prolongation of scrapie incubation period by an injection of dextran sulphate 500 within the month before or after infection. *Journal of General Virology*, **67**, 463–73.

Fischer, M. *et al.* (1996). Prion protein (Prp) with amino-proximal deletions restoring susceptibility of Prp knockout mice to scrapie. *EMBO Journal*, **15**, 1255–64.

Foote, W. C. *et al.* (1993). Prevention of scrapie transmission in sheep, using embryo transfer. *American Journal of Veterinary Research*, **54**, 1863–8.

Forloni, G. *et al.* (1993). Neurotoxicity of a prion protein-fragment. *Nature*, **362**, 543–6.

Foster, J. D. *et al.* (1992). Studies on maternal transmission of scrapie in sheep by embryo transfer. *Veterinary Record*, **130**, 341–3.

Foster, J. D., Hope, J., and Fraser, H. (1993). Transmission of bovine spongiform encephalopathy to sheep and goats. *Veterinary Record*, **133**, 339–41.

Foster, J. D. *et al.* (1996). Observations on the transmission of scrapie in experiments using embryo-transfer. *Veterinary Record*, **138**, 559–62.

Fraser, H. (1976). The pathology of a natural and experimental scrapie. *Frontiers of Biology*, **44**, 267–305 [Review].

Fraser, H. and Dickinson, A. G. (1978). Studies of the lymphoreticular system in the pathogenesis of scrapie: the role of spleen and thymus. *Journal of Comparative Pathology*, **88**, 563–73.welcome datacomp

Fraser, H. and Foster, J. D. (1993). Transmission to mice, sheep and goats and bioassay of bovine tissues. In *Transmissible spongiform encephalopathies*, (ed. R. Bradley and B. Marchant), Commission of the European Communities, Brussels, Belgium. pp. 145–59.

Fraser, H., McConnell, I., Wells, G. A. H., and Dawson, M. (1988). Transmission of bovine spongiform encephalopathy to mice. *Veterinary Record*, **123**, 472.

Goldfarb, L. G. *et al.* (1992). Fatal familial insomnia and familial Creutzfeldt–Jakob disease: disease phenotype determined by a DNA polymorphism. *Science*, **258**, 806–8.

Goldfarb, L. G., Brown, P., Cervenakova, L., and Gajdusek, D. C. (1994). Genetic-analysis of Creutzfeldt–Jakob-disease and related disorders. *Philosophical Transactions of the Royal Society of London Series B-Biological Sciences*, **343**, 379–84.

Goldmann, W. (1993). *Prp* gene and its association with spongiform encephalopathies. *British Medical Bulletin*, **49**, 839–59.

Goldmann, W., Hunter, N., Smith, G., Foster, J., and Hope, J. (1994). *Prp* genotype and agent effects in scrapie—change in allelic interaction with different isolates of agent in sheep, a natural host of scrapie. *Journal of General Virology*, **75**, 989–95.

Goldmann, W., Hunter, N., Somerville, R. A., and Hope, J. (1996). Prion phylogeny revisited. *Nature*, **382**, 32–3.

Hadlow, W. J. (1995). Neuropathology and the scrapie–kuru connection. *Brain Pathology*, **5**, 27–31.

Hadlow, W. J., Kennedy, R. C., and Race, R. E. (1982). Natural infection of Suffolk sheep with scrapie virus. *Journal of Infectious Diseases*, **146**, 657–64.

Harris, D. A., Falls, D. L., Johnson, F. A., and Fischbach, G. D. (1991). A prion-like protein from chicken brain copurifies with an acetylcholine receptor-inducing activity. *Proceedings of the National Academy of Sciences, USA*, **88**, 7664–8.

Harris, D. A., Gorodinsky, A., Lehmann, S., Moulder, K., and Shyng, S. L. (1996). Cell biology of the prion protein. *Current Topics In Microbiology and Immunology*, **207**, 77–93.

Herms, J. W., Kretzschmar, H. A., Titz, S., and Keller, B. U. (1995). Patch-clamp analysis of synaptic transmission to cerebellar Purkinje-cells of prion protein knockout mice. *European Journal of Neuroscience*, **7**, 2508–12.

Hogan, R. N. and Cavanagh, H. D. (1995). Transplantation of corneal tissue from donors with diseases of the central-nervous-system. *Cornea*, **14**, 547–53.

Hope, J. (1995). Mice and beef and brain diseases. *Nature*, **378**, 761–2.

Hope, J., Morton, L. J. D., Farquhar, C. F., Multhaup, G., Beyreuther, K., and Kimberlin, R. H. (1986). The major polypeptide of scrapie-associated fibrils (SAF) has the same size, charge-distribution and N-terminal protein-sequence as predicted for the normal brain protein (PrP). *EMBO Journal*, **5**, 2591–7.

Hope, J., Multhaup, G., Reekie, L. J., Kimberlin, R. H., and Beyreuther, K. (1988*a*). Molecular pathology of scrapie-associated fibril protein (PrP) in mouse brain affected by the ME7 strain of scrapie. *European Journal of Biochemistry*, **172**, 271–7.

Hope, J., *et al.* (1988*b*). Fibrils from brains of cows with new cattle disease contain scrapie-associated protein. *Nature*, **336**, 390–92.

Hope, J., Shearman, M. S., Baxter, H. C., Chong, A., Kelly, S. M., and Price, N. C. (1996). Cytotoxicity of prion protein peptide (PrP106–126) differs in mechanism from the cytotoxic activity of the Alzheimers-disease amyloid peptide, α-Beta-25–35. *Neurodegeneration*, **5**, 1–11.

Hunter, N., Foster, J. D., and Hope, J. (1992). Natural scrapie in British sheep: breeds, ages and PrP gene polymorphisms. *Veterinary Record*, **130**, 389–92.

Hunter, N., Goldmann, W., Benson, G., Foster, J. D., and Hope, J. (1993). Swaledale sheep affected by natural scrapie differ significantly in PrP genotype frequencies from healthy sheep and those selected for reduced incidence of scrapie. *Journal of General Virology*, **74**, 1025–31.

Ingrosso, L., Ladogana, A., and Pocchiari, M. (1995). Congo red prolongs the incubation period in scrapie-infected hamsters. *Journal of Virology* **69**, 506–8.

Jeffrey, M., Goodsir, C. M., Bruce, M. E., McBride, P. A., Scott, J. R., and Halliday, W. G. (1992). Infection specific prion protein (PrP) accumulates on neuronal plasmalemma in scrapie infected mice. *Neuroscience Letters*, **147**, 106–9.

Jeffrey, M., Goodsir, C. M., Fowler, N., Hope, J., Bruce, M. E., and McBride, P. A. (1996). Ultrastructural immuno-localization of synthetic prion protein peptide antibodies in 87V murine scrapie. *Neurodegeneration*, **5**, 101–9.

Kaneko, K. *et al.* (1995). Prion protein (prp) synthetic peptides induce cellular prp to acquire properties of the scrapie isoform. *Proceedings of the National Academy of Sciences, USA*, **92**, 11160–4.

Kimberlin, R. H. and Walker, C. A. (1986). Suppression of scrapie infection in mice by heteropolyanion 23, dextran sulfate, and some other polyanions. *Antimicrobial Agents and Chemotherapy*, **30**, 409–13.

Kimberlin, R. H. and Walker, C. A. (1989*a*). Pathogenesis of scrapie in mice after intragastric infection. *Virus Research*, **12**, 213–20.

Kimberlin, R. H. and Walker, C. A. (1989*b*). The role of the spleen in the neuroinvasion of scrapie in mice. *Virus Research*, **12**, 201–11.

Kirkwood, J. K. and Cunningham, A. A. (1994). Epidemiologic observations on spongiform encephalopathies in captive wild animals in the British-Isles. *Veterinary Record*, **135**, 296–303.

Kirkwood, J. K., Cunningham, A. A., Wells, G. A., Wilesmith, J. W., and Barnett, J. E. (1993). Spongiform encephalopathy in a herd of greater kudu (*Tragelaphus strepsiceros*): epidemiological observations. *Veterinary Record*, **133**, 360–4.

Kirkwood, J. K., Cunningham, A. A., Austin, A. R., Wells, G. A. H., and Sainsbury, A. W. (1994). Spongiform encephalopathy in a greater kudu (*Tragelaphus strepsiceros*) introduced into an affected group. *Veterinary Record*, **134**, 167–8.

Kirschbaum, W. R. (1968). *Jakob–Creutzfeldt disease*. Elsevier, Amsterdam.

Kitamoto, T., Muramoto, T., Mohri, S., Dohura, K., and Tateishi, J. (1991). Abnormal isoform of prion protein accumulates in follicular dendritic cells in mice with Creutzfeldt-Jakob disease. *Journal of Virology*, **65**, 6292–5.

Kocisko, D. A. *et al.* (1994). Cell-free formation of protease-resistant prion protein. *Nature*, **370**, 471–4.

Kocisko, D. A., Priola, S. A., Raymond, G. J., Chesebro, B., Lansbury, P. T., and Caughey, B. (1995). Species-specificity in the cell-free conversion of prion protein to protease-resistant forms—a model for the scrapie species barrier. *Proceedings of the National Academy of Sciences, USA*, **92**, 3923–7.

Krakauer, D. C., Pagel, M., Southwood, T. R. E., and Zanotto, P. M. (1996). Prion phylogeny. *Nature*, **380**, 675.

Kretzschmar, H. A. *et al.* (1991). Prion protein mutation in family first reported by Gerstmann, Straussler, and Scheinker. *Lancet*, 337, 1160, [letter].

Ladogana, A. *et al.* (1992). Sulphate polyanions prolong the incubation period of scrapie-infected hamsters. *Journal of General Virology*, **73**, 661–5.

Lasmezas, C. I. *et al.* (1996). Immune system-dependent and system-independent replication of the scrapie agent. *Journal of Virology*, **70**, 1292–5.

Laszlo, L. *et al.* (1992). Lysosomes as key organelles in the pathogenesis of prion encephalopathies. *Journal of Pathology*, **166**, 333–41.

Liberski, P. P., Yanagihara, R., Gibbs, C. J. Jr, and Gajdusek, D. C. (1988). Tubulovesicular structures in experimental Creutzfeldt–Jakob disease and scrapie. *Intervirology*, **29**, 115–19.

Lledo, P. M., Tremblay, P., Dearmond, S. J., Prusiner, S. B., and Nicoll, R. A. (1996). Mice deficient for prion protein exhibit normal neuronal excitability and synaptic transmission in the hippocampus. *Proceedings of the National Academy of Sciences, USA*, **93**, 2403–7.

McKinley, M. P., Bolton, D. C., and Prusiner, S. B. (1983). A protease-resistant protein is a structural component of the scrapie prion. *Cell*, **35**, 57–62.

McKinley, M. P., Braunfeld, M. B., Bellinger, C. G., and Prusiner, S. B. (1986). Molecular characteristics of prion rods purified from scrapie-infected hamster brains. *Journal of Infectious Diseases*, **154**, 110–20.

Manson, J., West, J. D., Thomson, V., McBride, P., Kaufman, M. H., and Hope, J. (1992). The prion protein gene—a role in mouse embryogenesis. *Development*, **115**, 117–22.

Manson, J. C., Clarke, A. R., Hooper, M. L., Aitchison, L., McConnell, I., and Hope, J. (1994*a*). 129/ola mice carrying a null mutation in PrP that abolishes messenger-RNA production are developmentally normal. *Molecular Neurobiology* **8**, 121–7.

Manson, J. C., Clarke, A. R., McBride, P. A., McConnell, I., and Hope, J. (1994*b*). PrP gene dosage determines the timing but not the final intensity or distribution of lesions in scrapie pathology. *Neurodegeneration*, **3**, 331–40.

Manson, J., Hope, J., Clarke, A. R., Johnston, A., Black, C., and MacLeod, N. (1995). PrP gene dosage and long term potentiation. *Neurodegeneration*, **4**, 113–15.

Merz, P. A., Somerville, R. A., Wisniewski, H. M., and Iqbal, K. (1981). Abnormal fibrils from scrapie-infected brain. *Acta Neuropathologica*, **54**, 63–74.

Merz, P. A. *et al.* (1984). Infection-specific particle from the unconventional slow virus diseases. *Science*, **225**, 437–40.

Mimms, C. A. and White, D. O. (1984). *Viral pathogenesis and immunology*, (1st ed.) Blackwell Scientific Publications, Oxford.

Muller, W. E. G. *et al.* (1993). Cytoprotective effect of NMDA receptor antagonists on prion protein (prion (sc))-induced toxicity in rat cortical cell-cultures. *European Journal of Pharmacology-Molecular Pharmacology Section*, **246**, 261–7.

Narang, H. K. (1990). Detection of single-stranded-DNA in scrapie-infected brain by electron-microscopy. *Journal of Molecular Biology*, **216**, 469–73.

Ozel, M. and Diringer, H. (1994). Small virus-like structure in fractions from scrapie hamster brain. *Lancet*, **343**, 894–5.

Palmer, M. S., Dryden, A. J., Hughes, J. T., and Collinge, J. (1991). Homozygous prion protein genotype predisposes to sporadic Creutzfeldt–Jakob disease. *Nature*, **352**, 340–2. [Published erratum appears in *Nature* (1991) **352**, 547.]

Pattison, I. H., Hoare, M. N., Jebbett, J. N., and Watson, W. A. (1974). Further observations on the production of scrapie in sheep by oral dosing with foetal membranes from scrapie-affected sheep. *British Veterinary Journal*, **130**, 65–7.

Pearson, G. R. *et al.* (1992). Feline spongiform encephalopathy–fibril and prp studies. *Veterinary Record*, **131**, 307–10.

Perovic, S., Pergande, G., Ushijima, H., Kelve, M., Forrest, J., and Muller, W. E. G. (1995). Flupirtine partially prevents neuronal injury-induced by prion protein-fragment and lead acetate. *Neurodegeneration*, **4**, 369–74.

Prusiner, S. B., Hadlow, W. J., Eklund, C. M., and Race, R. E. (1977). Sedimentation properties of the scrapie agent. *Proceedings of the National Academy of Sciences, USA*, **74**, 4656–60.

Raymond, G. J. *et al.* (1997). Molecular assessment of the potential transmissibilities of BSE and scrapie to humans. *Nature*, **388**, 285–8.

Riek, R., Hornemann, S., Wider, G., Billeter, M., Glockshuber, R., and Wurthrich, K. (1996). NMR structure of the mouse prion protein domain PrP (121–231). *Nature*, **382**, 180–2.

Robinson, M. M. *et al.* (1994). Experimental infection of mink with bovine spongiform encephalopathy. *Journal of General Virology* **75**, 2151–5.

Rowher, R. G. (1991). The scrapie agent: 'A virus by any other name'. In *Transmissible spongiform encephalopathies: scrapie, BSE and related disorders*, (ed. B. W. Chesebro), pp. 195–232. Heidelberg. Springer-Verlag,

Sailer, A., Bueler, H., Fischer, M., Aguzzi, A., and Weissmann, C. (1994). No propagation of prions in mice devoid of prp. *Cell*, **77**, 967–8.

Sakaguchi, S. *et al.* (1996). Loss of cerebellar Purkinje-cells in aged mice homozygous for a disrupted Prp gene. *Nature*, **380**, 528–31.

Salvatore, M. *et al.* (1995). Apolipoprotein-e in sporadic and familial Creutzfeldt–Jakob- disease. *Neuroscience Letters*, **199**, 95–8.

Sarkozi, E., Askanas, V., and Engel, W. K. (1994). Abnormal accumulation of prion protein messenger-RNA in muscle-fibers of patients with sporadic inclusion-body myositis and hereditary inclusion-body myopathy. *American Journal of Pathology*, **145**, 1280–4.

Schatzl, H. M., Dacosta, M., Taylor, L., Cohen, F. E., and Prusiner, S. B. (1995). Prion protein gene variation among primates. *Journal of Molecular Biology*, **245**, 362–74.

Scott, J. R., Reekie, L. J. D., and Hope, J. (1991). Evidence for intrinsic control of scrapie pathogenesis in the murine visual system. *Neuroscience Letters*, **133**, 141–4.

Scott, J. R., Foster, J. D., and Fraser, H. (1993). Conjunctival instillation of scrapie in mice can produce disease. *Veterinary Microbiology*, **34**, 305–9.

SEAC (Spongiform Encephalopathy Advisory Committee) (1994). *Transmissible spongiform encephalopathies. A summary of present knowledge and research*. HMSO, London.

Stahl, N., Borchelt, D. R., Hsiao, K., and Prusiner, S. B. (1987). Scrapie prion protein contains a phosphatidylinositol glycolipid. *Cell*, **51**, 229–40.

Tateishi, J., Kitamoto, T., Ishikawa, G., and Manabe, S. I. (1993). Removal of causative agent of Creutzfeldt–Jakob disease (CJD) through membrane filtration method. *Membrane*, **18**, 357–62.

Tateishi, J. *et al.* (1995). First experimental transmission of fatal familial insomnia. *Nature*, **376**, 434–5.

Taylor, D. M. (1993). Inactivation of SE agents. *British Medical Bulletin*, **49**, 810–21.

Taylor, D. M. and Diprose, M. F. (1996). The response of the 22A strain of scrapie agent to microwave irradiation compared with boiling. *Neuropathology and Applied Neurobiology*, **22**, 256–8.

Taylor, D. M. *et al.* (1994). Decontamination studies with the agents of bovine spongiform encephalopathy and scrapie. *Archives of Virology*, **139**, 313–26.

Taylor, D. M., Ferguson, C. E., Bostock, C. J., and Dawson, M. (1995). Absence of disease in mice receiving milk from cows with bovine spongiform encephalopathy. *Veterinary Record*, **136**, 592.

Taylor, D. M., Ferguson, C. E., and Chree, A. (1996*a*). Absence of detectable infectivity in trachea of BSE-affected cattle. *Veterinary Record*, **138**, 160–1.

Taylor, D. M., McConnell, I., and Fraser, H. (1996*b*). Scrapie infection can be established readily through skin scarification in immunocompetent but not immunodeficient mice. *Journal of General Virology*, **77**, 1595–9.

Telling, G. C. *et al.* (1995). Prion propagation in mice expressing human and chimeric prp transgenes implicates the interaction of cellular prp with another protein. *Cell*, **83**, 79–90.

Tobler, I. *et al.* (1996). Altered circadian activity rhythms and sleep in mice devoid of prion protein. *Nature*, **380**, 639–42.

Weissmann, C., Bueler, H., Fischer, M., Sauer, A., and Aguet, M. (1994). Susceptibility to scrapie in mice is dependent on prpc. *Philosophical Transactions of the Royal Society of London Series B-Biological Sciences*, **343**, 431–3.

Wells, G. A. H. *et al.* (1987). A novel progressive spongiform encephalopathy in cattle. *Veterinary Record*, **121**, 419–20.

Wells, G. A. H. *et al.* (1994). Infectivity in the ileum of cattle challenged orally with bovine spongiform encephalopathy. *Veterinary Record*, **135**, 40–1.

Westaway, D. *et al.* (1994). Degeneration of skeletal-muscle, peripheral-nerves, and the CNS in transgenic mice over-expressing wild-type prion proteins. *Neurology*, **44**, 260.

Wilesmith, J. W., Wells, G. A. H., Cranwell, M. P., and Ryan, J. B. M. (1988). Bovine spongiform encephalopathy—epidemiological studies. *Veterinary Record*, **123**, 638–44.

Will, R. G. *et al.* (1996). A new variant of Creutzfeldt–Jakob-disease in the UK. *Lancet*, **347**, 921–5.

Wisniewski, H. M., Sigurdarson, S., Rubenstein, R., Kascsak, R. J., and Carp, R. I. (1996). Mites as vectors for scrapie. *Lancet*, **347**, 1114.

37 RABIES

A. A. King

SUMMARY

Rabies virus thrives in most parts of the world; it can replicate in all warm-blooded animals, within which it conceals itself from their immunological defences; almost invariably the resultant disease is fatal, yet the virus ensures its own survival by causing the afflicted, when close to death, to find another host and victim (Gardner and King 1991).

Rabies is a disease of animals, and infection of humans is, almost always, a 'spillover' event from an infected dog. Over 90 per cent of human deaths from the disease occur in the tropics. From regions where disease surveillance is thorough and reporting is reliable, the current disease picture is one of either canine (variously known as urban or street) rabies, with little or no rabies in wildlife species, or of wildlife (sylvatic) rabies with spillover into domesticated animals.

Throughout the near global extent of the disease various mammalian species other than the dog may act as principal hosts and vectors. The majority of rabies wildlife hosts are small to medium-sized omnivores that scavenge for food and/or prey on rodents, other small vertebrates, and invertebrates. Often their diet is supplemented by human refuse and such a bountiful food supply permits them to reach substantial population densities in and around human habitation. All have high intrinsic population growth rates, thus permitting rapid recovery from severe losses due to disease; this regenerative ability ensures survival of the species and continuation of a rabies epizootic despite high case density within it (Wandeler 1991).

Traditional surveillance, monoclonal antibody studies, and genome structure characterization confirm that some rabies virus biotypes posses unique speciation as a result of mutual adaptation of virus variant and host population. Within an affected area the disease is usually manifest by a single host reservoir and vector species, disease in other animals represents a spillover of infection from sporadic contact with the major host species.

This picture, however, does not apply to rabies in bats. Within the Chiroptera there is a tremendous diversity of social organizations, different species exploit different but specific resources and all have low intrinsic population growth rates (Wandeler *et al.* 1994*a*). Virus strains prominent in North American insectivorous bats and South American vampire bats are also of serotype 1 but are distinct from those of terrestrial animal origin; virus strains from African frugivorous and insectivorous bats are of different serotypes (serotypes 2 and 4 respectively), whereas the viruses from European insectivorous bats, though not as yet fully classified, are distinct from those of American and African origin. The epidemiology of rabies in bats is poorly understood and, with the exception of vampire bat rabies, poorly investigated.

The majority of rabies-free countries are islands ranging in size from continental Australia to tiny groups of islands in major oceans. They are able to remain rabies-free by the application of importation controls which usually include quarantine.

With a few notable exceptions, the control of canine rabies is an intractable problem and the disease is still epizootic in most countries of Africa, Asia, and South America. Most human deaths from rabies occur in these countries. Prevention of human rabies is dependent on the control of canine rabies and this can only be achieved by the control of stray dog populations and the mass immunization of the remainder.

In Africa, as human habitation has expanded, canine rabies has spread to wildlife species and some already endangered canids now face extinction from the disease. In North America and Europe, human deaths from rabies are now rare due to the control of, or absence of, canine rabies. However, rabies exacts a terrible toll of wildlife and while the disease exists in these species the threat to domesticated animals and to man persists.

THE RABIES VIRUS

TAXONOMY

Taxonomically, rabies viruses belong to the Rhabdoviridae family, a constituent of the order Mononegavirales in which the viruses are characterized by a non-segmented negative-sense genome. The family is divided into two serologically distinct genera,

Table 37.1 Lyssavirus serotypes and genotypes: their sources and geographic distribution (adapted and updated from King and Crick 1988)

Name Sero/genotype	Source(s) of virus in nature	Known geographic distribution
Rabies 1/1	Dog, cat, bat, human; wild carnivora, e.g. red, grey, bat-eared fox, skunk, raccoon, jackal; mongoose	Worldwide except Australia, New Zealand, Antarctica, parts of Scandinavia, United Kingdom, Japan, Hawaii, and some other islands
Lagos bat 2/2	Frugivorous bat, cat, dog	Nigeria, Ethiopia, Senegal Central African Republic, Zimbabwe, South Africa
Mokola 3/3	Shrew, cat, dog, rodent, human	Nigeria, Ethiopia, Cameroon, Central African Republic, Zimbabwe, South Africa
Duvenhage 4/4	Insectivorous bat, human	Zimbabwe, South Africa
EBL 1[a] /5	Insectivorous bat (chiefly serotines), human	Germany, Poland, Ukraine, Netherlands, Denmark, France, Spain
EBL 2[a] /6	Insectivorous bat (*Myotis* spp.), human	Netherlands, Denmark, Switzerland, Finland, United Kingdom

[a] EBL, European bat lyssaviruses (not serotyped).

Vesiculovirus and *Lyssavirus*. The *Vesiculovirus* genus includes the viruses causing vesicular stomatitis and antigenically related viruses and the *Lyssavirus* genus includes rabies, the rabies-related viruses, and many others which share only a distant relationship to rabies.

By use of serological and molecular techniques, four lyssavirus serotypes encompassing six genotypes are recognized currently. The distinction between viruses of serotype 1 (rabies), serotype 2 (Lagos bat), serotype 3 (Mokola), and serotype 4 (Duvenhage) (Table 37.1) was established by cross-immunization experiments in animals, and these serotypes were shown to correspond to four genotypes (1–4). Differences within the virus ribonuclear protein (RNP) of the serotype 4 members Duvenhage (Africa) and the European bat lyssaviruses EBL 1 and EBL 2, detected by monoclonal antibody antinucleocapsid (Mab-N) reaction patterns by King (1991), have been confirmed by molecular techniques, and thus the latter two viruses correspond to genotypes 5 and 6 respectively (Bourhy *et al.* 1993).

Rabies virions are bullet-shaped with an average length of 180 (130–300) nm and diameter of 75 (60–110) nm. The cylindrical symmetry of the virion is formed by the approximately 165 × 50 nm helical nucleocapsid of 30–35 coils with a periodicity of around 4.5 nm. The lipid-containing envelope is a bilayer surrounding the RNP. The matrix protein is thought to line the inner layer, although studies of vesicular stomatitis virus (VSV) by Barge *et al.* (1993) suggest that it could lie inside the RNP coil. The glycoprotein is transmembranic and anchored within the bilayer in such a way that the surface of the virion is covered by 9 nm 'spikes' or peplomers formed by trimers of G protein at 5 nm intervals. The frequently observed irregular shape of the planar end of the infectious virion may be due to the formation of a 'tail' during budding from the plasma membrane at the time of release from the infected host cell (Wunner 1991). Observed variations in virion length may be due to differences in virus strain or to the presence of defective interfering (DI) particles. Truncated DI particles, which vary in size from approximately one-third to two-thirds of the standard rabies particle length, lack portions of the virus genome RNA. They are incapable of self-replication and require the presence of wild-type virus to complement their deficient genes. Therefore, they are more frequently observed *in vitro* in persistently infected cultures and in repeated high-multiplicity passages (Holland 1987).

MOLECULAR BIOLOGY

The genome RNA of a sequenced rabies virus was shown to consist of 11 932 nucleotides. From the 3′ to the 5′ end the genomic RNA encodes a leader RNA of about 50 nucleotides, followed by genes which encode the nucleoprotein (N), phosphoprotein (M1), matrix protein (M2), glycoprotein (G), and polymerase (L) (Tordo and Kouknetzoff 1993) (Fig. 37.1). Each gene is composed of an internal protein-coding region flanked by non-translated regions. Genes are also separated by non-transcribed intergenic regions. The latter are generally short (less than 5 nucleotides) and are bordered by the start and stop signals (Fig. 37.1) consisting of nine-nucleotide consensus sequences that govern gene transcription. Despite the considerable length (450 nucleotides) of the G–L intergenic region, it encodes no substantial polypeptide and thus has been proposed to correspond to a remnant gene (pseudogene).

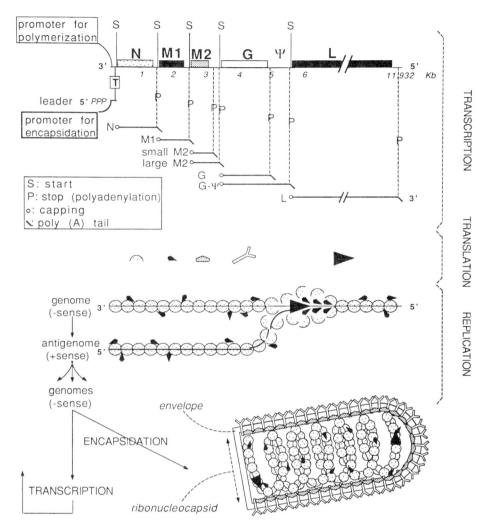

Fig. 37.1 Diagrammatic representation of the rabies virus genome, the process of transcription, translation, and replication of the structure of the complete virion (kindly supplied by Dr N. Todo, Laboratoire des Lyssavirus, Institut Pasteur, Paris).

Nucleotide sequence variation in the nucleoprotein, glycoprotein, and pseudogene regions of lyssavirus genomes has been used to infer epidemiological relationships. The nucleoprotein gene is highly conserved and strongly expressed and mutation rate within this gene is considered to be slow enough to enable epidemiological inferences to be made retrospectively for decades or even centuries. On the other hand, the pseudogene shows greatest variation without apparent selective pressure and, on this basis, has been suggested as an appropriate 'clock' for measuring virus evolution, particularly between closely related isolates (Sacramento *et al.* 1991).

The G and N are the two proteins which have been most extensively studied as immunogenic components of rabies virus. The G protein possesses the biological and immunological functions of cell surface receptor and antibody binding site. These functions reside in the 439 amino acid region of the G protein ecto-domain and this region defines the serotype. Variation in the amino acid sequence of this region may therefore alter the pathogenic, antigenic, or immunologic properties of the virus (Wunner 1991). The N protein is abundantly produced in infection; group specificity is determined by its cross-reactivity and it has an important role in diagnosis and virus identification by Mab-N techniques.

DISEASE MECHANISMS

Infection other than as a result of the bite of an infected animal is purported to be extremely rare and disease transmission occurs when virus present in the saliva of an infected animal contaminates the tissue cells of the bite victim. Rabies virus cannot penetrate unbroken skin but can enter the body across intact mucous membranes such as the conjunctivae and those lining the nose, mouth, anus, and external genital organs. Infection by inhalation of airborne rabies virus is extremely rare in humans but may be an important route of transmission in certain species of bats. Human to human transmission has not been reported in modern times, except for rare instances of mechanical transmission via corneal transplant surgery. In humans, the mortality rate following severe bites by infected dogs is about 45 per cent (Warrell 1988).

Cellular infection involves attachment of virus to the plasma membrane, entry of virus into the cell, replication, assembly of virions on intracytoplasmic membranes or plasma membrane, and release into intercellular spaces. Components of the plasma membrane which may be implicated in the virus attachment process include carbohydrate moieties, phospholipids, and gangliosides.

Following attachment, virus enters the host cell either by fusion of the viral envelope with the plasma membrane and extrusion of the ribonucleocapsid components into the cytoplasm, or by endocytosis followed by fusion of the viral envelope with the membrane of the endocytotic vesicle. Thereafter, replication and transcription of genomic RNA, translation of mRNA, and maturation take place. Budding of virions on neuronal plasma membrane in the CNS frequently occurs on dendritic plasma membrane at or adjacent to synapses. There is little evidence of cellular injury as determined by light microscopy.

Several reviews have been published (notably Charlton 1988; Baer and Lentz 1991; Tsiang 1992) of disease mechanisms involved in rabies and rabies-related virus infection.

The virus is neurotropic, and although there is good evidence that muscle at the inoculation site can be infected, there is no convincing evidence that such infection is a link in the pathogenesis—it may be merely incidental. Long-term retention, not necessarily with replication, of virus in myocytes at the site of infection may, however, explain the long incubation periods that occasionally occur in rabies; in addition, virus that is sequestered in tissue that is not part of the nervous system would theoretically permit more effective postexposure treatment than similar insulation within neuronal elements (Charlton 1994). Immunohistological or molecular biological techniques, such as the polymerase chain reaction, suggest that virus may enter the CNS and/or cerebrospinal ganglia before a cycle of virus replication in non-neural tissue has occurred. Rabies is an opportunistic virus and it may be that either of these pathways can be used.

There is substantial evidence that the nicotinic acetylcholine receptor (AChR) is a receptor for rabies virus and that virus uptake by either or both the axon terminal and myocyte is facilitated by the occurrence of nicotinic AChRs on postsynaptic membrane at the neuromuscular junction and on the sarcolemma. However, although the preponderance of evidence suggests a role for AChRs in the uptake of virus at the inoculation site, uptake *in vivo* may still be non-specific as it is *in vitro*, where the virus is able to infect many types of cultured cells, most of which do not possess AChRs.

Transport of rabies virus to the CNS as incomplete virions within endocytotic vesicles, occurs in axons of peripheral nerves and is by retrograde axoplasmic flow. Viral amplification may then occur in neuronal perikarya of either motor neurones in the brain stem or spinal cord, primary sensory neurones in cerebrospinal ganglia, or neurones in autonomic ganglia.

Dissemination of infection throughout the CNS is probably effected mainly by cycles of replication combined with intra-axonal (and to a lesser extent dendritic) transport and direct transneuronal transfer of virus. Electron microscopic evidence indicates the transcellular transfer of virions from the dendrite of one neurone to the axonal terminal of another.

Infection spreads from the entry site in the CNS to most areas of the brain and spinal cord. Spread can be extremely rapid and neurones with long axons may provide a means of 'leapfrogging' of infection to distant areas (Charlton 1988). Infection spreads to many motor neurones in the brain-stem/spinal cord and to neurones in cerebrospinal and autonomic ganglia. In natural infections, centrifugal neural transport leads to non-neural cell infection, and in the later stages of disease virus or antigen may be detected in several tissues. With the exception of salivary glands, such infection would appear to be incidental and is superfluous to disease transmission.

Infection of the salivary glands may lead to the secretion of virus in the saliva for many days before the onset of clinical signs. Reports of such preclinical periods range from 3 days in cats (Vaughn *et al.* 1963) through 10 days in vampire bats (Ruiz and Diaz 1990), 12 days in Mexican freetail bats (Baer and Bales 1967), 14 days in dogs infected with an Ethiopian virus isolate (Fekadu 1991), and 29 days in foxes (Aubert *et al.* 1991).

The mechanisms involved in the expression of clinical signs are largely unknown and, although the course of disease is unpredictable, the infecting virus strain may be a factor. For example, the paralytic form of human rabies is a more frequent outcome in persons infected with bat or fixed strains. Aggressive behaviour is a complex neurological phenomenon involving many regions of the brain and it may be that aggression in rabies is related to the presence of virus in the midbrain raphe nuclei and the medial hypothalamus, since these are inhibitory centres of aggressive behaviour. It may also be that the distribution of the virus within the brain has a bearing on whether the disease becomes manifest in the paralytic or furious form. The paralytic form of rabies in man is characterized by nerve cell destruction, microglial proliferation, and perivascular infiltration, mainly in the spinal cord and brain-stem, whereas in furious rabies the inflammatory reaction, vascular changes, and inclusion bodies are more widespread and include the thalamus, hypothalamus, cerebellum, and cerebral cortex. However, the visible histological change or damage to cellular organelles is usually far less obvious than that seen in, for example, poliomyelitis.

In most rabid animals the lesions are typical of a non-suppurative encephalomyelitis with ganglioneuritis and parotid adenitis, with the most significant lesions in the pons to hypothalamus and cervical spinal cord. Meningitis is usually present and perivascular cuffs contain lymphocytes, plasma cells, macrophages, and occasionally erythrocytes; the number of plasma cells present increases with the duration of clinical signs.

Spongiform lesions, which have been observed in naturally infected skunks, foxes, sheep, horses, cattle, and cats, but not in experimentally infected mice and rats, appear as vacuolation in the neuropil of the grey matter, with the thalamus and inner layers of the cerebral cortex being the most frequently and severely affected areas. The spongiform change occurs probably in less than 2–3 days and is not virus strain dependent; since most of the vacuoles begin in dendrites, it is likely that the lesions are due to an indirect effect of rabies infection.

Death results from the involvement of vital nerve centres leading to respiratory arrest. Although there is some experimental evidence of immunopathology and immunosuppression, host immune responses do not appear to influence the clinical course of the disease.

VIRUS GROWTH AND SURVIVAL

Following attempts by many workers to isolate virus in explant cultures, the susceptibility of primary mouse kidney cell cultures to rabies virus infection was reported (Vieuchange 1956) and 2 years later both street and fixed rabies viruses were serially passaged in primary hamster cells (Kissling 1958). In time, a multitude of cell types has been used for rabies virus cultivation, not only for diagnostic purposes but also for the production of vaccines and for research.

Baby hamster kidney (BHK-21) cells are now routinely used in many diagnostic laboratories. They are hardy, require a relatively simple medium supplemented with inexpensive bovine serum and, since they do not require additional carbon dioxide to support growth, they can be used in a closed and therefore safer culture system.

Neuroblastoma cells of human or murine origin are also widely used in rabies diagnosis, and in many laboratories their culture is used in the place of mouse inoculation as a method of virus isolation; they have been shown to be more susceptible to rabies virus infection than any other current cell line. Mouse neuroblastoma (NA-C1300) cells, which are hypoxanthine–guanine phosphoribosyl transferase-deficient, are especially useful, since they share a number of characteristics with human neurones, including gross microscopic and fine structural neurone-like morphology and the presence of microtubular protein, neurotransmitter synthetic enzymes, and electrically excitable cell membranes with acetylcholine receptors.

In many cell systems, considerable periods of adaptation and prolonged passaging may be required before substantial yields of virus can be obtained. However, high yields of virus can be obtained when fresh cells in suspension are infected and then allowed to form monolayers. The most rapid adaptation takes place when the monolayer is digested and a proportion (25 per cent) of the infected cells is passaged either daily or every 2 days, with or without the addition of further fresh cells. Not all viruses adapt at the same rate and two to five passages may be required before 100 per cent of the cells become infected and release virus into the supernatant. An advantage of the method is that a proportion of the infected cells can be used to seed multi-well plates for antigenic profile determination using monoclonal antibodies.

INCUBATION PERIOD

The wide variability of the incubation period of rabies in man was noted in early literature. Blancou (1994) has cited periods of between 7 and 100 days (Sun Si Miao of China, Sixth century), between 9 days and 7 years (Bernard de Gordon, thirteenth century), and between 20 days and several years (Fracastoro, sixteenth century). Similar variability noted in animals, however, may have been influenced by the difficulty of establishing the day on which the animal became infected. In modern times the incubation period in man, as defined by the interval between exposure and the first symptoms in the prodromal stage, is more variable than in any other acute infection. Fishbein (1991) has cited extremes from as short as 4 days to as long as 14 and 19 years, although in cases with very long incubation periods the possibility of an intervening second exposure often could not be ruled out. There is little doubt, however, that extraordinarily long incubation periods do occur: in a virological examination of unexplained rabies in three United States immigrants, the isolates were variants with distinctive antigenic or genetic characteristics which matched those found in specimens of rabid animals from or near the country in which the patient had lived prior to emigration; the migrants had not returned to their country of origin within 4 years, 6 years and 11 months, respectively (Smith *et al.* 1991).

Analysis of the incubation periods of 1555 patients revealed that although none was shorter than 10 days', 29.8 per cent were of 10–30 days'. 54.4 per cent were of 31–90 days', 14.6 per cent were of 91–365 days' and 1.2 per cent were of >365 days' duration (Fishbein 1991). Factors which may influence the length of the incubation period include the site of the bite (in general, the nearer the head, the shorter the period) and its severity, the degree of innervation of the bite site (bites on the face, neck, and hands are more dangerous, presumably because of their rich nerve supply), the quantity of virus 'inoculated', and the age and immune status of the host. The incubation period in children is purported to be shorter than that in adults and is probably associated with their infant stature and unusually severe or multiple bites on the face, head, and neck.

THE HOSTS

CLINICAL SYMPTOMS IN MAN

Rabies should be suspected when neurological symptoms follow an animal bite. The incubation period is followed by a 2–10 day prodromal period of non-specific symptoms, during which the patient may feel altogether unwell with tiredness, weakness, loss of appetite, headache, fever, and other aches and pains. The variety of conditions may suggest involvement of the respiratory or gastrointestinal systems or of the CNS. Paraesthesia or itching at the site of the bite is common during this stage. There may then be a period of acute nervous system dysfunction and this may lead to paralytic rabies or, in about 80 per cent of cases, furious rabies. Warrell (1986), from long experience of diagnosis in humans, summarized furious rabies symptoms thus: 'This short and horrifyingly hectic clinical course is characterized initially by hydrophobia, aerophobia and periods of extreme excitement, interspersed with intervals of lucidity and full comprehension; and finally by unconsciousness and complete paralysis'. In the absence of intensive care, coma may last for hours or days before respiratory arrest.

CLINICAL SIGNS IN ANIMALS

Clinical signs of rabies in animals are manifest by behavioural changes and unexplained paralysis.

Normally, domestic pets are friendly, are not easily disturbed, look healthy, and exhibit a predictable behavioural pattern. Wild animals also exhibit characteristic behavioural patterns—normally they are afraid of man and in a free environment they usually prefer to slip away unseen and to avoid contact. Exceptions to this retiring behaviour may occur: normally shy wild animals may become semi-tame as a result of protection and feeding, especially in parks and campsites, where, in close contact with man, their normal character may be abandoned as they learn to take food from holiday-makers.

Rabid animals do not behave normally. The signs of disease are quite variable and duration of illness may range from less than 1 day to a week or more; death often intervenes 2–7 days after onset of illness. Clinical disease may take either the dumb or furious form or most often a combination of the two. In dumb rabies, hypersensitivity is not readily apparent, although it may occur as a minor and transient manifestation. The first changes seen in a normal, healthy animal are somewhat benign, the animal is lethargic, appears unhealthy, with some slight incoordination. This condition may remain stable for about 12 hours then deteriorate rapidly as quadriplegia develops; mandibular paralysis with loss of swallowing reflex may be observed (dogs do not exhibit hydrophobia) and the animal may die without other signs.

In the prodromal stage of furious rabies, the pet animal appears unusually alert and responsive and the owner may interpret this as the pet being unusually well. This slight behavioural change would not be readily recognized in a wild animal. The abnormally alert pet, however, soon shows discreet changes of discomfort and uneasiness. Cats in particular show an uneasy facial expression and frequently mew, repeatedly extend and retract their claws, and exhibit a restless dancing movement of the front feet. They may respond to prodding, showing impatience and intolerance of minor irritations.

Rabid wild animals show similar signs of sensitivity and discomfort and may bite at a source of irritation as hypersensitivity to external irritation increases; they will snap at anything within reach and in biting they may hold tenaciously, making them particularly dangerous vectors. Irritation at the site of virus inoculation (bite) may result in their constant licking and chewing of the infected area. Compulsive seizures may then develop; these may become almost continuous until death, usually from respiratory arrest.

Confusion and disorientation are consistent signs of rabies in both domestic and wild animals. Wild animals may lose their normal caution and wander into farmyards, suburbs, and campsites. Such aberrant behaviour is common and may be considered almost pathognomonic in some areas.

Early signs in dogs last 2–5 days and are followed by paralytic rabies in 75 per cent of cases, or furious rabies in the remainder. Paralysis and death occurs in both paralytic and furious forms of the disease 4–8 days after the onset of symptoms. However, virus may be present in the saliva of rabid animals for many days before clinical signs appear and it may be steadily or intermittently secreted until just before death. Cats usually develop furious rabies and are especially dangerous to man since, as lap animals, they are more likely to strike at the face and neck.

One of the most consistent signs of rabies in animals is motor paralysis. Usually an ascending paralysis develops, the first signs being some weakness or incoordination in the hind limbs. As the paralysis becomes more extensive the locomotor dysfunction becomes more pronounced. This development of paraplegia without a history of compatible traumatic injury is highly suspicious of rabies. Ascending paralysis is commonly seen in wild as well as domestic animals.

As infection spreads through the CNS, cranial nerve involvement becomes apparent. Dysfunction in areas innervated by cranial nerves V, VII, IX, and XII leads to extension of the nictitating membrane across the eye and facial and lingual paralysis; paralysis of pharyngeal muscles frequently results in altered phonation. Both anorexia and pica are common signs—dogs may eat wood, straw, stones, etc. An animal infected with rabies may show any one, all, or none of these signs.

DIAGNOSIS

Unfortunately, in some countries where there is the most frequent need for accurate diagnosis, clinical diagnosis with or without an examination for Negri bodies is all that is attempted. However, whenever possible clinical suspicions should be confirmed by laboratory tests. The development of these tests has paralleled advances in microscopy, cellular theory, histopathology, and molecular biology, and early diagnosis now plays an important role in the organization of treatment of victims of the bites of possibly rabid animals and in the control of epizootics. Speed of confirmation is important since delay may lead to an increased number of contacts with the victim and a consequent increase in requirement for postexposure treatments.

In rabies endemic areas, when neurological symptoms of unexplained origin are present, the possibility of a rabies virus infection should always be considered. Lack of history of a biting incident should not eliminate rabies from consideration, since such bites may have appeared trivial or have occurred many months before and been forgotten by the patient. Even in areas where rabies is not endemic, rabies should be considered if there is a history of travel to rabies-endemic areas. Possible contact with insectivorous bats should not be ignored. Brass (1994) has cited 20 case histories of patients who have died in the United States since 1951 from rabies of insectivorous bat origin. In 10 of these cases where bat virus origin was confirmed by monoclonal antibody techniques, there was no record of a bat bite, although in three cases bats were implicated during the course of the investigations. Non-specific early symptoms in the 10 cases included headache, feverishness, sore throat, difficulty of swallowing, sleeplessness, and hallucination.

Other early symptoms in rabies patients may resemble those of tetanus, typhoid, and malaria, or of viral encephalitides caused by measles, mumps, herpesvirus, or enteroviruses. A paralytic rabies diagnosis may be confused with poliomyelitis, acute inflammatory polyneuropathy (Guillain–Barré syndrome), or with post-vaccinal encephalitis (PVE) due to the presence of myelin in brain-tissue vaccines.

Virus isolation

The earliest experimental diagnosis of rabies is attributed to Zinke (1804), who demonstrated the transmission of the disease to dogs and rabbits through the infection of cutaneous wounds with the saliva of rabid animals. Three-quarters of a century later, Gaultier (1879) achieved improved reproducibility by the use of subcutaneous inoculation. Pasteur, however, using the intracerebral route introduced to his laboratory by Roux, demonstrated that intracerebral inoculation was the method of choice for rabies virus propagation in the rabbit (Pasteur et al. 1882). Animal inoculation (using suckling or weaned mice) by this route remains a practical and reliable method, and in some countries is the only laboratory method of rabies diagnosis. The clinical disease in mice is brief but the incubation periods of street strains are typically long and may vary from 7 to 28 days. Diagnosis time may be shortened by using a method in which individuals of a series of inoculated mice are killed at daily intervals and their brains examined using immunofluorescence techniques.

With few exceptions rabies-infected primary cells and cell lines exhibit no obvious cytopathic changes. The introduction of the fluorescent antibody test (FAT) to the rabies field revolutionized diagnosis by permitting the visualization of rabies antigen present in cell cultures, as well as in smears and frozen sections. Although the test requires special microscopic techniques, it is now regarded as superior to all others in speed and accuracy and, apart from its immediate diagnostic function, has also helped to elucidate the pathogenesis of rabies.

Intra-vitam diagnosis in humans

Cell culture virus isolation techniques are most frequently used for specimens obtained at necropsy, but a rabies infection may be detected antemortem. During the first week of illness virus may be isolated, in suckling mice or neuroblastoma cells, from saliva, throat swabs, eye swabs, brain biopsy, or from the CSF. Antigen may be detected by FAT in 4 or 6 mm skin biopsies, including hair follicles taken from the neck and from the bitten limb. Although it may be necessary to examine 50 or more 7 mm frozen sections from each biopsy, the test is 60–100 per cent sensitive (Warrell *et al.* 1988).

In regions where vaccines of nervous tissue origin (NTO) are still used, rabies and PVE can present indistinguishable clinical pictures. However, neutralizing antibody is not detectable in unvaccinated patients during the first week of illness and it has been proposed that a diagnosis of PVE is strongly suggested in patients at risk if antibody is detected in the serum and no rabies antigen is detected in the skin biopsy. Antibody in unvaccinated patients frequently appears during the second week of illness and may be detected within 2 days by a neutralization test carried out in neuroblastoma cells, or in mice, although results may not be available in under 2 weeks.

Post-mortem diagnosis

In humans, a full post-mortem is not needed, a needle biopsy of the brain via the foramen magnum or superior orbital fissure provides sufficient material for FAT and/or virus culture. In animals and in ideal circumstances, the entire head and neck of a suspect animal should be sent to the laboratory for diagnosis, since brain sampling by opening the skull is hazardous when practised outside of the laboratory. However, a method of sampling without opening the skull has found favour in hot or tropical countries. A straw or plastic 2 ml pipette is passed either through the occipital foramen heading in the direction of an eye, or, after making an entry through the posterior wall of the orbit with a trocar, screwing the straw through the brain in the direction of the occipital foramen. One straw sample can be used for histological examination, in which case the straw contents are expelled into a formalin fixative; a second straw sample can be taken for FAT and/or virus isolation, in which case the brain tissue is retained in the straw in glycerol-saline during despatch to the laboratory.

Brain smears of the thalamus, pons or medulla, hippocampus and cerebellum, or spinal cord are made on glass slides, allowed to air-dry at room temperature, inactivated for 2 min under a UV light about 20 cm above the slides and then fixed in acetone at −20 °C for 1–2 h. Upon removal from acetone, the slides are again air-dried, rabies-specific conjugate containing Evan's blue as a counterstain is added to the smears and, after incubation at 37 °C for 30 min, the slides are washed in one or two changes of phosphate-buffered saline, air-dried and, depending upon the power of the microscope, the smears are examined either dry or mounted in buffered glycerine. Rabies antigen appears as apple-green fluorescent particles ranging in size from Negri bodies to 'star-dust', against a red background. Specificity can be enhanced by using as the conjugant either a monoclonal antibody 'cocktail' or an antiserum prepared in goats by immunization with purified N-protein.

Histopathology

Although inflammatory lesions found in the brain during rabies diagnosis may be common to other viral infections, the specific round to oval inclusions described by Negri (1903), usually found in the cytoplasm of undamaged nerve cells and particularly in the hippocampus, may be identified by histological and immunological techniques. In sections which have been wax-embedded, the refractory, acidophilic, RNP-containing 'Negri bodies', which consist of a reticulo-granular matrix containing tubular structures contiguous with maturing virus particles, are regarded as pathognomonic for rabies; their absence, however, does not exclude the disease. They may be found in almost any region of the brain, but they are seen in greater numbers in the central pyramidal layer of Ammon's horn of the hippocampus, in the lower loop and the middle layer of the ganglioneurones and in the neurones of the cerebellum, the motor area of the cerebral cortex, and in the medulla. Their frequency of occurrence, size, and shape may be influenced by the host species, the infecting virus strain, and the clinical phase period.

Other methods

FAT staining can be used on formalin-fixed tissue which has been wax-embedded. Pieces (of about 2 cm^3) from Susa-fixed cerebral cortex, basal ganglia, hippocampus (Ammon's horn), midbrain, and medulla are pre-treated by emulsification, washing with buffered saline, and digestion with trypsin. The method is claimed to markedly enhance the staining of rabies inclusions and to eliminate non-specific staining of formalin-preserved brain. As an alternative to the FAT, a streptavidin–biotin complex (ABC) immunoperoxidase test on formalin-fixed paraffin-embedded brain tissues has been described. Specificity of the test was claimed to be high, but more corroborative results are required before the test can be used as a routine diagnostic procedure.

An enzyme-linked immunosorbent assay (ELISA) has also been developed for the diagnosis of rabies. This rapid rabies enzyme immunodiagnosis (RREID) technique, which is based on the detection of virus nucleocapsid antigen in brain tissue, does not require microscopy and, with the aid of a special kit, can be used under field conditions. The test can be used to examine partially decomposed tissue specimens for evidence of rabies infection but it cannot be used with specimens that have been fixed in formalin, and there may be occasions when the FA test is positive but the RREID is negative. The test is said to be about 3 per cent less sensitive than FAT (Perrin *et al.* 1986).

At the molecular level, rabies RNA can be detected following reverse transcription and cDNA amplification by polymerase chain reaction (PCR). Molecular techniques for rabies diagnosis, however, need further refinement, particularly if they are to be used in countries where sample degradation is a problem because of the climatic conditions. Nevertheless, at the Pasteur Institute in Paris, 100 suspect samples checked in systematic blind trials by PCR and by three routine techniques (FAT, RTCIT, and RREID) gave 100 per cent correlation of the results (Tordo *et al.* 1994).

DISEASE TRANSMISSION

Worldwide, the vast majority of people who die from rabies do so following the bite of an infected dog. Equally, the vast majority of cases in domesticated animals (other than cats and dogs) arise via the bite of a rabid wild animal. Unusually, non-bite transmission of rabies virus by respiratory infection is found in wildlife and laboratory workers handling infected material. Ingestion (including milk during suckling) and the transplacental route are also cited, and evidence of natural infection in animals by these routes has been supported by animal experimentation.

Airborne transmission, which may be a significant route in the case of insectivorous bats, has been reviewed by Brass (1994). The precise source of airborne virus in bat caves is unknown but it is presumed to be from infective saliva generated as bats emit their high-pitched sounds.

The deaths from rabies in the 1950s of an entomologist and a mining engineer, both of whom had denied being bitten by bats during their time spent working in bat-infested caves, are generally accepted as examples of airborne infection, although proof is unobtainable. There is, however, a considerable volume of experimental evidence (cited by Brass 1994) which supports inhalation as a route of infection in animals exposed to the atmosphere in the Frio cave, Texas. Human rabies following exposure to an aerosol of virus in the laboratory has also been reported; in these accidental exposures, one veterinarian died and a previously vaccinated laboratory technician survived, although he sustained considerable neurological impairment.

Virus of bat origin was implicated in an epizootic in experimental animals at a Public Health Investigation station in New Mexico in 1967. Circumstantial evidence suggested that the source of infection for the 39 animals which died was from other animals intentionally infected with a bat virus sometime previously; an aerosol of the virus may have been generated by the water sprayer used to clean cages and its spread compounded by a malfunctioning air-exchange system (Winkler *et al.* 1972).

VACCINES AND VACCINATION

The control and worldwide eradication of rabies depends on the development of safe, effective, and economical vaccines that might be used in pre-exposure vaccination programmes for humans and animals (Prevec *et al.* 1990). The following vaccines are now available.

Vaccines of nervous tissue origin (NTO)

Following the production of Pasteur's prototype vaccine, which was composed of crude suspensions of desiccated brain and spinal cord, a number of vaccines were prepared in rabbit, sheep, or goat brain. They contained residual live virus which occasionally led to vaccine-induced rabies, although the introduction of inactivation by phenol and, later, beta-propiolactone (BPL) increased safety. The multidose schedules considered necessary to obtain adequate responses enhanced the possibility of allergic neurological reactions. Nevertheless, these 'Semple-type' vaccines are still used in vast quantities in developing countries because they are cheap and easy to prepare. Estimates of the number of people receiving the vaccine annually vary from 500 000 to 3 000 000 (Dutta *et al.* 1994). Vaccines prepared from brains of suckling mice of less than 9 days of age and inactivated with ultraviolet light or BPL (Fuenzalida and Palacios 1955) have significantly reduced the incidence of neuroallergenic side-effects and are still widely used in Latin America. WHO recommends the discontinuation of the use of other NTO vaccines for humans (WHO 1992).

Embryo vaccines

Vaccine prepared from virus propagated in duck embryos was used for almost 20 years in Europe and the United States, but specific responses to its recommended schedule of 14 to 20 doses were poor and its production has been abandoned. A new Swiss vaccine contains only about 1 per cent of the protein of previous duck embryo vaccines and is considerably more potent.

Modified live virus (MLV) vaccines prepared from the Flury strain of virus grown in chick embryos, were once used for human vaccination but are now confined to animals. Low egg passage (LEP) vaccine prepared at the fiftieth passage in chick embryos is safe for adult dogs but not for cattle, cats, or puppies. Flury high egg passage (HEP), harvested at the eightieth passage, is more attenuated and can be used for cattle, but neither LEP nor HEP is recommended for exotic pets or zoo animals.

Cell culture vaccines for animals

Pasteur's 'fixed' virus was maintained for many years by passage in rabbits and mice and provides the Challenge virus standard (CVS) strain. It was adapted to primary hamster kidney cells by Kissing in 1958. After numerous passages in a baby hamster kidney (BHK) cell line the virus (CVS-11) was used as an MLV to vaccinate dogs but was not considered safe for use in other species.

The Street Alabama Dufferin (SAD) rabies virus was isolated from a rabid dog in Alabama in 1935 and adapted to hamster kidney cells (Fenje 1960). Fenje's virus was passaged in chicken embryos and then in porcine kidney cells, leading to the production of ERA strain (named after the developers **E**velyn Gaynor, A. **R**ockitnicki and M. K. **A**belseth). The ERA-SAD strain, which produced long-term immunity in cattle, dogs, and cats (Lawson *et al.* 1967) has been used to prepare potent vaccines including SAD Berne (Steck *et al.* 1982), the oral vaccine that has been successful in controlling fox rabies in Switzerland, and SAD B19, which is widely used in oral vaccination of foxes in a number of other European countries.

The live attenuated rabies vaccine strain SAG-2 was prepared by a sophisticated two-step process in which anti-G monoclonal antibodies (Mab-Gs) were used to remove any residual pathogenicity caused by the amino acid arginine at position 333 of antigenic site III (330–338) of SAD Berne virus (Schumacher *et al.* 1993). Incubation of SAD Berne with the first Mab-G yielded an escape mutant in which arginine (encoded by AGA) was replaced by lysine (encoded by AAA); incubation of the escape mutant with the second Mab-G yielded a further escape mutant in which lysine was replaced by glutamic acid (encoded by GAA). Thus SAG-2 differs from SAD Berne by one amino acid in position 333 but by two nucleotides from any of six possible triplets encoding for arginine. SAG-2 is a genetically stable vaccine which is apathogenic for adult mice, foxes, cats, and dogs and, when distributed within a fox-bait, has been used successfully as one of the oral vaccines in the control of fox rabies in France. Preliminary trials of freeze-dried SAG-2 presented in a matrix attractive to dogs have given promising results.

Genetically engineered vaccines

A vaccinia-rabies glycoprotein (V-RG) recombinant vaccine has also been used widely in fox rabies control. The 1572 nucleotides which encode the 524 amino acid secondarily glycosylated glycoprotein of the ERA strain was inserted into a depleted region of the thymidine kinase (*tk*) gene of the Copenhagen strain (ts26) of vaccinia virus. Removal of a small proportion of the *tk* gene and replacement by the rabies glycoprotein gene and regulatory sequences rendered the *tk* gene non-functional, thus removing the vaccinia virus pathogenicity. V-RG has been shown to elicit high antibody levels when given parentally to a wide variety of species and was used widely in the European oral vaccination campaigns in a fish-meal polymer bait.

Human adenoviruses (HAVs) have a number of physical and biological properties that make them ideal for use as delivery system for genes smaller than 8 kb. The ubiquitous nature of HAV5 (over 70 per cent of the post-puberty population carries antibodies to the virus), the normal ability of the virus to infect by the mucosal route, and the relatively benign nature of the infection, make it an ideal candidate for an oral vaccine. The HAV5 virion can package a genome which contains up to 2 kb more than the normal virus and this can be increased to 8 kb and provide sites for gene insertion by deletions of up to 2.5 kb of the E3 region and of some 3.5 kb of the E1 region.

A recombinant (AdRG1) in which the glycoprotein gene of the ERA strain of rabies virus was inserted into the deleted E3 region of HAV5 has been constructed. When administered by either the parenteral or oronasal route, AdRG1 was highly efficient in eliciting good levels of rabies neutralizing antibodies in the sera of dogs and mice, and the latter were protected from lethal intracerebral challenge with rabies virus (Prevec *et al.* 1990). When it was administered by the oral route, foxes, skunks, and raccoons were immunized (Wandeler *et al.* 1994*b*).

Cell culture vaccines for humans

The human diploid cell vaccine (HDCV) developed in 1964 (Wiktor *et al.* 1964) was a landmark in the immunoprophylaxis of rabies and millions of doses have been administered; neurological side-effects have been exceptionally rare. There are now a number of other cell lines and cell strains available for vaccine production, but because of their heteroploid characteristics and oncogenic potential only a few of these have been used for the production of human vaccines. New vaccines include purified chick embryo cell vaccine (PCECV) and purified Vero rabies vaccine (PVRV). In Thailand, these purified vaccines have replaced NTO vaccines since 1990. In terms of safety and antigenicity, there is nothing to choose between these vaccines (Nicholson 1990). Although they are tolerated very well, late booster injections in particular do sometimes cause allergic reactions which range from urticaria to anaphylaxis and are seemingly unrelated to age, route of primary or booster immunization, timing of booster, history of allergies, or history of immunization with vaccines other than HDCV. The reactions are probably caused by the BPL used to inactivate the virus, which may render the human albumin, used as a stabilizer in the vaccine, antigenic. Persons who have experienced such reactions should receive no further HDCV unless they are actually exposed to rabies virus (Nicholson 1990).

Human pre-exposure immunization

All persons who work with rabies virus, who may come into contact with rabid animals (particularly in rabies endemic areas) or nurse patients with rabies should receive rabies pre-exposure immunization. The current recommended immunization schedule consists of three doses of cell-cultured rabies vaccine of potency at least 2.5 IU/dose, given intramuscularly in the deltoid area of the arm on days 0, 7, and 28 (WHO 1992). For young children the anterolateral area of the thigh is acceptable, but in no case should the gluteal area be used since administration of vaccine in this area has resulted in lower neutralizing antibody titres. Neutralizing antibody titres need not be confirmed with cell culture vaccines but should be checked regularly (every 6 months) for those working with live rabies virus. If the titre falls below 0.5 IU/ml, a booster vaccine dose is recommended. In practice, this is seldom necessary until 3–5 years after the initial immunizing schedule.

The use of cell-culture vaccines of similar potency given according to the same schedule induces comparable titres when carefully administered intradermally in 0.1 ml volumes. Vaccination costs are greatly reduced by this method and it is recommended except when combined with antimalarial prophylaxis. Virus-neutralizing antibody titres have been shown to be lower in patients receiving chloroquine phosphate, so these patients should be given 1.0 ml of vaccine intramuscularly (WHO 1992).

Human post-exposure treatment

Following exposure to a suspect rabid animal, or to a recognized vector in a rabies endemic area, post-exposure treatment should be commenced as soon as possible. To await the results of laboratory tests may prove fatal; pregnancy and infancy are never contraindications. The wound should be thoroughly washed immediately with soap and water or detergent and then, if available, either 70 per cent ethanol or an aqueous solution of iodine should be applied. The purpose of this vital aspect of treatment is to remove or inactivate infectious virions (and/or other potential pathogens) from the site before they have an opportunity to replicate or to reach the nerve endings. Wound suturing should be delayed or avoided. A physician should be consulted urgently. In all bite/mucous membrane contamination, anti-rabies immunoglobulin should be used, although in practice it is given to less than 5 per cent of post-exposure treated patients. Either human or equine rabies immunoglobulin (HRIG or ERIG) may be applied. A skin test prior to the administration of ERIG does not predict reactions and should not be used. Adrenaline should always be at hand in case of anaphylaxis. The purpose of RIG is to neutralize rabies virions and prevent them from entering the nerve endings; it is possible that it also participates in the destruction of infected cells by antibody-dependent cellular cytotoxicity. As much as possible of the recommended does (20 IU/kg bodyweight of HRIG or 40 IU/kg ERIG) should be infiltrated around the wound and the remainder administered intramuscularly into the gluteal region in a single dose (WHO 1992). Cell-cultured vaccine should be administered at the same time but in a different region (deltoid or, in children, anterolateral area of the thigh muscle). One dose of the vaccine should be administered on days 0, 3, 7, 14, and 30 days. In an abbreviated multiple-site schedule (the 2–1–1 regimen) one dose is given in the right arm and one in the left arm at day 0 and one dose applied intramuscularly in the deltoid region on days 7 and 21. This schedule induces an early antibody response and may be particularly effective when post-exposure treatment does not include administration of RIG (WHO 1992).

Vaccines of nervous tissue origin are still widely used in tropical endemic areas, but in China and the Russian Federation they have been replaced by cell culture vaccines produced locally. In parts of Asia and Africa, multiple-site intradermal regimens using imported European cell-culture vaccines are in routine use. The methods have proved effective, economical, and safe, reducing the cost of cell-culture post-exposure treatment by 60 per cent (Warrell *et al.* 1985; Suntharasamai *et al.* 1994).

IMMUNOLOGY

In a non-vaccinated, untreated subject exposed to rabies, the virus evades the host immune response because of its intrinsic neurotropism. The infectious virus needs time to enter the nerve endings and this period may offer the only opportunity for post-exposure treatment. The initial infecting dose of virus is unlikely to be large enough to provide sufficient antigen to stimulate an early immune response and after possible amplification in muscle or epithelial cells may be sufficient to invade nerve endings, but again insufficient to be antigenic. Late in infection, when virus has reached and multiplied in the brain, antigen is released in quantity and neutralizing antibody becomes detectable, usually in the terminal days of the illness. When survival is prolonged, antibody in serum, brain, and CSF may reach very high titres and virus may no longer be detectable, but death nevertheless ensues.

T lymphocytes are the effectors of cell-mediated immunity and monitor other cells for virus-induced changes on their surfaces; provided that the latter carry the same major histocompatability (MHC) antigens, they are destroyed by cytotoxic T cells. T cells or their subsets regulate antibody production by B lymphocytes, and rabies vaccines are among the antigens that were classified as T-cell dependent. Recent experiments (cited by Lafon 1994) have demonstrated the critical role of CD4[+] T lymphocytes in protection, and established their role in controlling rabies-specific antibody production. On the other hand, the role of CD8[+] cytotoxic T cells remains unclear. In mice, CD8[+] T-lymphocyte production affords a non-dose-dependent protection against the intracerebral inoculation of live attenuated rabies vaccines but not against fully virulent viruses. It may be that in natural infections CD8[+] T lymphocytes have a role, but only in combination with other immune effector mechanisms and dependent on the infecting virus strain.

The use of interleukin-2 (IL-2) to enhance rabies vaccination has been investigated and has been shown to improve the resistance of mice to an intracerebral challenge. The effect is not mediated by an increase in virus-neutralizing antibody titres, rather it appears to be dependent on T-cell cytotoxicity. Interferon inhibits the growth of street and fixed rabies virus *in vitro* and *in vivo*. Those viruses that multiply locally, such as attenuated vaccine strains, induce more interferon than do virulent strains. High-dose α-interferon therapy has not been successful in the treatment of human rabies encephalitis.

Neutralizing antibodies under the control of T-helper cells are regarded as a key factor in rabies protection, but protection does not always correlate with the level of neutralizing antibody in the serum. Despite the production of high-titred neutralizing antibodies against vaccine virus, protection against serotypes 2, 3 and 4 (Table 37.1) is variable and may be proportional to the degree of homology between the vaccine and the challenge virus. For example, vaccine-induced antibodies give no protection against serotype 3 Mokola virus, the most distantly related of the rabies-related viruses (Wiktor *et al.* 1984). Moreover, certain epitopes

in vaccine strains are critical for protection; Lafon *et al.* (1988) showed that while vaccine strains ERA, PV, PM, and LEP all produced high titres of circulating neutralizing antibodies in mice, those immunized with ERA or PV vaccines were fully protected against challenge with an EBL1 virus, whereas those immunized with PM and LEP vaccines were not.

In rabies post-exposure treatment, replacement of HRIG or ERIG with monoclonal antibodies of human or murine origin (to obviate accidental transmission of human blood-borne pathogens) has been proposed. Such antibodies are easily standardized, are efficient at low protein concentrations, and they can be selected to adapt treatment to the nature of the infecting virus (Montano-Hirose *et al.* 1993). Although the mechanisms have yet to be elucidated, some monoclonal antibodies can abrogate virus infection, even after CNS invasion, by inhibiting virus spread and blocking viral replication (Levine *et al.* 1991; Dietzschold *et al.* 1992).

Immunogenicity of rabies virus proteins

Rabies virus glycoprotein is responsible for the induction of virus neutralizing antibody and the stimulation of T-helper and cytolytic lymphocytes. Most of the antigenic determinants responsible for the induction of neutralizing antibody depend on the three-dimensional 58 amino acid protein structure at the G protein COOH terminus. Linear epitopes have been described (Benmansour *et al.* 1991) and their synthesis raises the possibility of using peptides of G protein as immunogens.

N protein, the main component of the nucleocapsid, has been shown to be a target antigen for T-helper cells that cross-react with the different rabies serotypes (Ertl *et al.* 1989). The protective activity of the N protein has been shown in experiments using purified N protein or live poxvirus recombinants expressing the N protein (Lodmell *et al.* 1991). The NS protein appears to have little or no role in protection.

EPIDEMIOLOGY

RABIES IN ASIA

Vulpine rabies in the arctic fox (*Alopex lagopus*) and the red fox (*Vulpes vulpes*) predominates in the Russian Federation, although within recent decades the raccoon dog (*Nyctereutes procyonoides*) has become a vector and victim since it became established in Eastern Europe after being transported westwards from Siberia for fur and hunting purposes. Canine rabies occurs over the length of the Asiatic continent, from the Sea of Japan to the Red Sea. The division between canine and fox rabies follows approximately the line between Belgrade and Khabarovsk, passing through Baku, Tashkent, and Irkutsk (Blancou 1988). Along the southern borders of the Russian Federation with Iraq, Iran, and Afghanistan the wolf is an important vector, together with the dog.

Rabies is vastly under-reported in Asia. For example, in India in 1991 only two human and 156 animal cases were confirmed in the laboratory, although a further 32 human cases were confirmed on clinical grounds (WHO 1993). These figures are in marked contrast to those from Sri Lanka, an island to the south which shares geographical, ecological, ethnic, and cultural features with India. Here and during the same period, 134 human and 819 animal cases were recorded. Unofficial estimates put the annual total for human rabies in India at 25 000 or more; Bögel and Motschwiller (1986) give a precise figure of 28.8 cases/million inhabitants, whereas the comparable figure for China in 1985, when 4109 human cases were recorded, was 3.97/million inhabitants. Human rabies cases reported from five other Asian countries are recorded in Table 37.2. Dogs account for the greatest proportion of animal cases, while foxes in the Middle East form a wildlife reservoir. Bat rabies is rarely reported, although it should be noted that bats are not examined unless captured following human exposure.

RABIES IN EUROPE

Great Britain had a long history of canine rabies (summarized by King and Turner 1993) and in 10 years from 1889, over 160 human cases were recorded. However, with the exception of two outbreaks in deer, in 1856 and 1886, the disease was rarely reported in wildlife species and canine rabies was finally eradicated in 1922. Import regulations, which included quarantine of imported dogs and cats, kept Britain free of animal rabies until two dogs which later developed the disease were released from quarantine, in 1969 and 1970. Both dogs were killed without rabies sequelae.

The introduction in 1971 of vaccination of dogs and cats on arrival in quarantine has resulted in no deaths from rabies in nearly 200 000 imported dogs and cats subsequently released from quarantine (King 1992). The last indigenously acquired human rabies case occurred in Wales in 1902 but a further 21 recorded human deaths have resulted from infection acquired abroad.

Canine (and less frequently wildlife) rabies was widely recognized in Central Europe during the middle of the 1800s but by the turn of the century it had virtually disappeared. However, from an initial focus near the Russo-Polish border at the beginning of the Second World War, fox-mediated rabies spread at 25–60 km/year towards the west and south-west until it reached central France and Italy in the mid-1980s, whereupon the epizootic came to a standstill. Spread was characterized by high case density in the front wave which lasted 1–2 years, followed by in-filling behind the wave-front. In the 10 most severely affected countries during the 1980s, over 137 000 foxes were confirmed rabid (Table 37.3). It has been estimated (Blancou et al. 1988), that only 10–20 per cent of foxes which die from the disease in the wild are submitted for diagnostic tests. The impact of the epizootic on the species, though clearly enormous, has not been catastrophic since in some countries of western Europe, fox populations have reached higher densities than were recorded before the epizootic and, as in the United Kingdom, the species has become highly urbanized. The impact on other wildlife species is less well documented. For example, badgers, the only species other than the fox that has been perceptibly reduced in population density, are able to repair their losses far more slowly; stoats, weasels, and free-roaming cats reach population densities that locally exceed fox densities, but none of these species appear to support independent rabies epizootics (Wandeler 1991).

During the epizootic, almost 15 per cent of the cases reported were in domesticated animals. Surprisingly,

Table 37.2 Human rabies cases reported in five Asian countries[a]

	1983	1984	1985	1986	1987	1988	1989	1990	1991	1992
Bangladesh										2000[b]
Cambodia	6	3	10	9	2	1	0	12	2	[c]
Laos							69	96	356	242[d]
North Vietnam					261	349	317	396	425	285
Sri Lanka								154	134	112
Thailand	288	288	210	179	212	213	212	185	159	96[e]

[a] Figures derived from WHO/Rabies Research/93.44.
[b] Approximate figure for that year.
[c] No figure stated for 1992.
[d] Recorded as number of positive tests.
[e] As of March 1993.

Table 37.3 Animal rabies in 10 European countries 1980–89[a]

	Domesticated animals				Wild animals					Total
	Dog	Cat	Other	Total	Fox	Deer	Badger	Other[c]	Total	
Aus.	47	236	383	666	11 355	543	747	391	13 036	13 702
Bel.	51	181	1473	1705	2471	23	35	67	2596	4301
Cze.	315	591	97	1003	14 267	243	118	325	14 953	15 956
Fra.	519	986	3627	5132	19 844	188	254	465	20 751	25 883
Ger.	1375	2959	7714	12 048	56 027	3892	1241	2951	64 111	76 159
Hun.	340	581	336	1257	10 044	82	10	50	10 186	11 443
Lux.	3	25	341	369	423	11	11	20	465	834
Pol.	536	865	876	2277	7602	584	131	1011	9328	11 605
Swi.	48	423	631	1102	4485	231	308	284	5308	6410
Yug.	175	232	192	599	10 673	44	63	211	10 991	11 590
Total	3409	7079	15 670[b]	26 158	137 191	5841	2918	5775	151 725	177 883

Aus., Austria; Bel., Belgium; Cze., Czechoslovakia; Fra., France; Ger., Germany; Hun., Hungary; Lux., Luxembourg; Pol., Poland; Swi., Switzerland + Liechtenstein; Yug., Yugoslavia.

[a] Figures derived from *Rabies Bulletins Europe* 1980–89.
[b] Includes cattle, 9291; sheep/goat, 5416; horse/donkey, 773; other, 190.
[c] Includes black rat, brown bear, chamois, dormouse, hare, hedgehog, martens, mouflon, muskrat, raccoon, raccoon-dog, squirrel, stoat, weasel, wild boar, wild cat, wolf.

many of the countries involved had compulsory vaccination policies for dogs and cats within rabies-infected areas and strongly recommend vaccination in other areas, yet over 10 000 of these two species died of the disease. There is no suspicion of vaccine failure, the high number of casualties is more a reflection of the difficulty of implementing statutory policies in the field. This is particularly so with regard to cats, and it may be noted (Table 37.3) that the death rate in cats was twice that in dogs.

Rabies in European bats was first recognized in the early 1950s but by early 1985 only 14 cases had been reported. During 1985 to 1987 a further 278 cases were reported and thereafter the number of reports quickly declined to an average of 19 over the past 3 years. In almost all of the 11 countries that reported bat rabies, the disease came to light when a member of the public was exposed to rabies through contact with an infected bat. Human death from European bat rabies was reported from Finland, Kiev (Ukraine), and from Belgorod in the Russian Federation. The bat species most frequently affected are *Eptesicus serotinus* (serotines) and *Myotis* spp. The disease has been reported in eight other species but it should be noted that, on occasions, the species remained unidentified, the bat infection was not independently confirmed by virus isolation, and/or the isolate was not antigenically characterized.

RABIES IN AFRICA

Urban rabies has been present in North Africa for centuries, although its history prior to 1900 is fragmentary and largely anecdotal. In sub-Saharan Africa, disease recognition only followed establishment of diagnostic laboratories at the turn of the twentieth century. Here, where humans and animals are more widely distributed than in northern Africa, there has been a greater tendency for epidemics of dog rabies to spread over large areas and for the disease to be observed in domestic herbivores and wild vertebrates (Blancou 1988). A proposition that rabies viruses evolved in West Africa (Swanepoel *et al.* 1993) is supported by the presence of three of the four serotypes and the historical occurrence of rabies viruses in dogs which are less virulent than conventional street viruses (Blancou 1988). However, it may be that rabies was introduced to West Africa some time after AD 1500 by slave-trading Europeans, since nucleotide sequencing has shown similarities between European, New World, and some West African isolates (Smith *et al.* 1993). Although it is unlikely to have been the first incidence of rabies in southern Africa, the first irrefutable diagnosis was made in 1893 during an epizootic involving dogs, cats, and domestic ruminants in the vicinity of Port Elizabeth on the south-east coast of South Africa (Hutcheon 1894). Today, biological variations among African serotype 1 lyssavirus infections are more apparent in southern Africa than elsewhere on the continent. Apart from domestic dogs and cats, representatives of at least 30 different species belonging to all five families of carnivore native to southern Africa have been diagnosed with rabies (Thomson and Meredith 1993). Some species, notably the jackal, bat-eared fox, and mongoose, are afflicted more frequently than others.

Table 37.4 Human and animal rabies in southern and eastern Africa 1987–91[a]

	Human	Domesticated animals				Wild animals						Total
		Dog	Cat	Other	Total	Jack	BEF	HYA	VIV	Other	Total	
Ken.	8	637	43	348	1028						30	1058
Zam.	67	117	1	41	159						5	164
Mal.	1	640	16	69	725	16		14	1	6	37	762
Moz.	73				60							60
Zim.	28	715	30	556	1297	224		1	6	18	249	1546
Bot.	6	91	4	526	621	87	5	2	15	15	124	745
Nam.		152	23	384	559	93	24		5	17	139	698
Swa.		17			17							17
Les.	17	15	1	8	24							24
Nat.	80	1062	21	84	1167	1			5	2	8	1175
SAT.	7	1232	68	493	1793	59	70		472	68	669	2462
Total	287	4678	197	2509[b]	7450	480	99	17	504	226[c]	1261	8711

Ken., Kenya; Zam., Zambia; Mal., Malawi; Moz., Mozambique; Zim., Zimbabwe; Bot., Botswana; Nam., Namibia; Swa, Swaziland; Les., Lesotho; Nat., Natal/KwaZulu; SAT., South Africa/Transkei. Jack, jackal; BEF, bat-eared fox; HYA, hyaena; VIV, viverrid.
[a] Figures derived from *Proceedings of the International Conference on Epidemiology Control and Prevention of Rabies in Southern and Eastern Africa, Lusaka, Zambia* (1992) (ed. A. King). Editions Foundation, Marcel Mérieux.
[b] Includes cattle, 1975; sheep/goat, 426; horse/donkey, 100; pig, 14.
[c] Includes wild cat, fox, hyrax, ground squirrel, badger, game.

In many countries of Africa information on rabies is still rather fragmented, since a lack of rural communication leads to difficulties in getting samples to the laboratory. A striking feature is the nature of rabies within southern Africa. In general terms, the more northerly countries report almost exclusively canine rabies, whereas further south, wildlife rabies plays the dominant role (Table 37.4). Whether this apparent difference is real is not clear, it may be that better communication and available facilities in the more southernly countries provide a more accurate reflection of the true picture. A second striking and inexplicable feature is the virtual absence of rabies within national game reserves, although the disease may be reported in surrounding areas.

RABIES IN THE AMERICAS

Canada

Although rabies was recognized in Canada during the late eighteenth and early nineteenth centuries, outbreaks were few and sporadic and involved mainly domestic animals. However, during the 1940s rabies in foxes spread into the Canadian provinces from the Arctic regions and, although in most of these regions it later died out, the disease has persisted in foxes in Ontario. Rabies in skunks spread from North Dakota into the prairie provinces during the late 1950s and 1960s. Since 1958 rabies has been confirmed in over 40 000 wild and domestic animals, mainly from the prairie provinces and southern Ontario (Rosatte

1988). About 1 per cent ($n = 402$) of these cases have been in insectivorous bats. Human rabies is reported infrequently (21 cases during 1925–86).

USA

Rabies has also been present in the United States for over 200 years. In the mid-1900s canine rabies predominated and over 100 000 cases of dog rabies were reported from 1940 to 1960. Wildlife accounted for an average of 2.8 per cent of cases from 1936–50 but since 1960, and in parallel with a reduction of canine rabies by pet animal vaccination and stray dog control, the number of cases reported in wildlife has steadily increased. Since 1990, however, the number of wildlife cases has dramatically doubled and wildlife species now account for more than 90 per cent of all reported cases (Table 37.5).

Unlike the situation in Europe, where there is a single vector species (the red fox), in the United States there are four terrestrial vector species (red fox, *Vulpes fulva*; grey fox, *Urocyon cineroargenteus*; skunks, *Mephitis mephitis, Spilogale putorius*; and raccoon, *Procyon lotor*) and insectivorous bats. Foxes provide only a small proportion of the total wildlife cases (Table 37.5) although the disease is enzootic in red foxes in northern New York State bordering Ontario and the disease persists in the grey foxes of Central Texas and Arizona. Skunks, however, are important reservoirs of rabies in the Midwestern States and California, and it is probable that the Midwest band of skunk rabies has resulted from the coalescence of two separate foci, an older

Table 37.5   Animal Rabies in the USA 1983–93[a]

	Domesticated animals				Wild animals						Total
	Dog	Cat	Other	Total	Fox	Skunk	Racc.	Bat	Other	Total	
1983	132	168	284	584	111	2285	1906	910	82	5294	5878
1984	97	140	216	453	139	2082	1820	1038	94	5173	5626
1985	113	130	260	503	180	2507	1487	830	98	5103	5606
1986	95	166	255	516	207	2379	1576	788	85	5035	5551
1987	170	166	223	559	119	2033	1311	629	77	4169	4728
1988	128	192	230	550	183	1791	1463	638	99	4174	4724
1989	160	212	212	584	207	1657	1544	720	96	4224	4808
1990	148	176	229	552	197	1579	1821	637	93	4327	4880
1991	155	189	27	618	318	2073	3079	690	194	6354	6972
1992	182	290	260	732	397	2334	4311	647	223	7912	8644
1993	130	291	185	606	361	1640	5912	759	217	8889	9495
Total	1510	2120	2628[b]	6258	2420	22 360	26 230	8286	1358[c]	60 654	66 912

[a] Figures derived from Eng *et al.* (1989) Reid-Sanden *et al.* (1990), Uhaa *et al.* (1992), Krebs *et al.* (1992, 1993, 1994) Racc., raccoon.
[b] Includes cattle, 1968; sheep/goat, 110; horse/mule, 519; other 31.
[c] Includes coyote, bobcat, ringtail, beaver, otter, groundhog, squirrel, rabbit, mongoose (in Puerto Rico).

focus in Minnesota/Iowa and a newer one in Texas (Smith and Baer 1988).

Raccoon rabies has become a growing urban threat. Although the disease was first identified in raccoons in California in 1936, subsequent reports of infection in this species across the United States were sporadic until the mid-1950s, when the disease became a major problem in Florida. In the late 1970s a further outbreak occurred in the mid-Atlantic states and this has continued to spread northward and westward to encompass New England, Ohio, Pennsylvania, New York, and New Hampshire; southern Ontario in Canada is under threat.

The most likely cause of spread of the epizootic from Florida to south-west Virginia was the illegal transportation of the species for hunting purposes; between 1977 and 1981 more than 3500 raccoons were translocated (Jenkins *et al.* 1988). The danger to public health lies in the fact that raccoons are highly urbanized and contact between rabid raccoons and dogs frequently occurs.

Insectivorous bat rabies was first reported in the United States in 1953 when a yellow bat, *Lasiurus intermedius*, later shown to be rabid, attacked a 7-years-old boy who was given post-exposure treatment and did not develop rabies. This episode was quickly followed by another in which a 39-year-old woman was attacked, possibly by a hoary bat *Lasiurus cinereus*, and, after post-exposure treatment, she suffered only local symptoms from the bat bite on her arm. Within a short period it became clear that rabies in bats was not a new phenomenon and in subsequent years the disease has been reported from all states, except Hawaii, and in most species that have been adequately sampled (Brass

1994). During 1983–93 the 8286 cases of bat rabies accounted for approximately 12 per cent of all rabies cases reported in the United States (Table 37.5).

Central and South America

In Central and South America rabies continues to cause serious public health and economic problems. For example, in the 10 countries (Argentina, Bolivia, Brazil, Colombia, Equador, Guatemala, Honduras, Mexico, Peru, and Venezuela) most seriously affected during the decade 1976–1985, 2641 human and 172 263 dog rabies cases were recorded (PAHO/WHO/CEPANZO, cited by Larghi *et al.* 1988). The situation is probably more serious than is reported since data from most of the countries were incomplete. Bovine paralytic rabies is of significant economic importance, 31 363 cases being reported from the same 10 countries in the 10 years 1982–91 (Table 37.6). Again, the data are incomplete. Although dogs are likely to have been the vector in some of these cases, vampire bats were responsible for the vast majority. The annual cost to the 10 countries of vampire bat rabies is estimated to be more than US$40 million.

PREVENTION AND CONTROL

PREVENTION

In countries with no land borders, rabies-free status is an asset that has been maintained by importation controls that include quarantine. The purpose of quarantine is to prevent the spread of rabies by allowing a period of time in which an imported animal which was

Table 37.6   Reported cases of bovine paralytic rabies in the 10 most affected Latin American countries, 1982–91[a]

	1982	1983	1984	1985	1986	1987	1988	1989	1990	1991	Total
Argentina	92	18	3	3	5	1	–	0	–	0	122
Bolivia	159	82	9[b]	151	8	65	82	24	0	0	580[b]
Brazil	5900	7959	1875	2990	2740	1825	1311	501	883	1205	27 189
Colombia	139	–	105	93	76	46	75	42	44	28	648
Equador	45	31	29[b]	12[b]	7	14	–	20	27	36	221[b]
Guatemala	22	6	14[b]	16	14[b]	8	46	28	20	24	198[b]
Honduras	19	26	36	20[b]	32[b]	4[b]	34	39	1	3	214[b]
Mexico	35	43	66[b]	27[b]	–	–	–	–	898[c]	0	1069[b, c]
Peru	32	32	30	44	18	11	16	7	30	18	238
Venezuela	54	50	60	90	112	67	80	36	51	26	626
Totals	6497	8247	2227	3446	3012	2041	1644	697	1954	1340	31 105[b, c]

[a] Figures derived from PAHO, cited by Brass (1994).
[b] Information incomplete.
[c] May include cases in foxes and vampire bats.

incubating the disease would develop obvious signs. Areas of the world which have included quarantine as a measure to maintain freedom from rabies include Australia, where an outbreak of disease considered likely to have been rabies occurred in Tasmania in 1866–67 (Doyle 1994), New Zealand, Hawaii, Sweden, where the last documented case was a dog originating from Russia in 1886 (Klintevall 1994), Norway (except the islands of Svalbard/Spitzbergen), where the last reported case was a human case in 1815 (Bakken 1994) and the United Kingdom where the last indigenously acquired human case was in Wales in 1902 and the last animal case was a dog which developed rabies after release from quarantine in 1970 (Gardner and King 1991).

Between 1922 and 1970, quarantine alone was at least 93.5 per cent effective in detecting animals which were incubating the disease when imported into the United Kingdom and has been 100 per cent effective since vaccination on the day of arrival was introduced in 1971 (King 1992). Apart from preventing the disease from entering its own animal population, quarantine has an important role in the prevention of spread of rabies to other countries; for example, many do not allow the importation of cats and dogs from rabies endemic areas unless they have first undergone vaccination and quarantine in the United Kingdom.

European Union (EU) intracommunity relaxation of border controls and a substantial reduction in the weight of infection throughout EU wildlife has permitted some changes to the strict importation regulations of the United Kingdom. Traded dogs and cats can now be imported without the 6 months quarantine period, provided that all of the wide-ranging terms of legislation are met. These terms include importation only from Member State-registered premises, health checks, identifying microchip implantation, vaccination (and,

for dogs, vaccination against distemper) and blood tests. Quarantine with vaccination is retained for any dog or cat that does not meet all of these requirements, for pet dogs and cats, and for animals which are imported to any Member State from rabies-endemic areas. It is likely, however, that the regulations will be modified to allow free movement of dogs and cats within the EU.

CANINE RABIES CONTROL

On introduction to a susceptible population, rabies spreads quickly and may reach an annual rate of 0.22–14.5 cases/1000 in unvaccinated dogs (Beran 1991). Numerous inactivated rabies vaccines have been shown to be efficacious in dogs, and the constraints to effective dog rabies control are economic and logistical rather than technical. It has been proposed (WHO 1984) that an immunization level of 70 per cent is required to control epidemic dog rabies. In economic environments characterized by severely limited resources, the cost-effectiveness of dog rabies vaccination could be improved considerably by concentrating on the identification of high-risk subpopulations (e.g. in high-density urban suburbs) where close proximity between households and minimal dog movement restriction result in high dog to dog contact rates (Perry 1993). These measures, however, are likely to lead to a temporary reduction in the rabies incidence rate rather than the long-term goal of disease elimination.

Nevertheless, canine rabies control measures should be applied even where wildlife rabies persists. Spillover of a wildlife rabies virus into the canine population may occur from time to time, but the tendency to spread within the canine population is less than that of a virus originating from canine rabies reservoirs (Perry 1993).

Parenteral vaccination of dogs is a well-tested method of rabies control in many countries, but the degree of success is diminished by an inability to vaccinate an acceptable proportion (60–80 per cent) of the dogs, particularly stray, unowned, or feral dogs. Consequently, attention has been focused on the development of oral vaccines, baits, and bait delivery systems appropriate to the dog. A number of vaccines, most of which are already in use in field trials of wildlife vaccination, have been tested. The vaccinia rabies glycoprotein recombinant (V-RG) and human adenovirus 5 recombinant (HAV5) both immunized dogs (WHO 1992), as did modified live vaccines SAD B19 and SAG-2. However, some work is still required on safety for non-target species, baits and bait acceptability, but with a concerted effort and the continued backing of international bodies such as WHO, the elimination of canine rabies would appear to be a realistic goal.

WILDLIFE RABIES CONTROL

Attempts to control wildlife rabies represent unprecedented international co-operation between veterinary public health authorities and have made an enormous contribution to understanding rabies epidemiology, virology, ecology, and vaccine technology. Early attempts included costly and culturally unacceptable wildlife population reduction by trapping, poisoning, den-gassing, and bounty payments, and were followed by the invention of devices such as 'Vac-Traps' and 'Coyote-Getters' to vaccinate wildlife parenterally with conventional vaccines or to explode vaccine into the oropharangeal cavity of target animals. All were universally unsuccessful (Winkler 1990).

Baer, perhaps influenced by the discovery by Correa-Giron and his colleagues (1970) that rabies could be transmitted to rodents if live virus was pipetted on to mucous membranes of the mouth, is credited with the oral vaccine idea. Winkler and Baer proved in the laboratory that animals could be vaccinated and protected against challenge using a field-applicable oral vaccine system (Winkler and Baer 1976). Following preliminary trials in 1977 on a river island and then near a rabies-infected area of Switzerland in 1978 (Steck *et al.* 1982) it was concluded that, provided the attenuated live rabies vaccine could be properly applied and controlled, trials under certain very strict preconditions could be initiated in other countries. The ensuing history of oral vaccination has been extensively and eloquently reviewed (Winkler 1990).

An important advance in the technological acceptability of oral vaccination trials was the development of Mabs which distinguished between rabies vaccine virus and the local field strain. Other research was directed towards the development of vaccines efficacious for the target species and towards the development of baits and bait delivery systems applicable to a variety of target species and ecological habitats. Research was also concerned with baiting campaign strategies—the number of campaigns required, the intervals between them, seasonality (with regard to vaccine and bait stability), and bait distribution techniques.

Wildlife rabies control in Africa

An oral vaccination system which will control the large rabies epidemics that occur in jackals in Zimbabwe is being investigated. The candidate vaccine (SAD Berne), however, proved lethal for Chacma baboons, a prominent non-target species (Bingham *et al.* 1992). On the other hand, Chacma baboons and civets, another non-target species, were immunized by SAG-2 vaccine and efficacy trials of this vaccine in black-backed and side-striped jackals are underway. Chicken-head baits have proved to be both attractive to and 'chewey' for jackals, whereas they did not readily consume baits composed of materials unfamiliar to them (Bingham *et al.* 1993).

Wildlife rabies control in the Americas

Despite the early interest in oral vaccination and the energy devoted to bait configurations and baiting strategies, wildlife rabies control in the Americas has only recently been put into practice. Rabies in foxes has been virtually eliminated from a 30 000 km^2 area in eastern Ontario (Garscadden *et al.* 1994). In the autumn of 1994, 1.45 million baits at 20–100 baits/km^2 were dropped from aircraft over an area of 62 425 km^2. The cost of the exercise was Cdn\$4.6/km^2 (MacInnes *et al.* 1994). Between 1991 and early 1994, material from about 1900 diagnosed rabid animals was subjected to Mabs analyses. The viruses isolated from three animals (skunk, red fox, and raccoon) were indistinguishable from ERA virus; all three animals originated from the vaccination area in Ontario (Wandeler *et al.* 1994c).

A novel approach was taken to prevent raccoon rabies from becoming established in Canada. During May to October 1994, over an area of 700 km^2, trappers live-trapped raccoons and then vaccinated, tagged, and released them; any foxes and skunks caught incidentally were also vaccinated and released. The costs of the trap–vaccinate–release (TVR) control tactic were estimated to be no higher than those for aerial baiting (Rosatte *et al.* 1994).

In order to prevent the spread of raccoon rabies in New Jersey, a V-RG vaccination zone of 55 917 ha, forming a band approximately 18 km wide, was placed across the northern Cap May peninsular. The raccoon epizootic, moving at a rate of approximately 50 km/

year, reached the northern border of the zone in April 1993, but the V-RG vaccine substantially inhibited its movement and incidence in the zone (Roscoe *et al.* 1994).

Attempts to control vampire bat rabies, which commenced in the 1950s, have met with variable success rates. In general, early methods, which included smoke, fire, or explosion in the refuges, were expensive and non-selective—bats of other species were similarly destroyed. Control by topical treatment of captured vampires with anticoagulants was specific, selective, and relatively inexpensive when warfarin was used. The treatment involved vampire capture, painting the chest with warfarin suspended in vaseline, then release, allowing conspecifics to become treated through grooming of the released bat. A variation of the method, in which the anticoagulant compound was painted on old wounds of cattle was equally successful. Thompson *et al.* (1972) introduced a method of control in which cattle were given anticoagulant via the intraruminant route, releasing anticoagulant into the bloodstream. Later it was found that the intramuscular route was as efficacious, simpler to apply and cheaper (Flores-Crespo *et al.* 1979).

Although vampiricidal methods of rabies control are claimed to be very effective (Flores-Crespo and Arellano-Sota 1991), vampire bat rabies continues to cause severe cattle losses in Central and South America. As in terrestrial animal rabies, control by population reduction has a poor record. It has been shown (Rupprecht and Kieny 1988) that cattle can be vaccinated with V-RG.

Wildlife rabies control in Europe

Early intervention in the European rabies epizootic by host species population control (shooting, poisoning, and den-gassing) was highly controversial and of limited success. Factors that militate against control by vector species depopulation include the difficulties of accurate population census, the reproductive potential of those that are spared, the unforeseen results of upsetting the balance of nature, and, not least, the lack of public support in developed countries for methods which decimate wildlife populations (King and Turner 1993).

After nearly a decade of relatively small-scale field trials, during which about 1.6 million 'chicken-head' vaccine baits were laid, predominantly by hand, attention turned to the large-scale manufacture of vaccine encased in, for example, fish-meal polymer baits and to their widespread distribution by fixed-wing aircraft or helicopters. Since 1985–86 the number of countries participating in control programmes has increased to 14, plus Russia, Estonia, and Belarus. Over 70 million vaccine baits, costing US$83 million have been distributed over an area of 4.5 million km^2 (Stohr and Meslin, 1996). The rabies incidence has fallen markedly in all countries where vaccine baits have been distributed, although no country so far has succeeded in eradicating the disease and remaining rabies-free for a long period. However, in the past 5 years, Germany and France, the two countries to have reported the highest incidence of the disease (Table 37.3) have made remarkable progress (Table 37.7). There is great optimism that rabies will

Table 37.7 Animal rabies in Germany and France 1989–94[a]

	Domesticated animals				Wild animals					Total
	Dog	Cat	Other[b]	Total	Fox	Deer	Badger	Other[c]	Total	
Germany										
1989	163	329	754	1246	4855	316	128	278	5577	6823
1990	192	267	523	1082	3937	242	94	216	4489	5571
1991	153	189	282	624	2665	130	48	132	2975	3599
1992	59	77	138	274	1011	56	24	60	1151	1425
1993	6	25	110	141	636	28	16	24	704	845
1994[d]	4	15	66	85	515	11	20	11	557	642
France										
1989	53	117	554	724	3341	28	35	86	3490	4214
1990	50	82	331	463	2406	19	37	59	2521	2984
1991	38	83	269	390	1663	24	23	45	1755	2165
1992	30	49	138	217	1000	16	16	35	1067	1284
1993	4	11	26	41	198	1	6	15	220	261
1994[d]	0	1	13	14	55	0	0	2	57	71

[a] Figures derived from *Rabies Bulletins Europe* 1989–June 1994.
[b] Includes cattle, sheep, goats, horses.
[c] Includes wild cat, raccoon, raccoon-dog, wild boar, squirrel.
[d] 1 January 1994–30 June 1994.

be eradicated from the EU within the next 2 or 3 years; success would be a remarkable achievement.

ACKNOWLEDGEMENT

This chapter contains contributions by a number of colleagues and friends in the rabies field. I wish to place on record my thanks to Dr N. Tordo for advice on molecular biology and permission to use Fig. 37.1; to Dr K. M. Charlton for advice on disease mechanisms, Dr W. G. Winkler on clinical disease in animals, Dr M. Lafon on immunobiology, and to Drs M. J. and D. A. Warrell, G. S. Turner and A. I. Wandeler for their helpful comments and suggestions for improvement. I also thank the Directorate of the Central Veterinary Laboratory, Weybridge, for the provision of library, copying, and communications facilities.

REFERENCES

Aubert, M. F. A., Blancou, J., Barrat, J., Artois, M. and Barrat, M. J. (1991). Transmissibility and pathogenicity of two isolates of rabies virus collected from red foxes at a 10-year interval. *Annales de Recherches Veterinaires*, **22**, 77–93.

Baer, G. M. and Bales, G. L. (1967). Experimental rabies infection in the Mexican freetail bat. *Journal of Infectious Diseases*, **177**, 82–90.

Baer, G. M. and Lentz, T. L. (1991). Rabies pathogenesis to the central nervous system. In *The Natural History of Rabies*, (2nd edn), (ed. G. M. Baer), pp. 105–32. CRC Press, Boca Raton.

Bakken, G. (1994). Rabies vaccination and antibody testing in lieu of quarantine—new requirements for dogs and cats imported to Norway and Sweden from European countries of the EU/EFTA. In *Expert consultation on the technical bases for recognition of rabies-free areas and animal quarantine requirements, Santo Domingo, Pan American Health Organization*, in press.

Barge, A., Gaudin, Y., Coulon, P., and Ruigrok, R. W. H. (1993). Vesicular stomatitis virus M protein may be inside the ribonucleocapsid core. *Virology*, **67**, 7246–53.

Benmansour, A. *et al.* (1991). Antigenicity of rabies virus glycoprotein. *Journal of Virology*, **65**, 4198–203.

Beran, G. W. (1991). Urban Rabies. In *The natural history of rabies*, (2nd edn), (ed. G. M. Baer), pp. 427–43. CRC Press, Boca Raton.

Bingham, J. *et al.* (1992). The pathogenicity of SAD rabies vaccine given by the oral route in Chacma baboons (*Papio ursinus*). *Veterinary Record*, **131**, 55–6.

Bingham, J. *et al.* (1993). Oral rabies vaccination of jackals: progress in Zimbabwe. *Onderstepoort Journal of Veterinary Research*, **60**, 477–8.

Blancou, J. (1988). Epizootiology of rabies: Eurasia and Africa. In *Rabies*, (ed. J. B. Campbell and K. M. Charlton), pp. 243–65. Kluwer Academic Publishers, Boston

Blancou, J. (1994). Early methods for the surveillance and control of rabies in animals. *Review Scientifique et Technique. Office International des Epizooties*, **13**, 363–71.

Blancou, J., Pastoret, P.-P., Brochier, B., Thomas, I., and Bogel, K. (1988). Vaccinating wild animals against rabies. *Revue Scientifique et Technique. Office International des Epizooties*, **7**, 1005–13.

Bögel, K. and Motschwiller, E. (1986). Incidence of rabies and post-exposure treatment in developing countries. *Bulletin of the World Health Organization*, **64**, 883–7.

Bourhy, H., Kissi, B., and Tordo, N. (1993). Taxonomy and evolutionary studies on lyssaviruses with special reference to Africa. *Onderstepoort Journal of Veterinary Research*, **60**, 277–82.

Brass, D. A. (1994). *Rabies in bats—natural history and public health implications*. Livia Press, Ridgefield, Connecticut, USA

Charlton, K. M. (1988). The pathogenesis of rabies. In *Rabies*, (ed. J. B. Campbell and K. M. Charlton), pp. 101–50. Kluwer Academic, Boston.

Charlton, K. M. (1994). The pathogeneses of rabies and other lyssaviral infections: recent studies. In *Lyssaviruses*, (ed. C. E. Rupprecht, B. Dietzschold, and H. Koprowski), pp. 95–119. Springer-Verlag, New York.

Correa-Giron, E. P., Allen, R., and Sulkin, S. E. (1970). The infectivity and pathogenesis of rabies virus administered orally. *American Journal of Epidemiology*, **91**, 203–15.

Dietzschold, B. *et al.* (1992). Delineation of putative mechanisms involved in antibody-mediated clearance of rabies virus from the central nervous system. *Proceedings of the National Academy of Science USA*, **89**, 7252–6.

Doyle, K. (1994). Maintenance of rabies-free status and quarantine requirements—Australia. In *Expert consultation on the technical bases for recognition of rabies-free areas and animal quarantine requirements, Santo Domingo*. Pan American Health Organization, in press.

Dutta, J. K., Warrell, M. J., and Dutta, T. K. (1994). Intradermal rabies immunization for pre- and post-exposure prophylaxis. *The National Medical Journal of India*, **7** (4), 119–22.

Eng, T. R., Hamaker, T. A., Dobbins, T. C., Bryson, J. H., and Finsky, P. F. (1989). Rabies surveillance, United States, 1988. *Morbidity and Mortality Weekly Report*, **38**, (SS-1), 1–21.

Ertl, H. C. J. *et al.* (1989). Induction of rabies virus-specific T-helper cells by synthetic peptides that carry dominant T-helper cell epitopes of the viral ribonucleoprotein. *Journal of Virology*, **63**, 2885–92.

Fekadu, M. (1991). Latency and aborted rabies. In *The Natural History of Rabies*, (2nd edn), (ed. G. M. Baer), pp. 191–8. CRC Press, Boca Raton.

Fenje, P. (1960). Propagation of rabies virus in cultures of hamster kidney cells. *Canadian Journal of Microbiology*, **6**, 479–84.

Fishbein, D. B. (1991). Rabies in Humans. In *The Natural History of Rabies*, (2nd edn), (ed. G. M. Baer), pp. 519–49. CRC Press, Boca Raton.

Flores-Crespo, R. and Arellano-Sota, C. (1991). Biology and control of the vampire bat. In *The Natural History of Rabies*, (2nd edn), (ed. G. M. Baer), pp. 461–76. CRC Press, Boca Raton.

Flores-Crespo, R., Said, F. S., de Anda, L. D., Ibarra, V. F., and Anaya, R. M. (1979). Nueva técnica para el combate de los vampiros, Warfarina por via intramuscular al ganado bovino. *Bol Of Panam*, **86**, (4), 283–285.

Fuenzalida, E. and Palacios, R. (1955). Un metodo mejorado para la preparacion de la vacuna antirabica. *Bulletin of the Institute of Bacteriology, Chile*, **8**, 3.

Gardner, S. and King, A. (1991). Rabies—recent developments in research and human prophylaxis. In *Current Topics in Clinical Virology*, (ed. P. Morgan-Capner), pp. 141–63. Public Health Laboratory Service.

Garscadden, M. D. *et al.* (1994). The Ontario baiting service. *Fifth Annual International Meeting, Rabies in the Americas*, Abstract, p. 15. Rabies Research Unit, Ontario Ministry of Natural Resources.

Gaultier, P. V. (1879). Etudes sur la rage. Rage du lapin. *Comptes Rendus de 1' Academie des Sciences, Paris*, **89**, 444–46.

Holland, J. J. (1987). Defective interfering rhabdoviruses. In *The Rhabdoviruses*, (ed. R. R. Wagner), pp. 297–360. Plenum Press, New York.

Hutcheon, D. (1894). *Reports of the colonial veterinary surgeon and assistant veterinary surgeons for the year 1893*. Department of Agriculture. Cape of Good Hope.

Jenkins, S. R., Perry, B. D., and Winkler, W. G. (1988). Ecology and epidemiology of raccoon rabies. *Review of Infectious Diseases*, **10**, S620–625.

King, A. A. (1991). Studies of the antigenic relationships of rabies and rabies-related viruses using anti-nucleocapsid monoclonal antibodies. Thesis. University of Surrey, Guildford, UK.

King, A. A. (1992). Current application of quarantine measures worldwide—new trends. *Report of the meeting of the OIE ad hoc group on rabies control, Paris, 21–23 April 1992*.

King, A. and Crick, J. (1988). Rabies-related viruses. In *Rabies*, (ed. J. B. Campbell and K. M. Charlton), pp. 177–99. Kluwer Academic, Boston.

King, A. A. and Turner, G. S. (1993). Rabies: a review. *Journal of Comparative Pathology*, **108**, 1–39.

Kissling, R. E. (1958). Growth of rabies virus in non-nervous tissue culture. *Proceedings of the Society of Experimental Biology*, **98**, 223–5.

Klintevall, K. (1994). Rabies vaccination and antibody testing in lieu of dog quarantine in Sweden. In *Expert consultation on the technical bases for recognition of rabies-free areas and animal quarantine requirements, Santo Domingo*. Pan American Health Organization, in press.

Krebs, J. W., Holman, R. C., Hines, U., Strine, T. W., Mandel, E. J., and Childs, J. E. (1992). Rabies surveillance in the United States during 1991. *Journal of the American Veterinary Medical Association*, **201**, (12), 1836–48.

Krebs, J. W., Strine, T. W., and Childs, J. E. (1993). Rabies urveillance in the United States during 1992. *Journal of the American Veterinary Medical Association*, **203**, (12), 1718–31.

Krebs, J. W., Strine, T. W., Smith, J. S., Rupprecht, C. E., and Childs, J. E. (1994). Rabies surveillance in the United States during 1993. *Journal of the American Veterinary Medical Association*, **205**, 1695–709.

Lafon, M. (1994). Immunobiology of lyssaviruses: the basis for immunoprotection. In *Lyssaviruses*, (ed. C. E. Rupprecht, B. Dietzschold, and H. Koprowski), pp. 145–60. Springer-Verlag, New York.

Lafon, M., Bourhy, H., and Sureau, P. (1988). Immunity against the European bat rabies (Duvenhage) virus induced by rabies vaccines: an experimental study in mice. *Vaccine*, **6**, 362–8.

Larghi, O. P., Arrosi, J. S., Nakajata-A, J., and Villa-Nova, A. (1988). Control of urban rabies. In *Rabies*, (ed. J. B. Campbell and K. M. Charlton), pp. 407–22. Kluwer Academic, Boston.

Lawson, K. F., Walker, V. C. R., and Crawley, J. F. (1967). ERA strain rabies vaccine, duration of immunity in cattle, dogs and cats. *Veterinary Medicine Small Animal Clinic*, **62**, 1073–4.

Levine, B., Hardwick, J. M., Trapp, B. D., Crawford, T. O., Bollinger, R. C., and Griffin, D. E. (1991). Antibody-mediated clearance of alphavirus infection from neurons. *Science*, **254**. 856–60.

Lodmell, D. L., Sumner, J. W., Esposito, J. J., Bellini, W. J., and Ewalt, L. C. (1991). Raccoon poxvirus recombinants expressing the rabies virus nucleoprotein protect mice against lethal rabies virus infection. *Journal of Virology*, **65**, 3400–5.

MacInnes, C. D. *et al.* (1994). The Ontario-vaccine-baiting system. *Fifth Annual International Meeting, Rabies in the Americas*, Abstracts, p. 22. Rabies Research Unit, Ontario Ministry of Natural Resources.

Montano-Hirose, J. A., Lafage, M., Weber, P., Badrane, H., Tordo, N. and Lafon, M. (1993). Protective activity of a murine monoclonal antibody against European bat lyssavirus 1 (EBL1) infection in mice. *Vaccine*, **11**, 1259–66.

Negri, A. (1903). Beitrag zum studium der aetiologie der tollwut. *Zeitschrift für Hygiene und infektionskrankheiten*, **43**, 507–28.

Nicholson, K. G. (1990). Modern vaccines: rabies. *Lancet*, **335**, 1202–5.

Pasteur, L., Chamberland, M. M., and Roux, M. (1882). Nouveaux faits pour servir a la connaissance de la rage. *Comptes Rendus de 1' Academie des Sciences*, **95**, 1187–92.

Perrin, P., Rollin, P. E., and Sureau, P. (1986). A rapid rabies enzyme immunodiagnosis (RREID): a useful and simple technique for the routine laboratory diagnosis of rabies. *Journal of Biological Standardization*, **14**, 217–22.

Perry, B. D. (1993). Dog ecology in eastern and southern Africa: implications or rabies control. *Onderstepoort Journal of Veterinary Research*, **60**, 429–36.

Prevec, L., Campbell, J. B., Christie, B. S., Belbeck, L., and Graham, F. L. (1990). A recombinant human adenovirus vaccine against rabies. *Journal of Infectious Diseases*, **161**, 27–30.

Reid-Sanden, F. L., Dobbins, J. G., Smith, J. S., and Fishbein, D. B. (1990). Rabies surveillance in the United States during 1989. *Journal of the American Veterinary Medical Association*, **197**, (12), 1571–83.

Rosatte, R. C. (1988). Rabies in Canada: history, epidemiology and control. *Canadian Veterinary Journal*, **29**, 362–5.

Rosatte, R. C. *et al.* (1994). Trap-vaccinate-release (T-V-R) as a tactic to prevent raccoon rabies from becoming established in the Niagara frontier: cost effectiveness of T-V-R versus oral vaccination with baits. *Fifth Annual International Meeting, Rabies in the Americas*, Abstracts, p. 32. Rabies Research Unit, Ontario Ministry of Natural Resources.

Roscoe, D. E., Holste, W., Niezgoda, M., and Rupprecht, C. E. (1994). Efficacy of the V-RG oral rabies vaccine in blocking epizootic raccoon rabies. *Fifth Annual International Meeting, Rabies in the Americas*, Abstracts, p. 33. Rabies Research Unit, Ontario Ministry of Natural Resources.

Ruiz, A. and Diaz, A. M. (1990). Epidemiology of rabies transmitted by vampire bats. In *Wildlife rabies control*, (ed. K. Bögel, F. X. Meslin, and M. Kaplan), pp. 57–64. Wells Medical, Kent, UK.

Rupprecht, C. E. and Kieny, M.-P. (1988). Development of a vaccinia-rabies glycoprotein recombinant virus vaccine. In *Rabies*, (ed. J. B. Campbell and K. M. Charlton), pp. 335–64. Kluwer Academic.

Sacramento, D., Bourhy, H., and Tordo, N. (1991). PCR technique as an alternative method for diagnosis and molecular epidemiology of rabies virus. *Molecular and Cellular Probes*, **5**, 229–40.

Schumacher, C. L. *et al.* (1993). SAG-2 oral rabies vaccine. *Onderstepoort Journal of Veterinary Research*, **60**, 459–62.

Smith, J. S. and Baer, G. M. (1988). Epizootiology of rabies: the Americas. In *Rabies*, (ed. J. B. Campbell and K. M. Charlton), pp. 267–99. Kluwer Academic, Boston.

Smith, J. S., Fishbein, D. B., Rupprecht, C. E., and Clark, K. (1991). Unexplained rabies in three immigrants in the United States. A virologic investigation. *New England Journal of Medicine*, **324**, 205–11.

Smith, J. S., Yager, P. A., and Ociari, L. A. (1993). Rabies in wild and domestic carnivores of Africa: epidemiological and historical associations determined by limited sequence analysis. *Onderstepoort Journal of Veterinary Research*, **60**, 307–14.

Steck, F., Wandeler, A., Bischel, P., Capt, S., and Schneider, L. G. (1982). Oral immunization of foxes against rabies: a field study. *Zenblat. Veterinarmed. B*, **29**, 372–96.

Stohr, K., Meslin, F. M. (1996). Progress and setbacks in the oral immunization of foxes against rabies in Europe. *Veterinary Record*, **139**, 32–35.

Suntharasamai, P. *et al.* (1994). A simplified and economical regimen of purified chick embryo cell rabies vaccine for postexposure prophylaxis. *Vaccine*, **12**, (6), 508–12.

Swanepoel, R. *et al.* (1993). Rabies in southern Africa. *Onderstepoort Journal of Veterinary Research*, **60**, 325–46.

Thompson, R. D., Mitchel, G. C., and Burns, R. J. (1972). Vampire bat control by systemic treatment of livestock with an anticoagulant. *Science*, **177**, 806.

Thomson, G. R. and Meredith, C. D. (1993). Rabies in bat-eared foxes in South Africa. *Onderstepoort Journal of Veterinary Research*, **60**, 399–403.

Tordo, N. and Kouknetzoff, A. (1993). The rabies virus genome: and overview. *Onderstepoort J. Vet. Res.*, **60**, 263–9.

Tsiang, H. (1992). Pathogenesis of rabies virus infection of the nervous system. *Advances in Virus Research*, **42**, 375–412.

Uhaa, I. J., Mandel, E. J., Whiteway, R., and Fishbein, D. B. (1992). Rabies surveillance in the United States during 1990. *Journal of the American Veterinary Medical Association*, **200**, (7), 920–9.

Vaughn, J. B., Gerhardt, P., and Paterson, J. C. (1963). Excretion of street rabies virus in saliva of cats. *Journal of the American Medical Association*, **184**, 705–8.

Vieuchange, J. (1956). Multiplication du virus rabique, (virus fixé et virus des rues) dans les cultures de tissus en dialyse. *Comptes Rendus de l' Academie des Sciences*, **242**, 201–3.

Wandeler, A. I. (1991). Carnivore rabies: ecological and evolutionary aspects. *Hystrix*, **3**, 121–35.

Wandeler, A. I., Nadin-Davis, S. A., Tinline, R. R. and Rupprecht, C. E. (1994a). Rabies epidemiology: some ecological and evolutionary perspectives. In *Lyssaviruses*, (ed. C. E. Rupprecht, B. Dietzschold, and H. Koprowski), pp. 297–324. Springer-Verlag, New York.

Wandeler, A. I. *et al.* (1994b). Human adenovirus type 5 rabies-glycoprotein recombinant vaccines: an update. *Fifth Annual International Meeting, Rabies in the Americas*, Abstracts, p. 44. Rabies Research Unit, Ontario Ministry of Natural Resources.

Wandeler, A. I., Armstrong, J., Elmgren, L. D., Casey, G. A., and Nadin-Davis, S. (1994c). ERA induced rabies in Ontario wildlife. *Fifth Annual International Meeting, Rabies in the Americas*, Abstracts, p. 43–44. Rabies Research Unit, Ontario Ministry of Natural Resources.

Warrell, D. A. (1986). Rabies in man; natural history, pathology and illustrative case histories. In *Rabies the facts*, (2nd edn), (ed. C. Kaplan, G. S. Turner, and D. A. Warrell), pp. 21–48. Oxford University Press, Oxford.

Warrell, M. J. (1988). Rabies. *Current Opinion in Infectious Diseases*, **1**, 704–12.

Warrell, M. J. *et al.* (1985). Economical multiple-site intradermal immunization with human diploid-cell-strain vaccine is effective for post-exposure rabies prophylaxis. *Lancet*, May 11, 1059–62.

Warrell, M. J. *et al.* (1988). Rapid diagnosis of rabies and post-vaccinal encephalitides. *Clinical Experimental Immunology*, **71**, 229–34.

WHO (World Health Organization) (1984). *Guidelines for dog rabies control*. WHO VPH/83.43, Geneva.

WHO (World Health Organization) (1992). *Expert Committee on Rabies. Eighth Report*. WHO Technical Report Series 824. WHO, Geneva.

WHO (World Health Organization) (1993). *World Survey of Rabies 27 (for year 1991)*. WHO/Rabies/93.209. WHO, Geneva.

Wiktor, T. J., Fernandes, M. V., and Koprowski, H. (1964). Cultivation of rabies virus in human diploid cell strain WI-38. *Journal of Immunology*, **93**, 353–66.

Wiktor, T. J., Macfarlan, R. I., Foggin, C. M., and Koprowski, H. (1984). Antigenic analysis of rabies and Mokola virus from Zimbabwe using monoclonal antibodies. International symposium on monoclonal antibodies standardization and their characterization and use, Paris. *Developments in Biological Standardization*, **57**, 199–211.

Winkler, W. G. (1990). A review of the development of the oral vaccination technique for immunizing wildlife against rabies. In *Wildlife rabies control*, (ed. K. Bögel, F. X. Meslin, and M. Kaplan), pp. 82–96. Wells Medical, Kent, UK.

Winkler, W. G. and Baer, G. M. (1976). Rabies immunization of red fox (*Vulpes fulva*) with vaccine in sausage baits. *American Journal of Epidemiology*, **103**, 408–15.

Winkler, W. G., Baker, E. F., and Hopkins, C. C. (1972). An outbreak of non-bite transmitted rabies in a laboratory animal colony. *American Journal of Public Health*, **95**, (3), 267–77.

Wunner, W. H. (1991). The chemical composition and structure of rabies viruses. In *The natural history of rabies*, (2nd edn), (ed. G. M. Baer), pp. 31–67. CRC Press, Boca Raton.

Zinke, G. G. (1804). *Neue Ansichten der Hundswuth, ihrer Ursachen und Folgen, nebst einer sichern Behandlungsart der von tollen Tierhen gebissenen Menschen*. C. E. Gabler, Jena.

38 RIFT VALLEY FEVER

R. Swanepoel

SUMMARY

Rift Valley fever (RVF) is an acute disease of domestic ruminants in mainland Africa and Madagascar, caused by a mosquito-borne virus and characterized by necrotic hepatitis and a haemorrhagic state. Large outbreaks of the disease in sheep, cattle and goats occur at irregular intervals of several years when exceptionally heavy rains favour the breeding of the mosquito vectors, and are distinguished by heavy mortality among newborn animals and abortion in pregnant animals. Humans become infected from contact with tissues of infected animals or from mosquito bite, and usually develop mild to moderately severe febrile illness, but severe complications, which occur in a small proportion of patients, include ocular sequelae, encephalitis, and fatal haemorrhagic disease. Modified live and inactivated vaccines are available for use in livestock, and an inactivated vaccine is made available on an experimental basis for use in humans with regular occupational exposure to infection. The literature on the disease has been the subject of several extensive reviews from which the information presented here is drawn, except where indicated otherwise (Henning 1956; Weiss 1957; Easterday 1965; Peters and Meegan 1981; Shimshony and Barzilai 1983; Meegan and Bailey 1989; Swanepoel and Coetzer 1994).

HISTORY

The disease was first recognized in sheep in the Rift Valley in Kenya at the turn of the century, but the causative agent was not isolated until 1930. Over the next four decades, epizootics were recorded only in eastern and southern Africa, where they tended to occur in association with population explosions of floodwater-breeding aedine mosquitoes following heavy rains. Large outbreaks affecting sheep and cattle occurred in Kenya in 1930–31, 1968, and 1978–79, and lesser outbreaks at irregular intervals in the intervening years. A major epizootic, which caused an estimated 500 000 abortions and 100 000 deaths of sheep, occurred in South Africa in 1950–51; a second major

and more widespread outbreak caused extensive losses of sheep and cattle in 1974–76, while lesser outbreaks were recorded in 1952–53, 1955–59, 1969–71, and 1981. Severe outbreaks occurred in the predominantly sheep-farming areas of southern Namibia in 1955 and 1974–76. Further extensive outbreaks of the disease in southern Africa occurred in areas where cattle farming predominates, in Zimbabwe in 1955, 1957, 1969–70, and 1978, in Mozambique in 1969, and in Zambia in 1973–74, 1978, and 1985. In addition, evidence of the occurrence of the infection was recorded in many other southern and East African countries.

It was realized from the time of the original investigations in Kenya that febrile illness in humans accompanied outbreaks of disease in livestock, and that some patients experienced transient loss of visual acuity, but the occurrence of serious ocular sequelae was first recognized in the 1950–51 epizootic in South Africa. The first known human fatality was recorded in 1934 in a laboratory worker in the United States, but since the infection was complicated by thrombophlebitis and the patient died from pulmonary embolism, the potential lethality of the virus for man was overlooked until seven deaths from encephalitis and/or haemorrhagic fever with necrotic hepatitis were ascribed to RVF during the 1974–76 epizootic in South Africa. Subsequently deaths were also observed in Zimbabwe.

Prior to the 1970s, the presence of the virus was known for decades in the Sudan and certain West African countries from antibody studies, and there were periodic isolations of the virus in West Africa, where it was sometimes reported as Zinga virus, which is now known to be identical to RVF virus. In 1973 and 1976, outbreaks of RVF affecting livestock were reported in the Sudan. These epizootics were followed in 1977–78 by a major outbreak which occurred along the Nile delta and valley in Egypt, causing an unprecedented number of human infections and deaths, as well as numerous deaths and abortions in sheep and cattle and some losses in goats, water buffaloes, and camels. Estimates of the number of human cases of disease range from 18 000 to more than 200 000, with at least 598 deaths occurring from encephalitis and/or haemorrhagic fever. Thereafter, a severe epizootic was reported in 1987 in the Senegal River basin of southern Mauritania and northern Senegal. In Mauritania alone an estimated 224 human patients died of the disease, and there was a high rate of abortion in sheep and goats. These outbreaks in North and West Africa differed in several respects from the pattern of disease which had hitherto been observed in sub-Saharan Africa; in particular they occurred independently of rainfall in arid countries, apparently in association with vectors which breed in large rivers and dams (Jouan *et al.* 1989).

Since the virus is capable of utilizing a wide range of mosquitoes as vectors, the occurrence of the outbreak in Egypt raised the possibility that RVF could be introduced to the mainland of Eurasia, and extensive preventive vaccination of livestock was undertaken at the time in the Sinai peninsula and Israel. Fears were also expressed that the virus could be transported to Saudi Arabia with animals exported from Africa for ritual slaughter on the annual Islamic pilgrimage to Mecca. In the event, only isolated outbreaks of RVF were recorded in Egypt in 1979 and 1980, and thereafter the country remained free of the disease for 12 years until it was again recognized in the Aswan Governate in May 1993. On this occasion there was not the same tendency for an explosive outbreak of the disease to occur as in 1977–78, but by October 1993 infections of humans and livestock, including sheep, cattle, and water buffalo, had also been recognized in Sharqiya, Giza, and El Faiyum Governates (Anonymous 1993, 1994).

The Smithburn strain of RVF virus, which had been isolated from mosquitoes in Uganda in 1944 and passaged intracerebrally in mice, was subjected to further passaging in embryonated chicken eggs and mice in South Africa, and issued in the form of freeze-dried infected mouse brain for use as a partially attenuated vaccine for livestock from 1951 onwards. In 1958, reversion was made to the use of a lower mouse passage level of the virus, and since 1971 the virus has been grown in cell cultures for the preparation of freeze-dried vaccine, recommended particularly for use in non-pregnant sheep (the virus retains abortigenic and teratogenic properties for a proportion of pregnant ewes). The same strain of virus is used at a slightly different level of mouse passage for the preparation of veterinary vaccine in Kenya when demand arises. The Smithburn virus was found to be inadequately immunogenic for cattle, and since 1975 a wild strain of virus grown in cell cultures has been used in South Africa for the preparation of a formalin-inactivated vaccine for use in cattle. An inactivated cell culture vaccine for veterinary use was also developed in Egypt in 1981. An experimental formalin-inactivated cell culture vaccine for use in humans was developed in the United States in 1962, and improvements to the vaccine were made in 1981.

THE VIRUS

TAXONOMY AND MOLECULAR BIOLOGY

The virus has the morphological and physicochemical properties typical of a member of the *Phlebovirus* genus of the family Bunyaviridae. It is spherical, approximately 100 nm in diameter, and has a host cell derived bilipid-layer envelope through which virus-coded glycoprotein spikes project. The genome comprises three segments of single-stranded RNA with a total molecular weight of 4×10^6 Da, and is in the negative sense (complementary to mRNA), except that the small segment consists of ambisense RNA, i.e. has bidirectional coding. Each of the three RNA segments, L (large), M (medium) and S (small), is contained in a separate nucleocapsid within the virion. In common with other bunyaviruses, phlebovirus virions contain three major structural proteins: two envelope glycoproteins, G1 and G2, and a nucleocapsid protein, N, plus minor quantities of viral transcriptase or L (large) protein, as it is termed. The L RNA segment codes for the viral transcriptase, the M segment for the G proteins and a non-structural protein, NS_m, and the S segment for the N protein and a non-structural protein, NS_s. The glycoproteins are responsible for recognition of receptor sites on susceptible cells, manifestation of viral haemagglutinating ability, and inducing protective immune response. The N protein induces production of and reacts with complement-fixing antibody. The non-structural NS_s protein synthesized during the replication of RVF virus, enters the cell nucleus to form intranuclear inclusions which are seen histologically in infected tissues. Virus which attaches to receptors on susceptible cells is internalized by endocytosis and replication occurs in the cytoplasm. Virions mature primarily by budding through endoplasmic reticulum in the Golgi region into cytoplasmic vesicles which are presumed to fuse with the plasma membrane to release virus, but particles can also bud directly from the plasma membrane.

No significant antigenic or genetic differences have been detected between RVF isolates and laboratory passaged strains originating from widely separated countries, but differences have been demonstrated in pathogenicity for laboratory rodents (Battles and Dalrymple 1988). However, it is uncertain whether this finding is reflected in differences in virulence for humans and livestock. Zinga virus, originally isolated in the Central African Republic in 1969 and long thought to be a distinct virus, and Lunyo virus, isolated in Uganda in 1955 and described as a variant of RVF virus, have both been found to be indistinguishable from RVF virus.

PATHOGENESIS

By analogy with the course of events believed to follow natural infection with other arthropod-borne viruses, it can be surmised that the pathogenesis of the disease may involve some replication of virus at the site of inoculation, conveyance of infection by lymphatic drainage to regional lymph nodes where there is further replication with spillover of virus into the circulation to produce primary viraemia, which in turn leads to systemic infection, and that intense viraemia then results from release of virus following replication in major target organs such as the liver and spleen (Peters and Anderson 1981). Wild RVF virus, which has not been subjected to serial passaging in laboratory host systems, is described as being hepato-, viscero-, or pantropic, and immunofluorescence studies in laboratory animals indicate that replication occurs in littoral macrophages of lymph nodes, most areas of the spleen except T-dependent periarteriolar sheaths, foci of adrenocortical cells, virtually all cells of the liver, most renal glomeruli and some tubules, lung tissue and scattered small vessel walls, as well as in necrotic foci in the brains of individuals which develop the encephalitic form of the disease. These sites correspond to the lymphoid necrosis in lymph nodes and spleen, hepatic necrosis and adrenal, lung and glomerular lesions seen in humans and livestock, and the brain lesions in humans (encephalitis has not been described in natural disease of ruminants). Cell damage is ascribed directly to the lytic effects of the virus, but the inflammatory response seen in human brain tissue suggests that there may also be an immunopathological element to the pathogenesis of encephalitis. The same may be true for ocular lesions. Recovery is mediated by non-specific and specific host responses, and the clearance of viraemia correlates with the appearance of neutralizing antibody. Immunity appears to be lifelong.

The mechanisms involved in the pathogenesis of the haemostatic derangement which occurs in RVF remain speculative. It is postulated that the critical lesions are vasculitis and hepatic necrosis. Destruction of the antithrombotic properties of endothelial cells is thought to trigger intravascular coagulation, and the widespread necrosis of hepatocytes and other affected cells to result in the release of procoagulants into the circulation. Severe liver damage presumably limits or abolishes production of coagulation proteins and reduces clearance of activated coagulation factors, thereby further promoting the occurrence of disseminated intravascular coagulopathy, which in turn augments tissue injury by impairing blood flow. Vasculitis and haemostatic failure result in purpura and widespread haemorrhages.

CULTURE OF THE VIRUS

The virus can be grown in, and readily produces cytopathic effect and plaques in, virtually all common continuous line and primary cell cultures, including Vero and BHK-21 line cells, primary calf and lamb kidney or testis cells; the only exceptions being primary macrophages and lymphoblastoid cell lines. It can be grown in embryonated chicken eggs and a variety of laboratory animals, including suckling or weaned mice and hamsters inoculated by intracerebral or intraperitoneal routes. Some laboratory strains of rat are resistant, as are rabbits, guinea-pigs, chickens, and African primates, but a proportion of rhesus monkeys manifests severe or fatal disease.

STABILITY

The virus is stable in serum and can be recovered after several months' storage at 4 °C or after 3 h at 56 °C; viraemic blood collected in an oxalate–carbol–glycerin preservative retained its infectivity after 8 years of storage under a variety of conditions of refrigeration, and the virus is very stable at temperatures lower than −60 °C or after freeze-drying, and in aerosols at 23 °C and 50–85 per cent relative humidity. It is inactivated by lipid solvents, such as ether and sodium deoxycholate, and low concentrations of formalin, and infectivity is rapidly lost below pH 6.8.

LIVESTOCK DISEASE

Newborn lambs and goat kids are extremely susceptible to the disease (Coetzer 1977), and the incubation period is short, in the range of 12–36 hours. The disease is marked by the development of fever which may be biphasic, listlessness, hyperpnoea, and disinclination to move or feed. Evidence of abdominal pain can be elicited. The course is usually peracute and lambs rarely survive longer than 24–36 hours after the onset of illness; many are simply found dead. Mortality may exceed 90 per cent in animals less than a week old. Lambs and kids older than 2 weeks and mature sheep and goats are significantly less susceptible to the disease. Nevertheless, following an incubation period of 24–72 hours, a few animals may die peracutely without exhibiting noteworthy signs of illness. Most develop an acute disease with fever of up to 42 °C that lasts for 24–96 hours, anorexia, weakness, listlessness, and hypernoea. Some animals may regurgitate ingesta, and develop melaena or fetid diarrhoea and a blood-tinged, mucopurulent nasal discharge. A few animals may be icteric. Many sheep and goats undergo inapparent infection. Reported death rates vary from 5 to

60 per cent for sheep, with highest mortality generally occurring in pregnant animals. Non-pregnant goats were described as resistant to the disease in some outbreaks, but suffered similar mortality to sheep in other instances.

The disease in calves resembles that in lambs and sheep, with occurrence of fever, inappetence, weakness, and a bloody or fetid diarrhoea, but a higher proportion of calves may develop icterus (Easterday *et al.* 1962*a*, *b*, *c*, Coetzer 1982). Death generally occurs 2–8 days after infection, and estimates of mortality range from less than 10 per cent in some outbreaks to 70 per cent in experimentally infected 1-week-old calves. Infection is frequently inapparent in adult cattle, but some animals develop acute disease characterized by fever of 24–96 hours duration, anorexia, staring coat, lachrymation, salivation, nasal discharge, dysgalactia, and a bloody or fetid diarrhoea. The death rate in cattle does not generally appear to exceed 5–10 per cent, but was reported to be 30 per cent among cattle which aborted in Egypt. Illness tended to run a prolonged course of 10–20 days in cattle in the Sudan in 1973, with severe icterus being a marked feature of the disease, although most animals recovered spontaneously.

Abortion appears to be the usual, if not invariable, outcome to infection in pregnant sheep, goats, and cattle. Animals may abort at any stage of gestation, and the fetuses generally have an autolysed appearance. However, abortion rates vary with epidemiological circumstances, and have ranged from 15 to 100 per cent in different outbreaks, or in separate herds and flocks in a single outbreak. Frequently, abortion may be the only overt manifestation of disease in a herd or flock. Factors determining the pattern of disease which occurs include the immune status of the animals, the challenge rate in the particular locality (mosquito biting frequency), and timing of the outbreak relative to the livestock breeding cycle. The offspring of immune ruminants acquire protective maternal immunity through the uptake of antibody from colostrum, but it was observed in South Africa that lambs were sometimes subjected to attack by large numbers of mosquitoes as soon as they were born, and could undergo irreversible infection before colostral immunity became effective.

Viraemia is generally demonstrable in domestic ruminants at the onset of fever and may persist for up to a week, with maximum titres of infectivity recorded being $10^{10.1}$ mouse intraperitoneal 50 per cent lethal doses/ml (MIPLD$_{50}$/ml) in lambs, $10^{8.2}$ in kids, and $10^{7.5}$ in calves, with somewhat lower maximum titres being recorded in adult animals.

Inoculation of pregnant ewes with the live Smithburn vaccine virus between about 5 and 10 weeks of gestation may result in the occurrence of a range of

anomalies of the central nervous system, including porencephaly, hydranencephaly and micrencephaly, as well as arthrogryposis and other defects in fetuses, and prolonged gestation and *hydrops amnii* in the ewes (Coetzer and Barnard 1977). Inoculation at an earlier stage of pregnancy may result in unnoticed early loss of the conceptus, while inoculation at a later stage may result in abortion, still birth or birth of immune or viraemic progeny. Teratology following vaccination has been recorded in the progeny of up to 15 per cent of pregnant ewes in flocks, but on average it appears to affect less than 2 per cent of ewes and abortion probably occurs in less than 10 per cent of pregnant ewes.

High prevalences of antibody were found in domesticated Asian water buffaloes during the 1977–78 epizootic in Egypt, and abortion and mortality rates of 7–12 per cent were recorded on some farms. Horses develop only low-grade viraemia following experimental infection, but during the Egyptian epizootic there was one isolation of virus from a horse, and four abortions in donkeys were ascribed to RVF, while a low prevalence of antibody to the virus was detected in the two species. No pathogenicity tests have been conducted on camels, but antibody was detected in camels in Kenya. Although there was only one isolation of RVF virus from a camel during the 1977–78 Egyptian outbreak, 56 deaths and one abortion were ascribed to the disease on the basis of circumstantial evidence. Pigs and dogs are resistant to infection, i.e. undergo inapparent infection, and birds are refractory to the virus.

Experimental RVF infection of African buffaloes (*Syncerus caffer*) in Kenya resulted in transient fever and viraemia, and one of two pregnant females aborted. It was noted on some properties involved in the 1950–51 epizootic in South Africa that abortion occurred in farmed springbok (*Antidorcas marsupialis*) and blesbok (*Damaliscus dorcas phillipsi*) antelope, but this was not confirmed to be due to RVF. A low prevalence of antibody to RVF virus was found in African buffaloes and a few species of antelopes in Zimbabwe, but no evidence of disease was recorded. Some species of wild myomorph rodents (rats and mice) exhibit transient viraemia following peripheral infection, and those that circulate the highest levels of virus succumb to the disease.

Although age and underlying illness undoubtedly influence the course of infection, it has been shown in cross-breeding experiments with inbred strains of laboratory rodent that there is a genetic basis to susceptibility to RVF, and it was postulated that the innate mechanisms involved also operate in humans and livestock to determine the manifestation of disease. It has been suggested that indigenous African breeds of livestock may be more resistant to RVF than exotic breeds, possibly through natural selection, but it was shown in limited experiments in Nigeria that local sheep were highly susceptible, and indigenous sheep, cattle, and goats were severely affected in the epizootics in Egypt and West Africa.

HUMAN DISEASE

SIGNS AND SYMPTOMS

The majority of RVF infections in humans are inapparent or associated with moderate to severe, non-fatal, febrile illness (Laughlin *et al.* 1979). After an incubation period of 2–6-days, the onset of the benign illness is usually very sudden and the disease is characterized by rigor, fever that persists for several days and is often biphasic, headache with retro-orbital pain and photophobia, weakness, and muscle and joint pains. Sometimes there is nausea and vomiting, abdominal pain, vertigo, epistaxis, and a petechial rash. Viraemia in humans lasts for up to a week, with a maximum recorded intensity of $10^{8.6}$ mouse intracerebral 50 per cent lethal doses/ml ($MICLD_{50}$/ml). Defervescence and symptomatic improvement occur in 4–7 days in benign disease and recovery is often complete in 2 weeks, but in a minority of patients the disease is complicated by the development of ocular lesions at the time of the initial illness or up to 4 weeks later. Estimates for the incidence of ocular complications range from less than 1 per cent to 20 per cent of human infections, and possibly the differences stem from failure to record mild cases in populations where illiterate persons are less likely to report minor disturbances of vision. The ocular disease usually presents as a loss of acuity of central vision, sometimes with development of scotomas. The essential lesion appears to be focal retinal ischaemia, generally in the macular or paramacular area, associated with thrombotic occlusion of arterioles and capillaries, and is characterized by retinal oedema and loss of transparency caused by dense white exudate and haemorrhages. Sometimes there is severe haemorrhage and detachment of the retina. The lesions and the loss of visual acuity generally resolve over a period of months with variable residual scarring of the retina, but in instances of severe haemorrhage and detachment of the retina there may be permanent uni-or bilateral blindness (Siam *et al.* 1980; Deutman and Klomp 1981)

Probably less than 1 per cent of human patients develop the haemorrhagic and/or encephalitic forms of the disease. Underlying liver disease may predispose to the haemorrhagic form of the illness. The haemorrhagic syndrome starts with sudden onset of febrile illness similar to the benign disease, but within 2–4 days there may be development of a petechial rash, purpura, ecchymoses and extensive subcutaneous haemorrhages, bleeding from needle-puncture sites, epistaxis, haematemesis, diarrhoea and melaena, sore and inflamed throat, gingival bleeding, epigastric pain, hepatomegaly or hepatosplenomegaly, tenderness of the right upper quadrant of the abdomen and deep jaundice. This is followed by pneumonitis, anaemia, shock with racing pulse and low blood pressure, hepatorenal failure, coma, and cardiorespiratory arrest. Factors contributing to fatal outcome in the hepatic form of the disease include anaemia, shock, and hepatorenal failure, with the kidney lesions possibly being as important as shock in producing anuria. A proportion of the less severely affected patients may make a protracted recovery without sequelae.

Encephalitis may occur in combination with the haemorrhagic syndrome. Otherwise, signs of encephalitis in humans may supervene during the acute illness, or up to 4 weeks later and include severe headache, vertigo, confusion, disorientation, amnesia, meningismus, hallucinations, hypersalivation, grinding of teeth, choreiform movements, convulsions, hemiparesis, lethargy, decerebrate posturing, locked-in syndrome, coma, and death. A proportion of patients may recover completely, but others may be left with sequelae, such as hemiparesis.

An attempt to relate the occurrence of abortion in humans to serological evidence of RVF infection in Egypt produced inconclusive results.

CLINICAL PATHOLOGY

The little information that is available on clinical pathology findings in humans is compatible with observations made in haematological and coagulation studies on rhesus monkeys (Peters *et al.* 1980), except that leucocytosis and anaemia may be more marked in severe human disease. Rhesus monkeys may have prolonged activated partial thromboplastin times and prothrombin times even in benign infection, and in severe liver disease there may be depletion of coagulation factors II, V, VII, IX, X and XII, thrombocytopenia and platelet dysfunction, increased schistocyte counts, and depletion of fibrinogen together with raised fibrin degradation product levels (Cosgriff *et al.* 1989). Raised serum aspartate aminotransferase and alanine aminotransferase levels have been recorded even in benign disease in humans.

DIAGNOSIS

The disease may be suspected when there is a sudden outbreak of febrile illness with headache and myalgia in humans, in association with the occurrence of abortions in domestic ruminants and deaths of young animals. Sometimes the human disease is only recognized from the occurrence of ocular complications, or haemorrhagic or encephalitic manifestations, and this is especially true in the rare instances where residents of other continents develop the illness following a visit to Africa. Frequently, outbreaks of RVF in livestock only become evident after investigations have been triggered by the recognition of the disease in humans.

Specimens to be submitted for laboratory confirmation of the diagnosis include blood from live patients, and tissue samples, particularly liver, but also spleen, kidney, lymph nodes, and heart blood of deceased patients. Tissue samples should be submitted in duplicate in a viral transport medium, and in 10 per cent buffered-formalin for histopathological examination (Shope and Sather 1979).

Viral antigen can often be detected rapidly in blood and other tissues by a variety of immunological methods, including immunodiffusion, complement-fixation, immunofluorescence, and enzyme-linked immunoassay. The virus is cytopathic and can be isolated readily in almost all cell cultures commonly used in diagnostic laboratories, and identified rapidly by immunofluorescence. Virus can also be isolated in suckling or weaned mice, or hamsters, inoculated intracerebrally or intraperitoneally, and antigen can be identified in harvested brain or liver by the immunological methods mentioned above. Definitive identification of isolates is achieved by performing neutralization tests with reference antiserum.

Antibody to RVF virus can be demonstrated in complement-fixation, enzyme-linked immunoassay, indirect immunofluorescence, haemagglutination-inhibition, or neutralization tests. Diagnosis of recent infection is confirmed by demonstrating seroconversion or a fourfold or greater rise in titre of antibody in paired serum samples, or by demonstrating IgM antibody activity in an enzyme-linked immunoassay (Niklasson *et al.* 1984).

Benign RVF in humans must be distinguished from other febrile zoonotic diseases such as brucellosis and Q fever which can be acquired from contact with livestock carcasses, while the fulminant hepatic disease must be distinguished from the so-called formidable viral haemorrhagic fevers of Africa: Lassa fever, Crimean–Congo haemorrhagic fever, Marburg disease, Ebola fever, and, theoretically, the haemorrhagic fever with renal syndrome associated with hantavirus infections (there has been serological evidence of, but no virologically confirmed case of, the latter syndrome in Africa).

PATHOLOGY

Histopathological lesions, particularly those in the liver, are considered to be pathognomonic, and are essentially similar in humans and domestic ruminants. The severity of the lesions varies from primary foci of coagulative necrosis, consisting of clusters of hepatocytes with acidophilic cytoplasms and pyknotic nuclei, multifocally scattered throughout the parenchyma, to massive liver destruction in which the primary foci comprising dense aggregates of cytoplasmic and nuclear debris, some fibrin and a few neutrophils and macrophages, can be discerned against a background of parenchyma reduced by nuclear pyknosis, karyorrhexis, and cytolysis to scattered fragments of cytoplasm and chromatin, with only narrow rims of degenerated hepatocytes remaining reasonably intact close to portal triads. Intensely acidophilic cytoplasmic bodies which resemble the Councilman bodies of yellow fever are common, and rod-shaped or oval eosinophilic intranuclear inclusions may be seen in intact nuclei. Icterus may be evident.

TREATMENT

Treatment is essentially symptomatic, and supportive therapy in the haemorrhagic disease includes replacement of blood and coagulation factors (Peters and Shelokov 1990). Results obtained in animal models suggest that the administration of immune plasma from recovered patients may be beneficial. The antiviral drug ribavirin inhibits virus replication in cell cultures and laboratory animals, and it has been suggested that it could be used even in benign disease in order to obviate the potentially serious complications which may occur in humans (Peters *et al.* 1986).

PROGNOSIS

Despite the sudden and dramatic change perceived in the nature of the human disease in the mid-1970s, it was deduced from the 598 reported deaths and 200 000 estimated cases of disease that RVF had a case fatality rate of less than 1 per cent in Egypt where a high prevalence of schistosomiasis may have predisposed the population to severe liver disease. The fatality rate may even have been lower in relation to total infections, since an antibody prevalence rate of approximately 30 per cent was detected and the human population estimated at 1 to 3 million in the areas affected by the epizootic. Remarkably high estimates of approximately 5 and 14 per cent were made for case fatality rates in two separate populations in the 1987 epizootic in Mauritania, on the basis of the proportion of IgM antibody-positive persons who actually reported illness considered to be compatible with RVF, but it can be deduced that the fatality rates in terms of total IgM antibody-positive persons are much closer to the corresponding fatality rate in Egypt.

EPIDEMIOLOGY

FACTORS AFFECTING THE OCCURRENCE OF EPIZOOTICS

Kenya, South Africa, Namibia, Mozambique, Zimbabwe, Zambia, Sudan, Egypt, Mauritania, and Senegal have experienced large outbreaks of RVF as outlined above, while lesser outbreaks, periodic isolations of virus or serological evidence of infection have been recorded in Angola, Botswana, Burkina Faso, Cameroon, Central African Republic, Chad, Gabon, Guinea, Madagascar, Malawi, Mali, Nigeria, Somalia, Tanzania, Uganda, and Democratic Republic of the Congo.

Outbreaks of RVF in eastern and southern Africa have tended to occur at irregular intervals of up to 15 years or longer, and the fate of the virus during inter-epizootic periods has long constituted a central enigma in the epidemiology of the disease. On the basis of early observations made in Uganda, Kenya, and South Africa, it was accepted for decades that the virus was enzootic in indigenous forests which extend in broken fashion from East Africa to the eastern and southern coastal regions of South Africa. The virus was thought to circulate in *Eretmapodites* spp. mosquitoes and unknown vertebrates in the forests, and to spread in seasons of exceptionally heavy rainfall to livestock-rearing areas where the vectors were believed to be floodwater-breeding aedine mosquitoes of the sub-genera *Aedimorphus* and *Neomelaniconion*, which attach their eggs to vegetation at the edge of stagnant surface water. In contrast to other culicine mosquitoes, it is obligatory that the eggs of aedines be subjected to a period of drying as the water recedes before they will hatch on being wetted again when next the area floods. Thus, the aedine mosquitoes overwinter as eggs which can survive for long periods in dried mud, possibly for several seasons if the area remains dry.

On the inland plateau of South Africa, where sheep rearing predominates, surface water gathers after heavy rains in undrained shallow depressions (pans) and farm dams which afford ideal breeding environments for aedines. On the watershed plateau of Zimbabwe, where cattle farming predominates, aedines breed in *vleis*, low-lying grassy areas which constitute drainage channels for surrounding high ground, and which are flooded by seepage after heavy rains. *Vleis* correspond to what are termed *dambos* in the livestock-rearing areas of central and eastern Africa. Sustained monitoring in Zimbabwe revealed that a low level of virus transmission to livestock occurred each year in the same areas where epizootics occurred. The generation of epizootics, therefore, was associated with the simultaneous intensification of virus activity over vast livestock-rearing areas where it was already present,

rather than lateral spread from cryptic enzootic foci: examination of satellite images and aerial photographs revealed that the enzootic areas coincided with savannah and grasslands with a high density of *vleis*, and not with canopy forests. Subsequently, RVF virus was isolated from unfed *Aedes mcintoshi* mosquitoes (= *Aedes lineatopennis sensu lato*) hatched in *dambos* on a ranch in Kenya during inter-epizootic periods in 1982 and 1984, confirming that the virus is enzootic in livestock-rearing areas and indicating that it appears to be maintained by transovarial transmission in aedines (Linthicum *et al.* 1985). The available evidence suggests that in Zimbabwe, as in Kenya, *Aedes* mcintoshi is the most important maintenance vector of the virus while *Aedes dentatus* is probably also a maintenance vector; the same two species and possibly *Aedes unidentatus* and *Aedes juppi* are maintenance vectors on the inland plateau of South Africa. An attempt has been made to utilize satellite imaging for the prediction of RVF outbreaks through the development of a green vegetation index as a marker of *dambo* or pan flooding, but it remains to be determined whether the technique finds application and proves to be reliable (Linthicum *et al.*, 1987).

In contrast to countries such as Zimbabwe and Kenya, or even the coastal areas of South Africa, the inland plateau of South Africa has harsh winters, and prolonged droughts are not uncommon, with pans and small dams remaining dry for many years or even decades at a time, so it is possible that aedine mosquito populations could decline to the point where RVF virus activity becomes virtually undetectable or the virus entirely disappears from the area. Indeed, no outbreaks of RVF have been recorded on the interior plateau of South Africa since the major epizootic of 1974–76, although a small outbreak was recognized in a coastal bush area in northern Natal in 1981. This suggests either that virus activity has declined on the inland plateau to a level where considerable amplification must occur before the disease again becomes evident, or that the virus has disappeared from the area and must be reintroduced through a mechanism permitting its long-range dispersal, as discussed below in relation to the appearance of the disease in Egypt in 1977.

Epizootics generally become evident in late summer after there has been an initial increase in vector populations and in circulation of the virus. Heavy rainfall and the humid conditions which prevail during epizootics favour the breeding of other biting insects besides aedine mosquitoes. Following extensive flooding of aedine breeding sites, significant numbers of livestock become infected and circulate high levels of virus in their blood during the acute stage of infection. Other culicines and anopheline mosquitoes then become infected and serve as epizootic vectors, particularly *Culex theileri* in southern Africa, and biting flies such as midges, phlebotomids, stomoxids, and simulids serve as mechanical transmitters of infection. Although contagion has been demonstrated on occasion under artificial conditions, non-vectorial transmission is not considered to be important in livestock, as opposed to humans. Outbreaks generally terminate in late autumn when the onset of cold weather depresses vector activity, or when most animals are immune following natural infection, or after there has been successful intervention with vaccine.

It can be deduced, and in some instances has been demonstrated directly, that the intensity of viraemia attained in domestic ruminants, humans, and many rodents is adequate for the infection of the mosquito vectors of RVF virus through the ingestion of blood meals: estimated threshold levels of viraemia required to infect 50 per cent of mosquitoes range from $10^{5.7}$ to $10^{8.7}$ MICLD$_{50}$/ml for the various putative vectors of southern Africa. Although extensive studies have failed to prove that the virus is maintained in natural transmission cycles in rodents, birds, or other wild vertebrates, it is felt that wild ruminants could play a role similar to their domestic counterparts in areas where they predominate. Furthermore, it is believed that the possibility that the virus is also maintained by circulation in forest mosquitoes and unidentified vertebrates, cannot be dismissed entirely and merits further investigation.

In retrospect, it can be surmised that the occurrence of the massive epizootic in Egypt in 1977–78 was probably facilitated by an increase in mosquito breeding sites brought about by agricultural developments which followed the building of the Aswan dam, although it remains necessary to explain the mechanisms responsible for the introduction of the virus into the country. Various theories were advanced to account for the first known appearance of the virus in Egypt in 1977, including the long-distance carriage of infected vectors at high altitude by prevailing winds associated with the inter-tropical convergence zone; a mechanism which has been invoked to explain the spread of many other arboviruses in the past (Sellers *et al.* 1982). The introduction of the virus through the transportation of infected sheep and cattle on the Nile or overland from northern Sudan to markets in southern Egypt was also considered to have been a strong possibility, and the movement of slaughter animals by sea could account for the evidence of infection detected in the northern and eastern coastal areas of Egypt. Although transportation on some routes would take a long time in relation to the course of the infection, RVF virus has been shown to persist for prolonged periods in various organs of sheep, particularly the spleen, for up to 21 days after infection. The same could be true for goats and cattle, or even the camels brought in by overland caravan routes. It is believed that humans slaughtering

or handling the tissues of such animals could have become infected and served as the amplifying hosts for the infection of mosquitoes since the main vector in the Egyptian epizootic, *Culex pipiens*, is known to be peridomestic and anthropophilic. In at least one instance there were indications that human infections centred on a location where introduced camels were slaughtered. The incidence of the disease declined with the onset of the cool season in 1977, but it is thought that hibernation of infected adult *Culex pipiens* or other vector species, or a continued low level of biting activity by a proportion of the mosquito population, could account for the overwintering of the virus and the continuance of the epizootic into 1978.

In West Africa, the construction of the large Manantali dam on the Senegal River in Mali and the Diama dam downstream on the border between Mauritania and Senegal increased potential mosquito breeding sites in an area where the virus was already known to active, and prevailing drought conditions led to the concentration of nomadic people and their livestock in proximity to the dams. However, virus activity has declined in the arid 'Sahelian' region since the epizootic of 1987, and RVF is thought to be enzootic in the more humid 'Guinean' areas of West Africa, where *Aedes mcintoshi*, *Aedes dalzieli*, and *Aedes vexans* are considered to be potentially important vectors.

FACTORS AFFECTING THE OCCURRENCE OF HUMAN INFECTION

In contrast to the main vector in the Egyptian epizootic of 1977–78, the principal mosquito vectors of RVF virus in sub-Saharan Africa tend to be zoophilic and sylvatic, with the result that humans become infected mainly from contact with animal tissues, although there are instances where no such history can be obtained and it must be assumed that infection has resulted from mosquito bite. Occasional infections diagnosed in tourists from abroad who have visited countries in Africa fall into this category. Generally, persons who become infected are involved in the livestock industry, such as farmers who assist in dystocia of livestock, farm labourers who salvage carcasses for human consumption, veterinarians and their assistants, and abattoir workers. The virus is notorious as a cause of laboratory infections, and there are numerous reports of humans becoming infected while investigating the disease in the field. The results of surveys following epizootics in southern Africa indicated that 9–15 per cent of farm residents became infected, with a slight preponderance of adult males, although it appeared that housewives also gained infection from handling fresh meat.

No outbreaks of the disease have been recognized in urban consumer populations and it is surmised that the fall in pH associated with the maturation of meat in abattoirs is deleterious to the virus. Moreover, highest infection rates were found in workers in the by-products sections of abattoris in Zimbabwe and the implication is that the carcasses of infected animals which reach abattoirs are generally recognized as being diseased and are condemned as unfit for human consumption, and are then sterilized in the process of preparing carcass meal which is incorporated in fertilizers.

Human infection presumably results from contact of virus with abraded skin, wounds, or mucous membranes, but aerosol and intranasal infection have been demonstrated experimentally and circumstantial evidence suggests that aerosols have been involved in some human infections in the laboratory, and in the field during the Egyptian outbreak of 1977–78. Many infections in Egypt are thought to have resulted from the slaughter of infected animals outside of abattoirs, and the fact that the mosquito vector was anthropophilic is thought to explain the high incidence of infection which occurred in people of all ages and diverse occupations. Low concentrations of virus have been found in milk and body fluids such as saliva and nasal discharges of sheep and cattle, and it appears that there may have been a connection between human infection and consumption of raw milk in Mauritania. In view of the intense viraemia which occurs in humans and the fact that virus has been isolated from throat washings, it is curious that there are no records of person to person transmission of infection.

PREVENTION AND CONTROL

Measures such as biological or chemical control of vectors, movements of livestock from low-lying areas to well-drained and wind-swept pastures at higher altitudes, or confining of animals to mosquito-proof stables, are usually impractical or at best palliative in the face of a RVF epizootic, and immunization remains the only effective method of controlling the disease.

In addition to the modified live Smithburn strain and the formalin-inactivated vaccines referred to above, trials have been reported with small plaque variant and mutagen-derived candidate veterinary vaccines (Caplen *et al.* 1985), but these have not been brought into commercial production. The Smithburn vaccine strain confers life-long immunity in sheep and goats, and it is recommended that they should be immunized on a single occasion in the first year of life, preferably at 6 months of age after maternal immunity has waned. The Smithburn strain protects cattle against infection, but does not induce adequate humoral response to ensure transfer of colostral immunity to calves. Cattle and other domestic ruminants can be immunized at any age after maternal immunity has waned with inactivated vaccine, but the

immunity is not durable and the animals should receive a second dose of vaccine 3–6 months later, plus annual boosters. It is, however, usually very difficult to persuade farmers to vaccinate livestock during long interepizootic periods, and the occurrence of outbreaks is difficult to predict. The result is that vaccine has almost invariably been used too late in the course of outbreaks to be fully effective. A further problem is that during outbreaks there is a chance of spreading infection with wild virus through transferring viraemic blood on needles used to inoculate different animals in succession. Nevertheless, in the past it has been practice in Kenya and South Africa to vaccinate all livestock, including pregnant ewes, with the Smithburn strain in the face of outbreaks, since it is deemed that the abortigenic and teratogenic effects of the vaccine are outweighed by the potentially severe consequences of allowing the disease to run its natural course. It is considered theoretically possible, although not proven, that live vaccine strains could revert to full virulence if passaged through hosts, as for instance through mosquitoes which become infected as a result of feeding on animals in the viraemic stage following administration of the vaccine. Hence, it is advised that only the inactivated vaccine should be used in situations where it is considered necessary to immunize animals in countries where the presence of RVF virus has not been proven.

Veterinarians and others engaged in the livestock industry should be made aware of the potential dangers of exposure to zoonotic agents in handling tissues of diseased animals, and precautions should be heightened during RVF epizootics. These should include the use of suitable protective clothing, such as an impervious gown or apron, gloves, and face mask or visor. The carcasses of sick animals should not be utilized for human consumption. No registered vaccines are available for mass use on susceptible human populations, nor would their use be practicable in view of logistic problems and the essentially unpredictable occurrence and variable nature of outbreaks of the disease. A formalin-inactivated cell culture vaccine produced in the United States is made available for use on an experimental basis, with the informed consent of recipients, to immunize persons such as veterinarians and laboratory workers who are regularly exposed to RVF infection (Eddy *et al.* 1981).

REFERENCES

Anonymous (1993). Rift Valley fever. *Weekly Epidemiological Record*, **68**, 300–1.
Anonymous (1994). Rift Valley fever. *Weekly Epidemiological Record*, **69**, 74–5.
Battles, J. K. and Dalrymple, J. M. (1988). Genetic variation among geographic isolates of Rift Valley fever virus. *American Journal of Tropical Medicine and Hygiene*, **39**, 617–31.

Caplen, H., Peters, C. J., and Bishop, D. H. L. (1985). Mutagen directed attenuation of Rift Valley fever as a method of vaccine development. *Journal of General Virology*, **66**, 2271–7.

Cash, P., Robeson, G., Erlich, B. J., and Bishop, D. H. L. (1981). Biochemical characterization of Rift Valley fever virus. *Contributions to Epidemiology and Biostatistics*, **3**, 1–20.

Coetzer, J. A. W. (1977). The pathology of Rift Valley fever. I. Lesions occurring in field cases in new-born lambs. *Onderstepoort Journal of Veterinary Research*, **44**, 205–12.

Coetzer, J. A. W. (1982). The pathology of Rift Valley fever. II. Lesions occurring in field cases in adult cattle, calves and aborted foetuses. *Onderstepoort Journal of Veterinary Research*, **49**, 11–17.

Coetzer, J. A. W. and Barnard, B. J. H. (1977). *Hydrops amnii* in sheep associated with hydranencephaly and arthrogryposis with Wesselsbron disease and Rift Valley fever viruses as aetiological agents. *Onderstepoort Journal of Veterinary Research*, **44**, 119–26.

Cosgriff, T. M. *et al.* (1989). Hemostatic derangement produced by Rift Valley fever virus in rhesus monkeys. *Reviews of Infectious Diseases*, **11**, S807–14.

Deutman, A. F. and Klomp, H. J. (1981). Rift Valley fever retinitis. *American Journal of Ophthalmology*, **92**, 38–42.

Easterday, B. C. (1965). Rift Valley fever. *Advances in Veterinary Science*, **10**, 65–127.

Easterday, B. C., McGavran, M. H., Rooney, J. R., and Murphy, L. C. (1962*a*). The pathogenesis of Rift Valley fever in lambs. *American Journal of Veterinary Research*, **23**, 470–8.

Easterday, B. C., Murphy, L. C., and Bennett, D. G. (1962*b*). Experimental Rift Valley fever in calves, goats and pigs. *American Journal of Veterinary Research*, **23**, 1224–30.

Easterday, B. C., Murphy, L. C., and Bennett, D. G. (1962*c*). Experimental Rift Valley fever in lambs and sheep. *American Journal of Veterinary Research*, **23**, 1231–40.

Eddy, G. A., Peters, C. J., Meadors, G., and Cole, F. E. Jr (1981). Rift Valley fever vaccine for humans. *Contributions to Epidemiology and Biostatistics*, **3**, 124–41.

Henning, M. W. (1956). Rabies. In *Animal Diseases in South Africa* (3rd edn), pp. 974–1022. Central News Agency, Cape Town.

Jouan, A. *et al.* (1989). Analytical study of a Rift Valley fever epidemic. *Research in Virology*, **40**, 175–86.

Laughlin, L. W., Meegan, J. M., Strausbaugh, L. J., Morens, D. M., and Watten, H. (1979). Epidemic Rift Valley fever in Egypt: observations of the spectrum of human illness. *Transactions of the Royal Society of Tropical Medicine and Hygiene*, **73**, 630–3.

Linthicum, K. J., Davies, F. G., Kairo, A., and Bailey, C. L. (1985). Rift Valley fever virus (family Bunyaviridae, genus *Phlebovirus*). Isolations from Diptera collected during an inter-epizootic period in Kenya. *Journal of Hygiene, Cambridge*, **95**, 197–209.

Linthicum, K. J., Bailey, C. L., Davies, F. G., and Tucker, C. J. (1987). Detection of Rift Valley fever viral activity in Kenya by satelite remote sensing imagery. *Science*, **235**, 1656–9.

Meegan, J. M. and Bailey, C. L. (1989). Rift Valley fever. In *The arboviruses: epidemiology and ecology*, Vol. IV, (ed. T. P. Monath), 51–76. CRC Press, Boca Raton, Florida.

Niklasson, B., Peters, C. J., Grandien, M., and Wood, O. (1984). Detection of human immunoglobulins G and M antibodies to Rift Valley fever virus by enzyme-linked immunosorbent assay. *Journal of Clinical Microbiology*, **19**, 225–9.

Peters, C. J. and Anderson, G. W. (1981). Pathogenesis of Rift Valley fever. *Contributions to Epidemiology and Biostatistics*, **3**, 21–41.

Peters, C. J. and Meegan, J. M. (1981). Rift Valley fever. In *CRC Handbook Series in Zoonoses*, Sect. B1, (ed. G. Beran), pp. 403–19. CRC Press, Boca Raton, Florida.

Peters, C. J. and Shelokov, A. (1990). Viral hemorrhagic fever. *Current Therapy in Infectious Disease*, **3**, 355–60.

Peters, C. J., Reynolds, J. A., Slone, T. W., Jones, D. E., and Stephen, E. L. (1986). Prophylaxis of Rift Valley fever with antiviral drugs, immune serum, interferon inducer and a macrophage activator. *Antiviral Research*, **6**, 285–97.

Peters, C. J. *et al.* (1988). Experimental Rift Valley fever in rhesus macaques. *Archives of Virology*, **99**, 31–44.

Rice, R. M., Erlick, B. J., Rosato, R. R., Eddy, G. A., and Mohanty, S. B. (1980). Biochemical characterization of Rift Valley fever virus. *Virology*, **105**, 256–60.

Sellers, R. F., Pedgley, D. E., and Tucker, M. R. (1982). Rift Valley fever, Egypt–1977: disease spread by wind-borne insect vectors? *Veterinary Record*, **110**, 73–7.

Shimshony, A. and Barzilai, R. (1983). Rift Valley fever. *Advances in Veterinary Science and Comparative Medicine*, **27**, 347–425.

Shope, R. E. and Sather, G. E. (1979). Arboviruses. In *Diagnostic procedures for viral, rickettsial and chlamydial infections*, (5th edn), (ed. E.H. Lennette and N. J. Schmidt), pp. 767–814. American Public Health Association, Washington.

Siam, A. L., Meegan, J. M., and Gharbawi, K. F. (1980). Rift Valley fever ocular manifestation: observations during the 1977 epidemic in the Arab Republic of Egypt. *British Journal of Ophthalmology*, **64**, 366–74.

Swanepoel, R. (1994). Bunyaviridae. In *Principles and practice of clinical virology* (3rd edn), (ed. A. J. Zuckerman, J. R. Pattison, and J. E. Banatvala), *in press*. Wiley, Chichester.

Swanepoel, R. and Coetzer, J. A. W. (1994). Rift Valley fever. In *Infectious Diseases of Livestock with Special Reference to Southern Africa* (ed. J. A. W. Coetzer, G. R. Thomson, and R. C. Tustin), 663–70. Oxford University Press Southern Africa, Cape Town.

Weiss, K. E. (1957). Rift Valley fever—a review. *Bulletin of Epizootic Diseases of Africa*, **5**, 431–58.

39 TICK-BORNE ENCEPHALITIDES

Patricia A. Nuttall and Milan Labuda

SUMMARY

Tick-borne encephalitides are caused by several different viruses belonging to the tick-borne encephalitis (TBE) subgroup, a distinct antigenic complex of the virus family, Flaviviridae. Encephalitic members of the complex are represented by the several subtypes of tick-borne encephalitis virus (including Russian spring–summer encephalitis virus), louping ill virus, and Powassan virus. They cause encephalitis affecting humans in Eurasia and North America. The TBE subgroup has been one of the most intensely studied groups of tick-borne pathogens.

INTRODUCTION

Tick-borne encephalitides affecting humans are caused by several different members of the tick-borne encephalitis (TBE) serocomplex in the virus family, Flaviviridae (Table 39.1). The most important of these are the Far Eastern and Western subtypes of TBE virus (FETBE and WTBE viruses, respectively). Louping ill (LI) and Powassan (POW) virus also cause encephalitis in humans but the disease incidence is much lower than for TBE viruses. LI virus is more commonly associated with an encephalomyelitic disease of sheep. Similar diseases affecting sheep are caused by Turkish sheep encephalitis virus and Spanish sheep encephalitis virus. In addition to FETBE and WTBE viruses, two other important human pathogens belonging to the TBE serocomplex are Omsk haemorrhagic fever (OHF) virus and Kyasanur forest disease (KFD) virus, both of which give rise to haemorrhagic disease (for reviews see Kharitonova and Leonov 1985; Lvov 1988; Banerjee 1988).

Several tick-borne viruses that primarily infect seabirds are thought to be human pathogens but appear to cause only mild symptoms. These include Tyuleniy and Saumarez Reef flaviviruses, and nairo-

Table 39.1 Arthropod-borne viruses causing encephalitis in humans

Virus	First isolated	Geographical distribution	Host range	Vector
Far Eastern tick-borne encephalitis	1937	Eastern CIS	Rodents, humans	Ixodid ticks
Western tick-borne encephalitis	1940	Europe	Rodents, humans	Ixodid ticks
Louping ill	1930	Europe	Sheep, humans	Ixodid ticks
Powassan	1952	N. America, East CIS	Rodents, humans	Ixodid ticks
West Nile	1937	Africa, Europe, Asia	Birds, humans	Mosquitoes (ixodid and argasid ticks)
Japanese encephalitis	1935	Asia	Birds, pigs, humans	Mosquitoes
Kunjin	1960	Australia, Borneo	Birds, humans	Mosquitoes
Murray Valley encephalitis	(1917)[a] 1951	Australia, New Guinea	Birds, humans	Mosquitoes
Rocio encephalitis	1975	Brazil	Birds, humans	Mosquitoes
St Louis encephalitis	1933	North and South America	Rodents, humans	Mosquitoes
Eastern equine encephalomyelitis	1933	North America	Birds, horses, humans	Mosquitoes
Venezuelan equine encephalomyelitis	1938	South and North America	Rodents, birds, horses, humans	Mosquitoes, (cliff swallow bugs)
Western equine encephalomyelitis	1930	North and South America	Birds, humans	Mosquitoes

[a] The agent isolated in 1917 was lost before its identity was established.

viruses (family, Bunyaviridae) of the Hughes sero-group, including Soldado and Zirqa virus. Kemerovo virus, a tick-borne member of the Reoviridae virus family in the genus *Orbivirus*, has been isolated from the blood and spinal fluid of patients with a suspected febrile form of TBE.

West Nile (WN) virus is regarded as a mosquito-borne flavivirus but in some localities the virus is transmitted by ticks. Typically, infections are asymptomatic or cause a febrile illness in humans. However, in 1957 severe meningoencephalitis was reported during an outbreak in Israel and more cases were recorded in 1962 and 1981. In India, four cases of encephalitis were reported in children infected with WN virus, three of which were fatal (George *et al.*, 1984). The largest outbreak of WN encephalitis to date, and the first urban outbreak of the disease, occurred in 1996 in southern Romania. The main vector was *Culex pipiens*. Several other mosquito-borne flaviviruses cause encephalitis in humans but they have no additional tick vector (Table 39.1).

This chapter focuses on tick-borne encephalitides associated with flaviviruses of the TBE serocomplex, with emphasis on the Far Eastern and Western sub-types of TBE virus.

HISTORY

As early as the eighteenth century, descriptions suggestive of TBE were noted in church registers on the Åland islands, Finland. During the summer of 1927, Schneider, working in a hospital in the Neunkirchen area in Lower Austria, recognized that several patients with encephalitis showed a similar clinical picture. He discovered that this condition occurred regularly, although the numbers of cases varied, and that the peak incidence occurred during the summer months. On the basis of clinical and epidemiological observations, the condition was named 'meningitis serosa epidemica' (Schneider 1931) and later, Sneider's disease. Several other synonyms for TBE have been used (Table 39.2).

Tick-borne encephalitis was recognized clinically in the Far East of the former USSR in the early 1930s.

Table 39.2 Synonyms for TBE

Bi-undulant meningo-encephalitis	Forest spring encephalitis
Biphasic meningoencephalitis	Früh–Sommer–Meningo–Enzephalitis (FSME)
Central European Encephalitis (CEE)	Kumlinge disease
Diphasic milk fever	Russian spring–summer encephalitis (RSSE)
Far Eastern encephalitis	Schneider's disease

The disease was known by several names, including Russian spring–summer encephalitis (RSSE). In 1939, Pavlovsky described the main characteristics of TBE and how the agent was maintained in nature.

A less severe form of encephalitis, affecting humans residing in central Bohemia, Czech Republic, was recorded in 1948. The virus recovered from the blood of a patient and from *I. ricinus* ticks was related to isolates from RSSE cases. In the following year, similar or milder forms of the disease, called biphasic meningo-encephalitis, were observed in other central and eastern European countries. In 1951, an outbreak of TBE was recorded in southern Slovakia associated with consumption of unpasteurized goat milk. The outbreak led to extensive ecological research on TBE virus in Central Europe.

In Finland, a form of aseptic encephalitis affecting the inhabitants and visitors of the islands in the Baltic Sea has been known for several decades. The disease was first observed in the 1940s in the small island parish of Kumlinge and became known as Kumlinge disease. The causative agent, Kumlinge virus, was isolated in 1959 and later found to be an isolate of central European TBE virus. In Sweden, the first case of TBE was described in 1954; the virus was isolated in 1958 from a patient and from *I. ricinus* ticks. Owing to the seasonal occurrence of the disease, Moritsch and Krausler in 1957 coined the name 'Früh-Sommer-Meningo-Enzephalitis' (FSME).

TBE virus was first isolated in 1937 from *I. persulcatus* ticks and the blood of patients in Far Eastern regions

Table 39.3 First TBE virus isolations and numbers of human cases

Country	First virus isolation	Number of cases/year
Albania	?	3–25
Austria	1957	90–300[a]
Bulgaria	1958	?
Czech Republic	1949	80–180
Denmark	1963	0–2
Finland	1959	2–11
France	1969	0–3 (10 in total)
Germany	1960	50–240
Greece	1964	0–1
Hungary	1952	200–300
Italy	1978	0–3
Norway	1976	(antibody only)
Poland	1953	17–54
Romania	1957	?
Slovakia	1953	10–25
Sweden	1958	40–70
Switzerland	1969	7–55
USSR (former)	1937	5000–7000
Yugoslavia (former)	1955	90–250

[a] During 1972–1982, the annual incidence in Austria was 300–700 cases (WHO 1986).

of the former USSR. In the following years (1938–39), numerous isolates of TBE virus were obtained from various geographical areas of the former USSR and the first evidence of their heterogeneity was reported. The first strains of TBE virus from outside the former USSR were obtained from *I. ricinus* ticks collected in former Czechoslovakia. TBE virus has now been isolated from most European countries, although, epidemiologically, the virus is most important in central and eastern Europe (Table 39.3).

The Far Eastern form of TBE (RSSE) was investigated extensively from 1937 to 1939 in the Central Virus Laboratory and the Institute of Experimental Medicine, Moscow. The clinical picture was reviewed by Smorodintsev (1944). The disease was characterized by an incubation period of 8–18 days, a temperature rise to 38–40 °C, violent headaches, pains in the nape of the neck, vertigo, and vomiting. The predominant signs were meningitis and focal lesions of the central nervous system, rapidly followed by paresis and paralysis of the limbs, neck, and back. Occasionally there were epileptic seizures and transitory mental confusion. The duration of the acute stage averaged 5–6 days but sometimes ran its course in 2–10 days. Pareses and paralyses appeared on the second or third day and were followed by an acute involvement of the cervical muscles ('drop neck') and of the shoulder girdle. In severe cases an ascending paralysis occurred, involving the cervical segments of the spinal cord and reaching the medulla, resulting in bulbar palsy associated with dyspnoea, cardiac arrhythmia, dysphagia, and aphonia. The predominant lesions occurred in the brain and spinal cord. The mortality rate ranged from 20 to 30%. Death usually occurred between the third and the eighth day of the disease. Many convalescents were physically disabled by paralysis and atrophy of the cervical muscles and shoulder girdle.

Preventative measures were reviewed by Smorodintsev (1944) who recommended:

1. Regular examination twice a day of forest dwellers to detect and to remove the ticks. (Experiments revealed that no infection of mice occurred when the ticks sucked blood for 2–4 hours, but a latent or clinical form of mouse encephalitis appeared when the ticks fed for 2–4 days.)
2. Protection of workers by adequate coveralls which shut out crawling ticks.
3. Application of repellents such as preparation SK (a heavily chlorinated product of turpentine oil) with which the coveralls were impregnated.
4. Efficient construction of military barracks and adequate preparation of the ground (removal of grass, irrigation of the camp territory with anti-tick disinfectant solutions, such as naphtholysol, lysol, and carbolic acid).
5. Drainage and forest clearance (the ticks cannot survive in dry places).
6. Eradication of rodents and tick control of domestic animals. (Both groups of animals are vitally important as hosts of ticks.)
7. Immunization of workers with an inactivated vaccine prepared from the brains of affected animals. (This was considered one of the most reliable methods.)

Louping-ill (LI) virus derived its name from the disease of sheep which has been recognized in southern Scotland for at least two centuries (reviewed by Smith and Varma 1981). 'Louping' refers to the characterisitic of 'leaping' shown by sheep infected with LI virus. It was, however, an ill-defined condition until 1913 when the specific histopathological lesions of the CNS were described. Subsequent attempts to determine the cause of the condition were confounded by another common infection of sheep, tick-borne fever. However, in 1931 the aetiological agent of louping ill was established as a filterable virus transmitted by the so-called sheep tick, *I. ricinus*. In the 1930s, LI was identified as a problem throughout much of the hill sheep farming areas of Scotland and northern England. Subsequently, the disease was recognized in Ireland, Wales and, in 1978, in south-western England. Louping ill also affects sheep in Norway but similar conditions in Spain and Turkey are caused by distinct viruses in the TBE serocomplex.

Powassan (POW) virus derives its name from the town in Northern Ontario where the first fatal case of the disease was recognized (reviewed by Artsob 1988). A virus was isolated from the patient, a 5-year-old boy who developed encephalitis and died in September 1958. In fact, the virus had been isolated previously from a pool of ticks collected in May 1952 in Colorado but specific identification of this virus was made subsequent to that from the fatal case in the town of Powassan. The first isolation of POW virus from the Asian continent was from a pool of ticks collected in the Southern Primor'ye of the CIS in 1972.

THE AGENT

Members of the TBE serocomplex are flaviviruses, consisting of a spherical ribonucleoprotein core surrounded by a lipoprotein envelope with small surface projections. Viral envelope lipids are derived from the host cell lipids. Virions contain three structural proteins: a nucleocapsid or core protein (C), a non-glycosylated membrane protein (M), and an envelope protein (E) which is usually glycosylated (Monath and Heinz 1996).

TAXONOMY

The TBE virus complex is a subgroup of the *Flavivirus* genus in the virus family, Flaviviridae. Most members of this virus family are arthropod-borne viruses (arboviruses), transmitted by either mosquitoes or ticks. Medically important mosquito-borne flaviviruses are dengue, yellow fever, and Japanese encephalitis virus. The name of the virus family and genus derives from yellow fever virus (*L. flavus*, yellow), the type species of the Flaviviridae and the first virus isolated from humans.

Tick-borne encephalitis flaviviruses were originally classed as a distinct serocomplex (TBE virus serocomplex) based on their antigenic cross-reactivity in neutralization tests. Initially they were placed in the so-called Group B of the arboviruses, and subsequently in the genus *Flavivirus* of the family Togaviridae, prior to their current classification within the family Flaviviridae. Based on cross-neutralization tests using specific polyclonal antiserum or mouse ascitic fluid, nine serologically defined groups and one 'unassigned' group of flaviviruses have been distinguished (Murphy *et al.* 1995). Further analyses of their interrelationships were undertaken using monoclonal antibodies, RNA–DNA hybridization, and nucleotide sequencing. For example, the use of monoclonal antibodies specific for LI virus, and subsequent sequence analysis, demonstrated that Negishi virus is a strain of LI virus (Venugopal *et al.* 1992).

MOLECULAR BIOLOGY

Flaviviruses are roughly spherical, enveloped viruses, 40–50 nm in external diameter with a 20–30 nm capsid. The viral genome is a single molecule of single-stranded RNA of approximately 11 kilobases which is positive-sense and infectious. The 5′ terminus is capped and at the 3′ end of the RNA molecule there is an untranslated region which forms a stem-loop structure of variable length. The virion RNA appears to be identical to the mRNA. Three structural proteins and seven non-structural (NS) proteins are encoded by the genome in the order:

5′-C-prM (M)-E-NS1-NS2A-NS2B-NS3-NS4A-NS4B-NS5-3′.

The characteristics of these viral proteins are summarized in Table 39.4.

The major surface glycoprotein (E) carries epitopes detected by neutralization and haemagglutination-inhibition tests that have been used to identify different flaviviral serological groups and species. Furthermore, three genetic markers have been identified in the sequence of the E protein: a type-specific hypervariable region which provides a unique genetic signature for individual flaviviruses; a subgroup-specific pentapeptide motif; and a hexapeptide insertion typical of TBE serocomplex viruses.

Determination of the crystallographic structure of a soluble form of the E protein of a European isolate of TBE virus revealed that, unlike the spikes seen on the surface of many viruses, the flavivirus envelope protein lies prone, parallel to the viral membrane, as an elongated dimer (Rey *et al.* 1995). Residues that influence binding of monoclonal antibodies occur on the outward-facing surface of the protein. Acidic pH in the cytoplasmic endosomes triggers dramatic structural changes of the protein E dimer that appear to be necessary for virus infectivity.

Comparative analyses of the nucleotide and amino acid sequence of the *E* gene have been used to investigate the phylogeny of flaviviruses. Cell fusing agent (CFA) *E* gene was used as the outgroup based on the distant relationship of CFA virus to tick- and mosquito-borne flaviviruses. The resulting phylogenetic tree was consistent with the serological classification of flaviviruses. Tick- and mosquito-borne viruses were separated into two major branches (Fig. 39.1). The TYU virus group appeared as a monophyletic sister of the TBE virus complex. Analyses of the *E* and *NS5* gene

Table 39.4 *Flavivirus proteins*

Protein	Molecular weight	Features	Function
C	12–14 kDa	Basic	Core protein
prM	18–19 kDa	Glycosylated	Precursor of M
M	8 kDa	In mature virions	Membrane protein
E	50–60 kDa	Glycosylated	Envelope protein
NS1	40 kDa	Dimer	? Virus maturation
NS2A	24–25 kDa	Hydrophobic	Processing of NS1
NS2B	12–15 kDa	Hydrophobic	Accessory function to NS3
NS3	70 kDa	Hydrophilic	Protease and helicase
NS4A	16 kDa	Hydrophobic	Accessory function to NS3
NS4B	27 kDa	Hydrophobic	Replicase component
NS5	103–105 kDa	Basic	Polymerase

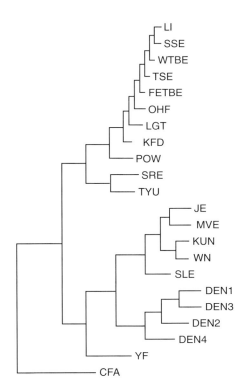

Fig. 39.1 Phylogenetic tree of flaviviruses based on the envelope gene. Maximum parsimony analysis of the nucleotide *E* gene sequence of 22 viruses (modified from Marin *et al.* 1995).

sequences to compare mutational regimes indicated that mosquito-borne flaviviruses are evolving almost twice as fast as tick-borne flaviviruses (Marin *et al.* 1995).

A detailed analysis of the branching pattern of the flavivirus phylogentic tree revealed a major difference between tick-borne and mosquito-borne viruses (Zanotto *et al.* 1996). Whereas tick-borne flaviviruses show a continual and highly asymmetric branching process over an estimated period of 2000 years, mosquito-borne dengue viruses have undergone a two-phase pattern in which a slow growth phase was followed by an explosive radiation in the past 200 years. This difference is thought to reflect the different ecologies of tick-borne and mosquito-borne flaviviruses. In particular, demographic changes in human populations may have had a major influence on dengue viral lineages.

DISEASE MECHANISMS

The greatest body of information about tick-borne flavivirus pathogenesis is derived from experiments on

mice and other laboratory rodents. Neurotropism and neurological disease, including encephalitis, are common denominators linking the flaviviruses of the TBE serocomplex. In humans, KFD and OHF viruses, which are associated with generalized infections and haemorrhagic fevers, occasionally cause neurological disease. All tick-borne flaviviruses are neurotropic in laboratory rodents, natural hosts, and even tick vectors, in which brain/ganglia are major sites of replication. However, invasion of the nervous system has generally been viewed as a 'dead end' for the virus, inconsequential to transmission or perpetuation in nature. Most natural hosts involved in transmission cycles probably escape brain infections.

Tick-borne flavivirus infections result in a wide spectrum of manifestations. At one extreme there is fatal encephalitis accompanied by high viraemia and extensive extraneural replication. Less severe is subclinical encephalitis with low viraemia, late establishment of brain infection, and clearance with minimal destructive pathology. At the other end of the spectrum there is inapparent infection with trace viraemia, limited extraneural replication, and no neuroinvasion. The outcome of infection depends on the specific virus–host pairing, location of infected tick bite, virus dose, and multiple host factors that influence the host response.

Following natural tick-transmitted infections, TBE virus first replicates in the skin site of inoculation (i.e. the feeding site of an infected tick) and in lymph nodes that drain the site. Studies in mice revealed that neutrophils, monocytes/macrophages and Langerhans cells that are attracted to the tick feeding site become infected (Labuda *et al.* 1996). In animals that develop viraemia, virus is carried via lymphatics to the thoracic duct and into the bloodstream. The primary viraemia seeds extraneural tissues which, in turn, support further viral replication and serve as a source for release of virus into the circulation. The level of viraemia is modulated by the rate of clearance by macrophages, and it is terminated by the appearance of humoral antibodies, approximately 1 week after infection. However, key natural hosts of the virus in nature do not exhibit patent viraemia.

Major extraneural sites of virus replication include connective tissue, skeletal muscle and myocardium, smooth muscle, lymphoreticular tissues, and endocrine and exocrine glands. Viral antigen has been demonstrated repeatedly in the muscularis of arteries and arterioles and occasionally in capillary walls, but the contribution of vascular endothelium as a source of viraemia and invasion of the CNS remains uncertain.

Studies of experimental TBE virus encephalitis in mice have shown a relationship between the level of viraemia, development of brain infection, and widespread or multisite simultaneous appearance of viral antigen in nervous tissue. These observations support the concept of haematogenous spread to the CNS, at least in an artificial laboratory model. Knowledge of the route of virus dissemination in humans is limited. The process by which the virus crosses the blood–brain barrier is unknown.

GROWTH AND SURVIVAL REQUIREMENTS

Experiments comparing different methods of infecting ticks have demonstrated the presence of a 'gut barrier' to virus infection. For example, Dhori and Dugbe viruses replicated in *Rhipicephalus appendiculatus* ticks after inoculation into the tick haemocoel, a route of infection bypassing the tick gut through which the virus would normally pass following an infective blood meal. However, neither Dhori nor Dugbe virus established an infection when the ticks were fed on an infective blood meal (the normal peroral route of infection). The presence of a gut barrier in ticks indicates that there is a specific interaction between virus (imbibed in the blood meal) and midgut cells. Although the nature of the gut barrier has not been determined, it appears to vary for different virus–tick systems.

The susceptibility of arthropod midgut cells to virus infection is one of the most important determinants of vector competence, 'the combined effect of all the physiological and ecological factors of vector, host, pathogen, and environment that determine the vector status of members of a given arthropod population' (McKelvey *et al.* 1981). Understanding the determinants of vector competence is important in explaining why certain tick-borne viruses have many tick vectors (e.g. Crimean–Congo haemorrhagic fever virus) whereas others have few (e.g. Nairobi sheep disease virus).

A feature that distinguishes tick-borne from insect-borne viruses is the comparative longevity of their vectors. The life cycle of ticks is usually measured in years rather than weeks or months, and individual stages can survive several years without a blood meal. Experimental data indicate that virus infections persist in ticks for the duration of the tick's life span. Ecological and epidemiological data also support the observation that tick-borne virus survival is greatly dependent on persistent infections in tick populations (WHO 1986).

One method of arbovirus persistence in the vector population is via vertical transmission in which virus from the infected parent, usually the female, is transmitted via the egg to the succeeding generation. Although evidence of vertical transmission has been recorded for numerous tick-borne viruses, including members of the TBE serocomplex (except POW

virus), the levels of vertical transmission and filial infection in nature generally appear low.

The introduction of salivary gland secretions into the feeding lesion is a potent mediator of host reactions. To counteract these reactions, tick saliva possesses pharmacologically active substances that have anti-haemostatic, vasodilatory, anti-inflammatory, and immunosuppressive activities. Thus, a virus transmitted by a tick during feeding enters a skin site that is profoundly altered by the effects of tick saliva (Titus and Ribeiro 1990).

Comparison of different methods of infecting ticks with viruses demonstrates clearly that co-feeding uninfected ticks with infected ticks is the most efficient means of virus transmission. For example, nearly all the uninfected *R. appendiculatus* nymphs, placed on an uninfected guinea-pig, became infected when they fed together with (though physically separated from) Thogoto virus-infected *R. appendiculatus* adult ticks (Jones *et al.* 1987). In contrast, fewer than 10 per cent of the nymphs became infected when fed on guinea-pigs inoculated with the virus by needle and syringe; however, when salivary gland extract was included in the virus inoculum, an average of 60 per cent of ticks were infected (Jones *et al.* 1989). Similar observations have been made for TBE and Dhori virus. The phenomenon has been termed saliva-activated transmission (SAT) because a protein(s) secreted in tick saliva potentiates virus transmission. The SAT factor modulates the skin site of tick attachment, presumably to facilitate feeding, and this modulation is exploited by the virus. However, the mode of action of the SAT factor is unknown but, at least for Thogoto virus, lymphoid tissues may be involved (Jones *et al.* 1992*b*).

Saliva-activated transmission is believed to be the mechanism underlying 'non-viraemic transmission,' the transmission of arboviruses between infected and uninfected ticks co-feeding on a vertebrate host that has no detectable (or very low levels of) viraemia (Nuttall *et al.* 1991). If such is the case, SAT has significant implications for virus transmissibility and virus virulence in the vertebrate host. A study of TBE virus transmission provides a graphic illustration of this (Labuda *et al.* 1993*c*). Uninfected and infected *Ixodes ricinus*, the primary vector species of TBE virus in Europe, were allowed to feed together on different uninfected wild-caught vertebrate species. Pine voles (*Pitymys subterraneus*) developed a highly virulent infection but yielded few infected ticks. In contrast, field mice (*Apodemus flavicollis* and *A. agrarius*) had low or undetectable viraemias, low titres of virus in target organs (spleen and lymph node), and no clinical signs of infection; however, they gave rise to the highest numbers of infected ticks. Based on the results of these studies, three hypotheses were proposed:

(1) low viraemia (synonymous with low virulence) ensures that the host remains alive for at least the duration of the relatively long tick feeding period;

(2) non-viraemic transmission is not delayed by the time taken for a viraemia to develop and, consequently, non-viraemic transmission maximizes the chances of transmission between co-feeding ticks; and, most important,

(3) non-viraemic transmission is an important mechanism for the survival of tick-borne viruses in nature.

Thus, by adapting to and exploiting the saliva-induced changes that occur in the skin site of tick feeding, tick-borne viruses possess a novel means of increasing their chances of survival in natural ecosystems. Indeed, estimations of the relative basic reproductive number (R_0) of TBE virus indicate that non-viraemic transmission between co-feeding infected and uninfected ticks is more important than classical viraemic transmission for the survival of TBE virus in nature (Randolph *et al.* 1996).

Non-viraemic transmission also has important implications for vertical transmission. Vertical transmission is common among tick-borne viruses but occurs at an apparently low level. This has led several authors to claim that vertical transmission is not a significant factor in the ecology and epidemiology of tick-borne viruses (Burgdorfer and Varma 1967). A recent study demonstrated that a low level of TBE virus infection in a population of larval ticks (detectable only by polymerase chain reaction) can be amplified by non-viraemic co-feeding to yield a significant number of infected nymphal ticks (Labuda *et al.* 1993*d*). Similar results have been reported for Crimean–Congo haemorrhagic fever virus. Because larvae quest in clusters, there are many opportunities for amplication of vertically acquired tick-borne virus infections in the vector population through non-viraemic transmission between co-feeding larvae. As a result of such amplification, vertical transmission might be the difference between survival and extinction of certain tick-borne virus infections in nature.

THE HOSTS

Arboviruses are transmitted to humans by blood feeding of infected mosquitoes or ticks. Members of the TBE serocomplex rely on two different types of host for their survival: invertebrates (ticks) which act as both biological virus vectors and reservoir hosts, and vertebrates that amplify the virus infection by acting as a source of infection for ticks. Humans are not normally a source of infection for ticks and consequently

they represent dead-end hosts in that their infection is not usually passed on to a new host.

Ticks are blood-sucking arachnids that comprise two major families: the Ixodidae (ixodid or hard ticks) and the Argasidae (argasid or soft ticks). The tick hosts and vectors of encephalitic TBE group viruses are all ixodid species, primarily of the genus *Ixodes*. They are three-host ticks: the larva, nymph, and adult each feed on a different individual vertebrate host (often a wide range of species) for a period of a few days. In general, immature stages (larvae and nymphs) feed on small mammals and birds, and adults on larger species. Such trophic relationships are a deterministic feature of enzootic transmission cycles. Larger mammals (deer, goats, cows, and sheep) become infected, but levels of viraemia may be low; consequently, they are considered as hosts sustaining vector tick populations rather than as hosts of the virus. The obvious exception is LI virus infection of sheep.

Transmission cycles are determined by the interactions between tick-borne viruses, their vectors and their vertebrate hosts. Such interactions are governed by the biology and population dynamics of the tick and vertebrate hosts, which in turn are strongly influenced by environmental factors (Nuttall 1984). These factors combine to determine the basic reproductive rate (R_0) of the virus infection, i.e. the number of new infections that arise from a single current infection (Dietz 1988; Hasibeder and Dye 1988).

One or two primary tick vectors, that play a crucial role in maintaining the transmission cycle of tick-borne flaviviruses, can be identified. Their host preferences determine which vertebrates are natural hosts of the virus. In addition to the primary vector, a few or several tick species may act as secondary vectors. Such vectors are probably not able to circulate the virus without the participation of the primary vector(s), but they can help to maintain the transmission cycle. Environmental changes, including changes in climate, may increase the role of secondary vectors in the virus transmission cycle. Similarly, ancillary vectors may act as the primary vector species in certain specific biotopes.

Evidence that a particular tick species is a primary vector of a TBE group virus is based mostly on virus isolation from field-collected ticks. Since the expedition of Zilber and colleagues, repeated field studies have identified *I. persulcatus* as the principal vector of the Far Eastern TBE viral subtype. Similarly, following the first isolation of TBE virus from *I. ricinus* ticks in the Czech Republic, large number of isolates have been obtained from *I. ricinus* in various countries of Europe, reflecting the primary role of *I. ricinus* as a vector of the European TBE viral subtype.

The epizoology of LI virus implicates *I. ricinus* as the sole vector of this virus (Reid 1988). In North America, most isolations of POW virus have been from *Ixodes cookei* (Artsob 1988). This tick is found throughout the east and midwest and feeds on mammals of many species, particularly groundhogs (*Marmota monax*). The greatest number of POW virus isolates in the Primor'ye region of south-east CIS were recorded from *Ixodes persulcatus* (Hoogstraal 1980).

All competent tick species occurring in sufficiently high numbers and having a sympatric distribution with the primary tick vector may become infected and subsequently transmit a member of the TBE virus complex. However, although experimental studies have shown that numerous tick species are competent vectors, their ecological roles have not been determined. For example, the vector competence of *I. hexagonus* for TBE virus has been demonstrated in the laboratory, including transmission of TBE virus to hedgehogs, the principal host of this tick species, and TBE virus has been isolated from field-collected *I. hexagonus*. *Ixodes arboricola*, a bird tick, was shown to be a competent vector in the laboratory. Similarly, *Haemaphysalis concinna*, *H. inermis* and *H. punctata* are competent vectors, and TBE virus has been isolated from field-collected specimens. In the Khabarovsk region (near the Sea of Japan), *Haemaphysalis* rather than *Ixodes* ticks may be the primary vector of the Far Eastern subtype (Hoogstraal 1966). The relative roles of *Ixodes ricinus* and *I. persulcatus* as primary and/or secondary vectors of the two TBE viral subtypes are undetermined for parts of Europe where the two species are sympatric.

In contrast to TBE virus, the epizootiology of LI virus implicates *I. ricinus* as the exclusive vector even though *Dermacentor reticulatus* and *Haemaphysalis punctata* are present in the United Kingdom. For POW virus, a few ixodid tick species have been implicated as alternative vectors (Artsob 1988). The evidence is based on virus isolations from field-collected specimens of *I. marxi* collected in Ontario and associated with red squirrels (*Tamiasciurus hudsonicus*), and from *D. andersoni* and *I. spinipalpus* in western North America. Field data indicate that the primary enzootic tick vectors and vertebrate hosts of POW virus vary according to the biotope and geographical area (Hoogstraal 1966). Experimental studies have demonstrated virus transmission by *D. andersoni* and *I. pacificus*, although *I. pacificus* appears to be an inefficient vector. In the CIS, POW virus has been isolated from *Haemaphysalis longicornis*, *I. persulcatus*, and *D. silvarum* ticks, and also from *Aedes togoi* and *Anopheles hyrcanus* mosquitoes. However, experimental studies failed to demonstrate POW virus replication following inoculation of *Aedes aegypti* and *Culex fatigans* mosquitoes.

There is little published information on the density-dependent mortality factors that regulate tick populations. The population dynamics of *I. ricinus* and *I. persulcatus* are determined by the availability of large mammalian species that support the adult stages (Milne 1949*a,b*), although fluctuations in the numbers of small mammals and gamebirds have been correlated with the population dynamics of *I. ricinus* (Smith and Varma 1981). The immature stages have a more catholic host range than the adults, feeding on most warm-blooded animals as well as reptiles. However, nymphs are less successful than larvae in feeding on small mammals. In western Slovakia there were about 20 times more *I. ricinus* larvae than nymphs on small mammals (Labuda *et al.* 1991); larva to nymph ratios on birds were almost equal. The height above ground at which each developmental stage quests for a host is an important determinant of the species infested. Nymphs are probably the most important vector stage in the transmission of TBE virus because they are more numerous than adults and are less host-specific. Since vertical transmission is rare, larvae are probably more important as acquirers (recipients) of the virus than as transmitters (donors), although amplification of vertically acquired infections may occur during co-feeding of infected and uninfected larvae.

Like ticks, certain vertebrate species play a crucial role in maintaining the transmission cycles of TBE group viruses. In addition, some species may be important in amplifying the number of infected ticks within an infection focus, though their role may be insufficient *per se* to maintain the virus transmission cycle. Such amplifying hosts are highly susceptible to the virus and infection may result in high mortality. In general, however, it is difficult to distinguish between maintenance and amplifying hosts.

The population dynamics of vertebrate hosts are an important factor in determining the number of susceptible maintenance and amplifying hosts that contribute to the enzootic or epizootic transmission cycle. Most TBE group viruses utilize rodents as maintenance and amplifying hosts. Such species have high reproductive rates, and life spans that are often less than that of the tick vector. Fluctuations in transmission dynamics are correlated with changes in rodent populations. Increases in rodent populations are followed within 1–2 years by increased tick populations and a higher risk of human infections.

At least 10 species of rodents have been implicated as maintenance hosts of TBE virus in Central Europe. The most important are probably field mice, *Apodemus flavicollis* and *A. sylvaticus*. They are generally abundant in infection foci and are readily infested with *I. ricinus* ticks (mostly larvae). Bank voles (*Clethrionomys glareolus*) were also considered to be important hosts because of their abundance although viraemia in adult *C. glareolus* was found to be below the infection threshold for ticks.

However, a wide range of viraemic titres (0.4–4.5 log$_{10}$LD$_{50}$/0.03 ml or 1.1–6.0 log$_{10}$LD$_{50}$/ml) was detected in adult *C. glareolus* infected with different TBE virus isolates. During a longitudinal study (1981 to 1986) of natural foci of TBE virus in West Slovakia, the importance of the most abundant rodent species, *C. glareolus* (52.9 per cent) and *A. flavicollis* (22.5 per cent), was demonstrated (Kozuch *et al.* 1990). The highest prevalence of neutralizing antibody to the virus was found in sera of *A. flavicollis* (18.1 per cent), followed by *C. glareolus* (15.1 per cent). The European mole (*Talpa europaea*) is also an important host of *I. ricinus* and is naturally infected with TBE virus in the Czech and Slovak Republics.

A problem in assessing the relative roles of different host species in the transmission cycles of arthropod-borne viruses is that studies are based largely on artificial infection of vertebrate hosts by syringe inoculation. A recent investigation mimicked natural conditions of transmission by allowing TBE virus-infected and uninfected *I. ricinus* ticks to feed together on wild vertebrate hosts (field mice, *A. flavicollis* and *A. agrarius*; bank vole; pine vole, *Pitymys subterraneus*; hedgehog, *Erinaceus europaeus*; and pheasant, *Phasianus colchicus*) (Labuda *et al.* 1993c). The greatest numbers of infected ticks were obtained from field mice, susceptible hosts that had undetectable or very low levels of viraemia. By contrast, fewer infected ticks were obtained from hosts that had significant (bank voles) or substantial (pine voles) levels of viraemia. The results suggest that non-viraemic transmission plays an important role in the ecology of TBE virus.

The role of birds in the ecology of TBE viruses has not been resolved. Birds belonging to more than 100 species have been associated with infections of the Far Eastern subtype, as determined by serology or virus isolations. A serological study of the fledglings of female thrushes (*Turdus pilaris*) with high antibody levels to TBE virus (Far Eastern subtype) showed that one-third of the progeny had received antibodies to the virus transovarially from the parent. In a disease focus in former Czechoslovakia, sera from birds of 15/20 species were positive and pheasants were identified as important hosts of the European subtype. However, when TBE virus-infected and uninfected *I. ricinus* ticks experimentally were fed together on pheasants, none of the uninfected ticks became infected. TBE virus was recovered from mallards (*Anas platyrhynchos*) following either virus inoculation or exposure to infected *I. ricinus* nymphs. Some of these viraemic ducks did not develop antibody to TBE virus and, conversely, some produced antibody but had no detectable viraemia. Considering the seemingly limited opportunities for tick infestation of ducks, the ecological significance of these results is unclear.

Experimental and epizoological studies indicate that sheep are the most significant maintenance host of LI virus (Reid 1984). They consistently exhibited viraemia above the infection threshold for ticks during a period of 2–3 days after virus inoculation. Sheep develop complete immunity to LI virus and consequently experience only one active infection with LI virus during their lifetime. Considering the turnover in sheep populations per year, the minimum proportion of sheep susceptible in each spring to LI virus infection is one-fifth of the adult flock which, in Scotland, represents about 0.5 million sheep. In contrast to domestic species, only two of eight native mammals developed viraemic titres that exceeded the threshold: in five of 59 field voles (*Microtus agrestis*) the titre exceeded 10^4 plaque-forming units (PFU)/0.2 ml, and one of three roe deer (*Capreolus capreolus*) had a titre of 10$^{3.2}$ PFU/0.2 ml on one day only (Reid 1988). Red grouse were highly susceptible to infection but showed high mortality; they may act as amplifying rather than maintenance hosts of LI virus. Thus, only sheep were considered to be important in virus transmission, based on artificial infection studies. However, attempts to control LI in grouse by immunizing sheep were not entirely successful, suggesting that either immune sheep can still support LI virus transmission or sheep are not the sole hosts involved in maintaining LI virus infections in nature. Experimental evidence that hares can support non-viraemic transmission of LI virus (Jones *et al.* 1997), together with the relatively high numbers of *I. ricinus* ticks that feed on hares, indicate that hares are a key maintenance host of LI virus. Formerly, hares were discounted from playing a role in the LI virus transmission cycle because they do not develop a patent viraemia. The experimental and field data contradicting this long-held dogma illustrate the need to reassess the host species considered not to support tick-borne virus infections. Indeed, any host that feeds large numbers of ticks should be considered a potential amplifying host of viruses vectored by the ticks.

INCUBATION PERIOD

The incubation period of TBE varies between 2 and 28 days, most often 7–14 days. Approximately two out of three TBE viral infections run a subclinical course with no or mild symptoms. The incubation period following tick-borne transmission of LI virus to sheep varies from 2 to 5 days; in humans, the incubation period is 4–7 days.

SIGNS AND SYMPTOMS

Typically, TBE in humans has a biphasic course. The initial stage, lasting 1–8 days, includes moderate fever, headache, and myalgia. These symptoms correspond to the viraemic phase of the disease when the virus can be isolated from systemic blood. About one-third of cases develop the second phase of the disease after an asymptomatic interval of 1–20 days, most often about 1 week. This second phase corresponds to the spread of TBE virus to the CNS, resulting in meningoencephalitis of varying severity. The CSF shows pleocytosis with a mononuclear dominance. Elevated protein levels are usually seen. The most serious cases of encephalitis are seen in adults, especially among persons more than 60 years old, whereas in children the disease more often runs a milder course. About 10 per cent of those afflicted develop cranial or peripheral paresis. The period of hospitalization varies from a few days to several months. Most patients recover completely. However, in some patients, sequelae such as headache, impaired power of concentration, decreased vitality or remaining paresis, persist for years.

Louping ill in humans is biphasic, resembling the European form of TBE. After an influenza-like phase, lasting 2–11 days, there is a period of remission of 5–6 days and then the reappearance of fever and a meningoencephalitis syndrome lasting 4–10 days. Leucopenia occurs during the first phase and leucocytosis during the encephalitic phase. No deaths have been reported. In one laboratory-acquired case, a haemorrhagic diathesis developed, and the disease closely resembled Kyasanur forest disease.

Powassan virus infections are characterized by a variable period of fever and non-specific symptoms, followed by neurological signs which are often severe. Of the 19 recognized cases of human disease associated with POW virus infection in North America, 13 were diagnosed as encephalitis, four as meningoencephalitis, and two as aseptic meningitis. Two cases terminated fatally during the acute phase of illness, and two patients died 1 and 3 years, respectively, after the onset of sequelae. In cases reported from the Primor'ye Region, a characteristic syndrome with prominent cerebellar signs differentiated the disease from the Far Eastern form of TBE.

DIAGNOSIS

Clinical manifestations of TBE are non-specific, hence diagnosis must rely on laboratory findings. Diagnosis is by virus isolation from blood during the first phase of illness, from CSF during the early encephalitic phase, or by serological methods. Serological techniques, such as the complement fixation test (CF), neutralization test (NT), and haemagglutination inhibition (HI) test for detecting antibodies to TBE virus, have been used. Similar tests, based on detection of a rise in HI or CF antibody titre, have been used to diagnose LI and POW infections in humans. Antibodies are pro-

duced locally in the CSF. The serum/CSF antibody ratio has been employed for diagnosing infections. Latterly, detection of IgM antibodies in serum using a μ-capture ELISA has proved a reliable method in most cases for diagnosing TBE already at the onset of CNS symptoms. IgM antibodies may remain and be detected in serum up to 9 months after infection with TBE virus. The polymerase chain reaction (PCR) may have applications for detecting evidence of TBE virus in blood or the CSF.

The tests used to evaluate the antibody response after immunization against TBE virus are the NT or HI test. Previously used IgG ELISA methods were found to give false-positive reactions (Kunz 1991, cited by Gustafson 1993).

PATHOLOGY

The extent, character, and distribution of lesions in the CNS vary with host and virus strain. By light microscopy, inflammatory changes in meninges and along Virchow–Robin spaces of penetrating vessels are characterized by infiltration of lymphocytes, macrophages, and plasma cells. In the brain parenchyma, perivascular infiltrates surround small vessels and also contain mainly small lymphocytes as well as moderate numbers of monocytes. Cellular aggregations or nodules in brain parenchyma consist of infiltrating mononuclear cells and possibly also activated resident microglial cells. Autopsy of the index case of POW encephalitis revealed inflammation in all areas of the brain, although the cerebellum and spinal cord were somewhat less affected. Endothelial cell proliferation and necrosis, perineural and perivascular oedema, spongy degeneration, and focal haemorrhages are evident in mice infected with TBE virus.

The comparative pathology of tick-borne encephalitides in various clinical hosts reveals interesting differences. LI virus causes neuronal degeneration and inflammatory changes in brain-stem and cerebellum of sheep, producing a characteristic ataxic disease. In the red grouse, however, lesions localize in the forebrain. WN encephalitis in horses is characterized by a poliomyelitis-like illness with prominent lesions restricted to the spinal cord. The molecular basis for the selective vulnerability of neuronal subsets to viruses remains largely unknown. The possible involvement of differences in virus–receptor interactions, particularly those involving neurotransmitter molecules, has been suggested.

Subacute and chronic forms of encephalitis have been described in association with FETBE in humans and LI in sheep. Hamsters given Langat virus (another member of the TBE serogroup) by various routes develop a subacute sclerosing disease characterized by typical inflammatory changes early on, followed by a progressive degeneration over 3 months with astrocyte proliferation, perivascular granulomatous infiltrates, and neuronal vacuolation. Chronic encephalitis with similar pathological lesions was found in monkeys surviving acute infection with TBE virus.

TBE viral strains vary in their capacity to produce chronic encephalitis. In monkeys surviving encephalitis, virus was recovered for as long as 2 years. Changes in phenotypic markers of strains recovered from chronically infected monkeys have been reported. Some, but not all strains, exhibited reduced mouse neurovirulence or absence of haemagglutinating antigen, or both.

TREATMENT

A curative treatment for TBE is not available. Care given to patients must therefore be based on treating symptoms. However, there are definite prospects open for prophylaxis and treatment of encephalitis as indicated by the use of sera from convalescent or hyperimmunized animals. Intramuscular or subcutaneous inoculation of mice with immune horse serum protected them during the following 10–14 days after subcutaneous infection. Seroprophylaxis was effective during the incubation period provided the interval between subcutaneous injection of a minimal virus dose to mice and inoculation of serum was not greater than 1–4 days. Sera obtained from human convalescents or hyperimmunized horses produced favourable results in a number of human cases when endospinal injection of 10–15 ml was supplemented with intramuscular injection of 30–50 ml of serum. Immediate intramuscular injection of 40–50 ml serum has been given to humans bitten by ticks in endemic encephalitic areas or following laboratory infection. Serotherapy, to be successful, had to be administered on the first or second day of the disease and followed by two or three additional injections. Patients thus treated with repeated injections of the convalescent serum showed a critical drop in temperature and a marked improvement in their general condition. IgG preparations for treatment of TBE virus infections are commercially available. The ability to engineer humanized antibodies now offers a more acceptable means of preparing immunoprotective sera.

EPIDEMIOLOGY

The occurrence of tick-borne encephalitic viruses is determined by the distribution of their tick vectors which, in turn, is governed by ecological conditions. *Ixodes persulcatus* is taxonomically closely related to

I. ricinus, which it replaces in the north-east of Europe, from the Baltic Sea shore and extending across northern Asia to Japan. The northern border of its distribution extends across the forests of the central taiga. The developmental biology of *I. persulcatus* is very similar to that of *I. ricinus*, though the seasonal activity of *I. persulcatus* may be shorter, lasting only from the end of April to the beginning of June in colder biotopes.

Ixodes ricinus is a tick of temperate regions in Europe, found within the latitudes 39° and 65° and extending east of the Caspian Sea as far as 60° longitude. This species has even been recorded in North Africa. *Ixodes ricinus* is of considerable importance in both medical and veterinary medicine. The main diseases caused by pathogens transmitted (or exacerbated) by *I. ricinus* are TBE, LI, Lyme disease, tick pyaemia, tick-borne fever, and babesiosis. Detailed studies on the ecology of *I. ricinus* were undertaken in Britain between 1932 and 1955 (reviewed by Arthur 1962), and were followed by research in Europe (reviewed by Hoogstraal 1966). Despite these studies, a recent overview of *I. ricinus* concluded that much of the ecology and biology of this tick species remains undetermined (Gray 1991). Each stage of *I. ricinus* takes approximately 1 year to develop to the next, so the life cycle takes 3 years to complete, though it may vary from 2 to 6 years throughout the geographical range. Unfed ticks can quest for several weeks but do not usually survive from one season to the next.

The incidence of TBE virus infection in *I. ricinus* varies from 0.1 per cent or less to about 5 per cent, depending on the geographic location and particular focus. By comparison, active foci of the Far Eastern subtype of TBE virus contain a comparatively high prevalence of infected ticks (Table 39.5). For example, in the Krasnojarsk region of Siberia the incidence of infection varied from 5 to 43 per cent, with a mean of

Table 39.5 Prevalence of *Ixodes ricinus* ticks infected with TBE virus (from Gustafson 1993)

Country	Prevalence	References
Czechoslovakia (former)	0.3–4.5%	Heinz *et al.* (1979)
Finland	0.1–2.6%	Brummer-Korvenkontio *et al.* (1973); Saikku (1975)
Germany	0.2–2.0%	Ackermann and Rehse Küpper (1979)
Italy	0.05%	Verani *et al.* (1979)
Sweden	0.1–1.0%	von Zeipel *et al.* (1959)
Switzerland	0.1–1.4%	Matile *et al.* (1979)
USSR (former)	3.0–40.0%	Kunz (1969)

16 per cent (Cirkin *et al.* 1968), and it was estimated as 40 per cent in western Siberia. The difference in infection prevalence may compensate for the shorter seasonal activity of *I. persulcatus* and consequent reduced period for active virus transmission. Variations in annual prevalence of infected ticks and in the virus titre in individual ticks have been recorded, but reasons for these differences are unknown. A number of countries, notably the Czech and Slovak Republics and Sweden, have reported increases in the incidence of TBE in the past few years. The increases may be explained partly by the increase in surveillance for tick-borne infections, especially Lyme disease.

The endemicity of TBE is focal (Table 39.6). For example, a study of 346 non-immunized individuals living on the Lisö peninsula, south of Stockholm, revealed that 12 per cent were seropositive for TBE virus and 3 per cent had a history of previous serologically confirmed TBE (with encephalitis) (Gustafson *et al.* 1990). Compared with previous serosurveys in Sweden and other European countries, the finding for Lisö indicates an area of relatively high endemicity. However, Gustafson and colleagues noted that only about half the population sampled responded to the questionaire. If these were the individuals at greatest risk from tick bite then the results may overestimate the seroprevalence. Hence a survey was initiated over a 2-year period (September 1987 to August 1989) of the selected Lisö population (Gustafson *et al.* 1992). One case of TBE was seen in each year, and seroconversion for TBE virus was found in 3/258 (1.2 per cent) subjects in the first year and 5/211 (2.4 per cent) in the second year, excluding subjects who had been immunized or developed TBE. The risk of contracting TBE after a single tick bite was estimated as below 1 in 600. During the period 1956–89 in Sweden, 5/1116 (0.5 per cent) cases were fatal (Holmgren and Forsgren 1990).

Foci of FETBE virus are found within the geographical distribution of *I. persulcatus*. They occur mostly in the taiga landscape which consists of mixed broad-leaved forests of the Manchurian type where the humidity is very high, and in coniferous forests with predominately Okhots conifers. Sporadic foci occur in river valleys covered with marshy meadows, and on undulating plains where suitable habitats overgrown with bushes are scattered among cultivated valleys.

Field investigations have revealed an aggregated distribution of TBE virus-infected ticks. The non-random distribution consists of 'elementary foci' which comprise many 'microfoci' associated with the feeding or resting places of maintenance. Several factors may contribute to the clumped distribution of TBE virus-infected ticks. These include the different spatial distribution of questing ticks (clumped for larvae and random for nymphs and adults), the enhanced efficiency of virus transmission between co-feeding ticks, and tick drop-off in the resting sites of small mammals. Models of vector-borne diseases predict that the basic reproductive number, R_0, of infections that show a clumped distribution can exceed the rate expected for a homogeneous distribution, while equilibrium disease prevalence may be lowered or raised (Hasibeder and Dye 1988). This is because within at least one elementary focus there are sites that have a higher vector-to-host ratio than in the homogeneous situation with the same total numbers of vectors and hosts. Such sites become microfoci or 'hot spots' in which the virus can persist and from which it can spread. An important consequence of an aggregated infection distribution is the increased difficulty of eradicating the disease.

Unlike TBE virus, LI virus infections of humans are largely an occupational health hazard confined to laboratory workers, veterinarians, farmers, and abbatoir workers (Reid 1988). Serosurveys of patients with aseptic meningitis or encephalitis of unknown aetiology identified 5/35 positive sera of patients in Ireland; examination of 775 sera from Scottish patients identified one case of LI encephalitis in a farmer and one fatal case in a slaughterman. However, 8 per cent of sera from abbatoir workers were positive despite the fact that only two clinical cases have been reported in

Table 39.6 Prevalence of antibodies to TBE virus in human populations (from Gustafson 1993)

Country	Prevalence	References
Austria	4–8%	Ackermann and Rehse Küpper (1979)
Czechoslovakia (former)	2–38%[a]	Ackermann and Rehse-Küpper (1979)
Denmark	1.4%	Ackermann and Rehse-Küpper (1979)
Germany	4–8%	Ackermann and Rehse-Küpper (1979); Roggendorf (1983)
Hungary	17%	Ribiczey *et al.* (1979)
Italy	1.5%	Verani *et al.* (1979)
Sweden	0.1–1.0%	von Zeipel (1959)
Switzerland	1.4%	Matile *et al.* (1979)
USSR (former)	30–100%	Ackermann and Rehse-Küpper (1979)

[a] In risk groups such as farmers and forestry workers, up to 50 per cent of the individuals were seropositive.

this occupational health group. In total, only 39 human cases have been reported, of which 26 resulted from laboratory exposure.

In the natural foci of LI virus in northern England and south-west Scotland, 94 to 99 per cent of the tick population is supported by sheep. Indeed, the distribution of infected ticks corresponds better with the distribution of sheep-farming areas in the United Kingdom than with the distribution of the vector, *I. ricinus*. In certain areas of the United Kingdom, red deer (*Cervus elaphus*) or hares (*Lepus europaeus, L. timidus*) may be important maintenance hosts of the ticks (Smith and Varma 1981). As for TBE virus (European subtype), comparatively few infected ticks (about 0.1 per cent) have been found in the field (Reid 1988). If LI virus is maintained solely in a sheep–tick cycle, adult ticks are probably the principal transmitters of the virus to livestock: *I. ricinus* can acquire the infection as a feeding larva and/or nymph and most adults parasitize susceptible hosts. Furthermore, since nymphs, more than larvae, seem to prefer livestock, the nymph is more likely to acquire the infection and the adult more likely to transmit the virus. Given the narrow time-window in which sheep are infective for ticks, the role of different tick stages in virus transmission dynamics depends on the overlap in both seasonal activity of the different tick instars and their host utilization. However, when sheep are treated against ticks, hares (*Lepus timidus*) may feed 95 per cent of the tick population, and recent studies have shown that hares can support non-viraemic transmission of LI virus (Jones *et al.* 1997).

Nineteen cases of clinical POW virus infection have been recognized in North America plus one probable but unconfirmed case (Artsob 1988). Antibody surveys in the United States and Canada have generally shown prevalences of 0.5–4 per cent. Both symptomatic and asymptomatic POW virus infections have been recorded in the former USSR but, as in North America, the incidence is very low. A study of 386 sera from patients in the Primor'ye region identified 15 patients with neutralizing antibodies specific for POW virus.

TRANSMISSION

Members of the TBE virus serocomplex are true arboviruses, relying on biological transmission by the tick vector for survival. The virus is imbibed during feeding, undergoes replication within tick cells, disseminates from the gut to the salivary glands, and is subsequently transmitted in tick saliva when the next tick instar takes a blood meal (Nuttall *et al.* 1994). The ability of a tick to support virus replication and transmit the virus determines the vectorial competence of a particular tick species. Potential restrictions to infec-

tion within the tick are the gut infection barrier, gut escape barrier, salivary gland infection barrier, and salivary gland release barrier (Nuttall *et al.* 1991). Few studies have been undertaken to define these potential barriers to infection by TBE group viruses. Indeed, the wide range of ixodid tick species that can be infected and transmit TBE group viruses under experimental conditions suggests that most, if not all, ixodid species are potential vectors of TBE serocomplex viruses.

Despite the vector potential of many ixodid ticks for TBE group viruses, only a few primary vectors are apparent. The reasons for this have not been fully defined. Obviously, virus and tick must be sympatric in their distribution. However, this is not the complete story as many competent tick vectors are found within the geographical range of TBE group viruses but virus transmission cycles (and R_0) depend on comparatively few species. Two parameters are particularly significant: vector efficiency and vertebrate host preferences.

Vector efficiency is the major determinant of vector status. The efficiency of a tick vector is reflected in the infection threshold and the transmission rate. Infection threshold is defined as the lowest amount of virus capable of causing an infection in approximately 1–5 per cent of the vector population (Chamberlain *et al.* 1954). Thus the lower the infection threshold, the less virus is required to infect the vector and hence the greater the probability of infection of the vector in nature.

Data on the infection thresholds of different tick species for TBE group viruses are limited. Furthermore, the data are difficult to compare because of differences in the experimental methods employed, the means of expressing the infection threshold, and the tick stage examined. For example, the infection threshold for POW virus was determined by feeding ticks on a rabbit inoculated with a high dose of virus. Direct comparison of *D. andersoni* and *I. pacificus* revealed a 100-fold difference in the susceptibility to POW virus. The infection threshold of *I. cookei*, the principal vector of POW virus, has not been reported. Similarly, the apparent difference in infection thresholds of *I. ricinus* and *I. persulcatus* for TBE virus needs critical examination.

Estimates of infection threshold are affected by the vertebrate host species used in experiments. Initial investigations of the infection threshold of *I. ricinus* for LI virus, in which larvae were fed on laboratory mice, indicated that viraemic titres of 2.0 to greater than 4.0 $\log_{10}$PFU/0.2 ml (2.7 to greater than 4.7 $\log_{10}$PFU/ml) blood were insufficient to establish infection in larval ticks (Beasley *et al.* 1978). However, using infected chicks, the threshold levels for larvae and nymphs were approximately 4.0 and 3.0 $\log_{10}$PFU/0.2 ml (4.7 and 3.7 $\log_{10}$PFU/ml), respectively (Reid 1988). This was in agreement with a threshold of 3.2 $\log_{10}$ PFU/0.2 ml (3.9 $\log_{10}$PFU/ml) for nymphs fed on viraemic sheep (Swanepoel 1968, cited by Reid 1984).

The concept of infection threshold has been challenged by the results of experimental studies demonstrating efficient transmission of Thogoto virus (family, Orthomyxoviridae) between infected and uninfected ticks co-feeding on non-viraemic guinea-pigs (Jones *et al.* 1987). In contrast to guinea-pigs, hamsters are highly susceptible to Thogoto virus, developing levels of viraemia of up to 8.0 $\log_{10}$PFU/ml blood. The 5 per cent infection thresholds of *Rhipicephalus appendiculatus* and *Amblyomma variegatum* determined by feeding nymphs on viraemic hamsters were 2.8 and 2.7 $\log_{10}$PFU/ml blood, respectively (Davies *et al.* 1990). These levels are in sharp contrast to the infection threshold of less than 1.0 $\log_{10}$PFU/ml blood (i.e. undetectable viraemia) determined using guinea-pigs (Jones *et al.* 1990). Experimental studies to elucidate the mechanism of non-viraemic transmission revealed that a protein, secreted in the saliva of feeding ticks, enhanced virus transmission (Jones *et al.* 1992*a*). The saliva-activated transmission (SAT) factor was demonstrated in the salivary glands of competent vectors of the virus but not in a limited number of non-competent vectors (Jones *et al.* 1992*b*).

A transmission strategy similar to that observed with Thogoto virus has been reported for TBE virus. The relevance of infection thresholds was questioned in studies of TBE virus infection of *I. persulcatus* that were fed on non-viraemic rabbits (Galimov *et al.* 1989). Similar studies using *I. persulcatus, I. ricinus, Dermacentor marginatus, D. reticulatus*, and *R. appendiculatus*, demonstrated TBE virus transmission between infected and uninfected ticks feeding either in contact with each other, or physically separated on non-viraemic guinea-pigs (Alekseev and Chunikhin 1990; Labuda *et al.* 1993*a*). Non-viraemic transmission of TBE virus was shown to be mediated by a factor associated with tick salivary glands (Labuda *et al.* 1993*b*). Saliva-activated transmission of TBE virus shows several differences from that of Thogoto virus, probably reflecting different infection strategies of the two viruses in the vertebrate host. Nevertheless, SAT may play an important role in determining vector efficiency of ticks species that transmit TBE group viruses.

The latent period between virus acquisition and the time at which the tick becomes infective is known as the extrinsic incubation period (EIP) (Hardy 1988). During this period the tick is incapable of virus transmission. It is unlikely that EIP is important in the ecology of TBE group viruses because of the relatively long developmental period between tick blood-meals.

Besides the infection threshold (whether apparent or subliminal), the transmission rate is also important in determining vector efficiency. Owing to the long feeding period of tick vectors of TBE group viruses, the true rate (i.e. as a function of time) of transmission is probably irrelevant. Of greater significance is the effectiveness of the tick vector in transmitting the virus to the vertebrate host (and thence to other tick vectors). As expected, tick-borne transmission of TBE group viruses appears to be an efficient process when the vertebrate host is susceptible to infection. For example, under experimental conditions, three TBE virus-infected larvae of *I. ricinus* or *I. persulcatus* that fed for 2 days on mice induced encephalitis; one TBE virus-infected female *I. ricinus* was sufficient to transmit the virus to a mouse (Benda 1958). Thus it seems likely that one infected tick is sufficient to infect a susceptible host. However, transmission efficiency may vary between tick species and between tick instars, and thus influence the role of a species/stage in the enzootic cycle. Experimental studies demonstrated that nymphs of *I. ricinus* were more efficient than either nymphs or larvae of *Haemaphysalis inermis*, or larvae of *D. reticulatus*.

Transmission cycles of Far Eastern and European subtypes of TBE viruses involve ixodid ticks and rodents. The most important rodents usually are those that are most abundant within a focus of infection (generally *Apodemus, Clethrionomys*, or *Microtus* species). In contrast to TBE viruses, the transmission cycle of LI virus is highly dependent on sheep farming and land management. Besides vector density, factors determining the prevalence of LI virus within enzootic areas are clearly influenced by the access of sheep to pasture during periods of tick activity, and vaccination regimes for sheep. The proportion of grouse that survive epizootics of LI appears to be insufficient to maintain the virus transmission cycle (Reid *et al.* 1978).

Powassan virus is transmitted in an enzootic cycle involving ixodid ticks, and rodents and carnivores. Lagomorphs and birds (the latter in the CIS) may also be involved (Artsob 1988). Although the virus has been isolated from mosquitoes in the Far East, including larvae of *Aedes togoi*, no insect vectors of POW virus have been identified in North America and the role of mosquitoes in the enzootic cycle is unclear.

The response of susceptible vertebrate hosts to tick-borne virus transmission depends on immune status. In nature, infected ticks feed on vertebrate hosts that are immune to the virus and/or develop a resistance response to tick infestation. Previously, virus-immune animals were considered to be 'dead-end' hosts, incapable of supporting transmission of the virus. However, recent studies have demonstrated efficient transmission of TBE virus between infected and uninfected *I. ricinus* nymphs feeding closely together on TBE virus-immune wood mice (*A. sylvaticus*). The ability of virus-immune natural hosts to support the transmission of TBE virus has important implications for virus survival (Labuda *et al.* 1997). Results of experimental studies indicate that the uptake of virus-specific antibodies by infected ticks has no effect on the infection in ticks other than a possible inhibitory effect on vertical transmission.

In a study of tick-host immunity, laboratory animals immunized with uninfected tick salivary glands were protected against infection when exposed to TBE virus-infected ticks, but were susceptible to challenge by syringe inoculation of TBE virus (Mishaeva, 1990). However, attempts to confirm this intriguing result were unsuccessful (M. L., unpublished data). The ability of vertebrate hosts to reject natural tick infestations has not been examined with regard to virus ecology.

Most TBE group viruses are transmitted vertically from the infected female via the egg to the succeeding generation. The significance of vertical transmission in the ecology of these viruses is undetermined. The frequency of vertical transmission generally appears to be low, indicating that vertical transmission is not important at the population level of virus infections (Burgdorfer and Varma 1967). However, results of modelling the relative contribution of transovarial transmission to the maintenance of tick-borne disease suggests that even a low level of vertical transmission can be significant (Randolph 1993). Furthermore, virus transmission between co-feeding infected and uninfected larvae may amplify the number of infections in the tick population.

Although ticks are the primary route of transmission of TBE group viruses, virus transmission via milk and milk products has been demonstrated for most members of the TBE virus serocomplex. In 1951 to 1952, an outbreak of TBE affecting at least 600 persons was recorded in the Roznava district of Slovakia. Milk of infected goats was incriminated as the probable source of infection. Milk-borne transmission to humans is more common in Europe than in the Far East. Experimental studies have demonstrated TBE virus in the milk of goats, sheep, and cattle for up to 8 days after infection (Grešiková and Calisher 1988). Although LI has not been reported in naturally infected goats, during experimental studies five kids acquired the infection after ingesting infected milk and all developed severe disease. Secretion of POW virus in goats' milk has been demonstrated experimentally.

PREVENTION

The most effective preventive measure is to avoid tick bites. Protective clothing, preferably light-coloured for easier detection of ticks, is effective. This may be unde-sirable during hot weather and reliance should then be placed on a thorough search of the body, at least daily, after exposure to tick-infested habitat. Ticks that have attached to the skin should be removed carefully using tweasers or forceps to grasp the mouthparts that are buried in the skin. Remember that tick mouthparts have backward pointing barbs so the action of removal should be like removing a fishing hook from a fish. Several tick repellents are available but their efficacy in preventing infection with TBE virus has not been fully elucidated.

The most common vaccine used in Europe is FSME-Immun®, prepared by Immuno AG, Austria. This vaccine is a suspension of purified viral antigen derived from TBE virus grown in chick embryo cells and inactivated with formaldehyde. Three doses, given intramuscularly (preferably in the musculus deltoideus for adults), give a protective effect persisting for at least 3 years. The seroconversion rate after active immunization with one, two, and three doses of the Immuno vaccine was greater than 70 per cent, 95 per cent and greater than 99 per cent, respectively (Kunz *et al.* 1980). Studies in Sweden revealed lower seroconversion rates although sample sizes were small (Gustafson *et al.* 1990, 1992). A booster dose is recommended every third year to maintain protective immunity. A protective rate of more than 97 per cent is achieved after the third dose and cases of TBE among persons fully immunized are rare (Kunz 1993, cited by Gustafson 1993). Adverse reactions are usually mild.

Passive immunization, using specific IgG antibodies against TBE virus as pre- or post-exposure prophylaxis, is available (FSME-Bulin®, Immuno AG, Austria) (Kunz 1977) and can be used in selected cases.

Vaccination of laboratory personnel is strongly recommended and in some countries is mandatory for anyone working with TBE virus. Vaccination of high-risk groups, e.g. forestry and agricultural workers, and people living in endemic areas, is recommended in several countries.

A vaccine to protect sheep against LI was developed soon after the isolation of the aetiological agent. The vaccine now in general use is grown in sheep kidney cell cultures, is formalin-inactivated, and is concentrated by methanol precipitation. Control of the disease in sheep also includes acaricide treatment (by dipping or application of pour-ons) of animals to control tick infestations. Sheep vaccination not only protects sheep but has helped to diminish the intensity of virus circulation. The other general important preventive measures are: avoidance of tick bite by use of repellents and protective clothing, health education, disease foci marked with warning signs, and pasteurization or boiling of raw milk. In the past, widespread use of pesticides, including aerial application of

DDT, has been undertaken in some areas in attempts to interrupt the transmission cycle.

REFERENCES

Ackerman, R. and Rehse-Küpper, B. (1979). Die Zentraleuropäische Enzephalitis in der Bundesrepublik Deutschland. *Fortschritte de Neurologie und Psychiatrie*, **47**, 103–22.

Alekseev, A. N. and Chunikhin, S. P. (1990). Exchange of the tickborne encephalitis virus between Ixodidae simultaneously feeding on the animals with subthreshold levels of viraemia. *Meditsinskaya Parazitologiya*, **1**, 28–31.

Arthur, D. R. (1962). *Ticks and disease*. Pergamon Press, Oxford.

Artsob, H. (1988). Powassan encephalitis. In *The arboviruses: epidemiology and ecology*, Vol. IV, (ed. T. P. Monath), pp. 29–49. CRC Press, Boca Raton, Florida.

Banerjee, K. (1988). Kyasanur forest disease. In *The arboviruses: epidemiology and ecology*, Vol. III, (ed. T. P. Monath), pp. 93–116. CRC Press, Boca Raton, Florida,

Beasley, S. J., Campbell, J. A., and Reid, H. W. (1978). Threshold problems in infection of *Ixodes ricinus* with the virus of louping ill. In *Tick-borne diseases and their vectors*, (ed. J. K. H. Wilde), pp. 487–500, Proceedings of the International Conference Edinburgh, 1976. Edinburgh University Press.

Benda, R. (1958). The common tick, *Ixodes ricinus* L. as a reservoir and vector of tick-borne encephalitis. II. Experimental transmission of encephalitis to laboratory animals by ticks at various stages of development. *Journal of Hygiene, Epidemiology, Microbiology and Immunology*, **2**, 331–44.

Brummer-Korvenkontio, M., Saikku, M., Korhonen, P., and Oker-Blom, N. (1973). Arboviruses in Finland. 1. Isolation of tick-borne encephalitis (TBE) virus from arthropods, vertebrates and patients. *American Journal of Tropical Medicine and Hygiene*, **22**, 382–9.

Burgdorfer, W. and Varma, M. G. R. (1967). Trans-stadial and transovarial development of disease agents in arthropods. *Annual Review of Entomology*, **12**, 347–76.

Chamberlain, R. W., Sikes, R. K., Nelson, D. B., and Sudia, W. D. (1954). Studies on the North American arthropod-borne encephalitides. Part VI: Quantitative determinations of virus-vector relationships. *American Journal of Hygiene*, **60**, 278–85.

Cirkin, Ju. M., Krasovskij, M., and Fastovskaja, E. I. (1968). Virophory of *Ixodes persulcatus* ticks in Krasnojarsk region. In *Questions on the epidemiology of tick-borne encephalitis and the biology of its natural focus*, (ed. M. V. Pospelovoy-Shtrom and M. G. Rashinoy), pp. 204–12. 'Meditsina' Moscow.

Davies, C. R., Jones, L. D., and Nuttall, P. A. (1990). A comparative study of the infection thresholds of Thogoto virus in *Rhipicephalus appendiculatus* and *Amblyomma variegatum*. *American Journal of Tropical Medicine and Hygiene*, **43**, 99–103.

Dietz, K. (1988). Density-dependence in parasite transmission dynamics. *Parasitology Today*, **4**, 91–7.

Galimov, V. R., Galimova, E. Z., Katin, A. A. and Kolchanova, L. P. (1989). The transmission of TBE virus to adult taiga ticks when virusaemia in their hosts is absent. In *Proceedings of the XII All-Union Conference on Natural Focality of Diseases, 10–12 October 1989, Novosibirsk*, pp. 43–4.

George. S., Gourie-Devi, M., Rao, J. A., Prasad, S. R., and Pavri, K. M. (1984). Isolation of West Nile virus from the brains of children who had died of encephalitis. *Bulletin WHO*, **63**, 879.

Gray, J. S. (1991). The development and seasonal activity of the tick *Ixodes ricinus*: a vector of Lyme borreliosis. *Reviews of Medical and Veterinary Entomology*, **79**, 323–33.

Grešiková, M. and Calisher, C. H. (1988). Tick-borne encephalitis. In *The arboviruses: epidemiology and ecology*, Vol. IV, (ed. T. P. Monath), pp. 177–202. CRC Press, Boca Raton, Florida.

Gustafson, R. (1993). *Epidemiological studies of Lyme borreliosis and tick-borne encephalitis*. Department of Infectious Diseases, Karolinska Institute at Huddinge University Hospital, Stockholm, Sweden.

Gustafson, R., Svenungsson, B., Gardulf, A., Stiernstedt, G., and Forsgren, M. (1990). Prevalence of tick-borne encephalitis and Lyme borreliosis in a defined Swedish population. *Scandinavian Journal of Infectious Diseases*, **22**, 297–306.

Gustafson, R., Svenungsson, B., Forsgren, M., Gardulf, A., and Granström, M. (1992). Two-year survey of the incidence of Lyme borresliosis and tick-borne encephalitis in a high risk population in Sweden. *European Journal of Clinical Microbiology of Infectious Diseases*, **11**, 894–900.

Hardy, J. L. (1988). Susceptibility and resistance of vector mosquitoes. In *The arboviruses: epidemiology and ecology*, Vol. I, (ed. T. P. Monath), pp. 87–126. CRC Press, Boca Raton, Florida.

Hasibeder, G. and Dye, C. (1988). Population dynamics of mosquito-borne disease: persistence in a completely heterogeneous environment. *Theoretical Population Biology*, **33**, 31–53.

Heinz, F., Asmera, J., and Januska, J. (1979). Present activity in natural foci of tick-borne encephalitis in the CSSR. *Tick-Borne Encephalitis, International Symposium Baden/Vienna*, pp. 279–81. Facultas Verlag, Wien.

Holmgren, B. Forsgren, M. (1990). Epidemiology of tick-borne encephalitis in Swedan 1956–1989: a study of 1116 cases. *Scandinavian Journal of Infectious Diseases*, **22**, 287–95.

Hoogstraal, H. (1966). Ticks in relation to human diseases caused by viruses. *Annual Review of Entomology*, **11**, 261–308.

Hoogstraal, H. (1980). Established and emerging concepts regarding tick-associated viruses, and unanswered questions. In *Arboviruses in the Mediterranean countries*, (ed. J. Vesenjak-Hirjan, J. S. Porterfied, and I. E. Arslanagic). Zentrbl. Bakt. Mikro. Hyg. I. Abt., Suppl. 9. pp. 49–62, Gustav Fischer Verlag, Stuttgart.

Jones, L. D., Davies, C. R., Steele, G. M., and Nuttall, P. A. (1987). A novel mode of arbovius transmission involving a nonviraemic host. *Science*, **237**, 775–7.

Jones, L. D., Hodgson, E., and Nuttall, P. A. (1989). Enhancement of virus transmission by tick salivary glands. *Journal of General Virology*, **70**, 1895–8.

Jones, L. D., Davies, C. R., Hodgson, E., Williams, T., Cory, J., and Nuttall, P. A. (1990). Non-viraemic transmission of Thogoto virus: vector efficiency of *Rhipicephalus appendiculatus* and *Amblyomma variegatum*. *Transactions of the Royal Society of Tropical Medicine and Hygiene*, **84**, 846–84.

Jones, L. D., Kaufman, W. R., and Nuttall, P. A. (1992a). feeding site modification by tick saliva resulting in enhanced virus transmission. *Experientia*, **48**, 779–82.

Jones, L. D., Hodgson, E., Williams, T. Higgs, S., and Nuttall, P. A. (1992b). Saliva-activated transmission (SAT) of Thogoto virus: relationship with vector potential of different haematophagous arthropods.*Medical and Veterinary Entomology*, **6**, 261–5.

Jones, L. D. *et al.* (1997). Transmission of louping ill virus between infected and uninfected ticks co-feeding on mountain hares. *Medical and Veterinary Entomology*, **11**, 172–76.

Kharitonova, N. N., Leonov, Y. A. (1985). The agent and epizootiology, in, *Omsk Haemorrhagic Fever* (Ed. P. M. P. Chumakov) New Delhi: Science (Nanka) Publishers.

Kožuch, O., Labuda, M., Lysy, J., Weismann, P., and Krippel, E. (1990). Longitudinal study of natural foci of Central European encephalitis virus in West Slovakia. *Acta Virologica*, **34**, 537–44.

Kunz, C. (1969). Arbovirus-B-Infektionen. In Vol. Bd II, pp. 1595–629. *Die Infectionskrankheiten des menschen und ihre Erreger*, Thieme-Verlag, Stuttgart.

Kunz, C. (1977). Die Fruhsommer-Meningoenzephalitis (FSME) in Osterreich und Ihre Verhütung. *Acta Medica Austriaca*, **4**, 90–2.

Kunz, C., Hofmann, H., and Heinz, F. (1980). Immunogenicity and reactogenicity of highly purified vaccine against tick-borne encephalitis. *Journal of Medical Virology*, **6**, 103–9.

Labuda, M., Lys'y, M., and Kožuch, O. (1991). On virus-vector relationships in the Central European tick-borne encephalitis foci (West Slovakia). In *Modern acarology*, Vol. 2, (ed. F. Dusb'-bek and V. Bukva), pp. 29–33. SPB Academic Publishing, Prague and Academia, The Hague.

Labuda, M., Jones, L. D., Williams, T., Danielova, V., and Nuttall, P. A. (1993*a*). Efficient transmission of tick-borne encephalitis virus between co-feeding ticks. *Journal of Medical Entomology*, **30**, 295–9.

Labuda, M., Jones, L. D., Williams, T., and Nuttall, P. A. (1993*b*). Enhancement of tick-borne encephalitis virus transmission by tick salivary gland extracts. *Medical and Veterinary Entomology*, **7**, 193–6.

Labuda, M. *et al.* (1993*c*). Non-viraemic transmission of tick-borne encephalitis virus: a mechanism for arbovirus survival in nature. *Experientia*, **49**, 802–5.

Labuda, M., Danielova, V., Jones, L. D., and Nuttall, P. A. (1993*d*). Amplification of tick-borne encephalitis virus infection during co-feeding of ticks. *Med. Vet. Ent.* 7: 339–342.

Labuda, M., Austyn, J. M., Zuffová E., Kozuch, O., and Nuttall, P. A. (1996). Importance of localised skin infection in tick-borne encephalitis virus transmission. *Virology*, **219**, 357–366.

Labuda, M., Kožuch, O., Zuffová, E., Elecková, E., Hails, R. S. and Nuttall, P. A. (1997). Tick-borne encephalitis virus transmission between ticks cofeeding on specific immune natural rodent hosts. *Virology*, **235**, 138–43.

Lvov, D. K. (1988). Omsk haemorrhagic fever. In *The Arboviruses: Epidemiology and Ecology*, Vol III, (ed. T. P. Monath), pp. 205–216. Boca Raton, Florida, CRC Press, Inc..

McKelvey, J. J., Jr., Eldridge, B. F. and Maramorosch, K. [eds]. (1981). Vectors of disease agents. Praeger, New York.

Marin, M. S., Zanotto, P. M. de A., Gritsun, T. S., and Gould, E. A. (1995). Phylogeny of TYU, SRE, and CFA virus: Different evolutionary rates in the genus Flavivirus. Virology **206**, 1133–1139.

Matile, H., Aeschlimann, A. and Wyler, R. (1979). Sero-epidemiological investigations on the incidence of TBE in man and dog in Switzerland. In: Kunc C, ed. International Symposium on Tick-Borne Encephalitis. Baden/Wienna, Austria: Facultas Verlag, Wien.

Milne, A. (1949*a*). The ecology of the sheep tick *Ixodes ricinus* L. Host relationships of the tick. Part I. Review of previous work in Britain. *Parasitology*, **39**, 167–72.

Milne, A. (1949*b*). The ecology of the sheep tick *Ixodes ricinus* L. Host relationships of the tick. Part II. Observations on hill and moorland grazing in northern England. *Parasitology* **39**, 173–97.

Mishaeva, N. P. (1990). Protection of vertebrates from experimental tick-borne encephalitis in active and passive immunization against *Ixodes* antigens. *Voprosy Virmologia*, **35**, 93–98.

Monath, T. P. and Heinz, F. X. (1996). Flaviviruses. In *Fields Virology*, (ed. B. N. Fields *et al.*), pp. 961–1034. Lippincott–Raven, Philadelphia.

Murphy, F. A., Fauquet, C. M., Bishop, D. H. L., Ghabrial, S. A., Mayo, M. A., and Summers, M. D. (ed.) (1995). Virus Taxonomy. Sixth Report of the International Committee on Taxonomy of Viruses. *Archives of Virology*. (Suppl. 10)

Nuttall, P. A. (1984). Transmission of viruses to wild life by ticks. In *Vectors in virus biology*, (ed. M. A. Mayo and K. A. Harrap), pp. 135–59. Academic Press, New York.

Nuttall, P. A., Jones, L. D., and Davies, C. R. (1991). The role of arthropod vectors in arbovirus evolution. *Advances in Disease and Vector Research*, **8**, 15–45.

Nuttall, P. A., Jones, L. D., Labuda, M., and Kaufman, W. R. (1994). Adaptations of arboviruses to ticks. *Journal of Medicine Entomology*, **31**, 1–9.

Randolph, S. E. (1993). The relative contributions of transovarial and transtadial transmission to the maintenance of tick-borne diseases. In *Lyme Borreliosis*, NATO ASI Series in Life Sciences (ed. J. S. Axford and D. H. E. Rees), pp. 131–8. Plenum Press, New York.

Randolph, S. E., Gern, L., and Nuttall, P. A. (1996). Co-feeding ticks: epidemiological significance for tick-borne pathogen transmission. *Parasitology Today*, **12**, 472–9.

Reid, H. W. (1984). Epidemiology of louping-ill. In *Vectors in virus biology*, (ed. M. A. Mayo and K. A. Harrap), pp. 161–78. Academic Press, London.

Reid, H. W. (1988). Louping -ill. In *The arboviruses: epidemiology and ecology*, Vol. III, (ed. T. P. Monath), pp. 117–35. CRC Press, Boca Raton, Florida.

Reid, H. W., Duncan, J. S., Phillips, J. D. P., Moss, R., and Watson, A. (1978). Studies on louping-ill virus (Flavivirus group) in wild red grouse (*Lagopus lagopus scoticus*). *Journal of Hygiene Cambridge*, **81**, 321–30.

Rey, F. A., Heinz, F. X., Mandl, C. W., Kunz, C., and Harrison, S. C. (1995). The envelope glycoprotein from tick-borne encephalitis virus at 2A resolution. *Nature*, **375**, 291–8.

Ribiczey, P., Sipos, J., Gabor, V., Bartok, K., and Toth, Z. (1979). Detection of specific and non-specific immunological parameters in the course of TBE, Tick-borne encephalitis. *International Symposium Baden/Vienna*, pp. 112–21. Facultas-Verlag, Wien.

Roggendorf, M. (1983). Zur Häufigkeit der Frühsommermeningoenzephalitis in Bayern. *Bayerische Ärzeblatt*, **H.5**, 306–8.

Saikku, P. (1975). Tick-borne viruses. *Medical Biology*, **53**, 317–20.

Schneider, H. (1931). Über epidemische akute 'Meningitis serosa' *Wiener Klin. Wschr*, **44**, 350–2. Wiener Khinische Workenschift.

Smith, C. E. G. and Varma, M. G. R. (1981). Louping ill. In *CRC Handbook Series in Zoonoses*, (ed. in chief J. H. Steele), *Section B: Viral zoonoses*, (ed. G. W. Beran), Vol. I, pp. 191–200. CRC Press, Boca Raton, Florida.

Smorodintsev, A. (1944). Tick-borne encephalitis. *American Review of Soviet Medicine*, **1**, 400–8.

Titus, R. G. and Ribeiro, J. M. C. (1990). The role of vector saliva in transmission of arthropod-borne disease. *Parasitology Today*, **6**, 157–60.

Venugopal, K., Buckley, A., Reid, H. W., and Gould, E. A. (1992). Nucleotide sequence of the envelope glycoprotein of Negishi virus shows very close homology to louping ill virus. *Journal of General Virology*, **190**, 515–21.

Verani, P. *et al.* (1979). Circulation of TBE virus in Italy: Seroepidemiological and ecovirological studies. *Tick-borne encephalitis, International Symposium. Baden/Vienna'*, Wien, pp. 265–72. Facultas-Verlag.

von Zeipel, G. (1959). Isolation of viruses of the Russian spring–summer encephalitis-louping ill group from Swedish ticks and from a human cases of meningoencephalitis. *Archir für die Virusforsching*, **9**, 460–9.

WHO (1986). *Tick-borne encephalitis and haemorrhagic fever with renal syndrome*, Report on a WHO Meeting, Baden, 3–5 October, 1983. EURO Reports and Studies 104.

Zanotto, P. M. de A., Gould, E. A., Gao, G. F., Harvey, P. H., and Holmes, E. C. (1996). Population dynamics of flaviviruses revealed by molecular phylogenies. *Proceedings of the National Academy of Sciences, USA*, **93**, 548–53.

40 YELLOW FEVER

Thomas P. Monath

SUMMARY

Yellow fever is an acute mosquito-borne flavivirus infection characterized in its full-blown form by fever, jaundice, albuminuria, and haemorrhage. Two forms are distinguished: *urban* yellow fever in which the virus is spread from person to person by peridomestic *Aédes aegypti* mosquitos and *jungle (sylvan)* yellow fever transmitted by tree-hole breeding mosquitoes between non-human primates and sometimes humans. Yellow fever is endemic and epidemic in tropical areas of the Americas and Africa but has never appeared in Asia or the Pacific region. Control is through vector control, prevention of mosquito bites, and yellow fever vaccination.

HISTORY

The earliest probable account of the disease was during an epidemic in the Yucatan Peninsula in 1648. In Africa, the disease was first recognized during an epidemic in 1778. During the eighteenth and nineteenth centuries, yellow fever was a major threat to human health in the Americas and Africa, and it invaded Europe on numerous occasions. For many years the disease was attributed to the spread of airborne miasmas. Although mosquitoes were suspected to be implicated in transmission as early as 1848, it was Carlos Finlay, a Cuban physician, who in 1881 promulgated the theory of mosquito transmission. Spurred by Finlay's suggestion, Walter Reed and his colleagues conducted studies in Cuba in 1900–1901 that proved transmission by *Aedes aegypti* mosquitoes, demonstrated that an extrinsic incubation period in the mosquito was required prior to transmission by bite, and showed that the disease was caused by a filtrable virus. Isolation of the virus proved an elusive goal until 1927, when workers at the Rockefeller Foundation laboratory in Nigeria isolated the agent by passage of human blood to rhesus macaques. The virus, recovered from a patient named Asibi, is the parent of the attenuated 17D strain now used as a vaccine.

For many years, *Ae. aegypti* was thought to be the only vector, and humans the only host for yellow fever virus. In 1932, 'jungle yellow fever' was described in an area of Colombia free from *Ae. aegypti*, and by 1938, yellow fever transmission by tree-hole breeding *Haemagogus* mosquitoes was documented. Field studies in South America and East Africa during the 1930s and 1940s unravelled many complexities of yellow fever as a zoonotic disease, demonstrating the role of sylvatic vectors in virus transmission between non-human primates and spillover of the infection to the urban cycle involving *Ae. aegypti* and humans. Research on virus survival across the long tropical dry season and on the recrudescence of epizootics/epidemics continued for several decades. In 1977, workers at the Pasteur Institute in Dakar obtained field evidence for transovarial transmission of the virus in the sylvatic vector *Ae. furcifer-taylori*. Subsequent field and experimental studies have implicated vertical transmission in vector mosquitoes as a viral maintenance mechanism.

In the Americas, control of urban yellow fever centred on the elimination of *Ae. aegypti*. Successful vector eradication programmes were undertaken in Cuba, Panama, Brazil, and other areas. The last *Ae. aegypti*-borne outbreaks in South America were in Brazil in 1942 and (possibly) in Trinidad in 1954. However, control efforts were never seriously undertaken in Africa, where *Ae. aegypti*-borne epidemic continue to occur. Efforts to develop a vaccine began in the 1930s in Senegal and the United States, and were spurred on by the recognition of yellow fever as a zoonotic disease. Field trials of the French neurotropic vaccine began in 1934 in West Africa and of the 17D vaccine in 1937 in Brazil. These vaccines came into widespread use in the 1940s. Yellow fever epidemics continue to occur (Monath 1991). The greatest impact of the disease is currently in Africa, but recent changes in the ecology and distribution of *Ae. aegypti* in the Americas raise the spectre of future urban outbreaks.

AETIOLOGICAL AGENT

TAXONOMY

Yellow fever virus is the prototype of the family Flaviviridae, a group of 69 viruses that includes a number of other important arthropod-borne diseases, such as dengue, St Louis encephalitis, Japanese encephalitis, and tick-borne encephalitis. By the neutralization test, yellow fever virus is antigenically distinct, but appears to be more closely related to Banzi, Wesselsbron, Bouboui, Zika, and Uganda S viruses than to other flaviviruses. Cross-protection between yellow fever and other flaviviruses can be demonstrated in animals. Prior immunization with Wesselsbron, Zika, and dengue viruses causes a significant reduction in viraemias in monkeys challenged with virulent yellow fever virus. Cross-protection may explain certain epidemiological events, including a lower incidence of clinical yellow fever infections in adult African populations with a background of heterologous flavivirus immunity. Immunity to dengue may be a barrier to the introduction of yellow fever into Asia.

MOLECULAR BIOLOGY AND BASIS FOR VIRULENCE

Yellow fever is a single-strand positive polarity RNA-containing virus of small size (35–45 nm in diameter), consisting of a nucleocapsid approximately 30 nm in diameter, surrounded by a lipid bilayer envelope (Chambers *et al.* 1990). Replication occurs in the cytoplasm, and mature virus particles accumulate in endoplasmic reticulum and are released by host cell lysis. After adsorption, entry, and uncoating, the genome is translated to yield viral replicases and serves as a template for transcription of minus-strand complementary RNA. In turn, progeny plus-strand RNAs are synthesized. These serve as mRNA for translation of viral proteins and incorporation into new virions.

The linear yellow fever genome has been completely sequenced and shown to contain 10 862 nucleotides with a single long open reading frame encoding, in order, the three structural proteins (C, capsid; M, membrane, and E, envelope) and seven non-structural proteins, designated NS1, NS2a, NS2b, NS3, NS4a, NS4b, and NS5. The gene products result from proteolytic processing of a polyprotein precursor. The E glycoprotein, a dimeric molecule composed of a 170 Å-long curved rod that is anchored to the viral membrane at its basal end, is involved in attachment of virus to cell receptors, and contains functional antigenic determinants, including those for haemagglutination and neutralization. Epitopes are clustered in three spatially distinct domains (domains A, B, and C) on the glycoprotein rod and biological activity (e.g. neutralization) is dependent on the native conformation of the protein. The NS1 glycoprotein, while not incorporated in the mature virion, is expressed on the surface of infected cells and elicits complement-fixing antibodies that may play a role in protection against yellow fever infection. As for protein E, most NS1 epitopes are conformation-dependent. The functions of

the other non-structural proteins are less well understood. NS3 functions as a protease in post-translational processing, and NS5 as the RNA polymerase.

Attenuation by serial passage led to the development of the yellow fever 17D vaccine. Nucleotide sequencing of the virulent, parental Asibi virus and 17D vaccine provided clues to the molecular basis of virulence (Hann *et al.* 1987), but the large number of mutations and their localization in many parts of the genome complicate interpretation of these comparative data. Sixty-seven nucleotide and 31 amino acid differences distributed across the genome were noted between vaccine and parental Asibi virus. Subsequent analyses of other vaccine strains derived from the 17D lineage and additional wild-type yellow fever viruses have significantly reduced the mutations that may explain attenuation. Thirteen non-conservative amino acid substitutions are specific to the vaccine strains, five of which occur in the E gene. Five of the changes in the E gene occur at sites (amino acids 52, 173, 200, 305, and 380) that are conserved in virulent yellow fever viruses from both Africa and South America isolated many years apart. Thus these mutations are likely to be implicated in yellow fever virulence.

Yellow fever virus exhibits two distinct virulence factors reflecting its capability to induce encephalitis (neurotropism) and hepatitis (viscerotropism). The attenuated 17D virus has lost its capacity to cause hepatitis, while retaining a reduced degree of neurotropism, particularly for the immature brain. A single fatal case of human encephalitis due to 17D virus has been reported. Sequencing of the E glycoprotein and comparison with other substrains of 17D vaccines revealed a single amino acid change at position 303 that could be correlated with the increased neurovirulence of the virus recovered from brain tissue (Jennings *et al.* 1994). Presumably this mutation arose during replication of the vaccine in the human host. Interestingly, this mutation is spatially close to two other mutations distinguishing wild-type from vaccine virus, suggesting that this region, which lies in antigenic domain B, may represent an important locus defining neurovirulence. The B domain contains an RGD sequence and is believed to represent part of the cell receptor binding site for flaviviruses.

ROLE OF YELLOW FEVER PROTEINS IN THE IMMUNE RESPONSE

The E protein plays the dominant role in the genesis of neutralizing antibodies and the induction of protective immunity. The prM protein also contains neutralizing and protective domains. prM is part of immature virions and is proteolytically cleaved in the trans-Golgi region to generate M protein in mature virions. If this cleavage is incomplete, prM protein in the virion can serve as a target for neutralizing protective antibodies.

The non-structural glycoprotein NS1 is expressed on the surface of infected cells and is also secreted into the circulation of the infected host as 'soluble complement fixing' (SCF) antigen. Although antibodies to NS1 do not react with the virion and exhibit no neutralizing activity, they confer protection against yellow fever virus infection in experimental animals. This phenomenon is dependent on the Fc portion of antibodies and appears to be due to complement-mediated cytotoxicity, although other mechanisms may contribute as well.

The immunological role of the other non-structural proteins appears to be limited to cellular immunity. Studies with dengue and other flaviviruses have demonstrated epitopes for CD4+ and CD8+ T-lymphocytes on NS1, NS3, NS4A, and NS4B as well as on the E glycoprotein.

Antibody-dependent enhancement of flavivirus replication in peripheral blood monocytes and macrophage-like cell lines has been demonstrated *in vitro* with a number of flaviviruses, including yellow fever. The mechanism involves attachment of complexes of virus and subneutralizing heterologous antibodies to Fc receptors on macrophage–monocytes, with increased virus uptake and replication. Antibody-dependent enhancement may explain the increased immunological response to attenuated dengue vaccines in persons previously vaccinated with yellow fever. Immune enhancement has been proposed as a pathogenetic mechanism in dengue haemorrhagic fever. However, there is no evidence to suggest that prior exposure to heterologous flaviviruses enhances or exacerbates clinical yellow fever infection; indeed, experimental and epidemiological studies suggest that cross-protection occurs in the presence of heterologous immunity.

DIVERSITY OF YELLOW FEVER VIRUS STRAINS: MOLECULAR EPIDEMIOLOGY

Antigenic differences have been shown between strains of yellow fever virus, and virus strains from tropical America and Africa may be readily distinguished by cross-absorption. By RNA oligonucleotide fingerprinting and nucleotide sequencing three genotypes are distinguished that segregate geographically—one in South America and two in Africa (Deubel *et al.* 1986; Lepiniec *et al.* 1994). E protein gene sequences of virus strains from West Africa (E-genotype IA) and tropical America (E-genotype IB) are distinguishable, but are more similar to each other than those in Central and East Africa (E-genotype II). The east–west dividing line between genotypes IA and II falls at a longitude sepa-

rating Nigeria/Cameroon and the Central African Republic. By RNA oligonucleotide fingerprinting and sequencing, West African strains (genotype IA) have been separated into two geographic subgroups, one representing Senegal–Gambia–western Ivory Coast–Mali and the other representing eastern Ivory Coast–Burkina Faso–Nigeria. Overall, the yellow fever gene pool appears to be quite stable, with genetic drift within each genotype occurring at a random mutation rate of 2.2 bases/year in the envelope gene. The stability of the viral genome suggests that gene flow is occurring over relatively wide geographic areas. In practice, it has sometimes been useful to determine viral genotype, as a means of confirming that an outbreak arose from recrudescence of a regional strain rather than importation from afar.

GROWTH *IN VITRO* AND HOST RANGE

Yellow fever virus can be propagated in a wide variety of primary and continuous cell cultures, including monkey kidney (MA-104, Vero, LLC-MK2), rabbit kidney (MA-111), baby hamster kidney (BHK), and porcine kidney (PS-2 and PK-15) cell lines, as well as in primary chick and duck embryo fibroblast monolayers, in which the virus causes cytopathic effects and plaque formation. Mosquito cells, particularly the *Ae. pseudoscutellaris* (AP61) cell line, are highly sensitive for primary isolation of wild-type yellow fever virus. Intrathoracic inoculation of *Toxorhynchites* or *Ae. aegypti* mosquitoes may be used for primary isolation or virus titration. After an appropriate incubation period, mosquitoes can be examined directly by immunofluorescence or subpassaged to a susceptible host such as suckling mice.

In vertebrate hosts, wild-type yellow fever virus produces both neurotropic and viscerotropic patterns of infection. Viscerotropism reflects the pathogenesis of yellow fever virus in human or non-human primates, in which disease is characterized by hepatic pathology. The European hedgehog (*Erinaceus europaeus*) and Sudanese hedgehog (*E. pruneri*) are the only non-primate species that develop viscerotropic infections (hepatitis). Infant mice are susceptible to neurotropic infection (encephalitis) after peripheral or intracerebral inoculation, whereas older mice and guinea-pigs develop encephalitis only after intracerebral inoculation. Monkeys develop encephalitis after intracerebral inoculation of wild-type virus but die of acute visceral yellow fever. Adaptation of wild-type virus by brain passage in mice reduces viscerotropism, and was the basis for development of the French neurotropic vaccine.

The host range for wild vertebrate species is described below.

THE HOSTS

INTERMEDIATE AND RESERVOIR HOSTS AND VECTORS

Maintenance of yellow fever virus in nature depends upon cyclic transmission between vertebrate hosts and mosquito vectors (Figure 40.1). In both Africa and tropical America, monkeys are the principal wild vertebrate hosts and aedine mosquitoes are the principal vectors. Humans are also important intermediate hosts in situations where *Ae. aegypti* is responsible for transmission (urban yellow fever) or where interhuman transmission is sustained by sylvatic vectors. For a more detailed summary of the role of vertebrate hosts and vectors in yellow fever ecology, see Monath (1988).

Tropical America

In South America, tamarins, marmosets, howling monkeys (*Alouatta* spp.), spider monkeys (*Ateles* sp.),

squirrel monkeys (*Saimiri* sp.), and owl monkeys (*Aotus* sp.) are effective viraemic hosts and may develop fatal infections. Monkey deaths in nature (particularly of howling monkeys) are an early sign of a yellow fever epizootic in progress. In contrast, capuchin monkeys (*Cebus* sp.), widow monkeys (*Callicebus* sp.), and wooly monkeys (*Lagothrix* sp.), are susceptible to viraemic infection but usually do not develop clinical signs. In non-human primates, viraemias at levels above the threshold for vector infection generally last several days.

Although South American marsupials have been suspected to play a role in virus transmission, they have not been clearly implicated by field studies. Experimental infection of *Didelphis marsupialis* with some yellow fever strains resulted in viraemic infections, but titres were generally low. Infection of *Marmosa cinerae* and *Metachirus nudicaudatus*, however, resulted in prolonged viraemias sufficient to infect *Haemagogus* mosquitoes. Further studies of the role of these vertebrates in yellow fever ecology are warranted. Rodents,

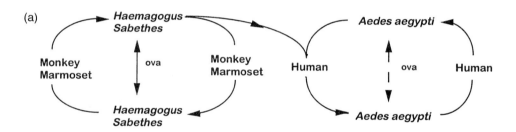

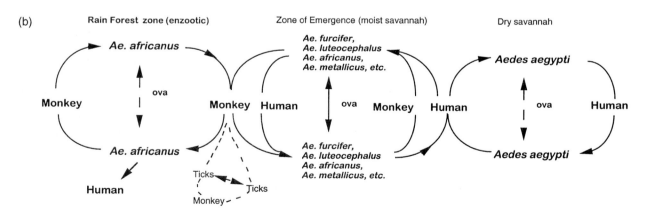

Fig. 40.1 Transmission cycles of yellow fever virus in South America (a) and Africa (b). Yellow fever virus has an enzootic maintenance cycle involving tree-hole breeding mosquito vectors and non-human primates. In tropical America, human yellow fever cases derive from contact with forest mosquito (*Haemagogus* spp.) vectors, and no urban (*Ae. aegypti*-borne) yellow fever has occurred for over 50 years. In Africa, sylvatic vectors are responsible for monkey–monkey and interhuman virus transmission, and there is frequent involvement of *Ae. aegypti* in urban areas and in the dry savannah vegetational zone. The maintenance mechanism for virus survival across the prolonged dry season (when adult mosquitoes are absent or reduced) is believed to involve vertical passage of virus in mosquito ova. Alternate mechanisms may occur, including survival of drought-resistant adult mosquitoes or secondary cycles of transmission involving ticks.

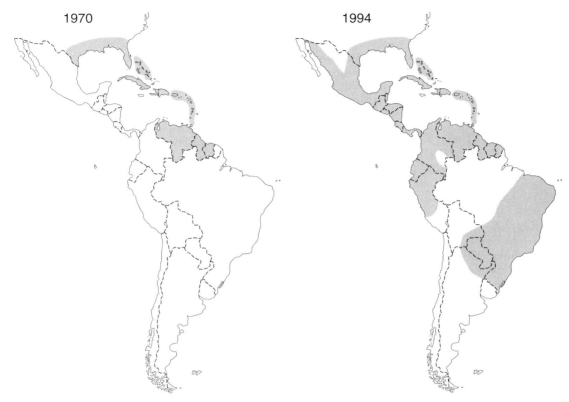

Fig. 40.2 Distribution of *Aedes aegypti* in the Americas (shaded areas). Re-invasion of the South American continent by *Ae. aegypti* occurred in the late 1970s and 1980s due to collapse of vector control programmes, the increase in breeding sites due to urbanization, and other factors, raising the risk of renewed urban outbreaks of yellow fever. (Figure kindly provided by Dr D. J. Gubler, Centers for Disease Control, Fort Collins, CO.)

ungulates, birds, reptiles, and amphibia are not efficient viraemic hosts. Most carnivores have been found refractory to experimental infection, an exception being the kinkajou (*Potos flavus*), but no evidence exists for a role in natural virus cycles.

Haemagogus mosquitoes (principally *Hg. janthinomys*) are the principal vectors of jungle yellow fever in tropical America. *Haemagogus* spp. breed in tree holes and feed in the forest canopy during the midday hours, but they also bite humans in forest clearings and even inside houses near the forest. In some circumstances, these mosquitoes exist in relatively high densities in neotropical forests, with documented biting rates as high as 140 per man-hour in the canopy. Vertical transmission of yellow fever virus by *Haemagogus equinus* has been demonstrated experimentally and provides a logical mechanism for maintenance of the virus during prolonged dry seasons, when adult mosquito populations are low or absent. *Sabethes chloropterus*, a drought-resistant vector species, may also play a role in virus maintenance across the dry season.

Aedes aegypti was responsible for frequent urban epidemics in the Americas through the 1930s. This highly anthropophilic mosquito reaches high densities in densely populated areas, breeds in man-made receptacles indoors and out, and has biting habits, including interrupted feeding, that favour virus transmission. In large cities in tropical America, endemic interhuman transmission of yellow fever was maintained by this mosquito in the past. Anti-*Ae. aegypti* campaigns in Latin America between the 1930s and the early 1970s led to eradication from most countries surrounding the Amazon Basin. Beginning in the late 1970s, however, *Ae. aegypti* re-invaded many areas of Brazil, Paraguay, Bolivia, Peru, Ecuador, and Colombia, so that infested towns and villages are again at risk of virus incursions from the jungle yellow fever cycle (Fig. 40.2). The threat of urbanization of yellow fever in South American cities and potential for spread to the Caribbean, Central America, and the United States have significantly increased in the past decade.

Africa

Non-human primates also serve as principal vertebrate hosts for yellow fever viruses in Africa. In some areas of Africa, monkey populations have been reduced and their range restricted due to human modification of their habitat. Thus, humans play an increasingly important role in the transmission cycle of yellow fever in Africa.

All species of cercopithecid and colobid monkeys, baboons, and lemurs appear to be effective viraemic hosts, circulating virus for several days at sufficient titres to infect vectors. Galagos do not play a major role in yellow fever transmission cycles. Infection rarely causes illness or death in African primates, indicating a balanced parasite–host relationship, and supporting the notion that yellow fever virus evolved in the continent.

Experimental studies have shown the Sudanese hedgehog to be susceptible to viraemia and hepatitis, but this creature has not been implicated in natural virus transmission. Other insectivores are refractory to infection. Most rodents and carnivores tested are also resistant. Yellow fever virus was isolated from an insectivorous bat (*Epomophorus* sp.) in Ethiopia, but the role of bats in natural transmission cycles has not been confirmed.

In the equatorial forests of Africa, *Ae. africanus* mosquitoes are responsible for year-round virus transmission. Tree holes serve as oviposition sites, and biting activity is largely in the canopy, although in some areas *Ae. africanus* may also breed and bite at ground level around human habitations. The level of viral activity in the enzootic high-forest zone is generally low, reflected by low immunity rates in human and monkey populations and absence of large epidemics. This is largely due to the extreme dilution of vectors and hosts in a continuous, uniformly favourable forest environment.

The *zone of emergence* of yellow fever in Africa is a term used to refer to the savannah–forest mosaic and Guinean and southern Sudan savannah vegetational zones, including riverine (gallery) forests, that support concentrated populations of monkeys and vector mosquitoes. In the moist savannah zones, yellow fever virus transmission intensifies during the rainy season and wanes during the dry season when vector populations decline. During the dry season, vertical transmission ensures virus survival in the egg stage. The principal species involved in virus transmission in West Africa are *Ae. africanus*, *Ae. furcifer*, and *Ae. luteocephalus*. It is not unusual for these species to penetrate into villages and even to bite indoors. Endemic transmission occurs annually and human immunity rates are high. Intense epidemics may occur at the limits of the zone, where viral activity may subside for intervals of several years or more and reappear during periods of increased or prolonged rainfall. In such fringe areas, the prevalence

of human immunity is low in the younger age groups and children sustain the highest incidence of disease. Other vector species which play a secondary or accessory role in the zone of emergence are: *Ae. opok*, *Ae. neoafricanus*, *Ae. vittatus*, and *Ae. metallicus*. In East Africa, *Ae. simpsoni gr.* mosquitoes have been responsible for interhuman transmission; this species complex is not anthropophilic in West Africa.

In areas of Africa subject to extreme drying, e.g. in the dry northern Sudan and Sahel savannah zones of western Africa, yellow fever occurs in intermittent epidemic form, and human immunity patterns indicate a low incidence of infection during interepidemic periods. In these areas, domestic water storage is intensively practiced, often with clay water storage jars being buried in the ground so that they cannot be cleaned or emptied. These receptacles are permanent breeding sites for domestic *Ae. aegypti*. Vector densities are high, and introduction of yellow fever virus into such an area (usually by a viraemic human) may result in an explosive outbreak. In 1987, for example, yellow fever was introduced into large towns of western Nigeria from a remote area undergoing a sylvatic outbreak. An explosive *Ae. aegypti*-borne epidemic followed and continued for over 5 years. *Aedes aegypti* density as measured by the Breteau index (number of infested breeding sites/100 houses) provides an estimate of the risk of urban yellow fever. An index of 5 is considered to constitute a low risk, and an index of 50 or greater a high risk of transmission. During the Nigerian epidemic in 1987, Breteau indices exceeded 600 in some affected localities.

Experimental studies show variation among geographical populations of *Ae. aegypti* in their vector competence for yellow fever virus. West African *Ae. aegypti* strains involved in epidemic transmission have proved to be biologically poor vectors; in this region high vector density compensated for low susceptibility, permitting reproduction of the epidemic. It has been suggested that low vector competence may select virus strains that elicit high viraemias and that may have high human virulence (Miller *et al.* 1989).

Yellow fever virus has been isolated from ticks (*Amblyomma variegatum*) in the Central African Republic, raising the possibility that alternate vectors play a role in dispersal or maintenance of the virus. Yellow fever virus is also transovarially transmitted in *Amblyomma* ticks.

Yellow fever virus has been isolated from other arthropods, including *Ae. dentatus*, *Coquilletidia fuscopennata*, and phlebotomine flies. In some areas (e.g. northern Nigeria and northern Kenya) *Mansonia africana* mosquitoes have been suspected to play a role in transmission. These observations are probably peripheral to the ecology of yellow fever, but are worthy of further study.

HUMANS

Clinical infection varies from a mild undifferentiated febrile illness to a fulminating fatal disease with pathognomonic features. The incubation period is usually 3–6 days. Abortive infections are not recognizable except in the setting of an epidemic. In its mildest form, yellow fever is a self-limited infection characterized by sudden onset of fever and headache without other symptoms. In other patients, fever and headache are more severe and accompanied by myalgia, albuminuria, and bradycardia in relation to the height of fever (Faget's sign). In such cases, the illness lasts several days, with uneventful recovery. Severe yellow fever begins abruptly with fever to 40 °C, chills, severe headache, lumbosacral pain, and generalized muscle aches. The patient appears toxic, the conjunctiva congested, the face and neck flushed, the tongue reddened at the tip and edges, and the heart rate slow despite fever. Anorexia, nausea and vomiting, and minor gingival haemorrhages or epistaxes are common. This syndrome lasts approximately 3 days and is named the *period of infection*, since yellow fever virus is present in the blood. A *period of remission* follows, with defervescence and mitigation of symptoms, lasting up to 24 h. Fever and symptoms then recur with more intense vomiting, epigastric pain, prostration, and the appearance of jaundice (*period of intoxication*). Viraemia is generally absent, and antibodies appear during this phase. A bleeding diathesis may be evident, with haematemesis (black vomit), melena, metorrhagia, petechiae, ecchymoses, and oozing blood from the gingival membranes and needle-puncture sites. Bleeding is occasionally life-threatening. Dehydration results from vomiting and increased insensible losses. Renal dysfunction is marked by a sudden increase in albuminuria and by diminishing urine output. Physical findings include scleral and dermal icterus, haemorrhages, and epigastric tenderness without hepatic enlargement. Oedema and ascites are not present. The patient recovers either rapidly after a period of intoxication of 3–4 days or over a protracted course of up to 2 weeks. Death occurs during the second week and is heralded by intensifying jaundice, haemorrhage, rising pulse, shock, oliguria, and azotaemia. Hypothermia, agitated delirium, intractable hiccup, stupor, and coma are terminal signs. The case fatality rate in patients who develop jaundice is 20–50 per cent.

Convalescence is often prolonged, with aesthenia lasting several weeks. Late death, occurring at the end of convalescence or even weeks after complete recovery from the acute illness, is a rare phenomenon attributed to yellow fever myocardial damage and cardiac arrythmia. Secondary bacterial infections, such as pneumonia or parotitis, may complicate recovery. The duration of icterus in surviving cases is poorly established, but jaundice has been observed for up to 3 months after recovery from serologically documented yellow fever.

Leucopenia (white cell counts as low as 1.5×10^9 cells/l) occurs during the first week of illness. Differential counts show an absolute neutropenia and lymphopenia. Leucocytosis often occurs during the terminal stage of the disease. Prolongation of the clotting, prothrombin, and partial thromboplastin times, decreased platelet count and presence of fibrin-split products may be found. Hyperbilirubinaemia may be present as early as the third day, with a peak on the sixth to eighth day at average levels of 9–10 mg/dl, but in fatal cases it may reach 48 mg/dL. Serum glutamic oxaloacetic, and pyruvic transaminase levels are markedly elevated in icteric patients, with elevation on the second day and peak values between days 5 and 10 of the illness. Elevations of serum transaminase levels have been documented to persist for at least 2 months after onset. The alkaline phosphatase level is generally normal. Hypoglycaemia has been noted in patients with severe hepatic damage. Plasma protein (especially gamma globulin) concentration may fall during the acute illness. During the period of infection, the urine may contain a small amount of albumin, which then increases during the period of intoxication, reaching levels of up to 5 g/l (rarely up to 40 g/l). The cerebrospinal fluid is clear and does not contain cells, but may be under increased pressure and may contain elevated protein.

Diagnosis

Mild yellow fever cannot be clinically distinguished from a wide array of other infections. Cases of yellow fever with jaundice must be differentiated from viral hepatitis (particularly hepatitis E), falciparum malaria, leptospirosis, Congo–Crimean haemorrhagic fever, Rift Valley fever, typhoid, Q fever, typhus, and surgical, drug-induced, and toxic causes of jaundice. The other viral haemorrhagic fevers, which usually present without jaundice, include dengue haemorrhagic fever, Lassa fever, Marburg and Ebola virus diseases, and Bolivian, Argentinian, and Venezuelan haemorrhagic fevers.

Specific diagnosis is made by histopathology, detection of the virus in blood, or demonstration of a specific antibody response. The virus may be isolated from serum during the first 3 or 4 days of illness and occasionally as late as 12 days. During epidemics, patients with fever and generalized, non-specific symptoms may provide useful specimens for virus isolation attempts. Proper handling and cold transport of specimens is essential to avoid bacterial contamination and to preserve virus. Virus isolation from clinical specimens can be made by intracerebral inoculation of infant mice, by intrathoracic inoculation of *Toxorhynchites* mosquitoes, or by use of cell cultures, the most sensitive being AP61 mosquito cells. Type-specific monoclonal antibodies may be used for viral identification by immunofluorescence. An antigen-capture enzyme immunoassay (ELISA) employing monoclonal antibodies provides a means of rapid, early diagnosis applicable under field conditions but is somewhat less sensitive than virus isolation (Saluzzo *et al.* 1985). The polymerase chain reaction has potential as a sensitive means of detection of virus in blood specimens (Brown *et al.* 1994). Virus may be occasionally isolated from postmortem liver specimens, or viral antigen detected by ELISA. Antigen in formalin-fixed material may be detected by immunoperoxidase staining, nucleic acid hybridization (Monath *et al.* 1989), or potentially by polymerase chain reaction.

Pathology

Gross pathological lesions include bile staining of tissues; cardiac enlargement; swelling and congestion of the kidneys; haemorrhages or petechiae of the mucous membranes, stomach, duodenum, renal capsule, and urinary bladder; and presence of bloody pleural and peritoneal effusions. The liver is usually normal in size, red or yellow in colour, and shows obliteration of normal lobular pattern and a greasy consistency.

Histopathological changes in the liver include coagulative necrosis of hepatocytes in the midzone of the liver lobule, sparing cells bordering the central vein. Eosinophilic degeneration of hepatocytes results in the formation of Councilman bodies and intranuclear eosinophilic granular inclusions (Torres bodies). Multi- and microvacuolar fatty changes is nearly always present, especially after the eighth day of illness. An inflammatory response is absent or mild, and the reticulin framework is preserved, so that healing is complete in surviving cases. Typical changes are seen in biopsy specimens taken as early as the third day of illness, while interpretation of necropsy material obtained after the tenth day is often difficult. It should be emphasized that biopsy during life is contraindicated as a diagnostic procedure, due to the high risk of haemorrhage. Deaths have resulted from this procedure.

Renal glomerular changes are insignificant compared to the marked acute tubular necrosis and fatty change. The myocardial fibres show cloudy swelling, degeneration, and fatty infiltration. The brain may show oedema and petechial haemorrhages. Lymphocytic elements in the spleen and lymph nodes are depleted, and large mononuclear or histocytic cells accumulate in the splenic follicles.

Treatment

Because medical services are rudimentary in areas where the disease occurs, most patients with yellow fever have not benefited from the intensive care required for management of this complex disease. Approaches to the management of patients are summarized in Monath (1987). The patient should be hospitalized and closely monitored. Isolation is not required, but precautions should be taken with sharp objects potentially contaminated with infectious blood, and a bed net or screened room should be used to limit access to vector mosquitoes. Temperature, pulse, blood pressure, respiratory rate, fluid intake, urine output, and other gastrointestinal losses should be closely monitored. Analgesics (acetaminophen) may be used to reduce headache and myalgia. Antiemetics (piperazine, phenothiazines) may be used sparingly to control nausea and vomiting, but should be avoided if hepatic dysfunction worsens or stupor appears. Patients who enter the period of intoxication should be frequently evaluated for cardiovascular status, renal function, and electrolyte and acid–base balance. Oxygen should be administered, nutrition maintained, and 10–20 per cent glucose solution given intravenously with care to avoid fluid overload. Nasogastric suction should be used to monitor haemorrhage and to prevent gastric distension and aspiration. Although no studies have been performed, it would seem logical to reduce the risk of gastric haemorrhage by suppressing gastric acid with parenteral H_2-receptor antagonists. If severe bleeding occurs, fresh-frozen plasma or fresh whole blood may be required to maintain adequate blood volume. In cases with strong laboratory evidence for disseminated intravascular coagulation, the use of heparin may be considered. In those with signs of progressive acute renal failure, haemodialysis may be required. Secondary bacterial infections or concurrent infections (including malaria) should be treated by the usual appropriate means. Antiviral chemotherapy with ribavirin or α-interferon have not proved useful in preclinical studies. There is no indication for treatment with antibodies (or pooled gamma globulin), corticosteroids, or immunosuppressive agents. Research is needed on the role of cytokines in the pathogenesis of shock in yellow fever, and may lead to specific means of intervention.

EPIDEMIOLOGY

TRANSMISSION AND COMMUNICABILITY

Yellow fever virus is acquired by the bite of an infected mosquito, and is not transmissible by contact with infected individuals. Inanimate sharp objects contaminated with blood pose a theoretical risk of accidental

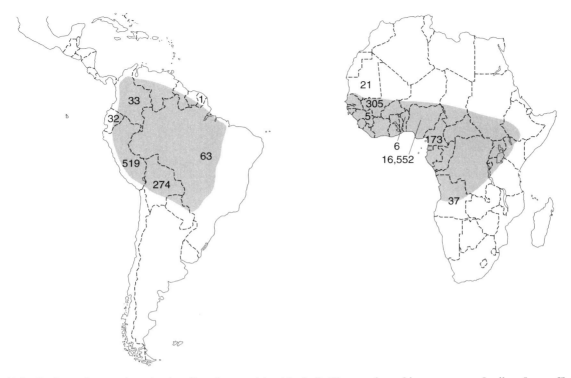

Fig. 40.3 Regions of enzootic-endemic yellow fever activity (shaded). The number of human cases of yellow fever officially notified to the World Health Organization during the 5-year interval 1987–91 is shown by country. Epidemics of yellow fever occurred in Ghana and western Kenya in 1993.

infection in the hospital setting. Laboratory infections have occurred, some possibly by the aerosol route. However, droplet or aerosol transmission between humans does not occur.

DISTRIBUTION AND INCIDENCE

Yellow fever occurs in tropical South America and sub-Saharan Africa (Fig. 40.3), where virus activity may be focal and intermittent. The distribution of reported human cases gives an incomplete picture of the natural circulation of yellow fever virus. Vaccination, inadequate reporting systems, low human population density, and other factors may result in an apparent absence of disease from areas with a high level of zoonotic viral transmission.

The annual incidence of officially reported yellow fever cases is between 50 and 300 in tropical America, and between 5 and 5000 in Africa (Fig. 40.4). However, the true morbidity may greatly exceed the reported incidence, as shown by investigations of various epidemics, especially in Africa. In South America, the incidence of jungle yellow fever is highest in the Amazon

region of Brazil and in areas of eastern Bolivia, Peru, Ecuador, and Colombia which encircle the Amazon Basin. The disease occurs principally during months with peak rainfall, humidity, and temperature—January to March in the Amazon Basin. Occasionally, epizootic waves and attendant human cases have swept outside the traditional enzootic zone in eastern Panama, Central America, Paraguay, northern Argentina, and south-eastern Brazil (Minas Gerais, Sao Paulo, Parana, and Santa Catarina states).

Outbreaks occur at intervals of 5–10 years, for reasons that are poorly understood, but may be due in part to the cycle of reconstitution of susceptible monkey populations after epizootic waves. Human cases occur in rural areas, among persons living near and working in the forest. The opening of forested areas to agricultural exploitation, oil exploration, and road construction has led to an influx of unvaccinated persons, with ensuing epidemics. It is estimated that 1 in 10 cases of jungle yellow fever are recognized and reported in tropical America. A system of viscerotomy (collection and pathological examination of liver samples from suspect fatal cases) has been used successfully for surveillance.

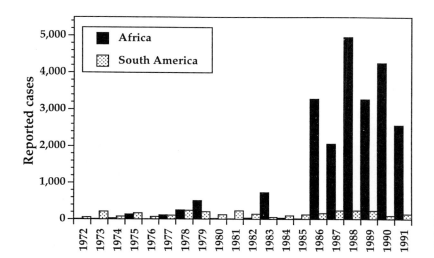

Fig. 40.4 Incidence of yellow fever by continent reported to the World Health Organization, 1972–91.

In Africa, sporadic cases are rarely recognized, due to confusion with other diseases and the lack of organized surveillance. It is likely that endemic yellow fever actually constitutes an important public health problem in many parts of Africa. In Nigeria, for example, the annual incidence of endemic disease with jaundice is estimated to be 1.1–2.4 cases per 1000, and of the incidence of yellow fever death at 0.2–0.5 per 1000, rates below the threshold of detection of medical surveillance but constituting a significant health problem (Monath and Nasidi 1993). Epidemics have occurred at irregular intervals, principally in West Africa and in the southern Sudan and Ethiopia. These outbreaks have sometimes involved large areas and affected hundreds of thousands of people. The epidemic in Nigeria, which began in 1986, ultimately spread throughout the country, to Cameroun and Niger (DeCock *et al.* 1988; Nasidi *et al.* 1989). Between 1986 and 1991, over 15 000 cases and 4000 deaths were officially notified (WHO 1993), but the true morbidity was undoubtedly many times higher. Investigations in one region documented an incidence of human infection of 20 per cent. Approximately 3 per cent of the affected population developed clinical disease (jaundice). In 1993, a yellow fever epidemic occurred in Kenya for the first time in history and for the first time in East Africa in 27 years.

In Africa, epidemics spread by tree-hole breeding mosquitoes peak during the late rainy season and early dry season. Where domestic *Ae. aegypti* is present, transmission may occur at any time of year, but is enhanced during the rainy season, when artificial containers around houses provide additional breeding sites.

AGE, SEX, AND OCCUPATION

In tropical America, jungle yellow fever principally affects young adult males, the male–female case ratio being 10 : 1, reflecting the higher incidence of exposure of males to *Haemagogus* vectors during wood-cutting and forest-clearing activities in the forest. In Africa, background immunity is the principal factor determining the age distribution of cases. In outbreaks affecting immunologically virgin populations (e.g. in Ethiopia, 1960–62), all ages were equally affected, whereas in West Africa, where endemic flavivirus and yellow fever transmission occurs, the highest rates in epidemics are in immunologically susceptible children. An excess of cases in males has been observed in some African outbreaks, possibly indicating greater exposure of males to sylvatic vectors.

INAPPARENT INFECTION

Inapparent, abortive, or clinically mild infections with yellow fever are frequent. In endemic areas of West Africa subject to yearly wet season recrudescence and amplification of yellow fever, the mean annual incidence of infection may be as high as 1.7 per cent and the prevalence of immunity in young adults in such areas reaches 20–40 per cent. The ratio of inapparent to apparent yellow fever infection has not been definitely established. In one study, a low ratio (2 : 1) was found in children who sustained primary yellow fever infections, whereas individuals with serological patterns indicating yellow fever infection after prior exposure to one or more hererologous flaviviruses (of which Zika virus was the most prominent), an inapparent: apparent infection ratio of 22 : 1 was found (Monath *et a.* 1980).

PREVENTION AND CONTROL

VACCINES

Travellers to endemic areas and persons working with yellow fever virus or vaccine in the laboratory should be immunized. The risk is greatest to persons visiting rural or forested areas, and individuals who plan only brief visits (of several days) to large urban centres can be exempted from vaccination. Preventive yellow fever vaccination is a highly effective public health measure. In South America, many nations promulgate control through mass immunization campaigns, and a high level of vaccine immunity has been achieved. In Africa, the approach in some countries has been to undertake mass immunization in response to the occurrence of disease outbreaks, whereas others have incorporated yellow fever vaccine in the expanded programme of immunization of children. The latter strategy is a cost-effective measure (Monath and Nasidi 1993; Robertson 1993).

Yellow fever 17D is one of the safest, most effective live viral vaccines. It is prepared from infected chicken embryos under standards developed by WHO. The 0.5 ml dose, delivered subcutaneously by syringe and needle or jet injector, results in a demonstrable immune response in over 95 per cent of vaccinees within 7–10 days. For the purposes of international certification, immunization is valid for 10 years, but studies have shown persistence of neutralizing antibodies for 35 years or more, and immunity is probably life-long. The vaccine requires cold storage and a cold chain for delivery to remote areas.

Serious adverse reactions to 17D vaccine are extremely uncommon. Some vaccinees experience inconsequential and mild headache and malaise. Allergic reactions, including skin rash, urticaria and asthma, are very infrequent (1 case per million vaccinations), predominantly in persons with allergy to eggs. Neurological accidents are also extremely uncommon; 19 cases of encephalitis and one fatality have been reported, all but three such cases being in infants less than 1 year of age. Because of the increased risk of neurotropic side-effects in infants, the vaccine should not be given to those under 6 months of age. In West Africa, at least four outbreaks have been recorded of severe bacterial (presumably clostridial or anaerobic streptococcal) infection at the inoculation site, leading in some cases to shock and death. These episodes underscore the need to handle and administer the vaccine with careful attention to recommended practices.

During mass vaccination campaigns, pregnant women have been immunized without recognized untoward effects (Nasidi et al. 1993; Tsai et al. 1993). On theoretical grounds, however, pregnant women should be excluded from vaccination unless there is a significant risk of acquiring yellow fever. Pregnant women that have received the vaccine have shown significantly reduced immune responses. Persons with known immunodeficiency states, including AIDS, or those taking immunosuppressive drugs should also not receive yellow fever vaccine. Current recommendations are for vaccination of HIV-infected persons without clinically significant immunosuppression who are at risk of yellow fever infection. However, studies are needed of the reactogenicity and immunogenicity of 17D vaccine in populations with a high prevalence of HIV infection undergoing mass yellow fever immunization.

Factors that may affect seroconversion to 17D vaccine include (1) nutritional state; (2) simultaneous administration of other vaccines; (3) pregnancy or immunosuppression; and (4) pre-existing heterologous flaviviral immunity. Children with kwashiorkor show marked impairment in antibody production after 17D vaccination. Other vaccine combinations have not shown interference, including yellow fever and BCG, measles, oral cholera, hepatitis A, typhoid and hepatitis B. In persons given 17D vaccine by the subcutaneous route, pre-existing heterologous immunity did not interfere with seroconversion.

The French neurotropic vaccine, produced from the brains of infected mice, is no longer manufactured. This vaccine had the advantage of high stability and ease of administration (by scarification). However, approximately 20 per cent of vaccinees developed systemic symptoms 3–4 per cent meningeal signs, and 0.5–1.3 per cent post-vaccinal encephalitis. Neurological accidents were more frequent in children than in adults.

PREVENTIVE VECTOR CONTROL

Areas infested with domestic *Ae. aegypti* are at risk of the introduction and interhuman spread of yellow fever. The threat of urban yellow fever (and epidemic dengue) has been the rationale for *Ae. aegypti* eradication programmes. Elimination of breeding sites (tires, artificial containers, etc.) and insecticidal treatments in the context of a well-administered programme have been successful in some areas, but have often been difficult to sustain.

EPIDEMIC CONTROL

The occurrence of epidemic yellow fever with its high case-fatality rate, constitutes a major public health emergency, particularly in Africa where intense interhuman transmission and high attack rates are the rule. Emergency mass vaccination has generally been the principal approach to control. Such campaigns have often been initiated after the epidemic peak, because of delays in disease recognition and in mobilization of teams for mass vaccination. The effective use of mass vaccination to abort a yellow fever epidemic depends upon early recognition, epidemiological investigation, and rapid deployment of vaccination teams. After inoculation of 17D vaccine, individuals may remain susceptible to infection with wild-type virus for an undetermined period, perhaps up to a week.

Emergency vector control is aimed at rapid reduction of the adult female mosquito population. Aerial ultra-low volume (ULV) application of insecticides may be used, but because they are not effective against immature stages, the applications must be repeated to achieve suppression of biting vectors across two incubation periods in humans (12 days). The control of yellow fever epidemics involving wild vector species requires aerial treatment of large forested areas. In experimental trials, ULV application of malathion was effective against *Ae. simpsoni* breeding in plantations in Ethiopia. Ground and aerial applications of malathion rapidly suppressed populations of *Ae. africanus* in forest habitats in West Africa for a period of time sufficient to interrupt virus transmission (Bang *et al.* 1980). Aerial ULV was also used to attempt control of *Haemagogus* vectors in forested areas in eastern Panama in 1974.

REFERENCES

Bang, Y. H. *et al.* (1980). Ground application of malathion thermal fogs and cold mists for the control of sylvatic vectors of yellow fever in rural communities near Enugu, Nigeria. *Mosquito News*, **40**, 541–50.

Brown, T. M. *et al.* (1994). Detection of yellow fever virus by polymerase chain reaction. *Clinical and Diagnostic Virology* **2**, 41–51.

Chambers, T. J. *et al.* (1990). Flavivirus genome organization, expression, and replication. *Annual Review of Microbiology* **44**, 649–88.

DeCock, K. M. *et al.* (1988). Epidemic yellow fever in eastern Nigeria, 1986. *Lancet*, **i**, 630–3.

Deubel, V. *et al.* (1986). Genetic heterogeneity of yellow fever virus strains from Africa and the Americas. *Journal of General Virology*, **67**, 209–13.

Hahn, C. S. *et al.* (1987). Comparison of the virulent Asibi strain of yellow fever virus with the 17D vaccine strain derived from it. *Proceedings of the National Academy of Science, USA*, **84**, 2019–23.

Jennings, A. D. *et al.* (1994). Analysis of a yellow fever virus isolated from a fatal case of vaccine-associated human encephalitis. *Journal of Infectious Diseases*, **169**, 512–18.

Lepiniec, L. *et al.* (1994). Geographic distribution and evolution of yellow fever viruses based on direct sequencing of genomic cDNA fragments. *Journal of General Virology*, **75**, 417–23.

Miller, B. M. *et al.* (1989). Epidemic yellow fever caused by an incompetent mosquito vector. *Tropical Medicine and Parasitology*, **40**, 396–9.

Monath, T. P. (1987). Yellow fever: a medically neglected disease. *Reviews of the Infectious Diseases*, **9**, 165–75.

Monath, T. P. (1988). Yellow fever. In *The arboviruses: ecology and epidemiology*, (ed. T. P. Monath), vol. V, pp. 89–231. CRC press, Boca Raton, Florida.

Monath, T. P. (1991). Yellow fever: *Victor, Victoria*? Conqueror, Conquest? Epidemics and research in the last forty years and prospects for the future. *American Journal of Tropical Medicine and Hygiene*, **45**, 1–43.

Monath, T. P. and Nasidi, A. (1993). Should yellow fever vaccine be included in the Expanded Program of Immunization in Africa? A cost-effectiveness analysis for Nigeria. *American Journal of Tropical Medicine and Hygiene*, **48**, 274–99.

Monath, T. P. *et al.* (1980). Yellow fever in the Gambia, 1978–1979: epidemiologic aspects with observations on the occurrence of Orungo virus infections. *American Journal of Tropical Medicine and Hygiene*, **29**, 912–28.

Monath, T. P. *et al.* (1989). Detection of yellow fever viral RNA by nucleic acid hybridization and viral antigen by immunocytochemistry in fixed human liver. *American Journal of Tropical Medicine and Hygiene*, **40**, 663–8.

Nasidi, A. *et al.* (1989). Urban yellow fever epidemic in western Nigeria, 1987. *Transactions of the Royal Society of Tropical Medicine and Hygiene*, **83**, 401–6.

Nasidi, A. *et al.* (1993). Yellow fever vaccination and pregnancy: a four-year prospective study. *Transactions of the Royal Society of Tropical Medicine and Hygiene*, **87**, 337–9.

Robertson, S. E. (1993). Yellow fever. Module 8, in *The Immunological Basis for Immunization*, Expanded Programme on Immunization, pp. 1–14. WHO, Geneva.

Saluzzo, J. -F. *et al.* (1985). Comparison de différences techniques pour la détection du virus de la fièvre jaune dans les prélèvements humains et des lots de moustiques: intérêt d'une méthode rapide de diagnostic par ELISA. *Annales de Virologie*, (*Institut Pasteur*), **136E**, 115–24.

Tsai, T. F. *et al.* (1993). Congenital yellow fever virus infection after immunization in pregnancy. *Journal of Infectious Diseases*, **168**, 1520–23.

WHO (1993). Yellow fever in 1991. *WHO Weekly Epidemiological Record*, **68**, 209–15.

PART 3   PARASITIC ZOONOSES

41 AFRICAN TRYPANOSOMOSIS

W. Gibson

SUMMARY

The African trypanosomoses are diseases of both man and his livestock. There are two forms of human trypanosomosis or sleeping sickness: Gambian or Rhodesian sleeping sickness, roughly corresponding to a West/Central or East African distribution respectively. Gambian sleeping sickness runs a more protracted and chronic course than the Rhodesian form; nevertheless, human trypanosomosis is invariably fatal if not treated. Animal reservoir hosts, both wild and domestic, assume greater importance for Rhodesian sleeping sickness than Gambian sleeping sickness, and the former is often an occupational hazard of those working in wildlife areas, e.g. hunters. Animal trypanosomosis transmitted by tsetse is generally referred to as *Nagana*.

Trypanosomosis is caused by obligate parasitic protozoan flagellates of the genus *Trypanosoma*. *Trypanosoma brucei gambiense* and *T. b. rhodesiense* are the causative organisms of Gambian and Rhodesian human trypanosomosis respectively. The third subspecies, *T. b. brucei*, is not infective to man. All three subspecies are morphologically indistinguishable. Several other trypanosome species cause *Nagana* besides *T. b. brucei*, but none is infective to man.

About 200 endemic foci of sleeping sickness are spread through 36 countries in sub-Saharan Africa (see Fig. 41.1). The annual incidence is about 25 000, but this figure is thought to be a gross underestimate due to difficulties of obtaining accurate figures from remote foci. Epidemics flare up in the endemic foci usually as a result of failure of control measures; however, new outbreaks can also occur in areas of resettlement. Sleeping sickness is largely restricted to rural areas by the distribution of its vector, the tsetse fly; however, both the fly and animal trypanosomosis have a far wider distribution than the human disease.

Sleeping sickness is transmitted by an insect vector, the tsetse fly (genus *Glossina*). Several species of the *palpalis* and *morsitans* groups are involved, which live in a variety of habitats and show different host preferences. Adults of both sexes suck blood and thereby transmit trypanosomes. The trypanosomes undergo a

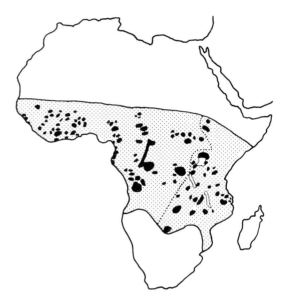

Fig. 41.1 Distribution of foci of human trypanosomiosis (black areas) and tsetse (dotted area) in Africa; dotted line divides foci of Gambian sleeping sickness to the west from those of Rhodesian sleeping sickness to the east (after Kuzoe 1993).

multiplicative and developmental cycle in the fly, taking about 4 weeks. Individual flies can remain infective all their life span—several months under favourable conditions. Other routes of transmission are relatively unimportant epidemiologically, e.g. via infected blood, raw meat or mechanically vector borne.

Sleeping sickness control measures are aimed either at the trypanosome or the fly. Human cases are detected by active or passive surveillance and cured by treatment with trypanocidal drugs. Control of the tsetse vector is by application of residual insecticides or bush clearing and, more recently, by traps or insecticide-impregnated targets. Tsetse control is more widely employed for the control of animal trypanosomosis than sleeping sickness.

HISTORY

DISCOVERY OF THE DISEASE

Sleeping sickness aroused the curiosity and wonder of visitors to tropical Africa long before its cause was discovered, because of the extraordinary comotose state characteristic of the late stage of the disease. The first mention of sleeping sickness is by a fourteenth century Arab scholar, al-Qalqashandi (Hoare 1972). In the eighteenth and nineteenth centuries, European slave traders working on the West African coast were sufficiently aware of the disease to avoid buying Africans showing enlarged cervical lymph nodes, an early sign of the disease. Despite such precautions many people in the early stages of sleeping sickness were transported to the West Indies during the years of the slave trade, but the disease never became established there, presumably because a suitable vector was lacking.

Various causes for sleeping sickness were put forward, mostly relating to the African way of life, since Europeans appeared not to be susceptible. However, the scientific search for a causative agent became imperative at the turn of the twentieth century as a series of major epidemics began to threaten European trade and colonization in Africa. At the request of the British Foreign Office, the Royal Society sent two Sleeping Sickness Commissions to investigate a major epidemic in Uganda. The second commission, under the leadership of David Bruce, swiftly revealed the cause of the disease, a discovery considered to be one of the greatest triumphs of tropical medicine, which was also sadly not without controversy (Davies 1962).

DISCOVERY OF THE CAUSATIVE ORGANISMS

Trypanosoma gambiense Dutton, 1902 was initially described from the blood of a patient with 'trypanosoma fever', a mild disease of the West African Coast (Hoare 1972). Soon after this, Castellani, a member of the Royal Society Commission on sleeping sickness in Uganda, found trypanosomes in the CSF of sleeping sickness patients, and suggested trypanosoma fever to be the early stage of sleeping sickness, before the trypanosomes had infiltrated the CNS from the bloodstream. Bruce and his wife, fresh from their discovery in South Africa that tsetse flies transmitted the pathogenic trypanosomes which caused Nagana in livestock, quickly grasped the significance of Castellani's findings and demonstrated that the vector of sleeping sickness was a tsetse fly. These results were published in 1903.

Subsequently, a second human trypanosome was isolated in Zambia and named as a distinct species, *T. rhodesiense* Stephens and Fantham, 1910, on the basis of its morphology and virulence to experimental rodents. Cases of Rhodesian sleeping sickness were sporadic at first, but once the disease assumed epidemic form, its acute and rapid nature compared to Gambian sleeping sickness was appreciated.

PATHOGENESIS

The pathogenesis of sleeping sickness was greatly clarified once it was discovered to be caused by a tsetse-transmitted protozoan parasite in 1903. The bouts of fever of the early stage of the disease were associated with parasitaemic waves of trypanosomes in the circulation, while the enlarged lymph glands (notably those of the neck—Winterbottom's sign), showed infiltration of parasites. The onset of mental symptoms in the late stage of the disease was associated with parasite invasion of the CNS and subsequent cellular infiltration. Further than this, the actual mechanisms by which trypanosomes cause disease remained obscure.

EPIDEMIOLOGY

Gambian sleeping sickness originally appears to have been a widespread endemic disease in West Africa, but with the opening up of Africa to trade and colonization at the turn of the twentieth century came a series of devastating epidemics, notably in the Congo River basin and Uganda. Rhodesian sleeping sickness later appeared to spread in a series of focal epidemics throughout East Africa, possibly associated with movements of troops, refugees, and migrant workers (Fig. 41.1) (Mulligan 1970).

From its discovery, Rhodesian sleeping sickness was always considered to be a zoonotic infection, since it could be contracted in areas inhabited only by wild animals (Ashcroft 1959). The proof of this came in 1958 when a human volunteer was infected with trypanosomes from a bushbuck in East Africa (Heisch *et al.* 1958). Subsequently, various wild and domestic animals have been incriminated as reservoir hosts of the disease by *in vitro* methods (Onyango *et al.* 1966; Rickman and Robson 1970; Geigy *et al.* 1975; Brun and Jenni 1987). By contrast, Gambian sleeping sickness was held to be a disease of man alone, until evidence for the existence of animal reservoirs (pigs, dogs, and antelope) was obtained in West Africa in the 1970s (Gibson *et al.* 1978; Mehlitz *et al.* 1982).

Initially it was believed that the Gambian and Rhodesian forms of sleeping sickness were associated with different vector species: the Gambian disease was believed to be transmitted only by tsetse flies of the *palpalis* group and the Rhodesian disease by flies of the *morsitans* group (Buxton 1955). However, *palpalis*

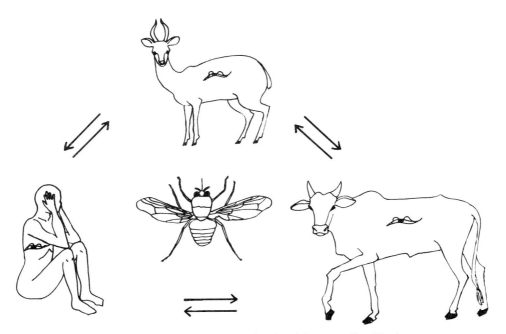

Fig. 41.2   Cycle of transmission of Rhodesian sleeping sickness mediated by the tsetse vector.

group flies were found to be vectors of *T. b. rhodesiense* in outbreaks of sleeping sickness in Kenya and Ethiopia in the 1960s and 1970s, and it is now accepted that either or both fly groups may transmit each species.

CONTROL

Before the cause of sleeping sickness was discovered, control measures involved the natural movement of populations away from tsetse-infested zones as unhealthy settlements were abandoned, or isolation measures, such as quarantine and restricted movement, enforced by various colonial governments. Once the tsetse fly was realized to be the transmitting agent, evacuation of tsetse-infested areas was instituted. This was a practical measure for control of Gambian sleeping sickness, where the vector species were *palpalis*-group tsetse occupying limited areas of riverine or lakeshore vegetation. The first trypanocidal drugs became available soon after the turn of the twentieth century, thanks to Ehrlich's work (atoxyl, 1905; suramin, 1920) and drugs effective against parasites in the CNS followed in the 1940s (Melarsen, 1940; Mel B, 1947), allowing effective programmes of surveillance and treatment (Mulligan 1970).

Early control measures against *morsitans*-group tsetse involved bush clearance to destroy their habitat and game eradication to remove their food source. These measures were employed more widely to control animal trypanosomosis than the human disease. Bush clearance was effective but labour intensive and required continu-

ous maintenance of cleared areas by settlement and farming to prevent reinvasion. Game eradication was first tried in a huge natural experiment brought about by rinderpest, which swept southern and eastern Africa in 1896. This dramatically reduced tsetse numbers by destroying large numbers of their favourite wild hosts. Later shoot-out campaigns failed to remove small, more secretive animals such as bushbuck and bushpig, which by themselves are capable of maintaining large tsetse populations, and the strategy lost favour as concern for wildlife conservation grew (Ford 1971).

Insecticides came into widespread use in the 1950s to control both *palpalis*- and *morsitans*-group flies. Residual insecticides could be applied locally by knapsack sprayers to tsetse resting sites on vegetation fringing lakeshores and rivers or surrounding settlements. Widescale coverage from the air was only suitable for conditions of flat terrain and light vegetation, besides being costly. Again, environmental concerns now discourage large-scale insecticide use.

THE AGENT

TAXONOMY

Kingdom: Protista; phylum: Sarcomastigophora; order: Kinetoplastida; family: Trypanosomatidae; genus: *Trypanosoma*; subgenus: *Trypanozoon*; species: *T. brucei*; subspecies: *T. b. gambiense, T. b. rhodesiense, T. b. brucei*.

All three subspecies are indistinguishable both by morphology (Fig. 41.3) and their life cycle in the fly (Hoare 1972). All infect a wide range of mammalian hosts, including wild and domestic animals, but only *T. b. rhodesiense* and *T. b. gambiense* are capable of infecting man. The present subspecies all originally had species status, which can be confusing in older literature.

The relationship between the three subspecies has always engendered heated debate. Some workers have proposed that *T.b. gambiense* and *T. b. rhodesiense* represent the same parasite under different epidemiological conditions, while others have argued that *T. b. rhodesiense* and *T. b. brucei* are one species (Ashcroft 1959). Long term transmission experiments demonstrated that *T. b. rhodesiense* retained infectivity to man despite extended sojourn in other animal hosts, while the fact that *T. b. brucei* had a far wider distribution than sleeping sickness indicated its separate identity. Extensive biochemical characterization data and the demonstration of genetic exchange now argues that *T. b. rhodesiense* and *T. b. brucei* represent a genetic continuum in East Africa, differentiated only by the trait of man-infectivity. *Trypanosoma b. gambiense*, although closely related, has distinct biochemical and biological features, which make this homogeneous group of strains easily recognizable throughout its range.

MOLECULAR BIOLOGY

Trypanosoma b. brucei has become a favourite laboratory organism for molecular biologists: not only is it easy to grow and purify, but it has a number of biochemical peculiarities, some of which challenge textbook orthodoxy (Opperdoes 1985). The order Kinetoplastida is named after the densely staining kinetoplast, a unique organelle containing the mitochondrial DNA. Kinetoplast DNA consists of a network of interlinked DNA circles of two sizes: about 5000 mini-circles, and 50 larger maxi-circles, carrying genes for mitochondrial function. Recent work has shown that maxi-circle transcripts are edited, rather than being faithfully transcribed as dogma would dictate. This has clarified the role of the mini-circles, now known to encode some of the short RNAs which guide the editing process. This helps explain the close association of mini-and maxi-circles, but the benefit of RNA editing to the trypanosome remains obscure. Kinetoplast DNA is one target for trypanocidal drugs such as isometamidium and homidium which bind to DNA, possibly interfering with its replication or resulting in damage by double-strand breakage.

The surface of trypanosomes in the mammalian host is covered by a dense coat consisting of a single protein, the variant surface glycoprotein (VSG). The VSG is highly antigenic, but by changing its protein coat, the trypanosome can evade the immune response of the host, and this leads to characteristic waves of parasitaemia in the infected host as antibody production catches up with each succeeding antigenic variant. Since each trypanosome has a repertoire of an estimated 1000 genes coding for different VSGs, which also have a high mutation rate, the trypanosome has also managed to evade the development of a vaccine by this means. The trypanosome only expresses one VSG gene at a time in an expression site located at the end of a chromosome (telomere). The mechanism of antigenic variation is complex (Borst and Rudenko 1994), but in essence, antigenic switching is brought about when the active gene is displaced from the expression site by one of the silent ones. In general, nothing is lost during the switch, since both VSG genes involved in the switch are simply copies of original

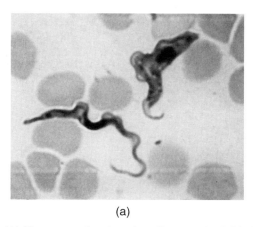

(a)

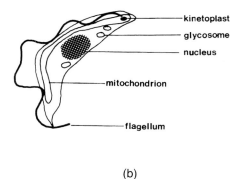

(b)

Fig. 41.3   (A) *Trypanosama brucei* ssp. in a Giemsa-stained thin blood smear, showing two extremes of morphological range. (B) Cross-section of trypanosome.

genes which remain in place. Study of the transcription of VSG genes led to the discovery of discontinuous transcription in trypanosomes, a mechanism whereby a short (39 nucleotide) RNA leader sequence is spliced on to the 5′ end of all messenger RNAs.

Trypanosome chromosomes do not condense during the cell cycle, but intact chromosomal DNA molecules can be separated by pulsed field gel electrophoresis. In this way *T. b. brucei* was estimated to have at least 100 chromosomes ranging in size from 50 kb to several Mb. VSG genes together with housekeeping genes are found on chromosomes of all sizes, but only VSG genes are found on the smaller chromosomes. In particular, the 100 or so mini-chromosomes—small linear chromosomes of 50–150 kb—constitute a reservoir of telomeric VSG genes, which may serve to promote rapid evolution of the antigenic repertoire.

Two other molecular features of trypanosomes may also provide new therapeutic avenues. Kinetoplastids are unique among eukaryotes in that glycolysis takes place inside a specialized organelle, the glycosome, which also contains enzymes for (parts of) other metabolic pathways. Gene sequencing has demonstrated that the glycosomal glycolytic enzymes are significantly different from their mammalian counterparts. Glutathione is an essential metabolite of eukaryote cells, which is reduced by glutathione reductase. In trypanosomes this enzymes was found to have a unique cofactor, trypanothione, a novel glutathione–spermidine conjugate. Inhibition of trypanothione synthesis or its dependent oxidation–reduction system would be expected to upset glutathione metabolism. This knowledge has already led to rational attempts at combination chemotherapy using existing drugs. Elfornithine (DFMO) inhibits ornithine decarboxylase, an enzyme in the polyamine biosynthetic pathway leading to trypanothione. The action of elfornithine can be augmented by combination chemotherapy with other drugs that interfere with this pathway, e.g. diminazene aceturate (Berenil). In the short term, this approach may well dramatically improve the efficacy of existing drugs, with the benefit of reduced dosage and hence toxicity, while the long-term search for new trypanocidal compounds continues.

DISEASE MECHANISMS

Trypanosoma brucei ssp. trypanosomes do not just circulate in the bloodstream, but invade various tissues, most importantly the CNS, where they can more effectively evade the immune system (Greenwood and Whittle 1980). Trypanosomes multiply initially at the site of the fly bite and local inflammation may result in the first sign of the disease, the chancre. From here the trypanosomes invade the bloodstream and lymphatic system, causing generalized febrile attacks. The trypanosomes have a complex interaction with cells of the immune system, which has yet to be fully unravelled. Each parasitaemic wave is associated with expression of a limited number of VSGs. Trypanosomes expressing these antigens are cleared from the blood by a specific antibody response, releasing further internal antigens. Subsequent parasitaemic cycles are initiated by residual trypanosomes that have switched to expression of new surface antigens (VSGs). Sequential parasitaemic waves give rise to high levels of IgM and in a chronic infection, exhaustion of the immune system, and immunosuppression. The latter effect is observed on both T- and B-cell responses, and interactions between macrophages and CD8+T cells appear to play a role, but the whole picture is by no means understood. Release of proinflammatory cytokines results in tissue damage and systemic effects. In animal models, the catabolic effects of cachectin (TNF) give rise to anorexia, fever, and weight loss, suggesting that it alone could be responsible for much of the clinical picture of trypanosomosis.

Invasion of the CNS leads to progressive damage and is now believed to commence at an earlier stage of infection than previously thought. In experimental animals dye-tracer studies show that the blood–CSF barrier is compromised within a few days of infection. An early change is the breakdown of the choroid plexus allowing infiltration of trypanosomes and lymphocytes into the circumventricular regions. No toxins are known to be released from the trypanosomes themselves; rather it appears to be the interactions of the parasites with the immune system that manifest disease. In particular, the cytokine/prostaglandin network appears to play a key role in the inflammatory processes in the brain, and also may be influencing wider physiological abnormalities such as somnolence and fever. Levels of the somnogenic prostaglandin PGD_2, but not interleukin-1 (IL-1) or PGE_2, were found to be markedly elevated in CSF from late-stage patients with Gambian sleeping sickness. Activated astrocytes within the CNS, as well as invading lymphocytes, are capable of producing cytokines and prostaglandins, and unravelling this complex series of interactions will doubtless clarify late-stage pathogenesis.

GROWTH AND SURVIVAL REQUIREMENTS

Trypanosomes are obligate parasites, which have no survival stages outside their hosts. In the mammalian host, trypanosome metabolism is dependent on high levels of glucose, as found in the bloodstream and CNS, while in the fly the main energy source is proline. Trypanosomes can survive for a limited time in samples of body fluids, e.g. blood, CSF, but are easily destroyed by heat, desiccation, detergents, and disinfectants.

THE HOSTS

GENERAL

Besides man, *T. brucei* ssp. can infect a wide variety of domestic and wild animal species. In general *T. b. rhodesiense* and *T. b. brucei* are more virulent than *T. b. gambiense* and produce more rapid and severe symptoms. Animal trypanosomosis is also caused by other tsetse-transmitted trypanosome species in Africa, notably *T. vivax*, *T. congolense*, and *T. simiae*, which are considered to be of far greater veterinary importance than *T. brucei* ssp., except perhaps for dogs, horses, and camels (Stephen 1986; Brown *et al.* 1990). Mixed infections of two or more trypanosome species occur frequently in livestock kept in endemic zones.

INCUBATION PERIOD

The incubation period in both man and animals is highly variable due to differences in trypanosome virulence and number of organisms inoculated, besides individual and species differences in susceptibility and previous exposure to tsetse challenge. It is also difficult to measure in an endemic area where fly bite is frequent. For the most virulent strains in susceptible hosts, the incubation period is probably as little as a week, but may be several weeks or much longer; prolonged incubation periods of several years are on record for Gambian sleeping sickness. Trypanosome infection in animals may remain cryptic for years, as evidenced by zoo animals.

SYMPTOMS AND SIGNS

Generally the early symptoms of Rhodesian sleeping sickness tend to be more severe and acute than those of the Gambian form, and the early and late stages are less clearly demarcated (WHO 1986). The early stage is characterized by intermittent fever, weakness, headache, backache, joint pains, oedema, pruritis, and enlargement of the lymph glands and spleen, while the late stage is marked by neurological symptoms and endocrine disorders, e.g. amenorrhoea or impotence. However, due to the early invasion of the CNS, neurological signs, such as facial ticks and mood and appetite changes, may be present at an early stage.

Two of the first signs of sleeping sickness are the chancre, an indurated swelling at the site of fly bite which may be present in early cases of Rhodesian sleeping sickness, but is seldom observed for Gambian sleeping sickness, and swelling of the lymph nodes, particularly the cervical glands—'Winterbottom's sign'. The eponymous sleep disorders include nocturnal insomnia and daytime somnolence, and classically sleeping sickness manifests itself finally in coma. Cerebral involvement may also be evident from psychiatric disturbances, ranging in severity from behavioural changes, often increased aggression or violence, to frank psychosis. Late-stage patients have ended up in mental institutions or even prison for these reasons.

Some animals infected with *T. brucei* ssp. (e.g. horses, dogs) may be obviously ill, but others, particularly bovids and wild animals, may remain asymptomatic, possibly showing disease only if stressed (Brown *et al.* 1990). There is the added complication that when a mixture of trypanosome species is present, the presence of *T. brucei* ssp. may be easily missed. Early infection is characterized by intermittent parasitaemia associated with bouts of fever. Clinical features of the chronic disease include anaemia, fever, cachexia, lymphadenopathy, and oedema. *Nagana* was the Zulu name for animal trypanosomosis and means 'a state of depressed spirits', which sums up the clinical picture quite well. Lameness of the hindquarters is characteristic of infection in dogs and horses, as is corneal opacity—so-called 'white eyes'—in dogs. There may also be disorders of reproduction, particularly sterility and abortion.

DIAGNOSIS

For human patients parasite demonstration is generally required before treatment commences as drug treatment is not without risk. For animal trypanosomosis, this is not always necessary and for example, herd treatment may be carried out after demonstration of trypanosomes in some individuals only. Much the same diagnostic methods are used for both human and animal trypanosomosis, but levels of parasitaemia may often be very low and fluctuating. Parasitaemias tend to be higher in Rhodesian sleeping sickness and therefore it is usually possible to find motile trypanosomes by simple microscopic examination of wet blood films. A trypanosome concentration method is usually necessary for demonstration of *T. b. gambiense*, the simplest being thick blood film stained with Giemsa or Field's stain. Other methods include mini anion-exchange columns (Lumsden *et al.* 1979), haematocrit buffy coat (WHO 1970) and QBC (quantitative buffy coat technique). If enlarged lymph glands are present, trypanosomes can often success-fully be demonstrated by gland puncture; this method has also been used for cattle. However, trypanosome numbers may be extremely low and the most reliable and sensitive means of demonstrating parasites is then by inoculation of rodents, which can also be immuno-suppressed in the case of *T. b. gambiense*.

Serological tests such as the CATT (card agglu-tination test for trypanosomiasis) (Magnus *et al.* 1978), which rely on antibody detection, are useful for pre-liminary screening in endemic areas of Gambian sleep-ing sickness, but suspects require parasitological confirmation before treatment. New diagnostic methods are constantly being sought: an ELISA test for antigen detection has been developed (Nantulya 1989) and the possibility of using PCR (polymerase chain reaction) is also being examined. The cost and ease of use of any new diagnostic test in the field are factors always to be borne in mind, however.

In man, CNS involvement is assessed by microscopic examination of centrifuged CSF withdrawn by lumbar puncture. If no parasites can be demonstrated, then high numbers of cells (more than 5/ml) or high levels of protein (greater than 37 mg/100 ml) indicate CNS involvement (WHO 1986). In exceptional cases, where trypanosomes can neither be demonstrated in the blood or CSF, diagnosis may be made on clinical grounds only.

PATHOLOGY

Much of the recent work has been carried out in animal models, which appear to share similar patho-logy with man. *Trypanosoma brucei* ssp. trypanosomes invade the intercellular fluids of various tissues, as well as the bloodstream and extracellular fluids. In the early haemolymphatic stage of sleeping sickness, the lymph nodes and spleen are enlarged and infiltrated with lymphocytes, plasma cells, and monocytes (Greenwood and Whittle, 1980). Later the lymph nodes become shrunken and atrophied with progres-sive exhaustion of the immune system. Anaemia is haemolytic and large numbers of reticulocytes are present. There is also thrombocytopenia. The inter-cellular spaces of various tissues are invaded, notably the heart, with resultant myocarditis and pericardial effusions. Invasion of the CNS begins with congestion of the meninges and infiltration of lymphocytes and large vesiculated cells. These are the so-called morular cells originally observed by Mott in 1905, which are plasma cells containing huge amounts of immuno-globulin. Inflammation extends into the brain tissue and blood vessels show perivascular cuffing. There is proliferation of neuroglial cells (astrocytes and microglia) associated with diffuse meningo-encephalitis.

TREATMENT

Unfortunately, all the drugs used for treatment of human sleeping sickness are rather toxic and cause side-effects ranging from unpleasant to severe (WHO, 1986). Early cases without CNS involvement are treated with suramin or, for Gambian sleeping sickness only, pentamidine (Lomidine). Some use has also been made of diminazene aceturate (Berenil), although this drug is not registered for human use. None of these drugs crosses the blood–brain barrier to any extent and late-stage cases require one or more courses of the arsenical melarsoprol (Arsobal). This drug is dissolved in propylene glycol and leakage into the tissues at the injection site causes severe irritation. Relapses following melarsoprol treatment are problem-atic as the patient may already be in a poor state. Some success has been achieved for relapsed cases of Gambian sleeping sickness with oral nifurtimox (Lampit) or elfornithine (DFMO; Ornidyl) given IV or orally (Pepin *et al.* 1987), but both drugs show adverse effects. Elfornithine is not effective against *T. b. rhode-siense* and there is insufficient data on nifurtimox; therefore at present there is no alternative drug in cases of arsenical-resistant Rhodesian sleeping sickness.

For animal trypanosomosis, three drugs are in common use for treatment of ruminants—Berenil, isometamidium (Samorin, Trypamidium) and homid-ium salts (Ethidium, Novidium) (Stephen 1986; Brown *et al.* 1990). Of these only Berenil and Samorin are re-commended for treatment of *T. b brucei* ssp. infections. For horses and camels, Samorin, suramin (Naganol) or quinapyramine sulphate (Antrycide, Trypacide) are the drugs of choice and Samorin is recommended for treatment of dogs. Samorin and Trypacide Prosalt (quinapyramine sulphate together with the more insoluble chloride salt) are recommended for pre-vention as well as cure in cattle and horses, the effects lasting 3–6 months. There is some degree of drug resistance to all veterinary trypanocidal drugs and the small number available make this possibility a constant concern.

PROGNOSIS

Untreated sleeping sickness is fatal, with death result-ing in 3–9 months with Rhodesian sleeping sickness and possibly a matter of years with Gambian sleeping sickness. In cases without CNS involvement, prognosis is generally good; however, such cases may relapse if CNS involvement was unrecognized at the time of treatment. The state of some patients admitted with late-stage disease may already be so poor that they require general nursing and supportive therapy before commencement of treatment (WHO 1986). The most severe complication of treatment in late-stage patients is so-called reactive encephalopathy, which occurs in 5–10 per cent of cases and leads to high mortality. In the past, this syndrome was considered to be a severe side-effect of arsenical treatment. However, it also occurs when other drugs are used for treatment of late-stage disease. This could indicate that it is a reaction to the rapid release of trypanosomal antigens in the CNS as the trypanosomes are killed, but work in an experimental mouse model suggests the cause to be the persistence of small numbers of live trypanosomes in the brain. The latter would indicate the beneficial effect of aggressive rather than gradual drug therapy. The results of reactive encephalopathy can be ameliorated by supportive treatment with anti-inflammatory drugs.

All patients need to be followed up after treatment for at least a year to ascertain whether cure has taken place. WHO (1986) recommends follow-up examinations at 6-monthly intervals for 2 years. A full parasitological and clinical examination is necessary, including lumbar puncture.

In animals the course and outcome of *T. brucei* ssp. infection is highly variable, depending on the subspecies and strain of infecting trypanosomes, the species and breed of mammalian host and its previous exposure to trypanosomes. In horses and dogs the disease may take an acute and fatal course within a few weeks. Severe chronic trypanosomosis leads to progressive debility and emaciation and death in a matter of months. Alternatively, infection may be transient. Drug therapy is generally curative, but relapses may arise from residual parasites hidden in the tissues or from drug resistance.

EPIDEMIOLOGY

OCCURRENCE

Incidence

Approximately 25 000 new cases of sleeping sickness are reported annually, but this is considered to be a gross underestimate, due to difficulties in collecting accurate information (Kuzoe 1993). Many endemic foci are located in remote and inaccessible areas, with poor health facilities. It is costly to maintain surveillance in such regions, but control programmes may also fail for other reasons. For example, until recently about half the annual total of sleeping sickness cases were reported from Zaire, but control programmes have almost ceased due to economic and political problems.

Prevalence

Accurate data would need to be gathered over a period of years to gain a true picture of the prevalence of sleeping sickness in an endemic focus. As noted above, such data is hard to come by for humans, and even harder to obtain for potential animal reservoir hosts. The activity and distribution of tsetse flies varies according to wet or dry seasons, with consequent effects on transmission rates and presumably prevalence (Buxton 1955). There may also be seasonal movements of domestic stock or wildlife. On top of this, survey work may be restricted, if not impossible, during the wet season in remote areas.

Sampling from animal species present in a focus is often unrepresentative, depending on the ease with which they can be caught. Conservation measures in some countries mean that a license is required to sample wild animals. Some information on prevalence can be obtained from tsetse flies caught in an endemic area by examining trypanosome infection rates, together with blood meal identification.

Epidemics

Most endemic foci smoulder on with a low annual incidence and occasional flare-ups (Kuzoe 1993). The usual reason for recrudescence of foci is breakdown of routine control measures. Sometimes control programmes are discontinued because the economic costs of control appear to outweigh the benefits of dealing with relatively few cases or small numbers of flies. This can be a false economy due to the high cost of controlling any ensuing epidemic. Some outbreaks result from prolonged civil disruption, when routine control measures break down and aid agencies withdraw financial and technical resources. Reliable statistics are then hard to come by. This is the current situation in Liberia, Mozambique, Rwanda, southern Sudan, and Zaire, and present epidemics in south-eastern and north-western Uganda and Angola reflect past civil wars. Recrudescence of old foci and geographic spread has been reported in Cameroon, Chad, Congo, and Central African Republic in recent years. In Malawi, government resettlement schemes adjacent to designated wildlife areas have resulted in new outbreaks.

Risk groups

There are considered to be 50 million at risk living in endemic areas (Kuzoe 1993). Occupational risk groups include hunters and tourists to wildlife parks in endemic areas in East Africa, who may contract sporadic Rhodesian sleeping sickness from wild animal reservoirs. No specific occupational groups, except perhaps fishermen, are at risk for Gambian sleeping sickness, since all sectors of the population come into contact with the fly in its riverine/lakeshore habitat during daily activities such as bathing and collecting water.

Population movements may also increase risk (Ford 1971). For example, resettlement schemes may bring people into close contact with flies which previously fed on wild animal reservoir hosts. Refugees fleeing from one country may move into an endemic focus in another, as has recently happened on the Sudan–Uganda–Zaire border spanned by an endemic focus of Gambian sleeping sickness. Immigrants are at no greater risk of infection than the indigenous population, since exposure does not confer immunity to reinfection. Returning refugees may find their abandoned farmland overgrown with bush and infested with tsetse, giving rise to new outbreaks.

Geography

Sleeping sickness has been reported in 36 countries in sub-Saharan Africa between latitudes 14°N and 29°S in the past 10 years (Kuzoe 1993). The distribution of the disease is restricted by that of the tsetse fly, which needs the right conditions of humidity and temperature for survival. *Palpalis*-group flies, which are the main vectors of Gambian sleeping sickness, need high humidity and are found in the forested zones of West and Central Africa, Uganda, and southern Sudan; their range also extends northwards through more arid country, following the lines of fringing vegetation on river and lakeshore. *Morsitans*-group flies can tolerate drier conditions and are found throughout the wooded savannah regions; they inhabit the vast tracts of mopane woodland in parts of East Africa (Buxton 1955; Mulligan 1970).

SOURCES

The source of infection is always another infected mammalian host. In an epidemic, other infected humans are generally thought to be the major source of infection, although it is acknowledged that a high infection rate in domestic livestock could boost transmission, if flies take a significant proportion of feeds from both hosts. At the other end of the spectrum, sporadic infections can be contracted when man breaks into a wild animal–tsetse cycle. This occurs most frequently in East Africa, where there are large concentrations of wild animals in uninhabited bush, but this possibility cannot be ruled out in some areas of West and Central Africa with plentiful wildlife. Domestic livestock will probably become increasingly important in disease transmission, either acting as an intermediary in transferring trypanosome strains from wild animals to man, or by replacing wild animal reservoirs altogether.

TRANSMISSION

The usual mode of transmission is via the bite of an infected tsetse fly, as can be deduced from the restriction of the disease to the area of tsetse infestation.

Trypanosomes undergo a developmental and multiplicative cycle in the fly, first in the midgut and then in the salivary glands, from whence they are conveyed to new hosts with the saliva (Hoare 1972). Flies are relatively refractory to infection, only readily becoming infected at the first blood meal after emergence from the puparium (Maudlin 1991); consequently much less than 1 per cent of flies are found infected with *T. brucei* ssp. in the wild. The cycle takes approximately 4 weeks to complete. With a life span of 2–3 months under favourable conditions and a requirement to feed every few days, an individual fly could infect at least 20 new hosts. It is for this reason that close man–fly contact, rather than sheer numbers of flies, is so important in the epidemiology of sleeping sickness: for example, one resident infected fly at the village water hole has the potential to cause a small epidemic in the dry season when people spend more time there (Nash 1969). By contrast, large concentrations of flies feeding predominantly on wild animals pose very little risk.

Other modes of transmission are possible, but depend on relatively high parasitaemia in the donor and a susceptible recipient, e.g. contaminative transmission by tsetse or other biting flies such as tabanids; direct transmission via fresh infected blood or raw meat (Moloo *et al.* 1973). Congenital transmission has rarely been recorded.

COMMUNICABILITY

The main route of sleeping sickness transmission is via the tsetse fly. Laboratory studies have shown not only that different trypanosome subspecies and strains vary in infectivity to flies, but also that the flies themselves differ in susceptibility to trypanosome infection (Maudlin 1991). In fact it appears that most flies are refractory to infection, and transmission appears to be sustained by relatively few flies. The long-term stability of endemic foci is evidence that this minimalist strategy is successful and further emphasizes the fundamental importance of the behaviour of individual flies rather than populations in transmission of the disease.

Establishment of infection in a new host following fly bite will depend on several factors: the number of trypanosomes inoculated with the saliva; the virulence of the trypanosome subspecies or strain; the level of intrinsic resistance of the host.

PREVENTION AND CONTROL

PREVENTION

The risk of contracting human trypanosomosis outside the 200 or so known foci of the disease is minimal, although sporadic infections could potentially be acquired in some tsetse-infested wildlife areas. Animal trypanosomosis caused by non-man-infective trypanosomes exists throughout the tsetse belt, however.

Even in an endemic area, the risk of being bitten by an infected fly is small. The risk of infection can be lowered by avoiding tsetse fly bite, easier said than done in the African bush. All tsetse species require some degree of shade and habitats vary from light bush to dense forest and even conifer plantations. Tsetse can be found in the peridomestic environment if there is suitable cover and those species favoring a riverine habitat may also be encountered at waterholes, river crossing points, and bathing places. Tsetse feed during the day and find their hosts by sight as well as smell. They are attracted to large moving objects, particularly vehicles, and also dark colored clothing. Clothing is no barrier to tsetse bite, but insect repellents might be of limited use if practical. Animals could be treated with pour-on residual insecticide, but this might not prevent fly bite and the possibility of infection.

Prophylactic drugs for human use cannot be recommended, although pentamidine was widely used in the past (Mulligan 1970). There would be too great a risk of masking early infection, giving the parasites time to invade the CNS. For animals, various drugs can be given prophylactically, but there could be toxic effects from long-term use and prophylaxis would probably be ineffectual in areas of high challenge.

CONTROL STRATEGIES

There are two current strategies for control: control of the parasite by regular medical surveillence of the population at risk or control of the fly. The parasite is targeted by drug therapy of its human host; there have been few, if any, attempts to eliminate trypanosomes in reservoir hosts, other than early attempts to destroy the wild animal reservoir. Eradication of tsetse flies in Africa is now realized to be a vain hope. Despite their slow breeding cycle—each female produces only a single larva every 9 days or so—and the various measures used to combat them, tsetse flies have actually increased in distribution since the turn of the century. Present environmental concerns favour limited use of insecticides and low-tech methodologies that can be widely and cheaply applied at local level (Dransfield *et al.* 1991).

METHODS AND PROGRAMMES

Sleeping sickness control is usually organized at governmental level; however, other organizations, such as aid agencies and missions, may be involved, especially during epidemics. For example, besides local govern-

ment, several European governments, United Nations organizations and charities have all provided financial or technical aid for control of the recent epidemic in south-eastern Uganda. International organizations such as OAU and WHO take responsibility for co-ordination of control measures between African countries. This is especially important where foci span borders and for communication between French-and English-speaking countries.

Control of the parasite

Case detection and treatment is possible at a number of organizational levels, with various degrees of cost-effectiveness (WHO 1986). At one extreme mobile teams can be used to survey endemic areas, screening the whole population every year. Active surveillance like this is very costly, but also fulfils the requirement for patient follow-up to assess cure. Such programmes are necessary to cover large areas of endemic Gambian sleeping sickness. At the other extreme, patients can be left to report to their local health centre. This is so-called passive surveillence and is adequate for small outbreaks of Rhodesian sleeping sickness.

Individual governments must decide the level of resources to devote to sleeping sickness surveillance on the basis of the population at risk, the level of endemicity and their own health priorities. Present pressures on health budgets and the relatively small number of cases, means that sleeping sickness is increasingly seen as a low priority (Kuzoe 1993). However, since it is simpler and less expensive to undertake regular surveillance than to deal with an explosive epidemic, the risk of epidemics makes sleeping sickness a major public health problem in Africa. Epidemics cause fear in local populations, since the aetiology of the disease is still mysterious, and have both social and economic consequences, such as depopulation and abandonment of farmland.

Tsetse control

Methods for controlling tsetse flies currently comprise insecticide application by knapsack sprayers or by air, trap/target technology, bush clearance, or sterile male release. In planning an insecticide campaign, both adult flies and offspring must be considered. Females deposit their fully grown larvae on the ground in suitable sites where the soil is loose and moist (Buxton 1955). This is to facilitate rapid burrowing of the larva into the ground, where it pupates. Survival of pupae depends greatly on humidity and temperature and adult flies emerge roughly 3 weeks later. Thus, a single application of non-residual insecticide will have little effect on the tsetse population. Aerial spraying of insecticide (e.g. endosulphan) necessitates several spray cycles at weekly intervals. Effective knapsack spraying uses residual insecticides (e.g. dieldrin) applied to tsetse resting sites on foliage and branches. In the dry season tsetse populations retreat to the most favourable parts of their range, making control far more cost-effective. Thorough knowledge of the distribution and habits of the tsetse species to be controlled is invaluable.

Environmental concerns have put widespread insecticide use into disfavour and promoted the development of trap and target technology (Fig. 41.4). Traps were originally used as a sampling method for tsetse populations and work on the principle that tsetse are attracted by sight to large, dark objects. Whether this is in order to seek shade or a host is unclear, as one optimum but curious design is a biconical trap made of dark blue cloth. The tsetse enter at the bottom and move upwards through the trap towards the light, where they are imprisoned in a small cage and soon succumb to death by desiccation or hunger. Targets consisting of simple square sheets of the same colour cloth are also attractive and can be impregnated with insecticide (e.g. deltamethrin) to kill the flies as they land. Odour attractants (constituents of cow breath or urine) can be used in combination with traps or targets to increase the catch. These methodologies, although environmentally sound and low cost, are labour intensive. Large numbers of traps/targets need to be deployed to give adequate coverage and they require regular repair and replenishment of odour baits or insecticide. For these reasons, trap/target methodology is well suited to programmes involving community participation (Dransfield *et al.* 1991). Ideally traps or targets are constructed locally out of indigenous or cheap materials and are maintained by the community.

Bush clearance permanently destroys the habitat of tsetse and is cost effective when new farmland is gained. Sometimes, though, farming practices actually create new tsetse habitats: for example, the widespread introduction of lantana hedges or plantations of conifers, coffee, or cocoa.

Control by sterile male release depends on the fact that females mate once only and store the sperm until required. Sufficiently large numbers of sterile males in competition with wild males will thus reduce the population density over time. This technique is essentially long-term and requires high capital input initially to set up facilities for rearing and irradiating large numbers of male tsetse. The area of release needs to be isolated by geographical features or bush clearance in order to prevent re-invasion, and other techniques such as trapping or insecticides may need to be used in conjunction to push the tsetse population below recoverable levels. Despite these strictures, programmes of sterile male release are operative in Burkina Faso, Nigeria, and Tanzania.

Control of tsetse is often of both medical and veterinary concern, and this can lead to problems of communication if more than one government department is involved. Sustained control programmes will be more cost-effective than emergency action in the long run. For example, regular application of insecticide by teams with knapsack sprayers or schemes to involve rural communities in making and maintaining tsetse traps are long-term, low-cost methods of control; application of insecticide from the air can rapidly and dramatically reduce transmission, but is a short-term, costly measure, unless the spraying successfully eliminates tsetse from the area.

EVALUATION

The success of control programmes should be measurable by a decreasing incidence of sleeping sickness. In practice, with health resources strained to the limits and political disruption widespread, regular surveillence and fly control has broken down in many endemic areas. This is sure to require expensive interventions by international organizations in the future in order to control epidemic disease.

In principle, community participation schemes should devolve responsibility for control activities to local level, thereby rendering them sustainable. In practice, without continued technical input, communities lose interest in control schemes as the problem becomes less acute.

LEGISLATION

There is no legislation to control sleeping sickness in most endemic countries and cases are not adequately reported. Within tropical Africa it is potentially

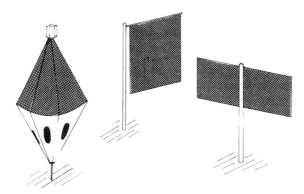

Fig. 41.4 Trap and targets for control of tsetse flies. Biconical trap (left), flies enter via holes at base and emerge into box cage at top; insecticide-impregnated simple screen target (centre); and pivoted target (right).

possible that movement of infected livestock between countries in the tsetse-infested zone could create new foci of disease. The translocation of wildlife species from endemic to non-endemic areas is a case in point. Infection with tsetse-transmitted trypanosomes is generally not considered to be a risk outside tropical Africa, since the chance of transmission is minimal. Cases are imported into Europe from time to time, usually in those who have visited wildlife areas.

REFERENCES

Ashcroft, M. T. (1959). The importance of African wild animals as reservoirs of trypanosomiasis. *East African Medical Journal*, **36**, 289.

Borst, P. and Rudenko, G. (1994). Antigenic variation in African trypanosomes. *Science*, **264**, 1872–3.

Brown, C. G. D., Hunter, A. G., and Luckins, A. G. (1990). Protozoa. In *Handbook on animal diseases in the tropics*, (ed. M. M. H. Sewell and D. W. Brocklesby), (4th edn). Baillière Tindall, London.

Brun, R. and Jenni, L. (1987). Human serum resistance of metacyclic forms of *Trypanosoma brucei brucei, T. brucei rhodesiense* and *T. brucei gambiense*. *Parasitology Research*, **73**, 218–23.

Buxton, P. A. (1955). *The natural history of tsetse flies*. Memoir 10, London School of Hygiene and Tropical Medicine. H. K. Lewis, London.

Davies, J. N. P. (1962). The cause of sleeping sickness. Parts I and II. *East African Medical Journal*, **39**, 81–99 and 145–60.

Dransfield, R. D., Williams, B. G., and Brightwell, R. (1991). Control of tsetse flies and trypanosomiasis: myth or reality. *Parasitology Today*, **7**, 287–91.

Ford, J. (1971). *The role of the trypanosomiases in African ecology. A study of the tsetse fly problem*. Clarendon Press, Oxford.

Geigy, R., Jenni, L., Kauffmann, M., Onyango, R. J., and Weiss, N. (1975). Identification of *Trypanosoma brucei* subgroup strains isolated from game. *Acta Tropica*, **32**, 190–205.

Gibson, W. C., Mehlitz, D., Lanham, S. M., and Godfrey, D. G. (1978). The identification of *Trypanosoma brucei gambiense* in Liberian pigs and dogs by isoenzymes and by resistance to human plasma. *Tropenmedizin und Parasitologie*, **29**, 335–45.

Greenwood, B. M. and Whittle, H. C. (1980). The pathogenesis of sleeping sickness. *Transactions of the Royal Society of Tropical Medicine and Hygiene*, **74**, 716–725.

Heisch, R. B., McMahon, J. P., and Manson-Bahr, P. E. C. (1958). The isolation of *Trypanosoma rhodesiense* from a bushbuck. *British Medical Journal*, **2**, 1203–4.

Hoare, C. A. (1972). *The trypanosomes of mammals*. Blackwell Scientific Publications, Oxford.

Kuzoe, F. A. S. (1993). Current situation of African trypanosomiasis. *Acta Tropica*, **54**, 153–62.

Lumsden, W. H. R., Kimber, C. D., Evans, D. A., and Doig, S. J. (1979). *Trypanosoma brucei*: Miniature anion exchange centrifugation technique for detection of low parasitaemias–adaptation for field use. *Transactions of the Royal Society of Tropical Medicine and Hygiene*, **73**, 312–17.

Magnus, E., Vervoort, T., and van Meirvenne, N. (1978). A card agglutination test with stained trypanosomes (CATT) for the serological diagnosis of *Trypanosoma brucei gambiense* trypanosomiasis. *Annales de la Société belge de Médecin Tropicale*, **58**, 169–76.

Maudlin, I. (1991). Transmission of African trypanosomiasis: Interactions among tsetse immune system, symbionts and parasites. *Advances in Disease Vector Research*, **7**, 117–48.

Mehlitz, D., Zillmann, U., Scott, C. M., and Godfrey, D. G. (1982). Epidemiological studies on the animal reservoir of gambiense sleeping sickness. III. Characterisation of Trypanozoon stocks by isoenzymes and sensitivity to human serum. *Tropenmedizin und Parasitologie*, **33**, 113–18.

Moloo, S. K., Losos, G. J., and Kutuza, S. B. (1973). Transmission of *Trypanosoma brucei* to cats and dogs by feeding on infected goats. *Transactions of the Royal Society of Tropical Medicine and Hygiene*, **67**, 287.

Mulligan, H. W. (ed.) (1970). *The African trypanosomiases*. George Allen and Unwin, London.

Nantulya, V. M. (1989). An antigen detection immunoassay for the diagnosis of *rhodesiense* sleeping sickness. *Parasite Immunology*, **11**, 69–75.

Nash, T. A. M. (1969). *The tsetse fly—Africa's bane*. Collins, London.

Onyango, R. J., Van Hoeve, K., and De Raadt, P. (1966). The epidemiology of *Trypanosoma rhodesiense* sleeping sickness in Alego location, Central Nyanza, Kenya. I. Evidence that cattle may act as reservoir hosts of trypanosomes infective to man. *Transactions of the Royal Society of Tropical Medicine and Hygiene*, **60**, 175–82.

Opperdoes, F. R. (1985). Biochemical peculiarities of trypanosomes, African and South American. *British Medical Bulletin*, **41**, 130–6.

Pepin, J., Guern, C., Milord, F., and Schecter, P. J. (1987). Difluoromethylornithine for arseno-resistant *Trypanosoma brucei gambiense* sleeping sickness. *Lancet*, **ii**, 1431–3.

Rickman, L. R. and Robson, J. (1970). The testing of proven *Trypanosoma brucei* and *T. rhodesiense* strains by the blood incubation infectivity test. *Bulletin of the World Health Organization*, **42**, 911–16.

Stephen, L. E. (1986) *Trypanosomiasis, a veterinary perspective*. Pergamon Press, Oxford.

WHO (1986). *Epidemiology and control of African trypanosomiasis*. Technical Report Series 739. WHO, Geneva.

Woo, P. T. K. (1970). The haematocrit centrifugation technique for the diagnosis of African trypanosomiasis. *Acta Tropica*, **35**, 384–6.

42 AMERICAN TRYPANOSOMOSIS

Philip Davis Marsden

SUMMARY

Trypanosoma cruzi infection is an ancient zoonosis of the New World. It is usually transmitted by faecal soiling of the mammalian integument during the act of feeding of blood-sucking triatomine bugs. Such transmission occurs from New York State to the Argentine pampas including all countries within this wide range. Chagas disease is the term applied to syndromes caused by human infection. *Trypanosoma cruzi* is the commonest cause of myocarditis in the world. The tissue amastigote phase of the parasite destroys cardiac and gut smooth muscle. This process can cause cardiomyopathy and gut megasyndromes depending on the degree of damage to the heart muscle and conducting system and the parasympathetic ganglia in the smooth muscle of the gut. Infection usually occurs in childhood, is usually incurable and is life long. In areas where bug transmission has been controlled other forms of transmission (blood transfusion, congenital, and oral) assume greater importance. *Trypanosoma cruzi* cannot resist desiccation. Control is by eradication of domiciliated vector bugs. Due to their slow life cycle they remain vunerable to many residual insecticides. In the past decade Brazil has successfully initiated a control programme against the principle vectors using National Health insurance funds. Other Latin American countries will follow suit since Chagas disease prejudices any health service. Unfortunately the affected population is the families of poor farmers, who have no political voice and often no official identity. Thus the most important endemic disease of the New World persists into the twenty-first century.

INTRODUCTION

Eponyms are common in traditional academic medicine because the precise cause was rarely known (e.g. Argyll Robertson pupils). Carlos Chagas found the cause of the disease he later described in the insect vector. His years of work in the field also incriminated animal reservoirs. Few in medicine reach his stature but Stockholm was asleep and he did not get a Nobel prize. An immediate distinction must be made between *T. cruzi* infection of man and Chagas disease. The former is widespread, reaching 50 per cent in some endemic areas. The latter, when the heart muscle fails or gut aperistalsis develops, is only detected in a small percentage of infected individuals.

Chagas disease is man's retribution for colonizing the New World. For millennia *T. cruzi* transmission was maintained among lower mammals. Marsupials (genus *Didelphis*) are among the oldest mammals in the Americas (Fig. 42.1). They show great tolerance to *T. cruzi* with little pathology and prolonged patent parasitaemia. They remain the most important sylvatic mammalian reservoir. Man, killing the wild animal blood sources for triatominae bugs and destroying the ecological balance, drove certain vector Triatominae into his own home in search of a blood meal.

All present Hemiptera of the subfamily Triatominae are blood suckers but they are probably derived from other members of the family Reduviidae which feed on plants and insects. Metacyclic trypanosomes of *T. cruzi* in bug faeces infect man and round up to form intracellular amastigotes. Division only occurs in this phase in mammalian tissues. Fresh trypomastigoles are released into the circulation as a result of rupture of pseudocysts containing numerous amastigotes. The time of pseudocyst rupture depends on the strain of

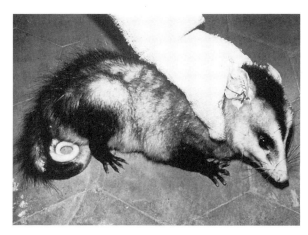

Fig. 42.1 Marsupial of the genus *Didelphis* the most important sylvatic mammalian reservoir of *T. cruzi* in the New World.

T. cruzi, the type of host cell invaded, and the immune response. *Trypanosoma cruzi* is highly antigenic, stimulating a marked immune response which controls detectable parasitaemia in man in a matter of weeks. However, host evasion mechanisms at an intracellular level mean some amastigotes always survive and infection is life long. Discompensation of heart or gut function as a result of tissue damage usually occurs only decades after initial infection in childhood. There are geographical differences in the behaviour of *T. cruzi* infection in man. Brasília is in the center of the greatest focus of pathogenic Chagas disease known, embracing the states of Bahia, Goiás, and Minas Gerais. Here gut megasyndromes and progressive cardiac failure are common, in contrast to Venezuela where megasyndromes are unknown. Response to specific chemotherapy in Brasília is also poor compared to Argentina.

Domiciled vector Triatominae determine the geographical distribution of Chagas disease. Of the 140 known species only six are of great importance in human transmission. Being true bugs they have an incomplete metamorphosis with five immature instars before achieving the status of winged adults (Fig. 42.2). Each instar needs an adequate blood meal to moult. A first instar can acquire *T. cruzi* infection which will persist for life. If it reaches adulthood it will have had a minimum of five opportunities to transmit the infection.

Triatomines are geared to two major activities. Rapid blood feeding and avoidance of their many predators. In nature they have long life cycles (over a year) and can resist starvation well. Domiciliated bugs are vunerable to control because they are house-bound, colonizing the fabric. Following Mueller's discovery of residual insecticides, Emmanuel Dias applied such insecticide spraying in control attempts in field studies in Brazil with remarkable success. However, the Brazilian National Control Programme was only initiated in 1984. At the time of writing the worst affected country is Bolivia where *Triatoma infestans* rules. This is the most successful house invader. It originated in the Cochabamba Valley in Bolivia where it can still be found in sylvatic habitats. From there it spread through the Cone Sul countries and up through southern and central Brazil as far as Maranhão State. It is an excellent passive migrator in clothing, umbrellas, railway carriage upholstery, etc. Why it has never colonized houses in the Amazon is a mystery, for lorries must have carried it up the Belém–Brasília highway many times. A possible explanation is that the enviromental temperatures of equatorial Amazon are too high for *T. infestans*. Many sylvatic cycles of *T. cruzi* transmission involving local Triatominae have been described from the Amazon. The Amazon Indian sleeps in a hammock in a house without walls. Very few cases of Chagas disease have been recorded in this racial group.

Table 42.1 gives some general idea of the dimension of the problem in the various South American countries. Figure 42.3 confirms that in Brazil Chagas disease is mainly a problem of the central and southern states. In my hospital in Brasília on the Central Plateau surgeons operate on many patients with megasyndromes. Chronic chagasic cardiomyopathy is a common cause of admission with a fatal outcome for over 50 per cent of patients presenting with congestive cardiac failure within 2 years.

THE AGENT

Trypanosoma cruzi is a polymorphic trypanosome characterized by a kinetoplast at its posterior end which is so large as to distort the cell membrane. This differentiates it from *Trypanosoma rangeli*, the other American trypanosomosis infecting man which has a small subterminal kinetoplast. No human pathology has been attributed to *T. rangeli*. It is a common infection in many South American mammals so its identification is important in epidemiological work. This is easily made by xenodiagnosis (a technique described by Brumpt where clean triatomines are fed on the suspect host

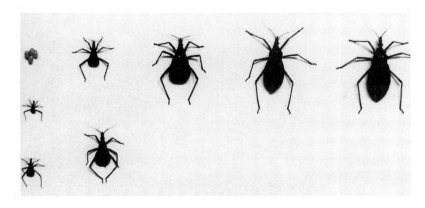

Fig. 42.2 *Dipetalogaster maximus*, showing all stages.

Table 42.1 Chagas disease in Latin America[a]

Country	Total population (millions)	% Rural	Estimated cases (millions)	Main vector
Argentina	26.393	21	2.640	*Triatoma infestans*
Belize	0.145	ND	0.003	*Triatoma dimidiata*
Bolivia	4.647	77	1.858	*Triatoma infestans*
Brazil	119.024	36	6.300	*Triatoma infestans*
Chile	10.857	20	0.367	*Triatoma infestans*
Colombia	26	29	0.217	*Rhodnius prolixus*
Costa Rica	2.110	59	0.130	*Triatoma dimidiata*
Ecuador	6.521	58	0.180	*Triatoma dimidiata*
El Salvador	4.300	60	0.322	*Triatoma dimidiata*
French Guiana	0.080	ND	0.021	*Rhodnius pictipes?*
Guatemala	7.110	64	0.730	*Triatoma dimidiata*
Guyana	0.835	73	0.208	*Rhodnius prolixus?*
Honduras	3.400	68	0.213	*Rhodnius prolixus*
Mexico	69.900	34	3.798	*Triatoma barberi*
Nicaragua	2.400	52	0.114	*Triatoma dimidiata*
Panama	1.630	49	0.226	*Rhodnius pallescens*
Paraguay	2.880	56	0.397	*Triatoma infestans*
Peru	16.800	42	0.643	*Triatoma infestans*
Suriname	0.352	ND	0.147	*Rhodnius pictipes?*
Uruguay	2.886	17	0.278	*Triatoma infestans*
Venezuela	13.913	30	4.865	*Rhodnius prolixus*
Total	322.233	36	24.697	

[a] From Schofield (1985).

and their rectal contents subsequently examined). *Trypanosoma cruzi* is restricted to the bug gut while *T. rangeli* invades the haemocoele and metacyclic trypanosomes are found in the salivary glands. Bug faeces contain trypanosomes of both species but they are morphologically distinct. *Trypanosoma rangeli* causes frequent death of its triatomine host. *Trypanosoma cruzi* does not shorten bug life.

Early *T. cruzi* amastigote nests or pseudocysts have no surrounding inflammatory infiltrate but many parasites fail to transform to trypomastigotes and promote a strong immune reaction. So subsequent pseudocysts are surrounded by an intense round cell infiltrate of lymphocytes and plasma cells. Several pathogenic mechanisms have been implicated apart from direct tissue cell destruction, including an autoimmune inflammatory cell response stimulated by *T. cruzi* antigens shared with host tissue cells. Such a mechanism could explain the tropism for cardiac and smooth muscle. Over decades heart muscle fibre destruction leads to pump failure which is irremedial. The Purkinje fibre conducting system of the heart is also involved, accounting for frequent arrhythmias. Parasympathetic ganglia destruction in the gut muscle gives rise to peristaltic wave incoordination, resulting in dilatation of the lumen of the oesophagus and colon (megasyndromes); the gut parts, with solid food residues. No mammalian host is insusceptible to *T. cruzi*. Birds cannot be infected possibly due to their higher body temperature. A complex of factors determine infection and its outcome. These include dose and type of inoculum, route, integrity of the integument, and microclimate, etc. A massive intravenous dose in a beagle dog will even produce amastigotes in the pituitary. Animals with patent parasitaemia may secrete trypanosomes in body fluids since these protozoa have great powers of tissue penetration. *Trypanosoma cruzi* is most infectious and there have been over 50 accidental human laboratory infections.

Trypanosoma cruzi stimulates antibody production by the end of the first month of infection. Today these antibodies are usually detected by the indirect fluorescent antibody test, haemagglutination, or enzyme-linked immunoassay techniques. These have tended to supersede the complement fixation test. Polymerase chain reaction technology is being introduced at the time of writing. Several of these reactions are often used, and serological reference laboratories play an important role in doubtful reactions. There are numerous cross-reactions with other Trypanosomatidae, mycobacteria, treponemes, malaria, collagenoses, etc. One of xenodiagnoses most important applications is to confirm serology. This technique depends on the exquisite sensitivity of vector bugs to *T. cruzi*. *Dipetalogaster maximus* is the best xenodiagnostic agent (Fig. 42.2). This is the most reliable test in chronic infections to recover the organism. The alternatives, culture or mouse inoculation, are less sensitive but usually positive in acute infections. *Trypanosoma cruzi* will grow *in vitro* on an agar slant of 10 per cent defibrinated rabbits' blood held at 26 °C. Defined and monophasic media are available. It has been shown that cloned populations of *T. cruzi* from a single isolate have different biological, pathological, and biochemical natures. *Trypanosoma cruzi* has survived in a drawn blood sample for a year. One of the main uses of serology in endemic areas is to screen blood transfusion samples if positive blood has to be used. Gentian violet (1 in 4000) must be added 24 hours before use. This is uniformly effective but blue blood is not well accepted by patients. Congenital infections in chronically infected parturients does not reach 2 per cent in Brazil but a much higher incidence has been recorded from Santa Cruz, Bolivia. Oral transmission can be easily shown in laboratory animals. Small epidemics in man have been caused by ingesting infected bug products or food contaminated with opposum urine.

Over 200 naturally infected animal species are recorded, especially insectivores. Eradication of *T. cruzi* is not feasible and the aim should be to reduce the possibility of human contamination. Most sylvatic cycles occur distant from human contact. For this reason *T. cruzi* human infection is rare in North America where houses will only be invaded by flying adult Triatominae and, due to good house structure, colonization will not occur.

THE VECTOR

This section is essential for it is by vector combat that control is achieved. Although acute disease then ceases (in Brasília we have not seen an acute case due to natural transmission for 8 years), the incidence of chronic chagasic cardiomyopathy takes decades to diminish due to the long genesis of the disease. Natural transmission from bug contact has always been a chance affair. Take the hypothetical case of a feeding infected bug defaecating on the face of a sleeping child (the only exposed part) at 4.0 a.m. Waking with the sun at 6 a.m. the child rubs the still-liquid infected faeces into its eye and infection ensues. Any part of the integument may be the site of entry and bug saliva is often allergic, causing scratching. Bug defaecation is governed by crop stretch receptors; a mechanism to ensure a maximal meal. Defaecation is early in successful vectors (*Rhodnius prolixus, Triatoma infestans*): later in others (*Triatoma protracta*). Triatomines are usually adventitious feeders, drawing blood from any host available by direct capillary penetration and rapid syringe-like engorgement. They take many times their body weight in a single meal but rapidly reduce this

volume by passing clear urine. Studies using manual demolition of infested houses shows the majority of the bug population is close to blood meal sources. Thus many are found in the wall adjacent to the conjugal bed, other beds, resting sites of bugs and chickens, pigs, and goats sleeping against outside walls. A chicken house annexed to an external wall many support a thriving colony. The bugs feed at night. Attempts to generate a risk factor for individual houses rely heavily on estimations of bug load. This is calculated from the number of bugs withdrawn from the fabric in unit time (usually 1 man hour); however, demolition data where total bug populations are known do not show a good correlation with man hour data. This is because collectors vary in efficiency, and distribution of bugs in the fabric is not uniform. Not only as a result of blood availability but also the presence of many intramural enemies (ants, spiders, lizards, mice, etc.). More than one bug vector in a house is common, but where *T. infestans* is present it dominates, probably by more efficient competition for blood meals.

Figure 42.3 shows the geographical distribution of the main domiciliary vectors and therefore reflects the distribution of human *T. cruzi* infection. Each species has many characteristics, learnt by watching their behaviour in laboratory colonies and in the field. Only a few can be mentioned. *T. infestans* has a great dominance in the south of the continent. In most areas it is restricted to the domicile in the upper wall and roof, and is vunerable to insecticide control. Such a control programme covering Cone Sul countries is currently in progress.

Panstrongylus megistus is a Brazilian problem and the bug that Carlos Chagas initially investigated. It has been controlled in the Brazilian north-east where it is only found in the houses, mainly in the first 1.5 m of wall and the beds. In central and southern Brazil this bug maintains sylvatic cycles. *Rhodnius prolixus* is a problem in Venezuela, Colombia, and eastern Central America. It merits its name because it is prolific, with several generations a year. This is the only important vector to have developed insecticide resistance in the field, first to benzene hexachloride (BHC) and then to Dieldrin. An aggressive feeder, it is also widely distributed in vegetation around houses, especially palm trees. *Triatoma dimidiata* and *T. braziliensis* are also common in the peridomicile and sylvatic ecotopes. Apart from these major vector there are several secondary vectors waiting to invade the domicile when the major vector has been controlled.

Far more triatomines are closely associated with their wild animal reservoirs. For example *Panstrogylus geniculatus* is found in armadillo burrows. Chagas himself implicated the armadillo as the first sylvatic

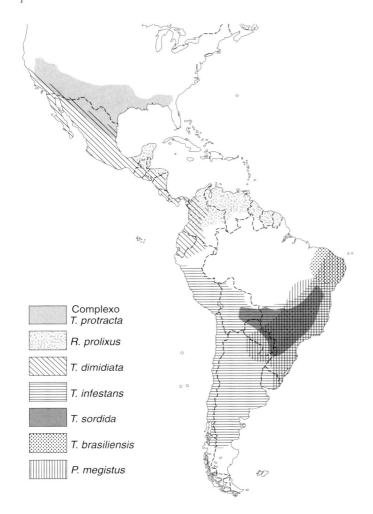

Complexo
T. protracta

R. prolixus

T. dimidiata

T. infestans

T. sordida

T. brasiliensis

P. megistus

Fig. 42.3 Geographical distribution of the principal species of triatomine vectors of *T. cruzi.*

reservoir. Yet other bugs are associated with wild bird or lizard feeds. The urge to feed and complete the life cycle is dramatically illustrated by demolishing a bug-infested house abandoned by the occupants a few weeks earlier. In such a case the adults have already flown and only starved wingless instars can be found disseminated throughout the fabric and walking into the peridomicile in search of blood.

HUMAN INFECTION

Most acute-phase disease passes unnoticed or is interpreted as a mild non-specific infection. The best definition of this phase is visible parasitaemia on fresh blood film examination, since all other signs are variable. The site of entry of *T. cruzi* or chagoma is evident in less than half the patients. If it is conjunctival a unilateral, brawny, bipalpebral oedema develops which is slow to resolve (Romana's sign). Step sections of the orbit show rapid amastigote invasion of the orbital tissues, especially the external ocular muscles. Trypanosomes may be present in tears, as the lacrimal gland and preauricular lymph node are involved. Within a week circulating trypanosomes reach the heart muscle. Peripheral inoculation chagomas (Fig. 42.4) may show trypanosomes if needled; a situation similar to the trypanosomal chancre of African trypanosomosis.

Acute disease may be associated with variable fever, tachycardia hepatosplenomegaly, lymphadenopathy, subcutaneous nodules, and a skin rash resembling measles. In less than 5 per cent of acute disease, death results either from acute heart failure due to overwhelming myocarditis or meningoencephalitis (trypanosomes may be present in the cerebrospinal fluid). Animal experiments suggest that the inoculating dose of flagellates and the host response are major factors

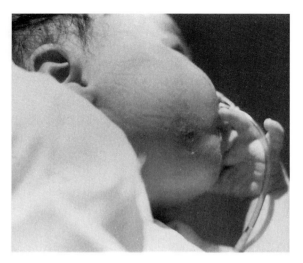

Fig. 42.4 Chagoma on the face at a site of inoculation. A needle aspiration may show trypanosomes.

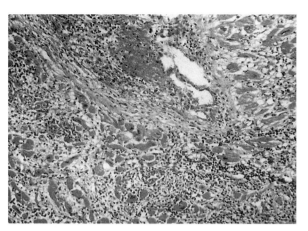

Fig. 42.5 Pancarditis with muscle fibre degeneration and destruction.

determining the gravity of the acute phase. Similar factors must govern the development of the rather rare subacute phase where progressive cardiomyopathy is accelerated and grave cardiac arrythmias develop.

After a few weeks of the acute phase, immunocompetent patients pass into the so-called indeterminate phase where positive serology remains a life-long marker of occult infection. About half the patients will show intermittent positive xenodiagnosis, showing that trypanomastigotes are still circulating in small numbers. Recent Brazilian work has suggested that the origin of these trypanosomes is amastigote nests in the smooth muscle in the wall of the suprarenal vein. This vein carries a high dose of corticoids which may favour *T. cruzi* multiplication.

Usually decades after infection in a minority of those infected, signs of Chagas disease appears. The early signs of cardiomyopathy are electrocardiographic and mild at first, such as extra systoles or first-degree atrioventricular block. In some instances these progress to complete right bundle branch block with left anterior hemiblock and eventually complete atrioventricular block with consequent Stokes–Adams attacks. More common is simple pump failure due to the extensive pancarditis with muscle fibre destruction (Fig. 42.5). The heart chambers are dilated and the muscle wall thinned. It pulsates weakly on screening and, if the great musculospiral bundles of the heart unwind, produces a small apical aneurysm. This heart fails on both sides so acute pulmonary oedema is rare. Valvular incompetence at the mitral and tricuspid values is functional due to valve ring dilatation. Such a weak heart is subject to mural eddies and thrombosis. Pulmonary and systemic emboli are common. Often combinations of ventricular muscle and conduction defects occur.

Such patients improve on bed rest and conventional therapy, but relapse. Death occurs in a few years depending on the quality of care. Men are more affected than women due to the factor of harder physical work. For a poor rural farmer the effect on family life is catastrophic as the breadwinner is a cardiac invalid. The pathogenesis of such a malignant course is still under discussion. The relative roles of the severity of the initial acute phase, the smouldering progressive cardiomyopathy, and the possible role of auto-immunity in this inflammation remain undefined. Positive xenodiagnosis is not associated with this bad prognosis which doesn't reach 10 per cent of the chronically infected, even in central Brazil.

It is also in this area that the highest frequency of megasyndromes is encountered. The oesophagus becomes dilated with solid residues due to aperistalsis and spasm of the cardiac sphincter. The symptoms of *entalo*, or difficulty in swallowing, are well known to local people. They often have to swallow water to assist the passage of dry food. Four degrees of oesophageal dilatation are described (Fig. 42.6). Spillover from the distended oesophagus may cause a secondary inhalation bronchopneumonia.

Megacolon is associated with persistent constipation requiring manual evacuation. Again it is usually the sigmoid colon containing solid residue. Surgical excision results in good success. Autonomic ganglia destruction in smooth muscle have resulted in mega gall bladder, mega urinary bladder, and mega duodenum. Half the patients with megasyndromes will have signs of chronic chagasic cardiomyopathy. Megasyndromes can be produced in experimental animals with certain strains of *T. cruzi*. Megasyndromes are described in children but are more common with longevity. Endocrine and exocrine gland dysfunction, the result of autonomic denervation, are documented.

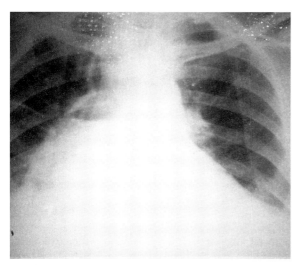

Fig. 42.6 Mega-oesophagus: the lumen of the oesophagus is dilated with solid material due to aperistalsis, as outlined by the barium meal.

The increasing use of immunosuppressive therapy in modern medicine is opening a new chapter in the clinical story of Chagas disease. Reactivation of latent infections has produced bizarre overwhelming disease. Over 20 such cases reported are associated with the aquired immunodeficiency syndrome (AIDS). Cardiac transplantation has been unsuccessful in chagasics because the necessary immunosuppression reactivates latent infection even after specific treatment.

Reliable serology and sensitive xenodiagnosis are the mainstays of accurate diagnosis in the chronic phase. Xenodiagnosis is much used to evaluate chemotherapy. Specific therapy with benzimidazole (Rochagan) in an oral dose of 10 mg/kg body weight for 30 days is only partially successful in parasite sterilization in central Brazil. Lampit (a nitrofurozone) is less effective and no longer produced, but is the only drug available from the Centers for Disease Control, Atlanta, Georgia. A call to have Rochagan available at one centre on each continent passed unheeded. The author could give little help for a transfusion acute case acquired from transfusion of Bolivian blood in Australia. Rochagan is mandatory in the acute phase to reduce tissue damage. The drug is not approved for general distribution in most countries outside South America. In the chronic phase, long-term benefit is still debatable and based on the ill-understood parameter of xenodiagnosis as serology does not convert. The author does not recommend specific chemotherapy in chronic-phase patients, due to side-effects and lack of proof of efficacy.

There is still no way of measuring the activity of myocardial inflammation. Auto-antibodies in the sera have not proved reliable. Repeated heart failure,

severe arrythmia and emboli are signs of a poor prognosis. Sudden death due to cardiac arrest or ventricular fibrillation is well documented.

ANIMAL HOSTS

Variable susceptibility in genetically defined mice is well known, but no wild animal is known to be insusceptible. Ancient hosts such as marsupials and armadillos show high tolerance. Most South American rodents have been found to be naturally infected, using xenodiagnosis. *Didelphis* sp. are dangerous sylvatic reservoirs for establishing a domiciliary transmission cycle, with their high parasitaemia, nocturnal habits, tendency to build roof nests, and habit of invading the kitchen. House mice and rats are usually infected by eating infected bugs. They in turn infect domestic cats, but the Felidae hunt at night and thus pose little risk. Dogs are a different matter; good reservoirs sleeping in the house can be the key in initiating a bug—*T. cruzi* cycle that ends in infecting man. Chickens are immune to infection but are sharp-eyed and eat many bugs; however, we never had any luck in reducing populations of *P. megistus* using chickens. Guinea-pigs are a special case among Indians, for they are often reared under the bed for food. High bug concentrations occur since *Cavia* sp. incubate infections well. Bed occupants are at great risk. Pigs and goats can be infected experimentally when young, but have low parasitaemias. The author knows of no good studies with horses and cows. Sometimes when you see a saddle on the wall with a lot of bugs behind it, you wonder.

Certain domestic environmental conditions influence domiciliated bug behaviour. If you sleep in a hammock, bugs congregate in the wall behind the hooks and run along the net at night. Pyrethroid-impregnated hammocks could be useful in such circumstances. In the cold high Andes, the author has seen *T. infestans*, like the human occupants, huddled round the fire. Normally they don't like kitchens and smoke. In Venezuela *R. prolixus* is present in the fresh palm fronds thrown on the roof to cover a leak. Our group showed that houses receiving more visitors had more bugs, due to the risk of passive introduction.

The author has infected a wide range of experimental mammals in pursuit of clarification of animal reservoir roles. For an animal reservoir to be a effective instrument for *T. cruzi* transmission it must have close proximity to man (dog) and maintain an adequate parasitaemia to infect bugs (opossum). Isolates from different geographical locations in South America show different pathology in mice and monkeys. Much relating to the pathogenicity, pathology, diagnosis, and treatment has been elucidated in such animal models. Critics of adequately controlled experiments have no case considering the dangerous unpredictable nature of *T. cruzi* infections.

EPIDEMIOLOGY

Many aspects under this title have already been mentioned. The figures of numbers of infected people per country in Table 42.1 are guesstimates but are useful to try and stimulate public health control programmes. New foci of *T. cruzi* infection are still being found. A recent example is in the south of Mexico. A Brazilian nationwide serological test programme estimated that 11 million rural Brazilians lived in bug-infested houses and were at risk. This was a major factor stimulating the national control programme. The people at risk are poor subsistence farmers who do not even own the land they cultivate. They have large families and move frequently. The men build the family house of local materials in a matter of weeks. Such homes are made of stout wooden uprights, walls of lath and mud and, for the very poor, a palm roof (Fig. 42.7). Bugs prefer such houses with abundant hiding places but, like the climicidae can be found in more sophisticated dwellings. An underinvestigated area is the capacity of other blood-sucking insects in the home (bed bugs, fleas), which often increase after a control programme, to transmit *T. cruzi*. *Trypanosoma cruzi* will develop in a wide variety of arthropods but to prove field transmission is a complex problem. Factors which favour bug presence in high density and increase the human risk of transmission are suitable house construction for colonization, poor lighting, poor domestic hygiene, intradomiciliary animals, large families, frequent visitors, and old houses. The aim of any control programme is to reduce the chance of contact between the sleeping child and the infected bug. Recently in Brazil there has been some evidence of urban transmission in favelas. However, the tendency of the modern Brazilian to urbanize is likely to reduce transmission risk. We have calculated the amount of money spent on hospital admissions, pacemaker implants, and gut surgery for megasyndromes in our hospital: it is crippling our service capacity.

Only one triatomine species has become tropicopolitan, namely *Triatoma rubrofasciata*. This was carried to distant ports from South America by the old wooden sailing ships which it colonized. A rodent trypanosome (*T. conorrhini*) transmitted by this bug was first described in Japan. Triatominae can harbour other flagellates, of which *Blastocrithidia triatominae* is the best known. This has caused great confusion in the interpretation of xenodiagnosis in the past. It is transmitted between bugs by resistant spores. Any xenodiagnostic colony with this problem must be destroyed.

PREVENTION AND CONTROL

Finally after all this preamble we come to the crunch— control of *T. cruzi* transmission is feasible by eradicating domiciliary vectors. House construction plays an

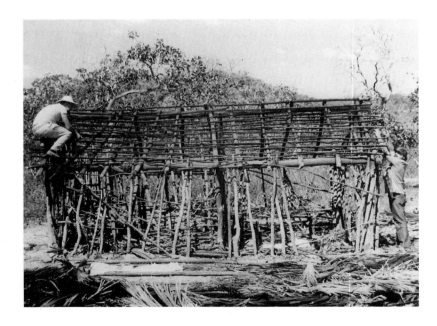

Fig. 42.7 Rural house constructed of wooden upright lathes and mud and often a palm roof. Such dwellings provide abundant opportunities for colonization by triatomes.

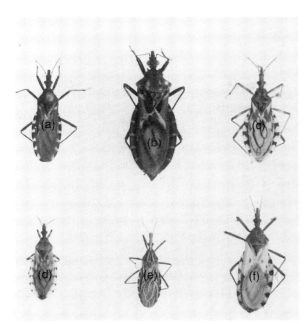

Fig. 42.8 Important vectors of *T. cruzi*: (a) *T. infestans*; (b) *P. megistus*; (c) *T. brasiliensis*; (d) *T. sordida*; (e) *R. prolixus*; (f) *T. dimidiata*.

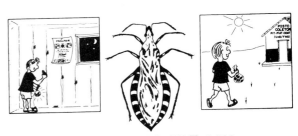

Fig. 42.9 Informative poster and calendar as a 'vigilance unit'.

important part in control. For instance, Brazilian constructions tend to be flimsy because of the heat and are easily penetrated by the insecticide spray. But what about a Bolivian Andean Indian house made of stone with a multilayered thatched roof to keep out the cold? A different proposition and one where an initial house demolition study after spraying is essential (Fig. 42.7). Such demolition studies should be done for all important vectors, (Fig. 42.8) but unfortunately good data are only available for *P. megistus* and *T. infestans* provided by the authors own teams. Also the Andean Indian seems to the author to be less accessible to community participation programmes. Could memories of the catastrophic Spanish conquest still linger? Such community participation is essential to ensure adequate vigilance in the long term.

In Brazil such control programmes on a state-wide scale have been in progress for decades. The first state to initiate such a programme was São Paulo—the richest state. Paulistas controlled *T. infestans* many years ago and the programme is well documented. Another rich cattle-rearing area, the Triângulo Mineiro, also anticipated the national control initiated in 1984. Our pilot study in the municipality of Mambaí was accepted for spraying by the Ministry of Health in 1980. The expense involved was quite beyond our slender research resources. The initial spray cost 5 dollars per house. We had evidence that the sole important vector, *T. infestans* was on the increase and

this study will serve as an example of field control procedure.

After contact with the local administration (mayor's office) the ministry personnel make their own maps of all farms in the municipality and the town. Each house is marked and whether it contained triatomines indicated. In all localities where a house is found to be infested all the houses will be sprayed. Then at local headquarters calculations are made regarding costs; the amount of transport and petrol, number of spray teams, and equipment including insecticide. In 1980 in Mambaí benzene hexachloride (BHC) was the insecticide used for the attack phase. Today this insecticide, which is not biodegradable, has been replaced by pyrethroids. Operational costs are similar and pyrethroids have a longer residual effect on a variety of surfaces and little residual smell.

In the attack phase house owners are warned beforehand of the arrival of the spray team so that they can lodge their animals. Before spraying all furniture is removed and the bed mattresses turned. Every square metre of wall inside and outside the house is sprayed and the inside of the roof. Appropriate protective clothing is worn (see Fig. 42.10). All out-houses are also sprayed. We have checked the throughness of this procedure using a biological test kit of triatomines in a flat metal tin exposed for unit time to the wall. Results

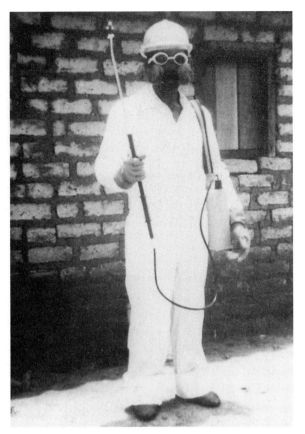

Fig. 42.10 Protective clothing worn by member of a spray team.

usually show effective application. It is the third phase of vigilance, to prevent re-invasion by bugs, where difficulties arise, since the ministry effector arm (SUCAM or FNS) has to move on to other areas. Our research over recent years has concentrated on this aspect recent (Garcia-Zapata and Marsden 1993). The following points are listed for brevity:

1. We found the people themselves only had a vague idea of the threat of *T. cruzi* to their family and little notion of how to collaborate with control personnel.

2. Mambaí showed that one well-conducted insecticide application will eliminate *T. infestans* from the great majority of houses and a second spraying after 6 months is not justified.

3. Due to the demands of a national programme vigilance tends to be neglected. In 1983 little fieldwork was possible by the ministry and even insecticide for residual spraying in houses where bugs were found was unavailable. A great advantage of the Mambaí yearly data is that they were

independently confirmed by the ministry and the University of Brasília.

4. For every house where you achieve bug capture another exists more lightly infected where only evidence of bug presence is found. Isolated visits by bug capture personnel are not sufficiently sensitive. That is why all houses are sprayed in an affected farm in the Brazilian regulation. We devised an individual family vigilance unit. Especially valuable in remote homes, it is a sensitive form of longitudinal vigilance. Initially this consisted of a Gomez Nuñes trap (a cardboard box with entry holes adjacent to the wall which acts as a wall extension and is colonized by bugs). A warning notice and diagram on the front of the box and a self-sealing plastic bag with the name and address completed the unit.

5. It is most important that the field worker visits the house and sits down with the mother to explain the unit. The father is out but she tells him when he comes in at night. The notice is read and explained, for most are illiterate. The function of plastic bag is demonstrated. Any bug found is put in the bag and sent to our notification centre. Once a year the vigilance units are examined. The unit is nailed to the wall over the conjugal bed (the largest blood mass) by the cardboard panels used for its eventual closure before examination. The children do not touch it.

6. Over the years our investigations have modified this unit to the minimal vigilance unit. The box, which is difficult to read, has been replaced by an informative poster and calender (Fig. 42.9). We found that faecal streaking was such a dominant sign of bug presence that it could replace the more expensive box and was easier to read using our faecal key. Bugs have projective defaecation that is different to other wall inhabitants. If bug presence is confirmed in the house, insecticide spraying is programmed.

7. Plastic bags coming into the notification centre containing Hemiptera other than Triatominae are simply discarded and the plastic bag replaced.

8. It has been suggested that such londitudinal vigilance only functions well in Mambaí because we have conditioned community participation. We have recently published similar success with these techniques from an adjacent area without such a service. Our work is suitable for national programmes and a year's longitudinal vigilance costs a fraction of a dollar per house.

9. The most observant bug vigilators are children, not their parents. So we lay emphasis on school children and their teachers—giving informative lectures. It is here that our peripheral vigilance

units are based (PITS—Postos de Informacão Triatomínica).

10. For remote farms, often inaccessible due to rain, we have established a number of information and attack posts (Piats). Here a responsible community member is trained to recognize *T. infestans*, equipped with suitable clothing and equipment, and is shown how to spray the infested house. This has worked well (Fig. 42.10).

Triatoma infestans has not been recorded in Mambaí for 3 years, though there are signs of its presence in neighbouring municipalities. Vigilance cannot be relaxed. We have captured 12 triatomine species in the area, among them four known house colonizers (Fig. 42.8). Though these have not presented a problem to date, they are briefly discussed below:

1. *Triatoma sordida.* A common frequenter of the peridomicile, it is mainly located in chicken houses. Families with a low hygiene standard passively transfer young instars to their beds in the feathers of live chickens. However, the incidence of *T. cruzi* infection is low in this species (<1 per cent) because of its preference for chicken blood, and the risk is slight. In some areas of central Brazil this species is thought to pose more of a threat to establishing transmission.

2. *R. neglectus* is present in animal nests in many palm trees. We have found a domiciliary colony of this species in Goiás but not in Mambaí.

3. *Triatoma pseudomaculata* established one colony in an outhouse in the peridomicile.

4. *P. megistus* is a bit of a mystery. It was the original house-dwelling vector in Mambaí before being displaced by *T. infestans*; occasionally heavily infected adults are still captured at night, probably from *Didelphis* nests. Our vigilance, however, has yet to detect domiciliation of this species in Mambaí.

The other bug species captured pose no threat since they are involved in purely sylvatic cycles, with only occasional adults flying into houses. This phenomenon occurs especially on sultry humid nights. This really does not justify residual spraying, although this is often done.

With the ecological variations among important vectors, each control programme must be tailored to the principal vector bug. Those present in the peridomicile and in nature may prove difficult to control. Broadcast insecticide application in the peridomicile is hardly justified. Better knowledge of bug ecology is the first step in control planning.

A further aspect of triatomine vector control is house improvement. We have much experience of various methods from the construction of totally new

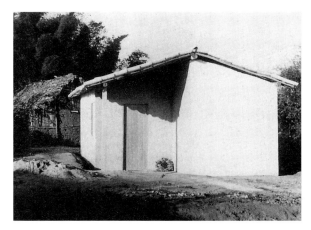

Fig. 42.11 New house construction to reduce or eliminate colonization by triatomes.

houses (Fig. 42.11) to the replastering of old houses. This expensive intervention is best reserved for houses persistently infested after repeated insecticide application. The house owner should be actively involved in the venture as this stimulates interest and better maintenance. It is cheaper to replaster and reroof than to build, and often more acceptable to the house owner. Initial research has to be done on the best formulations of local materials available. We have found in Mambaí that two parts of soil, two of and, are of lime, and are of cow faeces produces a plaster that resists cracking in the hot sun and driving rain. A binding agent is key (cow faeces). Examination of old plastered constructions in Brazil and England show that hair, wool, animal fat, whale oil, and molasses were all used as binding agents. We are currently investigating bagasse and corn husks in experimental walls. The plaster is applied by hand to inside and outside walls, with particular attention to close the space around the uprights to wall in the bugs. Fired Portuguese tiles laid on a wooden frame provide a ventilated roof. Reformed houses must be checked periodically. For example a relatively rich man with a persistent *T. infestans* colony and a uniformly infected family promised but failed to re-form his roof.

There is still a *laisser faire* attitude to triatomines among many farmers. The reasoning runs that his father always had them in his house and lived to ninety. So what's the fuss? The peridomicile must not be neglected. Garcia-Zapata has designed an ingenious bamboo trap for chicken houses. We are attempting to design a bug-proof chicken house acceptable to the people.

Although triatomine vigilance techniques have been in place for 13 years, the acid test is to show that children born in the rural area since the year of the massive attack phase (1980) are seronegative. This we have recently done and seropositivity has fallen to less than 1 per cent. The few positive sero-reacting children correlated with observations of special infectious risk during the first decade of life.

A factor which is difficult to evaluate and which favourably influences any control programme is the gradual development of the society under study. When we arrived in Mambaí in 1973 we had to ford a river on foot. There was no electric light and only one school in the town. Having established that the Chagas disease problem was in the farms, we spent many days driving the jeep over the bush and walking sandy paths from house to house. Today there is a bridge over the river, passable roads, rural schools and school teachers, and even a hospital in the town of Mambaí.

A final point is the need to train Latin American personnel. All afflicted countries are sensitive to comments on the Chagas disease problem. Success requires tact and their personnel—after all, it is their problem.

REFERENCES

Anonymous (1975). *American trypanosomiasis research.* PAHO Sc. Pub. No. 318, Washington DC.

Anonymous (1994). *Control de Doenca de Chagas.* Diretrizes Tecnicas, la edn, Fundação Nacional da Saude, Brasília.

Barreto, M. P. (1963). Reservatórios e vetores de *Trypanosoma cruzi* no Brasil. *Arq. Hig. Saude Publica*, **28**, 43–66.

Brener, Z. and Andrade, Z. (ed.) (1979). *Trypanosoma cruzi e Doença de Chagas.* Guanabara Koogan, Rio de Janeiro.

Brenner, R. R. and Stoka, A. M. (ed.) (1988). *Chagas' Disease Vectors*, Vols 1–3. CRC Press, Boca Raton.

Briceno L. R. (1940). *La Casa Enferma. Sociologia de la Enfermedad de Chagas.* Ediciones Caprales, Caracas.

Camargo, M. E., Da Silva, G. R., Castilho, E. A., and Silveira, A. C. (1984). Inquérito sorológico da prevaléncia de infecçáo chagásica no Brasil. 1975–1980. *Revista do Instituto de Medicina Tropical de São Paulo*, **26**, 192–204.

Cançado, J. R. (ed.) (1968). *Doença de Chagas.* Belo Horizonte.

Carneiro, M. and Antunes, C. M. F. (1994). A quasi experimental epidemiological model for evaluating public health programmes: efficacy of a Chagas' disease control programme in Brazil. *Bulletin of the World Health Organization*, **72**, 721–8.

Chagas, C. (1921). American trypanososmiasis study of the parasite and the transmitting insect. *Proceedings of the Institute of Medicine, Chicago*, **3**, 220–42.

D'Alessandro-Bacgalupo, A. and Saravia, N. G. (1992). *Trypanosoma rangeli.* In Vol. 2. *Parastic protozoa* (2nd edn), Ed. Vol. 2, (ed. J. P. Krier and J. R. Baker), pp. 1–54. Academic Press, San Diego.

Dias, E. (1945). *Um Ensaio de Profilaxia da Moléstia de Chagas.* Imprensa Nacional, Rio de Janeiro.

Dias, E. and Pellegrino, J. (1948). Alguns ensaios com a gammexane no combate de transmissores da doença de Chagas. *Brazil Médico*, **62**, 185–91.

Dias, J. C. P. (1987) Control of Chagas' disease in Brazil. *Parasitology Today*, **3**, 336–47.

Dvorak, J. A., Gibson, C. C., and Markelt, A. (1985). Chagas' disease: a medlars-based computer processed bibliography. (1968–1984). NIH/PAHO Ref. RD 24/1.

Emmans, L. H. and Feer, F. (1990). *Neotropical rainforest mammals.* University of Chicago Press, Chicago.

Forattini, O. P. (1980). Biografia, origem e distribuição de triatomíneos no Brasil. *Revista de Saúde Pública São Paulo*, **14**, 265–99.

Garcia-Zapata, M. T. A. and Marsden, P. D. (1986). *Chagas' disease.* In *Epidemiology and control of tropical diseases*, (ed. H. M. Gilles, pp. 557–85. Saunders, London.

Garcia-Zapata, M. T. A. and Marsden, P. D. (1993). Chagas' disease: Control and surveillance through use of insecticides and community participation in Mambaí, Goiás, Brazil. *Bulletin of the Pan American Health Organization*, **27**, 265–79.

Hoare, C. A. (1972). *The trypanosomes of mammals.* Blackwell, Oxford.

Lent, H. and Woygodzinsky, P. (1979). Revision of the Triatominae (Hemiptera, Reduviidae) and their significance as vectors of Chagas' disease. *Bulletin of the American Museum of Natural History*, **163**, 3.

Le Ray, D. and Recacoehea, M. (1985). Enfermedad de Chagas. Coloquio Internacional. *Annales de la Societe Belge de Medicina Tropical*, **65**, (Suppl. 1), 107–13.

Marsden, P. D. (1971). South American Trypanosomiasis (Chagas' Disease). In *International Review of Tropical Medicine*, Vol. 4, –121, (ed. D. C. Lincicome, and A. W. Woodruff) pp. 97–121. Academic Press, London.

Marsden, P. D. (1983). The transmission of *Trypanosoma cruzi* to man and its control. In *Human ecology and infectious disease*, (ed. N. A. Croll and J. M. Cross), pp. 253–89. Academic Press, New York.

Marsden, P. D. (1986). *Dipetalogaster maxima or Dipetalogaster maximus* as a xenodiagnostic agent. *Revista da Sociedade Brasileira de Medicina Tropical*, **19**, 205–7.

Marsden, P. D. (1994). The control of *Triatoma infestans* in Mambaí-Goiás, Brazil. P. 151–160. In *Progress in clinical parasitology*, Vol. 4, (ed. T. Sun), pp. 151–60. CRC Press, Boca Raton.

Miles, M. A. (1979). Transmission cycles and the heterogenicity of *Trypanosoma cruzi.* p. 117–196. In *Biology of the Kinetoplastidae*, Vol. 2, (ed. W. H. R. Lumsden and D. A. Evans) pp. 117–96. Academic Press, London.

Miles, M. A. and Rouse, J. E. (1970). Chagas' disease (South American Trypanosomiasis). A bibliography. *Tropical Diseases Bulletin* (Supplement), **67**.

Minter, D. M. (1977). Triatomine bugs and household ecology. *Royal Society for Tropical Medicine and Hygiene Medical Entomology Centenary Proceedings*, pp. 85–93.

Oliveira Filho, A. M. (1984). New alternatives for Chagas' disease control. *Memories do Instituto Oswalds Cruz*, **79**, (suppl), 117–23.

Prata, A. (1981). Carlos Chagas. Coletânea de Trabalhos Científicos. *Coleção Temas Brasileiros*, No. 6, Fundação Universidade de Brasília, Brasil.

Prata, A. and Sant' Anna. E. P. (1983). Bibliografia Brasileira sobre Doença de Chagas (1909–1979). *Coleção Temas Brasileiros*, No. 55. Fundação Universidade de Brasília, Brasil.

Rabinovitch, J. E., Wisniversky Colli, C., Solarz, N. D., and Guntler, R. E. (1990). Probability of transmission of Chagas' disease by *Triatoma infestans* (Hemiptera, Reduviidae) in an endemic area of Santiago del Estero Argentina. *Bulletin of the World Health Organization*, **68**, 737–46.

Rocha D, Silva, E. O., Guarita, O. F., and Ishihata, G. K. (1979). Doença de Chagas: atividades de controle dos transmissores no Estado de São Paulo, Brasil. *Revista Brasileira de Malariologia e Doencas Tropical*, **31**, 99–119.

Romana, C. (1968). *Enfermedad de Chagas*. Lopes Libreros, Buenos Aires.

Schofield, C. J. (1979). The behaviour of Triatominae (Hemiptera, Reduviidae). A review. *Bulletin of Entamological Research*, **69**, 363–79.

Schofield, C. J. (1985). Control of Chagas' disease vectors. *British Medical Bulletin*, **41**, 189–94.

Schofield, C. J. (1994). Triatominae biology and control. *Eurocommunica*, p. 76.

Schofield, C. J. and Dias, J. C. P. (1991). A cost benefit analysis of Chagas' disease control. *Memories de Instituto Oswalds Cruz*, **86**, 285–95.

Silveria, A. C. and Rezende, D. F. (1994). Epidemiologia e controle da transmissão vetorial da doença de Chagas no Brasil. *Revista da Sociedade Brasileira de Medicina Tropical*, **27**, (Suppl. III), 11–22.

World Health Organization (1991). *Control of Chagas' disease*. Technical Report Series No. 811, p. 95. WHO, Geneva.

Zeledon, R. (1981). Triatoma dimidiata. Universidade San José, Costa Rican.

43   THE LEISHMANIASES

R. W. Ashford

SUMMARY

The leishmaniases are a complex group of diseases ranging from the simple cutaneous lesions of oriental sore which self-cure, to the potentially fatal visceral leishmaniasis known as kala-azar and grossly disfiguring espundia which may erode the mucous membranes, destroying much of the patient's face. Although all the parasites have similar life cycles and are difficult to distinguish morphologically, they belong to more than 20 species, each with its own distinctive ecological requirements, vector, and reservoir hosts. More than 100 countries are affected and the 400 000 cases reported annually are a small proportion of those occurring.

Reservoir systems vary from purely anthroponotic to purely zoonotic, and illustrate almost every variety in between. Mammal reservoir hosts belong to the marsupalia, edentata, carnivora, hyracoidea, and rodentia, maintaining sylvatic zoonotic foci in the deserts of Africa and Asia, the forests of South and Central America, as well as synanthropic foci in the Mediterranean basin and much of South America.

Although the known vectors are all phlebotomine sandflies, these have a wide range of specific habits and habitats. The complexity of this group of infections has only recently been appreciated and is still being worked out. Control measures will depend on a detailed qualitative description of each focus separately and it is unlikely that any general guidelines will be widely applicable.

HISTORY

DISCOVERY OF THE DISEASES

While it may be that some of the biblical plagues refer to leishmaniasis, the earliest clear reference to cutaneous leishmaniasis or oriental sore is by Ibn Sina (Avicenna) who wrote of Balkh sore. To this day, the people of Balkh Province in northern Afghanistan suffer annual outbreaks of oriental sore caused by *Leishmania major*. Other cities of west and central Asia: Delhi, Sart, Kandahar, and Aleppo, and colonial outposts in North Africa: Biskra, Gafsa, and Mil (commonly misinterpreted as Nil), have given their names to the disease.

The earliest records of visceral leishmaniasis are possibly those of the fever epidemic in Bengal, which started around 1824 at Jessore and spread to Burdwan by 1865. The Dum-Dum military camp in the suburbs of Calcutta became notorious for this disease and, as it spread into Assam with the opening of trade routes and tea plantations it became known as British Government Disease. Early references to kala-azar in Ceylon relate to an alternative spelling for Shillong in Assam, not to Sri Lanka. The disease in India was known as kala-azar which may be equated with 'black fever' and was thought throughout the nineteenth century to be either hookworm disease or a particularly malignant form of malaria. The latter mistake was 'confirmed' by both Rogers and Ross, leaders of early tropical medicine, who thereby contributed to the low priority which has been attributed to leishmaniasis ever since.

Meanwhile, in the Mediterranean basin infantile visceral leishmaniasis was known as infantile splenomegalic anaemia.

Early records of cutaneous and mucocutaneous leishmaniasis (espundia) in the Americas are difficult to identify, though the pre-Columban *huacos*, pottery jugs made as burial offerings by the Mochica people of Peru, commonly in the form of erotic or pathological figurines, occasionally show lesions resembling those of both cutaneous and mucocutaneous leishmaniasis. The latter disease was well described by the earliest European invaders.

DISCOVERY OF THE ORGANISM

In the first few years of the twentieth century, in a rush of discovery, it was found that this diverse set of diseases, oriental sore, kala-azar, infantile splenomegaly, and espundia, were all caused by indistinguishable organisms. During the same period Nicolle, working in Tunis, found dogs to be infected with similar parasites, and postulated the zoonotic origin of infantile kala-azar. As the human diseases already had adequate vernacular names, the term leishmaniasis (*leishmaniose canin*) was initially applied only to the canine disease and only became widely used for the human diseases in the 1930s.

PATHOLOGY AND PATHOGENESIS

The taxonomic difficulties have delayed understanding of the pathology and pathogenesis. Early descriptions generally assumed that a given pathological presentation was caused by a given parasite species and vice versa, that a given parasite caused a given disease. Only recently have the tools of molecular biochemistry and genetics become available to allow an understanding of the spectrum of disease caused by each parasite. One important feature, only recently demonstrated, is that many infections cause no detectable disease or, alternatively, only cause disease after a delay of many years. The facility with which most *Leishmania* species can be maintained in culture or in laboratory animals has encouraged much work on leishmaniasis in unnatural hosts such as the golden hamster or domestic mouse. For these reasons much of the early comparative pathology, as well as more recent studies, are of limited significance; these are areas for current and future research.

EPIDEMIOLOGY AND TRANSMISSION

Epidemiological study was hampered by the similarity between the parasites in their various mammalian hosts and vectors, and in culture. As early as 1915, Yakimov used morphological and epidemiological evidence to distinguish urban anthroponotic cutaneous leishmaniasis from the rural, zoonotic form in central Asia, but this was an isolated and remarkable work. Adler developed a serological agglutination test which was of some value in distinguishing species, and some of the South American forms could be distinguished by their behaviour in culture and in vectors, but it was not till the 1970s that Chance and his colleagues developed biochemical markers which could reliably describe and identify large numbers of strains. The classification of the numerous species which have subsequently been described and our understanding of the relationships between parasite identity, clinical presentation, and ecology depends greatly on the isoenzyme markers developed by these workers. Probes using monoclonal antibodies or specific DNA sequences, with or without PCR amplification, are currently of value in identification but not for classification.

Throughout the history of the leishmaniases the problem of vector incrimination has been exacerbated by the difficulty of rearing phlebotomine sandflies. The first successful transmission experiments were in 1931 and human transmission was not achieved till 1941. To this day, laboratory transmission remains difficult, due mainly to the unexplained tendency of female sandflies to die during their first oviposition. The other outstanding question regarding sandflies is that of their breeding sites. Though Grassi, in the nineteenth century did discover larvae and pupae in drains in Rome, the early stages have only very rarely been found. Without this information it is impossible to determine the factors defining the geographical or ecological distribution of the various vectors and, therefore, of the diseases.

CONTROL

Even before the organisms had been recognized, measures were taken on an empirical basis to attempt to control the devastating plagues of visceral leishmaniasis in the north-east Indian provinces of Bengal and Assam. Control depended largely on the burning of homes and the resettlement of labourers.

In much of India, visceral leishmaniasis almost disappeared following the widespread use of insecticides for malaria control; in the Mediterranean basin infantile visceral leishmaniasis became very rare around the same time. While the malaria campaigns no doubt had a major effect, the enormous post-war increase in living standards, especially in the Mediterranean countries, probably contributed significantly.

The major attempts to control cutaneous leishmaniasis were in the USSR. *Leishmania tropica* infection was eradicated in Azerbaijan by a combination of insecticide application in houses and treatment of patients; military and scientific expeditions to areas of Turkmenia, Uzbekistan, and Khasakstan where zoonotic *L. major* occurs were protected by deliberate inoculation of viable parasites; Soviet health engineers redesigned the million-hectare Karshi Steppe irrigation scheme such that when the reservoir hosts for cutaneous leishmaniasis *Rhombomys opimus* had been eradicated within the scheme they could not re-invade (WHO 1986). In China a concerted effort to eliminate infected dogs, combined with insecticide application, led to the almost complete control of visceral leishmaniasis.

These examples show how control has sometimes been purely serendipitous and sometimes based on detailed knowledge of the natural history of the infection. More entensive reviews of leishmaniasis can be found in Rioux (1977), and Molyneux and Ashford (1983), Chang and Bray (1985), Peters and Killick-Kendrick (1987), Hart (1989), Killick-Kendrick (1990), Rioux *et al.* (1990a,b), Dedet (1992), Liew and O'Donnell (1993).

TREATMENT

Treatment depended on arsenicals and tartar emetic until the effectiveness of pentavalent antimony compounds was discovered in the 1920s. These last remain the treatment of choice, though recent developments give hope for new drugs or formulations and improved delivery. Treatment of domestic dogs still requires to be repeated frequently and does not usually lead to cure; canine leishmaniasis remains a mainstay of the veterinary profession in much of southern Europe.

THE AGENT

TAXONOMY

The genus *Leishmania* belongs to the protozoan flagellate family Trypanosomatidae, other members of which include monoxenous parasites of invertebrates (*Leptomonas, Crithidia, Herpetomonas, Blastocrithidia*), heteroxenous parasites of plants and insects (*Phytomonas*), and parasites of vertebrates transmitted by a wide range of haematophagous invertebrates (*Trypanosoma, Endotrypanum, Sauroleishmania*) (WHO 1984; Rioux 1986; Grimaldi *et al.* 1989; Rioux *et al.* 1990b). All known *Leishmania* species are parasites of the reticuloendothelial cells of mammals and are transmitted by the bite of phlebotomine sandflies of the genera *Phlebotomus* or *Lutzomyia*.

A comprehensive and closely argued classification of the genus is given by Lainson and Shaw (1987). These authors listed two subgenera, 22 named species, and 24 probable species which were unnamed. The species were mostly grouped in four complexes which, though they had no taxonomic validity, were held to be useful.

In a field where many workers are making new discoveries it is not to be expected that any such classification would be universally accepted or that it would remain stable. Nevertheless, it forms a valuable framework for further developments.

Fortunately, it is possible to simplify the system considerably for most practical purposes: the subgenera and complexes can be conveniently ignored, lesser-known forms can be grouped with named species, and subspecific categories can be used for closely related forms which show consistent biological differences and have allopatric distributions.

As will be seen, the different species may cause various disease spectra and the different diseases can be caused by various species of *Leishmania*. From the clinical point of view the new taxonomy is almost as confusing as it is useful. It is the ecological and therefore public health and control aspects of the leishmaniases which correlate well with the taxonomy

LIFE CYCLE

All *Leishmania* species have basically similar life cycles (Fig. 43.1) and are morphologically difficult to distinguish. In the mammal host the parasites are spherical or fusiform bodies between 2 and 5 μm in length, termed amastigotes. In the phlebotomine sandfly they become elongate, motile, flagellate bodies termed promastigotes. Both amastigotes and promastigotes divide repeatedly by longitudinal binary fission. Transmission depends on the uptake of amastigotes by a feeding sandfly and their inoculation to a new host at a subsequent meal.

Amastigotes contain two concentrations of DNA, in the nucleus and in a modified mitochondrion, the kinetoplast. A rudimentary flagellum occupies an indentation of the surface, the flagellar pocket. Amastigotes are intracellular, and are restricted to cells of the macrophage-monocyte series. Disruption of the host cell, which may contain as many as 50 organisms allows the parasites to be phagocytosed, thereby infecting new cells. Infected cells may be restricted to the dermis, where they may or may not be restricted to a discrete lesion. Alternatively, they may circulate throughout the body in lymph or blood, and infect the spleen, liver, bone marrow, lymph nodes, or mucosa. In these organs they are distributed throughout, not restricted to discrete lesions. Restriction to the skin may be explained in part by the temperature sensitivity of certain species.

On being ingested by a sandfly and released from the host cell the amastigotes continue to divide, at the same time elongating, and the flagellum extends greatly. These motile promastigotes divide repeatedly in the mid-gut of the sandfly as the blood meal is digested. After a series of morphological, behavioural, and biochemical changes they congregate in the cardiac valve, where the chitinous foregut projects into the midgut. The attachment of hundreds of parasites in this area impedes ingestion of a subsequent blood meal. A possibly distinct series of parasites become free-swimming infective forms with short bodies and long flagellae. These metacyclic promastigotes may enter the foregut and mouthparts, and are inoculated into a new mammalian host when the sandfly next feeds on blood.

In the subgenus *L. (Leishmania)* the parasites penetrate the peritrophic membrane surrounding the blood meal, and become attached to the microvilli of the enterocytes by insertion of their flagellae. In this way they are not expelled when the sandfly defecates.

In the subgenus *L. (Viannia)* promastigotes do not attach in the midgut, but invade the hindgut where they attach to the cuticular lining of the pyloric valve during defecation. Then they are thought to migrate forward to become attached to the cardiac valve.

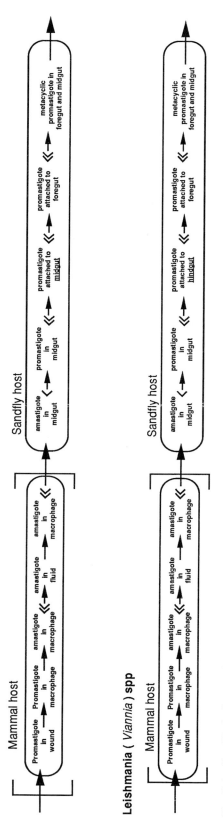

Fig. 43.1 Simplified schematic life history of *Leishmania*. →, Transformation or change of habitat; ⇢, change of host; [ ], host within brackets is eaten by that outside; <, division. (Style of diagram based on that of Combes 1995.)

MOLECULAR BIOLOGY

Molecular biochemical and genetic methods were first applied to the taxonomy of the genus *Leishmania* in the 1970s as described above. The main method which emerged as correlating with known biological features was that of isoenzyme analysis, and this remains the method of choice for the classification of these organisms.

While analysis of isoenzyme results by various techniques of purely numerical or cladistic cluster analysis is essential for the elaboration and maintenance of a useful classification, methods of nucleic acid and monoclonal antibody analysis have proved useful where simple identification is required.

Pulse–field gel electrophoresis shows a group of minichromosomes whose configuration is extremely labile: considerable variation occurs within isoenzymatically and biologically homogeneous groups of strains, even where these are sympatric. The same is true of restriction length fragment polymorphisms (RFLP), which have the potential for the detailed study of population genetics. For instance, a study of numerous stocks of parasites from visceral leishmaniasis of humans and dogs in South America showed astonishing RFLP uniformity, which indicates their recent common origin, supporting the supposition that the parasites were introduced in post-Columban times. A classification based on RFLP results agreed closely with those based on isoenzymes (Beverley *et al.* 1987).

The analysis of DNA fragments amplified by the polymerase chain reaction has allowed the detection and identification of parasites under difficult circumstances and in minute numbers. Isolation of cultured stocks in the field may be impossible in conditions where a 'squash blot' of tissue or of a sandfly, on cellulose paper may suffice to provide a specimen for identification.

While the qualitative description of the structure of leishmaniasis foci still depends on isoenzyme analysis of isolated strains from vertebrate and vector hosts, once the natural history is firmly established, newer methods become applicable for quantitative study.

The important question of cryptic or asymptomatic infection, which may last for many years but is poorly understood, will certainly benefit from the application of PCR techniques, as will other aspects of the 'spectral' pathology of leishmaniasis.

DISEASE MECHANISMS

There is relatively little direct effect of *Leishmania* parasites on their hosts. In cutaneous leishmaniasis, in the absence of effective immune response, as in diffuse cutaneous leishmaniasis, the parasites multiply in histiocytes in the lesions, forming raised nodules or plaques which, though unsightly and somewhat delicate are not associated with necrosis, toxicity, or other major pathogenic process. Only when effective cell-mediated immune response causes the foci of infected skin to be isolated by adventitious lymphocytes and other cells, is there necrosis of the infected area with ulceration, followed by granuloma formation, scarring, and cure. Cutaneous leishmaniasis is usually followed by long-lasting immunity to subsequent infection.

Even with visceral leishmaniasis much of the disease is caused by the immune response to the parasite. The anaemia may be the result of direct destruction of bone marrow or of spleen function, and the fever may result from toxins released by cells disrupted by the parasite. The splenomegaly and life-threatening cachexia, however, probably result from excessive stimulation of immune responses, especially TNF production. Hyperglobulinaemia is characteristic of visceral leishmaniasis and is a non-protective response, whose function is probably to protect parasites.

Mucocutaneous leishmaniasis is certainly caused by excessive allergic response to the small numbers of parasites present in the affected mucous membranes.

In domestic dogs, visceral leishmaniasis caused by *L. d. infantum* is rather different. An initial cutaneous ulcer some 1 cm diameter may or may not be produced at the site of the infective bite (Vidor *et al.* 1991). Visceralization of the parasites follows but the parasites are concentrated in lymph nodes and bone marrow; there is less sign of splenomegaly. The parasites later invade the skin where they may be very numerous but cause no necrosis or ulceration. The skin becomes dry and hypertrophic; there is considerable depilation which, together with the cachexia gives the appearance of a very sick animal. The dermal hypertrophy is particularly marked in the claws which become excessively elongate, adding to the sorry sight.

Recent evidence shows that dogs may self-cure following early stages of infection but the fully developed disease is fatal and treatment can only delay death.

The various wild animals which are natural hosts to *Leishmania* spp. respond in various ways to infection but, in general, they have mild, long-lasting disease, or show no disease at all. Most studies on the disease mechanisms of the leishmaniasis have been carried out on laboratory mice and golden hamsters, neither of which is a natural host and are, therefore, unlikely to be relevant to the human situation or to that in natural hosts. Experimental infections are surprisingly difficult to reproduce in natural hosts.

Survival of the parasites in the insect host seems to depend not so much on general physiological conditions, as amastigotes can transform to successfully dividing promastigotes under a wide range of conditions, including culture media. The first challenge to survival seems to come when the sandfly voids the digested remains of its blood meal, including any parasites which are not attached to the gut wall. As described above, *L. (Leishmania)* species require to attach to the microvilli of the midgut, especially the narrow thoracic midgut. *L. (Viannia)* species attach to the chitinous lining of the anterior hindgut, especially the so-called hindgut triangle. While attachment to cuticle seems to be fairly non-specific, as it can be mimicked with various plastics and glass, attachment to the microvillar surface possibly depends on a specific match between surface molecules on the flagellum and receptors on the midgut cell surface. It has recently been suggested that this match may be responsible for the host specificity of promastigotes in their insect hosts.

Exposure to various plant lectins promotes specific aggregation of promastigotes. This may be specific even to the stage of development: 'metacyclic' forms do not agglutinate in the presence of PNA as earlier stages do (Sacks and Perkins 1984). It has therefore been suggested that the sugar meal taken by sandflies before or after a blood meal might affect the survival of the parasites. Sugar meals are thought to be obtained from plant sap, extrafloral nectaries, and honeydew secreted by aphids or other plant-sucking insects.

THE HOSTS

HUMAN CUTANEOUS AND MUCOCUTANEOUS LEISHMANIASIS

Ulcerating cutaneous lesions ('Oriental sore') may be caused by all of the *Leishmania* species listed under the following section. The lesions differ in their duration and in their severity, but all are basically similar in their pathology. Those caused by *L. major* are frequently numerous, as many as 150 being recorded in a single patient, while those caused by other species are frequently single. Each lesion is thought to be caused by a single bite or probe of an infected sandfly. The multiplicity of lesions of *L. major* is thought to be due to the blockage of the gut of the vector, causing it to probe many times.

The lesions usually start with an erythematous swelling of the bitten area. This may ulcerate when less than 1 cm in diameter or may grow considerably before ulcerating. A necrotic area at the centre of the lesion becomes ulcerous and the parasites become restricted to the periphery. Subsequently the granulomatous base of the ulcer produces a characteristic scar which lasts for life. Cure of lesions is associated with long-lasting immunity against reinfection with homolo-

gous parasites and with a positive delayed hypersensitivity reaction (leishmanin skin test) against crude antigen from any *Leishmania* species.

Incubation periods vary from probably a few days in *L. major* to a few months in *L. tropica* and *L. d. infantum.* The ulcers of *L. major* generally cure completely in 3 months while those of the other species are more indolent, lasting anything up to 3 years. Serum antibodies are not easily detectable in the Old World species but are useful for confirmation of diagnosis of primary lesions of *L. braziliensis*.

Cutaneous leishmaniasis is generally distinguishable from other ulcers by their general appearance and painlessness but these are far from pathognomonic and diagnosis can only be confirmed by the detection of parasites. Parasites may be seen on Giemsa-stained microscope preparations, or in culture on blood-agar slopes prepared from biopsies or scrapings taken from the edge of a lesion.

The lesions caused by *L. braziliensis*, the African strains of *L. tropica* and *L. aethiopica* tend to be particularly large, indolent and long lasting. The last two forms are frequently very slow to ulcerate.

Leishmania tropica and *L. aethiopica* lesions are notable for the very large numbers of parasites they contain, while in infections with the other species parasites are sometimes difficult to detect. Haematoxylin and eosin (H & E) stained sections of biopsy material are very difficult to interpret but impression smears of a cut surface are useful.

'Leishmaniasis recidivans' is a specific sequel of *L. tropica* infection in which satellite lesions develop at the edges of a healed or healing lesion. This condition sometimes lasts for years, causing extensive disfiguration and scarring.

Pian bois and forest yaws are the names given to lesions caused by *L. guyanensis* when, instead of ulcerating and curing, the parasites spread along the lymphatics, producing linear arrays of nodules which eventually ulcerate and cure.

Chiclero ulcer is a very long-lasting erosion of the pinna of the ear caused when *L. mexicana* lesions occur at that site; *L. mexicana* lesions in other areas may resemble oriental sore or diffuse cutaneous leishmaniasis.

Diffuse cutaneous leishmaniasis (DCL) is caused by *L. mexicana, L. amazonensis,* or *L. aethiopica.* This condition, initially confused with lepromatous leprosy, is associated with a specific immunological anergy: the initial lesion fails to ulcerate or cure and spreads, sometimes over the whole body, in severely disfiguring raised nodules and plaques. These lesions are delicate, but do not ulcerate spontaneously. While treatment may alleviate DCL temporarily, it seems basically incurable. Repeated heat treatment using sauna or hot baths alleviates the condition temporarily.

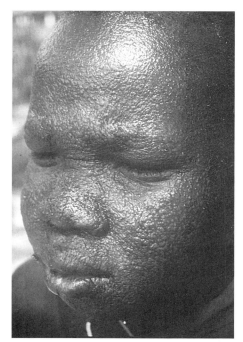

Fig. 43.2 Post kala-azar dermal leishmaniasis appeared in many patients following cure of visceral leishmaniasis in the recent devastating epidemic in southern Sudan.

Combination of chemotherapy with γ-interferon has had some success experimentally.

Post kala-azar dermal leishmaniasis (PKDL) is a frequent sequel of *L. donovani* infection in India and Sudan (Fig. 43.2), but rarely in Kenya. Following cure of the visceral infection, usually with chemotherapy, a mottling of the skin appears, followed by the development of large areas resembling allergic pustular dermatitis. Alternatively, the condition superficially resembles DCL. It can persist for years; reports vary on the ease of detecting parasites, on immunological responses, and the effect of treatment.

Mucocutaneous leishmaniasis (MCL) is occasionally caused by various species of *Leishmania* when primary lesions are on the mucosa, usually of the nose or mouth; more rarely the infection is in the pharynx. This form occurs particularly in Sudan where the causative organisms have not been identified.

Classically, however, mucocutaneous leishmaniasis is caused by *L. braziliensis* and is a sequel to a primary lesion which may have been cured many years previously. If left untreated, the lesion gradually erodes the mucosa and underlying tissues, including cartilage, so that the entire front of the face and soft palate may be destroyed. This condition is usually curable by intensive chemotherapy followed if necessary by reconstructive surgery, but presents a major occupational hazard to people working in endemic forests. In MCL the parasites may be very scanty; diagnosis frequently depends on clinical assessment, serological tests, and leishmanin skin test.

HUMAN VISCERAL LEISHMANIASIS

Kala-azar is the name given in India to the fever caused by *L. donovani* infection. The fever is occasionally preceded by an ulcerating 'eschar' at the site of the infective bite. The proportion of infections which lead to a positive delayed hypersensitivity reaction without fever has been estimated at between 25 and 31 per cent in an epidemic area of southern Sudan (Seaman *et al.* 1992, Zijlstra *et al.* 1994), and around 80 per cent in an endemic area of Ethiopia (Ali and Ashford 1994). Comparable figures are not available for India. The incubation period varies from a few weeks to many years and onset of disease is probably precipitated by external events.

Once the full syndrome has developed, it is thought almost invariably to be fatal if untreated, though the time to death varies from a few weeks to several months.

The condition starts insidiously with intermittent mild fever, classically with twice-daily peaks. The affected individual gradually loses weight, becoming extremely emaciated but with a protuberant abdomen due to the enlarged liver and spleen. The patient becomes progressively weaker and more emaciated and develops bleeding tendency with often persistent diarrhoea and dehydration but feels remarkably well considering his condition. Eventual death is thought usually to be due supervening septicaemic infection.

The principal signs are anaemia with leucopenia and highly raised serum proteins with reversed albumin/globulin ratio, but none of these is pathognomonic. The increased serum proteins are sometimes used in simple diagnostic tests, where a drop of formalin is found to coagulate 1 ml of serum to a solid mass resembling boiled egg-white, but this formal gel test is by no means specific and is only positive at a late stage (Kar 1995). Serological tests are useful from an early stage, especially a direct agglutination test (DAT) which is positive at very high dilutions.

Demonstration of parasites by rapidly executed spleen puncture with a narrow but long needle is widely practised in Africa but rarely in India. Only a minute amount of material is aspirated but this is sufficient to demonstrate parasites in a Giemsa-stained smear or in culture. Bone marrow or lymph node aspirates are also used but are less reliable.

Treatment involves daily injections of pentavalent antimony compounds over a long period, normally 30

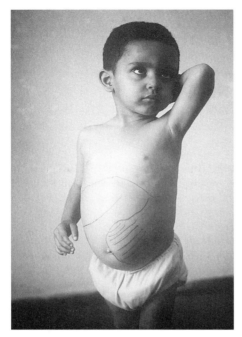

Fig. 43.3 Infantile zoonotic visceral leishmaniasis caused by *L. infantum* in Libya.

days and is usually supported by a rich diet and antibiotics. The diarrhoea may be a problem.

Infantile visceral leishmaniasis (Fig. 43.3) is caused by *L. infantum* (sometimes termed *L. chagasi* in the Americas). Classically this was predominantly a disease of children aged less than 2 years, but in some areas the age profile has changed considerably. The causes of the former restriction to infants and the subsequent changes are unclear, but must have little to do with selective exposure to infection or to acquired immunity: even in areas where transmission among dogs remains intense, and people are frequently bitten by the sandfly vector, human infection is very rare, and still restricted to infants. It seems that, in enzootic areas, people of all ages are frequently exposed to infection; only a small (and declining) fraction of children are susceptible; in addition, a very small (but increasing) proportion of older people are susceptible. The decline in susceptibility of infants may be due to increased living standards, while the increase in susceptibility of adults may be due to immunodepression caused by concomitant HIV infection (Peters *et al.* 1990; Pratlong *et al.* 1995), by transplant surgery, or by chemotherapy for malignant disease. This partly hypothetical account is supported by studies in Brazil which show a clear relation between both age and nutritional status, and susceptibility to disease in the presence of infection (Badaro *et al.* 1986).

The enormous variation in prepatent period is illustrated by the occasional occurrence of visceral leishmaniasis in people who only visited the enzootic areas many years previously.

The disease in children, once fully developed, is fatal if not treated. The pathology and symptomatology are similar to those of *L. donovani* infection but there is less cachexia and more involvement of lymph nodes.

LEISHMANIASIS IN NATURAL RESERVOIR HOSTS

In natural hosts the parasites generally cause little or no detectable disease. In gerbils *Rhombomys opimus* and *Psammomys obesus* only the margins of the ears are affected by *L. major* infection. These are slightly swollen, then become depilated and there is gradual mild erosion of the pinna. *Arvicanthis* spp. and other rodents infected with *L. major* in sub-Saharan Africa show no outward signs of disease, though parasites have been isolated from the viscera rather than the skin. This led some authors to suspect *A. niloticus* as the reservoir host of *L. donovani* in Africa but only in Sudan has this been tentatively confirmed.

Hyraxes in Africa (Fig. 43.4) and sloths in South and Central America are true reservoir hosts of *L. aethiopica*, *L. panamensis*, and *L. guyanensis* but show no external signs. In some studies parasites were isolated from the skin of sloths and, in others, from the viscera.

The forest rodent hosts of *L. mexicana* similarly rarely show any external signs, the parasites being isolated from unaltered skin.

CANINE LEISHMANIASIS

Cutaneous leishmaniasis has occasionally been recorded in dogs, caused by *L. tropica*, *L. major*, and *L. braziliensis*. The lesions are usually few in number

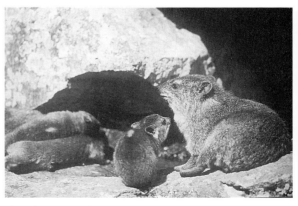

Fig. 43.4 Rock hyrax *Procavia* sp., reservoir host of both *L. aethiopica* and African zoonotic *L. tropica*.

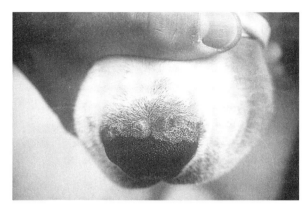

Fig. 43.5 The first sign of canine visceral leishmaniasis caused by *L. infantum* is sometimes a series of inconspicuous cutaneous lesions.

and restricted to the muzzle or ears where sandflies tend to bite. These lesions generally resemble homologous lesions in humans but are of little significance and have not been widely studied.

Of much greater significance is canine leishmaniasis caused by *L. infantum*. A recent experiment in France gives important insight into the early natural history of natural infection (Vidor *et al.* 1991). Among 50 naive male beagles exposed in an area of high transmission, 39 showed signs of infection after one transmission season. The first indication of infection was sometimes a small chancre on the ear or nose which reached almost 1 cm in diameter then cured after a few weeks (Fig. 43.5). Alternatively, serological (ELISA) positivity developed in the absence of any initial chancre. Seropositivity titres generally increased gradually over a period of 2–3 months then either declined below the threshold of positivity or continued to increase. Those dogs which 'cured' serologically during the winter remained healthy until the following transmission season. Those dogs whose serological titre continued to rise became sick and died or were sacrificed in anything from 2 to 12 months. The apparently resistant dogs which became reinfected in the second year were similarly divided in two groups: some recovered a second time and some became progressively sicker. There was no clear correlation between the occurrence of an initial chancre and the eventual outcome.

More generally, canine visceral leishmaniasis is associated with depilation which starts round the eyes as 'spectacles', wasting, lethargy, and lymph node enlargement. The disease may have an insidious onset and progress slowly with regression and relapse, or may proceed rapidly to death.

Diagnosis by serology is specific and sensitive in fully developed cases but can only be confirmed by aspiration of infected material and microscopic examination

of slides or cultures. The popliteal lymph nodes are a useful source of aspirate; alternatively sternal bone marrow may be taken.

Treatment, as with humans, is with pentavalent antimony compounds which, however, do not produce complete cure and may require repetition on at least an annual basis for the remaining life of the dog.

EPIDEMIOLOGY

In 1992 leishmaniasis was known or suspected to occur in 97 countries, with 100 000 visceral cases and 300 000 cases of cutaneous disease reported annually. Only a small proportion of cases are ever reported (Ashford *et al.* 1992a).

One of the main consequences of recent advances in the taxonomy of the genus has been the demonstration that each species of *Leishmania* has distinctive epidemiological features, which may vary geographically with different vectors or reservoir hosts. With reliable and repeatable methods of identification, vectors and reservoir hosts can be accurately associated with given parasites even when several forms are sympatric. One of the many generalizations is that transmission tends to be focalized in both space and time. The complete spectrum of zoonotic systems, from purely animal infection though purely human infection to secondary animal infection in new areas is illustrated by the various *Leishmania* species.

LEISHMANIA DONOVANI DONOVANI INFECTION

Classical kala-azar caused by *L. donovani* infection occurs in northern India, in Bihar and West Bengal and in Bangladesh, where the devastating historical epidemics occurred (Dye and Wolpert 1988). There are probably hundreds of thousands of human cases annually (77000 officially reported in Bihar State in 1993) but only a small proportion are officially recorded. When the disease reappeared in Bihar State around 1980 after a 30-year period of almost complete absence, epidemic conditions involved around six cases per 1000 population per year in some villages. The epidemics of the late nineteenth century were much more severe. The disappearance of the disease from India in the 1950s has been attributed to a side-effect of malaria control activities and its reappearance to the cessation of these activities.

The disease is largely restricted to the flood plains of the Ganges and Brahmaputra but extends into the southern lowlands of Nepal. In this area the vector, *P. argentipes* is a strictly synanthropic species; it is rarely found more than a few metres from a homestead. Unlike almost all other sandflies, its larval requirements are quite well known and it has frequently been found breeding in the accumulated straw and manure in the cattle byres which adjoin many village houses.

In India this parasite is thought not to be zoonotic. The human cases can generally be explained by anthroponotic transmission; cattle which are the preferred blood-meal source for *P. argentipes*, are not susceptible, and blood-meal analysis shows that dogs, which may be susceptible, are rarely bitten by this sandfly species.

People of all ages are susceptible and there is little evidence of infection without disease. However, epidemics have been associated with natural disaster and with population movement so, as with related diseases, susceptibility may be increased by physiological stress such as undernutrition.

The parasites causing visceral leishmaniasis in Kenya, Ethiopia, and Sudan are very similar to *L. donovani* of India and it may be reasonably be postulated that they were taken to India from East Africa early in the nineteenth century (Seaman *et al.* 1992). In East Africa there are foci where the disease is endemic and where a large proportion of infections lead to fleeting self-curing disease or none at all. Such foci have been described in southern Ethiopia and northern Kenya. Elsewhere in Kenya and in southern Sudan, foci tend to be unstable and epidemics occur. While those in Kenya have been relatively mild, with an incidence around 10 per 1000 per year over a 5-year period, some of the Sudanese epidemics have been far more intense. It is estimated that in around 5 years, between 1988 and 1993, more than half the population died in an area some 100 km diameter—a total of perhaps 250 000 people (Ashford *et al.* 1992c, Seaman *et al.* 1992).

In the southern parts of its East African range, *L. donovani* is transmitted by *Phlebotomus martini* and is

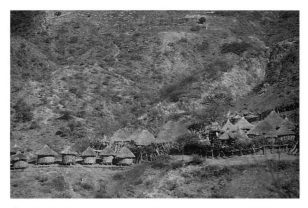

Fig. 43.6 Konso, southern Ethiopia, habitat of *Phlebotomus martini* and endemic visceral leishmaniasis.

restricted to semi-arid areas of laterite clays, characterized by large termitaria in which the flies rest (Fig. 4 3 .6). Further north, *P. orientalis* is the vector. This species is associated with mixed woodland of *Acacia seyal* and *Balanites aegyptiaca* on alluvial silty soils, mainly of the Niles and their tributaries. Both these vectors are strongly seasonal as well as being ecologically restricted, so transmission is also seasonal.

Despite extensive searches there is limited information on reservoir hosts. A small number of dogs were found infected in Kenya, and in Sudan up to 4 per cent of the Nile grass rat *Arvicanthis niloticus* were infected. Unfortunately, the latter study predated modern methods of identification and there is some doubt about the identity of the parasites.

East African kala-azar does, however, probably have some zoonotic source. While epidemics must be anthroponotic there are certain sparsely inhabited areas, for instance Dinder National Park in Sudan and the Segen River Valley in Ethiopia, where access during the sandfly season is associated with a high risk of infection.

Post kala-azar dermal leishmaniasis (PKDL)

In both India and East Africa a varying proportion of human cases develop diffuse infection of the dermis following cure. This may resemble an extensive allergic rash in which parasites may be sparse or numerous. The condition may last for years and is thought to provide a reservoir of infection between epidemic periods (Addy and Nandy 1992).

LEISHMANIA DONOVANI INFANTUM INFECTION

Parasites termed *L. infantum* are very close to *L. donovani* but are consistently distinguishable by certain isoenzyme patterns and generally have very different ecological features. (Fig. 43.7) *Leishmania infantum* is widely distributed in the Mediterranean basin, both in southern Europe and North Africa, as well as West Africa. The distribution includes southern Saudi Arabia and Yemen and extends through Iraq, Iran, and Pakistan to north-west India. Foci in the deserts of Central Asia are now largely inactive and the disease is almost completely controlled in China where it was a major problem until the 1950s. Visceralizing leishmaniasis is widely distributed in South and Central America where the parasites are not readily distinguishable from *L. infantum*, though some authors use the name *L. chagasi*.

Human infection is nowhere common and the disease is classically restricted to children aged 2 years or less. In southern Europe, where it has become even less common, the age distribution has also changed and adult cases are now the majority. The restriction of

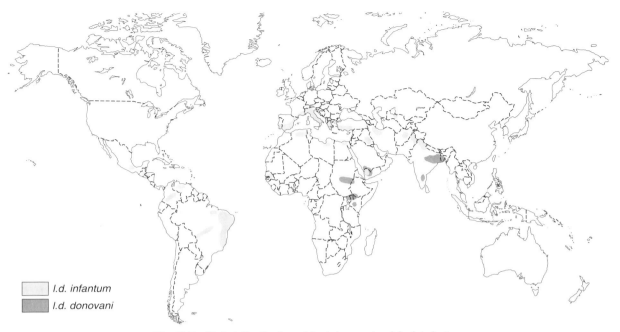

Fig. 43.7   Global distribution of *L. d. donovani* and *L. d. infantum.*

the disease to young children must be due to the innate resistance of adults; the vast majority of healthy children must also be naturally resistant as even in areas of intense transmission human cases are extremely rare. In Brazil undernourished children are particularly susceptible; many otherwise healthy children develop serological changes indicating infection, but develop little or no disease. The increase in adult cases in recent years is associated with HIV infection which may reactivate latent infection or promote susceptibility to new infection. The fact that most HIV *L. infantum* co-infection is in drug abusers raises the question of possible needle transmission (Peters *et al.* 1990; Altes *et al.* 1991).

In many parts of its range, particular strains of *L. infantum* cause a simple cutaneous lesion resembling that of *L. tropica*. HIV infection sometimes causes these dermotropic strains to visceralize. PKDL is unknown in *L. infantum* infection.

The ecological distribution of *L. infantum* infection is closely associated with the distribution of the vector sandflies. *Phlebotomus ariasi* in south-west France is concentrated in mixed oakwoods of *Quercus ilex* and deciduous *Quercus* species, which occur mainly between 300 m and 800 m above sea-level; in this region transmission is therefore concentrated at this level. *Phlebotomus perniciosus* is more widespread, in more arid regions mainly with natural or artificial outcrops of limestone. This explains the transmission of *L. infantum* in much of southern Europe and North

Africa, where it is concentrated in suburbs and villages close to the coast, with dry stone walls and terraces frequently protecting olive or fig trees. Other Mediterranean vectors such as *P. major* are less well known but no doubt each has its own story. The vector throughout South America is *Lutzomyia longipalpis*, chiefly known as a synanthropic species in semi-arid areas. *Leishmania infantum* in South America is concentrated in the degraded lands of north-east Brazil.

There is no evidence that *L. infantum* is transmitted from man to man. The predominant reservoir host is the domestic dog and transmission among dogs may be very intense. The experiment, described above, in southern France, where 50 naive beagles were held in open-air pens for 2 years, showed that many dogs self-cure but are not then resistant to reinfection. More than 20 per cent of dogs in highly enzootic areas may be seropositive at any one time, and in some places it is very difficult to maintain dog populations.

Leishmania infantum has been isolated from many species of wild canid, rats, and opossums. The role of these animals in maintaining the parasite supra-populations is controversial. Generally, carnivores live at densities which are too low for the maintenance of parasites transmitted by free-flying vectors. On Marajao Island in Brazil, a large proportion of the foxes *Cerdocyon thous* are infected but, even there, it seems probable that it is the foxes which visit farmyards with infected dogs and *L. longipalpis* which become

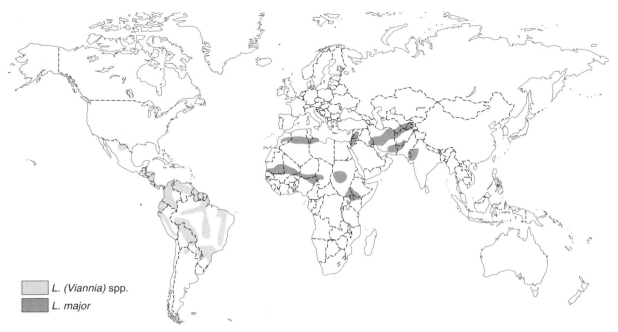

L. *(Viannia)* spp.

L. *major*

Fig. 43.8 Global distribution of *L. major* and *L. (Viannia)* spp.

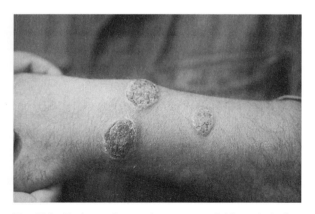

Fig. 43.9 Lesions of zoonotic cutaneous leishmaniasis due to *L. major* are commonly multiple and disabling, but usually cure within 3 months.

infected. Circumstantial evidence has been presented in favour of various other reservoir host systems but none of these is fully substantiated.

LEISHMANIA MAJOR INFECTION

Leishmania major occurs over a wide geographical area from central Asia to Morocco, extending south to sub-Saharan Africa (Fig. 43.8). Throughout this range it occurs in sparsely or newly inhabited areas in arid but hot desert bioclimatic zones of the Saharo-Sindian,

Irano-Turanian, and Sahelian belts also known as the Triad Zone. This relatively uniform ecological range is reflected by the small variety of closely related sandflies, *P. papatasi*, *P. duboscqi*, and *P. salehi* which are known as vectors.

The human disease (Fig. 43.9) is characteristically epidemic, sometimes with thousands of construction workers or agricultural labourers becoming infected simultaneously. Many programmes designed to develop arid areas have been severely disrupted by these epidemics of cutaneous leishmaniasis. The few people resident in these areas are usually infected at an early age and are not seriously affected.

In central Asia in north-eastern Iran, northern Afghanistan, Uzbekistan, and Turkmenia the disease occurs where the distribution of *P. papatasi* coincides with that of the chief reservoir host, the great gerbil *Rhombomys opimus*. In the same area, but extending further north, *R. opimus* is infected with another species, *L. turanica* which rarely, if ever, infects humans and is transmitted by sandflies of another subgenus, *P. (Paraphlebotomus)* spp. A third species, *L. gerbilli*, infects *R. opimus* but not humans in Mongolia and western China.

Great gerbils live in colonies, in extensive burrow systems which persist for centuries and provide uniform temperature and humidity in these regions of extreme climate. This provides an ideal habitat for the sandflies also. These colonies are most highly developed in areas of loess deposits on alluvial fans; the risk of human infection is thereby concentrated according to landscape features.

Elsewhere in Asia, including north-eastern India, other gerbils, *Meriones lybicus* and *M. hurrianae*, maintain the parasite. These have less specific habitat requirements and their populations fluctuate greatly. The foci maintained by *Meriones* spp. tend to be unstable as a result.

Another well-characterized situation occurs in west Asia and north Africa and has been described in Syria, Jordan, Saudi Arabia, Israel, Palestine, Sinai, Libya, Tunisia, and Algeria. Here the main reservoir host is another gerbil, the fat sand rat, *Psammomys obesus*, which is dependent on halophilic succulent plants of the family Chenopodiaceae. The rodent, and therefore the infection, are restricted to areas of salt-flat vegetation, usually in alluvial depressions. These are precisely the areas most suitable for modern irrigation schemes, many of which have been seriously affected. *Psammomys obesus* is also the host of *L. arabica* which has not been found in humans.

Elsewhere in North Africa outbreaks have occurred in areas with no *P. obesus*; in at least one of these *Meriones shawi* was the source of the outbreak.

In sub-Saharan Africa the picture is more complicated. The human disease is widespread in Mali, Niger, Nigeria, and Sudan, and coincides with the distribution of *P. duboscqi*, the proven vector. Parasites have been isolated from the viscera of rodents, including *Arvicanthis* spp., *Tatera* spp., and *Mastomys* sp. Most of these isolations were made in Senegal where there are occasional outbreaks of human disease and in Kenya where human infection is extremely rare.

The source of an outbreak which occurred in the city and suburbs of Khartoum in the late 1980s remains to be explained. It has been suggested that displaced people from endemic areas in the west of the country brought it with them. This would imply anthroponotic transmission, which is unsuspected elsewhere for *L. major*.

LEISHMANIA TROPICA INFECTION

Leishmania tropica is much less widely distributed than was originally thought, being largely restricted to the densely populated cities of central and west Asia from north-western India to Syria. Outposts in Azerbaijan have been eradicated and most cutaneous leishmaniasis in southern Europe and north Africa is now known to be caused by variants of *L. infantum* or *L. major*. On the other hand, it is now thought that certain apparently zoonotic parasites from Tunisia, Kenya, and Namibia are sufficiently close to *L. tropica* to be possibly included in that species. The Tunisian form has been called *L. killicki*.

The vector of urban *L. tropica* is *P. sergenti* which can be highly synanthropic but can also occur far from human habitation. The lesion caused by *L. tropica* contains abundant parasites close to the surface but it has been estimated that around 50 sandfly bites per person per night during the sandfly season are required to maintain a stable endemic (Ashford *et al.* 1992b). This is rarely achieved, and more commonly the infection moves in epidemics between suburbs or between cities, as cohorts of non-immune young people join the population. Alternatively, a high rate of immigration and emigration may maintain sufficient non-immunes to produce a semblance of endemic stability. Transmission is predominantly in densely populated outskirts of cities, whether in old houses or new housing estates.

There is no evidence that *L. tropica* in Asia depends on zoonotic sources. Domestic dogs have been found infected in India, Afghanistan, and Iran but the density of infected dogs is far less than that of humans and it is more likely that humans are the source of canine infection.

Since human *L. tropica* infection lasts, on average, 1 year and leads to protective immunity, point prevalence approximates annual incidence; in a stable population even with low annual incidence, immunity will develop in most individuals and only newcomers, by birth or immigration, will be susceptible. In the absence of immigration not more than around 6 per cent of people can be infected annually over a long period.

The parasites resembling *L. tropica* which have been found in Africa (Tunisia, Kenya, Namibia) have been from isolated rural areas and have been associated with shifting human populations among whom incidence was sometimes much higher than 6 per cent annually. In Namibia and Kenya similar parasites have been isolated from rock hyraxes, *Procavia* spp., and in Tunisia they have been tentatively identified from the gundi, *Ctenodactylus gundi*, a rodent which is ecologically similar to a hyrax. This appears to be a phylogenetically compact group of parasites with a wide geographical range which illustrates the remote origin of the anthroponotic forms in the cities of Asia.

Extraordinary cases of visceral leishmeniasis putatively caused by *L. tropica* were recorded in Desert Storm veterans. These require to be confirmed and explained (Magill *et al.* 1993).

LEISHMANIA AETHIOPICA INFECTION

Leishmania aethiopica is only known from the highlands of Ethiopia and Kenya (Fig. 43.10), in both of which countries human infection (Fig. 43.11) is focalized and

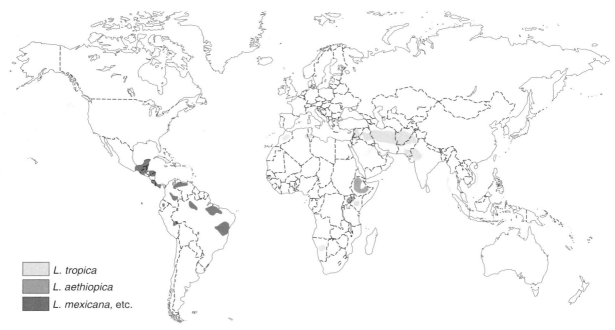

Fig. 43.10   Global distribution of *L. tropica*, *L. aethiopica*, and *L. mexicana* etc.

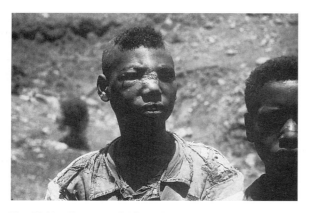

Fig. 43.11   Cutaneous leishmaniasis caused by *L. aethiopica* is sometimes very slow to ulcerate and cure.

generally uncommon. The altitudinal range of the parasite, between about 1500 and 2700 metres above sea-level seems to be determined by that of the two sandfly vectors, *P. longipes* and *P. pedifer*. The sandflies have wide habitat ranges, living in tree holes, rock crevices, and houses, where they feed preferentially on cattle. Within the requisite altitude, the parasite is limited to habitats shared by one or other vector and the reservoir hosts which are rock hyraxes *Procavia* spp., the 'bush' hyrax, *Heterohyrax brucei*, and the tree hyrax, *Dendrohyrax* sp. (The taxonomy of these ancient paenungulate mammals is in hopeless confusion: authors

list anything between four and 50 or so species!) These animals are gregarious herbivores living in rocks or trees which provide the deep crevices they require for shelter. Their faeces accumulate in latrines which probably provide the organic matter required for the sandflies to breed. People are at special risk of infection if they live close to hyrax colonies, though infection can be transmitted as far as 1 km from the nearest colony, due to the considerable flight range of the vector.

LEISHMANIA MEXICANA, L. AMAZONENSIS, ETC.

There are many parasites close to *L. mexicana* with disjunct geographical distributions and causing various clinical disease. However, as far as is known, all these forms share somewhat similar ecological requirements and are transmitted by closely related sandfly species. Human infection is everywhere sporadic and generally uncommon but has been recorded in most territories from southern Mexico to southern Brazil, with outlying populations in Trinidad and the Dominican Republic. Transmission is characteristically in areas of secondary forest and woodland, where *Lutzomyia flaviscutellata* or close relatives of this species are vectors. The list of recorded natural hosts of this group of species is long and includes many orders of mammal. However, ground-dwelling forest rodents of the genera *Ototylomys* (*L. mexicana*, Belize) and *Proechimys* (*L. amazonensis*, Brazil; *Leishmania* sp., Trinidad) seem to be

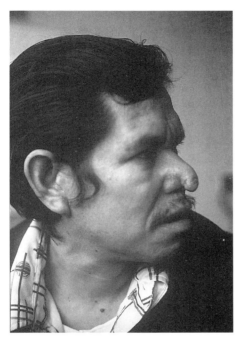

Fig. 43.12 Disfiguring mucocutaneous leishmaniasis due to *L. braziliensis* is a major occupational hazard for migrant workers in the upper Amazon basin. The reservoir host is unknown.

the most important hosts. In a few areas, notably the Dominican Republic, only human cases are known, but even there it is likely that the infection is zoonotic. Other related *Leishmania* species are known only from animals, notably the distinctive *L. hertigi* from the porcupines *Coendou* spp.

LEISHMANIA PANAMENSIS AND L. GUYANENSIS

These parasites are mainly found in Panama and the Guyanas, extending to Brazil but not south of the Amazon. The main hosts of both parasites are sloths, *Choloepus didactylus* and *C. hoffmanni*, both of which are specialized arboreal folivores whose preferred food is *Cecropia* spp. *Cecropia* trees grow in mature secondary forest and forest edges. The vectors are *Lu. umbratilis* for *L. guyanensis* and probably mainly *Lu. trapidoi* for *L. panamensis*. The former vector seems to be a specialized canopy feeder, resting during the day in sheltered buttresses close to ground level, but migrating to the canopy at night to feed. This specialization, along with the facts that sloths are long-lived and that the parasites persist in healthy skin, combine to allow persistence of the parasite population despite the low density of the host (4/ha is normal). Various other mammals have been found to be infected but are not thought to

play an important role in the maintenance of parasite suprapopulations.

LEISHMANIA BRAZILIENSIS AND L. PERUVIANA

Leishmania braziliensis is a heterogeneous species with many local variants, widely distributed, mainly in primary forest areas of Brazil and surrounding countries, including Bolivia, Ecuador, and Colombia. *Leishmania peruviana* is closely similar, but has very different ecology, being distributed in the high arid valleys of the western slopes of the Andes of Peru and probably Ecuador. Stocks isolated from the northern limits of *L. peruviana*, in the wetter, forested highlands of Ecuador are difficult to distinguish from *L. braziliensis*.

Throughout their range both species are probably at least partially zoonotic; *L. braziliensis* has been isolated from a few wild mammals and both species from domestic dogs but the primary reservoir hosts remain unknown. The altitudinal range of vectors of *L. peruviana*, *Lu. verrucarum*, and *Lu. peruensis* is coincident of that of the human infection, between 500 and 2800 above sea-level. The vectors of *L. braziliensis* are less well known; *Lu. (Psychodopygus) wellcomei* is fully incriminated in Serra dos Carajas, Brazil, but is much less widely distributed than the parasite. Other putative vectors include species of *Lu. (Nyssomyia)* and *Lu. (Psychodopygus)*.

Considering that *L. braziliensis* causes severely disfiguring disease (Fig. 43.12) it is surprising that its ecology remains so poorly known. This is partly due to the difficulty of growing the parasites in culture.

Human infection is associated with life in the rain forest, where miners, settlers, and military expeditions are affected. Indigenous people are much less severely affected, possibly because they are infected mildly at an early age, but they may be seriously affected if they move from their native lands.

PREVENTION AND CONTROL

The World Bank, UNDP, WHO Special Programme for Tropical Diseases has highlighted the public health importance of the leishmaniasis but this is still not fully recognized by national health services in many endemic nations. This is in part due to the focality of the diseases in both space and time and also to their generally rural distribution. Increasing health expectations among rural people, as well as improvements in potential control measures, are changing this attitude.

Prevention and control depend on the collection and maintenance of good records. In many countries this is the responsibility of malaria departments eager to diversify their activities in the aftermath of failed malaria eradication programmes. Because of the diverse expertise required for leishmaniasis control, WHO (1990) has recommended the establishment of a multi-disciplinary committee of public health officers, entomologists, and veterinarians to co-ordinate activities.

PREVENTION

There is as yet no fully effective vaccine available against any of the leishmaniases. Trials are in progress for vaccines against cutaneous leishmaniasis in Iran, and a product is available in Brazil whose effectiveness is in question. The latter product is also being tried against visceral leishmaniasis in dogs. Prophylactic chemotherapy is not feasible due to the toxicity and expense of available products. Experimentally, collars and topical insecticide application have been tried for the protection of individual dogs.

The traditional prevention of the harmful effects of *L. major* and *L. tropica* infection in West Asia was by deliberate inoculation of live virulent organisms to produce a single lesion in an inconspicuous place. This procedure prevents subsequent natural infection with multiple lesions or disfiguration. Difficulties in standardizing the product and the occasional occurrence of complications led to the withdrawal of this procedure in military groups entering endemic areas in the USSR and Israel but it was used to protect millions of Iranian recruits in the Iran–Iraq war.

Personal protection may be achieved by avoiding the bites of phlebotomine sandflies. As these almost invariably occur at night, small-mesh window or bed nets are partially effective for *L. tropica* and *L. d. donovani* where these are transmitted by endophagic sandflies. Chemical repellents on skin or clothing are effective for nocturnal activities out of doors; usually these are used to prevent the irritation of insect bites in general rather than leishmaniasis.

CONTROL

Epidemiological models show that if transmission is reduced, the initial effect is to increase the mean age at which people become infected. Only when transmission is almost halted does incidence decrease. With cutaneous leishmaniasis, which is more of a problem in teenagers than young children, partial control may even be counterproductive. Further, there are very recent indications that cutaneous leishmaniasis may protect against kala-azar: this could have very serious implications where transmission of both diseases is possible. Control of transmission depends on the identification of foci of infection, the vectors, and any reservoir hosts. As described above, the basic structure of the most serious leishmaniasis foci is fairly well described, but many minor systems remain to be fully understood.

Phlebotomine sandflies are susceptible to most insecticides so spraying of houses is very effective for *L. tropica* and *L. d. donovani* where these are transmitted by endophilic sandflies. Most sandflies are, however, exophilic and are difficult to control. Fogging with ultra low volume insecticides in the period of still air at dusk is sometimes used to control *P. papatasi* in small towns where it is a serious nuisance. This is not applicable in sylvatic sites, where no form of sandfly control is readily available. Pheromone traps or the destruction of larval sites are potential methods at an early stage of development.

Control of reservoir hosts is an option in certain circumstances. In China, elimination of dogs appeared to be highly effective, but attempts to identify infected dogs and destroy them selectively have largely failed due to popular antagonism or to the inefficiency of diagnostic methods.

Among desert rodents, *Rhombomys opimus* is relatively easy to control in the vicinity of habitations and in development projects by comprehensive mapping of their burrows then destruction by deep ploughing or by a combination of anticoagulants and poison placed deep in the burrow entrances. *Psammomys obesus*, the other important reservoir host for *L. major*, has very specific habitat requirements and can be eliminated by the removal of the succulent vegetation on which it depends. This can be achieved by ploughing, and the environmental change can be maintained by planting salt-tolerant trees. Control of *L. aethiopica* infection by destruction of hyraxes in the neighbourhood of affected villages has yet to be tested.

Little can be done to control transmission of cutaneous leishmaniasis in South and Central American forests. Clearing of forest around new housing estates has been effective in preventing much infection, but may have led to the expansion of visceral leishmaniasis.

EVALUATION

From the time when leishmaniasis largely disappeared from many places in the 1950s, few if any control programmes have been accompanied by effective evaluation. Methods of evaluation have not been developed to any degree of sophistication. The idea of a controlled experiment at a scale larger than that of a small pilot trial is inconceivable and the concentration of cases in both space and time tends to invalidate the use of historical data.

LEGISLATION

With the exception of the compulsory reporting of cases, which applies in an increasing number of countries on the recommendation of WHO (Desjeux 1991), legislation is inappropriate in leishmaniasis.

REFERENCES

Addy, M. and Nandy, A. (1992). Ten years of kala azar in West Bengal. Part 1. Did post kala azar dermal leishmaniasis initiate the outbreak in 24 Parganas? *Bulletin of the World Health Organization*, **70**, 341–6.

Ali, A. and Ashford, R. W. (1994). Visceral leishmaniasis in Ethiopia 4. Prevalence and incidence, and relationship between infection and disease in an endemic area. *Annals of Tropical Medicine and Parasitology*, **88**, 289–93.

Altes, J. *et al.* (1991). Visceral leishmaniasis: another HIV-associated opportunistic infection? Report of eight cases and review of the literature. *AIDS*, **5**, 201–7.

Ashford, R. W., Desjeux, P., and De Raadt, P. (1992*a*). Estimation of population at risk of infection and numbers of cases of leishmaniasis. *Parasitology Today*, **8**, 104–5.

Ashford, R. W., Kohestany, K. A., and Karimzad, M. A. (1992*b*). Cutaneous leishmaniasis in Kabul, Afghanistan: observations on a 'prolonged epidemic'. *Annals of Tropical Medicine and Parasitology*, **86**, 361–71.

Ashford, R. W., Seaman, J., Schorscher, J., and Pratlong, F. (1992*c*). Epidemic visceral leishmaniasis in southern Sudan: Identity and systematic position of the parasites from patients and vectors. *Transactions of the Royal Society of Tropical Medicine and Hygiene*, **86**, 379–80.

Badaro, R. *et al.* (1986). A prospective study of visceral leishmaniasis in an endemic area of Brazil. *Journal of Infectious Diseases*, **154**, 639–49.

Beverley, S. M., Ismach, R. B., and McMahon-Pratt, D. (1987). Evolution of the genus *Leishmania* as revealed by comparisons of nuclear DNA restriction fragment patterns. *Proceedings of the National Academy of Sciences USA*, **84**, 484–8.

Chang, K. -P. and Bray, R. S. (ed.) (1985). *Leishmaniasis*. Elsevier, Amsterdam.

Comber, C. (1995). *Interactions Durables*. Ecologie ct Evolution du Parasitisme Masson, Paris.

Dedet, J. -P. (1992). *Leishmania* et leishmaniases du continent americain. *Annales de l'Institut Pasteur*, **4**, (1), 3–25.

Desjeux, P. (1991). *Information on the epidemiology and control of the leishmaniases by country and territory. WHO/LEISH/91.30.* WHO, Geneva.

Dye, C. and Wolpert, D. M. (1988). Earthquakes, influenza and cycles of Indian Kala-azar. *Transactions of the Royal Society of Tropical Medicine and Hygiene*, **82**, 843–50.

Grimaldi, G., Tesh, R. B., and McMahon-Pratt, D. (1989). A review of the geographic distribution and epidemiology of leishmaniasis in the New World. *American Journal of Tropical Medicine and Hygiene*, **41**, 687–725.

Hart, D. T. (ed.) (1989). *Leishmaniasis. Strategies for Control, Proceedings of NATO Advanced Study Institute, Zakinthos, 1987.* Plenum, New York.

Kar, K. (1995). Serodiagnosis of leishmaniasis. *Critical Reviews in Microbiology*, **21**, 123–52.

Killick-Kendrick, R. (1990). Phlebotomine vectors of the leishmaniases: a review. *Medical and Veterinary Entomology*, **4**, 1–24.

Lainson, R. and Shaw, J. J. (1987). Evolution classification and geographical distribution. In: *The Leishmaniases in Biology and Medicine* Eds. W. Peters and R. Killick-Kendrick. Academic Press, London.

Liew, F. Y. and O'Donnell, C. A. (1993). Immunology of leishmaniasis. *Advances in Parasitology*, **33**, 161–259.

Magill, A. J., Grogl, M., Gasser, R. A., Sun, W., and Oster, C. N. (1993). Viscerotropic leishmaniasis caused by *Leishmania tropica* in veterans of Operation Desert Storm. *New England Journal Medicine*, **328**, 1383–7.

Molyneux, D. H. and Ashford, R. W. (1983). *The biology of Trypanosoma and Leishmania, parasites of man and domestic animals.* Taylor and Francis, London.

Peters, W. and Killick-Kendrick, R. (1987). *The leishmaniases in biology and medicine.* Academic Press, London.

Peters, B. S., Fish, D., Golden, R., Evans, D. A., Bryceson, A. D., and Pinching, A. J. (1990). Visceral leishmaniasis in HIV infection and AIDS: Clinical features and response to therapy. *Quarterly Journal of Medicine*, **77**, 1101–11.

Pratlong, F. *et al.* (1995). *Leishmania*—human immunodeffiency virus coinfection in the Mediterranean basin: isoenzymatic characterization of 100 isolates of the *Leishmania infantum* complex. *Journal of Infectious Disease*, **172**, 323–7.

Rioux, J. -A. (ed.) (1977). *Ecologie des Leishmaniases.* Colloques Internationaux du CNRS No. 239 CNRS, Paris.

Rioux, J. -A. (ed.) (1986). *Leishmania, Taxonomie et Phylogenese.* Institut Mediterraneen d'Etudes Epidemiologiques et Ecologiques, Montpellier.

Rioux, J. -A., Dereure, J., and Perieres, J. (1990*a*). Approche ecologique du 'risque epidemiologique'. L'exemple des leishmaniases. *Bulletin d'Ecologie*, **21**, 1–9.

Rioux, J. -A., Lanotte, G., Serres, E., Pratlong, F., Bastien, P. and Perieres, J. (1990*b*). Taxonomy of *Leishmania*, use of isoenzymes. Suggestions for a new classification. *Annales de Parasitologie Humaine et Comparee*, **65**, 111–25.

Sacks, D. L. and Perkins, P. V. (1984). Identification of an infective stage of *Leishmania* promastigotes. *Science*, **223**, 1417–19.

Seaman, J., Ashford, R. W., Schorscher, J., and Dereure, J. (1992). Visceral leishmaniasis in southern Sudan: status of healthy villagers in epidemic conditions. *Annals of Tropical Medicine and Parasitology*, **86**, 481–6.

Vidor, E. *et al.* (1991). Le chancre d'inoculation dans la leishmaniase canine a *Leishmania infantum*. Etude d'une cohorte en region cevenole. *Pratique Medicale et Chirurgicale de l'Animal de Compagnie*, **26**, 133–7.

WHO (1984). *The leishmaniases.* Technical Report Series, 701. World Health Organisation, Geneva.

WHO (1986). Report of a Training Seminar on Epidemiological Methods for the Leishmaniases, (prepared by R. W. Ashford and V. N. Vioukov). *TDR/LEISH-SEM/ 80.3.*

WHO (1990). *Control of the leishmaniases.* Technical Report Series, 793. World Health Organisation, Geneva.

Zijlstra, E. E., El-Hassan, A. M., Ismael, A., and Ghalib, H. W. (1994). Endemic kala-azar in eastern Sudan: a longitudinal study on the incidence of clinical and subclinical infection and post-kala-azar dermal leishmaniasis. *American Journal of Tropical Medicine and Hygiene*, **51**, 826–36.

44 *GIARDIA* INFECTIONS

R. C. A. Thompson

SUMMARY

Giardia infection is an intestinal disease of humans and other vertebrates caused by infection with the flagellate protozoan *Giardia*. It is the most common pathogenic intestinal parasite of humans and has a worldwide distribution including both temperate and tropical regions. It is a cause of both sporadic outbreaks of disease and epidemics (Lederberg *et al.* 1992).

The parasite colonizes anterior regions of the small intestine, where it adheres to the epithelial mucosa as the flagellated trophozoite form. The trophozoites multiply rapidly using predominantly asexual reproduction by a process of binary fission, and massive numbers of trophozoites can build up rapidly. As trophozoites pass through posterior regions of the small intestine, some will encyst. Quadrinucleate cysts which are passed in the faeces are the major transmissible stage and are a relatively resistant form in the life cycle. Infection is acquired by the ingestion of viable cysts. Transmission is primarily through faecal–oral contamination, although water-borne, food-borne, and zoonotic transmission may also be of significance.

A limited number of effective antigiardial agents are available for the treatment of clinical infections. However, in highly endemic areas, control is chiefly a question of improved hygiene, sanitation, and education. In addition, measures may need to be taken in certain areas to avoid the contamination of drinking water.

HISTORY

There is, today, general agreement that *Giardia* was first observed in 1681 by Antony van Leeuwenhoek in his own faeces (Dobell 1920; Kulda and Nohynkova 1978; Farthing 1994). However, the first detailed description of the parasite was not given until two centuries later by Lambl (1859). Koch's postulation was proven by Rendtorff in 1954 when he successfully transmitted symptomatic *Giardia* infection to human volunteers following ingestion of cysts. The first symptoms of clinical giardiasis were first reported in the early 1920s, although the significance of *Giardia* as a cause of diarrhoeal disease was controversial for many years (see Farthing 1994), and it is only recently that the significance of *Giardia* as a cause of chronic disease in children has been fully realized (reviewed in Islam 1990; Thompson *et al.* 1993; Farthing 1994; Gracey 1994; Hall 1994; Rabbani and Islam 1994).

The question of *Giardia*'s role as a source of zoonotically transmitted disease has not been fully resolved (see Bemrick and Erlandsen 1988; Faubert 1988; Connaughton 1989; Thompson *et al.* 1990*a*, 1993*a*). The World Health Organization recommended that *Giardia* infection should be considered as a zoonosis in 1979 (Anonymous 1979). Since that time, increasing circumstantial epidemiological evidence from water-borne outbreaks, the results of some cross-infection experiments and molecular characterization studies of *Giardia* isolates from humans and other animals has led most authorities to conclude that *Giardia* infection should be considered a zoonosis (Acha and Szyfres 1987; Meyer 1990*a*; Schantz 1991; Thompson 1992*a*,b; Thompson *et al.* 1990*a*, 1993*a*; Majewska 1994; and see Erlandsen 1994; Thompson and Boreham 1994).

THE AGENT

TAXONOMY

Giardia is a member of the phylum Sarcomoastigophora and the class Zoomastigophorea which also contains the medically important flagellates *Trichomonas*, *Trypanosoma*, and *Leishmania*. Species of the genus are classified in the order Diplomonadida and family Hexamitidae. As such, they are characterized by a duplication of organelles, bilateral symmetry, and an oval shape. Almost all members of the family are parasites of the intestinal tract of vertebrates and invertebrates.

The characteristics of the genus *Giardia* are clearly defined and well accepted (reviewed by Kulda and Nohynkova 1978; Meyer 1990*b*; Thompson *et al.* 1990*a*, 1993*a*) although the phylogenetic position of *Giardia* is a subject of much current debate (see below). The motile, intestinal stage, the trophozoite, is binucleate and has a distinctive morphology with characteristic ventral adhesive disc, eight flagellae, and a pair of distinctive median bodies (Fig. 44.1).

Although over 50 species have been described in the genus *Giardia* (Thompson *et al.* 1990*a*, 1993*a*), only five species are currently recognized as valid and their characteristics are summarized in Table 44.1.

Descriptions of the majority of species in the genus *Giardia* were primarily on the basis of host occurrence, but the lack of distinguishing morphological features (Thompson *et al.* 1990*a*; Majewska *et al.* 1993) and increasing evidence that *Giardia* is not host specific has resulted in the present classification (reviewed in Thompson *et al.* 1990*a*, 1993*a*). Unfortunately, this apparently simple scheme fails to reflect the considerable phenotypic and genetic heterogeneity that exists within the species *G. duodenalis* (Table 44.2 and see below). This species is the most widespread and is known to affect at least 40 species of vertebrates, including humans (Kulda and Nohynkova 1978; Thompson *et al.* 1990*a*, 1993*a*).

Table 44.2 Intraspecific variation in *Giardia*

Phenotypic differences	Genetic differences
Morphology	Molecular karyotyping
Host specificity and experimental cross-transmission	Electrophoresis of proteins and enzymes
Growth and development *in vito* and *in vitro*	Restriction site analysis and DNA hybridization
Course of infection: Infectivity Virulence Pathogenicity Sensitivity to drugs Antigenic characteristics	RAPDs and DNA profiling, DNA sequencing

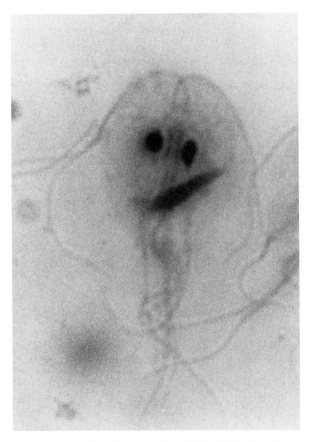

Fig. 44.1 A cultured trophozoite of *Giardia duodenalis* isolated from a human patient in Western Australia stained with Giemsa (×100). Note darkly stained paired nuclei and median bodies, and flagella. (courtesy of Dr Nicolette Binz).

Table 44.1 Recognized species/species groups in the genus *Giardia*

Species	Host	Morphological characteristics	Trophozoite dimensions
G. duodenalis	Mammals (possibly also birds and reptiles)	Pear-shaped trophozoites with claw-shaped median bodies	12–15 μm long 6–8 μm wide
G. agilis	Amphibians	Long, narrow trophozoites with club-shaped median bodies	20–30 μm long 4–5 μm wide
G. muris	Rodents (possibly also birds and mammals)	Rounded trophozoites with small, round median bodies	9–12 μm long 5–7 μm wide
G. psittaci	Birds (budgerigar or parakeet)	Pear-shaped trophozoites, without ventrolateral flange, claw-shaped median bodies	Approx 14 μm long Approx 6 μm wide
G. ardeae	Birds (herons)	Rounded trophozoites, with prominent notch in ventral disc and rudimentary caudal flagellum, median bodies round–oval to claw-shaped	Approx 10 μm long Approx 6.5 μm wide

For source of information, see Thompson *et al.* (1990*a*, 1993*a*, 1994).

The nature of the differences which have been found between isolates of *G. duodenalis* will have a significant influence on the epidemiology and control of *Giardia* infections, particularly differences in host specificity, growth and development, virulence, drug sensitivity, and antigenicity (Hopkins *et al.* 1993*a*; Thompson and Meloni 1993). In addition, it is now clear that much of this variation has a genetic basis and the extent of this variation indicates the existence of a number of species within the *G. duodenalis* morphological group (Meloni *et al.* 1998*a*, 1989, 1992, 1995; Andrews *et al.* 1989; Thompson and Meloni 1993; Thompson *et al.* 1993*a*). There is no evidence that these species are associated with different hosts, or that they are morphologically distinguishable (Thompson *et al.* 1990*a*, 1993*a*; Majewska *et al.* 1993). The source of genetic diversity in *Giardia* is uncertain and will not be resolved until a clearer understanding of the reproductive mechanisms of this parasite is obtained (see below).

MOLECULAR BIOLOGY

The molecular biology of *Giardia* has been reviewed in depth (Adam 1991; Thompson *et al.* 1993*a*). Major deficiencies exist in our understanding of certain fundamental aspects of the biology of this organism, including nucleic acid biochemistry, nuclear function and genomic organization, translational processes, and transcriptional characteristics. Recent research in these areas has revealed some unusual features about *Giardia* of particular interest to evolutionary biologists and molecular epidemiologists.

Phylogenetic relationships

As outlined above, *Giardia* has been classified traditionally in the mastigophoran order Diplomonadida along with *Spironucleus* and *Hexamita* and has been assumed to be closely related to the trichomonads. However, the relationship of *Giardia* to other flagellates, and its phylogenetic affinities in general with respect of eukaryotes, may have to be reappraised in view of recent studies of its ribosomal RNA. Sogin *et al.* (1989) estimated evolutionary distances on the basis of sequence comparisons between the 16S-like rRNAs of *Giardia* and some other eukaryotes and found the distances to be greater than between *Giardia* and several prokaryotes. They concluded that *Giardia* must have separated very early in the evolution of eukaryotes so that it is further removed from its presumed eukaryotic relatives than it is to several of its prokaryotic relatives. Most recently, van Keulen *et al.* (1991, 1994) similarly concluded that *Giardia* was one of the most primitive eukaryotes studied to date, based on the structure of the large and small subunit rRNA of *G. duodenalis*, *G. muris*, and *G. ardeae*. However, transla-

tion and transcription appear to be more similar to what is seen in other eukaryotes than in prokaryotes, although the translation apparatus of *Giardia* is quite different from that of other eukaryotes (reviewed by Adam 1991; Thompson *et al.* 1993*a*). Before we draw definitive conclusions on the phylogenetic position of *Giardia* on the basis of this molecular data, more comparative studies should be carried out using a greater range of flagellates, including other diplomonads. In this respect, Siddall *et al.* (1992) have questioned the method of distance analysis used by Sogin *et al.* (1989) and found no evidence to support *Giardia*'s presumed pivotal position in the evolution of eukaryotes following a detailed phylogenetic analysis of diplomonads using ultrastructural characteristics.

Nuclear function and ploidy

Each nucleus in a *Giardia* trophozoite appears to be derived from the division of its corresponding parent nucleus (Filice 1952). However, it is still not clear whether the nuclei are functionally and morphologically identical (Lymbery and Tibayrenc 1994; Tibayrenc 1994). *In situ* hybridization studies by Kabnick and Peattie (1990) suggested that the nuclei are equivalent and that each nucleus is haploid. However, estimates of DNA content, genome complexity, and karyotype have provided conflicting data (reviewed in Thompson *et al.* 1993*a*; Lymbery and Tibayrenc 1994). Genetic analysis of *Giardia* populations has suggested that *Giardia* may be haploid with two functional nuclei or diploid (or polyploid) with either one or both nuclei functional (Thompson and Meloni 1993; Meloni *et al.* 1995). Further studies using *in situ* approaches are urgently required as well as direct measurements of DNA content using cytometric techniques as applied to other protozoa (Mackenstedt *et al.* 1990*a*,*b*), if we are to understand the complexities of genome structure in *Giardia*. Such information is essential in determining the mode of reproduction and transmission dynamics of this organism.

Mode of reproduction

Giardia has always been presumed to reproduce entirely asexually by a process of binary fission with genetic diversity arising solely by mutation. Recent analyses of isoenzyme data support mutation and clonal selection as the mechanism maintaining genetic diversity (Tibayrenc *et al.* 1990; Thompson and Meloni 1993; Meloni *et al.* 1994, 1995; Tibayrenc 1994). Studies using isoenzyme and DNA analyses found that zymodeme classification of *G. duodenalis* was strongly correlated with schizodeme and rapdeme groupings of the same isolates (Meloni *et al.* 1989; Morgan *et al.* 1993*a*). Such a correlation between two independent sets of genetic markers supports a clonal theory of reproduction (Tibayrenc *et al.* 1990, 1993). However, detailed examination of genetic variation in natural populations of *G. duodenalis* from remote, localized endemic areas has suggested, for the first time, that a sexual phase may be present in *Giardia* (Meloni *et al.* 1988*a*, 1989, 1994, 1995).

Knowledge of the mode of reproduction in *Giardia* will not only help in determining the source and maintenance of genetic diversity exhibited by this organism, but will also have a profound effect on our understanding of the epidemiology of *Giardia* infections and attempts to control the causative agents. The clonal model of asexual reproduction has significant implications with respect to drug development, diagnosis and treatment (Tibayrenc and Ayala 1991), because of the predictability and stability inherent in such a model. However, occasional bouts of sexual recombination in a normally asexual organism can have a major effect on the extent of genetic diversity (Meloni *et al.* 1995).

Thus, current opinion considers *Giardia* to be predominantly clonal with the possibility of sporadic sexual reproduction (Thompson and Meloni 1993; Lymbery and Tibayrenc 1994; Meloni *et al.* 1994, 1995). Certain clonal lineages of *Giardia* are geographically widely distributed whereas others appear to be restricted to certain highly endemic foci. The existence of multiple clones in such areas is a cause for concern, since such genetic diversity will give rise to phenotypic differences which may manifest in features of clinical and epidemiological significance such as variability in virulence, drug sensitivity, and host specifity (Thompson and Meloni 1993; Thompson and Lymbery 1996).

DISEASE MECHANISMS

The mechanisms by which *Giardia* causes disease have been largely unknown and it is only recently that a coordinated picture has emerged of the factors involved in the disease process. Epithelial damage, increased epithelial cell turnover, villous shortening, disaccharidase deficiency, and impaired absorption have all been reported as manifestations of *Giardia* infection (Yardley *et al.* 1964; Ament and Rubin 1972; Gillon and Ferguson 1984; Buret *et al.* 1990*a,b*, 1992; Buret 1994).

Using rodent models, it has been possible to study in detail these clinical manifestations during the course of infection. Villous atrophy and damage to the microvilli have been correlated with brush border enzyme deficiencies which return to normal levels of activity following infection (Buret *et al.* 1990*b*, 1991). Brush border injury is expressed as lowered disaccharidase activity and decreased microvillous surface area which, in turn, result in impaired digestion and malabsorption, which lead to reduced growth (Buret *et al.* 1991,

1992). The loss of brush border thickness was directly correlated with observed decreases in disaccharidase activity, malabsorption, and weight gain (Buret *et al.* 1990*b*, 1991, 1992). The degree of brush border injury and loss of surface area of the microvillous border are the limiting factors for disaccharidase activity and appear to be dependent on the number of trophozoites present (Buret *et al.* 1991). Such a mechanism of pathogenesis could account for both of the major clinical features of *Giardia* infection: diarrhoea and failure to thrive. However, the roles of the parasite and host in inducing these changes remain to be established (see Buret 1994).

The physical damage inflicted by the adherence of *Giardia* to the gut is likely to play some part in the disease process, but the role of other factors such as toxins is uncertain. Proteolytic enzyme activity has been demonstrated in *Giardia* (Parenti 1989) and two major cysteine proteases have been characterized (Hare *et al.* 1989), although there is no evidence for the involvement of these proteases in pathogenesis.

The characteristics of both parasite and host most probably determine the outcome of infection with *Giardia*. The fact that symptomatic *Giardia* infection is more likely to occur in patients who are immunocompromised, malnourished, or very young is a clear indication that host factors are important. However, in other cases, there is increasing evidence of variable virulence between strains (for example, see Romia *et al.* 1990) and thus a particular strain, or isolate, of *Giardia* may have a greater potential to cause disease in a particular host (reviewed by Thompson *et al.* 1990*a*). The nature and competence of immune mechanisms are likely to be central in both cases, particularly in view of mounting evidence that differing virulence between *Giardia* isolates is related to the expression of different surface antigens (Nash *et al.* 1991).

GROWTH AND SURVIVAL REQUIREMENTS

Trophozoites colonize the duodenum and jejunum of their host, where they attach to the intestinal mucosa. Attachment is an essential feature of the relationship between *Giardia* and its host, and the ability to attach *in vitro* is an important indicator of viability (Meloni *et al.* 1990; Crouch *et al.* 1991*a,b*; Magne *et al.* 1991; Hernandez-Sanchez and Ortega-Pierres 1993). Trophozoites may detach intermittently but periods of detachment are likely to be of minimal duration since the parasite may be in danger of losing its position in the gut and being swept away as the result of peristalsis. A number of mechanisms have been proposed to explain how *Giardia* attaches to intestinal epithelial cells, but most evidence indicates that the ventral disc plays the major role in attachment and that the cytoskeletal elements of the disc are the major mediators in this process. This is indicated by the fact that microtubule inhibitors, including known β-tubulin antagonists, have been shown to inhibit adherence *in vitro* (Edlind *et al.* 1990; Meloni *et al.* 1990; Magne *et al.* 1991).

Trophozoites multiply rapidly in the small intestine of their host, although the growth rate has been shown to vary between different strains of *G. duodenalis* (Binz *et al.* 1992). In addition, strains have been shown to vary in their pH requirements and site localization in the small intestine (Binz *et al.* 1992; McInnes 1994; Thompson and Lymbery 1996). Recent research has also led to a reappraisal of *Giardia*'s basic energy requirements and whether amino acid substrates are more important than glucose (reviewed in Schofield and Edwards 1994). In this respect, evidence has shown that some strains are more reliant on glucose for metabolism than others (Hall *et al.* 1992).

Relatively little is known about how the host responds to the presence of *Giardia* and how the parasite survives host resistance mechanisms. Specifically induced IgA and thymus-dependent T lymphocytes both appear to be important components of host immunity (reviewed in Thompson *et al.* 1993*a*), although their role with respect to the outcome of infection is uncertain. However, the fact that symptomatic *Giardia* infection is more likely to occur in patients who are immunocompromised, malnourished, or very young is a clear indication that host factors are important. In other cases, there is increasing evidence that a particular strain, or isolate, of *Giardia* may have a greater potential to cause disease in a particular host. The nature and competence of immune mechanisms are likely to be central in both cases, particularly in view of mounting evidence that differing virulence between *Giardia* isolates is related to the expression of different surface antigens (Nash *et al.* 1991). As with host resistance mechanisms, the biological relevance of antigenic variation is uncertain (Hopkins *et al.* 1993*a*), although a protective function seems likely (Nash *et al.* 1991; Nash 1994).

During the course of infection, trophozoites will encyst in the posterior small intestine. The trigger for trophozoites to encyst is not completely understood but appears to be initiated by the presence of bile salts (Gillin *et al.* 1988). It is not clear whether all cysts are immediately infective when passed, since there is evidence that some undergo a maturation period of up to 7 days before becoming infective (Grant and Woo 1978; Bingham *et al.* 1979). Cysts are resistant and can survive for at least 2 months in suitable temperature and moisture conditions (Meyer and Jarroll 1980).

Excystation follows ingestion and takes place shortly after cysts leave the stomach. The low pH of the stomach environment appears to be the major factor which initiates the excystation process (Bingham and Meyer 1979; Boucher and Gillin 1990). Excystation leads to rapid colonization of the small intestine, and subsequent cyst production commencing after a further 4–15 days (Swan 1984). Trophozoites may also intermittently be passed in the faeces, particularly during acute infection, and could be a source of infection, especially in situations where direct transmission between individuals is likely to occur.

Some isolates of *G. duodenalis* can be cultured axenically in monophasic culture conditions. The development of a bile supplemented medium for cultivating *Giardia* (Keister 1983) and techniques for the excystation *in vitro* of trophozoites from cysts has enabled the isolation, amplification, and maintenance of a large number of different isolates in the laboratory, and has greatly facilitated investigations into trophozoite metabolism and growth requirements, biochemical, antigenic and molecular characteristics, and drug sensitivity (reviewed by Radulescu and Meyer 1990; Thompson *et al.* 1990*a*). Two recent developments will enhance the research value of *in vitro* cultivation of *Giardia*. Boucher and Gillin (1990) succeeded in inducing encystation of *Giardia in vitro* and demonstrated that cysts derived *in vitro* could excyst, thus enabling the complete life cycle to be completed in axenic culture. In addition, a simple reproducible method has recently been developed for establishing cloned lines of *G. duodenalis* from either single trophozoites or single cysts (Binz *et al.* 1991).

Not all isolates of *G. duodenalis* can be established and amplified *in vitro*. Thus much of our knowledge of the biochemistry and genetics of *Giardia* is based on cultivated varieties and thus may not reflect accurately the total gene pool, and indeed may be the result of laboratory-induced artificial selection.

THE HOSTS

The species of *Giardia* which affects humans and other animals, *G. duodenalis* (Table 44.1) has a broad host range, including numerous mammalian species such as rodents, ungulates, and carnivores and possibly some birds and reptiles (Thompson *et al* 1990*a*).

INCUBATION PERIOD

The first appearance of any symptoms usually coincides with the onset of cyst excretion. This incubation period may be short in both humans and other animals, commencing as early as 3 days after infection but can range up to 6 weeks (Rendtorff 1954; Swan 1984; Hopkins and Juranek 1991; Flanagan 1992; Lederberg *et al.* 1992). Very few cysts appear to be required to initiate an infection (De Carneri *et al.*

1977). The duration of infection may vary from a few days to several months, and cyst excretion is characteristically intermittent in both humans and other animal species.

SYMPTOMS AND SIGNS

Humans

The clinical signs associated with *Giardia* infections in humans vary greatly (Smith 1985; Farthing 1986, 1994; Wolfe 1990; Flanagan 1992; Table 44.3). There may be total latency, acute short-lasting diarrhoea, or chronic syndromes associated with nutritional disorders, weight loss, and failure to thrive.

In the majority of untreated patients, infection resolves spontaneously and symptoms usually disappear in a few weeks (Moore *et al.* 1969; Brodsky *et al.* 1974; Wolfe 1990). Occasionally, symptoms may persist for reasons that are not entirely clear and certain patients, such as those with hypogammaglobulinaemia, are at increased risk of chronic clinical giardiasis associated with malabsorption syndromes (Ament *et al.* 1973; Perlmutter *et al.* 1985). The pronounced variability in symptomatology that is so characteristic of *Giardia* infections is the result of a myriad of factors, including host immune and nutritional status, concurrent infections and heterogeneity in infectivity, virulence, and pathogenicity of strains of *G. duodenalis*.

Children appear to be at most risk of contracting clinical *Giardia* infection, particularly those from developing countries and from disadvantaged groups such as Australian Aborigines (Gracey 1983, 1994; Farthing 1986, 1994; Meloni *et al* 1988*b*, 1993; Islam 1990;

Table 44.3 Symptoms and signs of *Giardia* infection

Asymptomatic and/or latent

Acute or chronic
  Nausea
  Headache
  Bloating
  Anorexia
  Cramps
  Fever
  Diarrhoea
  Constipation
  Weight loss
  Flatulence
  Vomiting
  Heartburn
  Abdominal pain
  Fatigue/lethargy
  Foul-smelling stool
  Mucus in stool
  Malabsorption syndromes
  Protein–calorie malnutrition
  Failure to thrive

Sawaya *et al.* 1990; Kaminsky 1991; Rabbani and Islam 1994). In such children, *Giardia* is of particular concern in the aetiology of protein–calorie malnutrition and the retardation of growth and development. *Giardia* is most common in children under 10 years of age (Dupont and Sullivan 1986; Speelman and Ljungström 1986; Meloni *et al.* 1993; Hopkins *et al.* 1997*a*). Severe forms of the disease affecting growth appear to occur most frequently in the second year of life (Farthing *et al.* 1986). It has also recently been proposed that children with giardiasis may be exposed to greater amounts of intestinally absorbed antigens, leading to allergic disease (Di Prisco *et al.* 1993).

Other animals

Little attention has been given to the clinical effects of *Giardia* infection in animals other than humans. *Giardia* is common in dogs and cats, yet is rarely associated with overt symptoms or clinical disease (Simpson *et al.* 1988; Stevenson and Hughes 1988; Thompson 1992*a*). However, it appears likely that giardiasis is probably an underestimated cause of malabsorption and diarrhoea in many species of immature mammals (Kirkpatrick 1989). In dogs and cats, when clinical giardiasis has been reported, albeit rarely, it is usually associated with kennel or cattery situations, and young animals are more likely to show symptoms of *Giardia* infection (Thompson 1992*a*). Adult dogs are usually asymptomatic carriers (Barr *et al.* 1993). Clinical signs are considered to be rare in domestic livestock (Stevenson and Hughes 1988) although, when they do occur, they have been reported to be similar to those in humans (Buret *et al.* 1990*c*). However, establishing the cause of disease in animals is very difficult (Thompson 1992*a*). Concurrent infections are often present and, since diarrhoea is the most common symptom of *Giardia* infection in dogs and cats, a variety of nutritional factors must also be considered. The potential role of *Giardia* as a possible cause of disease in birds was highlighted recently with a report of infection in sick and dying nestling straw-necked ibis (*Threskiornis spinicollis*) by Forshaw *et al.* (1992). Although no other obvious pathogen was present in these birds, further investigations are required to determine the role, if any, of *Giardia* in such avian disease outbreaks.

DIAGNOSIS

Diagnosis of *Giardia* by traditional microscopic methods remains a reliable indicator of infection despite the intermittent nature of cyst excretion in humans and other animals (Baker *et al.* 1987; Simpson *et al.* 1988; Wolfe 1990). Consequently, at least three faecal samples taken on non-consecutive days are required for reliable determination of the presence of *Giardia* since a single sample identifies only 50–75 per cent of positive patients (Heymans *et al.* 1987; Goka *et al.* 1990; Wolfe 1990; Adam 1991). Accurate faecal examination relies on visual identification of cysts following concentration using zinc sulphate or formol-ether which may be facilitated with the use of trichrome or iron haematoxylin stains (Baker *et al.* 1987). Other methods such as duodenal fluid aspirate, duodenal biopsy, or the Entero-Test[R] are far more invasive and costly (Beal *et al.* 1970; Hall *et al.* 1988).

The greatest advances in detection of *Giardia* infection have come from recent research on immunological diagnostic tests (reviewed in Thompson *et al.* 1993*a*). Most success has come from the development of coproantigen detection systems based on the use of enzyme-linked immunosorbent assay (ELISA). Such techniques have been adopted for use in both clinic and field diagnostic situations as well as for water and other environmental samples (reviewed in Thompson *et al.* 1993*a*). ELISA antigen detection kits have now reached high levels of sensitivity, specificity, and reproducibility, and excellent commercial kits are now available for field and laboratory use (Hopkins *et al.* 1993*b*).

PATHOLOGY

Abnormalities in mucosal morphology and villous shortening have been reported and a mild chronic inflammatory response has been observed during resolution of infection (Adam 1991; Buret 1994). Mucosal injury is most severe in the upper small intestine (Buret 1994). In contrast to some early studies, it is now generally agreed that *Giardia* is not an invasive parasite (Buret 1994). The contributions of parasite and host factors to the variable pathological sequelae of *Giardia* infection in humans and other mammals remains to be determined (see above).

TREATMENT

A number of antigiardial drugs are available for treatment of humans and other animals with *Giardia* infections. These include quinacrine, the nitroimidazoles—metronidazole and tinidazole, furazolidone, paromomycin and, more recently, benzimidazoles such as albendazole. The efficacy and mode of action of these drugs has been reviewed in detail (Adam 1991; Reynoldson *et al.* 1992*a*,*b*; Thompson *et al.* 1993*a*; Jarroll 1994; Reynoldson 1994).

The nitroimidazoles are the most widely used drugs for the treatment of *Giardia* infection and are generally effective (reviewed in Thompson *et al.* 1993*a*). However, treatment failures do occur and variability in sensitivity between strains of *G. duodenalis* may be a lim-

iting factor in treatment, particularly on a community basis. Side-effects have been reported and compliance is often poor, particularly in children, which may reduce the effectiveness of treatment when multiple doses are required.

Benzimidazole drugs, particularly albendazole, may offer an alternative approach to antigiardial chemotherapy in the future (Reynoldson *et al.* 1992*b*). *In vitro* studies have shown that albendazole is more potent than metronidazole, and successful clinical trials in humans have been reported (Meloni *et al.* 1990; Hall and Nahar 1993; Morgan *et al.* 1993*b*). Albendazole has fewer side-effects than the nitroimidazoles and is much more palatable, which is an important consideration, since *Giardia* infection is most significant as a childhood disease (Reynoldson *et al.* 1992*a*,*b*).

PROGNOSIS

The prognosis is usually good in patients (both human and animal) once infection has been diagnosed. In patients who fail to respond to treatment, a second course of the same drug or an alternative compound usually results in cure. Combination therapy with two drugs may be advocated in patients who failed to respond to treatment with a single compound.

Chronic *Giardia* infection may be a problem in highly endemic foci of infection where environmental contamination is high and hygiene standards are poor. Under such circumstances, re-infection after treatment is common, especially in children, and thus the prognosis must be considered to be poor in the absence of measures to prevent reinfection.

EPIDEMIOLOGY

OCCURRENCE

Humans

Giardia is ubiquitous and is the most common pathogenic intestinal parasite of humans worldwide. *Giardia* infection is today well recognized as one of the most prevalent intestinal diseases of humans in both temperate and tropical areas, with prevalence rates varying between 2 and 7 per cent in Europe, United States of America, Canada, and Australia (Acha and Szyfres 1987; Schantz 1991; Eckert 1993; Thompson *et al.* 1993*a*; Farthing 1994), to over 40 per cent in developing areas where living conditions are poor, nutritional levels are often inadequate, and concurrent infections are common (Chunge *et al.* 1991; Torres *et al.* 1991; Meloni *et al.* 1993; Thompson *et al.* 1993*a*; Farthing 1994; Hopkins *et al.* 1997*a*). There is also evidence that the levels of infection in humans in developed countries such as the United States and United Kingdom may be increasing (Schantz 1991; Flanagan 1992).

Groups at particular risk of *Giardia* infection include inhabitants of developing countries or disadvantaged groups within developed countries. *Giardia* infection is one of the common causes of acute or persisting diarrhoea in developing countries (Anonymous 1987) and is a major health problem (Islam 1990). Within these countries, the incidence of *Giardia* infection is often over four times higher than in the United States (7.4 per cent; Quinn 1971) or the rest of the world (7.4 per cent, Nikolic *et al.* 1990), and it varies considerably between regions in the same country (3.9–18.2 per cent in Ghana; Annan *et al.* 1986). Children are more often affected (Gracey 1983, 1994; Farthing 1986; Meloni *et al.* 1988*b*, 1993; Islam 1990; Chunge *et al* 1991; Kaminsky 1991; Torres *et al.* 1991; Hopkins *et al.* 1997*a*), and this is of particular concern because of the repeated exposure to potentially toxic drugs in some regions. Furthermore, Sullivan *et al.* (1991) emphasized the high prevalence of *Giardia* in children with chronic diarrhoea in Gambia and the fact that infection often fails to respond to standard therapeutic measures. The higher prevalence of *Giardia* infection in children is likely to be a consequence of a greater risk of infection, as protective immunity is acquired with age and multiple exposure (Farthing 1986; Islam 1990).

Infection varies inversely with socio-economic status and is high in regions where water supplies are poor or non-existent and sanitation and hygiene standards are poor (Knight 1980; Islam 1990; Anonymous 1993; Meloni *et al.* 1993). Risk factors identified as important in facilitating emergence of *Giardia* infection include high environmental faecal contamination, lack of potable water, inadequate education and housing, overcrowding and high population density, and animal reservoirs of infection (Islam 1990; Kaminsky 1991; Lederberg *et al.* 1992).

High-risk groups also include children in day-care centres, pre-school children, and inmates of nursing homes and, in these situations, levels of infection are often close to those found in developing countries. *Giardia* is responsible for a significant number of outbreaks of diarrhoea in day-care centres, where giardiasis is often identified as an epidemic either alone or in association with other intestinal pathogens (Black *et al.* 1977; Keystone *et al.* 1978; Pickering *et al.* 1981; Boreham and Shepherd 1984; Sullivan *et al.* 1984; Bartlett *et al.* 1985*a*,b). Indeed, *Giardia* infection is now regarded as a 're-emerging' infection as a result of the increased use of child-care Facilities (Anonymous, 1995). The major factors involved in epidemics in these institutions are presence of young non-toilet-trained children, contamination of hands, communal classroom objects, and lack of infection control measures (Sullivan

et al. 1984). A proportion of each group is asymptomatic and can act as carriers of infection to relatives and the community (Pickering *et al.* 1981; Bartlett *et al.* 1985*a,b*), together with transmission by affected children (Polis *et al.* 1986). The public health problem of transmission to the community from these centres is a significant one and needs further evaluation and control through infection control measures and education.

Similar problems may be encountered in nursing homes. In one case from a nursing home, which also served as a day-care centre for children, 88 cases of *Giardia* infection were identified in a population of 312 in a period of 6 weeks, involving transmission by multiple routes including food-borne and person to person transmission (White *et al.* 1989).

Giardia is a common cause of 'travellers' diarrhoea' and is often associated with episodes of diarrhoea contracted by tourists. Individuals with immunodeficiency are also at risk of persistent *Giardia* infection and chronic disease occurs in individuals with immunoglobulin deficiency and in male homosexuals both with and without HIV infection (Webster 1980; McGowan and Weller 1990; Farthing 1994).

Animals

Giardia duodenalis is a common parasite of vertebrate animals, apart from humans (Thompson *et al.* 1990*a*, 1993*a*). Of particular concern from a zoonotic standpoint are potential reservoirs of infections in pets and livestock, and the occurrence of *G. duodenalis* in other animals and birds that may constitute a source of transmission and/or contamination in surface water supplies.

Numerous surveys of dogs and cats have been carried out in urban and rural areas of the world, and all have found *Giardia* to be common with prevalence rates from 7 per cent to over 50 per cent in dogs and from 3 to 50 per cent in cats (Swan and Thompson 1986; Baker *et al.* 1987; Collins *et al.* 1987; Kirkpatrick 1988; Simpson *et al.* 1988; Winsland *et al.* 1989; Castor and Lindquist 1990; Asano *et al.* 1991; Tonks *et al.* 1991; Arashima *et al.* 1992; Collyer *et al.* 1992; Jafri *et al.* 1993; Thompson *et al.* 1993*b*).

Giardia is prevalent in domestic ruminants (reviewed in Xiao, 1994). For example, a recent study in Canada found 17.7 per cent of sheep and 10.4 per cent of cattle to be infected with *Giardia*, although much higher prevalence rates were recorded in lambs (35.6 per cent) and calves (27.7 per cent) (Buret *et al.* 1990*c*). Similarly, in Switzerland, Taminelli and Eckert (1989) found 26.6 per cent of calves and 29.8 per cent of lambs to be infected with *Giardia*.

Small rodents, beavers, and other mammals have also been found to be infected with *G. duodenalis* on numerous occasions (see Pacha *et al.* 1987; Thompson *et al.* 1990*a*; Marino *et al.* 1992; Erlandsen 1994; Wallis 1994).

SOURCES

The sources of infection include other infected individuals and infected animals. Environmental sources are also very important and, in particular, water in certain geographical areas. Food-borne outbreaks have also been reported. Investigations of outbreaks of *Giardia* infection and transmission patterns are made difficult by the genetic heterogeneity of *G. duodenalis* isolates and the lack of appropriate molecular markers to 'type' *Giardia* cysts and trophozoites (see below). Lederberg *et al.* (1992) consider that four factors will facilitate the emergence of *Giardia* infection : (1) infection in animal populations (beavers and dogs); (2) capability of the organism to survive in water supply systems that use superficial water; (3) immunosuppression; and (4) international travel.

TRANSMISSION

Faecal–oral transmission

Transmission of *Giardia* is predominantly by faecal–oral contamination and levels of infection are therefore highest under conditions of poor hygiene and sanitation, particularly in tropical and subtropical environments. Most authorities consider that direct person to person transmission is more important in this respect than water-borne, food-borne, or zoonotic transmission (Pawlowski *et al.* 1987; Eckert 1989; Schantz 1991). Other predisposing factors which may enhance the frequency of faecal–oral transmission include day-care centres where conditions conducive to faecal–oral contamination are common and high prevalence rates of *Giardia* infection have often been observed (see above). Direct transmission between homosexual men is being increasingly recognized as significant in the epidemiology of *Giardia* infection (Phillips *et al.* 1981).

Water-borne transmission

Numerous cases of *Giardia* infection have been associated with contaminated water, and there is evidence that water-borne outbreaks are increasing in the United States (Malloy *et al.* 1993). *Giardia* infection is the most frequently diagnosed water-borne disease (Levine *et al.* 1990). Water-borne outbreaks of *Giardia* infection have also been reported in Canada (Wallis *et al.* 1986; Moorehead *et al.* 1990; Wallis 1994) and Europe (Jephcott *et al.* 1986; Neringer *et al.* 1986). *Giardia* cysts are widely dispersed in the aquatic environment in Canada, with higher levels of contamination in water

receiving sewage effluent (LeChevallier *et al.* 1991). The potential for water-borne transmission has also been recognized in Australia (Wade and Yapp 1989), and in New Zealand recent surveys have identified *Giardia* in a number of water supplies (Ampofo *et al.* 1991; Fraser and Cooke 1991). Water-borne transmission is also a well-documented cause of *Giardia* infection in travellers, who usually contracted infection from drinking local tapwater (Jokipii and Jokipii 1974). Investigations of endemic water-borne *Giardia* infection in the United States have usually found contamination of the water supply to have resulted from inadequate water treatment, ineffective filtration, or contamination with human sewage (Craun 1986, 1990; Schantz 1991). Filtration is necessary to remove *Giardia* as chlorination alone is insufficient without high concentrations of chlorine and long contact times (Schantz 1991).

However, the fact that human infections with *Giardia* have been traced to the consumption of water from streams in rural areas well away from urban environments has implicated a number of species of wild animals, particularly beavers and muskrats, as reservoirs of infection (Davies and Hibler 1979; Pacha *et al.* 1987; Craun 1990; Marino *et al.* 1992). However, the role of animals in water-borne transmission is controversial (see Thompson *et al.* 1990*a*; Erlandsen 1994; Thompson and Boreham 1994; Wallis 1994). Whether animals serve as the original source of contamination or amplify the numbers of the originally contaminating isolate, or both, remains to be determined (Bemrick and Erlandsen 1988; Thompson *et al.* 1990*a*).

Food-borne transmission

Food-borne transmission, usually as a result of contamination during food preparation, is also a well-recognized source of *Giardia* infection (Barnard and Jackson 1984; Petersen *et al.* 1988; Mintz *et al.* 1993).

Zoonotic transmission

The significance and interpretation of the results obtained from experimental infections of animals with human isolates of *Giardia* have been controversial (reviewed by Thompson *et al.* 1990*a*). However, there is sufficient evidence to show that at least some isolates of *Giardia* are not host specific and that humans and a variety of other animals naturally share the parasite. Most authorities therefore regard *Giardia* infection as a zoonosis (Acha and Szyfres 1987; Meyer 1990*b*; Schantz 1991; Thompson 1992*b*; Eckert 1993; Thompson *et al.* 1993*a*), although humans are likely to be the main reservoir of human *Giardia* infection with animals constituting an additional source of infection.

Studies of the prevalence of *Giardia* in a variety of mammals and birds (see above) underlie the fact that a potential reservoir of human infection exists. Thus treatment of *Giardia*-infected dogs and cats may be advocated, whether or not they are clinically ill, because of the potential zoonotic risk (Kirkpatrick 1984; Hoskins 1990; Thompson 1992*a*; Barr *et al.* 1993). If both family members and their pets are found to be infected with *Giardia*, as recently reported from Canada (Cribb and Spracklin 1986), or zoo handlers and their charges (Armstrong *et al.* 1979), this must be strong circumstantial evidence of zoonotic transmission, although the converse of *Giardia* infection in pets but not in their owners (Asano *et al.* 1991; Arashima *et al.* 1992; Pospisilova and Svobadova 1992) is not necessarily an indicator that humans are not susceptible to *Giardia* in their companion animals.

Very few studies of the occurrence of *Giardia* have been undertaken in domestic ruminants, although recent surveys in north America and Switzerland have found *Giardia* to be prevalent in sheep and cattle, particularly in young animals (Taminelli and Eckert 1989; Buret *et al.* 1990*c*; Xiao 1994; see above).

Some authors consider that birds may be a source of zoonotic contamination of open water with *Giardia* (Bemrick 1984). *Giardia* in a blue heron was suggested as a possible source of water-borne *Giardia* infection in humans, but not confirmed (Georgi *et al.* 1986), although the species of *Giardia* involved was not determined. Cross-infection experiments with the avian species *G. psittaci* and *G. ardeae* were taken to indicate that birds should not be considered as likely potential reservoirs of infection for mammalian hosts (Erlandsen *et al.* 1991), at least in the United States. The zoonotic significance of avian outbreaks in Australia (Forshaw *et al.* 1992) is not known but the isolates which have been characterized are quite distinct to those affecting humans (McRoberts *et al.* 1996).

Although the potential for zoonotic transmission of *Giardia* is now well accepted, irrefutable evidence for such transmission outside the laboratory has been difficult to obtain. Because all isolates of *G. duodenalis* are morphologically indistinguishable, and since some are more host specific than others (Thompson *et al.* 1990*a*), it has not yet been possible to prove that a particular outbreak of infection in humans was contracted from an animal source, or vice versa. The situation is compounded by the enormous genetic heterogeneity of *G. duodenalis*. Molecular characterization procedures such as enzyme electrophoresis and the use of DNA hybridization using specific probes have found some mammalian isolates to be very similar to human ones (Thompson *et al.* 1988*a*, b; Meloni *et al.* 1989). However, cat isolates of *Giardia* from Western Australia, for example, are quite different from isolates of *Giardia* infecting cats in Europe (Meloni *et al.* 1992). As a consequence, an indication of genetic identity between

isolates of *Giardia* from humans and other animals in one endemic area cannot be extrapolated to the situation in another endemic area (Thompson *et al.* 1990*a,b*). The isolates of *Giardia* involved may have quite different host specifities. For example, the conclusion that *Giardia* from dogs in England is not infective to their owners (Hay *et al.* 1990) is erroneous since it was based on a genetic comparison of canine isolates from England and human isolates from America (Thompson *et al.* 1990*b*, 1993*a*; Thompson 1992*a*). Comparative studies which utilize molecular characterization techniques for 'biotyping' and to provide evidence of zoonotic transmission must therefore compare isolates at a local level (Isaac-Renton *et al.* 1993; Thompson and Meloni 1993; Thompson and Lymbery 1996).

The most appropriate techniques to apply in such molecular epidemiological studies remain to be determined. Enzyme electrophoresis has been shown to be of value (Meloni *et al.* 1988*a*, 1989), but may not provide the level of genotypic discrimination necessary for differentiating and demonstrating affinities between closely related individuals. However, such techniques require the *in vitro* amplication of *Giardia* isolates. Since not all isolates can be grown in culture, non-culture-based techniques are required (Isaac-Renton *et al.* 1993) to avoid laboratory selection and to provide an accurate method of characterizing isolates of *Giardia* from the field (Thompson and Lymbery 1996). In this respect, PCR-based techniques will be the tools of choice in future studies (Morgan *et al.* 1993*a*). In particular, DNA profiling using mini- or microsatellites will be of value and should be applied to the study of *Giardia* transmission in the field (Thompson and Meloni 1993; Thompson *et al.* 1993*a*; Thompson and Lymbery 1996).

For example, studies on the molecular epidemiology of *Giardia* infection in remote Aboriginal communities in the north of Western Australia where *Giardia* is prevalent in humans and dogs (Meloni *et al.* 1993; Thompson *et al.* 1993*b*; Hopkins *et al.* 1997*a*) suggest that zoonotic transmission is infrequent (Hopkins *et al.* 1997*b*). Comparative sequence analysis of the 300 bp region of the small subunit of rDNA indicates that dogs in the communities rarely harbour isolates of *Giardia* which occur in humans from the same communities and similarly, dog-'type' *Giardia* has not been recovered from humans (Hopkins *et al.* 1997*b*).

PREVENTION AND CONTROL

With the widespread distribution of numerous species of potential animal reservoirs of infection and the fact that *Giardia* may survive for extended periods outside the host as resistant cysts in the environment, the possibility of human infection is unlikely to be eliminated.

Several cases of families with affected pets and symptomless carrier relatives have been reported and highlight the need to undertake therapy in these situations in order to prevent repeated infections (Pancorbo *et al.* 1985; Cribb and Spracklin 1986). In contrast, the value of treatment in some hyperendemic communities is questionable since treatment is soon followed by re-infection (Aplogan *et al.* 1990; Sullivan *et al.* 1991) and perhaps should only be considered when clinically indicated (Gilman *et al.* 1988). In many developing countries, the prevailing socio-economic conditions make it difficult to prevent infection, especially in children (Acha and Szyfres 1987).

The control of endemic gastrointestinal parasitic infections, such as *Giardia* infection , which are primarily transmitted in conditions of poor hygiene and sanitation, calls for other primary health-care activities such as health promotion and education which should ecompass both hygiene aspects and nutrition, and should include appropriate evaluation procedures to determine the success of such interventions. Intestinal parasite control programmes are regarded as highly desirable since the recipients see the beneficial effects of intervention and learn basic health-care facts, and sectors of the health-care services become integrated (Anonymous 1987). Public health measures are also clearly required to protect water supplies against contamination by human or animal faeces. Attention to personal hygiene in high-risk situations such as day-

care centres and residential institutions should minimize person to person transmission (Farthing 1994). Tourists should not drink tap water in places where its purity cannot be guaranteed.

The costs of not having a control programme for *Giardia* infection include those related to nutrition, growth and development, work and productivity, and medical care (Anonymous 1987). Strategies used to control *Giardia* infection are usually based on epidemiology providing basic information on transmission, the reduction of incidence rates with control of transmission and health education, and a reduction in number of infections through therapy (Anonymous 1987).

Control measures to counter the high infection rates with *Giardia* in developing regions include those listed in Table 44.4 (Anonymous 1987; Boreham 1987; Islam 1990; Lederberg *et al.* 1992; Rabbani and Islam 1994). Practical approaches are mainly centred on sanitation control and education about indiscriminate defaecation and on personal hygiene concerning the handling of domestic animals (Anonymous 1987). The central role of health education in prevention and control programmes should be adapted for each target community with education as a primary focus in each phase of a programme, including preparation, implementation, and follow-up involving all sectors of the community and health workers (Anonymous 1987; Halloran *et al.* 1989; Rabbani and Islam 1994).

Table 44.4 Desired results and practical approaches to controlling transmission of *Giardia*

Desired result	Practical approach
Reduction of overall prevalence in community	Health education and non-specific hygienic approach re: faecal–oral transmission, water quality, hand washing, sanitation, food handling
Prevention and control of epidemics	Quality of health education Treatment of wastes used as fertilizer Improved personal hygiene Improved water quality
Prevention of water-borne transmission	Disinfection of local water supplies Treatment of wastes used as fertilizer
Prevention of food-borne transmission	Effective surveillance and hygiene instruction Screening of food handlers
Reduced morbidity	Individual chemotherapeutic treatment
Elimination of reservoirs of *Giardia* infection	Treatment of people, pets and livestock with infection who are asymptomatic cyst passers

REFERENCES

Acha, P. N. and Szyfres, B. (1987). *Zoonoses and communicable diseases common to man and animals*. Scientific Publication No. 503. Pan American Health Organization, Washington.

Adam, R. D. (1991). The biology of *Giardia* spp. *Microbiological Reviews*, **55**, 706–32.

Ament, M. E. and Rubin, C. E. (1972). Relation of giardiasis to abnormal intestinal structure and function in gastrointestinal immunodeficiency syndromes. *Gastroenterology*, **62**, 216–26.

Ament, M. E., Ochs, H. D., and Davis, S. D. (1973). Structure and function of the gastrointestinal tract in primary immunodeficiency syndromes: a study of 39 patients. *Medicine*, **52**, 227–48.

Ampofo, E., Fox, E. G., and Shaw, C. P. (1991). *Giardia and giardiasis in New Zealand*. Environmental Health Unit, Department of Health, Wellington.

Andrews, R. H., Adams, M., Boreham, P. F. L., Mayrhofer, G., and Meloni, B. P. (1989). *Giardia intestinalis*: electrophoretic evidence for a species complex. *International Journal for Parasitology*, **19**, 183–90.

Annan, A., Crompton, D. W. T., Walters, D. E., and Arnold, S. E. (1986). An investigation of the prevalence of intestinal parasites in pre-school children in Ghana. *Parasitology*, **92**, 209–17.

Anonymous (1979). *Parasitic zoonoses*. Report of a WHO Expert Committee with the participation of FAO. Technical Report Series No. 637. World Health Organization, Geneva.

Anonymous (1987). *Report of a WHO Expert Committee: Prevention and control of intestinal parasitic infections.* Technical Report Series No. 749. World Health Organization, Geneva.

Anonymous (1993). Intestinal parasitic infections. *Weekly Epidemiological Record*, **7**, 43–4.

Anonymous (1995). *Infectious disease – a global health threat.* Report of the National Science and Technology Council Committee on International Science, Engineering, and Technology Working Group on Emerging and Re-emerging Infectious Diseases. Office of Science and Technology Policy, Washington, DC, USA.

Aplogan, A., Schneider, D., Dyck, J. L., and Berger, J. (1990). Parasitoses digestives chez le jeune enfant en milieu extra-hospitalier tropical. *Annalles de Pediatrics*, **37**, 677–81.

Arashima, Y. *et al.* (1992). Studies on the giardiasis as the zoonosis. III. Prevalence of *Giardia* among the dogs and the owners in Japan. *Kansenshogaku Sasshi*, **66**, 1062–6 [in Japanese].

Armstrong, J., Hertzog, R. E., Hall, R. T., and Hoff, G. L. (1979). Giardiasis in apes and zoo attendants, Kansas City, Missouri. *CDC Veterinary Public Health Notes*, January 1979.

Asano, R., Hokari, S., Murasugi, E., Arashima, Y., Kubo, N., and Kawano, K. (1991). Studies on the giardiasis as the zoonosis. II. Giardiasis in dogs and cats. *Kansenshogaku Sasshi*, **65**, 157–61.

Baker, G., Donald, B. S., Strombeck, D. R., and Gershwin, L. J. (1987). Laboratory diagnosis of *Giardia duodenalis* infection in dogs. *Journal of the American Veterinary Medical Association*, **190**, 53–6.

Barnard, R. J. and Jackson, G. J. (1984). *Giardia lamblia*. The transfer of human infections by food. In *Giardia and giardiasis*, (ed. S. L. Erlandsen and E. A. Meyer), pp. 365–78. Plenum Press, New York.

Barr, S. C., Bowman, D. D., Heller, R. L., and Erb, H. N. (1993). Efficacy of albendazole against giardiasis in dogs. *American Journal of Veterinary Research*, **54**, 926–8.

Bartlett, A. V., Moore, M., Gary, G. WS., Starko, K. M., Erben, J. J., and Meredith, B. A. (1985*a*). Diarrheal illness among infants and toddlers in day care centers. I. Epidemiology and pathogens. *Journal of Pediatrics*, **107**, 495–502.

Bartlett, A. V., Moore, M., Gary, G. W., Starko, K. M., Erban, J. J., and Meredith, B. A. (1985*b*). Diarrheal illness among infants and toddlers in day care centers. II. Comparison with day care homes and households. *Journal of Pediatrics*, **107**, 503–9.

Beal, C. B., Viens, P., Grant, R. G. L., and Hughes, J. M. (1970). A new technique for sampling duodenal contents—demonstration of upper small-bowel pathogens. *American Journal of Tropical Medicine and Hygiene*, **19**, 349–52.

Bemrick, W. J. (1984). Some perspectives on the transmission of giardiasis. In *Giardia and giardiasis* (ed. S. L. Erlandsen and E. A. Meyer), pp. 379–400. Plenum Press, New York.

Bemrick, W. J. and Erlandsen, S. L. (1988). Giardiasis—is it really a zoonosis? *Parasitology Today*, **4**, 69–71.

Bingham, A. K. and Meyer, E. A. (1979). *Giardia* excystation can be induced *in vitro* in acidic solutions. *Nature*, **277**, 301–2.

Bingham, A. K., Jarroll, E. L., Meyer, E. A., and Radulescu, S. (1979). *Giardia* sp.: physical factors of excystation *in vitro*, and excystation *vs* eosin exclusion as determinants of viability. *Experimental Parasitology*, **47**, 284–91.

Binz, N., Thompson, R. C. A., Meloni, B. P., and Lymbery, A. J. (1991). A simple method for cloning *Giardia duodenalis* from cultures and faecal samples. *Journal of Parasitology*, **77**, 627–31.

Binz, N., Thompson, R. C. A., Lymbery, A. J., and Hobbs, R. P. (1992). Comparative studies on the growth dynamics of two genetically distinct isolates of *Giardia duodenalis in vitro*. *International Journal for Parasitology*, **22**, 195–202.

Black, R. E., Dykes, A. C., Sinclair, S. P., and Wells, J. G. (1977). Giardiasis in day care centers: evidence of person to person transmission. *Pediatrics*, **60**, 486–91.

Boreham, P. F. L. (1987). Transmission of *Giardia* by food and water. *Food Technology in Australia*, **39**, (2), 61–3.

Boreham, P. F. L. and Shepherd, R. W. (1984). Giardiasis in child-care centres. *Medical Journal of Australia*, **141**, 263.

Boucher, S. E. M. and Gillin, F. D. (1990). Excystation of *in vitro*-derived *Giardia lamblia* cysts. *Infection and Immunity*, **58**, 3516–22.

Brodsky, R. E., Spencer, H. D. Jr, and Schultz, M. G. (1974). Giardiasis in American travelers to the Soviet Union. *Journal of Infectious Diseases*, **130**, 319–23.

Buret, A. (1994). Pathogenesis—how does *Giardia* cause disease? In *Giardia: from molecules to disease*, (ed. R. C. A. Thompson, J. A. Reynoldson, and A. J. Lymbery), pp. 293–315. CAB International, Wallingford.

Buret, A., Gall, D. G., Nation, P. N., and Olson, M. E. (1990*a*). Intestinal protozoa and epithelial cell kinetics, structure and function. *Parasitology Today*, **6**, 375–80.

Buret, A., Gall, D. G., and Olson, M. E. (1990*b*). Effects of murine giardiasis on growth, intestinal morphology and disaccharidase activity. *Journal of Parasitology*, **76**, 403–9.

Buret, A., den Hollander, N., Wallis, P. M., Befus, D., and Olson, M. E. (1990*c*). Zoonotic potential of giardiasis in domestic ruminants. *Journal of Infectious Diseases*, **162**, 231–7.

Buret, A., Gall, D. G., and Olson, M. E. (1991). Growth activities of enzymes in the small intestine, and ultrastructure of microvillous border in gerbils infected with *Giardia duodenalis*. *Parasitology Research*, **77**, 109–14.

Buret, A., Hardin, J. A., Olson, M. E., and Gall, D. G. (1992). Pathophysiology of small intestinal malabsorption in gerbils infected with *Giardia lamblia*. *Gastroenterology*, **103**, 506–13.

Castor, S. B. and Lindquist, K. B. (1990). Canine giardiasis in Sweden: no evidence of infectivity to man. *Transactions of the Royal Society of Tropical Medicine and Hygiene*, **84**, 249–50.

Chunge, R. N. *et al.* (1991). Longitudinal study of young children in Kenya: intestinal parasitic infection with special reference to *Giardia lamblia*, its prevalence, incidence and duration, and its association with diarrhoea and with other parasites. *Acta Tropica*, **50**, 39–49.

Collins, G. H., Pope, S. E., Griffin, D. L., Walker, J., and Connor, G. (1987). Diagnosis and prevalence of *Giardia* spp. in dogs and cats. *Australian Veterinary Journal*, **64**, 89–90.

Collyer, R., Lim, K. H., and Tang, R. (1992). Suburban dogs—a reservoir of human giardiasis. *Medical Journal of Australia*, **156**, 814–15.

Connaughton, D. (1989). Giardiasis—zoonosis or not? *Journal of the American Veterinary Medical Association*, **194**, 447–51.

Craun, G. F. (1986). Waterborne giardiasis in the United States 1965–1984. *Lancet*, **ii**, 513–14.

Craun, G. F. (1990). Waterborne giardiasis. In *Giardiasis*, (ed E. A. Meyer), pp. 267–93. Elsevier, Amsterdam.

Cribb, A. E. and Spracklin, D. (1986). Giardiasis in a home. *Canadian Veterinary Journal*, **27**, 169.

Crouch, A. A., Seow, W. K., Whitman, L. M., and Thong, Y. H. (1991*a*). Effect of human milk and infant milk formulae on adherence of *Giardia intestinalis*. *Transactions of the Royal Society of Tropical Medicine and Hygiene*, **85**, 617–19.

Crouch, A. A., Seow, W. K., Whitman, L. M., Smith, S. E., and Thong, Y. H. (1991*b*). Inhibition of adherence of *Giardia intestinalis* by human neutrophils and monocytes. *Transactions of the Royal Society of Tropical Medicine and Hygiene*, **85**, 375–9.

Davies, R. B. and Hibler, C. P. (1979). Animal reservoirs and cross-species transmission of *Giardia*. In *Waterborne transmission of giardiasis* (ed. W. Jakubowski and J. C. Hoff), pp. 104–26. Environmental Protection Agency, Cincinnati, USA.

De Carneri, I., Trane, F., and Mandelli, V. (1977). *Giardia muris*: oral infection with one trophozoite and generation time in mice. *Transactions of the Royal Society of Tropical Medicine and Hygiene*, **71**, 438.

Di Prisco, M. C., Hagel, I., Lynch, N. R., Barrios, R. M., Alvarez, N., and Lopez, R. (1993). Possible relationship between allergic disease and infection by *Giardia lamblia*. *Annals of Allergy*, **70**, 210–13.

Dobell, C. (1920). The discovery of the intestinal protozoa of man. *Proceedings of the Royal Society of Medicine*, **13**, 1–15.

Dupont, H. L. and Sullivan, P. S. (1986). Giardiasis: the clinical spectrum, diagnosis and therapy. *Pediatric Infectious Disease*, **5**, 131–8.

Eckert, J. (1989). New aspects of parasitic zoonoses. *Veterinary Parasitology*, **32**, 37–55.

Eckert, J. (1993). Carriers and excretors of protozoa. *Zentralblatt für Hygiene Umweltmedizine*, **194**, 173–85.

Edlind, T. D., Hang, T. L., and Chakraborty, P. R. (1990). Activity of anthelmintic benzimidazoles against *Giardia lamblia in vitro. Journal of Infectious Disease*, **162**, 1408–11.

Erlandsen, S. L. (1994). Biotic transmission—is giardiasis a zoonoses? In *Giardia: from molecules to disease*, (ed. R. C. A. Thompson, J. A. Reynoldson, and A. J. Lymbery), pp. 83–97. CAB International, Wallingford.

Erlandsen, S. L., Bemrick, W. J., and Jakubowski, W. (1991). Cross-species transmission of avian and mammalian *Giardia* spp.: inoculation of chicks, ducklings, budgerigars, mongolian gerbils and neonatal mice with *Giardia ardeae*, *Giardia duodenalis* (*lamblia*), *Giardia psittaci* and *Giardia muris*. *International Journal of Environmental Health Research*, **1**, 144–52.

Farthing, M. J. G. (1986). Clinical impact of giardiasis. In *Interactions of parasitic diseases and nutrition: clinical impact of giardiasis*, (ed. C. Chagas and G. T. Keusch), pp. 185–202. Pontificia Academia Scientiarum, Rome.

Farthing, M. J. G. (1994). Giardiasis as a disease. In *Giardia: from molecules to disease*, (ed. R. C. A. Thompson, J. A. Reynoldson, and A. J. Lymbery), pp. 15–37. CAB International, Wallingford.

Farthing, M., Mata, L., Urrutia, J., and Kronmal, R. (1986). Natural history of *Giardia* infection of infants and children in rural Guatemala and its impact on physical growth. *American Journal of Clinical Nutrition*, **43**, 395–405.

Faubert, G. M. (1988). Evidence that giardiasis is a zoonosis. *Parasitology Today*, **4**, 66–8.

Filice, F. P. (1952). Studies on the cytology and life history of a *Giardia* from the laboratory rat. *University of California Publication on Zoology*, **57**, 53–146.

Flanagan, P. A. (1992). *Giardia*—diagnosis, clinical course and epidemiology. A review. *Epidemiology and Infection*, **109**, 1–22.

Forshaw, D., Palmer, D. G., Halse, S. A., Hopkins, R. M., and Thompson, R. C. A. (1992). *Giardia* infection in straw necked ibis (*Threskiornis spinicollis*). *Veterinary Record*, **131**, 267–8.

Fraser, G. G. and Cooke, K. R. (1991). Endemic giardiasis and municipal water supply. *American Journal of Public Health*, **81**, 760–2.

Georgi, M. E., Carlisle, M. S., and Smiley, L. E. (1986). Giardiasis in a great blue heron (*Ardea herodias*) in New York State: another potential source of waterborne giardiasis. *American Journal of Epidemiology*, **123**, 916–17.

Gillin, F. D., Reiner, D. S., and Boucher, S. E. (1988). Small intestinal factors promote encystation of *Giardia lamblia in vitro. Infection and Immunity*, **56**, 705–7.

Gillon, J. and Ferguson, A. (1984). Changes in the small intestinal mucosa in giardiasis. In *Giardia and giardiasis*, (ed. S. L. Erlandsen and E. A. Meyer), pp. 163–83. Plenum Press, New York.

Gilman, R. H., Marquis, G. S., Miranda, E., Vistegui, M., Miranda, E., and Montinez, H. (1988). Rapid reinfection by *Giardia lamblia* after treatment in a hyperendemic Third World community. *Lancet*, **i**, 343–5.

Goka, A. K. J., Rolston, D. D. K., Mathan, V. I., and Farthing, M. J. G. (1990). The relative merits of faecal and duodenal juice microscopy in the diagnosis of giardiasis. *Transactions of the Royal Society of Tropical Medicine and Hygiene*, **84**, 66–7.

Gracey, M. (1983). Enteric disease in young Australian Aborigines. *Australian and New Zealand Journal of Medicine*, **3**, 576–9.

Gracey, M. (1994). The clinical significance of giardiasis in Australian Aboriginal children. In *Giardia: from molecules to disease*, (ed. R. C. A. Thompson, J. A. Reynoldson, and A. J. Lymbery), pp. 281–91. CAB International, Wallingford.

Grant, D. R. and Woo, P. T. K. (1978). Comparative studies of *Giardia* spp. in small mammals in southern Ontario. II. Host specificity and infectivity of stored cysts. *Canadian Journal of Zoology*, **56**, 1360–6.

Hall, A. (1994). *Giardia* infections: epidemiology and nutritional consequences. In *Giardia: from molecules to disease*, (ed. R. C. A. Thompson, J. A. Reynoldson, and A. J. Lymbery), pp. 251–80. CAB International, Wallingford.

Hall, A. and Nahar, W. (1993). Albendazole as a treatment for infections with *Giardia duodenalis* in children in Bangladesh. *Transactions of the Royal Society of Tropical Medicine and Hygiene*, **87**, 84–6.

Hall, E. J., Rutgers, H. C., and Batt, R. M. (1988). Evaluation of the peroral string test in the diagnosis of canine giardiasis. *Journal of Small Animal Practice*, **29**, 177–83.

Hall, M. L., Costa, N. D., Thompson, R. C. A., Lymbery, A. J., Meloni, B. P., and Wales, R. G. (1992). Genetic variants of *Giardia duodenalis* differ in their metabolism. *Parasitology Research*, **78**, 712–14.

Halloran, M. E., Bundy, D. A. P., and Pollitt, E. (1989). Infectious disease and the Unesco basic education initiative. *Parasitology Today*, **5**, 359–62.

Hare, D. F., Jarroll, E. L., and Lindmark, D. G. (1989). *Giardia lamblia*: characterization of proteinase activity in trophozoites. *Experimental Parasitology*, **68**, 168–75.

Hay, D. C., Savva, D., and Nowell, F. (1990). Characterisation of *Giardia* species of canine and human origin using RFLPs. *Veterinary Record*, **126**, 274.

Hernandez-Sanchez, J. and Ortega-Pierres, M. G. (1993). Isolation of adhesion deficient *Giardia lamblia* clones with a reduced ability to establish infection in Mongolian gerbils. *Journal of Parasitology*, **79**, (Suppl.), 287.

Heymans, H. S. A., Aronson, D. C., and van Hooft, M. A. J. (1987). Giardiasis in childhoold: an unnecessarily expensive diagnosis. *European Journal of Pediatrics*, **146**, 401–3.

Hopkins, R. M., Thompson, R. C. A., Hobbs, R. P., Lymbery, A. J., Villa, N., and Smithyman, T. M. (1993*a*). Differences in antigen expression within and between 10 isolates of *Giardia duodenalis*. *Acta Tropica*, **54**, 117–24.

Hopkins, R. M., Deplazes, P., Meloni, B. P., Reynoldson, J. A., and Thompson, R. C. A. (1993*b*). A field and laboratory evaluation of a commerical ELISA for the detection of *Giardia* coproantigens in humans and dogs. *Transactions of the Royal Society of Tropical Medicine and Hygiene*, **87**, 39–41.

Hopkins, R. M., Gracey, M., Spargo, R. M., Yates, M. and Thompson, R. C. A. (1997*a*). The prevalence of hookworm (*Ancylostoma duodenale*) infection, iron deficiency and anaemia in an Aboriginal community in north-west Australia. *Medical Journal of Australia*, **166**, 241–4.

Hopkins, R. M., Meloni, B. P., Groth, D. M., Wetherall, J. D., Reynoldson, J. A. and Thompson, R. C. A. (1997*b*). Ribosomal RNA sequencing reveals differences between genotypes of *Giardia* isolates recovered from humans and dogs living in the same locality. *Journal of Parasitology*, **83**, 44–51.

Hopkins, R. S. and Juranek, D. D. (1991). Acute giardiasis: an improved clinical case definition for epidemiologic studies. *American Journal of Epidemiology*, **133**, 402–7.

Hoskins, J. D. (1990). *Giardia*: a common invader. *Veterinary Technician*, **11**, 379–83.

Isaac-Renton, J. L., Cordeiro, C., Sarafis, K., and Shahriari, H. (1993). Characterization of *Giardia duodenalis* isolates from a waterborne outbreak. *Journal of Infectious Diseases*, **167**, 431–40.

Islam, A. (1990). Giardiasis in developing countries. In *Giardiasis*, (ed. E. A. Meyer), pp. 235–66. Elsevier, Amsterdam.

Jafri, H. S. *et al.* (1993). Detection of pathogenic protozoa in fecal specimens from urban dwelling dogs. *Journal of Parasitology*, **79**, 361.

Jarroll, E. L. (1994). Biochemical mechanisms of antigiardial drug action. In *Giardia: from molecules to disease*, (ed. R. C. A. Thompson, J. A. Reynoldson, and A. J. Lymbery), pp. 329–37. CAB International, Wallingford.

Jephcott, A. E., Begg, N. T., and Baker, I. A. (1986). Outbreak of giardiasis associated with mains water in the United Kingdom. *Lancet*, **i**, 730–2.

Jokipii, L. and Jokipii, A. M. M. (1974). Giardiasis in travelers: a prospective study. *Journal of Infectious Diseases*, **130**, 295–9.

Kabnick, K. S. and Peattie, D. A. (1990). *In situ* analyses reveal that the two nuclei of *Giardia lamblia* are equivalent. *Journal of Cell Science*, **95**, 353–60.

Kaminsky, R. G. (1991). Parasitism and diarrhoea in children from two rural communities and marginal barrio in Honduras. *Transactions of the Royal Society of Tropical Medicine and Hygiene*, **85**, 70–3.

Keister, D. B. (1983). Axenic culture of *Giardia lamblia* in TYI-S-33 medium supplemented with bile. *Transactions of the Royal Society of Tropical Medicine and Hygiene*, **77**, 487–8.

Keystone, J. S., Krajden, S., and Warren, M. R. (1978). Person-to-person transmission of *Giardia lamblia* in day care nurseries. *Canadian Medical Journal*, **119**, 241–8.

Kirkpatrick, C. E. (1984). Enteric protozoal infections. In *Clinical microbiology and infectious diseases of the dog and cat*, (ed. C. E. Greene), pp. 806–23. W. B. Saunders, Philadelphia.

Kirkpatrick, C. E. (1988). Epizootiology of enteroparasitic infections in pet dogs and cats presented to a veterinary teaching hospital. *Veterinary Parasitology*, **30**, 113–24.

Kirkpatrick, C. E. (1989). Giardiasis in large animals. *Compendium for Continuing Education for Practicing Veterinarians*, **11**, 80–4.

Knight, R. (1980). Epidemiology and transmission of giardiasis. *Transactions of the Royal Society of Tropical Medicine and Hygiene*, **74**, 433–6.

Kulda, J. and Nohynkova, E. (1978). Flagellates of the human intestine and of intestines of other species. In *Parasitic protozoa*, (ed. J. P. Kreier), Vol. II, pp. 2–139. Academic Press, New York.

Lambl, W. (1859). Mikroskopische Untersuchungen der Darm-Excrete. *Vierteljahtsschrift fur die praktisch Heilkunde (Prag)*, **61**, 1–58.

LeChevallier, M. W., Norton, W. D., and Lee, R. G. (1991). Occurrence of *Giardia* and *Cryptosporidium* spp. in surface water supplies. *Applied and Environmental Microbiology*, **57**, 2610–16.

Lederberg, J., Shope, R. E., and Oaks, S. C. (ed.) (1992). *Emerging infections: microbial threats to health in the United States*. National Academy Press, Washington.

Levine, W. C., Stephenson, W. T., and Craun, G. F. (1990). Waterborne disease outbreaks, 1986–1988. *Morbidity and Mortality Weekly Report*, **39**, 1–13.

Lymbery, A. J. and Tibayrenc, M. (1994). Population genetics and systematics: how many species of *Giardia* are there? In *Giardia: from molecules to disease*, (ed. R. C. A. Thompson, J. A. Reynoldson, and A. J. Lymbery), pp. 71–9. CAB International, Wallingford.

McGowan, I. and Weller, I. (1990). AIDS and the gut. In *Recent advances in gasteroenterology*, (ed. R. E. Pounder), pp. 133–56. Churchill Livingston, London.

McInnes, L. M. (1994). Phenotypic characterisation of the differential sensitivity of *Giardia* Isolated to drugs. Honours Thesis, Murdoch University, Western Australia

Mackenstedt, U., Gauer, M., Mehlhorn, H., Schein, E., and Hauschild, S. (1990*a*). Sexual cycle of *Babesia divergens* confirmed by DNA measurements. *Parasitology Research*, **76**, 199–206.

Mackenstedt, U., Wagner, D., Heydorn, A. O., and Mehlhorn, H. (1990*b*). DNA measurements and ploidy determination of different stages in the life cycle of *Sarcocystis muris*. *Parasitology Research*, **76**, 662–8.

McRoberts, K. M. *et al.* (1996). Morphological and molecular characterisation of *Giardia* isolated from the straw-necked ibis (*Threskiornis spinicollis*) in Western Australia. *Journal of Parasitology*, **82**, 711–8.

Magne, D. *et al.* (1991). Role of cytoskeleton and surface lectins in *Giardia duodenalis* attachment to Caco2 cells. *Parasitology Research*, **77**, 659–62.

Majewska, A. C. (1994). Successful experimental infections of a human volunteer and Mongolian gerbils with *Giardia* of animal origin. *Transactions of the Royal Society of Tropical Medicine and Hygiene*, **88**, 360–2.

Majewska, A. C., Kasprzak, W., and Kaczmarek, E. (1993). Comparative morphometry of *Giardia* trophozoites from man and animals. *Acta Protozoologica*, **32**, 191–7.

Malloy, D. C., Groves, C., and Schwartz, D. A. (1993). Giardiasis: a case report and discussion of outbreaks in the United States. *Maryland Medical Journal*, **42**, 43–6.

Marino, M. R., Brown, T. J., Waddington, D. C., Brockie, R. E., and Kelly, P. J. (1992). *Giardia intestinalis* in North Island possums, house mice and ship rats. *New Zealand Veterinary Journal*, **40**, 24–7.

Meloni, B. P., Lymbery, A. J., and Thompson, R. C. A. (1988*a*). Isoenzyme electrophoresis of 30 isolates of *Giardia* from humans and felines. *American Journal of Tropical Medicine and Hygiene*, **38**, 65–73.

Meloni, B. P., Lymbery, A. J., Thompson, R. C. A., and Gracey, M. (1988*b*). High prevalence of *Giardia lamblia* in children from a WA Aboriginal community. *Medical Journal of Australia*, **149**, 715.

Meloni, B. P., Lymbery, A. J., and Thompson, R. C. A. (1989). Characterisation of *Giardia* isolates using a non-radiolabelled DNA probe, and correlation with the results of isoenzyme analysis. *American Journal of Tropical Medicine and Hygiene*, **40**, 629–37.

Meloni, B. P., Thompson, R. C. A., Reynoldson, J. A., and Seville, P. (1990). Albendazole: a more effective antigiardial agent *in vitro* than metronidazole or tinidazole. *Transactions of the Royal Society of Tropical Medicine and Hygiene*, **84**, 375–9.

Meloni, B. P., Thompson, R. C. A., Stranden, A. M., Kohler, P., and Eckert, J. (1992). Critical comparison of *Giardia duodenalis* from Australia and Switzerland using isoenzyme electrophoresis. *Acta Tropica*, **50**, 115–24.

Meloni, B. P., Thompson, R. C. A., Hopkins, R. M., Reynoldson, J. A., and Gracey, M. (1993). The prevalence of *Giardia* and other intestinal parasites in children, dogs and cats from Aboriginal communities in the Kimberley. *Medical Journal of Australia*, **158**, 157–9.

Meloni, B. P., Lymbery, A. J., Binz, N., and Thompson, R. C. A. (1994). Genetic structure and reproductive strategies in *Giardia*. In *Giardia: from molecules to disease*, (ed. R. C. A. Thompson, J. A. Reynoldson, and A. J. Lymbery), pp. 49–50. CAB International, Wallingford.

Meloni, B. P., Lymbery, A. J., and Thompson, R. C. A. (1995). Genetic characterization of isolates of *Giardia duodenalis* by enzyme electrophoresis: implications for reproductive biology, population structure, taxonomy and epidemiology. *Journal of Parasitology*, **81**, 368–83.

Meyer, E. A. (1990*a*). Preface. In *Giardiasis*, (ed. E. A. Meyer). pp. v–vi. Elsevier, Amsterdam.

Meyer, E. A. (1990*b*). Taxonomy and nomenclature. In *Giardiasis*, (ed. E. A. Meyer), pp. 51–60. Elsevier, Amsterdam.

Meyer, E. A. and Jarroll, E. J. (1980). Giardiasis. *American Journal of Epidemiology*, **111**, 1–12.

Mintz, E. D., Hudson-Wragg, M., Mshar, P., Cartter, M. L., and Hadler, J. L. (1993). Foodborne giardiasis in a corporate office setting. *Journal of Infectious Diseases*, **167**, 250–3.

Moore, G. T. *et al.* (1969). Epidemic giardiasis at a ski resort. *New England Journal of Medicine*, **281**, 402–7.

Moorehead, P., Guasparini, R., Donovan, C. A., Mathias, R. G., Cottle, R., and Baytalan, G. (1990). Giardiasis outbreak from a chlorinated community water supply. *Canadian Journal of Public Health*, **81**, 358–62.

Morgan, U. M., Constantine, C. C., Greene, W. K., and Thompson, R. C. A. (1993*a*). RAPD (random amplified polymorphic DNA) analysis of *Giardia* DNA and correlation with isoenzyme data. *Transactions of the Royal Society of Tropical Medicine and Hygiene*, **87**, 702–5.

Morgan, U. M., Reynoldson, J. A., and Thompson, R. C. A. (1993*b*). Activities of several benzimidazoles and tubulin inhibitors against *Giardia* spp. *in vitro*. *Antimicrobial Agents and Chemotherapy*, **37**, 328–31.

Nash, T. E. (1994). Imunology: the role of the parasite. In *Giardia: from molecules to disease* (ed. R. C. A. Thompson, J. A. Reynoldson, and A. J. Lymbery), pp. 139–154. CAB International, Wallingford.

Nash, T. E., Merritt, J. W., and Conrad, J. T. (1991). Isolate and epitope variability in susceptibility of *Giardia lamblia* to intestinal proteases. *Infection and Immunity*, **59**, 1334–40.

Neringer, R., Andersson, Y., and Baker, I. A. (1986). A waterborne outbreak of giardiasis in Sweden. *Scandinavian Journal of Infectious Disease*, **19**, 85–90.

Nikolic, A., Petrovic, Z., and Radovic, M. (1990). Prevalence of *Giardia lamblia* in school children in Serbia, Yugoslavia. *Epidemiology of Directly Transmitted Parasites*, **S6.D 25**, 755.

Pacha, R. E., Clark, G. W., Williams, E. A., Carter, A. M., Scheffelmaier, J. J. and Debusschere, P. (1987). Small rodents and other mammals associated with mountain meadows as reservoirs of *Giardia* spp. and *Campylobacter* spp. *Applied and Environmental Microbiology*, **53**, 1574–9.

Pancorbo, J. M. C., Munoz, M. T. G., and Badia, J. L. S. (1985). Giardiasis: treatment of carriers. *Lancet*, **ii**, 984.

Parenti, D. M. (1989). Characterization of a thiol proteinase in *Giardia lamblia*. *Journal of Infectious Diseases*, **160**, 1076–80.

Pawlowski, Z., Kasprzak, W., Kociecka, W., and Lisowska, M. (1987). Epidemiological studies on giardiasis in Poznan Province—a review. *Wiadomosci Parasitologica*, **33**, 593–613.

Perlmutter, D. H., Leichtner, A. M., Goldman, H., and Winter, H. S. (1985). Chronic diarrhea associated with hypogammaglobulinemia and enteropathy in infants and children. *Digestive Disease Science*, **30**, 1149–55.

Petersen, L. R., Carter, M. L., and Hadler, J. L. (1988). A food-borne outbreak of *Giardia lamblia*. *Journal of Infectious Disease*, **157**, 846–8.

Phillips, S. C., Mildvan, D., Williams, D. C., Gelb, A. M., and White, M. C. (1981). Sexual transmission of enteric protozoa and helminths in a venereal-disease clinic population. *New England Journal of Medicine*, **305**, 603–6.

Pickering, L. K., Evans, D. G., Du Pont, H. L., Vollet, J. J., and Evans, D. J. (1981). Diarrhea caused by *Shigella*, rotavirus, and *Giardia* in day care centers: prospective study. *Journal of Pediatrics*, **99**, 51–6.

Polis, M. A., Tuazon, C. U., Alling, D. W., and Talmanis, E. (1986). Transmission of *Giardia lamblia* from a day care center to the community. *American Journal of Public Health*, **76**, 1142–4.

Pospisilova, D. and Svobodova, V. (1992). Giardiasis in dog and cat owners. *Microbiology and Immunology*, **41**, 106–10.

Quinn, R. W. (1971). The epidemiology of intestinal parasites of importance in the United States. *Southern Medical Bulletin*, **59**, 29–30.

Rabbani, G. H. and Islam, A. (1994). Giardiasis in humans: populations most at risk and prospects for control. In *Giardia: from molecules to disease*, (ed. R. C. A. Thompson, J. A. Reynoldson, and A. J. Lymbery), pp. 217–49. CAB International, Wallingford.

Radulescu, S. and Meyer, E. A. (1990). *In vitro* cultivation of *Giardia* trophozoites. In *Giardiasis*, (ed. E. A. Meyer) pp. 99–110. Elsevier, Amsterdam.

Rendtorff, R. (1954). The experimental transmission of human intestinal protozoan parasites. II. *Giardia lamblia* cysts given in capsules. *American Journal of Hygiene*, **59**, 209–20.

Reynoldson, J. A. (1994). New approaches in chemotherapy. In *Giardia: from molecules to disease*, (ed. R. C. A. Thompson, J. A. Reynoldson, and A. J. Lymbery), pp. 339–55. CAB International, Wallingford.

Reynoldson, J. A., Thompson, R. C. A., and Meloni, B. P. (1992*a*). The potential and possible mode of action of the benzimidazoles against *Giardia* and other protozoa. *Journal of Pharmaceutical Medicine*, **2**, 35–50.

Reynoldson, J. A., Thompson, R. C. A., and Horton, R. J. (1992*b*). Albendazole as a future antigiardial agent. *Parasitology Today*, **8**, 412–13.

Romia, S. A., Abou-Zakham, A. A., Gamil, R., and El-Khouly, E-S.I. (1990). Virulence of *Giardia lamblia* isolates. *Journal of the Egyptian Society of Parasitology*, **20**, 633–9.

Sawaya, A. L., Amigo, H., and Sigulem, D. (1990). The risk approach in preschool children suffering malnutrition and intestinal parasitic infection in the city of Sao Paulo, Brazil. *Journal of Tropical Pediatrics*, **36**, 184–8.

Schantz, P. M. (1991). Parasitic zoonoses in perspective. *International Journal for Parasitology*, **21**, 161–70.

Schofield, P. J. and Edwards, M. R. (1994). Biochemistry—is *Giardia* opportunistic in its use of substrates? In *Giardia: from molecules to disease*, (ed. R. C. A. Thompson, J. A., Reynoldson, and A. J. Lymbery), pp. 171–83. CAB International, Wallingford.

Siddall, M. E., Hong, H., and Desser, S. S. (1992). Phylogenetic analysis of the diplomonadida (Wenyon, 1926) Brugerolle, 1975: evidence for heterochrony in protozoa and against *Giardia lamblia* as a 'missing link'. *Journal of Protozoology*, **39**, 361–7.

Simpson, J. W., Burnie, A. G., Miles, R. S., Scott, J. L., and Lindsay, D. I. (1988). Prevalence of *Giardia* and *Cryptosporidium* infection in dogs in Edinburgh. *Veterinary Record*, **123**, 445.

Smith, P. D. (1985). Pathophysiology and immunology of giardiasis. *Annual Reviews of Medicine*, **36**, 295–307.

Sogin, M. L., Gunderson, J. H., Elwood, H. J., Alonso, R. A., and Peattie, D. A. (1989). Phylogenetic meaning of the kingdom concept: an unusual ribosomal RNA from *Giardia lamblia* Science, **243**, 75–7.

Speelman, P. and Ljungström, I. (1986). Protozoal enteric infections among expatriates in Bangladesh. *American Journal of Tropical Medicine and Hygiene*, **35**, 1140–5.

Stevenson, W. J. and Hughes, K. L. (1988). *Synopsis of zoonoses in Australia*. Australian Government Publishing Service, Canberra.

Sullivan, P., Woodward, W. E., Pickering, D. G., and DuPont, H. L. (1984). Longitudinal study of diarrheal disease in day care centers. *American Journal of Public Health*, **74**, 987–91.

Sullivan, P. B. *et al.* (1991). Prevalence and treatment of giardiasis in chronic diarrhoea and malnutrition. *Archives of Disease of Childhood*, **66**, 3–6

Swan, J. M. (1984). Giardiasis in dogs and cats in Western Australia. Honours Thesis, Murdoch University, Western Australia.

Swan, J. M. and Thompson, R. C. A. (1986). The prevalence of *Giardia* in dogs and cats in Perth, Western Australia. *Australian Veterinary Journal*, **63**, 110–12.

Taminelli, V. and Eckert, J. (1989). Haufigkeit und geographische verbreitung des *Giardia* Befalls bei Wiederkauern in der Schweiz. *Schweizer Archiv für Tierheilkunde*, **131**, 251–8.

Thompson, R. C. A. (1992*a*). Giardiasis. In *Zoonoses*, Proceedings 194, pp. 88–91. Postgraduate Committee in Veterinary Science, University of Sydney.

Thompson, R. C. A. (1992*b*). Parasitic zoonoses—problems created by people, not animals. *International Journal for Parasitology*, **22**, 555–61.

Thompson, R. C. A. and Boreham, P. F. L. (1994). Biotic and abiotic transmission. In *Giardia: from molecules to disease*, (ed. R. C. A. Thompson, J. A. Reynoldson, and A. J. Lymbery), pp. 131–6. CAB International, Wallingford.

Thompson, R. C. A. and Lymbery, A. J. (1996). Genetic variability in parasites and host–parasite interactions. *Parasitology*, **112**, 57–522.

Thompson, R. C. A. and Meloni, B. P. (1993). Molecular variation in *Giardia* and its implications. *Acta Tropica*, **53**, 167–84.

Thompson, R. C. A., Meloni, B. P. and Lymbery, A. J. (1988*a*). Humans and cats have genetically-identical forms of *Giardia*: evidence of a zoonotic relationship. *Medical Journal of Australia*, **148**, 207–9.

Thompson, R. C. A., Lymbery, A. J., and Meloni, B. P. (1988*b*). Giardiasis: a zoonosis in Australia? *Parasitology Today*, **4**, 201.

Thompson, R. C. A., Lymbery, A. J., and Meloni, B. P. (1990*a*). Genetic variation in *Giardia* Kunstler, 1882: taxonomic and epidemiological significance. *Protozoological Abstracts*, **14**, 1–28.

Thompson, R. C. A., Lymbery, A. J., Meloni, B. P., and Binz, N. (1990*b*). The zoonotic transmission of *Giardia* species. *Veterinary Record*, **126**, 513–14.

Thompson, R. C. A., Reynoldson, J. A., and Mendis, A. H. W. (1993*a*). *Giardia* and giardiasis. *Advances in Parasitology*, **32**, 71–160.

Thompson, R. C. A., Meloni, B. P., Hopkins, R. M., Deplazes, P., and Reynoldson, J. A. (1993*b*). Observations on the endo-and ectoparasites affecting dogs and cats in Aboriginal communities in the north-west of Western Australia. *Australian Veterinary Journal*, **70**, 268–9.

Thompson, R. C. A., Reynoldson, J. A., and Lymbery, A. J. (ed.) (1994). *Giardia: from molecules to disease and beyond*. CAB International, Wallingford.

Tibayrenc, M. (1994). How many species of *Giardia* are there? In *Giardia: from molecules to disease*, (ed. R. C. A. Thompson, J. A. Reynoldson, and A. J. Lymbery), pp. 41–8. CAB International, Wallingford.

Tibayrenc, M. and Ayala, F. J. (1991). Towards a population genetics of micro-organisms: the clonal theory of parasitic protozoa. *Parasitology Today*, **7**, 228–32.

Tibayrence, M., Kjellberg, F., and Ayala, F. J. (1990). A clonal theory of parasitic protozoa: the population structures of *Entamoeba*, *Giardia*, *Leishmania*, *Naegleria*, *Plasmodium*, *Trichomonas* and *Trypanosoma* and their medical and taxonomical consequences. *Proceedings of the National Academy of Sciences*, **87**, 2414–18.

Tibayrenc, M., Neubauer, K., Barnabe, C., Guerrini, F., Skarecky, D., and Ayala, F. J. (1993). Genetic characterisation of six parasitic protozoa: parity between random-primer DNA typing and multilocus enzyme electrophoresis. *Proceedings of the National Academy of Sciences*, **90**, 1335–9.

Tonks, M. C., Brown, T. J., and Ionas, G. (1991). *Giardia* infection of cats and dogs in New Zealand. *New Zealand Veterinary Journal*, **39**, 33–4.

Torres, D. M., Chieffi, P. P., Costa, W. A., and Kudzielics, E. (1991). Giardiase em creches mantidas pela prefeitura do Municipiode Sao Paulo. *Reviews Instituto Medicine Tropicale Sao Paulo*, **33**, 137–42.

Van Keulen, H., Horvat, S., Erlandsen, S. L., and Jarroll, E. L. (1991). Nucleotide sequence of the 5.8S and large subunit rRNA genes and the internal transcribed spacer and part of the external spacer from *Giardia ardeae*. *Nucleic Acids Research*, **19**, 6050.

Van Keulen, H., Gutell, R. R., Erlandsen, S. L., and Jarroll, E. L. (1994). In *Giardia: from molecules to disease*, (ed. R. C. A. Thompson, J. A. Reynoldson, and A. J. Lymbery), pp. 68–9. CAB International, Wallingford.

Wade, A. and Yapp, G. (1989). *Giardia: an emerging issue in water management.* Centre for Continuing Education, Australian National University, Canberra.

Wallis, P. M. (1994). Abiotic transmission—is water really significant? In *Giardia: from molecules to disease,* (ed. R. C. A. Thompson, J. A. Reynoldson, and A. J. Lymbery), pp. 99–122. CAB International, Wallingford.

Wallis, P. M., Zammuto, R. M., and Buchanan-Mappin, J. M. (1986). Cysts of *Giardia* spp. in mammals and surface waters in southwestern Alberta. *Journal of Wildlife Diseases,* **22**, 115–18.

Webster, A. D. B. (1980). Giardiasis and immunodeficiency diseases. *Transactions of the Royal Society of Tropical Medicine and Hygiene,* **74**, 440–8.

White, K. E., Hedberg, C. W., Edmonson, L. M., Jones, D. B. W., Osterholm, M. T., and MacDonald, K. L. (1989). An outbreak of giardiasis in a nursing home with evidence of multiple modes of transmission. *Journal of Infectious Diseases,* **160**, 298–304.

Winsland, J. K. D., Nimmo, S., Butcher, P. D., and Farthing, M. J. G. (1989). Prevalence of *Giardia* in dogs and cats in the United Kingdom: survey of an Essex veterinary clinic. *Transactions of the Royal Society of Tropical Medicine and Hygiene,* **83**, 791–2.

Wolfe, M. S. (1990). Clinical symptoms and diagnosis by traditional methods. In *Giardiasis,* (ed. E. A. Meyer), pp. 175–85. Elsevier, Amsterdam.

Xiao, L. (1994). *Giardia* infection in farm animals. *Parasitology Today,* **10**, 436–8.

Yardley, J. H., Takano, J., and Hendrix, T. R. (1964). Epithelial and other mucosal lesions of the jejunum in giardiasis: jejunal biopsy studies. *Bulletin of Johns Hopkins Hospital,* **115**, 389–406.

45 CRYPTOSPORIDIOSIS

R. L. Coop, S. E. Wright, and D. P. Casemore

INTRODUCTION

Although there are at least six species of *Cryptosporidium* (*C. baileyi* and *C. meleagridis* in birds; *C. muris* and *C. parvum* in mammals; *C. nasorum* in fish and *C. serpentis* in reptiles) it is *Cryptosporidium parvum* which is responsible for zoonotic infections, causing neonatal diarrhoea in lambs and calves and self-limited diarrhoea in immunocompetent human beings, but severe, persistent or chronic life-threatening diarrhoea in immunocompromised patients, particularly those with acquired immunodeficiency syndrome (AIDS).

This chapter focuses on *C. parvum* and refers to other *Cryptosporidium* species only where relevant.

HISTORY

Cryptosporidium is a small protozoan coccidian obligate parasite which infects mainly the apical region of epithelial cells lining the gastrointestinal tract of vertebrates, sometimes the respiratory tract and also can involve associated organs such as the biliary tract.

Tyzzer first formally described a small protozoan in the gastric epithelium of laboratory mice in 1907 which he named *C. muris*. In 1912 Tyzzer identified a second species of *Cryptosporidium* from the small intestines of mice. The oocysts of this species were smaller and the species was therefore named *C. parvum*. Although similar to that of other coccidia of the genus *Eimeria* the life cycle of *Cryptosporidium* has several different features:

(1) the microgametes do not have flagellae;
(2) the oocyst has a suture and does not have a sporocyst surrounding the sporozoites (Current and Reese 1986);
(3) sporulation occurs within the host.

A new family was therefore created, the Cryptosporidiiae, which includes the single genus *Cryptosporidium*.

Until the 1970s *C. parvum* was generally considered as an unimportant commensal. Veterinary and medical interest was stimulated (Reese *et al.* 1982) only after Panciera *et al.* (1971) described an episode of diarrhoea in a heifer which was associated with *Cryptosporidium* and, subsequently, the first cases of human infection were reported (Miesel *et al.* 1976; Nime *et al.* 1976). The involvement of *C. parvum* as an opportunist pathogen in immunocompromised patients with AIDS (Anon 1982) has resulted in an exponential increase in research activity over the past decade and *Cryptosporidium* has been the subject of a number of comprehensive reviews (Fayer and Ungar 1986; Chermette and Boufassa-Ouzrout 1988; Crawford and Vermund 1988; Angus and Blewett 1988; Naciri 1989; Casemore 1990*a*; Current and Blagburn 1990; Dubey *et al.* 1990; Current and Garcia 1991; O'Donoghue 1995; Meinhardt 1996).

THE AGENT

Cryptosporidium parvum infects primarily the small intestine of mammals and man and is the most frequently isolated cryptosporidial species. The oocysts are small (average diameter 4.5–5 μm) and *C. parvum* infection is responsible for diarrhoea in neonates or immunocompromised host animals. Human infection is not age limited and occurs in otherwise healthy immunocompetent but susceptible adults as well as the immunocompromised. Neonatal infection is uncommon even in underdeveloped countries.

TAXONOMY

Cryptosporidium follows the general classification of small intracellular protozoa; it belongs to the phylum, Apicomplexa; subclass, Coccidiasina; suborder, Eimeriorina; and family Cryptosporidiidae, which contains one genus, *Cryptosporidium* (Current, 1987). It can be differentiated from other coccidia by its size, structure, and by its development in the brush border region of epithelial cells where it has a superficial intracellular but extracytoplasmic location. Cross-transmission experiments have demonstrated the lack of host specificity of mammalian isolates of *Cryptosporidium* and this led Tzipori *et al.* (1980) to consider it as a single-species genus. This was subsequently disputed by Levine (1984) who rationalized the parasites into four species, *C. muris*, *C. meleagridis*, *C. crotali*, and *C. nasorum*, respectively, in mammals, birds, reptiles, and fish. However, a detailed examination of *C. crotali* has indicated that this is incorrect and that it is considered to be a species of *Sarcocystis*. At least two species have been shown to affect birds, *C. meleagridis* and *C. baileyi* (Current *et al.* 1986) and a minimum of two species infecting mammals, *C. parvum* (small intestine) and *C. muris* (stomach) (Upton and Current 1985). There is a single report in the literature of *C. baileyi* infection in an immunocompromised human (Ditrich *et al.* 1991) but the identification was uncertain (Ditrich, personal communication). Current (1988) suggested that species producing clinical disease in man and other mammals (with oocysts in the range 4–5 μm) should be referred to as *C. parvum* or, if insufficiently definitive details are available, as *Cryptosporidium* sp. He also suggested that the term 'isolate' rather than 'strain' be used for material recovered from mammalian hosts until further information is available on the taxonomy of *Cryptosporidium* spp.

LIFE CYCLE

The direct life-cycle of *C. parvum* is generally similar in all mammalian hosts and differs from that of other coccidia (*Eimeria* and *Isospora* spp.) in several respects:

(1) there is re-cycling from type I meronts;
(2) the production of thin-walled auto-infective oocysts;
(3) the sporulation of oocysts occurs within the host cells;
(4) the parasitophorous vacuole containing the intracellular stage of *C. parvum* is located superficially in the brush border region of the enterocyte.

The life-cycle (Fig. 45.1) is based on the proposal by Current (1988) and Current and Garcia (1991).

Sporulated thick-walled oocysts are ingested by the host from the environment and undergo excystation within the intestine to release four motile infective sporozoites. These invade the microvillous border region of the enterocytes, without penetrating the cytoplasm, and develop within the parasitophorous vacuole into trophozoites which undergo merogony and produce mature type I meronts containing eight merozoites. These can undergo re-cycling by liberating merozoites which invade new enterocytes, producing second-generation type I meronts. Merozoites can also enter enterocytes and mature to produce type II meronts containing four merozoites which do not recycle but develop and differentiate to either microgamonts containing 12–16 microgametes or to macrogamonts which mature into macrogametes. The

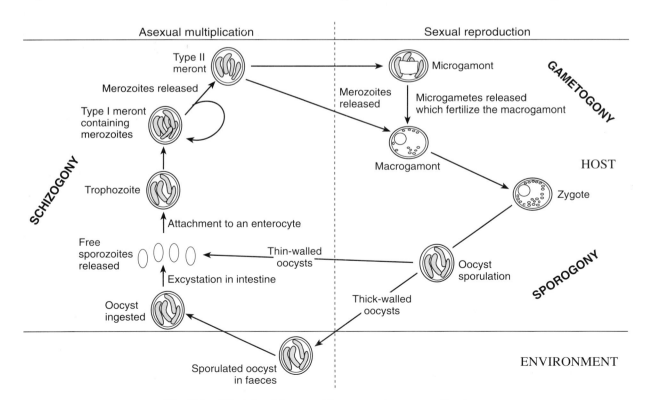

Fig. 45.1 Life cycle of *Cryptosporidium parvum* in a mammalian host.

microgamont releases free microgametes which fertilize the macrogamete to form a zygote. The majority (approximately 80 per cent) of these form thick-walled oocysts which undergo sporulation in the enterocyte and are passed into the faeces as the resistant sporulated infective oocyst containing four naked sporozoites. A minority of zygotes (approximately 20 per cent) are surrounded only by a unit membrane and these thin-walled oocysts rupture and release sporozoites which then recommence the infective cycle by invading other enterocytes (endogenous autoinfection). These two multiplicative stages (thin-walled oocysts and type I meronts) allow *C. parvum* to multiply rapidly and colonize the intestine of the host, even when the intake of infective oocysts from the environment is low.

MOLECULAR BIOLOGY

Despite the importance of *C. parvum*, infection studies at the genetic level have been undertaken only recently. The application of recombinant DNA technology and electrophoretic gel techniques, coupled with the ability to harvest and purify large numbers of oocysts and sporozoites, have begun to yield information on structure and function at the molecular level and to clarify relationships between isolates and species and improve the sensitivity of detection. However, much of the current information is conflicting or contradictory, mainly due to methodological or interpretative differences. Chromosomes have been identified but the number found also varies in different reports (Petersen 1993).

Protein and non-protein antigens and some enzymes have been characterized and some of their encoding genes have been cloned and sequenced (Petersen 1993; O'Donoghue 1995). In addition, some genes coding for structural proteins and proteins associated with biomechanical contractile functions have been characterized, including actin and tubulin, both of which are considered important in parasite motility and penetration, and hence invasion (Nelson *et al.* 1991; Kim *et al.* 1992). These may prove useful target molecules for the development of anti-cryptosporidial compounds. A detailed study of the human humoral immune response to *Cryptosporidium* in the crew of an American Coast Guard cutter, using Western blotting, has shown that a small molecular weight antigen may be of use as a diagnostic marker (Moss *et al.* 1995).

Nucleic acid sequences, isoenzymes, and other molecular structures have indicated both similarities and differences between isolates, within and between species (Morgan *et al.* 1995; Leng *et al.* 1996). Some molecular studies have shown differences between isolates of *C. parvum* from different sources, suggesting that those derived from different animal and human

hosts may differ (Awad-el-Kariem *et al.* 1993, 1995; McDonald and Kariem 1995; Moran *et al.* 1995; Spano *et al.* 1996). These findings, which contradict some epidemiological evidence, are yet to be resolved.

Techniques have been developed for the detection and characterization of cryptosporidial components, such as SDS–PAGE and Western blotting for proteins, and for nucleic acid sequences using PCR (reviewed by Webster 1993; Petersen 1993; McDonald and Kariem 1995; Moran *et al.* 1995). Sensitive genetically based probes have been developed which may be applied to the detection of the parasite in clinical and environmental samples (Webster *et al.* 1993; Johnson *et al.* 1995; O'Donoghue, 1995; Wagner-Wiening and Kimmig 1995). It is probable that some of these techniques will lead to the development of epidemiologically useful typing systems. Molecular methods are now also being applied to sero-prevalence studies (Moss *et al.* 1995; Patel *et al.* 1997).

LOCATION IN THE HOST AND DISEASE MECHANISMS

Cryptosporidium parvum generally infects the ileum, particularly in the region of the epithelial domes of the Payer's patches (Marcial and Madara 1986; Landsverk 1987) but it can be found also in other regions of the intestine. Involvement of crypts may indicate immunodeficiency (Phillips *et al.* 1992). It rarely occurs outside the digestive tract but occasionally has been found in associated organs such as the pancreas, liver, bile duct, gallbladder, and salivary glands. In immunodeficient hosts it may cause a disseminated infection and involve the respiratory tract.

Cryptosporidium maintains an intimate relationship with the host, developing within a parasitophorous vacuole in the brush border of the enterocyte. The vacuolar membrane appears to be host-derived. Electron microscopy has demonstrated fusion between the parasite and the microvilli and the creation of an electron-dense zone of attachment. At the base of the endogenous stages there is a folded lamellar structure which is thought to be a feeder organelle. *Cryptosporidium* is described as being 'intracellular' (being within a host-derived parasitophorous vacuole) but 'extracytoplasmic' (being superficially attached to the microvillous region). However, Marcial and Madara (1986) showed that it can be found also within the cytoplasm of membraneous epithelial cells in Peyer's patches and in macrophages. *Cryptosporidium* infection results in villous atrophy and hyperplasia of the crypt epithelium with infiltration of inflammatory cells.

The underlying mechanisms whereby *Cryptosporidium* causes diarrhoea are largely unknown (Casemore 1989*a*). Studies involving experimental infection of neonatal pigs (Argenzio *et al.* 1990) or gnotobiotic calves (Heine *et al.* 1984) with *C. parvum* suggest that the extent of the damage to the villous epithelium and reduction in absorptive surface area result in impaired digestion and malabsorption in the intestine. There is also widespread interference with brush border enzymes such as disaccharidases (Casemore 1989*a*). A further consequence may be protein-losing enteropathy with efflux of fluid from the mucosa into the intestinal lumen. Similar pathophysiological features are believed to occur in human infection; an enterotoxin may be involved also but this has not been confirmed (Crawford and Vermund 1988; Casemore 1989*a*; Phillips *et al.* 1992).

GROWTH AND SURVIVAL REQUIREMENTS

Limited information has come from attempts to grow and maintain *Cryptosporidium* isolates *in vitro*. Early studies showed that it was possible to infect the chorioallantoic membrane of chicken embryos with sporozoites of either calf or human isolates of *C. parvum* and that they completed their development to form sporulated oocysts (Current and Long 1983). The conditions required for parasite growth appear exacting, as results vary between *in ovo* cultivation systems and various tissue culture systems. The need to produce large numbers of oocysts, free from host contamination, has stimulated the search for more effective culture systems. There are several reports of incomplete development of *C. parvum* in a variety of cultured cell lines. Complete development was first achieved using a human fetal lung cell line (Current and Haynes 1984) but the recovery of oocysts was lower than from *in ovo* methods. Encouraging results have been reported using a human colon carcinoma cell line (Daltry *et al.* 1989; Buraud *et al.* 1991) or canine kidney cells (Gut *et al.* 1991) and recently, Rasmussen *et al.* (1993) have confirmed the complete development and replication of *C. parvum* within a human endometrial carcinoma cell line where production of both asexual and sexual intracellular stages occurred. In these studies there was no long-term proliferation, mainly because of poor sexual cycle development, thus limiting their use as a culture system. *In vitro* cultivation, even if incomplete, provides a useful tool for evaluation of anticryptosporidial drugs (McDonald *et al.* 1990).

THE HOSTS

ANIMAL

Cryptosporidium parvum infection has been recorded in a wide range of mammalian species, including non-human primates, cattle, sheep, goats, horses, pigs, camelids, cats, dogs, deer, antelope, rodents, rabbits, hamsters, and guinea-pigs (Fayer and Unger 1986; O'Donoghue 1995). Clinical disease occurs primarily in neonates, or immunologically compromised animals, older animals being less severely affected. Neonates can experience severe disease after infection and suffer a more protracted illness than older animals (Tzipori *et al.* 1981). An apparent age-related resistance to infection has been demonstrated in mice, calves, and lambs (Sherwood *et al.* 1982; Harp *et al.* 1990; Ortega-Mora and Wright 1994).

Incubation period, symptoms, and signs

The prepatent period (time between ingestion of oocysts and their appearance in faeces) varies between 2 and 12 days, depending on host species. There is also evidence that the size of the infective dose may influence the prepatent period, larger inocula producing earlier shedding of oocysts (Blewett *et al.* 1993). In a completely susceptible host, such as a gnotobiotic lamb, the minimum infective dose capable of initiating a clinical infection may be as low as a single oocyst (Blewett *et al.* 1993).

Onset of clinical symptoms usually coincides with onset of oocyst shedding. Profuse watery diarrhoea, abdominal tension and inappetance, resulting in dehydration, are all symptomatic of clinical cryptosporidiosis. In young domesticated ruminants (cattle, sheep, and goats), a prepatent period, usually of 2–5 days, is followed by a profuse diarrhoea which may persist for 7 days, before symptoms decline and the infection resolves. Excretion of large numbers of oocysts may continue for several days after the clinical symptoms have ceased. Total parasite production during a clinical infection may exceed 10^{10} oocysts, shed over a 7–10 day period. Infection in horses seldom results in clinical symptoms (Xiao *et al.* 1994), although they may contribute to the severity of mixed infections (Browning *et al.* 1991) and there are reports of fatal infections in Arabian foals with severe combined immunodeficiency (Snyder *et al.* 1978; Gibson *et al.* 1983). Infection in pigs is not normally associated with clinical disease, although experimental infections have produced a range of clinical responses, the most severe reactions occurring with the larger infective doses (Vitovec and Koudela 1992). Infection in companion animals or pets (dogs, cats, small rodents, rabbits, hamsters, and guinea-pigs) do not normally result in clinical symptoms, unless present in conjunction with other infections (Fayer and Unger 1986; Mtambo *et al.* 1991; Vitovec *et al.* 1991). While suckling rodents are readily infected and may shed large numbers of oocysts, they show no symptomatic reaction. By 3–4 weeks of age they are more difficult to infect, producing a low-grade infection and shed only small numbers of oocysts.

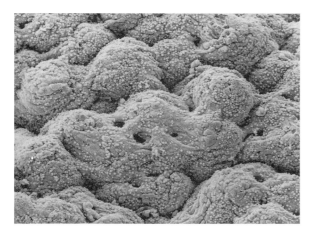

Fig. 45.2 Scanning electron micrograph of ovineileum showing blunt and fused villi covered with endogenous stages of *C. parvum* (×200).

Pathology and pathogenesis

The terminal ileum is the principal focus of infection, being the site where ingested oocysts excyst. Infection can also spread down into the caecum and colon. At necropsy, the small and large intestine may be distended with gas and contain watery yellow fluid. Enteritis and colitis may be apparent. Histopathological changes include blunting and fusion of the villi, which may be covered with endogenous stages of the parasite (Fig. 45.2). Infected epithelial cells can be low columnar, cuboidal, or squamous. The lamina propria may be mildly hypercellular, often infiltrated with mononuclear cells, oedematous with congestion of the vessels. Crypts are often elongated and contain neutrophils and sometimes eosinophils; apoptotic bodies may be present (Casemore 1989*a*). In some instances the mesenteric lymph nodes are oedematous, and reticuloendothelial cell hyperplasia evident.

Diagnosis

Diagnosis of infection is normally by microscopic examination of faecal smears stained most commonly by modified Ziehl-Neelsen (MZN), phenol auramine (PA) or fluorescein isothiocyanate (FITC) labelled monoclonal antibody (MAb) (Casemore 1991). MZN gives characteristic variable pale rose pink to deep-red staining bodies in a dark green ground, while PA and FITC Mab are both fluorescent stains, giving yellow/green or apple green fluorescence, respectively. Oocysts are 4.5–5.5 μm in diameter and often appear more densely stained at the edge, giving an erythrocyte-like effect.

If oocyst numbers are low, as at the end of an infection, concentration techniques can be employed to improve detection. Flotation in Sheather's sucrose

solution, zinc sulphate (specific gravity 1.18–1.20) or saturated sodium chloride (specific gravity 1.27) are all effective. Sedimentation by formalin–ether or formalin–ethyl acetate are also useful although a modified method is preferable (Casemore 1991). It is advisable when using flotation techniques to examine the samples as soon as possible, or dilute the flotation medium, as prolonged exposure to high osmotic pressures will cause the oocysts to collapse and make identification more difficult. Enzyme-linked immunosorbent (ELISA) methods have also been described (Chapman *et al.* 1990; Robert *et al.* 1990) for detection of antigen in faeces, while more recently PCR has been demonstrated as a very sensitive detection technique for oocysts in faeces (Leng *et al.* 1996).

Histological examination of ileal sections stained with haematoxylin and eosin reveals endogenous stages of the parasite as small spherical bodies, 2–5.5 μm in diameter in the microvillous region of the intestinal mucosa. Cryptosporidial infection in monkeys with simian AIDS may have extensive extraintestinal involvement similar to that seen in humans (Baskerville *et al.* 1991).

Serological studies may be used to determine background levels of infection within a population but are of little value for diagnostic purposes. Copro-antibody (IgA) (Hill *et al.* 1990) or the inducing antigen (Reperant *et al.* 1992) have been shown to be important in immunity to infection. Both IFAT (indirect immunofluoroscent antibody technique) and ELISA methods have been described (Current and Bick 1989).

TREATMENT AND PROGNOSIS

No effective therapy exists for cryptosporidiosis, although treatment of the symptoms is possible. Fluid replacement therapy and maintenance in warm conditions until the animal recovers are usually successful. Treatment with antibiotics may prevent bacterial overgrowth of damaged portions of the gut, but it is not always necessary. Colostrum does not appear to provide protection against cryptosporidial infection (Harp *et al.* 1989), although some reports indicate that hyperimmune bovine colostrum may limit the severity of the infection and reduce oocyst shedding in some animal models (Fayer *et al.* 1989*a,b*, 1990).

Numerous drugs have been tested in animal models, but all have failed to provide adequate control of the parasite. Lasalocid (a polyether ionophore antibiotic) was reported as being effective for prophylaxis in calves against experimental infection, but appeared to be toxic at the concentration required (Moon *et al.* 1982). Spiromycin failed to protect calves when administered at appropriate dosages (Blewett, unpublished data) and has been found also to have toxic side-effects on the intestinal epithelial cells (Weikel *et al.* 1991). Prophylactic treatment of goat kids with paromomycin sulphate has been demonstrated to reduce oocyst output and clinical symptoms, but not to effect a complete cure (Chartier *et al.* 1996).

Prognosis is generally good and with adequate supportive treatment bovine calves usually recover completely. Mortality in lambs and goat kids is often higher, but these animals are subjected also to greater environmental stresses than calves, being raised on more marginal lands where climatic changes can be more extreme, resulting in heat stress or hypothermia in an already weakened, inappetant young animal. Mortality rates in red deer calves (*Cervus elaphus*) can also be high, infected animals becoming dull and wasted, and dying within 1–2 days of becoming ill, sometimes in the absence of scouring (Simpson 1992).

HUMAN CRYPTOSPORIDIOSIS

Human infection was first recognized in 1976 (Meisel *et al.* 1976; Nime *et al.* 1976) but became more widely acknowledged as a potentially serious enteric pathogen with the recognition of AIDS and its associated infections in the early 1980s. It was also recorded amongst some occupational groups such as veterinary students and research workers (Reese *et al.* 1982; Currrent *et al.* 1983; Reif *et al.* 1989). Early reports referred to the organism as an opportunist zoonosis for which the major reservoir was believed to be scouring calves. As the early stages of the AIDS pandemic involved mainly urban adult males, this suggested the possibility of other reservoirs or routes of transmission. Subsequently, the parasite was found to be the cause of acute infectious gastroenteritis, worldwide, amongst otherwise healthy populations, especially young children, who may acquire the infection zoonotically or through non-zoonotic (person to person) transmission (Casemore 1990*a*; Hart and Baxby 1987; Ungar 1990; Cordell and Addis 1994; Juranek 1995). Outbreaks have increasingly been associated with open farms (Casemore 1989*b,c*; Shield *et al.* 1990; Anon 1994; Dawson *et al.* 1995; Evans and Gardner 1996). Infection may also be acquired indirectly through the environment, including drinking water and food (Anon 1990, 1995; Casemore 1990*a,b*; Millard *et al.* 1994; Juranek *et al.* 1995; MacKenzie *et al.* 1995; Goldstein *et al.* 1996; Meinhardt *et al.* 1996). It is now apparent that the distinction between zoonotic and non-zoonotic transmission is difficult and may reflect more the potential range of hosts rather than defining a necessary source and route of transmission. A small number of zoonotically acquired or water-borne infections may thus lead, particularly in an urban setting, to widespread propagated (person to person) transmission (Casemore 1990*a*, 1993, 1995*a*; MacKenzie *et al.* 1995). Human-adapted strains may also account for some infections (Awad-el-Kariem *et al.* 1993; McDonald and Kariem 1995; Spano *et al.* 1996).

Incubation period, symptoms, and signs

Cryptosporidiosis in the otherwise healthy patient

The incubation period appears to be about a week (range 2–14 days, although wider ranges have been cited; Jokipii and Jokipii 1986). Infection in immunocompetent humans causes an acute self-limiting gastroenteritis. There is often a prodromal malaise, nausea, and loss of appetite followed by an acute onset of diarrhoea and other symptoms. These include loose or watery stools typical of an excretory diarrhoea, anorexia, vomiting (especially in children), weight loss, and abdominal pain. Some patients may continue to experience mild intermittent symptoms and weight loss for some weeks following resolution of acute symptoms (Casemore 1989*a*). A detailed study of the clinical presentation of cases during a water-borne outbreak (Aston *et al.* 1991) produced a list of 12 symptoms of varying frequency of occurrence, the modal figure for the range of symptoms being seven symptoms (Table 45.1); the mean duration of acute symptoms was 13 days, range 2 to more than 31 days; 10 per cent required hospital admission, mainly for intravenous rehydration. The infection is normally limited by the immune system involving both humoral and cellular responses. Asymptomatic infection appears to be generally uncommon but has been reported in some studies, and probably often reflects hyperendemicity (animal or human) with recurrent exposure and transient reinfection in the 'immune' patient. Subchronic or recurrent infection may contribute to enteropathy and to the

Table 45.1 Cryptosporidiosis outbreak—North Humberside (Dec. 1989/Jan. 1990); symptoms experienced by 83 identified primary cases

Symptom	Frequency	%
Diarrhoea (three or more loose stools in 24 hours)	79	93
Loss of appetite	71	84
Abdominal pain	69	81
Loss of weight	63	74
Offensive-smelling stools	62	73
Headache/muscle aches/ flu-like symptoms	46	54
Nausea (feeling sick)	45	53
Feeling feverish	41	48
Vomiting (being sick)	37	44
Cough	30	35
Blood in stools	10	12
Loose stools (1 or 2 loose stools in 24 hours)	4	5

effects of malnutrition, especially in developing countries (Anon 1993; Molbak *et al.* 1993, 1994).

There is no evidence of transplacental transmission,
but infection during late pregnancy may result in
metabolic distress in the mother leading to complications including subsequent failure of the infant to
thrive. The latter syndrome has also been noted in
older infants and children and may be associated with
enteropathy even in developed countries (Phillips *et al.*
1992; Molbak *et al.* 1993, 1994). Severe abdominal pain
sometimes occurs and may be associated with evidence
of pancreatitis. Other sequelae including toxic megacolon and reactive arthritis have been described but
are thought to be uncommmon (Casemore 1989*a*).
Attributable death in the immunocompetent is
uncommon and results from failure to maintain home-
ostasis rather than to any specific effect. Cough is
a common symptom during cryptosporidiosis in
the non-immunocompromised but direct evidence is
lacking for respiratory tract infection in such cases.

Infection in immunocompromised humans

Intact humoral and cellular responses seem to be
essential for limiting the infection. Severe but none
the less self-limited infection may be seen in those with
concurrent or intercurrent viral infection, e.g. measles
or chickenpox, in whom there may be some natural
suppression of immune function. The infection is
usually more severe and protracted, and may be life-
threatening in those who are severely immunocompromised, especially those with AIDS. Abdominal
pain is often severe, due probably to involvement of
extraintestinal sites such as the biliary tract (Soave and
Armstrong 1986; Vakil *et al.* 1996). Cholera-like diarrhoea and vomiting are uncommon and tend to occur
during the terminal stages of AIDS (Connolly *et al.*
1988; Casemore *et al.* 1994). The occurrence and severity of the infection reflects the total level of immunosuppression, although the nature of the immune
deficit is also important; the risk of serious infection is
greatest in those with CD4 T-cell counts of below
200/mm^3 (Anon. 1991; Blanshard *et al.* 1992; Petersen
1992). AIDS patients sometimes show fluctuation of
oocyst excretion and clinical severity of infection;
recrudescence and remission, and apparently asymptomatic infection, have all been described (Casemore
1989*a*; Goodgame *et al.* 1993) and may reflect fluctuations in levels of immune function. The severe disease
seen in terminal AIDS is very distressing and may be
refractory to symptomatic or palliative treatment. The
lack of tissue specificity of *C. parvum* is of particular
importance in AIDS patients in whom the infection
may be found extending beyond the enteric tract.

Some transplant patients, for example those who
have had bone-marrow transplants, may suffer severe
infection which may reflect the high degree of
immunosuppression involved. However, a study of
renal transplant and AIDS patients, following a widespread outbreak resulting from water contamination in
the UK, suggested that renal patients are no more
likely to be infected nor to have more severe infection
than normal subjects (Clifford *et al.* 1990; Richardson
et al. 1991). AIDS patients, in contrast, were found to
be more prone to acquire cryptosporidiosis and to
suffer severe infection. In the large water-borne outbreak in Milwaukee in 1993 there were a number of
deaths from cryptosporidiosis, especially in AIDS
patients (MacKenzie *et al.* 1994).

The incidence of cryptosporidiosis in AIDS patients
differs in different centres but in some it exceeds 20
per cent and *Cryptosporidium* is often the most common
single cause of gastrointestinal disease in these
patients. Infections in AIDS patients may result from
sexual risk behaviour (Pedersen *et al.* 1996). The incidence of cryptosporidiosis in AIDS patients in the
London area appears to have fallen in recent years.
This may reflect improvements to water quality since
the Oxford/Swindon outbreak (Richardson *et al.*
1991), but may also reflect growing awareness among
such patients of the potential danger of consuming
unboiled water (Anon. 1995; Casemore 1992*a*). In
leukaemic patients, cryptosporidial infection can be
severe, especially if it coincides with or provokes an
aplastic crisis. Under such circumstances, interruption
of chemotherapy may be required to permit resolution
of the infection (Casemore 1989*a*; Foot *et al.* 1990).

Pathology and pathogenesis

Histopathology in man

The histological changes associated with human cryptosporidiosis are similar to those described for animals
(p. 629). The effects seen are those of a mucosal infection affecting primarily the small bowel, although
infection may extend throughout the gastroenteric
tract; rectal biopsy may reveal mild, non-specific proc-
titis. Infection sometimes extends to the bile duct and
gallbladder where extensive and chronic involvement
is seen in some AIDS patients. Respiratory tract infection also occurs, particularly in AIDS patients, and
oocysts and endogenous stages attached to exfoliated
cells in sputum may be an indication of probable AIDS,
if this has not already been diagnosed (Casemore
1989*a*, 1991; Moore and Frenkel 1991).

Pathogenesis

The mechanism by which the parasite causes symptoms in man have not been fully identified but would
appear to be multifactorial (Casemore 1989*a*; Zu *et al.*
1992; Guarino *et al.* 1995). The factors involved include

malabsorption of water, loss of brush-border enzymes with consequent osmotic effects, and probably also a so-far-unidentified secretagogue. Vomiting is a common feature of human cryptosporidiosis, especially in children but also in terminal AIDS infection. The parasite has been identified in vomit, possibly derived from regurgitated small bowel contents, although no emetic factor has been identified (Casemore *et al.* 1994). Respiratory tract infection probably occurs as a result of aspiration during vomiting but the haematogenous route has also been suggested (Gentile *et al.* 1987).

The immunological response in man

An immune response has been demonstrated in each of the four main immunoglobulin classes (Casemore *et al.* 1986; Casemore 1987; Ungar *et al.* 1988; Groves *et al.* 1994; Kuhls *et al.* 1994; Moss *et al.* 1995; Patel *et al.* 1997). Limited seroprevalence studies indicate that the infection is common (*c.* 30 per cent seroprevalence), even in developed countries. Antibody seroprevalence in dairy farmers has been shown to exceed 40 per cent (Lengerich *et al.* 1993). Detailed humoral antibody studies in a selected group involved in the outbreak in Milwaukee clearly showed seroconversion and provided useful epidemiological information (Moss *et al.* 1995). The variety of immunodeficiency conditions in which cryptosporidiosis has been reported to show increased severity suggests that both humoral and cellular factors have a role in limiting infection. Animal model studies confirm the role of CD4 cells and their cytokines in limiting or resolving infection (Ungar 1990; Petersen 1992; Enriquez and Sterling 1993). Reports differ on the effect of breast-feeding on incidence in infancy but some studies suggest a protective effect; it is not possible to say whether this is due to immunological factors or to protection from the environment, or both.

Laboratory detection and diagnosis for human infection

Diagnosis depends primarily upon the detection of oocysts in stools, as described for animals (p. 629) (Casemore 1991) but may also be made by examination of histological sections for the characteristic endogenous stages (Current and Reese 1986; Casemore 1989*a*, 1991) (Fig. 45.2). Concentration of stool specimens is not usually required for diagnosis in acute cases although oocyst excretion does fluctuate as the infection progresses. Patients may continue to excrete oocysts, usually in low numbers, for a variable period after resolution of symptoms. Detection of low-level excretion is difficult with the diagnostic laboratory methods currently in use. A variety of microscopic structures in human stools may readily be mistaken for oocysts, leading to delay in reaching a correct diagnosis and even to pseudo-outbreaks with consequent

unnecessary investigation (Casemore 1991, 1992*b*, 1995*a*). Serological methods have little value in diagnosis for individual cases. Environmental detection methods have been developed especially for water and associated samples (Anon. 1990; Casemore 1994*a*; Fricker 1995; Watkins *et al.* 1995), the lack of enrichment culture techniques is a constraint on efficient detection, especially in food.

Treatment

Effective specific therapy has not been identified despite trials of numerous compounds (Dubey *et al.* 1990; Anon. 1991; Rehg, 1994; White *et al.* 1994; Casemore and Warrell 1996). Rehydration and electrolyte supplementation should be given as required; opiates and antiemetics may be used to provide symptomatic relief. Many antibiotics and chemotherapeutics have been evaluated for treatment, both *in vivo* and *in vitro*, without any real success, although some reports suggest possible activity with paromomycin (Humatin), letrazuril, somatostatin, azidothymidine, diloxanide furoate, furazolidone, amprolium, macrolides, and immunotherapy (e.g. hyperimmune immunoglobulin, interleukin-2). The macrolide, spiramycin, showed early promise which has not been confirmed; the drug, as with some others reported to have a therapeutic effect, has little or no direct effect on the parasite itself although some patients may have amelioration of their symptoms (Casemore and Warrell 1996). Zidovudine therapy may also result in some amelioration of symptoms (Blanshard *et al.* 1992). It is difficult in such cases to separate the effect of drugs from that of fluctuations in immunocompetence, including that resulting from antiviral therapy, which may result in remission of the HIV infection. Symptoms sometimes result from the effects of multiple infecting agents, including viruses such as cytomegalovirus (CMV), and may thus respond to specific therapy aimed at those agents.

EPIDEMIOLOGY

ANIMAL

Occurrence and distribution

Cryptosporidium parvum infections have been identified in animals worldwide, particularly in Europe, North and South America, Africa, Asia, and Australia, but data on prevalence are limited. In the United States, a survey of 73 Idaho dairy farms revealed at least one calf infected on 56 per cent of farms—38 per cent of all faecal samples taken were positive (Anderson and Hall 1982). Of 12 Maryland dairy farms, selected at random within a 60 mile radius, nine had cryptosporidial infections in their calves, with between 8.3 and 75 per cent of animals examined shedding oocysts (Leek and Fayer 1984). In the United Kingdom, the veterinary investigation service recorded 10 789 cases of cryptosporidiosis in bovine calves in England and Wales between 1984 and 1994 (Veterinary Investigation Diagnosis Analysis—VIDA II).

Risk groups

Neonatal animals are most at risk, although immunologically compromised older animals may also be susceptible. Intensification of farming, with synchronized calving/lambing periods, ensures that large populations of susceptible hosts are available in small areas, facilitating transmission (Blewett 1989*a*). Year-round calving on dairy farms ensures a sequential supply of susceptible hosts.

Sources, transmission, and communicability

Cryptosporidium is an obligate parasite, and infection results from the ingestion of environmentally resistant oocysts shed in the faeces of an infected individual. This may be as the result of direct contact, or from environmental contamination with infected faecal material. Uncooked, contaminated foodstuffs may transmit infection, as can contaminated water supplies. *Cryptosporidium parvum* oocysts are being increasingly detected in both raw and treated water supplies (Anon. 1990, 1995; Dawson and Lloyd 1994; Juranek 1995; Meinhardt *et al.* 1996). The small size of the oocysts (5 μm) allows them to pass through some treatment systems, and their resistance to chlorination enables them to enter the distribution system in a viable state. The stable, cool conditions found in water courses favour survival of the oocyst which may be viable for many months (Robertson *et al.* 1992).

Recent studies suggest that although adult animals may not be clinically affected, they may shed small numbers of oocysts over prolonged periods (Scott *et al.* 1994). Further, it has been suggested that a periparturient rise in oocyst shedding may occur, providing the potential for the dam to infect her offspring (Xiao and Herd 1994). Adult rodents have also been observed to shed small numbers of oocysts in their faeces, another potential source of infection on farms (Klesius *et al.* 1986; Chalmers *et al.* 1994; Webster and MacDonald 1995; Webster 1996). The small numbers of oocysts required to initiate a clinical infection make these 'low-grade' sources of infection possible starting points for neonatal infections, which may then progress from neonate to neonate, resulting in the very high infection rates often observed on affected farms (Blewett 1989*a*). *Cryptosporidium parvum* infection is not a notifiable disease in livestock.

HUMAN

Occurrence and distribution

Geographical temporal distribution

The organism has been detected in man worldwide in both urban and rural settings (Reinthaler 1989; Casemore 1990*a*; Ungar 1990). In the United Kingdom, there is a pattern of peaks in the spring and in late autumn or early winter. However, these peaks do not necessarily both occur in any one locality, nor recur year by year. They have generally been shown to reflect rainfall, farming events and practices, such as lambing, calving, and muck-spreading (Casemore 1990*a*). Such peaks are seen in both temperate and some tropical countries and are often associated with similar factors. Conversely, in some localities rates have been seen to increase during or following extended dry periods, possibly because of the need to draw upon less satisfactory water sources. These various peaks therefore emphasize the importance of livestock as reservoirs and of water as a vehicle of infection for man.

Frequency of occurrence

It is difficult to be certain how reported figures reflect true incidence and prevalence because of a variety of factors, particularly related to variable clinical and laboratory diagnostic practice, leading to very variable ascertainment (Casemore and Roberts 1993). Laboratory rates of detection in non-immunocompromised subjects average about 2 per cent of samples submitted to the laboratory (range below 1 per cent to *c.* 5 per cent) in developed countries and about 8 per cent in developing countries (range 2 per cent to more than 30 per cent). Published reports show that the infection ranks about fourth or fifth in the list of pathogens detected in stools submitted to the laboratory, and in the United Kingdom represents about 6–8 per cent of the positive findings. Amongst young children in the United Kingdom, cryptosporidiosis is more common than salmonella, and during peak periods detection rates may exceed 20 per cent (Casemore 1990*a*; Palmer and Biffin 1990). This varies, however, from year to year and from locality to locality, depending upon the population sampled and on the criteria used for selection of specimens for screening. Mixed infections are seen, most commonly with *Campylobacter* and *Giardia*, probably reflecting common epidemiology (Casemore 1990*a*).

Risk groups

Unlike infection in animals, human infection is not age limited, although the incidence rates in the young may be higher because opportunities for exposure are greater and they are less likely to have any immunity from prior exposure. In developing countries, infection has been found to be common in children aged less than 1 year and asymptomatic infection to be common, especially among animal handlers (Nouri and Karami 1991; Molbak *et al.* 1993, 1994). This probably reflects their greater frequency of exposure. In developed countries, infection is uncommon in younger infants. This has been attributed in some surveys, even in some underdeveloped areas, to the effects of breast-feeding, although it is not possible to separate out the effects of immunological factors from limited environmental exposure in this age group. The infection is generally most common in children aged from 1 to 5 years. In a survey in the United Kingdom in which over 60 000 diagnostic specimens were screened (Palmer and Biffin 1990), two-thirds of cases were in this age group and nearly a third of cases found were in young adults; the infection was uncommon in adults over 45 years old. Reports from Finland (Vuorio *et al.* 1991) suggest differences in age-specific incidence, with the infection occurring mainly in adults who have travelled abroad. The reason for the apparent relative absence of symptomatic infection among young children has not been reported.

The age range for infection in the immuno-compromised is generally higher, reflecting the higher mean age of this group. For reasons related to the dynamics of transmission, a relative increase in otherwise healthy adult cases is often seen in water-borne outbreaks (Casemore 1994*b*; Meinhardt *et al.* 1996). There is usually no significant difference in distribution of cases by sex. It is probable, however, that if denominator figures (from samples submitted to the laboratory) were used to provide age- and sex-specific positivity rates then the younger adults are likely to show a preponderance of females, reflecting the higher proportion having greater contact with children at home and in day-care facilities.

Sources, transmission, and communicability

Human infection may be zoonotic or acquired by person to person transmission, for example within families and in day-care centres, and may be direct or indirect (Casemore 1990*a*; Cordell and Addiss 1994). Zoonotic exposure has generally been attributed to contact with farm animals, for example among veterinary students and animal research workers. Household pets do not seem to be a significant source of infection. Increasingly, open or educational farms are being associated with outbreaks and sporadic infection among visitors, many of whom are from urban areas (Casemore 1989*b,c*; Shield *et al.* 1990; Anon. 1994; Dawson *et al.* 1995). Thus, they may lack the immunity to the infection enjoyed by the farm staff, who may fail to appreciate the danger to their visitors. This may

have repercussions under Health and Safety legislation, under local authority by-law, and in their common law responsibility and duty of care.

There are a number of reports of nosocomial (hospital acquired) transmission to health-care staff from immunosuppressed and immunocompetent patients, and between patients (Casemore *et al.* 1994). Evidence from some case reports supports the view that disinfection is difficult and that the minimum infective dose is small, as is the case for animals (p. 628) (Blewett *et al.* 1993; Dupont *et al.* 1995; Chappell *et al.* 1996).

The source of many sporadic infections, particularly in urban areas, is unknown and is the subject of ongoing study. Some of the answers may be forthcoming as the improvement of molecular biological techniques enables typing of isolates, an advance required for more detailed epidemiological studies.

PREVENTION AND CONTROL

ANIMAL

Prevention is difficult since exclusion of the parasite from the farm is almost impossible; the resistance of *Cryptosporidium* oocysts to disinfection makes it difficult to treat the environment, and the absence of effective chemotherapy precludes treatment of new stock. Maintenance of closed herds/flocks may reduce transmission but is not effective against parasite ingress via water, or against a parasite reservoir in indigenous wild animals. Ensuring that all young stock receive an adequate feed of colostrum does not appear to protect them against infection with *Cryptosporidium*.

Following an outbreak, disinfection of buildings and fitments will reduce environmental contamination, but cannot remove any low-grade infections in adult animals. Ammonia-based disinfectants are currently the only practical solution on the farm (hydrogen peroxide-based disinfectants are inactivated by excessive organic material), but are unpleasant to use and cannot be employed until buildings are completely cleared of stock. Commercial ammonia-based disinfection kits are available for decontamination of agricultural buildings, having been developed to control the build-up of *Eimeria* spp. in poultry houses. Steam cleaning can also be effective, particularly for gates, pens, and utensils, since the parasite cannot survive exposure to temperatures in excess of 60 °C for more than a short period (Blewett 1989*b*).

Control of an outbreak can be attempted by rigorous separation of clean and infected stock, which should then be treated as two separate groups. Individual housing of young animals, especially calves, has been favoured, with scrupulous attention to hygiene regarding feeding utensils. However, for many farms this is not practicable, and the ease with which this parasite can be spread via protective clothing and equipment tends to limit the success of such containment measures (Angus 1992; Biewett 1989*a*). Removal of contaminated bedding from pens and cleaning between groups of animals is obviously a sensible measure. There are no official control programmes and legislation is concerned only with prevention of contamination of water supplies by *C. parvum*—catchment control—through more general regulations on the spreading of farm wastes to agricultural land.

Water suppliers are legally obliged to prevent ingress of *Crytosporidium* oocysts into the final potable supply although there are no agreed criteria for sampling or for detection levels (Dawson and Lloyd 1994; Meinhardt *et al.* 1996).

HUMAN

The results of preliminary human volunteer studies in the United States suggest a minimal infective dose for humans of fewer than 30 oocysts and an ID_{50} of 132 (Dupont *et al.* 1995; Chappell *et al.* 1996). This will probably vary according to the isolate or strain used and the previous history of exposure and immunological status of the individual concerned.

Control of infections within urban groups (families, day-care centres, etc. are those appropriate for any diarrhoeal disease (Anon. 1990; Cordell and Addiss 1994; MacKenzie *et al.* 1995). Aerosol or droplet transmission, from fluid faeces, vomit, or sputum, are possible means of transmission (Casemore *et al.* 1994). It is not known to what extent asymptomatic cases represent a risk of transmitting infection to third parties.

Contaminated water supplies will inevitably occur from time to time, even in developed countries, and may be the source of some sporadic cases as well as outbreaks. Current water treatment processes are unable to guarantee control (Anon. 1990, 1995; Rose 1990; Smith and Rose, 1990; MacKenzie *et al.* 1994; Casemore 1995*b*). This may lead to sporadic cases and to small clusters which are hard to identify, or to large outbreaks; the largest on record, in the United States, involved some 403 000 people and resulted in a number of deaths (MacKenzie *et al.* 1994). Water-initiated outbreaks often result in significant secondary (person to person) spread in the community (MacKenzie *et al.* 1994, 1995). Ozone shows some effect in laboratory studies but has so far not been shown to be as effective in practice (Casemore 1995*b*). High-risk subjects should be advised to avoid consumption of unboiled water as a control measure (Casemore 1992*a*; Centres for Disease Control and Prevention 1995). The origin and significance of oocysts in water is still a matter of debate and research but their detection is an indication for particular attention to water treatment process efficiency.

Within the hospital setting, the adequate disinfection of faecal contamination or of endoscopes, etc., is problematic (Casemore *et al.* 1989, 1994). Where such instruments have been used for patients known to have cryptosporidiosis then prolonged immersion in glutaraldehyde at elevated temperature (>37 °C), or with hydrogen peroxide, after thorough cleaning, may be required to ensure safety, despite the problems associated with use of this disinfectant (p. 634).

Guidelines have been issued for the control of infection resulting from visits to open farms (Casemore 1989*b*,*c*; Dawson *et al.* 1995). Legislation, or action under existing legislation, is needed to license and control the proliferation, and running, of open or educational farms and of the taking of livestock into urban sites such as schools.

REFERENCES

Anderson, B. C. and Hall, R. F. (1982). Cryptosporidial infection in Idaho dairy calves. *Journal of the American Veterinary Medical Association*, **181**, 484–5.

Angus, K. W. (1992). *Cryptosporidiosis of man and animals*, (ed. J. P. Dubey, C. A. Speer and R. Fayer), pp. 83–103. CRC Press, Boca Raton.

Angus, K. W. and Blewett D. A. (ed.) (1988). *Proceedings of the first international workshop on cryptosporidiosis*. Moredun Research Institute, Edinburgh.

Anon. (1982). Cryptosporidiosis: assessment of chemotherapy of males with acquired immune deficiency syndrome (AIDS). *Morbidity and Mortality*, **31**, 589–97.

Anon. (1990). *Cryptosporidium in water supplies*. Dept of Health/Dept of Environment. Report of the Group of Experts, Chairman, Sir John Badenoch. HMSO, London.

Anon. (1991). Feedback from the Sixth International AIDS Conference. San Francisco. *Genitourinary Med*, **67**, 162–71.

Anon. (1993). Intestinal malabsorption of HIV-infected children: relationship to diarrhoea, failure to thrive, enteric micro-organisms and immune impairment. *AIDS*, **7**, 1435–40.

Anon. (1994). Cryptosporidiosis associated with farm visits. *PHLS Communicable Disease Report*, **4**, 73.

Anon. (1995). *Cryptosporidium in water supplies*. Dept of Health/Dept of Environment. Second Report Report of the Group of Experts, Chairman, Sir John Badenoch. HMSO, London.

Argenzio, R. A., Liacos, J. A., Levy, M. L., Meuten, D. L., Lecce, J. G., and Powell, D. W. (1990). Villous atrophy, crypt hyperplasia, cellular infiltration and impaired glucose–Na absorption in enteric cryptosporidiosis in pigs. *Gastroenterology*, **98**, 1129–40.

Aston, R. *et al.* (1991). Report of the outbreak control group to coordinate the investigation and control of the outbreak of cryptosporidiosis in North Humberside. Formal report to the Local Authorities of Beverley and Kingstone-upon-Hull, UK.

Awad-el-Kariem, F. M., Robinson, H. A., McDonald V., Evans D., and Dyson D. A. (1993). Is human Cryptosporidiosis a zoonotic disease? *Lancet*, **341**, 1535.

Awad-el-Kariem, F. M., Robinson, H. A., Dyson, D. A., Evans, D., Wright, S., Fox, M. T., and McDonald, V. (1995). Differentiation between human and animal strains of *Cryptosporidium parvum* using isoenzyme typing. *Parasitology*, **110**, 129–32.

Baskerville, A., Ramsay, A. D., Millward-Sadler, G. H., Cook R. W., Cranage, M. P., and Greenaway, P. J. (1991). Chronic pancreatitis and biliary fibrosis associated with Cryptosporidiosis in Simian AIDS. *Journal of Comparative Pathology*, **105**, 415–21.

Blanshard, C., Jackson, A. M., Shanson, D. C., Francis, N., and Gazzard, B. G. (1992). Cryptosporidiosis in HIV-seropositive patients. *Quarterly Journal of Medicine*, **85**, 813–14.

Blewett, D. A. (1989*a*). Quantitative techniques in *Cryptosporidium* research. In *Cryptosporidiosis*, (ed. K. W. Angus and D. A. Blewett), pp. 85–95. Moredun Research Institute, Edinburgh.

Blewett, D. A. (1989*b*). Disinfection and oocysts. In *Cryptosporidiosis*, (ed. K. W. Angus and D. A. Blewett), pp. 107–15. Moredun Research Institute, Edinburgh.

Blewett, D. A., Wright, S. E., Casemore, D. P., Booth, N. E., and Jones, C. E. (1993). Infective dose size studies on *Cryptosporidium parvum* using gnotobiotic lambs. *Water Science and Technology*, **27**, 61–4.

Browning, G. F. *et al.* (1991). The prevalence of enteric pathogens in diarrhoeic thoroughbred foals in Britain and Ireland. *Equine Veterinary Journal*, **23**, 405–9.

Buraud, M., Forget, E., Favennec, L., Bizet, J., Gobert, J. G., and Deluol, A. M. (1991). Sexual stage development of *Cryptosporidia* in the Caco-2 cell line. *Infection and Immunity*, **59**, 4610–13.

Casemore, D. P. (1987). The antibody response to *Cryptosporidium*: development of a serological test and its use in a study of immunologically normal persons. *Journal of Infection*, **14**, 125–34.

Casemore, D. P. (1989*a*). Human cryptosporidiosis. In *Recent Advances in Infection*, (ed. D. S. Reeves and A. M. Geddes), pp. 209–36. Churchill Livingstone, Edinburgh.

Casemore, D. P. (1989*b*). Educational farm visits and associated infection hazards. *PHLS Communicable Disease Report*, **19**, 3.

Casemore, D. P. (1989*c*). Sheep as a source of human Cryptosporidiosis. *Journal of Infection*, **19**, 101–4.

Casemore, D. P. (1990*a*). Epidemiological aspects of human cryptosporidiosis. *Epidemiological Infections*, **104**, 1–28.

Casemore, D. P., (1990*b*) Foodborne illness: Foodborne protozoal infection. *Lancet*, **336**, 1427–32.

Casemore, D. P. (1991). ACP Broadsheet 128: Laboratory methods for diagnosing cryptosporidiosis. *Journal of Clinical Pathology*, **44**, 445–51.

Casemore, D. P. (1992*a*). Cryptosporidium—Detection and Control. *Journal of Sterile Services Management*, **3**, 14–17.

Casemore, D. P. (1992*b*). A pseudo-outbreak of cryptosporidiosis. *Communicable Disease Report; Review 2*, R66-70. Public Health Laboratory Service, London.

Casemore, D. P. (1993). Is human cryptosporidiosis a zoonotic disease? *Lancet*, **342**, 312.

Casemore, D. P. (1994*a*). Problems associated with sampling and examination for *Cryptosporidium* in water supplies. In *Proceedings of workshop on* Cryptosporidium *in water supplies*, (ed. A. Dawson and A. Lloyd), pp. 11–17. HMSO London.

Casemore, D. P. (1994*b*). Enteric protozoa and the water route of transmission-epidemiology and dynamics. In *Water and public health*, ed. A. M. B. Golding, N. Noah, and R. Stanwell-Smith) pp. 123–36. Smith Gordon Nishimura, London.

Casemore, D. P. (1995*a*). The problem with protozoan parasites. In *Protozoan parasites in water* (ed. B. Betts *et al.*), pp. 10–18. Royal Society of Chemistry, Cambridge.

Casemore, D. P. (1995*b*). Disinfection options. In *Proceedings of workshop on treatment optimisation for* Cryptosporidium *removal from water supplies*. (ed. P. A. West and M. S. Smith), 19–24. Department of Environment, Welsh Office, UK Water Industry Research Ltd. HMSO London.

Casemore, D. P. and Roberts, C. (1993). Guidelines for screening for *Cryptosporidium* in stools: Report of a joint working group. *Journal of Clinical Pathology*, **46**, 2–4.

Casemore, D. P., Jessop, E. G., Douce, D., and Jackson, F. B. (1986). *Cryptosporidium* plus *Campylobacter*: an outbreak in a semi-rural population. *Journal of Hygiene, Cambridge*, **96**, 95–105.

Casemore, D. P., Blewett, D. A., and Wright S. (1989). Cleaning and disinfection of equipment for gastrointestinal flexible endoscopy. *Gut*, **30**, 1156–7.

Casemore, D. P., O'Mahony, C., and Gardener, C. (1994). Cryptosporidial infection, with special reference to nosocomial transmission of *Cryptosporidium parvum*: a review. *Folia Parasitologica*, **41**, 17–21.

Casemore, D. P., and Warrell, D. A. (1996). Cryptosporidium and Cryptosporidiosis. In Oxford Textbook of Medicine, 3rd Edition (eds. D. Weatherall, J G G. Ledingham, D. A. Simpson). Oxford University Press, Oxford.

Centres for Disease Control and Prevention (1995). Assessing the public health threat associated with waterborne cryptosporidiosis: report of a workshop. *MMWR*, **44**, 1–19.

Chalmers, R. M. *et al* (1994). *Cryptosporidium muris* in wild house mice (*Mus musculus*): First Report in the UK. *European Journal of Protistology*, **30**, 151–5.

Chapman, P. A., Rush, B. A., and McClaughlin, J. (1990). An enzyme immunoassay for detecting *Cryptosporidium* in faecal and environmental samples. *Journal of Medical Microbiology*, **32**, 233–7.

Chappell C. L., Okhuysen, P. B., Sterling, C. R., and DuPont, H. L. (1996). *Cryptosporidium parvum*: Intensity of infection and occyst excretion patterns in healthy volunteers. *Journal of Infectious Diseases*, **173**, 232–6.

Chartier, C., Mallereau, M. P., and Nacriri, M. (1996). Prophylaxis using Paromomycin of Natural Cryptosporidial Infection in Neonatal kids. *Preventive Veterinary Medicine*, **25**, 357–61.

Chermette, R. and Boufassa-Ouzrout, S. (1988). *Cryptosporidiosis: A cosmopolitan disease in animals and in man*. Office International des Epizooties, Technical Series No. 5 (2nd edn), Paris.

Clifford, C. P., Crook, D. W. M., Conlon, C. P., Fraise, A. P., Day, D. G., and Peto, R. E. A. (1990). Impact of waterborne outbreak of cryptosporidiosis on AIDS and renal transplant patients. *Lancet*, **335**, 1455–6.

Connolly, G. M., Dryden, M. S., Shanson, D. C., and Gazzard, B. G. (1988). Cryptosporidial diarrhoea in AIDS and its treatment. *Gut*, **29**, 593–7.

Cordell, R. L. and Addiss, D. G. (1994). Cryptosporidiosis in child care settings: a review of the literature and recommendation for prevention and control. *Pediatric Infectious Diseases Journal*, **13**, 310–17.

Crawford, F. G. and Vermund, S. H. (1988). Human cryptosporidiosis. *Critical Reviews Microbiology*, **16**, 113–59.

Current, W. L. (1987). *Cryptosporidium*: Its biology and potential for environmental transmission. *CRC Critical Reviews in Environmental Control*, **17**, 21–51.

Current, W. L. (1988). *Cyptosporidium* and Cryptosporidiosis. In *Cryptosporidiosis, Proceedings of the first International Workshop, Edinburgh*, (ed. K. W Angus and D. A Blewett).

Current, W. L. and Bick, P. H. (1989). Immunobiology of *Cryptosporidium* spp. *Pathological Immunopathology*, **8**, 141–60.

Current, W. L. and Blagburn, B. L. (1990). *Cryptosporidium*: infections in man and domestic animals. In *Coccidiosis of man and domestic animals*, (ed. P. L. Long), pp. 155–85. CRC Press, Boca Raton.

Current, W. L. and Garcia, L. S. (1991). Cryptosporidiosis. *Clinical Microbiological Reviews*, **4**, 325–58.

Current, W. L. and Haynes, T. B. (1984). Complete development of *Cryptosporidium* in cell culture. *Science*, **224**, 603–5.

Current, W. L. and Long, P. L. (1983). Development of human and calf *Cryptosporidium* in chicken embryos. *Journal of Infectious Diseases*, **148**, 1108–13.

Current, W. L. and Reese, N. C. (1986). A comparison of endogenous development of three isolates of *Cryptosporidium* in suckling mice. *Journal of Protozoology*, **33**, (1), 98–108.

Current, W. L. *et al.* (1983). Human cryptosporidiosis in immunocompetent and immunodeficient persons. *New England Journal of Medicine*, **308**, 1252–7.

Current, W. L., Upton, S. J., and Haynes, T. B. (1986). The life-cycle of *Cryptosporidium baileyi* n.sp (Apicomplexa, Cryptosporidiidae) infecting chickens. *Journal of Protozoology*, **33**, 289–96.

Daltry, A., Danis, M., and Gentilini, M. (1989). Development complet de *Cryptosporidium* en culture cellulaire: applications. *Medecine Sciences*, **5**, 762–6.

Dawson, A. and LLoyd, A. (1994). *Proceedings of workshop on* Cryptosporidium *in Water Supplies*. The Drinking Water Inspectorate. Department of the Environment, Welsh Office Department of Health Publication (HMSO).

Dawson, A., Griffin., R., Fleetwood, A., and Barrett, N. J. (1995). Farm visits and zoonoses. *Communicable Disease Report*, Public Health Laboratory Service, R81–86.

Ditrich, O., Palkovic, L., Sterba, J., Prokopic, J., Loudova, J., and Giboda, M. (1991). The first finding of *Cryptosporidium baileyi* in man. *Parasitology Research* **77**, 44–7.

Dubey, J. P., Speer, C. A., and Fayer, R. (ed.) (1990). *Cryptosporidiosis of man and animals*. CRC Press, Boca Raton.

Dupont, H. L., Chappell, C. L., and Sterling, C. R. (1995). The infectivity of *Cryptosporidium parvum* in healthy volunteers. *New England Journal of Medicine*, **332**, 855–9.

Enriquez, F. J. and Sterling, C. R. (1993) Role of CD4+TH1- and TH2-cell-secreted cytokines in Cryptosporidiosis. *Folia Parasitologica*, **40**, 307–11.

Evans, M. R. and Gardner, D. (1996). Cryptosporidiosis outbreak associated with an educational farm holiday. *Communicable Diseases Report*, **6**, R50–51.

Fayer, R. and Ungar, B. P. L. (1986). *Cryptosporidium* spp. and Crytosporidiosis. *Microbiological Reviews*, **50** 458–83.

Fayer, R., Andrews, C., Ungar, B. L. P., and Blagburn, B. (1989*a*). Efficacy of hyperimmune bovine colostrum for prophylaxis of cryptosporidiosis in neonatal calves. *Journal of Parasitology*, **75**, 393–7.

Fayer, R., Perryman, L. E., and Riggs, M. W. (1989*b*). Hyperimmune bovine colostrum neutralises *Cryptosporidium* sporozoites and protects mice against oocyst challenge. *Journal of Parasitology*, **75**, 151–3.

Fayer, R., Guidry, A., and Blagburn, B. (1990). Immunotherapeutic efficacy of bovine colostral immunoglobulins from a hyperimmunised cow against *Cryptosporidium* in neonatal mice. *Infection and Immunity*, **58**, 2962–5.

Foot, A. B. M., Oakhill, A., and Mott, M. G. (1990). Cryptosporidiosis and acute leukaemia. *Archives of Diseases in Childhood*, **65**, 236–7.

Fricker, C. R. (1995). Detection of *Cryptosporidium* and *Giardia* in water. In *Protozoan parasites in water* (ed. B. Betts *et al.*), pp. 91–6. Royal Society of Chemistry Cambridge.

Gentile, G. *et al.* (1987). Colonic vascular invasion as a possible route of extraintestinal cryptosporidiosis. *American Journal of Medicine*, **82**, 574–5.

Gibson, J. A., Hill, H. W. M., and Huber, M. J. (1983). Cryptosporidiosis in Arabian foals with severe combined immunodeficiency. *Australian Veterinary Journal*, **60**, 378–9.

Goldstein, S. T. *et al.* (1996). Cryptosporidiosis: An outbreak associated with drinking water despite state-of-the-art water treatment. *Annals of Internal Medicine*, **124**, 459–68.

Goodgame R. W., Genta, R. M., White, A. C., and Chappell, C. L. (1993). Intensity of Infection in AIDS-Associated Cryptosporidiosis. *Journal of Infectious Diseases*, **167**, 704–9.

Groves, V. J., Lehman, D., and Gilbert, G. L. (1994). Seroepidemiology of cryptosporidiosis in Paua New Guinea and Australia. *Epidemiology and Infection*, **113**, 491–9.

Guarino, A. *et al.* (1995). Human intestinal cryptosporidiosis: secretory diarrhoea and enterotoxic activity in Caco-2 cells. *Journal of Infectious Diseases*, **171**, 976–83.

Gut, J., Petersen, C., Nelson, R., and Leech, J. (1991). *Cryptosporidium parvum*: *In vitro* cultivation in Madin–Darby canine kidney cells. *Journal of Protozoology*, **38**, 725–35.

Harp, J. A., Woodmansee, D. B., and Moon, H. W. (1989). Effects of colostral antibody on susceptibility of calves to *Cryptosporidium parvum* infection. *Americal Journal of Veterinary Research*, **50**, 2117–19.

Harp, J. A., Woodmansee, D. B., and Moon, H. W. (1990). Resistance of calves to *Cryptosporidium parvum*: Effects of age and previous exposure. *Infection and Immunity*, **58**, 2237–40.

Hart, C. A. and Baxby, D. (1987). Cryptosporidiosis in children. *Pediatric Reviews and Communications*, **1**, 311–41.

Heine, J., Pohlenz, J. F. L., Moon, H. W., and Wood, G. N. (1984). Enteric lesions and diarrhoea in gnotobiotic calves monoinfected with *Cryptosporidium* species. *Journal of Infectious Diseases*, **150**, 768–75.

Hill, B. D., Blewett, D. A., Dawson, A. M., and Wright, S. (1990). Analysis of the kinetics, isotype and specificity of serum and coproantibody in lambs infected with *Cryptosporidium parvum*. *Research in Veterinary Science*, **48**, 76–81.

Johnson, D. W., Pieniazek, N. J., Griffin, D. W., Misener, L., and Rose, J. B. (1995). Development of a PCR protocol for sensitive detection of *Cryptosporidium* oocysts in water samples. *Applied Environmental Microbiology*, **61**, 3849–55.

Jokipii, L. and Jokipii, A. M. M. (1986). Timing of symptoms and oocyst excretion in human cryptosporidiosis. *New England Journal of Medicine*, **315**, 1643–7.

Juranek, D. D. (1995). Cryptosporidiosis: Sources of infection and guidelines for prevention. *Clinical Infectious Diseases*, **21**, S57–61.

Juranek, D. D., Addiss, D. G., and Bartlett, M. E. (1995). Cryptosporiodosis and public health: workshop report. *Journal of American Water Works Association*, **87**, 69–80.

Kim, K., Gooze, L., Petersen, C., Gut, J., and Nelson, R. G. (1992). Isolation, sequence and molecular karyotype analysis of the actin gene of *Cryptosporidium parvum*. *Molecular Biochemistry and Parasitology*, **50**, 105–14.

Klesius, P. H., Haynes, T. B., and Malo, L. K. (1986) Infectivity of *Cryptosporidium* sp. isolated from wild mice for calves and mice. *Journal of the American Veterinary Medicine Association*, **189**, 192–3.

Kuhls, T. L., Mosier, D. A., Crawford, D. L., and Griffis, J. (1994). Seroprevalence of cryptosporidial antibodies during infancy, childhood and adolescence. *Clinical Infectious Diseases*, **18**, 731–5.

Landsverk, T. (1987). Cryptosporidiosis and the follicle-associated epithelium over the ileal Peyer's patch in calves. *Research in Veterinary Science*, **42**, 299–306.

Leek, R. G. and Fayer, R. (1984). Prevalence of infections, and their relation to diarrhoea in calves on 12 dairy farms in Maryland. *Proceedings of the Helminthological Society of Washington*, **51**, 360–1.

Leng, X. G., Mosier, D. A., and Oberst, R. D. (1996). Differentiation of *Cryptosporidium parvum*, *Cryptosporidium muris* and *Cryptosporidium baileyi* by PCR–RFLP analysis of the 19S ribosomal-RNA gene. *Veterinary Parasitology*, **62**, 1–7.

Lengerich, E. J., Addiss, D. G., Marx, J. J., Ungar, B. L. P., and Juranek, D. D. (1993). Increased exposure to Cryptosporidia among dairy farmers in Wisconsin. *Journal of Infectious Diseases*, **167**, 1252–5.

Levine, N. D. (1984). Taxonomy and review of the coccidian genus *Cryptosporidium* (Protozoa, Apicomplexa). *Journal of Protozoology*, **31**, 94–8.

McDonald, V. and Kariem, F. M. (1995). Strain variation in *Cryptosporidium parvum* and evidence for distinctive human and animals strains. In *Protozoan parasites in water*, (ed. B. Betts *et al.*), pp. 104–7. Royal Society of Chemistry, Cambridge.

McDonald, V. *et al.* (1990). *In vitro* cultivation of *Cryptosporidium parvum* and screening for anticryptosporidial drugs. *Antimicrobial Agents and Chemotherapy*, **34**, (8), 1498–500.

MacKenzie, W. R. *et al.* (1994). A massive outbreak in Milwaukee of *Cryptosporidium* infection transmitted through the public water supply. *New England Journal of Medicine*, **331**, (3), 161–7.

MacKenzie, W. R., Schell, W. L., and Blair, K. A. (1995). Massive outbreak of waterborne cryptosporidiosis infection in Milwaukee, Wisconsin: recurrence of illness and risk of secondary transmission. *Clinical Infectious Diseases*, **21**, 57–62.

Marcial, M. A. and Madara, J. L. (1986). *Cryptosporidium*: cellular localization, structural analysis of absorptive cell–parasite membrane—membrane interactions in guinea pigs, and suggestion of protozoan transport by M cells. *Gastroenterology*, **90**, 583–94.

Meinhardt, P., Casemore, D. P., and Miller, K. B. (1996). Epidemiology aspects of human cryptosporidiosis and the role of waterborne transmission. *Epidemiologic Reviews*, **18**, 118–36.

Miesel, J. L., Perera, D. R., Meligro, C., and Rubin, C. E. (1976). Overwhelming watery diarrhea associated with *Cryptosporidium* in an immunosuppressed patient. *Gastroenterology*, **70**, 1156–60.

Millard, P. S. *et al.* (1994). An outbreak of Cryptosporidiosis from fresh-pressed apple cider. *Journal of the American Medical Association*, **272**, 1592–6.

Molbak, K. *et al.* (1993). Cryptosporidiosis in infancy and childhood mortality in Guinea Bissau, West Africa. *British Medical Journal*, **307**, 417–20.

Molbak, K., Aaby, P., Hojlyng, N., and da Silva, A. P. J. (1994). Risk factors for *Cryptosporidium* diarrhea in early childhood: A case-control study from Guinea-Bissau, West Africa. *American Journal of Epidemiology*, **139**, 734–40.

Moon, H. W., Wood, G. N., and Ahrens, F. A. (1982). Attempted chemoprophylaxis of cryptosporidiosis in calves. *Veterinary Record*, **110**, 181.

Moore, J. A. and Frenkel, J. K. (1991). Respiratory and enteric cryptosporidiosis in humans. *Archieves of Pathology and Laboratory Medicine*, **115**, 1160–2.

Moran, S., Casemore, D. P., McLauchlin, J., and Nichols, G. L. (1995). Detection of *Cryptosporidium* antigens on SDS–PAGE Western blots using enhanced chemiluminescence. In *Protozoan parasites in water*, (ed. B. Betts *et al.*), pp. 168–71. Royal Society of Chemistry, Cambridge.

Morgan, U. M., Constantine, C. C., O'Donaghue, P., Meloni, B. P., O'Brien, P. A., and Thompson, R. C. (1995). Molecular characterisation of *Cryptosporidium* isolates from humans and other animals using random amplified polymorphic DNA analysis. *American Journal of Tropical Medical Hygiene*, **52**, 559–64.

Moss, D. M., Bennett, S. N., and Arrowood, M. J. (1995). Kinetic and isotypic analysis of specific immunoglobulins from the crew members with cryptosporidiosis on a US Coast Guard cutter. *Journal of Eukaryotic Microbiology*, **41**, 52S–55S.

Mtambo, M. M. A., Nash, A. S., Blewett, D. A., Smith, H. V., and Wright, S. (1991). *Cryptosporidium* infection in cats: prevalence of infection in domestic and feral cats in the Glasgow area. *Veterinary Record*, **129**, 502–4.

Naciri, M. (1989). Animal and human cryptosporidosis: opportunist infections? Pathogenicity of the genus *Cryptosporidium*. In *Coccidia and intestinal coccidiomorphs*, (ed. P. Yvore). Proceedings of V International Coccidiosis Conference, Tours, France.

Nelson, R. G., Kim, K., Gooze, L., Petersen, C., and Gut, J. I. R. G. (1991). Identification and isolation of *Cryptosporidium parvum* genes encoding microtubule and microfilament proteins. *Journal of Protozoology*, **38**, 52S–55S.

Nime, F. A., Burek, J. D., Page, D. L., Holscher, M. A., and Yardley, J. H. (1976). Acute enterocolitis in a human being infected with the protozoan *Cryptosporidium*. *Gastroenterology*, **70**, 592–8.

Nouri, M. and Karami, M., (1991) Asymptomatic Cryptosporidiosis in nomadic shepherds and their sheep. *Journal of Infection*, **23**, 331–3.

O'Donoghue, P. J. (1995). *Cryptosporidium* and Cryptosporidiosis in man and animals. *International Journal for Parasitology*, **25**, 139–95.

Ortega-Mora, L. M. and Wright, S. E. (1994). Age-related resistance in ovine Cryptosporidiosis: patterns of infection and humoral immune response. *Infection and Immunity*, **62**, 5003–9.

Palmer, S. R. and Biffin, A. (1990). Cryptosporidiosis in England and Wales: prevalence and clinical and epidemiological features. *British Medical Journal*, **300**, 774–7.

Panciera, R. J., Thomassen, R. W., and Gardner, F. M. (1971). Cryptosporidial infection in a calf. *Veterinary Pathology*, **8**, 479–84.

Patel, S., McLaughlin, J., and Casemore, D. P. (1997). A simple SDS–PAGE immunoblotting technique using an enhanced chemiluminescence detection system to identify polyclonal antibody responses to complex cryptosporidial antigen preparations. *Journal of Immunological Methods*, **205**, 157–61.

Pedersen, C. *et al.* (1996). Epidemiology of Cryptosporidiosis among European AIDS patients. *Genitourinary Medicine*, **72**, 128–31.

Petersen, C. (1992). Cryptosporidiosis in patients infected with the human immunodeficiency virus. *Clinical Infectious Diseases*, **15**, 903–9.

Petersen, C. (1993). Cellular biology of *Cryptosporidium parvum*. *Parasitology Today*, **9**, (3), 87–91.

Phillips, A. D., Thomas, A. G., and Walker-Smith, J. A., (1992). *Cryptosporidium*, chronic diarrhoea and the proximal small intestinal mucosa. *Gut*, **33**, 1057–61.

Rasumssen, K., Larsen, N. C., and Healey, M. C. (1993). Complete development of *Cryptosporidium parvum* in a human endometrial carcinoma cell line. *Infection and Immunity*, **61**, 1482–5.

Reese, N. C., Current, W. L., Ernst, J. V., and Bailey, W. S. (1982). Cryptosporidiosis of man and calf: a case report and results of experimental infections in mice and rats. *American Journal of Tropical Medicine and Hygiene*, **31**, 226–9.

Rehg, J. (1994). New potential therapies for cryptosporidiosis: an analysis of variables affecting drug efficacy. *Folia Parasitologica*, **41**, 23–6.

Reif, J. S., Wimmer, L., Smith, J. A., Dargatz, D. A., and Cheney, J. M. (1989). Human Cryptosporidiosis associated with an epizootic in calves. *American Journal of Public Health*, **79**, 1528–30.

Reinthaler, F. F. (1989). Epidemiology of cryptosporidisis in children in tropical countries. *Journal of Hygiene Epidemiology Microbiology and Immunology*, **33**, 505–13.

Reperant, J. M., Naciri, M., Chardes, T., and Bout, D. T. (1992). Immunological characterisation of a 17kDa antigen from *Cryptosporidium parvum* recognised early by mucosal IgA antibodies. *FEMS Microbiology Letters*, **78**, 7–14.

Richardson, A. R. *et al.* (1991). An outbreak of waterborne cryptosporidiosis in Swindon and Oxfordshire. *Epidemiology and Infection*, **107**, 485–95.

Robert, B., Ginter, A., Antoine, H., Collard, A., and Coppe, P. (1990). Diagnosis of bovine Cryptosporidiosis by an enzyme-linked immunosorbent assay. *Veterinary Parasitology*, **37**, 1–8.

Robertson, L. J., Campbell, A. T., and Smith, H. V. (1992). Survival of *Cryptosporidium parvum* oocysts under various environmental pressures. *Applied and Environmental Microbiology*, **58**, (11), 3494–500.

Rose, J. B. (1990). Occurrence and control of *Cryptosporidium* in drinking water. In *Drinking water microbiology: progress and recent developments* (ed. G. A. McFeters), pp. 294–321. Brock Springer Series in Contemporary Bioscience. Springer Verlag, New York.

Scott, C. A., Smith, H. V., and Gibbs, H. A. (1994). Excretion of *Cryptosporidium parvum* oocysts by a herd of beef suckler cows. *Veterinary Record*, **134**, 172.

Sherwood, D., Angus, K. W., Snodgrass, D. R., and Tzipori, S. (1982). Experimental Cryptosporidiosis in laboratory mice. *Infection and Immunity*, **38**, 471–5.

Shield, J., Baumer, J. H., Dawson, J. A., and Wilkinson, P. J. (1990). Cryptosporidiosis—an educational experience. *Journal of Infection*, **21**, 297–301.

Simpson, V. R. (1992). Cryptosporidiosis in newborn red deer (*Cervus elephus*). *Veterinary Record*, **130**, 116–18.

Smith, H. V. and Rose, J. B. (1990) Waterborne Cryptosporidiosis. *Parasitology Today*, **6**, (1), 8–12.

Snyder, S. P., England, J. J., and McChesney, A. E. (1978). Cryptosporidiosis is immunodeficient Arabian foals. *Veterinary Pathology*, **15**, 12–17.

Soave, R. and Armstrong, D. (1986). *Cryptosporidium* and cryptosporidiosis. *Reviews of Infectious Diseases*, **8**, 1012–23.

Spano, F., Putigaani, L., McLaughlin, J., Casemore, D. P., and Crisanti, A. (1996). A PCR–RFLP analysis of the *Cryptosporidium* oocyst wall protein (COWP) gene discriminates between *C. wrairi* and *C. parvum* and between *C. parvum* isolates of human and animal origin. *FEMS Microbiology Letters*, **150**, 209–17.

Tyzzer, E. E. (1907). A sporozoan found in the peptic glands of the common mouse. *Proceedings of the Society for Experimental Biology and Medicine*, **5**, 12–13.

Tyzzer, E. E. (1912). *Cryptosporidium parvum* (sp. nov.), a coccidium found in the small intestine of the common mouse. *Archiv fur Protistenkunde*, **26**, 394–412.

Tzipori, S., Angus, K. W., Campbell, I., and Gray, E. W. (1980). *Cryptosporidium* evidence for a single species genus. *Infection and Immunity*, **30**, 884–6.

Tzipori, S., Angus, K. W., Campbell, I., and Clerihew, L. W. (1981). Diarrhoea due to *Cryptosporidium* infection in artificially reared lambs. *Journal of Clinical Microbiology*, **14**, 100–5.

Ungar, B. L. P. (1990). Cryptosporidiosis in humans. In *Cryptosporidiosis of man and animals*, (ed. J. P. Dubey, C. A. Speer) pp. 59–84. CRC Press, Boca Raton.

Ungar, B. L. P., Gilman, R. H., Lanata, C. F., and Schael, P. (1988). I. Seroepidemiology of *Cryptosporidium* infection in two Latin American populations. *Journal of Infectious Diseases*, **157**, 551–6.

Upton, S. J. and Current, W. L. (1985). The species of *Cryptosporidium* (Apicomplexa: Cryptosporidiae) infecting mammals. *Journal of Parasitology*, **71**, 625–9.

Vakil, N. B. *et al.* (1996). Biliary Cryptosporidiosis in HIV-infected people after the waterborne outbreak of cryptosporidiosis in Milwaukee. *Massachusetts Medical Society*, **334**, 19–23.

Vitovec, J. and Koudela, B. (1992). Pathogenesis of intestinal cryptosporidiosis in conventional and gnotobiotic piglets. *Veterinary Parasitology*, **43**, 25–36.

Vitovec, J., Koudela, B., Vladik, P., and Hausner, O. (1991). Interaction of *Cryptosporidium parvum* and campylobacter jejuni in experimentally infected neonatal mice. *Zentoalblatt für Bakteriologie*, **274**, 548–59.

Vuorio, A. F., Jolipii, A. M. M., and Jokipii, L., (1991). *Cryptosporidium* in asymptomatic children. *Reviews of Infectious Diseases*, **13**, 261–4.

Wagner-Wiening, C. and Kimmig, P. (1995). Detection of viable *Cryptosporidium parvum* oocysts by PCR. *Applied Environmental Microbiology*, **61**, 4514–6.

Watkins, J., Kemp, P., and Shepherd, K. (1995). Analysis of water samples for *Cryptosporidium* including the use of flow cytometry. In *Protozoan parasites in water*, (ed. B. Betts *et al.*), pp. 115–21. The Royal Society of Chemistry, Cambridge.

Webster, J. P. (1996). Wild brown rats (*Rattus norvegicus*) as a zoonotic risk on farms in England and Wales. *Communicable Diseases Report*, **6**, R46–49.

Webster, J. P. and MacDonald, D. W. (1995). Cryptosporidiosis reservoir in wild brown rats (*Rattus norvegicus*) in the UK. *Epidemiological Infections*, **115**, 207–9.

Webster, K. A. (1993). Molecular methods for the detection and classification of *Cryptosporidium Parasitology Today*, **9**, 263–6.

Webster, K. A., Pow, J. D. E., Giles, M., Catchpole, J., and Woodward, M. J. (1993). Detection of *Cryptosporidium parvum* using a specific polymerase chain reaction. *Veterinary Parasitology*, **50**, 35–44.

Weikel, C., Lazenby, A., Belitsos, P., McDewitt, M., Fleming, H. E., and Barbacci, M. (1991). Intestinal injury associated with Spiramycin therapy of *Cryptosporidium* infection in AIDS. *Journal of Protozoology*, **38**, 147S.

White, A. C., Chappell, C. L., Hayat, C. S., Kimball, K. T., Flanigan, T. P., and Goodgame, R. W. (1994). Paromomycin for Cryptosporidiosis in AIDS: A prospective, double-blind trial. *Journal of Infectious Diseases*, **170**, 419–24.

Xiao, L. and Herd, R. P. (1994). Review of equine *Cryptosporidium* infection. *Equine Veterinary Journal*, **26**, 9–13.

Xiao, L., Herd, R. P., and McClure, K. E. (1994). Periparturient rise in the excretion of *Giardia* sp. cysts and *Cryptosporidium parvum* oocysts as a source of infection for lambs. *Journal of Parasitology*, **80**, 55–9.

Zu, S. X., Fang, G. D., Fayer, R., and Guerrant, R. L. (1992). Cryptosporidiosis: pathogenesis and immunology. *Parasitology Today*, **8**, 24–7.

46 TOXOPLASMOSIS, SARCOCYSTOSIS, ISOSPOROSIS, AND CYCLOSPOROSIS

J. P. Dubey

TOXOPLASMOSIS

SUMMARY

Toxoplasmosis is a protozoan disease caused by *Toxoplasma gondii*. It is widely prevalent in humans and animals throughout the world, especially in the western hemisphere. Virtually all warm-blooded animals can act as intermediate hosts but the life cycle is completed only in cats, the definitive host. Cats excrete the resistant stage of *T. gondii* (oocysts) in faeces, and oocysts can survive in the environment for months. Humans become infected congenitally, by ingesting undercooked infected meat, or by ingesting food and water contaminated with oocysts from cat faeces. It can cause mental retardation and loss of vision in congenitally infected children and deaths in immunosuppressed patients, especially those with AIDS. There is no vaccine to control toxoplasmosis in humans at the present time butone is available for sheep.

HISTORY

Toxoplasma gondii was discovered in 1908 in Tunisia in a rodent, *Ctenodactylus gundi*, and in a laboratory rabbit in São Paulo, Brazil (Table 46.1). The name *Toxoplasma* (*toxon* = arc, *plasma* = form) is derived from the crescent shape of the tachyzoite stage, and the host, gundi. The medical importance of *T. gondii* was not discovered until late 1930s. The development of a serological test for toxoplasmosis in 1948 led to the findings that it was a common infection of humans throughout the world (Table 46.1).

While considerable progress on the characterization of the disease in humans and animals was made between 1940 and 1960, the main routes of transmission remained a mystery. Congenital transmission occurred too rarely to explain widespread infection in humans and animals. In 1960s it was found that organisms from tissue cysts could survive digestive enzymes and that humans can become infected by ingesting undercooked infected meat.

While congenital transmission and carnivorism partially explain transmission of *T. gondii*, these routes cannot explain the widespread *T. gondii* infection in vegetarians and in herbivores. Prevalence rates for *T. gondii* in strict vegetarians were found to be similar to those in non-vegetarians. Fresh excretions and secretions of animals which had even overwhelming infections proved essentially negative for *T. gondii* when tested in mice. Attempts to transmit *T. gondii* via arthropods were essentially unsuccessful.

The mystery of transmission was resolved when a resistant form of *T. gondii* was discovered in feline faeces and the coccidian phase of its life cycle was discovered in 1970 (Table 46.1).

THE AGENT

CLASSIFICATION

Toxoplasma gondii (Nicolle and Manceaux 1908) Nicolle and Manceaux 1909 is a coccidian parasite of cats with warm-blooded animals as intermediate hosts. Coccidia are among the most important parasites of animals. Traditionally, all coccidia of veterinary importance were classified under the family Eimeriidae, Michin, 1903. Classification was based on the structure of the oocyst. Oocysts with four sporocysts, each with two sporozoites (total eight sporozoites) are classified as *Eimeria*. Oocysts containing two sporocysts, each with four sporozoites, were classified historically as *Isospora*. After the discovery of the life cycle of *T. gondii*, several other genera (*Sarcocystis, Besnoitia, Hammondia, Frenkelia*) were found to have isosporan oocysts with two sporocysts and eight sporozoites.

Toxoplasma gondii and related genera discussed in the chapter are classified as follows:

Table 46.1   History of *Toxoplasma gondii* and toxoplasmosis[a]

Contributions and year	Contribution
Nicolle and Manceau (1908)	Discovered in gundi
Splendore (1908)	Discovered in rabbit
Mello (1910)	Disease described in a domestic animal (dog)
Wolf and Cowen (1937)	Congenital transmission documented
Pinkerton and Weinman (1940)	Fatal disease described in adult humans
Sabin (1942)	Disease characterized in man
Sabin and Feldman (1948)	Dye test described
Siim (1952)	Glandular toxoplasmosis described in man
Weinman and Chandler (1954)	Suggested carnivorous transmission
Hartley and Marshall (1957)	Abortions in sheep recognized
Beverley (1959)	Repeated congenital transmission observed in mice
Jacobs *et al.* (1960)	Tissue cysts characterized biologically
Hutchison (1965)	Faecal transmission recognized, nematode eggs suspected
Hutchison *et al.* (1969, 1970, 1971); Frenkel *et al.* (1970); Dubey *et al.* (1970*a,b*); Sheffield and Melton (1970); Overdulve (1970)	Coccidian phase described
Frenkel *et al.* (1970); Miller *et al.* (1972)	Definitive and intermediate hosts defined
Dubey and Frenkel (1972)	Five *T. gondii* types described from feline intestinal epithelium
Wallace (1969); Munday (1972)	Confirmation of the epidemiological role of cats from studies on remote islands

[a] From Dubey (1993). For a complete bibliography see Dubey (1993).

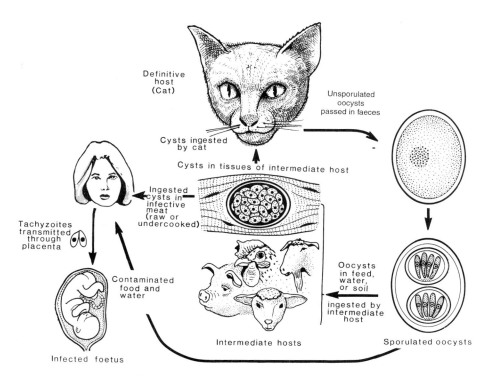

Fig. 46.1   Life cycle of *T. gondii*.

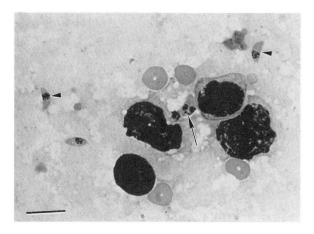

Fig. 46.2 Tachyzoites of *T. gondii*. Impression smear. Note individual crescentic (arrowheads) and dividing (arrow) tachyzoites. (Giemsa; bar = 10 μm.)

Phylum: Apicomplexa; Levine, 1970
Class: Sporozoasida; Leukart, 1879
Subclass: Coccidiasina; Leukart, 1879
Order: Eucoccidiorida; Leger and Duboseq, 1910
Suborder: Eimeriorina; Leger, 1911

Opinions differ regarding the further classification of *T. gondii* into families and subfamilies. It has been classified in the families Eimeriidae, Minchin 1903; Sarcocystidae, Poche 1913; or Toxoplasmatidae, Biocca 1956 by various authorities.

STRUCTURE AND LIFE CYCLE

There are three infectious stages of *T. gondii* (Fig. 46.1): the tachyzoites (in groups), the bradyzoites (in tissue cysts), and the sporozoites (in oocysts) (Frenkel 1973).

The tachyzoite is often crescent-shaped and is approximately 2 × 6 μm (Fig. 46.2). Its anterior (conoidal) end is pointed and its posterior end is round. It has a

pellicle (outer covering), polar ring, conoid, rhoptries, micronemes, mitochondria, subpellicular microtubules, endoplasmic reticulum, Golgi apparatus, ribosomes, rough surface endoplasmic reticulum, micropore, and a well-defined nucleus (Fig. 46.3). The nucleus is usually situated toward the posterior end or in the central area of the cell (Dubey 1977, 1993).

The pellicle consists of three membranes. The inner membrane complex is discontinuous at three points: the anterior end (polar ring), the lateral edge (micropore), and toward the posterior end. The polar ring is an osmiophilic thickening of the inner membrane at the anterior end of the tachyzoite. The polar ring encircles a cylindrical, truncated cone (the conoid) which consists of 6–8 fibrillar elements wound like a compressed spring. Twenty-two subpellicular microtubules originate from the anterior end and run longitudinally almost the entire length of the cell. Terminating within the conoid are 4–10 club-shaped organelles called rhoptries (Fig. 46.3). The rhoptries are gland-like structures, often labrinthine, with an anterior narrow neck up to 2.5 μm long. Their sac-like posterior end terminates anterior to the nucleus. Micronemes (also called toxonemes) are convoluted tube-like structures which occur at the anterior end of the parasite.

The functions of the conoid, rhoptries, and micronemes are not fully known. The conoid is probably associated with the penetration of the tachyzoite through the membrane of the host cell. It can rotate, tilt, extend, and retract as the parasite searches for a host cell. *Toxoplasma gondii* can move by gliding, undulating, and rotating. Rhoptries have a secretory function associated with host cell penetration, secreting their contents through the conoid to the exterior. The microtubules probably provide the cytoskeleton.

The tachyzoite enters the host cell by active penetration of the host cell membrane. After entering the host cell the tachyzoite becomes ovoid in shape and

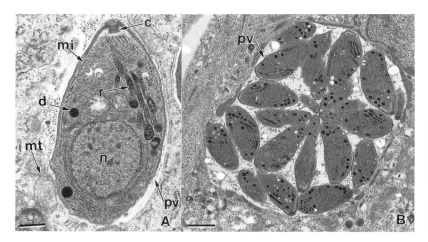

Fig. 46.3 Transmission electron micrographs of *T. gondii* tachyzoites in cell culture. (A) Tachyzoite in a parasitophorous vacuole (pv) in the cytoplasm of a host cell. Note conoid (c), rhoptries (r), micronemes (mi), nucleus (n), and dense granules (d). The host cell mitochondria (mt) are closely associated with the pv. (Bar = 0.5 μm.) (B) Several tachyzoites in pv. (Bar = 1.8 μm.)

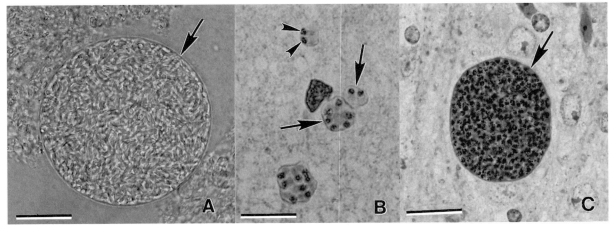

Fig. 46.4   Tissue cysts of *T. gondii* with thin cyst walls (arrows) in brain. (A) Impression smear, unstained. This tissue cyst was freed by grinding a piece of brain in a mortar with a pestle. (Bar = 20 μm.) (B) Impression smear. Four young tissue cysts with silver-positive cyst walls. Two tissue cysts each have two bradyzoites with terminal nuclei (arrowheads). (Silver stain, bar = 10 μm.) (C) Histological section. Note bradyzoites have PAS-positive red granules that appear black in this micrograph. (Periodic acid–Schiff haematoxylin; bar = 20 μm.)

becomes surrounded by a parasitophorous vacuole (PV). It has been suggested that the PV is derived from both the parasite and the host. Numerous intravacuolar tubules connect the parasitophorous vacuolar membrane to the parasite pellicle.

The tachyzoite multiplies asexually within the host cell by repeated endodyogeny. Endodyogeny (*endo* = inside, *dyo* = two, *geny* = progeny) is a specialized form of reproduction in which two progeny form within the parent parasite, consuming it in the process. Tachyzoites continue to divide by endodyogeny until the host cell is filled with parasites (Fig. 46.3B).

After a few divisions, *T. gondii* encysts to form tissue cysts (Fig. 46.4). Tissue cysts grow and remain intracellular as the bradyzoites (encysted *T. gondii*) divide by endodyogeny. Tissue cysts vary in size. Young tissue cysts may be as small as 5 μm and contain only two bradyzoites, while older ones may contain hundreds of organisms (Fig. 46.4). Tissue cysts in brain are often circular and rarely reach a diameter of 60 μm whereas intramuscular cysts are elongated and may be 100 μm long. Although tissue cysts may develop in visceral organs, including lungs, liver, and kidneys, they are more prevalent in the neural and muscular tissues, including the brain, eye, skeletal, and cardiac muscle. Intact tissue cysts probably do not cause any harm and can persist for the life of the host.

The tissue cyst wall is elastic, thin (<0.5 μm) and argyrophilic (Fig. 46.4B). The bradyzoites are approximately 7 × 1.5 μm. Bradyzoites differ structurally only slightly from tachyzoites. They have a nucleus situated toward the posterior end, whereas the nucleus in tachyzoites is more centrally located. The contents of rhoptries in bradyzoites in older tissue cysts are elec-

tron dense (Fig. 46.5). Bradyzoites contain several amylopectin granules which stain red with periodic acid–Schiff (PAS) reagent (Fig. 46.4C); such material is either in discrete particles or absent in tachyzoites. Bradyzoites are more slender than are tachyzoites. Bradyzoites are less susceptible to destruction by proteolytic enzymes than are tachyzoites.

Cats excrete oocysts after ingesting tachyzoites, bradyzoites, or sporozoites. Prepatent periods (time to the shedding of oocysts after initial infection) and frequency of oocyst shedding vary according to the stage of *T. gondii* ingested. Prepatent periods are 3–10 days after ingesting tissue cysts and 14 days or more after ingesting tachyzoites or oocysts. Fewer than 50 per cent of cats shed oocysts after ingesting tachyzoites or oocysts, whereas nearly all cats shed oocysts after ingesting tissue cysts.

After the ingestion of tissue cysts by cats, the cyst wall is dissolved by the proteolytic enzymes in the stomach and small intestine. The released bradyzoites penetrate the epithelial cells of the small intestine and initiate development of numerous generations of *T. gondii*. Five morphologically distinct types (A to E) of *T. gondii* develop in intestinal epithelial cells before gametogony begins. Types A to E divide asexually by endodyogeny, endopolygeny, or schizogony (division into more than two organisms).

The origin of gamonts has not been determined, probably the merozoites released from meronts of types D and E initiate gamete formation. Gamonts occur throughout the small intestine but most commonly in the ileum (Fig. 46.6), they are found 3–15 days after infection. They occur distal to the host epithelial cell nucleus near the tips of the villi of the

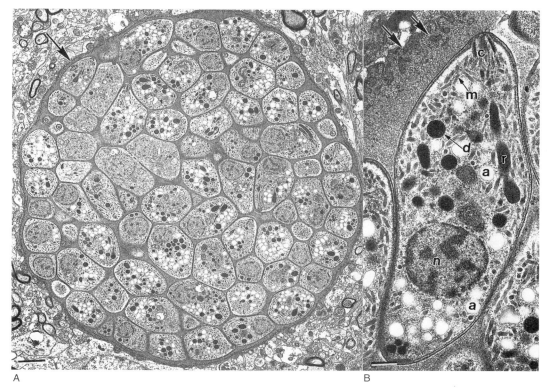

Fig. 46.5 Transmission electron micrographs of tissue cysts of *T. gondii* in brain. (A) Young cyst with well-developed cyst wall (arrow). The bradyzoites are plump (dividing or preparing to divide). (Bar = 3.4 μm.) (B) Longitudinally cut bradyzoite. Note electron-dense contents of rhopties (r), the subterminal nucleus (n), a conoid (c), numerous micronemes (m), and amylopectin granules (a) that appear as empty spaces here. The cyst wall (arrows) is convoluted. (Bar = 0.77 μm.)

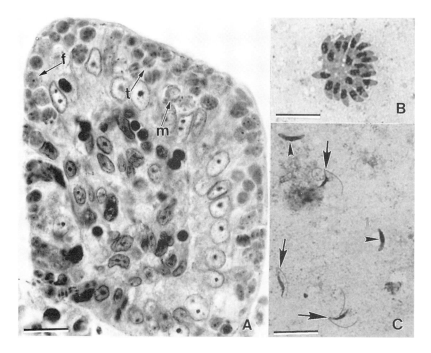

Fig. 46.6 Enteroepithelial stages of *T. gondii*, 6 days after feeding tissue cysts to a cat. (A) Histological section of a villus in small intestine. Note heavy infection of epithelial cells with *T. gondii* types (t), male gamonts (m), and numerous uninucleate female gamonts (f). Cells in the lamina propria are not infected. (Haematoxylin and eosin; bar = 15 μm.) (B) Impression smear. Note a type D schizont with 20 merozoites. (Giemsa; bar = 10 μm.) (C) Impression smear. Three biflagellate microgametes (arrows) and two free merozoites (arrowheads). (Giemsa; bar = 10 μm.)

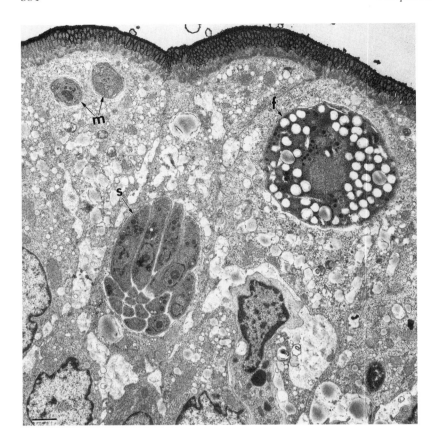

Fig. 46.7 Electron micrograph of coccidian stages of *T. gondii* in epithelial cells of ileum of a cat six days after ingesting tissue cysts. Note two merozoites (m), a female gamont (f) located just below the microvillus border, and a schizont(s) above the host cell nucleus. (Bar = 2.5 μm.)

small intestine (Fig. 46.6, 46.7). The female gamete is subspherical and contains a single, centrally located nucleus and several PAS-positive granules.

Mature male gamonts are ovoid to ellipsoidal in shape. Each microgamete has two flagella (Fig. 46.6C). The microgametes swim to and penetrate a mature macrogamete. After penetration, oocyst wall formation begins around the fertilized gamete. When they are mature, oocysts are discharged into the intestinal lumen by the rupture of intestinal epithelial cells.

Unsporulated oocysts are subspherical to spherical and are 10 × 12 μm in diameter (Fig. 46.8A). The oocyst wall contains two colourless layers. The sporont almost fills the oocyst, and sporulation occurs outside the cat within 1–5 days, depending upon aeration and temperature.

Sporulated oocysts are subspherical to ellipsoidal and are 11 × 13 μm in diameter. Each sporulated oocyst contains two ellipsoidal sporocysts without a Stieda body. Sporocysts measure 6 × 8 μm (Fig. 46.8B). There are four sutures with lip-like thickenings in the sporocyst wall (Fig. 46.8B); these sutures open during excystation of the sporozoites. A sporocyst residuum is present. There is no oocyst residuum. Each sporocyst contains four sporozoites. The sporozoites are 2 ×

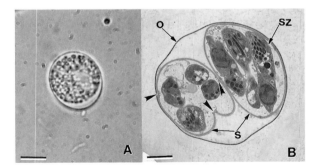

Fig. 46.8 Oocysts of *T. gondii*. (A) Unsporulated oocyst. Note sporont fills the oocyst. (Unstained; bar = 6 μm.) (B) Transmission electron micrograph of a sporulated oocyst. Note thin-walled oocyst (o) enclosing the two sporocysts (s) each with four sporozoites (sz). Each sporocyst has four lip-like thickenings (arrowheads). (Bar = 4.2 μm.) (Courtesy of Dr D. S. Lindsay.)

6–8 μm in size with a subterminal to central nucleus and a few PAS-positive granules in the cytoplasm (Fig. 46.8B).

As the enteroepithelial cycle progresses, bradyzoites penetrate the lamina propria of the feline intestine and multiply as tachyzoites. Within a few hours after infection of cats, *T. gondii* may disseminate to extra-intestinal tissues. *Toxoplasma gondii* persists in intestinal and extraintestinal tissues of cats for at least several months, if not for the life of the cat.

CULTIVATION

Toxoplasma gondii has not been grown in cell-free media. *Toxoplasma gondii* can be cultivated in laboratory animals, chick embryos, and cell cultures. Mice, hamsters, guinea-pigs, and rabbits are all susceptible but mice are generally used as hosts because they are more susceptible than the others and are not naturally infected when raised in the laboratory on commercial dry food free of cat faeces.

Tachyzoites of some strains of *T. gondii* grow in the peritoneal cavity of mice, sometimes producing ascites, and also grow in most other tissues after intra-peritoneal inoculation with any of the three infectious stages of *T. gondii*. Virulent strains usually produce illness in mice and sometimes kill them within 1–2 weeks. Most strains of *T. gondii* do not kill mice.

Toxoplasma gondii tachyzoites will multiply in many cell lines in cell cultures (Fig. 46.9). Although tissue cysts can develop in cell cultures with most strains of *T. gondii*, the yield is lower than that produced by infection in mice.

Tissue cysts are obtained by injecting tachyzoites, bradyzoites, or oocysts into mice. To obtain tissue cysts from mice inoculated with a virulent strain, it is necessary to administer anti-*T. gondii* chemotherapy to prevent death from acute toxoplasmosis before tissue cysts form. Sulphadiazine is effective in controlling the acute stages of toxoplasmosis in mice. Tissue cysts are prominent in the mouse brain about 8 weeks after infection (Fig. 46.10).

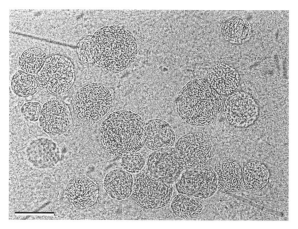

Fig. 46.10 Squash of a portion of brain of a mouse with numerous *T. gondii* tissue cysts. This mouse appeared clinically normal although it had many cysts. (Unstained; bar = 50 μm.)

Enteroepithelial stages of *T. gondii* have not yet been cultivated *in vitro*.

Oocysts can be obtained by feeding tissue cysts from infected mice to *T. gondii*-free cats.

MOLECULAR BIOLOGY

Toxoplasma gondii nucleus is haploid except during the sexual division in the intestine of the cat (Pfefferkorn 1990). Sporozoites are the results of meiosis and seem to follow classical Mendelian laws. The total haploid genome contains approximately 8×10^7 base pairs. There is also a 36 kb, circular mitochondrial DNA, which has been partly sequenced. Nine chromosomes have been identified by pulsed-field gel electrophore-

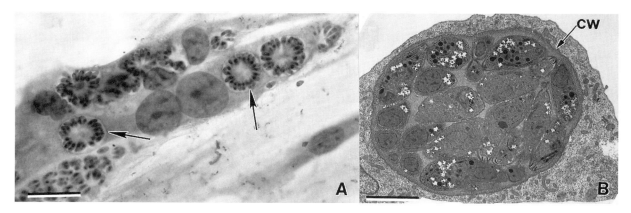

Fig. 46.9 *Toxoplasma gondii* in cell cultures. (A) Tachyzoites, some groups in rosettes (arrows). (Giemsa; smear; bar = 20 μm.) (B) Transmission electron micrograph of a tissue cyst. Note a well-developed cyst wall (cw) enclosing approximately 14 bradyzoites. The empty spaces in bradyzoites are amylopectin granules. (Bar = 3.6 μm.) (Courtesy of Dr D. S. Lindsay.)

sis. The karyotype has been studied using probes from low-copy number genes. Several virulent *T. gondii* strains have been characterized genetically, they are considered to have a common lineage. The *T. gondii* DNA has been characterized and a genetic nomenclature for *T. gondii* has been proposed (McLeod *et al.* 1991; Sibley *et al.* 1992).

Toxoplasma gondii rRNA has as usual a large and a small subunit. Sequence analysis of the small rRNA suggests that *T. gondii* is closely related phylogenetically to *Sarcocystis* but distant from *Plasmodium*. Although there are stage-specific proteins, all infective stages of *T. gondii* share common proteins. Most of the proteins that have been characterized are from tachyzoites. *Toxoplasma gondii* tachyzoites have four major surface proteins (22, 30, 35, and 43 kDa). Of these the p30 is the dominant protein and comprises 5 per cent of the total tachyzoite protein (Johnson 1989).

HOST—PARASITE RELATIONSHIP

Toxoplasma gondii usually parasitizes the host (both definitive and intermediate) without producing clinical signs. Only rarely does it cause severe clinical manifestations. The majority of natural infections are probably acquired by ingestion of tissue cysts in infected meat or oocysts in food or water contaminated with cat faeces. The bradyzoites from the tissue cysts or sporozoites from the oocyst penetrate the intestinal epithelial cells and multiply (Fig. 46.11A). *Toxoplasma gondii* may spread first to the mesenteric lymph nodes (Fig. 46.11B) and then to distant organs by invasion of lymph and blood. An infected host may die because of necrosis of intestine and mesenteric lymph nodes before other organs are severely damaged. Focal areas of necrosis may develop in many organs. The clinical picture is determined by the extent of injury to organs, especially vital organs such as the eye, heart, and adrenal glands. Necrosis is caused by the intracellular growth of tachyzoites. *Toxoplasma gondii* does not produce a toxin.

In those hosts which develop disease, the host may die of acute toxoplasmosis but much more often recovers with the acquisition of immunity (Frenkel 1973). In the recovering individual inflammation usually develops in sites where initially there was necrosis. By about the third week after infection, *T. gondii* tachyzoites begin to disappear the from visceral tissues and may localize in tissue cysts in neural and muscular tissues. *Toxoplasma gondii* tachyzoites may persist longer in the spinal cord and brain than in visceral tissues because immunity there is less effective than in neural organs. *Toxoplasma gondii* tachyzoites can persist in the placenta for months after the initial infection of the dam. How *T. gondii* is destroyed in immune cells is not completely known. All extracellular forms of the parasite are directly affected by antibody but intracellular forms are not. It is believed that cellular factors includ-

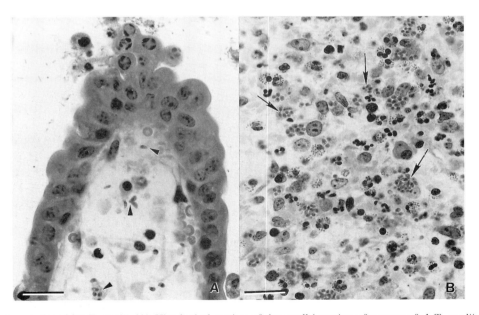

Fig. 46.11 Lesions induced by *T. gondii*. (A) Histological section of the small intestine of a mouse fed *T. gondii* oocysts. Note oedema (empty spaces), necrosis and tachyzoites (arrowheads) in the lamina propria, and desquamation of epithelial cells into the lumen. (Haematoxylin and eosin; bar = 20 μm.) (B) Section of mesenteric lymph node with numerous tachyzoites (arrows) destroying host cells. (Haematoxylin and eosin; bar = 20 μm.)

ing lymphocytes and lymphokines are more important than humoral ones in immune-mediated destruction of *T. gondii* (Frenkel 1973; Gazzinelli *et al.* 1993). Under experimental conditions, infection with avirulent strains protects the host from damage but does not prevent infection with more virulent strains. In most instances, immunity following a natural *T. gondii* infection persists for the life of the host.

Immunity does not eradicate infection. *Toxoplasma gondii* tissue cysts persist several years after acute infection. The fate of tissue cysts is not fully known. Whether bradyzoites can form new cysts directly without transforming into tachyzoites is not known. However, the finding of new cysts adjacent to old ones suggests that it might happen. It has been proposed that tissue cysts may at times rupture during the life of the host. The released bradyzoites may be destroyed by the host's immune responses. The reaction may cause local necrosis accompanied by inflammation. Hypersensitivity plays a major role in such reactions. After such events, inflammation usually again subsides with no local renewed multiplication of *T. gondii* in the tissue; however, occasionally there may be formation of new tissue cysts.

In immunosuppressed patients, such as those given large doses of immunosuppressive agents in preparation for organ transplants and in those with acquired immunodeficiency syndrome (AIDS), rupture of a tissue cyst may result in transformation of bradyzoites into tachyzoites and renewed multiplication (Fig. 46.12). The immunosuppressed host may die from toxoplasmosis unless treated. It is not known how corticosteroids cause relapse but it is unlikely that they directly cause rupture of the tissue cysts.

Pathogenicity of *T. gondii* is determined by the virulence of the strain and the susceptibility of the host species. *Toxoplasma gondii* strains may vary in their pathogenicity in a given host. Certain strains of mice are more susceptible than others and the severity of infection in individual mice within the same strain may vary. Certain species are genetically resistant to clinical toxoplasmosis. For example, adult rats do not become ill while the young rats can die because of toxoplasmosis. Mice of any age are susceptible to clinical *T. gondii* infection. Adult dogs, like adult rats, are resistant, whereas puppies are fully susceptible. Cattle and horses are among the hosts more resistant to clinical toxoplasmosis whereas certain marsupials and New World monkeys are the most susceptible to *T. gondii* infection. Nothing is known concerning genetic-related susceptibility to clinical toxoplasmosis in higher mammals, including humans.

Various factors vaguely classified as stress may affect *T. gondii* infection in a host. More severe infections are found in pregnant or lactating mice than in non-lactating mice. Concomitant infection may make the host more susceptible or resistant to *T. gondii* infection.

DISEASE IN HUMANS AND OTHER ANIMALS

INFECTION IN HUMANS

Toxoplasma gondii infection is widespread among humans and its prevalence varies widely from place to place (Dubey and Beattie 1988). In the United States and the United Kingdom it is estimated that about

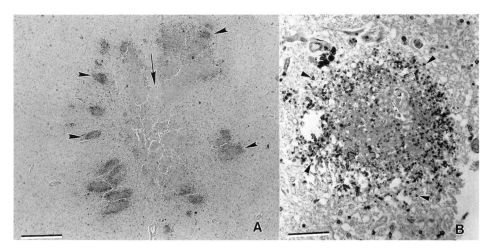

Fig. 46.12 Necrosis associated with *T. gondii* in an AIDS patient. Immunohistochemical stain with anti-*T. gondii* serum. (A) Central area of necrosis (arrow) and several satellite lesions (arrowheads). (Bar = 200 μm.) (B) Higher magnification of one of the satellite lesions. Note hundreds of tachyzoites (arrowheads, all black dots) at the periphery of the necrotic lesion. (Bar = 20 μm.)

Table 46.2 The relation of clinical toxoplasmosis in children to the time of infection in the mother[a]

Trimester infected	Children with toxoplasmosis (%)			
	Serious	Mild	Subclinical	Total No.
First	40	50	10	10
Second	17.7	45	37	62
Third	2.7	28.7	68.5	108
Undetermined	16.6	20.6	56.6	30

[a] From Couvreur *et al.* (1984).

16–40 per cent of people are infected, whereas in Central and South America and continental Europe estimates of infection range from 50 to 80 per cent.

Most infections in humans are asymptomatic but at times the parasite can produce devastating disease. Infection may be congenitally or postnatally acquired.

Congenital infection occurs only when a woman becomes infected during pregnancy and the severity of disease may depend upon the stage of pregnancy when the woman becomes infected (Table 46.2). While the mother rarely has symptoms of infection, she does have a temporary parasitaemia. Focal lesions develop in the placenta and the fetus may become infected. At first there is generalized infection in the fetus. Later,

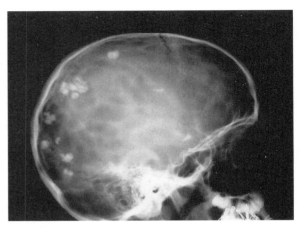

Fig. 46.14 Intracerebral calcification discovered fortuitously in a 10-year-old girl, on a dental panoramic X-ray asked by a dentist. The girl had unilateral retinochoroiditis and an IQ of 80. (Courtesy of Dr J. Couvreur.)

infection is cleared from the visceral tissues and may localize in the central nervous system. A wide spectrum of clinical disease occurs in congenitally infected children. Mild disease may consist of slightly diminished vision only, whereas severely diseased children may have the full tetrad of signs: retinochoroiditis, hydrocephalus (Fig. 46.13), convulsions, and intracerebral calcification (Fig. 46.14). Of these, hydrocephalus is the least common but most dramatic lesion of toxoplasmosis. This lesion is unique to congenitally acquired toxoplasmosis in humans and has not been reported in other animals.

By far the most common sequel of congenital toxoplasmosis is ocular disease (Guerina *et al.* 1994; McAuley *et al.* 1994; Remington *et al.* 1995). Except for the occasional involvement of an entire eye, in virtually all cases the disease is confined to the posterior chamber. *Toxoplasma gondii* proliferates in the retina and this leads to inflammation in the choroid. Therefore, the disease is correctly designated as retinochoroiditis. In humans the characteristic lesions of ocular toxoplasmosis in the acute or subacute stage of inflammation appear as yellowish-white, cotton-like patches in the fundus. The lesions may be single or multiple and may involve one or both eyes (Dutton 1989). During the acute stage, inflammatory exudate may cloud the vitreous fluid and may be so dense as to preclude visualization of the fundus by the examiner using an ophthalmoscope. As the inflammation subsides, the vitreous clears and the diseased retina and choroid can be seen through the ophthalmoscope. Retinal lesions may be single or multifocal, small, grey areas of active retinitis with minimal oedema and reaction in the vitreous humor. The punctate lesions are usually harmless unless they are located in a macular

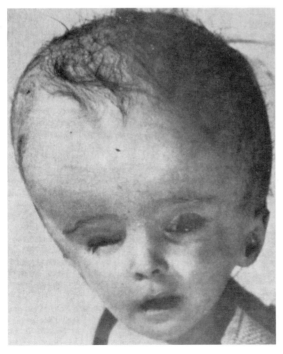

Fig. 46.13 Congenital toxoplasmosis in a child. Note hydrocephalus and microphthalmia. (Courtesy of Dr R. Belfort Jr and National Eye Institute, NIH, Bethesda, Maryland, USA.)

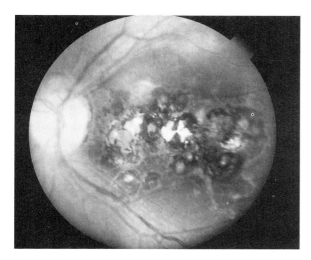

Fig. 46.15 Congenital toxoplasmosis. Retinochoroiditis in the macula of the left eye. (Courtesy of Dr R. Belfort Jr.)

Table 46.3 Frequency of symptoms in people with postnatally acquired toxoplasmosis

| Symptoms | Patients with symptoms (%) | |
	Atlanta outbreak[a] (35 patients)	Panama outbreak[b] (35 patients)
Fever	94	90
Lymphadenopathy	88	77
Headache	88	77
Myalgia	63	68
Stiff neck	57	55
Anorexia	57	NR[c]
Sore throat	46	NR
Arthralgia	26	29
Rash	23	0
Confusion	20	NR
Earache	17	NR
Nausea	17	36
Eye pain	14	26
Abdominal pain	11	55

[a] From Teutsch *et al.* (1979).
[b] From Benenson *et al.* (1982).
[c] Not reported.

area (Fig. 46.15). Although severe infections may be detected at birth, milder infections may go undetected until they flare up in adulthood.

The socio-economic impact of toxoplasmosis in human suffering and the cost of care of sick children, especially those with mental retardation and blindness, are enormous (Roberts and Frenkel 1990; Roberts *et al.* 1994). The testing of all pregnant women for *T. gondii* infection is compulsory in France and Austria. In Austria and France, all pregnant women are tested serologically on their first visit to their gynaecologist. Women with *T. gondii* antibodies are not tested further. Seronegative women are tested monthly and they are treated for toxoplasmosis if they acquire *T. gondii* antibodies during pregnancy. Studies from France and Austria indicate that treatment of women during pregnancy reduces fetal damage. The cost benefits of such mass screening are being debated in many countries (Dubey and Beattie 1988; Lebech and Petersen 1992; Remington *et al.* 1995).

Postnatally acquired infection may be localized or generalized (Teutsch *et al.* 1979; Benenson *et al.* 1982). Oocyst-transmitted infections may be more severe than tissue cyst-induced infections. Lymphadenitis is the most frequently observed clinical form of toxoplasmosis in humans (Table 46.3). Although any node may be involved, the most frequently involved are the deep cervical nodes. These nodes when infected are tender, discrete but not painful, and the infections resolve spontaneously in weeks or months. Lymphadenopathy may be associated with fever, malaise, fatigue, muscle pain, sore throat, and headache. Although the condition may be benign, its diagnosis is vital in pregnant women because of the risk to the fetus. Histologically, there is reticular cell hyperplasia whereas necrosis and

fibrosis are absent, the node architecture is preserved but only a few *T. gondii* are present. The diagnosis can be confirmed by bioassay of lymph node by injection into mice, by immunohistochemical staining with *T. gondii* antiserum, or by use of the polymerase chain reaction (PCR) to detect *T. gondii* DNA.

Toxoplasmosis ranks high in the list of diseases which lead to death of patients with AIDS; approximately 10 per cent of AIDS patients in the United States and up to 30 per cent in Europe are estimated to die from toxoplasmosis (Luft and Remington 1992; Luft *et al.* 1993; Rabaud *et al.* 1994). Clinically, patients may have headache, disorientation, drowsiness, hemiparesis, reflex changes, and convulsions, and many become comatose. Diagnosis is aided by serological examination. However, in immunosuppressed patients both inflammatory signs and antibody production may be suppressed, thus making the diagnosis very difficult. Although in AIDS patients any organ may be involved, including the testis, dermis, and the spinal cord, infection of the brain is most frequent. In the brain, the predominant lesion is necrosis, especially of the thalamus. In most AIDS patients, the disease is reactivation of latent *T. gondii* infection because of immunosuppressive effects of the human immunodeficiency virus infection.

INFECTION IN ANIMALS OTHER THAN HUMANS

Toxoplasma gondii is capable of causing severe disease in animals other than humans. Among livestock, great losses occur in sheep and goats. *Toxoplasma gondii* causes early embryonic death and resorption, fetal death and mummification, abortion, still birth, and neonatal death. Toxoplasmosis-induced abortion can occur in ewes of all ages. Infected lambs that survive the first week after birth grow normally. Abortion occurs in ewes that acquire infection during pregnancy. Therefore, ewes which have aborted should be saved for future breeding. Fatal toxoplasmosis has been reported in pigs, dogs, cats, rabbits, birds, and many species of wildlife (Dubey and Beattie 1988).

Cattle and horses are more resistant to clinical toxoplasmosis than any other species of livestock. Although both cattle and horses have been found infected with *T. gondii*, there is no documented report of clinical toxoplasmosis in horses or cattle. Toxoplasmosis is most severe in certain species of Australian marsupials and New World monkeys (Dubey and Beattie 1988).

DIAGNOSIS

Diagnosis is made by biological, serological, or histological methods or by some combination of them. Clinical symptoms of toxoplasmosis are non-specific and toxoplasmosis in fact mimics several other infectious diseases.

Toxoplasma gondii can be isolated from patients by inoculation of laboratory animals and tissue cultures with secretions, excretions, body fluids, and tissues taken by biopsy ante-mortem or tissues with macroscopic lesions taken post-mortem.

Detection of *T. gondii* antibody in patients may aid diagnosis. There are numerous serological procedures used to detect humoral antibodies; these include the Sabin–Feldman dye test, the indirect hemaglutination assay, the indirect fluorescent antibody assay (IFA), the direct agglutination test (DAT), the latex agglutination test, the enzyme-linked immunoabsorbent assay (ELISA), and the immunoabsorbent agglutination assay test (IAAT). The IFA, IAAT, and ELISA have been modified to detect IgM antibodies. The IgM antibodies appear sooner than the IgG antibodies but IgM antibodies also disappear faster than IgG antibodies.

The result of examining one positive serum sample only establishes that the host has been infected at some time in the past. It is best to collect two samples on the same individual. A 16-fold higher antibody titre in a serum taken 2–4 weeks after the first serum was collected indicates an acute acquired infection. A high antibody titre sometimes persists for months and a rise may not be associated with clinical symptoms. As indicated earlier, most acquired infections in humans are asymptomatic.

Diagnosis can be made by finding *T. gondii* in host tissue removed by biopsy or at necropsy. A rapid diagnosis may be made by making impression smears of lesions on glass slides. After drying for 10–30 minutes, the smears are fixed in methyl alcohol and stained with Giemsa. Well-preserved *T. gondii* are crescent-shaped and stain well with any of the Romanowsky stains (Fig. 4 6 .2). In sections, the tachyzoites usually appear as oval to round and only half the size of those in smears (Fig. 46. c.11). Electron microscopy can aid diagnosis. *Toxoplasma gondii* tachyzoites are always located in vacuoles and have rhoptries with honeycomb structure (Fig. 46.3). Tissue cysts are without septa and with a thin cyst wall butted against the host cell plasmalemma (Figs 46.4, 46.5). Occasionally, tissue cysts might be found in areas with lesions. The immunohistochemical staining of parasites with *T. gondii* antiserum can aid in diagnosis (Fig. 46.12).

TREATMENT

Sulphadiazine and pyrimethamine (Daraprim®) are two drugs widely used for therapy of toxoplasmosis. These two drugs act synergistically by blocking the metabolic pathway involving *p*-aminobenzoic acid and the folic–folinic acid cycle, respectively. These drugs are usually well tolerated but sometimes thrombocytopenia or leucopenia may develop. These effects can be overcome by administering folinic acid and yeast without interfering with treatment because the vertebrate host can utilize presynthesized folinic acid while *T. gondii* cannot (Frenkel 1973). While these drugs have a beneficial action when given in the acute stage of the disease process when there is active multiplication of the parasite, they will not usually eradicate infection. It is believed that these drugs have little effect on cysts. Sulfonamides are excreted within a few hours of administration; therefore, treatment has to be administered in daily divided doses (four doses of 500 mg each) usually for several weeks or months. A loading dose (75 mg) of pyrimethamine during the first 3 days has been recommended because it is absorbed slowly and binds to tissues. From the fourth day, the dose of pyrimethamine is reduced to 25 mg, and 2–10 mg of folinic acid and 5–10 g of bakers' yeast are added (Frenkel 1973; St. Georgiev 1994).

Certain other drugs, atovaquone, spiramycin, chlorinated lincomycin analogues, lasalocid, and monensin, piritrexim, and roxithromycin have been found effective in treatment of experimentally induced *T. gondii* infection in animals or cell cultures (St. Georgiev 1994). Spiramycin administration produces high tissue concentrations, particularly in the placenta, but does not cross the placental barrier, and has been used in humans without harmful effects. However, spiramycin, is a less effective antitoxoplasmicidal than is sulphadiazine and pyrimethamine. Clindamycin is reported to be effective against *T. gondii*, but may cause ulcerative colitis in humans. Among all of the drugs tested, atovaquone was the most cysticidal. Search for newer cysticidal drugs is continuing.

EPIDEMIOLOGY

Toxoplasma gondii infection in humans is widespread and occurs throughout the world. Approximately one-half billion humans have antibodies to *T. gondii*. Infection rates in humans and others animals differ from one geographical area of a country to another. The causes of these variations are not yet known. Environmental conditions, cultural habits of the people, and animal fauna are some of the factors that may determine the level of infection with *T. gondii*. Infection is more prevalent in hot and humid areas than in dry and cold climates. Only a small proportion (less than 1 per cent) of people acquire infection congenitally.

Women produce children with congenital infection only once. Mothers of congenitally infected children have not been known to give birth to infected children in subsequent pregnancies.

The relative frequency of acquisition of postnatal toxoplasmosis due to eating raw meat and that due to ingestion of food contaminated by oocysts from cat faeces is not known and is difficult to investigate. *Toxoplasma gondii* infection is common in many animals used for food. Sheep, pigs, and rabbits are commonly infected throughout the world. Infection in cattle is less prevalent than in sheep or pigs. Infection is common in many species of wildlife, especially in deer and bears (Dubey 1994). *Toxoplasma gondii* tissue cysts survive in live food animals for years. As stated earlier, humans can acquire infection by eating raw or undercooked meat.

Toxoplasma gondii organisms in meat are susceptible to extremes of temperatures. Tissue cysts are killed by cooking meat to 67 °C. *Toxoplasma gondii* in meat is killed by cooling to −13 °C. Tissue cysts are also killed by exposure to 0.5 kGy of gamma irradiation.

Cultural habits of people may play a role in acquiring *T. gondii* infections. For example, in France the prevalence of *Toxoplasma* antibody is very high. The higher incidence in France appears to be related in part to the French habit of eating some of their meat raw. The high prevalence of *T. gondii* infection in Central and South America is in part due to high levels of contamination of the environment by oocysts (Dubey and Beattie 1988).

Oocysts are shed by cats, not only the domestic cat but by other members of the Felidae as well. Widespread infection of the environment is possible because a cat may excrete millions of oocysts after ingesting one infected mouse. Oocysts are resistant to most ordinary environmental conditions and can survive in moist conditions for months and even years. Invertebrates, such as flies, cockroaches, dung beetles, and earthworms, can spread oocysts mechanically and even carry them on to food.

While only a few cats may be shedding *T. gondii* oocysts at any given time, the enormous numbers shed is important in the spread of *T. gondii*. Whether cats normally shed oocysts only once or several times during their lifetime is not known; however, under experimental conditions, cats develop good immunity to *T. gondii* against oocyst shedding but can reshed oocysts after re-inoculation of tissue cysts (Dubey 1995). Congenital infection can occur in cats and congenitally infected kittens can excrete oocyts. Infection rates of cats probably vary with the rate of infection in local avian and rodent populations because cats are thought to become infected in nature by eating these animals.

Theoretically, transmission of toxoplasmosis may be by sexual means, by ingestion of milk, saliva, or by eating of eggs. The stage most likely to be involved in these transmissions would be tachyzoites. Tachyzoites are delicate and do not survive outside the body for long. Therefore, there is practically no risk of transmission by kissing or by venereal transmission. There is little, if any, danger of *T. gondii* infection by drinking cow's milk and, in any case, milk is generally pasteurized or even boiled, but infection has followed drinking unboiled goat's milk. Raw hens' eggs, although an important source of *Salmonella* infection, are extremely unlikely to transmit *T. gondii* infection.

In recent years transmission by transplantation has become important (Wreghitt and Hakim 1989). Toxoplasmosis may arise in two ways in people undergoing transplantation: from implantation of an organ or bone marrow from an infected donor into a non-immune immunocompromised recipient, and from induction of disease in an immunocompromised latently infected recipient. In the later case, the immunosuppressive treatment activates the latent infection of the recipient. In these cases both tachyzoites and tissue cysts might be involved, but more probably tissue cysts. In both cases the cytotoxic and immunosuppressive therapy given to the recipient is the cause of induction of the active infection and the disease.

PREVENTION AND CONTROL

VACCINATION

The objectives of use of vaccines against toxoplasmosis include reducing fetal damage, reducing the number of *T. gondii* tissue cysts in animals, and preventing the formation of oocysts in cats (Araujo 1994; Dubey

1994). All of these objectives are not currently feasible with the use of a single vaccine. At present there are no effective subunit or killed vaccines for immunization against *T. gondii* but research is under way in many laboratories (Araujo 1994).

Prevention of oocyst shedding by cats is the key to controlling the spread of *T. gondii*. The oral ingestion of live bradyzoites is necessary to acquire immunity to oocyst shedding because parenterally administered *T. gondii* (of any stage) do not induce protective immunity to oocyst shedding in cats. A recently developed vaccine for use in cats contains live bradyzoites from the mutant strain (T-263) of *T. gondii*. After oral inoculation of T-263 bradyzoites, the coccidian cycle is arrested at the sexual stage because gamonts of a single sex develop; thus oocysts are not produced (Frenkel *et al.* 1991). In one trial, 84 per cent of cats vaccinated with T-263 bradyzoites did not shed oocysts following challenge (Frenkel *et al.* 1991). The duration of immunity in cats induced by the vaccine has not yet been determined.

The objectives of vaccination of farm animals are:

(1) to reduce abortions in sheep and goats resulting from transplacental infection of fetuses; and
(2) to reduce the risk of human exposure resulting from ingestion of infected meat (with the subsequent risk of fetal infection).

For these purposes, non-persistent strains of *T. gondii* are candidates for immunization. One vaccine that contains a strain (S48) of tachyzoites that does not persist in the tissues of sheep is available in Europe and New Zealand to reduce fetal losses attributable to toxoplasmosis (Buxton 1993). Ewes vaccinated with the S48 strain vaccine retain immunity for at least 18 months (Buxton 1993). Another strain of *T. gondii* (RH) does not persist in tissues of swine and induces immunity against *T. gondii* infection. A mutant (ts-4) of the RH strain is also a candidate for use in developing a vaccine for intermediate hosts, because it grows better at 33 °C than it does at 37 °C (body temperature). The ts-4 stain is non-pathogenic, even to nursing pigs. These non-persistent strains of *T. gondii* (S48, RH, ts-4) do not induce oocyst shedding in cats.

PREVENTION

To prevent infection of human beings by *T. gondii*, hands should be washed thoroughly with soap and water after handling meat. All cutting boards, sink tops, knives, and other materials coming in contact with uncooked meat should be washed with soap and water. This is effective because the stages of *T. gondii* in meat are killed by soap and water. Meat of any animal should be cooked to 67 °C before consumption, and tasting meat while cooking or seasoning home-made sausages should be avoided. Pregnant women, especially, should avoid contact with cats, soil, and raw meat. Pet cats should be fed only dry, canned, or cooked food. The cat litter box should be emptied every day, preferably not by a pregnant woman. Gloves should be worn while gardening. Vegetables should be washed thoroughly before eating because they may have been contaminated with cat faeces. Expectant mothers should be aware of the dangers of toxoplasmosis.

To prevent infection in cats, they should never be fed uncooked meat, viscera, or bones, and efforts should be made to keep cats indoors to prevent hunting. Trash cans also should be covered to prevent scavenging.

Cats should be neutered to control the feline population on farms. Dead animals should be removed promptly to prevent cannibalism by pigs and scavenging by cats. Sheep that have aborted due to toxoplasmosis usually do not have subsequent toxoplasmic abortions, and thus can be saved for future breeding. Fetal membranes and dead fetuses should be not be handled with bare hands and should be buried or incinerated to prevent infection of felids and other animals on the farm. Cats should not be allowed near pregnant sheep and goats. Grain should be kept covered to prevent oocyst contamination.

To prevent infection of zoo animals with *T. gondii*, cats, including all wild Felidae, should be housed in a building separate from other animals, particularly marsupials and New World monkeys. Cats as a rule should not be fed uncooked meat. However, if a choice has to be made, frozen meat is less likely to contain live *T. gondii* than fresh meat, and beef is less likely to contain *T. gondii* than is horse meat, pork, or mutton. Dissemination of *T. gondii* oocysts in the zoo should be prevented because of potential exposure of children. Brooms, shovels, and other equipment used to clean cat cages, and cat enclosures should be autoclaved or heated to 67 °C for at least 10 minutes at regular intervals. While cleaning cages, animal caretakers should wear masks and protective clothing. Feline faeces should be removed daily to prevent sporulation of oocysts.

SARCOCYSTOSIS

INTRODUCTION AND HISTORY

The *Sarcocystis* parasite was first found in the skeletal muscle of a house mouse, *Mus musculus* in Switzerland in 1843 (Table 46.4). Before 1972, many of these parasites were named based upon the finding of cysts in the muscles of a host. The true nature of these intramuscular cysts remained unknown until the discovery of the life cycle of *Sarcocystis* in 1972 (Table 46.4).

Table 46.4 Historical landmarks concerning *Sarcocystis*[a]

Year	Findings	Reference
1843	Sarcocysts found in muscles of a horse	Miesher (1843)
1882	Genus *Sarcocystis* introduced	Lankaster (1982)
1943	*Sarcocystis* not transmitted from sheep to sheep, role of carnivores suspected but not proven	Scott (1943)
1972	Sexual phase cultured *in vitro*	Fayer (1972)
1972	Two-host life cycle found	Rommel and Heydorn (1972); Rommel *et al.* (1972)
1973	Vascular phase recognized and pathogenicity demonstrated	Fayer and Johnson (1975)
1975	Multiple *Sarcocystis* species within a given host recognized	Heydorn *et al.* (1975)
1975	Chemotherapy demonstrated	Fayer and Johnson (1973)
1976	Abortion due to sarcocytosis is recognized	Fayer *et al.* (1979)
1981	Protective immunity demonstrated	Dubey (1980)
1986	Vascular phase cultured *in vitro*	Speer and Dubey (1986)

[a] From Dubey *et al.* (1989). For complete bibliography see Dubey *et al.* (1989).

CLASSIFICATION

Sarcocystis species are coccidian parasites, classified in the family Sarcocystidae, Poche, 1913; subfamily, Sarcocystinae, Poche, 1913; genus, *Sarcocystis*, Lankester, 1882.

STRUCTURE AND LIFE CYCLE

Sarcocysts (in Greek *sarkos* = flesh, *kystis* = bladder) are the terminal asexual stage of development of these parasites. They are found primarily in the striated muscles of mammals, including humans (Fig. 46.16), birds, marsupials, and poikilothermic animals.

Sarcocystis has an obligatory prey–predator two-host life cycle (Fig. 46.17). Asexual stages develop only in the intermediate host, which in nature is often a prey animal. Sexual stages develop only in the definitive host, which is carnivorous.

The intermediate host becomes infected by ingesting sporocysts in food or water. Sporozoites excyst from sporocysts in the small intestine and produce

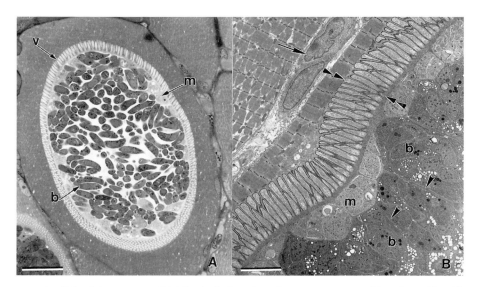

Fig. 46.16 Intramuscular *S. hominis* sarcocysts. (A) Histological section of a mature sarcocyst. Note finger-like villar protrusions on the cyst wall enclosing numerous bradyzoites (b) and a few metrocytes (m). (Toluidine blue; bar = 20 μm.) (B) Transmission electron micrograph. Note villar projections on the cyst wall (double opposing arrowheads), metrocytes (m), bradyzoites (b), and septa (arrowheads). Arrow points to the host cell nucleus. (Bar = 4.3 μm.)

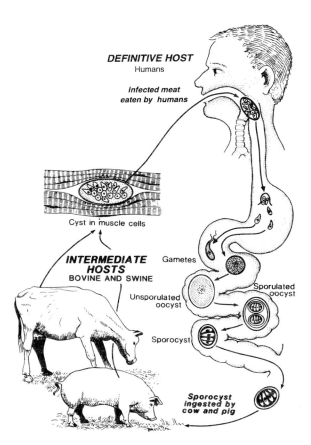

Fig. 46.17　Life cycle of *S. hominis* and *S. suihominis*.

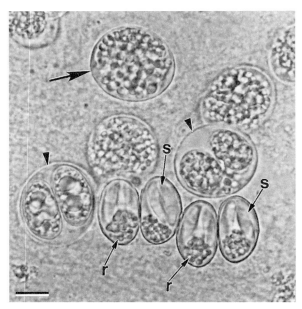

Fig. 46.18　Sporogony of *Sarcocystis* in the intestinal lamina propria of an infected animal. Note unsporulated oocyst (arrow), two partially sporulated oocysts (arrowheads), and two fully sporulated oocysts containing sporozoites (s) and residual body (r). (Unstained; bar = 10 μm.)

intravascular meronts that give rise to the encysted form (sarcocyst) in muscles. Sarcocysts become infectious only when they contain bradyzoites.

The definitive host become infected by ingesting tissues containing mature sarcocysts. Bradyzoites liberated from the sarcocyst by digestion in the stomach and intestine transform into male (micro) and female (macro) gamonts. After fertilization of macrogamete by microgamete, a wall develops around the zygote and the oocyst is formed. The entire process of gametogony and fertilization can be completed within 24 hours, and gamonts and oocysts may be found at the same time. *Sarcocystis* species oocysts sporulate in the lamina propria (Fig. 46.18). Sporulated oocysts are generally colourless, thin-walled (<1 μm), and contain two elongated sporocysts. Each sporocyst contains four elongated sporozoites and a residual body. The oocyst wall is thin and often ruptures. Free sporocysts, released into the intestinal lumen, are passed in the faeces.

Only certain species of *Sarcocystis* are pathogenic to intermediate hosts (Dubey *et al.* 1989). Generally species transmitted by canids are more pathogenic

than those transmitted by felids. *Sarcocystis* generally does not cause illness in definitive hosts.

SARCOCYSTOSIS IN HUMANS

There are two known species of *Sarcocystis* for which humans serve as the definitive host, *S. hominis* and *S. suihominis* (Murrell *et al.* 1985). Humans also serve as accidental intermediate hosts for several unidentified species of *Sarcocystis*. Symptoms in persons with intestinal sarcocystosis are different from those persons with muscular sarcocystosis and vary with the species of *Sarcocystis* causing infection.

INTESTINAL SARCOCYSTOSIS

Sarcocystis hominis (Railliet and Lucet 1891) Dubey 1976

Infection with this species is acquired by ingesting uncooked beef containing *S. hominis* sarcocysts. *Sarcocystis hominis* is only mildly pathogenic for humans. Volunteers who ate raw beef developed nausea, stomach ache, and diarrhoea 3–6 hours after ingesting the beef; these symptoms lasted 24–36 hours. The volunteers excreted *S. hominis* sporocysts between 14 and 18 days after ingesting the beef (Aryeetey and Piekarski 1976; Heydorn 1977).

Sarcocystis suihominis (Tadros and Laarman 1976) Heydorn 1977

This species, acquired by eating undercooked pork, is more pathogenic than *S. hominis*. Human volunteers developed hypersensitivity-like symptoms; nausea, vomiting, stomach ache, diarrhoea, and dyspnoea within 24 hours of ingestion of uncooked pork from naturally or experimentally infected pigs. Sporocysts were shed 11–13 days after ingesting pork (Dubey *et al.* 1989).

MUSCULAR SARCOCYSTOSIS

Sarcocysts have been found in striated muscles of human beings, mostly as incidental findings. Judging from the published reports, sarcocysts in humans are rare (Beaver *et al.* 1979). Most reported cases were from Asia and South-East Asia. Of the 40 histologically diagnosed reports that Beaver *et al.* (1979) reviewed and six additional cases since 1982 reviewed by Dubey *et al.* (1989) 15 were from South-East Asia, 11 from India, five from Central and South America, four from Europe, four from Africa, three from the United States, one from China, and the sources of two were undetermined. Of the 46 confirmed cases, sarcocysts were found in skeletal muscles of 35 and in the heart of 11. The clinical significance of sarcocysts and their life cycles in humans are unknown.

EPIDEMIOLOGY AND CONTROL

Poor hygiene paractised in underdeveloped countries during handling of meat from slaughterplace to kitchen can be a source of *Sarcocystis* infection. In one survey in India, *S. suihominis* oocysts were found in the faeces of 14 out of 20 3–12-year-old children (Banerjee *et al.* 1994), indicating that meat was consumed raw at least by some because *S. suihominis* can only be transmitted to humans by the consumption of raw pork. In another study, 3–5-year-old children from a slum area were found to consume meat scraps virtually raw, and many pigs from that area harboured *S. suihominis* sarcocysts (Solanki *et al.* 1991). In European countries where consumption of raw or undercooked meat is relatively high, humans are expected to have intestinal sarcocystosis (Dubey *et al.* 1989). To prevent intestinal infection, meat should be cooked thoroughly before human consumption.

DIAGNOSIS

The ante-mortem diagnosis of muscular sarcocystosis can only be made at present by histological examination of muscle collected by biopsy. The finding of immature sarcocysts with metrocytes suggests recently acquired infection. The finding of mature sarcocysts only indicates past infection. The diagnosis of intestinal sarcocystosis is easily made by faecal examination. As said earlier, sporocysts or oocysts are shed fully sporulated in faeces. It is not possible to distinguish species of *Sarcocystis* based on sporocyst morphology.

TREATMENT

There is no treatment known for *Sarcocystis* infections of humans.

ISOSPOROSIS

INTRODUCTION AND THE AETIOLOGICAL AGENT

Isospora belli Wenyon 1923, is the cause of coccidiosis in humans. It belongs to the family Eimeriidae and the genus, *Eimeria*. Most of the reported cases occurred in the tropics rather than in the temperate zone. Infection is now seen more frequently in immunocomprised patients, particularly those with AIDS (Restrepo *et al.* 1987; Dubey 1993; Michiels *et al.* 1994).

STRUCTURE AND LIFE CYCLE

Isospora belli oocysts are elongate, ellipsoidal, and are 20–33 × 10–19 μm (Fig. 46.19A). Sporulated oocysts contain two ellipsoidal sporocysts without a Stieda body. Each sporocyst is 9–14 × 7–12 μm and contains four crescent-shaped sporozoites and a residual body. Sporulation occurs within 5 days, both within the host and in the external environment (Trier *et al.* 1974). Thus, both unsporulated and sporulated oocysts may be shed in faeces.

Infection occurs by the ingestion of food contaminated by oocysts. Merogony and gametogony occur in

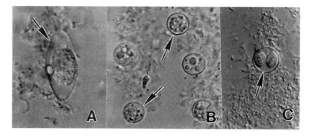

Fig. 46.19 *Isospora belli* and *Cyclospora cayetanensis* oocysts (arrows) in human faeces. (A) Unsporulated *I. belli*; (B) unsporulated *C. cayetanensis*; (C) sporulated *C. cayetanensis*. (Bar = 10 μm.) (Courtesy of Drs Y. Ortega and C. Sterling.)

the upper small intestinal epithelial cells, from the level of the crypts to the tips of the villi. The number of generations of merogony is unknown. In AIDS patients the parasite may be disseminated to extra-intestinal organs, including mesenteric and mediastinal lymph nodes, liver, and spleen (Michiels *et al.* 1994). Single zoites surrounded by a capsule (cyst wall) have a prominent refractile or crystalloid body, indicating that the encysted organisms are sporozoites. Organisms with a cyst wall are found only in extra intestinal organs.

SYMPTOMS

Isospora belli can cause severe clinical symptoms with an acute onset, particularly in AIDS patients. Infection has been reported to cause fever, malaise, cholecystitis, persistent diarrhoea, weight loss, steatorrhoea, and even death (Dubey 1993).

DIAGNOSIS

Diagnosis can be established by finding characteristic bell-shaped oocysts in the faeces (Fig. 46.19A) or coccidian stages in intestinal biopsy material. Affected intestinal portions may have a flat mucosa, similar to that occurring in sprue. The stools during infection are fatty and at times very watery.

TREATMENT

Sulphonamides are considered effective against coccidiosis (St. Georgiev 1993).

CYCLOSPOROSIS

INTRODUCTION AND AETIOLOGICAL AGENT

Cyclospora cayetanensis Ortega, Gilman, and Sterling 1994 is the cause of disease in humans. Ortega *et al.* (1994) identified this parasite and named it *Cyclospora cayetanensis*.

STRUCTURE AND LIFE CYCLE

Cyclospora cayetanensis oocysts are approximately 8 μm in diameter and they contain two ovoid 4 × 6 μm sporocysts (Fig. 46.19B,C). Each sporocyst has two sporozoites. Thus there are a total of four sporozoites in a sporulated oocyst. Unsporulated oocysts are

excreted in faeces. Sporulation occurs outside the body. Other stages in the life cycle are not known.

SYMPTOMS

Both immunocompetent and immunosuppressed patients of all ages may have diarrhoea, fever, fatigue, and abdominal cramps. Infection has been reported from several countries (Adal 1994; Ortega *et al.* 1993, 1994).

DIAGNOSIS

Diagnosis can be made by faecal examination. *Cyclospora* oocysts are approximately 8 μm, remarkably uniform, and contain a sporont (inner mass) that occupies most of the oocyst. They are acid-fast and need to be distinguished from *Cryptosporidium* oocysts. Unlike cryptosporidial oocysts, *C. cayetanensis* oocysts have a much thicker oocyst wall and their contents are more granular than are those of cryptosporidial oocysts.

TREATMENT

Treatment is unknown.

REFERENCES

Adal, K. A. (1994). From Wisconsin to Nepal: *Cryptosporidium*, *Cyclospora*, and microsporidia. *Current Opinion in Infectious Diseases*, **7**, 609–15.

Araujo, F. G. (1994). Immunization against *Toxoplasma gondii*. *Parasitology Today*, **10**, 358–60.

Aryeetey, M. E. and Piekarski, G. (1976). Serologische *Sarcocystis*-Studien an Menschen und Ratten. *Zeitschrift für Parasitenkunde*, **50**, 109–24.

Banerjee, P. S., Bhatia, B. B., and Pandit, B. A. (1994). *Sarcocystis suihominia* infection in human beings in India. *Journal of Veterinary Parasitology*, **8**, 57–8.

Beaver, P. C., Gadgil, R. K., and Morera, P. (1979). *Sarcocystis* in man: A review and report of five cases. *American Journal of Tropical Medicine and Hygiene*, **28**, 819–44.

Benenson, M. W., Takafuji, E. T., Lemon, S. M., Greenup, R. L., and Sulzer, A. J. (1982). Oocyst transmitted toxoplasmosis associated with ingestion of contaminated water. *New England Journal of Medicine*, **307**, 666–9.

Buxton, D. (1993). Toxoplasmosis: the first commercial vaccine. *Parasitology Today*, **9**, 335–7.

Couvreur, J., Desmonts, G., Tournier, G., and Szusterkac, M. (1984). Etude d'une série homogène de 210 cas de toxoplasmose congénitale chez des nourrissons âgés de 0 a 11 mois et dépistés de façon prospective. *Annales de Pediatric (Paris)*, **31**, 815–19.

Dubey, J. P. (1977). *Toxoplasma, Hammondia, Besnoitia, Sarcocystis*, and other tissue cyst-forming coccidia of man and animals. In *Parasitic protozoa*, (ed. J. P. Kreier), Vol. 3, pp. 1101–27. Academic Press, New York.

Dubey, J. P. (1993). *Toxoplasma, Neospora, Sarcocystis*, and other tissue cyst-forming coccidia of humans and animals. In *Parasitic protozoa*, (ed. Kreier J. P.), Vol. 6, pp. 1–158. Academic Press, New York.

Dubey, J. P. (1994). Toxoplasmosis. *Journal of the American Veterinary Medical Association*, **205**, 1593–8.

Dubey, J. P. (1995). Duration of immunity to shedding of *Toxoplasma gondii* oocysts by cats. *Journal of Parasitology*, **81**, 410–15.

Dubey, J. P. and Beattie, C. P. (1988). *Toxoplasmosis of animals and man*, pp. 1–220. CRC Press, Boca Raton, Florida.

Dubey, J. P., Speer, C. A., and Fayer, R. (1989). *Sarcocystosis of animals and man*, pp. 1–215. CRC Press, Boca Raton, Florida.

Dutton, G. N. (1989). Toxoplasmic retinochoroiditis—A historical review and current concepts. *Annals of Academy of Medicine*, **18**, 214–21.

Frenkel, J. K. (1973). Toxoplasmosis: parasite life cycle, pathology and immunology. In *The Coccidia. Eimeria, Isospora, Toxoplasma and related genera*, (ed. D. M. Hammond and P. L. Long), pp. 343–410. University Park Press, Baltimore, Maryland.

Frenkel, J. K., Pfefferkorn, E. R., Smith, D. D., and Fishback, J. L. (1991). Prospective vaccine prepared from a new mutant of *Toxoplasma gondii* for use in cats. *American Journal of Veterinary Research*, **52**, 759–63.

Gazzinelli, R. T., Denkers, E. Y., and Sher, A. (1993). Host resistance to *Toxoplasma gondii*: model for studying the selective induction of cell-mediated immunity by intracellular parasites. *Infectious Agents and Diseases*, **2**, 139–49.

Guerina, N. G., Hsu, H. W., Meissner, H. C., Maguire, J. H., Lynfield, R., and Stechenberg, B. (1994). Neonatal serologic screening and early treatment for congenital *Toxoplasma gondii* infection. *New England Journal of Medicine*, **330**, 1858–63.

Heydorn, A. O. (1977). Sarkosporidienifiziertes Fleisch als mögliche Krankheitsursache für den Menschen, *Arch. Lebensmittelhyg*, **28**, 27–31.

Johnson, A. M. (1989). *Toxoplasma* vaccines: biology, pathology, immunology, and treatment. In *Veterinary protozoan and hemoparasite vaccines*, (ed. I. G. Wright), pp. 177–202. CRC Press, Boca Raton, Florida.

Lebech, M. and Peterson, E. (1992). Congenital toxoplasmosis. *Scandinavian Journal of Infectious Diseases*, Supplement 84. pp. 5–96.

Luft, B. J. and Remington, J. S. (1992). Toxoplasmic encephalitis in AIDS. *Clinical Infectious Diseases*, **15**, 211–22.

Luft, B. J., Hafner, R., Korzun, A. H., Leport, C., Antonishkis, D., and Bosler, E. M. (1993). Toxoplasmic encephalitis in patients with the acquired immunodeficiency syndrome. *New England Journal of Medicine*, **329**, 995–1000.

McAuley, J., Boyer, K. M., Patel, D., Mets, M., Swisher, C., and Roizen, N. (1994). Early and longitudinal evaluations of treated infants and children and untreated historical patients with congenital toxoplasmosis—the Chicago collaborative treatment trial. *Clinical Infectious Diseases*, **18**, 38–72.

McLeod, R., Mack, D., and Brown, C. (1991). *Toxoplasma gondii*—new advances in cellular and molecular biology. *Experimental Parasitology*, **72**, 109–21.

Michiels, J. F., Hofman, P., Bernard, E., Saint-Paul, M. C., Boissy, C., and Mondain, V. (1994). Intestinal and extraintestinal *Isospora belli* infection in an Aids patient. A second case report. *Pathology Research Practice*, **190**, 1089–93.

Murrell K. D., Fayer R., and Dubey J. P. (1985). Parasitic organisms in meat and poultry. *Advances in Meat Research*, **2**, 311–77.

Ortega, Y. R., Sterling, C. R. (1993), Gilman, R. H., Cama, V. A. and Diaz, F. *Cyclospora* species: a new protozoan pathogen of humans. *New England Journal of Medicine*, **328**, 1308–12.

Ortega, Y. R., Gilman, R. H., and Sterling, C. R. (1994). A new coccidian parasite (Apicomplexa: Eimeriidae) from humans. *Journal of Parasitology*, **80**, 625–9.

PFefferkorn, E. R. (1990). Cell biology of *Toxoplasma gondii*, pp. 26–50, Freedman and Company, New York.

Rabaud, C., May, T., Amiel, C., Katlama, C., Leport, C., and Ambroise-Thomas, P. (1994). Extracerebral toxoplasmosis in patients infected with HIV. *A French National Survey, Medicine* **73**, 306–14.

Remington, J. S., McLeod, R., and Desmonts, G. (1995). Toxoplasmosis. In *Infectious diseases of the fetus and newborn infant*, (ed. J. S. Remington and J. O. Klein), (4th edn.), pp. 140–267. Saunders Company, Philadelphia.

Restrepo, C., Macher, A. M., and Radany, E. H. (1987). Disseminated extraintestinal isosporiasis in a patient with acquired immune deficiency syndrome. *American Journal of Clinical Pathology*, **87**, 536–42.

Roberts, T. and Frenkel, J. K. (1990). Estimating income losses and other preventable costs caused by congenital toxoplasmosis in people in the United States. *Journal of the American Veterinary Medical Association*, **196**, 249–56.

Roberts, T., Murrell, K. D., and Marks, S. (1994). Economic losses caused by foodborne parasitic diseases. *Parasitology Today*, **10**, 419–23.

St. Georgiev, V. (1993). Opportunistic infections: treatment and developmental therapeutics of cryptosporidiosis and isosporiasis. *Drug Development Research*, **28**, 445–59.

St. Georgiev, V. (1994). Management of toxoplasmosis. *Drugs*, **48**, 179–88.

Sibley, L. D., Pfefferkorn, E. R., and Boothroyd, J. C. (1991). Proposal for a uniform genetic nomenclature in *Toxoplasma gondii*. *Parasitology Today*, **7**, 327–8.

Sibley, L. D., LeBlanc, A. J., Pfefferkorn, E. R., and Boothroyd J. C. (1992). Generation of a restriction fragment length polymorphism linkage map for *Toxoplasma gondii*. *Genetics*, **132**, 1003–15.

Solanki, P. K., Shrivastava, H. O. P., and Shah, H. L. (1991). Prevalence of *Sarcocystis* in naturally infected pigs in Madhya-Pradesh with an epidemiological explanation for the higher prevalence of *Sarcocystis suihominis*. *Indian Journal of Animal Science*, **61**, 820–1.

Teutsch, S. M., Juranek, D. D., Sulzer, A., Dubey, J. P., and Sikes, R. K. (1979). Epidemic toxoplasmosis associated with infected cats. *New England Journal of Medicine*, **300**, 695–9.

Trier, J. S., Moxey, P. C., Schimmel, E. M., and Robles, E. (1974). Chronic intestinal coccidiosis in man: intestinal morphology and response to treatment. *Gastroenterology*, **66**, 923–35.

Wolf, A., Cowen, D., and Paige, B. (1939). Human toxoplasmosis: occurrence in infants as an encephalomyelitis verification by transmission to animals. *Science*, **89**, 226–7.

Wreghitt, T. G. and Hakim, M. (1989). Toxoplasmosis in heart and lung transplant recipients. *Journal of Clinical Pathology*, **42**, 194–9.

47 BABESIOSIS AND MALARIA

F. E. G. Cox

INTRODUCTION

Babesiosis and malaria are very rare zoonoses. Although some 350 million people are infected with one of four species of *Plasmodium*, all these infections are acquired from other humans through the agency of infected mosquitoes and the number of recorded infections from animals to humans is very small. Similarly *Babesia* species infect millions of cattle and unknown numbers of sheep, dogs, and horses, and transmission is usually from one member of the species to another member of the same species through the bite of a tick, and human infections are very rare. The parasites that cause malaria and babesiosis are protozoa classified in the same phylum, Sporozoa, but in different classes (Table 47.1). Both inhabit red blood cells during part of their life cycles and this is the stage that causes the signs of disease that are similar in many respects. The facts that humans can occasionally acquire malaria and babesiosis from animals, that both parasites appear similar when seen in blood films, and that both cause similar symptoms can cause problems

Table 47.1 Outline classification of the Sporozoa showing the taxonomic positions of the genera that affect humans and the species of *Babesia* and *Plasmodium* that can be transmitted from animals to humans

Kingdom Protista
Phylum Sporozoa
Class Gregarinea
   Order Archigregarinida
   Order Neogregarinida
   Order Eugregarinida
Class Coccidea
   Order Agamococcidiida
   Order Protococcidiida
   Order Adeleida
   Order Eimeriida (*Cryptosporidium, Isospora, Toxoplasma*)
Class Haemosporidea
   Order Haemosporidida (*Plasmodium*: *P. brasilianum, P. cynomolgi, P. eylesi, P. inui, P. knowlesi, P. schwetzi, P. simium*.
Class Piroplasmea
   Order Piroplasmida (*Babesia*: *B. divergens, B. microti, B. gibsoni*)
   Order Dactylosomida

in diagnosis are of interest to both clinicians and epidemiologists.

BABESIOSIS

SUMMARY

Babesia species are parasites of vertebrates and are transmitted by ticks. The form in the vertebrate is the trophozoite that infects red blood cells in which it divides by binary fission to produce two merozoites each of which invades a new cell. These blood stages cause serious diseases in domesticated animals including cattle, horses, and dogs, and the general name given to these is babesiosis (Zwart and Brocklesby 1979; Young, 1988). Nearly 100 species parasitic in mammals have been identified on the stages in the blood but, as there are few morphological characters to go on, this is not altogether satisfactory and new information based on DNA techniques is gradually reducing the number of species. In this chapter, the traditional classification will be used because it is more in line with what has been published in the past than some of the newer classifications and this makes it easier to cross-refer to the earlier literature.

The life cycles of all *Babesia* species are similar. The infection begins when sporozoites are injected through the bite of an infected tick. What happens next is unclear and it may be that there is some multiplication in cells other than red blood cells but this has been very difficult to demonstrate (Young, 1988). However, what is clear is that what follows is a phase of multiplication, usually by binary fission, within red blood cells and that this is the phase that causes the disease (Healy and Ristic 1988). The symptoms of babesiosis are fever, anaemia, jaundice, and haemoglobinuria, and the infections are often fatal (Telford *et al.* 1993). Eventually gametocytes are formed and these are taken up by a tick when it feeds. Within the gut of the tick, fertilization and the formation of zygotes occur followed by phases of multiplication in the intestinal cells and salivary glands, resulting in the production of many sporozoites that are injected into a new host. During their life cycle, ticks pass through three stages, larva, nymph, and adult. Each stage feeds on blood but the stage that becomes infected is never the stage that is infective. If the larva is infected then the nymph is infective and if the nymph is infected then the adult is infective. In addition, in some species of ticks, infected female adults may pass the infection on to their larvae.

The rodent babesia, *B. microti*, occasionally infects humans in North America and, to a lesser extent, elsewhere and in Europe, humans, particularly those that have been splenectomized, can be infected with the cattle species *B. divergens*, which can be fatal (Cox, 1982; Telford *et al.* 1993).

HISTORY

Babesias are conspicuous parasites in red blood cells in which they occur either singly or in pairs. They were recognized for the first time and associated with a disease in cattle by a Romanian scientist, Viktor Babes in 1888, who thought that they were bacteria (see Ristic, 1988). In 1893, Smith and Kilbourne, studying the cause of Texas fever in cattle in the United States, not only established the protozoan nature of these parasites but also demonstrated their transmission by ticks, predating the discovery of the transmission of malaria parasites by another arthropod by several years. Subsequently many other animals, wild and domesticated, were shown to be infected with these parasites which are now named *Babesia* after their discoverer. The first clues that humans could be infected with babesias came in 1904 when Wilson and Chowning found an organism that they named *Piroplasma hominis* in patients suffering from Rocky Mountain spotted fever but, although their drawings clearly show babesias, whether or not these were really babesias will never be known (see Telford *et al.* 1993). There then followed a number of isolated reports of human infections with babesias but these are now thought to be misidentifications of malaria parasites. It was not until 1957 that the first really well-documented case of human babesiosis, in a farmer in the former Yugoslavia, was reported and this was followed by a number of other cases in Europe. The importance of human babesiosis only became apparent from 1968 onwards when patients suffering from febrile illness from Nantucket Island, Massachusetts, were found to be harbouring the rodent malaria parasite *Babesia microti* (Healy and Ristic 1988). Since then numerous other cases have been recorded from Massachusetts and Connecticut and, to a lesser extent, elsewhere in the United States, and there have also been isolated reports from other parts of the world (Tabaoda and Merchant 1991).

Human babesiosis is rare and difficult to diagnose accurately because the different species of *Babesia* are morphologically very similar and also resemble malaria parasites. Thus many records, particularly earlier ones and ones from outside the recognized areas where the disease occurs, are largely based on guesswork.

When only the authenticated and well-documented cases are considered, human babesiosis is seen to fall into three categories, the European form, derived from cattle; the American form, derived from rodents; and a recently isolated form from the United States that has affinities with a canine species.

THE AGENTS

CATTLE-DERIVED BABESIOSIS

It is estimated that some 1.2 billion cattle all over the world are at risk from infection with babesiosis, and actual infections with *B. bovis*, *B. divergens*, *B. major*, and *B. bigemina* are very common (Kakoma and Mehlhorn 1994). *Babesia bovis* has a worldwide distribution and is transmitted by ticks of the genus *Boophilus*, which feed as larvae, nymphs, and adults on the same host and are rarely found on hosts other than cattle. *Babesia divergens*, once though to be the same as *B. bovis*, is a smaller parasite that occurs only in Europe and is transmitted by *Ixodes ricinus*, a three-host tick whose larvae, nymphs, and adults feed on different hosts which are virtually any warm-blooded animals. Typically, the larvae feed on small mammals while the nymphs and larvae feed on larger ones, but there is no rigidity about this pattern. In all species of *Babesia* transmission occurs in the spring and autumn when the larvae and nymphs are most active. In those species of *Babesia* that cause disease, the rapidly dividing parasites in the red blood cells cause the destruction of the cells, resulting in anaemia which is greater than can be accounted for by simple cell destruction. This is accompanied by fever, jaundice, and haemoglobinuria. In terms of virulence, *B. bovis* is regarded as being very virulent while *B. divergens* is moderately so. As far as human infections are concerned, it is unlikely that any of them have actually been *B. bovis* because the ticks involved seldom feed on humans and, in any case, this parasite is a southern European form. On the other hand, *I. ricinus*, the tick that transmits *B. divergens*, the species that occurs in northern Europe where most human cases have been reported, frequently feeds on humans. The approach taken here is that human babesial infections in Europe are all probably caused by *B. divergens*.

Since the first report in 1957, there have been a further 20 reports of human babesiosis in Europe (Table 47.2). All these cases occurred between May and October, and some, but not all, occurred in indi-

Table 47.2 Human *Babesia* infections acquired from cattle

Country of origin	Number of cases	Species	Outcome
France	11	*B. divergens*	2 fatal
			7 recovered[a]
			2 asymptomatic
Scotland	2	*B. divergens*	2 fatal
Northern Ireland	2	*B. divergens*	1 fatal
			1 unknown
Russia	1	*B. divergens*	1 fatal
Sweden	1	*B. divergens*	1 recovered
Yugoslavia	2	*B. divergens*[b]	2 fatal
Spain	2	*B. divergens*[b]	1 fatal
			1 recovered[c]

[a] Includes one unknown species and one reported as *B. canis*.
[b] Includes one reported as *B. bovis*.
[c] Unknown species.

viduals associated with farming, camping, or some other outdoor activity (Telford *et al.* 1993). Most recalled having been bitten by ticks. Although the vector is not known for certain, circumstantial evidence points to *I. ricinus*. When it has been done, the parasite reverts to a typical *B. divergens* form when passaged back into calves. The general pattern, therefore, seems to be one in which larval ticks become infected with *B. divergens* from cattle, drop off and moult, and infect individuals, such as farmers, campers, and hikers, that come in close contact with them. Not all individuals seem to be equally susceptible to infection and it is worth noting that all but one of the fatal cases occurred in patients that had been splenectomized, as did seven of those that recovered, but none of those that were asymptomatic had had their spleens removed.

Babesia divergens infections in cattle are relatively mild but in humans they are usually severe. After an incubation period of 1–3 weeks the patient begins to experience a range of rather vague symptoms, including headaches, muscle pains and weakness, and then develops a high fever, alternating sweating and chills, intestinal discomfort, vomiting and diarrhoea, and haemoglobinuria. In some cases the haemoglobin level drops catastrophically, there is renal failure, loss of consciousness, coma, and death.

RODENT-DERIVED BABESIOSIS

The first authenticated case of rodent-derived human babesiosis in the United States was from Nantucket Island Massachusetts, in 1969 and in the next 10 years there were over 40 similar cases from the coastal strip of New England, comprising islands off the Massachusetts

coast, Rhode Island, and Connecticut (Anderson *et al.* 1991; Telford *et al.* 1993). Since then, there have been numerous cases of babesiosis in these areas and also in inland Connecticut, and babesiosis is now a notifiable disease in the states of Massachusetts and New York. The causative agent is a common rodent babesia, *B. microti*, transmitted by the deer tick *Ixodes dammini* which feeds on small rodents and deer. Adult ticks feed on deer, *Odocoileus virginianis*, in the autumn and lay their eggs in the following spring. Larvae emerge in the autumn, feed on the white-footed mouse *Peromyscus leucopus*, from which they acquire their infections, then overwinter and moult into nymphs in the following spring. Humans are infected from nymphs and the first signs of the infection occur in early July, about 1–4 weeks after being bitten by a tick. The symptoms are at first rather vague, headaches, fever, sweating, muscle pains, malaise, and swings in mood, accompanied by clinical signs including splenomegaly, anaemia, thrombocytopenia. Parasitaemias tend to be between 1 and 20 per cent but can reach 85 per cent in splenectomized individuals.

Human infections with parasites that are probably *B. microti* have also recently been recorded from Washington State (Thomford *et al.* 1994). However, the parasite isolated produces fulminating infections in hamsters, something that the East Coast and European strains never do. It is possible that on the West Coast there is a completely different focus of infection.

Babesia microti is also a very common parasite in small mammals in Britain, where it is transmitted by *Ixodes trianguliceps*, and throughout Europe. However, *I. trianguliceps* rarely, if ever, feeds on humans, and cases of rodent-derived babesiosis in Europe are rare; there have only been three such records, two in Germany and one in Belgium, and none caused serious disease.

OTHER BABESIOSIS

There have also been a number of cases of human babesiosis in California, including the first case recorded in the United States in 1966 which was in a splenectomized individual. These Californian cases have been attributed to *B. equi*, a babesia of horses, or *B. canis* from dogs, but no unequivocal identification has been possible. Recent isolates from Washington State have been of a parasite morphologically similar to *B. microti* but genetically quite different as, with the aid of nucleic acid techniques, it can be distinguished from the rodent form and demonstrated to have affinities with the canine form, *Babesia gibsoni* (Thomford *et al.* 1994). This is interesting because *B. gibsoni* is thought to be related to *B. microti* and *B. equi* of horses. Dogs are reservoirs of a number of human parasitic diseases and the close contact between dogs, their ticks, and humans could facilitate accidental transmission to humans. Elsewhere, there have been reports from South America, China, Taiwan, and South Africa but there is no convincing evidence that any parasite other than *B. divergens* or *B. microti* has been responsible for any of these infections.

DIAGNOSIS

Babesiosis is very difficult to diagnose clinically partly because of its rarity and partly because of the inconclusive symptoms. Diagnosis is based on the detection of parasites in stained thin blood films but these must be interpreted with great caution because babesias are virtually indistinguishable from the ring stages of malaria parasites, particularly *Plasmodium falciparum*. In addition, the small size of the parasite and its lack of morphological characteristics means that it could be confused with other intraerythrocytic inclusions, and there has been a report of quinine-induced haemolysis as babesiosis. There are no records of human babesiosis from tropical countries, so anyone returning from such areas should be provisionally diagnosed as having malaria. For those who have not travelled to the tropics, particular attention should be paid to individuals whose activities have taken them into contact with infected ticks: farmers, hikers, and campers for example. Most people are aware that they have been bitten by a tick and the spread of Lyme disease has heightened the need to take tick bites seriously. Severe and unexplained thrombocytopenia in individuals who have been at risk is a useful indication of human babesiosis. For absolute certainty, suspected infected blood should be injected into susceptible hosts, calves or hamsters as appropriate, and the resulting infection monitored. Jirds, *Meriones unguiculatus*, can be infected with *B. divergens*. Serological tests, particularly the indirect immunofluorescent antibody test (IFAT), have proved to be useful, as has the quantitative buffy coat technique, devised for malaria diagnosis. The most promising diagnostic technique is the application of the polymerase chain reaction which can detect as few as three merozoites. However, it is important to point out that all these techniques, except stained blood films, are purely experimental at present (Telford *et al.* 1993).

TREATMENT

Human babesiosis, particularly in splenectomized individuals, must be considered as an emergency. Many antiprotozoal and antibacterial drugs have been tested and the current treatment is a combination of quinine and clindamycin. For *B. microti* infections, quinine may be given orally at a dose of 650 mg three times a day plus 1200 mg clindamycin intravenously twice a day (or 600 mg three times a day) for 7 days. For *B. divergens* infections, a blood exchange transfusion is recommended followed by 3 times daily oral 600 mg quinine and 3–4 times daily intravenous injections of 600 mg clindamycin until the parasitaemia resolves. Transfusion followed by treatment with quinine and clindamycin has been successful in treating splenectomized patients suffering from *B. divergens* infections in France and Sweden but the World Health Organization is still cautious about the use of these drugs, especially in uncomplicated cases (Telford *et al.* 1993).

EPIDEMIOLOGY

Human babesiosis is a real problem in restricted foci, particularly along the New England coast, and all those who camp or hike in these areas should be aware of the problem of tick-borne diseases, not only babesiosis but also Lyme disease, particularly when the nymphs are most active in late June. Tick bites can be avoided by the use of sensible clothing and repellents. Attached ticks that are removed within 48 hours are unable to transmit the infection. Elsewhere, the chances of acquiring human babesiosis are very remote but anybody who develops fevers, headaches, and malaise should be carefully screened for this infection, particularly those individuals who have had their spleens removed. Corticosteroids and other immunodepressants render natural and experimental hosts more susceptible to infection and, while there is no evidence that humans treated with such drugs are more susceptible to infection, those whose immune systems are compromised should take particular care. There is no evidence that those infected with the HIV virus are particularly susceptible to infection with babesiosis but the possibility exists that they might well be and such individuals should also be very careful about engaging in any activities that might bring them in contact with ticks. Human bebesiosis is never going to be a major health problem but those who intrude into any natural life cycle do put themselves at risk.

PREVENTION AND CONTROL

The best method of prevention is the avoidance of tick bites especially in tick-infested areas which, in the United States, are often clearly signposted. The removal of all ticks within 48 hours is usually sufficient to prevent infection. Campers, hikers, and others involved in outdoor pursuits should take particular care. Individuals without spleens are at particular risk. Babesiosis is difficult to diagnose and anyone who develops irregular fevers after being bitten by a tick in one of the endemic areas should obtain expert advice.

MALARIA

SUMMARY

Human malaria is caused by infection with one of four species of *Plasmodium*, *P. falciparum*, *P. vivax*, *P. ovale*, or *P. malariae*, which together affect over 350 million people in the tropics and subtropics, causing deaths in excess of 2 million each year and countless episodes of debilitating febrile disease (Bruce-Chwatt 1985). Humans are not the only hosts of malaria parasites which also occur in birds, rodents, and other primates (Garnham 1966, 1980). There are 25 species of *Plasmodium* in non-human primates and these occur in New World and Old World monkeys, gibbons, great apes, and lemurs. The malaria parasites belong to the same phylum as the coccidians such as *Toxoplasma*, *Sarcocystis*, and *Cryptosporidium* but to a different order, the Haemosporidida (Table 47.1). Members of the Haemosporidida, as the name implies, are parasitic in the red blood cells of vertebrates. All *Plasmodium* species have similar life cycles and are transmitted by female blood-sucking mosquitoes belonging to the genus *Anopheles*. The infection begins when the infective stages, sporozoites, are injected through the bite of an infected mosquito. The sporozoites enter liver cells where a massive phase of multiplication occurs, resulting in the production of thousands of merozoites. These merozoites invade red blood cells where they undergo another phase of multiplication during which they produce 8–16 merozoites every 24, 48 or 72 hours, depending on the species. This phase of erythrocytic multiplication is repeated indefinitely and is responsible for the disease which is characterized by periodic fevers coinciding with the liberation of merozoites and anaemia caused by the loss of red blood cells. However, some merozoites do not divide within the red cell but instead develop into male and female gametocytes which are taken up when another mosquito feeds. Within the mosquito, the male and female gametes fuse to produce a zygote which comes to lie on the outside of the gut wall where it forms an oocyst within which a third phase of multiplication occurs, resulting in the formation of many sporozoites which migrate to the salivary glands of the mosquito from which they are injected when the mosquito feeds. In the human malaria parasites *P. vivax* and *P. ovale*, some of the parasites in the liver lie dormant for months and subsequent infections due to the maturation of these forms are called relapses. *Plasmodium falciparum* causes malignant tertian malaria and is the most common and serious of all the forms of malaria. The infection is acute and the parasites tend to stick to endothelial cells, causing blockage and cerebral damage often resulting in death. *Plasmodium vivax* causes benign tertian malaria and is the second most serious infection. *Plasmodium ovale* causes ovale tertian malaria and is concentrated in West Africa. *Plasmodium malariae* causes quartan malaria and infections may last 30 years or more. Infections with these last three parasites, although debilitating, are seldom fatal in themselves (Wernsdorfer 1980).

The malaria parasites of humans, with the possible exception of *P. malariae*, are not naturally transmissible to other animals so the malaria parasites of non-human primates have received considerable attention both in their own rights and as models for the human infections. Of the 25 species of *Plasmodium* in non-human primates, *P. cynomolgi*, which resembles *P. vivax*, has been the most studied and another species from macaques, *P. knowlesi*, has been widely used in laboratory studies despite the fact that it has a 24-hour periodicity and does not closely resemble any of the human species. *Plasmodium knowlesi* and *P. simium* are known to infect humans naturally and *P. cynomolgi*, *P. schwetzi*, *P. brasilianum*, and *P. inui* can infect humans under experimental (or accidental) conditions (Collins and Aikawa 1993). The malaria parasites of rodents and birds have been studied extensively and none of them has ever been reported to infect humans.

HISTORY

The fevers characteristic of human malaria have been known since ancient times and the Greek and Roman physicians clearly recognized the various forms of the disease and its association with marshy areas. In keeping with contemporary ideas, the causes of malaria were variously ascribed to punishments by the gods, miasmas—the vapours rising from the marshes or unsanitary conditions—and it was not until 1880 that the French scientist, Laveran, first saw malaria parasites in the blood. In 1898 the British scientist, Ross, and the Italians Grassi, Bignami, and Bastianelli, established that the parasite was transmitted by mosquitoes but it was not until 1948 that other British scientists, Shortt and Garnham, completed our knowledge of the life cycle when they demonstrated the development of the parasite in the liver (Garnham 1966). Although malaria-like parasites belonging to the genus *Hepatocystis* had erroneously, but not surprisingly, been recognized since 1899 by German and French scientists, including Laveran himself, malaria parasites of non-human parasites were not identified with certainty until 1907, with the independent discoveries of *P. cynomolgi*, *P. inui*, and *P. pitheci* in monkeys imported into Germany from Java (Coatney *et al.* 1971). A number of reports of new species, many of them spurious, occurred throughout the 1920s and 1930s and, following their discovery of *P. knowlesi* in 1932, Sinton and Mulligan established order out of the existing chaos and set out a framework which was to accommodate the various new species that were recognized in the 1930s, 1950s, and 1960s and which persisted until the publication of Garnham's authoritative monograph in 1966 (Garnham 1966). Since then the only new records have been of *P. silvaticum* from an orang-utan and four new species from lemurs (Collins and Aikawa 1993).

During the 1960s, there were reports of a number of accidental human infections with primate malarias and this led to intensive efforts to determine whether or not primates could act as reservoirs for human malaria (Brack 1987). This was important because of the possible effect that the existence of any such reservoir infections might have on the malaria control and eradication schemes then in progress and also the potential complications that might affect the diagnosis of infections from blood films. In the event, it became clear that the chances of humans acquiring malaria from primates was very remote but that occasional accidental and natural infections could occur.

THE AGENTS

Primate malarias transmissible to humans

An outline classification of the malaria parasites is given in Table 47.1 and a list of the species that have been transmitted to humans is given in Table 47.3. Natural infections can only be acquired from infected mosquitoes but accidental and experimental infections can be acquired either from mosquitoes or from infected blood.

Plasmodium knowlesi occurs in South East Asia where its natural hosts are the macaque monkeys, *Macaca fascicularis* and *M. nemestrina*, but it also infects other macaques and leaf monkeys naturally and many other species of monkeys and higher primates experimentally. The natural mosquito host is *A. hackeri* which lives in forest canopies and feeds only on monkeys (Collins and Aikawa 1993). *Plasmodium knowlesi*, probably because of its very rapid erythrocytic multiplication, tends to be very pathogenic, especially in unnatural hosts such as rhesus monkeys which almost inevitably die with a fulminating parasitaemia, as do splenectomized kra monkeys. Fevers are difficult to measure

Table 47.3 Primate malarias naturally, accidentally, or experimentally transmitted to humans

	Human equivalent	Periodicity
Natural infections		
P. knowlesi	None	24 hours
P. simium		48 hours
P. eylesi	P. vivax	48 hours
Accidental infections		
P. cynomolgi	P. vivax	48 hours
Experimental infections		
P. knowlesi		
P. cynomolgi		
P. schwetzi		48 hours
P. inui		72 hours
P. brasilianum	P. malariae	72 hours
P. malariae		72 hours

in monkeys but there is a severe anaemia reminiscent of the fatal anaemia sometimes seen in children infected with *P. falciparum*. Humans are very susceptible to blood-induced but apparently not mosquito-transmitted infection with *P. knowlesi*. In humans, the infection is very variable, from mild to life-threatening, and in all cases there are the usual signs of malaria, fever, headaches, muscle pain, and anaemia. Caucasians and Negroes are equally susceptible to infection. For many years, *P. knowlesi* was used in Romania to induce fevers in patients suffering from general paralysis of the insane but this was discontinued when the parasite became too virulent after years of blood-passage from monkey to monkey. In passing, it should be mentioned that the treatment of paralysis with malaria is not as bizarre as it seems, and in Britain some 13 000 patients were therapeutically treated with *P. vivax*. There has only been one authenticated case of naturally acquired human infection with *P. knowlesi*, in 1965. The patient was an American surveyor working in the forests of Pahang in Malaysia who developed fever, fatigue, anorexia, and nausea and, later, sweating and rigor. He was initially diagnosed as suffering from *falciparum* malaria but when his blood was passaged into a monkey it developed a typical *knowlesi* infection. The patient recovered naturally without treatment. No other cases have been recorded and it is extremely unlikely that humans could become infected because the mosquito vectors rarely feed on any hosts other than monkeys and because contacts in the forest canopy are likely to be rare. Nevertheless, the fact that splenectomized kra monkeys rapidly succumb to infection suggests that it would be unwise for anybody without a spleen or on immunosuppressive therapy to venture into areas such as the Malaysian forests where *P. knowlesi* is known to exist (see Collins and Aikawa 1993).

Plasmodium simium is restricted to Brazil where it infects howler monkeys, *Alouatta fusca*, particularly younger animals, and the woolly spider monkey, *Brachyteles arachnoides*. Howler monkeys live in the forest canopy where they seldom come in contact with humans. Very little is known about this parasite except that the infections tend to be light and transient. The mosquito host is not known for certain but it is thought to be *Anopheles cruzi*. It was while looking for the mosquito host that the only recorded human infection occurred. An entomological assistant working near Sao Paulo became ill with a periodic 48-hour fever and was found to have, in his blood, small numbers of parasites which disappeared after a week. When his blood was injected into a splenectomized *Saimiri* monkey a typical *P. simium* infection resulted. There is no doubt that this infection occurred in a tree platform where the unusual circumstances brought infected monkeys, mosquitoes, and man together. This is the only record of a malaria zoonosis in the New World (see Collins and Aikawa 1993).

Plasmodium cynomolgi is found all over southern Asia, especially in Malaysia, its natural home. Several macaque monkeys, *Macaca* spp. especially *M. fascicularis*, harbour *P. cynomolgi*, as do leaf monkeys, *Presbytis* spp. Experimentally, *P. cynomolgi* can be transmitted to rhesus monkeys, in which it has been extensively studied, and baboons. Infections in monkeys cause anaemia, which can be quite severe, but otherwise tend to be mild and self-limiting within a few months, although relapses may occur up to 2 years later. Many Asian species of *Anopheles* can transmit this parasite naturally and over 60 *Anopheles* species can do so experimentally. *Plasmodium cynomolgi* can be transmitted to humans either through the bite of a mosquito or by infected blood. In 1960 there were the first reports of the accidental infection of laboratory workers and since then a number of accidental and experimental infections have been recorded (Eyles, *et al.* 1960). The infections, which last several weeks, are characterized by low parasitaemias and high fevers and an irregular 48-hour periodicity accompanied by headaches, anorexia, nausea, enlarged livers, and spleens. Observations on human infections indicate that Caucasians are more susceptible to infection than Negroes, something that also applies to infections with the human counterpart of *P. cynomolgi*, *P. vivax*. In this chapter *P. cynomolgi* has been treated as a single entity but it actually occurs as two subspecies, *P. c. cynomolgi* and *P. c. bastianelli*, which behave slightly differently from one another in the laboratory, but humans are equally susceptible to both. Because of the ease with which humans can be infected, the wide range of mosquito hosts, some of which are man-biting, and the relative frequency of contact between monkeys, mosquitoes, and humans,

the possibility that *P. cynomolgi* might be a zoonosis is a real one, although no authenticated cases have been recorded despite intensive investigations (Garnham 1966; Collins and Aikawa, 1993).

Plasmodium eylesi occurs in the forests of northern Malaysia where it is a parasite of the gibbon *Hylobates lar*. The natural vector is not known, but *P. eylesi* can develop in a number of anopheline mosquitoes. Infections in gibbons are characterized by high parasitaemias but few signs of disease. There have been reports that humans can be infected experimentally with sporozoites but the resulting parasitaemias are low and no signs of illness have been recorded (Collins and Aikawa 1993).

Plasmodium schwetzi occurs in forests in tropical Central and West Africa where it infects chimpanzees, *Pan troglodytes*, and, less frequently, gorillas, *Gorilla gorilla*. The natural vector is not known but *A. gambiae*, the main vector of human malaria in Africa, cannot be infected. Humans experimentally infected with parasitized blood develop transient febrile self-limiting infections. Negroes are not susceptible to infection (Collins and Aikawa 1993).

Plasmodium inui is the most widely distributed malaria parasite in Asian macaques (*Macaca iris* and other *Macaca* spp.) and leaf monkeys (*Presbytis* spp.). The mosquito hosts include *A. elegans* and *A. leucosphyrus*, neither of which bites humans. Infections in monkeys are usually mild and self-limiting but are virulent in splenectomized animals. In experimental human blood-induced infections the infection is mild with fever and scanty parasites in the blood. It should be mentioned here that the parasite isolated by Romanian workers and transmitted to humans in 1934 and identified as *P. inui* was almost certainly *P. knowlesi* (Collins and Aikawa 1993).

Plasmodium brasilianum occurs in tropical South America where it is a common parasite in several species of monkeys, including *Alouatta* spp., *Ateles* spp., *Brachyteles* spp., *Cebus* spp., and *Saimiri* spp. The natural vector is unknown. Experimentally, *P. brasilianum* can infect an even wider range of monkeys and is very pathogenic even in its natural hosts. Early attempts to infect humans with infected blood or mosquitoes failed but subsequent attempts using *A. freeborni* as a vector were successful. Parasitaemias were low and accompanied by quartan fevers and enlarged spleens. Caucasians and Negroes are equally susceptible to infection (Collins and Aikawa 1993).

Plasmodium malariae occurs throughout the tropical regions of the Old World and in scattered localities in the New World. *Plasmodium malariae* is the parasite that causes quartan malaria in humans and is the only species that is also found in non-human primates. At one time it was thought that the non-human form belonged to a different species, *P. rodhaini*, and it is interesting to note that the person responsible for syn-onymizing this name with *P. malariae* was Jerome Rodhain himself. *Plasmodium malariae* infects chim-panzees, *Pan troglodytes*, in tropical forests of Africa and, although known to infect a wide range of mosqui-toes, the natural vector of the chimpanzee form is not known. Although *P. malariae* could theoretically be transmitted from chimpanzees to humans, there is no evidence that this has ever occurred and such transmis-sion is unlikely given the probability that different vectors are involved in the human and in the sylvatic non-human cycles and the distances that chimpanzees maintain between themselves and humans. In human to human infections with *P. malariae*, Caucasians and Negroes are equally susceptible (Garnham 1996).

DIAGNOSIS

Although human malaria infections acquired from non-human hosts are rare, it is important that an accurate diagnosis should be made of any suspected cases. Because human and non-human parasites are so similar, the only ways to be certain that a parasite has been derived from an animal host is by careful examination of thin blood films, in which the morphology of the par-asite is maintained, and the passage of infected blood into the suspected natural host in which a characteristic infection should occur. The human malarias are very host specific and do not infect monkeys other than owl monkeys, *Aotus* spp., and squirrel monkeys, *Saimiri* spp. Immunological tests and DNA probes are unlikely to be of any help in the immediate diagnosis of an infection but could be invaluable in confirming the diagnosis.

TREATMENT

All malaria parasites respond to treatment with a variety of drugs, of which the most useful is the 4-aminoquino-line schizonticide, chloroquine, which should be given orally at a dose of 20–30 mg base/kg body weight for 3 days. Chloroquine resistance, which has threatened the use of this drug for human malaria in many parts of the world, does not occur naturally in non-human primates. The 8-aminoquinoline, primaquine, should be used for the elimination of the liver stages of the tertian malarias; 0.25 mg/kg body weight for 14 days is the standard treatment (Bruce-Chwatt 1985).

EPIDEMIOLOGY

Human malaria infections from animals are very rare but are known to occur and thus do present some risk, albeit very small. Non-human malarias tend to be cycled between monkeys in forest canopies by zoophilic and exophilic mosquitoes, thus the only people who have a chance of becoming infected are those who intrude into such habitats. Normally, only particular groups such as explorers, biologists, and surveyors are likely to be involved but, increasingly, military person-nel and refugees have tended to move into areas not normally populated by humans. Such individuals are at risk. Splenectomy and immunosuppressive drugs increase the chances of infection with unusual parasites and individuals so affected are at even greater risk. At present, it is not known whether or not HIV infections increase susceptibility to animal malaria infections, but this must be a real possibility. With increasing unrest in Africa coupled with the spread of AIDS, it is likely that more infections with animal malarias will occur but these will never create any real health problem.

PREVENTION AND CONTROL

Cases of human malaria acquired from animals are so rare that it is not necessary to suggest any control mea-sures. Those working with primate malarias should be very careful when working with infected blood and should avoid being bitten by mosquitoes. If anyone working with these malarias does become exposed to infection, any symptoms such as fever should be reported immediately and diagnosis made on blood films. If positive, expert advice should be taken and treatment with chloroquine begun immediately.

REFERENCES

BABESIOSIS

Anderson, J. F., Mintz, E. D., Gadbaw, J. J., and Magnarelli, L. A. (1991). *Babesia microti*, human babesiosis and *Borrelia burgdorferi* in Connecticut. *Journal of Clinical Microbiology*, **29**, 2779–83.

Cox, F. E. G. (1982). Babesiosis in rodents and humans. In *Animal models in parasitology*, (ed. D. G. Owen), pp. 83–91. Macmillan, London.

Healy, G. and Ristic, M. (1988). Human babesiosis. In *Babesiosis of domestic animals and man*, (ed. M. Ristic), pp. 209–25. CRC Press, Boca Raton.

Kakoma, I. and Mehlhorn, H. (1994). Babesia of domestic animals. In *Parasitic protozoa*, (2nd edn), Vol. 7, (ed. J. P. Kreier), pp. 141–216. Academic Press, San Diego.

Ristic, M. (ed.) (1988). *Babesiosis of domestic animals and man*. CRC Press, Boca Raton.

Tabaoda, J. and Merchant, S. R. (1991). Babesiosis of com-panion animals and man. In *Tick-transmitted diseases*, (ed. J. D. Hoskins). *Veterinary Clinics of North America, Small Animal Practice*, **21**, 103–23.

Telford, S. R., Gorenflot, A., Brasseur, P., and Spielman, A. (1993). Babesial infections in humans and wildlife. In *Parasitic protozoa*, (2nd edn), Vol. 5, (ed. J. P. Kreier), pp. 1–47. Academic Press, San Diego.

Thomford, J. W. *et al.* (1994). Cultivation and phylogenetic characterization of a newly discovered human pathogenic protozoan. *Journal of Infectious Diseases*, **169**, 1050–6.

Young, A. S. (1988). Epidemiology of babesiosis. In *Babesiosis of domestic animals and man*, (ed. M. Ristic), pp. 81–98. CRC Press, Boca Raton.

Zwart, D. and Brocklesby, D. W. (1979). Babesiosis: non-specific resistance, immunological factors and pathogenesis. *Advances in Parasitology*, **17**, 49–113.

MALARIA

Brack, M. (1987). *Agents transmissible from simians to man.* Springer-Verlag, Berlin.

Bruce-Chwatt, L. J. (1985). *Essential malariology*, (2nd edn). Heinemann, London.

Coatney, G. R., Collins, W. E., Warren, M., and Contacos, P. G. (1971). *The primate malarias.* US Government Printing Office, Washington.

Collins, W. E. and Aikawa, M. (1993). Plasmodia of non-human primates. In *Parasitic protozoa*, (2nd edn), Vol. 5, (ed. J. P. Kreier), pp. 105–33. Academic Press, San Diego.

Eyles, D. E., Coatney, G. R., and Getz, M. E. (1960). Vivax-type malaria parasite of macaques transmissible to man. *Science*, **132**, 1812–13.

Garnham, P. C. C. (1966). *Malaria parasites and other haemosporidia.* Blackwell, Oxford.

Garnham, P. C. C. (1980). Malaria in its various vertebrate hosts. In *Malaria*, Vol. 1, (ed. J. P. Kreier), pp. 95–144. Academic Press, New York.

Wernsdorfer, W. (1980). The importance of malaria in the wild. In *Malaria*, Vol. 1, (ed. J. P. Kreier), pp. 1–93. Academic Press, New York.

48 MICROSPORIDIOSIS

Elizabeth U. Canning

SUMMARY

Four microsporidia have been reported from mammals other than man. These are: *Encephalitozoon cuniculi*, causing disseminated infections in a wide range of rodents, lagomorphs, carnivores, and primates; *Thelohania apodemi*, giving rise to cysts in the brain of field mice, *Apodemus sylvaticus; Microsporidium buyukmichii* in the cornea of a cat; and *Microsporidium simiae* in the jejunal enterocytes of a *Callicebus* monkey, *Callicebus moloch cupreus*. Of these only *E. cuniculi* has also been reported from humans.

Thirteen species of microsporidia are known to infect man, occurring mainly in immunocompromised patients, but some have infected the eyes of otherwise healthy people. The species infecting AIDS patients are: *Enterocytozoon bieneusi*, the most commonly occurring species, with a primary site of infection in small intestinal enterocytes; *Encephalitozoon (Septata) intestinalis*, also infecting small intestinal enterocytes but disseminating more widely; *Encephalitozoon hellem*, infecting the urinary and respiratory systems but also infecting the corneal and conjunctival epithelia, possibly secondarily; *Encephalitozoon cuniculi*, reported from the liver, peritoneum and kidney; *Trachipleistophora hominis* and a *Nosema*-like species in skeletal muscle; *Vittaforma corneae* as a disseminated infection; and a *Trachipleistophora*-like species in brain, heart and kidney. A *Pleistophora*-like microsporidium, has also been recorded from an immunocompromised, HIV-negative man, and *E. cuniculi* has caused neurological diseases in two children, who were at most mildly immunocompromised. *Nosema connori* was found as a generalized infection in every organ of an athymic infant and *Vittaforma corneae* (*Nosema corneum*), *Nosema ocularum, Microsporidium ceylonensis*, and *Microsporidium africanum* all infected the deep corneal stroma of otherwise healthy people.

Growth of microsporidia in host cells causes hypertrophy and eventual death of the cells. Infection in epithelia usually results in hyperplasia. Villous atrophy is associated with *E. bieneusi* infection of the small intestine. Release of parasite antigens into tissues surrounding infected cells e.g. in kidney and brain, often results in an intense cellular reaction with infiltration of lymphocytes, plasma cells, macrophages, neutrophils, and eosinophils. The lesions are typically focal granulomata but perivascular cuffing and widespread inflammation are also characteristic.

Detection and identification can be achieved at the light microscopic level with classical stains but the introduction of a modified trichrome method, fluorescence brighteners (Uvitex 2B and Calcofluor M2R) and Warthin–Starry stain has greatly facilitated routine diagnosis in stool, urine, and biopsies. Serological identification of species has been hampered by cross-reactions. Sequencing of ribosomal RNA genes has thrown light on the relationship of species, and PCR amplification has been used to detect infections in tissue biopsies and most recently in stool.

The most valuable drug for treatment is albendazole, which will eliminate infections due to *Encephalitozoon* spp. and will sometimes ameliorate the diarrhoea associated with *E. bieneusi*, without reducing the parasite burden significantly. Infections of *E. hellem* have been treated successfully with broline and fumagillin applied topically but this form of treatment may not be necessary in the light of the known activity of albendazole.

Little is known of the source of infections to man. Transmission of most microsporidia is by the oral route and it is known that *E. cuniculi* can be transmitted transplacentally in non-human hosts. Differences have been observed between isolates of *E. cuniculi* of murine, canine, and human origin but cross-infectivity between animal species has been demonstrated and may also occur from animals to man. *Enterocytozoon bieneusi* has been reported from immunocompetent people and from pigs. It seems likely that this is a natural infection of man, not dependent on an animal reservoir and it may be that spores are water-borne.

HISTORY

The early history of microsporidial infections in mammals begins with the observation of Gram-positive spores in the brain of rabbits that were being used for investigations on poliomyelitis (Wright and Craighead 1922). References to the early history of microsporidial infections in mammals are given in Canning and Lom (1986). Over the period 1923–26 Levaditi and colleagues studied the organisms seen by Wright and Craighead, which they named *Encephalitozoon cuniculi*, recognizing them as microsporidia and demonstrating their lack of host specificity by transmitting infections from rabbits to mice, rats and a dog, but not to a monkey, *Macacus cynomolgus*. These cross-transmission experiments are significant in the light of recent discoveries of *E. cuniculi* in AIDS patients.

In this early era of investigation there were several reports of microsporidia in the neurones and salivary glands of dogs. New names, which have passed into obscurity, were given to these parasites and it was suggested that there was a causal relationship between them and rabies or canine encephalitis. Although these diseases are now known to be of viral origin, the parasites could have been *Encephalitozoon*.

Still in this early period in the history of mammalian microsporidioses were descriptions of other *Encephalitozoon* species: in a 2-day-old female baby who died, having suffered generalized muscle contractions and convulsions; in the cerebrospinal fluid of a 17-year-old youth, who had died after a short illness of fever, coma, and meningitis; and from the brain and spinal cord of a 4-week-old infant. It is known that the diagnoses in the latter two cases were incorrect, but material from the baby girl cannot be traced and confirmation or otherwise cannot be obtained.

The first confirmed report of a human infection with microsporidia is that of Matsubayashi *et al.* (1959). Microsporidian spores were detected in cerebrospinal fluid (CSF) and urine of a 9-year-old boy who suffered a severe but non-fatal convulsive illness of about 25 days duration, characterized by fever and vomiting and including a comatose period. After intraperitoneal inoculation of mice with blood and sediments from CSF and urine from the patient, ascites accumulated in the abdominal cavity of the mice, and spores were detected in macrophages or free in the peritoneal fluid. Some doubt may be cast on the validity of the transmission experiments because it had not been demonstrated that the mice were microsporidia-free before the inoculations, but there is little doubt that the organisms collected from the child's fluids were spores of *Encephalitozoon*. A similar case history of a child of about 2 years of age suffering a convulsive illness was reported by Bergquist *et al.* (1984). On this occasion encephalitozoonosis was confirmed when spores from the urine gave rise to infections when inoculated intraperitoneally into *Encephalitozoon*-free mice, and sera from the child were positive for IgG and IgM antibodies, when tested by indirect immunofluorescence against *E. cuniculi* spores.

Other reports of microsporidial infections in humans, linking microsporidia with multiple sclerosis and of infection in cells of a pancreatic adenocarcinoma have not stood up to further scrutiny. However, in recent years it has become clear that microsporidia are quite common, especially in immunocompromised patients but also in immunoprivileged sites of healthy people. Several species have been described infecting the corneal stroma, corneal and conjunctival epithelia, skeletal musculature, intestine and associated organs, and as generalized infections. Serological surveys have indicated that self-limiting, clinical, or subclinical infections are also common in immunocompetent people, but this has yet to be fully evaluated.

Microsporidia are small unicellular organisms with biological characters sufficiently distinctive for them to be classified in a separate phylum, the Microspora. They are obligate intracellular parasites which have a proliferative phase, termed merogony, during which they multiply extensively by binary or multiple fission. A spore-producing phase, sporogony, follows merogony or is concurrent with it. Sporonts, distinguished by the acquisition of a dense surface coat, divide by binary or multiple fission into sporoblasts, which mature into spores.

Microsporidia lack mitochondria and have ribosomes with prokaryotic characteristics but are otherwise typically eukaryotic in organization. The 70S ribosomes have rRNAs of 16S and 23S in the small and large subunits respectively, features which have been used to amplify the 16S rRNA genes for the diagnosis of infections in host tissues and stool and to aid in the differentiation of species. The nuclei of most genera are typical of eukaryotes but electron-dense centriolar plaques in nuclear pores are present at the poles of division spindles in place of centrioles. In several genera, including *Vittaforma*, which has been isolated from human corneal stroma, and *Nosema*, which has been found as a generalized infection in an athymic infant, the nuclei are unusual in being paired as diplokarya, the two nuclei lying closely appressed and dividing synchonously. In some genera the diplokaryotic condition is maintained throughout the life cycle but, in others, there is an alternation between unpaired and paired nuclei, meiosis occurring in each nucleus of the diplokaryon at the onset of sporogony, producing haploid spores. In a few genera alternation of hosts is an obligate part of the life cycle but, as far as is known, these complexities do not occur in the genera infecting humans.

The structure of the spores is quite unique and unmistakable at the ultrastructural level. Spores range from spherical forms, 1.0 μm diameter, to tubular structures up to 20 μm long. The species infecting man all have ovoid spores of 5.0 μm or less in length. By light microscopy they appear greenish and refractile when fresh. They stain blue with a reddish-purple nucleus with Giemsa, reddish with Ziehl–Neelsen and are Gram-positive. Three new methods which have been developed to aid the diagnosis of human infections are Chromotrope 2R which stains spores pinkish (Weber *et al.* 1992), Warthin–Starry, which stains them brownish-black and the fluorescence brighteners Uvitex 2B (Van Gool *et al.* 1993) and Calcofluor M2R (Vavra *et al.* 1993), which bind to the chitin in the spore wall and exhibit a brilliant blue-white fluorescence when exposed to light of wavelength about 350 nm.

The spore wall consists of an electron-dense proteinaceous exospore and an electron-lucent chitinous endospore. The wall encloses the cytoplasm and nucleus of the infective agent (sporoplasm) and an extrusion apparatus consisting of a polar tube inserted at the anterior pole into an anchoring disc within a sac (polar sac) shaped like a mushroom cap. The polar tube is coiled just beneath the wall in the posterior half of the spore and joins the anchoring disc after running forward along a straight course, where it is surrounded by folded membranes and vesicles comprising the polaroplast. In some genera there is a prominent vacuole at the posterior end of the spore.

Natural transmission occurs when spores are ingested. Upon stimulation in the intestine, an increase in internal pressure effected by changes in the polaroplast membranes, causes the polar tube to be everted through the anterior end of the spore. When fully everted the cytoplasm and nucleus pass through the hollow tube and, if the tip of the tube has penetrated an enterocyte, the sporoplasm is injected into the cytoplasm of the host cell. Cell to cell spread of infection is not fully understood but, in at least some species, it is effected by *in vitro* germination of spores and inoculation of sporoplasms into neighbouring cells via the polar tube. There is evidence of transplacental transmission of *Encephalitozoon cuniculi* from the presence of *E. cuniculi* infections in three rabbits that had been delivered by Caesarian section and reared in germ-free isolators (Hunt *et al.* 1972) and in four pairs of mice similarly delivered and fostered to germ-free rats (Innes *et al.* 1962). There are also many reports of infections developing in new-born animals so soon after birth that it is unlikely that infections could have been acquired postnatally, e.g. in squirrel monkeys (Zeman and Baskin 1985). Infection of an AIDS patient with *Encephalitozoon hellem* throughout the tracheobronchial tree was interpreted by Schwartz *et al.* (1992) as indicative of respiratory acquisition of infection.

Altogether in the phylum about 135 genera have been described, most of which have been accepted. Fortunately only six of the established genera, with eleven species and two species placed in the collective genus *Microsporidium* are known from man.

THE AGENTS

SPECIES OF *MICROSPORIDIA* DETECTED IN MAN

Encephalitozoon cuniculi Levaditi, Nicolau and Schoen, 1923

This species has a wide host range among mammals, and organisms with similar morphology occur in birds and lizards (Canning and Lom 1986). It has rarely been reported in man but has twice been found in children (Matsubayashi *et al.* 1959; Bergquist *et al.* 1984) and a few times in AIDS patients (Terada *et al.* 1987; Zender *et al.* 1989; Hollister *et al.* 1993a, 1995; De Groote *et al.* 1995; Deplazes *et al.* 1996a). As macrophages can be infected, foci of infection can be found in most organs but parasites are especially common in unidentified cells in the brain (likely but not investigated in human cases) and in tubule cells in the kidney. All stages have unpaired nuclei and development is within a parasitophorous vacuole in the host cell. The meronts are closely adherent to the vacuolar membrane and divide by binary fission of binucleate stages. As the surface coat is deposited to form the sporonts, these stages detach themselves from the vacuolar membrane and the typically disporoblastic sporogony is completed in the lumen of the vacuole, amid a finely granular matrix. Host cells become enlarged as the vacuole becomes packed with spores. Spores measure about 2.5×1.5 μm, are uninucleate and have a rugose exospore and 4.5–7 coils of the polar tube in a single rank.

Encephalitozoon hellem Didier *et al.* 1991

This species has only been found in AIDS patients. Although rarely diagnosed, it has a wide geographical distribution, having been found in patients in several continents. It was originally discovered in corneal and conjunctival epithelia only (Didier *et al.* 1991) but the infection appears to be systemic, as it has been found additionally in kidney tubule cells, epithelium of ureters, epithelium of the tracheobronchial tree (Schwartz *et al.* 1992) and in nasal sinus epithelium and nasal polyps (Hollister *et al.* 1993b). It develops in parasitophorous vacuoles and is ultrastructurally very similar to *E. cuniculi*. The two species can be differentiated by their protein profiles separated by SDS–PAGE and by immunoblotting of these profiles with specific antisera. Spores measure 1.5–2.0 μm $\times$ 1.0 μm and have 6–8 coils of the polar tube in a single rank.

Encephalitozoon intestinalis (Cali, Kotler and Orenstein, 1993)

This species has also been found only in AIDS patients, with a wide geographical distribution. It has a primary site of infection in enterocytes of the intestine (principally the small intestine) but passes into macrophages in the lamina propria and disseminates into other organs including the kidney and liver. *Encephalitozoon intestinalis* was originally placed in a new genus *Septata* (Cali *et al.* 1993). It has many features in common with *E. cuniculi* and *E. hellem*, including development in a parasitophorous vacuole and typically disporoblastic sporogony (occasionally tetrasporoblastic). The morphological similarity and the 90 per cent sequence identity of the 16S rRNA genes with the other *Encephalitozoon* spp. were used to suppress the genus *Septata* (Hartskeerl *et al.* 1995). It differs from the other *Encephalitozoon* spp. in that vacuoles containing sporogonic stages are characteristically divided into compartments by granular 'septa', which are formed by compression of the matrix in the vacuole as the parasites pack the lumen (Canning *et al.* 1994; Van Gool *et al.* 1994) and fusion of vacuoles is common (Canning *et al.* 1994). Tubules, whcih are expanded at intervals or at the termini arise from the exospore and weave in the septa. These also serve to differentiate this species. Spores measure 2.0×1.2 μm and have 4–7 coils of the polar tube in a single rank.

Enterocytozoon bieneusi Desportes *et al.* 1985

This is the most commonly occurring microsporidium in AIDS patients. It has a primary site of infection in small intestinal enterocytes (Desportes *et al.* 1985) but may spread to the epithelium of the bile duct and gallbladder and has been found also in bronchial, nasal, and nasal sinus epithelia. All stages lie in direct contact with host cell cytoplasm and have unpaired nuclei, the nuclei being irregular and elongate in meronts and rounded and compact in sporonts. Meronts and sporonts are both multinucleate and are traversed by electron-lucent clefts. Deposition of the surface coat is delayed until sporoblast separation but the initiation of sporogony is signalled by the appearance of electron-dense discs, which arise from the clefts and eventually fuse to form the polar tube. The characteristic spore organelles are formed precociously around each nucleus, so that at division of the sporont the products are virtually fully formed spores. Spores, which are dispersed in the host cell cytoplasm measure 1.0×1.5 μm, are uninucleate, have a thin endospore and about six coils of the polar tube in two ranks.

Nosema connori Sprague, 1974

One case only has been found, as a generalized infection involving all organs examined of an athymic infant in the USA (Margileth *et al.* 1973). Merogonic stages were not seen. Spores measuring 4.0×2.0 μm

have nuclei in diplokaryotic arrangement and a polar tube with about 11 coils in a single rank.

Vittaforma corneae (Shadduck et al. 1990)

This species was isolated into culture from the corneal stroma of an otherwise healthy man in the USA and was first assigned to the genus *Nosema* as *Nosema corneum* (Shadduck *et al.* 1990). All stages have diplokaryotic nuclei and are completely surrounded by a cisterna of host endoplasmic reticulum bearing ribosomes on the outer membrane. The cisterna divides with the parasites so that each stage is isolated in its own cisterna. Originally it was thought that sporogony was disporoblastic but Silveira and Canning (1995) have shown that sporonts are multinucleate and divide to produce several linearly arranged sporoblasts. On the basis of the multisporous sporogony and investment by host endoplasmic reticulum Silveira and Canning (1995) proposed that it should be transferred to a new genus as *Vittaforma corneae*. Spores measure about 3.7×1.0 μm and have 5–7 coils of the polar tube. Recently *Vittaforma* has been found as a disseminated infection in an AIDS patient, from whom it was isolated into culture. On ultrastructure, SDS PAGE protein profiles and nucleotide sequence of the 16S r RNA gene, the isolate was identified as *V. corneae* (P. Deplazes, personal communication).

Trachipleistophore hominis Hollister et al. 1996 and Pleistophora spp.

Cases of microsporidian myositis caused by *Pleistophora*—like species have been reported as *Pleistophora* sp. in an immunocompromised but HIV—negative man (Ledford *et al.* 1985) and in an AIDS patient (Chupp *et al.* 1993). In another case, parasites were detected in the cornea and nasal washings as well as in skeletal muscle. (Field *et al.* 1996). An *in vitro* isolation was made from this patient and development was studied in cultured cells and in muscle of athymic mice which were susceptible (Hollister *et al.* 1996). The parasite was named as a new genus and species *Trachipleistophora hominis*. The predominant feature of all these parasites is the presence of a thick surface coat on all stages, which finally separates from the plasma membrane to become an envelope (sporophorous vesicle) enclosing the spores in groups of two to many. It is likely t hat the parasite seen b Chupp *et al.* (1993) is also *T. hominis* but the one seen by Ledford *et al.* (1985) may be different. In *T. hominis* the surface coat extends into lysed host cell cytoplasm as complex networks and merogonic and sporogonic divisions are by repeated binary fissions. The sporophorous vesicle grows to accommodate the increasing number of uninucleate sporoblasts and spores. The spores measure

4.0 × 2.4 μm (fresh) and have about 11 coils of the polar tube. In *Pleistophora* the surface coat is thicker and more uniform, the sporonts are multinucleate plasmodia and the sporophorous vesicle size is fixed by the size of the plasmodium at the onset of sporogony.

Microsporidium ceylonensis Canning and Lom, 1986

Few details are available. Spores, measuring 3.5 × 1.5 μm in fixed tissue, were found free and in macrophages in the corneal stroma of a young Tamil boy in Sri Lanka (Ashton and Wirasinha 1973). No further details were given but examination of the original sections, by electron microscopy after re-embedding in resin, showed that the spores have up to 12 coils of the polar tube and possibly that there is a single nucleus lying laterally to the posterior region of the polaroplast which is lamellar (Canning and Curry, unpublished observations). Spores lie in direct contact with host cell cytoplasm.

Microsporidium africanum Canning and Lom, 1986

Few details are available of this infection from a 26-year-old woman in Botswana (Pinnolis *et al.* 1981). Spores, measuring about 4.5–5.0 × 2.5–3.0 μm in fixed tissue, were present mainly in the cytoplasm of histiocytes in the cornea and in direct contact with the stroma. The spores have a single nucleus and 11–13 coils of the polar tube.

Nosema ocularum Cali et al. 1991

Few details are available of this infection from the eye of a 39-year-old man in the USA. The parasite was observed in the corneal stroma of the patient, who had experienced visual problems and had a corneal ulcer but was otherwise healthy. Only spores were present, these being distributed in the host cell cytoplasm and in direct contact with it. Spores, measuring about 5.0 × 3.0 μm in fixed tissue, have diplokaryotic nuclei and 9–12 coils of the polar tube in a single rank. In size and number of coils of the polar tube this parasite resembles *M. africanum*. It is not certain from the published micrograph that the spore has more than one nucleus.

Trachipleistophora—like species of Vávra *et al.* 1997

A parasite found in the brain and other organs of two AIDS patients (Yachnis *et al.* 1996) has the generic characters of *Trachipleistophora* but differs from *Trachipleistophora hominis* in that two types of spore are formed. One type, formed in sporophorous vesicles with varying numbers of spores, often 8, measures 3.7 × 2.0 μm (fixed) and has a polar tube of about 7 thick coils and 2 narrower, posterior coils (anisofilar). Spores of the second type, of which only two are formed in each sporophorous vesicle, are nearly spherical 2.2–2.5 × 1.8–2.0 μm. They are thin walled and have

only 4–5 isofilar coils of the polar tube (Vávra *et al.* 1997). This is the first reported occurrence of a dimorphic microsporidium in mammals.

Nosema—like species of Cali *et al.* 1996

A case of microsporidian myositis in an AIDS patient, involving a *Nosema*—like species was described by Cali *et al.* 1996. The tentative generic assignment was based on the presence of diplokaryotic nuclei in all stages and the free distribution of spores in host cell cytoplasm. Pre-spore stages have thick surface coats apparently extending as complex tubular secretions into lysed host tissue and interspersed between these stages are irregularly–shaped cytoplasmic sections, also with a surface coat. Spores measure 2.5–2.9 × 1.9–2.0 μm (fixed) and have about 9 coils of the polar tube in 2 ranks. This species is distinguished from the others causing myositis in being diplokaryotic.

MOLECULAR BIOLOGY

The first molecular studies on microsporidia were those of Vossbrinck and Woese (1986) who reported, for *Vairimorpha necatrix* (a microspordium of Lepidoptera) that the sequence corresponding to the eukaryotic 5.8S rRNA formed part of the large subunit rRNA, i.e. the 5′ end of the 23S rRNA. It had previously been shown that the prokaryotic-like, 70S ribosomes of microsporidia are composed of 30S and 50S subunits, each with a single rRNA of 16S and 23S, respectively. Still using *V. necatrix*, Vossbrinck *et al.* (1987) found that the sequence of the 16S rRNA was unlike the sequence of known eukaryote 18S rRNA and proposed that microsporidia are extremely ancient eukaryotes, which branched at a very early stage from the line leading from the prokaryotes to eukaryotes.

Amplification by polymerase chain reaction (PCR) and sequencing of the ribosomal genes have been used to detect microsporidia in human tissues and determine the taxonomic relationships of microsporidian genera. Sequences for the 16S rRNA genes have been obtained for *E. cuniculi*, *E. hellem*, *E. intestinalis* (= *Septata intestinalis*), and *E. bieneusi* (Vossbrinck *et al.* 1993; Zhu *et al.* 1993, 1994; Hartskeerl *et al.* 1995). Vossbrinck *et al.* (1993) used a region spanning part of the small subunit, the spacer region, and part of the large subunit to assess the degree of relatedness of *E. cuniculi* and *E. hellem* in comparison with microsporidia of fish and insect origin. The high sequence homology between *E. cuniculi* and *E. hellem* confirmed their taxonomic position as different species of the same genus. Similar results with the *Encephalitozoon* spp. were obtained by Zhu *et al.* (1994) sequencing the genes for the 16S rRNA. These authors included *E. intestinalis* (known then as *Septata*) and *E. bieneusi* in the study (as well as species of non-human origin) finding that *Septata* was closer to the *Encephalitozoon* spp. than was *E. bieneusi*, thus justifying the placement by Cali *et al.* (1993) of *Septata* with *Encephalitozoon* in the family Encephalitozoonidae. Harlskeerl *et al.* (1995) found such close homology in the 16S rRNA gene sequences of *Septata* and *Encephalitozoon* that they considered *S. intestinalis* to be a species of *Encephalitozoon* (see above).

Differences between isolates of *E. cuniculi* from different host species have been revealed by SDS–PAGE, Western blotting, and sequences of the intergenic spacer between the 16S and 23S rRNA genes. Four repeats of a short sequence 5'-GTTT-3' were found in two dog isolates, three repeats in three rabbit isolates and one mouse isolate, and two repeats in two other mouse isolates (Didier *et al.*, 1995). Subtle differences in their protein profiles have been found between a human, a canine, and a murine isolate of *E. cuniculi* but the human isolate more closely resembled the canine than the murine by RAPD–PCR, using *Bam*HI as the primer (Hollister *et al.* 1995), and in having four repeats of 5'-GTTT-3' in the spacer region of the ribosomal genes (Hollister *et al.* 1996a). The techniques used by Didier *et al.* (1995), plus PCR amplification followed by restriction enzyme digestion and double-stranded DNA heleroduplex mobility shift analysis, were applied to isolates of *E. intestinalis* (Didier *et al.* 1996). The isolates were from stool, bronchoalveolar lavage, and nasal mucus aspirate from AIDS patients, but differences as found between isolates of *E. cuniculi* were not detected.

Baker *et al.* (1995) have analysed the 16S rRNA gene sequence data for 16 microsporidia of diverse origin, including those from insect, decapod, fish, and human hosts, to determine their phylogenetic relationships. As expected, the three *Encephalitozoon* spp. clustered together but, surprisingly, *Vittaforma corneae*, which has diplokaryotic nuclei and was isolated from human cornea, appeared most closely related to the insect-derived *Endoreticulatus schubergi*, which has isolated nuclei. *Vittaforma* and *Endoreticulatus* formed a group with *Enterocytozoon*.

TISSUE CULTURE

As all microsporidia are obligate intracellular parasites, growth outside the host can only be achieved in tissue culture. Growth of a microsporidium *in vitro* was first achieved by adding haemolymph of silkworms (*Bombyx mori*) extracted 2 days after they had ingested spores of *Nosema bombycis*, to cultures of silkworm cells. This was followed by infection of cultures using purified spores of *N. bombycis* primed for germination by suspension in 0.1 M KOH for 40 minutes before addition to the cultures. All stages of merogony and sporogony, including mature spores, developed in the cultures.

Numerous tissue culture systems have since been developed for microsporidia of invertebrate origin.

Encephalitozoon cuniculi, the first of the microsporidia from mammals to be established *in vitro* (Shadduck 1969), is particularly easy to culture. Cultures have been initiated from naturally infected host cells or by addition of mouse ascites, tissue homogenates, or purified spores to cell monolayers. It is not necessary to prime the spores for germination before addition to the cell cultures. Many cell types have been used (summarized by Canning and Lom 1986) with some supporting more prolific growth than others. Growth is particularly luxuriant in rabbit choroid plexus cells, but leads to destruction of cultures in a few weeks. Madin Darby canine kidney cells (MDCK) are more convenient, as destruction of infected cells is matched by replication of uninfected cells. Cultures in MDCK cells can be maintained at 37 °C with a gas mixture of 5 per cent CO_2 in air. Spores can be harvested from the supernatant and medium changed once weekly.

Microsporidia of human origin that have been established *in vitro* are *Vittaforma corneae* (*Nosema corneum*) (Shadduck *et al.* 1990), *E. hellem* (Didier *et al.* 1991; Hollister *et al.* 1993b), *E. cuniculi* (Hollister *et al.* 1993a 1995; De Groote *et al.* 1995), *E. intestinalis* (Van Gool *et al.* 1994), and *T. hominis* (Hollister *et al.* 1996b). Numerous attempts to culture *E. bieneusi* continuously have been unsuccessful, although Visvesvara *et al.* (1995) reported short-term growth. Material of the other species of mammalian origin, with which to seed cultures, has not been available.

THE HOSTS

ANIMAL

Apart from *E. cuniculi*, four microsporidia have been described from non-human mammals. *Thelohania apodemi* was found in the brain of field mice as 100 μm diameter colonies with no tissue reaction round them (Doby *et al.* 1963). *Microsporidium buyukmihcii* (named by Canning and Lom 1986) was found once in a domestic cat causing opacity with moderate inflammation of the cornea, conjunctiva, and anterior uvea (Buyukmihci *et al.* 1977). *Microsporidium simiae* (named by Canning and Lom 1986) parasitized a captive *Callicebus* monkey (*Callicebus moloch cupreus*) in the epithelial cells of the jejunum (Seibold and Fussell 1973). The monkey had lost weight over a period of 1 month before death. At post-mortem the jejunal epithelium was found to be totally desquamated. No further information is available about the progression of these isolated cases of infection. *Enterocytozoon bieneusi* has recently been reported from pigs (Deplazes *et al.* 1996b)

Encephalitozoon cuniculi is a common parasite of mammals and has a wide host range among rodents, lagomorphs, carnivores, and primates (reviewed by Canning and Lom 1986). Clinical signs of encephalitozoonosis vary markedly according to host species. Susceptibility of mice depends on strain, resistant strains showing few signs of infection while susceptible strains may develop ascites at about 14 days post-infection and there may be a 10 per cent mortality rate. Survivors return to normal over a period of weeks. Rabbits also vary in their response to infection. Seropositive individuals have been detected in laboratory rabbits which showed no outward signs of infection. Conversely, overt encephalitozoonosis has been detected in both laboratory and broiler rabbits, the clinical manifestations being mainly neurological, in the form of torticollis, ataxia, and paralysis, with mortality ranging from 15 to 50 per cent. The differences may be due in part to mode of transmission, whether oral or transplacental, as neonate animals are more severely affected.

Amongst carnivores, encephalitozoonosis has been most fully described in dogs (Van Dellen *et al.* 1978) and blue foxes (Nordstoga 1972). Clinical signs are most apparent in new born animals infected *in utero*. Again neurological signs predominate, such as ataxia, partial paralysis, blindness, convulsions, and aggressive behaviour. Affected animals are normally euthanized.

Encephalitozoon cuniculi has been incriminated several times in the death of neonate squirrel monkeys, *Saimiri sciureus*. In one report *E. cuniculi* was found at post-mortem in 22 monkeys that had died at a primate centre and was considered as a probable contributing cause of death in 13 of the 17 neonates and infants up to 9 months old (Zeman and Baskin 1985).

Microscopic lesions may be found in most organs but are most common in the brain and kidney. Breakdown of host cells, releasing spores into the surrounding tissue, stimulates an intense cellular reaction resulting in focal granulomata composed, according to site, of macrophages, plasma cells, lymphocytes, histiocytes, some neutrophils and, in the brain, microglia. In the kidney, release of spores from their site of development in the tubule cells, into the interstitium causes an interstitial nephritis which may be so severe that it can be recognized by indentation at the surface. Lesions are frequently associated with blood vessels, with thickening of the walls, and sometimes perivascular cuffing, causing occlusion of the vessels. Polyarteritis nervosa was a particular feature of encephalitozoonosis in neonate blue foxes. Infection has also been reported in the eyes, involving the retina, causing cataractal changes in the lenses and thickening of the arterial walls.

HUMAN

There have been several reports of demonstrable *E. cuniculi* parasites in man. The first cases were two otherwise healthy children, who suffered severe neurological illnesses manifested by convulsions, recurrent fever, loss of consciousness, headache, and vomiting. Both children made full recoveries (Matsubayashi *et al.* 1959; Bergquist *et al.* 1984). The other cases were AIDS patients. The first patient had a progressive hepatitis culminating in jaundice, fever, and diarrhoea before death: parasites were associated with focal granulomatous, suppurative necrosis, mainly in the portal area (Terada *et al.* 1987). In the second patient, who suffered peritonitis, parasites were found at post-mortem in an inflammatory mass on the omentum magnum (Zender *et al.* 1989). In these four cases the specific identification was based on morphology of the spores, although this was supported by serological evidence in the case of the child examined by Bergquist *et al.* There is no certainty that the specific identification was correct, i.e. that *E. cuniculi* rather than *E. hellem* or *E. intestinalis* was involved.

Microsporidia were isolated into culture from the urine of a third patient with AIDS. Identification of this parasite was assisted by a comparison of *Encephalitozoon* isolates by RAPD–PCR and by SDS–PAGE and Western blotting of protein profiles (Hollister *et al.* 1993*a*, 1995). The human isolate was differentiated as *E. cuniculi* rather than *E. hellem* but minor differences were found between it and murine and canine isolates of *E. cuniculi*. A renal biopsy showed a granulomatous infiltrate, mainly of macrophages and lymphocytes, in some glomeruli, infiltration of the interstitium by lymphocytes, plasma cells, neutrophils, and eosinophils, and the presence of microsporidian spores in vacuoles in the tubule cells and free in the tubule lumina and glomerular granulomata (Aarons *et al.* 1994). These histopathological changes are similar to those observed in renal encephalitozoonosis of animals. Another *in vitro* isolate of *E. cuniculi* was made from urine and sputum of an AIDS patient who had a disseminated infection causing keratoconjunctivitis, bronchiolitis, nephritis, sinusitis, and, probably, infection in the brain (De Groote *et al.* 1995). The species was identified by indirect immunofluorescence (IFAT) and by PCR with primers specific for *E. cuniculi*. The isolate gave an identical PCR amplification product with that of a rodent isolate of *E. cuniculi* but was not characterized further. These AIDS patients were in advanced renal failure when encephalitozoonosis was diagnosed. Several isolates from Switzerland were typed as of rabbit origin on the basis of sequences of the ITS region of the ribosomal genes (Deplazes *et al.* 1996*a*).

There is considerable evidence from serology that infections of *Encephalitozoon* are widespread (Hollister *et al.* 1991; Ombrouck *et al.* 1995*b*) but determination of the species involved is hampered by antigenic similarity and cross-reactivity. However, it is likely that a seropositive child in South Africa (McInnes and Stewart 1991) was infected with *E. cuniculi*, as this species had been diagnosed in a litter of heavily infected bull terrier puppies with which the child had had very close contact.

Encephalitozoon hellem has been found only in AIDS patients. It was originally detected in corneal and conjunctival epithelium only, causing keratoconjunctivitis (Didier *et al.* 1991). Several other cases of ocular infection have been reported. However, the systemic nature of the infection has been shown by Schwartz *et al.* (1992), who found it disseminated in kidney, urinary bladder, ureters, and throughout the tracheobronchial tree, as well as bilaterally in the eyes of patients. It has also caused respiratory problems by stimulating polyp formation of the nasal epithelium and hypertrophy of nasal sinus epithelium (Lacey *et al.* 1992; Hollister *et al.* 1993*b*). Histopathological changes in the kidney were similar to those caused by *E. cuniculi*. In the respiratory system, parasites were restricted to the epithelium which was hyperplastic in some areas, thinned in others, while the underlying tissue was acutely inflamed. Parasites were not present in the terminal bronchioles or alveoli. Symptoms include keratoconjunctivitis, bronchiolitis, sinusitis, and nephritis, with progressive respiratory and renal failure.

Encephalitozoon intestinalis has been found only in AIDS patients. It infects the small intestinal epithelium, rarely the large intestine, and is associated with chronic diarrhoea and malabsorption (Orenstein *et al.* 1992). Infection spreads to macrophages of the lamina propria and thence disseminates to the kidneys, where it causes a tubulointerstitial nephritis similar to that caused by the foregoing *Encephalitozoon* spp. Small numbers of spores have also been found in bronchial epithelial cells and in Kupffer and endothelial cells of the liver. Symptoms include diarrhoea, dysuria, haematuria, rhinosinusitis, and chronic cough.

Enterocytozoon bieneusi has been found mainly in AIDS patients. It has a primary site of infection in the small intestinal epithelium and differs from *E. intestinalis* in that it does not normally spread into the lamina propria. In most reports of its occurrence in AIDS patients, it has been linked with chronic diarrhoea, malabsorption, and weight loss, with several episodes of watery, non-bloody stools per day (Orenstein 1991). Villous atrophy, crypt hyperplasia, cell degeneration and sloughing and decreased xylose absorption have all been reported in AIDS patients with *E. bieneusi* (Dieterich *et al.* 1994). However, in a controlled study (Rabeneck *et al.* 1993), no significant difference was found in the occurrence of *E. bieneusi* microsporidiosis in patients with and without diarrhoea. In the two reported cases of *E. bieneusi* infection in HIV-negative patients, there was a strong correlation between diarrhoea and the transient presence of the organism (Sandfort *et al.* 1993; Sobottka *et al.* 1995*a*). There are several reports of sclerosing cholangitis of *E. bieneusi* origin caused by infection of the gallbladder and the bile duct, reached presumably by direct spread from the intestinal epithelium. The parasite has also been found in nasal sinus mucosa, causing chronic rhinosinusitis with nasal discharge, and in bronchial epithelium of a patient with chronic cough and dyspnoea. The occurrence of infections in patients who were immunosuppressed after organ transplantation (Sax and Rich quoted by Weber *et al.* 1994; Rabodonirina *et al.* 1996) demonstrates how exposed human beings are to multiplication of microsporidia when immune control is removed.

Vittaforma corneae (*N. corneum*) was isolated into culture from biopsy tissue removed from the eye of an HIV-negative patient with progressive keratitis, patchy stromal infiltration, and iritis (Shadduck *et al.* 1990). In a study of the development of this species in athymic mice (Silveira *et al.* 1993) infections spread systemically to involve all organs of the body, including the retina of the eye, after intraperitoneal inoculation of spores. However, infections were not established in the eyes by topical application of spores to the eyes of neonate mice. In general, ocular infections with microsporidia (*V. corneae, M. ceylonensis, M. africanum, N. ocularum*) in HIV-negative patients have involved the deep stromal tissue. *Encephalitozoon cuniculi* in animals has been found in the lenses, retina, and walls of the ciliary arteries. In contrast, ocular infections in AIDS patients have been due to *E. hellem*, which is restricted to the epithelium, where it causes punctate keratopathy and foreign body sensation, relieved by corneal scraping. *V. corneae* has recently been found as a disseminated infection in an AIDS patient (P. Deplazes, personal communication).

Nosema connori has been found just once in an immunocompromised infant, who was progressively incapacitated by diarrhoea, vomiting, fever, rash, bowel obstruction, and respiratory distress before death (Margileth *et al.* 1973). Microsporidia were found in all organs examined (the brain was excluded) and, apart from the muscularis of the diaphragm, where there was a marked inflammatory infiltrate, there was almost no host response. The massive extent of the microsporidian infection and the proliferation of *Pneumocystis carinii* (the principal cause of the respiratory distress) can be attributed to the minimal development of the thymus, lymph nodes, and lymphoid tissue of the spleen in this child.

Pleistophora-like infections have been diagnosed in three immunodeficient patients (two with AIDS) infecting the skeletal musculature (Ledford *et al.* 1985; Chupp *et al.* 1993; Field *et al.* 1996). The parasite involved in the last case has been described as a new genus and species, *Trachipleistophora hominis* (Hollister *et al.* 1996*b*), and it is likely that two of the three infections were due to this species. All patients exhibited progressive muscle weakness and tenderness due to degeneration of muscle fibres around foci of infection. An acute inflammatory reaction of plasma cells, lymphocytes, histiocytes, and eosinophils was reported in the first two cases but a minimal response, of macrophages only, was seen in the latter case. This latter infection was interesting in that infected cells were also present in conjunctival epithelium and spores were detected in nasopharyngeal washings.

Recently *Pleistophora*-like infections have been detected at autopsy in lesions in the brain of two AIDS patients, who also had significant renal and cardiac disease (Yachnis *et al.* 1996). The parasites had morphological features in common with *T. hominis*. *Trachipleistophora hominis* has been transmitted to athymic mice, in which infections developed in a variety of tissues as well as skeletal muscle, after intraperitoneal inoculation (Hollister *et al.* 1996*b*). It may be that myositis is only one of the manifestations of *T. hominis* infection and that myositis may not be as important as infection in other sites as an immediate cause of death.

DETECTION

When intestinal microsporidiosis (*E. bieneusi*) was first detected in AIDS patients, diagnosis depended on light- and electron-microscopic examination of small intestinal biopsies. Methylene blue/azur II/basic fuchsin on resin sections and Warthin–Starry stain on paraffin sections give good definition of microsporidia in tissues. However, the recognition of spores in Giemsa-stained smears of stool (Van Gool *et al.* 1990) has led to the development of more refined staining techniques for detection without resort to biopsy. Weber *et al.* (1992) introduced a modified trichrome stain which gave specific reddish-pink staining to the spores and facilitated routine screening of stool samples. A reduction in the level of phosphotungstic acid and substitution of an aniline blue for fast green as counterstain (Ryan *et al.* 1993) and a reduction in staining time by raising the temperature of the stain to 50 °C (Kokoskin *et al.* 1994) have been recommended as improvements of the trichrome method.

Van Gool *et al.* (1993) introduced fluorescence staining using Uvitex 2B as an extremely rapid method for spore detection. Vavra *et al.* (1993) have used Calcofluor M2R in a similar way and have shown that alkaline pretreatment of spore-containing material

enhances fluorescence. These fluorescence brighteners bind to chitin and will, thus, stain fungal spores and other chitin-containing material in stool as well as microsporidian spores. Nevertheless it is an extremely easy way to screen stool samples and confirmation of positives can be obtained by other methods. Ombrouck *et al.* (1996) have used a combination of Uvitex 2B and an immunofluorescence assay using polyclonal serum specific for *E. intestinalis* to differentiate this species from *E. bieneusi* in stool.

Staining methods, as described above, can be used to detect microsporidia in stool urine, nasal discharge, or in biopsies such as kidney and corneal scrapings. Specific identification is more difficult by light microscopy, although size and shape may be used. As identification is important in treatment, it may be necessary to resort to electron microscopy of tissues or stool, using characters such as the number and arrangement of polar tube coils to recognize the species.

At the time when only *E. cuniculi* of the microsporidia infecting mammals could be cultured, serological surveys based on *E. cuniculi* antigen indicated that microsporidian infections were common. After the discovery of *E. hellem* and *E. intestinalis* in man, it could no longer be assumed that the antibodies detected in the surveys were specific for *E. cuniculi*. Various refinements have been introduced, including preabsorption of the sera with the antigens of interest, but cross-reactions continue to be problematic. Monoclonal antibodies raised against *E. hellem* (Aldras *et al.* 1994) and polyclonal sera raised against *E. hellem*, *E. cuniculi*, and *N. corneum* (Zierdt *et al.* 1993; Aldras *et al.* 1994) have been found to cross-react with *E. bieneusi* and *E. intestinalis* in biopsies and formalin-fixed stool, and can thus be used to detect infections but not to differentiate species. In contrast to the other microsporidia infecting AIDS patients, *E. bieneusi* cannot be established *in vitro* and, thus, a supply of antigen for serology is not readily available. Ombrouck *et al.* (1995*a*) reported that antigens common to *E. bieneusi* were present in *Glugea atherinae* (a microsporidium of fish origin) so that Western blotting of *G. atherinae* antigens could be used to detect antibodies to *E. bieneusi*. However, extreme caution has to be used in interpretation of the results.

Considerable progress has been made towards diagnosis by PCR, which gives unequivocal identification of species. Primers can be selected from conserved sequences of the 16S rRNA genes, which will amplify from the DNA of all microsporidian species. This has been applied to the three *Encephalitozoon* spp. using spores from culture or infected biopsies (Weiss *et al.* 1993; Fedorko *et al.* 1995; Hartskeerl *et al.* 1995) and to *E. bieneusi* (Zhu *et al.* 1993). Identification of the species can then be achieved by restriction enzyme digestion of the amplification products. Fedorko *et al.* (1995) also obtained PCR products of *E. intestinalis* and *E. bieneusi* from sodium hypochlorite-treated stool but the procedure required both mechanical and chemical disruption of the spores over a 4-day period. This, however, represents the first step towards PCR diagnosis of intestinal microsporidiosis without recourse to tissue biopsies. As the sequences are known for the three *Encephalitozoon* spp. and *E. bieneusi*, species-specific primers have been designed to amplify fragments from DNA of *E. hellem* (Visvesvara *et al.* 1994), *E. cuniculi* (De Groote *et al.* 1995), *E. intestinalis* (Hartskeerl *et al.* 1995), and *E. bieneusi* (Franzen *et al.* 1995). Franzen *et al.* (1995) also developed a fluorescein-labelled *E. bieneusi* oligonucleotide probe based on an internal sequence of the 16S rRNA gene, which was used to confirm by Southern blotting that amplification products from human biopsy specimens were those of *E. bieneusi*.

TREATMENT

The intracellular location of developmental stages of microsporidia and the highly resistant nature of the spore wall are factors which render treatment and elimination of infections difficult. Prior to the recognition that microsporidial infections are common in AIDS patients (and probably occur at a subclinical level in immunocompetent people), the antimicrosporidial activity of benomyl, fumagillin, and itraconazole had been demonstrated on species of insect origin. Itraconazole 200 mg given orally twice daily, was later used, together with corneal scraping, in the resolution over a period of 6 weeks of a corneal infection of *E. hellem* (Yee *et al.* 1991). Fumagillin has also been used successfully on *E. hellem* (Rosberger *et al.* 1993). In this case 10 mg/ml of a suspension of fumagillin in saline was applied topically and the keratoconjunctivitis resolved promptly. Broline (propamidine isethionate) applied topically also cured the keratoconjunctivitis due to *E. hellem* in another AIDS patient, but the infection returned when the treatment was discontinued (Metcalfe *et al.* 1992).

The most promising antimicrosporidial drug at present is albendazole. Its activity was first noted in a pilot study of patients with *E. bieneusi* infection (Blanshard *et al.* 1992), when resolution of the diarrhoea was achieved in some patients but without elimination of the infection. In a follow-up study (Blanshard *et al.* 1993) again there was resolution of the diarrhoea in half of the patients, a reduction in parasite load, and abnormalities in the developmental stages and spores. Similar results were obtained with albendazole on *E. bieneusi* by Dieterich *et al.* (1994),

who found that the number of bowel movements decreased and that patients gained weight after treatment. In an *in vitro* study of albendazole on *E. cuniculi*, the drug prevented nuclear and cytoplasmic division and caused cytoplasmic leaching and formation of abnormal bundles of tubules (Colbourn *et al.* 1993). The inhibition of nuclear division is in keeping with the known activity of the drug, i.e. prevention of polymerization of microtubules in the mitotic spindle.

Albendazole is highly effective against the *Encephalitozoon* spp. (De Groote *et al.* 1995; Dore *et al.* 1995; Sobottka *et al.* 1995*b*) and is apparently able to eliminate these infections completely. It may be that the drug is concentrated in the parasitophorous vacuoles, thus being more effective against the *Encephalitozoon* infections than against the dispersed stages of *E. bieneusi*. Alternatively, the different microsporidian species may have different susceptibilities. The recommended dose is 400 mg twice daily for 1 month and can be continued for long periods.

Other drugs with some activity which have been tested *in vivo* but are considered less effective are metronidazole and octreotide.

EPIDEMIOLOGY

Encephalitozoon cuniculi has a wide host range among mammals (Canning and Lom 1986). Prevalences are probably quite low in wild animals but can be high in captivity, as revealed by serological surveys. Thus, in a study of wild rabbits no infections were found but in young broiler rabbits a 15 per cent morbidity was attributed to *E. cuniculi*, as was a 50 per cent mortality in the 0–16-week age group of rabbits in a laboratory colony. Among carnivores, an epidemic in blue foxes (*Alopex lagopus*) resulted in the death of 1500 cubs, and an outbreak of encephalitozoonosis in the Prague Zoo resulted in deaths among several carnivore species.

Encephalitozoon cuniculi is transmitted by ingestion of spores and, under certain circumstances, transplacentally. One of the principal sites of infection is the kidney, and spores are passed, at least sporadically, in urine. Thus, spread of infection under conditions of population density, e.g. rabbit farms, fur farms, laboratory colonies, primate centres, is likely to be by contamination of food or water by urine. The conditions under which infections are likely to be passed from infected mothers to the fetus *in utero* are not fully understood. It is not known whether the infections in the mother must be acute or chronic to be passed on, nor at what stage of development the fetus is most susceptible, nor indeed whether it is developmental stages or spores which effect the transmission. However, severe loss of condition and high mortality rates have been observed in neonate blue foxes and squirrel monkeys, although infections were not overt in the mothers (Mohn *et al.* 1974; Zeman and Baskin 1985). Clearly neonate animals which acquire the infection transplacentally or perinatally are at greatest risk.

In man high prevalences of microsporidia have only been recorded in AIDS patients. The most commonly reported species is *E. bieneusi*, with prevalences varying from about 15 to 30 per cent from different hospitals (Canning *et al.* 1993). The number of reported cases of *E. hellem* is increasing steadily as a result of greater clinical awareness. For example Schwartz *et al.* (1993) reported on seven cases presenting at four ophthalmology units in the United States, and Dore *et al.* (1995) reported on nine cases (8.0 per cent) of *E. intestinalis* in a cohort of 112 patients with microsporidiosis who were treated at one hospital in Australia. Light was shed on the prevalence of *E. intestinalis* by Van Gool *et al.* (1994). Previously thought to occur at much lower prevalence than *E. bieneusi*, it was established *in vitro* regularly from stool of patients with overt *E. bieneusi* infection but barely detectable *E. intestinalis*. Although only four patients were involved, the study suggests that *E. intestinalis* may be at least as common as *E. bieneusi* but at such low levels in most patients that spores are not detectable in stool. The reasons why some AIDS patients develop clinical infections are not known.

Little is known of the origin of human infections. The intestinal and disseminated infections (*E. bieneusi*, *E. intestinalis*, and *E. hellem*) have now been recorded from numerous places in several continents and it is likely that they have a universal distribution. Although *E. hellem* and *E. intestinalis* have only been reported from AIDS patients, there are three reports of *E. bieneusi* in apparently immunocompetent individuals. In a study of 990 children in Niger, microsporidial spores, identified as those of *E. bieneusi* by electron microscopy, were found in abundance in the stool of six children and more rarely in two others (Bretagne *et al.* 1993). The HIV status of the children was not known, but in any case it is unlikely that any of them had T-lymphocyte counts below $100 \times 10^6/1$, which is recognized as the threshold above which microsporidian infections are not normally detected in AIDS patients. Infection could not be correlated with any clinical condition, including diarrhoea, in these children. In contrast, a healthy immunocompetent adult male, who suffered a transient episode of severe diarrhoea when travelling in the Middle East, recovered completely when the spores were no longer detectable in his stool (Sandfort *et al.* 1993). Sobottka *et al.* (1995*a*) reported on a case of dual infection with *E. bieneusi* and *Cryptosporidium* in a child who suffered severe but transient diarrhoea. The limited data

available suggest that *E. bieneusi* is a natural parasite of man. Although E. bieneusi has been detected in pigs (Deplazes *et al.* 1996*b*), it is unlikely that these animals are the direct sources of infection to AIDS patients. Transmission is likely to be by the oral route and it may be that spores are water-borne as has been found for *Cryptosporidium*.

Of the ocular infections, there is evidence to suggest that those caused by *E. hellem* and probably also *V. corneae* (= *N. corneum*) are initiated by ingestion or inhalation, and that corneal infection may be secondary to systemic spread. Infection of *E. hellem* in the kidney, urinary bladder, ureters, throughout the epithelium of the tracheobronchial tree, and focally in the corneal epithelium but not in other organs, was found at an autopsy (Schwartz *et al.* 1992). In the same patient, renal infection was detected ante-mortem apparently without conjunctival or corneal infection. The authors suggested that the eyes may have been infected later by urine-contaminated fingers. Only two cases of *V. corneae* infection have been detected one involving the cornea (Shadduck *et al.* 1990). Organisms isolated into culture have been used to infect athymic mice (Silveira *et al.* 1993). In these mice developmental stages and spores were found in every organ but in the eyes infection was present in the retina not the cornea. Although athymic mice cannot be considered models for the original (human) infection, it is possible that there was a latent systemic infection in both patients and, again, that corneal infection was secondary.

Human infections with *E. cuniculi* appear to be rare. Four infections diagnosed parasitologically (Matsubayashi *et al.* 1959; Bergquist *et al.* 1984; Terada *et al.* 1987; Zender *et al.* 1989) were were identified before *E. hellem* had been distinguished from *E. cuniculi* on antigenic profiles (Didier *et al.* 1991). However, as the sites of infection included brain (probably, because of neurological disorders in two of the patients), liver, and peritoneum, all sites in which *E. hellem* infection has not been reported, it is possible that the identification as *E. cuniculi* was correct. *Encephalitozoon cuniculi* has been diagnosed several times in AIDS patients who were in severe renal failure before the diagnosis and treatment (Hollister *et al.* 1993*a*, 1995; De Groote *et al.* 1995; Deplazes *et al.* 1996*a*). The identifications were based on SDS–PAGE protein profiles, RAPD–PCR profiles, Western blotting, immunofluorescence, and PCR amplification with *E. cuniculi*-specific primers. The protein and RAPD profiles used by Hollister *et al.* (1995) indicated that the human isolate was close to, but not identical to a dog isolate but the dog profile was later confirmed by sequence of the ITS region of the ribosomal genes (Hollister *et al.* 1996*a*). The close association of people with dogs suggests that dogs may often be the source of infection. Some support for this comes from recent work with echinococcosis. Furuya *et al.* (1995*a*) identified *Encephalitozoon* developing in parasitophorous vacuoles in an *in vitro* culture set up from a human liver lesion infected with *Echinococcus multilocularis*. Four out of 10 echinococcal liver lesions were found to be positive for *Encephalitozoon*, and antibodies to *E. cuniculi* were found in 62/119 (52 per cent) of patients with alveolar hydatid disease. Additionally, Furuya *et al.* (1995*b*) found that primers designed for PCR amplification of *E. multilocularis* DNA would also amplify the DNA from purified, *in vitro*-derived spores of the *Encephalitozoon* isolated from hydatid tissue. This is of special epidemiological interest because a survey of 71 serum samples from the Turkana people of Kenya revealed that 47.9 per cent were positive by ELISA when *E. cuniculi* was used as antigen (W. S. Hollister and E. U. Canning, unpublished results). The Turkana people live in very close association with dogs and have a high prevalence of hydatid disease. (*Echinococcus granulosus*), for which dogs are the final hosts.

Trachipleistophora hominis, which infects the skeletal muscle and other tissues of AIDS patients, has some morphological characters in common with the genus *Pleistophora*, species of which are common in fish and decapod crustacea, but the differences are great enough to warrant generic separation. However, only a few species from the non-mammalian hosts have been studied by electron microscopy and some species of *Trachipleistophora* may be parasites of these hosts. It is not known whether spores from fish can pass unharmed through the stomach of mammals, germinate, and initiate infections. The only clue lies in the observation by McDougall *et al.* (1993) of microsporidian spores apparently intact within skeletal muscle in the faeces of an AIDS patient. The authors suggested that the microsporidia had been ingested with food and survived rapid passage in the gastrointestinal tract because the patient had diarrhoea. The genus in this case was thought to be *Nosema*, but it is likely that *Pleistophora* in muscle of fish or crustacea can also survive.

PREVENTION AND CONTROL

Preventive strategies for human microsporidioses are not obvious because very little is known about the origin of the human infections. Patients in the advanced stages of AIDS should perhaps avoid contact with pets but it may be that those patients who develop overt infections have already been harbouring subclinical infections, so that preventive measures at this stage are like shutting the stable door after the horse has fled.

In the case of epidemics of encephalitozoonosis in laboratory colonies or in valuable animals (fur bearing animals), latent infections could be detected and animals with chronic infections culled, to prevent morbidity and mortality in offspring. The use of albendazole may well prove advantageous in these settings.

ACKNOWLEDGEMENTS

The author acknowledges the generous financial support of the Medical Research Council and Wellcome Trust for her research quoted in this review.

REFERENCES

Aarons, E. J., Woodrow, D., Hollister, W. S., Canning, E. U., Francis, N., and Gazzard, B. G. (1994). Reversible renal failure caused by a microsporidian infection. *AIDS*, **8**, 1119–21.

Aldras, A. M., Orenstein, J. M., Kotler, D. P., Shadduck, J. A., and Didier, E. S. (1994). Detection of microsporidia by indirect immunofluorescence antibody test using polyclonal and monoclonal antibodies. *Journal of Clinical Microbiology*, **32**, 608–12.

Ashton, N. and Wirasinha, P. A. (1973). Encephalitozoonosis of the cornea. *British Journal of Ophthalmology*, **57**, 669–74.

Baker, M. D., Vossbrinck, C. R., Didier, E. S., Maddox, J. V., and Shadduck, J. A. (1995). Small subunit ribosomal DNA phylogeny of various microsporidia with emphasis on AIDS related forms. *Journal of Eukaryotic Microbiology*, **42**, 564–70.

Bergquist, N. R., Stintzing, G., Smedman, L., Waller, T., and Andersson, T. (1984). Diagnosis of encephalitozoonosis in man by serological tests. *British Medical Journal*, **288**, 902.

Blanshard, C., Ellis, D. S., Tovey, D. G., Dowell, S., and Gazzard, B. G. (1992). Treatment of intestinal microsporidiosis with albendazole in patients with AIDS. *AIDS*, **6**, 311–13.

Blanshard, C., Ellis, D. S., Dowell, S. P., Tovey, G., and Gazzard, B. G. (1993). Electron microscopic changes in *Enterocytozoon bieneusi* following treatment with albendazole. *Journal of Clinical Pathology*, **46**, 898–902.

Bretagne, S., Foulet, F., Alkassoum, W., Fleury-Feith, J., and Develoux, M. (1993). Prevalence of microsporidial spores in stools from children in Niamey, Niger. *AIDS*, **7** (Suppl. 3), S34–S35.

Buyukmihci, N., Bellhorn, R. W., Hunziker, J., and Clinton, J. (1977). *Encephalitozoon* (*Nosema*) infection of the cornea in a cat. *Journal of the American Veterinary Medical Association*, **171**, 355–7.

Cali, A. *et al.* (1991). Corneal microsporidioses: characterization and identification. *Journal of Protozoology*, **38**, 215S–217S.

Cali, A., Kotler, D. P., and Orenstein, J. M. (1993). *Septata intestinalis* n.g., n.sp., an intestinal microsporidian associated with chronic diarrhea and dissemination in AIDS patients. *Journal of Eukaryotic Microbiology*, **40**, 101–12.

Cali, A. *et al.* (1996). Identification of a new Nosema-like microsporidian associated with myositis in an AIDS patient *Journal of Eukaryotic Microbiology*, **43**, 108S.

Canning, E. U. and Lom, J. (1986). *The Microsporidia of Vertebrates*. Academic Press, London.

Canning, E. U., Hollister, W. S., Colbourn, N. I., Curry, A., and Göbel, U. B. (1993). Human microsporidioses: site specificity, prevalence and species identification. *AIDS*, **7**, (Suppl. 3), S3–S7.

Canning, E. U., Field, A. S., Hing, M. C., and Marriott, D. J. (1994). Further observations on the ultrastructure of *Septata intestinalis* Cali, Kotler and Orenstein, 1993. *European Journal of Protistology*, **40**, 414–22.

Chupp, G. L., Alroy, J., Adelman, L. S., Breen, J. C., and Skolnik, P. R. (1993). Myositis due to *Pleistophora* (Microsporidia) in a patient with AIDS. *Clinical Infectious Diseases*, **16**, 15–21.

Colbourn, N. I., Hollister, W. S., Curry, A., and Canning, E. U. (1994). Activity of albendazole against *Encephalitozoon cuniculi in vitro*. *European Journal of Protistology*, **30**, 211–20.

De Groote, M. A. *et al.* (1995). Polymerase chain reaction and culture confirmation of disseminated *Encephalitoon cuniculi* in a patient with AIDS: successful therapy with albendazole. *Journal of Infectious Diseases*, **171**, 1375–8.

Deplazes, P. *et al.* (1996*a*). Immunologic and molecular characteristics of *Encephalitozoon* microsporidia isolated from humans and rabbits indicated that *Encephalitozoon cuniculi* is a zoonotic parasite. *Clinical Infectious Diseases*, **22**, 557–9.

Deplazes, P., *et al.* (1996*b*). Molecular epidemiology of *Encephalitozoon cuniculi* and first detection of *Enterocytozoon biencusi* in faccal samples of pigs. *Journal of Eurkaryotic Microbiology*, **43**, 935.

Desportes, I. *et al.* (1985). Occurrence of a new microsporidian: *Enterocytozoon bieneusi* n.g., n. sp., in the enterocytes of a human patient with AIDS. *Journal of Protozoology*, **32**, 250–4.

Didier, E. S. *et al.* (1991). Isolation and characterization of a new human microsporidian *Encephalitozoon hellem* n. sp., from three AIDS patients with keratoconjunctivitis. *Journal of Infectious Diseases*, **163**, 617–21.

Didier, E. S., Vossbrinck, C. R., Baker, M. D., Rogers, L. B., Bertucci, D. C., and Shadduck, J. A. (1995). Identification and characterization of three *Encephalitozoon cuniculi* strains. *Parasitology*, **111**, 411–21.

Didier, E. S. *et al.* (1996). Characterization of *Encephalitozoon (Septata) intestinalis* isolates cultured from nasal mucosa and bronchoalveolar lavage fluids of two AIDS patients. *Journal of Eukaryotic Microbiology*, **43**, 34–43.

Dieterich, D. T., Lew, E. A., Kotler, D. P., Poles, M. A., and Orenstein, J. M. (1994). Treatment with albendazole for intestinal disease due to *Enterocytozoon bieneusi* in patients with AIDS. *Journal of Infectious Diseases*, **169**, 178–83.

Doby, J. -M., Jeannes, A., and Rault, B. (1963). *Thelohania apodemi* n. sp., première microsporidie du genre *Thelohania*, observée chez un mammifère. *Compte Rendu Hebdomadaire des Séances de l'Académie des Sciences*, **257**, 248–51.

Dore, G. J., Marriott, D. J., Hing, M. C., Harkness, J. L., and Field, A. S. (1995). Disseminated microsporidiosis due to *Septata intestinalis* in nine patients infected with the human immunodeficiency virus: response to therapy with albendazole. *Clinical Infectious Disease*, **21**, 70–6.

Fedorko, D. P., Nelson, N. A., and Cartwright, C. P. (1995). Identification of microsporidia in stool specimens by using PCR and restriction endonucleases. *Journal of Clinical Microbiology*, **23**, 1739–41.

Field, A. S. *et al.* (1996). Myositis associated with a newly described microsporidium *Trachipleistophora hominis* in a patient with AIDS. *Journal of Clinical Microbiology*, **34**, 2803–11.

Franzen, C. *et al.* (1995). Detection of microsporidia (*Enterocytozoon bieneusi*) in intestinal biopsy specimens from 18 human immunodeficiency virus-infected patients by PCR. *Journal of Clinical Microbiology*, **33**, 2294–6.

Furuya, K., Sato, C., Nagano, H., Sato, N., and Uchino, J. (1995*a*). *Encephalitozoon*-like organisms in patients with alveolar hydatid disease: cell structure, ultrastructure, histoimmunochemical localization and seroprevalence. *Journal of Eukaryotic Microbiology*, **42**, 518–25.

Furuya, K., Nagano, H., and Sato, C. (1995*b*). Primers designed for amplification of *Echinococcus multilocularis* DNA amplify the DNA of *Encephalitozoon*-like spores in the polymerase chain reaction. *Journal of Eukaryotic Microbiology*, **42**, 526–8.

Hartskeerl, R. A., Van Gool, T., Schuitema, A. R. J., Didier, E. S., and Terpstra, W. J. (1995). Genetic and immunological characterization of the microsporidian *Sepatata intestinalis* Cali, Kotler and Orenstein, 1993: reclassification to *Encephalitozoon intestinalis*. *Parasitology*, **110**, 277–85.

Hollister, W. S., Canning, E. U. and Anderson, C. L. (1996*a*). Identificaiton of microsoporidia causing human *disease Journal of Eukaryotic Microbiology*, **42**, 1045–55.

Hollister, W. S., Canning, E. U., and Willcox, A. (1991). Evidence for widespread occurrence of antibodies to *Encephalitozoon cuniculi* (Microspora) in man, indicated by ELISA and other serological tests. *Parasitology*, **102**, 33–43.

Hollister, W. S., Canning, E. U., and Colbourn, N. I. (1993*a*). A species of *Encephalitozoon* isolated from an AIDS patient: criteria for species differentiation. *Folia Parasitologica*, **40**, 293–5.

Hollister, W. S., Canning, E. U., Colbourn, N. I., Curry, A., and Lacey, C. J. N. (1993*b*). Characterization of *Encephalitozoon hellem* (Microspora) isolated from the nasal mucosa of a patient with AIDS. *Parasitology*, **107**, 351–8.

Hollister, W. S., Canning, E. U., Colbourn, N. I., and Aarons, E. J. (1995). *Encephalitozoon cuniculi* isolated from the urine of an AIDS patient, which differs from canine and murine isolates. *Journal of Eukaryotic Microbiology*, **42**, 367–72.

Hollister, W. S., Canning, E. U., Weidner, E., Field, A. S., Kench, J., and Marriott, D. J. (1996*b*). Development and ultrastructure of *Trachipleistophora hominis* n.g., n.sp. after *in vitro* isolation from an AIDS patient and inoculation into athymic mice. *Parasitology*, **112**, 143–54.

Hunt, R. D., King, N. W., and Foster, H. L. (1972). Encephalitozoonosis: evidence for vertical transmission. *Journal of Infectious Diseases*, **126**, 211–14.

Innes, J. R. M., Zeman, W., Frenkel, J., and Borner, G. (1962). Occult endemic encephalitozoonosis of central nervous system in mice (Swiss Bagg-O'Grady strain). *Journal of Neuropathology and Experimental Neurology*, **21**, 519–33.

Kokoskin, E., Gyorkos, T. W., Camus, A., Celidotte, L., Purtill, T., and Ward, B. (1994). Modified technique for efficient detection of microporidia. *Journal of Clinical Microbiology*, **32**, 1074–5.

Lacey, C. J. N., Clarke, A. M. T., Fraser, P., Metcalfe, T., Bonsor, G., and Curry, A. (1992). Chronic microsporidian infection in nasal mucosae, sinuses and conjunctivae in HIV disease. *Genitourinary Medicine*, **68**, 179–81.

Ledford, D. K., Overman, M. D., Gonzalvo, A., Cali, A., Mester, W., and Lockey, R. F. (1985). Microsporidiosis myositis in a patient with the acquired immunodeficiency syndrome. *Annals of Internal Medicine*, **102**, 628–30.

McDougall, R. J., Tandy, M. W., Boreham, R. E., Stenzel, D. J., and O'Donoghue, P. J. (1993). Incidental finding of a microsporidian parasite from an AIDS patient. *Journal of Clinical Microbiology*, **31**, 436–9.

McInnes, E. F., and Stewart, C. G. (1991). The pathology of subclinical infection of *Encephalitozoon cuniculi* in canine dams producing pups with overt encephalitozoonosis. *Journal of the South African Veterinary Medical Association*, **62**, 51–4.

Margileth, A. M., Strano, A. J., Chandra, R., Neafie, R., Blum, M., and McCully, R. M. (1973). Disseminated nosematosis in an immunologically compromised infant. *Archives of Pathology*, **95**, 145–50.

Matsubayashi, H., Koike, T., Mikata, I., Takei, H., and Hagiwara, S. (1959). A case of Encephalitozoon-like body infection in man. *Archives of Pathology*, **67**, 181–7.

Metcalfe, T., Doran, R., Rowland, P., Curry, A., and Lacey, C. J. N. (1992). Microsporidial keratoconjunctivitis in a patient with AIDS. *British Journal of Ophthalmology*, **76**, 177–8.

Mohn, S. F., Nordstoga, K., Krogsrud, J., and Helgebostad, A. (1974). Transplacental transmission of *Nosema cuniculi* in the blue fox (*Alopex lagopus*). *Acta Pathologica Microbiologica Scandinavica (B)*, **82**, 299–300.

Nordstoga, K. (1972). Nosematosis in blue foxes. *Norddisk Veterinaermedicin*, **24**, 21–4.

Ombrouck, C. *et al.* (1995*a*). Use of cross reactive antigens of the microsporidian *Glugea atherinae* for the possible detection of *Enterocytozoon bieneusi* by Western Blot. *American Journal of Tropical Medicine and Hygiene*, **52**, 89–93.

Ombrouck, C., Van Gool, T., Benhamou, Y., Datry, A., Desportes-Livage, I., and Gentilini, M. (1995*b*). Intestinal microsporidiosis: serological studies. *European Journal of Protistology*, **31**, 451 (abstract).

Ombrouck, C., Desportes-Livage, I., Achbarou, A., and Gentilini, M. (1996). Specific detection of the microsporidia *Encephalitozoon intestinalis* in AIDS patients. *Compte Rendu Hebdomadaire des Séances de l'Académie des Sciences*, **319**, 39–43.

Orenstein, J. M. (1991). Microsporidiosis in the acquired immunodeficiency syndrome. *Journal of Parasitology*, **77**, 843–64.

Orenstein, J. M., Dieterich, D. T., and Kotler, D. P. (1992). Systemic dissemination by a newly recognised intestinal microsporidia species in AIDS. *AIDS*, **6**, 1143–50.

Pinnolis, M., Egbert, P. R., Font, R. L., and Winter, F. C. (1981). Nosematosis of the cornea. Case report including electron microscopic studies. *Archives of Ophthalmology*, **99**, 1044–7.

Rabenek, L., Gyorkey, F., Genta, R. M., Gyorkey, P., Foote, L. W., and Risser, J. M. H. (1993). The role of microsporidia in the pathogenesis of HIV-related chronic diarrhea. *Annals of Internal Medicine*, **119**, 895–9.

Rabodonirina, M. *et al.* (1996). *Enterocytozoon bieneusi* as a cause of chronic diarrhoea in a heart-lung transplant recipient who was seronegative for human immunodeficiency virus. *Clinical Infectious Disease*, **23**, 114–17.

Rosberger, D. F. *et al.* (1993). Successful treatment of microsporidial keratoconjunctivitis with topical fumagillin in a patient with AIDS. *Cornea*, **12**, 261–5.

Ryan, N. J. *et al.* (1993). A new trichrome blue stain for detection of microsporidial species in urine, stool and nasopharyngeal specimens. *Journal of Clinical Microbiology*, **31**, 3264–9.

Sandfort, J., Hannemann, A., Gelderblom, H., Owen, R. L., Stark, D., and Ruf, B. (1993). *Enterocytozoon bieneusi* infection in an immunocompetent patient who had acute diarrhoea and who was not infected with the human immunodeficiency virus. *Clinical Infectious Diseases*, **19**, 514–16.

Schwartz, D. A. *et al.* (1992). Disseminated microsporidiosis (*Encephalitozoon hellem*) and acquired immunodeficiency syndrome. Autopsy evidence for respiratory acquisition. *Archives of Pathology and Laboratory Medicine*, **116**, 660–8.

Schwartz, D. A. *et al.* (1993). Pathologic features and immunofluorescent antibody demonstration of ocular microsporidiosis (*Encephalitozoon hellem*) in seven patients with acquired immunodeficiency syndrome. *American Journal of Ophthalmology*, **115**, 285–92.

Seibold, H. R. and Fussell, E. N. (1973). Intestinal microsporidiosis in *Callicebus moloch*. *Laboratory Animal Science*, **23**, 113–18.

Shadduck, J. A. (1969). *Nosema cuniculi*: *in vitro* isolation. *Science*, **166**, 516–17.

Shadduck, J. A., Meccoli, R. A., Davis, R., and Font, R. L. (1990). Isolation of a microsporidian from a human patient. *Journal of Infectious Diseases*, **162**, 773–6.

Silveira, H. and Canning, E. U. (1995). *Vittaforma corneae* N. Comb. for the human microsporidium *Nosema corneum* Shadduck, Meccoli, Davis and Font, 1990, based on its ultrastructure in the liver of experimentally infected athymic mice. *Journal of Eukaryotic Microbiology*, **42**, 158–65.

Silveira, H., Canning, E. U., and Shadduck, J. A. (1993). Experimental infection of athymic mice with the human microsporidian *Nosema corneum*. *Parasitology*, **107**, 489–96.

Sobottka, *et al.* (1995*a*). Self limited travellers diarrhoea due to a dual infection with *Enterocytozoon bieneusi* and *Cryptosporidium parvum* in an immunocompetent HIV-negative child. *European Journal of Clinical Microbiology and Infectious Disease*, **14**, 919–20.

Sobottka, I. *et al.* (1995*b*). Disseminated *Encephalitozoon* (*Septata*) *intestinalis* infection in a patient with AIDS: novel diagnostic approaches and autopsy—confirmed parasitological cure following treatment with albendazole. *Journal of Clinical Microbiology*, **33**, 2948–52.

Terada, S., Reddy, K. R., Jeffers, L. J., Cali, A., and Schiff, E. R. (1987). Microsporidian hepatitis in the acquired immune deficiency syndrome. *Annals of Internal Medicine*, **107**, 61–2.

Van Dellen, A. F., Botha, W. S., Boomker, J, and Warnes, W. E. J. (1978). Light and electron microscopical studies on canine encephalitozoonosis: cerebral vasculitis. *Onderstepoort Journal of Veterinary Medicine*, **45**, 165–86.

Van Gool, T. *et al.* (1990). Diagnosis of *Enterocytozoon bieneusi* microsporidiosis in AIDS patients by recovery of spores from faeces. *Lancet*, **336**, 697–8.

Van Gool, T. *et al.* (1993). Diagnosis of intestinal and disseminated microsporidial infections in patients with HIV by a new rapid fluorescence technique. *Journal of Clinical Pathology*, **46**, 694–9.

Van Gool, T. *et al.* (1994). *Septata intestinalis* frequently isolated from stool of AIDS patients with a new cultivation method. *Parasitology*, **109**, 281–9.

Vávra, J., Dahbiova, R., Hollister, W. S., and Canning, E. U. (1993). Staining of microsporidian spores by optical brighteners with remarks on the use of the brighteners for the diagnosis of AIDS associated human microsporidioses. *Folia Parasitologica*, **40**, 267–72.

Vávra, J. *et al.* (1997). A *Trachipleistoplora*-like microsporidium of man: its dimorphic nature and relationship to *Thclohania apodemi*. *Folia Parasitologica* (in press).

Visvesvara, G. S. *et al.* (1994). Polyclonal and monoclonal antibody and PCR-amplified small-subunit rRNA identification of a microsporidian *Encephalitozoon hellem* isolated from an AIDS patient with disseminated infection. *Journal of Clinical Microbiology*, **32**, 2760–8.

Visvesvara, G. S. *et al.* (1995). Short-term *in vitro* culture and molecular analysis of the microsporidian *Enterocytozoon bieneusi*. *Journal of Eukaryotic Microbiology*, **42**, 506–10.

Vossbrinck, C. R. and Woese, C. R. (1986). Eukaryotic ribosomes that lack a 5.8S RNA. *Nature*, **320**, 287–8.

Vossbrinck, C. R., Maddox, J. V., Friedman, S., Debrunner-Vossbrinck, B. A., and Woese, C. R. (1987). Ribosomal RNA sequence suggests microporidia are extremely ancient eukaryotes. *Nature*, **326**, 411–14.

Vossbrinck, C. R., Baker, M. D., Didier, E. S., Debrunner-Vossbrinck, B. A., and Shadduck, J. A. (1993). Ribosomal DNA sequences of *Encephalitozoon hellem* and *Encephalitozoon cuniculi*: species identification and phylogenetic construction. *Journal of Eukaryotic Microbiology*, **40**, 354–62.

Weber, R. *et al.* (1992). Improved light microscopical detection of microsporidia spores in stool and duodenal aspirates. *New England Journal of Medicine*, **326**, 161–5.

Weber, R., Bryan, R. T., Schwartz, D. A., and Owen, R. L. (1994). Human microsporidial infections. *Clinical Microbiology Reviews*, **7**, 426–61.

Weiss, L. M., Zhu, X., Keohane, E., Cali, A., Tanowitz, H. B., and Wittner, M. (1993). Polymerase chain reaction identification of microsporidia using ribosomal RNA. *AIDS*, **7** (Suppl. 3), S62–S63.

Wright, J. H. and Craighead, E. M. (1922). Infectious motor paralysis in young rabbits. *Journal of Experimental Medicine*, **36**, 135–40.

Yachnis, A. T. *et al.* (1996). Disseminated microsporidosis especially infecting the brain, heart and kidneys: report of a newly recognised pansporoblastic species in two symptomatic AIDS patients. *American Journal of Clinical Pathology*, **106**, 535–43.

Yee, R. W., Tio, F. O., Martinez, J. A., Held, K. S., Shadduck, J. A., and Didier, E. S. (1991). Resolution of microsporidial epithelial keratopathy in a patient with AIDS. *Ophthalmology*, **98**, 196–201.

Zeman, D. H. and Baskin, G. B. (1985). Encephalitozoonosis in squirrel monkeys (*Saimiri sciureus*). *Veterinary Pathology*, **22**, 24–31.

Zender, H. O., Arrigoni, E., Eckert, J., and Kapanci, Y. (1989). A case of *Encephalitozoon cuniculi* peritonitis in a patient with AIDS. *American Journal of Clinical Pathology*, **92**, 352–6.

Zhu, X., Wittner, M., Tanowitz, H. B., Kotler, D., Cali A., and Weiss, L. M. (1993). Small subunit rRNA sequence of *Enterocytozoon bieneusi* and its potential diagnostic role with the use of the polymerase chain reaction. *Journal of Infectious Diseases*, **168**, 1570–5.

Zhu, X., Wittner, M., Tanowitz, H. B., Cali, A., and Weiss, L. M. (1994). Ribosomal RNA sequences of *Enterocytozoon bieneusi*, *Septata intestinalis* and *Ameson michaelis*: phylogenetic construction and structural correspondence. *Journal of Eukaryotic Microbiology*, **41**, 204–9.

Zierdt, C. H., Gill, V. J., and Zierdt, W. S. (1993). Detection of microsporidian spores in clinical samples by indirect fluorescent-antibody assay using whole cell antisera to *Encephalitozoon cuniculi* and *Encephalitozoon hellem*. *Journal of Clinical Microbiology*, **31**, 3071–4.

49 BLASTOCYSTIOSIS

Peter F. L. Boreham and Deborah J. Stenzel

SUMMARY

Blastocystis is a poorly investigated member of the Protista and there are large gaps in our knowledge of all aspects of the parasite and the disease which it is reputed to cause. Vague gastrointestinal symptoms have been associated with infection but none of the putative symptoms are pathognomonic of the infection. There is debate as to whether *Blastocystis* is a zoonosis and can be acquired by humans from animals. Parasites morphologically similar to the human parasite are found in a wide range of animals and this led Garavelli and Scaglione (1989) to suggest that *B. hominis* is a zoonotic infection. The only data to support this conclusion are in a study by Doyle *et al.* (1990), which reported that 44 per cent of 121 patients infected with *B. hominis* had a history of exposure to domestic or farm animals. Only in the past few years has it been possible to suggest the life cycle for this organism based on detailed ultrastructural observations. The parasite is widespread in humans, other mammals, birds, and reptiles, but to date there have been few studies to determine whether this represents one or more species. The organism is most probably transmitted by faecal contamination, with the recently described cyst form as the infective agent.

HISTORY

The history of *Blastocystis* has been reviewed in detail by Zierdt (1991). However, the early reports often do not exclude the possibility that artefacts, such as degenerating tissues, organisms, or yeast cells, were being described. *Blastocystis* was first described as a distinct organism by Alexeieff (1911), who proposed the name *Blastocystis enterocola* and gave an extensive morphological description and a tentative life cycle which included multiple modes of division. Brumpt (1912) proposed the name *Blastocystis hominis* for the organism isolated from human faecal material, and this is the name now recognized. Although Alexeieff (1911) believed that only one species of *Blastocystis* was present in a variety of hosts, Brumpt (1912) concluded that several different species existed. This controversy

has still not been resolved and in this chapter we shall refer to the organism isolated from humans as *B. hominis* and that from other hosts, except where specific species names have been designated, as *Blastocystis* sp. Very few significant advances occurred in our knowledge of this organism until the work of Zierdt *et al.* (1967) which indicated that *Blastocystis* was indeed a protist. This observation renewed interest in *Blastocystis*. Since that time, a large number of case reports of *B. hominis* have been presented (see Boreham and Stenzel 1993*a*), but very few experimental studies have been conducted on the organism.

THE AGENT

TAXONOMY

The exact taxonomic status of *Blastocystis* remains unknown. The organism has variously been described as the cyst of a flagellate, protophyte, yeast, and fungus (see Zierdt 1991). The taxonomy of this organism was put on a sound footing in 1967 when it was assigned to the subkingdom Protista (Zierdt *et al.* 1967). In subsequent publications Zierdt classified it as belonging to the subphylum Sporozoa with a separate suborder, Blastocystina (Zierdt and Tan 1976), and then to the subphylum Sarcodina (Zierdt 1988). Molecular studies have provided some information on the taxonomy of *Blastocystis*, but to date the information is limited. Small subunit rRNA sequencing analysis of a single human isolate has indicated that the taxa *Blastocystis*, *Saccharomyces*, *Toxoplasma*, *Sarcocystis*, *Prorocentrum*, *Tetrahymena* and *Plasmodium* form a clade (Johnson *et al.* 1989). However, *B. hominis* was not monophyletic with *Saccharomyces* nor with any of the sporozoans or sarcodines for which data was examined. This suggests that *Blastocystis* is not closely related to any of these groups. Jiang and He (1993) argue that *Blastocystis* should be given its own subphylum (Blastocysta) in the Protista and it would seem preferable at this stage to classify *Blastocystis* as a genus of uncertain position within the subkingdom Protista (Boreham and Stenzel 1993*b*), a view confirmed by Hollebeke and Mayberry (1994).

In general, *Blastocystis* from all hosts has been classified as a single species, *B. hominis*, although there is now evidence to suggest that there are at least two other true species. A new species, *B. galli* (Belova and Kostenko 1990), first described from the caecum of chickens in the Commonwealth of Independent States, is probably a genuine species based on nuclear morphology (Stenzel *et al.* 1994). *Blastocystis lapemi* has been described from the sea snake (*Lapemis hardwickii*) collected off the coast of Singapore, based on different culture requirements and electrophoretic karyotype (Teow *et al.* 1991). Two other species, *B. anatis* from ducks (Belova 1991) and *B. anseri* from geese (Belova 1992*b*) have been proposed on morphological characteristics. In addition, the parasite found in turkeys was identified as *B. galli* (Belova 1992*a*). The work of Stenzel *et al.* (1994) indicates that the parasites isolated from ducks and geese cannot be consistently distinguished morphologically from *B. hominis*. They concluded that three morphologically distinct groups are represented among the birds studied, one from the chicken (*B. galli*), one from the ostrich, and another from ducks and geese. Thus, the exact speciation of *Blastocystis* among domestic birds and other animals remains unresolved.

At least two discrete groups of organisms were found among *B. hominis* stocks isolated from human stools by protein and DNA analysis (Boreham *et al.* 1992), while serological tests suggest up to four groups (Kukoschke and Müller 1991; Müller 1994). These results indicate that there may be more than one species of *Blastocystis* in humans, but until further work is conducted this cannot be confirmed. No information is available on speciation of *Blastocystis* from non-human mammals.

ANIMAL HOSTS

Blastocystis has been shown to be present in a wide variety of mammals, birds, reptiles and arthropods, although a number of the early records must be questioned because of confusion over the exact nature of the cells observed. Table 49.1 lists hosts where *Blastocystis* has been detected in recent studies. From our own wide-ranging observations, *Blastocystis* sp. has been found in all hosts examined, although often in very small numbers. The hosts include both native and domestic animals.

Only a few attempts have been made to infect experimental animals with *Blastocystis*. The original studies were conducted by Phillips and Zierdt (1976) in gnotobiotic guinea-pigs, using oral or intracaecal inoculations of *B. hominis* from cultured human isolates to produce infections. Approximately 30 per cent of animals became infected when a large inoculum was used. Guinea-pigs were symptomatic, with a watery diarrhoea. The parasite was most prevalent in the caecum, although smaller numbers were found in the ileum and colon. Amoeba-like forms were reported in the epithelial cells but ulceration, lesions, and inflammation were not present in the intestinal mucosa. The low rates of infection of the guinea-pigs may have resulted from the use of cultured vacuolar forms to infect the animals rather than the cyst form.

Suresh *et al.* (1993) showed that neonatal rats could be infected with partially encysted cultures of *B. hominis*, but not with unencysted cultured forms. Also domestic ducks were infected with the caecal contents from mallards and *Blastocystis* sp. was found in the caecum and cloaca up to 1 year after infection (Pakandl and Pecka 1992). No attempt was made in either case to examine possible pathological effects of the organism on the host.

LIFE CYCLE

The life cycle recently proposed by Boreham and Stenzel (1993*a*) for *B. hominis* is shown in Fig. 49.1. The form present in the colon of humans appears to be a small avacuolar cell without a surface coat. As this avacuolar form passes through the colon, the small vesicles present in the cytoplasm probably coalesce to give rise to the multivacuolar forms with a thick surface coat (Fig. 49.2) seen in faecal material. A cyst wall appears to form beneath the surface coat. The surface coat subsequently sloughs off, leaving the cyst form (Fig. 49.3). The cyst wall appears to be composed of chitin (Stenzel 1994) and thus is probably resistant to external environmental conditions. The cyst form is assumed to be the infective form of *B. hominis*. This hypothesis requires further experimental verification, although preliminary support has been provided by Suresh *et al.* (1993). Ingestion of the cyst by a new host and excystation of the cell in the gastrointestinal tract would complete the cycle. Excystation may occur as a result of exposure to gastric acid and intestinal enzymes, as has been described for *Giardia* (see Schaefer 1990).

Very little information is available on differentiation to the amoeboid form (Fig. 49.4), as few amoeboid cells have been found in any samples. However, since there are some morphological similarities, it is possible that the amoeboid form, as described by Dunn *et al.* (1989), arises from the *in vivo* avacuolar form.

The vacuolar form (Fig. 49.5) has been shown to arise in culture from the multivacuolar form, and this may occur by coalescence and enlargement of the smaller vacuoles to form the large central vacuole. Altered culture conditions have been demonstrated to initiate the transformation of the vacuolar form to the granular form (Fig. 49.6).

It seems probable that a continuum of morphological forms of *B. hominis* exists, with the appearance of the organism dependent upon environmental factors.

Table 49.1 Non-human hosts of *Blastocystis*[a]

Species		Comments	Reference
Monkey	*Macaca* sp.	Diarrhoea reported in pig-tail macaque. Large multinucleated cysts in some samples	McClure *et al.* (1980), Yamada *et al.* (1987), Boreham and Stenzel (1993*a*)
	Presbytis sp.	Cyst form uncommon. Vacuolar forms identical to *Blastocystis* from macaques	Boreham and Stenzel (1993*a*)
	Saimiri sp.		Yamada *et al.* (1987)
Pig	*Sus scrofa*	Found in pigs older than 2 days. Present in wild pigs	Burden *et al.* (1978/1979), Pakandl (1991), Stenzel and Boreham (unpublished)
Cattle	*Bos taurus*	Similar morhologically to human *Blastocystis*	Stenzel *et al.* (1993, unpublished)
Sheep	*Ovis aries*	Similar morphologically to human *Blastocystis*	Stenzel, Cassidy, and Boreham (unpublished)
Horse	*Equus caballus*	Similar morphologically to human *Blastocystis*	Stenzel, Boreham, and Gasser (unpublished)
Dog	*Canis familiaris*	43/60 positive from local pound	Duda, Boreham, and Stenzel (unpublished)
Cat	*Felis domesticus*	35/52 positive from local pound	Duda, Boreham, and Stenzel (unpublished)
Alpaca	*Lama pacos*	Exotic animal farm	Stenzel and Boreham (unpublished)
Llama	*Lama glama*	Travelling circus	Stenzel *et al.* (1993)
Camel	*Camelus dromedarius*	Travelling circus	Stenzel *et al.* (1993)
Lion	*Panthero leo*	Travelling circus	Stenzel *et al.* (1993)
Wombat	*Vombatus ursinus*	Veterinary pathology laboratory	Stenzel, Boreham, and Gasser (unpublished)
Eastern grey kangaroo	*Macropus giganteus*	Veterinary pathology laboratory	Stenzel, Boreham, and Gasser (unpublished)
Koala	*Phasolarctos cinereus*	Wildlife park	Stenzel, Cassidy, and Boreham (unpublished)
Guinea-pig	*Cavia porcellus*	Experimental infection of gnotobiotic animals	Phillips and Zierdt (1976), Molet *et al.* (1981)
Chicken	*Gallus gallus domesticus*	Distinct nuclear morphology. Species *Blastocystis galli*	Belova and Kostenko (1990), Yamada *et al.* (1987), Stenzel *et al.* (1994)
Duck	*Anas platyrhynchos*	Present in wild mallards and domestic ducks. Transmissible from wild to domestic animals	Belova (1991), Pakandl and Pecka (1992), Stenzel *et al.* (1994)
Goose	*Anser domesticus*		Belova (1992*b*) Stenzel *et al.* (1994)
Turkey	*Melagris gallopavo*		Lee (1970) Belova (1992*a*)
Ostrich	*Struthio camelus*	Zoological gardens and exotic animal farm. Distinct differences in nuclear morphology	Yamada *et al.* (1987) Stenzel *et al.* (1994)
Sea snake	*Lapemis hardwickii*	*Blastocystis lapemi* grows at 26 °C in culture	Teow *et al.* (1991)
Galapagos tortoise	*Geochelone elephantopus*	Singapore zoo	Teow *et al.* (1992)
Starred tortoise	*Geochelone elegans*	Singapore zoo	Teow *et al.* (1992)

Table 49.1   (Continued)

Species		Comments	Reference
Red-footed tortoise	*Geochelone carbonaria*	Singapore zoo	Teow *et al.* (1992)
Mangrove snake	*Boiga dendrophilla*	Singapore zoo	Teow *et al.* (1992)
Copperhead snake	*Elaphe radiata*	Singapore zoo	Teow *et al.* (1992)
Reticulated python	*Python reticulatus*	Singapore zoo	Teow *et al.* (1992)
Olive python	*Liasis olivaceus*	Veterinary pathology laboratory	Stenzel, Boreham, and Gasser (unpublished)
Esturine crocodile	*Crocodylus porosus*	Singapore zoo	Teow *et al.* (1992)
Rhinoceros iguana	*Cyclura cornuta*	Singapore zoo	Teow *et al.* (1992)
Skink	*Lampropholis delicata*	Queensland garden	Stenzel and Jones (unpublished)
Cockroach	*Periplaneta americana*	Sewers of Singapore	Zaman *et al.* (1993)

[a] Monroe and Lewis (unpublished) conducted a survey of animals at San Diego zoo and found *Blastocystis* in a range of mammals including non-human primates and the orders Artiodactyla, Rodentia, Hyracoidea, Carnivora, and Marsupialia, as well as in eight different orders of birds. Details of the species are not available.

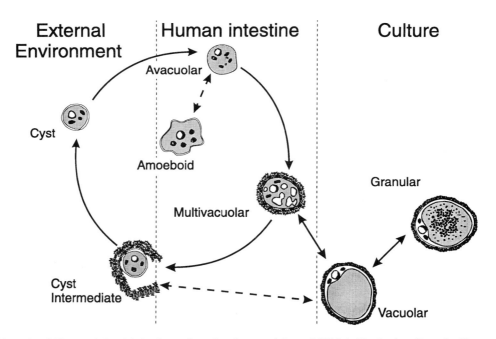

Fig. 49.1   Life cycle of *Blastocystis hominis* (redrawn from Boreham and Stenzel 1993*a*). The broken lines signify unproven pathways.

Physical factors such as osmotic changes or metabolic status may influence the morphology the organism, both *in vivo* and *in vitro*.

MORPHOLOGY OF *BLASTOCYSTIS*

Studies of the ultrastructure of *Blastocystis* have shown considerable heterogeneity of the forms, and the presence of organelles and structures of unknown function. Although *Blastocystis* is an obligate anaerobe, all forms except the amoeboid form contain large numbers of organelles which morphologically resemble mitochondria (Fig. 49.3, 49.5).

Ribosomes, rough endoplasmic reticulum, and lipid inclusions are seen in the cytoplasm of the cells. The Golgi complex is present in the vacuolar, granular, and

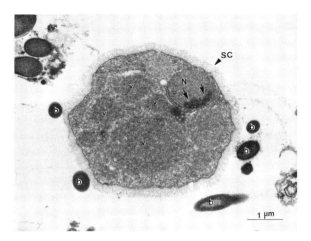

Fig. 49.2 TEM of multivacuolar form of *B. hominis* from human faecal material. A number of small vacuoles are present in the cell. The nucleus displays a crescentic band of condensed chromatin (as indicated by arrows). N, nucleus; v, vacuoles; SC, surface coat; b, bacterium

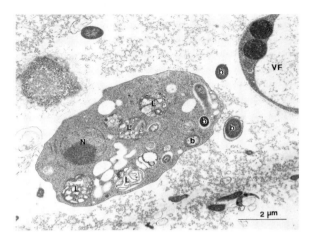

Fig. 49.4 TEM of amoeboid form of *B. hominis* from culture. Bacteria are present in lysosome-like organelles in the cell. N, nucleus; L, lysosome-like organelles; b, bacterium; VF, vacuolar form.

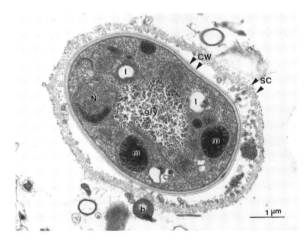

Fig. 49.3 TEM of cyst form of *B. hominis* from human faecal material. A multilayered cyst wall surrounds the cell. Lipid-like inclusions and glycogen are present. N, nucleus; m, mitochondrion; l, lipid-like inclusion; gly, glycogen; SC, surface coat; CW, cyst wall; b, bacterium.

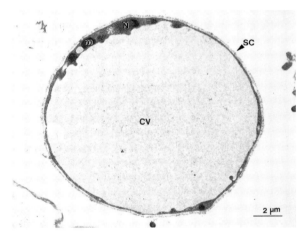

Fig. 49.5 TEM of vacuolar form of *B. hominis* from culture. Organelles are present in a thin peripheral band of cytoplasm surrounding the large central vacuole. N, nucleus; m, mitochondrion; CV, central vacuole; SC, surface coat.

multivacuolar forms. The cyst forms have a condensed cytoplasm, and often large glycogen inclusions (Fig. 49.3).

A thick surface coat is present on all multivacuolar forms of *Blastocystis* from faecal material, but is not found on *B. hominis* obtained directly from the colon of humans, or on the amoeboid form. The surface coat is decreased in thickness or lost entirely after culture of the multivacuolar cells.

The nucleus of *Blastocystis* from most hosts has a characteristic crescentic band of electron-opaque

material, of unknown composition. This structure has been suggested to be a nucleolus, but cytochemical data (Stenzel 1994) do not support this, and indicate that the material is condensed chromatin, containing histone proteins. Nuclear morphology was similar among isolates of *B. hominis* from humans and *Blastocystis* sp. from most animal hosts, except the *Blastocystis* sp. isolated from chickens which had discrete 'spots' of electron-opaque material in the nucleus (Fig. 49.7), rather than a crescentic band. The nuclei of *Blastocystis* from ostriches showed an elliptical rather than a crescentic band (Fig. 49.8).

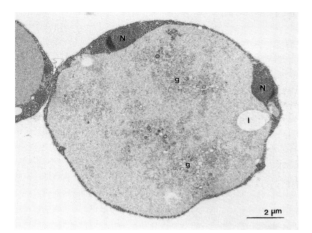

Fig. 49.6 TEM of granular form of *B. hominis* from culture. Granules and a lipid-like inclusion are present in the central vacuole. N, nucleus; g, granules; l, lipid-like inclusion.

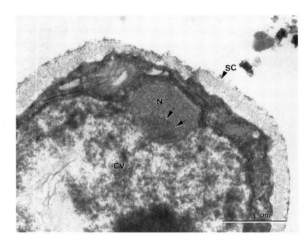

Fig. 49.8 TEM of nuclear region of *Blastocystis* sp. from ostrich faecal material. An elliptical band of condensed chromatin (as indicated by arrows) is seen in the nucleus. N, nucleus; CV, central vacuole; SC, surface coat.

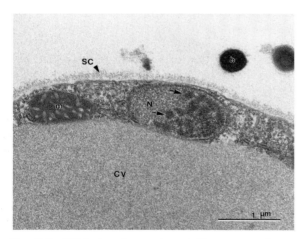

Fig. 49.7 TEM of nuclear region of *Blastocystis* sp. from a chicken. The nucleus displays 'spots' of condensed chromatin (as indicated by arrows). N, nucleus; m, mitochondrion; CV, central vacuole; SC, surface coat; b, bacterium

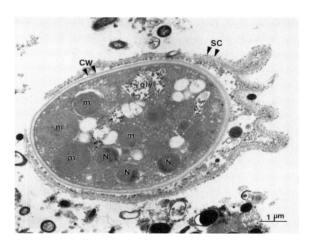

Fig. 49.9 TEM of multinucleated cyst of *Blastocystis* sp. from *Macaca* monkey faecal material. N, nucleus; m, mitochondrion; gly, glycogen; SC, surface coat; CW, cyst wall.

In other respects isolates of *Blastocystis* from animals are similar in morphology to *B. hominis* from humans. However, large multinucleated cysts (Fig. 49.9) have been found in isolates from *Macaca* monkeys. *Presbytis* monkeys housed in the same enclosure did not reveal these cysts.

The limited data currently available for *Blastocystis* sp. from non-human hosts are consistent with the suggested life cycle shown in Fig. 49.1.

GROWTH AND SURVIVAL *IN VITRO*

The culture medium of choice for *Blastocystis* is an inspissated egg slant overlaid with Ringer solution con-

taining 10 per cent horse serum (Boeck and Drbohlav 1925). Other media which have been shown to support the growth of *Blastocystis* include Loeffler medium covered with Ringer solution, containing 20 per cent human serum (Silard *et al.* 1983), Diamond's trypticase panmede serum (TP-S-1) monophasic medium (Molet *et al.* 1981), and minimal essential medium containing 10 per cent horse serum (MEMS), which has been pre-reduced for 48 h (Dunn and Boreham 1991).

Blastocystis hominis cannot be lyophilized but is readily cryopreserved using 7.5 per cent dimethyl-sulphoxide as a cryoprotectant (Zierdt 1991). Optimal results are obtained by controlled slow cooling, maintenance in liquid nitrogen, followed by rapid thawing of the cells at 37 °C. Before the cells are inoculated into a fresh culture tube of pre-reduced medium, they should be washed twice in Locke's solution (Dunn 1992).

THE HOST

DISEASE MECHANISMS

First of all it needs to be stated clearly that *Blastocystis* has not yet been proven to cause disease in either humans or animals. The current position is reviewed by Markell and Udkow (1986), Miller and Minshew (1988), *Lancet* (1991), Zierdt (1991), and Boreham and Stenzel (1993*a*). Evidence that *B. hominis* causes disease is based on observations that there are patients with diarrhoea and other gastrointestinal symptoms where *B. hominis* and no other pathogen or cause of the symptoms can be detected, and secondly, that the putative symptoms of blastocystosis disappear after treatment. However, these findings are disputed because all possible aetiological agents of the diarrhoea, especially viruses and non-infectious causes, are often not excluded and the drugs used to treat *Blastocystis* are not specific, acting on a range of protozoa and anaerobic bacteria.

A very recent study of a patient where no other cause could be found for the symptoms and who was shedding primarily cysts with an unusual morphology, rather than the usual multivacuolar forms, may perhaps suggest that there are some strains or species of *B. hominis* which are pathogenic. This remains to be proven (Boreham *et al.* 1996).

The possibility that *B. hominis* causes toxic–allergic reactions leading to a non-specific inflammation of the colonic mucosa has been raised (Garavelli *et al.* 1991), and oedema of the colonic mucosa with variable presence of lymphocytes and plasmocytes has been noted (Garavelli *et al.* 1992). The significance of these observations is unknown. No studies have been undertaken to determine whether *Blastocystis* contains any toxin or substance likely to be harmful to the host. There is no doubt that *Blastocystis* may be an opportunistic infection in immunosuppressed individuals, but whether as a commensal or pathogen is questionable (Henry *et al.* 1986; Church *et al.* 1992; Cegielski *et al.* 1993).

DIAGNOSIS

The only method currently available for the identification of *Blastocystis* in faeces is parasitological examination. Wet mounts of either fresh stools or concentrates are normally used, although staining with iodine or permanent trichrome mounts may be helpful. It is important to examine the sample for the small

(*c* 5 μm) multivacuolar forms as well as the larger vacuolar forms (10–15 μm) (Stenzel *et al.* 1991). Care must be taken not to confuse *Blastocystis* with leucocytes. Kukoschke *et al.* (1990) compared the effectiveness of microscopy and culture in the identification of positive stools, and found that culture had no benefit over microscopy. Invasive techniques such as endoscopy and 'enterotest' have occasionally been used in diagnosis, but have not been thoroughly evaluated and generally are not required (Matsumoto *et al.* 1987; Narkewicz *et al.* 1989).

TREATMENT

Treatment of *B. hominis* infections in humans is controversial. Many physicians express concern about the risk of unnecessary treatment with potentially dangerous drugs and the failure of physicians to investigate the true cause of symptoms (see Markell and Udkow 1986). However, others believe that if debilitating symptoms are present, and no other cause is obvious, treatment of *B. hominis* infection should be instigated (LeBar *et al.* 1985; Vanatta *et al.* 1985; Lambert *et al.* 1992).

Commonly, antiprotozoal drugs are recommended for treatment of *B. hominis* infections. Generally, metronidazole or iodoquinol (see Boreham and Stenzel 1993*a* for references) have been used. Dietary management also has been suggested, and found to be effective in two studies (Swellengrebel 1917; Kain *et al.* 1987).

The choice and dosage of drugs used is largely empirical, and there are very little experimental data to verify the efficacy of chemotherapy. Only two studies have examined the effects of drugs on *B. hominis in vitro* (Zierdt *et al.* 1983; Dunn and Boreham 1991). In addition, few clinical studies have attempted to determine the effectiveness of chemotherapy, either for reduction in parasite numbers or for alleviation of symptoms (Guirges and Al Waili 1987; Kain *et al.*, 1987; Hussain Qadri *et al.* 1989; Zaki *et al.* 1991). Conflicting results have been reported of the efficacy of both metronidazole and iodoquinol, and whether this reflects the existence of resistance strains of *B. hominis*, differing pharmacokinetic responses of the patients, or other factors remains unknown.

At the present time, the most appropriate drugs for chemotherapy of *B. hominis* would appear to be metronidazole or one of the other 5-nitroimidazoles. However, it should be noted that the infection may be self-limiting, and therapy may not be warranted (Babb and Wagener 1989; Sun *et al.* 1989; Doyle *et al.* 1990; Rosenblatt 1990; Zuckerman *et al.* 1990; Zaki *et al.* 1991). This is especially true in asymptomatic persons, and patients with mild or transient symptoms.

EPIDEMIOLOGY

The epidemiology of *B. hominis* is almost totally unknown. Speculative data have been presented on important factors such as prevalence, mode of transmission, and the importance of animal reservoirs, but studies have been hampered by misinformation and confusion over the status of *B. hominis*. It generally is assumed that *B. hominis* is transmitted by the faecal–oral route, in a manner similar to other gastrointestinal protozoa (Garcia and Bruckner 1988; Ash and Orihel 1990; Lambert *et al.* 1992), but this has not been confirmed.

Water-borne transmission has been reported (Kain *et al.* 1987), and food-borne transmission suggested (Garavelli and Scaglione 1989; Casemore 1990). These modes of transmission have not been proven. Garavelli and Scaglione (1989) suggested that *B. hominis* is a zoonotic infection, and this was supported by the study of Doyle *et al.* (1990), who reported patient histories of exposure to pets or farm animals. A recent report by Zaman *et al.* (1993) suggests that cockroaches may act as vectors for human infection.

Travel, predominantly to developing countries or to wilderness areas, has been implicated as a risk factor in acquiring *B. hominis* infections (Sheehan *et al.* 1986; Kain *et al.* 1987; Yamada *et al.* 1987; Doyle *et al.* 1990; Wittner and Tanowitz 1992). Immigrants and adopted children from developing countries also appeared to have higher incidences of *B. hominis* infection when compared with adults and children raised from birth in their new community (Guglielmetti *et al.* 1991, 1993; Lee 1991) Familial transmission (Guglielmetti *et al.* 1989; Sanad *et al.* 1991; Torres *et al.* 1992), transmission among mentally deficient people in institutions (Yamada *et al.* 1987; Hunt *et al.* 1990; Libanore *et al.* 1991), and in communities without sanitary facilities (Torres *et al.* 1992) have been documented.

Many reports indicate a higher prevalence in adults than in children (Kain *et al.* 1987; Hussain Qadri *et al.* 1989; Doyle *et al.* 1990; Senay and MacPherson 1990; Sanad *et al.* 1991; Ashford and Atkinson 1992). Prevalence rates in various communities are reviewed by Boreham and Stenzel (1993*a*) and are in the order of 1.5–10 per cent in developed countries and 30–50 per cent in developing countries.

PREVENTION AND CONTROL

Since the mode of transmission and risk factors for infection have not been clearly defined, it would appear reasonable to assume at the present time that *B. hominis* is transmitted via the faecal–oral route, and factors which reduce the incidence of ingestion of faecally contaminated material will probably reduce the transmission of *B. hominis*. Thus, the most important means of control would be good personal hygiene, including hand washing, education to prevent faecal contamination of the environment, and improvement in sanitary facilities.

ACKNOWLEDGEMENTS

The original research reported in this review has been supported by grants from the Australian National Health and Medical Research Council, the Australian Research Council and the Queensland University of Technology. We are grateful to Dr. R. Gasser, Mr M. Cassidy and Dr A. Duda for allowing us to quote unpublished data.

REFERENCES

Alexeieff, A. (1911). Sur la nature des formations dites kystes de *Trichomonas intestinalis*. *Comptes Rendus des Séances de la Société de Biologie*, **71**, 296–8.

Ash, L. R. and Orihel, T. C. (1990). *Blastocystis hominis* and fecal elements. In *Atlas of human parasitology*, No. 3, pp. 88–9. American Society of Clinical Pathologists Press, Chicago.

Ashford, R. W. and Atkinson, E. A. (1992). Epidemiology of *Blastocystis hominis* infection in Papua New Guinea: age-prevalence and associations with other parasites. *Annals of Tropical Medicine and Parasitology*, **86**, 129–36.

Babb, R. R. and Wagener, S. (1989). *Blastocystis hominis*—a potential intestinal pathogen. *Western Journal of Medicine*, **151**, 518–19.

Belova, L. M. (1991). *Blastocystis anatis* sp. n. (Rhizopoda, Lobosea) from *Anas platyrhynchos*. *Zoologicheskii Zhurnal*, **70**, 5–10.

Belova, L. M. (1992*a*). On the occurrence of *Blastocystis galli* (Rhizopoda, Lobosea) in turkey. *Parazitologiia*, **26**, 166–8.

Belova, L. M. (1992*b*). *Blastocystis anseri* (Protista: Rhizopoda) from domestic goose. *Parazitologiia*, **26**, 80–2.

Belova, L. M. and Kostenko, L. A. (1990). *Blastocystis galli* sp. n. (Protista: Rhizopoda) from the intestine of domestic hens. *Parazitologiia*, **24**, 164–8.

Boeck, W. C. and Drbohlav, J. (1925). The cultivation of *Entamoeba histolytica*. *American Journal of Hygiene*, **5**, 371–407.

Boreham, P. F. L. and Stenzel, D. J. (1993*a*). *Blastocystis* in humans and animals: morphology, biology and epizootiology. *Advances in Parasitology*, **32**, 1–70.

Boreham, P. F. L. and Stenzel, D. J. (1993*b*). The current status of *Blastocystis hominis*. *Parasitology Today*, **9**, 251.

Boreham, P. F. L., Upcroft, J. A., and Dunn, L. A. (1992). Protein and DNA evidence for two demes of *Blastocystis hominis* from humans. *International Journal for Parasitology*, **22**, 49–53.

Boreham, R. E., Benson, S., Stenzel, D. J., Boreham, P. F. L. (1996). *Blastocystis hominis* infection. *Lancet*, **348**, 272–73.

Brumpt, E. (1912). Côlite à *Tetramitus mesnili* (Wenyon 1910) et côlite à *Trichomonas intestinalis* Leuchart 1879. *Blastocystis hominis* n. sp. et formes voisines. *Bulletin de la Société de Pathologie Exotique*, **5**, 725–30.

Burden, D. J., Anger, H. S., and Hammet, N. C. (1978/1979). *Blastocystis* sp. infections in pigs. *Veterinary Microbiology*, **3**, 227–34.

Casemore, D. P. (1990). Foodborne protozoal infection. *Lancet*, **336**, 1427–32.

Cegielski, J. P. *et al.* (1993). Intestinal parasites and HIV infection in Tanzanian children with chronic diarrhea. *AIDS*, **7**, 213–21.

Church, D. L. *et al.* (1992). Absence of an association between enteric parasites in the manifestations and pathogenesis of HIV enteropathy in gay men. *Scandinavian Journal of Infectious Diseases*, **24**, 567–75.

Doyle, P. W., Helgason, M. M., Mathias, R. G., and Proctor, E. M. (1990). Epidemiology and pathogenicity of *Blastocystis hominis*. *Journal of Clinical Microbiology*, **28**, 116–21.

Dunn, L. A. (1992). Variation among cultured stocks of *Blastocystis hominis* (Brumpt 1912). Ph. D. Thesis, *The University of Queensland*.

Dunn, L. A. and Boreham, P. F. L. (1991). The *in-vitro* activity of drugs against *Blastocystis hominis*. *Journal of Antimicrobial Chemotherapy*, **27**, 507–16.

Dunn, L. A., Boreham, P. F. L., and Stenzel, D. J. (1989). Ultrastructural variation of *Blastocystis hominis* stocks in culture. *International Journal for Parasitology*, **19**, 43–56.

Garavelli, P. L. and Scaglione, L. (1989). Blastocystosis. An epidemiological study. *Microbiologica*, **12**, 349–50.

Garavelli, P. L., Scaglione, L., Bicocchi, R., and Libanore, M. (1991). Pathogenicity of *Blastocystis hominis*. *Infection*, **19**, 185.

Garavelli, P. L., Scaglione, L., Merighi, A., and Libanore, M. (1992). Endoscopy of blastocystosis (Zierdt–Garavelli Disease). *Italian Journal of Gastroenterology*, **24**, 206.

Garcia, L. S. and Bruckner, D. A. (1988). *Diagnostic Medical Parasitology*, (2nd edn). Elsevier, New York.

Garcia, L. S., Bruckner, D. A., and Clancy, M. N. (1984). Clinical relevance of *Blastocystis hominis*. *Lancet*, **1**, 1233–4.

Guglielmetti, P., Cellesi, C., Figura, N., and Rossolini, A. (1989). Family outbreak of *Blastocystis hominis* associated gastroenteritis. *Lancet*, **2**, 1394.

Guglielmetti, P., Sansoni, A., Fantoni, A., and Rossolini, A. (1991). Pathogenesis of blastocystosis. *Lancet*, **338**, 57.

Guglielmetti, P., Fantoni, A., Sansoni, A., and Rossolini, A. (1993). Prevalenza e significato clinico di *Blastocystis hominis* in bambini sintomatici e asintomatici autoctoni e provenienti da aree tropicali. *Revista Di Parassitologia*, **10**, 15–24

Guirges, S. Y. and Al-Waili, N. S. (1987). *Blastocystis hominis*: evidence for human pathogenicity and effectiveness of metronidazole therapy. *Clinical and Experimental Pharmacology and Physiology*, **14**, 333–5.

Henry, M. C. *et al.* (1986). Parasitological observations of chronic diarrhoea in suspected AIDS adult patients in Kinshasa (Zaire). *Transactions of the Royal Society of Tropical Medicine and Hygiene*, **80**, 309–10.

Hollebeke, N. L. and Mayberry, L. F. (1994). Taxonomic uncertainty and *Blastocystis* (Protista: Sarcodina). *Parasitology Today*, **10**, 64.

Hunt, A. L. C., Goldsmid, J. M., and Pasha, M. (1990). Enteric pathogens in mentally handicapped patients in hospital. *Medical Journal of Australia*, **152**, 277–8.

Hussain Qadri, S. M., Al-Okaili, G. A., and Al-Dayel, F. (1989). Clinical significance of *Blastocystis hominis*. *Journal of Clinical Microbiology*, **27**, 2407–9.

Jiang, J. B. and He, J. G. (1993). Taxonomic status of *Blastocystis hominis*. *Parasitology Today*, **9**, 2–3.

Johnson, A. M., Thanou, A., Boreham, P. F. L., and Baverstock, P. R. (1989). *Blastocystis hominis*: phylogenetic affinities determined by rRNA sequence comparison. *Experimental Parasitology*, **68**, 283–8.

Kain, K. C., Noble, M. A., Freeman, H. J., and Barteluk, R. L. (1987). Epidemiology and clinical features associated with *Blastocystis hominis* infection. *Diagnostic Microbiology and Infectious Disease*, **8**, 235–44.

Kukoschke, K. G. and Müller, H. E. (1991). SDS–PAGE and immunological analysis of different axenic *Blastocystis hominis* strains. *Journal of Medical Microbiology*, **35**, 35–9.

Kukoschke, K. G., Necker, A., and Müller, H. E. (1990). Detection of *Blastocystis hominis* by direct microscopy and culture. *European Journal of Clinical Microbiology and Infectious Diseases*, **9**, 305–7.

Lambert, M., Gigi, J., and Bughin, C. (1992). Persistent diarrhoea and *Blastocystis hominis*. *Acta Clinica Belgica*, **47**, 129–30.

Lancet (1991). Editorial: *Blastocystis hominis*: commensal or pathogen. *Lancet*, **337**, 521–2.

LeBar, W. D., Larsen, E. C., and Patel, K. (1985). Afebrile diarrhea and *Blastocystis hominis*. *Annals of Internal Medicine*, **103**, 306.

Lee, D. L. (1970). The fine structure of *Blastocystis* from the caecum of turkey. *Transactions of the British Mycological Society*, **54**, 313–17.

Lee, M. J. (1991). Pathogenicity of *Blastocystis hominis*. *Journal of Clinical Microbiology*, **29**, 2089.

Libanore, M., Rossi, M. R., Scaglione, L., and Garavelli, P. L. (1991). Outbreak of blastocystosis in institution for the mentally retarded. *Lancet*, **337**, 609–10.

McClure, H. M., Strobert, E. A., and Healy, G. R. (1980). *Blastocystis hominis* in a pig-tailed macaque: a potential enteric pathogen for nonhuman primates. *Laboratory Animal Science*, **30**, 890–4.

Markell, E. K. and Udkow, M. P. (1986). *Blastocystis hominis*: pathogen or fellow traveler. *American Journal of Tropical Medicine and Hygiene*, **35**, 1023–6.

Matsumoto, Y., Yamada, M., and Yoshida, Y. (1987). Light microscopical appearance and ultrastructure of *Blastocystis hominis*, an intestinal parasite of man. *Zentralblatt für Bakteriologie, Microbiologie and Hygiene*, **A264**, 379–85.

Miller, R. A. and Minshew, B. H. (1988). *Blastocystis hominis*: an organism in search of a disease. *Reviews of Infectious Diseases*, **10**, 930–8.

Molet, B., Werler, C. and Kremer, M. (1981). *Blastocystis hominis*: improved axenic cultivation. *Transactions of the Royal Society of Tropical Medicine and Hygiene*, **75**, 752–3.

Müller, H. (1994). Four serologically different groups within the species *Blastocystis hominis*. *Zentralblatt für Bakteriologie*, **280**, 403–8.

Narkewicz, M. R., Janoff, E. N., Sokol, R. J., and Levin, M. J. (1989). *Blastocystis hominis* gastroenteritis in a hemophiliac with acquired immune deficiency syndrome. *Journal of Pediatric Gastroenterology and Nutrition*, **8**, 125–8.

Pakandl, M. (1991). Occurrence of *Blastocystis* sp. in pigs. *Folia Parasitologica*, **38**, 297–301.

Pakandl, M. and Pecka, Z. (1992). A domestic duck as a new host of *Blastocystis* sp. *Folia Parasitologica*, **39**, 59–60.

Phillips, B. P. and Zierdt, C. H. (1976). *Blastocystis hominis*: pathogenic potential in human patients and in gnotobiotes. *Experimental Parasitology*, **39**, 358–64.

Rosenblatt, J. E. (1990). *Blastocystis hominis*. *Journal of Clinical Microbiology*, **28**, 2379.

Sanad, M. M., Darwish, R. M., Yousef, S. M., and Nassef, N. E. (1991). *Blastocystis hominis*: laboratory identification and clinical relevance. *Journal of Tropical Medicine*, **1**, 61–70.

Schaefer, F. W. (1990). Methods for excystation of *Giardia*. In *Giardiasis*, (ed. E. A. Meyer), pp. 111–36. Elsevier, Amsterdam.

Senay, H. and MacPherson, D. (1990). *Blastocystis hominis*: epidemiology and natural history. *Journal of Infectious Diseases*, **162**, 987–90.

Sheehan, D. J., Raucher, B. G., and McKitrick, J. C. (1986). Association of *Blastocystis hominis* with signs and symptoms of human disease. *Journal of Clinical Microbiology*, **24**, 548–50.

Silard, R., Panaitescu, D., and Burghelea, B. (1983). Ultrastructural aspects of *Blastocystis hominis*. *Archives Roumaines de Pathologie Experimentale et de Microbiologie*, **42**, 233–42.

Stenzel, D. J. (1995). Ultrastructural and cytochemical studies of *Blastocystis* sp. Ph.D. Thesis, Queensland University of Technology.

Stenzel, D. J., Boreham, P. F. L., and McDougall, R. (1991). Ultrastructure of *Blastocystis hominis* in human stool samples. *International Journal for Parasitology*, **21**, 807–12.

Stenzel, D. J., Cassidy, M. F., and Boreham, P. F. L. (1993). Morphology of *Blastocystis* sp. isolated from circus animals. *International Journal for Parasitology*, **23**, 685–7.

Stenzel, D. J., Cassidy, M. F., and Boreham, P. F. L. (1994). Morphology of *Blastocystis* sp. from domestic birds. *Parasitology Research*, **80**, 131–7.

Sun, T., Katz, S., Tanenbaum, B., and Schenone, C. (1989). Questionable clinical significance of *Blastocystis hominis* infection. *American Journal of Gastroenterology*, **84**, 1543–7.

Suresh, K., Ng, G. C., Ramachandran, N. P., Ho, L. C., Yap, E. H., and Singh, M. (1993). *In vitro* encystment and experimental infections of *Blastocystis hominis*. *Parasitology Research*, **79**, 456–60.

Swellengrebel, N. H. (1917). Observations on *Blastocystis hominis*. *Parasitology*, **9**, 451–9.

Teow, W. L. *et al.* (1991). A *Blastocystis* species from the seasnake *Lapemis hardwickii* (Serpentes: hydrophiidae). *International Journal for Parasitology*, **21**, 723–6.

Teow, W. L. *et al.* (1992). A survey of *Blastocystis* in reptiles. *Parasitology Research*, **78**, 453–5.

Torres, P. *et al.* (1992). Blastocystosis and other intestinal protozoan infections in human riverside communities from Valdivia River Basin, Chile. *Revista Do Instituto de Medicina Tropical de Sao Paulo*, **34**, 557–64.

Vannatta, J. B., Adamson, D., and Mullican, K. (1985). *Blastocystis hominis* infection presenting as recurrent diarrhea. *Annals of Internal Medicine*, **102**, 495–6.

Wittner, M. and Tanowitz, H. B. (1992). Intestinal parasites in returned travelers. *Medical Clinics of North America*, **76**, 1433–48.

Yamada, M. *et al.* (1987). Light microscopical study of *Blastocystis* spp. in monkeys and fowls. *Parasitology Research*, **73**, 527–31.

Zaki, M., Daoud, A. S., Pugh, R. N. H., Al-Ali, F., Al-Mutairi, G., and Al-Saleh, Q. (1991). Clinical report of *Blastocystis hominis* infection in children. *Journal of Tropical Medicine and Hygiene*, **94**, 118–22.

Zaman, V., Ng, G. C., Suresh, K., Yap, E. H., and Singh, M. (1993). Isolation of *Blastocystis* from the cockroach (Dictyoptera: Blattidae). *Parasitology Research*, **79**, 73–4.

Zierdt, C. H. (1988). *Blastocystis hominis*, a long-misunderstood intestinal parasite. *Parasitology Today*, **4**, 5–17.

Zierdt, C. H. (1991). *Blastocystis hominis*—past and future. *Clinical Microbiology Reviews*, **4**, 61–79.

Zierdt, C. H. and Tan, H. (1976). Endosymbiosis in *Blastocystis hominis*. *Experimental Parasitology*, **39**, 422–30.

Zierdt, C. H., Rude, W. S., and Bull, B. S. (1967). Protozoan characteristics of *Blastocystis hominis*. *American Journal of Clinical Pathology*, **48**, 495–501.

Zierdt, C. H., Swan, J. C., and Hosseini, J. (1983). *In vitro* response of *Blastocystis hominis* to antiprotozoal drugs. *Journal of Protozoology*, **30**, 332–4.

Zuckerman, M. J., Ho, H., Hooper, L., Anderson, B., and Polly, S. M. (1990). Frequency of recovery of *Blastocystis hominis* in clinical practice. *Journal of Clinical Gastroenterology*, **12**, 525–32.

50 CYSTICERCOSIS AND TAENIOSIS
TAENIA SAGINATA, TAENIA SOLIUM, AND ASIAN *TAENIA*

Sheelagh Lloyd

SUMMARY

This chapter reviews current knowledge of the taxonomy, epidemiology, diagnosis, therapeutic regimens, and potential control strategies for human *Taenia* spp. The recently identified Asian *Taenia* is compared with *Taenia saginata* and *Taenia solium*, both named in the eighteenth century. Sanitary and agricultural practices that lead to the infection of animal intermediate hosts are described; as are the socio-economic and cultural/dietary practices that lead to infection of humans as definitive hosts for adult tapeworms and as intermediate hosts for the metacestodes of *T. solium*. The relative merits and disadvantages of various diagnostic techniques are discussed. The development of coproantigen ELISA for adult tapeworms in man is a major advance but still is not species specific. Diagnosis of metacestode infections in animals still remains inefficient, with modern immunological techniques not yet showing any major advance over current meat inspection practices. While major advances have been made in diagnosis of neurocysticercosis in man, the merits and disadvantages of CT scan, MRI and antigen/antibody detection methods still mean that no single test should be used for diagnosis and/or prognosis. The advent of albendazole and praziquantel have greatly improved therapy of adult tapeworms and metacestodes in man, but surgery remains an important therapeutic regimen for ventricular, subarachnoid, and ocular cysts. The merits of each therapeutic regimen are discussed in relation to the viability, site, and intensity of infection with metacestodes. Finally, the value of different potential measures for control of the taeniid cestodes of man is discussed in relation to parasite biology and the social, cultural, economic, and agricultural practices that must be considered before implementation of control.

HISTORY

Tapeworm proglottids and metacestodes must have been known prehistory and were mentioned in the Papyrus and by Hippocrates, Aristotle, Galen, and possibly by Moses (Grove 1990). Aristotle compared the metacestodes to hailstones. Aristophanes in the fifth century BC referred to examinations made by cooks for *Taenia solium* in pigs' tongues to determine if the pig was measled. Interestingly, the means of ante-mortem diagnosis in pigs to this day remains palpation of the tongue! In the mid sixteenth and seventeenth centuries cysts were described in the brain of persons with epilepsy. It was not, however, until the eighteenth and nineteenth centuries that Göze and Leuckart distinguished *T. saginata* from *T. solium*. The life cycle of *T. solium* was demonstrated between 1853 and 1860 when Humbert conducted a self-infection and Küchenmeister gave cysts to prisoners about to be executed, while van Beneden in Belgium, Haubner, Küchenmeister, Leuckart, and others completed the life cycle, producing metacestodes in pigs. Details of the life cycle of *T. saginata* developed from the realization that it was common in those that ate raw beef, and Leuckart experimentally produced cysts of *T. saginata* in cattle in the 1860s. Control also was described at this time when Küchenmeister recommended thorough cooking of all pork to prevent infection.

THE AGENTS

Taenia solium Linnaeus, 1758, and *Taenia saginata* Göze, 1782, (= *Taeniarhynchus saginata*) were the taeniids described in man. However, Huang *et al.* (1966) questioned the identity of the *T. saginata* in Taiwan aborigines as they consumed pork and wild animals, ate little beef and raised no cattle. Recently, Fan (1988) and Fan *et al.* (1990, 1992*a,b*) demonstrated that the Taiwan *Taenia*/Asian *Taenia* has pigs as the main intermediate host, Eom and Rim (1993) proposed a new species name. *asiaticus.* It is genetically distinct from *T. solium* and *T. saginata,* but very closely related to *T. saginata* (Zarlenga *et al.* 1991; Bowles and McManus 1994), so McManus and Bowles (1994) suggested it more appropriate to designate the parasite a subspecies or strain.

TAENIA SAGINATA

Adult tapeworms

Adults are 4–8 m long and often occur singly in the small intestine. The scolex has four suckers and no rostellum or hooks. It is followed by the unsegmented neck (growth region), and then hundreds of immature, sexually mature, and gravid proglottids. In mature proglottids testes are scattered through the parenchyma, the ovary is posterocentral and bilobed. In gravid proglottids, the uterus has 14–32 lateral branches but conclusive differentiation from *T. solium* by this is not reliable. There is a vaginal sphincter muscle and the cirrus sac does not extend to the excretory vessels (Verster 1969). An important characteristic is that gravid proglottids leave the host singly and often spontaneously.

Metacestodes

These are cysticerci, fluid-filled bags about 0.5–1.0 cm, into which a single protoscolex (unarmed and without a rostellum) is invaginated.

ASIAN/TAIWAN TAENIA

Adult tapeworms

These are *T. saginata*-like with a similar ovary, vaginal sphincter muscle, cirrus sac, but they do have a rostellum, posterior protuberances on proglottids, and 11–32 uterine buds. Proglottids are passed singly and often spontaneously (Fan 1988; Fan *et al.* 1992*c*).

Metacestodes

These are smaller than *T. saginata* metacestodes. The protoscolex has a rostellum and two rows of primitive hooklets: Those of the outer row are numerous and tiny; those of the inner row number 13–24 (6–76) (Fan 1988; Fan *et al.* 1992*b*; Eom and Rim 1993).

TAENIA SOLIUM

Adult tapeworms

Adults are 3–5 m long with a rostellum carrying two rows of hooks 130–180 μm long. The ovary has a third (accessory) lobe, there is no vaginal sphincter muscle, the cirrus pouch extends to the excretory vessels, and gravid proglottids have 7–13 (<116) lateral branches. Gravid proglottids do not normally leave the host spontaneously but passively in chains.

Metacestodes

These are up to 2 cm in diameter have a rostellum with two rows of hooks. Some cysts, primarily in the subarachnoid space or basal cisterns in humans, evolve into a racemose form of hydropic degeneration, without a scolex, producing large bullae which can fill the cisterns or appear as clusters of grapes.

Eggs of all three taeniids are very similar in size and range from about 30 to 45 μm in diameter. The oncosphere carries three pairs of hooks. The embryophore (the so-called 'shell') is thick, brown, and striated, being composed of blocks. An outer thin capsule is present in eggs from fresh proglottids but lost from eggs in faeces.

HOSTS

1. *Taenia saginata*:
   Adult tapeworm: humans
   Metacestodes: cattle; reindeer; wild ruminants, but to what extent requires determination. Some mature, unarmed cysticerci have been recovered from the liver of pigs fed *T. saginata* eggs (Fan *et al.* 1992*d*)

2. *Taenia solium*:
   Adult tapeworm: humans; development to the sexual stages has been achieved in immunosuppressed hamsters (Allan *et al.* 1991).
   Metacestodes: domestic and wild pigs; humans; also, dogs; the identity of metacestodes in other species usually is not confirmed

3. Asian *Taenia*:
   Adult tapeworm: humans
   Metacestodes: domestic and wild pigs; also, cattle, goats, monkeys

LIFE CYCLE AND EPIDEMIOLOGY

TAENIA SAGINATA

Excretion of eggs

The prepatent period is 87–100 days. Gravid proglottids, 3–10 or more a day, separate individually from the end of the tapeworm; some migrate spontaneously from the anus and in the perianal region to drop off; others are passed passively in the faeces, usually on the surface, or may partially break down in the intestine. Proglottids will migrate a few centimetres. Eggs are released, from an opening created when segments break from the tapeworm, into the intestine, on the skin, or on the ground, by pressure of eggs in the uterus and muscular contractions of the crawling proglottid. Egg production may vary between 100 000 and 1 000 000 day. Periodically a variable length of mature/gravid proglottids is lost and gravid proglottids are not passed until this chain is replaced. The adult tapeworm survives up to 30 years.

Eggs in the environment

Desiccation is rapidly lethal to eggs, but they will survive for several weeks or months in sewage, river water, on pasture, etc. (Silverman 1956; Suvorov 1965). Eggs reach cattle in a variety of ways:

1. Eggs are sticky and contaminate hands and fingers. This is described as a route of infection for artificially reared calves when calves are taught to suck by *T. saginata*-infected handlers (Urquhart 1961; Khadaiberganun 1980).
2. The high prevalence of *T. saginata* in pastoralist grazing systems of Africa, etc., comes from cattle grazing around human habitations that have no sanitation.
3. 'Cysticercosis storms', where large groups of naive cattle become heavily infected, occur when an infected worker defaecates indiscriminately to contaminate food, or in silos of cattle feedlots or water supplies (Dewburst *et al.* 1967; Schultz *et al.* 1969; McAninch 1974; Slonka *et al.* 1978).
4. Most sewage treatment plants do not adequately remove taeniid eggs; irrigation/fertilization of pastures with relatively fresh sewage effluent, slurry, and sludge has been responsible for several outbreaks of cysticercosis in herds of cattle in the developed world (Rickard and Adolph 1977; Macpherson *et al.* 1978). Access to streams carrying effluent from sewage treatment plants was a major risk factor for cattle in Denmark (Kyvsgaard *et al.* 1991).
5. Increased travel and tourism and indiscriminate deposition of faeces on camp grounds, along main roads, and along rail tracks transfer infection to and from urban individuals (Pawlowski 1982).
6. Egg dispersal by flies to pastures at high intensity over 80 m and lower intensity for up to 10 km (Chapter 52) will transfer *T. saginata* from human faecal deposits to grazing cattle. Further examinations are required on the role of birds in dispersal, e.g. gull ingestion of segments from sewage (Silverman and Griffiths, 1955) and insectivorous bird–insect co-operation for long-distance, low-level contamination of pastures, as suggested for *T. hydatigena* (Torgerson *et al.* 1992).

Metacestodes in cattle

Eggs, ingested by cattle, produce metacestodes in skeletal and cardiac muscle and occasionally internal organs. Metacestodes are infective in 8–10 weeks. Predilection sites, or at least sites where the cysts are most obvious, are the masseters, heart, diaphragm, and tongue, but a high proportion of the cysticerci are found through all the musculature. Cyst viability seems to be higher in the skeletal musculature than in the more active muscles of predilection. A substantial number of cysticerci are dead and calcifying by 9 months. However, some infections, e.g. infections of neonatal calves, can survive for very prolonged periods (Urquhart 1961; Soulsby 1963). Strong immunity to re-infection does develop in cattle, largely antibody-mediated (Lloyd 1987).

Infection of humans with the adult tapeworm

Infection depends on the consumption of raw or lightly cooked meat. Infection is common in parts of Africa and Latin America where meat, which is unlikely to have undergone any meat inspection or freezing, is eaten raw and/or variably cooked on open fires. Food preparation, dietary habits, and preference of eating raw or rare beef delicacies (e.g. beef tartare in Europe and the CIS) are contributory factors to increased prevalence of *T. saginata* carriers.

Infection of humans with metacestodes

Man is not normally regarded as a host for the metacestodes of *T. saginata*. Rare reports of cysts have not been accompanied by strong documentation.

ASIAN *TAENIA*

Excretion of eggs and eggs in the environment

This part of the life cycle is similar to that of *T. saginata*. Close association between the intermediate host pigs (and other animals) and humans within habitations without sanitation, the pigs undoubtedly acting as sanitary policemen, must be important in transmission to pigs.

Metacestodes in pigs and other animals

Pigs are an important intermediate host, but the infection has been induced experimentally in wild boars, cattle, goats, and monkeys. The metacestodes develop primarily in the liver, with more in the parenchyma than on the surface. Up to 30 per cent of cysts have been found in the omentum, lungs, and colonic serosa (Eom *et al.* 1992). Development is rapid, mature metacestodes are seen as early as 27–43 days and survive at least 79 days after infection (Fan *et al.* 1990).

Infection of humans with the adult tapeworm

Dietary preferences that induce infection in South–East Asia are the raw or only lightly grilled meat and viscera of pigs and wild animals (Fan *et al.* 1992*e*).

Infection of humans with metacestodes

There is no evidence that humans are infected with metacestodes of Asian *Taenia*. Bowles and McManus (1994) disagree with Ito (1992) and consider that, as Asian *Taenia* is very closely related to *T. saginata*, it is unlikely to cause human cysticercosis. Further, adult tapeworms are common in South-East Asia, but cysticercosis is not and, as pork meat also is eaten raw, *T. solium* cysticercosis can occur. However, Asian *Taenia* has a wide intermediate host range, including monkeys, so human liver infection cannot yet be ruled out.

TAENIA SOLIUM

Excretion of eggs

Less is known about egg production and excretion in *T. solium*- than in *T. saginata*- infected persons. The prepatent period is about 9–10 weeks. Gravid proglottids, which contain about 50 000 eggs, do not leave the host spontaneously but passively in the faeces in a chain of about 5–6 a day (**1** in Fig. 50.1).

Eggs in the environment

Where *T. solium* is common free-ranging pigs act as 'sanitary policemen' to remove human faeces (**2** in Fig. 50.1) (Sarti-G *et al.* 1992). Pigs presumably can eat whole chains of proglottids in faeces and so massive numbers of eggs. Other means for dispersal of eggs have not been examined for *T. solium*, e.g. fly-borne transfer, carriage by birds, etc., from faecal deposits to areas where pigs graze/root.

Metacestodes in pigs

Metacestodes, infective about 10 weeks after infection, occur primarily in the skeletal and cardiac muscles of pigs and also in the brain. The length of cyst survival in pigs is not known, but this probably is not critical in limiting transfer as most pigs are slaughtered younger than cattle.

Infection of humans with adult tapeworms

Cultural dietary preferences which include eating of raw flesh, methods of cooking that include smoking, variable grilling on fires, cooking between hot stones in West Irian, Indonesia, and consumption of the delicacy of measly pork ('tomatillo') in Mexico, all ensure ingestion of viable metacestodes (**3** in Fig. 50.1). In many

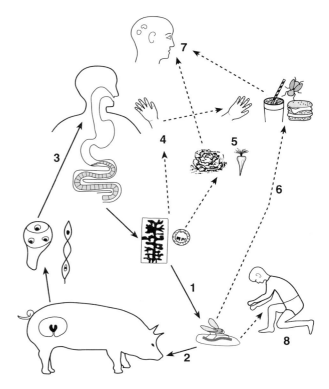

Fig. 50.1 Life cycle of *Taenia solium*. Solid line, human–pig–human transfer: **1**, chains of proglottids passed in faeces; **2**, proglottids or eggs eaten with faeces by pigs acting as sanitary policemen; flies harbouring eggs also could be eaten by pigs rooting in rubbish dumps, etc.; **3**, metacestodes eaten in pork that is raw or lightly smoked or cooked. Dashed line, human–human transfer to result in human cysticercosis: **4**, faeco-oral transfer of eggs, e.g. by contaminated hands; such persons then may contaminate the food of other people; **5**, contamination of vegetables, etc., for example through use of night soil for fertilization, faecal contamination of irrigation water, etc.; **6**, transfer of eggs from faeces to food in the vomitus, on the body and in faeces of lapping flies. These all result in: **7**, accidental oral infection of persons not concurrently infected with the adult tapeworm; and **8**, ingestion of eggs in contaminated soil, e.g. by children with geophagia.

rural communities no meat inspection is available and, where it is, antemortem diagnosis by palpation of cysts on the tongue will result in meat by-passing official inspection and being sold cheaply or illegally through unofficial meat channels to avoid condemnation. Some societies in the Far East consume dog meat, and dogs can act as an intermediate host, with cysts reported mainly in the brain but undoubtedly present in other tissues, to give another source of infection.

Infection of humans with metacestodes

Humans also act as intermediate hosts for the metacestodes of *T. solium* when they ingest eggs passed by a human carrier of the adult tapeworm. It is possible that tapeworm carrying humans may become infected by autoinfection, e.g. reverse peristalsis and vomiting, with internal hatching of eggs, but this is largely discounted (Webbe 1967). The metacestodes occur in the musculature, subcutaneous tissues, and occasionally viscera, but are most obvious in the brain, spinal cord, and eye.

Human–human transfer (**4** and **7**, Fig. 50.1) is common in rural areas with poor water supply and sanitation and where the man–pig–man cycle occurs. Also, where *T. solium* is endemic, meat that either has bypassed meat inspection or in which meat inspection has failed to detect the infection, will be sold in semi-urban and urban areas. Subsequent man–man transfer of infection acquired in this way can be quite high in urban areas. Finally, humans may be exposed to man–man transfer of infection even in non-endemic countries when infected immigrants/travellers contaminate food.

Poor personal hygiene with direct faeco-oral transfer of eggs or contamination of food is important in human cysticercosis (**4** Fig. 50.1). Risk factors for human infection with metacestodes have been recorded as a history of passing proglottids, frequent pork consumption, poor personal and household hygiene, and residence in a household of a person with a history of passing segments. Significant clustering of seropositive persons is described in village households in Mexico (Sarti *et al.* 1992). The importance of a carrier in the household increases when such a person prepares and serves food, with clustering of neurocysticercosis cases, e.g. in some Jewish families in New York where infected immigrants acted as household employees, e.g. housekeepers (Schantz *et al.* 1992; Sorvillo *et al.* 1992). However, this certainly is not the only route of infection in endemic areas and other potential routes require confirmation. Contamination of vegetables by fertilization with human faeces and by use of contaminated water must occur (**5**, Fig. 50.1). Indiscriminate defaecation with subsequent fly-borne deposition of eggs from faeces on to food (**6**, Fig. 50.1) as described for *T. hydatigena* and presumed for *E. granulosus* may occur (Chapter 52). Children in particular will acquire infection by geophagia (**8**, Fig. 50.1) (see *Toxocara*, Chapter 65).

GEOGRAPHIC DISTRIBUTION

TAENIA SAGINATA

Taenia saginata occurs worldwide. Virtually every country reports infection; exceptions are mainly islands in the West Indies and Pacific (*FAO/OIE/WHO Animal Health Yearbook* 1992). The infection is pre-valent throughout Africa, particularly in some Central and East African countries, in the Caucasian and south-central Asian countries, and in parts of the eastern Mediterranean (Syria, Lebanon, Bosnia, and Montenegro). Surveys in these countries have found infection in more than 10 per cent of humans and 10–80 per cent of cattle (Pawlowski and Schultz 1972). Infection rates are lower but the parasite is present in eastern Europe, Central and South America. Prevalence is very low in humans in North America, parts of western Europe, Australia, New Zealand, but remains sporadic detected, by meat inspection, in up to 0.5 per cent of cattle in countries such as the United Kingdom, The Neitherlands, Denmark, etc. The high prevalences described previously for *T. saginata* in South-East Asia must now be attributed to the Asian *Taenia*, but *T. saginata* remains present in these areas.

ASIAN/TAIWAN TAENIA

Infection rates in man of 2–18 per cent were described in 10 mountainous districts in Taiwan (Fan *et al.* 1992*e*) and it occurs in China, Korea, Thailand, Burma, Malaysia, the Philippines, and Indonesia. Infection studies suggest it might be present in East Africa (e.g. Madagascar, Ethiopia) and might account for liver cysticercosis in cattle in Kenya.

TAENIA SOLIUM

Taenia solium is important in pork-eating countries, usually of low social development with poor sanitation, where human faeces are an important part of the diet of free-ranging, scavenging pigs. Infection is common in Central and South America, Southern Africa, parts of the CIS and the People's Republic of China, and non-Islamic areas of Asia. Infection in man, usually imported, is reported occasionally in countries of North America, Europe, Australia/New Zealand. Some studies in Mexico and other areas in Latin America have shown a prevalence of 0.2–7.1 per cent in humans and 10–30 per cent in pigs in rural villages (Acha and Aguilar 1964; de Aluja 1982; Cruz *et al.* 1989; Sarti-G *et al.* 1994).

SYMPTOMS, CLINICAL SIGNS, AND PATHOGENESIS

TAENIOSIS

The most obvious symptom for *T. saginata* and Asian *Taenia* is the spontaneous migration of proglottids from the anus and in the perianal area giving a crawling/itching sensation for perhaps 5 min (Pawlowski and Schultz 1972; Fan *et al.* 1992*c*). Only 2–5 per cent those questioned did not describe this feature. Variable levels of pruritis ani are reported. Common symptoms are nausea and abdominal pain; others are dizziness, weakness, headache, increased appetite, feeling of hunger, diarrhoea or constipation, loss of weight, vomiting. The symptomatology of *T. solium* is less marked and, in particular, migration of proglottids and pruritis ani are not prominent features so *T. solium* is far more likely to go unnoticed.

CYSTICERCOSIS IN ANIMALS

The metacestodes of *T. solium* and *T. saginata* are unlikely to cause any clinical signs other than palpable cysts in the tongue. Experimental infections with several hundred thousand eggs, have produced muscle weakness and reluctance to move for several days, possibly related to the oncospheres settling in the muscles, and, rarely, death from myocarditis. As pigs might ingest a complete chain of proglottids, this might occur in the field. Pigs develop neurocysticercosis but whether these cysts produce neurological disease has not yet been determined, as many pigs are slaughtered young and older infected animals are unlikely to have close clinical examinations.

CYSTICERCOSIS IN HUMANS

Disseminated cysticercosis

Cysts in the tissues, at subcutaneous, intramuscular, and occasionally visceral sites, usually are asymptomatic, though the site may be tender and, in heavy infections, there may be muscle pain and weakness. The granulomatous, inflammatory infiltration of dead cysts may resolve completely or leave variable sized, oval/rounded areas of fibrosis and calcification.

Neurocysticercosis

Sixty to ninety per cent of cysticercosis infected persons also have metacestodes in the CNS (brain parenchyma, meninges, subarachnoid space, ventricles, spinal cord). Neurocysticercosis has clinical polymorphism described by Zenteno-Alanis *et al.* (1982) depending on the intensity of infection, site of cysts, and current viability of cysts plus immune response of the host. In a Mexican village study, half of those that were seropositive denied any clinical signs (Sarti-G *et al.* 1994). Commonly 1–5 cysts are present; means of 5 and 12 cysts were recorded in two recent studies (Vazquez and Sotelo 1992; Botero *et al.* 1993), but over 1000 have been described.

The proportion of neurocysticercosis patients that present as clinical cases is unknown and will depend on available medical facilities. Patients may present from a few months to perhaps 30 years after infection.

1. Viable cysts in the parenchyma or ventricular system are space-occupying lesions that, depending on site, may cause immediate symptoms. Alternately, cysts may remain viable without signs for many years. Reasons for death of cysts and the immune inflammatory response are still unknown.

2. Dying cysticerci (transitional lesions) are surrounded by strong, circular inflammatory lesions of plasma cells, lymphocytes, macrophages, and eosinophils, that subsequently will invade the cyst. Generally the inflammatory processes provoke more problems than the cyst itself and, in some previously asymptomatic patients, symptoms will be provoked.

3. In some patients, more commonly children and young women, there can be diffuse parenchymal involvement—cysticercosis encephalitis.

4. Finally, there can be either complete resolution of lesions or mineralization and persistence of calcified cysts. This may produce complete remission of symptoms or, alternately, partial or no improvement as some scars continue to provoke convulsions, etc.

The most common presenting sign in neurocysticercosis is seizures. Convulsions were recorded in 50 per cent of neurocysticercosis patients (Schenone *et al.* 1982) and in 82 and 88 per cent of patients with active or transitional lesions (Carpio *et al.* 1994). Neurocysticercosis was described as the aetiological agent in 50 per cent of cases of late-onset epilepsy in endemic areas (Medina *et al.* 1990). Other symptoms, varying with cyst site, are hemiparesis, visual tract damage, movement disorders, and numbness. Increased intracranial hypertension is common, recorded in 53 per cent of patients by Schenone *et al.* (1982), causing violent and chronic headache, vomiting, neurophsychiatric changes, and visual impairment. Papilloedema may occur. Ventricular cysts may be rapidly fatal if they cause complete sudden blockages of the CSF pathways. Alternately, they can cause intermittent increased cranial hypertension with hydrocephalus, violent headache, nausea, and movement disorders. Various localized syndromes from cysts in the subarachnoid space or ventricles are described (Schenone *et al.* 1982). A mesencephalic syndrome of abnormal movements, halting speech, ocular defects, and with poor prognosis, is seen in patients where arachnoiditis, arteritis, and granular ependymitis have occurred, possibly due to venous congestion induced by a cyst or hypertension. Meningeal cysts can produce meningitis. Intramedullary spinal cord cysts occur in up to 5 per cent of cases manifesting as motor or sensory disorders due to compression of tissue.

Ocular cysticercosis

Parasites are located in an eye in about 25 per cent of cases. These are diagnosed at a younger age, probably due to early effects of parasites on visual acuity with blurred vision, shadows, etc. (Cardenas *et al.* 1992). Most cysts are found in the subretinal tissues and vitreous humour, a few in the aqueous humour, supporting a migratory route of arrival in subretinal arteries, the cyst then breaking through the retina into the vitreous humor (Zenteno-Alanis *et al.* 1982; Cardenas *et al.* 1992). On cyst death, there can be severe chorioretinitis with complications such as retina detachment. Cysts in a subretinal or subconjunctival location may manifest as slowly growing nodules, potentially confused with tumours (Zenteno-Alanis *et al.* 1982).

DIAGNOSIS

TAENIOSIS

Symptoms, if any, induced by adult tapeworms are insufficiently specific for diagnosis. Carriers (>95 per cent) of *T. saginata* are likely to recognize the infection through the spontaneous migration of proglottids from the anus, so questioning is useful in surveys, but is not absolute as carriers may deny infection, recall previous infection, or confuse infection with *Enterobius vermicularis*. Perianal migration means eggs may be found on swabs or scotch tape applied to the perianal area, this and faecal examination (ethyl acetate extract or Kato thick smear) can reveal eggs in 60–90 per cent of carriers. However, proglottids are released intermittently, as are eggs from proglottids, so eggs are not evenly dispersed and easily missed or absent. These methods of diagnosis are not necessarily satisfactory for *T. solium*. Chains of proglottids passed passively in the faeces are less likely to be noticed and less likely to leave eggs in the perianal area, with fewer eggs released into faeces. Questioning of carriers infected mainly with *T. solium* revealed only 12–50 per cent positives (de Kaminsky 1991; Allan *et al.* 1993). Egg examination cannot differentiate species.

An important development has been antigen capture AG-ELISA to detect coproantigen in faeces. It is less subjective, more sensitive, and has recently been developed into a dipstick technique (Allan *et al.* 1992; 1993). Of 41 persons confirmed positive as they passed proglottids after treatment: the dot-AG-ELISA detected 76 per cent; microscopy 56 per cent; and questioning 12 per cent. This technique, therefore, is very useful for screening, but does not differentiate *T. saginata* and *T. solium*. DNA probes that differentiate *T. solium* and *T. saginata* have been developed (Harrison *et al.* 1990) but cannot be considered a survey technique and suffer from the fact that proglottids and eggs can be absent from faeces or aggregated. Ultimately, treatment to obtain the tapeworm for specific identification, preferably by the scolex, still is required. This is hazardous and known to give false negatives as treatment is not 100 per cent effective, while patients may deny passing a tapeworm (Hall *et al.* 1981).

CYSTICERCOSIS IN ANIMALS

Palpation of the tongue

This reveals nodules and still remains the technique used to detect infection in living pigs. It is extremely time consuming and is not sensitive, but is useful to define villages with high levels of transmission.

Meat inspection

This remains the most widely used method to detect and divert infected carcasses for treatment or condemnation. However, meat inspection detects only a proportion of infections and is particularly inadequate in light infections; the relatively few cuts that can be made without detracting from carcass value will miss infections, and cysts may not be present in predilection sites. Meat inspection can have an overall detection rate of only 32–38 per cent: 78 per cent of carcasses infected with more than 20 cysts were detected, but only 31 per cent of those with fewer cysts (Rickard and Adolph 1977; Walther and Koske 1980).

Immunodiagnosis

Serological tests, including ELISA, are not yet acceptable for diagnosis of infection in individual animals but may be useful on a herd basis when cysticercosis 'storms' occur. Specificity generally is low, particularly in animals with other metacestode or trematode infections, and live versus dead infections are not distinguished. Recently, monoclonal antibody based AG-ELISAs that detect only live infections have been described (Harrison *et al.* 1991; Brandt *et al.* 1992). Sensitivity needs improvement as AG-ELISA detected only more than 88 to 200 cysts, although Onyango-Abuje *et al.* (1993) have recently reported identification of 47 per cent of infected cattle and 43 per cent of 30 animals with up to 30 cysticerci.

CYSTICERCOSIS IN HUMANS

Disseminated cysticercosis

Cysts may be palpated and biopsied to differentiate them from tumours, abscesses, etc. Calcified cysts will be detected by radiography.

Neurocysticercosis

Computed tomography (CT scan)

This is particularly useful to determine site and intensity of infection and to differentiate between live, dying (transitional), and dead cysts in the brain parenchyma (Del Brutto *et al.* 1993; Carpio *et al.* 1994):

1. Live cysts in the parenchyma appear as rounded areas of low density with no perilesional oedema and show little or no contrast enhancement.

2. The image of transitional cysts in the parenchyma varies with the degree of host response and viability of the cyst. A colloidal phase, as the cyst fluid becomes gelatinous, may show as ill-defined hypo- or isodense lesions but the wall will be thickened by the inflammatory response and there is perilesional oedema and ring enhancement on contrast. The lesion becomes nodular or granular as the cyst is replaced with inflammatory tissue. This stage is the most difficult to differentiate from tuberculoma, astrocytoma, metastases, abscesses.

3. Dead cysts are apparent as annulated, rounded, or pedunculated areas of calcification usually of less than 10 mm.

4. CT scan is very useful for cysticercosis encephalitis, seen as diffuse cerebral oedema, small or collapsed ventricles with, on contrast, multiple nodular or annular images through the parenchyma. Differentiation from multiple tuberculoma, toxoplasmosis, and microabscesses, can be a problem.

5. CT scan is less useful for ventricular or subarachnoid cysts that occur in up to 25 per cent of patients. The cysts are often isodense, with the thin wall and scolex rarely visualized. Contrast ventriculography improves efficacy but this is an invasive technique and the cyst itself or ependymitis may occlude the CSF pathways to prevent diffusion of the contrast medium.

Magnetic resonance imaging (MRI)

This is as useful as CT scans for detecting parenchymal cysts (MRI can reveal the protoscolex within a cyst) and signs of cyst degeneration and surrounding inflammation, but MRI is inferior for detection of parenchymal calcification. MRI, particularly with Gd enhancement, is described as superior to CT scan for visualization of intraventricular/subarachnoid cysts (Zee *et al.* 1993). MRI is important before surgery to locate intraventricular/subarachnoid cysts as the cysts are motile.

Immunodiagnosis

Immunological tests under development are: ELISA using crude antigen to detect antibody in serum or CSF; AG-ELISA using polyclonal or monoclonal antibodies to detect *T. solium* antigen in CSF; and an enzyme-linked immunoelectrotransfer blot (EITB) assay to detect antibody (Diwan *et al.* 1982; Estrada *et al.* 1989; Garcia *et al.* 1994). Of these, EITB has shown the greatest sensitivity and specificity (Diaz *et al.* 1992; Garcia *et al.* 1994); 8 and 26 kDa antigen bands are specific for *T. solium* (Gottstein *et al.* 1987; Pilcher *et al.* 1991). In a group of 34 patients whose infection had been confirmed by biopsy, surgery, or ocular infection, EITB had a sensitivity and specificity of 94 and 100 per cent, respectively, and ELISA 65 and 63 per cent respectively, for serum samples. For CSF samples, sensitivity of EITB was 86 per cent: ELISA, 62 per cent; and AG-ELISA, 67 per cent.

When immunodiagnosis and CT scan have been compared there are reports of major discrepancies between the results (Ramoskuri *et al.* 1992; Garcia *et al.* 1994). For example, Garcia *et al.* (1994) diagnosed 32 of 383 persons positive on CT scan and 32 persons positive with EITB, but positives often were different patients, only 50 per cent of the CT positives being EITB positives. Each test has it advantages and disadvantages. On EITB, false-positive diagnoses of neurocysticercosis can be recorded in patients who have only muscular and no CNS lesions (10–40 per cent of patients with cysticercosis may not have CNS involvement). Also, the prevalence of abortive infections or those that resolve spontaneously but induce antibody responses is not known. False-negative EITB is likely where cysts have died but have left symptomatic, calcified lesions. Thus, Wilson *et al.* (1991) reported that 94 per cent of patients with one or more viable parasites were seropositive, but that only 40–70 per cent with single lesions or calcifications were likely to have antibody. Conversely, CT scan and even MRI may fail to detect ventricular cysts, particularly racemose cysts at the base of the brain which may appear only as hydrocephalus or deformation of the basal cisterns. CT scan and MRI both suffer from subjective evaluation of lesions when different readers ascribe different aetiologies (Garcia *et al.* 1994). EITB will be the most useful in surveys in terms of cost and transport. A combination of CT scan or MRI plus immunological testing, e.g. by EITB, is necessary if facilities and funds allow, as diagnosis requires not only identification of infection, but its viability, site, and intensity, for prognosis and therapeutic management.

TREATMENT

TAENIOSIS—ADULT TAPEWORMS

Treatment of adult tapeworms using an extract of male fern dates back to early Greek medicine; this and kamala, kousso, areca, or betel nuts (containing arecoline) from palms and a paste from pumpkin seeds, all have been used extensively, only dying out in this century (Grove 1990). Frequent culinary use of pumpkin and squash seeds in the diet in Mexico is thought to decrease tapeworm prevalence.

Currently, praziquantel, at 2.5–8.7 mg/kg is highly effective and the drug of choice for adult *Taenia* spp. (Cruz *et al.* 1989; Pawlowski 1991). It is very safe and, while occasional transient abdominal discomfort, nausea, headache, and dizziness have been reported, these are dose related and should not occur at the doses used for adult tapeworms. Pawlowski (1991) has reported that 2.5 mg/kg is highly effective against *T. saginata,* and a study in Ecuador described efficacy for a dose of between 3.4 and 8.7 mg/kg for *T. solium.* It is important that the minimum dose possible be given as Torres *et al.* (1992) demonstrated that a single dose of praziquantel at 25 mg/kg damaged the metacestodes in the brain of pigs, inducing an inflammatory response to kill them. As a result, until more information is available, clinical monitoring should accompany even the lower dose regimen used for adult tapeworms and should definitely accompany the higher dose treatments required for schistosomes if *T. solium* is endemic in the area.

Niclosamide is still used extensively as a safe and effective drug (usually >80 per cent efficacy) for treatment of adult *Taenia* (Pawlowski and Schultz 1972) at 2 g for adults 1 g for children of 11–35 kg and 0.5 g for children below 2 years of age. Side-effects are occasional abdominal upset, nausea, vomiting, and very rarely syncope. In some clinics a saline purgative is given after treatment, but this cannot be considered necessary. Albendazole given as a single dose of 400–800 g has shown greater than 85 per cent efficacy (Pamba and Bwibo 1987). Albendazole has efficacy against metacestodes also (below) but only at much higher doses.

Older drugs remain in use in some countries due to their low cost and availability, but have considerably more side-effects and cannot be recommended. Mepacrine HCl, at 0.6–1.0 g adult, is usually given orally followed an hour later by a saline purge. Diclorophen/ trichlorophen and bithionol all have given very variable results with several side-effects. Other products are being sought, e.g. in Thailand a crude extract of the wood of *Atrocarpus lakoocha* ('*Puag-Haad*') followed by a $MgSO_4$ purgative is described (Charoenlaep *et al.* 1989). Hypertonic salt solutions themselves have been used to eliminate tapeworms, although, at high doses (e.g. 60 g $MgSO_4$) toxicity is observed.

NEUROCYSTICERCOSIS—METACESTODES

A well-referenced review relating CT diagnosis to therapeutic approaches and current treatment regimens has been given by Del Brutto *et al.* (1993).

1. Dead cysts with brain calcification. No anthelmintic treatment is required. Antiepileptic drugs are required to control seizures if the lesions are symptomatic. Surgery may be considered.

2. Viable, vesicular cysts in the parenchyma. Information as to how many cyst-positive persons develop clinical disease in later life is not available. As a result, as the onset of disease cannot be predicted, anthelmintic therapy or surgery must be recommended to kill the cysts so that potential side-effects can be monitored and managed. Efficacy of anthelmintic therapy is good. Praziquantel or albendazole produced a decrease in seizures from a mean of 11.3 a year to 0.6, a decrease in cysts from 5.0 to 0.9, and 71 per cent of patients were free of cysts and 54 per cent seizure free. This compared with patients who also had viable cysts but remained untreated—all continued to have 10.9 seizures/year (Vazquez and Sotelo 1992). Surgical treatment also was efficacious, though in part this efficacy might be related to the lower number of cysts (usually only one) in the majority of these patients. Seizures decreased from 12.8 to 1.7/year and 40 per cent of patients were seizure free.

3. Transitional or colloidal (dying) cysts. There is no conclusive data as to the benefits of treating these cases. Without treatment, in the study described above, patients with degenerating cysts showed a spontaneous reduction in the number of seizures/year from 12.8 to 1.7, and cyst numbers declined from 2.5 to 0.7, with 83 per cent of patients free of cysts on follow-up. However, while only 20 per cent of cysts eliminated with anthelmintic therapy left residual granulomata, 81 per cent of cysts that underwent spontaneous inflammatory degeneration did, so fewer patients became seizure free in the latter group. Anthelmintic therapy therefore might speed up resolution of the granulomatous reaction and speed up subsequent re-evaluation of patients for lesions of other aetiologies (Del Brutto 1993).

4. Severe cysticercotic encephalitis, in which the brain is already severely damaged by a massive inflammatory reaction, could be exacerbated by anthelmintic therapy, management with high-dose anti-inflammatory drugs was recommended (Del Brutto *et al.* 1993).

5. Cysts in the CSF pathways probably are best managed by surgery. Albendazole has effect but, with the potential for acute onset blockage of the CSF pathways, surgical removal is recommended (Del Brutto *et al.* 1993).

6. Spinal cysts can be removed effectively by surgery. Swelling due to inflammation after anthelmintic

therapy, particularly if unaccompanied with corticosteroids, could affect cord function.

INTRAOCULAR CYSTS

These are usually removed surgically from the subretinal or intravitreal site. Intraocular efficacy of anthelmintics is not proven and inflammation provoked to a dying cyst may lead to complications, e.g. a detached retina. Cardenas *et al.* (1992) described surgical results as poor, but Lozano and Barbosa (1990) reported no side-effects when intravitreal cysts were treated with albendazole followed by aspiration.

ANTHELMINTIC THERAPY

Praziquantel (usually 15, but up to 50 mg/kg for 15 days) or albendazole (15 or 20 mg/kg for 8 or 30 days) are the regimens commonly recommended for parenchymal cysts. Reduced neurological manifestations usually are recorded in more than 83 per cent of patients. Cyst damage is evident soon after the beginning of albendazole therapy so that efficacies of 8 days' or 30 days' albendazole therapy were statistically similar (Botero *et al.* 1993). In most studies, albendazole has shown higher efficacy than praziquantel and usually is cheaper (Sotelo *et al.* 1988; Cruz *et al.* 1991; Takayanagui and Jardim 1992). Antiepileptic drugs decrease bioavailability of praziquantel—perhaps accounting for some failures (Bittencourt *et al.* 1992). As benzimidazoles may have hepatotoxicity in some individuals revealed early in the course of therapy, the patient must be monitored for liver function.

Side-effects, primarily headaches, nausea, and vomiting, occur in as many as 60 per cent of anthelmintic-treated patients, probably related to the inflammation around dying cysts. Some clinics recommend concurrent dexamethasone therapy to reduce severity. However, most report that side-effects are mild, transient, and usually can be controlled with analgesics/antiemetics, so concommitant dexamethasone therapy is instituted only if the side-effects become severe, e.g. increased cerebral hypertension. Also, dexamethasone decreased bioavailability of praziquantel but not albendazole (Vazquez *et al.* 1987; Jung *et al.* 1990*a*). Generally, cases with heavy parasite loads must be most at risk from a damaging inflammatory response. There are occasional reports of severe side-effects, even deaths, after anthelmintic therapy.

Less information is available on anthelmintic therapy for non-parenchymal cysts. Reports from a limited number of cases suggest that albendazole was highly effective for subarachnoid cysts and some ventricular cysts. Praziquantel seems to be less effective for these, probably as levels of praziquantel in the CSF are low (Groll and Merck 1986; Jung *et al.* 1990*b*).

SURGERY

Surgery is used for ventricular cysts and may be applied to accessible, usually single parenchymal cysts, although the excision itself carries the risk of tissue damage (Vazquez and Sotelo 1992). Various surgical approaches related to the site of the cyst to relieve pressure by decompression craniotomy, extirpation, or drainage are described by Escobedo *et al.* (1982).

PREVENTION AND CONTROL STRATEGIES

Control of *T. solium* is preferable to treatment. Despite new, more effective therapies, there can be adverse neurological sequelae during therapy and effective treatment is not achieved in all cases. Losses to the budget due to *T. solium* infection in countries where infection is common seem destined to increase. Increased health standards and expectations will increase costs to the health budget through increased access and expectations of the community. As increasing numbers of pigs enter official meat inspection channels, costs to the agricultural budget will increase for increased numbers of inspectors, inspection facilities, storage facilities, and condemnations. For *T. saginata*, although human health is not severely affected, costs to the agricultural budget from infected carcasses continue to be high and may restrict exports.

Control must be multifaceted, involving the public health and veterinary authorities. Changes in socioeconomic conditions are a most important factor in control complemented by treatment/elimination of infection in humans and pigs/cattle. Efficacy of this was seen in the massive reduction particularly in *T. solium*, but also *T. saginata*, infection in the Western world in the late nineteenth, early twentieth century. Cultural changes accepting and requiring improved sanitation were very important. Dietary changes reduced consumption of raw meat; the fear of acquiring trichinellosis from raw pork products played a major role. Movement of most animals through official meat inspection channels, emphasized to control trichinellosis in pigs, markedly reduced the amount of infected meat on the market. Retention and freezing of suspect carcasses (the centre must reach −10 °C for 48 h) is lethal to cysts. Indoor husbandry of pigs also separated them from many sources of infection.

BASELINE DATA

It is important that the biological parameters are defined in a mathematical model: including prevalence of infection, infection pressure on, and reinfection rate in, definitive and intermediate hosts, and importance of acquired immunity in constraining the infection. The reproduction ratio (R_0) to define stability (endemicity) must be determined (Roberts 1994). Only then can: (1) the costs versus benefits of control be predicted, and (2) the effects of control be monitored. The reproduction ratio (R_0) must be determined in different environments. Hughes *et al.* (1993) described higher prevalence of *T. saginata* in cattle in dry compared with wet zones in Swaziland and ascribed this either to differences in human behaviour or to a climatic constraint on the parasite, producing an unstable endemic state with loss of host immunity.

PUBLIC HEALTH EDUCATION

This always is considered a key factor but it is difficult to alter traditional cultural and behavioural factors in a population in order to accept dietary changes, sanitation, and compulsory treatment/vaccination. Often a rural population's greatest anxiety is food availability and their infected pigs or cattle will represent the means to allay this fear.

DIETARY CHANGES

Reduced consumption of rare/raw pork and beef is required (50–60°C will kill cysts), but ultimately can be difficult to achieve. There currently seems to be an increase in the prevalence of *T. saginata* in some Western countries, presumably associated with increased travel, exposure to different eating habits, and increased leisure time and travel at home.

SANITATION/SEWAGE FACILITIES

Considerable funds are required for latrines and sewage disposal systems, but without hygiene education, the facilities can be rejected through misuse. Even improved sanitation in areas where *T. solium* is common may not improve the situation markedly as disposal of sludge and slurry, much of it on farmland, and re-use of effluent for irrigation will need to continue. Some 1.3×10^6 tonnes of sludge was produced in United Kingdom in 1977, with 67 per cent of this disposed on the land (Pike 1986). Facilities must be costed and provided whereby sludge can be anaerobically digested, stored long term, to destroy eggs, or there should be a 6-month no-grazing period after application (Arundel and Adolph 1980; Pike 1986).

OFFICIAL MEAT INSPECTION

The facilities and personnel required to detect and withhold infected meat are expensive. Also, current meat inspection practices fail to detect a relatively high proportion of infected carcasses. Improved diagnosis, undoubtedly by immunodiagnosis, is required, but the high species specificity and high sensitivity needed to detect the low levels of infection that create most of the problems with current meat inspection practices, have not yet been achieved. The test must be automated for large facilities, but have a dipstick technology for sites where few animals are slaughtered, and not add significantly to the costs of slaughter. Further, in the developing world, the infected meat remains an important source of protein and/or cash to the family unit so continued avoidance of meat inspection (even using the diagnostic technique to do so!) may prevent change.

HUSBANDRY

Animals are herded together at night, usually close to human habitation, for protection. Also, human faeces and refuse supply an important part of the pigs' diet in villages and would need replacement. Changes in management to supply housing, food, and security would be expensive and difficult to achieve in village units in which each holding is inevitably small.

MASS TREATMENT OF HUMANS

This has been advocated by Pawlowski (1990) as not requiring major improvements in economics, sanitation, husbandry, or meat inspection. This vertical approach to control was adopted in Ecuador where 10 000 persons were treated, with effective removal of tapeworms, a reduction in prevalence in pigs, and an apparently low rate of reinfection (Cruz *et al.* 1989). However, considerable information is yet required. The number of persons examined for re-infection must be higher as prevalence of infection in man is low. Biological data are essential to determine that an unstable endemic steady state is not induced. Paradoxically, control by mass therapy could increase prevalence and disease incidence through loss of acquired immunity in the population, as demonstrated for dog/sheep taeniids and cattle *Babesia* (Smith 1983; Gemmell *et al.* 1987) and *T. solium* and *T. saginata* are as highly fecund as the sheep taeniids. This has been noted for one of two field trials in Mexico (Keilbach *et al.* 1989). It is important to consider whether mass chemotherapy of humans is ethically acceptable and to consider the costs of litigation at a later date for real or supposed side-effects; idiosyncratic reactions are almost invariable with any drug. Potential side-effects of treatment for adult tapeworms must be carefully evaluated in persons with cysticercosis.

VACCINATION OF INTERMEDIATE HOSTS

This also may not require major improvements in economics, sanitation, husbandry, or meat inspection. Prospects for vaccines against *T. saginata* and *T. solium* are excellent. Vaccination against Asian *Taenia* with its variety of intermediate hosts, some sylvatic, logistically is less feasible. Even relatively crude antigen vaccines have resulted in a very significant protection of pigs and cattle (Lloyd 1979; Rickard *et al.* 1982; Molinari *et al.* 1993) and there has been outstanding recent progress in the biotechnological development of vaccination against taeniid cestodes. A recombinant vaccine has been produced and has now being patented for *Taenia ovis* in sheep (Johnson *et al.* 1989; Lightowlers *et al.* 1992; Lightowlers and Rickard 1993). A number of questions remain, however. Antigens for *T. saginata* and *T. solium* have yet to be defined and examined for efficacy, vaccination intervals, etc. It is important to predict the impact of vaccination and the proportion of animals (which may be very high for these highly fecund taeniids) that must be vaccinated annually for extinction to be achieved (Roberts 1994). Some animals, high as well as low responders, fail to respond with protection after vaccination. A less than 100 per cent efficacy in individual animals will mean that low numbers of cysts, these the most difficult to detect, will remain in marketed carcasses. The importance of these in maintaining an endemic steady state must be determined; concurrent development of more effective meat inspection measures may be required to identify these animals. Acceptance of vaccination is important and legislation will be needed to ensure implementation and monitoring, and so success.

COST–BENEFIT ANALYSES

In order to develop and maintain the impetus for control/eradication, strict attention must be paid to analyses of the benefits compared with costs. It seems likely this ratio will be very favourable for control of *T. solium*, with its widespread prevalence and importance as a cause of severe human disease. A favourable ratio for control of *T. saginata* will depend more on the economic benefits accrued in reduced loss of income to farmers and reduced costs of meat inspection.

REFERENCES

Acha, P. N. and Aguilar, F. J. (1964). Studies on cysticercosis in Central America and Panama. *American Journal of Tropical Medicine and Hygiene*, **13**, 48–53.

Allan, J. C., Garciadominguez, C., Craig, P. S., Rogan, M. T., Lowe, B. S. and Flisser, A. (1991). Sexual development of *Taenia solium* in hamsters. *Annals of Tropical Medicine and Parasitology*, **85**, 573–6.

Allan, J. C. *et al.* (1992). Coproantigen detection for immunodiagnosis of echinococcosis and taeniasis in dogs and humans. *Parasitology*, **104**, 347–55.

Allan, J. C. *et al.* (1993). Dipstick dot ELISA for the detection of *Taenia* coproantigens in humans. *Parasitology*, **107**, 79–85.

Aluja, A. S. de (1982). Frequency of porcine cysticercosis in Mexico. In *Cysticercosis: present state of knowledge and perspectives* (ed. A. Flisser, K. Willms, J. P. Laclette, C. Larralde, C. Ridaura, and F. Beltrán), pp. 53–62. Academic Press, New York.

Arundel, J. H. and Adolph, A. J. (1980). Preliminary observations on the removal of *Taenia saginata* eggs from sewage using various treatment procedures. *Australian Veterinary Journal*, **56**, 492–5.

Bittencourt, P. R. M., Garcia, C. M., Martins, R., Fernandes, A. G., Diekmann, H. W., and Jung, W. (1992). Phenytoin and carbamazepine decrease oral bioavailability of praziquantel. *Neurology*, **42**, 492–6.

Botero, D. *et al.* (1993). Short course albendazole treatment for neurocysticerocosis in Columbia. *Transactions of the Royal Society of Tropical Medicine and Hygiene*, **87**, 576–7.

Bowles, J. and McManus, D. P. (1994). Genetic characterization of the Asian *Taenia*, a newly described taeniid cestode of humans. *American Journal of Tropical Medicine and Hygiene*, **50**, 33–44.

Brandt, J. R. E. *et al.* (1992). A monoclonal antibody based ELISA for the detection of circulating secretory antigens in *Taenia saginata* cysticercosis. *International Journal for Parasitology*, **22**, 471–7.

Cardenas, F., Quiroz, H., Plancarte, A., Meza, A., Dalma, A., and Flisser, A. (1992). *Taenia solium* ocular cysticercosis—findings in 30 cases. *Annals of Ophthalmology*, **24**, 25–8.

Carpio, A., Placencia, M., Santillan, F., and Escobar, A. (1994). A proposal for classification of neurocysticercosis. *Canadian Journal of Neurological Sciences*, **21**, 43–7.

Charoenlaep, P., Radomyos, P., and Bunnag, D. (1989). The optimum dose of Puag-Haad in the treatment of taeniasis. *Journal of the Medical Association of Thailand*, **72**, 71–3.

Cruz, M., Davis, A., Dixon, H., Pawlowski, Z. S., and Proana, J. (1989). Operational studies on the control of *Taenia solium* taeniasis/cyticercosis in Ecuador. *Bulletin of the World Health Organisation*, **67**, 401–7.

Cruz, M., Cruz, I., and Horton, J. (1991). Albendazole versus praziquantel in the treatment of cerebral cysticercosis—clinical evaluation. *Transactions of the Royal Society of Tropical Medicine and Hygiene*, **85**, 244–7.

Del Brutto, O. H. (1993). The use of albendazole in patients with single lesions enhanced on contrast CT. *New England Journal of Medicine*, **328**, 356–7.

Del Brutto, O. H., Sotelo, J., and Roman, G. C. (1993). Therapy for neurocysticercosis—a reappraisal. *Clinical Infectious Diseases*, **17**, 730–5.

Dewhurst, L. W., Cramer, J. D., and Sheldon, J. J. (1967). An Analysis of current inspection procedures for detecting bovine cysticercosis. *Journal of the American Veterinary Medical Association*, **150**, 412–17.

Diaz, J. F. *et al.* (1992). Immunodiagnosis of human cysticercosis (*Taenia solium*)—a field comparison of an antibody enzyme linked immunosorbent assay (ELISA), an antigen ELISA, and an enzyme linked immunoelectrotransfer blot (EITB) assay in Peru. *American Journal of Tropical Medicine and Hygiene*, **46**, 610–15.

Diwan, A. R. *et al.* (1982). Enzyme-linked immunosorbent assay (ELISA). for the detection of antibody to cysticerci of *Taenia solium*. *American Journal of Tropical Medicine and Hygiene*, **31**, 364–9.

Eom, K. S. and Rim, H. J. (1993). Morphologic descriptions of *Taenia asiaticus* sp. n. *Korean Journal of Parasitology*, **31**, 1–6.

Eom, K. S., Rim, H. J., and Geerts, S. (1992). Experimental infection of pigs and cattle with eggs of Asian *Taenia saginata* with specific reference to its extrahepatic viscerotropism. *Korean Journal of Parasitology*, **30**, 269–75.

Escobedo, F., González-Mariscal, G., Revuelta, R., and Ruben, M. (1982). Surgical treatment of cerebral cysticercosis. In *Cysticercosis: present state of knowledge and perspectives*, (ed. A. Flisser, K. Willms, J. P. Laclette, C. Larralde, C. Ridaura, and F. Beltrán), pp. 219–26, Academic Press, New York.

Estrada, J. J., Estrada, J. A., and Kuhn, R. E. (1989). Identification of *Taenia solium* antigens in cerebrospinal fluid and larval antigens from patients with neurocysticercosis. *American Journal of Tropical Medicine and Hygiene*, **41**, 50–5.

Fan, P. C. (1988). Taiwan *Taenia*, and taeniasis. *Parasitology Today*, **4**, 86–8.

Fan, P. C., Chung, W. C., Lin, C. Y., and Wu, C. C. (1990). The pig as an intermediate host for Taiwan *Taenia*, infection. *Journal of Helminthology*, **64**, 223–31.

Fan, P. C., Lin, C. Y., and Chen, L. M. (1992*a*). Experimental infection and morphology of *Taenia saginata* (Burma strain), in domestic animals. *Annals of Tropical Medicine and Parasitology*, **86**, 317–18.

Fan, P. C., Lin, C. Y., and Chung, W. C. (1992*b*). Experimental infection of Philippine *Taenia* in domestic animals. *International Journal for Parasitology*, **22**, 235–8.

Fan, P. C., Chung, W. C., Lin, C. Y., and Chan, C. H. (1992*c*). Clinical manifestations of taeniasis in Taiwan aborigines. *Journal of Helminthology*, **66**, 118–23.

Fan, P. C., Chung, W. C., Lin, C. Y., and Pawlowski, Z. S. (1992*d*). Experimental infection with *Taenia saginata* (Poland strain) in taiwanese pigs. *Journal of Helminthology*, **66**, 198–204.

Fan, P. C., Chung, W. C., Soh, C. T., and Kosman, M. L. (1992*e*). Eating habits of East-Asian people and transmission of taeniasis. *Acta Tropica*, **50**, 305–15.

Garcia H.H., *et al.* (1994). Discrepancies between cerebral computed-tomography and Western-blot in the diagnosis of neurocysticercosis. *American Journal of Tropical Medicine and Hygiene*, **50**, 152–7.

Gemmell, M. A., Lawson, J. R., Roberts, M. G., Kerin, B. R., and Mason, C. J. (1987). Population dynamics in echinococcosis and cysticercosis: comparison of the response of *Echinococcus granulosus*, *Taenia hydatigena* and *T. ovis* to control. *Parasitology*, **93**, 357–69.

Gottstein, B., Zini, D., and Schantz, P. M. (1987). Species-specific immunodiagnosis of *Taenia solium* cysticercosis by ELISA and immunoblotting. *Tropical Medicine and Parasitology*, **38**, 299–303.

Groll, E. and Merck, E. (1986). Praziquantel concentration in cerebral spinal fluid. In *Proceedings of the 2nd International Symposium on Taeniasis/Cysticercosis and Echinococcosis/Hydatidosis*, pp. 200–11.

Grove, D. I. (1990). *A history of human helminthology*, p. 848, CAB International, Wallingford.

Hall, A., Latham, M. C., Crompton, D. W. T., and Stephenson, L. S. (1981). *Taenia saginata* (Cestoda) in western Kenya: the reliability of faecal examinations in diagnosis. *Parasitology*, **83**, 91–101.

Harrison, L. J. S., Delgado, J., and Parkhouse, R. M. E. (1990). Differential diagnosis of *Taenia saginata* and *Taenia solium* with DNA probes. *Parasitology*, **100**, 459–61.

Harrison, L. J. S., Joshua, G. W. P., Wright, S. H., and Parkhouse, R. M. E. (1991). Specific detection of circulating surface/secreted glycoproteins of viable cysticerci in *Taenia saginata* cysticercosis. *Parasite Immunology*, **11**, 351–70.

Huang, S. W., Lin, C. Y., and Khaw, O. K. (1966). Studies on *Taenia*, species prevalent among the aborigines in Wulai District, Taiwan. Part I. On the parasitological fauna of the aborigines in Wulai District. *Bulletin of the Institute of Zoology, Academia Sinica*, **5**, 87–91.

Hughes, G., Hoque, M., Tewes, M. S., Wright, S. H., and Harrison, L. J. S. (1993). Seroepidemiological study of *Taenia saginata* cysticercosis in Swaziland. *Research in Veterinary Science*, **55**, 287–91.

Ito, A. (1992). Cysticercosis in Asian Pacific regions. *Parasitology Today*, **8**, 182–3.

Johnson, K. S. *et al.* (1989). Vaccination against ovine cysticercosis using a defined recombinant antigen. *Nature*, **338**, 585–7.

Jung, H., Hurtado, M., Medina, M. T., Sanchez, M., and Sotelo, J. (1990*a*). Dexamethasone increases plasma-levels of albendazole. *Journal of Neurology*, **237**, 279–80.

Jung, H., Hurtado, M., Sanchez, M., Medina, M. T., and Sotelo, J. (1990*b*). Plasma and CSF levels of albendazole and praziquantel in patients with neurocysticercosis. *Clinical Neuropharmacology*, **13**, 559–64.

Kaminsky, R. J. de. (1991). Albendazole treatment in human taeniasis. *Transactions of the Royal Society of Tropical Medicine and Hygiene*, **85**, 648.

Keilbach, N. Ma., Aluja, A. S. de, and Sarti-Guterriez, E. (1989). A programme to control taeniasis-cysticercosis (*T. solium*): experiences in a Mexican village. *Acta Liedensia*, **57**, 181–9.

Khadaiberganun, I. (1980). The transmission of *Taenia saginata* eggs to calves via the hands of farm workers. *Byulletyn' Vsesoyuznogo Instituta Gel'mintologii im K. I. Skryabina*, **7**, 87–90.

Kyvsgaard, N. C., Ilsoe, B., Willeberg, P., Nansen, P., and Henriksen, S. A. (1991). A case control study of risk factors in light *Taenia saginata* cysticercosis in Danish cattle. *Acta Veterinaria Scandinavica*, **32**, 243–52.

Lightowlers, M. W. and Rickard, M. D. (1993). Vaccination against cestode parasites. *Immunology and Cell Biology*, **71**, 443–51.

Lightowlers, M. W., Gemmell, M. A., Harrison, G. L. B., Heath, D. D., Rickard, M. D., and Roberts, M. G. (1992). Control of tissue parasites. II. Cestodes. In *Animal parasite control utilizing biotechnology*, (ed. W. K. Tong), pp. 171–98. CRC Press, Boca Raton.

Lloyd, S. (1979). Homologous and heterologous immunization against the metacestodes of *Taenia saginata* and *Taenia taeniaeformis* in cattle and mice. *Zeitschrift für Parasitenkunde*, **60**, 87–96.

Lloyd, S. (1987). Cysticercosis. In *Immune response in parasitic infections: immunology, immunopathology and immunoprophylaxis*. Vol. II. *Trematodes and Cestodes*, (ed. E. J. L. Soulsby) pp. 183–212. CRC Press, Boca Raton.

Lozano, D. and Barbosa, S. (1990). Tratamiento con albendazole de la cisticercosis intraocular. *Revista Mexicana Oftalmologia*, **64**, 15–28.

McAninch, A. (1974). Case report. An outbreak of cysticercosis in feedlot cattle. *Canadian Veterinary Journal*, **15**, 120–2.

McManus, D. P. and Bowles, J. (1994). Asian (Taiwan) *Taenia*: species or strain? *Parasitology Today*, **10**, 273–5.

Macpherson, R., Mitchell, G. B. B., and McCance, C. B. (1978). Bovine cysticercosis storm following the application of human slurry. *Veterinary Record*, **102**, 156–7.

Medina, M. T., Rosas, E., Rubiodonnadieu, F., and Sotelo, J. (1990). Neurocysticercosis as the main cause of late onset epilepsy in Mexico. *Archives of Internal Medicine*, **150**, 325–7.

Molinari, J. L. *et al.* (1993). Immunization against porcine cysticercosis in an endemic area in Mexico—a field and laboratory study. *American Journal of Tropical Medicine and Hygiene*, **49**, 502–12.

Onyango-Abuje, J. A. *et al.* (1993). Recent advances in diagnosis of bovine cysticercosis: detection of circulating antigen in live cattle. *East African Agriculture and Forestry Journal*. [Cited in Hughes *et al.* 1993.]

Pamba, H. O. and Bwibo, N. O. (1987). Open study in the treatment of *Trichuris trichiura* and *Taenia saginata* with 800 mg albendazole as a single dose. *East African Medical Journal*, **64**, 590–4.

Pawlowski, Z. (1982). Epidemiology and prevention of *Taenia saginata* infection. In *Cysticercosis: present state of knowledge and perspectives*, (ed. A. Flisser, K. Willms, J. P. Laclette, C. Larralde, C. Ridaura, and F. Beltrán), pp. 69–86. Academic Press, New York.

Pawlowski, Z. S. (1990). Perspectives on the control of *Taenia solium. Parasitology Today*, **6**, 371.

Pawlowski, Z. S. (1991). Efficacy of low doses of praziquantel in taeniasis. *Acta Tropica*, **48**, 83–8.

Pawlowski, Z. and Schultz, M. G. (1972). Taeniasis and cysticercosis (*Taenia saginata*). *Advances in Parasitology*, **10**, 269–343.

Pike, E. B. (1986). Recent UK research on incidence, transmission and control of *Salmonella* and parasitic ova in sludge. In *Epidemiological studies of risk associated with the agricultural use of sewage sludge: knowledge and needs*, (ed. J. C. Block, A. H. Havelaar, and P. L'Hermite), pp. 50–9, Elsevier Science Publishers, London.

Pilcher, J. B., Tsang, V. C., Gilman, R. H., Rhodes, M. L., and Pawlowski, Z. S. (1991). Further evidence of 100 per cent specificity in a recently developed *Taenia solium* (cysticercosis) immunoblot assay. *American Journal of Tropical Medicine and Hygiene*, **45**, (Suppl. 131).

Ramoskuri, M. *et al.* (1992). Immunodiagnosis of neurocysticercosis—disappointing performance of serology (enzyme-linked immunosorbent assay) in an unbiased sample of neurological patients. *Archives of Neurology*, **49**, 633–6.

Rickard, M. D. and Adolph, A. J. (1977). The prevalence of cysticerci of *Taenia saginata* in cattle reared on sewage-irrigated pasture. *Medical Journal of Australia*, **1**, 525–7.

Rickard, M. D., Brumley, J. L., and Anderson, G. A. (1982). Field trial to evaluate the use of antigens from *Taenia hydatigena* oncospheres to prevent infection with *T. saginata* in cattle grazing on sewage irrigated pastures. *Research in Veterinary Science*, **32**, 189–93.

Roberts, M. G. (1994). Modelling of parasitic populations: cestodes. In *Understanding and control of parasitic diseases of animals*, (ed. S. Lloyd and E. J. L. Soulsby). *Veterinary Parasitology*, **54**, 145–160.

Sarti, E. *et al.* (1992). Prevalence and risk factors for *Taenia solium* taeniasis and cysticercosis in humans and pigs in a village in Morelos, Mexico. *American Journal of Tropical Medicine and Hygiene*, **46**, 677–85.

Sarti-G, E., Schantz, P. M., Aguilera, J., and Lopez, A. (1992). Epidemiologic observations on porcine cysticercosis in a rural community of Michoacan State, Mexico. *Veterinary Parasitology*, **41**, 195–201.

Sarti-G, E. *et al.*. (1994). Epidemiologic investigation of *Taenia solium* taeniasis and cysticercosis in a rural village of Michoacan state, Mexico. *Transactions of the Royal Society of Tropical Medicine and Hygiene*, **88**, 49–52.

Schantz, P. M. *et al.* (1992). Neurocysticercosis in an orthodox Jewish community in New York city. *New England Journal of Medicine*, **327**, 692–5.

Schenone, H., Villarroel, F., Rojas, A., and Ramirez, R. (1982). Epidemiology of human cysticercosis in Latin America. In *Cysticercosis: present state of knowledge and perspectives*, (ed. A. Flisser, K. Willms, J. P. Laclette, C. Larralde, and F. Beltrán), pp. 25–38. Academic Press, New York.

Schultz, M. G., Halterman, L. G., Rich, A. B., and Martin, G. A. (1969). An epizootic of bovine cysticercosis. *Journal of the American Veterinary Medical Association*, **155**, 1708–17.

Silverman, P. H. (1956). The longevity of eggs of *Taenia pisiformis* and *Taenia saginata* under various conditions. *Transactions of the Royal Society of Tropical Medicine and Hygiene*, **50**, 8.

Silverman, P. H. and Griffiths, R. B. (1955). A review of methods of sewage disposal in Great Britain with special reference to the epizovtiology of *Cysticercus bovis Annals of Tropical Medicine and Parasitology*, **49**, 436–50.

Slonka, G. F., Matulich, W., Morphet, E., Miller, C. W., and Bayer, E. V. (1978). An outbreak of bovine cysticercosis in California. *American Journal of Tropical Medicine and Hygiene*, **27**, 101–5.

Smith, R. D. (1983). *Babesia bovis*: computer simulation of the relationship between the tick vector, parasite, and bovine host. *Experimental Parasitology*, **56**, 27–40.

Sorvillo, F. J., Waterman, S. H., Richards, F. O., and Schantz, P. M. (1992). Cysticercosis surveillance—locally acquired and travel-related infections and detection of intestinal tapeworm carriers in Los Angeles county. *American Journal of Tropical Medicine and Hygiene*, **47**, 365–71.

Sotelo, J., Escobedo, F., and Penagos, P. (1988). Albendazole vs praziquantel for therapy for neurocysticercosis—a controlled trial. *Archives of Neurology*, **45**, 532–4.

Soulsby, E. J. L. (1963). Immunological unresponsiveness to helminth infections in animals. In *Proceedings of the 17th International Veterinary Congress*, **1**, 761–7.

Suvorov, V. Y. (1965). Viability of *Taenia saginata* oncospheres. *Meditsinskaia Parazitologiia i Parazitarnye Bolezni*, **34**, 98–100.

Takayanagui, O. M. and Jardim, E. (1992). Therapy for neurocysticercosis: comparison between albendazole and praziquantel. *Archives of Neurology*, **49**, 290–4.

Torgerson, P. R., Gulland, F. M., and Gemmell, M. A. (1992). Observations on the epidemiology of *Taenia hydatigena* in Soay sheep on St Kilda. *Veterinary Record*, **131**, 218–19.

Torres, A., Plancarte, A., Villalobos, A. N. M., Dealuja, A. S., Navarro, R., and Flisser, A. (1992). Praziquantel treatment of porcine brain and muscle *Taenia solium* cysticercosis. 3. Effect of 1 day treatment. *Parasitology Research*, **78**, 161–4.

Urquhart, G. M. (1961). Epizootological and experimental studies on bovine cysticercosis in East Africa. *Journal of Parasitology*, **47**, 857–69.

Vazquez, M. L., Jung, H., and Sotelo, J. (1987). Plasma levels of praziquantel decrease when dexamethasone is given simultaneously. *Neurology*, **37**, 1561–2.

Vazquez, V. and Sotelo, J. (1992). The course of seizures after treatment for cerebral cysticercosis. *New England Journal of Medicine*, **327**, 696–701.

Verster, A. (1969). A taxonomic revision of the genus *Taenia* Linnaeus, 1758 s. str. *Onderstepoort Journal of Veterinary Research*, **37**, 3–58.

Walther, M. and Koske, J. K. (1980). *Taenia saginata* cysticercosis: a comparison of routine meat inspection and carcass dissection results in calves. *Veterinary Record*, **106**, 401–2.

Webbe, G. (1967). The hatching and activation of taeniid ova in relation to the development of cysticercosis in man. *Zeitschrift für Tropenmedizin and Parasitologie*, **18**, 354–69.

Wilson, M. *et al.* (1991). Clinical evaluation of the cysticercosis enzyme linked immunoelectrotransfer blot in patients with neurocysticercosis. *Journal of Infectious Disease*, **164**, 1007–9.

Zarlenga, D. S., McManus, D. P., Fan, P. C., and Cross, J. H. (1991). Characterization and detection of a newly described Asian taeniid using cloned ribosomal DNA fragments and sequence amplification by the polymerase chain-reaction. *Experimental Parasitology*, **72**, 174–83.

Zee, C. S., Segall, H. D., Destian, S., Ahmadi, J., and Apuzzo, M. L. J. (1993). MRI of intraventricular cysticercosis—surgical implications. *Journal of Computer Assisted Tomography*, **17**, 932–9.

Zenteno-Alanis, G. H. (1982). A classification of human cysticercosis. In *Cysticercosis: present state of knowledge and perspectives*, (ed. A. Flisser, K. Willms, J. P. Laclette, C. Larralde, C. Ridaura, and F. Beltrán) pp. 107–26. Academic Press, New York.

51 OTHER CESTODE INFECTIONS HYMENOLEPIOSIS, DIPHYLLOBOTHRIOSIS, COENUROSIS, AND OTHER ADULT AND LARVAL CESTODES

Sheelagh Lloyd

SUMMARY

This chapter examines a number of cestodes in diverse orders. Two of them are common in man, the other sporadic. *Hymenolepis (Vampirolepis) nana* is the only cestode that has a direct life cycle, both metacestodes and adults develop in the same host. As a result, direct human–human transfer is the most important route of infection and infection is common in man. The exact contribution to human infection by rodent hosts, and by the optional indirect life cycle through arthropods in food, has not been determined. Thus, education, public health, and improved sanitation are equally as important as rodent/arthropod control measures. Man is one of several definitive hosts for *Diphyllobothrium latum*, freshwater copepods and fish acting as intermediate hosts in its indirect life cycle. The risk factor for infection is consumption of fish by persons living around lakes/reservoirs, particularly in the Baltics and Russia, with foci of infection established elsewhere. A marine species, *D. klebanovskii* is common on the coast of Far-East Russia and is carried inland by migrating salmon. A number of other freshwater and marine *Diphyllobothrium* species occur sporadically throughout the world in humans who eat raw fish. Control measures have been implemented in Russia, but are complicated by the diverse definitive and intermediate hosts for the parasites, and our inability to differentiate between zoonotic and non-zoonotic *Diphyllobothrium* spp. The characteristics and geographic location of other sporadic infections of humans with adults of *Hymenolepis diminuta*, *Dipylidium caninum*, *Bertiella* spp., *Inermicapsifer* spp., *Raillietina* spp., *Mesocestoides* spp., and *Diplogonoporus grandis* are described. Man also acts as an intermediate host for some metacestodes. In many parts of the world, *Taenia multiceps*, *T. serialis*, and *T. brauni* are common in their normal host assemblages of canids/small ruminants, lagomorphs, rodents. Humans occasionally become infected accidentally with a space-occupying coenurus in the brain, subcutaneous tissues, or eye. *Spirometra* spp. are found particularly in Asia, but also occasionally in Australia and the Americas. Humans periodically acquire infection by ingestion of the copepod or reptile/amphibian/mammalian intermediate hosts, or by contact when these are used as poultices. The ribbon-like plerocercoids (spargana) are found in many tissues, particularly subcutaneous tissues, but also around the eye and in the brain. Little information is available on treatment for many of these infections. Praziquantal is the drug of choice for the adult tapeworms. Many of the metacestode infections are likely to be, or are best, managed surgically. In some instances, daily treatment with albendazole and praziquantal should be tested.

HYMENOLEPIS (VAMPIROLEPIS) NANA AND *HYMENOLEPIS DIMINUTA*

HISTORY

These two parasites were recognized from rats, mice, and humans in the nineteenth century (Grove 1990). *Hymenolepis diminuta* was described as *Taenia diminuta*, first from rodents by Rudolphi, 1819, and then from a child in the United States. Bilharz observed *Taenia*, later *Hymenolepis nana* in a child in Egypt in 1851, and soon afterwards it was described in mice. Discovery of the direct life cycle of *H. nana* in 1887 by Grassi pre-dated the demonstration by Grassi and Rovelli, 1892, of the obligate indirect life cycle of *H. diminuta*. The optional indirect life cycle of *H. nana* was described in 1911 by Nicholl and Minchin.

THE AGENTS

Hymenolepis nana (von Siebold, 1852), the dwarf tape-worm, is only 2.5–4 cm long. The scolex has four suckers and one row of 20–30 hooks on a retractable rostellum. A long neck is followed by about 200 proglottids that are wider than long, each having a single set of genital organs of three testes, a single ovary, and unilateral genital pores. The gravid proglot-tids have a sac-like uterus. Eggs are oval, 45 by 30 μm, and contain an oncosphere with three pairs of hooks, surrounded by two smooth membranes. The outer membrane is thin and clear, the inner has two polar thickenings (knobs) each of which bears 4–8 filaments.

Hymenolepis diminuta Rudolphi, 1819, may reach 20–60 cm long in man and has about 1000 proglottids. The rostellum lacks hooks. The proglottids are similar to *H. nana*, but eggs are larger, 60–70 μm long, the polar thickenings do not have filaments, and the outer membrane is thicker, darker, and may have striations.

THE HOSTS

1. *Hymenolepis nana*:
   adult tapeworm: man, rodents
   metacestode: man; rodents; stored food beetles (meal worms), *Tenebrio molitor*, *T. obscurus*, *Tribolium* spp.; flea larvae, *Ceratophyllus fasciatus*, *Xenopsylla cheopis*, *Pulex irritans*, *Ctenocephalides* spp.; moths
2. *Hymenolepis diminuta*:
   adult tapeworm: rodents, particularly rats; man
   metacestodes: stored food beetles (*Tenebrio* spp., *Tribolium* spp.) and at least 90 other arthropod species

LIFE CYCLE AND EPIDEMIOLOGY

Eggs shed from gravid proglottids and disintegrating proglottids are passed in the faeces. *Hymenolepis nana* is the only tapeworm that does not require an intermedi-ate host. Thus, faeco–oral contamination is very import-ant in human infection, so infection is common in institutions and in poor areas where direct human–human transfer can predominate. Further, in houses with poor hygiene/sanitation, infected rodents are

likely to be prevalent to contaminate food with eggs in their faeces. Eggs eaten by humans or rodents develop to metacestodes (cysticercoids) in the lymph vessels of the villi of the small intestine, emerge from the villous tissue in 5–6 days and then develop to adults in the intestinal lumen with a prepatent period of 16 days. Internal autoinfection, where eggs hatch within the host, accounts for the build up of very large numbers of worms (Heyneman 1961).

An indirect life cycle is optional for *H. nana* and required for *H. diminuta*. Houses where rodents have access to foods are likely also to have cereal foods infested with beetles; such houses also supply a good environment for other arthropods, e.g. fleas. Beetles in stored food are attracted to eat infected rodent faeces and, where there is poor sanitation and hygiene, flea larvae may eat rodent and possibly human faeces; cysticercoids develop in their haemocoels. Infection of human/rodent definitive hosts occurs by eating uncooked food contaminated with beetles or by accidental ingestion of fleas (see *Dipylidium caninum*). There is no general consensus as to the level of transfer of infection between rodents and humans. However, Saeki (1921, cited in Grove 1990) trans-ferred infection from mice to a child, and higher rates of infection were noted to derive from homologous rather than the heterologous infections (Pampiglione 1962).

Little is known about protection against infection or rejection of these parasites in man. *Hymenolepis dimin-uta* is rapidly expelled from non-permissive mouse hosts but persists for long periods in rats (Ito and Smyth 1987); infections in humans are sporadic and so compa-rable information is not available. While infection with *H. nana* is more common in children than in adults, there is no clear evidence that this is a result of protec-tive immunity and not improved hygiene; stage-specific immunity does, however, develop rapidly in mice.

GEOGRAPHIC DISTRIBUTION

Hymenolepis nana is cosmopolitan in distribution, but most common in South America, Africa, Asia and eastern and southern Europe. It is the most frequently encountered human cestode. Prevalence is highest in children, infection is common in institutions even in the Western world, and higher levels may occur in various groups, e.g. aborigines in Australia. Infections with *H. diminuta* are sporadic although they occur in many areas of the world.

Recent surveys for *H. nana* give prevalences of 2–28 per cent in children in various cities and villages in Chile, Brazil, Egypt, Ethiopia, Saudi Arabia, northern Iraq, Turkey, India, various regions of the CIS and eastern Europe, with prevalences highest in institutions, e.g. orphanages, and in 20.5 per cent of an aboriginal group in Australia. The potential for transfer of infection to food may be high: 5.8 per cent of food handlers in an Al-Medinah hospital in Saudi Arabia were infected (Ali *et al.* 1992); 8.9 per cent of students at a Health College were infected, as were 0.8–0.9 per cent of kitchen workers in Turkey (Babur *et al.* 1987). Clustering of cases in households may exist with contamination by food handlers (Chapter 51) and could occur in this way in the Western world as 5–7 per cent of immigrants/travellers from infected areas arriving in the United Kingdom carried *H. nana* (Chattopadhyay *et al.* 1988).

SYMPTOMS AND CLINICAL SIGNS

Hymenolepis nana infections, particularly light infections, and *H. diminuta* infections often produce no symptoms. However, heavy infections of many thousands of *H. nana* can develop in the intestine through autoinfection. In a study of children in Chile, abdominal pain was described by 74.5 per cent, bloating by 52.7 per cent, diarrhoea by 49 per cent, and poor weight gain and eosinophilia in 32.7 per cent and 49 per cent, respectively; nausea and vomiting can occur also (Noemi *et al.* 1991). In a Moscow study, 26 per cent of a group of adults reported symptoms, and clinicopathological examination showed intestinal malabsorption in 73 per cent, decreased numbers of T and B cells and levels of serum IgA and lysozyme, but increased IgE (Makarova and Astafev 1992).

DIAGNOSIS

Eggs are found in the faeces; ethyl acetate extraction is a common technique. An ELISA to detect serum antibody in humans showed sensitivity but very poor specificity (Gomez-Priego *et al.* 1991). A coproantigen test has been developed using experimental rat infections (Allan and Craig 1994) but requires clinical evaluation.

TREATMENT

Praziquantel is the preferred anthelmintic; a single dose of 15–25 mg/kg shows high efficacy (91–98 per cent) against both adult tapeworms and intestinal metacestodes (Ata *et al.* 1988; Khalil *et al.* 1991). Niclosamide has low efficacy against the metacestodes so the drug must be given daily for 5–7 days at 2 g for adults 1.5 g for children heavier than 35 kg and 1.0 g for children of 11–35 kg for about 70 per cent efficacy

(Noemi *et al.* 1991). Mebendazole and albendazole given for 3 days have lower recorded efficacies (50–60 per cent) (Ai-Issa *et al.* 1985; Amato Neto *et al.* 1990; Khalil *et al.* 1991) but give the advantage of broad-spectrum activity as patients infected with *H. nana* are likely to be infected concurrently with *Enterobius vermicularis*. Natural, indigenous products have been examined. Powdered *Nigella sativa* seeds at 40 mg/kg or an ethanol extract of this produced faecal egg count reductions comparable to those seen with niclosamide (Akhtar and Riffat 1991). A crude extract of garlic, *Allium sativum*, 5 ml twice a day, was reported to reduce symptoms in 8 of 10 children (Soffar and Mokhtar 1991) but information on egg counts is needed.

PREVENTION AND CONTROL

Sanitation and hygiene education will reduce transmission, sometimes markedly if accompanied by treatment. In a suburb of Azerbaijan, treatment with niclosamide plus improved sanitary measures and public health education reduced prevalence of infection in women and children from 5–9 to 0.5 per cent at 3 months and zero at 6 months (Chobanov and Guseinova 1987). Sanitary measures may reduce water contamination and water-borne infection; in Zimbabwe a piped water supply was associated with lower prevalences of *H. nana* in children (Mason *et al.* 1986).

Data are needed to ascertain the importance of the indirect life cycle and rodents for human infection. Rodent control measures are required. Large colonies of rodents must be exterminated. Also, a household with rodents invariably will have cereal foods infested with beetles. Cereals, grains, and other foodstuffs that are eaten uncooked must be protected from rodents and their droppings. Better storage facilities may reduce grain beetles which also might be controlled on a large scale with products such as *Bacillus thuringiensis*. The role of fleas from dogs, cats, and rodents in transmission should be lower but must be elucidated and flea control instituted if necessary.

DIPHYLLOBOTHRIUM LATUM AND OTHER *DIPHYLLOBOTHRIUM* SPECIES

HISTORY

The Swiss physician, Thaddeus Dunus, first drew attention to *Diphyllobothrium latum*, and Felix Platter of Basel in 1602 noted the difference in its genital pore from the taeniids. Eggs have since been found in archaeological sites dating back to AD 100–500. It was not until

1881/82, however, that Braun fed fish plerocercoids to dogs and man. Braun described the abdominal symptoms suffered by his experimentally infected patients and the relationship between pernicious anaemia and diphyllobothriosis was noted in 1886 in accounts by Reyher in Estonia and Runeberg in Finland. Finally Rosen, in 1917, completed the life cycle in *Cyclops* and fish (Grove 1990).

THE AGENTS AND TAXONOMY

The parasite, first named *Taenia lata* Linnaeus, 1758, then *Taenia vulgaris* and *Halysis lata*, then variously *Bothriocephalus latus*, *Dibothrium*, and *Dibothriocephalus* (Grove 1990), became *Diphyllobothrium latum* (Linnaeus, 1758) Lühe, 1910. *Diphyllobothrium nihonkaiense* Yamane, Kamo, Yazaki, Fukumoto and Maejima, 1981, was differentiated morphologically and antigenically from *D. latum* as the '*D. latum* of Japan'. Other species which infect man include *D. dendriticum* (Nitzsch, 1824), *D. klebanovskii* Muratov and Posakhov, 1988, and *D. pacificum* (Nybelin, 1931). *Diphyllobothrium orcini*, *D. yonagoense*, *D. comeroni*, *D. scoticum*, and *D. hians* have also been recorded. There is considerable structural plasticity in plerocercoids and adults of *Diphyllobothrium* (Devos *et al.* 1990) so genus only often is recorded. Keys and descriptions for some plerocercoids and adults have been given by Yamane *et al.* (1981). Muratov and Posokhov (1988), and Andersen and Gibson (1989). Gradually, molecular methods using antigenic differences, isoenzymes, restriction profiles, and ribosomal gene probes are being applied to differentiate species (Devos and Dick 1989; Devos *et al.* 1990).

Adult *D. latum* are ivory in colour, up to 10 m long. The spoon-shaped scolex, about 1×2.5 mm, has two long, weak grooves or bothria. Mature and gravid proglottids are broader than long, with numerous testes and vitellaria in the lateral edges. From the posterior ovary a central brown rosette is the uterus containing eggs that are released from a central genital pore. Eggs (light brown, operculate, with rounded ends and about 70×50 μm) are passed in the faeces. Proglottids usually disintegrate, but strings of proglottids, characterized by their brown, central rosette-like uterus, may be passed. Eggs in water develop and hatch to a ciliated, swimming coracidium. Procercoids in the haemocoel of copepods are about 500 μm long and retain the six oncospheral hooks at the posterior end. Plerocercoids in fish commonly are glistening and opaque with a rugose or furrowed body and 1–4 cm long; others are translucent bluish-white.

HOSTS

First intermediate hosts: copepods, including *Diaptomus gracilis*, *D. graciloides*, *D. oregonensis*, *Cyclops furcifer*, *C. abyssorum*, and *C. strenuus*.

1. *D. latum*:
   plerocercoid: freshwater fishes, including burbot, pike, river perch, ruff, salmon, trout
   adult tapeworm: piscivorous mammals, e.g. man, dog, cat, mongoose, fox, bear, pig, etc.
2. *D. dendriticum*:
   plerocercoid: freshwater fishes, primarily coregonids, salmonids, threespined stickleback.
   adult tapeworm: piscivorous birds, particularly seagulls and terns; mammals, e.g. dogs, man
3. *D. klebanovskii*:
   plerocercoid: *Onchorhynchus* salmon in marine littoral environment
   adult tapeworm: bear, man, dog, cat
4. *D. pacificum* and *Diphyllobothrium* spp.:
   plerocercoid: a variety of marine fishes
   adult tapeworm: sea lion, seal, other marine mammals; piscivorous birds; man

Immature adults of a number of *Diphyllobothrium* spp. have been established experimentally in hamsters, rats, and birds.

LIFE CYCLE AND EPIDEMIOLOGY

The prepatent period for *D. latum* is 4–6 weeks. In humans, infections may live 7–10 years, and produce up to 1 000 000 eggs/day. Little immunity develops so that high rates of re-infection and superinfection are possible (Bronshtein 1988). In chicks, *D. dendriticum* matured in 5–6 days, survived 3 weeks to 6 months, and average egg production/worm was 74×10^6 (Pronin *et al.* 1989a; Sharp *et al.* 1990). The epidemiology of these eggs has been studied in Russia. In one survey at a reservoir where *D. latum* was endemic, effluent from the town sewage plant contained 0.6–4.1 eggs/l, effluent from septic tanks at institutions contained 52.1 eggs/l and eggs were found in canals and ditches, all draining into the reservoir (Gerasimov 1987). However, the infection may not establish in water near large human settlements as industrial pollution can greatly decrease zooplankton levels.

Eggs hatch in as little as 5 days at 25 °C; *D. latum* and *D. dendriticum* survive in fresh water while *D. klebanovskii* was differentiated as its eggs/coracidia survive only in sea water. The coracidia ingested by copepods develop in 2–3 weeks to procercoids. Fish eat infected zooplankton and the plerocercoids are long-lived in either the viscera or musculature and can transfer from prey fish to predator fish, accumulating in the tissues of older, big predator fish. Humans with a dietary preference for raw, smoked, lightly salted or lightly pickled fish, and fish roe are at risk of infection. The most prevalent species in humans are those whose plerocercoid's predilection site is the musculature (e.g. *D. latum*, *D. klebanovskii*) rather than the viscera (e.g. *D. dendriticum*).

GEOGRAPHIC DISTRIBUTION

Diphyllobothrium latum is circumpolar and common in northern temperate and subarctic countries with many lakes where fish is eaten raw. Infection stretches from northern Italy through to the Baltic States, west from Lake Tiberius and the Danube Delta through northern European CIS, People's Republic of China, and Japan. There are several foci of infection in North America and infection has been introduced into South America, particularly Brazil and Chile. *Diphyllobothrium dendriticum* is common in many of the same areas as *D. latum*, particularly north-western Europe and North America; *D. klebanovskii* occurs in Far-East Russia; *D. pacificum* infects man in Peru and Chile but is found in other waters also. The other species are recorded in man, particularly in Japan and South-East Asia, but as these records are in seamen, infections probably were acquired elsewhere.

In 1880 one-quarter of the population of Geneva was reported to be infected with *D. latum*, but this prevalence has declined drastically. Recently, in various foci of infection around rivers and lakes in Russia, levels of *D. latum* reached 6–12 per cent in humans, 27 per cent in dogs, 90–95 per cent in pike, and 14 per cent in perch (Plyusheva *et al.* 1987; Zhuravlev and Puzyrev 1987). On the River Valdiva, Chile, 0–1.2 per cent of humans and 5–10 per cent of dogs were infected with *D. latum* (Torres *et al.* 1989). *Diphyllobothrium latum* and *D. dendriticum* were present in 28 per cent and 58 per cent, respectively, of rainbow trout in Lake Moreno, Argentina (Revenga 1993). *Diphyllobothrium dendriticum* has been recorded in 70–100 per cent of Arctic cisco and 30–50 per cent of pollan and Arctic grayling in Lake Baikal, Russia (Pronin *et al.* 1988), in 77–93 per cent of rockeye salmon smolts in Great Central Lake, Canada (Ching 1988), and in 45 per cent of dogs in Fort Chimo, Canada (Desrochers and Curtis 1987). In the coregonids, plerocercoids were found primarily in the viscera but those in rockeye salmon were in the muscles rather than viscera. In eastern Russia around the coast of the Okhotsk Sea, *D. klebanovskii* has been found in 1 per cent of humans and, in the south of the areas, in 3.3 per cent of humans, 3.1 per cent of dogs, and 10.5 per

cent of cats (Dovgalev 1988*a*). In the Amur Region inland from here, 0.4–4.2 per cent of people living along the rivers were infected; brown bear are a principal definitive host, 47 per cent being infected. Infection is acquired only in June to October when salmon, having acquired infection (30–46 per cent) in the marine littoral environment, migrate to spawn (Muratov and Posokhov 1989). Although *D. dendtriticum* was present in wild and not farmed salmon in the Puget Sound, Sharp (1991) reported that it can be prevalent in salmon farmed in Scotland. This will be true of many other fish farmed in lakes/reservoirs with an abundant zooplankton or where zooplankton is allowed to pass into hatchery raceways.

SYMPTOMS, CLINICAL SIGNS AND PATHOLOGY

Plerocercoids in the viscera usually are encysted in nodules, those in flesh often free. In many surveys 1–10 and occasionally more parasites are recorded. Heavily infected fish are said to die off more rapidly than uninfected fish, but clinical, subclinical, and economic effects are not documented.

In humans, many infections are asymptomatic, but abdominal symptoms were accurately described by Braun in 1881–82 as abdominal pain, dizziness, fatigue, transient diarrhoea, dyspepsia, and vomiting. A clear relationship exists between *D. latum* infection and pernicious anaemia due to competitive uptake and use of vitamin B_{12} by the worm; patients exhibit a megaloblastic anaemia. This is regarded as a classic sign of diphyllobothriosis but in fact occurs mainly on a genetic or familial basis in the Baltics and is now rare with improved winter diets in the areas where it occurred.

DIAGNOSIS

Diagnosis is made from eggs in the faeces. Sometimes chains of proglottids with their central, brown rosette will be noticed by the patient. A coproantigen test would be useful as Kamo *et al.* (1986) reported periodicity in egg production with quite long periods when eggs were not seen.

TREATMENT

The same drugs as used for *Taenia* (chapter 51) are effective, Praziquantel as a single oral dose of 10–25 mg/kg is highly effective and the drug of choice. Niclosamide as a single oral dose is useful (adults 2.0 g: children heavier than 35 kg, 1.5 g; lighter than 35 kg,

1.0 g). Other drugs, e.g. quinicrine (adults 1.0 g in five divided doses every 10 min; children 35–45 kg, 0.6 g; 18–35 kg; 0.4 g) are used, followed by a saline purgative after 2 hours if necessary, but are less effective and have side-effects. Vitamin B_{12} may be given as a precautionary treatment. Other anthelmintics that still are quite widely used in Russia, Japan, and South-East Asia include bithionol, paromomycin sulphate, and the contrast medium, intraduodenal gastrografin. These should be replaced in view of the very high efficacy and ease of administration of praziquantel.

PREVENTION AND CONTROL

Control of *D. latum* has been attempted in areas of Russia. Exponential models developed to approximate the situation in Russia pinpointed the importance of the lack of definitive host immunity when considering mass treatment of humans (Bronshtein 1988). Additional information is needed to ascertain stability of the cestode in fish. However, a major obstacle is the absence of tests with which to differentiate non-zoonotic or rarely zoonotic species of *Diphyllobothrium* in their wild animal definitive and fish intermediate hosts, e.g. *D. detrimum* in freshwater fish and the numerous species in marine fish that have marine birds, seals, porpoises, etc. as definitive hosts.

Culinary habits and the importance of fish in human diets in coastal areas of seas/lakes makes education on the correct processing of fish and reduced consumption of raw fish important to prevent infection, but it is difficult to alter cultural behaviour. Thorough cooking kills plerocercoids, freezing to −10 to −20 °C in the centre for at least 6 h is effective (Pronin *et al.* 1989*b*). Salt content of 7 per cent or more is lethal. Dry salting at 35–45 per cent salt = fish w/w kills plerocercoids in 4–8 days at 10–15 °C, cold salting with 35–40 per cent salt and 50–60 per cent ice to fish w/w at −3 to −5 °C is effective for 3 kg of fish in 7–10 days, but weights of more than 4 kg require 35–39 days (Dovgalev 1988*b*).

Improved sanitation and treatment of effluents would prevent human egg discharge into rivers. However, control is complicated by animal definitive hosts, e.g. the brown bear for *D. klebanovskii*, the dog for *D. latum*, whose role in water contamination could be greater than that of humans. Consideration must be given to these animals when inland bodies of water are developed because a wide variety of freshwater copepods and fish act as hosts, and foci of infection can develop rapidly. Ten years after a reservoir was built, infection was present in 90 per cent of pike, 14 per cent of perch, 27 per cent of dogs, and 8–12 per cent of humans (Plyusheva *et al.* 1987). Similarly, infection

imported from the Baltic into South America was able to establish in lakes and rivers.

OTHER ADULT CESTODE INFECTIONS

A number of tapeworms in other genera are found occasionally in humans. As with the more common tapeworm infections, most are asymptomatic, some may cause abdominal pain, nausea, hunger, diarrhoea. Praziquantel must be the drug of choice for treatment. Niclosamide has lower efficacy than praziquantel against most cestode species and, as the benzimidazoles have low efficacy against some tapeworms in animals, e.g. *Dipylidium caninum*, they cannot be recommended.

DIPYLIDIUM CANINUM (LINNAEUS, 1758) LEUCKART, 1863

The adult tapeworm in Canidae and Felidae is up to 50 cm long. Its acetabulate scolex has a protrusable rostellum and up to 150 rose-thorn shaped hooks, usually in 3–4 rows. The neck is thin and the subsequent strobila is made up of 'cucumber-seed', elongate oval proglottids. Each mature proglottid has two sets of genital organs opening in two lateral genital pores and ovaries and vitellaria are grouped on either side. In gravid proglottids, there are egg capsules or packets (each containing up to 30 thin-walled eggs) scattered through the parenchyma.

Proglottids detach and commonly migrate from the anus or may be passed in the faeces. They migrate on the faeces or in the perianal area and drop to the floor, particularly in the sleeping area of the dog/cat. Cat fleas, *Ctenocephalides felis*, parasitic on both cats and dogs, act as intermediate hosts. Experimentally, *Xenopsylla cheopis* can be infected, but not *Ctenocephalides canis* (Pugh 1987). The dog louse, *Trichodectes canis*, continues to be named as a host; additional studies would be appropriate.

Flea larvae, common in the area where the dog or cat sleeps, eat proglottids, and mature cysticercoids develop in as little as 9–15 days at 32 °C. At lower temperatures development is slow and metacestodes won't complete their development until after the adult flea has spent a period of a few days at above 32 °C in the coat of the final host animal (Pugh and Moorhouse 1985). Adult fleas are eaten accidentally as the dog or cat grooms its coat.

This tapeworm is the most common (1–88 per cent) in dogs and cats worldwide (Boreham and Boreham 1990). Prevalences tend to follow the expected prevalence of intermediate host fleas: usually higher in tropical, developing countries than in temperate, Western countries; in backyard cats and stray animals rather than in domestic pets. One to ten per cent of fleas have been reported infected with up to 82 metacestodes/flea.

INFECTION OF HUMANS

Considering the ubiquitous and prevalent nature of infection in dogs and cats, infection of humans is not common. There are about 200 reports of human infections from all around the world, this undoubtedly an underestimate. Infection usually is reported in children below 10 years with about one-third of cases in babies younger than 6–12 months, possibly due to an age resistance or to closer examinations of these young children. Fleas are accidentally ingested when a child is in close contact with an infested pet dog/cat. There are suggestions that metacestodes from a flea that is crushed in the mouth of a dog can be transferred in a saliva by dog(s) licking, but the probability of this transfer seems low.

In addition to the non-specific abdominal signs of infection, anal pruritis may occur in a child. Proglottids crawling in the anus and perineal region of a dog may cause it to sit and pull its anus along the ground ('scoot'). Infection must be differentiated from *Enterobius vermicularis* by cutting into a proglottid to see egg packets.

BERTIELLA STUDERI (BLANCHARD, 1891) AND *BERTIELLA MUCRONATA* (MEYNER, 1895)

The adults of these, common in primates, are unarmed and can reach 45 cm. Each proglottid is much wider than long, with a single set of genital organs, the uterus is a transverse tube. Eggs, about 50 μm in diameter, have a well-developed pyriform apparatus (the inner membrane is pear-shaped due to a pair of hooked projections on one side). Gravid proglottids are excreted in chains of 10–12. Oribatid mites that are free-living on vegetation eat eggs and act as the intermediate hosts.

INFECTION IN HUMANS

Many cases of human infections with *B. studeri* have been reported in Africa, the Pacific islands, and Asia—particularly India, and South-East Asia. *Bertiella mucronata* has been reported occasionally in man in South American countries and Cuba. Most cases occur in children, presumably through accidental ingestion of mites on food, on hands, or in soil (geophagia pica). Most patients come from villages where monkeys are bred in captivity.

INERMICAPSIFER MADAGASCARIENSIS (DAVAINE, 1870) AND *INERMICAPSIFER CUBENSIS* (KOURI, 1938)

The adults of these tapeworms are common in rodents and hyracoids and are unarmed and can reach 45 cm. Proglottids are wider than long and eggs are found in egg capsules of 6–10 eggs. The life cycle undoubtedly involves an arthropod, probably mite, intermediate host.

INFECTIONS IN HUMANS

These tapeworms have been reported sporadically in man in Africa and Central and South America.

RAILLIETINA FUHRMANN, 1920

A large number of different *Raillietina* spp. are described in rodents although they may in fact represent only a few species. Adults have a large rostellum armed with large numbers of small, hammer-shaped hooks in two rows; the four suckers are weak and armed with minute hooks. Eggs are found in egg capsules. As the better known *Raillietina* spp. of domestic birds use ants and beetles as intermediate hosts, similar life cycles are assumed for the rodent forms.

INFECTION IN HUMANS

Infections with these rodent *Raillietina* spp. have been recorded occasionally in humans in the People's Republic of China, the Asian Pacific region, and in South America.

MESOCESTOIDES LINEATUS (GÖZE, 1782) RAILLIET, 1893, AND *MESOCESTOIDES VARIABILIS* MUELLER, 1928,

While speciation of these is uncertain, adults are found in birds and mammals, particularly carnivores, e.g. dogs, cats, martens, polecats, foxes, wolves, racoons, coyotes, etc., in Asia, Europe, Africa, and North America. The scolex is unarmed. Proglottids have a central genital pore. Eggs enter a central paruterine organ which has a wall of dense fibrous-type tissue. The life cycle involves cysticercoids in mites, at least experimentally, as first intermediate hosts. Second intermediate hosts are amphibia, reptiles, birds, and mammals, including the dog and cat. In these a tetrathyridium which has an invaginated protoscolex with four suckers and which can multiply by asexual division occurs in the body cavities. When eaten by the definitive host, tetrathyridia can develop to adults, but also can again multiply asexually in the peritoneal cavity before entering the intestine to develop to adults.

INFECTION IN HUMANS

Adults of *M. lineatus* have been reported in humans, mainly in Japan and recently China and Korea, while records of *M. variabilis* have come from Europe, Africa, and the United States. Severe diarrhoea has been reported, while other patients described abdominal pain, hunger, and dizziness.

DIPLOGONOPORUS GRANDIS (BLANCHARD, 1894) LÜHE, 1899

This is a parasite of whales but in fact the tapeworm was described first by Blanchard from a human in Japan. It is closely related to *D. latum* with a relatively similar structure and life cycle. Adults of *D. grandis* differ from *D. latum* in that their bothria are keyhole shaped and, in particular, there are two sets of reproductive organs in each proglottid. Copepods act as the first intermediate hosts, with marine fish as the second intermediate host.

INFECTION IN HUMANS

Infection is reported primarily in Japan, related to the eating of raw fish, e.g. anchovies, sardines. Kochi Prefecture has the highest reported numbers—40 up until 1992 with about 200 cases recorded in Japan (Suzuki *et al.* 1993).

COENUROSIS: *TAENIA MULTICEPS*, *TAENIA SERIALIS*, AND *TAENIA BRAUNI*

HISTORY

The many protoscolices in the metacestode (coenurus) stage led to the species name *Taenia multiceps* (many-headed) by Leske. Cerebral coenurosis in ruminants, known since antiquity, was mentioned by Hippocrates and recognized in man in the seventeenth century (Bakay 1971). A full description of clinical neurocoenurosis in animals occurred when Wepfer described an epidemic of 'gid' in sheep and cattle in 1658, although 'gid' for giddiness in sheep is ascribed to Holland in 1601 (*Oxford English Dictionary*), (2nd edn), 1989). The first human case was reported in 1913 in France. Küchenmeister in 1853 connected the parasite in cattle, sheep, and goats and completed the life cycle in sheep and dogs. He also set out control

measures—feed dogs dry food; cook sheep heads before they are fed; restrain and purge dogs twice a year and burn the resultant faeces and worms. Wepfer recorded that peasants 'operated' to remove the cysts and Hogg in an 1807 Shepherd's Guide advocated crude perforation of the 'bag' with knitting wires passed through the nostrils to the brain. A few years later this was refined to the current penetration through a softening in the skull.

THE AGENTS

Taenia multiceps Leske, 1980, was also called *Multiceps multiceps*. The parasite in goats was named *Taenia gaigeri* but now differences seem to be specific for the host and not the parasite. It is difficult to differentiate related species but *Taenia serialis* (Gervais, 1847) Baillet, 1863, and *Taenia brauni* (Setti, 1897) Fain *et al.*, 1956, are described. Molecular methods will be needed to confirm their differences.

Adult *T. multiceps* reach 40–100 cm, have a scolex with four suckers and a double ring of rostellar hooks. The gravid uterus has 18–26 lateral branches that contain characteristic taeniid eggs (Chapter 51). *Taenia serialis* has 10–18 lateral branches and it has a well-developed vaginal sphincter while that of *T. multiceps* is only a pad (Verster 1969). Protoscolices are found within cysts at 2 months. The coenurus of *T. multiceps* can reach 5 or more centimetres in diameter with 70–100, but up to 400, protoscolices clustered in groups on the wall. In general the total number of protoscolices and in particular the average number of protoscolices in a cluster increase with age of the coenuri (Willis and Herbert 1987). The coenurus of *T. serialis* is similar but smaller and has protoscolices in radiating rows. *Taenia brauni* is very similar to *T. serialis*.

HOSTS

1. *Taenia multiceps*:
   adult tapeworm: dog and other Canidae (fox, wolf, etc.)
   metacestode: sheep, goat, cattle, chamois, gazelle, and other ruminants; man
2. *Taenia serialis*:
   adult tapeworm: dog and other Canidae
   metacestode: lagomorphs and rarely rodents and the cat; man
3. *Taenia brauni*:
   adult tapeworm: dog and other Canidae
   metacestode: rodents; it has been described in primates; man

LIFE CYCLE AND EPIDEMIOLOGY

The life cycle of *Taenia multiceps* has been described by Willis and Herbert (1984, 1987) and Herbert *et al.* (1984). The prepatent period of infection in dogs is 38–43 days. There is evidence, at least experimentally, for the gradual development of resistance to reinfection. Gravid proglottids contain 37 000 eggs, but there is scanty information on intensity of infection, fecundity, and infection pressure so the reproduction ratio of *T. multiceps* cannot yet be compared with the hierarchy of the other canine taeniids (Gemmell 1990). Eggs remain viable on pasture for at least several weeks and fly-borne transfer of infection to pasture at high intensity for up to 80 m from dog faecal deposits, as described for *Taenia hydatigena* (Chapter 51) should occur. Ingested oncospheres migrate in all tissues, but usually only those in the CNS develop, although cysts can mature intramuscularly and subcutaneously in the goat. Cysts in the brain of sheep undoubtedly debilitate or kill them, thereby increasing the chances of being scavenged by dogs. *Taenia serialis* and *T. brauni* occur intramuscularly and subcutaneously and may restrict the activity of rabbits and hares, thereby increasing their likelihood of capture by hunting dogs.

INFECTION IN HUMANS

The species in man is still questioned and commonly is not identified. In the United States only *T. serialis* is encountered to account for mainly subcutaneous/intramuscular cysts. However, as *T. serialis* is described in the brain of monkeys and cats (Smith *et al.* 1988), it presumably could account for CNS lesions in humans. Infections in Europe are largely in the brain and usually are *T. multiceps*, some are subcutaneous and often ascribed to *T. serialis*. Intraocular cases could be due to either species. Infections in Africa are primarily subcutaneous or intraocular and largely ascribed to *T. brauni*. CNS involvement is rare in Africa.

Infection in man is rare with fewer than 100 cases in the literature, although many tissue nodules undoubtedly remain undiagnosed and unreported. This is probably true for some neurological cases also. Infectivity for man of the eggs seems low to account for the very low incidence of *T. multiceps* compared with the higher human prevalence of *E. granulosus* which has the same dog–sheep/man assemblage.

GEOGRAPHIC DISTRIBUTION

Taenia multiceps is common in many mountainous or range areas where ready access of unsupervised dogs to sheep is possible. However, *T. multiceps* has disappeared from some countries, e.g. the United States and New Zealand. *Taenia serialis* is recorded worldwide, *T. brauni* is described in Africa. Surveys which examine prevalence of helminths in dogs usually record only *Taenia* spp., so information is scanty. Prevalence of infection has been described as 0.4–26.6 per cent for *T. multiceps* and 4.0–7.0 per cent for *T. serialis* in dogs in Wales (Williams 1976; Hackett and Walters 1980). In Pakistan and Uruguay, 0.5 per cent and 0.3 per cent, respectively, of dogs were infected with *T. multiceps*. *Taenia multiceps* was reported to have a prevalence of up to 5.8 per cent in slaughtered sheep in Wales (Williams and Boundy 1983) and to cause 5 per cent mortality in sheep in Ethiopia (Njua *et al.* 1988).

SYMPTOMS, CLINICAL SIGNS, AND PATHOGENESIS

ANIMALS

Acute coenurosis

Experimental infection with 1000–5000 eggs in lambs produces acute coenurosis manifest, in the field, as a 'storm' (Edwards and Herbert 1982; Doherty *et al.* 1989). Acute disease is reported in 25 per cent or more of animals receiving large experimental or field infections, with fatalities in 25 per cent or more of these. It is predictable 1–5 weeks after infection when the large numbers of immature protoscolices migrate in the brain (Edwards and Herbert 1982) causing neurological signs, pyrexia, and retinal haemorrhages, presumably due to physical destruction of tissues. Sinuous tracts with larvae in the centre of some are seen in the CNS. Degenerate larvae and tracts might be seen in other tissues. Retinal haemorrhage is assumed to be from the route of entrance for intraocular cysts; from ciliary arteries into the subretinal space and then perforation of the retina. Animals that recover from acute coenurosis go into a quiescent period but these, and those more lightly infected, then develop the chronic form of the disease.

Chronic coenurosis

As far as is known, most sheep with viable coenuri will develop clinical signs of chronic coenurosis. There may be one or more coenuri and possibly one or more caseous lesions also. The cysts cause a space-occupying lesion in the brain. Clinical signs, seen 1.5 to 13 or more months after infection, depend on the site and size of the cyst, and are paresis, ataxia, blindness, nystagmus, leaning, circling, pushing head against objects, etc.; papilloedema is common. Individual subcutaneous/intramuscular cysts usually cause no overt changes in the health of goats or lagomorphs, but several hundred cysts in a goat resulted in a 'puffed up' appearance, disturbances in gait, inappetence, and retarded growth (Dey *et al.* 1988). Little attention has been paid to ocular coenurosis in animals.

The prolonged survival of the coenuri may be related to their elaboration of two immunosuppressive factors, TMCF F24 and F7 (Rakha *et al.* 1991, 1992). The first modifies accessory cells to inhibit their helper activity; the second, a mitogen, acts on CD4+T cells to intensify the inhibition induced by the accessory cells.

HUMAN COENUROSIS

Subcutaneous/intramuscular nodules normally are painless or only slightly tender. Organisms in the eye are unilateral, are usually found in the vitreous and affect visual acuity with blurring of the vision, shadows, and perhaps pain. Cyst death has been associated with severe endophthalmitis (Junior 1949; Ibechukwu and Onwukeme 1991). In the brain, cysts have a predilection for the subarachnoid space, basal cisterns, and ventricular cavities, so that a main presenting sign is disturbance in the cerebrospinal fluid pathways (Schellhas and Norris 1985, Pau *et al.* 1987). The fourth ventricular foramina are particularly prone to blockage. Ventricular cysts can be rapidly fatal if they cause sudden blockage. Alternately, there can be increased cranial hypertension, hydrocephalus, violent headache, nausea, and movement disorders. There may be subsequent arachnoiditis or diffuse ependymitis, depending on the location of the cyst. Occasionally cysts will be found in the parenchyma of the brain and symptoms then vary with site of the lesion, e.g. seizures, weakness of a limb, paralysis, etc. (Pau *et al.* 1987). Spinal cysts have been recorded.

DIAGNOSIS AND TREATMENT

Subcutaneous cysts are palpable and recognition of intramuscular cysts is aided by radiology and ultrasound. Where medical and veterinary services are freely available, individual cysts in humans or pet animals, e.g. rabbits, goats, are likely to be removed surgically for differentiation from 'tumours'.

Intravitreal cysts in man are visible on detailed funduscopy which shows the outline of the cyst and possibly its scolices as white spots. Vitreal inflammation, if present, will obscure the cyst. In these cases, diagnostic tests comparable to those used for ocular larva migrans (Chapter 65) may be useful; eosinophils should be present in the humour; ecography could outline a cyst. The cyst then can be removed by closed vitrectomy (Kruger-Leite *et al.* 1985). As severe endophthalmitis

has been observed on death of the cyst, the cyst should be removed immediately on diagnosis without anthelmintic treatment (Junior 1949; Ibechukwu and Onwukeme 1991).

Metrizamide-enhanced computed tomography (CT) scan and magnetic resonance imaging (MRI) have proved valuable in patients presenting with cerebral coenurosis. These can allow precise evaluation of size and location of the cyst(s) (Pau *et al.* 1987). Nevertheless, as most coenuri locate in the ventricular system, there may be problems with diagnosis, as with neurocysticercosis (Chapter 51). Intraventricular cysts often will be isodense and there may be problems in visualizing the cyst wall. MRI may reveal protoscolices and contrast ventriculography may be useful, although blockage of CSF pathways may prevent diffusion of the medium. Immunodiagnostic tests are not yet available.

Surgical removal of the coenurus is an important therapeutic regimen due to the potential for a cyst to move and cause acute onset blockage of CSF pathways. Surgery also is used for parenchymal cysts, particularly as these usually occur singly. There is some evidence to suggest efficacy of anthelmintics for coenurosis in animals. Praziquantel in high doses (50 mg/kg for 3 days) killed the mature coenurus in some animals, reducing the clinical signs (Arkhipova *et al.* 1986). Praziquantel and fenbendazole (25 mg/kg or 0.75 g/ lamb, respectively, for 6 days at 20-day intervals) was used prophylactically with apparent success to control experimentally induced acute disease and levels of disease in sheep in a flock with a history of disease (Azimzhanov *et al.* 1988). However, unlike sheep which have parenchymal cysts, in humans coenuri most commonly lie in the ventricular system. Thus, the information obtained with *T. solium* (Chapter 51) would suggest that praziquantel therapy of human intraventricular *T. multiceps* is unlikely to be successful. Although albendazole might well have a better effect, additional data is required.

PREVENTION AND CONTROL

Measures that curb the freedom of and numbers of dogs, control disposal of sheep carcasses and ensure regular anthelmintic treatments of dogs will curb transmission of *T. multiceps*. Where these measures have been applied successfully for the control of echinococcosis/ hydatidosis (National Hydatids Control Programme in New Zealand and South Powys Hydatidosis Control Scheme in Wales) (Chapter 52; Walters 1986; Gemmell 1990; Lloyd *et al.* 1991) outbreaks of *T. multiceps* either declined or were eliminated. The exact treatment interval required to control *T. multiceps* has not been determined, however, and when previously successful control measures directed against hydatidosis in Wales were reduced to voluntary owner purchase of drug, outbreaks of neurocoenurosis returned (Walters and Lloyd 1992).

OTHER TISSUE METACESTODE INFECTIONS

SPIROMETRA (*DIPHYLLOBOTHRIUM*) *MANSONI* JOYEUX AND HOUDEMER, 1927, *SPIROMETRA ERINACEI* FAUST, CAMPBELL, AND KELLOG, 1929, AND *SPIROMETRA MANSONOIDES* MUELLER, 1935

Plerocercoids were first described in the peritoneal cavity of a Chinaman by Manson (Grove 1990). Now plerocercoids are described in humans periodically through most of the world. *Spirometra mansoni* is dominant in Asia and South America, *S. erinacei* in Asia and Australia, and *S. mansonoides* in the Americas. There have been a few records of adult *S. erinacei* in humans in Japan.

The life cycle was described by Yoshida and Yamara in 1916 and then Okumura in 1919 (Grove 1990). Adult tapeworms resemble *Diphyllobothrium* but there is both a vaginal and a uterine pore, the uterus takes the form of a spiral not a rosette, and eggs have pointed rather than rounded ends. Adults occur in wild carnivores and in the dog and cat (but not usually man) in many parts of the world. Procercoid larvae are found in *Cyclops* inhabiting small ponds; plerocercoids in amphibia, reptiles, small mammals, birds, e.g. ducks, chickens, and large game animals in Africa, that all act as second intermediate and paratenic hosts. The plerocercoids, known as spargana, are ribbon-like, white, wrinkled and can reach 30–40 cm. They can transfer from one to another intermediate host. Man can act as a second intermediate host.

INFECTION IN HUMANS

Humans acquire infection with the plerocercoid in a number of ways:

(1) by ingesting infected *Cyclops* in water;
(2) by eating plerocercoids in raw flesh of snakes, tadpoles, frogs, etc.; wild pigs can be an important source (Corkhum 1966); and
(3) in China and South-East Asia, muscles of split amphibia often are applied as a poultice to an ulcer, infected eyes, or an infected vagina; spargana then wander across to the human tissues.

Ingested procercoids or spargana penetrate the intestine, wander through deep tissues and may be found intraperitoneally and in the viscera or may migrate to subcutaneous sites where they either elicit a recurrent inflammatory response or encyst in a fibrous nodule of about 2 cm diameter. A sparganum can persist in the tissues for 20–30 years.

As the sparganum grows and elicits the inflammatory response, the site is painful. Ocular sparganosis can cause intense pain, oedema, and ulceration. Occasionally proliferating spargana, where the parasite breaks up into segments each capable of further development, have been seen and can be serious and fatal. There have been several cases of cerebral sparganosis presenting primarily as headaches and seizures. In one, CT scan revealed a contrast-enhanced mass that was avascular on angiography (Fan and Pezeshkpour 1986). Other cases showed migratory tracts and inflammation as unilateral areas of low density along white matter bundles with nodular or irregular enhancement. Changes in location suggested their sparganum aetiology (Chang *et al.* 1987).

Diagnosis is made after surgical removal or biopsy of the organism. The sparganum can be identified as cestode in origin by its laminated, basophilic calcareous corpuscles which characterize cestode tissues. Individual or small numbers of spargana will be treated by surgery. Little information is available on anthelminitic therapy but, in heavy or cerebral infections, albendazole or praziquantel should be considered.

There have been rare reports of *Taenia crassiceps* (Zeder, 1800) Rudolphi 1810 in the human eye in Europe and America and *Taenia taeniaeformis* (Batsch, 1786) in the liver of humans.

REFERENCES

Ai-Issa, T., Jafar, T., and Idan, H. (1985). A field study in the treatment of intestinal helminths by the drug Zentel. *Bulletin of Endemic Diseases*, **26**, 81–91.

Akhtar, M. S. and Riffat, S. (1991). Field trial of *Saussurea lappa* roots against nematodes and *Nigella sativa* seeds against cestodes in children. *Journal of the Pakistan Medical Association*, **41**, 185–7.

Ali, S. A., Jamal, K., and Quadri, S. M. H. (1992). Prevalence of intestinal parasites among food handlers in Al-Medinah. *Annals of Saudi Medicine*, **12**, 63–6.

Allan, J. C. and Craig, P. S. (1994). Partial characterization and time course analysis of *Hymenolepis diminuta* coproantigens. *Journal of Helminthology*, **68**, 97–103.

Amato Neto, V. *et al.* (1990). Evaluation of therapeutic activity of albendazole in experimental and human infection with *Hymenolepis nana*. *Revista do Instituto de Medicina Tropical de São Paulo*, **32**, 185–8.

Andersen, K. I. and Gibson, D. I. (1989). A key to 3 species of larval *Diphyllobothrium* Cobbold, 1858 (Cestoda, Pseudophyllidea) occurring in European and North American fresh water fishes. *Systemic Parasitology*, **13**, 3–9.

Arkhipova, N. S., Bessenov, A. S., Malakova, E. I., Movsesyan, S. O., Stepanyan, S. G., and Sogomonyan, A. S. (1986). Praziquantel therapy of coenuriosis in sheep. *Byulletyn'*

Vsesoyuznogo Instituta Gel'mintologii im K. I. Skryabina, **43**, 13–16.

Ata, A. A., El-Khashab, M. N., Mourad, A. A., and Soliman, H. M. (1988). The effect of praziquantel on *Heterophyes heterophyes*, *Hymenolepis nana* and *Fasciola* sp. infections. *Journal of the Egyptian Society of Parasitology*, **18**, 243–6.

Azimzhanov, M., Musinov, M., and Baratov, V. A. (1988). Chemoprophylaxis of *Coenurus cerebralis* infestation in sheep using fenbendazole and praziquantel. *Veterinariya, Moscow*, **10**, 46–7.

Babur, C., Kabasolak, B., and Seckin, M. (1987). A coprological investigation in a health college. *Turk Hijyen Deneysel Biyoloji Dergisi*, **44**, 109–12.

Bakay, L. (1971). *The treatment of head injuries in the Thirty Years' War*. Charles C. Thomas, Illinois.

Boreham, R. E. and Boreham, P. F. L. (1990). *Dipylidium caninum*, life cycle epizootiology and control. *Compendium of Continuing Education for the Practicing Veterinarian*, **12**, 667–74.

Bronshtein, A. M. (1988). Analysis of the prevalence of opisthorchiasis and diphyllobothriasis in the local and the indigenous populations of endemic foci, using 3 exponential models with determination of transmission potentials. *Meditsinskaia Parazitologiia i Parazitarnye Bolezni*, **2**, 14–18.

Chang, K. H. *et al.* (1987). Cerebral sparganosis, CT characteristics. *Radiology*, **165**, 505–10.

Chattopadhyay, B., Fricker, E. and Gelia, C. B. (1988). Incidence of parasitic infestations in minority group travellers to and new immigrants arriving from the third world countries. *Public Health*, **102**, 245–50.

Ching, H. L. (1988). The distribution of plerocercoids of *Diphyllobothrium dendriticum* (Nitzsch) in rockeye salmon (*Onchorhynchus nerka*) smolts from Great Central Lake, British Columbia. *Canadian Journal of Zoology*, **66**, 850–2.

Chobanov, R. E. and Guseinova, A. S. (1987). Control strategies in foci of hymenolepiasis. *Meditsinskaia Parazitologiia i Parazitarnye Bolezni*, **2**, 46–7.

Corkhum, K. C. (1966). Sparganosis of some vertebrates of Louisiana and observations of human infection. *Journal of Parasitology*, **52**, 444–8.

Desrochers, F. and Curtis, M. A. (1987). The occurrence of gastrointestinal helminths in dogs from Kuujjuaq (Fort Chimo), Quebec, Canada. *Canadian Journal of Public Health*, **78**, 403–6.

Devos, T. and Dick, T. A. (1989). Differentiation between *Diphyllobothrium dendriticum* and *Diphyllobothrium latum* using isozymes, restriction profiles and ribosomal gene probes. *Systemic Parasitology*, **13**, 161–6.

Devos, T., Szalai, A. J., and Dick, T. A. (1990). Genetic and morphological variability in a population of *D. dendriticum* (Nitzsch, 1824). *Systemic Parasitology*, **16**, 99–105.

Dey, P. C., Nayak, D. C., Mohanty, D. N., Nayak, S., and Pattanayak, G. M. (1988). A brief note on massive infection of *Coenurus gaigeri* cysts in a desi goat. *Indian Veterinary Journal*, **65**, 166.

Doherty, M. L., Bassett, H. F., Breathnach, R., Monaghan, M. L., and McErlean, B. A. (1989). Outbreak of acute coenurosis in adult sheep in Ireland. *Veterinary Record*, **125**, 185.

Dovgalev, A. S. (1988*a*). Diphyllobothriasis in the western coastal region of the Okhotsk Sea. *Meditsinskaia Parazitologiia i Parazitarnye Bolezni*, **4**, 67–71.

Dovgalev, A. S. (1988*b*). Decontamination of Pacific salmon from type F plerocercoids. *Meditsinskaia Parazitologiia i Parazitarnye Bolezni*, **5**, 88–91.

Edwards, G. T. and Herbert, I. V. (1982). Observations on the course of *Taenia multiceps* infections in sheep, clinical signs and post-mortem findings. *British Veterinary Journal*, **138**, 489–500.

Fan, K. J. and Pezeshkpour, G. H. (1986). Cerebral sparganosis. *Neurology*, **36**, 1249–51.

Gemmell, M. A. (1990). Australasian contributions to an understanding of the epidemiology and control of hydatid disease caused by *Echinococcus granulosus*—past, present and future. *International Journal for Parasitology*, **20**, 431–56.

Gerasimov, I. V. (1987). Establishing the routes of contamination of the water of the Krasnoyarsk reservoir by *Diphyllobothrium latum* ova as a basis for elaborating prophylactic measures. *Meditsinskaia Parazitologiia i Parazitarnye Bolezni*, **5**, 72–5.

Gomez-Priego, A., Godinezhana, A. L., and Gutierrezquiroz, M. (1991). Detection of serum antibodies in human *Hymenolepis* infection by enzyme immunoassay. *Transactions of the Royal Society of Tropical Medicine and Hygiene*. **85**, 645–7.

Grove, D. I. (1990). *A history of human helminthology*, p. 848. CAB International, Wallingford.

Hackett, F. and Walters, T. M. H. (1980). The prevalence of cestodes in farm dogs in mid-Wales. *Veterinary Parasitology*, **7**, 95–101.

Herbert, I. V., Edwards, G. T., and Willis, J. M. (1984). Some host factors which influence the epidemiology of *Taenia multiceps* infections in sheep. *Annals of Tropical Medicine and Parasitology*, **78**, 243–8.

Heyneman, D. (1961). Studies on helminth immunity. III. Experimental verification of autoinfection from cysticercoids of *Hymenolepis nana* in the white mouse. *Journal of Infectious Diseases*, **109**, 10–18.

Ibechukwu, B. I. and Onwukeme, K. E. (1991). Intraocular coenurosis—a case report. *British Journal of Ophthalmology*, **75**, 430–1.

Ito, A. and Smyth, J. D. (1987). Adult cestodes—immunology of the lumen-dwelling cestode infections. In *Immune Responses in Parasitic Infections: Immunology, Immunopathology and Immunoprophylaxis*. Vol. II, *Trematodes and Cestodes*, (ed. E. J. L. Soulsby). pp. 115–82. CRC Press, Boca Raton.

Junior, L. (1949). Ocular cysticercosis. *American Journal of Ophthalmology*, **32**, 523–47.

Kamo, H., Yazaki, S., Fukumoto, S., Maejima, J., and Kawasaki, H. (1986). Evidence of egg-discharging periodicity in experimental human infection with *Diphyllobothrium latum*. *Japanese Journal of Parasitology*, **35**, 53–7.

Khalil, H. M., El-Shimi, S., Sarwat, M. A., Fauzy, A. F. A., and El-Sorougy, A. O. (1991). Recent study of *Hymenolepis nana* infection in Egyptian children. *Journal of the Egyptian Society of Parasitology*, **21**, 293–300.

Kruger-Leite, E., Jalkh, A. E., Quiroz, H., and Schepens, C. L. (1985). Intraocular cysticercosis. *American Journal of Ophthalmology*, **99**, 252–7.

Lloyd, S., Martin, S. C., Walters, T. M. H., and Soulsby, E. J. L. (1991). Use of sentinel lambs for early monitoring of the South Powys Hydatidosis Control Scheme, prevalence of *Echinococcus granulosus* and some other helminths. *Veterinary Record*, **129**, 73–6.

Makarova, I. A. and Astafev, B. A. (1992). Clinical and immunological characteristics of hymenolepidiosis. *Meditsinskaia Parazitologiia i Parazitarnye Bolezni*, **3**, 40–3.

Mason, P. R., Patterson, B. A., and Loewenson, R. (1986). Piped water supply and intestinal parasitism in Zimbabwean children. *Transactions of the Royal Society of Tropical Medicine and Parasitology*, **80**, 88–93.

Muratov, I. V. and Posokhov, P. S. (1988). *Diphyllobothrium klebanovskii* sp. n. a parasite of man. *Parazitologiia*, **22**, 165–70.

Muratov, I. V. and Posokhov, P. S. (1989). Aspects of the epidemiology of diphyllobothriasis in the lower Pri-Amur region. *Meditsinskaia Parazitologiia i Parazitarnye Bolezni*, **4**, 53–7.

Njau, B. C., Kasali, O. B., Scholtens, R. G., and Degefa, M. (1988). *ICLA Bulletin, International Livestock Centre for Africa*, **31**, 19–22.

Noemi, I. *et al.* (1991). Clinical characteristics of *Hymenolepis nana* infection in children. *Parasitologia Dia*, **15**, 32–6.

Pampliglione, S. (1962). Indagine sulla diffusione dell'imenolepiasi nella Sicilia occidentale. *Parassitologia*, **4**, 49–58.

Pau, A., Turtas, S., Brambilla, M., Leoni, A., Rosa, M., and Viale, G. L. (1987). Computed-tomography and magnetic-resonance imaging of cerebral coenurosis. *Surgical Neurology*, **27**, 548–52.

Plyusheva, G. L. *et al.* (1987). Establishment of diphyllobothriasis foci on the Krasnoyarsk reservoir. *Meditsinskaia Parazitologiia i Parazitarnye Bolezni*, **1**, 64–7.

Pronin, N. M., Pronin, S. V., and Sanzhieva, S. D. (1988). Prevalence of *Diphyllobothrium dendriticum* plerocercoids in fish in the Lake Baikal Basin. *Meditsinskaia Parazitologiia i Parazitarnye Bolezni*, **4**, 64–7.

Pronin, N. M., Timoshenko, T. M., and Sanzhieva, S. D. (1989*a*). Dynamics of egg production and fecundity of the cestode *Diphyllobothrium dendriticum* (Cestoda., Pseudophyllidea). *Parazitologia*, **23**, 146–52.

Pronin, N. M., Pronin, S. V., Voronov, M. G., and Timoshenko, T. M. (1989*b*). Survival of *Diphyllobothrium dendriticum* plerocercoids during processing of fish, sanitary and helminthological evaluation of production. *Meditsinskaia Parazitologiia i Parazitarnye Bolezni*, **4**, 57–60.

Pugh, R. E. (1987). Effects on the development of *Dipylidium caninum* and on the host reaction to this parasite in the adult flea (*Ctenocephalides felis felis*). *Parasitology Research*, **73**, 171–7.

Pugh, R. E. and Moorhouse, D. E. (1985). Factors affecting the development of *Dipylidium caninum* in *Ctenocephalides felis felis*. *Zeitschrift für Parasitenkunde*, **71**, 765–75.

Rakha, N. K., Dixon, J. B., Jenkins, P., Carter, S. D., and Skerritt, G. C. (1991). Modification of cellular immunity by *Taenia multiceps* (Cestoda)—accessory macrophages and CD4+ lymphocytes are affected by 2 different coenurus factors. *Parasitology*, **103**, 139–47.

Rakha, N. K., Dixon, J. B., Skerritt, G. C., Carter, S. D., and Jenkins, P. (1992). Modification of accessory activity of sheep monocytes *in vitro* by a coenurus antigen from *Taenia multiceps*. *Veterinary Immunology and Immunopathology*, **30**, 293–304.

Revenga, J. E. (1993). *Diphyllobothrium dendriticum* and *Diphyllobothrium latum* in fishes in southern Argentina, asso-

ciation, abundance, distribution, pathological effects, and risk of infection. *Journal of Parasitology*, **79**, 379–83.

Schellhas, K. P. and Norris, G. A. (1985). Disseminated human subarachnoid coenurosis—computed tomographic appearance. *American Journal of Neuroradiology*, **6**, 638–40.

Sharp, G. J. E. (1991). Worms—a further cause for concern? *Fish Farmer*, **14**, 42–3.

Sharp, G. J. E., Secombes, C. J., and Pike, A. W. (1990). On the laboratory maintenance of *Diphyllobothrium dendriticum* (Nitzsch, 1824). *Parasitology*, **101**, 153–61.

Smith, M. C., Bailey, C. S., Baker, N., and Kock, N. (1988). Cerebral coenurosis in a cat. *Journal of the American Veterinary Medical Association*, **192**, 82–4.

Soffar, S. A. and Mokhtar, G. M. (1991). Evaluation of the antiparasitic effect of aqueous garlic (*Allium sativum*) extract in hymenolepiasis *nana* and giardiasis. *Journal of the Egyptian Society of Parasitology*, **21**, 497–502.

Suzuki, N., Imamura, K., and Kumazawa, H. (1993). Diplogonoporiasis in Kochi Prefecture between 1991–2. *Japanese Journal of Parasitology*, **42**, 123–7.

Torres, P., *et al.* (1989). Epidemiology of *Diphyllobothrium* spp. in the Valdava river basin, Chile. *Revista de Saúde Pública*, **23**, 45–57.

Verster, A. (1969). A taxonomic revision of the genus *Taenia* Linnaeus, 1758 s. str. *Onderstepoort Journal of Veterinary Research*, **37**, 3–58.

Walters, T. M. H. (1986). Echinococcosis/hydatidosis and the South Powys Control Scheme. *Journal of Small Animal Practice*, **27**, 693–703.

Walters, T. M. H. and Lloyd, S. (1992). Hydatidosis control scheme. *Veterinary Record*, **130**, 18.

Williams, B. M. (1976). The epidemiology of adult and larval (tissue) cestodes in Dyfed (U. K.). 1. The cestodes of farm dogs. 2. The cestodes of foxhounds. *Veterinary Parasitology*, **1**, 271–6, 277–80.

Williams, B. M. and Boundy, T. (1983). Coenurosis. In *Diseases of Sheep*, (1st edn), (ed. W. B. Martin), pp. 621–41. Blackwell Scientific Publications, Oxford.

Willis, J. M. and Herbert, I. V. (1984). Some factors affecting the eggs of *Taenia multiceps*—their transmission onto pasture and their viability. *Annals of Tropical Medicine and Parasitology*, **78**, 236–42.

Willis, J. M. and Herbert, I. V. (1987). A method for estimating the age of coenuri of *Taenia multiceps* recovered from the brains of sheep. *Veterinary Record*, **121**, 216–18.

Yamane, Y., Kamo, H., Yazaki, S., Fukumoto, S., and Maejima, J. (1981). On a new marine species of the genus *Diphyllobothrium* (Cestoda, Pseudophyllidea) found from a man in Japan. *Japanese Journal of Parasitology*, **30**, 101–11.

Zhuravlev, S. E. and Puzyrev, V. P. (1987). Human helminthiasis in northern Ob'region. *Meditsinskaia Parazitologiia i Parazitarnye Bolezni*, **5**, 64–6.

52 CYSTIC ECHINOCOCCOSIS (*ECHINOCOCCUS GRANULOSUS*)

M. A. Gemmell and M. G. Roberts

SUMMARY

This chapter summarizes the contributions made by natural scientists during the nineteenth century that led workers in zoology, molecular biology, ecology, epidemiology, mathematical modelling, medicine, and veterinary science in the twentieth century to :

(1) define the systematics and some of the factors concerned, with infraspecific variation within the genus *Echinococcus*;

(2) develop surgical and diagnostic techniques and chemotherapy for treating cystic echinococcosis (CE) caused by *Echinococcus granulosus*;

(3) introduce a highly effective drug for treating dogs infected with this parasite;

(4) elucidate its transmission dynamics; and

(5) compare cost-effective options and predict their outcome, before control is introduced.

Such studies have identified gaps in knowledge that will generate further research in the twenty-first century.

Current knowledge indicates that there are four species of the genus *Echinococcus*. These are *E. granulosus*, *E. multilocularis*, *E. oligarthrus*, and *E. vogeli*. For *E. granulosus* two biotypes with a rank higher than 'strain' have now been proposed. These are the northern ancient form with a relatively strong genetic uniformity and the European biotype which, having evolved through a wide range of hosts following domestication of animals, tends to form 'strains'.

With respect to current status of diagnosis and treatment of *E. granulosus* in animals, arecoline hydrobromide is still the only practical diagnostic test for dogs, but progress in research suggests a coproantigen test will be developed that will be able to replace it in most circumstances. Praziquantel has been used in millions of doses and has been shown to be highly effective and safe for treating dogs. Diagnostic tests with high specificity and sensitivity and drugs to kill the larval phase of *E. granulosus* have yet to be developed.

During the past two decades, improvements in surgical procedures have been made with a high cure rate for CE, and chemotherapy has assisted with the introduction of mebendazole and, more particularly, albendazole. Current experiences suggest that these have parasitostatic and parasitocidal properties. Highly sensitive serodiagnostic tests for CE have yet to be developed, but considerable progress has recently been made in non-invasive diagnostic methods. Here, sonography and computed tomography have largely replaced older procedures. Mass ultrasonography with or without radiography is now a relatively common procedure for use in field surveys.

Until recently it was considered that CE was contracted in childhood. Investigations have now shown that it can be contracted at any age and both rapid development and long periods of latency may occur. The factors involved in cyst growth and regression are not yet understood. It is now known that taeniid eggs disperse rapidly over long distances from the site of deposition. Experimental research has clearly demonstrated that blowflies can act as transport hosts and that taeniid eggs can be deposited by them on to human foodstuffs (vegetables and meat) by their normal activities of vomiting and defaecation. It seems that CE may result not only from direct contact with dogs, but may also be food-borne.

With respect to epidemiological research undertaken to assist in planning control, it is now known that the factors that most contribute to stability are the biotic potential of the parasite in the definitive host and acquired immunity in the intermediate animal host. Where stability has been measured for *E. granulosus*, no detectable density-dependent constraint was invoked, implying that this parasite is normally in the endemic steady state and susceptible to control in the farm situation. Based on this research and the evaluation of the outcome of field trials and control programmes, it is clear that a vigorous control effort benefits the whole community, including the elderly. Moreover, it is now possible through mathematical modelling to:

(1)   quantify the stability of the system,
(2)   determine the effective and cost-effective options, and
(3)   predict the outcome before a control programme is introduced.

INTRODUCTION AND HISTORICAL CONSIDERATIONS

Hydatid disease has been recognized in humans and animals since ancient times. Perhaps one of the first references may be that of Hippocrates (379 BC) in his 55th Aphorism, Section VII, 'when the liver is filled with water and bursts into the epiploon, in this case the belly is filled with water and the patient dies'.

Other early references would include the works of Galen (AD 139–200), Aretaeus (AD 7–79), and Rhazes (AD 860–932). The cyst was often regarded as enlarged degenerating glands, pus, or end blood vessels (reviewed in Dew 1928; Schwabe 1986).

DISCOVERY AND INVESTIGATIONS OF THE LIFE CYCLE FROM THE SEVENTEENTH CENTURY

Recognition that the cyst was of animal origin may be attributed to Redi (1624–94), followed by Pallas who considered them to be a bladder forming parasite. Goeze recognized the tapeworm heads and divided this genus into visceral and intestinal taeniasis and nominated the former as *Taenia visceralis socialis granulosa*. The name *Echinococcus* was introduced into zoology by Rudolphi in 1801. In 1808, Rudolphi described three species within the genus *Echinococcus*: *E. hominis*, *E. simiae*, and *E. veterinorum*. In 1855, Kuchenmeister described two forms of *Echinococcus*: *E. scolicipariens* and *E. altricipariens* in which proto-scolices and daughter cysts were formed, respectively. Credit is due to Von Siebold for experimentally infecting dogs with *Echinococcus veterinorum=Taenia echinococcus* (Von Siebold, 1853). This was followed by Naunyn in 1863 in Berlin and Krabbé in Iceland who independently infected dogs with adult worms derived from human protoscolex material. Haubner in 1855 first infected sheep. At that time, Virchow recognized that the condition known as colloid carcinoma was caused by a larval cestode. Subsequently, Leuckart described a form nominated as *Taenia multilocularis*, but did not regard it as a distinct species. At about this time also a hydatid-type parasite *Taenia oligarthra* from the cat was described by Diesing. Although Leuckart provided the first clear account of the life cycle before the end of the nineteenth century, speciation within the genus *Echinococcus* (Rudolphi, 1801) was not solved until the mid-twentieth century.

EPIDEMIOLOGY AND CONTROL UP TO THE FIRST HALF OF THE TWENTIETH CENTURY

Sufficient knowledge of the life cycle of *E. granulosus* was known by the 1860s for Krabbé to recommend in 1864 that control should be undertaken in Iceland. He wrote a 16-page pamphlet which explained the life cycle and this was distributed free to every householder. This, together with the Bible and Icelandic Sagas were the only pieces of literature written in the Icelandic tongue. This pamphlet was read avidly during the long winter nights by a literate community with a prevalence of 25 per cent CE. Control was initiated in 1869. Dog numbers were limited by taxation and some were treated with areca nut, but the two most important factors in reducing prevalence were a change from wool to lamb production and the reading of Krabbé's article. Of 15 888 autopsies carried out between 1932 and 1982, 214 had CE. However, all but eight were born before 1900. The last non-latent case was found in 1960 in a 23-year-old woman, but the last two latent cases were found in 1984 and 1988. These were born in 1905 and 1920. The last two cases of ovine echinococcosis were observed in 1979, (Dungal 1957; Schwabe 1969; Beard 1973*a*,*b*; Palsson, 1995, personal communication).

The introduction of *E. granulosus* into Australia preceded knowledge of the life cycle, and it was considered prior to about 1867 that 'hydatids' in humans was caused by eating undercooked sheep meats. From that time, however, information from Europe spread rapidly and it was recommended in 1898 in the sixth Annual Report of the New Zealand Department of Agriculture that all dogs should be treated with areca nut. Several attempts were made to introduce control there and elsewhere, but except for Iceland, they were without success until the second half of the twentieth century (Gemmell 1990).

SYSTEMATICS AND BIOLOGY IN THE TWENTIETH CENTURY

For the first half of the twentieth century, an academic controversy existed (often known as the unicist and duelist theories) as to whether or not the alveolar form of *Echinococcus* was in fact a separate species as supported by Posselt or a pleomorphic form of *E. granulosus*, as subsequently supported by Dévé in the 1930s. It was not until the 1950s that the cestode observed in a rodent on St Lawrence Island by Rausch and Schiller (1951) was considered to be conspecific with the parasite causing alveolar hydatid disease in Eurasia (Rausch 1953) and then nominated as *E. sibericensis* Rausch and Schiller, 1954. In collaboration with Vogel (1955) in Europe, this was renominated as *E. multilocularis* Leuckart, 1863. Two further species have been regarded as valid. *Taenia oligartha* Diesing, 1863 was transferred to the genus *Echinococcus* in 1910 by Lühe and the life cycle of *E. oligarthrus* was determined experimentally by Sousa and Thatcher (1969) A fourth species, *E. vogeli*, was subsequently described by Rausch and Bernstein (1972) in Ecuador.

Several species were nominated during the first half of the twentieth century, such as *E. longimanubrius* Cameron, 1926; *E. lycaontis* Ortlepp, 1934; *E. cameroni* Ortlepp, 1934; *E. felidis* Ortlepp, 1937; *E. intermedius* Lopez-Neyra et Soler, 1943 and *E. ortleppi* Lopez-Neyra et Soler, 1944. All have now been placed in synonymy with *E. granulosus* by Rausch (1953) and Rausch and Nelson (1963). Subsequently, other species were nominated, including *E. patagonicus* Szidat, 1960 and *E. cepanzoi* Szidat, 1971. It is now considered that these also are synonymous with *E. granulosus* (Schantz *et al.* 1975, 1976). Indeed, from the second half of the twentieth century, the taxonomy and speciation of this genus began to change dramatically following the introduction of biochemical, developmental, and behavioural studies, including *in vitro* culture, to characterize the various hydatid populations (Smyth and Smyth 1964; Smyth 1969; Howell 1986).

THE AGENTS OF ECHINOCOCCOSIS

Since the early 1960s there has been a rapid increase in information on taxonomy, speciation, biology, molecular biology, and host–parasite relationships, much of which has a bearing on control.

CURRENT CONCEPTS IN SYSTEMATICS OF THE GENUS *ECHINOCOCCUS*

Systematics

The suborder Taeniata Skriabin and Schults, 1937 (subclass Eucestoda, order Cyclophyllidae) consists of a single family, Taeniidae Ludwig, 1886, to which belong the eucestodes of the greatest medical significance (Rausch 1993). Two monotypic subfamilies, Taeninae Stiles, 1896 and Echinococcinae Abuladze, 1960, are recognized. The latter subfamily contains a single genus *Echinococcus* Rudolphi, 1801. Within this genus on account of biological isolation and distinctive ecological and biological characteristics, four species are recognized. These are *E. granulosus* (Batsch, 1786), *E. multilocularis* Leuckart, 1863, *E. oligarthrus* (Diesing, 1863), and *E. vogeli*, Rausch and Bernstein, 1972.

Host range

Echinococcus spp. are very small tapeworms of about 2–7 mm in length and rarely possess more than five proglottids. They require two mammalian hosts: a definitive (final) host in which the adult develops in the small intestine of carnivores, and an intermediate host in which the cystic larval stage or metacestode usually develops in the visceral organs. There is also a free-living egg phase. Definitive hosts of *E. granulosus*, *E. multilocularis*, and *E. vogeli* are canids, but *E. multilocularis* can and *E. oligarthrus* must develop in felids. The principal intermediate hosts for the first two named are ungulates and arvicoline rodents, respectively, and caviomorph rodents for the last two named. (Rausch 1967*a,b*, 1986, 1993; Thompson 1986; Thompson and Allsop 1988). The principal definitive host of *E. granulosus* is the domestic dog with domestic animals, such as sheep, pigs, cattle, camels, and pigs, as intermediate hosts. Several wild life cycles exist, including for example the dingo (*Canis familiaris dingo*) and wallaby *Wallabia* spp.

Infraspecific variation

Considerable infraspecific variation (as well as host susceptibility exists) in the globally important *E. granulosus*. These variants were until recently given subspecific rank, such as *E. g. canadiensis* Webster and Cameron, 1961 and *E. g. borealis* Sweatman and Williams, 1963. However, due to lack of evidence of ecological segregation they are now regarded as strains or forms of *E. granulosus* (Rausch 1967*b*).

Two major biotypes of *E. granulosus* have now been defined with a higher rank than 'strain' (Rausch 1967*a*). The northern ancient type with a relatively strong genetic uniformity is indigenous to boreal regions throughout the holarctic, with wolf *Canis lupus*, reindeer *Rangifer tarandus* and elk (= moose) *Alces alces* as the principal hosts. The European biotype has a cosmopolitan distribution and from the time of domestication of animals about 10 000 years ago (Rausch 1967*a*, 1986) has evolved through a wide range of synanthropic hosts and been dispersed globally during colonization from the Old to the New World. It is this biotype that forms locally genetically diverse populations and the term 'strain' is used informally (e.g. the horse, cattle, pig, sheep strains). This genetic diversity may be greater within than between strains of the European biotype and must be taken into account in any evaluation of the transmission dynamics in each ecological niche. Strain identification is complex and is based on a combination of criteria, notably morphological, histological, biochemical, and epidemiological features, including characteristics of the genome using molecular techniques for DNA analysis (Verster 1965; Rausch 1967*a,b*, 1986, 1993; Kumarilake and Thompson 1982; McManus and Bryant 1986; Thompson 1986, 1988; Thompson and Lymbery 1988, 1990; McManus and Rishi, 1989; Lymbery *et al.* 1990; McManus 1990; Bowles *et al.* 1992; Bowles and McManus 1993*a,b,c*).

THE LIFE CYCLE OF *E. GRANULOSUS*

Definitive host

Infection with *E. granulosus* is acquired by ingestion of protoscolices. These evaginate with the aid of intestinal enzymes, establish and then develop as tapeworms in the small intestine. Reproduction is sexual. Development involves proglottidization and formation of new reproductive units or proglottids and their maturation. The onset of egg production varies from 34 to 58 days. Apolysis usually occurs within 42–56 days, but may be delayed. It has been estimated that gravid proglottids are shed every 7–14 days. The number of eggs per proglottid is highly variable, with the number ranging from as low as 100 to as high as 1500. On average it is possibly about 600 eggs. No definitive studies have been recorded on the longevity of the worms in the dog, but this may be 1–2 years (Gemmell and Lawson 1986; Heath 1986; Thompson 1986).

The egg

Taeniid eggs are similar in size (30–40 μm), shape, and structure, and cannot be differentiated morphologically. Embryos of *E. granulosus* hatch in the small intestine and rapidly and actively penetrate it, aided by hook movement and possibly secretions. The factors that determine the site for the development of the cyst are not yet known. It has been suggested that transfer may occur via lymphatic or venous migration (Heath 1971). Once established, the oncosphere rapidly undergoes a series of changes to develop into a metacestode. (Lethbridge 1980; Thompson 1986).

The metacestode

The developed metacestode of *E. granulosus* is typically unilocular, subspherical in shape and fluid-filled. It consists of a thin germinal layer supported by a strong acellular laminated layer of variable thickness. Asexual proliferation of the germinal layer and brood capsule formation takes place endogenously. Pouching of the wall may give rise to secondary chambers and a multi-locular appearance. In some cases especially in humans (CE), daughter cysts may develop within the primary cyst. Reproduction is asexual and thus has an almost unlimited generative capacity (Whitfield and Evans 1983). Brood capsules develop in the perinuclear layer and within them protoscolices are generated. Fertile cysts may occur in about 195 days in mice, 10–12 months in pigs, or 2–4 years in sheep, but only about 50 per cent of *E. granulosus* cysts are fertile by 6.65 years (Gemmell *et al.* 1986*a*).

ANIMAL HOSTS

CLINICAL ASPECTS

There is no evidence for clinical signs or symptoms of *E. granulosus* in dogs. There is also little evidence that food animals show any disease syndromes. This may be accounted for in one respect by truncation of life expectancy (Schwabe 1986). Cysts are found more frequently in the lungs of ruminants and liver of non-ruminants. In wild hosts, large cysts may render them susceptible to predation.

DIAGNOSIS IN DEFINITIVE HOSTS

Chemical

Testing dogs with arecoline hydrobromide has the advantage that if a purge is induced there is a high probability that some of the worm burden will be expelled. Further, if positive, quantitative data for epidemiological studies and for education can be obtained. It has a serious disadvantage that up to 25 per cent of dogs may not be purged and it should not be used on pregnant bitches, aged dogs, or young puppies. Safety precautions must be taken when collecting and examining these purges (Gemmell 1968, 1973; FAO/UNEP/WHO 1981; Schantz 1993).

Immunological

An extensive programme has been initiated to develop immunodiagnostic tests for use against canine echinococcosis (Rickard and Lightowlers 1986; Lightowlers 1990; Craig 1993; Lightowlers *et al.* 1993; Schantz 1993). Following ingestion of a cyst, dogs will be exposed at the intestinal level to various antigens during the establishment of the parasite and its development and oogenesis. Oncosphere and protoscolex antibodies can be readily detected in the serum of infected dogs (Jenkins and Rickard 1986; Gasser *et al.* 1988). This has not yet reached a practical stage, as it does not differentiate between current and previous infections (Jenkins *et al.* 1990). An alternative approach based on faecal antigen detection antibody sandwich ELISA technique has recently been developed and has shown particular promise because antigen can be detected shortly after infection and the level declines rapidly following expulsion of the worms. The sensitivity and specificity of the test was estimated at 87.5 per cent and 96.5 per cent, respectively (Allan *et al.* 1992; Deplazes *et al.* 1992; Craig *et al.* 1994).

Chemical v. immunological

The advantage of the coproantigen-ELISA test, like the arecoline test, over the serum antibody test is that a positive means the animal is infected at the time of testing. Arecoline testing is qualitative and quantitative and is most useful for base-line epidemiological studies on the comparative rates of infection among Taeniidae. Further work may show that the coproantigen test will be more cost-effective than arecoline surveillance during routine surveillance of the dog population during control programmes.

The method that is essential for base-line surveys and for surveillance of control programmes is autopsy of intermediate hosts (FAO/UNEP/WHO 1981; Gemmell 1987). A refinement includes the use of 'sentinel animals' (Lloyd *et al.* 1991). Immunological tests, useful in humans, are less sensitive and specific in live-stock and at present cannot replace autopsy (Schantz and Gottstein 1986; Schantz 1993).

Definitive host

At the end of the nineteeth century, the only drug available to treat dogs for tapeworms was *Areca catechu*. In 1924 a synthetic salt, arecoline hydrobromide, was developed and used for treating dogs. However, up to 11 treatments may be needed to free some dogs from worms. Praziquantel was evaluated in the 1970s and found to be highly effective. The single dose ED90 with 95 per cent confidence intervals for *E. granulosus* ranged between 2.3 (1.5–3.7), 2.7 (2.1–3.5), and 3.2 (1.8–5.6) mg/kg, and the recommended dose rate is 5.0 mg/kg. Praziquantel was of similar efficacy against *E. granulosus* when administered by the intramuscular and oral routes, but was lower when given subcuta-neously with an ED90 and 95 per cent confidence intervals of 7.6 (3.1–18.6) mg/kg (Gemmell and Johnstone 1981c). The drug is equally effective when given with or without food and can be successfully incorporated into a medicated dog food of high acceptability (Chi-pu-sheng 1993). The drug does not have a practical ovacidal effect. Praziquantel has now been used in millions of doses without toxicity or drug resistance (FAO/UNEP/WHO 1981; Gemmell and Johnstone 1981c).

Intermediate hosts

Mebendazole in micronized form has been tested for efficacy against *E. granulosus* in food animals. Young experimental infections in sheep and pigs with thin-walled cysts survived daily treatments for 5–14 days. With naturally acquired thick-walled cysts in aged sheep, daily treatments at 50 mg/kg for 5 days was

without effect; at one month considerable damage was observed, but some protoscolices survived and were infective to dogs. None, however, survived daily treat-ment for 3 months (Gemmell *et al.* 1981; Eckert 1986). Praziquantel given at 50 mg/kg for 6 weeks to sheep had little effect on the survival of cysts (Morris *et al.* 1990). There is as yet no chemotherapeutic approach to control through the metacestode stage in the inter-mediate animal host.

Definitive hosts

While considerable research has been undertaken with crude antigens to protect dogs from echinococcosis, no real success has so far been demonstrated (Gemmell and Lawson 1986; Gemmell *et al.* 1986a; Heath 1986; Gemmell and Roberts, 1995).

Intermediate hosts

A vaccine, based on a single polypeptide antigen derived from oncospheres and produced in *Eschericia coli* using recombinant DNA technology, has been developed successfully for use against *Taenia ovis* in sheep (Johnson *et al.* 1989). This technology is now being applied to *E. granulosus* (Lightowlers *et al.* 1992).

HUMAN HOST

Cystic echinococcosis may be diagnosed at any age and has been recorded at 1 and 2 years of age and more than 80 years of age (Drolshammer *et al.* 1973; Chaouachi *et al.* 1989; Utrilla *et al.* 1991). The peak age at the time of diagnosis of CE is about 30–40 years (range 8–75), the sex distribution is about equal in most areas, but in Kenya and China, for example, the rate was greater in females than males (Romig 1990; Chai-Jun-jie, 1993). To an extent the incubation period and clinical picture is dependent on the organ involved (Grossi *et al.* 1991). The proportion of cysts in the various organs were: hepatic 52–77 per cent, pulmonary 8–44 per cent and 13–19 per cent in other organs (Schantz 1972). The sites of predilection of 1802 cysts recorded in the Australian Hydatid Register were liver (63 per cent), lung (25 per cent), muscles, (5 per cent), bones (3 per cent), kidney (2 per cent); spleen, brain (1 per cent), and heart, breast, prostate, parotid and pancreas (<1 per cent) (Grove *et al.* 1976). Most patients have single cysts and the right lobe is more commonly affected than the left lobe of the liver (Reeder and Palmer 1981; Gloor 1988; Romig 1990; Amman and Eckert 1995).

Growth and formation of protoscolices is variable (Amman and Eckert 1995). 'Collosal' cysts have been recorded, but the average size may be 1–10 cm (Todorov *et al.* 1992*c*). In one study, 30 per cent of cysts grew slowly (1–5 mm/year), 43 per cent showed moderate growth (6–15 mm), and 11 per cent a rapid increase (>30 mm), with a maximum growth of 160 mm/year, and 4 of 75 cysts collapsed (Romig *et al.* 1986). Protoscolices may be found in daughter cysts of diameter 0.5 cm (Alvarez *et al.* 1991). Both parasite and host factors may modify clinical disease. For example, the northern biotype is likely to be relatively benign (Wilson *et al.* 1968; Pinch and Wilson 1973).

SYMPTOMS, SIGNS, AND COMPLICATIONS

Symptomatology of CE is variable and rarely pathogonomic (Amman and Eckert 1995). Since almost any organ can be invaded, the spectrum depends on:

1.   the organ involved;
2.   the size of the cyst and its location;
3.   pressure induced within that organ, and
4.   complications such as rupture and spread of larval tissue with formation of secondary cysts and possible bacterial infections.

Leakage following diagnostic puncture or rupture may induce mild or serious complications, such as urticaria, asthma, anaphylaxis, or membrane nephropathy. Cysts may rupture in almost all sites of predilection with varying consequences. Secondary peritoneal echinococcosis may result from spontaneous, traumatic rupture, or rupture during surgery of a hepatic cyst, but is rare from a pulmonary cyst (Vara Thorbeck and Vara Thorbeck 1986, Kitani *et al.* 1992; Amman and Eckert 1995). The consequences of secondary CE are recognized several years later. Cysts that become encapsulated and calcified, although potentially viable, may remain asymptomatic indefinitely. This may account for a relatively high proportion of cases being asymptomatic during ultrasound surveys (Caremani *et al.* 1991; Grossi *et al.* 1991; Pawlowski 1993; Amman and Eckert, 1995). Spontaneous cure of CE does occur due to collapse and resolution, calcification, or cyst rupture into the bronchial tree or bile ducts (Van Steenbergen *et al.* 1987; Bernardini and Valle 1991; Amman and Eckert, 1995).

DIAGNOSIS

Non-invasive methods

Pulmonary CE is detected on chest radiographs as sharply demarcated large cysts with fluid, or as thin-walled empty cystic structures. With hepatic cysts, ultrasonography (US) and computed tomography (CT)

have a comparable sensitivity and have largely replaced diagnostic angiography and scintigraphy (Beggs 1983, 1985). With US a spherical smooth rim of calcification (egg-shell pattern) is a typical sign of an inactive liver or intra-abdominal cyst. Echodense structures are observed when the cyst is filled with folded membranes. Differential diagnosis from benign cysts and abscesses may be difficult. A 'cart-wheel' sign is indicative of multiple daughter cysts. An 'egg-shell' pattern can be expected if the cyst is inactive (Jain *et al.* 1989; Reeder and Palmer 1981; Romig 1990; Caratozzolo *et al.* 1991; Caremani *et al.* 1991; Xu Ming-quian 1991, 1993; Morris and Richards 1992; Pawlowski 1993; Amman and Eckert 1995).

Ultrasonography is relatively easy to perform and portable units, with and without portable X-ray equipment and or serodiagnosis, is now frequently used in surveys of *E. granulosus*. These include, for example, surveys undertaken in Kenya (Macpherson *et al.* 1987, 1989; Romig 1990), in Libya (Shambesh *et al.* 1992), Tunisia (Bchir *et al.* 1991), and Uruguay (Perdomo *et al.* 1990; Paolillo *et al.* 1991). It has an overall diagnostic accuracy of between 83 and 93 per cent (Frider *et al.* 1990; Guerra *et al.* 1990). It seems, therefore, that ultrasonography is an efficient mass-screening method and additional serological examination is indicated for the diagnosis of doubtful cysts (Amman and Eckert 1995).

Computed tomography and magnetic resonance imaging (MRI) are costly, but do allow the detection of very small cysts and are of value for the differential diagnosis of *E. granulosus* from non-parasitic lesions in almost all organs (Marani *et al.* 1990; Di Palma *et al.* 1991; Munzer 1991; von Sinner 1991; Pawlowski 1993; Amman and Eckert 1995).

Laboratory tests

Routine laboratory tests, including for example eosinophilia, have little value in the diagnosis of CE (Pawlowski 1993; Amman and Eckert 1995).

Immunological methods

Antibody immunodiagnostic tests for CE are employed for mass screening of communities as well as for detection of cysts in individual patients before and after surgery. Extensive research has resulted in the characterization of numerous antigens for surveys and clinical diagnosis of CE and differentiation from AE (Gottstein *et al.* 1983, 1986; Schantz and Gottstein 1986; Gottstein 1992). It seems that about 10 per cent of patients with hepatic CE and 40 per cent with pulmonary CE may not produce detectable serum antibodies. False negatives and positives reduce the predictive value for both sensitivity and specificity.

Thus, tests for confirming CE should be based on highly specific criteria. These include *Echinococcus-specific* arc 5 by gel diffusion or the 8–12 or 116 kDa band in immunoblot assays (McManus 1990; Kanwar *et al.* 1992). Techniques to assist clinical diagnosis using antibody detection and detection of circulating antigens and immune complexes are reviewed in Craig (1993) and Pawlowski (1993).

SURGICAL TREATMENT AND PROGNOSIS

There are numerous important reviews on the surgical management of CE. The principal methods include hepatic resection; polycystectomy and cystectomy for hepatic cysts and extrusion of cysts; percystectomy and lobectomy for pulmonary cysts (Morris and Richards 1992; Xu Ming-quian 1993). Nowadays, surgical intervention when indicated, should be possible in about 90 per cent of cases. However, recurrence rates vary from 2 to 25 per cent (Romig 1990; Soleto Saez 1991; Morris and Richards 1992; Todorov *et al.* 1992*c*). In an extensive review in China, it was determined that 92, 7, 0.8 and 0.2 per cent had 1, 2, 3, and 4 or more operations (Luo Menghebat *et al.* 1993). Postoperation complications may occur in between 10 and 25 per cent of cases (Bernardini and Valle 1991; Perdomo *et al.* 1991; Kammerer and Schantz 1993). Some of the untoward sequelae that may be expected are summarized in Table 52.1. Lethality associated with the first operation is about 2 per cent (Soleto Saez 1991; Kammerer and Schantz 1993), but this may increase after subsequent surgery (Amir-Jahed *et al.* 1975).

Pre-operative treatment and non-surgical management

Preoperative cyst inactivation with hypersaline solution or hydrogen peroxide prior to surgery is preferable to formalin, but even these are not always safe. Indeed it is now considered that the application of scolicidal chemicals should be avoided (Teres *et al.* 1984; Prasad *et al.* 1991; Morris and Richards 1992; Kammerer and Schantz 1993; Pawlowski 1993; Amman and Eckert

Table 52.1 Prevalence of postoperative complications in 63/212 patients with cystic echinococcosis (CE) (after Barros 1978)

Complication	Number of cases	%
Death	8	3.8
External bile fistula	8	3.8
Infection of residual cavity	3	1.4
Intraperitoneal abscess	5	2.8
Wound infection	10	4.7
Pneumonia	11	5.2
Recurrent CE	18	8.5

1995). This is because such syndromes as sclerosing cholangitis may occur (Belghiti *et al.* 1986; Houry *et al.* 1990; Morris and Richards 1992; Pawlowski 1993; Amman and Eckert 1995). Recently, percutaneus puncture (PAIR) for inoperable cases has been advocated. This includes puncture of the cyst, introduction of a protoscolicide, such as hypertonic saline or alcohol and re-aspiration. This is carried out under ultrasonic guidance (Morris and Richards 1992; Kammerer and Schantz 1993; Pawlowski 1993; Amman and Eckert, 1995). Prior to, and for a period following this procedure, benzimidazoles should be administered. Success has been reported in most but not all cases after a prolonged follow-up period (Ben Amor 1986; Gargouri *et al.* 1990; Filice *et al.* 1991; Khuroo *et al.* 1991; 1993). This method requires further study before being considered as an alternative for surgery of hepatic CE (Pawlowski 1993; Amman and Eckert 1995).

CHEMOTHERAPY AND PROGNOSIS

The first drug to be evaluated for activity against CE was mebendazole (Bekhti *et al.* 1977; Osborne 1980). This drug is poorly absorbed, even when given with food, and serum, drug levels are variable; it is also rapidly metabolized in the liver and excreted in bile and urine. While there is evidence that efficacy is related to serum drug concentrations and duration of treatment, the effective serum drug levels are not well defined (Bryceson *et al.* 1982; Luder *et al.* 1985, 1986; Eckert 1986; Todorov *et al.* 1990, 1992*a,b,c*; Pawlowski 1993; Amman and Eckert 1995). Serum blood levels should be monitored 1 month after commencement of treatment and then every 3 months (WHO 1992). Daily doses at 50 mg/kg for at least 3 months, but doses as high as 100–200 mg/kg, have been suggested for pulmonary echinococcosis in children (Messariticas *et al.* 1991; Pawlowski 1993). Due to its low level of absorption, this drug is now mainly recommended, subject to no adverse reactions, for use in long-term chemotherapy of inoperable CE, but even then the results are not always encouraging (Davis *et al.* 1986, 1989; Pawlowski 1993).

Albendazole lacks the absorption problems encountered with mebendazole (Morris *et al.* 1985, 1987; Wen *et al.* 1990), but is also rapidly metabolized in the liver. The main metabolite and active component is albendazole sulphoxide (ABX), the serum concentration of which is also highly variable between individuals, but is higher with long-term than short-term treatment schedules (Saimot *et al.* 1983; Okela 1986; Morris *et al.* 1987; Cotting *et al.* 1990; Wen *et al.* 1990; Tan Jia-zhong *et al.* 1993; Amman and Eckert 1995). The treatment schedule recommended is a daily dose of 10–15 mg/kg (maximum 400 mg twice daily) in 3–4 week cycles with 2-week intermission periods (Davis *et al.* 1989; Horton 1989).

Praziquantel has been tested for scolicidal efficacy *in vitro*. In one *in vivo* study involving 101 patients, there was very little difference in the viability of protoscolices between the treated and untreated patients as determined at surgery (Tan Jia-zhong *et al.* 1993). Further extensive studies would be needed before a prediction on its value, if any, in the chemotherapy of CE can be defined.

Current status of the chemotherapy of CE

Most studies have used echographic methods to assess efficiency (Morris *et al.* 1984, 1985; Singcharoen *et al.* 1985; De Rosa and Teggi 1990; Todorov *et al.* 1990; El Mufti *et al.* 1993; Wen *et al.* 1993). Difficulties have been found in ascribing death of cysts to the treatment. In a study to evaluate the effect of albendazole on cyst viability, patients received either no treatment (controls) or treatment at 10 mg/kg for 1 month or 3 months. At surgery, it was found that 50, 72, and 94 per cent were non-viable in the three groups, respectively, as determined by protoscolex viability and mouse tests. Treatment was also associated with total cyst membrane disintegration. Only one patient had a viable cyst after 3 months of treatment. The drug was well tolerated by most patients (Gil-Grande *et al.* 1993).

These results suggest that albendazole treatment may be a valuable safety precaution when used presurgically to reduce the risk of recurrence (Morris 1987, 1989) and back-up after surgery to deal with spillage of protoscolices during surgery or after the use of PAIR (Morris and Taylor 1988; Pawlowski 1993; Amman and Eckert 1995). Although surgery is the first choice for treating CE (WHO 1992), further work may also show that chemotherapy may sometimes take the place of surgery in uncomplicated hepatic CE (El-Mufti *et al.* 1993). In this regard, the addition of cimetidine (an anti-peptic ulcer drug), possibly by suppressing drug metabolism, may allow a higher serum concentration of albendazole sulphoxide and possibly a higher therapeutic value (Wen *et al.* 1994). This has also been observed with mebendazole (Luder *et al.* 1986; Bekhti and Pirrotte, 1987). It follows that during the past decade, remarkable progress has been made, but trials are still needed to define the full value and limitations of chemotherapy in the treatment of CE.

EPIDEMIOLOGY OF ECHINOCOCCOSIS

GEOGRAPHICAL OCCURRENCE

Echinococcus granulosus can be regarded as a cosmopolitan parasite, being present to a greater or lesser extent on all occupied continents (Fig. 52.1). In general, it is

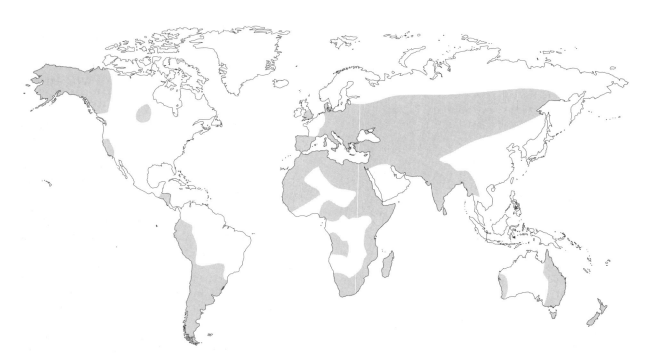

Fig. 52.1 Geographical distribution of *Echinococcus granulosus*.

a recognizable health problem in all sheep-rearing communities, with its greatest prevalence where relatively low standards of hygiene and development exist. Among the most important foci are the sheep-rearing countries of South America: Argentina, Brazil. Chile, Peru, and Uruguay. As far as has been determined, it is in an endemic steady state, except in Cyprus, the Falkland Islands, New Zealand, and Tasmania, and possibly Regions 11 and 12 in Chile, where it has been transformed to extinction status.

In the CIS and parts of Eurasia vast endemic areas occur. In most, both synanthropic and sylvatic life cycles coexist. CE also occurs throughout western Europe, but transmission is highest in countries bordering the Mediterranean and on the Iberian Peninsula. In Africa, two major foci exist. The first includes the countries of the Maghreb, while south of the Sahara, the focus involves the Turkana in Kenya. High transmission rates also occur in some southern and northern regions of India as well as in Nepal. CE has been recorded in 21 of China's 31 provinces and autonomous regions, representing 87 per cent of its territory, and is regarded as one of the most important infectious diseases in the vast pastoral regions of north-western China. It is also prevalent in the northern, central and southern tablelands of New South Wales, in Victoria and South Australia, and was, until recently, in Tasmania and New Zealand.

QUANTIFYING THE HOST–PARASITE RELATIONSHIPS

Biological data needed to quantify the transmission dynamics of echinococcosis in any given situation include a definition of contributions made to the stability of the system by:

(1)   the parasite;
(2)   each host population;
(3)   intrinsic and extrinsic factors impinging on the free-living egg phase; and
(4)   socio-economic factors modifying the system.

Parasite populations are subject to two types of constraint. Density-dependent constraints include parasite-induced host-mortality (not important for taeniids) and the acquisition of immunity to infection or super-infection by one or another of the hosts. Density-independent constraints, on the other hand, such as the action of weather on free-living stages and the mortality of hosts due to reasons unconnected with their parasite burdens, may modify transmission, but do not regulate the parasite population. Research, quantifying the transmission dynamics of the dog–sheep taeniids has now been reviewed extensively (Gemmell and Johnstone 1977, 1981*a,b*; Gemmell and Lawson 1986,

1989; Gemmell *et al.* 1986*a*, *b*, 1987*a*; Roberts *et al.* 1986, 1987; Gemmell 1990, 1993; Tolley and Ming, 1993; Roberts 1994; Roberts and Gemmell 1994; Gemmell and Roberts 1995).

Contributions by the parasite

Echinococcus granulosus has an overdispersed distribution that fits a series of negative binomial distributions in both hosts with only a small number of animals harbouring large numbers of worms or larvae (Roberts *et al.* 1986). There is neither a 'crowding effect' nor a parasite-induced host-mortality and this distribution does not contribute to the regulation of either the adult or larval subpopulations. The parasite's major contribution is its biotic potential. This can be defined as the potential number of viable cysts, which could be established in a susceptible intermediate host per day by the egg output from an infected dog. This is very low in most dog–sheep assemblages and has been estimated at only 28 for *E. granulosus*, which is less than five per cent of that of *T. hydatigena* (2698) and *T. ovis* (644) in the same host assemblages (Gemmell *et al.* 1986*a*, 1987*a*; Roberts *et al.* 1986, 1987). With such highly susceptible hosts as dingoes in Australia and Turkana dogs in Kenya, where very high burdens are the rule, this may be substantially increased (Rausch and Nelson 1963; Macpherson *et al.* 1985; Jenkins 1992).

Contributions by the hosts

Considerable knowledge has now been gained on the 'protective immune' response to adult and larval cestode infections. (Rickard and Williams 1982; Rickard 1983; Harrison and Parkhouse 1985; Gemmell and Lawson 1986; Heath 1986, Gemmell *et al.* 1987*a*; Gemmell 1990). In epidemiological terms, acquired immunity is a negative feedback system operating as a density-dependent constraint to limit population abundance.

Dogs by their lingual-anal grooming habits have abundant access to tapeworm eggs, but appear only to acquire immunity to *E. granulosus* from protoscolices. Each dog remains susceptible to infection for varying numbers of challenges, with about 50 per cent of the population showing reduced susceptibility by the sixth infection. An extrapolation suggests that 99 per cent may do so by the twelfth infection (Gemmell *et al.* 1986*a*). Although immunity acquired by dogs could act as a density-dependent constraint, it would only operate at high infection pressures, where acquired immunity in the intermediate host would be more important as a regulator of the parasite population.

Immunity to superinfection with *E. granulosus*, *T. ovis*, and *T. hydatigena* can be acquired or induced in sheep (Gemmell *et al.* 1986*a*, 1987*a*). Passive immunity operates in some systems (Gemmell *et al.* 1990). Based on studies with *T. hydatigena* and *T. ovis* in sheep, the property of this immunity appears to be:

(1) acquired within 7–14 days by the ingestion of as few as 10 eggs;
(2) life-long in the presence of eggs;
(3) lost between 6 and 12 months in the absence of eggs; and
(4) not dependent on the presence of larvae from a previous infection (Gemmell and Johnstone 1981*a*; Gemmell *et al.* 1987*a*).

Without doubt this is the density-dependent constraint that regulates taeniid populations (Roberts *et al.* 1986, 1987; Gemmell 1990; Ming *et al.* 1992*a,b*).

Contributions by the environment

Environmental factors operate as density-independent constraints on the survival and dispersal of the free-living egg phase, but do not regulate the parasite population (Gemmell and Johnstone 1977; Gemmell 1978, 1990; Lawson and Gemmell 1983; Gemmell and Lawson 1986, 1989). Eggs on expulsion are at various stages of development and are then subjected to a maturation–senescence process by climate. The higher the temperature, the more rapidly this proceeds. Desiccation is lethal (Laws 1968) and the endpoints for temperature are of the order +40 °C to −70 °C. Between these extremes, temperature regulates this process. For example, eggs of *E. granulosus* survived for more than 200 days at 7 °C, but only 50 days at 21 °C (Gemmell 1977).

IMMIGRATION, EMIGRATION, AND EGG-DISPERSAL MECHANISMS

Most of the early studies considered that hydatid eggs were dispersed by wind and water. There is very little evidence for this. More recent studies on egg survival and dispersion have been undertaken using *T. hydatigena*, *T. ovis*, and *T. pisiformis* as models for *E. granulosus*. Although most eggs remain within 180 m of the site of deposition, some may rapidly disperse over an area of up to 30 000 ha (Gemmell and Johnstone 1981*b*). Losses of eggs from the environment occur by death of the embryo (see above) or physical removal, such as high rainfall or high winds (Sweatman and Williams 1963). Experimental and field evidence is now available that blowflies (particularly Calliphoridae) are important transport hosts for taeniid eggs (Lawson and Gemmell 1985, 1990). Birds have been reported as transport hosts of *T. saginata* (Crewe and Crewe 1969). It has been reported that eggs of *T. hydatigena* regularly disperse some 60 km upwind from the mainland of Scotland to an uninhabited island. This occurs through co-operation between birds and insects (Torgerson *et al.* 1992, 1994).

DETERMINING THE STABILITY OF TAENIID SYSTEMS

Considerable advances have been made in quantifying the transmission dynamics of *E. granulosus*, *T. hydatigena*, and *T. ovis* by mathematical modelling Roberts 1994; Roberts and Gemmell 1994; Gemmell and Roberts, 1995). This approach not only identifies the research still needed, but also allows a prediction of the outcome of control strategies in both epidemiological and economic terms.

Stability

Stability is an essential part of the description of host/parasite systems. It describes the ability of biological systems in equilibrium to withstand perturbation, such as might be encountered in a control programme, and after that perturbation has ceased to return to the previous equilibrium or reach a new one. In general, a parasite system is asymptotically stable if the parasite population returns to that state, following a temporary perturbation away from it. It is locally asymptotically stable if a population will return to its original state over time if it were originally in that state but has been perturbed by a small amount. A parasite system is structurally stable if its dynamics are qualitatively unchanged by perturbations in its parameters.

Basic reproduction ratio

The concept of the basic reproduction ratio (R_0) of a parasite population is central to an understanding of the transmission dynamics, stability in the environment, and control and eradication of parasites (Anderson and May 1978; Anderson 1982). It is the potential ratio of the number of adults in the 'next generation' to the number of parasites in this generation in the absence of density-dependent constraints. For a review of its definition and application see Heesterbeek and Roberts (1995).

A parasite population that is neither decreasing nor increasing in size is in a steady state and the *effective reproduction ratio* (R) is unity. To distinguish steady states for taeniids, a parasite population is said to be in an endemic steady state if the population size is constant ($R = 1$) and the effects of density-dependent constraints are insignificiant (R_0 is greater than but near to 1), and in an hyperendemic steady state when $R = 1$ and the population is strongly regulated by density-dependent constraints ($R_0 \gg 1$). The extinction steady state is identified as that when no parasite is present.

Methods for determining the equilibrium steady state

Provided that the infection pressure has remained constant throughout the lifetime of the host animals, the steady state of *E. granulosus* can be defined by determining the intensity of infection in relation to their age. A linearly increasing age–intensity prevalence curve indicates endemicity, but if the curve is depressed below the straight line, hyperendemicity is indicated.

A mathematical method for quantifying the basic reproduction ratio has been developed by Roberts *et al.* (1986, 1987) using an integrodifferential equation of the form:

$$h' = -\mu h + \lambda f * (Sh)$$

where:

- h = infection pressure;
- μ = rate of loss of parasites from the system;
- λ = rate of transmission of parasites through the system in the absence of density-dependent constraints, $R_0 = \lambda/\mu$;
- f = probability density function for delays;
- S = proportion of intermediate hosts that are susceptible to infection;
- $*$ = denotes convolution representing delays in the system.

A non-linear form is used for parasites with high biotic potentials, such as the ovine cysticercoses (*T. hydatigena* and *T. ovis*), and a linear form (with $S = 1$) is used for *E. granulosus*. If the parasite is in a steady state, R_0 can be estimated from:

$$R_0 = 1 + \frac{\text{(mean duration of immunity in the host population)}}{\text{(mean time to immunity in that population)}}.$$

If the infection pressure is so high that acquired immunity lasts for life, then this formula is equivalent to:

$$R_0 = \frac{\text{(mean life expectancy of the host)}}{\text{(mean age at which immunity is acquired)}}.$$

HOW OFTEN DO SHEEP INGEST HYDATID EGGS IN THE FIELD?

Age–intensity prevalence was obtained in New Zealand prior to the introduction of control. There it was estimated that R_0 for *E. granulosus* in male and female sheep was 1.3 and 1.6, respectively, and that they were subjected to 0.4 infections/year. Using an estimate for the overall proportion of eggs that develop into cysts as 0.0087 (Gemmell *et al.* 1986a), the former ingested per infection 155 and latter 373 eggs (Roberts *et al.* 1986). A similar evaluation was made in a county in the People's Republic China. This study also showed that the infection pressure on female sheep was 0.44 infections/year and the mean number of cysts increased by 0.88 per cent

of per year, implying that each infection produced 2.0229 cysts/year. Using the same estimate of the overall proportion of eggs that developed into cysts as in New Zealand, each infection consisted of 232 eggs (Ming *et al.* 1992b). A similar evaluation in Uruguay, implied that the infection pressure on sheep was 0.1743 infections/year and the mean number of cysts increased by 6.03 cysts and that each infection consisted of 693.6 eggs (Cabrera *et al.* 1995). It seems that sheep in Uruguay received fewer infections per year, but a higher number of eggs/infection than occurred in New Zealand or China. This may have a seasonal climatic explanation (Gemmell 1978). Clearly in each situation, the interval between each infection was too long to invoke a strong acquired immunity and the equilibrium steady state was endemic and the parasite was susceptible to attack (see below).

FIELD TRIALS MEASURING STABILITY

The Styx field trial, undertaken in an isolated valley in New Zealand, compared the stability of *E. granulosus* and *T. hydatigena*, when a 3-monthly dog-testing programme with arecoline hydrobromide was applied in an educational approach to control (Gemmell *et al.* 1986b). Stability was determined by changes in the prevalence of the larval forms in sheep. The weak force used against *E. granulosus* was sufficient to drive this system from endemic to extinction status ($R_0 = 1.3$ to $R_0 = 0.4$); B to C in Fig. 52.2. In contrast, this force had no effect against *T. hydatigena*, which was hyperendemic and remained at A throughout the trial. When, however, a strong force of 4-weekly dog-dosing with bunamidine was introduced, *T. hydatigena* paradoxically increased in the adult sheep. This resulted from the transformation of the parasite from hyperendemic to endemic status (from A to B in Fig. 52.2) with a loss of acquired immunity and superinfection. It should be noted that a control programme in New Zealand had the effect of increasing the larval population of *T. ovis* in the national sheep flock through loss of acquired immunity when it was driven from hyperendemic to endemic status with a 6-weekly dog-dosing programme with praziquantel. In other words, following the introduction of a strong force directed against a highly stable parasite, too few eggs become available to retain an acquired immunity to superinfection (Gemmell *et al.* 1986b; Gemmell 1990; Lawson 1994).

EPIDEMIOLOGY OF ECHINOCOCCOSIS

TRANSMISSION DYNAMICS

Until quite recently, it was assumed that CE 'hydatids' was a rural health problem caught in childhood either

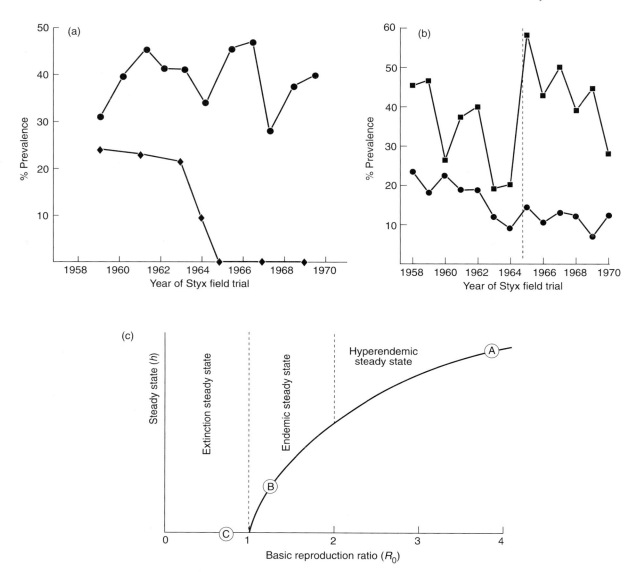

Fig. 52.2 *Force required to* drive endemic and hyperendemic taeniid systems towards extinction. (a) *Echinococcus granulosus* (◆) and *Taenia hydatigena* (●) in aged sheep. The force used was a 3-monthly arecoline testing programme with a high educational component. This drove endemic *E. granulosus* to extinction status (B to C in the bifurcation diagram (c)) and *T. hydatigena* remained hyperendemic (A). (b) *T. hydatigena* in adult sheep (■) and lambs (●) remained at (A) until in 1963 the force was changed to a 4-weekly dog dosing programme with bunamidine. This drove the system from hyperendemic to endemic status (A to B) with an increase in cysts in adult sheep through loss of immunity and superinfection. (c) Bifurcation diagram showing possible steady state values of *h*, the measure of parasite abundance, for different values of R_0. To drive the system from endemic ($R_0 > 1$) or hyperendemic ($R_0 \gg 1$) to extinction status, the force applied must be strong enough to drive it from B to C and A to C, respectively.

by direct transfer of eggs from dog to mouth (disease of dirty hands), from dogs contaminating the water supply with eggs or defaecating on vegetables. While not disputing these and other possibilities, such as coprophagia or geophagia, experiments suggest that echinococcosis is likely to occur from eating eggs deposited by flies on foodstuffs (Lawson and Gemmell 1983, 1985, 1990).

Experimental evidence

Blowflies (*Calliphora maculata*) were first allowed to feed on dog faeces containing proglottids of *T. pisiformis* or *T. hydatigena* and then on to grass or cooked meats, respectively, that were then fed to rabbits and pigs, appropriately, (Lawson and Gemmell 1990). The results demonstrated that:

(1) taeniid eggs remain viable after passage through the gut of flies, and

(2) that flies transmit eggs indirectly to animals by their normal activities of vomiting and defaeca- tion. If it is assumed that the grass and cooked meat used in these experiments represent the normal vegetable and meat diets of humans, then these results imply that where there is an abun- dance of blowflies, together with opportunies to contact dog faeces and human foodstuffs, flies would provide a practical way to transmit CE.

AGE SUSCEPTIBILITY OF HUMANS TO INFECTION

Until quite recently, it was assumed that CE was acquired in childhood (Dew 1928) Intensive studies were made during the control programmes in New Zealand and Tasmania on changes in the age pre- valence of CE in humans (Anon. 1961–1989; Anon. 1965–1991; Beard, 1969, 1978, 1984, 1987, 1988). Both programmes were regarded as being in the endemic steady state ($R_0 > 1$) prior to control. The former was initiated in 1959 and the latter in 1965. The data for New Zealand were collected only from public hospi- tals, but those in Tasmania included all hospitals con- ducting surgery using the criteria:

(1) cyst confirmed at operation, or

(2) cyst confirmed at necropsy as a cause of symp- toms or death, not as incidental findings. Only new cases were collected for surgical incidence (Tables 52.2 and 52.3).

In Tasmania, incidences were collected annually and the most important were those for the first two 5-year periods 1966–1970 and 1971–1975 (Table 52.3), during which time the incidence halved. Age-specific rates were calculated from the estimated populations in each age group at the midpoint of each period. Of the 87 new patients, 77 (89 per cent) were autochthonus. The incidence in the second period declined to about half without a significant change in the age dis-

Table 52.2 Age distribution of new hospital cases of CE in New Zealand 1958–1962 and 1963–1967 (adapted from Anon. 1961–1989; Beard 1987)

Age Groups	Number of cases 1958–1962	1963–1967	Total cases	% reduction
0–4	19	3	22	84.2
5–14	98	35	133	64.3
15–24	82	46	128	43.9
25–44	112	64	176	42.9
45–64	98	48	146	51.0
>65	44	25	69	43.2
Total	453	221	674	51.2

Table 52.3 Age-specific annual surgical incidence (per 100 000) of CE in Tasmania 1966–1970 and 1971–1975 with the percentage reduction in the second 5-year period (adapted from Anon. 1965–1991; Beard 1987, 1988)

	All ages	0–4	5–14	15–24	25–44	45–64	>65
1960–1970	3.1	1.5	2.7	2.9	3.2	4.4	3.4
1971–1975	1.4	0.0	1.0	2.0	1.5	2.0	1.3
Percentage reduction	55	100	63	31	53	55	62

tribution. This was also the case in New Zealand (Table 52.2). This means that adults are susceptible and com- monly have a short latency of CE. The discovery of adult susceptibility with a short latency is still compati- ble with long latency in individuals. What these data show is that childhood infections (as proposed by Dew 1928) can no longer be regarded as the rule. This casts no doubt on the existence of exceptions to long-term latency before clinical symptoms occur and there is no inconsistency with the fact that silent infections can still be discovered at autopsy.

DOES CONTROL IN ANIMALS BENEFIT THE HEALTH OF THE WHOLE COMMUNITY?

The results obtained in Tasmania show that the preva- lence of echinococcosis declined rapidly in both young and adult sheep (Fig. 52.3). This was also the case for transmission to children and young adults (<19 years). In this group, transmission ceased within about 7–12 years of the start of the programme, even though trans- mission was still occurring at a low level between dogs and sheep. There was also a decline in CE in adults (>19 years), but as expected, these would include persons with a long latency who were infected prior to, but came to surgery after, the initiation of control. The decline in sheep and humans of all age groups pro- vides clear evidence that a vigorous control effort benefits the whole community, including the elderly (Beard 1978, 1984, 1987, 1988).

PREVENTION AND CONTROL

Some experience has now been gained on applying control based on studies of field trials, control pro- grammes and, more recently, mathematical modelling (Gemmell and Varela Diaz 1973; Gemmell and Lawson 1986; Gemmell *et al.* 1986*c*, 1987*b*; Gemmell 1987, 1990; Lawson *et al.* 1988; Lawson and Gemmell 1989; Tolley and Ming 1993; Lawson 1994; Roberts 1994;

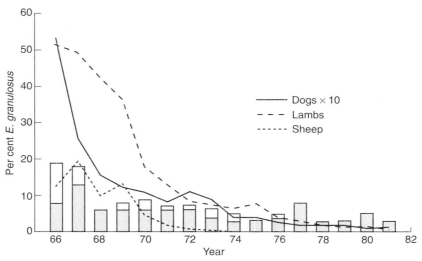

Fig. 52.3 The rate of decline of *Echinococcus granulosus* in dogs, sheep, and humans during the control programme in Tasmania. This island model applied an educational control approach (Option 3) with transformation from the 'attack' to the 'consolidation' phase within 10 years, with potential to achieve the 'maintenance of eradication' phase. Number of new surgical cases of CE in persons aged 1–19 years □ and >19 years ▨. (Modified from Beard 1987, 1988.)

Roberts and Gemmell 1994; Gemmell and Roberts 1995).

Control describes the 'active implementation of a programme by a recognized authority on an instruction from the legislature to limit prevalence of a specific disease'.

Eradication, on the other hand, describes the 'purposeful reduction of a specific disease prevalence to the point of continued absence of transmission within a specific area by means of a time-limited campaign'.

PRIORITY STATUS FOR CONTROL

Many factors may influence the human health priority for control of echinococcosis as well as the decision to adopt a control or an eradication policy. These include:

(1) prevalence of disease;
(2) morbidity or severity of disability;
(3) risk of mortality;
(4) feasibility of control or eradication, including relative efficiency and cost of intervention;
(5) absence of adverse ecological factors;
(6) adequate administration, operational and financial resources;
(7) availability of effective tools;
(8) favourable epidemiological features;
(9) socio-economic importance;

(10) specific reasons for preferring eradication over control.

It should always be remembered that these two goals are not the same.

LEGISLATION, ADMINISTRATION AND FUNDING

There are two models. The first creates, through specific legislation, a national or regional executive authority with responsibility for the control programme, The second utilizes an existing government organization (e.g. Ministry of Health or Agriculture). To an extent, the former is likely to be funded through a dog tax and latter through the legislature.

Depending on the programme to be adopted, areas in which legislation may be needed include:

(1) meat inspection and effective disposal of offal at abattoirs and prevention of clandestine leakage of offals;
(2) banning dogs from abattoirs and closure if necessary;
(3) prevention of feeding raw offal to dogs, including inspection of offal disposal facilities on farms or other premises where sheep are killed;
(4) control of dogs, including registration, submission of dogs for dosing, and elimination of unwanted dogs; and
(5) quarantine of premises with infected livestock.

OPTIONS AND PHASES OF CONTROL

Options

Based on the results of several control programmes, five options can be discerned. These are summarized below with the potential minimum time in the 'attack' phase.

Option 1 consists of deciding not to proceed with any specific measures, either because there is a recognizable health problem, but no suitable infrastructure or funding for control, or there is insufficient infection vis-à-vis other diseases to warrant setting up a specific control programme.

Option 2 consists of introducing a positive long-term horizontal approach with the introduction of educational materials, particularly for, schools, upgrading of water supplies, meat inspection, etc., and possibly supplying drugs for owners to treat their dogs (say 50–100 years).

Option 3 involves introducing a vertical approach, with the adoption of arecoline hydrobromide to test dogs in an educational approach to control with a relatively 'slow-track', to complete the 'attack' phase (say 15–30 years).

Option 4 is similar to Option 3, but includes a positive euthanasia policy for dogs (say 10–15 years).

Option 5 involves treating all dogs at specified periods with praziquantel and is also a fast-track approach (say 10–15 years).

Phases

Four phases can be recognized. These include a 'preparatory' and/or 'planning' phase; 'attack' 'consolidation' and, where appropriate, 'maintenance of eradication' phase (Yekutiel 1980; Gemmell 1987). During the costly 'attack' phase, the control measures are applied non-discriminately to the entire host population at risk. Examples of this include mass dog-dosing. As soon as the parasite reaches a certain low level it becomes more cost-effective to cease the overall attack and to target control in the 'consolidation' phase. If appropriate, once the parasite has been almost eliminated, the 'maintenance of eradication' phase may be entered. Here all specific activities are suspended or disbanded and 'vigilence' is permanently maintained through the normal meat inspection services.

REVIEW OF CURRENT CONTROL PROGRAMMES

The control programmes selected for review in this section, differ from one another in administration, resources used, methods applied, and rate of decline in transmission. The changes that occurred in the prevalence of *E. granulosus* in adult sheep are illustrated in Fig. 52.4.

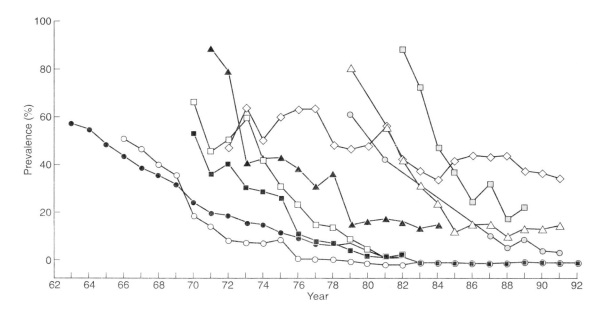

Fig. 52.4 Changes in the prevalence of *Echinococcus granulosus* in adult sheep during control in Uruguay (◇, Option 2); New Zealand (●) and Tasmania (○) (Option 3); Cyprus (□, Option 4); and the Falkland Islands (■), Argentina (Neuquén; ▲; Rio Negro, ◉), and Chile (Region 11, ▨; Region 12, △) (Option 5).

Option 2 with evidence of success over 100 years

The successful programme initiated in the nineteenth century in Iceland has been described previously.

Option 2 with no evidence of success over 20 years

Island model

In New Zealand in 1908, it was made compulsory for owners to register their dogs. In 1935, a strong educational campaign was introduced. In 1937 by an ammendment to the Dog Act (1908), all owners who registered their dogs received sufficient arecoline hydrobromide to treat them four times a year. In 1940, it was made illegal to feed raw offal to dogs. No change was detected in the prevalence of echinococcosis in animals or humans 20 years later (Gemmell 1987, 1990).

Continental model

Control in Uruguay was initiated in 1965 with the creation of a National Commission (Commission Honoraria de Lucha Contra la Hidatidosis). Funding was provided *ab initio* by a dog tax and owners were also expected to purchase tablets and treat their dogs. No evidence could be found that any of the activities attempted between 1965 and 1991 modified the level of transmission of echinococcosis between dogs and sheep (Cabrera *et al.* 1995; Parada *et al.* 1995). Recent evidence from serological and ultrasound surveys also suggests that in some departments, up to 2 per cent of the rural population may have asymptomatic CE (Perdomo *et al.* 1990; Bonifacino *et al.* 1991; Cohen *et al.* 1991; Paolillo *et al.* 1991). Since 1990, the programme has been transformed to Option 5).

Option 3 with evidence of success within 30 years

Island models

Two programmes using a 'slow-track' approach have been almost completed; namely the national programme of New Zealand and the Australian state programme of Tasmania (Anon. 1961–1989; Anon. 1965–1991, McConnell and Green 1979; McConnell 1987; Gemmell 1987, 1990).

Administration was undertaken in New Zealand by a council (National Hydatids Council; see Uruguay above) under an Act of Parliament (Hydatids Act 1959). Funding resources were derived from the dog registration system (about 400 000 dogs) administered by the local county councils. In contrast, in Tasmania administration was undertaken by the Department of Agriculture through the State legislature with funding supplied by the legislature (about 40 000 dogs). Technical differences included:

(1) application of laboratory and field testing of dogs in New Zealand and Tasmania, respectively;

(2) introduction of a 6-weekly dosing programme to combat *T. ovis* in New Zealand; and

(3) gradual transfer from the 'attack' to the 'consolidation' phase with quarantine of infected farms in Tasmania.

In both programmes, transmission of CE (Tables 52.2 and Fig. 52.3) ceased to children within about 7–12 years of their introduction, although the 'maintenance of eradication' phase was not reached until about 35 years of their introduction.

Option 4 with evidence of success within 15 years

Island model

Cyprus, using the resources of the Ministry of Agriculture, initiated stray dog euthanasia (about 80 000 animals) in 1970 and a dog-testing programme with arecoline surveillance in 1972 as an educational measure. In 1974, partition occurred, but control continued in the government-controlled area. There, transmission between animals rapidly ceased and in 1985 eradication was assumed (Polydorou 1971, 1974, 1976, 1977, 1980, 1981, 1984). More recently, small foci have reappeared confirming the need to maintain 'vigilance' even when the parasite becomes difficult to find with current diagnostic tools.

Option 5 with evidence of success within 15 years

Island model

The Falkland Islands also used the resources of the Ministry of Agriculture and introduced a 6-weekly dog-dosing programme in 1970 with praziquantel. Here the slope of the decline in the prevalence of *E. granulosus* in sheep and duration of the 'attack' phase was similar to that in Cyprus without a dog euthanasia programme. In this programme, due to distances, farm owners assumed responsibility for regular dog treatments. While transmission of CE to humans has ceased, it is not yet known whether or not eradication has been achieved (Gemmell *et al.* 1986*c*; Sommers 1955, personal communication).

Continental model

In Chile, programmes with Option 5 were introduced in Region 12 in 1979 and Region 11 in 1982. Both used the administrative and veterinary resources of the Ministry of Agriculture (SAG) at national and regional levels. The results obtained are illustrated in Fig. 52.5 and show clearly that this option is being successfully pursued (Vidal Ogueta 1989, Vidal Ogueta *et al.* 1989; Anon. 1994) and should lead to the transformation from the costly 'attack' programme to a permanent 'consolidation' phase within 20 years.

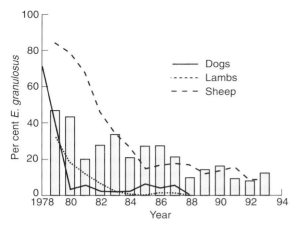

Fig. 52.5 The rate of decline of *Echinococcus granulosus* in dogs, sheep, and humans during the control programme in Region 12, Chile. This continental model applied a 6-weekly dog-dosing programme (Option 5) with a plateau of prevalence in the sheep due to premature increase in intervals between treatments in the 'attack' phase, resulting in a delay in reaching the permanent 'consolidation' phase. Human data show decline in the number of surgical cases in all age groups/100 000 population. (From Vidal Ogueta 1989; Vidal Ogueta *et al.* 1989; Anon. 1994.)

Table 52.4 Changes in the prevalence of *Echinococcus granulosus* in dogs, sheep, and humans in the control programme in Rio Negro Province (source: Larrieu *et al.* 1989)

		Base-line surveys 1980	Continuing surveillance 1987	% reduction
Dogs	(%)	41.5	3.1	92
Sheep	(%)	61.0	12.0	80
Humans	(%)	1.5	0.4	76
Children	(%)	2.1	0.2	88
New cases	(*n*)	65	45	31
children	(*n*)	10	2	80

Table 52.5 Changes in the prevalence (notifications) of CE in humans in the Province of Chubut (source: Iriate, personal communication)

Year	Total	Incidence/100 000	Children
1984	241	67.5	30
1985	146	40.9	15
1986	139	38.9	8
1987	156	43.1	10
1988	106	29.7	9
1989	96	26.9	6
1990	76	21.3	5

Option 5 with limited evidence of success within 15 years

Continental models

In Argentina, control programmes using Option 5 have been funded by provincial ministries of health (Gemmell and Varela Diaz 1973). Few have been sustained, but three have demonstrated that control is feasible. For example, in a pilot trial in the Province of Neuquén in 1970, 28 per cent of the dogs, 71.4 per cent of sheep, and 90 per cent of cattle harboured *E. granulosus*, but 17 years later when the trial was terminated, these prevalences were 2.1, 6.9, and 13.8, per cent respectively, and transmission of CE to children had almost ceased (Kaczorkiewiecz 1988). Similar programmes have been undertaken in the Provinces of Rio Negro (Larrieu *et al.* 1989) and Chubut (J. Iriate, personal communication) with evidence of a reduction in prevalence in humans or animals or both (Tables 52.4, 52.5). However, no evidence is available demonstrating that the 'attack' phase can be transformed by a ministry of health to the 'Consolidation' phase using animal movement legislation with surveillance and quarantine.

EVALUATION OF CONTROL POLICIES

In the past, control programmes have been introduced and funded with little idea of their duration and the costs involved. Some have succeeded, others have not. Important conclusions can be drawn from them.

Comparing the results obtained from programmes using Options 2 with 3, it seems that little progress is likely to be made in echinococcosis control simply by introducing legislation directing owners to treat their dogs and preventing them from gaining access to raw offal, even if a substantial educational programme is involved. From the results of the island programmes using Option 3, it is clear that control and even eradication is not only feasible, but also rapidly benefits the whole community. The important contributing factors in this vertical approach include:

(1) adequate funding;
(2) education of the public through community participation; and
(3) supervision of the dog population, their treatment, and prevention of access to raw offal by technical personnel.

Comparing results obtained from programmes selecting Options 3, 4, and 5, it is clear that the costly 'attack' phase may be shorter with options 4 and 5 than with 3, provided that this phase can be transformed to the 'Consolidation' phase. It seems that this can only readily be achieved if effective survey and surveillance policies and animal health movement legislation can be applied. In their absence, there may be a trend to relax the dosing programme with unpredictable results. It seems that the most rapid progress can best be achieved by using animal health rather than human health administrations. Advantages also include:

(1) experience with control of other animal diseases;
(2) use of established laboratory and field services;
(3) access to specialized services;
(4) uniformity in staff training;
(5) establishment of effective trace-forward and trace-back surveillance systems.

In conclusion, control is expensive and long-term and the 'planning' phase is now regarded as essential if the legislature is to be expected to support a programme financially. The mathematical framework now available provides a method for determining the characteristics of the dynamics of cestode populations. It provides a criterion for deciding if a control programme can succeed in eradicating a parasite and underpins a benefit–cost analysis of control options. It follows that an intervention can now be assessed for epidemiological and economic merit before it proceeds (Lawson *et al.* 1988; Lawson 1994). Several indicators of economic performance are available, including the net present value and the internal rate of return, but the most usual method is the benefit–cost ratio. This is calculated as the total discounted benefit over a fixed time period. If the benefit–cost ratio is greater than unity, then the benefits of a control action outweigh its costs and the programme can be recommended to the legislature as efficient from an economic point of view, with a relatively high priority as control has now been shown to be feasible

REFERENCES

Allan, J. C. *et al.* (1992). Coproantigen detection for immunodiagnosis of echinococcosis and taeniasis in dogs and humans. *Parasitology*, **104**, 347–55.

Alvarez, C., Latourette, F., Geninazzi, H., and Perdomo, R. (1991). True and false relapses in hepatic hydatid disease. Usefulness of per-operatory control of parasitary sterilization. *Archivos de la Hidatidosis*, **30**, 599–607.

Amir-Jahed, A. K., Fardin, R., Farzad, A., and Bakshandeh, K. (1975). Clinical echinococcosis. *Annals of Surgery*, **182**, 541–6.

Amman, R. W. and Eckert, J. (1995). Clinical diagnosis and treatment of echinococcosis in humans. In *Echinococcus and hydatid disease*, (ed. R. C. A. Thompson and A. J. Lymbery). CAB International, Wallingford, pp. 411–63.

Anderson, R. M. (1982). *Transmission dynamics of infectious disease agents. Dahlem Konferenzen*, (ed. R. M. Anderson and R. M. May), pp. 149–76. Springer Verlag, New York.

Anderson, R. M. and May, R. M. (1978). Regulation and stability of host–parasite interactions. 1. Regulatory processes. *Journal of Animal Ecology*, **7**, 219–47.

Anon. (1961–1989). *Annual Reports of the National Hydatids Council*, Ministry of Agriculture and Fisheries, Wellington, New Zealand.

Anon. (1965–1991). *Annual Reports and Accounts.* Tasmanian Hydatids Eradication Council, Hobart, Tasmania.

Anon. (1994). *Evaluacion proyecto de control de la hidatidosis en la X11 Region de Chile, periodo 83/87.* Servicio d'Agricola y Ganadero, Ministerio de Agricultura, Santiago, Chile.

Barros, J. L. (1978). Hydatid disease of the liver. *American Journal of Surgery*, **135**, 597–600.

Bchir, A. *et al.* (1991). Echotomographic and serological population-based study of hydatidosis in central Tunisia. *Acta Tropica*, **49**, 149–53.

Beard, T. C. (1969). Hydatid control: a problem in health education. *Medical Journal of Australia*, **2**, 456–9.

Beard, T. C. (1973*a*) Observations for Icelanders on hydatids and precautions against them. *Australian Veterinary Journal*, **49**, 396–401.

Beard, T. C. (1973*b*). The elimination of echinococcosis from Iceland. *Bulletin of the World Health Organization*, **48**, 653–60.

Beard, T. C. (1978). Evidence that a hydatid cyst is seldom as old as the patient. *Lancet*, **2**, 30–2.

Beard, T. C. (1984). Changing rural behaviour: two campaigns that worked. *Hygie*, **111**, 9–13.

Beard, T. C. (1987). Human hydatid disease in Tasmania. In *Epidemiology in Tasmania* (ed H. King), pp. 77–88. Brolga Press, Canberra.

Beard, T. C. (1988). Human behaviour and the ethics of coercion. *Medical Journal of Australia*, **148**, 82–5.

Beggs, J. (1983). The radiological appearances of hydatid disease of the liver. *Clinical Radiology*, **34**, 555–63.

Beggs, J. (1985). The radiology of hydatid disease. *American Journal of Roentgenology, Radium Therapy and Nuclear Medicine*, **145**, 639–48.

Bekhti, A. and Pirotte, J. (1987). Cimetidine increases serum mebendazole concentrations: implications for treatment of hepatic hydatid cysts. *British Journal of Clinical Pharmacology*, **24**, 390–2.

Bekhti, A., Schaaps, J. P., Capron, M., Dessaint, J. P., Santoro, F., Capron, A. (1977). Treatment of hepatic hydatid disease with mebendazole: preliminary results in four cases. *British Medical Journal*, **ii**, 1047–51.

Belghiti, J., Benhamou, J. P., Houry, S., Grenier, P., Huguier, M., and Fekete, F. (1986). Caustic sclerosing cholangitis. A complication of the surgical treatments of hydatid disease of the liver. *Archives of Surgery*, **121**, 1162–5.

Ben Amor, N., Gargouri, M., Gharbi, H. A. Golvan, Y. J., Ayachi, K., and Kchouck, H. (1986). Essai de traitment par ponctio des kystes hydatiques abdominaux inoperables. *Annales de Parasitologie Humaine et Comparee*, **61**, 689–92.

Bernadini, P. and Valle, M. (1991). Complicaciones biliares de la hidatidosis hepatica: problems para el chirurgianos. *Archivos de la Hidatidosis*, **30**, 643–8.

Bonifacino, R. *et al.* (1991). Seroprevalence of *Echinococcus granulosus* infection in a Uruguayan rural population. *Transaction of the Royal Society of Tropical Medicine and Hygiene*, **85**, 769–72.

Bowles, J. and McManus, D. P. (1993*a*). Rapid discrimination of *Echinococcus* species and strains using a polymerase chain reaction-based RFLP method. *Molecular Biology and Parasitology*, **57**, 231–9.

Bowles, J. and McManus, D. P. (1993*b*). NADH hydrogenase 1 gene sequences compared for species and strains of the genus *Echinococcus*. *International Journal for Parasitology*, **23**, 969–72.

Bowles, J. and McManus, D. P. (1993*c*). Molecular variation in echinococcus. *Acta Tropica*, **53**, 291–305.

Bowles, J., Van Knapen, F., and McManus, D. P. (1992). Genetic variants within the genus *Echinococcus* identified by mitochondrial DNA sequencing. *Molecular Biochemistry and Parasitology*, **54**, 163–73.

Bryceson, A. D. M. *et al.* (1982). Experience with mebendazole in the treatment of inoperable hydatid disease in England. *Transactions of the Royal Society of Tropical Medicine and Hygiene*, **76**, 501–18.

Cabrera, P. A. *et al.* (1995). Transmission dynamics of *Echinococcus granulosus*, *Taenia hydatigena* and *Taenia ovis* in sheep in Uruguay. *International Journal for Parasitology*, **25**, 807–13.

Caratozzolo, M., Scardella, L., Grossi, G., and Angelini, L. (1991). Diagnostic approach of abdominal hydatidosis by ultrasonography. *Archivos de la Hidatidosis*, **30**, 531–44.

Caremani, M. *et al.* (1991). Detection of hydatid cysts with echography: survey on 249, 299 patients. *Archivos de la Hidatidosis*, **30**, 277–307.

Chai Jun-jie (1993). Sero-epidemiological surveys for cystic echinococcosis in the Xinjiang Uygur Autonomous Region PRC. In *Compendium on Cystic Echinococcosis*, (ed. F. L. Andersen), pp. 153–61. Brigham Young University Print Services, Provo, Utah.

Chaouachi, B., Ben Salah, S., Lakhoua, R., Hammou, A., Gharbi, H. A., and Saied. H. (1989). Hydatid cysts in children. Diagnostic and therapeutic aspects. A propos of 1195 cases. *Annales de Pediatrie*, **36**, 441–4.

Chi pu-sheng (1993). Use of praziquantel-medicated tablets for control of cystic echinococcosis in the Xinjiang Uygur Autonomous Region, P. R. C. In *Compendium on Cystic Echinococcosis*, (ed. F. L. Andersen), pp. 190–5. Brigham Young University Print Services, Provo, Utah.

Cohen, H. *et al.* (1991). Hidatidosis en area rural: estudio simultaneo en tres hospederos. Capitulo seres humanos. *Archivos de la Hidatidosis*, **30**, 935–6.

Cotting, J., Zeugin, T., Steiger, U., and Reichen, J. (1990). Albendazole kinetics in patients with echinococcosis: delayed absorption and impaired elimination in cholestasis. *European Journal of Clinical Pharmacology*, **38**, 605–8.

Craig, P. S. (1993). Imunodiagnosis of *Echinococcus granulosus*. In *Compendium on Cystic Echinococcosis*, (ed. F. L. Andersen), pp. 85–118. Brigham Young University Print Services, Provo, Utah.

Craig, P. S. *et al.* (1994), Diagnosis of canine echinococcosis: comparison of coproantigen and serum antibody test with arecoline purgation in Uruguay. *Veterinary Parasitology*, **56**, 293–301.

Crewe, W. and Crewe, S. M. (1969) Worm eggs found in gull droppings. *Transactions of the Royal Society of Tropical Medicine and Hygiene*, **63**, 17.

Davis, A., Pawlowski, Z. S., and Dixon, H. (1986). Multicentre clinical trials of benzimidazole carbamates in human echinococcosis. *Bulletin of the World Health Organization*, **64**, 383–8.

Davis, A., Dixon, H., and Pawlowski, Z. S. (1989). Multicentre clinical trials of benzimidazole-carbamates in human echinococcosis (2). *Bulletin of the World Health Organization*, **67**, 503–8.

Deplazes, P., Gottstein, B., Eckert, J., Jenkins, D. J., Wald, D., and Jimenez-Palacios, S. (1992). Detection of *Echinococcus* coproantigens by enzyme linked immunosorbent assay in dogs, dingoes, and foxes. *Parasitological Research*, **78**, 303–8.

De Rosa, F. and Teggi, A. (1990). Treatment of *Echinococcus granulosus* hydatid disease with albendazole. *Annals of Tropical Medicine and Parasitology*, **84**, 467–72.

Dew, H. R. (1928). *Hydatid disease.* Australian Medical Publishing Company, Sydney.

Di Palma, A., Ettorre, G. C., and Scapati, C. (1991). The role of computerized tomography in the diagnosis of hydatid disease. *Radiologica Medica* (Torino), **82**, 430–6.

Drolshammer, I., Wiesmann, E. and Eckert, J. (1973). Echinokokkose beim Menschen in der Schweiz 1956–1969. *Schweizerische Medizinische Wochenschrift*, **103** 1337–92.

Dungal, N. (1957). Eradication of hydatid disease in Iceland. *New Zealand Medical Journal*, **56**, 213–22.

Eckert, J. (1986). Prospects for treatment of the metacestode stage of *Echinococcus*. In *The Biology of Echinococcus and Hydatid Disease*, (ed. R. C. A. Thompson), pp. 250–84. George Allen and Unwin, London.

El Mufti, M. *et al.* (1993). Albendazole therapy of hydatid disease: 2-year follow-up of 40 cases. *Annals of Tropical Medicine and Parasitology*, **87**, 241–6.

FAO/UNEP/WHO (1981). *Guidelines for surveillance, prevention and control of echinococcosis/hydatidosis*, (ed. J. Eckert, M. A. Gemmell, and E. J. L. Soulsby) VPH/81.28 p. 147. World Health Organization, Geneva, Switzerland.

Filice, C., Stroesseli, M., Brunetti, E., Colombo, P., Emmi, E., and D'Andrea, F. (1991). P. A. I. R (Puncture, reaspiration, introduction, respiration) with alcohol under US guidance of hydatid liver cysts. *Archivos de la Hidatidosis*, **30**, 811–17.

Frider, B., Ledesma, C., Odriozzola, M., and Larrieu, E. (1990). Echographic specificity in the early diagnosis of human hydatidosis. *Acta Gastroenterologica Latinamericana*, **20**, 13–5.

Gargouri, M. *et al.* (1990). Percutaneous treatment of hydatid, cysts (*Echinococcus granulosus*), *Cardiovascular and Interventional Radiography*, **13**, 169–73.

Gasser, R. B., Lightowlers, M. W., Obendorf, D. L., Jenkins, D. J., and Rickard, M. D. (1988). Evaluation of a serological test system for the diagnosis of natural *Echinococcus granulosus* infections in dogs using *E. granulosus* protoscolex and oncosphere antigens. *Australian Veterinary Journal*, **65**, 369–73.

Gemmell, M. A. (1968). Safe handling of infected definitive hosts and eggs of *Echinococcus*. *Bulletin of the World Health Organization*, **89**, 122–5.

Gemmell, M. A. (1973). Surveillance of *Echinococcus granulosus* in dogs with arecoline hydrobromide. *Bulletin of the World Health Organization*, **48**, 649–52.

Gemmell, M. A. (1977) Taeniidae: Modification to the life span of the egg and the regulation of tapeworm infections. *Experimental Parasitology*, **41** 314–28.

Gemmell, M. A. (1978). The effect of weather on tapeworm eggs and its epidemiological implications. In *Weather and Parasitic Animal disease.* (ed. T. E. Gibson), pp. 83–94. World Meteorological Organization, Technical Notes, **159**, 83–94.

Gemmell, M. A. (1987). A. critical approach to the concepts of control and eradication of echinococcosis/hydatidosis and taeniasis/cysticercosis. *International Journal for Parasitology* **17**, 465–72.

Gemmell, M. A. (1990). Australasian contributions to an understanding of the epidemiology and control of hydatid disease caused by *Echinococcus granulosus*; past, present and future. *International Journal for Parasitology*, **20**, 431–56.

Gemmell, M. A. (1993). Quantifying the transmission dynamics of the family Taeniidae, with particular reference to *Echinococcus* spp. In *Compendium on Cystic Echinococcosis*, (ed. F. L. Andersen), pp. 57–73. Brigham Young University Print Services, Provo, Utah.

Gemmell, M. A. and Johnstone, P. D. (1977). Experimental epidemiology of hydatidosis and cysticercosis. *Advances in Parasitology*, **15**, 311–69.

Gemmell, M. A. and Johnstone, P. D. (1981a). Factors regulating tapeworm populations: estimation of the duration of acquired immunity by sheep to *Taenia hydatigena*. *Research in Veterinary Science*, **30**, 53–6.

Gemmell, M. A. and Johnstone, P. D. (1981b). Factors regulating tapeworm populations: dispersion of eggs of *Taenia hydatigena* on pasture. *Annals of Tropical Medicine and Parasitology*, **70**, 431–4.

Gemmell, M. A. and Johnstone, P. D. (1981c). Cestodes. *Antibiotics and Chemotherapy*, **30**, 54–114.

Gemmell, M. A. and Lawson, J. R. (1986). Epidemiology and control of hydatid disease. In *The biology of echinococcus and hydatid disease*, (ed. R. C. A. Thompson), pp. 189–216. George Allen & Unwin, London.

Gemmell, M. A. and Lawson, J. R. (1989). The ovine cysticercoses as models for research into the epidemiology of the human and porcine cysticercosis: Epidemiological considerations. *Acta Leidensia*, **57**, 165–72.

Gemmell, M. A. and Roberts, M. G. (1995). Modelling echinococcus life cycles. In *Echinococcus and hydatid disease*, (ed. R. C. A. Thompson and A. J. Lymbery), pp. 333–54. CAB International, Wallingford.

Gemmell, M. A. and Varela Diaz, V. M. (1973). *Review of Programs for the Control of Hydatidosis/Echinococcosis up to 1974*. Series of Scientific Technical Monographs, CPZ 8, pp. 91. Pan American Zoonoses Center, Buenos Aires, Argentina.

Gemmell, M. A., Parmeter, S. N., Sutton, R. J., and Khan, N. (1981). Effect of mebendazole against *Echinococcus granulosus* and *Taenia hydatigena* cysts in naturally infected sheep and relevance to larval tapeworm infections in man. *Zeitschrift für Parasitenkunde*, **64**, 135–47.

Gemmell, M. A., Lawson, J. R., and Roberts, M. G. (1986a). Population dynamics in echinococcosis and cysticercosis: biological parameters of *Echinococcus granulosus* in dogs and sheep. *Parasitology*, **92**, 599–620.

Gemmell, M. A., Lawson, J. R Roberts, M. G., Kerin, B. R., and Mason, C. J. (1986b). Population dynamics in echinococcosis and cysticercosis. Comparison of the response of *Echinococcus granulosus* and *Taenia hydatigena* and *T. ovis* to control. *Parasitology*, **93**, 357–69.

Gemmell, M. A., Lawson J. R., and Roberts, M. G. (1986c). Control of echinococcosis/hydatidosis: present status of worldwide progress. *Bulletin of the World Health Organization*, **64**, 333–9.

Gemmell, M. A., Lawson, J. R., and Roberts, M. G. (1987a). Population dynamics in echinococcosis and cysticerosis: biological parameters of *Taenia hydatigena*. and *T. ovis* and comparison with those of *Echinococcus granulous*. *Parasitology*, **94**, 161–80.

Gemmell, M. A., Lawson, J. R., and Roberts, M. G., (1987b). Towards global control of cystic and alveolar hydatid diseases. *Parasitology Today*, **3**, 144–51.

Gemmell, M. A., Lawson, R. J., Roberts, M. G., and Griffin, J. F. T. (1990). Population dynamics in echinococcosis and cysticercosis: regulation of *Taenia hydatigena* and *T. ovis* in lambs through passively transferred immunity. *Parasitology*, **101**, 145–51.

Gil-Grande, L. E. *et al.* (1993). Randomised controlled trial of efficacy of albendazole in intra-abdominal hydatid disease. *Lancet*, **342**, 1269–72.

Gloor, G. (1988). Echinokokkose beim Menschen in der Schweiz 1970–83. Medical Dissertation, University of Zurich (cited in Amman and Eckert 1995).

Gottstein, B. (1992). Molecular and immunological diagnosis of echinococcosis. *Clinical Microbiological Reviews*, **5**, 248–61.

Gottstein, B., Eckert, J., and Fey, H. (1983). Serological differentiation between *Echinococcus granulosus* and *E. multilocularis* infections in humans. *Zeitschrift für Parasitenkunde*, **69**, 347–56.

Gottstein, B., Schantz, P. M., Todorov, T., Saimot, A. G., and Jacquier, P. (1986). An international study on the serological differential diagnosis of human cystic and alveolar echinococcosis. *Bulletin of the World Health Organization*, **64**, 101–5.

Grossi, G. *et al.* (1991). 420 patients with hydatid cysts: observations on the clinical picture. *Archivos de la Hidatidosis*, **30**, 1021–43.

Grove, D. I., Warren, K. S. and Mahmoud, A. A. F. (1976). Algorithms in the diagnosis and management of exotic disease: Echinococcosis. *Journal of Infectious Disease*, **133**, 354–8.

Guerra, M., Arroyo, A., and Ubilla, R. (1990). Hepatic hydatid cyst. Ultrasonograph study. *Boletin Chileno de Parasitologia*, **45**, 35–8.

Harrison, L. J. and Parkhouse, R. M. (1985). Antigens of taeniid cestodes in protection. *Current Topics in Microbiology and Immunology*, **120**, 159–72.

Heath, D. D. (1971). The migration of oncospheres of *Taenia pisiformis*, *T. serialis* and *Echinococcus granulosus* within intermediate hosts. *International Journal for Parasitology*, **1**, 145–52.

Heath, D. D. (1986). Immunobiology of echinococcus infections. In *The biology of echinococcus and hydatid disease*, (ed. R. C. A. Thompson), pp. 164–88. George Allen & Unwin, London.

Heesterbeek, J. A. P. and Roberts, M. G. (1995). Threshold quantities for helminth infections. *Journal of Mathematical Biology*, **33**, 415.

Horton, R. J. (1989). Chemotherapy of echinococus infection in man with albendazole. *Transactions of the Royal Society of Tropical Medicine and Hygiene*, **83**, 97–102.

Houry, S., Languielle, O., Hugnier, M., Benhamou, J. P., Belghiti, J., and Msika, S. (1990). Sclerosing cholangitis induced by formaldehyde solution injected into the biliary tree of rats. *Archives of Surgery*, **125**, 1059–61.

Howell, M. J. (1986). Cultivation of *Echinococcus* species *in vitro*. In *The biology of echinococcus and hydatid disease*, (ed. R. C. A. Thompson ed), pp. 143–63. George Allen & Unwin, London.

Jain, A. K., Gupta, P. D., and Saha, M. M. (1989). Membraneous glomerunephritis secondary to hydatid disease. *Australian Radiology*, **33**, 373–5.

Jenkins, D. J. (1992). Epidemiology of *Echinoccus granulosus* in wildlife in South Eastern Australia. In: *Epidemiological survey on the new unilocular echinococcosis occurring in tropical Queensland of Australia*, (ed. T. Sakamoto), pp. 75–86. Yamaguti-Hokushyu, Japan.

Jenkins, D. J. and Rickard, M. D. (1986). Specificity of scolex and oncosphere antigens for the serological diagnosis of taeniid cestodes of dogs. *Australian Veterinary Journal*, **63**, 40–2.

Jenkins, D. J., Gasser, R. B., Romig, T., and Macpherson, C. N. L. (1990). Assessment of a serological test for the detection of *Echinococcus granulosus* infection in dogs in Kenya. *Acta Tropica*, **47**, 245–8.

Johnson, K. S. *et al.* (1989). Vaccination against ovine cysticercosis using a defined recombinant antigen. *Nature (London)*, **338**, 585–7.

Kaczorkiewicz, A. (1988). Lineamientos generales del Ministerio de Salud Publica del Neuquen en materia de control de la hidatidosis. *Boletin International Asociacion de la Hidatidosis*, **11**, 53–7.

Kammerer, W. S. and Schantz, P. M. (1993). Echinococcal disease. *Infectious Disease Clinics of North America*, **7**, 605–18.

Kanwar, J. R., Kaushik, S. P., Sawhney, I. M. S., Kamboj, M. S., Mebta, S. K., and Vinayak, V. K. (1992). Specific antibodies in serum of patients with hydatidosis recognised by immunoblotting. *Journal of Medical Microbiology*, **36**, 16–51.

Khuroo, M. S., Zargar, S. A., and Mahajan, R. (1991). *Echinococcus granulosus* cysts in the liver: management with percutaneous drainage. *Radiology*, **180**, 141–5.

Khuroo, M. S. *et al.* (1993). Percutaneous drainage versus albendazole therapy in hepatic hydatidosis: a prospective randomized study. *Gastroenterology*, **104**, 1452–9.

Kitani, T., Horchani, H., and Daoues, A. (1992). Secondary bronchogenic pulmonary hydatidosis. *Annales de Chirurgie*, **46**, 160–4.

Kumaratilake, L. M. and Thompson, R. C. A. (1982). A review of the taxonomy and speciation of the genus *Echinococcus* Rudolphi 1801. *Zeitschrift für Parasitenkunde*, **68**, 121–46.

Larrieu, E., De la Fuente, R., Aquino, A., Costa, M. T., and Vargas, F. (1989). Control of hydatidosis in the Rio Negro Province of Argentina. *Veterinary Medical Reviews*, **60**, 54–9.

Laws, G. F. (1968). Physical factors influencing the survival of taeniid eggs. *Experimental Parasitology*, **22**, 227–39.

Lawson, J. R. (1994). Hydatid disease and sheep measles: the history of their control and the economics of a recent change of control policy. *New Zealand Journal of Zoology*, **21**, 83–9.

Lawson, J. R. and Gemmell, M. A. (1983). Hydatidosis and Cysticercosis: the dynamics of transmission. *Advances in Parasitology*, **22**, 261–308.

Lawson, J. R. and Gemmell, M. A. (1985). The potential role of blowflies in the transmission of taeniid eggs. *Parasitology*, **91**, 129–43.

Lawson, J. R. and Gemmell, M. A. (1989). The ovine cysticercoses as models for research on the epidemiology and control of the human and porcine cysticercosis *Taenia solium* ii. The application of control. *Acta Leidensia*, **57**, 173–80.

Lawson, J. R. and Gemmell, M. A. (1990). Transmission of taeniid tapeworm eggs via blowflies to intermediate hosts. *Parasitology*, **100**, 143–6.

Lawson, J. R., Roberts, M. G., Gemmell, M. A., and Best, S. J. (1988). Population dynamics in echinococcosis and cysticercosis: economic assessment of control strategies for *Echinococcus granulosus*, *Taenia ovis* and *T. hydatigena*. *Parasitology*, **97**, 1–15.

Lethbridge, R. C. (1980). The biology of the oncosphere of cyclophyllidean cestodes. *Helminthological Abstracts*, **49**, 59–72.

Lightowlers, M. W. (1990). Cestode infections in animals: immunological diagnosis and vaccination. *Revue Scientifique et Technique. Office International des Epizooties*, **9**, 463–87.

Lightowlers, M. W., Gemmell, M. A., Harrison, G. L. B., Heath, D. D., Rickard, M. D., and Roberts, M. G. (1992). Control of tissue parasites. 11. cestodes. In) *Animal parasite control utilizing biotechnology*, (ed. W. K. Yong), pp. 171–98. CRC Press, Boca Raton.

Lightowlers, M. W., Mitchell, G. F., and Rickard, M. D. (1993). Cestodes. In *Immunology and molecular biology of parasitic infections*, (ed. K. S. Warren and N. Agabian), pp. 438–72. Blackwell Scientific Press, Oxford.

Lloyd, S. S., Martin, S. C., Walters, T. M. H., and Soulsby, E. J. L. (1991). Use of sentinel lambs for early monitoring of the South Powys hydatidosis control scheme prevalence of *Echinococcus granulosus* and some other helminths. *Veterinary Record*, **129**, 73–6.

Luder, P. J., Witassek, F., Weigand, K., Eckert, J., and Bircher, J. (1985). Treatment of cystic echinococcosis (*Echinococcus granulosus*) with mebendazole: Assessment of bound and free drug levels in cyst fluid and of parasite vitality in operative specimens. *European Journal of Clinical Pharmacology*, **28**, 279–85.

Luder, P. J., Siffert, B., Witassek, F., Meister, F., and Bircher, J. (1986). Treatment of hydatid disease with high oral doses of mebendazole. Long-term follow-up of plasma mebendazole levels and drug interactions. *European Journal of Clinical Pharmacology*, **31**, 443–8.

Luo Menghebat, Li Jiang, and Jun-jie Chai (1993). A retrospective survey for surgical cases of cystic echinococcosis in the Xingjiang Uygur Autonomous Region, P. R. C. (1951–90). In *Compendium on cystic echinococcosis*, (ed. F. L. Andersen), pp. 135–45. Brigham Young University Print Services, Utah.

Lymbery, A. J., Thompson, R. C. A., and Hobbs, R. P. (1990). Genetic diversity and genetic differentiation in *Echinococcus granulosus* (Batsch, 1786) from domestic and and sylvatic hosts on the mainland of Australia. *Parasitology*, **101**, 283–9.

McConnell, J. D. (1987). Hydatid disease in Tasmania: control in Animals. In *Epidemiology in Tasmania* (ed. H. King), pp. 61–75. Brolga Press, Canberra, Australia.

McConnell, J. D. and Green, J. (1979). The control of hydatid disease in Tasmania. *Australian Veterinary Journal*, **55**, 140–5.

McManus, D. P. (1990). Characterisation of taeniid cestodes by DNA analysis. *Revue Scientifique et technique de l'Office International des Epizooties*, **9**, 489–510.

McManus, D. P. and Bryant, C. (1986). Biochemistry and physiology of *Echinococcus*. In *The Biology of Echinococcus and hydatid disease* (ed. R. C. A. Thompson), pp. 114–42. George Allen & Unwin, London.

McManus, D. P. and Rishi, A. K. (1989). Genetic heterogeneity with *Echinococcus granulosus*: isolates from different hosts and geographical areas characterized with DNA probes. *Parasitology*, **99**, 17–29.

Macpherson, C. N. L., French, C. M., Stevenson, P., Karstad, L. and Arundel, J. H. (1985). Hydatid disease in the Turkana district of Kenya. (iv) the prevalence of *Echinococcus granulosus* infections in dogs and observations on the role of the dog in the lifestyle of the Turkana. *Annals of Tropical Medicine and Parasitology*, **79**, 57–61.

Macpherson, C. N. L., Romig., T., Zeyhle, E., Rees, P. H., and Were, J. B. O. (1987). Portable ultrasound scanner versus serology in screening for hydatid cysts in a nomadic population. *Lancet*, **ii**, 259–61.

Macpherson, C. N. L., Spoerry, A., Zeyhle, E., Romig, T., and Gorfe, M. (1989). Pastoralists and hydatid disease: an ultra-sound scanning prevalence survey in East Africa. *American Journal of Tropical Medicine and Hygiene*, **83**, 243–7.

Marani, S. A. D., Camossi, G. C., Nicoli, F. A., Alberti, G. P., Monni, S. G., and Casolo, P. M. (1990). Hydatid disease. M. R. Imaging study. *Radiology*, **175**, 701–6.

Messaritakis, J. *et al.* (1991). High mebendazole doses in pulmonary and hepatic hydatid disease. *Archives of Diseases of Childhood*, **66**, 532–3.

Ming, R., Tolley, H. D., Andersen, F. L., Chai, J., and Chang, Q. (1992*a*). Frequency distribution of *Echinococcus granulosus* in dog populations in the Xinjiang Uygur Autonomous Region, China. *Veterinary Parasitology*, **44**, 223–41.

Ming, R., Tolley, H. D., Andersen, F. L., Chai, J., and Sultan, Y. (1992*b*). Frequency distribution of *Echinococcus granulosus* hydatid cysts in sheep populations in the Xinjiang Uygur Autonomous Region, China. *Veterinary Parasitology*, **44**, 67–75.

Morris, D. L. (1987). Preoperative albendazole therapy for hydatid cyst. *British Journal of Surgery*, **74**, 805–6.

Morris, D. L. (1989). Albendazole treatment of hydatid disease: follow-up at five years. *Tropical Doctor*, **19**, 179–80.

Morris, D. L. and Richards, K. S. (1992). *Hydatid disease Current medical and surgical management*. Butterworth-Heinemann, Oxford.

Morris, D. L. and Taylor, D. (1988). Optimal timing of post-operative albendazole prophylaxis in *E. granulosus*. *Annals of Tropical Medicine and Parasitology*, **82**, 65–6.

Morris, D. L., Skene-Smith, H., Haynes, A., and Burrows, F. G. O. (1984). Abdominal hydatid disease: computed tomographic and ultrasound changes during albendazole therapy. *Clinical Radiology*, **35**, 297–300.

Morris, D. L. *et al.* (1985). Albendazole: objective evidence of response in human hydatid disease. *Journal of the American Medical Association*, **253**, 2053–7.

Morris, D. L., Chinnery, J. B., Georgiou, G., Stamatakis, G., and Golematis, B. (1987). Penetration of albendazole sulphoxide into hydatid cysts. *Gut*, **28**, 75–80.

Morris, D. L., Richards, K. S., Clarkson. M. J., and Taylor, D. H. (1990). Comparison of albendazole and praziquantel therapy of *Echinococcus granulosus* in naturally infected sheep. *Veterinary Parasitology*, **36**, 83–90.

Munzer, D. (1991). New perspectives in the diagnosis of *Echinococcus* disease. *Journal of Clinical Gastroenterology*, **13**, 415–23.

Okela, G. B. A. (1986). Hydatid disease research and control in Turkana: 111—Albendazole in the treatment of inoperable hydatid disease in Kenya: a report on 12 cases. *Transactions of the Royal Society of Tropical Medicine and Hygiene*, **80**, 193–5.

Osborne, D. R. (1980). Mebendazole and hydatid disease. *British Medical Journal*, **280**, 183.

Paolillo, E. *et al.* (1991). Hidatidosis un problema de attencion primaria de salud. *Revista Medicina del Uruguay*, **7**, 32–7.

Parada, L. *et al.* (1994). *Echinococus granulosus* infections of dogs in three areas of the Durazno Region of Uruguay. *Veterinary Record*, **136**, 389–391.

Pawlowski Z. S. (1993). Critical points in the clinical management of cystic Echinococcosis. In *Compendium on cystic echinococcosis*, (ed. F. L. Andersen), pp. 119–31. Brigham Young University Print Services, Utah, U.S.A.

Perdomo, R. *et al.* (1990). Estudio epidemiologico de hidatidosis. Deteccion precoz por ultrasonido en areas de alto riesgo. *Revista Medicina del Uruguay*, **4**, 34–47.

Perdomo, R. *et al.* (1991). Estenosis biliares posthidaticas y sus complicaciones. *Archivos de la Hidatidosis*, **30**, 635–42.

Pinch, L. W. and Wilson, J. F. (1973). Non-surgical management of cystic hydatid disease in Alaska: review of 30 cases of *Echinococcus granulosus* infection treated without operation. *Annals of Surgery*, **178**, 45–8.

Polydorou, K. (1971). Hydatid disease in Cyprus. *Bulletin de l'Office International des Epizooties*, **76**, 611–9.

Polydorou, K. (1974). The sanitary position and methods of control in Cyprus. *Bulletin de l'Office International des Epizooties*, **82**, 379–84.

Polydorou, K. (1976). The control of the dog population as the first objective of the anti-echinococus campaign in Cyprus. *Bulletin de l'Office International des Epizooties*, **86**, 705–15.

Polydorou K. (1977). Anti-echinococcosis campaign in Cyprus. *Tropical Animal Health and Production*, **9**, 141–6.

Polydorou, K. (1980). The control of echinococcosis in Cyprus. *FAO World Animal Revue*, Issue No. 33, 19–25.

Polydorou, K. (1981). The national-echinococcosis campaign in Cyprus. Infection in dogs: according to use, age, sex and breed. *Bulletin de l'Office International des Epizooties*, **93**, 1303–7.

Polydorou, K. (1984). How echinococcosis was conquered in Cyprus. *World Health Forum*, **5**, 160–4.

Prasad, J., Bellamy, P. R., and Stubbs, R. S. (1991). Instillation of scolicidal agents into hepatic hydatid cysts: can it any longer be justified? *New Zealand Medical Journal*, **104** 336–7.

Rausch, R. L. (1953). The taxonomic value and variability of certain structures in the cestode genus *Echinococcus* (Rud., 1801) and a review of recognized species. In *Thapar Commemorative Volume, Lucknow University*, (ed. J. Dayal and S. Singh), pp. 233–46. Prem Printing Press, Lucknow.

Rausch, R. L. (1967*a*). On the ecology and distribution of *Echinococcus* spp. (Cestoda: Taeniidae), and characteristics of their development in the intermediate host. *Annals Parasitologie Humaine et Comparee*, **42**, 16–93.

Rausch, R. L. (1967*b*). A consideration of infraspecific categories in the genus *Echinococcus* Rudolphi, 1801 (Cestoda: Taeniidae). *Journal of Parasitology*, **53**, 484–91.

Rausch, R. L. (1986). Life cycle patterns and geographical distribution of *Echinococcus* species. In *The biology of echinococcus and hydatid disease*, (ed. R. C. A. Thompson), pp. 44–80. George Allen and Unwin, London.

Rausch, R. L. (1993). The biology of *Echinococcus granulosus*. In *Compendium of cystic echinococcosis. With special reference to the Xinjiang Uygur Autonomous Region, the People's Republic of China*, (ed. F. L. Andersen), pp. 27–56. Brigham Young University Print Services, Provo, Utah

Rausch, R. L. and Bernstein, J. J. (1972). *Echinococcus vogeli* sp. n. (Cestoda: Taenidae) from the Bush Dog, *Spethyos venaticus* (Lund). *Zeitschrift für Tropenmedizin und Parasitologie*, **23**, 25–34.

Rausch, R. L. and Nelson, G. S. (1963). A review of the genus *Echinococcus Rudolphi, 1801. Annals of Tropical Medicine and Parasitology*, **57**, 127–35.

Rausch, R. L. and Schiller, E. (1951). Hydatid disease (echinococcosis) in Alaska and the importance of rodent intermediate hosts. *Science*, **113**, 58.

Reeder, M. M. and Palmer, P. E. S. (1981). *The radiology of tropical diseases with epidemiological, pathological and clinical correlation*. Williams & Wilkins, Baltimore.

Rickard, M. D. (1983). Immunity. In *Biology of the Eucestoda*, (ed. C. Arme and P. W. Pappas), pp. 539–79. Academic Press, London.

Rickard, M. D. and Lightowlers, M. W. L. (1986). Immunodiagnosis of hydatid disease. In *The biology of echinococcus and hydatid disease*, (ed. R. C. A. Thompson), pp. 217–49. George Allen and Unwin, London.

Rickard, M. D. and Williams, J. F. (1982). Hydatidosis and cysticercosis. Immune mechanisms and immunization against infection. *Advances in Parasitology*, **21**, 229–96.

Roberts, M. G. (1994). Modelling of parasitic populations: cestodes *Veterinary Parasitology*, **54**, 145–60.

Roberts, M. G. and Gemmell, M. A. (1994). Echinococcosis. In *Parasite ecology* (ed. M. E. Scott and G. Smith), pp. 249–62. Academic Press, San Diego. York, Boston, London, Sydney, Tokyo, Toronto.

Roberts, M. G., Lawson, J. R., and Gemmell, M. A. (1986). Population dynamics in echinococcosis and cysticercosis: mathematical model of the life cycle of *Echinococcus granulosus*. *Parasitology*, **92**, 621–41.

Roberts, M. G., Lawson, J. R., and Gemmell, M. A. (1987). Population dynamics in echinococcosis and cysticercosis: mathematical model of the life cycle of *Taenia hydatigena* and *T. ovis*. *Parasitology*, **94**, 181–97.

Romig, T. (1990). Beobachtungen zur zystischen Echinokokkose des Menschen im Turkana-Gebiet, Kenia, Dissertation, Faculty, 11 (Biology) University of Hohenheim (cited in Amman and Eckert 1995).

Romig, T., Zeyhle, E., Macpherson, C. N. L., Rees, P. H., and Were, J. B. O. (1986). Cyst growth and spontaneous cure in hydatid disease. *Lancet*, **i**, 861.

Saimot, A. G. *et al.* (1983). Albendazole as a potential treatment for human hydatidosis. *Lancet*, **ii**, 652–6.

Schantz, P. M. (1972). Hidatidosis: magnitud del problema perspectivas de control. *Boletin Oficina Sanitaria Panamericano*, **63**, 198–202.

Schantz, P. M. (1993). Surveillance and surveys for cystic echinococcosis. In *Compendium on Cystic Echinococcosis*, (ed. F. L. Andersen), pp. 74–84. Brigham Young University Print Services, Provo, Utah, USA

Schantz, P. M. and Gottstein, B. (1986). Echinococcosis (hydatidosis). In *Immunology of Parasitic Diseases*, Vol. 1 (ed. K. W. Walls and P. M. Schantz), pp. 69–107. Academic Press, Orlando.

Schantz, P. M., Cruz-Reyes, A., Colli, C., and Lord, R. D. (1975). Sylvatic echinococosis in Argentina. 1. On the morphology and biology of strobilar *Echinococcus granulosus* (Batsch, 1786) from domestic and sylvatic animal hosts. *Tropenmedizin und Parasitologie*, **26**, 334–44.

Schantz, P. M., Colli, C., Cruz-Reyes, A., and Prezioso, U. (1976). Sylvatic echinococcosis in Argentina. 11. Suspectibility of wild carnivores to *Echinococcus granulosus* (Batsch, 1786) and host-induced morphological variation. *Tropenmedizin und Parasitologie*, **27**, 70–8.

Schwabe, C. W. (1969). *Veterinary medicine and human health*, (2nd edn.). Williams and Wilkins, Baltimore.

Schwabe, C. W. (1986). Current status of hydatid disease: a zoonosis of increasing importance. In *The biology of echinococcus and hydatid disease*, (ed. R. C. A. Thompson), pp. 81–113. George Allen and Unwin, London.

Shambesh, M. K., Macpherson, C. N., Beesley, W. N., Gusbi, A., and Elsonosi, T. (1992). Prevalence of human hydatid disease in northwestern Libya: a cross sectional ultrasound study. *Annals of Tropical Medicine and Parasitology*, **86**, 381–6.

Singharoen, T., Mahandona, N., Powell, L. W., and Baddeley, H. (1985). Sonographic changes of hydatid cyst of the liver after treatment with mebendazole and albendazole. *British Journal of Radiology*, **58**, 905–7.

Smyth, J. D. (1969). Parasites as biological models. *Parasitology*, **59**, 73–91.

Smyth, J. D. and Smyth, M. M. (1964). Natural and experimental hosts of *Echinococcus granulosus* and *E. multilocularis*, with comments on the genetics of speciation in the genus *Echinococcus*. *Parasitology*, **54**, 493–514.

Soleto Saez, E. (1991). Recidivas de la hidatidosis hepatica: problemas de tratamiento quirurgico. *Archivos de la Hidatidosis*, **30**, 609–16.

Sousa, O. E. and Thatcher, V. E. (1969). Observations on the life cycle of *Echinococcus oligarthrus* (Diesing, 1863) in the Republic of Panama. *Annals of Tropical Medicine and Parasitology*, **63**, 165–75.

Sweatman, G. K. and Williams, R. J. (1963). Survival of *Echinococcus granulosus* and *Taenia hydatigena* eggs in two extreme climatic regions in New Zealand. *Research in Veterinary Science*, **4**, 199–216.

Tan Jia-Zhong, Pan Wei, and Quing Chang (1993). Recent investigations on the pharmacotherapy of cystic echinococcosis in the Xingjiang Uygur Autonomous Region, P. R. C. In *Compendium on Cystic Echinococcosis*, (ed. F. L. Andersen), pp. 162–7. Brigham Young University Print Services, Utah.

Teres, J., Gomez, J., Bouguera, M., Visa, J., Bordas, J. M., and Pera, C. (1984). Sclerosing cholangitis after surgical treatment of hepatic echinococcal cysts. Report of three cases. *American Journal of Surgery*, **148**, 694–7.

Thompson, R. C. A. (1986). Biology and systematics of Echinococcus. In *The biology of echinococcus and hydatid disease*, (ed. R. C. A. Thompson) pp. 5–43. George Allen and Unwin, London.

Thompson, R. C. A. (1988). Infraspecific variation and epidemiology. In *Parasitology in focus*, (ed. H. Mehlhorn), pp. 391–411. Springer Verlag, Berlin.

Thompson, R. C. A. and Allsop, C. E. (1988). *Hydatidosis: veterinary perspectives and annotated bibliography*, pp. 246. Commonwealth Agricultural Bureau, Wallingford.

Thompson, R. C. A. and Lymbery, A. J. (1988). The nature, extent and significance of variation within the genus *Echinococcus*. *Advances in Parasitology*, **27**, 209–63.

Thompson, R. C. A. and Lymbery, A. J. (1990). *Echinococcus*: Biology and strain variation. *International Journal for Parasitology*, **20**, 457–70.

Todorov, T., Vutova, K., Mechkov, G., Petkov, D., Nedelkov, G., and Tonchev, Z. (1990). Evaluation of response to chemotherapy of human cystic echinococcosis. *British Journal of Radiology*, **63**, 523–31.

Todorov, T. *et al.* (1992*a*). Chemotherapy of human cystic echinococcosis: comparative efficiency of mebendazole and albendazole, *Annals of Tropical Medicine and Parasitology*, **86**, 59–66.

Todorov, T. *et al.* (1992*b*). Factors influencing the response to chemotherapy in human cystic hydatid disease. *Bulletin of the World Health Organization*, **70**, 347–58.

Todorov, T., Vutova, K., Mechkov, G., Tonchev, Z., Georgiev, P., and Lazarova, I. (1992*c*). Experience in the chemotherapy of severe, inoperable echinococcosis in man. *Infection*, **20**, 19–24.

Tolley, H. D. and Ming, R. (1993). Applying a stochastic model to *Echinococcus granulosus* data. In *Compendium on cystic echinococcosis*, (ed. F. L. Andersen), pp. 211–20. Brigham Young University Print Services, Provo, Utah.

Torgerson, P. R., Gulland, F. M. D., and Gemmell, M. A. (1992). Observations on the epidemiology of *Taenia hydatigena* on St Kilda. *Veterinary Record*, **131**, 218–19.

Torgerson, P. R., Pilkington, J., Gulland, F. M. D., and Gemmell, M. A. (1995). Further evidence for long distance dispersal of taeniid eggs. *International Journal for Parasitology*, **25**, 265–67.

Utrilla, J. G., Eyre, F. P., Muguerza, R., Alami, H., and Bueno, J. (1991). Hidatidosis en la infancia. *Archivos de la Hidatidosis*, **30**, 721–30.

Van Steenbergen, W. *et al.* (1987). Hepatic echinococcosis rupture into the biliary tract. Clinical, radiological and therapeutic features during five episodes of spontaneous rupture in three patients with hepatic hydatidosis. *Journal of Hepatology*, **4**, 133–9.

Vara Thorbeck, C. and Vara Thorbeck, R. (1986). Peritoneal echinococcosis. *Zentralblatt für Chirurgie*, **111**, 980–6.

Verster, A. J. M. (1965). Review of *Echinococcus* species in South Africa. *Onderstepoort Journal of Veterinary Research*, **23**, 43–61.

Vidal Ogueta, M. (1989). Control de la hidatidosis in Chile. *Archivos Internacionales de la Hidatidosis*, **XX1**, 180–92.

Vidal Ogueta, M., Chacon Guinez, S., and Bonilla, C. (1989). Diagnostico de situacion de hidatidosis ovina y echinococcosis canina, X1 Region, Chile. *Archivos Internacionales de la Hidatidosis*, **XX1**, 38.

Vogel, H. (1955). Über den Entwicklungszyklus und die Artzugehörigkeit des Europäischen Alveolarechinococcus. *Deutsche Medizinische Wochenschrift*, **80**, 931–2.

von Sinner, W. N. (1991). New diagnostic signs in hydatid disease: radiography, ultrasound, CT and MRI cor- related to pathology. *European Journal of Radiology*, **12**, 150–9.

Wen, H., Zou, P. F., Yao, P. L., and Lu, J. (1990). Research on chemotherapy of hydatidosis with albendazole. *Chinese Medical Journal*, **70**, 47–9.

Wen, H., New, R. R. C., and Craig, P. S. (1993). Diagnosis and treatment of human hydatidosis. *British Journal of Clinical Pharmacology*, **35**, 565–74.

Wen, H., Zhang, H. W., Muhmut, M., Zou, P. F., New, R. R. C., and Craig, P. S. (1994). Initial observation on albendazole in combination with cimetidine for the treatments of human cystic echinococcosis. *Annals of Tropical Medicine and Parasitology*, **88**, 49–52.

Whitfield, P. J. and Evans, N. A. (1983). Pathogenesis and asexual multiplication among parasitic platyhelminths. *Parasitology*, **86**, 121–60.

WHO (1992). *Report of the working group meeting on clinical medicine and chemotherapy of alveolar and cystic echinococcosis* (WHO/CDS/VPH. 93.118). World Health Organization, Geneva.

Wilson, J. F. A., Diddams, A. C., and Rausch, R. L. (1968). Cystic hydatid disease in Alaska. A review of 101 cases. *American Journal of Respiratory Diseases*, **98**, 1–15.

Xu Ming-quian (1991). Image diagnosis of hydatidosis of the liver. *Archivos de la Hidatidosis*, **30**, 501–19.

Xu Ming-quian (1993). Diagnosis and complications of cystic echinococcosis, and surgical procedures for removal of hydatid cysts in the Xinxiang Uygur Autonomous Region, PRC. In *Compendium on cystic echinococcosis*, (ed. F. L. Andersen), pp. 146–52. Brigham Young University Print Services, Utah.

Yekutiel, P. (1980). Eradication of infectious disease: a critical study. In *Contribution to epidemiology and biostatistics*, (ed. M. A. Klingsberg). Karger Basel.

53 ALVEOLAR ECHINOCOCCOSIS (*ECHINOCOCCUS MULTILOCULARIS*) AND OTHER FORMS OF ECHINOCOCCOSIS (*ECHINOCOCCUS VOGELI* AND *ECHINOCOCCUS OLIGARTHRUS*)

J. Eckert

INTRODUCTION

At present four species of the genus *Echinococcus* are recognized as valid, namely *Echinococcus granulosus* (Batsch 1786), *Echinococcus multilocularis* Leuckart, 1863, *Echinococcus oligarthrus* (Diesing 1863), and *Echinococcus vogeli* Rausch and Bernstein, 1972 (Thompson 1995). Larval forms, the metacestode stages, of all four species may establish and develop in the human host and cause various forms of echinococcosis (hydatid disease) (Table 53.1). This chapter deals with *Echinococcus multilocularis, E. vogeli,* and *E. oligarthrus.* In order to reduce the number of references, review articles are preferentially cited.

HISTORY

ECHINOCOCCUS MULTILOCULARIS

A first case of human alveolar echinococcosis (AE) was described in 1852 by Buhl in Munich (southern Germany) as a tumour-like lesion of the liver which he designated as 'alveolar colloid' (Posselt 1928). In 1855, the German pathologist Virchow identified the lesion

as a 'multilocular and ulcerating echinococcosis tumour' of the liver (Posselt 1928). At this time, it was unclear whether this form of echinococcosis was caused by *E. granulosus* or another *Echinococcus* species. In 1901 Posselt in Austria infected a dog with alveolar parasite material containing protoscolices from a human liver and found in the dog's intestine small tapeworms clearly differing from *E. granulosus* and showing characteristics of another species described as *Echinococcus multilocularis* by Leuckart in 1863 (named by Posselt as *Taenia echinococcus alveolaris*). Posselt (1928) and some other authors provided further biological, clinical, and epidemiological evidence for a 'dualistic' aetiology of cystic and alveolar echinococcosis opposing the 'unicistic' view of Dévé and adherents that only a single species, *E. granulosus,* caused both forms of echinococcosis (Rausch 1986). About 100 years after the detection of the first human cases of AE the 'dualistic' view was finally accepted, based on results of the classical studies by Rausch and Schiller (1954) in Alaska and by Vogel (1957) in Germany which unequivocally demonstrated that *E. granulosus* and *E. multilocularis* are separate species and that the latter is the causative agent of human AE.

Table 53.1 Forms of echinococcosis (hydatid disease) in humans

Echinococcus species	Name (abbreviation) and synonym of disease	Geographical distribution
Echinococcus granulosus	Cystic echinococcosis (CE), hydatid disease	Cosmopolitan
Echinococcus multilocularis	Alveolar echinococcosis (AE), alveolar hydatid disease	Northern hemisphere (Eurasia, North America)
Echinococcus vogeli	*E. vogeli* echinococcosis (VE)	Central and South America
Echinococcus oligarthrus	*E. oligarthrus* echinococcosis (OE)	Central and South America

ECHINOCOCCUS OLIGARTHRUS

Taenia oligarthrus, from the cougar (*Felis concolor* L.) in Brazil originally identified by Diesing in 1863 was redescribed by Lühe in 1910 and transferred to the genus *Echinococcus*. The life cycle of *E. oligarthrus* was experimentally determined by Sousa and Thatcher in 1969 (Rausch 1986). A first human case of an infection with *E. oligarthrus* was reported in 1989 from Venezuela (Lopera *et al.* 1989).

ECHINOCOCCUS VOGELI

This species was first recovered from a bush dog, *Speothos venaticus*, kept in the Los Angeles Zoo and originally captured in Ecuador (Rausch and Bernstein 1972). This species is known as causative agent of a polycystic form of echinococcosis occurring in humans in several Central and South American countries (Schantz *et al.* 1995).

ALVEOLAR ECHINOCOCCOSIS

THE AGENT (*ECHINOCOCCUS MULTILOCULARIS*)

BASIC LIFE CYCLE

The adult (strobilar) stage of *E. multilocularis* inhabits the small intestine of definitive hosts, primarily of foxes (genera *Vulpes* and *Alopex*), but also of other canids and cats (Table 53.2, Fig. 53.1). The adult worms produce eggs which are released to the environment, either enclosed in the terminal segment of the parasite or free in the intestinal content. Upon release from the final host the eggs normally contain a fully developed larval stage, the oncosphere, and are infective to susceptible hosts.

If mature eggs are ingested by susceptible intermediate host animals, primarily arvicolid and cricetid rodents, oncospheres hatch in the small intestine, they become activated by certain physiological factors, attach to the microvillus border of the intestinal villi in the jejunal and upper ileal region, penetrate the epithelial layer, and migrate to the lamina propria within 30–120 min after hatching (Thompson 1995). After penetration of venous or lymphatic vessels, the oncospheres migrate to the liver which is a primary site of further development to another larval stage, the metacestode. In highly susceptible intermediate hosts mostly large numbers of protoscolices are formed by asexual proliferation within 40–45 days (Bosch 1982) or later. If an intermediate host containing metacestodes with mature protoscolices is eaten by a definitive host, the cycle of development is closed. After establishment in the small intestine protoscolices develop to adult strobilated (segmented) stages which start to

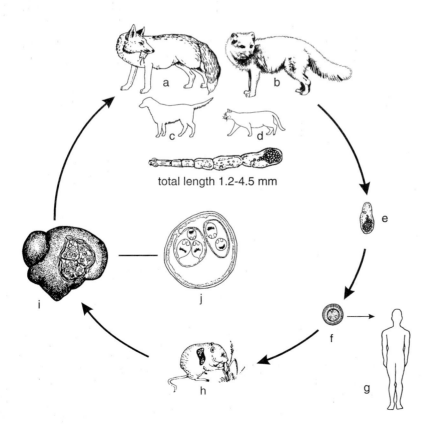

total length 1.2-4.5 mm

Fig. 53.1 Life cycle of *Echinococcus multilocularis*. (a) Red fox (*Vulpes vulpes*) and (b) arctic fox (*Alopex lagopus*) as important definitive hosts; (c) domestic dog and (d) domestic cat as occasional definitive hosts; (e) terminal segment of the parasite with eggs; (f) egg; (g) man as accidental host; (h) common vole (*Microtus arvalis*) as representative of many species of intermediate hosts; (i) liver of a rodent with metacestodes of the parasite; (j) magnification of (i), showing one cyst with two brood capsules and protoscolices. (J. Eckert and H. Bucklar, Institute of Parasitology, Zurich©.)

Table 53.2   *Echinococcus multilocularis*: selected examples of definitive and intermediate host animals in various geographical regions and of parasite prevalence rates in some regions[a] (names in bold letters: animals known to be of special significance in the cycle)

Region	Definitive hosts	Intermediate hosts
Western and central Europe	**Red fox** (*Vulpes vulpes*) Domestic dog (*Canis familiaris*) Domestic cat (*Felis catus*) *Prevalence rates*: Foxes: < 1– < 60% Dogs and cats: generally low: from 0 to around 1%, rarely higher	**Common vole** (*Microtus arvalis*) Snow vole (*Microtus nivalis*) Earth vole (*Pitymys subterraneus*) Red-backed vole (*Clethrionomys glareolus*) **Water vole** (*Arvicola terrestris*) **Muskrat** (*Ondatra zibethicus*) House mouse (*Mus musculus*) *Prevalence rates*: generally low: < 1% to 6%, rarely higher, notably in muskrats
States of former Soviet Union	Arctic fox (*Alopex lagopus*) Red fox (*Vulpes vulpes*) Corsac fox (*Vulpes corsac*) Wolf (*Canis lupus*) Wildcat (*Felis silvestris*) Domestic dog (*Canis familiaris*)	Northern vole (*Microtus oeconomus*) Common vole (*Microtus arvalis*) Voles (*Microtus* spp.) Brown lemming (*Lemmus sibiricus*) Red-backed voles (*Clethrionomys* spp.) Jirds (*Meriones* spp.) Muskrat (*Ondatra zibethicus*) and others
China	Red fox (*Vulpes vulpes*) Wolf (*Canis lupus*) Domestic dog (*Caynis familiaris*) and others	**Brandt's vole** (*Microtus brandti*) **Pika** (*Ochotona* sp.) Jird (*Meriones unguiculatus*) and others
Japan	**Red fox** (*Vulpes vulpes*) Domestic dog (*Canis familiaris*) Domestic cat (*Felis catus*) Raccoon dog (*Nyctereutes procynoides*) *Prevalence rates*: (averages 1965–1991): Foxes: 14% Dogs: 1% Cats: up to 5.5%	Red-backed vole (*Clethrionomys glareolus*) **Grey red-backed vole** (*C. rufocanus*) Red-backed vole (*Clethrionomys rutilus*) *Prevalence rates*: (averages 1965–1991): generally low with average around 1%
North America: • Northern tundra zone	**Arctic fox** (*Alopex lagopus*) **Domestic dog** (*Canis familiaris*) *Prevalence rates*: Arctic foxes: 40–100% Dogs: 12%	**Northern vole** (*Microtus oeconomus*) **Brown lemming** (*Lemmus sibiricus*) Red-backed vole (*Clethrionomys rutilus*) and others *Prevalence rates*: generally high: 42–83%
• Central North America	**Red fox** (*Vulpes vulpes*) **Coyote** (*Canis latrans*) Grey fox (*Urocyon cineroargentus*) *Prevalence rates*: Foxes: < 1–> 65% Coyotes: 6–35% Cats: focally 1–5%	**Deer mouse** (*Peromyscus maniculatus*) **Meadow vole** (*Microtus pennsylvanicus*) Muskrat (*Ondatra zibethicus*) Woodrat (*Neotoma cinerea*) House mouse (*Mus musculus*) *Prevalence rates*: generally low: about 0.5–6%, rarely higher

[a] Data from Schantz (1993), Rausch (1995), Schantz *et al.* (1995), Eckert (1996*a*), Ohbayashi (1996), Schantz *et al.* (1996) and other sources.

produce mature eggs after a prepatent period which may be as short as 26–28 days (Thompson and Eckert 1983; Yagi *et al.* 1996).

Humans and several mammalian animal species may accidentally acquire the infection, and metacestodes may develop in their internal organs (Fig. 53.1). If such hosts do not play a role in the transmission of the infec-

tion, they may be distinguished from the natural intermediate hosts and denominated as 'accidental' hosts.

MORPHOLOGY

Morphologically the various developmental stages of *E. multilocularis* can be characterized as follows:

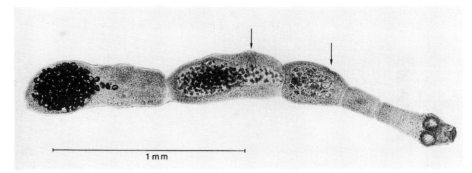

Fig. 53.2 Adult stage of *Echinococcus multilocularis* with sack-like uterus in the terminal segment containing eggs. Arrows point to genital pores. (Photograph: Institute of Parasitology, Zurich©.)

Adult stage

Echinococcus multilocularis is a very small tapeworm with a total body length between 1.2 and 4.5 mm and typically five (2–6) segments (Thompson 1995) (Fig. 53.2). The scolex is equipped with four suckers and a double row of large and small hooks with a mean length of 31.0 μm (range: 24.9–34.0 μm) and 27.0 μm (range: 20.4–31.0 μm), respectively. In comparison to *E. granulosus*, characteristic diagnostic features of *E. multilocularis* are the sac-like uterus without lateral sacculations in the gravid (terminal) segment and the position of the genital pore anterior to the middle of both the mature and the gravid segments (for details see Vogel 1957; Thompson 1995). Gravid segments contain between 200 and 300 eggs. The various stages of development from protoscolices to adult stages have been described by Kamiya and Sato (1990*a,b*).

Egg

The eggs released from gravid segments are spherical in shape and range in size from 30–40 × 28–39 μm (Vogel 1957) (Fig. 53.1f). The egg is composed of a centrally located oncosphere and is surrounded by a thick-walled embryophore. The oncosphere is a spherical, fully differentiated, infective larval stage, about 25 μm in diameter. As documented for *E. granulosus* (Swiderski 1983), the oncosphere is armed with three pairs of hooks, and it contains various groups of cells, including two binucleate medullary cells, several penetration gland and secretory cells, muscle cells and 10 germinative cells. The outer vitelline layer ('egg shell') is normally lost during egg release. In the light microscope the embryophore has a striped appearance due to its composition of blocks of a keratin-like protein which are held together by a cementing substance (Thompson 1995). By light or electron microscopy the eggs of *E. multilocularis* are indistinguishable from eggs of the other *Echinococcus* species and of *Taenia* species.

This fact causes considerable problems in diagnosis and differential diagnosis (p. 690).

Metacestode

In experimental animals perivascular leucocyte infiltrations and oncospheres of *E. multilocularis* can be microscopically detected in the liver as early as 4 h and 8 h, respectively, after peroral inoculation with eggs, and macroscopic foci are visible after 2 days (Bosch 1982). These foci are found nearby the branches of the portal vein, indicating the invasion of the liver by the portal circulation (Yamashita 1960). After an oncosphere has attained a site of predilection unilocular vesiculation (vesicle diameter between 15 and 70 μm) occurs within 1–7 days by central cavity formation and a ring-shaped arrangement of germinal cells in one layer (Sakamoto and Sugimura 1970; Bosch 1982). Multilocular vesiculation starts within 5–7 days after inoculation. At this stage the metacestode is formed by vesicles made up of a thin layer of germinal cells. Light-microscopically, an outer acellular laminated ('cuticular') layer can be detected by periodic acid Schiff (PAS) reaction in parts of the cysts 14 days after infection (Sakamoto and Sugimura 1970). Evidence from recent studies suggests that the laminated layer is—at least in part—produced by the parasite, as it is also formed *in vitro* in the absence of host tissue (Gottstein *et al.* 1992; Howell and Smyth 1995). Formation of brood capsules and protoscolices begins about 20–35 days after infection, and mature protoscolices are found 40–60 days or later after infection, depending on the species and susceptibility of the intermediate host (Sakamoto and Sugimura 1970; Bosch 1982). It has to be underlined that time and type of metacestode development and protoscolex production is highly variable in various intermediate and accidental hosts. For example, many protoscolices may be formed in highly susceptible intermediate host animals (Figs. 53.1i–j and 53.3) while formation of

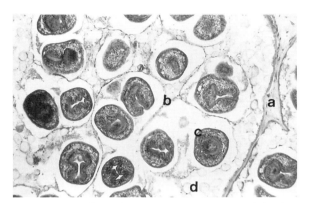

Fig. 53.3 Histological section of *Echinococcus multilocularis* metacestode from a rodent: (a) cyst wall; (b) wall of brood capsule; (c) protoscolex; (d) calcareous corpuscle. (Photograph: Institute of Parasitology, Zurich©.)

├───────┤ 100 μm

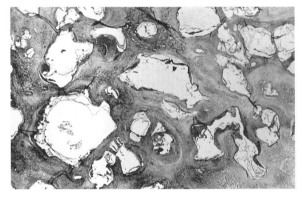

Fig. 53.4 Histological section of *Echinococcus multilocularis* metacestode in a human liver: cysts without brood capsule and protoscolex formation. (Photograph: Institute of Parasitology, Zurich©.)

├───────┤ 100 μm

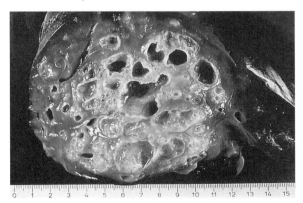

Fig. 53.5 Macroscopic appearance of human liver with *Echinococcus multilocularis*: multiple small and larger cysts (maximum diameter of 3 cm). (Photograph: Institute of Parasitology Zurich©.)

scale: cm

protoscolices in the human liver is rare (see p. 694) (Fig. 53.4).

The fully developed metacestode stage of *E. multilocularis* is quite different from that of *E. granulosus*. In macroscopic sections of the liver of an infected intermediate or accidental host, the metacestode of *E. multilocularis* exhibits an alveolar structure composed of numerous cysts of irregular shapes and sizes between less than 1 mm and 30 mm (Ammann and Eckert 1995) (Fig. 53.5). From the cystic cavities small cyst vesicles can be isolated which contain a jelly-like mass rather than fluid. Due to peripheral proliferation and reduced supply of nutrients in the inner parts of the metacestode, central parts of the parasite may become necrotic so that cavities containing necrotic and liquid masses may be formed, notably in the human liver. Histologically, the cysts are composed of a relatively thin acellular outer laminated (PAS-positive) layer and an inner cellular germinative layer.

A special feature of the *E. multilocularis* metacestode is its capacity for progressing proliferation and metastasis formation (Fig. 53.6). Various forms of proliferation have been described, namely the exogenous and endogenous budding of cysts and the production of solid, filamentous protrusions of the germinal layer which are extruded out of cysts to the surrounding tissue. These protrusions may transform to tube-like and cystic structures which may be interconnected in a network-like structure (Vogel 1978; Eckert *et al.* 1983; Mehlhorn *et al.* 1983) (Fig. 53.7).

There is evidence that detachment of germinal cells from protrusions of the germinal layer and their dissemination via the lymph and blood may lead to formation of metastases in distant organs, such as the lung, brain, or bone. Furthermore, metastases may be formed by infiltrative proliferation of metacestode tissue to adjacent organs (for example, from liver to other abdominal organs) (Ammann and Eckert 1995, 1996).

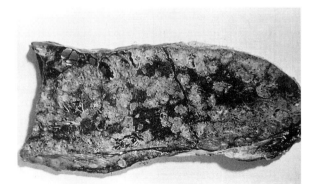

Fig. 53.6 Macroscopic appearance of human lung with multiple metastases of *Echinococcus multilocularis*. (Photograph: Dept. of Surgery, University Hospital Zurich©.)

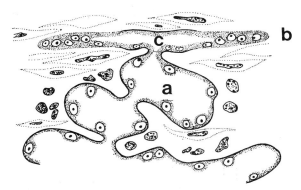

Fig. 53.7 Scheme of proliferation of *Echinococcus multilocularis* metacestode: (a) cyst with inner nucleated germinal and outer laminated layer; (b) solid protrusion of the germinal layer (devoid of laminated layer) infiltrating surrounding host tissue; (c) formation of central lumen and outer laminated layer in a protrusion. (After Vogel 1978; Eckert *et al.* 1983; Mehlhorn *et al.* 1983. Institute of Parasitology, Zurich©.)

MOLECULAR BIOLOGY

The present status of knowledge on molecular biology and biochemistry has recently been reviewed by Frosch and Lucius (1994) and McManus and Bryant (1995). Only some selected aspects can be discussed here.

Genes and gene products

For *E. multilocularis* and *E. granulosus* a chromosome number of $2n = 18$ has been described, with two larger rod-like and 16 smaller dot-like chromosomes (Frosch and Lucius 1994). Several genes of *E. multilocularis* have been cloned and sequenced. Some of the gene products will be mentioned in the following sections.

Molecular characterization of the genome and genetic variation

Molecular techniques allow a direct characterization of the genome of parasite species and strains and can be used for identification of *Echinococcus* species and of intraspecific variants (reviewed by Bowles *et al.* 1995; Lymbery 1995; McManus and Bryant 1995; Thompson *et al.* 1995).

All four species of *Echinococcus* (*E. granulosus*, *E. multilocularis*, *E. oligarthrus*, *E. vogeli*) are clearly distinguishable by sequence comparison of a 366 bp-fragment of the mitochondrial cytochrome oxidase subunit 1 DNA (CO1), and of a 471 bp region in the mitochondrial NADH dehydrogenase gene, by analysis of a ribosomal (r) DNA fragment (ITS2) or by the random amplified polymorphic DNA–PCR (RAPD–PCR) method (Bowles *et al.* 1995; Gasser and Chilton 1995).

Echinococcus granulosus is not a uniform species, and various strains, differing in morphology, infectivity to intermediate hosts, and other biological features have been identified using a combination of criteria, notably morphological, biological, biochemical, epidemiological features and, more recently, a variety of molecular techniques (Bowles *et al.* 1995; McManus and Bryant 1995; Thompson *et al.* 1995; Eckert and Thompson 1997). There is some evidence of morphological and biological differences between *E. multilocularis* isolates from North America and Eurasia, but genetic differences found to date appear to be very small. These two populations may be regarded as strains but further studies are required, especially on the status of isolates from Japan and China (Thompson *et al.* 1995).

Diagnostic probes

A cloned 2.6 kb fragment of genomic DNA of *E. multilocularis*, pAL1, has been characterized and sequenced. Species-specific identification of *E. multilocularis* material (adult worms, metacestodes) was achieved using pAL1 as a probe in Southern blots and using its sequence to design primers for PCR (Gottstein and Mowatt 1991). The gene encoding the U1 snRNA of *E. multilocularis* has been cloned, sequenced, and used for detection of parasite DNA in fox faeces using PCR amplification (Bretagne *et al.* 1993). Recently, Gasser and Chilton (1995) demonstrated that *E. granulosus*, *E. multilocularis* and several *Taenia* species can be distinguished by sequence differences in the second internal transcribed spacer rDNA (ITS2) using the RFLP–PCR technique (restriction fragment length polymorphism–polymerase chain reaction).

IMMUNOLOGY

The immunology of the *E. multilocularis* infection in definitive, intermediate, and accidental hosts (humans) has been reviewed by Gottstein (1992), Frosch and Lucius (1994), Gottstein and Felleisen (1995), and Lightowlers and Gottstein (1995). Some aspects will be discussed in context with the various hosts (see below).

PARASITE MAINTENANCE *IN VIVO* OR *IN VITRO* AND CRYOPRESERVATION

Serial passages of metacestodes in rodents

Rodents, such as jirds (*Meriones unguiculatus*), cotton rats (*Sigmodon hispidus*), or susceptible strains of mice (for example AKR, BALB/c or C57BL/6J) are infected by intraperitoneal injection of a suspension containing minced metacestode material (Howell and Smyth 1995) or by surgical transplantation of metacestode tissue. The transfer of germinal layer fragments is essential as after injection of purified protoscolices of *E. multilocularis* metacestodes do not develop (Gottstein *et al.* 1992). After transfer of infective material, the parasites primarily develop within the peritoneal cavity but they may also infiltrate the liver, the spleen, the lungs, and other organs. The production of protoscolices in the metacestodes is variable and depends on the isolate of the parasite, the susceptibility of the hosts, and the duration of the infection. In susceptible hosts mature protoscolices are found within 40–60 days (p. 684). *Echinococcus multilocularis* metacestodes can be transferred between individuals of homologous or heterologous rodent species or even from other host groups (for example man) to rodents (Eckert and Jacquier 1991). Serial passage of metacestodes is a rather safe method, but certain precautions should be observed (Howell and Smyth 1995).

Infection of rodents with eggs

For some purposes it is necessary to infect rodents perorally with infective eggs of *E. multilocularis*, for example to produce liver infections with metacestodes comparable to those after natural infections. Doses of about 100–10 000 eggs per rodent have been used for these purposes, but in highly susceptible rodents (*Microtus arvalis*) as few as five eggs may result in the development of metacestodes (Veit *et al.* 1995). For viability testing the eggs can also be applied by intraperitoneal injection as the oncospheres hatch and develop in the environment of the peritoneal cavity. Handling of infective eggs requires strict safety precautions.

Infection of natural definitive hosts

For chemotherapeutic trials, immunological studies, etc. working with definitive hosts infected with immature or mature intestinal stages is unavoidable. For such studies dogs are the preferred hosts as they are regularly highly susceptible whereas cats are more variable in susceptibility (Thompson and Eckert 1983). Helminth-free, young (about 3–4-month-old) dogs are perorally infected with large numbers of protoscolices (at least 5000–15 000 per animal). If the dogs are maintained under routine conditions, the experiment has to be terminated at the latest on day 24 after infection, i.e. before the end of the minimum prepatent period of 26–28 days. In this way dispersion of eggs and accidental infections of humans can be avoided. Experiments with patent infections require isolation units for dog maintenance and special safety precautions.

Infection of experimental definitive hosts

Successful infections with intestinal stages of *E. multilocularis* in immunosuppressed experimental definitive

hosts, i.e. in golden hamsters and jirds, were achieved by Kamiya and Sato (1990*a*,*b*). The pattern of development and maturation was generally comparable to that in dogs (reviewed by Howell and Smyth 1995).

In vitro cultivation

Maintenance of the whole cycle of *E. multilocularis* is not yet possible as the parasite fails to undergo insemination *in vitro*. However, the development of viable metacestode cysts, containing protoscolices, from fragments of germinal layer, cyst tissue, and protoscolices has been achieved (Howell and Smyth, 1995). Further, metacestode vesicles could be cultivated from oncospheres on a monolayer of mouse embryo cells in tissue-culture medium (DMEM with 10 per cent fetal calf serum (FCS)) (Deplazes and Gottstein 1991). Parasite vesicles derived from metacestode tissue multiply and grow if cultivated in a suspension culture with fluid medium (RPMI 1640 with 10 per cent FCS) in the presence of human colon carcinoma cells (CACO 2) as feeder cells (Hemphill and Gottstein 1995). Cysts obtained from mice and maintained *in vitro* in CMRL 1066 culture medium for about 10 days may be useful for drug testing (Emery *et al.* 1995). Cultures of hepatic cells from rats were used for assaying transferrin and albumin secretion of these cells in the presence of *E. multilocularis* protoscolices (Gabrion *et al.* 1995) or for other studies (Jura *et al.* 1996). On the other hand, immature unsegmented or segmented intestinal stages of *E. multilocularis* could be produced *in vitro* from protoscolices (Thompson *et al.* 1990; Howell and Smyth 1995). Further, maturation of the parasites with development of thick-shelled eggs was achieved by cultivation of intestinal stages following partial development in the dog for 20–21 days (Thompson and Eckert 1982).

Cryopreservation

Metacestodes of *E. multilocularis* can be cryopreserved and maintained in a viable state for at least 1–2 years by appropriate deep-freezing and storage in liquid nitrogen (Eckert 1988). This method can—at least partially—replace serial passages of the parasites in laboratory rodents for maintenance of parasite isolates.

THE HOSTS

Infections of final hosts with intestinal (immature and/or mature) stages of *E. multiloculoris* and of intermediate or accidental hosts with the metacestode stage differ significantly in their consequences. While the former are typically asymptomatic, the latter may lead to severe and often lethal disease in intermediate or accidental hosts, including man.

FINAL HOST ANIMALS

Biology

Foxes, domestic dogs, and other canids (Table 53.2) are highly susceptible to the infection with *E. multilocularis*, whereas cats are generally poor hosts, as indicated by lower infection rates after experimental infections, retardation of worm development, and lower egg production (Thompson and Eckert 1983). However, susceptibility of cats is variable and they may well harbour parasites producing mature eggs, but their significance as sources of infection is apparently much lower than that of canids.

In foxes and dogs *E. multilocularis* can attach to the intestinal mucosa of any region but the site of predilection of the mature parasites is the posterior region of the small intestine, while *E. granulosus* prefers the anterior part (Thompson and Eckert 1983). In 72 per cent of about 900 naturally infected foxes *E. multilocularis* was localized in the posterior third of the intestine, and in 28 per cent the parasites inhabited also the middle and anterior parts, notably in heavy infections (Ewald 1993). Natural mixed infections of *E. multilocularis* with other helminths occur quite frequently (up to 15 per cent in Europe), particularly with other cestodes (*Taenia, Mesocestoides*, etc.) and nematodes (*Toxocara*, ancylostomes, etc.) but less frequently with trematodes (for example *Alaria alata*) and protozoa (Rausch *et al.* 1990; Ballek *et al.* 1992; Ewald 1993). The other parasites apparently do not significantly influence the development of *E. multilocularis* (Ewald 1993). It was shown by experimental infections of dogs that *E. multilocularis* and *E. granulosus* may establish and develop in the intestine of the same host animal (Thompson and Eckert 1983).

Natural infections of canids with *E. multilocularis* may be heavy. For example, mean infection rates of about 7400–59 000 with a range of 1–184 000 have been observed in 138 arctic foxes on St Lawrence Island, Alaska. In this area 57 per cent of the foxes had average worm burdens of about 7400 and 43 per cent had higher burdens of about 44 000 or more (Rausch *et al.* 1990). In Europe (Germany and Switzerland) 66–90 per cent of the foxes had estimated worm burdens below 1000 per animal and a smaller proportion was infected with more than 1000 up to more than 50 000 parasites (Ballek *et al.* 1992; Ewald 1993; Eckert, unpublished observations).

After infections of dogs with protoscolices, development of *E. multilocularis* and production of thick-shelled eggs take a minimum of 26–28 days (Thompson and Eckert 1983; Yagi *et al.* 1996). Egg excretion in faeces is high 4–5 weeks after the end of the prepatent period and may reach egg counts of more than 100 000 per gram. Duration of egg excretion is variable, between about 1.5 and 6 months (Yagi *et al.*

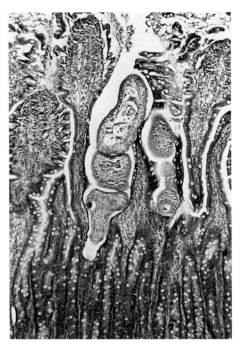

Fig. 53.8 Histological section of dog intestine with immature stages of *Echinococcus multilocularis* penetrating between villi. (Photograph: Institute of Parasitology, Zurich©.)

├────────────┤ 1 mm

1996). The life span of *E. multilocularis* in the final host is estimated to be 2–5 months (Ishige *et al.* 1990).

Pathology and clinical aspects

In the intestine of dogs, *E. multilocularis* attaches between the villi, and worms extend the apical region of the rostellum deeply into crypts of Lieberkühn (Thompson and Eckert 1983) (Fig. 53.8). The hooks superficially penetrate the epithelium, and the suckers may grasp substantial plugs of host tissue. Although the epithelium of parasitized crypts is commonly flattened, no evidence of breakdown in the integrity of the crypts is normally seen (Thompson and Eckert 1983). Typically, relevant inflammatory reactions do not occur so that infections of definitive hosts—even with heavy worm burdens—are asymptomatic (Fig. 53.9).

Immunity

Little is known of immune responses of final hosts against the *E. multilocularis* infection. In some regions young foxes (< 1 year) had significantly higher infection prevalences than older foxes, for example: 82 per cent versus 58 per cent in Alaska (Rausch *et al.* 1990), 46 per cent versus 26 per cent in Germany (Ballek *et al.* 1992), 30 per cent versus 21 per cent in Switzerland

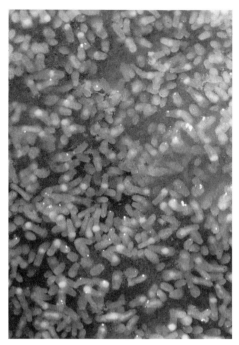

Fig. 53.9 Massive natural infection of the small intestine in a Swiss dog with *Echinococcus multilocularis* (about 45 000 specimens). Aggregations of eggs in the sack-like uterus are visible as white spots. (Photograph: Institute of Parasitology, Zurich©.)

⊢————⊣ 2 mm

(Ewald 1993). However, this has not been found in other studies. Young foxes may also have higher worm burdens than older animals (Ewald 1993). Reduced infection rates and lower worm burdens in older foxes may be an expression of acquired immunity, but supporting data and information on the potential role of protective immunity are lacking. Experimental data suggest that dogs may acquire immunity with frequencies of ingestion of *E. granulosus* protoscolices, and that by the sixth infection about 50 per cent of the animals are less susceptible (Gemmell and Lawson 1986).

Immunological responses to protoscolex, adult worm, and oncospheral antigens of *E. granulosus* have been observed in dogs (Gasser *et al.* 1993; Deplazes *et al.* 1994*b*, Lightowlers and Gottstein 1995). After primary infection of dogs with *E. granulosus* protoscolices, significant cell proliferation was demonstrated, using an *in vitro* assay, in Peyer's patches as well as in mesenteric and popliteal lymph nodes in response to protoscolex and adult homologous antigen. In the same animals specific circulating antibodies were detected (Deplazes *et al.* 1994*b*). From other studies it is known that a proportion of dogs naturally or experimentally infected with *E. granulosus* produces antibodies of various subclasses (IgG, IgE,

IgM, IgA). Foxes in endemic areas have been shown to produce circulating antibodies against a specific antigen of *E. multilocularis* (Em2 antigen) (Gottstein *et al.* 1991) (see also below).

Diagnosis

The diagnosis of the *E. multilocularis* infection in final hosts is difficult and associated with infection risk for the laboratory personnel. Therefore, safety precautions have to be observed during handling of potentially infected animals and diagnostic materials.

At present the most reliable technique for the diagnosis of *E. multilocularis* infections in foxes and other final hosts is the parasitological examination of the small intestine at necropsy (Eckert *et al.* 1991; Ewald, 1993; Deplazes and Eckert 1996; Eckert and Deplazes 1996). Recently, some alternative techniques have been evaluated. Among them, coproantigen detection by an enzyme-linked immunosorbent assay (ELISA) is most promising.

Necropsy and parasitological examination

The following technique is employed in our laboratory (Eckert and Deplazes 1996): Using microscopic slides ($75 \times 25 \times 1$ mm each) five deep mucosal scrapings are made at nearly equal distances from the proximal, middle, and posterior third of the small intestine. The material adhering to the slide is transferred to a square plastic Petri dish (9×9 cm, Falcon®, No. 1012) and squashed to a thin layer by means of pressure on the slide. The mucosal squashes are then examined in transmitted light under a stereomicroscope at ×120 magnification. With this technique 44 per cent more infected foxes were detected than by macroscopic examination alone (Ewald 1993). The sensitivity of a very similar technique has been estimated to about 96 per cent even in infections with low worm numbers of fewer than 10 specimens (Ballek *et al.* 1992), but sensitivity estimates of 85 per cent may be more realistic for routine examinations (Deplazes and Eckert 1996).

In order to reduce or exclude an infection risk for laboratory personnel, the carcasses or intestines of the final hosts should—if possible—be deep-frozen at –70 °C to –80 °C for one week prior to necropsy (Eckert and Deplazes 1996). This procedure kills eggs of *E. multilocularis* if the temperature is retained in all parts of the material for at least 4 days at –70 °C (Blunt *et al.* 1991) or for 2 days at –80 °C to –83 °C (Frank 1989; Eckert *et al.* 1991; Veit *et al.* 1995). Strict safety precautions should be observed during the whole necropsy procedure (Ewald 1993; Eckert and Deplazes 1996). They are indispensable if fresh material is handled but they are also recommended when the material has previously been deep-frozen as described above.

Detection of eggs and proglottids of E. multilocularis

Eggs of *E. multilocularis* can be detected in faeces of final hosts during patency using flotation techniques. However, egg excretion may be low and irregular (Yagi *et al.* 1996). In dogs with *Taenia* infection anal-skin swabs proved to be more reliable for egg detection than examination of faecal samples using a flotation technique (Eckert and Deplazes 1996). The main problem is that eggs of *E. multilocularis* are morphologically indistinguishable from eggs of *E. granulosus* and *Taenia* species. Therefore, confirmatory tests are needed (see below) once eggs have been detected.

As shown in *Taenia*, proglottids may be released from the host with or without defaecation. Proglottids of *E. multilocularis* may be detected if they are numerous on the surface of fresh faeces or on anal swabs as tiny, whitish, elongated particles of about 1 mm length. In most cases, they are overlooked. Therefore, the diagnosis based on detection of eggs and proglottids is highly unsatisfactory.

Detection of coproantigens

A new approach to the diagnosis of intestinal cestode infections is the detection of antigens released by the parasites into the intestinal fluid. Several groups have developed enzyme-linked immunosorbent assays (ELISAs) for the detection of such antigens released in faecal material (= coproantigens) in carnivores harbouring *Taenia* or *Echinococcus* species (Deplazes *et al.* 1994*a*; Craig *et al.* 1995; Lightowlers and Gottstein 1995; Deplazes and Eckert 1996; Eckert and Deplazes 1996). A recent, well-controlled study (Deplazes *et al.* 1994*a*) involving a total of 229 dogs has shown that a sandwich-ELISA based on protein-A-purified polyclonal catching antibodies (produced in rabbit and directed against adult *E. granulosus* excretory/secretory antigens) exhibits a very high specificity of 96 per cent in dogs infected with *Taenia* spp. and of 98 per cent in dogs with non-taeniid helminths. The sensitivity was also high (92 per cent) in 25 dogs with more than 100 *E. granulosus*, but it was much lower (29 per cent) in 21 dogs with *E. granulosus* burdens less than 100, resulting in an average sensitivity of 63 per cent.

Coproantigens of *E. multilocularis* could also be detected by this ELISA in experimentally infected dogs and in naturally infected foxes (Deplazes *et al.* 1992). However, the sensitivity of this test was unsatisfactory. By using polyclonal antibodies against *E. multilocularis* the test could be recently improved to an overall sensitivity of 80 per cent and even to 93 per cent in foxes harbouring more than 55 *E. multilocularis*; specificity was also high at 95 per cent (Deplazes and Eckert 1996; Eckert and Deplazes 1996). Very promising results on the detection of heat-resistant coproantigens were reported by Nonaka *et al.* (1996).

Detection of circulating antibodies

In dogs and foxes infected with *E. granulosus* and *E. multilocularis*, respectively, circulating (serum) antibodies can be detected (reviewed by Lightowlers and Gottstein 1995; Deplazes and Eckert 1996; Eckert and Deplazes 1996).

In most fox populations infected with *E. multilocularis* specific antibodies against the Em2-antigen are present (Gottstein *et al.* 1991). However, on an individual or population basis there is no correlation between the prevalence rate of circulating antibodies and the prevalence rates of *E. multilocularis* in the intestines of foxes. Therefore, the test may be used for pre-screening of fox populations for the presence of intestinal *E. multilocularis* and the discrimination of infected and uninfected populations. However, final proof that fox populations free of *E. multilocularis* are negative in the Em2-ELISA is still not available (Deplazes and Eckert 1996; Eckert and Deplazes 1996).

DNA detection

Genomic DNA could be specifically identified in adult *E. multilocularis* isolated from intestines of naturally infected foxes by the polymerase chain reaction (PCR) (Gottstein and Mowatt 1991). Furthermore, a PCR-technique was described for the detection of *E. multilocularis* DNA in faecal samples of foxes (Bretagne *et al.* 1993). In our hands this test system was useful in identifying *E. multilocularis* (DNA from proglottids or isolated eggs) but it did not provide reliable results with faecal samples (Mathis, personal communication). Recently, the PCR technique of Bretagne *et al.* (1993) was adapted to the examination of faecal samples from foxes by a preceding step of concentrating eggs employing sequential sieving with a step of flotation in zinc chloride solution (Mathis *et al.* 1996). Compared to parasitological findings from 55 foxes, the specificity of this PCR was 100 per cent and the sensitivity 94 per cent (Deplazes and Eckert, 1996; Mathis *et al.* 1996).

Selection of techniques for diagnosis in individual cases and in populations

In our laboratory a combination of techniques is presently used for the *in vivo* diagnosis of *E. multilocularis* infections in individual dogs and cats or in dog/cat populations, including examination of faeces for eggs and coproantigen detection. In special cases species identification with PCR using eggs isolated from the faeces or excreted proglottids is performed (Mathis *et al.* 1996).

Treatment

Chemotherapy against intestinal infections with *E. multilocularis* may be indicated in individual dogs or cats or in dog/cat populations for control purposes. Mass treatment of fox populations has been considered.

Treatment of individual dogs and cats

Dogs and cats with patent intestinal E. multilocularis burdens represent an infection risk for humans, notably to owners and to other persons handling such animals. Chemotherapy may lead to a short-term increase of the infection risk due to the release of large numbers of infective E. multilocularis eggs in the faeces of treated animals. Therefore, treatment should always be carried out under special safety precautions. If such precautions are unfeasible, infected animals should be euthanized.

Drugs with high efficacy against intestinal E. multilocularis infections are praziquantel (Droncit® and other trade names) and epsiprantel (Cestex®).

Praziquantel This isoquinoline derivative is given to dogs and cats at doses of 5.0 mg/kg body weight (b.w.) perorally or of 5.7 mg/kg b.w. intramuscularly. A single oral dose of 5.0 mg/kg b.w. eliminated 100 per cent of immature or mature stages of E. multilocularis from dogs and cats (Rommel et al. 1976). The drug is well tolerated.

Epsiprantel This is also an isoquinoline derivative with similar high efficacy against E. multilocularis as praziquantel. In our trials (unpublished) a single oral dose of 5 mg/kg b.w. eliminated on average 99.6 per cent of E. multilocularis from dogs with very heavy infections.

Since there is no guarantee that a single-dose treatment will eliminate 100 per cent of the parasites from a dog or cat we recommend repetition of treatment after 1–2 days. The result of treatment should be checked by faecal examination for taeniid eggs and if possible by coproantigen detection (Eckert 1996b; Deplazes and Eckert 1996).

Treatment of dog and cat populations

In endemic areas dogs and cats may acquire the infection by ingestion of E. multilocularis-infected intermediate hosts. A possibility to prevent the establishment of egg-producing intestinal populations of E. multilocularis is the regular treatment of the animals with praziquantel or epsiprantel (see above) at intervals of 3–4 weeks (minimum prepatent period: 26–28 days). However, the implementation of such a programme is difficult in practice.

Mass treatment of dog populations was evaluated in a 10-year field trial in a village on St Lawrence Island, Alaska, where E. multilocularis occurs in an intermediate cycle regularly involving domestic dogs as final hosts (Schantz et al. 1995). All dogs of this village were treated with praziquantel at 5 mg/kg b.w. at monthly intervals. Infection rates of voles with E. multilocularis metacestodes declined from 29 per cent to less than 5 per cent but the infection rate rebounded rapidly toward pretreatment levels after discontinuation of mass treatment (Schantz et al. 1995).

Treatment of fox populations

Control of E. multilocularis in sylvatic cycles with foxes as final hosts appears to be extremely difficult for various reasons (Schantz et al. 1995). In southern Germany 'baits' containing 50 mg praziquantel were placed in the environment at a density of 15–20 per km². In an area of 566 km² after delivery of baits six times during a period of 14 months the infection prevalence rate of E. multilocularis in foxes decreased from 32 to 4 per cent (Schelling et al. 1997). However, more studies are needed for careful evaluation of efficacy, practicability, cost–benefit ratio, and other factors (Roming et al. 1996).

INTERMEDIATE AND ACCIDENTAL HOST ANIMALS

Biological and immunological aspects

It is well documented that various species of natural intermediate hosts differ in their susceptibility to E. multilocularis infection (Obayashi et al.. 1971). This applies also to laboratory rodents. For example, jirds (Meriones unguiculatus), cotton rats (Sigmodon hispidus), and some strains of mice (AKR, BALB/c, C57BL/6J) are particularly susceptible, while some other mouse strains (C57BL/10, C3H/HeJ, CB-17) are relatively resistant (Playford et al. 1993; Gottstein and Felleisen 1995). Control of parasite growth in resistant mice is regulated by granulomatous inflammation and modified lymphoid cell functions (Playford et al. 1993; Gottstein and Felleisen 1995).

Under natural conditions, intermediate host populations exhibit variable levels of infection with E. multilocularis which are rather low in many areas. For example, in an endemic area of southern Germany (Reutlingen) where 28 per cent of the foxes were infected with intestinal stages of E. multilocularis only 1 per cent of microtine rodents (Microtus arvalis) harboured metacestodes of the parasite (Zeyhle 1982). Whether the infection level of rodent populations is regulated by the degree of exposure to infective eggs of E. multilocularis and/or by mechanisms of innate resistance and acquired immunity is an open question.

Pathology

Two principal types of response of rodents to infection with E. multilocularis can be distinguished (Yamashita 1960):

1. In highly susceptible rodents: rapid cystic development of the metacestode with protoscolex formation in about 1.5–2 months and slight host tissue reaction.
2. In more resistant rodents: prolonged development of the the metacestode with protoscolex formation after 5 months or later, complicated cyst structure, severe host reaction with intensive formation of connective tissue and tendency of parasite necrosis in central parts.

This infection, either induced by peroral inoculation of eggs or by intraperitoneal transplantation of metacestode material, may lead to parasite infiltration of the liver, the peritoneal cavity and abdominal organs, the lung and other organs, associated with severe organ dysfunctions. In experimentally infected *Meriones*, parasite masses may reach 30–50 per cent of the animal's body weight, inducing reduced mobility. Under natural conditions heavily infected rodents are an easy prey of carnivores.

Regarding the pathology of the *E. multilocularis* infection of accidental hosts (see below) special references should be consulted.

Diagnosis

Intermediate hosts of *E. multilocularis* are mainly arvicolid rodents and other small mammals (Table 53.2). Such animals have to be collected for epidemiological studies by specific methods of trapping under consideration of national regulations of animal protection. At necropsy of small mammals metacestodes of *E. multi-*

locularis can often be detected visually in organs, notably in the liver. In doubtful cases the macroscopic observations have to be complemented by histology and/or careful parasitological and pathological differential diagnosis of lesions caused by other parasites. Furthermore, for parasite identification immunohistology with monoclonal antibodies (Deplazes and Gottstein 1991), PCR (Gottstein and Mowatt 1991), or other DNA techniques can be used, but great care should be taken for specificity evaluation of the test system.

Domestic and wild pigs, horses, dogs, monkeys, and some other animal species have been described as accidental hosts of the metacestode stage of *E. multilocularis* (Eckert 1996*a,b*; Ohbayashi 1996). The diagnosis of the infection is possible by post-mortem examination. Furthermore, in living larger animals, such as dogs and monkeys, the diagnosis can be based on ultrasound detection of lesions in the liver, in combination with detection of circulating antibodies.

Treatment

Dogs, monkeys, or other accidentally infected animals should not be treated because of the uncertain prognoses and the difficulties of therapy (see pp. 695–7).

HUMANS AS ACCIDENTAL HOSTS

In humans the metacestodes of *E. multilocularis* may cause the alveolar form of echinococcosis, a chronic cancer-like disease with high mortality rates in untreated patients. Clinical aspects of the disease have

Table 53.3 Sites of *Echinococcus multilocularis* metacestodes in Swiss patients with single and multiple or only with single organ involvement

Patients with single and multiple organ involvement ($n = 70$)[a]		Patients with single organ involvement ($n = 251$)[b]	
Organ	Number (%) cases	Organ	Number (%) cases
Liver only	47 (67%)	Liver only	248 (98.8%)
Liver and adjacent organs:	14 (20%)		
abdominal	1		
retroperitoneal	4		
thoracic	6		
thoracic and abdominal	1		
Liver and distant metastases:	9 (13%)		
brain	3		
lungs	4		
bones	2		
		Bones only	2 (0.8%)
		Muscles only	1 (0.4%)

[a] Ammann and Eckert (1995).
[b] Accumulated data from Drolshammer *et al.* (1973), Gloor (1988), and Eckert *et al.* (1995).

recently been summarized in publications by Morris and Richards (1992), Uchino and Sato (1993, 1996), Ammann and Eckert (1995, 1996) and Wilson *et al.* (1995).

Biological and clinical aspects

Organ localization of metacestodes

After peroral infection with eggs of *E. multilocularis*, metacestodes almost exclusively develop primarily in the liver. Primary extrahepatic sites of metacestodes are rare (Table 53.3). In the liver only one lobe (predominantly the right lobe), both lobes, only the hilus, or the hilus and one or two lobes may be affected by the parasite (Sato *et al.* 1993*a*; Ammann and Eckert 1995). From the primary site of development, the liver, metacestodes tend to spread to adjacent and distant organs by continuous proliferation or by metastasis formation. Therefore, about one-third of patients have metacestode lesions in the liver and simultaneously in one ore more extrahepatic organs at the time when the cases reach medical attention (Sato *et al.* 1993*a,b*; Amman and Eckert 1995, 1996) (Table 53.3).

Course of infection and symptomatology

In the course of the infection three main clinical stages (Sato *et al.* 1993*a*) and several pathological entities (Nakajima *et al.* 1993) can be distinguished.

The *initial phase* is always asymptomatic. Estimates of the incubation period vary between less than 5 and 15 years (Sato *et al.* 1993*a*; Ammann and Eckert 1995, 1996). The shortest time of seroconversion after peroral infection with *E. multilocularis* eggs is unknown (Ammann and Eckert 1995). The infection may be cured spontaneously (see below) or may turn to a progressive phase.

In the *progressive period* symptoms occur due to dysfunctions caused by the parasite, mainly in the liver. The ages of the patients at diagnosis range from 5 to 89 years, with means in a Japanese series of 45 (± 15) years (Sato *et al.* 1993*a*) and a Swiss series of 52 (±17) years (Eckert *et al.* 1995). Peak ages at diagnosis range between 35 and 65 years (Sato *et al.* 1993*a*; Eckert *et al.* 1995). The ratio of male : female patients varies between 1 : 0.7 and 1 : 0.9 (Ammann and Eckert 1995).

As the disease progresses symptoms may occur, including hepatomegaly, abdominal pain, jaundice, sometimes fever and anaemia (Sato *et al.* 1993*a*). Among 70 Swiss patients 36 per cent presented as initial symptoms abdominal pain, 27 per cent jaundice, and 21 per cent other signs (weight loss, neurological symptoms, pleural pain, etc.); 16 per cent were asymptomatic and detected incidentally (Mesarini-Wicki 1991).

The *advanced stage* is characterized by severe hepatic dysfunction and often associated with portal hypertension (Sato *et al.* 1993*a*).

The duration of the disease is variable, between weeks and years. In an older Swiss study of 64 patients the mean duration was 3.7 years (2 weeks to 18 years) (Drolshammer *et al.* 1973). Mortality rates in untreated or inadequately treated patients are high and may reach 94–100 per cent within 10–15 years after diagnosis (Ammann and Eckert 1995, 1996). As survival rates depend on the stage of disease at the time of hospitalization, early diagnosis is extremely important (Nakajima *et al.* 1993).

Immunity and natural resistance

The following account is a brief summary of some relevant aspects. For further information the reader is referred to reviews (Gottstein 1992; Gottstein and Felleisen 1995; Lightowlers and Gottstein 1995).

The majority of patients with alveolar echinococcosis respond to the infection with the production of antibodies of all isotypes, which can be detected in serological tests. Most of the diagnostic tests are based on IgG detection. A direct role of antibodies in controlling metacestode proliferation has not been demonstrated, but they may be involved in immunopathological processes (Gottstein and Felleisen 1995).

Accumulating evidence suggests that modulation of T-lymphocyte responses plays an important role regarding the outcome of the infection. It has been found that patients with the 'abortive' form of the infection, or patients after radical resection of the lesions, had high lymphoproliferative and low antibody responses, while in patients in advanced stages of the disease lymphoproliferative reactions were low and antibody responses high. This may be interpreted as an indication that in advanced stages of the disease lymphoproliferative responses are increasingly suppressed (Gottstein and Felleisen 1995). In patients with active metacestode infection the numbers of CD8+ cells were increased whereas in patients with the abortive form CD4+ lymphocytes prevailed (Vuitton *et al.* 1984). The presence of elevated numbers of CD8+ cells may be indicative for a local immunosuppression (Gottstein and Felleisen 1995). A recent study provides evidence that a T_{H2} immune response is gradually activated during the course of infection, indicating a critical role for interleukin-5 (IL-5) in the manifestation of human alveolar echinococcosis (Sturm *et al.* 1995)

As indicated by the slow development of the metacestode, the histopathological reaction, the very limited capacity of protoscolex formation, and other features, humans have a relatively low susceptibility to *E. multilocularis* and therefore a high natural resistance. Markers of the degree of resistance are possibly lymphoid cell-surface proteins encoded in the HLA region. Preliminary studies have shown in patients with alveolar echinococcosis a higher frequency of certain HLA antigens (Gottstein and Bettens 1994; Scherbakov 1996).

Pathology

Lesions of the liver

The lesions caused by the metacestodes in the human liver vary from minor foci of a few millimetres in size up to extensive areas of infiltration occupying large parts of the liver (Ammann and Eckert 1995, 1996).

In macroscopic sections of the human liver, the metacestodes of *E. multilocularis* exhibit an alveolar spongy structure composed of numerous irregular cysts with diameters between less than 1 mm and 30 mm (see also p. 685) (Fig. 53.5). Due to necrosis, cavities filled with liquid and necrotic material may be formed in central parts of the parasite, reaching diameters of 15–20 cm or more (Ammann and Eckert 1995, 1996).

Microscopically, cysts of *E. multilocularis* in the human host have a relatively thin laminated layer. The germinal layer of cysts in the human liver is a thin and delicate layer with only a few nuclei or is not discernible in light microscopy (Ammann and Eckert 1995, 1996). Brood capsules and protoscolices are rarely formed (about 10–15 per cent of cases) (Fig. 53.4). The cysts within those parts of the metacestode actively infiltrating the liver parenchyma are surrounded by an inner necrotic zone and outer layers of histiocytes and lymphocytes. In later phases, tissue reactions of chronic inflammation, often with giant-cell foreign body reaction, fibrous tissue, calcifications, or necrotic areas are seen around cysts (Fujioka *et al.* 1993). In the human liver fibrous proliferation is often so intense that cysts are embedded in a very dense and hard fibrous stroma (Ammann and Eckert 1995, 1996). However, the metacestode as a whole is not demarcated at its outer limits by a fibrous capsule like cysts of *E. granulosus*, except in cases of abortive lesions (see below).

Lesions of other organs and metastases formation

The metacestode of *E. multilocularis* is characterized by a tumour-like proliferation and the potential of metastasis formation (see above). In the human host metastases may be formed in organs adjacent to the liver (gallbladder, pancreas, diaphragm, etc.) or in distant localizations (lungs, bones, muscles, skin, brain, spine, etc.) (Posselt 1928). In a series of 70 Swiss patients 13 per cent had distant metastases (Table 53.3) and 11 per cent of 156 Japanese patients (Sato *et al.* 1996*b*). The morphological structure of *E. multilocularis*

metacestodes in other organs is essentially similar to those in the liver, but may differ in certain localizations. In bones it might be especially difficult to distinguish *E. granulosus* and *E. multilocularis* infections, as the former may exhibit an unusual small-vesicular structure if the parasite is restricted to the network of the spongiosa of the bones.

Abortive lesions

During the course of infection active metacestodes of *E. multilocularis* can partially degenerate centrally and calcify, but it was believed that they would retain an unlimited proliferative capacity. Several years ago spontaneous death of *E. multilocularis* metacestodes in the human liver was documented in five asymptomatic patients in Alaska (Rausch *et al.* 1987) with calcified dead parasite lesions (diameters 0.5–9.0 cm), a mineralized wall of the lesions and a cavity filled with amorphous necrotic material, and in some cases also with folded parasite membranes. Later such cases were also observed in other countries.

Diagnosis

Clinical diagnosis

The clinical diagnosis of alveolar echinococcosis is based on the following triad: (1) clinical findings and anamnestic epidemiological data; (2) lesion morphology reviewed by imaging techniques; and (3) immunological and other laboratory tests. Details have been reviewed by Morris and Richards (1992), Uchino and Sato (1993), Ammann and Eckert (1995, 1996) and WHO (1896), and only some aspects are discussed here.

Imaging L. Lesions of the liver are best visualized by ultrasonography (US) and computed tomography (CT). Pulmonary lesions can be detected by radiography.

Diagnostic puncture of liver lesions. This should be avoided in any case as it may possibly lead to dissemination of parasite material and local metastases formation (Ammann and Eckert 1995, 1996). However, it may be necessary in seronegative cases with unclear imaging results. A polymerase chain reaction for detection of *E. multilocularis* specific messenger RNA from fine-needle biopsy specimens was recently developed (Kern *et al.* 1995).

Immunodiagnostic tests. These tests, for primary diagnosis or confirmation of imaging results, are more reliable in the diagnosis of alveolar echinococcosis than of cystic echinococcosis. Sensitivity and specificity of tests are high if purified and specific antigens are used (Auer *et al.* 1988; Gottstein *et al.* 1993). For example, the so-called Em2plus-ELISA using a mixture of affinity-purified *E. multilocularis* metacestode antigens (Em2-Antigen) and of a recombinant antigen (EmII/3-10) had a diagnostic sensitivity for alveolar echinococcosis of 97.1 per cent and an overall specificity of 98.9 per cent (Gottstein *et al.* 1993). Serodiagnosis by Western blot analysis is also highly sensitive and specific (Ito 1996; Sato *et al.* 1996*a*; Nagano *et al.* 1996).

Routine laboratory tests. These do not yield specific aetiological findings (Ammann and Eckert 1995, 1996) but they have to be performed for diagnosing the general clinical condition of the patient and to identify certain pathological changes, such as cholestasis or bilirubinaemia.

Early detection of the infection

If the *E. multilocularis* infection in humans is detected in an early stage, the prospects for complete cure by surgical resection of liver lesions are favourable (Sato *et al.* 1993*b*). Certain techniques have been used for screening of populations of individuals with the aim of early detection of the infection.

Screening of populations. Screening of populations for alveolar echinococcosis (AE) has been reported from various countries, including Alaska, Austria, China, France, Japan, Switzerland L, and others.

In all recent studies ELISAs alone or in combination with Western blot analysis have been used for serological primary screening. For such studies, test systems with high sensitivity and specificity are required. The method of choice for secondary screening is ultrasound examination of the liver, possibly followed by other imaging procedures and further laboratory tests in suspected cases (Sato *et al.* 1993*b*; Bresson-Hadni *et al.* 1994).

Special experience with mass screening programmes exists in Japan (Sato *et al.* 1993*b*). In Hokkaido a total of 542 520 persons were submitted to primary screening during 1984–91, with annual ranges between 26 356 and 96 152 persons. Overall 4509 persons had a positive ELISA reaction (0.83 per cent of the total), 4055 persons underwent secondary US screening, and finally 54 persons (0.01 per cent of total) were detected with asymptomatic alveolar echinococcosis (Sato *et al.* 1993*b*). This figure corresponds to an annual incidence rate of 1.2 AE cases per 100 000 inhabitants. In these patients liver lesions were small, ranging from 8 to 50 mm in diameter. Most important was that in this group of screened patients the rate of complete surgical excision of liver lesions was 100 per cent as compared to a resectability rate of only 20 per cent in non-screened patients with AE detected at a later stage (Sato *et al.* 1993*b*).

In the Doubs Department in France 7884 subjects were primarily screened by ELISA and 140 of 152 seropositive persons were secondarily screened by US and other imaging techniques (Bresson-Hadni *et al.* 1994). Among the total, 13 cases with asymptomatic alveolar echinococcosis were detected, among them five patients with the abortive form of the infection. The authors indicated that costs for screening are rather low but high for the diagnosis, follow-up, and treatment of detected cases.

Screening of individuals See pp. 694–695.

Treatment

A summary of the current status of knowledge is presented below. For more detailed information see Morris and Richards (1992), Sato *et al.* (1993*c*), Uchino and Sato (1993), Ammann and Eckert (1995, 1996), Uchino and Sato (1996), and WHO (1996).

Surgical treatment

Surgical *resection* of the involved liver lesions (subsegmentomy, segmentomy, lobectomy, trisegmentomy) and of lesions in other affected organs is indicated in all operable cases (Ammann and Eckert 1995, 1996; WHO 1996). Depending on the stage of the disease, radical resection can be carried out in 20–40 per cent of symptomatic cases (Ammann and Eckert 1995, 1996) but in up to 100 per cent of cases if the infection had been diagnosed in an early stage (Sato *et al.* 1993*b*, Uchino *et al.* 1993). *Palliative* surgery (i.e. partial resection, marsupialization, bile drainage, and other measures) is indicated in certain inoperable cases (Uchino *et al.* 1993; WHO 1996). Another option for severe inoperable cases is liver transplantation (see below).

In many cases it is difficult or impossible to predict whether or not an operation has eliminated all parts of the metacestode tissue. Therefore, postoperative chemotherapy should be carried out for (at least) 2 years after surgery with careful monitoring of the patient during a minimum of 10 years for possible recurrence (Ammann and Eckert 1995, 1996; WHO 1996).

Liver transplantation

This has been performed in France from 1986 to 1992 in 21 patients suffering from severe alveolar echinococcosis. Eight patients died, and 6 year survival of patients was 66 per cent; in 10 of 13 patients (77 per cent) growth of parasite remnants or metastases were observed (Bresson-Hadni 1990; Bresson-Hadni *et al.* 1991, 1992; Vuitton 1995, personal communication). It appears that proliferation of remnants of metacestode tissue under immunosuppression after transplantation is a major problem in liver transplantation.

Chemotherapy

Long-term chemotherapy of human alveolar echinococcosis with benzimidazole derivatives was introduced in 1976, based on animal studies (Eckert 1986; Wen *et al.* 1994; Amman and Eckert 1995, 1996; Horton 1996). Chemotherapy is still developing but it represents a valuable adjuvant therapy in some of the cases. At present, mebendazole (Vermox®, 500 mg, Janssen) and albendazole (Zentel®, Eskazole®, Smith Kline Beecham) are routinely used for chemotherapy of human alveolar echinococcosis. Data presented below refer to these drugs if not otherwise indicated.

Indications and contraindications for chemotherapy. Chemotherapy is indicated for the following cases of alveolar echinococcosis:

(1) inoperable cases;
(2) cases after incomplete surgical resection of parasitic lesions;
(3) cases after anticipated radical surgery and after liver transplantation (dosages and duration, see below).

In view of the severeness of alveolar echinococcosis and the relative low toxicity of mebendazole and albendazole, there are only a few contra-indications or limitations of chemotherapy (WHO 1996). Careful monitoring of the patients is necessary in all cases of chemotherapy (Ammann and Eckert 1995, 1996; WHO 1996).

Selection of drugs, dosage, and duration of chemotherapy. For chemotherapy of human AE only two benzimidazole derivatives, namely mebendazole and albendazole, are commercially available in a limited number of countries. These drugs are generally administered as follows:

Mebendazole (Vermox® 500 mg, Janssen) is given perorally in tablets of 500 mg continuously at daily doses of 30–50 mg/kg body weight (b.w.). (in three divided doses postprandially). After initial treatment of 4 weeks it is advisable to adjust the oral doses in order to obtain plasma drug levels of greater than 250 nmol/l (= 74 ng/ml). In special situations the daily dosage may then exceed the normal daily dosage, but a daily dose over 6 g is not recommended.

Duration of treatment is at least 2 years in cases after radical surgery, or continuously for many years in inoperable cases, in cases with incomplete resection, and after liver transplantation. In some cases mebendazole has been administered for more than 11 years.

Albendazole (Zentel®, Eskazole®, SmithKline Beecham) is given as 400 mg tablets for repeated cycles of 28 days at daily doses of 10–15 mg/kg b.w. (two divided doses) with intervals of 14 days (WHO 1996). The number of necessary cycles has not yet been determined, and it is not known whether this drug can be given for long periods of many years. In cases of cystic echinococcosis it has been administered for 2 years.

In China 11 patients with AE have been treated *continuously* with *20 mg/kg* b.w./day (two divided doses) for about 1–5 years. The treatment was well tolerated (Liu *et al.* 1991).

Praziquantel, an isochinoline derivative, has been used for treatment of human AE, but experimental data obtained from animal models indicate that efficacy against the metacestode stage of *E. multilocularis* is far less pronounced than in the benzimidazole derivatives mentioned above, even if praziquantel is given in excessively high doses (Ammann and Eckert 1995).

Drug efficacy. The substances with antiparasitic properties are mebendazole and the main metabolite of albendazole, albendazole sulphoxide. Animal experiments have shown that long-term treatment with mebendazole, albendazole, fenbendazole, and some other benzimidazoles has the following effects against metacestodes of *E. multilocularis* (Eckert 1986; Ammann and Eckert 1995):

(1) inhibition of metacestode proliferation, resulting in reduction of parasite masses;
(2) destruction of protoscolices and partial destruction of the germinal layer and of the cystic structure of the metacestode;
(3) prevention or suppression of metastasis formation;
(4) prolongation of animal host survival.

The parasites are normally not killed but only inhibited in proliferation during treatment. The effect of the drugs in animals is therefore not parasiticidal but parasitostatic.

Several well-controlled studies with a total of more than 150 patients with AE have shown that long-term treatment with mebendazole was beneficial in a proportion of patients (Ammann and Eckert 1995, 1996). About 60 per cent of the patients under treatment showed clinical improvement, 20 per cent stabilization, and 20 per cent progression. In a large series, 61 per cent of 52 patients showed increased body weight, 90 per cent of 52 patients regression of cholestasis, and 16 per cent of 51 patients decrease of liver lesion size. The most convincing effect of chemotherapy with mebendazole in two independent long-term studies was a significant prolongation of survival time. In a

Swiss study the 10-year survival rate in a group of 70 treated patients was 89 per cent as compared to 6 per cent in untreated patients (historical controls); and in an Alaskan series, 90 per cent of 12 patients had survived at 10 years, as compared to 25 per cent of untreated patients. A second reliable criterion of therapeutic efficacy is the marked response on the parasitic mass which is, however, observed only in patients after long-term treatment (37 patients treated for an average of 6.4 years; decrease of lesions in 49 per cent, stabilization in 35 per cent, and progression in 16 per cent). Data on albendazole are also favourable but do not yet allow definitive conclusions (Horton 1996). In a recent Japanese study, 55 per cent of 20 patients with AE showed favourable response to albendazole treatment with a cumulative survival rate of 87 per cent, 15 years after operation (Ishizu *et al.* 1996).

Adverse reactions. Mebendazole and albendazole are generally well tolerated. Two-thirds of the patients experienced one or more side-effects, but they were mostly of minor importance and reversible. Permanent discontinuation of chemotherapy was indicated only in rare cases. Monitoring of serum drug levels is mandatory to avoid toxic adverse reactions (Ammann and Eckert 1995, 1996; WHO 1996).

EPIDEMIOLOGY

GEOGRAPHICAL DISTRIBUTION AND PREVALENCE

Echinococcus multilocularis occurs in the northern hemisphere within a large belt stretching from the northern tundra zone southward to some regions around 40°–45°N. The currently known endemic areas include regions in western and central parts of Europe, in eastern Europe and Asia, and in North America. A few cases were also reported from northern Africa (Fig. 53.10) (reviewed by Rausch 1995; Schantz *et al.* 1995; Eckert 1996*a,b*; Schantz *et al.* 1996). Some data on the prevalence rates of *E. multilocularis* in definitive and intermediate hosts are presented in Table 53.2; selected incidence rates of AE in humans are given in Table 53.4.

Western and central Europe

Echinococcus multilocularis has a geographical range extending further north, east, and south than previously anticipated. Currently, the parasite is known to occur in 10 European countries (sequence of order from west to east): Belgium (southern part), France (Massif Central and eastern regions), Duchy of Luxembourg, Germany (12 of 16 provinces), Switzerland (21 of 26 cantons), Principality of Liechtenstein, Austria (6 of 9 provinces), Poland, Czech Republic, and Turkey (including the

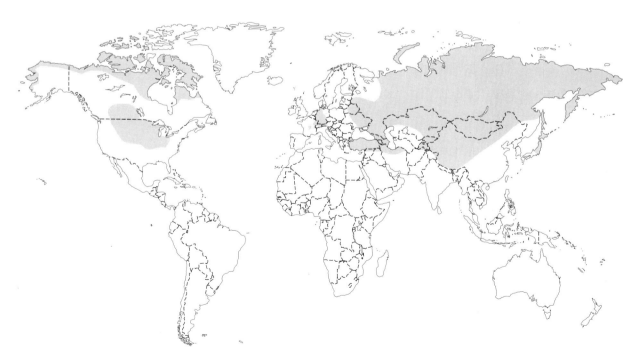

Fig. 53.10 Approximate geographic distribution of *Echinococcus multilocularis* (shaded areas). (Modified after Schantz *et al.* (1995). J. Eckert and H. Bucklar, Institute of Parasitology, Zurich©.)

Table 53.4   Selected incidence data on clinical cases of alveolar echinococcosis in humans

Region, country	Period	Number of new cases	Average per year	Incidence rate per year and per 100 000 inhabitants	Reference
Eurasia					
Switzerland	1956–69	122	8.7	–	Drolshammer *et al.* (1973)
(whole country)	1970–83	145	10.4	0.18	Gloor (1988)
	1984–92	65	7.2	0.10	Eckert *et al.* (1995)
Austria					
(whole country)	1983–90	14	1.8	0.024	Auer and Aspöck (1991)
Germany					
(Bavaria)	1985–89	50	10	0.03	Nothdurft *et al.* (1995)
France					
(whole country)	1975–83	97	10.7	–	WHO (1984)
(Franche Comté)	1971–89	85	4.5	0.5	Bresson-Hadni (1980)
Turkey					
(whole country)	1934–83	157	3.1	–	Uysal and Paksoy (1986)
China					
(whole country)	To 1992	500	–	–	Schantz *et al.* (1995)
Japan					
(whole country)	1965–91	314	12	–	Ohbayashi (1996)
(Hokkaido)	1984–91	82[a]	9.1[a]	1.2[b]	Sato *et al.* (1993*b*)
Northern America					
Alaska					
(St Lawrence Island)	1947–90	53	–	7–98[c]	Schantz *et al.* (1995)
Central North					
America	1937–95	2	–	–	Schantz *et al.* (1995)

[a] Cases detected by serological screening or without screening; figures calculated from graph.
[b] Data calculated from seroepidemiological survey.
[c] Data refer only to villages where cases have been diagnosed.

Asian part) (Malczewski *et al.* 1995; Kolarova *et al.* 1996; Schantz *et al.* 1995, 1996; Eckert 1996*a,b*).

Eastern Europe and Asia

In northern Eurasia the geographic range of *E. multilocularis* includes the tundra zone of Russia extending from the White Sea in the west to the Bering Strait in the east. Further south the parasite is found in a broad belt stretching from the Ukraine and Moldavia through most of Russia to its eastern borders, including the islands of Sakhalin and Kuriles and to some Japanese islands. The known southern limit of this belt includes Turkey, northern Iraq and Iran, Georgia, Armenia, Azerbaijan, Kazakhstan, Uzbekistan, Tajikistan, Kyrgtstan, and parts of China. In China there are two major endemic areas, namely in central China (south Gansu, southern Ningxia Hui AR, eastern Qinghai, and northern Sichuan) and in northern Xinjiang Uygur AR. The endemic area in Japan includes the northern island Hokkaido and parts of Honshu island (Schantz *et al.* 1995, 1996).

Northern Africa

Two human cases of the *E. multilocularis* infection have been reported from northern Tunisia (Schantz *et al.*

1995), but it is unclear whether the parasite is endemic or not.

North America

In North America the geographical range of *E. multilocularis* extends from some islands in the Bering Sea (Saint George Island [Pribilof group], Nunivak Island, St Lawrence Island) along the Alaskan coast from the mouth of the Kuskokwim River north-, east- and southward to Canada (Fig. 53.10) (Schantz *et al.* 1995, 1996). Prior to the 1960s *E. multilocularis* apparently spread from the northern tundra zone to southern Manitoba (Canada) and North Dakota (USA). Today, the parasite is known to occur in the Canadian provinces of Manitoba, Saskatchewan, and Alberta, and in the following states of the USA (west to east): Montana, Wyoming, North Dakota, South Dakota, Nebraska, Minnesota, Iowa, Missouri, Wisconsin, Michigan, Illinois, Indiana and Ohio (Rausch 1995; Schantz *et al.* 1995, 1996; Kazacos and Storandt 1997).

LIFE CYCLE PATTERNS

The natural cycle of *E. multilocularis* is based upon the predator–prey relationship between carnivores and small mammals. The natural definitive hosts are wild canids, mainly foxes of the genera *Vulpes* and *Alopex*. In some regions other wild canids (coyotes, raccoon dogs, wolves, etc.) or domestic dogs and cats may also serve as definitive hosts. Metacestodes of *E. multilocularis* have been reported from mammals representing eight families, but genera and species from the family Arvicolidae (voles and lemmings) (seven genera) and Cricetidae (hamsters, gerbils, 'mouse-like' rodents) (six genera) are the most important intermediate hosts (Rausch 1995). Definitive host species and particularly intermediate host species involved in the cycle may differ in various endemic regions and even within smaller areas (Rausch 1995). Examples are presented in Table 53.2.

Epidemiologically, several types of life cycles have to be considered, namely the sylvatic (or wildlife) cycle, the intermediate cycle, and the synanthropic (or domestic) cycle.

Sylvatic cycle

In the sylvatic cycle *E. multilocularis* is restricted to wild animal hosts and is therefore to some degree ecologically separated from humans (Schantz *et al.* 1995). This may be one of the factors responsible for restricting the infection risk for humans to generally low levels (Table 53.4). However, evidence suggests that in most endemic regions infections of humans are mainly acquired from the sylvatic cycle, with foxes as a source of infective *E. multilocularis* eggs. For example, in western and central Europe red foxes (*Vulpes vulpes*) have to be regarded as the most important definitive hosts as population densities of foxes and prevalence rates of *E. multilocularis* in these animals are high, other wild carnivores do not play a role, and domestic dogs and cats are far less frequently infected (Schantz *et al.* 1995, 1996; Eckert 1996*a*,*b*). In France, the sylvatic cycle was shown to exist very close to a village where human cases of alveolar echinococcosis occurred (Pétavy *et al.* 1991). In Hokkaido (Japan) with a similar epidemiological situation as in western and central Europe, the dominating role of foxes as potential sources of infections for humans is well documented: during 1965–91 the average rate of infection with *E. multilocularis* was 14 per cent in 18 073 foxes and only 1.0 per cent in 9742 dogs (Ohbayashi 1996).

Intermediate cycle

Domestic dogs and cats may be involved as definitive hosts in an intermediate cycle. Dogs having regular access to metacestode-infected rodents may frequently become infected with *E. multilocularis*. Under these special circumstances they may represent a major source of infection for humans. For example, on St Lawrence Island (Alaska) numerous infected voles are an easy prey for dogs maintained in the villages. In

1951, 12 per cent of dogs in one of the villages were infected with *E. multilocularis*, and 22–35 per cent of the voles trapped in the years 1980–83 harboured metacestodes (Schantz *et al.* 1995). A study in an area of the north-western coast of Alaska with a similar epidemiological situation revealed that Eskimo patients with alveolar echinococcosis were more likely than controls to have owned dogs for their entire lives, tethered their dogs near the house, and lived in houses built directly on the tundra. Interestingly, trapping or skinning of foxes was not associated with higher infection risk (Stehr-Green *et al.* 1988). High prevalence rates of *E. multilocularis* in dogs (10–14 per cent) were also reported from various provinces of China (Schantz *et al.* 1995).

Cats are less susceptible to *E. multilocularis* than dogs (Thompson and Eckert 1983) but they may harbour egg-producing intestinal stages. Therefore, they have to be regarded as potential sources of human infections but their importance is probably much lower than that of foxes and dogs (Eckert 1996*b*).

Synanthropic cycle

Infrequently metacestodes of *E. multilocularis* have been found in house mice (Table 53.2). A cat/house mouse cycle is theoretically possible but of very minor, if any, importance as a risk factor for humans.

INFECTION RISK OF HUMANS

Infection route of humans

It is generally assumed that humans can become exposed to the eggs of *E. multilocularis* by handling of infected definitive hosts, or by food contaminated with eggs. Some reports suggested that egg transmission may occur by water-borne routes (Schantz *et al.* 1995). However, studies on the epidemiological significance of the various potential ways of transmission are lacking.

In relation to the high prevalence rates of *E. multilocularis* in definitive hosts (Table 53.2) the incidence rates of alveolar echinococcosis in humans are low in most of the endemic areas (Table 53.4). This discrepancy is still unexplained. Several aspects have to be considered and should be further studied, including exposure of humans to eggs of *E. multilocularis* and the resistance/immunity of humans to infection.

Exposure of humans to eggs of E. multilocularis

Echinococcus multilocularis is mainly restricted to the sylvatic cycle and thereby to some degree ecologically separated from humans. However, the degree of separation may vary from region to region, from high in isolated and sparsely populated areas to moderate or low where infected foxes or other definitive hosts live in close proximity, or even within villages and cities, for example in Europe or in Hokkaido (Japan). Ecological separation does not exist if infected dogs or cats live in close association with humans (see above).

Exposure to eggs may be influenced by occupational and behavioural factors. Hunters, trappers, and persons who work with fur may frequently be exposed to eggs of *E. multilocularis* but there is little evidence that these groups are at increased risk (Schantz *et al.* 1995). On the other hand, data from Austria (Auer and Aspöck 1991), France (Bresson-Hadni 1990), and Switzerland (Gloor 1988) indicate that persons working in agriculture are at increased risk of infection. Living in the countryside in close proximity to infected foxes and/or frequent contacts with egg-contaminated food or soil may be the reasons for a higher infection risk, but exact information is not available. There are indications that high prevalence rates of *E. multilocularis* in the fox population are correlated with an increased infection risk for humans (Nothdurft *et al.* 1995) but this needs further evaluation.

Resistance and immunity to infection

Apparently, humans have a relatively high degree of innate resistance to infection with eggs of *E. multilocularis*, as indicated by the slow development of the metacestode stage in the liver and other organs, the reduced capacity of protoscolex formation, and the degree and type of histopathological reaction. The reasons for this resistance are not well understood but recent preliminary studies have shown that in patients with alveolar echinococcosis the frequency of certain HLA antigens was increased (Gottstein and Bettens 1994; Scherbakov 1996), implying the possibility of a immunogenetic predisposition for susceptibility or resistance to alveolar echinococcosis (Gottstein and Felleisen 1995). The potential role of acquired immunity for the regulation of the metacestode population in humans is still obscure, but cases of self-cure from the infection indicate that immunity may play a role (p. 694).

TRANSMISSION DYNAMICS

The regulation of the cycle of *E. multilocularis* depends upon various factors, such as species and numeric density of definitive and intermediate hosts, interactions between these populations, egg dispersion, and others. According to Gemmell and Roberts (1995) parasite populations are subject to density-independent and density-dependent constraints. For *E. granulosus* it has been found that the acquisition of immunity of intermediate hosts against the infection is an important factor of density-dependent population regulation (Gemmell and Roberts 1995). In this respect little is known on *E. multilocularis*. Therefore, the data discussed below have to be regarded as preliminary.

Role of final hosts

Immunity acquired by foxes, dogs, etc. following single or repeated infections may be important as a factor of population regulation. Experiments with *E. granulosus* in dogs have shown that the animals remain susceptible to infection with protoscolices for a varying number of challenges, with about 50 per cent of the dog population showing reduced susceptibility by the sixth infection. It was concluded that immunity acquired by dogs to *E. granulosus* does not play a role for population regulation (Gemmell and Roberts 1995). Infection intensities may be higher in young foxes than in older foxes (p. 688). This may be an expression of immunity or of other factors with potential to influence egg production and egg release in fox populations.

Role of intermediate hosts

Immunity to superinfection with eggs of *E. granulosus*, *Taenia hydatigena*, and *T. ovis* can be naturally acquired or experimentally induced in sheep and cattle. The immune status of the intermediate host population represents an important density-dependent constraint in the cycle of *E. granulosus* (Gemmel and Roberts 1995). Regarding the intermediate hosts of *E. multilocularis*, it is known from experimental studies that various rodent species and strains vary in susceptibility and resistance to the infection, respectively (see p. 691). Although some protection against superinfection with *E. multilocularis* in rodents has been demonstrated, the role played by acquired immunity as a regulatory factor in the epidemiology of the infection has not yet been evaluated (Gemmel and Roberts 1995). Parasite-induced mortality in intermediate host populations does not represent a constraint in the regulation of the *E. granulosus* population (Gemmel and Roberts 1995). In contrast, infections with *E. multilocularis* metacestodes in rodents may cause disease and high mortality rates but it is not known whether this factor is important for parasite population regulation.

Role of eggs

Eggs of *E. multilocularis* deposited with droppings of foxes or other final hosts may remain an important reservoir of the infection for intermediate and accidental hosts during prolonged periods of time due to their considerable resistance to environmental conditions. In southern Germany maximum survival of *E. multilocularis* eggs under natural conditions was 8 months in the period between August and May with air temperature extremes of −15 °C and +27 °C (Veit *et al.* 1995). Fox faeces collected in the Alaskan tundra and subsequently stored at room temperature still contained infective *E. multilocularis* eggs after 24 months (Thomas and Babero 1956). Eggs suspended in tap water at +4 °C survived for almost 16 months (478 days) (Veit *et al.* 1995). The eggs are highly resistant to lower temperatures. For example, −18 °C for 240 days or −27 °C for 54 days are not lethal, but they are killed at −70 °C within 4 days (Blunt *et al.* 1991) and at −80 °C to −83 °C within 2 days (Eckert *et al.* 1991; Veit *et al.* 1995).

At higher temperatures of +60 °C to +80 °C eggs of *E. granulosus* are killed within 5 minutes, and this most likely applies also for the eggs of *E. multilocularis* (Eckert *et al.* 1992). Like eggs of various *Taenia* species and of *E. granulosus* (Gemmell and Lawson 1986), the eggs of *E. multilocularis* are sensitive to desiccation. Eggs in air of 27 per cent relative humidity (r.h.) at +25 °C lost infectivity within 24 hours, and at 15 per cent r.h. at +43 °C within 2 hours (Veit *et al.* 1995).

In this connection it should be mentioned that the eggs of *E. multilocularis* are resistant to a variety of commercially available disinfectants containing phenol derivatives, aldehydes, or ethanol (Veit *et al.* 1995). Sodium hypochlorite (NaOCl) was shown to kill eggs of *E. granulosus* within 10 min if applied at room temperature in concentrations of at least 3.75 per cent NaOCl (Craig and MacPherson 1988). One should be aware, however, that the effect of this disinfectant may vary (Craig and MacPherson 1988; Veit *et al.* 1995). Eggs of *E. multilocularis* were not killed in 10–40 per cent ethanol within 24 hours (Veit *et al.* 1995), and eggs of *Taenia pisiformis* survived in 10 per cent formalin for 3 weeks (Eckert *et al.* 1992).

Egg dispersal is epidemiologically important. *Echinococcus multilocularis*-infected foxes disperse eggs with their droppings in their territories, which in Europe may vary in size between about 18 ha and 16 km² (Labhardt 1990). In some regions (Europe, Japan) foxes have tended to invade cities in increasing numbers during recent years. In the USA *E. multilocularis*-infected foxes have been transported from endemic areas to hunting enclosures of non-endemic regions (Schantz *et al.* 1995). This practice poses the risk of long-distance dispersal of eggs and of establishment of the parasite cycle in previously non-endemic areas.

Eggs of *Taenia* species from dogs spread up to 80 m from the site of deposition withing 10 days (Gemmel and Lawson 1986). *Taenia* and *Echinococcus* eggs can be dispersed by flies which may travel several kilometres (Gemmel and Lawson 1986). Evidence from an island off the west coast of Scotland suggests that eggs of *T. hydatigena* may have been transported by birds over 60 km (Torgerson *et al.* 1995). It is assumed that eggs of *E. multilocularis* can be transported with plants contaminated with droppings of infected definitive hosts. We have observed *E. multilocularis* infections in domes-

tic pigs and in monkey colonies in a zoo after feeding of grass harvested from meadows accessible to infected foxes (unpublished).

Role of population dynamics

This complex matter can only be discussed here in very general terms. A comparatively clear situation exists on St Lawrence Island, Alaska, characterized by rather uniform biotope conditions, high population densities of voles (*Microtus oeconomus*), and relatively high prevalence rates of *E. multilocularis* both in arctic foxes and voles which, however, underlie regular seasonal variations (Rausch 1986). In other regions, such as Europe, the situation is far more complex as the biotopes of foxes and of several species of intermediate hosts (Table 53.2), geographical distribution, population densities, and dynamics of both definitive and intermediate hosts, feeding habits of foxes, macro–and microclimatic conditions, and other factors may vary significantly from region to region, and even within smaller areas. While the prevalence rates of *E. multilocularis* in foxes may reach high levels, infection rates of intermediate hosts in some regions are typically low (Table 53.2). Some seasonal variations in prevalence rates of *E. multilocularis* in foxes have been described. There are some indications that prevalence rates of *E. multilocularis* in foxes are positively correlated with fox densities (Ewald 1993) but the reasons are unknown. Profound regional variations are indicated by large differences of the infection rates of foxes (Table 53.2). Giraudoux (1991) in France has hypothesized that the *E. multilocularis* infection in foxes and rodents exists in 'patches' and persists in a region by shifting to non-endemic patches with foxes being the main vector.

As our present epidemiological knowledge is insufficient, the development of mathematical models of the *E. multilocularis* infection (Roberts and Aubert 1995) and attempts to control the infection in the sylvatic cycle (p. 691) remain on an uncertain basis.

PREVENTION AND CONTROL

ANIMALS

Wild carnivores

Echinococcus multilocularis is mainly perpetuated in a sylvatic cycle with foxes or other wild carnivores as definitive hosts. Therefore, control appears to be especially difficult. Treatment of fox populations with baits containing praziquantel has been attempted in a preliminary trial in southern Germany, but this method needs further evaluation regarding efficacy, practicability, and costs (p. 691). The statement that such treatment could possibly eradicate the parasite in areas of low endemicity (Roberts and Aubert 1995) is deduced from a theorethical mathematical model based on several uncertain assumptions. In any plans of *E. multilocularis* control, experiences with *E. granulosus* should be considered. This parasite, with its synanthropic cycle, is relatively easy to control by treatment of dogs with drugs, but the 'attack phase' of control may last for 10–15 years, or even for 30–50 years (PAHO 1995). In view of the apparently low degree of immunity acquired by foxes during natural *E. multilocularis* infections, prospects for developing a vaccine against the infection in definitive hosts are rather uncertain. Reduction of fox population densities as a control measure has to be considered. However, the influence upon regulation of the parasite cycle is still unclear. Reduction of fox populations by hunting alone is mostly unsatisfactory, the development of new methods which are both effective and humane, is therefore necessary.

Dogs and cats

In situations where dogs and cats are under close supervision by their owners, the risk of acquiring *E. multilocularis* infections can be reduced by preventing the animals preying on small mammals, by training (dogs) and/or adequate feeding (dogs and cats). Another and safer option is regular treatment with praziquantel or epsiprantel at intervals of 3–4 weeks (see p. 691). In endemic areas this treatment has to be carried out permanently in animals at risk. It cannot exclude human infections from eggs dispersed by foxes, other wild carnivores, or untreated domestic carnivores.

Mass treatment of dogs which were involved in an intermediate type of cycle on St Lawrence Island (Alaska) with praziquantel at monthly intervals reduced the infection rates significantly during a 10-year trial, but infection rates rebounded toward pre-treatment levels after discontinuation of treatment (Schantz *et al.* 1995).

HUMANS

Control of *E. multilocularis* in the sylvatic cycle, the main source of human infections, is especially difficult and at present not feasible. Therefore, some measures are recommended aiming at the reduction of the infection risk and of morbidity/mortality in humans. These measures refer to individuals or populations. For both groups education is an essential part of prevention.

Measures for individuals

The Swiss National Centre for Echinococcosis in Zurich recommends the following measures for individuals:

1. In endemic areas where *E. multilocularis* is known to occur in foxes, wild berries, mushrooms, other plants or fruits from locations accessible to contamination with fox droppings should be thoroughly washed or, better, boiled before consumption. Deep-freezing at −18 to −20 °C does not kill eggs of *E. multilocularis* (they can only be killed at −70 to −80 °C; see also p. 701).

2. Foxes or other final hosts potentially infected with *E. multilocularis* should be handled with great care, always using disposable plastic gloves.

3. Special recommendations have been worked out for laboratory workers concerned with examinations of foxes for *E. multilocularis* (Eckert *et al.* 1991; Ewald 1993; Eckert and Deplazes 1996). In endemic areas similar measurers may be applied to all laboratories in which necropsies of foxes are carried out, for example for rabies.

4. After agricultural or gardening work including contact with potentially egg-contaminated soil, hands should be thoroughly washed.

5. Persons who had single contact with infected final hosts or egg-contaminated materials (for example fox faeces) can be submitted to serological examinations for specific antibodies against *E. multilocularis* antigens at the following intervals after the suspected contact: 4 weeks; 6, 12, and 24 months. Highly sensitive and specific tests have to be employed for this purpose (p. 694).

Individuals with repeated infection risk (for example fox hunters, laboratory personnel, etc.) should be serologically examined once or twice per year.

Measures for populations

In Japan and some other endemic areas population screening by serology and US examination of human populations has been used successfully for early detection of cases. This can reduce morbidity and mortality considerably (p. 695).

ECHINOCOCCUS VOGELI
ECHINOCOCCOSIS (VE)

THE AGENT (*ECHINOCOCCUS VOGELI*) AND LIFE CYCLE

Echinococcus vogeli has typically three segments, the total length varies between 3.9 and 5.5 mm. The gravid segment is very long in relation to the anterior part of the strobila and contains a long, tubular and sac-like uterus (Thompson 1995) (Fig. 53.11). The metacestode stage is characterized by a polycystic structure and development in visceral organs.

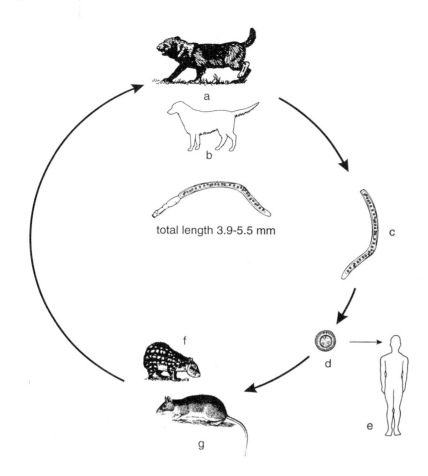

total length 3.9-5.5 mm

Fig. 53.11 Life cycle of *Echinococcus vogeli*. (a) Bush dog (*Speothos venaticus*) as major definitive host; (b) domestic dog as occasional definitive host; (c) terminal segment with eggs; (d) egg; (e) man as accidental host; (f) paca (*Cuniculus paca*) and (g) spiny rat (*Proechimys* sp.) as representatives of intermediate hosts. (Modified after Schantz *et al.* (1995). J. Eckert and H. Bucklar, Institute of Parasitology, Zurich©.)

Under natural conditions *E. vogeli* is typically perpetuated in a life cycle with the bush dog (*Speothos venaticus*) as definitive host and the paca (*Cuniculus paca*) as intermediate host (Rausch 1995) (Fig. 53.11). Natural infections with intestinal stages were also found in a hunter's dog in Brazil and with metacestodes in spiny rats (*Proechimys* spp.) in Columbia (Rausch 1986). Furthermore, rodents of other species and mammals of other orders (for example monkeys) are also susceptible to *E. vogeli*.

HUMANS AS ACCIDENTAL HOSTS

To date 36 cases of human VE have been diagnosed and confirmed by parasitological examinations (D'Alessandro *et al.* 1995). Polycystic metacestode proliferation has been shown to involve liver, pancreas, mesentery, spleen, peritoneal cavity, and lung (Ammann and Eckert 1995). Clinical and radiological presentation is very similar to infection with multiple cysts of *E. granulosus,* and differential diagnosis depends on isolation of protoscolices and morphological hook

characteristics (Meneghelli *et al.* 1992). Albendazole has been used for chemotherapy in six cases with success of treatment in four (Meneghelli *et al.* 1992).

EPIDEMIOLOGY AND PREVENTION

Echinococcus vogeli is known to occur in countries of Central and South America, including Panama, Columbia, Ecuador, Brazil, and Venezuela (Schantz *et al.* 1995). Special methods of prevention or control are not known but similar measures as for *E. multilocularis* may be considered.

ECHINOCOCCUS OLIGARTHRUS *ECHINOCOCCOSIS* (OE)

THE AGENT (*ECHINOCOCCUS OLIGARTHRUS*) AND LIFE CYCLE

The adult stage of *E. oligarthrus* is tiny, only 2.2–2.9 mm long, typically composed of three segments, with a sac-

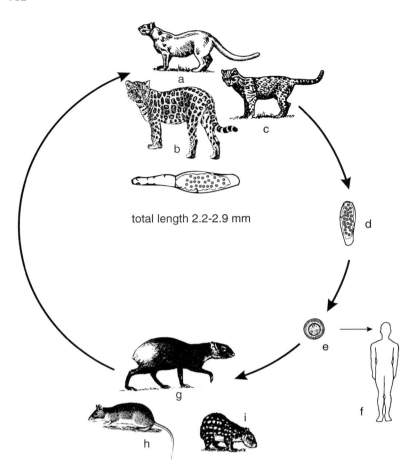

total length 2.2-2.9 mm

Fig. 53.12 Life cycle of *Echinococcus oligarthrus*. (a) Cougar (*Felis concolor*) as type definitive host; (b) jaguar (*Panthera onca*) and (c) ocelot (*Felis pardalis*) as representatives of other definitive hosts; (d) terminal segment of the parasite with eggs; (e) egg; (f) man as accidental host; (g) agouti (*Dasyprocta* sp); (h) spiny rat (*Proechimys guayannensis*) and paca (*Cuniculus paca*) as intermediate hosts. (Modified after Schantz *et al.* (1995). J. Eckert and H. Bucklar, Institute of Parasitology, Zurich©.)

like uterus in the gravid segment (Thompson 1995) (Fig. 53.12).

The life cycle involves carnivores of the family Felidae and rodents, with the cougar (*Felis concolor*) as the type host (Rausch 1995). Some further felids have also been found to serve as final hosts, such as jaguar (*Panthera onca*), ocelot (*Felis pardalis*), jaguarundi (*F. yagouaroundi*), and others. The main intermediate hosts are agoutis (*Dasyprocta* spp), paca (*Cuniculus paca*), and spiny rat (*Proechimys guyannensis*).

HUMANS AS ACCIDENTAL HOSTS

The metacestode of *E. oligarthrus* is polycystic in structure, and in naturally infected animals it has been most commonly found in the musculature and the skin, but also in viscera (D'Alessandro *et al.* 1995). Only two human cases have been reported to date, one with a retro-ocular cyst (2 cm diameter) in Venezuela (Lopera *et al.* 1989) and a second in Brazil with two

cysts (1.5 cm diameter) in the heart (D'Alessandro *et al.* 1995). The diagnosis was mainly based on morphological features of hooks and protoscolex. For differential diagnosis of VE and OE from cystic echinococcosis molecular techniques may be of special interest in the future.

REFERENCES

Ammann, R. W. and Eckert, J. (1995). Clinical diagnosis and treatment of echinococcosis in humans. In *Echinococcus and hydatid disease*, (ed. R. C. A. Thompson and A. J. Lymbery), pp. 411–63. CAB International, Wallingford, Oxon.

Amman, R. W. and Eckert, J. (1996). Parasitic diseases of the liver and intestines: Cestodes: *Echinococcus*. *Gastroenterology Clinics of North America*, **25**, 655–89.

Auer, H. and Aspöck, H. (1991). Incidence, prevalence and geographic distribution of human alveolar echinococcosis in Austria from 1854 to 1990. *Parasitology Research*, **77**, 430–6.

Auer, H., Hermentin, K., and Aspöck, H. (1988). Demonstration of a specific *Echinococcus multilocularis* antigen in the supernatant of *in vitro* maintained protoscolices. *Zentralblatt für Bakteriologie, Mikrobiologie und Hygiene (A)*, **268**, 416–23.

Ballek, D., Takla, M., Ising-Vollmer, S., and Stoye, M. (1992). Zur Helminthenfauna des Rotfuchses (*Vulpes vulpes* LINNE 1758) in Nordhessen und Ostwestfalen. Teil 1: Zestoden. *Deutsche tierärztliche Wochenschrift*, **99**, 362–65.

Blunt, G., Gubrud, J. D., and Hildreth, M. B. (1991). Lethal effects of freezing *Echinococcus multilocularis* eggs at low temperatures. *Proceedings of the 66th Meeting of the American Society of Parasitologists, Madison, Wisconsin, 4–8 August,* Abstract No. 205.

Bosch, D. (1982). Tierexperimentelle Untersuchungen zur Entwicklung von *Echinococcus multilocularis*. In *Probleme der Echinokokkose unter Berücksichtigung parasitologischer und klinischer Aspekte*, (ed. R. Bähr), pp. 36–40. H. Huber, Bern.

Bowles, J., Blair, D., and McManus, D. P. (1995). A molecular phylogeny of the genus *Echinococcus*. *Parasitology*, **110**, 317–28.

Bresson-Hadni, S. (1990). L'infection humaine par *Echinococcus multilocularis*: du depistage a la transplantation hepatique. Thesis, Université de Paris XII Val-de-Marne.

Bresson-Hadni, S., *et al.* (1991). Orthotoptic liver transplantation for incurable alveolar echinococcosis of the liver; report of 17 cases. *Hepatology*, **13**, 1061–70.

Bresson-Hadni, S., *et al.* (1992). Recurrence of alveolar echinococcosis in the liver graft after liver transplantation (letter). *Hepatology*, **16**, 279–80.

Bresson-Hadni, S., *et al.* (1994). Seroepidemiologic screening of *Echinococcus multilocularis* infection in a European area endemic for alveolar echinococcosis. *American Journal of Tropical Medicine and Hygiene*, **51**, 837–46.

Bretagne, S., Guillou, J. P., Morand, M., and Houin, R. (1993). Detection of *Echinococcus multilocularis* DNA in fox faeces using DNA amplification. *Parasitology*, **106**, 193–9.

Craig, P. S. and Macpherson, C. N. L. (1988). Sodium hypochlorite as an ovicide for *Echinococcus*. *Annals of Tropical Medicine and Parasitology*, **82**, 211–13.

Craig, P. S. *et al.* (1995). Diagnosis of canine echinococcosis: comparison of coproantigen and serum antibody tests with arecoline purgation in Uruguay. *Veterinary Parasitology*, **56**, 293–301.

D'Alessandro, A., Ramirez, L. E., Chapadeiro, E., Lopes, E. R., and de Mesquita, P. M. (1995). Second recorded case of human infection by *Echinococcus oligarthrus*. *American Journal of Tropical Medicine and Hygiene*, **52**, 29–33.

Deplazes, P. and Eckert, J. (1996). Diagnosis of the *Echinococcus multilocularis* infection in final hosts. *Applied Parasitology*, **37**, 245–52.

Deplazes, P. and Gottstein, B. (1991). A monoclonal antibody against *Echinococcus multilocularis* Em2 antigen. *Parasitology*, **103**, (Pt 1), 41–9.

Deplazes, P., Gottstein, B., Eckert, J., Jenkins, D. J., Ewald, D., and Jimenez Palacios, S. (1992). Detection of *Echinococcus* coproantigens by enzyme-linked immunosorbent assay in dogs, dingoes and foxes. *Parasitology Research*, **78**, 303–8.

Deplazes, P., Jimenez Palacios, S., Gottstein, B., Skaggs, J., and Eckert, J. (1994a). Detection of *Echinococcus* coproantigens in stray dogs of northern Spain. *Applied Parasitology*, **35**, 297–301.

Deplazes, P., Thompson, R. C., Constantine, C. C., and Penhale, W. J. (1994b). Primary infection of dogs with *Echinococcus granulosus*: systemic and local (Peyer's patches) immune responses. *Veterinary Immunology and Immuno-pathology*, **40**, 171–84.

Drolshammer, I., Wiesmann, E., and Eckert, J. (1973). Echinokokkose beim Menschen in der Schweiz 1956–1969. *Schweizerische Medizinische Wochenschrift*, **103**, 1337–41, 1386–92.

Eckert, J. (1986). Prospects for treatment of the metacestode stage of *Echinococcus*. In *The biology of* Echinococcus *and hydatid disease*, (ed. R. C. A. Thompson), pp. 250–84. Allen and Unwin, London.

Eckert, J. (1988). Cryopreservation of parasites. *Experientia*, **44**, 873–7.

Eckert, J. (1996a). *Echinococcus multilocularis* and alveolar echinococcosis in Europe (except parts of Eastern Europe). In *Alveolar echinococcosis*, (ed. J. Uchino and N. Sato), pp. 27–43. Fuji Shoin, Sapporo, Japan.

Eckert, J. (1996b). Der 'gefährliche Fuchsbandwurm' (*Echinococcus multilocularis*) und die alveoläre Echinokokkose des Menschen in Mitteleuropa. *Berliner und Münchener Tierärztliche Wochenschrift*, **109**, 202–10.

Eckert, J. and Deplazes, P. (1996). Methods for surveys on *Echinococcus multilocularis* infections in final hosts. In *Alveolar echinococcosis*, (ed. J. Uchino and N. Sato), pp. 151–63. Fuji Shoin, Sapporo, Japan.

Eckert, J. and Jacquier, P. (1991). Viability testing of *Echinococcus multilocularis* metacestodes from untreated and treated patients. *Archivos de la Hidatidosis*, **30**, 863–7.

Eckert, J. and Thompson, R. C. A. (1997). Intraspecific variation of *Echinococcus granulosus* and related species with emphasis on their infectivity to humans. *Acta Tropica* **64**, 19–34.

Eckert, J., Thompson, R. C. A., and Mehlhorn, H. (1983). Proliferation and metastases formation of larval *Echinococcus multilocularis*. I. Animal model, macroscopical and histological findings. *Zeitschrift für Parasitenkunde*, **69**, 737–48.

Eckert, J., Deplazes, P., Ewald, D., and Gottstein, B. (1991). Parasitologische und immunologische Methoden zum Nachweis von Echinococcus multilocularis bei Füchsen. *Mitteilungen der Österreichischen Gesellschaft für Tropenmedizin und Parasitologie*, **13**, 25–30.

Eckert, J., Kutzer, E., Rommel, M., Bürger, H.-J., and Körting, W. (1992). *Veterinärmedizinische Parasitologie*, (4th edn)., P. Parey, Berlin.

Eckert, J., Jacquier, P., Baumann, D., and Raeber, P. A. (1995). Echinokokkose des Menschen in der Schweiz, 1984–1992. *Schweizerische Medizinische Wochenschrift*, **125**, 1989–98.

Emery, I., Bories, C., Liance, M., and Houin, R. (1995). *In vitro* quantitative assessment of *Echinococcus multilocularis* metacestode viablity after *in vivo* and *in vitro* maintenance. *International Journal for Parasitology*, **25**, 275–8.

Ewald, D. (1993). Prävalenz von *Echinococcus multilocularis* bei Rotfüchsen (*Vulpes vulpes* L.). in der Nord-, Ost-und Südschweiz sowie im Fürstentum Liechtenstein. Ph.D. Thesis, Phil. II, University of Zürich.

Frank, W. (1989). *Survival* of *Echinococcus multilocularis* eggs in the environment and potential modes of transmission. WHO Informal Consultation on Alveolar Echinococcosis, 14–16, August 1989, Hohenheim (WHO/VPH/ECHIN. RES./ WP/89).

Frosch, M. and Lucius, R. (1994). Echinokokkose. In *Immunologische und molekulare Parasitologie*, (ed. M. Röllinghoff and M. Rommel), pp. 187–206. Gustav Fischer Verlag, Jena.

Fujioka, Y., Hobi, S., Sato, N., and Uchino, J. (1993). Pathology. In *Alveolar echinococcosis of the liver*, (ed. J. Uchino and N. Sato), pp. 51–62. Hokkaido University School of Medicine, Sapporo, Japan.

Gabrion, C., Walbaum, S., Al Nahhas, Mesnil, M., and Petavy, A. F. (1995). *Echinococcus multilocularis* protoscoleces and hepatic cell activity *in vitro*. *International Journal for Parasitology*, **25**, 127–30.

Gasser, R. and Chilton, N. B. (1995). Characterisation of taeniid cestode species by PCR-RFLP of ITS2 ribosomal DNA. *Acta Tropica*, **59**, 31–40.

Gasser, R. B., Jenkins, D. J., Paolillo, E., Parada, L., Cabrera, P., and Craig, P. S. (1993). Serum antibodies in canine echinococcosis. *International Journal for Parasitology*, **23**, 579–86.

Gemmell, M. A. and Lawson, A. J. R. (1986). Epidemiology and control of hydatid disease. In *The biology of* Echinococcus *and Hydatid Disease*, (ed. R. C. A. Thompson), pp. 189–216. Allen and Unwin, London.

Gemmell, M. A. and Roberts, M. G. (1995). Modelling of *Echinococcus* life cycles. In *Echinococcus and hydatid disease*, (ed. R. C. A. Thompson and A. J. Lymbery), pp. 333–54. CAB International, Wallingford, Oxon.

Giraudoux, P. (1991). Utilisation de l'espace par les hotes du Tenia multiloculaire (*Echinococcus multilocularis*): conséquences épidémiologiques. Thesis, Université Dijon.

Gloor, B. (1988). Echinokokkose beim Menschen in der Schweiz 1970–1983. Medical Dissertation, University of Zurich.

Gottstein, B. (1992). *Echinococcus multilocularis* infection: immunology and immunodiagnosis. *Advances in Parasitology*, **31**, 321–80.

Gottstein, B. and Bettens, F. (1994). Association between HLA-DR13 and susceptibility to alveolar echinococcosis (letter). *Journal of Infectious Diseases*, **169**, 1416–17.

Gottstein, B. and Felleisen, R. (1995). Protective immune mechanisms against *Echinococcus multilocularis*. *Parasitology Today*, **11**, 320–6.

Gottstein, B. and Mowatt, M. R. (1991). Sequencing and characterization of an *Echinococcus multilocularis* DNA probe and its use in the polymerase chain reaction. *Molecular and Biochemical Parasitology*, **44**, 183–93.

Gottstein, B. *et al.* (1991). Serological (Em2-ELISA) and parasitological examinations of fox populations for *Echinococcus multilocularis* infections. *Journal of Veterinary Medicine B*, **38**, 161–8.

Gottstein, B., Deplazes, P., and Aubert, M. (1992). *Echinococcus multilocularis* immunological study on the 'Em2-positive' laminated layer during *in vitro* and *in vivo* post-oncospheral and larval development. *Parasitology Research*, **78**, 291–7.

Gottstein, B., Jacquier, P., Bresson-Hadni, S., and Eckert, J. (1993). Improved primary immunodiagnosis of alveolar echinococcosis in humans by an enzyme-linked immunosorbent assay using the Em2 plus antigen. *Journal of Clinical Microbiology*, **31**, 373–6.

Hemphill, A. and Gottstein, B. (1995). Immunology and morphology studies on the proliferation of *in vitro* cultivated *Echinococcus multilocularis* metacestodes. *Parasitology Research*, **81**, 605–14.

Horton, J. (1996). Albendazole: A review of the pharmacology, pharmacokinetics, clinical efficacy and safety in hydatid disease. In *Alveolar echinococcosis*, (ed. J. Uchino and N. Sato), pp. 261–82. Fuji Shoin, Sapporo, Japan.

Howell, M. J. and Smyth, J. D. (1995). Maintenance and cultivation of *Echinococcus* species *in vivo* and *in vitro*. In *Echinococcus and hydatid disease*, (ed. R. C. A. Thompson and A. J. Lymbery), pp. 201–32. CAB International, Wallingford, Oxon.

Ishige, M., Yagi, K., and Itoh, T. (1990). Egg production and life span of *Echinococcus multilocularis* in dogs, Hokkaido, Japan. *International Workshop on Alveolar Hydatid Disease, 7–8 June 1990, Anchorage, Alaska.* Abstracts, pp. 14–15.

Ishizu, H. *et al.* (1996). Adjuvant chemotherapy for alveolar echinococcosis: Complete response of residual alveolar echinococcosis by albendazole administration. In *Alveolar echinococcosis* (ed. J. Uchino and N. Sato), pp. 293–7. Fuji Shoin, Sapporo, Japan.

Ito, A. (1996). Serodiagnosis of alveolar and cystic echinococcosis by Em18 and Em16 Western blot analysis. In *Alveolar echinococcosis*, (ed. J. Uchino and N. Sato), pp. 139–46. Fuji Shoin, Sapporo, Japan.

Jura, H., Bader, A., Hartmann, M., Maschek, H. and Frosch, M. (1996). Hepatic tissue culture model for study of host-parasite interactions in alveolar echinococcosis. *Infection and Immunity* **64**, 3484–90.

Kamiya, M. and Sato, H. (1990*a*). Complete life cycle of the canid tapeworm, *Echinococcus multilocularis*, in laboratory rodents. *FASEB Journal*, **4**, 3334–9.

Kamiya, M. and Sato, H. (1990*b*). Survival, strobilation and sexual maturation of *Echinococcus multilocularis* in the small intestine of golden hamsters. *Parasitology*, **100**, 125–30.

Kazacos, K. R. and Storandt, S. T. (1997). *Echinococcus multilocularis* in North America. *Proceedings 42nd Annual Meeting of the American Association of Veterinary Parasitologists, July 19–22, 1997, Reno, Nevada (Abstract No. 131).*

Kern, P. *et al.* (1995). Diagnosis of *Echinococcus multilocularis* infection by reverse-transcription transcription polymerase chain reaction. *Gastroenterology*, **109**, 596–600.

Kolarova, L., Pavlasek, I. and Chalupsky, J. (1996). *Echinococcus multilocularis* Leuckart, 1863 in the Czech Republic. *Helminthologia* **33**, 59–65.

Labhardt, F. (1990). *Der Rotfuchs*. P. Parey, Hamburg.

Lightowlers, M. W. and Gottstein, B. (1995). Echinococcosis/hydatidosis: antigens, immunological and molecular diagnosis. In *Echinococcosis and hydatid disease*, (ed. R. C. A. Thompson and A. J. Lymbery), pp. 355–410. CAB International, Wallingford, Oxon.

Liu, Y. H., Wang, X. G., and Chen, Y. T. (1991). Preliminary observation of continuous albendazole therapy in alveolar echinococcosis. *Chinese Medical Journal*, **104**, 930–3.

Lopera, R. D., Melendez, R. D., Fernandez, I., Sirit, J., and Perera, M. P. (1989). Orbital hydatid cyst of *Echinococcus oligarthrus* in a human in Venezuela. *Journal of Parasitology*, **75**, 467–70.

Lymbery, A. J. (1995). Genetic diversity, genetic differentiation and speciation in the genus *Echinococcus* Rudolphi 1801. In *Echinococcus and hydatid disease*, (ed. R. C. A. Thompson and A. J. Lymbery), pp. 51–87. CAB International, Wallingford, Oxon.

McManus, D. P. and Bryant, C. (1995). Biochemistry, physiology and molecular biology of *Echinococcus*. In *Echinococcus and hydatid disease*, (ed. R. C. A. Thompson and A. J. Lymbery), pp. 135–81. CAB International, Wallingford, Oxon.

Malczewski, A., Rocki, B., Ramisz, A., and Eckert, J. (1995). *Echinococcus multilocularis* (Cestoda), the causative agent of alveolar echinococcosis in humans: First record in Poland. *Journal of Parasitology*, **81**, 318–21.

Mathis, A., Deplazes, P., and Eckert, J. (1996) improved test system for PCR-based specific detection of *Echinococcus multilocularis* eggs. *Journal of Helminthology*, **70**, 219–22.

Mehlhorn, H., Eckert, J., and Thompson, R. C. A. (1983). Proliferation and metastases formation of larval *Echinococcus multilocularis*: II. Ultrastructural investigations. *Zeitschrift für Parasitenkunde*, **69**, 749–63.

Meneghelli, U. G., Martinelli, A. L., Bellucci, A. D., Villanova, M., and Magro, J. E. (1992). Polycystic hydatid disease (*Echinococcus vogeli*). Treatment with albendazole. *Annals of Tropical Medicine and Parasitology*, **86**, 151–6.

Mesarina-Wicki, B. (1991). Long-term course of alveolar echinococcosis in 70 patients treated by benzimidazole derivatives (mebendazole and albendazole), (1976–1989). Medical Dissertation, University of Zurich.

Morris, D. L. and Richards, K. S. (1992). *Hydatid disease. Current medical and surgical management.* Butterworth-Heinemann, Oxford.

Nagano, H., Sato, C., and Furuya, K. (1996). Seroprevalence of human alveolar echinococcosis demonstrated by Western blotting in Hokkaido. In *Alveolar echinococcosis*, (ed. J. Uchino and N. Sato), pp. 135–8. Fuji Shoin, Sapporo, Japan.

Nakajima, Y., Sato, N., and Uchino, J. (1993). Stage of the disease. In *Alveolar echinococosis of the liver*, (ed. J. Uchino and N. Sato), pp. 115–19. Hokkaido University School of Medicine, Sapporo, Japan.

Nonaka N., *et al.* (1996). A diagnostic method for the definitive host of *Echinococcus multilocularis* by coproantigen detection. In *Alveolar echinococcosis*, (ed. J. Uchino and N. Sato), pp. 147–9. Fuji Shoin, Sapporo, Japan.

Nothdurft, H. D., Jelinek, T., Mai, A., Sigl, B., von Sonnenburg, F., and Löscher, T. (1995). Epidemiology of alveolar echinococcosis in Southern Germany (Bavaria). *Infection*, **23**, 85–8.

Obayashi, M., Rausch, R. L., and Fay, F. H. (1971). On the ecology and distribution of *Echinococcus* spp. (Cestoda: Taeniidae), and characteristics of their development in the intermediate host. II. Comparative studies on the development of larval *E. multilocularis* Leuckart, 1863, in the intermediate host. *Japanese Journal of Veterinary Research*, **19**, suppl., 1–63.

Ohbayashi, M. (1996). Host animals of *Echinococcus multilocularis* in Hokkaido. In *Alveolar echinococcosis*, (ed. J. Uchino and N. Sato), pp. 59–64. Fuji Shoin, Sapporo, Japan.

PAHO (1995). *Proceedings of the Scientific Working Group on the Advances in the Prevention, Control and Treatment of Hydatidosis, Pan American Health Organization, Montevideo, 26–28 October, 1994.*

Pétavy, A. F., Deblock, S., and Walbaum, S. (1991). Life cycles of *Echinococcus multilocularis* in relation to human infection. *Journal of Parasitology*, **77**, 133–7.

Playford, M. C., Ooi, H. K., Oku, Y., and Kamiya, M. (1993). Rodent intermediate host models for alveolar echinococcosis: biology and immunology. In *Alveolar echinococcosis of the liver*, (ed. J. Uchino and N. Sato), pp. 33–49. Hokkaido University School of Medicine, Sapporo, Japan.

Posselt, A. (1928). Der Alveolarechinokokkus und seine Chirurgie. In *Die Echinokokkenkrankheit*, (ed. G. Hosenmann, E. Schwarz, J. C. Lehmann, and A. Posselt), pp. 305–418. F. Enke, Stuttgart.

Rausch, R. L., (1986). Life-cycle patterns and geographic distribution of *Echinococcus* species. In *The biology of Echinococcus and hydatid disease*, (ed. R. C. A. Thompson). pp. 44–80. George Allen and Unwin, London.

Rausch, R. L. (1995). Life cycle patterns and geographic distribution of *Echinococcus* species. In *Echinococcus and hydatid disease*, (ed. R. C. A. Thompson and A. J. Lymbery), pp. 88–134. CAB International, Wallingford, Oxon.

Rausch, R. L. and Bernstein, J. J. (1972). *Echinococcus vogeli* sp. n. (Cestoda: Taeniidae) from the bush dog, *Speothos venaticus* (Lund). *Zeitschrift für Tropenmedizin und Parasitologie*, **23**, 25–34.

Rausch, R. and Schiller, E. L. (1954). Studies on the helminth fauna of Alaska: XXIV. *Echinococcus sibiricensis* n. sp., from St. Lawrence Island. *Journal of Parasitology*, **40**, 659–62.

Rausch, R. L., Wilson, J. F., Schantz, P. M., and McMahon, B. J. (1987). Spontaneous death of *Echinoccocus multilocularis*: cases diagnosed serologically (by Em2 ELISA) and clinical significance. *American Journal of Tropical Medicine and Hygiene*, **36**, 576–85.

Rausch, R. L., Fay, F. H., and Williamson, F. S. (1990). The ecology of *Echinococcus multilocularis* (Cestoda: Taeniidae) on St. Lawrence Island, Alaska. II. Helminth populations in the definitive host. *Annales de Parasitologie Humaine et Comparée*, **65**, 131–40.

Roberts, M. G. and Aubert, M. F. A. (1995). A model for the control of *Echinococcus multilocularis* in France. *Veterinary Parasitology*, **56**, 67–74.

Romig, T. *et al.* (1996). Ein Pilotprojekt zur Bekämpfung von *Echinococcus multilocularis* in Baden-Württemberg. 17. *Tagung der Deutschen Gesellschaft für Parasitologie, 27–29 March 1996, München* (Abstract).

Rommel, M., Grelck, H., and Hörchner, F. (1976). Zur Wirksamkeit von Praziquantel gegen Bandwürmer in experimentell infizierten Hunden und Katzen. *Berliner und Münchener Tierärztliche Wochenschrift*, **89**, 255–7.

Sakamoto, T. and Sugimura, M. (1970). Studies on echinococcosis: XXIII. Electron microscopical observations on histogenesis of larval *Echinococcus multilocularis*. *Japanese Journal of Veterinary Research*, **17**, 131–44.

Sato, C., Nagano, H., and Furuya, K. (1996a). A diagnostic polysaccharide antigen in human alveolar hydatid disease. In *Alveolar echinococcosis*, (ed. J. Uchino and N. Sato), pp. 129–34. Fuji Shoin, Sapporo, Japan.

Sato, N., Uchino, J., Aoki, S., Katayama, F., Kon, H., Ishizu, H. and Yamashita, K. (1996b). Metastases in human alveolar echinococcosis of the liver. In: *Alveolar echinococcosis* Uchino, J. and Sato, N. (Eds.), pp. 219–223. Fuji Shoin: Sapporo, Japan.

Sato, N., Aoki, S., Matsushita, M., and Uchino, J. (1993a). Clinical features. In *Alveolar echinococcosis of the liver*, (ed. J. Uchino and N. Sato), pp. 63–8. Hokkaido University School of Medicine, Sapporo, Japan.

Sato, N. *et al.* (1993b). Mass screening. In *Alveolar echinococcosis of the liver*, (ed. J. Uchino and N. Sato), pp. 121–9. Hokkaido University School of Medicine, Sapporo, Japan.

Sato, N., Uchino, J., and Suzuki, K. (1993c). Chemotherapy. In *Alveolar echinococcosis of the liver*, (ed. J. Uchino and N. Sato), pp. 151–66. Hokkaido University School of Medicine, Sapporo, Japan.

Schantz, P. M. (1993). Echinococcus multilocularis in North America. In *Alveolar echinococcosis of the liver*, (ed. J. Uchino and N. Sato), pp. 11–20. Hokkaido University School of Medicine, Sapporo, Japan.

Schantz, P. M. *et al.* (1995). Epidemiology and control of hydatid disease. In *Echinococcus and hydatid disease*, (ed. R. C. A. Thompson and A. J. Lymbery), pp. 233–331. CAB International, Wallingford, Oxon.

Schantz, P. M., Eckert, J., and Craig, P. S. (1996). Geographic distribution, epidemiology, and control of *Echinococcus multilocularis* and alveolar echinococcosis. In *Alveolar echinococcosis*, (ed. J. Uchino and N. Sato), pp. 1–25. Fuji Shoin, Sapporo, Japan.

Schelling, U., Frank, W., Will, R., Romig, T. and Lucius, R. (1997). Chemotherapy with praziquantel has the potential to reduce the prevalence of *Echinococcus multilocularis* in wild foxes (*Vulpes vulpes*). *Annals of Tropical Medicine and Parasitology* **91**, 179–186.

Scherbakov, A. (1996). Human echinococcosis: role of histocompatibility antigens in the realization of invasions and specific features of their course. In *Alveolar echinococcosis*, (ed. J. Uchino and N. Sato), pp. 115–21. Fuji Shoin, Sapporo, Japan.

Stehr-Green, J. K., Stehr-Green, P. A., Schantz, P. M., Wilson, J. F., and Lanier, A. (1988). Risk factors for infection with *Echinococcus multilocularis* in Alaska. *American Journal of Tropical Medicine and Hygiene*, **38**, 380–5.

Sturm, D., Menzel, J., Gottstein, B., and Kern, P. (1995). Interleukin-5 is the predominant cytokine produced by peripheral blood mononuclear cells in alveolar echinococcosis. *Infection and Immunity*, **63**, 1688–97.

Swiderski, Z. (1983). *Echinococcus granulosus*: hook-muscle systems and cellular organisation of infective oncospheres. *International Journal for Parasitology*, **13**, 289–99.

Thomas, L. J. and Babero, B. B. (1956). Observations on the infectivity of *Echinococcus* eggs obtained from foxes (*Alopex lagopus* Linn.) on St. Lawrence Island, Alaska. *Journal of Parasitology*, **42**, 659.

Thompson, R. C. A. (1995). Biology and systematics of *Echinococcus*. In *Biology and hydatid disease*, (ed. R. C. A. Thompson and A. J. Lymbery), pp. 1–50. CAB International, Wallingford, Oxon.

Thompson, R. C. A. and Eckert, J. (1982). The production of eggs by *Echinococcus multilocularis* in the laboratory following *in vivo* and *in vitro* development. *Zeitschrift für Parasitenkunde*, **68**, 227–34.

Thompson, R. C. A. and Eckert, J. (1983). Observations on *Echinococcus multilocularis* in the definitive host. *Zeitschrift für Parasitenkunde*, **69**, 335–45.

Thompson, R. C. A. Deplazes, P., and Eckert, J. (1990). Uniform strobilar development of *Echinococcus multilocularis* in vitro from protoscolex to immature stages. *Journal of Parasitology*, **76**, 240–7.

Thompson, R. C. A., Lymbery, A. J., and Constantine, C. C. (1995). Variation in *Echinococcus*: Towards a taxonomic revision of the genus. *Advances in Parasitology*, **35**, 145–76.

Torgerson, P. R., Pilkington, J., Gulland, F. M. D., and Gemmell, M. A. (1995). Further evidence for the long distance dispersal of taeniid eggs. *International Journal for Parasitology*, **25**, 265–7.

Uchino, J. and Sato, N. (ed.) (1993). *Alveolar echinococcosis of the liver*. Hokkaido University School of Medicine, Sapporo, Japan.

Uchino, J. and Sato, N. (ed.) (1996). *Alveolar echinococcosis*, pp. 1–327. Fuji Shoin, Sapporo, Japan.

Uchino, J., Sato, N., Nakajima, Y., Matsushita, M., Takahashi, M., and Une, Y. (1993). Treatment. In *Alveolar echinococcosis of the liver*, (ed. J. Uchino and N. Sato), pp. 137–49. Hokkaido University School of Medicine, Sapporo, Japan.

Uysal, V. and Paksoy, N. (1986). *Echinococcus multilocularis* in Turkey. *Journal of Tropical Medicine and Hygiene*, **89**, 249–55.

Veit, P., Bilger, B., Schad, V., Schäfer, J., Frank, W., and Lucius, R. (1995). Influence of environmental factors on the infectivity of *Echinococcus multilocularis* eggs. *Parasitology*, **110**, 79–86.

Vogel, H. (1957). Über den *Echinococcus multilocularis* Süddeutschlands. I. Das Bandwurmstadium von Stämmen menschlicher und tierischer Herkunft. *Zeitschrift für Tropenmedizin und Parasitologie*, **8**, 404–54.

Vogel, H. (1978). Wie wächst der Alveolarechinokokkus? *Tropenmedizin und Parasitologie*, **29**, 1–11.

Vuitton, D. *et al.* (1984). Humoral and cellular immunity in patients with hepatic alveolar echinococcosis. A 2 year follow-up with and without flubendazole treatment. *Parasite Immunology*, **6**, 329–40.

Wen, H. *et al.* (1994). Albendazole chemotherapy for human cystic and alveolar echinococcosis in north-western China. *Transactions of the Royal Society of Tropical Medicine and Hygiene*, **88**, 340–3.

Wilson, J. F., Rausch, R. L. and Wilson, F. R. (1995). Alveolar hydatid disease. Review of the surgical experience in 42 cases of active disease among Alaskan Eskimos. *Annals of Surgery*, **221**, 315–23.

WHO (1994). Parasitic disease surveillance. Alveolar echinococcosis. *Weekly Epidemiological Record*, **68**, 160–2.

WHO (1996). Guidelines for treatment of cystic and alveolar echinococcosis in humans. WHO Informal Working Group on Echinococosis. *Bulletin of the World Health Organization*, **74**, 231–42.

Yagi, K., Ito, T., and Ishige, M. (1996). A survival strategy of *Echinococcus multilocularis* presumed by experimental studies. In *Alveolar echinococcosis*, (ed. J. Uchino and N. Sato), pp. 97–9. Fuji Shoin, Sapporo, Japan.

Yamashita, J. (1960). On the susceptibility and histogenesis of *Echinococcus multilocularis* in the experimental mouse, with the state of echinococcosis in Japan. *Parassitologia*, **2**, 399–406.

Zeyhle, E. (1982). Die Verbreitung von *Echinococcus multilocularis* in Südwestdeutschland. In *Probleme der Echinokokkose unter Berücksichtigung parasitologischer und klinischer Aspekte*, (ed. R. Bähr), pp. 26–33. H. Huber, Bern.

54   SCHISTOSOMOSIS

M. G. Taylor

SUMMARY

Schistosomosis remains one of the great endemic diseases of the tropics and subtropics, with more than 200 million people infected in 74 countries and a further 400 million at risk of infection. The disease is also of veterinary significance, with high prevalences of infection being reported from many countries, particularly those in tropical areas, though in very few instances are accurate epidemiological data available for the animal disease.

Schistosomosis is caused by blood flukes (trematodes) of many different species: the majority of human cases are due to *S. mansoni*, *S. haematobium*, and *S. japonicum*, while the animal disease is caused by a large number of different species, such as *S. spindale*, *S. indicum*, *S. nasale* and *S. japonicum* in Asia and *S. bovis* and *S. mattheei* in Africa. *Schistosoma japonicum* is a major zoonosis, with a large variety of domestic and wild mammals found naturally infected, and contributing substantially to transmission. *Schistosoma mansoni* also quite frequently infects rodents and non-human primates but these hosts are believed not to contribute in a major way to transmission of the disease to man. *Schistosoma haematobium* is found occasionally in non-human primates in Africa but these infections seem to be of no epidemiological significance.

In all cases the intermediate host is an aquatic or amphibious snail and man and animals become infected when their skin is penetrated directly by the cercaria larvae produced by infected snails. Most of the pathology of schistosome infections is caused by the parasite eggs. When these exit the body they cause haemorrhage in the target organs (the bladder in the case of *S. haematobium*, since the adult worms are found in the vesical plexus; the nasal mucosa in the case of the bovine parasite, *S. nasale*, the adult worms of which live in the veins of the submucosa of the nose; the intestine wall in all other instances, since the worms inhabit the mesenteric veins). Most of the pathology of human schistosomosis is due to fibro-obstructive lesions associated with eggs trapped in the tissues, while in the animal disease the major signs are due to loss of blood from the gut caused by exit of the eggs from the tissues. In addition, penetration of the human skin by cercariae of animal or bird schistosomes can cause a severe form of dermatitis.

The outcome of schistosome infection is influenced by many factors, such as the species of infecting parasite, the intensity and duration of infection, host genetic make-up, and acquired immunity. In endemic areas, prevalence of schistosomosis is often very high, with essentially all young individuals being infected, but even so, because the adult worms do not multiply in the body, most infections are light, and only in the case of the heavily infected minority does significant disease occur. Occasionally, however, epidemics occur due to exacerbation of transmission by ecological factors or the exposure of large numbers of non-immune individuals.

Control of human schistosomosis has been attempted for many years and has usually been based on a mixture of measures directed against the snail hosts and chemotherapeutic treatment of man and reservoir hosts, together with environmental management and public health measures. For the past 15 years such efforts have been greatly facilitated by the availability of a highly effective oral schistosomicide, praziquantel. Control programmes have achieved the complete eradication of the disease in Japan, and a great reduction in China and in several other countries formerly of major endemicity. However, little has been achieved in vast regions of sub-Saharan Africa, where, due to socioeconomic and demographic changes and the expansion of irrigation, transmission of schistosomosis persists unabated. As far as schistosomosis of farm animals is concerned, the disease has been eliminated in Japan and greatly reduced in China and the Philippines, but elsewhere has been largely ignored, although the situation may be changing now that the economic importance of the animal disease is becoming accepted, and effective treatment is available. Intensive research is continuing on the development of vaccines for both animal and human disease; the availability of cost-effective vaccines would revolutionize prospects for control.

HISTORY

As reviewed by Grove (1990) and Ouma and Fenwick (1991), it is clear from hieroglyphic records and from parasitological examination of mummified remains that human schistosomosis was endemic in Dynastic Egypt. Remarkably, schistosomosis has now been diagnosed in a 5000-year-old Predynastic mummy using an antigen-detection assay (Miller *et al.* 1992). It was not until 1852, however, that the adult worms were first recovered from a human body, while a further 65 years elapsed before the three main human schistosome species and their complex life cycles were clearly described (Taylor 1994). Subsequently, several other species were found in man, most recently the *S. japonicum*-like parasite *S. malayensis*, described in 1988 (Chen 1993). Schistosomes (*S. bovis*) were first discovered in livestock (also in Egypt) in 1876. Many other species of veterinary significance have since been discovered, the most recent being *S. curassoni*, the validity of which was established by Vercruysse *et al.* in 1984.

Following elucidation of the schistosome life cycle in the second decade of the twentieth century, knowledge of the biology, epidemiology, and pathogenesis of schistosomes grew rapidly. The efficacy of trivalent antimonial drugs as schistosomicides was soon discovered, and integrated control measures adopted in some heavily endemic areas. Globally, schistosomosis is recognized as being the most important human helminth infection, ranking second to malaria among parasitic causes of human ill-health. The first life cycle to be elucidated was that of *S. japonicum*, and it was realized from the outset that this was a major zoonosis, as well as being a cause of disease in domestic animals. Subsequently, many other 'animal' species of schistosomes were also found to be infective to man, though here the role of animals as reservoirs of human infection is less significant than for *S. japonicum*.

THE AGENT

TAXONOMY

Schistosomes are digenetic trematodes ('flukes') of the superfamily Schistosomatoidea of the phylum Platyhelminthes (Schmidt and Roberts 1989). They are dioecious worms living in the blood vascular system of reptiles, fish, birds, and mammals ('blood flukes').

All the schistosomes which mature in birds and mammals belong to the family Schistosomatidae, which contains 12 genera. The genera *Schistosoma* and *Orientobilharzia* contain the major species of medical and veterinary significance, but the other genera are of some medical importance as causes of cercarial dermatitis (Rollinson and Southgate 1987). By far the most important genus is *Schistosoma*, which contains 19 species, of which five (*S. haematobium*, *S. mansoni*, *S. japonicum*, *S. mekongi*, and *S. intercalatum*) are of prime medical importance while the others are essentially parasites of non-human mammals (although zoonotic transmission of some of these to man does occur) though they do cause cercarial dermatitis in man. Many of the 'non-human' species are of veterinary importance, including *S. bovis*, *S. japonicum*, *S. indicum*, *S. spindale*, *S. incognitum*, *S. mattheei*, *S. curassoni*, *S. margrebowiei*, *S. nasale*, *S. leiperi*, and *Orientobilharzia dattai*, *O. bomfordi*, *O. harinasutai*, and *O. turkestanicum* (Rollinson and Southgate 1987; Taylor 1987). Cercarial dermatitis in man is usually attributed to 'animal' species of *Schistosoma* and to bird and mammalian species in the genera *Trichobilharzia*, *Gigantobilharzia*, *Schistosomatium*, *Austrobilharzia*, *Microbilharzia*, and *Ornithobilharzia* (Hoeffler 1987).

Differentiation of schistosome species was classically based on morphological and biological criteria and isoenzyme comparisons (Rollinson and Southgate 1987) but is now being powerfully augmented by the use of molecular techniques such as mapping of restriction sites in the rRNA gene complexes, DNA sequence analysis, and the random amplification of polymorphic DNA using the polymerase chain reaction (Walker *et al.* 1986; Omer Ali *et al.* 1991; Barral *et al.* 1993; Johnston *et al.* 1993; Neto *et al.* 1993; Kane and Rollinson 1994; Kaukas *et al.* 1994).

STRUCTURE, BIOLOGY AND LIFE CYCLE

Unlike all other medically important trematodes, schistosomes are dioecious (rather than hermaphroditic). Adult *Schistosoma* are about 1 cm long and the male has a deep ventral groove or schist (hence 'schistosome') in which the female worm permanently resides *in copulo*. Each sex has a mouth at the anterior end which also serves as the anus since there is only a single gut opening. Around the mouth is the oral sucker while nearby more posteriorly is the ventral sucker. These suckers are much better developed in the male worms and it is the male worms which are mainly responsible for adhering to the venous epithelium and for conducting locomotion of the worm pair. Nearly all our detailed knowledge of schistosome biology is derived from work on human schistosomes, particularly *S. mansoni*, which is the species most readily passaged in the laboratory. To obtain amino acids for protein synthesis adult *S. mansoni* ingest red blood cells and break down the haemoglobin with a haemoglobinase. Small molecules (including glucose, amino acids, purines, and pyrimidines) are taken up via transtegumentary absorption and there is evidence that the female (who is largely enclosed in the schist of the male) derives much of her nutrition via transtegumentary absorption from the male worm. The metabolism of the adult schistosomes is largely anaerobic, by glycolysis (Rumjanek 1987).

Adult *Schistosoma* parasitizing man live a long time (up to 30 years, with a mean of 3–6 years (Anderson 1987) and produce a large number of eggs (300/female/day for *S. mansoni* and *S. haematobium* and 10 times as many for *S. japonicum*). These are large (e.g. 145 × 60 μm for *S. mansoni*) and consist of an egg shell of tanned protein containing, when laid, about 40 yolk cells and the oocyte. The eggs mature after about 1 week in the tissues to contain the large (150 × 70 μm) ciliated miracidium larva, which is the life-cycle stage which is infective to the snail host.

The adult worms are found either in the vesical plexus of the human bladder (*S. haematobium*), the nasal capillaries of bovines (*S. nasale*) or in the mesenteric veins (all the other species). The eggs are laid there and transit to the lumen of the bladder (*S. haematobium*), the nasal passages (*S. nasale*), or the intestine (other species) where they exit the body in urine, nasal discharge, or faeces, respectively. Eggs retained in the tissues induce granulomatous lesions and fibrosis. Eggs are the main cause of clinical disease, the adult worms themselves being essentially harmless (Warren 1978).

Embryonated eggs excreted from the body hatch if deposited in water, to liberate the free-swimming miradium larvae. If the miradia are able to locate an appropriate type of snail host within a few hours they penetrate the snail; otherwise the miracidia (which do not feed) will die.

Within the tissues of the snail the miracidium transforms into the mother sporocyst within which are formed several hundred daughter sporocysts. These migrate from the site of penetration to the digestive gland and reproductive tract of the snail, in which they proliferate internally to produce cercariae, the stage which is infective to man. This process takes about 1 month in the snail, and from one miracidium up to several million genetically identical cercariae may be produced by this asexual process during the life time of the infected snail.

The cercariae are shed from the snail in response to temperature and light stimuli and aggregate at the surface of the water ready to infect the human definitive host. They swim tail first and locate the host by responding to host chemical and temperature signals (Haas *et al.* 1994) and adhere to the skin using their suckers. The cercaria is approximately 0.5 mm long and consists of a head end bearing the oral and ventral suckers and a tail with a pronounced fork. Cercariae respire aerobically using glycogen as a substrate but do not feed, and if they do not penetrate the final host within a few hours they die.

The life cycle of *S. mansoni* has been worked out in great detail in the mouse model (the behaviour in the natural human host appears to be similar). Cercariae penetrate the skin rapidly, using proteolytic enzymes produced by the paired penetration glands at their anterior ends; the tail is discarded in the water. Within the skin a profound metamorphosis takes place and the cercaria is transformed into the 'skin-stage schistosomulum'. Metamorphosis includes shedding of the cercarial glycocalyx, transformation from the single lipid bilayer tegument of the cercaria into the double lipid bilayer of the schistosomulum, and various physiological changes such as a switch from aerobic to anaerobic respiration, and the acquisition of host molecules, particularly lipids, some of which are incorporated into the tegument (Wilson 1987).

The schistosomulum next penetrates the tough basement membrane of the epidermis, using proteinases secreted by the residual penetration glands of the cercaria stage. In mice this process takes about 3 days after which the schistosomulum enters a lymphatic or capillary in the dermis and is carried passively to the lungs via the right side of the heart (Wilson 1987). The young schistosomula embolize in the capillaries, being too wide to pass through to the pulmonary veins, whereupon they again metamorphose, this time to the 'lung-stage schistosomulum', which, unlike the skin stage, is capable of stretching out its body to become long and thin. Because of their newly acquired thin cross-section, the schistosomula are now able to cross the capillary bed of the lungs, taking 3–6 days to reach the left side of the heart (Wilson 1987). They are now distributed all over the body via the left ventricle, in proportion to cardiac output. Schistosomula embolizing in various capillary beds migrate through these to regain the heart and recirculate until they reach the hepatic portal system, a process usually completed within three recirculations. When the hepatic portal system is reached, a third metamorphosis takes place, the elongate migratory forms returning to the squat shape of the skin stage schistosomula. Blood feeding begins and this is followed by a growth spurt, organogenesis, and sexual maturation. The mature worms pair up (copulate) in the intrahepatic portal venules from about 4 weeks onwards and then migrate to the final sites of oviposition in the mesenteric veins.

The above account, derived from studies on *S. mansoni*, probably broadly holds also for all the other species of mammalian schistosomes which parasitize the mesenteric veins, though with some variations in timing of the various phases of migration. The route by which developing *S. nasale* reach the nasal capillaries of bovines is unknown; likewise it is unclear how *S. haematobium* reach the vesical plexus, though it seems likely that this is achieved via anastomoses between the inferior mesenteric veins and the rectal and vesical plexus.

THE HOST

HUMAN

Pathogenesis

The outcome of human schistosome infection is known to be affected by many factors, including: the species of schistosome; the intensity and duration of infection; host genetic make-up (Salam *et al.* 1979; Sasazuki *et al.* 1980; Kamel *et al.* 1984; Kojima *et al.* 1984; Wishashi *et al.* 1989; Ohta *et al.* 1990; Abel *et al.* 1991; Hafez *et al.* 1991), host immunological responses (Phillips and Lammie 1986; Boros 1989; Weinstock 1992), and concomitant infections, notably hepatitis viruses (Bassily *et al.* 1992; Uemura *et al.* 1992; Chen *et al.* 1993; Darwish *et al.* 1993). Therefore the manifestations of schistosomosis vary greatly from patient to patient and between different endemic areas.

Most of the pathology of schistosome infections is due to the eggs. When these escape from the body they cause polyposis and petechial haemorrhages in the epithelium of the bladder (*S. haematobium*) and haematuria; when they exit via the gut epithelium heavy egg excretion results in polyposis and colitis. When eggs are retained in the tissues granulomas and fibro-obstructive lesions result (Warren 1978; Abdel-Wahab and Mahmoud 1987; Olvedo and Domingo 1987; Prata 1987; von Lichtenberg 1987; Wilkins and Gilles 1987; Chen and Mott 1989; Chen 1993; Farid 1993; Lambertucci 1993). *Schistosoma haematobium* adult worms reside in the vesical plexus and ureteric veins, and the worst-affected organs are therefore the bladder and ureters, where egg deposition is heaviest. In contrast, the other schistosome species all live in the mesenteric veins, depositing their eggs in the intestine and liver.

The larval forms of the schistosomes are, however, also involved in the disease process. Repeated penetrations of the skin by cercariae (particularly of non-human species of schistosomes which die in the epidermis) can cause a severe form of dermatitis, which is known to be a complex, immunologically mediated reaction involving immediate, as well as delayed hypersensitivity components (Boros 1989).

The presence of maturing schistosome infections of *S. mansoni* or *S. japonicum* can cause an acute febrile illness called Katayama syndrome or acute schistosomosis. Although exact chronologies of cercarial exposure are usually difficult to establish, it appears that in most cases the onset of this syndrome coincides with the start of egg laying by the adult worms, which occurs approximately 3–4 weeks after exposure to cercariae (eggs do not appear in the faeces for at least 1 further week). Since the symptoms of acute schistosomosis resemble those of serum sickness, acute schistosomosis may also be a form of type III immune complex disease (von Lichtenberg 1987). The cercarial glycocalyx contains carbohydrate antigens which cross-react with antigens of the egg stage and small, soluble immune complexes may be formed in the period of initial egg laying when egg antigens are present in excess over the small amounts of low-affinity antibody then present. As antibody titre and affinity increase, larger, insoluble immune complexes would be phagocytosed and the symptoms would subside. Alternatively, chemotherapeutic removal of the worms will lead to resolution by removing the source of antigen.

Mature *S. haematobium* lay their eggs in the subepithelial tissues of the bladder and the ureters. Some of these eggs exit the body via the urine, causing petechial haemorrhages which, when sufficiently numerous, result in visually obvious haematuria. The aggregation of large numbers of eggs in the superficial tissues of the bladder and ureters can lead to filling defects in the bladder and obstruction of the ureters. Eventually inflammatory polyps may subside, leaving fibrous 'sandy patches' on the urothelium. Eggs retained in the subepithelial tissues live 3 weeks, and 'mineralize', acquiring calcium and magnesium salts, and subsequently persist for many years as 'calcified' black eggs. If these are very numerous, they form a ring of radio-opaque tissue clearly visible in an X-ray, the so-called 'calcified bladder'. The progressive accumulation of eggs and the attendant inflammatory and granulomatous host reactions usually affect bladder function, frequency of micturation and dysuria being common symptoms. Stenosis of the ureters causes hydroureter and hydronephrosis, and failure of the ureteric sphincter can lead to ascending bacterial infection of the ureters and kidneys (pyelonephritis). Chronic *S. haematobium* infections have been associated with bladder cancer in some, but not all endemic areas (von Lichtenberg 1987; Wilkins and Gilles 1987; Farid 1993).

Schistosoma haematobium often migrate to the veins of pelvic organs other than the bladder and ureters to produce eggs with their attendant inflammatory/granulomatous reactions. Dead (calcified) eggs are frequently seen in the submucosa of the colon (though are rarely excreted in the faeces), where they are of little pathological consequence. More important are the reactions to eggs in the tissues of the reproductive tract: ectopic schistosomosis of the vagina, uterus, Fallopian tubes, and ovaries can result in sterilization or misdiagnosis as cancer (Berry 1966; El-Maraghy *et al.* 1982). Similarly, schistosomal orchitis can simulate malignancy (Bambirra *et al.* 1986; Mikhail *et al.* 1988). Many eggs failing to lodge in the pelvic organs are shunted to the lungs, where they cause granulomatous reactions. Central nervous system involvement is, perhaps surprisingly, rare in *S. haematobium* infection.

Mature worms of the other species, such as *S. mansoni* and *S. japonicum* deposit their eggs in the distal branches of the mesenteric veins in the submucosa of the intestine. Some eggs transit the bowel and exit the body via the faeces, causing as they do so petechial haemorrhages which may often give rise to visible traces of blood in the faeces. Large clusters of eggs in the mucosa can cause the formation of haemorrhagic polyps and colitis with resulting serious blood loss and colonic dysfunction (El Masry *et al.* 1986; Mohamed *et al.* 1990).

Many eggs are retained in the tissues, fail to lodge in the submucosa and are swept downstream to the intrahepatic branches of the hepatic portal vein. Being too large (approximately 45 μm in diameter) to enter the sinusoids they embolize and elicit granulomatous reactions. Large granulomas are formed in sensitized individuals, 100 times the volume of the eggs themselves. The granulomas consist of a complex mixed population of cell types, mostly lymphocytes, monocytes, macrophages, eosinophils, epithelioid cells, and fibroblasts. Collagen deposition occurs in granulomas both directly in response to antigens produced by the miracidium and in response to cytokines produced by granuloma lymphocytes. When the miracidium dies (after 3 weeks) further fibrosis ('scar tissue formation') may occur, although sometimes the granulomas are completely resorbed. The gradual accumulation of granulomas in the liver tissue can cause hepatomegaly and portal hypertension. Fibrosis occurs not only within the periovular granulomas but also at distant sites, around large branches of the intrahepatic portal vein, probably in response to cytokine action. In prolonged infections significant periportal fibrosis ('Symmers' fibrosis') often develops and is associated with severe portal hypertension, development of gastrooesophageal varices, and haematemesis. Splenomegaly is present, enlargement of the spleen being caused partly by congestion and partly by a reactive hyperplasia (Abel-Wahab and Mahmoud 1987; Prata 1987; von Lichtenberg 1987; Farid 1993; Lambertucci 1993).

Chronic *S. mansoni* and *S. japonicum* infections are usually well tolerated by the patients for many years because the liver lesions are restricted to the portal triads and hepatocytes function normally. However, fibrosis and collateral circulation development may progress insidiously and fatal haematemesis may occur without warning. Also, some patients develop liver failure, perhaps caused by concomitant infection with hepatitis viruses (von Lichtenberg 1987).

If collateral circulation is present, many eggs bypass the liver and instead embolize in the lungs, where progressive accumulation, granuloma formation, and fibrosis develop, leading to pulmonary arteritis and cor pulmonale (right ventricular hypertrophy). The development of collateral circulation also predisposes

to an immune complex-mediated glomerulonephritis (Andrade and Van Marck 1981).

Schistosoma mansoni and *S. japonicum*, but rarely *S. haematobium*, sometimes reach the central nervous system and cause significant disease. For unknown reasons, some eggs are usually found in the spinal cord, whereas *S. japonicum* eggs tend to localize to the brain (Norfray *et al.* 1978; El-Rooby 1985; Scrimageour and Gadjusek 1985).

Particularly when infection intensity is high, schistosomosis can lead to a decrease in working capacity (Parker 1992, 1993), and there is increasing evidence that *S. japonicum* (McGarvey *et al.* 1993), *S. haematobium* (Stephenson 1993; Stephenson *et al.* 1985, 1989) and *S. mansoni* (Jordan and Randall 1962; de Lima e Costa *et al.* 1988; Corbett *et al.* 1992) can each adversely affect child growth and nutritional status. It has been shown recently (Kimura *et al.* 1992) that *S. haematobium* infection depresses cognitive function in children.

Diagnosis

The 'gold standard' method for patent infections (i.e. infections with mature, egg-producing adult worms) is to demonstrate the presence of eggs in the urine (*S. haematobium*) or faeces (other species). In routine medical practice diagnosis is usually qualitative, rather than quantitative, but usually employs some form of concentration technique to increase sensitivity. Thus, urine samples may be centrifuged or filtered to concentrate the eggs, while eggs in faecal samples are frequently concentrated by the formol–ether technique. For most epidemiological purposes, however, quantitative egg counts are required. For this, the most popular techniques are membrane (cellulose acetate or nylon) filtration in filter holders attached to a syringe (for *S. haematobium*) and the Kato technique for eggs in faeces, which involves clearing a measured volume (weight) of faeces using a glycerine-impregnated cellophane coverslip (Feldmeier and Poggensee 1993).

In very old (chronic) or very light infections eggs may be difficult to demonstrate using the above techniques and in such cases rectal biopsy is sometimes used, followed by microscopic examination of the compressed mucosal specimens for eggs. Sometimes eggs (or adult worms) are found by histopathology during examination of biopsied lesions from other anatomical sites, or in cytological smears: *S. haematobium* eggs are frequently reported from diverse parts of the urogenital system while 'ectopic' lesions of the central nervous system, caused by *S. japonicum* or *S. mansoni* are also quite common (Chen and Mott 1989).

Schistosomosis is a protean, multisystem disease, and clinical signs and symptoms are often non-specific (Abdel-Wahab and Mahmoud 1987; Olvedo and

Domingo 1987; Prata 1987; von Lichtenberg 1987; Wilkins and Gilles 1987; Chen and Mott 1989). Thus, multiple abdominal symptoms are found in *S. mansoni*, *S. japonicum*, and *S. intercalatum* patients, of which only bloody diarrhoea is significantly associated. Other symptoms such as splenomegaly are often due to other causes, such as malaria, while hepatomegaly only occurs in 50 per cent of *S. mansoni* or *S. japonicum* cases. Schistosome eggs and associated granulomas and fibrosis are frequently detected by liver biopsy. The degree of periportal fibrosis can now be accurately assessed by ultrasonography of the liver (*S. mansoni*, *S. japonicum*, *S. intercalatum*) or urinary tract (*S. haematobium*), the latter having replaced intravenous pyelography, which was formerly the standard method of assessment (Hatz *et al.* 1992*a,b,c,d*; Jenkins and Hatz 1992; Wei-win *et al.* 1992).

In *S. haematobium* infection, presence of macroscopic or microscopic haematuria is a highly sensitive and specific diagnostic sign in some (Savioli and Mott 1989; Savioli *et al.* 1990; Lengeler *et al.* 1993), but apparently not all (Eltoum *et al.* 1992) endemic areas. For preliminary surveys, simple questionnaires eliciting a history of haematuria have been accurate enough to form the basis of subsequent control programmes in Tanzania (Lengeler *et al.* 1991*a,b*).

Cercarial dermatitis is usually diagnosed by a combination of typical appearance of the lesions, a history of probable exposure to schistosome cercariae, and immunodiagnosis (Abdel-Wahab and Mahmoud 1987).

Acute schistosomosis (Katayama syndrome) presents difficult problems of differential diagnosis because usually its onset precedes passage of eggs in the faeces and the clinical features of the disease cannot readily be distinguished from those of other acute febrile illnesses, although the presence of eosinophilia is suggestive (Abdel-Wahab and Mahmoud 1987; Prata 1987).

Particularly for *S. mansoni* and *S. japonicum* infections (on which research has concentrated) many immunodiagnostic techniques have been described in the scientific literature, although no tests are actually commercially available. This is largely because of the competition from the simple microscopic tests for egg detection, but immunodiagnostic techniques are now attracting increased attention because although microscopy is 100 per cent specific, it is insensitive (De Vlas and Gryseels 1992; De Vlas *et al.* 1993), missing many light infections (due to presence of immature worms, only a single sex of worms, or perhaps 'sterile' female worms). Further disadvantages of the parasitological techniques are that they are slow, labour intensive, require trained microscopists, are expensive, and may be hazardous (fresh urine or faeces are usually examined). In contrast, immunological tech-

niques may be more cost-effective, especially for screening large populations. In the early days, immediate hypersensitivity based intradermal testing was widespread, but this was largely abandoned in favour of more sensitive and specific tests for specific antibodies. Many of these tests have performed well in blinded multicentre trials (Mott and Dixon 1982; Mott *et al.* 1987). Purified (rather than crude) schistosome antigens are now also being evaluated and some of these, e.g. the 31/32 kDa antigens of *S. mansoni*, are available in recombinant form (Götz and Klinkert 1993). Keyhole limpet haemocyanin (KLH) shares epitopes with schistosomes and appears to have considerable diagnostic potential for *S. mansoni* (Mansour *et al.* 1989; Alves–Brito *et al.* 1992; Rabello *et al.* 1993) and *S. japonicum* infections (particularly for acute infections, Zheng *et al.* 1992) and for *S. haematobium* infections (Xue *et al.* 1993). Because this antigen is commonly used as 'carrier' by immunologists it is cheaply available in a highly purified form.

Even when the problem of sensitivity has been solved, antibody detection assays suffer from the fault of giving too many 'false positive' reactions. In many cases these may in fact be true results—it is the parasitological techniques which are giving a 'false negative' result through their inherent lack of sensitivity. But there are many cases where the immunological test is falsely positive due to the presence of residual antibody from a previous, now cured infection. This is a particular disadvantage now that large-scale chemotherapy campaigns are so frequently carried out (Bergquist 1992). A further drawback of antibody-detection methods is that the readouts (e.g. ELISA Optical Density), being determined by antibody affinity and titre, bear no simple relationship to the number of parasites present.

Antigen detection assays may solve these problems. Several systems are being developed, the most advanced being those of Deelder and colleagues using the circulating anodic and cathodic antigens CAA and CCA of *S. mansoni*. These glycoconjugate antigens are produced by the gut epithelial cells of adult schistosomes and are absent in the other life-cycle stages. They are continually excreted by adult schistosomes in their vomitus and are present in diagnostically useful amounts in both serum and urine. Some but not all epitopes of these antigens appear to be present only in schistosomes, and assays based on such epitopes are thus 100 per cent specific, but CAA and CCA are not schistosome-species specific. Sensitivity was a problem in the early days but is now essentially solved since serum levels of 1 ng/ml can now be reliably detected using a monoclonal antibody double-sandwich ELISA. Further attractions of these assays are that they can be performed on urine samples instead of serum, that they rapidly (within 6 weeks) become negative post-treatment, and that they can be presented in a user-friendly 'dipstick' format (De Jonge 1992; Deelder 1994).

Treatment

Safe and effective chemotherapy is available for all the schistosomes affecting man (Davis 1993). The most versatile drug is praziquantel, which is effective in a single oral dose against all species of schistosomes (plus some other trematodes and cestodes). It is expensive, however, and in pure *S. haematobium* areas the much cheaper metrifonate may be preferred, though this has to be given in two or three doses 2 weeks apart. Metrifonate is only effective against *S. haematobium*, while the third available drug, oxamniquine, is only effective against *S. mansoni*, for which it provides safe and effective treatment in single oral doses. None of these drugs is significantly effective against prepatent infections of immature worms, so prophylactic treatment is not available. Usually, Katayama syndrome is treated symptomatically for the hypersensitivity reactions but praziquantel is also given to kill the adult worms as these mature. In advanced or ectopic disease, surgery for anatomical consequences and complications of infection may be necessary, but even in advanced cases, antischistosomal drug therapy usually produces great improvement. It is now believed that the liver fibrosis of *S. mansoni* and *S. japonicum* disease is usually arrested by the treatment and that it may even be reversed. Similarly, in *S. haematobium* infection, it has been discovered that many cases of hydroureter and hydronephrosis are reversible by treatment (Mohamed-Ali *et al.* 1991; Hatz *et al.* 1992*a,b,c,d*; Mott *et al.* 1992; Wei-min *et al.* 1992).

ANIMAL

Pathogenesis

The pathogenesis of the various species causing domestic animal schistosomosis has been reviewed in detail (Taylor 1987; see also Yason and Novilla 1984; Vercruysse *et al.* 1985*a*; Kassuku *et al.* 1986; de Bont *et al.* 1989). *Schistosoma nasale* is unique, in that the adult schistosomes inhabit the nasal capillaries, causing a haemorrhagic, mucopurulent, nasal discharge associated with periovular granulomas. The other schistosome species all parasitize the mesenteric veins, thus causing lesions in the intestine and associated organs, the outcome depending principally on the intensity and duration of infection. The best-studied species are the African ruminant parasites *S. mattheei* and *S. bovis*, but the limited available evidence suggests that findings from these two species are representative of

animal schistosomosis in general. In a typical case of heavy primary experimental infection with *S. bovis*, calves became clinically ill around the seventh week after exposure to cercariae and during the following 2–3 months showed intermittent diarrhoea and inappetence, becoming progressively anaemic, hypoalbuminaemic, and hyperglobulinaemic, developed a marked eosiophilia, and either lost weight or failed to maintain the rate of growth recorded in uninfected animals. Subsequently, there was a slow but pronounced improvement in clinical condition of these animals and in their blood indices, but in a minority of cases the disease was fatal. The development of the anaemia and hypoalbuminaemia coincided closely with the first appearance of eggs in the faeces and was maximal when faecal egg counts and worm burden were highest. Conversely, both indices improved only after faecal egg counts had been markedly reduced and a large proportion of the initially established worms eliminated. Studies on red cell kinetics and albumin metabolism, which showed that the anaemia was basically due to an accelerated rate of loss of red cells from the circulation, which became evident around the seventh week of infection, increased in severity during the following 2 months, and subsequently subsided. In view of its close similarity to the pattern of faecal egg excretion, it was concluded that haemorrhage into the intestine caused by the exit of eggs was the prime cause: haemolysis was excluded by the absence of splenomegaly and hyperferraemia. Anaemia was exacerbated by a poor erythrokinetic response, particularly initially, and haemodilution was involved, but not to a significant extent. The hypoalbuminaemia associated with infection was caused by an increased rate of albumin catabolism and a plasma volume expansion and was accompanied by a marked depletion of all albumin pools, but particularly the extravascular pool. The pattern of albumin catabolism closely followed that of the red blood cells, suggesting that passage of plasma as whole blood was the basic cause of hypoalbuminaemia (Taylor 1987).

Most cases of naturally occurring clinical schistosomosis in animals take the form of this 'intestinal syndrome'. As in human schistosomosis, heavy involvement of the liver is present, but in animals there is no evidence of portal hypertension or its complications, such as congestive splenomegaly or gastro-oesophageal varices. It therefore seems that animals develop efficient collateral channels and thereby succeed in bypassing the portal obstruction. Another distinctive feature of the animal disease, associated with the ability of the host to mount an immune response sufficient to eliminate large numbers of established adult worms (which does not appear to be a feature of the human disease) is the development of large lymphoid nodules around dead parasites (Taylor *et al.* 1991).

Diagnosis

In Japan, China, and the Philippines, where the importance of a domestic animal reservoir of human *S. japonicum* infection has long been obvious, very large-scale diagnostic surveys of livestock have been carried out by examining faecal samples qualitatively for eggs or by carrying out miracidial hatching tests on faecal samples (Cheng 1971; Anon. 1992; Chen, 1993). Elsewhere, diagnosis has usually only been attempted when epizootics of schistosomosis are suspected. For example in Africa, when cattle or sheep develop a typical group of signs including haemorrhagic diarrhoea, inappetance, weakness, and emaciation, post-mortem examination for worms and faecal examinations are carried out to determine whether a species of *Schistosoma* is responsible (McCauley *et al.* 1983*a*,*b*). Prevalence rates are usually determined by abattoir surveys, since the adult worms can readily be found by inspection of the mesenteric veins, but quantitative faecal examination has been used in epidemiological observations on *S. bovis* infection in cattle and sheep and in monitoring field trials of *S. bovis* and *S. japonicum* vaccines in bovines (Taylor 1987).

Treatment

Schistosomicidal treatment of *S. japonicum*-infected livestock has been practised for many years and on a wide scale in China, Japan, and the Philippines, originally with trivalent antimonials, and subsequently with praziquantel (Cheng 1971; Anon. 1992; Chen 1993). Elsewhere, drug treatment of livestock has rarely been attempted, because of the unavailability of cost-effective schistosomicides (Taylor 1987). However since praziquantel has now been shown to be effective against *S. bovis* (and is likely to be effective against other schistosome species too) and because the price of this compound has fallen dramatically in recent years, drug treatment of schistosome-infected livestock is likely to become much more widespread, now that the economic impact of the animal disease is at last being recognized (McCauley *et al.* 1983*b*, 1984).

EPIDEMIOLOGY

WHO (1993) estimates that over 600 million people are exposed to the risk of schistosome infection in 74 countries, and that 200 million of these are currently infected. Schistosomosis may be the second most important parasitic disease of man, after malaria. About 95 per cent of the cases are of *S. mansoni* or *S. haematobium*, the remainder *S. japonicum*, *S. intercalatum*, and *S. mekongi*. The geographical distribution of the schistosomes roughly corresponds to the distribution of susceptible snail hosts, which are present in many tropical and subtropical regions. *Schistosoma mansoni* is the most widespread species, being prevalent in 52 countries in Africa, the Middle East, and South and Central America. *Schistosoma haematobium* has a similar distribution to *S. mansoni* in the Old World, but is absent from South America, where *Bulinus* snails do not occur. Apart from a possible small focus of *S. haematobium* in India, neither *S. mansoni* nor *S. haematobium* occurs in central or east Asia. Here, *S. japonicum* is endemic in three countries (China, the Philippines, and Indonesia) whereas the related *S. mekongi* distribution is restricted to the Mekong River basin countries of Laos and Kampuchea. In Africa, *S. mansoni* and *S. haematobium* often coexist, and mixed infections are common. *Schistosoma intercalatum*, a much rarer species than *S. mansoni* or *S. haematobium*, is restricted to limited foci in 10 central and west African countries.

Of the major schistosome species parasitizing humans, *S. japonicum* is by far the least host-specific, with 40 species of wild and domesticated mammals found naturally infected in China and being of major significance in transmission of the parasite to man (Chen 1993). Animal reservoirs are much less important for *S. mansoni* or *S. haematobium* infection. Infection of non-human primates and rodents is sometimes recorded for *S. mansoni*, but natural infection of non-human hosts with *S. haematobium* is rare, and in neither case do animal reservoirs usually contribute significantly to transmission to man (Hillyer 1982; Ouma and Fenwick 1991). Hybridization between closely related human and animal schistosome species is readily achieved in the laboratory and may be of some epidemiological significance (Taylor 1970; Southgate and Rollinson 1987; Basch 1991).

Within the different endemic areas, prevalence of infection varies greatly from area to area, being determined by many factors such as the type and size of snail populations present, human population size and behaviour, and geographical, climatic, and hydrological features, with exposure to cercaria-infested water of course being the major risk factor (Jordan and Webbe 1993). In the absence of control campaigns, prevalence is often high, with essentially all young children being infected. In common with other worm infections, however, schistosomes are not evenly distributed among infected cases, but highly aggregated in 'wormy' individuals in a manner best described by the negative binomial distribution. Since the amount of tissue damage caused by a schistosome infection is roughly proportional to the numbers of worms present, it is this heavily infected segment of the population who manifest most disease and who contribute most to the transmission of the parasite. Since schistosomes, like most other helminths, do not multiply in man, it is therefore a striking feature of schistosomal epidemiology that, though prevalence of infection may be very high, significant symptoms are only present in the small segment who are most heavily infected. Susceptibility/resistance is believed to be at least in part determined by one, or a few, major co-dominant genes (Abel *et al.* 1991).

Another important feature of schistosome epidemiology is that peak prevalence and intensity of infection usually occur in the second decade of life, after which prevalence and (even more strikingly) intensity decline significantly. This is believed to be mainly due to the gradual acquisition of immunity, although other age-related factors such as decreasing contact with infected waters and physiological changes associated with the onset of puberty also may be important (Hagan *et al.* 1991; Rihet *et al.* 1991; Dessein *et al.* 1992; Dunne *et al.* 1992).

EPIZOOTIOLOGY

Although at least 14 species of schistosomes commonly infect domestic animals, often over wide geographical ranges, the geographical distribution of very few of these species has been precisely mapped, and very few epizootiogical data are available. Most of our knowledge derives from work on the African species *S. mattheei* and *S. bovis* (reviewed by Taylor 1987; see also Majid *et al.* 1980*a*; Vercruysse *et al.* 1985; Kassaku *et al.* 1986) and more recently also on *S. curassoni* (Vercruysse *et al.* 1984, 1985*b*) and on the Asian species *S. nasale* (de Bont *et al.* 1989) and *S. spindale* (de Bont *et al.* 1991). As for human schistosomosis prevalence rates are frequently very high, but intensity of infection is usually low, except when epizootics occur. For *S. mattheei* and *S. bovis* naturally acquired immunity has been shown to be of great importance in the host–parasite relationship, with clinical disease usually only being evident in young animals. As with human schistosomosis, transmission frequently shows seasonal variations in response to climatic changes which affect the snail intermediate hosts.

PREVENTION AND CONTROL

Detailed knowledge of the life cycle of schistosomes has been available to public health workers for 80 years and from the beginning it was clear that control of schistosomosis in the community might in practice be achievable by removing the adult worms by chemotherapy, by eliminating the snail intermediate hosts by habitat modifications or chemical attack, by changing human behaviour by health education, and by providing safe water supplies and sanitation so that excreta containing live eggs do not reach water containing snails and people avoid water contaminated with cercariae.

Effective drugs indeed soon became available: trivalent antimonials were introduced in 1918, although these toxic compounds were far from ideal for control programmes, requiring repeated intravenous injections. Chemical control of snails by molluscicides became available in the 1920s, when copper sulphate was introduced for the control of the aquatic vectors of *S. mansoni* and *S. haematobium* and lime was first used to attack the amphibious vectors of *S. japonicum*.

Using integrated control measures, beginning in the 1920s, the Japanese eventually eradicated schistosomosis by the end of the 1970s (Kitani and Iuchi 1990). Similarly, in the much more extensive endemic areas of *S. japonicum* in China, unremitting integrated control measures over a 40-year period have reduced the prevalence of human schistosomosis by 90 per cent, and prevalence in cattle by 92 per cent (Chen 1989; Anon 1992; Chen 1993). In two other countries, of minor endemicity, eradication has also been achieved: *S. haematobium* has been eliminated in Tunisia, and *S. mansoni* in Monserrat. In several countries, particularly those where schistosomosis was early on identified as a major public health problem, such as Egypt, Brazil, Philippines, Venezuela, and Iran, significant reductions in disease prevalence have been achieved, usually by national control programmes incorporating integrated measures. Even in cases where prevalence of infection has remained high, prevalence of serious disease manifestations (such as Symmers' fibrosis or fibro-obstructive lesions of the urogenital tract) has often been reduced, largely by the use of population-based chemotherapy campaigns (WHO 1993; Webbe and Jordan 1993).

Set against this, however, the demographic increases in the younger age groups (who are most affected by the disease) has increased the susceptible populations, and this has been combined with expansion of water resource developments and irrigation, leading to a spread of the disease to new areas and to an intensification of transmission in existing endemic areas. Overall, WHO concluded in its 1993 report on schistosomosis control that the global number of infected cases shows no reduction from its 1984 estimates. Furthermore, in only a very few areas has the snail vector been eradicated, so if control measures break down or are relaxed, the disease will rapidly sweep back, and may in fact become worse than before because of the loss of immunity by the population.

Currently, no antischistosome vaccine for humans is available, though intensive research efforts are being made to produce these, and the first clinical trials of recombinant-derived antigens and chemically synthesized antigens are expected to start soon (Capron *et al.* 1992; Taylor 1994). A major stimulus to this work has been the general acceptance that endemic communities do gradually develop an effective acquired immunity to *S. mansoni* and *S. haematobium* (Hagan *et al.* 1991; Rihet *et al.* 1991; Dunne *et al.* 1992; Demeure *et al.* 1993). Parallel efforts to develop vaccines for the important schistosome parasites of domestic livestock have already led to field trials in Sudan against *S. bovis* (Majid *et al.* 1980*b*) and in China against *S. japonicum* (Hsu *et al.* 1984; Xu *et al.* 1993). These trials, which employed live, irradiation-attenuated schistosomula (and in some of the experiments of Xu *et al.* 1993 and Xu *et al.* 1994 also a crude, non-live schistosomular vaccine with BCG as adjuvant), showed unequivocally that schistosome vaccines can confer benefit even under conditions of intense natural exposures in the field. Currently, the first trials of recombinant-derived vaccines for *S. bovis* and *S. japonicum* are being carried out in both Sudan and China (Taylor 1994).

ACKNOWLEDGEMENTS

Our research on schistosomiasis vaccines is supported by the Science and Technology for Development Programme of the Commission of the European Communities. I am most grateful to Angel Hathaway for her help in preparing this review.

REFERENCES

Abdel-Wahab, M. F. and Mahmoud, S. S. (1987). Schistosomiasis mansoni in Egypt. In *Ballière's Clinical Tropical Medicine and Communicable Diseases*, Vol. 2. *Schistosomiasis*, (ed. A. A. F. Mahmoud), pp. 371–95. Ballière Tindall, London.

Abel, L., Demenais, F., Prata, A., Souza, A. E., and Dessein, A. (1991). Evidence for the segregation of a major gene in human susceptibility/resistance to infection by *Schistosoma mansoni*. *American Journal of Human Genetics*, **48**, 959–70.

Alves-Brito, C. F., *et al.* (1992). Analysis of anti-keyhole limpet haemocyanin antibody in Brazilians supports its use for the diagnosis of acute schistosomiasis mansoni. *Transactions of the Royal Society of Tropical Medicine and Hygiene*, **86**, 53–6.

Anderson, R. M. (1987). Determinants of infection in human schistosomiasis. In *Ballière's Clinical Tropical Medicine and Communicable Diseases*, Vol. 2, *Schistosomiasis*, (ed. A. A. F. Mahmoud), pp. 279–300. Ballière Tindall, London.

Andrade, Z. A. and Van Marck, E. (1984). Schistosomal glomerular disease (a review). *Memórias do Instituto Oswaldo Cruz*, **79**, 499–506.

Anon. (1992). *Parasitic Diseases in China*, pp. 1–102, Ministry of Health, Department of Health and Endemic Prevention, Division of Parasitic Diseases, Beijing.

Bambirra, E. A. *et al.* (1986). Testicular schistosomiasis mansoni: a differential diagnostic problem with testicular neoplasias. *American Journal of Tropical Medicine and Hygiene*, **35**, 791–2.

Barral, V., This, P., Imbert-Establet, D., Combes, C., and Delseny, M. (1993). Genetic variation and evolution of the *Schistosoma* genome analysed by using random amplified polymorphic DNA markers. *Molecular and Biochemical Parasitology*, **59**, 211–22.

Basch, P. F. (1991). *Schistosomes: Development, Reproduction, and Host Relations*, pp. 1–248. Oxford University Press.

Bassily, S. *et al.* (1992). Efficacy of hepatitis B vaccination in primary school children from a village endemic for *Schistosoma mansoni*. *Journal of Infectious Diseases*, **166**, 265–8.

Bergquist, N. R. (1992). Present aspects of immunodiagnosis of schistosomiasis. *Memórias do Instituto Oswaldo Cruz*, **87**, (Suppl. IV), 29–38.

Berry, A. (1966). A cytopathological and histopathological study of Bilharziasis of the female genital tract. *Journal of Pathology and Bacteriology*, **91**, 325–38.

Boros, D. L. (1989). Immunopathology of *Schistosoma mansoni* infection. *Clinical Microbiology Reviews*, **2**, 250–69.

Capron, A., Dessaint, J. P., Capron, M., and Pierce, R. J. (1992). Schistosomiasis: from effector and regulation mechanisms in rodents to vaccine strategies in humans. *Immunological Investigations*, **21**, 409–22.

Chen, M. G. (1989). Progress and problems in schistosomiasis control in China. *Tropical Medicine and Parasitology*, **40**, 174–6.

Chen, M. G. (1993). *Schistosoma japonicum* and *S. japonicum*-like infections: epidemiology, clinical and pathological aspects. In *Human Schistosomiasis*, (ed. P. Jordan, G. Webbe, and R. Sturrock), pp. 237–70. CAB International, Wallingford.

Chen, M. G., and Mott, K. E. (1989). *Progress in assessment of morbidity due to schistosomiasis. R1-R45, R1-R56, R1-R36, R1-R18.* Bureau of Hygiene and Tropical Diseases, Wallingford.

Chen, M. G., Mott, K. E., Wang, Q. H., and Kane, M. (1993). Hepatitis B and schistosomiasis: interaction or no interaction? *Tropical Diseases Bulletin*, **90**, R97–R115.

Cheng, T. H. (1971). Schistosomiasis in mainland China. A review of research and control since 1949. *American Journal of Tropical Medicine and Hygiene*, **20**, 26–53.

Corbett, E. L., Butterworth, A. E., Fulford, A. J. C., Ouma, J. H., and Sturrock, R. F. (1992). Nutritional status of children with schistosomiasis mansoni in two different areas of Machakos District, Kenya. *Transactions of the Royal Society of Tropical Medicine and Hygiene*, **86**, 266–73.

Darwish, M. A., Raouf, T. A., Rushdy, P., Constantine, N. T., Rao, M. R., and Edelman, R. (1993). Risk factors associated with a high seroprevalence of hepatitis C virus infection in Egyptian blood donors. *American Journal of Tropical Medicine and Hygiene*, **49**, 440–47.

Davis, A. (1993). Antischistosomal drugs and clinical practice. In *Human Schistosomiasis*, (ed. P. Jordan, G. Webbe, and R. F. Sturrock), pp. 367–404, CAB International, Wallingford.

de Bont, J., van Aken, D., Vercruysse, J., Fransen, J., Southgate, V. R., and Rollinson, D. (1989). The presence and pathology of *Schistosoma nasale* Rao, 1933 in cattle in Sri Lanka. *Parasitology*, **98**, 197–202.

de Bont, J., Vercruysse, J., van Aken, D., Southgate, V. R., Rollinson, D., and Mancrieff, C. (1991). The epidemiology of *Schistosoma spindale* Montgomery, 1906 in cattle in Sri Lanka. *Parasitology*, **102**, 237–41.

Deelder, A. M. *et al.* (1994). Quantitative diagnosis of *Schistosoma* infections by measurement of circulating antigens in serum and urine. *Tropical and Geographical Medicine*, **46**, 233–8.

de Jonge, N. (1992). Detection of the circulating anodic antigen for immunodiagnosis of *Schistosoma* infections. In *Immunodiagnostic Approaches in Schistosomiasis*, (ed. N. R. Bergquist), pp. 111–24. Wiley, New York.

de Lima e Costa, M. F. F., Corrèa Leite, M. L., Rocha, R. S., de Almeida Maglhaes, M. H., and Katz, N. (1988). Anthropometric measures in relation to schistosomiasis mansoni and socioeconomic variables. *International Journal of Epidemiology*, **17**, 880–6.

Demeure, C. E., Rihet, P., Abel, L., Ouattara, M., Bourgois, A., and Dessein, A. J. (1993). Resistance to *Schistosoma mansoni* in humans: influence of the IgE/IgG4 balance and IgG2 in immunity to reinfection after chemotherapy. *Journal of Infectious Diseases*, **168**, 1000–8.

Dessein, A. J., Abel, L., Carballo, E. M., and Prata, A. (1992). Environmental, genetic and immunological factors in human resistance to *Schistosoma mansoni*. *Immunological Investigations*, **21**, 423–53.

de Vlas, S. J. and Gryseels, B. (1992). Underestimation of *Schistosoma mansoni* prevalences. *Parasitology Today*, **8**, 274–7.

de Vlas, S. J., Gryseels, B., van Oortmarssen, G. J., Polderman, A. M., and Habbema, J. D. F. (1993). A pocket chart to estimate true *Schistosoma mansoni* prevalences. *Parasitology Today*, **9**, 305–6.

Dunne, D. W., *et al.* (1992). Immunity after treatment of human schistosomiasis: association between IgE antibodies to adult worm antigens and resistance to reinfection. *European Journal of Immunology*, **22**, 1483–94.

El-Maraghy, M. A. *et al.* (1982). Bilharziasis of the female genital tract: new concepts. *Journal of the Egyptian Society of Parasitology*, **12**, 179–86.

El-Masry, N. A., Farid, Z., Bassily, S., Kilpatrick, M. E., and Wattern, R. H. (1986). Schistosomal colonic polyposis: clinical, radiological and parasitological study. *Journal of Tropical Medicine and Hygiene*, **89**, 13–17.

El-Rooby, A. (1985). Management of hepatic schistosomiasis. *Seminars in Liver Diseases*, **5**, 263–76.

Eltoum, I. A., Sulaiman, S., Ismail, B. M., Ali, M. M. M., Elfatih, M., and Homeida, M. M. A. (1992). Evaluation of haematuria as an indirect screening test for schistosomiasis haematobia: a population-based study in the White Nile Province, Sudan. *Acta Tropica*, **51**, 151–7.

Farid, Z. (1993). Schistosomes with terminal-spined eggs: pathological and clinical aspects. In *Human Schistosomiasis*, (ed. P. Jordan, G. Webbe, and R. F. Sturrock), pp. 87–158. CAB International, Wallingford.

Feldmeier, H. and Poggensee, G. (1993). Diagnostic techniques in schistosomiasis control. *Acta Tropica*, **55**, 205–20.

Götz, B. and Klinkert, M.-Q. (1993). Expression and partial characterization of a cathepsin B-like enzyme (Sm31) and a proposed 'haemoglobinase' (Sm32) from *Schistosoma mansoni*. *Biochemical Journal*, **260**, 801–6.

Grove, D. I. (1990). *A History of Human Helminthology*, pp. 1–848, CAB International, Wallingford.

Haas, W., Haberi, B., Schmalfuss, G., and Khayyal, M. (1994). *Schistosoma haematobium* cercarial host-finding and host-recognition differs from that of *S. Mansoni*. *Journal of Parasitology*, **80**, 345–53.

Hafez, M. *et al.* (1991). Immunogenetic susceptibility for post-schistosomal hepatic fibrosis. *American Journal of Tropical Medicine and Hygiene*, **44**, 424–33.

Hagan, P., Blumenthal, U. J., Dunn, D., Simpson, A. J. G., and Wilkins, H. A. (1991). Human IgE, IgG4 and resistance to reinfection with *Schistosoma haematobium*. *Nature*, **349**, 243–5.

Hatz, C., Jenkins, J. M., Meudt, R., Abdel-Wahab, M. F., and Tanner, M. (1992*a*). A review of the literature on the use of ultrasonography in schistosomiasis with special reference to its use in field studies. 1. *Schistosoma haematobium*. *Acta Tropica*, **51**, 15–28.

Hatz, C., Jenkins, J. M., Ali, Q. M., Abdel-Wahab, M. F., Cerni, C. G., and Tanner, M. (1992*b*). A review of the literature on the use of ultrasonography in schistosomiasis with special reference to its use in field studies. 2. *Schistosoma mansoni*. *Acta Tropica*, **51**, 15–28.

Hatz, C., Murakami, H., and Jenkins, J. M. (1992*c*). A review of the literature on the use of ultrasonography in schistosomiasis with special reference to its use in field studies. 3. *Schistosoma japonicum*. *Acta Tropica*, **51**, 29–36.

Hatz, C., Jenkins, J. M., Morrow, R. H., and Tanner, M. (1992*d*). Ultrasound in schistosomiasis—a critical look at methodological issues and potential applications. *Acta Tropica*, **51**, 89–97.

Hillyer, G. V. (1982). Schistosomiasis. In *CRC Handbook Series in Zoonoses Section C: Parasitic Zoonoses, Vol. III*, (ed. G. V. Hillyer and C. E. Hopla), pp. 177–210. CRC Press, Boca Raton.

Hoeffler, D. F. (1987). Cercarial dermatitis. In *Immunology, Immunoprophylaxis and Immunotherapy of Parasitic Infections*, Vol. II, *Trematodes and Cestodes*, (ed. E. J. L. Soulsby), pp. 7–15. CRC Press, Boca Raton.

Hsu, S. Y. L. *et al.* (1984). Vaccination of bovines against schistosomiasis japonica with highly irradiated schistosomula in China. *American Journal of Tropical Medicine and Hygiene*, **33**, 891–8.

Jenkins, J. M. and Hatz, C. (1992). The use of diagnostic ultrasound in schistosomiasis—attempts at standardization of methodology. *Acta Tropica*, **51**, 45–63.

Johnston, D. A., Kane, R. A., and Rollinson, D. (1993). Small subunit (18S) ribosomal RNA gene divergence in the genus *Schistosoma*. *Parasitology*, **107**, 147–56.

Jordan, P. and Randall, K. (1962). Bilharziasis in Tanganyika: observations on its effects and the effects of treatment in schoolchildren. *Journal of Tropical Medicine and Hygiene*, **65**, 1–6.

Jordan, P. and Webbe, G. (1993). Epidemiology. In *Human Schistosomiasis*, (ed. P. Jordan, G. Webbe, and R. Sturrock), pp. 87–158. CAB International, Wallingford.

Kamel, M. A., Zakaria, E., Mabrouk, M. A., Zakaria, S., Hgazi, A. R. M., and El Raziky, E. H. (1984). HLA antigen frequencies in Egyptian patients with complicated schistosomiasis mansoni. *Transactions of the Royal Society of Tropical Medicine and Hygiene*, **78**, 850–1.

Kane, R. A. and Rollinson, D. A. (1994). Repetitive sequences in the ribosomal DNA internal transcribed spacer of *Schistosoma haematobium*, *Schistosoma intercalatum*, and *Schistosoma mattheei*. *Molecular and Biochemical Parasitology*, **65**, 153–6.

Kassuku, A., Christensen, N. Ø., Nansen, P., and Monrad, B. J. (1986). Clinical pathology of *Schistosoma bovis* infection in goats. *Research in Veterinary Science*, **40**, 44–7.

Kassuku, A., Christensen, N. Ø, Morrad, J., Nansen, P., and Knudsen, J. (1986). Epidemiological studies on *Schistosoma bovis* in Iringa Region, Tanzania. *Acta Tropica*, **43**, 153–63.

Kaukas, A., Neto, E. D., Simpson, A. J. G., Southgate, V. R., and Rollinson, D. (1994). A phylogenetic analysis of *Schistosoma haematobium* group species based on randomly amplified polymorphic DNA. *International Journal for Parasitology*, **24**, 285–90.

Kimura, E. *et al.* (1992). Effects of *Schistosoma haematobium* infection on mental test scores of Kenyan school children. *Tropical Medicine and Parasitology*, **43**, 155–8.

Kitani, K. and Iuchi, M. (1990). Schistosomiasis japonica: a vanishing endemic in Japan. *Journal of Gastroenterology and Hepatology*, **5**, 160–72.

Kojima, S., Yano, A., Sasazuki, T., and Ohta, N. (1984). Associations between HLA and immune responses in individuals with chronic schistosomiasis japonica. *Transactions of the Royal Society of Tropical Medicine and Hygiene*, **78**, 325–9.

Lambertucci, J. R. (1993). *Schistosoma mansoni*: pathological and clinical aspects. In *Human Schistosomiasis*, (ed. P. Jordan, G. Webbe, and R. F. Sturrock), pp. 195–235. CAB International, Wallingford.

Lengeler, C. *et al.* (1991*a*). Community-based questionnaries and health statistics as tools for the cost-efficient identification of communities at risk of urinary schistosomiasis. *International Journal of Epidemiology*, **20**, 769–807.

Lengeler, C., Kilima, P., Mashinda, H., Morona, D., Hatz, C., and Tanner, M. (1991*b*). Rapid, low-cost, two-step method to screen for urinary schistosomiasis at the district level: the Kilosa experience. *Bulletin of the World Health Organization*, **69**, 179–89.

Lengeler, C., Mshinda, H., Morona, D., and de Savigny, D. (1993). Urinary schistosomiasia: testing with urine filtration and reagent sticks for haematuria provides a comparable prevalence estimate. *Acta Tropica*, **53**, 39–50.

McCauley, E. H., Majid, A. A., Tayeb, A., and Bushara, H. O. (1983*a*). Clinical diagnosis of schistosomiasis in Sudanese cattle. *Tropical Animal Health and Production*, **15**, 129–36.

McCauley, E. H., Tayeb, A., and Majid, A. A. (1983*b*). Owner survey of schistosomiasis mortality in Sudanese cattle. *Tropical Animal Health and Production*, **15**, 227–33.

McCauley, E. H., Majid, A. A., and Tayeb, A. (1984). Economic evaluation of the production impact of bovine schistosomiasis and vaccination in the Sudan. *Preventive Veterinary Medicine*, **2**, 735–54.

McGarvey, S. T. *et al.* (1993). Child growth, nutritional status, and schistosomiasis japonica in Jiangxi, People's Republic of China. *American Journal of Tropical Medicine and Hygiene*, **48**, 547–53.

Majid, A. A. *et al.* (1980*a*). Observations on cattle schistosomiasis in the Sudan, a study in comparative medicine. I. Epizootiological observations in the White Nile Province. *American Journal of Tropical Medicine and Hygiene*, **29**, 435–41.

Majid, A. A., Bushara, H. O., Saad, A. M., Hussein, M. F., Taylor, M. G., and Dargie, J. D. (1980*b*). Observations on cattle schistosomiasis in the Sudan, a study in comparative medicine. III. Field testing of an irradiated *Schistosoma bovis* vaccine. *American Journal of Tropical Medicine and Hygiene*, **26**, 452–5.

Mansour, M. M., Ali, P. O., Farid, Z., Simpson, A. J. G., and Woody, J. W. (1989). Serological differentiation of acute and chronic schistosomiasis mansoni by antibody responses to keyhole limpet haemocyanin. *American Journal of Tropical Medicine and Hygiene*, **26**, 338–44.

Mikhail, N. E., Tawfic, M. I., Abel Hadi, A., and Akl, M. (1988). Schistosomal orchitis stimulating malignancy. *Journal of Urology*, **140**, 147–8.

Miller, R. L., Armelagos, G. J., Ikram, S., de Jonge, N., Krijger, F. W., and Deelder, A. M. (1992). Palaeoepidemiology of *Schistosoma* infection in mummies. *British Medical Journal*, **304**, 555–6.

Mohamed, A. R. E.-S., Karawi, M. A. A., and Yasawy, M. I. (1990). Schistosomal colonic disease. *Gut*, **31**, 439–42.

Mohamed-Ali, Q. *et al.* (1991). Utrasonographical investigation of periportal fibrosis in children with *Schistosoma mansoni* infection: reversibility of morbidity seven months after treatment with praziquantel. *American Journal of Tropical Medicine & Hygiene*, **44**, 444–51.

Mott, K. E. and Dixon, H. (1982). Collaborative study on antigens for immunodiagnosis of schistosomiasis. *Bulletin of World Health Organization*, **60**, 729–53.

Mott, K. E., *et al.* (1987). Collaborative study on antigens for immunodiagnosis of *Schistosoma japonicum* infection. *Bulletin of World Health Organization*, **65**, 233–44.

Mott, K. E. *et al.* (1992). Liver ultrasound findings in a low prevalence area of *S. japonicum* in China: comparison with history, physical examination, parasitological and serological results. *Acta Tropica*, **51**, 65–84.

Neto, E. D., de Souza, C. P., Rollinson, D. A., Katz, N., Pena, S. D. J., and Simpson, A. J. G. (1993). The random amplification of polymorphic DNA allows the identification of strains and species of schistosome. *Molecular and Biochemical Parasitology*, **57**, 83–8.

Norfray, J. F., Schlachter, L., Heiser, W. J., Weinberg, P. E., Jerva, M. J., and Wizgird, J. P. (1978). Schistosomiasis of the spinal cord. *Surgical Neurology*, **9**, 68–71.

Ohta, N., Edahiro, T., Ishii, A., Yasukawa, M., and Hosaka, Y. (1990). HLA-DQ-controlled T cell response to soluble egg antigen of *Schistosoma japonicum* in humans. *Clinical and Experimental Immunology*, **79**, 403–8.

Olvedo, R. M. and Domingo, E. O. (1987). Schistosomiasis japonica. In *Schistosomiasis. Ballière's Clinical and Tropical Medicine and Communicable Diseases*, Vol. 2, (ed. A. A. F. Mahmoud), pp. 397–417. Ballière Tindall, London.

Omer Ali, P. *et al.* (1991). Sequence of a small subunit rRNA gene of *Schistosoma mansoni* and its use in phylogenetic analysis. *Molecular and Biochemical Parasitology*, **46**, 201–8.

Ouma, J. H. and Fenwick, A. (1991). Animal reservoirs of schistosomiasis. In *Parasitic Helminths and Zoonoses in Africa*, (ed. C. N. C. Macpherson and P. S. Craig), pp. 224–36. Unwin Hyman, London.

Parker, M. (1992). Re-assessing disability: the impact of schistosomal infection on daily activities among women in Gezira Province, Sudan. *Social Science and Medicine*, **35**, 877–90.

Parker, M. (1993). Bilharzia and the boys: questioning common assumptions. *Social Science and Medicine*, **37**, 481–92.

Phillips, S. M. and Lammie, P. J. (1986). Immunopathology of granuloma formation and fibrosis in schistosomiasis. *Parasitology Today*, **2**, 296–301.

Prata, A. (1987). Schistosomiasis mansoni in Brazil. In *Ballière's Clinical and Tropical Medicine and Communicable Diseases*, Vol. 2, *Schistosomiasis*, (ed. A.A.F. Mahmoud), pp. 349–69. Ballière Tindall, London.

Rabello, A. L. T., Garcia, M. M. A., Dias Neto, E., Rocha, R.S., and Katz, N. (1993). Dot-dye-immunoassay and dot-ELISA for the serological differentiation of acute and chronic schistosomiasis mansoni using keyhole limpet haemocyanin as antigen. *Transactions of the Royal Society of Tropical Medicine and Hygiene*, **87**, 279–81.

Rihet, P., Demeure, C. E., Bourgois, A., Prata, A., and Dessein, A. J. (1991). Evidence for an association between human resistance to *Schistosoma mansoni* and high antilarval IgE levels. *European Journal of Immunology*, **21**, 2679–86.

Rollinson, D. and Southgate, V. R. (1987). The genus *Schistosoma*: a taxonomic appraisal. In *The Biology of Schistosomes. From Genes to Latrines*. (ed. D. Rollinson and A. J. G. Simpson), pp. 1–49. Academic Press, London.

Rumjanek, F. D. (1987). Biochemistry and Physiology. In *The Biology of Schistosomes. From Genes to Latrines*, (ed. D. Rollinson and A. J. G. Simpson), pp. 163–83. Academic Press, London.

Salam, E. A., Ishaac, S., and Mahmoud, A. A. F. (1979). Histocompatibility-linked susceptibility for hepatospleno megaly in human schistosomiasis mansoni. *Journal of Immunology*, **123**, 1829–31.

Sasazuki, T., Kaneoka, H., Nishimura, Y., Kaneoka, R., Hayama, M., and Ohkuni, H. (1980). An HLA-linked immune suppression gene in man. *Journal of Experimental Medicine*, **152**, 297s–313s.

Savioli, L. and Mott, K. E. (1989). Urinary schistosomiasis on Pemba Island: low-cost diagnosis for control in a primary health care setting. *Parasitology Today*, **5**, 333–7.

Savioli, L., Hatz, C., Dixon, H., Kisumku, U. M., and Mott, K. E. (1990). Control of morbidity due to *Schistosoma haematobium* on Pemba Island: egg excretion and haematuria as indicators of infection. *American Journal of Tropical Medicine and Hygiene*, **43**, 289–95.

Schmidt, G. D. and Roberts, L. S. (1989). *Foundations of Parasitology*, (4th edn). pp. 1–750. Times Mirror/Mosby College Publishing, St, Louis.

Scrimageour, E. M. and Gadjusek, D. G. (1985). Involvement of the central nervous system in *Schistosoma mansoni* and *S. haematobium* infection. A review. *Brain*, **108**, 1023–38.

Southgate, V. R. and Rollinson, D. (1987). National history of transmission and schistosome interactions. In *The Biology of Schistosomes—from Genes to Latrines*, (ed. D. Rollinson and A. J. G. Simpson), pp. 346–78. Academic Press, London.

Stephenson, L. (1993). The impact of schistosomasis on human nutrition. *Parasitology*, **107**, S107–S123.

Stephenson, L. S., Latham, M. C., Kurz, K. M.,Kinoti, S. N., Oduris, M. L., and Crompton, D. W. T. (1985) Relationships of *Schistosoma haematobium*, hookworm and malarial infections and metrifonate treatment to growth of Kenyan school children. *American Journal of Tropical Medicine and Hygiene*, **34**, 1109–18.

Stephenson, L. S., Latham, M. C., Kurz, K. M., and Kinoti, S. N. (1989). Single dose metrifonate or praziquantel treatment in Kenyan children. II. Effects of growth in relation to *Schistosoma haematobium* and hookworm egg counts. *American Journal of Tropical Medicine and Hygiene*, **41**, 445–53

Taylor, M. G. (1970). Hybridisation experiments on five species of African schistosomes. *Journal of Helminthology*, **44**, 253–314.

Taylor, M. G. (1987). Schistosomes of domestic animals: *Schistosoma bovis* and other animal forms. In *Immunology, Immunoprophylasix and Immunotherapy of Parasitic Infections*, (ed. E. J. L. Soulsby), pp. 50–90. CRC Press, Boca Raton.

Taylor, M. G. (1994). Schistosomiasis vaccines: Farewell to the God of Plague? *Journal of Tropical Medicine and Hygiene*, **97**, 257–68.

Taylor, M. G., Hussein, M. F., and Harrison, R. A. (1991). Baboons, bovines and bilharzia vaccines. In *Parasitic Helminths and Zoonosis in Africa*, (ed. C. N. L. Macpherson and P. S. Craig), pp. 237–59. Unwin Hyman, London.

Uemura, K., Kawaguchi, T., Sodeyama, T., and Kiyosawa, K. (1992). Antibody to hepatitis C virus in patients with chronic schistosomiasis. *Annals of Tropical Medicine and Parasitology*, **86**, 257–62.

Vercruysse, J., Southgate, V. R., and Rollinson, D (1984). *Schistosoma curassoni* Brumpt 1931 in sheep and goats in Senegal. *Journal of Natural History*, **18**, 969–76.

Vercruysse, J., Fransen, J., Southgate, V. R., and Rollinson, D. (1985*a*). Pathology of *Schistosoma curassoni* in sheep. *Parasitology*, **91**, 291–300.

Vercuysse, J., Southgate, V. R., and Rollinson, D. (1985*b*). The epidemiology of human and animal schistosomiasis in the Senegal River Basin. *Acta Tropical*, **42**, 249–59.

von Lichtenberg, F. (1987). Consequences of infections with schistosomes. In *The Biology of Schistosomes. From Genes to Latrines*, pp. 185–232, Academic Press, London.

Walker, T. K., Rollinson, D., and Simpson, A. J. G. (1986). Differentiation of *Schistosoma haematobium* from related species using cloned ribosomal RNA gene probes. *Molecular and biochemical Parasitology*, **20**, 123–31.

Warren, K. S. (1978). Hepatosplenic schistosomiasis: a great neglected disease of the liver. *Gut*, **19**, 572–7.

Webbe, G. and Jordan, P. (1993). Control. In *Human Schistosomiasis*, (ed. P. Jordan, G. Webbe, and R. F. Sturrock), pp. 367–404. CAB International, Wallingford.

Weinstock, J. V. (1992). The pathogenesis of granulomatous inflammation and organ injury in schistosomiasis: interactions between the schistosome ova and the host. *Immunological Investigation*, **21**, 455–75.

Wei-win, C., Dong-chuan, Q., and Hatz, C. (1992). Studies on ultrasonographic diagnosis of schistosomiasis japonica in China—a review of selected Chinese studies. *Acta Tropica*, **51**, 37–43.

WHO (1993). *The Control of Schistosomiasis. Second Report of the WHO Expert Committee* pp. 1–86, (WHO tech. Rep. Ser.). WHO, Geneva.

Wilkins, A. and Gilles, H. (1987). Schistosomiasis haematobia. In *Ballière's Clinical and Tropical Medicine and Communicable diseases*, Vol.2, *Schistosomiasis*, (ed. A. A. F. Mahmoud), pp. 333–48. Ballière Tindall, London.

Wilson, R. A. (1987). Cercariae to liver worms: development and migration in the mammalian host. In *The Biology of Schistosomes. From Genes to Latrines*, (ed. D. Rollinson and A. J. G. Simpson), pp. 115–46. Academic Press, London.

Wishashi, M., El-Baz, H. G., and Shaker, Z. A. (1989). Association between HLA-A, B, C and DR antigens and clinical manifestations of *Schistosoma haematobium* in the bladder. *European Journal of Urology*, **16**, 138–43.

Xu, S. *et al.* (1993). Vaccination of bovines against Schistosomasis Japonica with cryopreserved-irradiated and freeze-thaw schistosomula. *Veterinary Parasitology*, **47**, 37–50.

Xu, S. *et al.* (1994). Vaccination of sheep against *Schistosoma japonicum* with either glutathione S-transferase, Keyhole Limpet Haemocyanin, or the freeze/thaw schistosomula/BCG vaccine. *Veterinary Parasitology*, **58**, 301–312.

Xue, C. G, Taylor, M. G., Bickle, Q. D., Savioli, L., and Renganathan, E.A. (1993). Diagnosis of *Schistosoma haematobium* infection: evaluation of ELISA using keyhole limpet haemocyanin or soluble egg antigen in comparison with detection of eggs or haematuria. *Transactions of the Royal Society of Tropical Medicine and Hygiene*, **87**, 654–8.

Yason, C. V. and Novilla, M. N. (1984). Clinical and pathologic features of experimental *Schistosoma japonicum* in pigs. *Veterinary Parasitology*, **17**, 47–64.

Zheng, F., Wang, S., Lai, W., Xiang, X., and Yi, X. (1992). Studies on the KLH-ELISA and KLH-IHA for diagnosis of schistosomiasis japonica. *Chinese Journal of Schistosomiasis Control*, **4**, 57–8.

55   OTHER TREMATODE INFECTIONS

S. Lloyd and E. J. L. Soulsby

SUMMARY

A large variety of zoonotic trematodes produce at least 40 million human infections worldwide. Most infections occur in Asia, particularly the Far East and South-East Asia. Man may be an important definitive host or acquire infection only rarely. The life cycle involves an egg from which the miracidium hatches either into water or after ingestion by the first intermediate host, a snail. Snails are aquatic in fresh or brackish water, occasionally they are semiaquatic (*Fasciola*) or land (*Dicrocoelium*) snails. Released cercariae encyst on plants (*Fasciola, Fasciolopsis*) or on or in the tissues usually of fishes, crustacea, or molluscs. Dietary customs are the most important determining factor for infection of man. Raw or undercooked watercress (*Fasciola*), water tubers (*Fasciolopsis*), fish (*Clonorchis, Opisthorchis, Heterophyes*), crabs/crayfish (*Paragonimus*), snails (*Echinostoma*), or occasionally insects are the offending foods. Adult flukes are found in the biliary system, lungs, or intestine although infections at ectopic sites do occur. Inflammation and chronic fibrosis of the biliary system and complications thereof occur in response to the liver flukes; cholangiocarcinoma is associated with heavy infections of some. Heavy infections with the intestinal flukes cause mucoid enteritis, diarrhoea, and protein loss. The drug of choice for most of these flukes is praziquantel. Treatment of humans and improved human sewage disposal to prevent contamination of water may not be sufficient for control as many of these flukes have important animal reservoir hosts. Education to change dietary habits must be a major effort in control programmes.

HISTORY

Fasciola hepatica was described in 1379 when de Brie, commissioned to write on sheep husbandry by Charles V of France, described 'liver rot' resulting from consumption of a plant that corrupted the liver to produce a type of worm (Grove 1990). Fitzherbert, an English lawyer, referred to 'flokes' in the liver in 1523. In 1760, Pallas described *Fasciola* from a patient in Berlin. Animals were assumed to acquire infection from contaminated pastures, but understanding of the life cycle was delayed due to its complexity. While cercariae in water were discovered by Müller in 1773, Nitzsch described their similarity to flukes, Bojanus described rediae and Creplin hatching of the eggs, they all recorded these as separate organisms. It wasn't until the late nineteenth century that Lutz, Leuckart, and Thomas described development in the snail, and infected guinea-pigs. De Brie had described seasonality of infection on damp pastures and advocated grazing control, while Thomas later defined the environmental conditions necessary for the life cycle, but not until 1959 was meteorological forecasting to predict times of high risk developed by Ollerenshaw and Roland.

Oriental liver flukes, first described in Western literature in the nineteenth century might be recorded earlier in oriental literature even though the Chinese were prejudiced against mutilation of dead bodies (Grove 1990). *Clonorchis sinensis* was first described in the 1870s from autopsies on Chinese workers in India and Mauritius; 'putrid, half-raw' fish, vegetables, or snails were suggested as the vehicle. *Opisthorchis* spp. were first described in man at the end of the nineteenth and early twentieth centuries, and Japanese scientists described the life cycle when Kobayashi infected cats with metacercariae from fish and Muto transferred infection from snails to fish to dogs; but not until 1940 were eggs shown to hatch only after ingestion by snails. *Fasciolopsis buski* was first described in an Indian in 1843. When Lankester named the parasite he predicted a life cycle similar to *F. hepatica* and lower animals as main hosts (Grove 1990), but the life cycle was completed and published only in 1921 by Nakagawa in Taiwan. *Paragonimus westermani* adults and eggs in reddish sputum were first described in 1879/80 and, in 1915, Nagakawa in Japan determined the significance of the snail host and metacercariae in crabs.

AETIOLOGICAL AGENTS AND THEIR STRUCTURE

Over 100 species in 40 genera and 19 families of the Digenea infect man. They are hermaphrodites, usually dorsoventrally flattened and have an oral (anterior) sucker and an acetabulum (ventral sucker). Eggs, usually operculate, are passed daily through the genital pore. Many infections are very rare so details will not be given for all. Common or cosmopolitan infections and examples in different groups will be described (Table 55.1).

OPISTHORCHIIDAE

Clonorchis sinensis (Cobbold 1875) Blanchard, 1895, the Chinese or Oriental liver fluke, is pinkish, of variable size up to 25 × 5 mm, transparent and spatulate. Young flukes are spiny, adults are smooth. The testes are much branched and lie in tandem in the posterior of the body. The uterus is obvious and ascends in loops from the pretesticular, small, three-lobed ovary to the acetabulum. Vitelline follicles are confined to the level of the uterus.

Eggs are yellowish-brown, 26–30 by 15–17 μm, and pyriform. The convex operculum fits into a unique, prominent rim in the shell and there is a knobbed, abopercular protuberance. The egg contains a miracidium with asymmetrical internal structure.

Opisthorchis viverrini (Poirier 1886) Stiles and Hassall, 1896 and *Opisthorchis felineus* (Rivolta 1884) Blanchard, 1895 are very similar to *C. sinensis*. They measure 7–12 by 1.5–2.5 mm. Testes are lobed, not branched. The small ovary lies in the midline at the beginning of the posterior third of the body, with the uterine coils in front of this. Vitellaria lie in the middle third of the lateral fields.

Eggs are 22–32 by 10–22 μm and many have a tubercular, abopercular appendage. The ratio of length to breadth of *O. viverrini* is 1.75, that for *O. felineus* 2.75.

Other Opisthorchiidae found occasionally in man, primarily in the liver, include *Metorchis albidus* and *M. conjunctus* in Alaska, Canada, Greenland, France, and Russia, acquired from cyprinid and sucker fish; and *Pseudamphistomum truncatum* and *P. aethiopicum* in Europe, Russia, India, and Africa.

FASCIOLIDAE

Fasciola hepatica Linnaeus, 1758 is leaf-shaped, grey-brown, broad anteriorly with a cone-shaped projection followed by broad 'shoulders', a spiny tegument and reaches 30 by 13 mm. The suckers are powerful. Testes are highly branched occupying the middle half of the body. The ovary is anterior to these, branched and to the right of centre, the uterus coils to the acetabulum. Vitellaria fill the lateral fields. The caeca are highly branched.

Eggs measure 130–150 by 63–90 μm, are yellowish-brown, have an indistinct operculum, thin shell, and are filled with cells.

Fasciola gigantica Cobbold, 1885 is very similar, but larger and narrower and has larger eggs, 156–197 by 90–104 μm. The adults, in domestic and wild ruminants, horse, camel, donkey, etc., and occasionally in man, are widespread in Africa, Asia, Pacific Islands, southern USA, southern Europe, the Middle East. The snails, and so infection, are commonly associated with ponds.

Fasciolopsis buski (Lankester 1857) Odhner, 1902 is large, thick, elongate-oval and pinkish, up to 75 by 20 mm, with a large acetabulum. Large, much branched testes in tandem occupy most of the posterior two-thirds. The ovary and uterus are anterior. Caeca are unbranched. Vitellaria almost fill the lateral fields. The eggs are similar to those of *F. hepatica* but are wider, 80–85 μm.

PARAMPHISTOMATIDAE

Gastrodiscoides hominis (Lewis and McConnell 1876) Leiper, 1913, is red in colour, 5–14 mm long and pear-shaped, having a discoidal posterior (up to 14 mm wide) and conical anterior. The acetabulum is very large and posterior.

Eggs are large, 160 by 65 μm, and similar to those of *Fasciola*, but relatively colourless.

DICROCOELIIDAE

Dicrocoelium dendriticum (Rudolphi 1819) Looss, 1899 is elongate, 6–10 by 2 mm. The testes are slightly lobed and in tandem in the anterior of the body just behind the acetabular sucker. The ovary is behind this and the posterior half of the worm is filled with eggs in the coiled uterus. Vitelline glands are in the middle third of the lateral fields.

Eggs are brown, 36–45 by 20–30 μm, operculate and embryonated.

Dicrocoelium hospes has been reported from man in Africa. *Eurytrema pancreaticum*, which uses a land snail but then a grasshopper second host, has been reported from the pancreatic ducts of man in Asia and South America.

HETEROPHYIDAE

These minute, tear-drop-shaped flukes are less than 2 mm long. The body is scaled especially on the tapering anterior end. The suckers usually are weak, but

Table 55.1 Some trematodes causing infection in man

Parasite	Definitive host	Site of infection	First intermediate host snail	Second intermediate host or metacercariae on	Geographic distribution
Clonorchis sinensis	Man, other fish-eating mammals, e.g. dog, pig, cat, badger, marten, mink, rat, etc.	Biliary system, occasionally pancreatic ducts	*Parafossalurus manchouricus, Allocinma longicornis, Bulimus* spp., e.g. *B. striatulus, Melania tuberculata, Hemiculter* spp.	>100 spp. of fish, primarily Cyprinidae: *Pseudorasbora parva, Ctenopharyngodon idellus, Mylopharyngodon aethiops, Cutter abumus?*	From Indo China to Japan
Opisthorchis viverrini	Man, fish-eating mammals, e.g. wild and domestic cat, dog, etc.	Biliary system, occasionally pancreatic ducts and intestine	*Bithynia inflata, B. siamensis, B. goniomphalus, B. funiculata, B. laevis,* slow-flowing streams	Primarily Cyprinidae: *Cyclocheilichthys siaja, Hampala dispar, Puncitus orphoides*	South-East Asia, particularly north-eastern, northern, central Thailand and Laos
Opisthorchis felineus	Fish-eating mammals, e.g. wild and domestic cat, dog, etc.; man.	Biliary system, occasionally pancreatic ducts and intestine	*Bithynia (Codiella) leachi, B. tentaculata;* slow-flowing streams	Cyprinidae: *Tinca tinca, Idus melanotis, Barbus barbus, Abramis brama,* etc.	Southern, central and eastern Europe from Spain into European CIS countries including the Caucasus and Siberia
Dicrocoelium dendriticum	Domestic and wild ruminants, lagomorphs, donkey, etc.; man	Biliary system	*Cochlicopa lubrica, Helicella corderoi, Zebrina detrita, Z. hohenacheri,* etc., dry pastures	Ants: *Formica fusca, F. cunicularia, F. gagati,* etc.	Europe, Asia, China, northern half of Africa, North America
Fasciola hepatica	Domestic and wild ruminants, horse, donkey, camel, etc.; man	Biliary system, liver, immature stages, ectopic: lungs, brain	Lymnaeidae: *Lymnaea truncatula L. columnella, . L. bulimoides, L. cubensis, L. viridis,* etc., damp pasture	Metacercariae encyst on vegetation or in water, watercress	Cosmopolitan
Fasciolopsis buski	Man; pig; dog	Small intestine	Planorbidae: *Segmentina hemisphaerula, Hippeutis cantori,* ponds	Metacercariae encyst on water caltrop, water chestnuts, roots of other edible aquatic plants	Indochina, Japan, South-East Asia
Gastrodiscoides hominis	Man; pig, monkey	Caecum, upper colon	*Helicorbis coenosus,* ponds	Metacercariae encyst on water caltrop, water chestnuts, etc.	South-East Asia, Philippines, Indian sub-continent, European Russia

Table 55.1 (Continued)

Parasite	Definitive host	Site of infection	First intermediate host snail	Second intermediate host or metacercariae on	Geographic distribution
Heterophyes heterophyes, H. nocens	Piscivorous birds and mammals: dog, cat, fox, wolf, weasel, etc. *Milvus, Pelicanus,* man	Small intestine	*Pirenella conica, Cerithidea cingulata, Tympanotomus micropter, Melania tuberculata,* etc.; lakes, ponds, streams	*Mugil,* including *M. cephalus, M. capito, Tilapia nilotica, Lichia, Barbus,* etc.	Middle East, Indochina, Japan, South-East Asia, southern provinces of Russia, France, Brazil, parts of Africa
Haplorchis yokogawai	Heron, egret, dog, cat, cattle, macaque; man	Small intestine	*Melanoides tuberculata, Stenomelania newcombi*	*Cirrhina, Puntius, Ophicephalus*	South-East Asia, southern China, India, Middle Philippines, Middle East, Australia, USA, Hawaii
Metagonimus yokogawai	Dog, cat, pig, heron, egret, mink, fox; man	Small intestine	*Semisulcospira libertina, S. coreana;* lakes, ponds, streams	Many species of freshwater fish, particularly Cyprinidae	East, and South-East Asia, Philippines, and areas such as Azerbaidzhan, Ukraine, Balkans
Echinostoma, Echinochasmus, Echinoparyphium, Euparyphium, Hypoderaeum spp.	Dog, cat, pig, rat, wild birds, man	Small intestine	Lymnaeidae and Planorbidae: *Lymnaea, Physa, Helisoma, Stagnicola, Segmentina, Planorbis,* etc.; ponds, lakes	Freshwater molluscs (snails, mussels, clams), fish, tadpoles	Asia, particularly the Far-East and South-East Asia, Europe; but very cosmopolitan
Nanophyetus salmincola	Wild piscivorous mammals and birds, cat, dog; man	Small intestine	*Oxytrema silicula, Goniobasis, Semisulcospira* spp.	*Oncorhynchus, Hucho* salmon, *Cargonus, Cyprinus,* etc.	Western USA, eastern Russia
Paragonimus westermani/ P. pulmonalis, Paragonimus spp.	Man; canines, felines, opossum, pig, monkey, etc.	Lungs; ectopic, subcutaneous, brain	lakes, rivers *semisulcospira libertina, Brotia costula, B. asperata, Assiminea, Tricula, Potamiopsis, Aroapyrgus;* fast-flowing streams	Crab, shrimp, crayfish: *Eriocheir japonicus, E. sinensis, Pseudothelphusa, Cambaroides, Geothelphusa, Sinopotamon, Potamon, Sudanautes, Liberonautes,* etc., paratenic hosts, e.g. wild boar, carrying immature stages in the tissues	Asia, particularly Far-East and South-East Asia, West and Central Africa, the Americas

there is a sucker-like genital sinus. Testes are oval, slightly lobed and horizontal or diagonal in the posterior of the body. The ovary is slightly lobed, anterior to the testes. Vitellaria are lateral, usually in the posterior of the body with the uterus. The eggs of all the species are similar and small.

Heterophyes heterophyes (v. Siebold, 1852) Stiles and Hassall, 1900 is very small, 1–1.7 by 0.3–0.7 mm. The morphologically similar species in Asia usually is called *Heterophyes nocens* Onji and Nishio, 1916. The ventral sucker is large, the genital sinus immediately behind it has a conspicuous sucker and 70–80 toothed spines. The testes are oval and posterior.

Eggs are light brown, 26–30 by 15–17 μm, slightly pointed at both ends and the operculum fits into a slightly thickened rim. The miracidium is bilaterally symmetrical.

Metagonimus yokogawai (Katsurada 1912) Katsurada, 1913 can be differentiated from *H. heterophyes* by a very poorly developed genital sucker anterior to the ventral sucker and the eggs lack a rim.

A large number of other heterophyids and some microphallids that occur in piscivorous birds and mammals may be found in dogs and cats, particularly strays, and occasionally man. Essentially all heterophyids should be considered potential parasites of man. Differentiation of them is difficult but descriptions of many are given by Pearson and Ow-Yang (1982). *Haplorchis yokogawai, H. pumilio*, and *H. taichui* described in South-East Asia, the Philippines, Egypt, Tunisia, acquired particularly from *Puntius* spp. fish, can be common in man. *Heterophyes disbar* in Greece, Turkey, Sardinia, the Middle East and *Heterophyopsis continua* in Japan, Korea, Tunisia, come from fresh/brackish water fish, mullet, barbel, perch, etc.; *Stellantchasmus falcatus* in Japan, South-East Asia, Australia, Egypt, from fish such as mullet; *Centrocestus armatus* and *C. formosanus* in China, Far-Eastern Russia, Japan, Korea, Laos, India, from metacercariae on the gills of fish and probably also frogs and toads. Other species described in man are *Procerovum varium Pygidiopsis summa, Stictodora fuscata, Microcephalus minus* in Japan and Korea; *Isoparorchis hypselobagri* in China and India; *Carneocephallus brevicaeca* in the Philippines; *Apophallus donicus* and *Cryptocotyle lingua* in Canada and Greenland; and *Ascocotyle (Phagicola)* spp. in Brazil; but the species are much more widespread than this.

NANOPHYETIDAE

Nanophyetus salmincola (Chapin 1927) is better known for transmitting the 'salmon poisoning' rickettsia to dogs. It is reported in man occasionally in northwestern USA and commonly in eastern Russia. Adults are white/cream and reach 2.5 by 0.5 mm. The testes are large, oval, and side by side in the posterior third. Eggs, 52–82 by 32–56 μm, are unembryonated, yellowish-brown, have an indistinct operculum and a small blunt, abopercular knob.

ECHINOSTOMATIDAE

The flukes in this family are not specific to definitive hosts and so infect a broad spectrum of mammals and aquatic birds. They are elongate with a strong ventral sucker placed anteriorly. The oral sucker is surrounded by a conspicuous 'head-collar' bearing large spines.

Echinostoma revolutum (Frolich 1802) Looss, 1899 is 10–22 by 2 mm with a spiny tegument anteriorly. The head collar has 37 spines including a group of five corner spines on either side. It cannot be differentiated morphologically from other 37-spined species (Kanev 1994). The testes are tandem, oval or slightly lobed, the ovary is anterior to them at about the midline, and the uterus coils forward to a large acetabulum. Vitellaria fill the lateral fields. The eggs are large, 90–126 by 54–71 μm, unembryonated, and operculate.

At least 15 species of *Echinostoma, Echinochasmus*, and *Echinoparyphium*, some of which may be synonyms, infect man in China, the Far East and South-East Asian countries, with infections recorded elsewhere, e.g. Brazil, India, Europe. Many species are widespread and include *Echinostoma cinetorchis, E. macrorchis, E. hortense, E. echinatum (E. lindoense), E. ilocaninum, E. (Artyfechnostomum) malayanum, Echinoparyphium recurvatum, Echinochasmus perfoliatus, E. japonicus, Euparyphium melis*, and *Hypoderaeum conoideum*. Species differ particularly in the number of collar spines. All have eggs greater than 90 μm long. Infections are acquired from raw freshwater fish, e.g. loach, perch, etc., snails and tadpoles.

PARAGONIMIDAE

Paragonimus contains over 10 species that infect man. Their morphological similarity means identification and delineation of the geographical distribution of species can be difficult.

Paragonimus westermani (Kerbert 1878) Braun, 1899, reddish-brown, 7.5–16 by 4–8 mm, and thick, up to 5 mm, has large spines with bifid tips. The ventral sucker lies just anterior to the midline. The rounded testes are placed slightly posterior. The lobed ovary is left of the midline. Vitellaria are extensive in the lateral fields. Triploid and diploid *P. westermani* have been described in Japan and also Korea, Taiwan and China (Hirai and Agatsuma 1991). Triploids have larger adults and eggs than diploids; triploids do not contain sperm and are considered to have parthenogenetic reproduction; and hosts and geographic distribution in Japan differ (triploid, *Eriocheir japonicus* and south-west; diploid, *Geothelphusa dehaani* and north-east), so the triploid has been suggested as a sibling species, *P. pulmonalis* (Baelz 1883) (Miyazaki 1979).

Eggs, 75–118 by 42–67 μm, with a flattened operculum fitted into a slight rim and thickened opposite pole, are unembryonated and yellowish-brown.

Human infections are most frequently due to *P. westermani*. In China, Japan and South-East Asia, *P. skrjabini*, *P. miyazakii*, *P. heterotremus*, *P. iloktsuensis*, *P. siamensis*, and *P. ohirai* in canines, felines, rodents, and man are acquired from *Eriocheir*, *Sinopotamon*, *Parathelphusa* crabs. In tropical West and Central Africa, *P. africanus* and *P. uterobilateralis* in man, civet cat, dog, cat, mongoose, are acquired from crabs, e.g. *Sudanautes africanus*, *S. pelli*, and *Liberonautes latidactylus*. *Paragonimus kellicotti* in North America is acquired from *Cambarus* spp. crayfish by mink, dog, cat, raccoon. *Paragonimus mexicana* (*P. peruvianus*, *P. ecuadoriensis*) occurs in Mexico, Central America, and the north-west of South America in the opossum, cat, dog, raccoon, and occasionally man.

Other flukes recorded in man include: *Fibricola seoulensis* (intestine, Korea, from amphibia), various *Plagiorchis* spp. (intestine, East and South-East Asia, from insects—mayflies, dragonflies), *Watsonius watsoni* (intestine, Nigeria), *Phaneropsolus bonnei* and *Prosthodendrium molenkampi* (intestine, Thailand, ?from metacercariae in dragon- and other flies), *Philophthalmus lacrymosus* (conjunctival sac, former Yugoslavia, Sri Lanka, ?cercaria while bathing).

LIFE CYCLE AND EPIDEMIOLOGY

The life cycles of all these flukes require one or two intermediate hosts (Fig. 55.1). Common hosts and their habitats are presented in Table 55.1, but this list certainly is not exhaustive.

Eggs are passed in the faeces either partly differentiated or containing a miracidium. Development and hatching of miracidia from eggs and development of snails and the parasites within them all require temperatures greater than 10 °C. Eggs may take one to

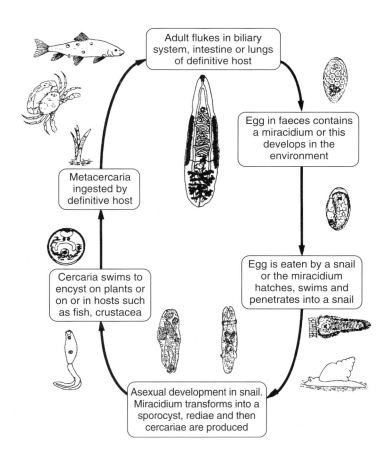

Fig. 55.1 Life cycle of a digenetic trematode.

Adult flukes in biliary system, intestine or lungs of definitive host

Egg in faeces contains a miracidium or this develops in the environment

Egg is eaten by a snail or the miracidium hatches, swims and penetrates into a snail

Asexual development in snail. Miracidium transforms into a sporocyst, rediae and then cercariae are produced

Cercaria swims to encyst on plants or on or in hosts such as fish, crustacea

Metacercaria ingested by definitive host

several weeks to develop, depending on temperature. While eggs of some species must be ingested by the snail host (e.g. *Dicrocoelium*, *Clonorchis*), for many, the ciliated mirachidium hatches and needs to detect and penetrate a snail host within 2–24 hours. Miracidia may show positive or negative phototropism and geotropism and recognize chemoattractants from the snail host. Water biology must be suitable for development of eggs, survival of the miracidia, and development of snails (Potseluev 1991). Thus, depending on species, snails will occur in fast-flowing, oxygenated streams, or in fresh or brackish water in slow-flowing streams and canals, or ponds. Man is an important definitive host for *C. sinensis*, *Opisthorchis* spp., *G. hominis*, and *F. buski*, so sanitary habits, sewage facilities, and customs of the people determine the level of contamination of the water with eggs. Even where sewage facilities are provided, studies with *Diphyllobothrium latum*, which has a very similar operculate egg, show that effluent from sewage plants and septic tanks can be heavily contaminated to contaminate canals, ditches, ponds, and lakes (see Chapter 49). In many areas, human faeces are used as fertilizer, not only for land from which eggs might be washed into ditches, but to fertilize ponds and canals growing edible water bulbs for man, or plants and algae as food for pigs or fishes, and the faeces supply food for fishes. Pigs are important reservoir hosts for *C. sinensis*, *G. hominis,* and *F. buski*, and their faeces also are used as fertilizer. Animals, e.g. Canidae and Felidae, also are contributors to maintain infections such as *C. sinensis*, *O. felineus*, and heterophyids where humans consume little or no raw fish (Posokhov *et al.* 1987). Piscivorous birds carry many fluke infections, e.g. heterophyids, echinostomes, to contaminate water. Finally, cattle and other ruminants, and even lagomorphs, provide the source of infection on to swampy or dry pastures for infection of snails with *F. hepatica* and *D. dendriticum*, respectively.

Development in the snail is temperature dependent and at above 10 °C varies from weeks to several months. At high and low temperatures development is inhibited but resumes, provided the snail survives, when favourable conditions return. *Fasciolopsis buski* develops in 4–8 weeks in the snail; development of *F. hepatica* can occur in 5 weeks in a tropical, humid climate. Usually the miracidium transforms into a sporocyst which produces rediae, perhaps daughter rediae, and in turn cercariae. *Dicrocoelium dendriticum* cercariae are excreted in groups in slime balls, but most cercariae are liberated into water. Cercariae show taxis and attraction to detect and produce a protective cyst wall on plants or on or in the muscles or viscera of fish, crustacea, or molluscs. The metacercariae mature to become infective (up to 12 hours for *F. hepatica*; longer periods, perhaps 3–4 weeks or more, for many other species).

Fasciola hepatica and *F. buski* cercariae encyst on plant matter, e.g. for *F. hepatica*, herbage on damp pastures or watercress, etc.; for *F. buski*, aquatic plants, including water caltrops and water chestnuts. Cercariae of *D. dendriticum* are passively acquired by ant second intermediate hosts that ingest slime balls. Some cercariae enter the suboesophageal ganglion of the ant to cause tetanic spasm of the mouthparts at low temperatures, so affected ants are more likely to be eaten as they attach to herbage surrounding the nest until morning temperatures increase. Other cercariae have only a limited time and use behavioural patterns to detect and enter an aquatic fish, crustacean, or molluscan second host. *Opisthorchis viverrini* cercariae show swimming behaviour and positive phototactic orientation to find plant-free microhabitats and are stimulated to attach and penetrate the fish by water currents and hydrophilic components of fish skin (Haas *et al.*, 1990). Cercariae of *Paragonimus* creep over rocks in inchworm fashion to attack crabs and crayfish; these also ingest cercariae and cercaria-infected snails (Shibahara 1991).

Dietary habits, particularly a preference for raw, salted, pickled, or undercooked fish, shellfish or snails, then become a most important risk factor for human infection. Further, fish are an important source of protein and many fish that are fast-growing, e.g. grass carp (*Ctenopharyngodon idellus*), can be 'farmed' in ponds fertilized by human or pig faeces. These factors combine in areas such as north-east Thailand—small cyprinid fish develop well in areas of water including rice paddies, and the Thai descendants of Laotians favour a variety of raw fish dishes. Equally, in Far-East Russia, 92 per cent of indigenous inhabitants, compared with 44 per cent of non-indigenous inhabitants, ate uncooked fish and this was reflected in 69 per cent compared with 37 per cent infection in the two groups. Even occasional consumption of inadequately prepared fish can be important; in the Komi-Permyak region high prevalence but low intensity of infection in man was related to occasional, 2–3 times a year, consumption of lightly salted fish (Bronshtein *et al.* 1989*a*). Wild and domestic pigs, cats, dogs, etc., that eat fish can maintain the cycle. Thus, high levels of *C. sinensis* infection in the south of Khabarovsk Territory, Russia, occur in cats (75 per cent), snails (3 per cent), and fish (10 per cent), yet infection in humans is rare as the inhabitants of the area do not eat raw fish (Posokhov *et al.* 1987).

Ethnic dishes of fish eaten raw, marinated, smoked, fermented, or lightly salted, favour infection and are popular in north-east Thailand, in the Philippines, and in Canton. Sliced raw fish is common in Japan. A salted fish delicacy in Egypt favours infection with *H. heterophyes* from mullet. *Paragonimus westermani* metacercariae are consumed when crabs or crayfish are eaten lightly cooked as crab soup or as 'drunken crab', marinated in brine, vinegar, soy, or wine. Children in Liberia chew on or eat the legs of crabs whose cephalothorax and leg muscles can be heavily infected (Sachs and Cumberlidge 1990). People may contaminate their hands and mouth accidentally in preparing fish or shellfish. Juice extracted from shellfish is used as an oral medicant for diarrhoea or measles in some countries and in a Philippine food dish. *Paragonimus westermani* can also be acquired from paratenic hosts that have eaten infected crabs or crayfish. Thus, the ingestion of wild boar sliced raw was incriminated in transmission in Japan. Flukes migrate to the muscles of paratenic hosts, boar, frogs, rodents, but remain immature until eaten by a definitive host (Shibahara and Nishida, 1986). As many of the raw meat and fish dishes are eaten on ceremonial occasions at which men predominate, this can account for the higher prevalence of infection often seen in men compared with women.

Metacercariae of *F. hepatica* are eaten on semiaquatic plants, watercress, water dandelions, grasses, or occasionally herbs or salad plants. Metacercariae of *F. buski* are eaten when water chestnuts, lotus tubers, bamboo, etc., grown in ponds or canals contaminated with faeces are cracked with the teeth to peel, particularly by children, or are eaten raw. Cercariae, that do not find a plant, encyst in water and may be swallowed in unfiltered water. Weng *et al.* (1989) estimated that 11 per cent of human and 37 per cent of pig infections with *F. buski* were due to drinking contaminated water.

Metacercariae excyst in the stomach and small intestine. Intestinal flukes do not undergo further migration. Juvenile *F. hepatica* migrate across the peritoneal cavity into the liver parenchyma where they migrate, feed, and grow for about 8 weeks before finally entering the bile ducts. The other liver flukes migrate from the small intestine through the common bile duct directly into the bile ducts. *Paragonimus* spp. are assumed to migrate across the peritoneal cavity, into the skeletal, e.g. abdominal muscles, diaphragm, and pleural cavity into the lungs (Sugiyama *et al.* 1990). In the lungs flukes usually pair and lie in cysts with openings to the bronchi.

PREVALENCE OF INFECTION

Infection with *C. sinensis* and *Opisthorchis* spp. is highly aggregated in a small proportion of individuals. Prevalence and intensity of infection usually increase with age, being lowest in the 0–10 years group, reach maxima between 30 and 50 years, often with a decline thereafter. Some recent surveys show a plateau at above 20 years but this may be related not to immunity but to periodic treatments and changes in customs as education and health care improve (Haswell-Elkins *et al.* 1991; Sithithaworn *et al.* 1994). Although prevalences have declined in many areas, infection remains widespread and common.

Clonorchis sinensis occurs in nine Asian countries and areas of the former Soviet Union. Recent studies examining prevalence include: 5–28 per cent of residents in endemic areas in Vietnam and China and 10–11 per cent in areas of Korea, with 0.5 per cent of snails and 13–85 per cent of fish infected and an intensity of 8–35 metacercariae/g of fish (Joo and Hong 1991).

Opisthorchis viverrini remains a problem in Thailand, particularly the north-east region, where one-third of the population is infected, with pockets of infection of 80 per cent (Sithithaworn *et al.* 1994) and infection is present in Laos. *Opisthorchis felineus* is more widespread through Asia into Europe. Prevalences and the participation of man decline from being high in central Russia to low in the Middle East and central Europe. Up to 95 per cent of the population in the Ob'-Irtysh basin, Siberia, were infected, with infection levels declining upstream and with man least involved in the cycle at the periphery of the basin (Zavoikin *et al.* 1991). In other endemic areas of central Russia, *O. felineus* can be found in 2–55 per cent of humans, and up to 50 per cent of cats, 1 per cent of snails, and 50 per cent of cyprinid fish.

About 28 countries, these primarily in Asia, regularly report infections with intestinal flukes. In different surveys in South Korea, 0.5–22 per cent of persons were infected with *E. hortense* and 2–41 per cent of fish contained metacercariae (Lee *et al.* 1988); in a tribal community in Bandipore, India, 10 per cent of persons were passing echinostome eggs (Bandyopadhyay and Nandy 1986). In the Far East of Russia *Nanophyetus* has been described in 10–68 per cent of the indigenous peoples while up to 17 per cent of humans, 30 per cent of pigs, and 63–77 per cent of dogs and cats were infected with *Metagonimus*. A nationwide survey in Korea in 1981 showed at least 1.2 per cent prevalence of *Metagonimus*, and in various endemic areas up to 42 per cent of individuals and a high proportion of fish were infected (Chai *et al.* 1993). Infections can be very common (59 per cent) in areas of Japan where raw fish is eaten, each *Plecoglossus* ayu or sweetfish containing averages of 2000–22 000 metacercariae (Ito *et al.* 1991). Where raw intermediate hosts are consumed habitually, mixed infections with a variety of flukes occur. The following parasites were recovered after treatment of a population in 16 provinces in north-east Thailand: *E. malayanum*, 8.3 per cent *E. ilocanum*, 8.1 per cent; *E. revolutum*, 0.8 per cent; *H. taichui*, 7.8 per cent; *H. pumilio*, 6.2 per cent;

H. yokogawai, 2.9 per cent; *P. bonnei* 15 per cent, *P. harinasutai*, 0.7 per cent; *P. molenkampi*, 19.4 per cent; *S. falcatus*, 0.3 per cent (Radomyos *et al.* 1994).

Paragonimus is common in man in China and the Far East and South-east of Asia. For example, in endemic areas of Hunan Province, China, up to 100 per cent of the crayfish, 94 per cent of the dogs and cats, and 15 per cent of humans were positive. In three countries in Taiwan, 17–79 per cent of patomid crabs each contained 1–5 metacercariae. Pockets of high prevalence are reported in West Africa. In endemic areas of Nigeria, Cameroon, and Liberia up to 10–17 per cent of inhabitants and 7–45 per cent of *Sudanautes* and *Liberonautes* spp. may be infected (Moyou *et al.* 1983; Udonsi 1987; Sachs and Cumberlidge 1990). Occasionally infections are described from India and the Americas.

Fasciola hepatica is reported at least sporadically in man in some 50 countries worldwide, particularly in South America and parts of Africa, Asia, and Europe. Recent surveys in Uruguay, Chile, Peru, etc., suggest that infection is more common than realized. For example, a survey in the province of Curico, Chile, found a series of foci where 0.6 per cent of persons were infected, far greater than the number of infections normally diagnosed (Alcaino 1990). Infections recently have been shown to be very common in Bolivia.

PATHOGENESIS, PATHOLOGY, AND CLINICAL SYMPTOMS

LIVER FLUKES

Migrating immature *F. hepatica* cause traumatic destruction of the liver parenchyma, particularly 6–8 weeks after infection, followed by inflammatory cell infiltration and fibrosis. Usually this is asymptomatic but large numbers migrating can cause acute disease, with abdominal pain, biliary colic, fever, hepatomegaly, elevated liver enzymes, eosinophilia, and, in children, anaemia and even deaths.

Fasciola hepatica, *C. sinensis*, *O. felineus* and less commonly *D. dendriticum*, induce changes in the bile ducts, the extent depending on the intensity and duration of infection. Mechanical irritation by the powerful suckers and spines of feeding flukes and the immune response to them result in proliferation and desquamation of bile duct epithelium, inflammatory cell infiltration into and degranulation in the bile duct wall. Released inflammatory mediators produce damage, tissues in the portal triads become oedematous, there is hyperplasia of the bile duct wall, cholangitis, and gradual healing with widespread fibrosis of the bile ducts. This and dead worms may cause biliary obstruction, diverticula, duct dilation, cholelithiasis

and, in prolonged heavy infections, portal hypertension may produce splenomegaly. Infection may manifest as acute or chronic disease with accompanying symptoms, pathology, and physical changes (Chen *et al.* 1989). Varying with the stage of the infection, heavy infections with hundreds or thousands of worms will produce fever, upper abdominal pain, hepatomegaly, eosinophilia, diarrhoea; in chronic infections there will be recurrent cholangitis, cholecystis, and possibly biliary colic, obstructive jaundice, dyspepsia, vomiting, eosinophilia, and hepatosplenomegaly. Anaemia and hypoalbuminaemia may be present.

Opisthorchis viverrini infection differs. There are fewer reports of acute disease but, in the later stages, gallbladder enlargement and dysfunction may be common. Most important is the striking association between *O. viverrini* and an increased incidence of bile duct cancer, cholangiocarcinoma (CHCA), which is an important cause of death after 20–40 years of infection. Although no correlation between infection and CHCA was shown in some hospital-based studies, the cancer might have prevented egg excretion through bile duct blockage. Parkin *et al.* (1991) did show a significantly higher frequency of antibody to *O. viverrini* in CHCA cases; consumption of sticky rice and betel nut chewing, which are common in northern Thailand, were also correlated with CHCA. Persons with long-standing, heavy infections are the most likely to develop CHCA and a much higher prevalence of early, presymptomatic CHCA was detected in persons with heavy infections (>6000 eggs/g) (Elkins *et al.* 1990; Sithithaworn *et al.* 1994). Patients with *C. sinensis* occasionally develop CHCA.

The mechanisms for enhancement of carcinogenesis are not understood. There might be synergism between the fluke and co-carcinogens, dietary *N*-nitroso compounds, particularly dimethylnitrosamine and nitrites, which occur in fermented fish sauce. Recently, however, an important role for nitric oxide and other reactive oxygen intermediaries that can induce DNA damage has been suggested. The vigorous immune response and production of endogenous oxygen metabolites in the bile ducts could represent an endogenous source of genotoxic substances in the vicinity of the infection. Thus, the parasites might induce DNA damage and mutations as a consequence of cellular proliferation of the bile duct epithelium and the formation of carcinogens/free-radicals (Parkin *et al.* 1993; Sithithaworn *et al.* 1994; Oshima and Barlsch 1995).

INTESTINAL FLUKES

Most infections are asymptomatic. *Gastrodiscoides hominis* and echinostomes seem well tolerated.

Fascrolopsis buski in the duodenum causes traumatic damage with its suckers, there is excessive mucus production ulceration, haemorrhage at the site of attachment, and abscess formation. It is said to interfere with vitamin B_{12} absorption. Particularly in children, heavy infections of 100 to more than 1000 worms produce a protein-losing enteropathy. The small heterophyids and *Nanophyetus* penetrate between the villi, producing inflammation and necrosis of the mucosa. Heterophyids penetrate into the crypts inducing, in heavy infections, inflammation, oedema, superficial congestion, villous atrophy, ulceration, and petechial haemorrhages. All these trematodes may present as mild digestive disturbances to intermittent or continuous usually mucoid, but occasionally bloody, diarrhoea. There may be eosinophilia, nausea, and severe colicky pain, possibly relieved by food. 'Flu-like' symptoms are described in heavy *Nanophyetus* infections. Ascites and facial oedema may be due to loss of albumen while 'toxaemia' from heavy *F. buski* infection has been described.

Some heterophyids may penetrate the intestinal mucosa and enter the circulation to embolize in various organs of the body. Granulomatous lesions have been particularly noticeable in the brain and heart, e.g. lesions on the mitral valves have caused cardiac failure.

LUNG FLUKES

Paragonimus migration in the lungs produces focal haemorrhagic pneumonia with pain, cough, fever, fatigue, and marked eosinophilia. Those migrating in the pleural cavity induce profuse pleural effusions, adhesions, pneumothorax, and chest pain. Migration is followed by fibrous encapsulation enclosing pairs of worms in greyish-white cysts about 1–3 cm in diameter, opening into a bronchus and containing yellow-brown purulent fluid. There is chronic cough, chest pain, and rust-coloured sputum with a 'fish-taste'. Secondary bacterial pneumonia and haemoptysis are complications. Pulmonary and pleural paragonimosis are reviewed by Shim *et al.* (1991) and Nana and Bovornkitti (1991).

ABERRANT MIGRATION

Paragonimus spp. may be found in various organs in the abdominal cavity, in subcutaneous tissues and the brain. *Paragonimus skrjabini*, in particular, has been shown to migrate in the liver to produce hepatic dysfunction from marked adhesions surrounding the liver, spleen and duodenum, and eosinophilic abscesses and cysts containing worms in the liver (Xiaosu *et al.* 1982). *Paragonimus skrjabini*, *P. heterotremus*, and *P. mexicana* usually do not cause lung lesions, man

apparently not being a suitable host, but are found subcutaneously on the chest, abdominal wall, or extremities. The nodule or mass produced often is a very painful and migrating lesion inducing marked eosinophilia.

Cerebral migration of *Paragonimus* causes oedema, haemorrhage, and meningitis. The lesions and symptoms may be confused with a cerebral tumour; severe headache, seizures, and hemiparesis are common signs. Cerebral paragonimosis is reviewed by Kusner and King (1993). *Fasciola hepatica* also may be found in the brain, or encapsulated in a nodule in the lungs or other organs.

DIAGNOSIS

EXAMINATIONS FOR EGGS

Faecal samples are normally examined for *Clonorchis, Opisthorchis,* and the small intestinal flukes by formalin-ether/ethyl acetate concentration methods or Stoll technique. These have proved superior to Kato thick smears (Sithithaworn *et al.* 1994). Modifications of the methods continue to be suggested. Overall sensitivity of 85–90 per cent for *O. viverrini* and *C. sinensis* is described, reduced to 70 per cent on a single evaluation of persons harbouring fewer than 20 worms. For a number of the liver flukes, duodenal aspiration may detect scarce eggs and swallowing a brushed nylon string can concentrate eggs (Enterotest). Canulation of the bile duct has been carried out in cases of blockage, but this is invasive and not a simple procedure. The eggs of many of the liver and small intestinal flukes are very similar; skilful and time-consuming examinations are required for their differentiation. Size and shape have considerable intraspecific variability such that biometrical analysis may only divide eggs into groups (Xu 1980; Lee *et al.* 1984). Eggs of the Fasciolidae and echinostomes are detected with detergent/sedimentation techniques and iodine staining. If *G. hominis* is suspected a methylene green/blue stain is substituted so the relatively colourless eggs will appear silvery compared with the yellowish *Fasciola*. *Paragonimus* eggs in the sputum or faeces may be scarce in chronic infections so concentration techniques are useful.

Not all surveys show correlations between egg and worm numbers. A recent survey showed that infections of fewer than 1000 to more than 15 000 *O. felineus* produced an irregular distribution of eggs (Bychkov *et al.* 1990). However, a strong correlation was described between egg numbers, IgG, and post-mortem worm numbers for *O. viverrini*, though fecundity was negatively associated with total worm burden (Elkins *et al.* 1991; Sithithaworn *et al.* 1994).

Spurious infections from eating infected liver are not uncommon, particularly for *D. dendriticum*. Spurious infections can be ruled out after several days on a controlled diet.

ULTRASOUND, RADIOGRAPHY, ETC.

Radiography for *Paragonimus* shows nodular or soap bubble-shaped shadows that must be differentiated from tuberculosis lesions. Fibrous or calcified cysts of *Paragonimus* may be seen in the brain. Cerebral eosinophilia is a useful indicator. Contrast media may outline liver flukes and damaged bile ducts (irregular filling defects and dilated). Persons heavily infected with *O. viverrini* on ultrasonography and CT scan frequently showed increased size of the left liver lobe and gallbladder dysfunction (fasting and post-meal), an indistinct gallbladder wall, sludge in the gallbladder, and enhanced portal vein radical echoes (Mairiang *et al.*, 1992, 1993). Biliary stones and flukes can be confused on ultrasonography but M-mode sonogram may detect fluke movement. CT scan has been used to diagnose acute fasciolosis which manifested as hypodense areas in the liver, indicative of hepatic destruction, accompanied by eosinophilia, fever, pain, and a recent history of eating watercress (Loutan *et al.*, 1989).

IMMUNODIAGNOSIS

Skin tests have long been used in Asia in surveys and as an aid to diagnosis and remain a common method of diagnosis for *C. sinensis* and *Paragonimus*. These now are being superseded by serological tests.

Serology

ELISA diagnosis has been developed for the liver flukes. That for *O. viverrini* showed 87 per cent sensitivity (Chen 1988) and, for *C. sinensis*, 79–95 per cent sensitivity. Nevertheless, specificity can be poor and positive titres can remain for some time after apparently successful treatment—50 per cent of light infections became negative only after 6 months and after 24 months for heavy infections (Chen 1988). Chen *et al.* (1989) have, however, suggested division of clonorchosis patients into three clinical stages based on antibody isotype: acute stage, recently infected patients being IgM, IgA, and IgG positive; subacute, IgA and IgG positive; and the chronic infections, IgG positive. *Fasciola* is diagnosed using tests developed for the normal ruminant hosts. ELISA and haemagglutination, particularly with E/S antigens, have shown good sensitivity (about 90 per cent) and high specificity in Western patients (Ambroise-Thomas *et al.* 1980; Alcaino 1990). The positive predictive value of the serological

tests still is such that corroborating clinical and/or parasitological evidence must be obtained. Nevertheless, serological assays are very useful in confirmation of a diagnosis and particularly in surveys.

Tests for circulating antigen of liver and lung flukes are being examined experimentally and show promise. A dot-ELISA using a monoclonal antibody to adult worm antigen was positive in all persons with parasitologically confirmed *P. westermani* and also in a high proportion of suspected cases. It showed high specificity against infections with other helminths and pulmonary tuberculosis (Zhang *et al.* 1993). In experimentally infected dogs circulating antigen peaked 5–6 days after praziquantel treatment and declined over the next 2 months.

Coprological diagnosis

Techniques to detect trematode coproantigen are being developed. Monoclonal antibody against an E/S antigen of *O. viverrini* showed a sensitivity of 57 per cent. Improvements in the antibodies and possibly detection of multiple E/S antigens should increase sensitivity. An *O. viverrini*-specific probe also has been developed (Sirisinha *et al.* 1991).

TREATMENT

Praziquantel is the drug of choice for most of these trematode infections. 75 mg/kg divided into three doses given 5–6 hours apart on 1 day or repeated on a second day shows greater than 90 per cent efficacy against *Clonorchis* and *Opisthorchis* spp. and is needed for moderate and heavy infections. Light infections can often be treated with 40 mg/kg given once, which produces fewer side-effects (Jong *et al.* 1985; Bronshtein *et al.* 1989*b*). Vertigo, headache, weakness, nausea, and a pruritic rash, although common side-effects, are mild and transient and usually occur within 2–3 hours and last less than 24 hours. Severity should be reduced if patients eat before treatment (Bronshtein *et al.* 1989*b*). Praziquantel at a 14 mg/kg dose repeated three times a day for 5 days also has been highly effective. Improvement in gallbladder status (size and function) has been reported after successful praziquantel treatment. However, long-standing, particularly heavy infections would have produced permanent damage and resultant sequelae in the portal triads. Thus, symptoms of digestive dysfunction can continue in a proportion of patients despite successful treatment for liver flukes, while malignancy with *O. viverrini*, once initiated, was not reversible (Mairiang *et al.* 1993).

Albendazole given at 5 mg/kg/day or 10 mg/kg twice a day, both for 7 days, was 90–92 per cent and 100 per cent effective, respectively, when judged by faecal egg examinations. Albendazole has the advantage of clearing concurrent nematode infections, has relatively low cost, and only mild and transient side-effects, but it does require the 7-day course for *Clonorchis* (Liu *et al.* 1991).

Bithionol, 100 mg/kg every second day for 2–3 weeks has been used with effect for the Opisthorchiidae and intestinal flukes but has largely been superseded by praziquantel. Hexachloroparaxylene (60 mg/kg for 5 days) has been used, particularly in the former USSR, with reasonable effect but its side-effects are too severe. Praziquantel in its liposomal form showed higher efficacy experimentally than did praziquantel alone. Triclabendazole has been used experimentally for *Clonorchis* and *Opisthorchis* infections.

Praziquantel, 60–75 mg/kg in three divided doses, has been used with effect to treat both pulmonary and ectopic *Paragonimus*. Sixty mg/kg given for three consecutive days was effective in 87 per cent of patients (Moyou *et al.* 1983). Generally a single dose of 10–15 mg/kg praziquantel is effective against *F. buski* and other gastrointestinal flukes. In some clinical trials 20 mg/kg three times a day has been used.

Praziquantel is less effective for *F. hepatica* in man. Bithionol, at approximately 100 mg/kg every second day for 2–3 weeks, effective only against the adult stages, is used with effect. Recently, triclabendazole given as a single dose or two doses of 10 mg/kg showed good effect in acute fasciolosis in man; it is known to kill both immature and adult *Fasciola* in animals (Loutan *et al.* 1989). Dehydroemetine and even emetine (usually at 60 mg/day for 10 days for adult patients) still remain drugs used, often legally authorized, for *F. hepatica*. However, the immediate problems of pain or abscess at the site of injection and severe toxicity (nausea, vomiting, cardiac alterations requiring hospitalization and ECG monitoring) mean they should be superseded by triclabendazole.

CONTROL

Baseline data on the biology of each trematode, both in the field and from experimental studies, must be collected before control measures are instituted. Only with this information can the costs and feasibility of control, the difficulty in attaining and maintaining control, and the potential for maintenance of eradication, if feasible, be predicted mathematically. The data are needed also to monitor efficacy of the decisions made. The data required include: age-related prevalence and intensity of infection, longevity of infection, fecundity of the parasite, immunity to infection (if any) in the intermediate and definitive hosts, and rates of re-infection in the human population. Food

supply, sanitation, social and cultural customs, and sources of food (fish, crustaceans, and molluscs), whether farmed or wild-caught, and food preferences (methods of preparation, preferred species eaten and/or fed to domestic animals) all must be identified. In addition, farming practices (fish farming), including methods of fertilization and the costs and feasibility of alternate methods, must be considered. Most important is knowledge as to the variety and numbers of reservoir hosts. The extent of their involvement in the transmission dynamics varies greatly with the species of parasite; if important, feasibility of control in these must be determined.

Surveys to identify foci of infection, to identify areas where transmission could occur if there were immigration of an infected human population, and to monitor control, all require collaboration between public health personnel, the veterinary department, malacologists, and ichthyologists. Some diagnostic techniques for surveys of snail-borne diseases are reviewed by Impand *et al.* (1989). Immunodiagnosis will gradually replace labour-intensive parasitological diagnosis in surveys of definitive hosts for many of the liver and lung flukes but predictive values must be determined for these analyses. Differentiation of adult parasites recovered after treatment and identification of infections in snails, metacercariae in fish, etc., also require considerable technical skills for morphometric differentiation of the fluke species. Species-specific techniques suitable for use in field laboratories are an urgent need. Recently, a DNA probe and a reverse transcriptase–polymerase chain reaction have been developed to detect *F. hepatica* infection in snails, and the latter should detect *F. buski* (Rognlie *et al.* 1994).

Changes in the environment and their impact (favourable or otherwise) on transmission must be considered also. An increase in the price of fish (export or poor supply) may decrease levels of infection in an indigenous population. Conversely, increased wealth and standard of living could increase incidence. A period of famine may ensure consumption of more fish/shellfish versus meat, fish might be only lightly cooked due to lack of fuel, or fish species that normally are not eaten or are fed to animals are eaten by man. Water biology will determine the development of the free-living stages and proliferation of snails and fish. Pollution may in fact affect water biology unfavourably for transmission. Thus, an increase in water pollution with insecticides and from factories has been linked to a decline in *C. sinensis* in Japan. A decline in infection with *H. heterophyes* along the Nile, e.g. in Mataria, Egypt, has been attributed to a change in water nutrients due to the Aswan Dam. Conversely, a consequence of construction of the Diama dam on the Senegal river was the production of conditions suitable for a rapid rise in *Lymnaea natalensis* and *F. gigantica* in sheep; this could spill-over into the human population. Chefranova (1989) delineated factors to be considered in forecasting changes in foci of *Opisthorchis* induced by dam construction, emphasizing the need to consider changes in water flow in the network of water bodies and not just in the immediate vicinity. Data on technical characteristics of reservoirs, copepods, molluscs, fish, parasite infection levels, collated at Martsinovskii Institute of Medical Parasitology and Tropical Medicine, Moscow, will aid forecasting of parasitological changes for recommendations at the planning and construction stages of reservoirs (Plyushcheva *et al.* 1986).

Control programmes in which man is the most important definitive host have shown considerable success in reducing prevalence of infection for *Opisthorchis* and *Clonorchis*. Treatment alone was considered insufficient due to rapid re-infection after treatment (Sornmani *et al.* 1984; Upathan *et al.* 1988; Saowakontha *et al.*, 1993). However, when combined with public health education, praziquantel treatments showed considerable success for control of *O. viverrini* in north-east Thailand (Saowakontha *et al.*, 1993). Infected village inhabitants were treated every 6 or 12 months with praziquantel. This was combined with education of the inhabitants aimed at changing raw-fish eating habits and to encourage construction and use of latrines. Prevalence of infection, intensity of infection, incidence, and rate of reinfection all declined significantly over a period of 3 years. Knowledge on *Opisthorchis* among individuals increased from 5 per cent of the population to as high as 80 per cent and there was a rapid drop, from 80 per cent to zero by 3 years, in the numbers of persons reporting raw fish consumption in the 2 months prior to questioning.

Targeting of populations for treatment might be cost-effective. Haswell-Elkins *et al.* (1991) have suggested targeting for *O. viverrini* as 74 per cent of infections were aggregated in 10 per cent of individuals. Targeting is likely to prevent severe disease and associated CHCA due to *O. viverrini*. In this regard, Markin (1991) has prepared a multi-factor, mathematically based table for better identification of groups at risk of *O. felineus* as an aid for questionnaire screening of populations. Data would be required, however, to delineate the relevance of the infection pressure generated by the remaining untreated, albeit lower, levels of human infection with *Opisthorchis* or other trematodes and the relevance of reservoir hosts with regard to control.

Treatment could be targeted to season. Forecasting emergence of cercariae of *F. hepatica* was described in 1959 by Ollerenshaw and Roland and many mathe-

matical models now delineate times for prophylactic treatments to limit transmission and prevent disease in animals. Infection with trematodes, e.g. *Metagonimus* in Korea, is acquired from early June when fishing for sweetfish begins, the infection rate being highest in July and August when the fish is eaten raw (Kim *et al.* 1979). Such knowledge can target treatments. Times at risk do vary, however, with geographic area and terrain. Thus, *F. buski* was at its highest level from November/December onwards on the coast of Fujian Province, China, but at its lowest levels from November in the north-east Montane, Meghalaya, India, even though these areas are at the same latitude (Wang *et al.* 1977; Roy and Tandon 1992).

Targeting important reservoir hosts can be effective. Human fasciolosis occurs most commonly when cercariae/metacercariae flood from wet and swampy animal pastures on to watercress beds. Regulations in France require that no animals graze around commercial watercress beds and that production is restricted to authorized growers and sellers. Methods for detection of infection in beds are given by Rondelaud and Mage (1990). This does not, however, prevent people picking watercress from wild beds. In a study in Puerto Rico none of the snails on commercial farms harboured *Fasciola*, no metacercariae were detected on the watercress, and no susceptible animals were observed near the establishments. This was not true of natural beds where infected snails and metacercariae in the beds and infected cattle nearby were identified (Bendezu *et al.* 1988). Alteration in farming methods can reduce levels of infection. Heat treatment of faeces used as fertilizer in fish ponds has been used to break the cycles of *C. sinensis* and *F. buski* in China. Even simple composting can suffice. Water plants should be dried before feeding to pigs. Other methods to reduce infection still are largely experimental. Some copepods and fish prey on cercariae. Predator aquatic snails/ducks/geese, etc., can reduce numbers of snails, but predators must be introduced with care as they themselves can be destructive to plants.

The most important risk factors for infection are faecal contamination of water, fishing, and inadequate preparation of fish for eating. Cessation in consumption of raw or lightly pickled fish/shellfish will prevent both common and occasional infections. Regular health education and sanitation improvement to change the customs of the population are the most important aspects of a control programme. Thus, design and implementation of programmes must be undertaken with the co-operation of educationalists, and the funding authorities must be aware that such programmes must be long-lived. There is evidence for a decline in levels of infection among populations as education and the standard of living increase and the population becomes aware of the diseases and their transmission.

With the increased trade in chilled fish, infected fish is transported throughout the world. This fish may be favoured and used in ethnic dishes among emigrant populations, but also increased travel has altered food habits among indigenous peoples. Consideration must be given to inspection of fish. Information is needed on methods of preparation that kill the metacercariae. Heterophyid metacercariae dissected from Nile fish are killed when marinated in 5 per cent lemon juice and more than 1.5 per cent acetic acid in vinegar (Mahmoud *et al.* 1988). In Russia, salting of fish to high salt concentration (10 per cent saline solution) can kill the metacercariae, but the traditional methods using lower concentrations, i.e. 3-day wet salting or dry salting to 1.7 per cent salt content fail to kill metacercariae, although infectivity does decline with time (Kotel'nikov and Malkov 1992). Potentially useful for the future transport of fish is irradiation or freezing. Metacercariae may be killed by freezing of fish at –10 °C for 5–70 days (depending on species) or within 24 hours at –28 °C. Irradiation of fish at 0.15 kGy controlled infectivity of *C. sinensis* metacercariae in the muscles of fish and could be adopted as a control measure (Song *et al.* 1992). Metacercariae of *F. hepatica* and *F. buski* can remain viable on plants, even dried plants, for prolonged periods, perhaps 2–3 months. Irradiation of fresh or dried produce could be successful.

REFERENCES

Alcaino, H. (1990). Epidemiology of fascioliasis in Chile. In *Basic Research in helminthiasis*, (ed. R. Ehrlich, A. Nieto, and L. Yarzabal), pp. 11–30. Ediciones LOGOS, Montevideo.

Ambroise-Thomas, P., Desgeorges, P. T., and Bouttaz, M. (1980). Diagnosis of human and bovine fascioliasis by means of enzyme-linked immunosorbent assay (ELISA). Detection of circulating antibodies and/or antigens. *Annales de la Societe Belge de Medicine Tropicale*, **60**, 47–60.

Bandyopadhyay, A. K. and Nandy, A. (1986). A preliminary observation on the prevalence of echinostomes in a tribal community near Culcutta. *Annals of Tropical Medicine and Parasitology*, **80**, 373–5.

Bendezu, P., Frame, A. D., Frame, E. L., and Bonilla, C. (1988). Watercress cultivation sites and their relationships to fascioliasis in Puerto Rico. *Journal of the Agricultural University of Puerto Rico*, **72**, 405–11.

Bronshtein, A. M., Uchuatkin, E. A., Romanenko, N. A., Kantsan, S. N., Veretennikova, N. L., and Sabgaida, T. P. (1989 *a*). Complex evaluation of a focus of opisthorchiasis in the Komi-Permyats Autonomous Region. *Meditsinskaya Parazitologiya i Parazitarnye Bolezni*, No. 4, 66–72.

Bronshtein, A. M., Merzlova, N. B., Veretennikova, N. L., and Dmitrieva, A. M. (1989*b*). Treatment of patients with praziquantel in out-patient conditions in a focus of opisthorchiasis in the Komi-Permyats Autonomous Region. *Meditsinskaya Parazitologiya i Parazitarnye Bolezni*, No. 2, 30–3.

Bychkov, V. G., Ivanskikh, V. I., Molokova, O. A., and Prokopenko, V. I. (1990). Comparison of the number of *Opisthorchis* worms in the host with the number of eggs present in the faeces. *Meditsinskaya Parazitologiya i Parazitarnye Bolezni*, No. 2, 14–16.

Chai, J. Y., *et al.* (1993). An epidemiological study of metagonimiasis along the upper reaches of the Namhan river. *Korean Journal of Parasitology*, **31**, 99–108.

Chefranova, Y. F. (1989). Forecasting the status of opisthorchiasis in zones affected by hydrological plants. *Meditisinskaya Parazitologiya i Parazitarnye Bolezni*, No. 6, 60–3.

Chen, C. Y. (1988). Clinical study of treatment and immunodiagnosis in patients with clonorchiasis. *Journal of the Formosan Medical Association*, **87**, 1170–5.

Chen, C. Y., Shin, J. W., Chen, S. N., and Hsieh, W. C. (1989). A preliminary study of clinical staging in clonorchiasis. *Chinese Journal of Microbiology and Immunology*, **22**, 193–200.

Elkins, D. B. *et al.* (1990). A high frequency of hepatobiliary disease and suspected cholangiocarcinoma associated with heavy *Opisthorchis viverrini* infection in a small community in Northeast Thailand. *Transactions of the Royal Society of Tropical Medicine and Hygiene*, **84**, 715–19.

Elkins, D. B., Sithithaworn, P., Haswell-Elkins, M. R., Kaewkes, S., Awacharagan, P., and Wongratanacheewin, S. (1991). *Opisthorchis viverrini*—relationships between egg counts, worms recovered and antibody levels within an endemic community in Northeast Thailand. *Parasitology*, **102**, 283–8.

Grove, D. I. (1990). *A history of human helminthology*. CAB International, Wallingford.

Harai, H. and Agatsuma, T. (1991). Triploidy in *Paragonimus westermani Parasitology Today*, **7**, 16–18.

Hass, W., Grazner, M., and Brockelman, C. R. (1990). *Opisthorchis viverrini*: finding and recognition of the fish host by the cercariae. *Experimental Parasitology*, **71**, 422–31.

Haswell-Elkins, M. R., Elkins, D. B., Sithithaworn, P., Treesarawat, P, and Kaewkes, S. (1991). Distribution patterns of *Opisthorchis viverrini* within a human community. *Parasitology*, **103**, 97–101.

Impand, P., Kitikoon, V., and Sormani, S. (1989). Diagnostic techniques for the survey of snail-borne parasitic diseases. In *Proceedings SEAMEO-TROPMED Seminar, Surat Thani, Thailand*, (ed. T. Bunnag and S. Sornmani), pp. 269–74.

Ito, J., Mochizuki, H., Ohno, Y., and Ishiguro, M. (1991). On the prevalence of *Metagonimus* sp. among the inhabitants at Hamamatsu Basin in Shizuoka Prefecture, Japan. *Japanese Journal of Parasitology*, **40**, 274–8.

Joo, C. Y. and Hong, Y. A. (1991). Epidemiological studies of *Clonorchis sinensis* in the vicinity of River Ahnseong, Kyungpook Province, Korea. *Japanese Journal of Parasitology*, **40**, 542–52.

Jong, E. C. *et al.*, (1985). Praziquantel for treatment of *Clonorchis–Opisthorchis* infections—report of a double blind, placebo controlled trial. *Journal of Infectious Diseases*, **152**, 637–40.

Kanev, I. (1994). Life-cycle, delimitation and redescription of *Echinostoma revolutum* (Froelich, 1802) (Trematoda, Echinostomatidae). *Systematic Parasitology*, **28**, 125–44.

Kim, D. C., Lee, O. Y., Jeong, E. B., and Han, E. J. (1979). Epidemiological conditions of *Metagonimus yokogawai* in Hadong Gun, Gyeongsang, Nam Do. *Korean Journal of Parasitology*, **17**, 51–9.

Kotel'nikov, G. A. and Malkov, S. N. (1992). Sanitary helminthological evaluation of various methods of salting fish in the basins of the rivers Vyatka and Kama. *Meditsinskaya Parazitologiya i Parazitarnye Bolezni*, No. 2, 28–9.

Kusner, D. J. and King, C. H. (1993). Cerebral paragonimiasis. *Seminars in Neurology*, **13**, 201–8.

Lee, S. H., Hwang, S. W., Chai, J. Y., and Seo, B. S. (1984). Comparative morphology of eggs of heterophyids and *Clonorchis sinensis* causing human infections in Korea. *Korean Journal of Parasitology*, **22**, 171–180.

Lee, S. K., Chung, N. S., Ko, I. H., and Sohn, W. M. (1988). An epidemiological survey of *Echinostoma hortense* infection in Chongsong-gun, Kyongbuk Province. *Korean Journal of Parasitology*, **26**, 199–206.

Liu, Y. H., Wang, X. G., Gao, P., and Qian, M. X. (1991). Experimental and clinical trial of albendazole in the treatment of clonorchiasis sinensis. *Chinese Medical Journal*, **104**, 27–31.

Loutan, L. *et al.* (1989). Single treatment of invasive fascioliasis with triclabendazole. *Lancet*, **2**, 383.

Mahmoud, N. A. M., El-Salam, F. A. A., and El-Gawad, A. F. A. (1988). Some studies on the metacercarial infection in *Schilbe mystis* fresh water Nile fish at Sohag Province, Egypt. The effect of household diluted acids on the viability and infectivity of the metacercariae of *Stictodora tridactyla* Martin & Kuntz, 1955 and *Prohemistomum vivax* Sonsind, 1892. *Assiut Veterinary Medical Journal*, **38**, 63–7.

Mairiang, E. *et al.* (1992). Relationship between intensity of *Opisthorchis viverrini* infection and hepatobiliary disease detected by ultrasonography. *Journal of Gasroenterology and Hepatology*, **7**, 17–21.

Mairiang, E., Haswell-Elkins, M. R., Mairiang, P., Sithithaworn, P., and Elkins, D. B., (1993). Reversal of biliary tract abnormalities associated with *Opisthorchis viverrini* infection following praziquantel treatment. *Transactions of the Royal Society of Tropical Medicine and Hygiene*, **87**, 194–7.

Markin, A. V. (1991). Questionnaire screening in opisthorchiasis. *Zhurnal Mikrobiolgii, Epidemiologii i Immunobiologii*, No. 11, 30–3.

Miyazaki, I. (1979). On the newly proposed lung fluke, *Paragonimus pulmonalis* (Baelz, 1880). *Medical Bulletin of Fukuoka University*, **6**, 267–76.

Moyou, S. R. *et al.* (1983). Study of paragonimiasis in five villages of the Department of Meme (south-western Cameroon). Results of praziquantel treatment. *Revue Science Technique, Science Sante*, No. 6/7, 125–9.

Nana, A. and Bovornkitti, S. (1991). Pleuropulmonary paragonimiasis. *Seminars in Respiratory Medicine*, **12**, 46–54.

Ollerenshaw, C. B. and Roland, L. P. (1959). A method for forecasting the incidence of fascioliasis in Anglesey. *Veterinary Record*, **71**, 591–8.

Oshima, H. and Barlsch, H. (1995). Infections and inflammatory processes as cancer risk factors: possible role of nitric oxide in carcinogenesis. *Mutation Research*, Fundamental + Molecular Mechanisms of Mutagenesis, **305**, 253–64.

Parkin, D. M. *et al.* (1991). Liver cancer in Thailand. 1. A case-control study of cholangiocarcinoma. *International Journal of Cancer*, **48**, 323–8.

Parkin, D. M., Ohshima, H., Srivatanakul, P., and Vatanasapt, V. (1993). Cholangiocarcinoma—epidemiology, mechanisms of carcinogenesis and prevention. *Cancer Epidemiology, Biomarkers and Prevention*, **2**, 537–44.

Pearson, J. C. and Ow-Yang, C. K. (1982). New species of *Haplorchis* from Southeast Asia, together with keys to the *Haplorchis*-group of heterophyid trematodes of the region. *Southeast Asian Journal of Tropical Medicine and Public Health*, **13**, 35–60.

Plyushcheva, G. L., Yarotskii, L. S., and Gerasimov, I. V. (1986). Forecasting the parasitological situation in zones affected by reservoirs. *Meditsinskaya Parazitologiya i Parazitarnye Bolezni*, No. 5, 78–82.

Posokhov, P. S., Dovgalev, A. S., and Bryunetkina, N. M. (1987). A case of chlonorchiasis unrecognized during life. *Meditsinskaya Parazitologiya i Parazitarnye Bolezni*, No. 5, 45–6.

Potseluev, A. N. (1991). The role of small hydro-engineering installations in changing the habitat of molluscs, intermediate hosts of *Opisthorchis*. *Meditsinskaya Parazitologiya i Parazitarnye Bolezni*, No. 5, 32–4.

Radomyos, P., Radomyos, B., and Tungtrongchitr, A. (1994). Multi-infection with helminths in adults from Northeast Thailand as determined by post-treatment fecal examination of adult worms. *Tropical Medicine and Parasitology*, **45**, 133–5.

Rognlie, M. C., Dimke, K. I., and Knapp, S. E. (1994). Detection of *Fasciola hepatica* in infected intermediate hosts. *Journal of Parasitology*, **80**, 748–55.

Rondelaud, D. and Mage, C. (1990). Human fasciliasis and watercress beds. *Point Veterinaire*, **21**, 899–903.

Roy, B. and Tandon, V. (1992). Seasonal prevalence of some zoonotic trematode infections in cattle and pigs in the North-east Montane Zone, Meghalaya, India. *Veterinary Parasitology*, **41**, 69–76.

Sachs, R. and Cumberlidge, N. (1990). Distribution of metacercariae in freshwater crabs in relation to *Paragonimus* infection of children in Liberia, West Africa. *Annals of Tropical Medicine and Parasitology*, **84**, 277–80.

Saowakontha, S., Pipitgool, V., Pariyanonda, S., Tesana, S., Rojsathaporn, K., and Intarakhao, C. (1993). Field trials in the control of *Opisthorchis viverrini* with an integrated programme in endemic areas of Northeast Thailand. *Parasitology*, **106**, 283–8.

Shibahara, T. (1991). The route of infection of *Paragonimus westermani* (diploid type) cercariae in the freshwater crab, *Geothelphusa dehaani*. *Journal of Helminthology*, **65**, 38–42.

Shibahara, T. and Nishida, H. (1986). Studies on the lung fluke, *Paragonimus westermani*—diploid type—in the northern part of Hyogo Prefecture, Japan. VI. Experimental oral infection of wild boars and pigs with metacercariae. *Japanese Journal of Parasitology*, **35**, 303–11.

Shim, Y. S., Cho, S. Y., and Han, Y. C. (1991). Pulmonary paragonimiasis: a Korean perspective. *Seminars in Respiratory Medicine*, **12**, 35–45.

Sirisinha, S., Chawengkirttkul, R., Sermswan, R., Amornpant, S., Mongkolsuk, S., and Panyim, S. (1991). Detection of *Opisthorchis viverrini* by monoclonal antibody-based ELISA and DNA hybridization. *American Journal of Tropical Medicine and Hygiene*, **44**, 140–5.

Sithithaworn, P. *et al.* (1994). Parasite associated morbidity—liver fluke infection and bile duct cancer in Northeast Thailand. *International Journal for Parasitology*, **24**, 833–43.

Song, C. C., Duan, Y. F., Shou, G. C., and Zhu, H. (1992). Studies on the use of cobalt-60 gamma irradiation to control infectivity of *Clonorchis sinensis* metacercariae. *Southeast Asian Journal of Tropical Medicine and Public Health*, **23**, 71–6.

Sornmani, S., Vivatanasesth, P., Impand, P., Phatihatakorn, W., and Sitabutra, P. (1984). Infection and re-infection rates of opisthorchiasis in the Water Resource Development Area of Nam Pong Project, Khon Kaen Province, northeast Thailand. *Annals of Tropical Medicine and Parasitology*, **78**, 649–56.

Sugiyama, H., Matsumoto, M., Horiuchi, T., and Tomimura, T. (1990). Migration route of flukes in cats experimentally infected with the diploid type of *Paragonimus westermani* metacercariae. *Journal Japan Veterinary Medical Association*, **43**, 808–11.

Udonsi, J. K. (1987). Endemic *Paragonimus* infection in Upper lgwun Basin, Nigeria: a preliminary report on a renewed outbreak. *Annals of Tropical Medicine and Parasitology*, **81**, 57–62.

Upatham, E. S., Viyanant, V., Brockelman, W. Y., Kurathong, S., Lee, P., and Kraengraeng, R. (1988). Rate of reinfection by *Opisthorchis viverrini* in an endemic northeast Thai community after chemotherapy. *Transactions of the Royal Society of Tropical Medicine and Hygiene*, **83**, 241–2.

Wang, P., Zhang, K., Wu, F., and Yao, T. (1977). Studies on the life history of *Fasciolopsis buski* (Lankester, 1857) with consideration of its seasonal infection in pigs. *Acta Zoologica Sinica*, **23**, 88–96.

Weng, Y. L., Zhuang, Z. L., Jiang, H. P., Lin, G. R., and Lin, J. J. (1989). Studies on ecology of *Fasciolopsis buski* and control strategy of fasciolopsiasis. *Chinese Journal of Parasitology and Parasitic Diseases*, **7**, 108–11.

Xiaosu, H., Ruiyuan, F., Zhiren, Z., Jinzhong, L., Hanxun, W., and Jianhua, L. (1982). Hepatic damage in experimental and clinical paragonimiasis. *American Journal of Tropical Medicine and Hygiene*, **31**, 1148–55.

Xu, B. K. (1980). The identification of *Clonorchis sinensis* ova found in human faeces and tissues. *National Medical Journal of China*, **60**, 33–5.

Zavoikin, V. D., Darchenkova, N. N., and Zelya, O. P. (1991). Territorial structure of opisthorchiasis in the Ob'-Irtysh basin. *Meditsinskaya Parazitologiya i Parazitarnye Bolezni*, No. **6**, 25–8.

Zhang, Z. H. *et al.* (1993). Diagnosis of active *Paragonimus westermani* infections with a monoclonal antibody-based antigen detection assay. *American Journal of Tropical Medicine and Hygiene*, **49**, 329–34.

56 STRONGYLOIDOSIS

T. J. Nolan, R. M. Genta, and G. A. Schad

SUMMARY

Strongyloidiosis is normally an intestinal parasitism caused by the threadworm, *Strongyloides stercoralis*. The parasite, occurring in dogs, primates, and man, is distributed throughout the moist tropics, as well as in temperate areas where poor sanitation or other factors facilitate the occurrence of faecally transmitted organisms. In some parts of the world, notably Africa and New Guinea, human infections caused by *S. fulleborni* have been reported. In Africa, the latter is primarily a parasite of primates, but in New Guinea, no animal host is known. *Strongyloides stercoralis* is unique among zoonotic nematode species, in that larvae passing in the faeces can give rise to a free-living generation of worms which, in turn, give rise to infective larvae. This life history alternative (i.e. heterogonic development) acts as an amplification mechanism, increasing the population of infective larvae in the external environment. The infective larvae are active skin penetrators; infection *per os*, while possible, is probably of limited importance, the acidity of the stomach serving as a barrier. Because the parasite's eggs hatch internally, a potential for autoinfection exists when precociously developing larvae attain infectivity while still in the host. This is another virtually unique feature of *S. stercoralis* infections in both its human and animal hosts. When, opportunistically, the rate of autoinfection escapes control by the host, massive larval migration may result, causing pulmonary or cerebro spinal strongyloidiasis as well as fulminant intestinal parasitism. Control of canine strongyloidiasis has been achieved in kennels by strategic use of anthelmintics. Given the lack of epidemiological information and the lack of specific highly effective anthelmintics, community-based programme to control human strongyloidosis have not been attempted. The growing importance of human strongyloidosis depends upon the unique ability of *S. stercoralis* to replicate within its host and behave as a potentially fatal opportunistic pathogen in immunocompromised hosts, particularly in those receiving corticosteroids.

HISTORY

The history of strongyloidosis and of its aetiological agent, *Strongyloides stercoralis*, is presented in great scholarly detail by Grove (1989). Therefore, only a brief account is presented here. The disease, originally called Cochin China diarrhoea, was discovered by the French naval physician Louis Normand in 1876. Meanwhile, in the same year, the parasite, known only on the basis of the rhabditiform pre-infective larvae passing in the faeces, was described by Bavay, Normand's colleague and professor of pharmacy at the naval hospital in Toulon. Bavay named the nematode *Anguillula stercoralis* and recognized that when the larvae were kept in faeces for a few days under favourable conditions, they developed into free-living adult male and female worms. Subsequently, in autopsies of soldiers returning from duty in Cochin China (presently Vietnam), Normand found larvae throughout the intestines, bile, and pancreatic ducts and adult parasitic females in the intestines. Not surprisingly, given that the parasitic females differ markedly from the free-living adults in morphology, the former were considered a different species and named *Anguillula intestinalis*. Giving further credence to this deduction was the additional discovery of a second kind of larva, a filariform larva (subsequently recognized as the infective stage) which at that point in the history of strongyloidiasis could logically be considered the larva of the putative second species, *A. intestinalis*. Thus, in the years immediately following the recognition of the disease and of the parasite, all the stages in the life of the parasite became known, but their relationship was confused because it appeared that there were two species with different life cycles, namely, *A. stercoralis* whose rhabditiform larva occurred in the stools and whose adults occurred in the external environment, and *A. intestinalis* whose adults were intestinal parasites and whose progeny were filariform larvae.

Remarkably, Grassi and Parona almost immediately resolved some of the confusion and explained much of the unusual and complex life cycle of the parasite. They found that the parasitic female named *A. intestinalis* laid eggs which hatched rapidly, giving rise to the rhabditiform larvae that were known as *A. stercoralis*. Apparently, they had a homogonic strain of the parasite because all of the rhabditiform larvae developed to infective filariform larvae such as had been described for *A. intestinalis*. It remained for Perroncito in 1881 to complete the free-living part of the life cycle by showing that the rhabditiform larvae, as originally observed in faeces by Normand, do indeed develop into free-living males and females and, furthermore, that these in turn produce filariform larvae, the infective stage of the parasite. Perroncito, however, did not realize that the various life history stages he and others had observed were parts of a complex life cycle having facultatively alternating parasitic and free-living generations.

The French workers, Normand and Bavay, discovered the disease and described the parasite; the Italian workers, Perroncito and Grassi and Parona, elucidated the free-living life cycle; and, subsequently, the German parasitologists Loss, in 1905, and Fulleborn in 1914, found, respectively, that infection occurred by skin penetration, and that larvae could migrate from the skin to intestines via the circulation, lungs, and trachea. Finally, Gage (1911) reported the occurrence of autoinfection, i.e. that larvae hatching from eggs laid in the host can develop to infectivity precociously and re-infect the same host in which they were hatched. The host, parasite, and environmental factors that determine the alternative developmental pathways of *S. stercoralis* in both man and animals remain poorly understood but are under active investigation (see below).

THE AGENT

TAXONOMY

The family Strongyloididae (class Secernentea, order Rhabditida, superfamily Rhabditoidea) is constituted of three genera, *Strongyloides* Grassi, 1879; *Parastrongyloides*, Morgan, 1928; and *Leipernema* Singh, 1976. The members of the genus *Strongyloides*, also called threadworms, are heterogenetic, with both free-living and parasitic generations. The genus includes 52 named species. The majority of these are parasites of mammals, but some can be found in birds, reptiles, and amphibians. The only species dealt with in detail in this chapter is *Strongyloides stercoralis* Bavay, 1876 (synonyms: *Anguillula stercoralis*, *S. intestinalis*, *S. canis*, *S. felis*) an intestinal parasite of dogs, primates, and man. *Strongyloides fulleborni* von Linstow, 1905, is usually considered a parasite of primates that also infects humans, but, at least in some parts of its range, is transmitted in the absence of primates (Hira and Patel 1980). Thus, its zoonotic status is presently uncertain and it is omitted here. Several species are important parasites of livestock (*S. ransomi*, *S. westeri*, *S. papillosus*) or are laboratory models of human strongyloidiasis (*S. ratti*, *S. venezuelensis*).

LIFE HISTORY

The life history of *S. stercoralis* is made extraordinarily interesting, as well as complicated, by a number of facultative alternatives. These alternatives include:

(1) direct (or homogonic) development with parasitic parthenogenetic females and only larval stages occurring in the free-living phase of the life cycle;

(2) indirect (or heterogonic) development with the inclusion of one generation of free-living adult worms (i.e. with an alternation of parasitic and free-living generations); and, finally,

(3) autoinfective development, with some of the larval progeny of the parasite population developing to infectivity precociously, while still in the intestines, and after parenteral migration returning to the intestines mature.

The latter pathway, when constrained by still poorly understood host and/or parasite factors, is thought to lead to a slow turnover in the adult worm populations, thus maintaining highly persistent chronic infection. When these constraints fail, autoinfection is explosive, forming the basis for the fulminant hyper- and disseminated forms of the infection.

In its simplest homogonic form, the life cycle involves parthenogenetic females lying embedded in the crypts of the intestinal mucosa where they deposit their eggs. The egg hatches giving rise to a first-stage larva (L1), known as a rhabditiform larva in the parasitological literature. This actively feeding, microbiverous form leaves the crypts and moves down the intestines and exit the body while still a pre-infective rhabditiform larva. During intestinal passage and in faecal deposits, these larvae feed, grow, and moults, so that two rhabditiform stages occur (L1, L2). Under favourable environmental conditions, including a suitable faecal flora, warmth, and moisture, the L2 grows and moults, giving rise to an infective filariform larva (L3), a long slender form, with a long slender oesophagus, hence the name filariform larva. It invades the host by active skin penetration.

In the heterogonic cycle, as in homogonic cycle, the larval progeny of the parthenogenetic parasitic females exit the host in the faeces. However, instead of developing directly to infective third-stage (filariform larvae), they develop to free-living adult male and female worms. These give rise to infective larvae (L3) via the usual two rhabditiform stages. The infective forms leave the faeces or polluted soil in which they have developed and ascend surface particles to the extent permitted by soil or faecal moisture films. Here the larvae are positioned for contact with a host. After contact and percutaneous entry into a host, the larvae enter the circulation and migrate to the intestines. It is generally accepted that the migratory route involves the lung, trachea, and oesophagus (pulmotracheal migration), but this route has recently been challenged by Schad and colleagues (1989). After percutaneous infection of dogs, some larvae do follow the pulmonary route but most do not. In fact, studies with radiolabelled larvae have indicated that no predominant migratory route exists and that larvae reach the intestines via a number of different pathways.

Autoinfection is the third life history alternative. In this case, eggs hatch in the intestines as they normally do, but the larvae develop to infectivity precociously while still in the host (Schad *et al.* 1993). They penetrate the wall of the large intestine and from here migrate to many organs of the body, again, some use pulmonary migration, but others return to the intestine, by other pathways (Genta and Caymmi-Gomes 1989). Upon return to the intestine, the third-stage larvae give rise to a fourth larval stage which in turn moults to give rise to the adult worm.

MORPHOLOGY

The parasitic female is one of the stages found in tissue sections of the small intestine; it is rarely seen in the stools of infected hosts. It measures 2.0–2.8 mm in length and 37 μm in width (Schad 1989). It has a long, cylindrical oesophagus, an intestine constituted of dorsal and ventral rows of 20 cells each. The tail is a short cone. The vulva is ventrally situated at two-thirds the body length from the anterior tip. Eggs are present in two single rows, one to either side of the vulva. The cuticle of the female worm is finely striated and, in tissue sections, is often wrinkled. In cross-section, depending on the level, one may see a muscular oesophagus, intestine, ovaries, and eggs. Reproduction is by parthenogenesis and, hence, there are no parasitic males.

The rhabditiform larva, the stage that hatches from the egg, is the form most commonly identified in faecal samples. It measures approximately 250 μm in length and 17 μm in diameter when passed in faeces, and is characterized by a bulbed oesophagus and a thinner, longer intestine (Schand, 1989). In intestinal aspirates, the newly hatched larva is smaller, measuring 180–240 μm in length and 14–15 μm in width. In tissue sections they are often found in the intestinal submucosa and within small intestinal crypts, but only exceptionally in the lungs; they cannot be specifically identified based on their morphological characteristics. The filariform (third stage) larva of autoinfective origin is the stage most frequently identified in parenteral tissues and body fluids (most often the sputum) in patients with disseminated infections. They are longer and more slender than rhabditiform larvae and have a cylindrical oesophagus that occupies one-half the body length. In transverse sections the cuticle shows four characteristic lateral alae, which can be used for species identification. Filariform infective larvae arising as progeny of free-living adults are even longer and more slender, measuring up to 700 μm in length and 20 μm in width.

DISEASE MECHANISMS

Chronic infections are probably sustained by a relatively low number of adult worms, many of which may be barren (the so-called post-reproductive females), which reside in relative harmony within their hosts intestine and the infection is believed to persist by means of periodic bouts of autoinfection. The occurrence and rate of autoinfection is generally believed to be regulated by the host's cell-mediated immunity. When this regulatory function becomes impaired during immunosuppression, increasing numbers of autoinfective larvae complete the cycle, and the population of parasitic adult worms increases (hyperinfection) (Genta 1992). Eventually, with extraordinary numbers of larvae migrating, large numbers deviate from the generally presumed route (intestine → venous bed → lungs → trachea → intestine) and disseminate to other organs, including meningeal spaces and brain, liver, kidneys, lymph nodes, cutaneous, and subcutaneous tissues. In these organs the larvae cause haemorrhage by breaking capillaries, elicit inflammatory responses, and implant Gram-negative bacteria carried from faecal material. The resulting syndrome, known as disseminated strongyloidosis, is nearly always fatal.

The validity of the migratory pathways in the above widely accepted model has been questioned by Schad *et al.* (1989), who used an experimental canine model of disseminated strongyloidosis to show that only a few larvae could be recovered from the lungs of dogs with massive hyperinfection. In studies based on the organ-specific distribution of radiolabelled larvae and compartmental analysis of the data, these authors presented strong evidence that, in young dogs, the pulmonary route was not used by the majority of the migrating larvae. Larvae that began their migration in the skin (primary infection) or in the distal ileum (autoinfection) were not more likely to pass through the lungs than through any other organ, suggesting that the migratory pathway involved random dissemination throughout the body. However, this conclusion has not been fully accepted because large numbers of larvae are frequently identified in bronchoalveolar lavage fluid from hyperinfected human patients (Genta *et al.* 1989). It may be that in hyperinfection, as distinct from a primary infection, pulmonary migration is more frequent.

Recently also, the accepted paradigm that host mechanisms regulate hyperinfection and dissemination has been challenged (Genta 1992). The theory that host immunity controls the rate and mode of parasite development fails to consider the role that parasites may play in this regulation. The adverse impact of increased parasite density on egg production and growth ('crowding effect') has been demonstrated for several intestinal nematodes. Although it may be difficult to distinguish between host resistance and direct parasite to parasite effects, it seems clear that in a normal host–parasite relationship, the parasite may reach a particular population size or a critical biomass, after which yet unknown regulatory mechanisms intervene to limit the population. As yet unpublished results of investigations using a new gerbil-based model of strongyloidosis has failed to provide support for self-regulation of worm burden by the parasite.

One of us (RMG) has proposed that, during the parallel evolution of humans and their parasites, *S. stercoralis* developed the ability to reach an optimal population size in the duodenum of a human. If the initial infective dose of larvae is low, a higher rate of intraluminal moulting occurs, enabling the parasite to attain the infective stage internally, reinfect and multiply (Genta 1992). This occurs until the 'optimal' size of the adult population is reached. In this model, it is assumed that *S. stercoralis*, similar to other nematodes, transmit their moulting signal by moulting hormones (ecdysteroids). As the size of the parasite population reaches a certain level, adult females decrease their production of ecdysteroids, resulting in a lowered moulting rate, i.e. just sufficient to replace the dying adults. During the initial phase of infection, the host mounts humoral and cellular immune responses directed at all tissue stages of the parasite. These well-characterized responses do not eradicate all the parasites, but limit the size of the parasite population. Impaired immune responses may allow the growth of larger numbers of parasites, as reported in agammaglobulinaemic patients, but total dysregulation of the parasite population does not occur since worms, in part, regulate their own growth. Conversely, the presence of intact immune responses is not sufficient to prevent dissemination should the parasites' own regulatory mechanisms fail.

The level of ecdysteroid-like substances are generally negligible in healthy subjects. The administration of exogenous, or endogenous, corticosteroids may result in increased amounts of ecdysteroid-like substances in the host's tissues, including in the intestinal wall, where adult females reside. These substances may act as moulting signals for the eggs or rhabditiform larvae, which transform intraluminally into excessive numbers of filariform larvae. Available data are not sufficient to prove a dose-dependent effect, but it is indeed remarkable that patients who develop fulminating hyperinfection after only a few days of steroid administration are usually those who have received intravenous methylprednisone. Once a population has become very large (for example 100 000 adult worms) it may continue to expand rapidly, even at low moulting rates, and the discontinuation of steroids may not be sufficient to arrest the relentless growth process which leads to the host's death.

GROWTH AND SURVIVAL REQUIREMENTS

Attempts to cultivate the parasitic stages of *S. stercoralis in vitro* have been unsuccessful. Infective larvae have been maintained for months under host-like conditions in tissue culture media (Chapman *et al*. 1994), but the larvae failed to grow or develop. Free-living stages are easily reared in standard parasitological coprocultures. These stages can also be raised on agar plates seeded with bacteria or in liquid cultures consisting of bacteria in a nematode saline (Schad *et al*. 1989).

HOSTS

These include dogs, various primates, and humans (Chandler 1925). Cats have been infected experimentally (Sandground 1928). Transmissibility of *S. stercoralis* between host species varies geographically (Galliard 1950). The canine strain from North America is transmissible to humans (Georgi and Sprinkle 1974).

ANIMAL HOSTS

Prepatent period

In both primates and dogs the prepatent period is short, rhabditiform larvae appearing in the faeces in 1–2 weeks.

Symptoms and signs

Symptoms and signs of infection vary markedly with respect to the individual. In primates there is also marked interspecific variation, monkeys being less susceptible than the anthropoid apes (Harper *et al*. 1982). Most cases in dogs are asymptomatic and become occult in 2–3 months (Grove *et al*. 1983; Genta *et al*. 1986). Although larvae disappear from the faeces, barren adult females may survive embedded in the intestinal mucosa for several months after the infection becomes inapparent. These infections can be reactivated by immunosuppression attributable to either chemotherapy or concurrent disease. Dogs that have expelled an infection are resistant to reinfection.

In young pups, hyperinfective strongyloidosis occurs spontaneously (Schad *et al*. 1993). Although these infections are usually mild and self-limiting, in some animals the worm burden may increase to clinically significant levels associated with watery or mucus diarrhoea and with signs of bronchopneumonia. Older dogs rarely become severely infected.

Strongyloides stercoralis occurs commonly in various monkeys (Faust 1933). It is usually well tolerated, but in young Patas monkeys (*Erythrocebus patas*) it may produce severe hyperinfective strongyloidosis (Harper *et al.* 1982). These severely affected animals have diarrhoea, lose weight, and may die suddenly. Larvae may or may not be found in the faeces even in severely affected cases. Severe, often fatal strongyloidosis occurs even more frequently in young anthropoid apes (Penner 1981). Gibbons are particularly susceptible to sudden death without a history of previous illness (De Paoli and Johnsen 1978).

Diagnosis

Diagnosis of *S. stercoralis* infection is complicated by the fact that larvae may be absent from the faeces even in symptomatic cases. Additionally, larvae (not eggs) pass in the faeces, making concentration techniques using high density flotation solutions somewhat difficult to use. The Baermann apparatus is commonly used for finding larvae in faeces. The first-stage larvae are easily recognized, their genital primordium being exceptionally prominent. Many cases of this infection are probably first suspected when larvae are seen either in a direct smear or in a saturated salt flotation. The Baermann funnel is then used to obtain clean, intact larvae for a definitive diagnosis. However, faecal flotations done with zinc sulfate yield readily identifiable larvae provided that the preparation is examined promptly before the larvae shrink. In animals showing respiratory symptoms, a transtracheal wash may reveal migrating third-stage larvae. This stage is easily identifiable by its long filariform oesophagus and its notched tail. A small percentage of the larvae present in a faecal sample may be third-stage larvae, particularly in recently acquired infections. Infectious stools held at room temperature for 24 hours or more may contain a variety of stages, including free-living adults.

Pathology

Intestinal pathology varies with intensity of the infection, which in turn varies with the strain of organism and the age and species of host. In asymptomatic infected dogs, the intestinal tissues may be grossly normal and worms and larvae exceedingly difficult to find by histological methods (Genta *et al.* 1986). In symptomatic cases, gross intestinal changes range from congestion of mucosal surface with an abnormal abundance of luminal mucus to confluent ulceration that may penetrate to the muscular layer. In cases of severe infection, parasites in great abundance will be present in the intestinal walls.

In primates a similar range of lesions has been observed; however, severe strongyloidiasis with significant ulcerative enteritis is rare in monkeys but well known in gibbons and orang-utans. Complicated

strongyloidosis with severe hyperinfection occurs spontaneously in young Patas monkeys, gibbons, and orang-utans. Characteristic pathological lesions include the presence of the full spectrum of parasite life history stages in the gastrointestinal tract and the presence of filariform larvae in the lungs associated with pulmonary haemorrhage. The number of migrating larvae frequently does *not* correlate with the amount of pulmonary haemorrhage (Genta *et al.* 1984; Kerlin *et al.* 1995).

Treatment

Treatment of dogs with an active hyperinfection is difficult because available drugs do not kill the migrating autoinfective L3. However, unless a dog is very young or immunosuppressed, it is unlikely to have numerous migrating autoinfective larvae at any one time. The following anthelmintic treatments will remove adult *S. stercoralis* from dogs: albendazole, twice daily for three consecutive days at 100 mg/kg; thiabendazole, once a day for three consecutive days at 50 mg/kg; fenbendazole, once a day for 3 days at 50 mg/kg; ivermectin, one dose at 200 μg/kg. In all cases, follow-up faecal examinations should be done weekly for 2–3 weeks to verify that no migrating larvae survived the treatment and matured. In cases where hyperinfection is suspected the following treatments can be used: fenbendazole, once daily for 7–14 days at 50 mg/kg or ivermectin once every 4 days for 3 or 4 doses at 200 μg/kg (Mansfield and Schad 1992). Although these treatments will not kill migrating larvae, they will remove adults as they mature in the small intestine and therefore prevent new autoinfective larvae from being produced. The problem is that the life-span of migrating autoinfective larvae is unknown, and, therefore, recommended treatments may continue for longer than necessary. Again, follow-up faecal examinations should be done to confirm that a parasitological cure has been achieved. Ivermectin and fenbendazole should also be effective against *S. stercoralis* infections in cats.

The possible occurrence of migrating autoinfective larvae must also be considered in treating primates for a *S. stercoralis* infection. In most animals, unless immunosuppressed, it is unlikely that numerous autoinfective larvae will be present, and, therefore, a single course of treatment should be curative. The following treatment regimes, each repeated after 2 weeks, have been used in primates: thiabendazole, 50–100 mg/kg, orally (PO), once a day for 2 days; mebendazole, 50 mg/kg, PO, twice a day for 3 days; fenbendazole, 25 mg/kg, PO, once a day for 3 days; ivermectin, 0.2 mg/kg, PO, as a single dose. However, in the anthropoid apes, i.e. gibbons, chimpanzees, gorillas, and the orang-utan, fatal infections have occurred, especially in juveniles in the absence of immuno-suppression. Fatal hyperinfections are also seen in otherwise normal Patas monkeys. Thus, in these animals a more extended course of treatment may be advisable. In all cases, follow-up faecal examinations should be done for an extended period to verify that treatment has completely eliminated the parasites.

Prognosis

The prognosis for dogs infected with *S. stercoralis* is good. Except in dogs infected with the South-East Asian (Indochinese) strain of the parasite, the infection is usually self-limiting and infrequently attains a clinical level of intensity. The prognosis for infections in primates varies with the species of host. Most monkeys carry easily treated asymptomatic infections. Anthropoid apes, on the other hand, are more suscept-ible to severe strongyloidosis, and young gibbons and orang-utans, in particular, may die suddenly without apparent previous illness. In anthropoid apes, partial clearing of the infection by most anthelmintics occurs, resulting in low-grade, sometimes occult, chronic infection which may be seriously exacerbated by subsequent immunosuppression.

HUMAN HOSTS

Prepatent period

The prepatent period for experimental infection with *S. fulleborni* in man has been reported to be 28 days (Pampiglione and Ricciardi 1972). This is at least a week longer than the prepatent period in animals and may be a misleading estimate based on limited observations.

Symptoms and signs

No other nematode has been associated with as broad a spectrum of manifestations or implicated as the cause of so many different clinical syndromes as *S. stercoralis*. Although some of these manifestations are dramatic, the majority of persons with chronic infection are either asymptomatic or have mild, non-specific symptoms (Genta *et al.* 1984; Genta 1992, 1993).

Gastrointestinal manifestations

The gastrointestinal manifestations of chronic strongy-loidosis are usually non-specific. Epigastric abdominal pain, post-prandial fullness or bloating, and heartburn are among the symptoms most commonly reported. Brief episodes of diarrhoea alternating with constipa-tion may also occur. The diarrhoea usually consists of semi-formed non-bloody stools. Occultly bloody stools occasionally occur in persons with chronic infections, and even massive colonic haemorrhage has been

reported. A severe, cholera-like diarrhoea with elec-trolyte imbalance and cardiac arrest has been reported in two patients, but this is exceedingly uncommon (Silva *et al.* 1981).

Physical examination of chronically infected patients is normal or reveals only mild abdominal tenderness on palpation. Less commonly, chronic strongyloidosis resembles inflammatory bowel disease, particularly ulcerative colitis, and the endoscopic appearance may be that of pseudopolyposis (Carp *et al.* 1987). Rarely, patients have undergone surgery for 'chronic colitis', the correct diagnosis being established by pathological examination of the resected colon. Malabsorption fre-quently occurs in patients with strongyloidosis. The majority of these patients, however, are from areas of the world where tropical sprue and sprue-like condi-tions are widespread, making a clear relationship of cause and effect between *S. stercoralis* infection and malabsorption difficult to determine. Garcia *et al.* (1977) have argued convincingly that malnutrition was the cause rather than the effect of severe strongyloido-sis in a group of Colombian patients. Experimental work in rodents seems to support this conclusion (Weesner *et al.* 1988).

In contrast to the asymptomatic nature of chronic strongyloidosis, the gastrointestinal manifestations of disseminated strongyloidosis are dramatic and often catastrophic (Longworth and Weller 1986). Hyper-infection is often heralded by profuse diarrhoea, which may be watery, mucoid, and bloody. The diarrhoea is a consequence of the erosions, ulcerations, and oedema caused by millions of adult worms and filariform larvae in the mucosa of small and large intestine. Depending on the extent, severity, and location of these lesions, malabsorption, exudation, and altered motility result. These mucosal changes predispose the patient to bac-terial enterocolitis and, after variable periods of diar-rhoea, paralytic ileus. Probably because of the large numbers of larvae migrating from the large intestine into the circulation, polymicrobial (predominantly Gram-negative) sepsis may occur with local infections and abscesses developing in virtually any organ (Igra-Siegman *et al.* 1981). Larvae have been identified in other gastrointestinal organs, including the liver, stomach, and pancreas of patients with overwhelming infections, but the presence of parasites in these loca-tions does not cause characteristic symptoms.

Pulmonary manifestations

Although patients with chronic obstructive pulmonary disease may have an increased risk of strongyloidiosis, no respiratory signs or symptoms are associated with acute or with chronic strongyloidiosis. In these infec-tions the number of larvae passing through the lungs is probably negligible. Occasionally, patients who presented with asthma and were treated with corticosteroids, have later developed disseminated strongyloidiosis, but these patients are often maintained on low-dose steroid therapy, which predisposes to strongloidiosis (Higenbottam and Heard 1987). Chronic obstructive pulmonary disease has been associated with strongyloidiosis in some series of American patients (Berk *et al.* 1987). Although peculiar microcalcifications have been observed in the lungs of chronically infected dogs (Caceres and Genta, 1988), a direct effect of parasites on the pulmonary parenchyma has not been documented in humans and appears unlikely. Among patients with disseminated strongyloidiosis, pulmonary manifestations are common, particularly diffuse bronchopneumonia. Pulmonary abscesses have also been reported. Intra-alveolar haemorrhage, often sufficiently severe to cause the patient's death, is a frequent event during the course of disseminated strongyloidiosis. In some cases, fatal pulmonary haemorrhages occur a few days after the apparently successful treatment of the parasite, suggesting an immunologically mediated mechanism of vascular damage (Berk and Verghese 1988).

Neurological manifestations

Gram-negative polymicrobial meningitis is the most frequent central nervous system manifestation of disseminated strongyloidiosis (Igra-Siegman *et al.* 1981; Longworth and Weller 1986). In some cases, larvae have been identified in the cerebrospinal fluid. Rarely, larvae have been found in the absence of bacteria in patients with signs of meningeal involvement, suggesting the possibility of parasitic (aseptic) meningitis. Eosinophilic meningitis has not been described in association with strongyloidiosis, possibly because most of these patients receive corticosteroids and their eosinophilic counts are generally low. A less common form of central nervous system involvement is the formation of cerebral and cerebellar abscesses containing *S. stercoralis* larvae (Masdeu *et al.* 1982).

Other systemic manifestations

Arthritis is an unusual manifestation of strongyloidiosis and is associated with the local deposition of immune complexes containing *S. stercoralis* antigens. Cardiac arrhythmias and arrest are rare and have been attributed to a direct myocardial damage caused by the migrating larvae or to electrolyte imbalance precipitated by severe intestinal strongyloidiosis. Depression and neurosis have been associated with chronic strongyloidiosis, but they likely represent reaction to the long duration of symptoms. The passage of larvae in the sperm and the presence of genital lesions in association with strongyloidosis have also been described.

Cutaneous manifestations

Three types of cutaneous manifestations have been described in patients with chronic strongyloidiosis (von Kuster and Genta 1989). Urticarial rashes, possibly caused by a sensitization to parasite antigens, have occurred sporadically in patients from all parts of the world. In contrast, a characteristic dermatitis caused by the subcutaneous migration of filariform larvae (larva currens), has been reported almost exclusively in Caucasian patients who acquired the infection in South-East Asia. In many of these patients, larva currens was the only sign of strongyloidiosis, and therapy with thiabendazole caused the permanent disappearance of the dermatitis. Finally, generalized cutaneous purpura has been recently described in several patients with leucopenia, various degrees of thrombocytopenia, and disseminated infection. In two of these cases the purpuric lesions were related to filariform larvae migrating in the dermis.

Diagnosis

Radiographic features of *S. stercoralis* infection of the gastrointestinal tract are non-specific. However, certain radiological patterns may suggest strongyloidiosis in patients at risk for the infection. When malabsorption is present, the radiographic findings are similar to those of tropical sprue, including increased diameter of the small intestinal lumen, generalized hypotonia, and oedema. Oedema and fibrosis may be associated with severe, long-standing infections. In hyperinfection and dissemination, complete disruption of the mucosal patterns, ulcerations, and paralytic ileus have been observed. In the presence of dissemination, pulmonary involvement may be heralded by bilateral oedema and patchy, often rapidly changing infiltrates.

The stage of *S. stercoralis* most commonly identified in faeces is the rhabditiform larva, but filariform larvae, adult females, and even eggs also may be identified. The sensitivity of a single stool examination for the detection of *S. stercoralis* ranges between 30 and 60 per cent. The method of Baermann allows a larger volume of faeces (up to several grams) to be examined, and is more sensitive than direct microscopy (Pereira-Lima and Delgado 1961). Culturing faeces mixed with charcoal or peat moss also increases the sensitivity of faecal examination. However, these procedures are not suited for routine diagnosis in the clinical laboratory. A detection method recently proposed by Koga involves the use of agar plates and appears to be very sensitive and easy to perform (Koga *et al.* 1992). Although the examination of duodenal aspirate is reportedly very sensitive, this invasive method is recommended only in the pediatric patient when it is necessary to achieve a rapid demonstration of parasites, as in an immunocompromised child with suspected overwhelming infection. The 'string test', a gelatin capsule containing a string swallowed by the patient and retrieved after a few hours, enjoyed some popularity a few years ago, but currently is infrequently used. In disseminated infections larvae of all stages and adult parasites have been found in specimens of sputum and bronchoalveolar lavage, ascitic fluid, pancreatic aspirates, and cerebrospinal fluid. In summary, stool examination is currently the primary technique for the detection of *S. stercoralis*. If special techniques are not available, several specimens collected on different days should be examined if the diagnosis is strongly suspected (Nielsen and Mojon 1987).

The only haematological abnormality associated with chronic, uncomplicated strongyloidiosis is eosinophilia. Although eosinophils may exceed 30 per cent of the total white blood cells, in most series between 70 and 80 per cent of the patients have values between 6 and 15 per cent (between 500 and 1500 eosinophils/mm^3). Considerable day-to-day variation in the degree of eosinophilia occurs so that it is not uncommon for infected subjects to have normal counts on some days, explaining why 20 or 30 per cent of the infected patients, studied at one point in time, do not have eosinophilia. Patients with disseminated strongyloidiosis usually have normal eosinophil counts, likely due to the immunosuppressive agent.

Total serum IgE levels are elevated (>200 IU/ml) in 50–70 per cent of the patients with strongyloidiosis. The diagnostic relevance of such elevation is similar to that of eosinophilia. Both eosinophilia and an elevated IgE level should be investigated, but the absence of elevation does not necessarily rule out strongyloidiosis. The other classes of immunoglobulins are not affected by the presence of *S. stercoralis*, except in infected children with malnutrition and protein-losing enteropathy in whom levels may be reduced.

Several immunoassays for the detection of serum antibodies against filariform larvae or larval antigens are now available. The most commonly used tests include an indirect immunofluorescence test, which detects serum IgG antibodies to surface antigens of fresh or formalin-fixed filariform larvae and an enzyme-linked immunosorbent assay (ELISA) which also detects parasite-specific IgG antibodies (Genta 1988; Bianco 1993). The latter has a sensitivity of approximately 90 per cent and a specificity approaching 100 per cent. The former has a lower sensitivity (<85 per cent) and a similar specificity. Serum from patients with filarial or *Ascaris lumbricoides* infections may, on rare occasions, give a false positive test for *S. stercoralis* infection. Assays for the detection of parasite-specific antibodies of the IgG$_4$ subclass of immunoglobulins and assays utilizing purified antigens have been developed to increase specificity

(Genta and Lillibridge 1989; Conway *et al.* 1993). Although immunoserology appears to be a promising tool for the diagnosis of strongyloidiosis, its widespread use has been limited by the insufficient availability of suitable antigens.

Pathology

The pathological lesions associated with chronic, uncomplicated *S. stercoralis* have received little attention, because only rarely have patients with such lesions come to autopsy. However, pathological descriptions of the lesions in a few patients in whom strongyloidiosis was an incidental finding and our own studies indicate that the worms can exist in the intestinal mucosa without causing significant inflammatory responses or tissue damage. The classic description of the pathology of strongyloidiasis was made by De Paola (1962), and later updated by Genta and Caymmi-Gomes (1989). These authors proposed the subdivision of the intestinal lesions into three distinct forms.

In 'catarrhal enteritis' (presumably associated with light infections), the small intestine is congested, the mucosa is covered with abundant mucoid secretions, and scattered petechial haemorrhages are present. The most remarkable histological feature is an increased mononuclear infiltrate in the submucosa, although parasites are rare. In the more severe 'oedematous enteritis', the intestinal wall is grossly thickened, the mucosal folds flattened, and the affected intestinal segments assume a rubbery consistency. Submucosal oedema, flattening of the villi, and parasites scattered throughout the lamina propria are observed microscopically. The most severe form 'ulcerative enteritis' is almost exclusively seen in association with hyperinfection. The intestinal walls may be rigid due to the oedema and fibrosis resulting from longstanding inflammation, the mucosa may be show atrophy, erosions, and ulcerations. An abundant inflammatory infiltrate, most often consisting of neutrophils, as well as all stages of *S. stercoralis*, are present throughout the intestinal mucosa. Jejunal perforation has been reported in patients with the ulcerative enteritis form of strongyloidiosis. Uncommonly, the mucosal damage occurs predominantly in the large intestine, simulating ulcerative colitis and pseudopolyposis. *Strongyloides stercoralis* larvae have been found in the appendix, and eosinophilic appendicitis apparently caused by this parasite has been reported. In patients with disseminated strongyloidiosis, the intestinal lesions reflect the large number of worms dwelling within the small intestinal mucosa and penetrating the intestinal walls. In addition, the stomach and the peritoneal cavity may be invaded by migrating parasites. However, because most of these patients are receiving immunosuppressive doses of corticosteroids, inflammatory responses are often minimal in spite of extensive tissue damage. The gastrointestinal pathology is often overshadowed by the lesions found in other organs, particularly in patients who receive antihelminthic therapy before succumbing to disseminated strongyloidiosis.

Migrating parasites may cause mechanical damage as well as inflammation. In human patients, the extra-intestinal organ most commonly affected by this migratory damage is the lung. In severe disseminated infection, when hundreds of thousands of adult parasites dwell in the intestine and millions of larvae migrate throughout the body, alveolar microhaemorrhages may result in massive pulmonary bleeding. As larvae penetrate the large intestine, they create small breaks in the mucosa that facilitate the invasion of the bloodstream by enteric bacteria. The larvae themselves carry bacteria on their cuticle to distant sites. Regardless of the mechanism, the widespread dissemination of larvae is frequently associated with polymicrobial sepsis, diffuse or patchy bronchopneumonia, pulmonary and cerebral abscesses, and meningitis. Filariform larvae, and occasionally rhabditiform larvae and adult worms, also may disseminate to mesenteric lymph nodes, the biliary tract, as well as the liver, pancreas, spleen, heart, endocrine glands, and ovaries. In these locations the parasite frequently induces a granulomatous response.

Treatment

The drug of choice for strongyloidiosis is thiabendazole. The recommended regimen is 25 mg/kg/day for 2 days, which appears to be effective in 80–90 per cent of patients with chronic, uncomplicated infections. Multiple courses of therapy may be necessary to eradicate the parasite in certain cases. Immuno-compromised patients appear not to respond as well to this regimen, and higher doses of thiabendazole (up to 50 mg/kg/day) for longer periods have been recommended. (For patients unable to take oral medications, thiabendazole may be administered per rectum. This may become an important route in small children). Thiabendazole side-effects include nausea, vomiting, foul-smelling urine, and dizziness in a high percentage of patients. In countries where thiabendazole is not available and in patients in whom thiabendazole therapy was unsuccessful, eradication of the parasites has been achieved with albendazole and mebendazole (Grove 1989). However, because the efficacy of these two agents is not always satisfactory and the regimens are not well standardized, the use of albendazole and mebendazole should only be considered in selected cases. Ivermectin, originally introduced for the treatment of onchocerciosis, has been used more recently to successfully treat strongyloidiosis in several trials conducted in Latin America, Asia, and Africa (Datry *et al.* 1994; Jorgenson *et al.* 1996). In the United States, ivermectin is not approved for the treatment of uncomplicated *S. stercoralis*. Compassionate use has occasionally been approved in patients with life-threatening disseminated infection, but the data are presently insufficient to determine whether it is more effective than thiabendazole.

Prognosis

Except in cases of hyperinfection, the prognosis is good. Many infected persons are asymptomatic or have non-specific minor complaints. In adults, these well-regulated infections may persist for decades without producing clinically significant strongyloidiosis, and most will respond to anthelmintic treatment. However, because the risk of developing severe, hyperinfective strongyloidiosis is always present, all infected persons must be considered at risk for fatal infection and treated with the goal of achieving a parasitological cure. Once hyperinfection occurs, the prognosis should be guarded; even when treatment is promptly administered the mortality is still greater than 70 per cent.

EPIDEMIOLOGY

Although information regarding the worldwide prevalence of strongyloidiosis is fragmentary, 3 million to 100 million are estimated to be infected worldwide (Genta 1989). The unreliability of these estimates is reflected in the wide range of prevalence rates, varying between less than 1 per cent and 85 per cent of populations living in adjacent regions of the same country. With these limitations in mind, one can assume that *S. stercoralis* is present in virtually all tropical and subtropical regions of the world. Pockets of low endemicity (less than 1 per cent to 3 per cent) exist in several industrialized countries of western Europe (e.g. Italy, France, and Switzerland), eastern Europe (e.g. Poland and many parts of the former Soviet Union), the United States (the Appalachian region and the southern states), Japan (Okinawa), and Australia (Aboriginal populations). Significant prevalence rates of strongyloidiosis have been found in institutionalized patients, even in Pennsylvania and British Columbia where the parasite is not known to be endemic in the general population. Considering the long persistence of this parasite in its host and its relatively high prevalence among some populations, physicians practising in industrialized countries should consider strongyloidiosis in immigrant or refugee patients born in tropical or subtropical regions, as well as in persons from local areas of endemicity.

STRONGYLOIDIASIS AND THE ACQUIRED IMMUNODEFICIENCY SYNDROME

Since cell-mediated immunity is thought to regulate *S. stercoralis* autoinfection, patients with the acquired immunodeficiency syndrome (AIDS) were expected to have more frequent and severe infections with *S. stercoralis* than the general population. However, in areas of the world where both *S. stercoralis* and AIDS are endemic, there does not appear to be a higher incidence of acute or chronic strongyloidiosis with AIDS (Lucas 1990). This has led several authors to speculate that strongyloidosis is regulated by other factors and that it will remain one of the missing infections in AIDS (Hunter *et al.* 1992). During the past few years, a very limited number of patients, almost exclusively from Western countries, with AIDS and extraintestinal strongyloidiosis have been reported. Although most of these patients had conditions that required corticosteroid treatment, in several the development of *S. stercoralis* hyperinfection was apparently spontaneous. Thus, although it is unlikely that strongyloidosis will become an important opportunistic infection associated with AIDS, the infection should be searched for and promptly treated in HIV-infected patients with a suggestive geographic history (Zumla and Croft 1992; Celedon *et al.* 1994).

PREVENTION AND CONTROL

Transmission of *S. stercoralis* among both humans and animals can be prevented by implementing measures aimed at ensuring proper disposal and treatment of excrement and by avoiding contact with contaminated substrata, i.e. soil, caging, etc. (Conway *et al.* 1995). The free-living larval stages are susceptible to desiccation. Thus, maintaining a clean, dry environment provides effective control. In human patients from endemic areas who may harbour asymptomatic chronic strongyloidiosis, life-threatening disseminated hyperinfection may be prevented by seeking and eradicating the parasite before corticosteroid, immunosuppressive, or antineoplastic therapy is started. Strongyloidiosis in animal populations has been a problem in canine breeding kennels and in the primate colonies of zoos and research organizations. Both death losses and occurrences of clinical strongyloidiosis can be reduced in breeding kennels by periodic mass treatment with thiabendazole, but this will not eradicate the parasitism in the dog population. Apparently, eradication has been achieved as a by-product of *Filaroides hirthi* control. This involved treating of brood bitches between pregnancies with albendazole given at the rate of 25 mg/kg orally twice daily for 5 days. Control of strongyloidiosis in primate colonies has depended on creating a clean, dry environment because

the free-living larvae of strongyloides are highly susceptible to desiccation. It also depends on the detection of infected individuals by faecal examination and their treatment. Thiabendazole given orally by stomach tube or in food as a single dose of 100 mg/kg and repeated after 2 weeks is effective for control.

REFERENCES

Berk, S. L. and Verghese, A. (1988). Parasitic pneumonia. *Seminars in Respiratory Infection* **3**, 172–8.

Berk, S. L., Verghese, A., Alvarez, S., Hall, K., and Smith, B. (1987). Clinical and epidemiologic features of strongyloidiasis. A prospective study in rural Tennessee. *Archives of Internal Medicine*, **147**, 1257–61.

Bianco, A. E. (1993). Immunodiagnosis of *Strongyloides stercoralis* infection: a method for increasing the specificity of the indirect ELISA. *Transactions of the Royal Society for Tropical Medicine and Hygiene*, **87**, 173–6.

Caceres, M. H. and Genta, R. M. (1988). Pulmonary microcalcifications associated with Strongyloides stercoralis infection. *Chest*, **94**, 862–5.

Carp, N. Z., Nejman, J. H., and Kelly, J. J. (1987). Strongyloidiasis. An unusual case of colonic pseudopolyposis and gastrointestinal bleeding. *Surgical Endoscopy*, **1**, 175–7.

Celedon, J. C., Mathur-Wagh, U., Fox, J., Garcia, R., and Wiest, P. M. (1994). Systemic strongyloidiasis in patients infected with the human immunodeficiency virus. A report of 3 cases and review of the literature. *Medicine*, **73**, 256–63.

Chandler, A. C. (1925). The species of *Strongyloides* (Nematoda). *Parasitology*, **17**, 426–33.

Chapman, M. R., Hutchinson, G. W., Cenac, M. J., and Klei, T. R. (1994). *In vitro* culture of equine strongylidae to the fourth larval stage in a cell free medium. *Journal of Parasitology*, **80**, 225–31.

Conway, D. J., Bailey, J. W., Lindo, J. F., Robinson, R. D., Bundy, D. A., and Bianco, A. E. (1993). Serum IgG reactivity with 41-, 31-, and 28-kDa larval proteins of *Strongyloides stercoralis* in individuals with strongyloidiasis. *Journal of Infectious Diseases* **168**, 784–7.

Conway, D. J., Lindo, J. F., Robinson, R. D., and Bundy, D. A. P. (1995). Towards effective control of *Strongyloides stercoralis*. *Parasitology Today*, **11**, 420–4.

Datry, A. *et al.* (1994). Treatment of *Strongyloides stercoralis* infection with ivermectin compared with albendazole: results of an open study of 60 cases. *Transactions of the Royal Society for Tropical Medicine and Hygiene*, **88**, 344–5.

De Paola, D. (1961). Patologia de estrongiloidiase. *Boletim do Centro de Estudios do Hospital dos Servidores do Estrado, Rio de Janeiro*, **14**, 3–98.

De Paola, A. and Johnsen, D. O. (1978). Fatal strongyloidiasis in gibbons (*Hylobates lar*). *Veterinary Pathology*, **15**, 31–9.

Faust, E. C. (1933). Experimental studies on human and primate species of *Strongyloides*, II. The development of *Strongyloides* in the experimental host. *American Journal of Hygiene*, **18**, 114–32.

Gage, J. G. (1911). A case of *Strongyloides intestinalis* with larvae in the sputum. *Archives of Internal Medicine*, **7**, 561–79.

Galliard, H. (1950). Recherches sur l'infestation experimentale a *Strongyloides stercoralis* au Tonkin (1re note). *Annales de Parasitologie*, **XXV**, 441–73.

Garcia, F. T. *et al.* (1977). Intestinal function and morphology in strongyloidiasis. *American Journal of Tropical Medicine and Hygiene*, **26**, 859–65.

Genta, R. M. (1988). Predictive value of an enzyme-linked immunosorbent assay (ELISA) for the serodiagnosis of strongyloidiasis. *Journal of Clinical Pathology*, **89**, 391–4.

Genta, R. M. (1989). Global prevalence of strongyloidiasis: critical review with epidemiologic insights into the prevention of disseminated disease. *Reviews of the Infectious Diseases*, **11**, 755–67.

Genta, R. M. (1992). Dysregulation of strongyloidiasis: a new hypothesis. *Clinical Microbiological Reviews*, **5**, 345–55.

Genta, R. M. (1993). Diarrhea in helminthic infections. *Clinics in Infectious Diseases*, **16**, (Suppl. 2); S 122–9.

Genta, R. M., and Caymmi-Gomes, M. (1989). Pathology. In (1989) *Strongyloidiasis, a major roundworm infection of man*, (ed. D. I. Grove) pp. 105–32. Taylor and Francis, London.

Genta, R. M. and Lillibridge, J. P. (1989). Prominence of IgG4 antibodies in the humoral responses to *Strongyloides stercoralis*. *Journal of Infectious Diseases*, **160**, 692–9.

Genta, R. M., Harper, J. S., Gam, A. A., London, W. J., and Neva, F. A. (1984). Experimental disseminated strongyloidiasis in *Erythrocebus patas*. Part II. Immunology. *American Journal of Tropical, Medicine and Hygiene*, **33**, 444–50.

Genta, R. M., Schad, G. A., and Hellman, M. E. (1986). *Strongyloides stercoralis*: parasitological, immunological and pathological observations in immunosuppressed dogs. *Transactions of the Royal Society for Tropical Medicine and Hygiene*, **80**, 34–41.

Genta, R. M., Miles, P., and Fields, K. (1989). Opportunistic *Strongyloides stercoralis* infection in lymphoma patients. Report of a case and review of the literature. *Cancer*, **63**, 1407–11.

Georgi, J. R. and Sprinkle, C. L. (1974). A case of human strongyloidosis apparently contracted from asymptomatic colony dogs. *American Journal of Tropical Medicine and Hygiene*, **23**, 899–901.

Grove, D. I. (ed) (1989). *Strongyloidiasis: a major roundworm infection of man*. Taylor and Francis, London.

Grove, D. I., Heenan, P. J., and Northern, C. (1983). Persistent and disseminated infections with *Strongyloides stercoralis* in immunosuppressed dogs. *International Journal of Parasitology*, **13**, 483–90.

Harper, J. S., Rice, J. M., London, W. T., Sly, D. L., and Middleton, C. (1982). Disseminated Strongyloidiasis in *Erythrocebus patas*. *American Journal of Primatology*, **3**, 89–98.

Higenbottam, T. W. and Heard, B. E. (1987). Opportunistic pulmonary strongyloidiasis complicating asthma treated with steroids. *Thorax*, **31**, 226–33.

Hira, P. R. and Patel, B. G. (1980). Human strongyloidiasis due to the primate species *Strongyloides fuelleborni*. *Tropical Geography and Medicine*, **32**, 23–9.

Hunter, G., Bagshawe, A. F., Baboo, K. S., Luke, R., and Prociv, P. (1992). Intestinal parasites in Zambian patients with AIDS. *Transactions of the Royal Society for Tropical Medicine and Hygiene*, **86**, 543–5.

Igra-Siegman, Y., Kapila, R., Sen, P., Kaminski, Z. C., and Louria, D. B. (1981). Syndrome of hyperinfection with *Strongyloides stercoralis*. *Reviews of the Infectious Diseases*, **3**, 397–407.

Jorgensen, T., Montresor, A., and Savioli, L. (1996). Effectively controlling Strongyloidasis. *Parasitology Today*, **12**, 164.

Kerlin, R. L., Nolan, T. J., and Schad, G. A. (1995). *Strongyloides stercoralis*: Histopathology of uncomplicated and hyper-

infective strongyloidasis in the Mongolian gerbil, a rodent model for human strongyloidiasis. *International Journal of Parasitology*, **25**, 411–20.

Koga, K., Kasuya, S., and Ohtomo, H. (1992). How effective is the agar plate method for *Strongyloides stercoralis*? *Journal of Parasitology*, **78**, 155–6.

Longworth, D. L. and Weller, P. F. (1986). Hyperinfection syndrome with strongyloidiasis. In *Current clinical topics in infectious diseases*, (ed. J. S. Remington and M. N. Schwartz), pp. 1–26. McGraw Hill, New York.

Lucas, S. B. (1990). Missing infections in AIDS. *Transactions of the Royal Society for Tropical Medicine and Hygiene*, **84**; (Suppl. 1), 34–8.

Mansfield, L. S. and Schad, G. A. (1992). Ivermectin treatment of naturally acquired and experimentally induced *Strongyloides stercoralis* infections in dogs. *Journal of the American Veterinary Medicine Association*, **201**, 726–30.

Masdeu, J. C., Tantulavenich, S., and Gorelick, P.P. (1982). Brain abscess caused by *Strongyloides stercoralis*. *Archives of Neurology*, **39**, 62–3.

Nielsen, P. B. and Mojon, M. (1987). Improved diagnosis of *Strongyloides stercoralis* by seven consecutive stool specimens. *Zentralblatt Fur Bakteriologie, Mikrobiologie, Und Hygiene - Series A*, **263**, 616–17.

Pampiglione, S. and Ricciardi, M. L. (1972). Experimental infestation with human strain *Strongyloides fulleborni* in man. *Lancet*, **1**, 663–5.

Penner, L. R. (1981). Concerning threadworm (*Strongyloides stercoralis*) in great apes-lowland gorillas (*Gorilla gorilla*) and chimpanzees (*Pantroglodytes*). *Journal of Zoo Animal Medicine*, **12**, 128–31.

Pereira-Lima, J. and Delgado, P. G. (1961). Diagnosis of strongyloidiasis: importance of the Baermann's method. *American Journal of Digestive Diseases*, **6**, 899–904.

Sandground, J. H. (1928). Some studies on susceptibility, resistance, and acquired immunity to infection with *Strongyloides stercoralis* in dogs and cats. *American Journal of Hygiene*, **8**, 507–38.

Schad, G. A. (1989). Morphology and life history of *Strongyloides stercoralis*. pp. 85–104. In *Strongyloidiasis: a major roundworm infection of man*, (ed. D. I. Grove), pp. 85–104. Taylor and Francis, London.

Schad, G. A., Aikens, L. M., and Smith, G. (1989). *Strongyloides stercoralis*: is there a canonical migratory route through the host? *Journal of Parasitology*, **75**, 740–9.

Schad, G. A., Smith, G., Megyeri, Z., Bhopale, V. M. Niamatali, S., and Maze, R. (1993). *Strongyloides stercoralis*: an initial autoinfective burst amplifies primary infection. *American Journal of Tropical Medicine a* **48**, 716–25.

Silva, O. A., Santos-Amaral, C. F., Bruno, J. C., Lopez, M., and Homem-Pittella, J. E. (1981). Hypokalemic respiratory muscle paralysis following *Strongyloides stercoralis* hyperinfection. A case report. *American Journal of Tropical Medicine and Hygiene*, **30**, 69–73.

von Kuster, L. and Genta, R. M. (1989). Cutaneous manifestations of strongyloidiasis. *Archives of Dermatology*, **124**, 1826–30.

Weesner, R. E., Kolinjivadi, J., Giannella, R. A., Huitger, O. T. and Genta, R. M. (1988). Effect of *Strongyloides ratti* on small bowel function in normal and immunosuppressed host rats. *Digestive Diseases and Sciences*, **33**, 1316–21.

Zumla, A. and Croft, S. L. (1992). Chemotherapy and immunity in opportunistic parasitic infections in AIDS. *Parasitology*, **105**, (Suppl.) S93–101.

57 CAPILLARIOSIS

John H. Cross

SUMMARY

Only four nematodes of the genus *Capillaria* are reported to be zoonotic; *Capillaria philippinensis*, *Capillaria hepatica*, *Capillaria aerophila*, and *Anatrichosoma cutaneum*. *Capillaria philippinensis* is a parasite of the small intestine and causes a severe enteropathy and at times death in humans. Over 2000 cases of intestinal Capillariosis have been reported from the Philippines and Thailand, with sporadic cases reported from Korea, Japan, Taiwan, India, Iran, Egypt, Italy and Spain. Small freshwater and brackish-water fish are the source of infection and probably fish-eating birds the reservoir host. Control measures in endemic areas should be treatment, education, avoidance of eating raw fish, and improved sanitation. Although *C. hepatica* is found in rodents worldwide, fewer than 30 cases of hepatic capillariosis have been reported in humans from Europe, Asia, Africa, North and South America. The infection is acquired by the ingestion of embryonated eggs from the soil. Female worms deposit eggs in the liver tissue and granulomas develop around the egg. The eggs are released after the rodent is eaten and the liver digested. Eggs pass in the faeces and are deposited in the soil where they embryonate. Avoidance of contaminated soil would prevent human infection and destruction of rodents would control animal infections. Only 11 cases of capillariosis aerophila have been reported, the majority from Russia. The parasite is found within tissue of the respiratory passages of canines and felines worldwide. The prevalence rates seem to be highest in foxes and the parasitosis is especially hazardous in foxes raised for fur on domestic farms. Eggs from infected animals are usually passed in faeces, then embryonate in the soil and become infective. Eggs ingested by earthworms hatch and the larvae become infective. The definitive host becomes infected when the earthworm is eaten or when eggs are eaten directly from the soil. Control is difficult in nature but on fox-raising farms the animals should be suspended in cages above the soil and given periodic anthelminthic treatment. *Anatrichosoma cutaneum* is primarily a subcutaneous parasite of monkeys, but there are two reports of cutaneous infections in humans. The parasite causes serpiginous lesions in the skin of the soles, palms, and nasal passages. Whole monkey colonies can be infected and control is difficult. Anthelminthic treatment and improved sanitation should help control the anatrichosomiosis.

INTRODUCTION

Although there are over 300 capillarid species infecting wildlife populations, only a few of these nematodes infect humans and cause disease. Three species of *Capillaria* (*C. philippinensis*, *C. hepatica*, and *C. aerophila*) and one species of *Anatrichosoma* (*A. cutaneum*) have been reported in humans. Only *C. philippinensis* is a serious human public health problem; the other species are rarely reported. Consequently emphasis in this chapter will be on *C. philippinensis* and the disease it causes, intestinal capillariosis.

CAPILLARIA PHILIPPINENSIS

HISTORY

The first case of capillariosis philippinensis was in a 29-year-old schoolteacher from Bacarra, a *barrio*, in the province of Ilocos Norte in northern Luzon in the Philippines. The man had suffered from an intractable diarrhoea for 3 weeks before admission to the Philippine General Hospital in Manila in 1963. He was a chronic alcoholic and manifested symptoms of ascites, emaciation, and cachexia, and died after 1 week in hospital. At autopsy a large number of tiny worms were found in the intestines (Chitwood *et al.* 1964). The worms were first thought to be *C. hepatica* but were later correctly classified as a new species (Chitwood *et al.* 1968). In an interview several years later with the physician who first saw the patient in Bacarra, it was learned that 13 others had similar symptoms and all had died.

During 1965 and 1966 in Pudoc West, a *barrio*, in Ilocos Sur province, approximately 150 km south of Bacarra, an alarming number of middle-aged males were found to be dying of what was termed gastroenteritis. A Catholic priest from the town of Tagudin, Ilocos Sur recognized the seriousness of the problem and notified the Philippine Health Department. Investigations of the epidemic began in early 1967. Initially it was believed that the increase in illness and deaths was due to an intoxication, but when a partial autopsy was done on one of the victims, a large number of worms were found in the small intestines. A hospital and a capillariosis research centre were established in Tagudin and patients with intestinal capillariosis began to be documented and treated. Cases continued to appear in Pudoc West and neighbouring *barrios* and a total of 1037 patients were seen from February to December 1967; 77 died. During 1968 and 1969 infections were found in people from other provinces, especially along the Philippine northern coast of the South China Sea. Eventually early case detection and treatment resulted in a decrease in infections and deaths. There were 291 new cases and 13 deaths in 1968, 74 cases and three deaths in 1969, and in 1970, 41 cases and two deaths (Cross and Bhaibulaya 1983). Cases continued to appear over the next 20 years and varied from 2 to 60, with only one or two deaths. Death is rare today if the diagnosis is made early and the parasitosis treated.

During the early years of the epidemic the pathophysiology of the disease and adequate treatment regimes were ascertained. The life cycle of the parasite was established in the laboratory and the means of infection determined. In 1973 the disease was recognized in Thailand and patients are now seen regularly in Thai hospitals. The next case reports were from the Middle East, Iran and Egypt, then Japan, Taiwan, and Korea (Cross 1992). Single cases have been recently reported from India and from Italy and Spain but in persons who were thought to acquired the infection in Indonesia and Columbia, respectively.

THE AGENT

The taxonomic status of the capillarids is in a state of confusion. Some authors place *Capillaria* spp. in the family Trichuridae in the superfamily Trichinelloidea, while others consider them in the family Capillaridea. To add to the confusion Moravec (1982) and Moravec *et al.* (1987) suggested that *C. philippinensis* be placed in the genus *Aonchotheca*, and in a more recent publication Anderson (1992) placed it into the genus *Calodium*. However, these genera are not well known or recognized by most parasitologists and biomedical scientists, and it seems prudent to continue to use the genus *Capillaria* since the name is hallowed in the scientific literature by tradition.

Chitwood *et al.* (1968) described the tiny nematode recovered from the first patient that died of intestinal capillariosis and worms obtained from several sub-

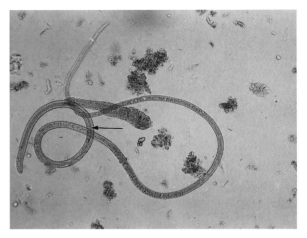

Fig. 57.1 Adult male *C. philippinensis* (×40), arrow indicates spicule. Male length varies from 1.5 to 3.9 mm.

sequent autopsies. The authors based speciation upon characteristics of its small size, the male caudal alae, a long, non-spiny spicular sheath. In the female the vulva is slightly salient without a flap. Other characteristics based upon those of Chitwood *et al.* (1968) and other investigators are as follows: male (Fig. 57.1) length 1.5–3.9 mm; width 3–5 μm at the head, 23–28 μm at the stichosome and 18 μm at the cloaca; spicule 230–300 μm, unspined spicular sheath may extend to 440 μm; anus subterminal and the tail has ventrolateral expansions containing two pairs of papillae. Females (Fig. 57.2) 2.3–5.3 mm; width 5–8 μm at the head, 25 μm at the widest part of the stichosome, 28–36 μm at the vulva and 29–47 μm post-vulva. The anus is subterminal. The vulva is located immediately

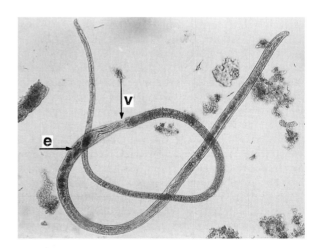

Fig. 57.2 Adult female *C. philippinensis* (×40), arrows indicate salient vulva (v) and eggs (e) in the uterus. Female length varies from 2.3 to 5.3 mm.

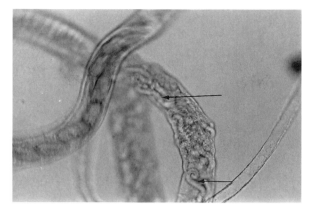

Fig. 57.3 Adult female *C. philippinensis* showing a larvae (arrow) in the uterus (×107).

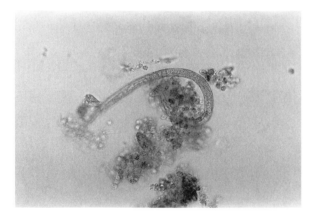

Fig. 57.4 Larva of *C. philippinensis* recovered from the intestinal content of a Filipino who died of capillariosis philippinensis (×100).

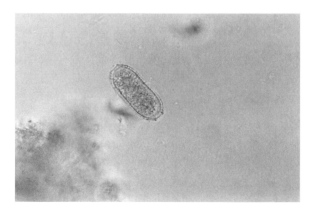

Fig. 57.5 Egg of *C. philippinensis* (×100) with flattened bipolar plugs and striated eggshell (36–45 by 20 μm).

behind the oesophagus and the uterus of the mature female may contain thick-shelled eggs (Fig. 57.2), thin-shelled eggs with or without embryos (Fig. 57.3), or larvae (Fig. 57.4). Eggs in faeces are usually thick-shelled, peanut-shaped with bipolar plugs, and measure 36–45 by 20 μm (Fig. 57.5).

The life cycles of relatively few capillarids have been determined. Some species have a direct, egg to egg, life cycle while others utilize an intermediate host. During the course of study on *C. philippinensis* attempts were made to transmit infections by introducing embryonated eggs into a variety of animals including human volunteers. None of the eggs hatched in these animals until eggs were introduced into freshwater fish from the lagoons of northern Luzon under laboratory condition (Cross *et al.* 1972). It was found that the eggs hatched within hours after ingestion and the larvae doubled in length in 3 weeks; no further growth occurred after this. When larvae were fed to monkeys the larvae matured and patient infections developed. The monkeys suffered no ill effects of infection even though some animals passed eggs for as long as 14 months. Mongolian gerbils were subsequently exposed to infection and details of the life cycle established (Cross *et al.* 1978). Larvae given to gerbils by stomach tube developed into sexually mature adults in 10–11 days and female worms release first-stage larvae in 13–14 days. In 22–24 days these larvae matured and the second-generation females produced eggs which passed in the faeces in 25–35 days. Most female worms produce eggs that pass in the faeces but there were always a few that continued to produce larvae. The worms in gerbils lived for 6–7 weeks but new generations maintained the infection until the gerbil died. It is believed that this life cycle also occurs in humans with autoinfection leading to hyperinfection.

Other laboratory and wild animals were exposed to experimental infections but only transient infections developed in some wild-caught rats (*Rattus* spp.) and multimammate rats (*Mastomys natalensis*) (Cross *et al.* 1978; Cross and Basaca-Sevilla 1983*a*). Fish-eating birds in Thailand (Bhaibulaya and Indra-Ngarm 1979) and Taiwan (Cross and Basaca-Sevilla 1983*b*) were also exposed to infection and patent infections developed. It is believed that fish-eating birds are important in the epidemiology and the spread of *C. philippinensis* in nature.

During the course of study over 150 000 animal specimens were examined for natural infections of *C. philippinensis*. While some capillarids were found, none were *C. philippinensis*. Some larval capillarids were also found, but species identification could not be determined. Once the life cycle was established, fish from lagoons were found to be infected and when fed to gerbils patent infections developed (Cross *et al.* 1978)

The disease caused by *C. philippinensis* can be attributed to the build up of massive numbers of parasites. At autopsy of one patient over 200 000 worms were estimated in 1 litre of bowel fluid. Most likely only a few parasites are initially acquired after the ingestion of fish containing larvae. The larvae mature, mate and females deposit both larvae and eggs. The larvae develop into adults and the process continues. The number of worms increases gradually and begins to cause early symptoms of diarrhoea, abdominal pain, and stomach gurgling. Eventually the intestinal tissue is severely damaged and the patients develop a protein losing enteropathy and electrolyte loss. There is some evidence that substances are produced by the parasite that damage the intestinal tissues (Sun *et al.* 1974).

THE HOST

ANIMAL

All information on the life cycle of *C. philippinensis* was obtained in the laboratory based upon experimental infections in animals. Monkeys infected with the parasite showed no signs of infections and most data resulted from infections in Mongolian gerbils. The prepatent period in gerbils averaged 27 days and the animals lived for an average of 45 days. The highest number of worms were found between 35 and 45 days postinfection. There usually were fewer worms after 45 days if the animal survived, but the numbers increased again until about 57 days when the animals died (Cross *et al.* 1978). Gerbils lost body weight and serum protein as the infection progressed. As reported by Sun *et al.* (1974) infection in gerbils led to intestinal mucosal changes, direct mechanical compression, microulceration of the epithelium due to lytic substances, and degeneration of cells. The life cycle of the parasite in birds was similar to that found in gerbils. However, some birds survived the infection and were immune to subsequent infection.

HUMAN

The incubation period in human infections has not been definitely determined but evidence suggests 3 weeks; i.e. time between ingestion of raw fish and the first symptoms of diarrhoea and borborygmus. This is followed by weight loss and intermittent diarrhoea for several weeks. Patients may have as many as 10 voluminous bowel movements per day, loss of body weight, and the development of malaise, vomiting, and anorexia. Whalen *et al.* (1969) reported physical findings of muscle wasting and weakness, borborygmus, distant heart sounds, hypotension, gallop rhythm, pulses alterans, abdominal distention and tenderness,

oedema, and hyporeflexia. Laboratory analysis showed a protein losing enteropathy, malabsorption of fats and sugars, decrease excretion of xylose and low levels of potassium, calcium, carotene, and total serum protein. Immunoglobulin IgE increased while IgG, IgM, and IgA decreased. Patients who are not treated before the irreversible effects of the disease develop usually die 4–7 months after the first symptoms.

Autopsies were conducted on 15 Filipinos who died of intestinal capillariasis (Canlas *et al.* 1967; Fresh *et al.* 1972). The bodies were usually dehydrated, pale, and emaciated with serous fluid in the pleural and peritoneal cavities. Hearts were within normal limits with little pericardial fat and the lungs were usually congested. Livers were yellow in colour and in the spleens white pulp was conspicuous. Kidney, liver, spleen, and pancreas weights were reduced. There was also cerebral vascular congestion.

Histological changes were more or less confined to the small intestines. The parasites, in amazingly large numbers, were found in all stages in the lumen, and crypts of Lieberkühn. Most worms were found in the jejunum, with some found throughout the digestive tract probably as a result of post-mortem migration. Worms were not found in any other location or tissue except once when sections of a worm with stichocytes were found in the liver. Histological findings were similar in animals infected with the parasite. Parasites were confined to the intestinal tract and no other organ.

Some changes, however, were seen in other human organs, probably because of physiological alterations. Fatty metamorphosis of the liver and vacuolization of the cytoplasm of the renal proximal convoluted tubular lining cells was found at autopsy in some patients. Haemoglobulin pigments were also found in the tubules. Myocardial cells showed vacuolization and concentrations of lipochrome pigments in the myocardium were also seen. The crypts of Lieberkühn of the intestines were atrophied and contained eosinophils, cellular debris, and at times *C. philippinensis*. The intestinal villi were often flattened and denuded and the mucosal glands dilated (Fig. 57.6). The lamina propria was infiltrated with macrophages, lymphocytes, neutrophils, a few eosinophils, and plasma cells. Intestinal material contained all stages of the parasite and mucosal fragments resulting from mucosal sloughing (Fig. 57.7).

In endemic areas of the Philippines the diagnosis is made from the symptoms of abdominal pain, borborygmus, diarrhoea, and weight loss. The parasitological diagnosis is made by finding eggs, larvae, and adults in the faeces. Speciation by larvae alone is difficult, but the adult characteristics are easy to identify. Eggs may be confused with eggs of *Trichuris*

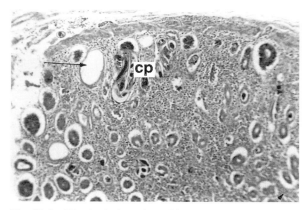

Fig. 57.6 Histological section of human intestine showing cellular infiltration, denuded gland (arrow), and sections of *C. philippinensis* (cp) in the crypts of Leiberkühn (×20).

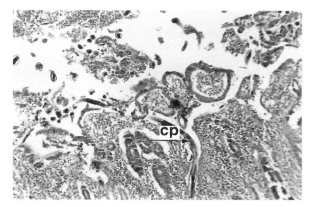

Fig. 57.7 Histological section of human intestine showing *C. philippinensis* (cp) in the tissue, mucosal fragments, and worm sections in the gut lumen (×20).

trichura by inexperienced technicians, but *T. trichura* eggs are larger (50–54 × 22–23 μm) and are barrel-shaped with bipolar mucoid plugs. *Capillaria philippinensis* eggs are peanut-shaped with a striated shell, the bipolar plugs are flattened and they measure 36–45 × 20 μm (Fig. 57.5). Several stools may have to be examined before finding the parasite. If intestinal capillariosis is suspected, an anthelminthic can be given which will stimulate the parasite, causing it to pass in the faeces in a day or two. Duodenal aspirates may also yield eggs, larvae, and adults of the parasite. Serologic testing is not reliable.

Patients with severe intestinal capillariosis should be given electrolyte replacement, an antidiarrhoeal agent and a high protein diet followed by an anthelminthic. Thiabendazole was found to be effective but caused side-effects; treatment was long term and relapses were common. Relapses at one time were more common

than new cases (Singsong 1974). Mebendazole became the drug of choice in dosages of 400 mg day in two divided doses for 20 days for new cases and 30 days for relapse cases. Albendazole is currently the drug of choice, at 400 mg day in divided doses for 10 days; relapses are rare with albendazole. The patients respond quickly to anthelminthic therapy with the symptoms abating in 4–5 days. It is important to continue full treatment otherwise relapses will occur.

Infections in gerbils responded to treatment with small doses of mebendazole. Abbreviated treatment was also given but resulted in reappearance of eggs in the faeces. Deaths in gerbils could be prevented by treatment with small doses of mebendazole.

Prognosis is good when the infection is treated before the devastating effects of the parasitosis occurs. Deaths are rare today because physicians, especially in the Philippines and Thailand, recognize the symptoms early and immediate treatment is initiated. Deaths have not been reported outside of Asia because the disease has been recognized early and treated.

EPIDEMIOLOGY

Three locations the Philippines were known endemic areas for capillariosis philippinensis; northern Luzon, central Luzon, and southern Leyte. A total of 1896 cases have been documented from northern Luzon but there are probably many more that have not been documented. Over 100 people are known to have died from the disease in northern Luzon; the numbers of cases from central Luzon and southern leyte are unknown. Cases in Thailand have been sporadic and the numbers of people infected are not known but in one epidemic over 100 people acquired the disease and nine died. As far as is known, four cases have been reported in Japan, at least seven cases in Taiwan, one and possibly two in Korea. Iran and India reported one case each and Egypt two. One case was reported from Italy in a person who visited Indonesia (Chichino *et al.* 1992) and in Spain a case is reported from a person who visited Columbia in South America (Drondra *et al.* 1993).

Since the extensive use of anthelminthic the incidence of intestinal capillariosis has decreased in northern Luzon. A total of 1896 cases have been recorded, most of which (1328) occurred during the epidemic of 1967–68. Throughout the years twice as many men (1345) as women (551) have been infected with the parasite, mostly middle-aged males between 20 and 40 years of age. The reason for more infection in males is not known, but it is believed that males eat raw fish more often than females. Males collect the fish from traps and eat them fresh. They also eat raw fish while drinking alcoholic beverages. As far as is known epidemics have occurred only in the three endemic areas of the Philippines, and in Sisakis province in northeastern Thailand.

Groups at risk of infection seem to be those who eat raw freshwater or brackish-water fish, mostly fishermen—farmers and their families. Population groups in the Philippines and Thailand consider raw fish an important part of their diet. Raw fish is also eaten by Koreans, Japanese, and some Taiwanese. Raw fish has also been implicated in cases in Iran and Egypt, but the source of infection for the reported cases from Italy and Spain is unknown. Small freshwater or brackish-water fish in the Philippines and Thailand have been experimentally infected when given embryonated eggs of *C. philippinensis*. The larvae from these fish developed into adults in monkeys and gerbils. In other studies in the Philippines, infections were established in laboratory animals given larvae recovered from fish caught in lagoons or purchased from the market; these fish were naturally infected.

The fish that are eaten whole by Asian populations are small (5–8 cm), the size that can easily be eaten by fish-eating birds. The fish found naturally infected in the Philippines (*Hypseleotris bipartita*) is eaten raw, especially when the females are graved. It is small and easily swallowed whole by birds. It is now believed that fish-eating migratory birds are the natural host of the parasite. Birds such as *Amaurornis phoenicurus* and *Ardeola baccus* in Thailand (Bhaibulaya and Indra-Ngarm 1979), and *Nycticorax nycticorax*, *Babulcus ibis*, *Ixobrychus sinensis*, *Gallinula chloropus*, and *A. phoenicurus* on Taiwan, were experimentally infected (Cross and Basaca-Sevilla 1983*b*). Furthermore, one *Ixobrychus* sp. was found naturally infected with a male *C. philippinensis*. Migratory fish-eating birds can easily disseminate the parasite along their flyways, dropping faeces with eggs into water bodies, providing exposure to fish. When humans eat these fish, infections develop.

PREVENTION AND CONTROL

Human infections with *C. philippinensis* can be prevented by avoiding the eating of small freshwater or brackish-water fish. The fish are too small to eviscerate and are eaten whole without cleaning. Cooking of fish would prevent infections. It would be impossible to control infections in the wildlife populations.

Epidemics in the human population could be controlled by careful disposal of faeces from infected persons. It is believed that the washing of faecally-laden capillarioasis patients' bed sheets in lagoons in the Philippines and indiscriminate defaecation contributed to the epidemic. Fish became infected by

ingesting embryonated eggs from the faeces and people in the *barrios* ate the fish from the lagoon uncooked.

Treatment of infected persons with anthelminthics should be included in a control programme. The decrease in the number of infected persons in the Philippines is attributed to the use of thiabendazole, mebendazole, and albendazole.

Educational programme warning of the dangers of eating raw fish would help in any control programme. Laws preventing the eating of raw fish maybe of some value but would be difficult to enforce among rural populations that customarily eat raw fish. Legislation against the washing of contaminated bed sheets or depositing faeces in natural waters may be enforceable.

CAPILLARIA HEPATICA

HISTORY

Capillaria hepatica was first reported in 1850 in a rat liver. In the ensuing years capillarids were discovered in the livers of rats and other animals (Skrjabin *et al.* 1957). Bancroft (1893) described the parasite as *Trichocephalus hepatica* from worm fragments in the liver, and noted the encapsulated eggs in the liver parenchyma. The nematode was subsequently placed into the genera *Trichosoma*, *Hepaticola*, *Eucoleus*, *Thominx* and *Capillaria*. Moravec (1982) placed it into the genus *Calodium* and Anderson (1992) concurred and consider it *Calodium hepaticum*. The parasitological and medical literature continue to refer to the parasite as *Capillaria hepatica*, consequently it will remain in use in this chapter.

Human hepatic capillarioasis was first reported by MacArthur (1924) in a English soldier who died after serving in India for 3 years. Eggs and adult worms were found in his liver at autopsy. McQuown (1950) discovered the parasitosis in a man who died in Louisiana, and Otto *et al.* (1954) found eggs and worms in a woman from Maryland. Human infection continued to be reported sporadically during the next 40 years and to date fewer than 30 cases of capillariasis hepatica have been documented worldwide. Spurious infections of eggs in human faeces are often reported, the eggs resulting from the ingestion of infected animal livers.

Hepatic capillarioasis is reported from rodents and other animals from all parts of the world; it is not uncommon, with prevalence rates varying from 0.7 to 85 per cent of rodents examined. The parasite has also been found in livers of other rodent species and other wild animals, dogs, cats, pigs, ungulates, and monkeys.

Adult *C. hepatica* mature and reproduce in the liver of animals, and eggs are deposited into the surrounding tissue. The adults eventually die and the eggs become encapsulated. Mild infections are subclinical but in heavy infections there is hepatitis, splenomegaly, ascites, and eosinophilia. The eggs may elicit granuloma formation and fibrosis. The eggs remain in the tissue until the animal dies or is consumed by another animal.

Eggs reaching the soil after release from liver tissue, embryonate and become infectious. Humans accidentally acquire infection probably through geophagy or eating contaminated food. Control measures are difficult except for rodent control and education.

THE AGENT

Capillaria hepatica has been placed in the superfamily Trichinelloidea, family Trichiuridae, subfamily Capillariinae. The adult worm is delicate when removed from the liver, is filariform and white. The cuticle is finely transversely striated. There are two wide bacillary bands, each occupying one-fifth of the circumference and dividing the muscle layer. The female is 5–8 cm long and 0.1 mm wide and the male about 2–4 cm long and 0.1 mm wide. The anterior of both sexes is narrow and is occupied by the oesophagus. The posterior and is wider and contains the intestines and reproductive organs. The oesophagus, like other members of the family, is surrounded by stichocytes. The vulva of the female opens near the end of the oesophagus. The male spicule is slightly chitinized and measures 0.4–0.5 mm in length; the sheath is membranous and without spines. Eggs are thick-shelled and minute pores give a striated appearance. There are two polar plugs and the eggs measure 50–68 by 30–35 μm (Fig. 57.10).

The eggs remain undeveloped while in the liver tissue. Adults in the liver parenchyma eventually die and are destroyed by the inflammatory reaction. When the infected animals is eaten by another animal the eggs are digested out of the liver and pass out with the faeces and are dispersed in the soil. In a moist environment with the right temperature the eggs mature and larvae develop in about 1 month. When the egg is ingested by a susceptible host it hatches in the intestines and the released larva (140–190 μm in length) penetrates the intestinal wall and is picked up by the hepatic portal system and carried to the liver. These larvae may reach the liver in 1 or 2 days and develop into adults within 18–20 days. Eggs are soon produced and the males die by 40 days and females live up to 59 days. The development maybe variable, depending on the host. The eggs and worms form yellow streaks or white patches on the liver surface. The liver becomes enlarged and soft in acute hepatic capillariosis and in chronic infection the liver becomes

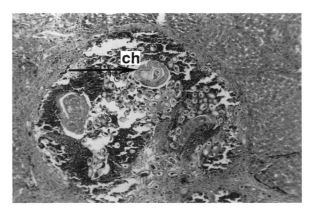

Fig. 57.8 Rodent liver showing *C. hepatica*, worm sections (ch) and eggs surrounded by an inflammatory reaction (×20).

fibrotic. In the acute infection focal parenchymal destruction and granulomas may develop with mononuclear cells and eosinophils. In older infections some adults and eggs are scattered throughout the liver tissue, causing granulomatous inflammation (Fig. 57.8). Eggs continue to be produced and group together with bundles of fibrous connective tissue and cellular infiltration with lymphocytes and polymorphonuclear cells, especially eosinophils. Eggs continue to build up and the fibrosis increases. Giant cells will destroy adult worms and some eggs.

Survival of the parasite in nature depends upon the presence of a rodent or other animal species, and cannibalism among the animal groups. The eggs also contaminate the environment following death and decomposition of infected animals. Temperature and humidity are also important to survival. However, eggs can withstand cold weather and infections can be acquired in the winter time.

THE HOST

ANIMAL

The disease in the rodent host as well as other animals depends upon the degree of infection; the greater the number of eggs ingested, the more severe the disease. Hepatitis and hepatomegaly develop soon after egg deposition. There is an early onset of granuloma formation and cellular infiltration. Parenchymal alterations are characterized by degeneration, pycnosis and karyorrhexis of liver cells, and loss of typical structure of the liver. Increasing egg deposition causes an increase in weight and size of the liver. The weight of the spleen also increases. A chronic granulomatous response occurs when egg deposition ceases. Calcification occurs at a later stage, with dead parasites in the centre of the lesion. At about 100 days most lesions are non-reactive and surrounded by a thin layer of connective tissue. Although large numbers of inflammatory and giant cells are evident in early lesions, these clear later in the infection. The acute inflammatory reaction is replaced by a relative normalization of remaining hepatic sections with the retention of atrophic changes. Animals usually die in the acute stage in heavy infections.

There are also changes in enzyme activity in the first few weeks of infection, with the maximum increase in transaminase and dehydrogenases in the third week. Activity continued but plateaus at a lower level into the chronic stage.

The only means of diagnosing animal infection is by examination of liver tissue by open biopsy or by autopsy and histological examination of the tissue. Serological testing using immunofluorescence technique, haemagglutination tests, or ELISA should be possible. Several drugs (febantel, albendazole, mebendazole, oxfendazole) were reported to be effective in preventing deposition of *C. hepatica* eggs in mouse livers (Cheetham and Markus 1991). However the value of treatment after egg deposition is questionable.

Animals may survive light infections, with the development of acquired immunity. However, with heavy infection death may readily occur.

HUMAN

People are accidental hosts of *C. hepatica* and usually the time of infection is not known. Many cases have been discovered at autopsy and ante-mortem by liver biopsy. Enlargement of the liver is first noticed by the patient. There may also be abdominal pain, fatigue, anorexia, high morning fever, nausea, and vomiting. Enlargement of the spleen, diarrhea or constipation, abdominal distension, oedema of the extremities, and sometimes pneumonia are reported.

Laboratory findings show marked leucocytosis with eosinophilia, and moderate hyperchromic anaemia, and bone marrow examination may reveal a cellular marrow with normoblastic erythropoiesis and a marked proliferation of the eosinophilic series of leucocytes. Liver function tests and serum proteins may be abnormal.

The diagnosis is made by finding eggs, and at times adults, in liver tissues taken by needle biopsy or at autopsy (Fig. 57.9). The lesions taken early in the infection will show worms and eggs and some liver fibrosis. The eggs can be identified by the thick striated shell, and two polar plugs (Fig. 57.10). The adult worms can be identified by the presence of stichocytes and other characteristics listed above. Serological tests

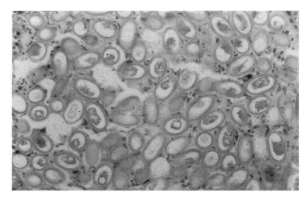

Fig. 57.9 Histological section of human liver taken at autopsy, showing cluster of *C. hepatica* eggs (×100).

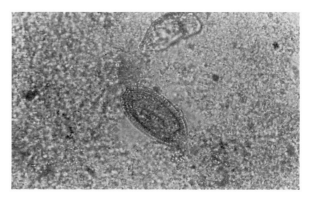

Fig. 57.10 Egg of *C. hepatica* (50–68 by 30–35 μm) recovered from human faeces from a spurious infection (×100).

are not readily available, but those indicated above for animal infections could be used in the presumptive diagnosis of human hepatic capillariosis.

The pathology associated with human infections is similar to that found in animals, such as white to greying nodules on the surface of the liver. Microscopically, the principal lesions consist of necrotic foci and granuloma consisting of numerous eosinophils. As the disease progresses inflammatory changes continue, with eggs grouping together within bundles of fibrous connective tissue and eosinophils. Eventually there is extensive fibrosis and the eggs may become phagocytosed by multinucleated giant cells and destroyed.

Treatment of human capillariosis hepatica is not well documented. Anthelminthics would have little action on eggs but could affect adult worms in the liver. Choe *et al.* (1993) used thiabendazole and albendazole and found the drugs to be ineffective against the eggs but effective against the adults. Sodium antimony gluconate may have some effect.

The prognosis is not good for hepatic capillariosis, most infections are fatal. The prognosis is good if the diagnosis is made early and treatment initiated.

EPIDEMIOLOGY

Capillaria hepatica has a worldwide distribution, being found in the liver of rodents and a myriad of other mammals. It lacks host specificity, having been found in the dog, cat, beavers, rabbits, hyrax, peccary, prairie dog, shrew, skunk, and opossum. It was found in 12 different species of *Rattus* on several islands of Indonesia (Brown *et al.* 1975) and *C. hepatica*-like eggs were found in the liver of a short-nosed fruit bat (*Cynoptrus brachyotis*) and a sheath-tailed bat (*Emballonura alectro*) from Kalimantan Island (Borneo) Indonesia (Brown *et al.* 1974). Monkeys and the chimpanzee among the primates, have also been reported with hepatic capillariosis. The prevalence of infections is variable. Although animals other than rodents have been found infected, the rates of infections have been low. However, in rodents, 90 per cent of the animals examined have been found to be infected in some areas of the world.

Capillariosis hepatic is rare in humans and, as far as it can be determined, only 28 cases are reported. Choe *et al.* (1993), starting with the first case, has summarized 26 cases from India, the United States, Turkey, South Africa, Mexico, Brazil, Italy, Czechoslovakia, Nigeria, Switzerland, Japan, and Korea. Additional cases are reported from Germany (Pannenbecker *et al.* 1990) and Yugoslavia (Kokai *et al.* 1990). Many spurious infections have also been reported with eggs being found in faeces (Fig. 57.10). *Capillaria hepatica*-like eggs were also found in the sputum of a woman on Taiwan (Liu *et al.* 1970). Spurious infections occur when the liver of infected animals is eaten raw or cooked. The eggs are digested out of the tissue and pass with the faeces.

Humans, as well as other animals, acquire hepatic infections by ingesting embryonated eggs in food or drink. The eggs are in the soil or on vegetation in areas where there is an abundance of rodents. Children more often than adults acquire infections because of their habit of geophagy. There is no known transmission of infections from humans to other animals.

PREVENTION AND CONTROL

Hepatic capillariosis is so rare that extensive control measures would be difficult. However, rodent control and sanitary disposal of dead animals would be recom-

mended. Education and improved hygiene would also be advisable and the training of children to avoid eating dirt.

CAPILLARIA AEROPHILA

HISTORY

Capillaria aerophila was described as *Trichosoma aerophila* by Creplin (1839) after finding the nematode in the trachea of a wolf in Germany. Dujardin (1845) placed it in the genus *Eucoleus* and Ramson (1911) referred to it as *Capillaria*. The name was changed many times over the years: *Capillaria, Thominx,* and *Eucoleus,* and Moravec (1982) and Anderson (1992) considered it *Eucoleus aerophilius*. However, most texts still refer to it as *Capillaria aerophila*.

It is a parasite of the respiratory tract of canines, felines, and mustellids. The parasite invades the respiratory mucosa causing irritation, increased mucosal secretion, and constriction of the lumen of the respiratory passages. There may be rhinitis, tracheitis, bronchitis, and bronchopneumonia. Secondary bacterial infection may cause death, especially in young animals.

The parasite has a widespread distribution in nature in North and South America, Europe, Russia, Asia, North Africa, and Australia. The prevalence of natural infection in wild and domestic animals is variable. Butterworth and Beverley-Burton (1981) reported prevalence rates of infection of 44 per cent and 15 per cent for the red fox and marten, respectively, and Skirnisson *et al.* (1993) found 6 per cent of arctic foxes passing *C. aerophila* eggs. Control of these lungworm infections is nearly impossible in nature, but on farms for fur-bearing animals infections can be kept at a minimum by raising animals in cages suspended from the floor.

THE AGENT

Capillaria aerophila is in the order Enoplida, superfamily Trichnelloidea, family Trichuridae, sub family Capillarinae. The males are 15–18 mm in length and 9 μm at the anterior end, 62 μm at the end of the oesophagus and 28 μm at the posterior end; the anus is subterminal; caudal alae absent; spicule moderately sclerotized, the spicular sheath long and densely covered with cuticular spines. The female is 18–20 mm in length with a maximum width of 96–105 μm; width at the anterior end, 12 μm; at the oesophagus, 86–99 μm; and at the posterior end, 27–49 μm. The anus is subterminal and the vulva is located behind the oesophagus and it is not elevated.

Eggs are deposited in the lungs, are coughed up, swallowed, and pass in the faeces. They are unsegmented but after 5–7 weeks in the soil become embryonated. The eggs maybe ingested by earthworms where they hatch and the infection acquired by an animal after eating the earthworm. Infection may also be trasmitted directly by the ingestion of embryonated eggs. Once in the host the larvae migrate to the respiratory passages and invade the mucosa. The migration route is not known but it is speculated that the larvae reach the respiratory passages via the blood and lymphatics. The parasite causes an increase in mucosal secretions by direct action on the tissue or provoked by products from the parasites metabolism. In addition the infection may also cause lobar, catarrhal purulent bronchopneumonia with mucosal haemorrhage of the respiratory tract. This occurs especially in young animals. The life span of *C. aerophila* in the fox is about 1 year.

THE HOST

ANIMAL

The prepatent period for capillariosis aerophila is variable, depending on the animal and may be 25–40 days, but the incubation period is not known. The most common symptoms are coughing, sneezing, rales, superficial respiration, weakness, loss of appetite, and progressive emaciation.

The parasite becomes established in tunnels in the respiratory mucosa, and there is leucocytosis and eosinophilia. At necropsy of infected animals the respiratory mucosa is swollen and covered with mucus and small haemorrhages. Some areas may be emphysematous and other areas in a state of atelectasis. The thoracic cavity may contain a brownish to red fluid containing fibrin. Abscesses sometimes occur in the

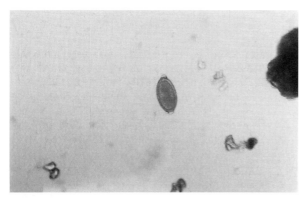

Fig. 57.11   Egg of *C. aerophila* (65 × 35 μm) recovered from the faeces of an arctic fox (×100). (courtesy of Dr K. Skirnisson. U. of Iceland).

lungs. Fatalities usually occur in animals less than 1 year of age, adults do not suffer as much and can be re-infected. The diagnosis is made by finding characteristic eggs in the faeces. The eggs are barrel-shaped and measure 65 × 35 μm, are thick-shelled with polar plugs (Fig. 57.11). Biopsy of respiratory tissue may also reveal the parasite.

Intratracheal injection of aqueous iodine alone or with potassium iodide have been used in the past to treat pulmonary capillariosis. Tracheal brushes have also been used. Currently anthelminthics are recommended; thiabendazole or ivermectin (Kazacos and Cantwell 1985) Steroids can also be used to relieve symptoms. The prognosis is good if infections are light. Young animals may die with heavy infection while adults survive and become re-infected.

HUMANS

Human capillariosis aerophila is very rare; only 11 cases have been reported—from Russia and Ukraine (8), Morocco (1), Iran (1), and France (1) (Vilella *et al.* 1986). The incubation period in humans is not known, but could be similar to the prepatent period in animals, 25–40 days. Most of the cases reported have been in adults and a few children. Infection in humans consist of bronchitis, coughing, mucoid or blood-tinged sputum, fevers, dyspnoea and eosinophilia. Some patients developed hepatomegaly, become cyanotic, and produced moist rales. Radiographs show infiltrates with reticulogranular patterns that progress to a honeycomb pattern. Lung biopsies have shown numerous granulomatous lesions with foreign body multinucleated giant cells containing the parasite surrounded by lymphocytes, plasma cells, eosinophils, and fibrin deposits.

The diagnosis of human pulmonary capillariosis is by finding characteristic eggs in sputum and or faeces. Eosinophils may also be present in the sputum. Biopsy of pulmonary tissue reveals the parasite.

Thiabendazole has been shown to be effective in treating human infections. Steroids may also be of value in relieving symptoms. Prognosis is good with treatment.

EPIDEMIOLOGY

Capillaria aerophila has been found in the respiratory passages of the dog, cat, wolf, marten, fox, ferret, opossum, badger, hedgehog, and humans in Europe, North and South America, Asia, Africa, and Australia. The prevalence rates are highly variable for species and geographic location. In the United States 0.8–9.6

per cent of dogs and nearly 10 per cent of the cats examined were found to be infected, while in Belgium 12 per cent of the cats examined were positive for infection, but no dogs were infected. In England 20 per cent of wild red foxes were positive, and on fur-breeding farms 30 per cent of the red foxes and 50–100 per cent of the silver foxes were infected. Epidemics of the parasitosis are serious problems on farms raising fur-bearing animals.

Infections are acquired by ingestion of embryonated eggs that are in the soil or by the ingestion of earthworms that have ingested embryonated eggs. The egg hatches in the earthworm and enters the body cavity. Transmission of the parasite to dogs, foxes, and cats has been accomplished by feeding infected earthworms. However, the major means of transmission is by ingestion of embryonated eggs since the susceptible animals usually do not include earthworms in their diets.

Human infections have been reported for the most part from the former USSR, Morocco, Iran, and France. The means of infection are unknown but most probably were through eating soil contaminated with embryonated eggs.

PREVENTION AND CONTROL

Infections of *C. aerophila* are difficult to control in nature. Infection in foxes and other animals raised for fur can be prevented by keeping the animals elevated above the floor and by maintaining good sanitary practices. Anthelminthics routinely administered to the animals would also be beneficial. Intratracheal injection with aqueous solutions of iodine and potassium iodide have also been used in the past. The use of thiabendazole or ivermectin would make this treatment obsolete, however.

Human infections could be prevented by avoiding the ingestion of contaminated soil and preventing children from playing in areas that may have been contaminated with wild animal faeces.

ANATRICHOSOMA CUTANEUM
HISTORY

Anatrichosoma species are found in the subcutaneous tissue of a number of animals. Swift *et al.* (1922) described *Trichosoma cutaneum* from skin lesion and nodules, and serpiginous tracts of the palms and soles of a *Macaca mulatta*. Smith and Chitwood (1954) and Chitwood and Smith (1958) described *A. cynamolae*. They transferred *T. cutaneum* to the genus *Anatrichosoma* and designated the species to *A. cutaneum*. Conrad and

Wong (1973) described two other species, *A. rhina* and *A. nadpoli* from *M. mulatta* and reported *Anatrichosoma* spp. from other Asian monkeys. In the meantime Orihel (1970) reported finding *Anatrichosoma* spp. in the nasal epithelium of several monkeys and baboons. Breznock and Pulley (1975) found *Anatrichosoma* sp. in ears, eyes, noses, and eyelids of adult gibbons (*Hylobates lar*) originally from Thailand. *Anatrichosoma* spp. have also been reported from the opossum, cat, and dog. Two human cases of creeping eruption have been reported with *A. cutaneum*.

THE AGENT

Anatrichosoma spp. are in the family Trichiuridae, subfamily Trichosomoidinae. The morphologic features are characteristic of the group: stichocytes surrounding the oesophagus, etc. The oesophagus extends from one-third to one-half of the body. Females measure 22–24 mm in length, width at the head 52 μm, at the oesophagus 100–110 μm, and at the posterior end 200 μm. The vulva is behind the oesophagus without a special appendage, the anus terminal. Very few worms have been extracted in their entirety. The males are about the same length as females but more slender. Males are without a spicule and spicular sheath, the posterior end has two subneutral papillae, and they have at least two pair of lateral papillae. During copulation the male inserts one-half of the posterior end of the spicule into the vagina of the female. Eggs produced by the females are ellipsoidal, thick walled, and have a smooth surface with polar plugs; they measure 56–70 by 37–42 μm and are embryonated when deposited (Fig. 57.12).

The worms are in serpiginous lesions in the subcutaneous tissue on the soles and palms and nasal mucosa of primates. The lesions may contain exudate

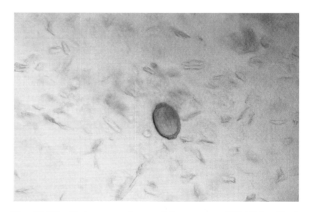

Fig. 57.12 Embryonated egg of *A. cutaneum* (56–70 by 42 μ) recovered from the skin of the palm of a monkey (×100).

and eggs are released in the exudate. The life cycle has not been determined but it is believed to be direct since the eggs are embryonated and an intermediate host has not been found. Eggs probably hatch after ingestion and the larvae migrate to the subcutaneous tissue to mature.

THE HOST

ANIMAL

Little is known about the details of the life cycle, prepatent period, or incubation period. Animals develop the infection and lesions begin to appear in the nasal tissue, feet, or palms. Swift *et al.* (1922) described the evolution of a nodule in the hands in which oedema first occurred with nodular thickening in the middle. The oedema disappeared and the nodule became more distinct. The nodules may or may not become tender. Aside from oedema there was little evidence of acute inflammation. These small nodules eventually decreased in size. Larger swellings of irregular size were found over the muscle of the arm, involving both skin and subcutaneous tissues. These lesions were flat, 5–10 by 8–20 mm in size, would persist for 2–5 days, and quickly disappeared. They resembled urticarial wheals. Lesions also developed on the ankles and wrists. Blisters, 3–5 by 2–10 cm, developed on the palms and soles, they were serpiginous and filled with blood-tinged serous fluid. Microscopic examination of lesions would reveal cross-sections of the worm surrounded by epithelial cells and leucocytes, especially eosinophils. Oedema, a perivascular reaction, and diffuse infiltration with eosinophils were present in the surrounding tissue. Eggs in the tissue were surrounded by a thick pink shinning hyaline structure two to three times the diameter of the egg.

In the nasal tissue the female worms become located in the squamous epithelial layer with eggs deposited in the epithelium and shed from the mucosal surface in plaques of exfoliating keratinized cells. Diffuse hyperplasia and parakeratosis are prominent changes in the mucosal epithelium (Allen 1960). Inflammatory reactions were also observed in the lamina propria with lymphocytes, plasma cells, and eosinophils. Some worms were within vessels of the lamina propria and the vessels exhibited focal necrosis and distension. Worms were also free in the connective tissue.

HUMAN

The two human cases of anatrichosomiosis cutaneum reported were from Japan and Vietnam. Morishita and Tani (1960) reported cutaneous creeping eruption in a finger and ankle of a Japanese male. The patient noted redness that moved 5–10 mm/day causing severe pruritis. One female worm was removed from each lesion. The pruritis ceased after the surgery. In the second case three adult female worms were removed from superficial galleries in the skin of the hand, foot, and scrotum of a Vietnamese male (Le-Van-Hoa *et al.* 1963).

In both monkeys and humans surgical removal of the worms is beneficial; however, anthelmintics such as thiabendazole, mebendazole, albendazole, and fenbendazole given daily for 10–14 days may also relieve symptoms and provide cure. The prognosis appears to be good with treatment.

EPIDEMIOLOGY

It appears that *Anatrichosoma* spp. are not uncommon parasites of non human primates. Orihel (1970) reported 29 per cent of 298 African monkeys belonging to five species infected with a species of *Anatrichosoma*. Conrad and Wong (1973) reported 5 per cent of nasal swabs and 17 per cent histological examinations of monkeys positive for *Anatrichosoma*, while in other studies (Wong and Conrad 1978) 18 per cent of 697 macaques were infected. Karr *et al.* (1979) examined 100 rhesus monkeys; 3 per cent were positive from one geographic site and 68 per cent from another site. Ulrich *et al.* (1981) found 54 per cent of wild-caught macaques positive, and within 3 years they were negative for the parasite. Infants born to these monkeys after captivity never developed infection. Eggs were collected from the nasal epithelium by cotton swabs. Long *et al.* (1976) found 3.6 per cent of 394 monkeys examined for *Anatrichosoma* sp. by nasal swab to be positive, and 13.9 percent positive by histological examination of tissue.

The means of transmission of *A. cutaneum* is not known but may be through the faecal–oral route, by fomites, or airborne. Captive primates should be maintained in clean cages and a clean environment. Infected animals should be isolated from uninfected ones and anthelminthics given. In the case of outbreaks, uninfected animals should be given prophylactic doses of an anthelminthic.

PREVENTION AND CONTROL

It is not known how human infections are acquired but animal caretakers should be examined periodically when monkeys in their charge are infected. However, there have been no known human infections among those working in animal care facilities.

REFERENCES

Allen, A. M. (1960). Occurrence of the nematode, *Anatrichosoma cutaneum* in the nasal mucosae of *Macaca mulatta* monkeys. *American Journal of Veterinary Research*, **21**, 389–92.

Anderson, R. C. (1992). *Nematode parasites of vertebrates: Their development and transmission*, pp. 540–61. C. A. B. International, Wallingford, Oxon.

Bancroft, T. L. (1893). On the whipworm of the rats liver. *Journal and Proceedings of the Royal Society of New South Wales*, **27**, 86–90.

Bhaibulaya, M. and Indra-Ngarm, S. (1979). *Amaurornis phoenicurus* and *Ardeola bacchus* as experimental definitive hosts for *Capillaria philippinensis* in Thailand. *International Journal of Parasitology*, **9**, 321–2.

Breznock, A. and Pulley, L. T. (1975). *Anatrichosoma* infection in two white-handed gibbons. *Journal of the American Veterinary Medical Association*, **167**, 631–3.

Brown, R. J., Cross, J. H., Van Peenen, P. F. D., and Carney, W. P. (1974). Capillarid-like eggs in livers of bats from Indonesia. *Southeast Asian Journal of Tropical Medicine and Public Health*, **4**, 599–600.

Brown, R. J., Carney, W. P., Van Peenen, P. F. D., and Cross, J. H. (1975). Capillariasis in wild rats in Indonesia. *Southeast Asian Journal of Tropical Medicine and Public Health*, **6**, 219–22.

Butterworth, E. W. and Beverley-Burton (1981). Observations on the prevalence and intensity of *Capillaria* spp. (Nematoda: Trichuroidea) in wild carnivora from Ontario, Canada. *Proceedings of the Helminthological Society of Washington*, **48**, 24–37.

Canlas, B. C., Cabrera, B. D., and Davis, U. (1967). Human intestinal capillariasis. II Pathological features. *Acta Medica Philippina*, **4**, 84–91.

Cheetham, R. F. and Markus, M. B. (1991). Drug treatment of experimental *Capillaria hepatica* infection in mice. *Parasitological Research*, **77**, 517–20.

Chichino, G. *et al.* (1992). Intestinal capillariasis (*Capillaria philippinensis*) acquired in Indonesia: A case report. *American Journal of Tropical Medicine and Hygiene*, **46**, 10–12.

Chitwood, M. G. and Smith, W. N. (1958). A redescription of *Anatrichosoma cynamolgi*, Smith and Chitwood, 1954. *Proceedings of the Helminthological Society of Washington*, **25**, 112–17.

Chitwood, M. B., Velasquez, C., and Salazar, N. G. (1964). Physiological changes in a species of *Capillaria* (Trichuroidea) causing a fatal case of human intestinal capillariasis. *Proceedings of the First International Congress of Parasitology*, **2**, 797.

Chitwood, M. B., Valasquez, C., and Salazar, N. G. (1968). *Capillaria philippinensis* sp. N. (Nematoda: Trichinellida) from intestine of man in the Philippines. *Journal of Parasitology*, **54**, 368–71.

Choe, C. Y. *et al.* (1993). Hepatic capillariasis: First case report in the Republic of Korea. *American Journal of Tropical Medicine and Hygiene*, **48**, 610–25.

Conrad, H. D. and Wong, M. M. (1973). Studies on *Anatrichosoma* (Nematoda: Trichinellida) with descriptions of *Anatrichosoma rhina* sp. N and *Anatrichosoma nacepobi* sp.n. from the nasal mucosa of Macaca mulatta. *Journal of Helminthology*, **47**, 289–302.

Creplin, F. C. H. (1839). Eingeweidewürmer, Binnenwüemer, Tierwürmer. *Allgemeine Encyclopaedie der Wissenschaften und Kunste*, **32**, 277–392.

Cross, J. H. (1992). Intestinal capillariasis. *Clinical Microbiology Reviews*, **5**, 120–9.

Cross, J. H. and Basaca-Sevilla, V. (1983*a*). Experimental infections of *Capillaria philippinensis* in multimammate rats (*Mastomys natalensis*). *Southeast Asian Journal of Tropical Medicine and Public Health*, **14**, 264.

Cross, J. H. and Basaca-Sevilla, V. (1983*b*). Experimental transmission of *Capillaria philippinensis* to birds. *Transactions of the Royal Society of Tropical Medicine and Hygiene*, **77**, 511–14.

Cross, J. H. and Bhaibulaya, M. (1983). Intestinal capillariasis in the Philippines and Thailand. In *Human ecology and infectious diseases*, (ed. N. Croll and J. H. Cross), pp. 103–36. Academic Press, New York.

Cross, J. H., Banzon, T. C., Clarke, M. D., Basaca-Sevilla, V., Watten, R. H., and Dizon, J. J. (1972). Studies on the experimental transmission of *Capillaria philippinensis* in monkeys. *Transactions of the Royal Society of Tropical Medicine and Hygiene*, **66**, 819–27.

Cross, J. H., Banzon, T. C., and Singson, C. M. (1978). Further studies on *Capillaria philippinensis*: development of the parasite in the Mongolian gerbil. *Journal of Parasitology*, **64**, 208–13.

Dronda, F., Chaves, F., Sanz, A., and Lopex-Velez, R. (1993). Human intestinal capillariasis in an area of nonendemicity: Case report and review. *Clinical Infectious Diseases*, **17**, 909–12.

Dujardin, F. (1845). *Histoire naturelle des helminthes ou vers intestinaux*. Paris XVI+654+15 pp.

Fresh, J. W., Cross, J. H. Reyes, V., Whalen, G. E., Uylangco, C. V., and Dizon, J. J. (1972). Necropsy findings in intestinal capillariasis. *American Journal of Tropical Medicine and Hygiene*, **21**, 169–73.

Karr, S. L., Henrickson, R. V., and Else, J. G. (1979). A survey for *Anatrichosoma* (Nematoda: Trichinellida) in wild caught *Macaca mulatta*. *Laboratory of Animal Science*, **29**, 789–90.

Kazacos, K. R. and Cantwell, H. D. (1985). Ivermectin for treatment of nasal capillariasis in a dog. *Journal of the American Veterinary Medical Association*, **186**, 174–5.

Kokai, G. K., Misic, S., Perisic, V. N., and Grujovska, S. (1990). *Capillaria hepatica* infestation in a 2-year-old girl. *Histopathology*, **17**, 275–7.

Le-Van-Hoa, Dong-Hong-Mo, and Nguyen-Luu-Vien. (1963). Premier cas de capillariose cutanée humaine. *Bulletin de la Société de Pathologie Exotique*, **56**, 121–6.

Liu, J. C., Whalen, G. E., and Cross, J. H. (1970). *Capillaria* ova in human sputum. *Journal of the Formosan Medical Association*, **69**, 80–2.

Long, G. G., Lichtenfels, J. R., and Stookey, J. L. (1976). *Anatrichosoma cynamolgi* (Nematoda: Trichinellida) in rhesus monkeys, *Macaca mulatta*. *Journal of Parasitology*, **62**, 111–15.

MacArthur, W. P. (1924). A case of infestation of the human liver with *Hepaticola hepatica* (Bancroft, 1893), Hall, 1916. *Proceedings of the Royal Society of Medicine*, **17**, 83–4.

McQuown, A. L. (1950). *Capillaria hepatica*. Report of genuine and spurious cases. *American Journal of Tropical Medicine*, **30**, 761–7.

Moravec, F. (1982). Proposal of a new systematic arrangement of nematodes of the family Capillariidae. *Folia Parasitologica*, **29**, 119–32.

Moravec, F., Prokopic, J., and Shlikas, A. V. (1987). The biology of nematodes of the family Capillariidae, Neveu-Lemaire, 1936. *Folia Parasitologica*, **34**, 39–56.

Morishita, K. and Tani, T. (1960). A case of *Capillaria* infection causing cutaneous creeping eruption in man. *Journal of Parasitology*, **46**, 79–89.

Orihel, T. C. (1970). *Anatrichosoma* in African monkeys. *Journal of Parasitology*, **56**, 982–5.

Otto, G. F., Berthrong, M., Appleby, R. D., Rawlings, J. C., and Wilber, D. (1954). Eosinophilia and hepatomegaly due to *Capillaria hepatica* (Bancroft, 1893) infection. *Bulletin of Johns Hopkins Hospital*, **94**, 319–36.

Pannenbecker, J., Miller, T. C., Muller, J., and Jeschke, R. (1990). Schwerer leberbefall durch *Capillaria hepatica*. *Monatsschrift Kinderheilkunde*, **138**, 767–71.

Ramson, B. H. (1911). *The nematodes parasitic in the alimentary tract of cattle, sheep, and other ruminants*. U S Department of Agriculture, Bureau of Animal Industry Bulletin 127.

Singson, C. N. (1974). Recurrences in human intestinal capillariasis. *Phillipine Journal of Microbiology and Infectious Diseases*, **3**, 7–13.

Skirnisson, K., Eydal, M., Gunnarsson, E., and Hersteinsson, P. (1993). Parasites of the Artic fox (*Alopex lagopus*) in Iceland. *Journal of Wildlife Diseases*, **29**, 440–6.

Skrjabin, K. I., Shikhobalova, N. P., and Orlon, I. V. (1957). *Essentials of nematology. Trichocephalidae and Capillariidae of animals and man and the disease caused by them*, Vol. VI. (Israel Program for Scientific Translations, Jerusalem, 1970). Academy of Sciences of the USSR.

Smith, W. M. and Chitwood, M. B. (1954). *Anatrichosoma cynamolgi*, a new trichiurid nematode from monkeys. *Journal of Parasitology*, **40**, Sect. 2, (Suppl.) p. 12. [absract].

Sun, S. C. *et al.* (1974). Ultrastructural studies of intestinal capillariasis *Capillaria philippinensis* in human and gerbil hosts. *Southeast Asian Journal of Tropical Medicine and Public Health*, **5**, 524–33.

Swift, H. F., Boots, R. H., and Miller, C. P. (1922). A cutaneous nematode infection in monkeys. *Journal of Experimental Medicine*, **35**, 599–620.

Ulrich, C. P., Henrickson, R. V., and Karr, S. L. (1981). A epidemiological survey of wild caught and domestic born rhesus monkeys (*Macaca mulatta*) for *Anatrichosoma* (nematoda: Trichinellida). *Laboratory of Animal Sciences*, **31**, 726–7.

Vilella, J. M., Desmaret, M. C., and Rouault, E. (1986). Capillariose a *Capillaria aerophila* chez un adulte? *Médecine et Maladies Infectienses*, **1**, 35–6.

Whalen, G. E. *et al.* (1969). Intestinal capillariasis—a new disease in man. *Lancet*, i, 13–16.

Wong, M. M. and Conrad, H. D. (1978). Prevalence of metazoan parasite infections in five species of Asian macaques. *Laboratory Animal Sciences*, **28**, 412–16.

58 ANGIOSTRONGYLOSIS

John H. Cross

SUMMARY

Although there are over 20 species of *Angiostrongylus* infecting the vascular system of a variety of vertebrates, only two species naturally found in rodents are known to infect humans and cause disease. *Angiostrongylus cantonensis* is found in the pulmonary arteries of rats worldwide and *A. costaricensis* is a parasite of cotton rats and a few other rodents predominently in America. The intermediate hosts for these parasites are terrestrial mollucs.

Angiostrongylus cantonensis is acquired by ingesting terrestrial snails infected with third-stage larvae. The larvae are released in the digestive tract and migrate to the central nervous system of rats. After a few weeks the young adult parasites migrate to the pulmonary arteries and reproduce. First-stage larvae develop in the lungs and migrate up the pulmonary tree are swallowed and pass in the faeces. The giant African snail (*Achatina fulica*) is a important intermediate host along with other terrestrial snails and slugs. Humans who eat infected snails uncooked acquire the infection. The infective-stage larvae migrate to the central nervous system and cause an eosinophilic meningitis. Major symptoms are headache, stiff neck, and paraesthesia. There may be paralysis of the internal rectus muscle and at times young adult worms are found in the eye. In most cases symptoms gradually disappear and death is rare. On one occasion adult worms were found in the lung of a child that died in Taiwan. The pathology in the central nervous system is attributed to dead worms. The use of anthelminthic is not recommended. Most human infections are reported from Taiwan and Thailand where indigenous populations eat snails uncooked. The diagnosis is bases upon symptoms, history of eating or an association with snails, and immunodiagnostic tests.

The slug, *Vaginulus plebius*, is the major source of infection of *A. costaricensis* in cotton rats (*Sigmodon hispidus*) and humans. Larvae released after digestion of the slugs migrate to the lymphatics and then to ileocaecal arteries where they mature and reproduce. Eggs are deposited in the intestinal tissue and larvae that develop migrate to the lumen and pass in the faeces of the rat. A similar development occurs in humans but the larvae usually do not reach the intestinal lumen and faeces. Although human infections are reported throughout the Americas and one case in Africa, most infections have been reported in children in Costa Rica. Clinical symptoms are usually that of an acute abdomin along with fever, anorexia, vomiting, diarrhoea, and abdominal rigidity. The diagnosis is difficult and is usually made at surgery. Anthelminthic treatment is not recommended.

Infections of angiostrongylosis could be prevented by eating only cooked terrestrial mollucs. Many populations enjoy eating snails but very few intentionally eat slugs. The parasitoses could be controlled by educational campaigns and snail and rodent control. The accidental ingestion of slugs on salad greens could be prevented by washing the vegetables thoroughly.

INTRODUCTION

There are approximately 21 species of *Angiostrongylus*, found primarily in the vascular system of carnivores, insectivores, rodents, and marsupials. A few species are found in the lungs or stomach. As far as it is known all have a molluscan intermediate host, especially gastropods, and some species also utilize paratenic hosts. Two species, *A. cantonensis* and *A. costaricensis* are known to cause disease in humans and two others, *A. mackerrasse* and *A. malaysiensis*, have the potential of causing human disease. This chapter will consider only the known human pathogens, *A. cantonensis* and *A. costaricensis*.

ANGIOSTRONGYLUS CANTONENSIS

HISTORY

The rat lung worm, *A. cantonensis* was first reported by Chen (1935) who found the nematode in the pulmonary arteries of *Rattus norvegicus* and *R. rattus* in Canton, China. He described the worm and named it *Pulmonema cantonensis*. In 1937 Matsumoto found the parasite in Taiwan (Formosa) rats and in the same year Yokogowa (1937) described it as *Hemostrongylus ratti*. Dougherty (1946) later synonymized the parasite and called it *Angiostrongylus cantonensis*. Some authors refer to it as *Parastrongylus cantonensis* but since *A. cantonensis* is well established in the literature it will be used here.

Ten years after being described as a parasite of rats, 10 *A. cantonensis* larvae were recovered from the spinal fluid of a 12-year-old boy from central Taiwan with meningitis. The report was published in a Japanese journal with limited distribution (Nomura and Lin 1945) but the parasite was not internationally recognized until Rosen and associates reported finding larvae in the brain of a Filipino who died in Hawaii (1962). Prior to this, outbreaks of an unusual type of meningitis of unknown aetiology were observed on Pacific Islands. The disease was characterized by a pleocytosis with large numbers of eosinophilic leucocytes and the disorders termed eosinophilic meningitis. Since these early reports, eosinophilic meningitis due to *A. cantonensis* has been documented from widespread areas of the world, however, the majority of cases continue to be reported from Asia, particularly from Taiwan and Thailand.

THE AGENT

Angiostrongylus cantonensis is in the superfamily Metastrongyloidea, family Angiostrongylidae. The family is characterized by the presence of three pairs of lobes in the bursa; dorsal ray long and digitiform; ventral, lateral, and externodorsal rays stout; spicules long and slender. Tails of female pointed; anus and vulva separated, not terminal; ovoviviparous.

Angiostrongylus cantonensis body is filariform tapered at both ends. Epidermis smooth with transverse striae. The mouth has three lips and is surrounded by papillae. Males are 16–19 mm in length and approximately 0.25 mm wide; females 21–25 mm and 0.30–0.36 mm wide. Male caudal bursa is well developed and kidney-shaped. The bursal rays are arranged as follows: ventral ray branched at a point two-thirds of its length into a small ventro-ventral and a large lateroventral ray. Lateral rays arise from a common trunk, the anterolateral is thicker than the others and projected like a thumb. The mediolateral ray and posterolateral ray usually originate as a common trunk. The posterolateral ray is usually shorter than the mediolateral ray and at times reduced to a stump. The externodorsal ray is simple and arises from between the lateral and dorsal rays. The dorsal ray is variable, emerging as a short trunk, terminating in several small digitations. Spicules are equal, slender with conspicuous striations and range from 1.00 to 1.46 mm in length. A gubernaculum is present (Bhaibulaya 1979).

Living females have white uterine tubules that wind around a blood-filled intestine, giving a characteristic 'barber's pole' appearance. The vagina (1.50–3.25 mm in length) at the junction of the uterine tubules extends posteriorly to open into the vulva. The vulva opening is anterior to the subterminal anus. There is no minute projection at the tip of the tail which is found in other *Angiostrongylus* species. Eggs are ovoid and measure 21–25 μm and are unembryonated when laid in the pulmonary arteries. The eggs pass to the capillaries of the lung and embryonate in 5–6 days. The first-stage larvae hatch from the eggs break through the capillaries into the alveoli, and migrate into the bronchioles, up the trachea, are swallowed and pass in the rat faeces.

A variety of snails and slugs serve as intermediate hosts. The first-stage larvae enter the molluscan host either by ingestion or direct penetration, migrate to the foot muscle and viscera and moult twice into second- and third-stage larvae in 7–9 and 12–16 days, respectively. The third-stage larvae retain the sheaths of the first and second stages and are infective for the definitive host (Bhaibulaya 1979) The larvae remain coiled in the molluscan tissue until freed after the mollusc is eaten and the tissue digested in the rats intestinal tract.

The freed larvae penetrate the rat stomach, enter the hepatic portal system and are carried to the liver, heart, and lungs. They pass through the alveoli, into the veins, back to the heart, and enter the arterial circulation to be distributed around the body. The larvae reach the central nervous system (CNS) in 1 or 2 days. The larvae move into the neural parenchyma and in 4–6 days moult into the fourth larval stage. The final moult occurs in 7–9 days and the young worms move into the subarachnoid space where they remain for 10–14 days before they invade the cerebral vein and migrate to the pulmonary arteries. The worms become sexually mature and reproduce; the prepatent period is 42–45 days postinfection.

THE HOST

ANIMAL

Rattus and *Bandicota* species are natural hosts for *A. cantonensis*. In other vertebrate species experimentally exposed to infection the parasite was unable to complete development (Anderson 1992). Only on rare occasions have adult worms been found in the lung of humans.

Rats usually manifest little disease when experimentally infected with small numbers of infective-stage larvae. However, when large numbers of the parasite are introduced, the animals develop symptoms and die. Upon entering the gastric wall the submucosa becomes oedematous with an eosinophilic infiltration. In the liver small necrotic foci develop and become infiltrated with eosinophils. In the lungs the larvae produce small foci of intra-alveolar haemorrhages and those that enter the pleural cavity provoke a seropurulent pleurisy. In early infections in the CNS small foci of oedema and haemorrhage develop, and as the parasites grow granulomatous reactions develop in all parts of the brain. Granulomas with giant cells and monocytes develop around moulted sheaths. Abscesses may develop with heavy infections. The subarachnoid space becomes dilated, accompanied by infiltration, and as the infection progresses there is massive haemorrhage from ruptured dilated cerebral veins in the subarachnoid space. Haemorrhage may also occur in the nerve roots of cranial and spinal nerves. When given thousands of worms rats develop coma, cerebral rigidity paralysis, and die. With 1000–1500 worms, rats show considerable weakness of the extremities and disordered gait. Subsequently the animals exhibit bloody nasal discharge, bloody tears, and ataxia.

As the worms accumulate in the lung arteries a rapid hypertrophy of the right heart ventricle takes place. The adventitia of the arteries and the bronchi become infiltrated by eosinophils and mononuclear cells. The intima of the arteries become hypertrophic and the arteries sometimes become partially thrombosed; the thrombi may encase adult parasites, eggs, and larvae. Nodules containing eggs may develop in the lung parenchyma and completely replace it (Fig. 58.1). In prolonged infections the lung parenchyma becomes increasingly firm. Pleural adhesions and lung abscesses may also develop. Symptoms of coughing, sneezing, and raspy breathing develop after the parasites become established in the lungs; episodes of dyspnoea and cyanosis sometimes develop (Alicata and Jindrak 1970).

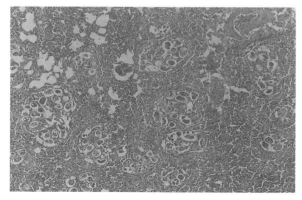

Fig. 58.1 Eggs of *Angiostrongylus cantonensis* scattered throughout the lung parenchyma of a rat (× 63).

HUMAN

When humans ingest an infected molluscan host, usually terrestrial snails, it is a dead end for the parasite. The third-stage larvae digested from snail tissue follow the same migratory pathways as in rats. A gastroenteritis and hepatomegaly is experienced after eating the snails. As the larvae traverse the lungs there maybe cough, rhinorrhoea, nasal obstruction, sneezing, sore throat, headache, malaise, and mild fever. Once in the CNS severe headache develops, along with nausea and vomiting, fever, and stiff neck. These symptoms are often abrupt and persistant (Yii 1976). Destruction and inflammation of the nerve fibres are responsible for further symptoms of myalgia, pain, and paraesthesia of the skin. Dead worms are associated with granuloma formation in the CNS. If the parasites live, they leave the brain parenchyma, reach the surface or subarachnoid space and develop into young adults. Worms on the brain surface illicit an eosinophilic inflammation of the meninges. Coma is associated with infections involving a large number of worms. In one death on Taiwan over 500 worms were recovered from the brain and spinal cord at autopsy. Adult worms were also found in the lung of this patient (Yii *et al.* 1968). Moving worms in the eye have also been reported in people on Taiwan and Thailand.

Punyagupta *et al.* (1975) and Yii (1976) reported on angiostrongylosis in 484 and 114 people, respectively, from Thailand and Taiwan. The most often reported symptoms were headache, neck stiffness, nausea, vomiting, anorexia, fever, cough, constipation, malaise, lethargy, blurred vision, paraesthesia, abdominal pain, weakness of extremities, and muscle twitching. These were signs of abnormal muscle reflexes, abnormal achilles reflex, positive Kernig sign, vision impairment, eye muscle paralysis, and impairment of sensorium. Death is rare, but will occur with the ingestion of extremely large numbers of worms.

At autopsy there is evidence of congestion in the brain and spinal cord and the leptomeninges show thickening at the basal portion of the brain. Subarachnoid haemorrhage may occur throughout the cord and brain (Kliks *et al.* 1982). Living worms do not provoke tissue reactions (Fig. 58.2), while dead worms elicit an eosinophilic inflammatory reaction, giant cell formation, necrosis, and granulomas (Fig. 58.3).

Worms are not always found in the tissues, but evidence of infection is demonstrated by glial scars containing haemosiderin, microscopic haemorrhages, eosinophils, and Charcot–Leyden crystals. Vascular dilatation, both arterial and venous, in the subarachnoid space may also be seen.

At autopsy of the patient on Taiwan, the leptomeninges were infiltrated with lymphocytes, pigment–

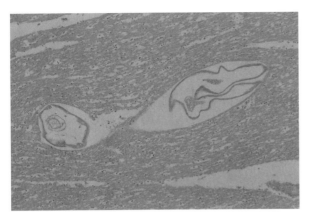

Fig. 58.2 Sections of *Angiostrongylus cantonensis* in the human brain without a cellular reaction (× 100). From a 5-year-old Taiwanese child who died of a massive infection.

laden macrophages and mononuclear cells and giant cells were found adjacent to degenerated worms (Fig. 5 8 .4). Cross-sections of viable parasites were found in the cerebral and cerebellar sulci. Parasites were also seen in the central canal of the spinal cord along with giant cells (Fig. 58.5). When the lungs were examined histologically there was congestion and pigment-laden macrophages, and sections of living worms were found in the pulmonary vessels (Fig. 58.6).

The diagnosis of angiostrongylosis cantonensis is based upon symptoms of headache, stiff neck, paraesthesia, paralysis of eye muscle, eosinophilic pleocytoses, and a history of eating snails uncooked or an association with terrestrial snails or paratenic hosts. Worms may be present in spinal fluid, especially in young children (Hwang and Chen 1991). Examination of cerebrol spinal fluid (CSF) may show increased pressure, an opalescent or turbid apearance, xantho-

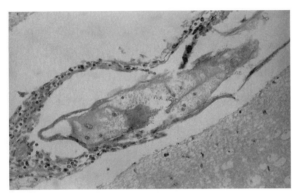

Fig. 58.3 Section of *Angiostrongylus cantonensis* in the brain of the Taiwanese child who died of angiostrongylosis, showing a cellular infiltration (× 100).

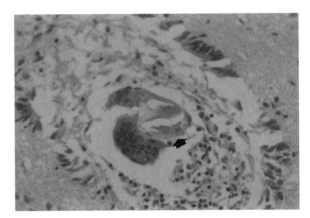

Fig. 58.5 *Angiostrongylus cantonensis* (arrow) in spinal cord canal, showing giant cell formation and other inflammatory cells (× 400).

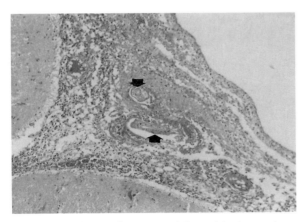

Fig. 58.4 *Angiostrongylus cantonensis* (arrow) in the meninges of the Taiwanese child that died of the infection, showing an intense inflammatory reaction (× 100).

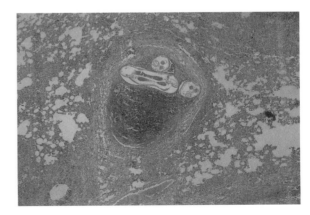

Fig. 58.6 *Angiostrongylus cantonensis* in the lung of the child that died in Taiwan (× 25).

chromia, and at times erythrocytes. Eosinophils as well as lymphocytes maybe present in the CSF and there may be an increase in protein content and at times low sugar. Peripheral blood usually shows a leucocytosis with eosinophilia of over 10 per cent (Punyagupta *et al.* 1975).

Immunological tests on sera and CSF may aid in a presumptive diagnosis (Cross and Chi 1982; Yen *et al.* 1991). Computed tomography (CT) and magnetic resonance imaging (MRI) may also aid in a presumptive diagnosis.

In a differential diagnosis, other helminthic infection such as paragonimosis, cysticercosis, echinococcosis, schistosomosis, and gnathostomosis must be considered.

Treatment of angiostrongylosis cantonensis is symptomatic. Anthelminthics are not recommended by most physicians, as dead worms are considered to be more pathogenic than living worms. However, mebendazole and albendazole have been used successfully to treat children on Taiwan (Hwang and Chen 1991).

EPIDEMIOLOGY

Angiostrongylus cantonensis, once considered a tropical Asian parasite, is now known to have a widespread distribution and, without question, it is spreading either by snails or stowaway rats. It is reported in rats from nearly all Asian countries except Korea, many of the Pacific Islands, Australia, India, and a few African countries. Several Caribbean islands are now known to be endemic and recently the parasite has been reported from New Orleans, Louisiana, in the continental United States. Human cases of angiostrongylosis are reported from most of these areas and was recently reported from New Orleans (New *et al.* 1995).

The natural definitive host includes many species of *Rattus*, including *R. rattus*, *R. novegicus*, *R. coxinga*, *R. diardi*, *R. exulans*, *R. argentiventer*, *R. losea*, *R. jalorensis*, *R. tiomanicus*, and *R. rattus midanensis* and *Bandicota indica* (Cross 1979). The parasite may develop partially in other rodents and other mammals but it fails to complete development. Some of these vertebrates, as well as invertebrates, may serve as paratenic hosts. Frogs and toads have been shown to harbour infective-stage *A. cantonensis* along with freshwater prawn, land and coconut crabs, and planarians. Not all of these, however, are associated with human infections. Infection rates are greatest in the intermediate and definitive hosts, as well as in humans during rainy seasons.

A large number of molluscs serve as intermediate hosts, mostly snails and slugs. The major sources of human infection in Asian countries are the snails *Achatina fulica*, *Pila scutata*, *P. ampullacea*, *Bradybaena similasis*, *Macrochlamys resplendens*, *Subulina octona*, and *Cipangopaludina chinensis*, and slugs *Vaginulus plebeus*, *Veronicella siamensis*, *Laevicaulis alte*, and *Microparmarion malayanus*.

Infections in humans are acquired by eating, intentionally or accidentally, an intermediate host uncooked. Snails eaten raw intentionally are usually chopped into small pieces and mixed with vegetables and seasoning. It is a custom among some groups to eat raw snails while drinking alcohol. Infection may also be acquired by drinking untreated water in which snails have died and released the infective larvae. Slugs can be accidentally ingested on leafy vegetables and there is evidence that larvae maybe shed from slugs into mucous trails while crawling on vegetation. Infected planarians may also be eaten accidentally with vegetables. Infected coconut crabs are eaten uncooked by Pacific islanders and some ethnic groups eat infected prawns or use juice extracted from the prawns for seasoning or medicinal purposes. The only case of angiostrongylosis reported from the continental United States was in a 11-year-old boy who ate a raw snail as a challenge (New *et al.* 1995) Similar transmission of the parasite to a group of US Marines occurred on Okinawa when they ate raw snails during a survival training exercise (Cross 1987).

PREVENTION AND CONTROL

Angiostrongylosis cantonensis is a food-borne parasitic zoonosis that would be difficult to control in nature. The elimination of rats and snails may be possible in some areas, but in most endemic areas a change in human eating habits would be a more realistic approach. However, changing eating habits that have existed in a population for generations would also be difficult. Cooking the molluscan host would eliminate human infection with the parasite. Freezing snails or snail meat at −15 °C for 12–24 hours would also kill the larvae. The thorough washing of vegetables that are eaten raw would eliminate slugs, tiny snails, and mucus containing larvae. Children should be educated not to handle snails, since hands could become contaminated with larvae. Paratenic host such as prawn, shrimp, and crabs should be cooked before eating. The juices from these animals should also be cooked before use

ANGIOSTRONGYLUS COSTARICENSIS

HISTORY

In the early 1950s surgical specimens in Costa Rica were found containing sections of nematodes. In later specimens from Costa Ricans the lesions were described and eggs, larvae, and adult worms were observed within the tissue and a few adult worms were recovered (Cespedes *et al.* 1967; Morera 1967) The aetiological agent responsible for the granulomatous lesion was described as a new species, *Angiostrongylus costaricensis*, in 1971 by Morera and Cespedes. Chabaud (1972) proposed a new genus for the parasite, *Morerastrongylus*; however, Anderson (1978) reduced this genus to synonymy with *Angiostrongylus*. The natural host of the parasite was unknown until 1971 when Morera reported finding the parasite in arteries and arterioles of cotton rats (*Sigmodon hispidus*) hispidus) and black rats (*Rattus rattus*). The intermediate host was identified in 1991 by Morera and Ash who found infective-stage larvae in tissue of the slug *Vaginulus plebeius*. Animal infections with the parasite have been reported throughout the Americas and human infections from Argentina to the United States; human infection has also been reported from Africa.

THE AGENT

The nematode resides in mesenteric arteries of the definitive host. It is filiform in shape and tapered at both ends. Males are approximately 17–22 mm in length; width at the base of the oesophagus 0.112–0.12 mm and a maximum width of 0.28–0.3 mm; oesophagus 0.182–0.225 mm in length. Spicules are slender, striated, equal, with rounded cephalic ends and the caudal tip is sharp. They measure 0.318–0.330 mm. A gubernaculum is present. The copulatory bursa is symmetrical; the ventral rays are fused except at the tips; the ventrolateral are longer than the ventroventral, lateral rays emerge from a common trunk separated from the ventrals; the medio lateral and the posterolaterals are fused in their proximal half. The anterolateral is thicker and separates from the common trunk after emergence from it. The externodorsal ray arises close to the lateral trunk and is separated from the dorsal ray with a knob-like distal end. The dorsal ray is short and bifuricates into arms, terminating in sharp tips, there are papillae on the ventral side behind the bifusication.

The female body length is 28–42 mm; width at base of oesophagus 0.135–0.15 mm; maximum width 0.322–0.35 mm; oesophagus 0.23–0.26 mm; caudal end conical with a minute projection at the tip. The anus is located 0.06 to 0.65 and the vulva 0.24 to 0.29 mm from the tip of the tail. In living specimens the uterine tubes wind around the blood-filled intestines and terminate into a short vagina close to the vulva (Morera 1973).

Females deposit ovoid, transparent, thin-shelled, unembryonated eggs into the mesenteric arterioles of

the rat hosts. These are then carried to the intestinal wall where they embryonate and develop into firststage larvae. The larvae migrate into the intestinal lumen and pass in the rat faeces. Larvae may also develop in the regional lymph nodes (Morera 1973). Veronicellid slugs eat the faeces, the larvae migrate to the fibromuscular tissues of the slug and after 16–19 days develop into third-stage infective larvae. The larvae remain in the tissue of the slug for months or emerge from the slug tissue and are released into mucous secretions which maybe deposited along mucous trails on to vegetation.

When ingested by rats either in slugs (or in mucous trails) the third-stage larvae are digested from the tissue and migrate through the intestinal tissue and travel to the lymphatics. The larvae moult into the fourth and fifth stages, and by the tenth day migrate to the ileocaecal vessels and subsequently to the arterioles and arteries where sexual reproduction begins by 18 days. Eggs, ovoidal in shape and measuring 90 μm embryonate, and first-stage larvae are found in the faeces in 22–24 days.

THE HOST

ANIMAL

A number of mammals have been found with natural infections of *A. costaricensis*, especially rodents, including the cotton rat, *Sigmodon hispidus*, *Rattus rattus*, *Zigodontomy microtinus*, and *Liomys adspersies* (Morera 1973). The coati-mundi *Nasua narica bullata* (Monge *et al.* 1978) is also reported as a definitive host, as well as the marmoset, *Saguinus mystax.* (Sly *et al.* 1987), and dogs, *Canis familiaris* (Arroyo *et al.* 1988).

In early infections larvae maybe found in lymphatic sinuses with an eosinophilic infiltration near the parasite. Multiple small haemorrhages may occur in the vessels with massive infections of adult worms in the mesenteric artery and there maybe obstruction and necrosis in the mesentery and intestinal wall. The accumulation of eggs in the capillaries of the intestinal wall, especially in the caecum, gives a yellowish appearance to the serosa. In heavy infections the rat may die with necrosis in the ileocaecal region. There is histological evidence that the capillaries of the wall are obstructed with eggs, indicating that the necrosis has a vascular origin and not inflammatory. In light infections rats pass larvae for months (Morera 1973)

HUMANS

Angiostrangylus costaricensis develops into adults in arteries in the ileocaecal region of humans as it does in the natural rodent host. Reproduction occurs and females

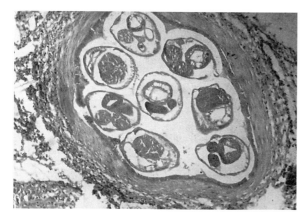

Fig. 58.7 *Angiostrongylus costaricensis* in an intestinal artery of a human from Costa Rica (× 25; courtesy of Dr Lawrence Ash).

deposit eggs into the intestinal wall via the mesenteric arterioles. Embryos develop and hatch from the eggs and some larvae may, on rare occasions, reach the lumen of the intestine. The eggs and larvae, along with secretions and excretions, cause a granulomatous inflmmatory reaction with oedema, thickening of the intestinal wall, and narrowing of the lumen. Adult worms in the arteries (Fig. 58.7) damage the endothelium, provoking thrombosis and necrosis. The blood vessels may become partially occluded and eosinophilic infiltration occurs in vessels harbouring the worms. Eggs and larvae may locate in the vessels and are often visualized within granuloma. The development of large areas of necrosis may lead to perforation of the bowel and peritonitis. The regional mesenteric lymph nodes may become hyperplastic and infiltrated with eosinophils. The granulomas containing eggs and larvae consist of histiocytes, a few mononuclear cells, and large numbers of eosinophils. Gross examination of surgical specimens reveals a rigid and thickened intestinal wall with yellowish foci on the serosal surface of the intestine and the mesentery (Morera 1995). Liver lesions, caused by migrating juvenile and adult worms and eggs carried into the liver, are reported. Testicular invasion by adult worms, causing necrosis, is also reported (Morera 1995).

Most infections have been reported in children, especially in Costa Rica; adult infections have also been documented. Since the parasite usually locates in the ileocaecal region, most patients complain of pain in the right iliac fossa. The clinical symptoms are those of an acute abdomen (Loria-Cortes and Lobo-Sanahuja 1980) Patients also report fever, anorexia, vomiting, diarrhoea, constipation, and abdominal rigidity. Pain is often experienced upon abdominal palpation, and tumour-like masses may be found in the lower right quadrant. Rectal examination may be painful in half of the patients (Morera 1995). Leucocytosis between 1000 and 40 000 mm³ and eosinophilia of 20–50 per cent are reported. Higher levels have also been reported (Morera 1987). The clinical findings are suggestive of appendicitis.

The diagnosis of angiostrongylosis costaricensis is difficult. Larvae are not found in the faeces. Radiological findings may show changes in the terminal ileum, caecum, appendix, and ascending colon. In radiographs the contrast medium shows incomplete filling and irritability of the involved area. The thickening of the intestinal wall causes a reduction in the lumen (Morera 1995). The liver is usually involved and laparoscopy reveals yellow spots on the liver surface; most patients have liver involvement (Morera 1995).

The parasitological diagnosis is generally made following histological examination of surgical specimens. Eggs, larvae, worms, and marked eosinophilia are usually found in the tissue.

Serological tests such as immunoelectrophoresis and Ouchterlony immunodiffusion are available (Sauerbrey 1977), as well as a latex bead agglutination test (Morera 1995).

The disease is often self-limiting and specific treatment is not required. Anthelminthics such as diethylcarbamazine, thiabendazole and albendazole (Morera 1995), and mebendazole (Hulbert *et al.* 1992) have been used but the results were not reliable. Chemotherapy is not recommended, however, since the worms are known to become excited when drugs are used in rodent infections (Morera 1987, 1995). Surgery is the treatment of choice in most cases.

EPIDEMIOLOGY AND EPIZOOLOGY

Angiostrongylus costaricensis is documented in rats throughout the Americas from Argentina to the United States. Human case reports are also from these areas, with most cases reported from Costa Rica. It was estimated that in 1993 there were 2116 human infections per 100 000 persons per year in Costa Rica (Morera 1995). Three children in the United States have also been infected (Silvera *et al.* 1989; Hulburt *et al.* 1992). The parasitosis is also reported in Africa (Baird *et al.* 1987).

Eleven species of rodents are reported as natural definitive hosts but the cotton rat, *S. hispidus*, is the most important. The reported infection rate in this rat was 43.2 per cent in Costa Rica (Morera 1995), and 35 per cent in Panama (Tesh *et al.* 1973). Naturally infected cotton rats have also be found in the United States (Uberlaker and Hall 1979). Two species of veronicellid slugs, *V. plebius* and *V. occidentalis*, are known intermediate hosts in Costa Rica; however, aquatic snails have also been infected (Uberlaker *et al.* 1980) and other molluscs are considered potential hosts. Fifty per cent of 6025 slugs from 20 locations in Costa Rica were found to be naturally infected; one harboured 16 000 infective larvae (Morera 1985).

Populations living in endemic areas usually do not include slugs in their diets. Tiny slugs could be innocently eaten on vegetables. Infective larvae secreted in mucous trails may also be ingested with unwashed salad greens. However, there are reports of infants eating slugs. The habit of putting things in their mouths may be responsible for the high number of cases of intestinal angiostrongylosis occurring in children (Morera 1995).

PREVENTION AND CONTROL

Human infection with *A. costaricensis* could be prevented by making populations in the endemic areas aware of the parasitosis. Education of parents to train children to avoid placing things in their mouths would be beneficial, but may be difficult to accomplish. Thorough washing of salad greens and cooking of vegetables should also be recommended. Rodent control measures and even control of slugs would also help to prevent infections.

REFERENCES

Alicata, J. E. and Jindrak, K. (1970). *Angiostrongylosis in the Pacific and Southeast Asia.* C. Thomas Publications, New York.

Anderson, R. C. (1978). No. 5. Keys to genera of the Superfamily Metastrongyloidea. In *CIH key to the nematode parasites of vertebrates*, (ed. R. C., Anderson, A. G. Chabaud, and S. Willmott), CAB International, United Kingdom.

Anderson, R. C. (1992). *Nematode parasites of vertebrates. Their development and transmission* pp. 175–82. CAB International, Wallingford, Oxon.

Arroyo, R., Rodriguez, F., and Berrocal, A. (1988). Angiostrongilosis abdominal en *Canis familiaris. Parasitologia al Dia*, **12**, 181–5.

Baird, J. K., Neafie, R. C., Lanoie, L., and Connor, D. H. (1987). Abdominal angiostrongyliosis in an African man: case study. *American Journal of Tropical Medicine and Hygiene*, **37**, 353–6.

Bhaibulaya, M. (1979). Morphology and taxonomy of major *Angiostrongylus* species of Eastern Asia and Australia. In *Studies in angiostrongyliasis in Eastern Asia and Australia*, (ed. J. H. Cross), Naval Medical Research Unit Special Publication—44, pp. 4–13. Taipei, Taiwan.

Cespedes, R., Salas, J., Mekbel, S., Troper, L., Mullner, F., and Morera, P. (1967). Granulomas entericos y linfatico con intensa eosinofilia tisular por un estrongilideo (Strongylata). *ACTA Medica Costarricense*, **10**, 235–55.

Chabaud, A. (1972). *Stefankostrongylus dubosti* n.sp. parasite du potamogales et essai de classification des Nematodes Angiostrongylinae. *Annales de Parasitologie Humaine et Comparee*, **47**, 735–44.

Chen, H. T. (1935). Un nouveau nematode pulmonaire, *Pulmonema cantonensis* n.g., n. sp. des rats de Canton. *Annals of Parasitology*, **13**, 312–17.

Cross, J. H. (ed.) (1979). *Studies on Angiostrongyliasis in Eastern Asia and Australia*, Naval Medical Research Unit No. 2 Special Publication—44. Taipei, Taiwan.

Cross, J. H. (1987). Public health importance of *Angiostrongylus cantonensis* and its relatives. *Parasitology Today*, **3**, 367–9.

Cross, J. H. and Chi, J. H. C. (1982). ELISA for the detection of *Angiostrongylus cantonensis* antibodies in patients with eosinophilic meningitis. *Southeast Asian Journal of Tropical Medicine and Public Health*, **13**, 73–7.

Dougherty, E. C. (1946). The genus *Aelurostrongylus* Cameron, 1927. (Nematoda: Metastrongylidae) and its relatives with description of *Parafiloroides* gen. nov and *Angiostrongylus gubernaculatus* sp. nov. *Proceeding of the Helminthological Society of Washington*, **13**, 16–26.

Hulbert, T. V., Larsen, R. A., and Chandrasoma, P. T. (1992). Abdominal angiostrongyliasis mimicking acute appendicitis and Meckel's diverticulum: Report of a case in the United States and review. *Clinical Infectious Diseases*, **14**, 836–40.

Hwang, K. P. and Chen, E. R. (1991). Clinical studies on angiostrongyliasis cantonensis among children in Taiwan. In *Proceedings of the 33rd SEAMEO-TROPMED Seminar on Emerging Problems in Food-borne Parasitic Zoonoses, November 1990, Chiang Mai, Thailand*, pp. 194–9.

Kliks, M. M., Kroenke, I., and Hardman, J. M. (1982). Eosinophilic radiculomyeloencephalitis: An angiostrongyliasis outbreak in American Samoa related to ingestion of *Achatina fulica* snails. *American Journal of Tropical Medicine and Hygiene*, **31**, 1114–22.

Loria-Cortes, R. and Lobo-Sanahuja, J. F. (1980). Clinical abdominal angiostrongylosis. A study of 116 children with intestinal eosinophilic granuloma caused by *Angiostrongylus costaricensis. American Journal of Tropical Medicine and Hygiene*, **19**, 538–44.

Matsumoto, T. (1937). On a nematode found in the lungs, especially in the pulmonary artery of the wild rat. *Journal of the Formosan Medical Association*, **36**, 2620–3.

Monge, E., Arroyo, R., and Salanp, E. (1978). A new definitive host of *Angiostrongylus costaricensis* Morera and Cespedes, 1971. *Journal of Parasitology*, **64**, 34.

Morera, P. (1967). Granulomas entericos y infaticos con intensa eosinofilia tisular producidos por un strongilideo (*Strongylata* Railliet y Henry, 1903). II. Aspecto parasitologico (NotaPrevia). *Acta Medica Costarricense*, **10**, 257–63.

Morera, P. (1973). Life history and redescription of *Angiostrongylus costaricensis* Morera and Cespedes, 1971. *American Journal of Tropical Medicine and Hygiene*, **22**, 613–21.

Morera, P. (1985). Abdominal angiostrongyliasis: A problem of public health. *Parasitology Today*, **6**, 173–75.

Morera, P. (1987). Abdominal angiostrongylosis: In *Clinical tropical medicine and communicable diseases: intestinal helminthic infections*, (ed. Z. S. Pawlowski), pp. 747–53. Bailliere, London.

Morera, P. (1995). Abdominal angiostrongylosis. In *Enteric infection 2: Intestinal helminths*, (ed. M. J. G. Farthing, G. T. Keusch, and D. Wakelin), pp. 225–30, Chapman & Hall, London.

Morera, P. and Ash, L. R. (1970). Investigacion del huesped intermediario de *Angiostrongylus costaricensis* (Morera y Cespedes, 1971). *Boletin Chileno de Parasitologia*, **25**, 135.

Morera, P. and Cespedes, R. (1971). *Angiostrongylus costaricensis* n.sp. (Nematoda: Metastrongylidae) a new lungworm occurring in man in Costa Rica. *Revista de Biologia Tropical (Costa Rica)*, **18**, 173–85.

New, D., Little, M. D., and Cross, J. H. (1995). *Angiostrongylus cantonensis* infection from eating raw snails. *New England Journal of Medicine*, **332**, 1105–6.

Noumura, S. and Lin, P. H. (1945). First case report of human infection with *Haemostrongylus ratti* Yokogawa in man. *Taiwan NO IKAI*, **3**, 589–92.

Punyagupta, S., Bunnag, T., Juttijudata, P., and Rosen, L. (1975). Eosinophilic meningitis in Thailand. Clinical studies on 484 typical cases probably caused by *Angiostrongylus cantonensis*. *American Society of Tropical Medicine and Hygiene*, **24**, 921–31.

Sauerbrey, M. (1977). A precipitin test for the diagnosis of human abdominal angiostrongyliasis. *American Journal of Tropical Medicine and Hygiene*, **26**, 1156–8.

Silvera, C. T., Ghali, V. S., Roven, S., Heimann, J., and Gelb, A. (1989). Angiostrongyliasis: A rare cause of gastrointestinal hemorrhage. *American Journal of Gastroenterology*, **84**, 329–32.

Sly, D. L., Toft, J. D., Gardiner, G. H., and London, W. T. (1982). Spontaneous occurrence of *Angiostrongylus costari-censis* in marmosets (*Saguinus mystax*). *Laboratory Animal Science*, **32**, 286–8.

Tesh, R., Ackerman, L., Dietz, W., and Williams, J. (1973). *Angiostrongylus costaricensis* in Panama. Prevalence and pathological findings in wild rodents infected with the parasite. *American Journal of Tropical Medicine and Hygiene*, **22**, 348–56.

Uberlaker, J. E. and Hall, N. M. (1979). First report of *Angiostrongylus costaricensis* Morera and Cespedes 1971 in the United States. *Journal of Parasitology*, **65**, 307.

Uberlaker, J. E., Bullick, G. R., and Caruso, J. (1980). Emergence of third-stage larvae of *Angiostrongylus costaricensis* Morera and Cespedes 1971 from *Biomphalaria glabrata* (Say). *Journal of Parasitology*, **66**, 856–7.

Yen, C. M. and Chen, E. R. (1991). Detection of antibodies to *Angiostrongylus cantonensis* in serum and cerebrospinal fluid of patients with eosinophilic meningitis. *International Journal of Parasitology*, **21**, 17–21.

Yii, C. Y. (1976). Clinical observations on eosinophilic meningitis and meningoencephalitis caused by *Angiostrongylus cantonensis* in Taiwan. *American Journal of Tropical Medicine and Hygiene*, **25**, 233–49.

Yii, C. Y., Chen, C. Y., Fresh, J. W., Chen, T., and Cross, J. H. (1968). Human angiostrongyliasis involving the lungs. *Chinese Journal of Microbiology*, **1**, 148–50.

Yokogawa, S. (1937). A new species of nematode found in the lungs of rats, *Haemostrongylus ratti* sp. nov. *Transactions of the Natural History Society of Formosa*, **27**, 247–50.

59 ZOONOTIC INFECTIONS WITH FILARIAL NEMATODES

D. A. Denham

SUMMARY

Lymphatic filariosis occurs widely in the wet tropics and subtropics, affecting some 200 000 000 people. In its chronic form the disease causes elephantiasis of the limbs and scrotum and hydrocoel. The disease is caused by two filarial nematodes, *Wuchereria bancrofti* and *Brugia malayi*. The large majority of cases are due to *W. bancrofti* which is strictly limited to humans and has no zoonotic reservoir. *Brugia malayi* exists in two forms, one of which is a zoonosis in Malaysia and Indonesia. Transmission of the zoonotic form is usually through mosquitoes of the genus *Mansonia*. Control is extremely difficult because the main zoonotic reservoir is the leaf-eating monkey, *Presbytis* spp. This animal is usually a protected species and lives in very close association with man.

Dirofilaria species are common parasites of a variety of mammals in the hot, wet areas of the world. Humans are not hosts to the full development of any *Dirofilaria* species but become zoonotically infected with two types of lesion.

Dirofilaria immitis is a very common parasite of dogs throughout the hot, wet areas. In dogs, its adult worms live in the right side of the heart and pulmonary arteries and produce a great deal of debilitating disease and frequent early death. In people the infection presents as a coin lesion in the lungs, usually detected in routine radiographic examination and frequently mistaken as a tumour. This has led to numerous, unnecessary, open chest surgical removals of the lump in the belief that it was a tumour.

Other *Dirofilaria* species infect dogs and other carnivora with subcutaneously dwelling adult worms. Zoonotic infection with these species produces subcutaneous lumps in humans. These parasites are transmitted by various mosquitoes. No control methods for human infection are practised. Dogs can be protected against *D. immitis* disease by the use of monthly prophylactic ivermectin treatment.

HISTORY

The older work on *Brugia malayi* is documented by Denham and McGreevy (1977). Brugian filariosis was first described by Dutch workers who noticed that in different areas of Indonesia people developed different forms of elephantiasis and other clinical signs of filarial disease.

The microfilariae were first shown to be different from those of *W. bancrofti* by Brug in Indonesia. The adult worm of the zoonotic form was isolated in mainland Malaysia. Domestic cats were infected with the human parasite by Edeson and Wharton. Since then this isolate has been maintained in several laboratories in dogs, cats, jirds, and multimammate rats.

THE AGENT

BRUGIA MALAYI

Brugia malayi occurs in at least two forms. Probably the most common form is that seen in India and China. This form shows strong nocturnal periodicity and is strictly limited to humans, having no zoonotic reservoir. The other form, which is common in South-East Asia, shows nocturnal subperiodicity (Fig. 59.1) and is strongly zoonotic.

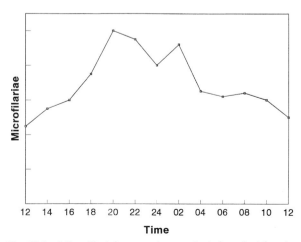

Fig. 59.1 Microfilarial counts in people infected with subperiodic *Brugia malayi*.

Zoonotic brugian filariosis is transmitted by *Mansonia* species mosquitoes; the periodic form is transmitted by *Mansonia* species in India and by *Anopheles* species in most other areas. The female mosquitoes ingest microfilariae (mf) while feeding. After being ingested they penetrate the midgut and migrate to, and penetrate, the flight muscles where they develop into infective larvae (L3). The L3 migrate to the mouthparts of the mosquito, emerge from her proboscis while she is feeding, and penetrate the puncture wound left by the mosquito. The L3 rapidly penetrate the lymphatics where they grow and mature into adult male and female worms. After about 2 months the female produces mf that migrate to the bloodstream. Mf cannot develop further unless they are ingested by a susceptible mosquito.

OTHER *BRUGIA* SPECIES FOUND IN MAN

There are numerous species of the genus *Brugia* in animals. In the USA several cases of biopsy lesions containing worms identified as *Brugia* have been reported. Most of these biopsy specimens were enlarged lymph nodes (Baird *et al.* 1986) but Beaver *et al.* (1971) found a *Brugia* sp. in the lung of a patient who had resided in India but in an area not endemic for *Brugia malayi*.

Simmons *et al.* (1984) reported an extraordinary case of a child from the USA with an immuno-deficiency disease, who became mf-positive with a *Brugia* infection and developed lymphoedema.

DIROFILARIA SPECIES

Dirofilaria immitis is a very common parasite of dogs where the mosquito vector can breed. It is very common in Australia, much of the United States, and southern Europe, as well as most of Asia, Africa, and South America. Although there are probably different geographical strains of *D. immitis*, this has no relevance from our point of view. The vectors are certainly different in different areas.

The situation with the subcutaneous *Dirofilaria* is much more complicated. In the Old World dogs are often infected with *Dirofilaria repens*. The adult of this parasite lives subcutaneously. *Dirofilaria repens* does not occur in the New World. In fact there was big problem after the USA–Vietnamese war because all the dogs used by the US forces were infected with *D. repens* and had to be treated before they could be repatriated to the United States.

In the southern United States the offending parasite is probably *Dirofilaria tenuis*, a parasite of racoons. Further north *Dirofilaria ursi*, a parasite of bears, and *Dirofilaria subdermata*, a parasite of porcupines, have been implicated (Beaver *et al.* 1987).

INTRAOCULAR FILARIAL INFECTIONS

There have been several reports of people with filarial worms inside their eyes. Beaver *et al.* (1980) reviewed the American cases, which are due to *Dipetalonema* spp. infection. Dissaniake *et al.* (1977) described a case from Malaysia and reviewed other cases.

THE HOSTS

As indicated above, zoonotic *B. malayi* is a natural parasite of humans and *Presbytis*. Although many other mammals can be found to be infected, it is probable that these are the victims of transmission from *Presbytis* and, possibly, people. In areas where people are infected with the periodic strain, which is man to man transmitted, low levels of infection can be found in feral monkeys, but these infections are most probably derived from people.

The source of infection with *D. immitis* and the other subcutaneous species is discussed above.

DIFFERENTIAL DIAGNOSIS

It is simple to differentiate the mf of *Wuchereria bancrofti* and *Brugia malayi*. However, there is some controversy about whether more than one species of *Brugia* occurs in people. Redington *et al.* (1975) claimed to be able to differentiate the mf of *B. pahangi* and *B. malayi* by staining the mf for alkaline phosphatase. Palmieri (1985) used this technique to examine blood from both humans and cats in Indonesia and claimed that nearly all mf from cats were *B. pahangi*. However, he also claimed that many mf in the blood of humans were also *B. pahangi*. At present the only certain way of identifying which species is present is to feed infected blood to laboratory mosquitoes, collect the L3 and inject them into the peritoneal cavity of jirds. Adult worms are then collected and the species identified by examination of the spicules of the male worms. Edeson (personal communication) says that his technicians in Malaysia could tell whether they were looking at the mf of *B. malayi* or *B. pahangi* but, although they were usually right, they could not say what criteria they used!

The coin lesions in the lungs, caused by *D. immitis*, are frequently removed on the suspicion that they are tumours. On histopathological examination the nematodes are very easily seen. Like all filarial nematodes they are essentially circular in cross-section, and internally the females contain three tubes. One of these is the intestine and the other two are the uteri. Other nematodes have only one uterus. Because they are in an abnormal host, and usually there is only one worm, they do not produce mf. Some worms have been extraordinarily large.

The subcutaneous lesions caused by *Dirofilaria* species are also often mistaken for tumours. Because of their position, they are easily removed. On histological examination the characteristic worms can be recognized using the criteria described above. It is probably of no clinical importance to identify them to species but, needless to say, parasitologists will always have their hypotheses. Luzi *et al.* (1982) reported on a subcutaneous nodule, from a patient in Italy, that contained *D. immitis*. Beaver has recorded several *D. immitis*-like parasites in subcutaneous lesions in patients in the United States and Canada. The two types can be differentiated by the facts that *D. immitis* is large (about 500 μm in diameter) and the cuticle is smooth without ridges, whereas the *D. repens* subcutaneous type is smaller and has longitudinal ridges on the cuticle.

We received a histopathological section of a lesion removed from the subcutaneous tissue of the breast of a girl aged 19. The accompanying letter stated that she had never lived outside England but the letter also gave her name and this indicated that she was of Greek origin. It is certain that she did not become infected in England, as the worm does not exist here, but, unfortunately, the doctor who sent in the specimen failed to reply to our enquiries as to whether she had visited her relatives in Greece, where *D. repens* is endemic in dogs.

EPIDEMIOLOGY

Much of our understanding of the epidemiology of brugian filariosis is intimately tied up with attempts at control. In Malaysia and Indonesia in villages where brugian filariosis is endemic, mf of *Brugia* can be found in the blood of people, cats, dogs, and *Presbytis*. Mf rates are high in cats and almost every *Presbytis* is mf-positive. However, the finding of the same parasite in man and animals in the same environment does not prove that it is a zoonosis. Amongst the filariae this is beautifully demonstrated by the work of Duke with *Loa loa*. He found that in Cameroon both monkeys and people were infected with *Loa loa* but that in monkeys the mf showed nocturnal periodicity whereas in humans there was diurnal periodicity. Human loiosis is transmitted by day-biting *Chrysops* that feed at ground level, whereas transmission of monkey loiosis is by canopy-dwelling, night-biting, *Chrysops*. Although the human parasite could experimentally infect monkeys, and vice versa, natural transmission was impossible due to the separation of the vectors and mammalian hosts.

In Malaysia, Wharton *et al.* (1958) attempted to control transmission of zoonotic brugian filariosis by either intense use of insecticides within the villages, thus effectively stopping mosquitoes from transmitting infection, or by using diethylcarbamazine (DEC) to treat the people, thus preventing mosquitoes from becoming infected. To test the effectiveness of the control measures, they collected mosquitoes coming to bite people and identified the L3 found in them.

In the villages studied by Wharton and his colleagues people were infected only with *B. malayi*. Cats were infected with *Brugia* (the problem of the species infecting cats is discussed below) and *Dirofilaria repens*. The *Presbytis* monkeys in the surrounding forest were infected with *B. malayi* and *Dirofilaria magnilarvatum*. The L3 of the two *Dirofilaria* species can be morphologically differentiated. Thus, mosquitoes that had fed on monkeys could be identified because they were infected with L3 of both *B. malayi* and *D. magnilarvatum*; those mosquitoes that had fed on cats were infected with *Brugia* and *D. repens*.

After DDT had been used in the villages (thus killing all mosquitoes that came to feed in the village) most of the infected mosquitoes coming to feed on people were infected with the monkey parasites and none with the cat parasites. This confirmed that people were being bitten by infected mosquitoes that had fed on monkeys.

If no antimosquito measures were taken but people were treated with DEC, mosquitoes coming to feed were infected with either both monkey or both cat parasites. This suggested that both mammals were acting as a reservoir. However, subsequent investigation suggested that cats were infected with *Brugia pahangi* rather than *B. malayi*. This additional information suggests that monkeys are almost certainly the main source of infection for humans. People may not be a major source of infection for people. Although *Mansonia* feed avidly on people, they then return to the surrounding forest, they may not return to the village but stay in the forest and subsequently feed on monkeys. Denham and McGreevy (1977) produced a diagram showing the likely pattern of infection based on the older data. If *Presbytis* is the main source of infection for people, then control is going to be very difficult.

If Palmieri is correct and *B. pahangi* can infect people, the epidemiological situation becomes much more complicated than that described above. My feeling is that the only way to test the validity of Palmieri's results is to feed mosquitoes on human blood containing the putative *B. pahangi* and to produce adult worms in jirds. Until this is done I cannot accept that people are commonly mf-positive with *B. pahangi*.

SIGNS AND SYMPTOMS

BRUGIAN FILARIOSIS

In an area endemic for *B. malayi* people usually become microfilaraemic during early life, but to start with have no clinical signs of infection.

Early clinical disease

The first signs of clinical disease are fevers, lymphadenitis, and lymphangitis, usually occurring together.

Filarial fever

This is either low- or high-grade fever (38–40 °C). It may be accompanied by rigor, chills, and sweating. Fever persists for 2–7 days and typically occurs 3–6 times per annum but occasionally much more frequently.

Acute lymphadenitis

This presents as enlarged painful lymph nodes. It is most common in superficial inguinal nodes, occasionally in the femoral nodes and rarely in deep inguinal nodes. Nodes are soft and lobulated. The skin above the nodes is free and non-adherent.

Acute lymphangitis

This presents as retrograde, cord-like, painful swellings of the lymph trunks and proceeds centrifugally from enlarged tender lymph nodes. Red congested streaks on superadjacent skin surfaces may be seen in the early phase in light-skinned people. Lymphangitis may also spread from the periphery if associated with pyogenic infection with streptococci or staphylococci. Acute lymphangitis occasionally results in abscess formation along the line of the lymphatic, and sometimes these abscesses break through to the surface to produce a painful ulcer. These occur especially on the inside of the thighs. Scars from these ulcers are often seen in patients from endemic areas.

Later developments

Filariosis is a progressive disease as long as infection continues. Fevers continue to occur and the lymphatic trunks become thickened and ropy as a sequel to frequent attacks of acute lymphangitis. Dilated varicosis (lymph varix) of the lymph trunks may follow recurrent lymphangitis. Repeated acute attacks commonly result in chronic lymphadenitis which produces enlarged lymph nodes but there is reduced or no tenderness.

Lymphoedema

Grade I lymphoedema is characterized by healthy skin overlying a soft pitting oedema. It is usually restricted to the lower limbs, especially around the ankle and upper surface of the foot. Grade I lymphoedema is intermittent and regresses completely within a few weeks without residual swelling between episodes. There is usually a history of intermittent fever with lymphadenitis and/or lymphangitis.

Grade II lymphoedema follows repeated attacks of acute lymphangitis and grade I lymphoedema. It is chronic with slight or no pitting. The skin is healthy but does not pinch up. It seldom extends above the knee.

Grade III lymphoedema exhibits as solid, non-pitting oedema. It is usually confined to the lower legs. The skin is often abnormal and may be rough, thickened, and lustreless. Hair is dry and sparse and there may be pachydermia. Pigmentation changes are common, with hyperpigmentation frequent. Depigmentation is less common. There is no clear demarcation of healthy and affected skin. Secondary fungal infections are common. Small skin wounds, caused by the clumsy limb being banged against objects, are frequent and may become infected with bacteria.

No clinical signs of infection have been reported in monkeys or cats and dogs in endemic areas. In the laboratory, beagle dogs often develop soft lymphoedema; this usually seen in dogs that are apparently naturally resistant to infection and that do not become mf-positive after L3 have been injected. Cats repeatedly infected with L3 of *B. pahangi* sometimes develop lymphoedema but this is usually mild and transient. Both cats and dogs develop lymphadenitis and lymphangitis and have been used to investigate the histopathology of these conditions.

DIROFILARIOSIS

Dirofilaria immitis produces coin lesions in human lung but these do not appear to cause any problem and are normally found during routine radiographic examination.

Dirofilaria spp. cause subcutaneous lesions but these are of little significance and are usually removed for histological analysis.

TREATMENT

Currently the only treatment for *B. malayi* infection is the drug DEC. Wilson (1950) was the first to use this drug in this infection. Figure 59.2a shows the mf counts of patients before and after treatment. Unfortunately, the death of such large numbers of mf (I calculate that about 250 000 000 mf die in 24 hours) cannot be without unpleasant side-effects due to the release of so much protein into a host with large amounts of antibody. Figure 59.2b shows the body temperature of some of their patients. Partono *et al.* (1981) were the first to demonstrate that treatment with DEC could reverse the clinical disease. Grade I and II lymphoedema are most susceptible to this treatment and affected legs often return to the normal state.

As the removal of the lesions caused by *Dirofilaria* species contain the offending worms this is also curative.

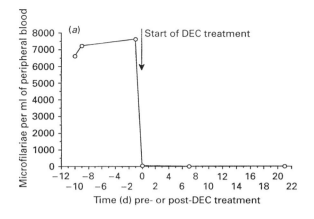

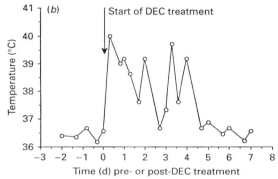

Fig. 59.2 Effect of treating *Brugia malayi*-infected patients with diethylcarbamazine. (a) Microfilarial counts; (b) body temperature. (Data from Wilson 1950.)

PREVENTION AND CONTROL

As the mosquitoes transmitting zoonotic Brugian filariosis bite nocturnally, the use of bed nets is a good personal way to prevent infection. Because the bites of *Mansonia* are painful, villagers frequently make bed nets for themselves. Unfortunately, the mosquitoes feed avidly in the evening. In Indonesia it is common for a village to have one television set and for the villagers to sit in the open watching the screen. They get bitten while watching the television; perhaps this is the first case of television-transmitted disease!

There is no point in using insecticides in the villages as the mosquitoes come from the forest. They may die but they will have fed first. The surrounding forests are a mass of breeding sites for *Mansonia* and it is not possible to stop them breeding.

Presbytis are protected species in many countries and, therefore, the zoonotic source of infection cannot be removed. It would certainly be regarded as grossly inhumane to suggest the elimination of these beautiful monkeys anyway. If the village cats and dogs are a source of infection it would be possible to treat them with a

subcutaneously injected benzimidazole carbamate. These drugs kill adult worms and for several weeks gives chemoprophylactic protection against infection. If cats were treated every 5 or 6 months they would probably never become mf-positive. If money were no object, the *Presbytis* could be trapped and treated with the same anthelmintic but this is most unlikely to happen.

The vector *Mansonia* are entirely dependent on the floating water plants, *Pistia*, etc., for oxygen during their larval stage and destruction of this plant has reduced transmission in areas of non-zoonotic transmission, such as Kerala State in India. Unfortunately, in the zoonotic areas there are huge areas of breeding sites and the wet forests interdigitate with the villages so there is little point in localized killing of the water weeds.

Currently, the only way in which human zoonotic brugian filariosis can be prevented is by the regular use of DEC. DEC is effective against *Brugia* species and has been shown to kill developing larvae in cats. Assuming that this is also true for humans, it should be possible to prevent the development of the pathology by regular use of DEC. A practical schedule would need to be devised but it is believed that a once-monthly regime of 6 mg/kg would be the easiest to apply. Propaganda could be used to link taking the drug to something like the full moon. A very useful side-effect would be the elimination of *Ascaris lumbricoides*. Salt-containing DEC would also be effective. The use of DEC for chemoprophylaxis would have no side-effects after the first use because the people would not have mf in their blood.

The only way in which humans can prevent themselves from becoming infected with *Dirofilaria* is to avoid being bitten by mosquitoes in endemic areas. This is easier said than done, as the mosquitoes transmitting these nematodes are normally diurnal biters. As someone who works on human filariosis, which is transmitted by night biting mosquitoes, I am more likely to become infected with these zoonoses rather than human infections. My personal prophylaxis is the use of repellants containing DEET (diethyltoluamide).

Canine heartworm disease can be prevented by the chemoprophylactic use of ivermectin (Blair and Campbell 1980). This drug is sold by Merck, Sharp and Dohme as Heartgard®. Presumably ivermectin could be used as a prophylactic in people but is unlikely to be licensed for this use.

PROGNOSIS

Without treatment, filarial lymphoedema is a progressive disease for patients who reside in endemic villages. They will be bitten every day by infected mosquitoes and although they become resistant to the development of the larvae into later stages they cannot prevent the L3 from penetrating into their bodies and probably cannot prevent them from entering the lymphatics. The subsequent death of the larvae and the inflammatory infiltration of granulocytes and macrophages is probably responsible for the progressive nature of the disease.

The lesions caused by *D. immitis* and *Nochtiella* are probably not progressive.

REFERENCES

Baird J. K., Alpert, L. I., Kriedman, R., Schraft, W. C., and Connor, D. H. (1986). North American brugian filariasis: report of nine infections of humans. *American Journal of Tropical Medicine and Hygiene*, **35**, 1205–9.

Beaver P. C., Fallon M., and Smith G. H. (1971). Pulmonary nodule caused by a living *Brugia malayi*-like filaria in an artery. *American Journal of Tropical Medicine and Hygiene*, **20**, 661–6.

Beaver P. C., Meyer, E. A., Jarroll E. L., and Rosenquist R. C. (1980). *Dipetalonema* from the eye of a man in Oregon, USA. *American Journal of Tropical Medicine and Hygiene*, **29**, 369–72.

Beaver, P. C., Wolfson, J. S., Waldron, M. A., Swartz, M. N., Evans, G. W., and Adler, J. (1987). *Dirofilaria ursi*-like parasites acquired by humans in the northern United States and Canada: report of two cases and brief review. *American Journal of Tropical Medicine and Hygiene*, **37**, 357–62.

Blair, L. S. and Campbell W. C. (1980). Efficacy of ivermectin against *Dirofilaria immitis* larvae in dogs 31, 60 and 90 days after infection. *American Journal of Veterinary Research*, **41**, 2108.

Denham D. A. and McGreevy P. B. (1977). Brugian filariasis: epidemiological and experimental studies. *Advances in Parasitology*, **16**, 243–309.

Dissaniake, A. S., Ramalingam, S, Fong, A., Pathmayokan, S., Thomas V., and Fan S. P. (1977). Filaria in the vitreous of the eye of man in peninsular Malaysia. *American Journal of Tropical Medicine and Hygiene*, **26**, 1143–7.

Luzi, P., Leoncini, L., and Lungarella, G. (1982). Human Subcutaneous Dirofilariasis in Italy. *Rivista Parasitologia*, **43**, 259–263.

Palmeri, J. R., Masbar, S., Purnomo, Marwoto, H. A., Tirtokusomo, S., and Darwis, F. (1985). The domestic cat as a host for Brugian filariasis in South Kalimantan (Borneo), Indonesia. *Journal of Heliminthology*, **59**, 277–81.

Partono, F., Purnomo, Oemijati, S., and Soewata, A. (1981). The long term effects of repeated diethylcarbamazine administration with special reference to microfilaraemia and elephantiasis. *Acta Tropica*, **38**, 217–25.

Redington, B. C., Montgomery, C. A., Jarvis, H. R., and Hockmeyer, W. T. (1975). Histochemical differentiation of the microfilariae of *Brugia pahangi* and sub-periodic *Brugia malayi*. *Annals of Tropical Medicine and Parasitology*, **69**, 489–92.

Simmons, C. F. *et al.* (1984). Zoonotic filariasis with lymphedema in an immunodeficient infant. *New England Journal of Medicine*, **310**, 1243–5.

Wharton, R. H., Edeson, J. F. B., Wilson, T., and Reid, J. A. (1958). Studies on filariasis in Malaya: pilot experiments in the control of filariasis due to *Wuchereria malayi*, *Transactions of the Royal Society of Tropical Medicine and Hygiene*, **52**, 93–102.

Wilson, T. (1950). Hetrazan in the treatment of filariasis due to *Wuchereria malayi*. *Transactions of the Royal Society for Tropical Medicine and Hygiene*, **44**, 49–66.

60   TRICHINELLOSIS

Inger Ljungström, Darwin Murrell, Edoardo Pozio, and Derek Wakelin

SUMMARY

Epidemiological evidence indicates that trichinellosis is a cosmopolitan infection, characterized by two main cycles, a synanthropic–domestic cycle, involving the species *T. spiralis*, and a sylvatic cycle involving *T. spiralis* and other members of the genus.

Trichinella is unusual among parasitic nematodes in that the worm undergoes a complete developmental cycle, from larva to adult to larva, in the body of a single host, which has a profound influence on the epidemiology of trichinellosis as a zoonosis. When the cycle is complete, the muscles of the infected animal contain a reservoir of larvae, capable of long-term survival. Humans and other hosts become infected by ingesting muscle tissues containing viable larvae.

The symptoms associated with trichinellosis vary with the severity of infection, i.e. the number of viable larvae ingested, and the time after infection. The capacity of the worm population to undergo massive multiplication in the body is a major determinant. Progression of disease follows the biological development of the parasite. Symptoms are associated first with the gastrointestinal tract, as the worms invade and establish in the small intestine, become more general as the body responds immunologically, and finally focus on the muscles as the larvae penetrate and develop there. Although *Trichinella* worms cause pathological changes directly by mechanical damage, most of the clinical features of trichinellosis are immunopathological in origin and can be related to the capacity of the parasite to induce allergic responses.

The main source of human infection is raw or undercooked meat products from pig, wild boar, walrus, and horses, but meat products from other animals have been implicated.

Diagnosis of infection is made by direct examination of muscle using microscopy or by recovery of larvae after artificial digestion; immunological tests are also available. Treatment requires both the use of anthelmintic drugs to kill the parasite itself and symptomatic treatment to minimize inflammatory responses.

Both pre-slaughter prevention and post-slaughter control can be used to prevent *Trichinella* infections. The first involves pig management control as well as continuous surveillance programmes. Meat inspection is a successful post-slaughter strategy. In countries where meat inspection is not mandatory, consumers/hunters must be advised on correct meat handling procedures.

HISTORY

DISCOVERY OF DISEASE, ORGANISM, PATHOGENESIS, EPIDEMIOLOGY, AND CONTROL

Trichinella spiralis was discovered and first described by James Paget in 1835. Paget was at that time a medical student in London, and he recorded finding larvae in the muscles of a 40-year-old Italian who died from pulmonary tuberculosis. Given that Paget had only the aid of a primitive microscope, the drawings he made are surprisingly accurate and show clearly the characteristic cysts (Campbell 1979). The parasite was first formally identified (and named *Trichinella spiralis*) in a paper published by Owen in the same year (Owen 1835).

Following these initial descriptions, there were many other reports of *Trichinella* infections in humans, although their origins and relationship to defined disease remained obscure for several years. The parasite was first found in animals by Leidy (1846), who identified larval cysts in muscles from a pig and realized that they were identical to those described in humans. Evidence that infection was acquired by ingestion of live larvae from infected muscles was obtained in the 1850s by feeding experiments using dogs and other animals (Virchow 1859). The first account of transmission to humans from infected pig meat, and association with a defined set of symptoms, was published by Zenker (1860) who made a detailed study of a patient who had been clinically diagnosed as having typhoid. Post-mortem examination of muscle tissue, however, confirmed the presence of a heavy infection of *Trichinella*, and the symptoms recorded before death (fatigue, fever, oedema, muscle and joint pain) are now recognized as characteristic of trichinellosis and largely immunopathological in origin. The patient had eaten infected ham and sausage shortly before the onset of her symptoms, and similar symptoms also occurred in other members of the household who had eaten these items. Zenker's association of a defined pathogen with a defined disease was a milestone in medical microbiology, though it rarely receives the recognition it deserves, being overshadowed by later discoveries in bacteriology.

Early accounts of the organism were confined to the larval stages in the muscle. The shape of the cyst, the coiled ('spiral') nature of the larvae and details of their internal organization were clearly described, although there was some confusion as to the orientation of the larvae, Owen considering the larger part of the body to represent the anterior end. It was quickly realized that the worms were similar to the related *Trichuris* (*Trichocephalus*) and it was initially believed that the larvae did in fact belong to this genus. However, Virchow's experiments, in which dogs were fed larvae from human origin, allowed the intestinal adult stages to be identified and the taxonomic separation from *Trichuris* to be established. The name *Trichinella spiralis* was given by Railliet in 1896, *Trichina* having been used much earlier for a dipteran genus, and the disease, should therefore, correctly be termed 'trichinellosis', although the earlier use of 'trichinosis' still persists. The work of Virchow and Zenker gave a remarkably accurate picture of the life cycle of the parasite and of the migration of larvae from the intestine to the muscles. As a result, much of the basic biology of *Trichinella* was defined by the 1870s, a truly remarkable achievement.

The recognition of trichinellosis as a clinical entity and elucidation of the mode of transmission led to a spate of reports of epidemics in Europe and America (see Gould 1945; Campbell 1983). One of the first concerned an outbreak in Germany, in 1863, in which 158 people became infected and 27 died. Trichinellosis was recorded in USA in 1864 and in Britain in 1871. In each case infection was acquired from pig meat. Inspection of pig meat by trichinelloscopy (microscopic examination of compressed tissue) became compulsory in many parts of Germany in the 1860s and 1870s, and large numbers of inspectors were appointed (more than 27 000 in Prussia alone). *Trichinella* infection in pigs was recognized as a major problem in the USA, and import of American pig meat products was banned in many European countries during the later years of the nineteenth century. Control by improved husbandry, regulation of feed sources, tighter meat inspection procedures, and freezing of carcasses after slaughter was introduced to reduce the problem.

Although consumption of raw or undercooked pig meat was identified as a major factor in the transmission of *Trichinella* to humans there was, and to some extent still is, debate about the means by which infection can be maintained in pigs. Leuckart's view that pigs became infected by eating rats carrying *Trichinella* larvae exerted a profound influence, although initially the evidence for this route was not strong. In the days when herds were maintained on feed containing waste pigmeat products it is clear that infection could easily be transmitted if the feed itself was infected. However, infections persisted even after the introduction of stringent feed controls. More recent studies (Hanbury *et al.* 1986; Schad *et al.* 1987) have shown not only that cannibalism alone can maintain transmission in infected herds, but that infected rats can also be an important additional source. Pigs readily eat both live and dead rats, and rats scavenge on pig carcasses. Where herds are heavily infected the local rat population is also likely to harbour significant *Trichinella* infections. Pigs are, however, not the only source of infection to humans. A variety of animals, whose meat is used, can transmit infection, including wild boar, bear, walrus, and horses. *Trichinella* occurs in many species of wild animals and it is clear that there are significant sylvatic cycles of infection, in many parts of the world, although these are now known to involve species in addition to *T. spiralis*. At the present time trichinellosis is still present in many countries, though much less important than it was earlier this century. However, increased incidences of human trichinellosis are being reported from former Soviet Republics such as Estonia and Lithuania and from Romania. Outbreaks are now primarily associated with consumption of meat from home-killed pigs or from animals killed during hunting and with ethnic preferences for eating raw or undercooked meat products.

THE AGENT

TAXONOMY

The taxonomy of the genus *Trichinella* is complex and a subject of much debate. However, there is a general agreement to consider the following classification as the most suitable to explain the molecular, biochemical, biological, immunological, pathological, clinical, and epidemiological differences observed among the nematodes of the genus. Five sibling species and three phenotypes of uncertain taxonomic level have been identified (Pozio *et al.* 1992*c*).

Trichinella spiralis s. str. (Owen 1835) characterized by high infectivity for rats and pigs, the highest female fertility in the genus, no resistance to freezing of muscle larvae, and a cosmopolitan distribution.

Trichinella nativa Britov and Boev, 1972, characterized by high resistance to freezing of muscle larvae, widespread in the wildlife of arctic and subarctic regions.

Trichinella britovi Pozio *et al.*, 1992*a*, characterized by low infectivity for rats and pigs and a low resistance to freezing of muscle larvae, present in temperate areas of the Palaearctic region.

Trichinella pseudospiralis Garkavi, 1972, in which non-encapsulation in host muscle is a hallmark, present in birds and marsupials of the Australian region and in carnivores and birds in the Palaearctic region.

Trichinella nelsoni Britov and Boev, 1972, characterized by a slow nurse cell development, no resistance to freezing, low infectivity for rats and pigs, widespread in wildlife south of the Sahara in Africa.

Trichinella T5, present in wildlife, could be considered a phenotype of *T. britovi* in the Nearctic region. *Trichinella* T6, present in wildlife of subarctic areas of the Nearctic region, is closely related to *T. nativa*. *Trichinella* T8, is closely related to *T. britovi*. Its presence in wildlife of South Africa is an enigma, but may be the result of man's movement of animals between regions.

LIFE CYCLE

Trichinella is unusual among parasitic nematodes in that the worm undergoes a complete developmental cycle, from larva to adult to larva, in the body of a single host (Fig. 60.1), a characteristic that has a profound influence on the epidemiology of trichinellosis as a zoonosis and on the pathology associated with infection. When the developmental cycle is complete, the muscles of infected animals contain a reservoir of larvae that can

then infect other hosts, and these larvae are capable of long-term survival. Hosts become infected by ingesting muscle tissues that contain viable larvae. Transmission of *Trichinella* to humans occurs when meat containing infective larvae is eaten raw or undercooked.

In most species of *Trichinella* the infective larvae are found encapsulated within cysts in the muscle, *T. pseudospiralis* is exceptional in having unencysted larvae. Larvae are released from the cysts by digestion in the stomach and pass into the small intestine, where they penetrate rapidly into the epithelial cells of the mucosa, occupying an intracellular niche. At this stage the larvae is about 1 mm long, and its body occupies some 40–50 enterocytes. Subsequent development is extremely rapid, the parasite undergoing four moults in about 30 hours to reach the immature adult stage and increasing in length 2–3 times. As with all nematodes, the sexes are separate, and the female is the larger, reaching 3 mm in length.

Males and females mate in the small intestine, the eggs of the female are fertilized, develop rapidly in the uterus, and the female then begins to release newborn larvae (the first larval stage) directly into the mucosa. In rodents, where experimental infections are possible, larval release is known to begin after 4 or 5 days, in humans it may take a little longer. Release continues for

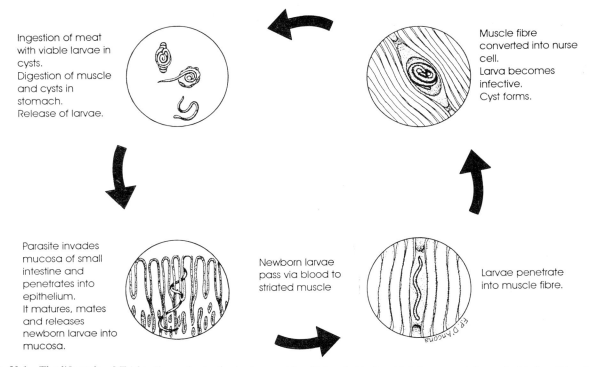

Ingestion of meat with viable larvae in cysts. Digestion of muscle and cysts in stomach. Release of larvae.

Muscle fibre converted into nurse cell. Larva becomes infective. Cyst forms.

Parasite invades mucosa of small intestine and penetrates into epithelium. It matures, mates and releases newborn larvae into mucosa.

Newborn larvae pass via blood to striated muscle

Larvae penetrate into muscle fibre.

Fig. 60.1   The life cycle of *Trichinella* species in the host except for *T. pseudospiralis*, which has no cyst forms, but is free-living in host muscle.

several days (rodents) or possibly weeks (humans), and is eventually terminated by the onset of immunity or by senility of the worm. The number of larvae produced during the lifetime of each female is dependent on many factors, and differs between the various species of *Trichinella*—it can be more than 1000 or fewer than 100. Survival of the worms in the intestine is likewise very variable, but clinical data suggest a life span of some weeks in humans. The severity of trichinellosis as a disease results largely from this capacity of the worm population to undergo massive multiplication in the body of the host.

After release from the female, the newborn larvae migrate into mucosal lymphatics, pass through the draining lymph nodes, enter blood vessels, and are carried around the body. Although they can complete development only in striated skeletal muscles, larvae may attempt to penetrate other tissues, including the brain, heart, and kidneys. After penetration into striated muscle fibres the larva lies free in the cytoplasm and induces a complex series of changes which result in the host cell becoming transformed into quite different structure—the nurse cell—that serves to ensure the growth, development, and survival of the parasite. With time the nurse cell becomes surrounded by a capsule and a network of capillaries to form the characteristic cyst. After 3–4 weeks the larva has grown considerably (from 100 μm to 1 mm), is resistant to digestion, and is capable of infecting another host to initiate a further infection cycle. With time the cysts become calcified and the larvae die, but they can remain infective for very long periods, in some hosts for many years (e.g. man and pigs). Larvae can remain viable in cysts for a considerable time after the death of the host, allowing transmission by scavenging. In the case of the Arctic species, larvae can also survive exposure to low temperatures, although this is to some extent also dependent upon the species of host animal concerned.

DISEASE MECHANISMS, IMMUNOPATHOLOGY

THE DISEASE

The symptoms associated with trichinellosis vary with the severity of infection (i.e. the number of viable larvae ingested) and with the time after infection. The progression of the disease follows the biological development of the parasite. Symptoms are associated first with the gastrointestinal tract, as the worms invade and establish in the small intestine, become more general as the body responds immunologically to the infection, and finally focus on the muscles as the larvae penetrate and develop there. A significant proportion of the symptoms characteristic of trichinellosis arise from strong immediate hypersensitivity responses to antigens of the parasite. Detailed accounts of the pathology of this disease are given by Castro and by Stewart in Campbell (1983).

Trichinellosis presents with a wide variety of signs and symptoms, but high eosinophilia and allergic symptoms after a period of gastrointestinal disturbance strongly suggest trichinellosis as a diagnosis, particularly if ingestion of a suspect meat product (raw or undercooked pork, boar, bear, horse) is implicated.

IMMUNOPATHOLOGY

Although it is certain that *Trichinella* worms cause pathological changes as a result of mechanical damage to the intestine and to muscle tissues, the majority of the clinical features of trichinellosis are immunopathological in origin and can be related to the capacity of *Trichinella* to induce allergic responses, a property shared by many species of worm parasites. The molecular basis of this allergenicity is still undefined, although clearly it must reflect particular characteristics of worm antigens and the manner in which they are presented to the host. Recent studies in mouse models show that *Trichinella* infections preferentially stimulate cells of the T helper 2 (Th2) subset of CD4+T lymphocytes (Grencis *et al.* 1991), which release the cytokines necessary for the development of many of the allergic components of the disease, and it can reasonably be assumed that a similar situation exists during human infections.

During the intestinal phase there is a marked infiltration of inflammatory cells, including neutrophils, eosinophils, and mast cells into the gut mucosa. Significant changes take place in mucosal architecture (e.g. villous atrophy), fluid flux across the mucosa is disturbed, mucus production is increased, and intestinal transit time is decreased (Castro, in Campbell 1983). All of these changes are the result of T-cell activity and all can be related to the symptoms appearing during the intestinal phase of infection, of which diarrhoea is the most characteristic. Eosinophilia is a consequence of T-cell responses to both the intestinal adult worms and the muscle larvae and is dependent upon release of the cytokine IL-5 (Herndon and Kayes 1992). It has been shown in rodents that infection stimulates both parasite-specific IgE and total IgE antibodies as well as IgG isotypes (IgG1) that are involved in hypersensitivity reactions (e.g. Gabriel and Justus 1979) and this is consistent with the dominance of the T-cell response by the Th2 subset. Although *Trichinella*-specific IgE responses have been detected in humans by some workers (e.g. Bruschi *et al.* 1990) but not by others (Ljungström *et al.* 1988*a*), may be due to the assays used, it does seem probable that many of the systemic allergic symptoms of the disease do reflect type-1 hypersensitivity responses.

Invasion of the muscles and formation of the characteristic cysts is accompanied by the development of intense inflammatory responses. These are again T-cell-dependent, involve accumulation of eosinophils and other leucocytes, and are maintained by continuous release of antigenic material from the larvae. This inflammation is the direct cause of the myositis that occurs at this stage of infection and which contributes, together with the physical disruption of muscle fibres, to the mechanical and electrophysiological disturbances associated with severe trichinellosis.

Although the major features of the immunopathological responses to *Trichinella* infections are now well defined, it seems clear that many other components of inflammatory responses (e.g. cytokines, acute-phase proteins, granulocyte and mast cell mediators, complement components) must also play an important part.

The importance of immunopathological events in trichinellosis means that treatment of infection requires both the use of antiparasitic drugs to kill the parasite itself and symptomatic treatment to minimize inflammatory responses, some of which can be aggravated by chemotherapy through the release of antigens from dead and dying parasites. A variety of anti-inflammatory compounds, primarily corticosteroids, are effective in this respect.

THE HOST

ANIMAL

Clinical aspects

As with humans, the degree of clinical disease that develops in an animal host generally depends on the number of muscle larvae ingested. During the first few weeks, if large numbers of worms are present in the intestine, illness may be characterized by gastrointestinal problems and diarrhoea. Subsequent to the production of the muscle-invading larval offspring, the acute muscle stage disease occurs. This is classically characterized by muscular pain, fever, and eosinophilia.

Infected pigs, because of their importance in the epidemiology of human trichinellosis, have been investigated frequently for development of clinical disease. In heavily *T. spiralis* infected young pigs, loss of appetite, malaise, hind limb paralyses, incontinence, and diarrhoea have been observed (Beck 1970). Older pigs, however, appear to be more tolerant. Schwartz (1937) reported that little or no symptoms could be expected in infected pigs which had fewer than 800–900 larvae per gram of diaphragmatic muscle, and that animals with up to 1215 larvae per gram could recover.

However, there is considerable individual variation in tolerance to heavy infection (Schwartz 1938). Campbell and Cuckler (1966) observed minimal effects of infection on growth rates in pigs receiving 10 000 larvae/kg body weight. This contrasts with the results of Schwartz (1938), but agrees with that of Olsen *et al.* (1964) in which dosages of 2000 to 7000 larvae/kg were used. In the experiments conducted by Campbell and Cuckler (1966), fever was not manifested, although this response was noted earlier by Schwartz (1938). Because the majority of naturally infected swine have infection levels far below these levels (Schad *et al.* 1985), it is not expected that clinical trichinellosis in swine will be observed in the field. Eosinophilia, however, was observed in all reported studies on pig infections.

In contrast to mice and rats, pigs appear to respond slowly to the enteral infection stage, and do not begin expelling adult worms until 3–4 weeks after initial exposure (Campbell and Cuckler 1966). Murrell (1985a) observed that in light to moderately infected pigs, adult worms may persist for 2 months or more, albeit in reduced numbers. Unlike in rodents, the intestinal immune response to secondary infection in pigs is moderate (Murrell 1985a). The major acquired immune barriers in pigs to re-infection with *T. spiralis* are effector mechanisms that act on the newborn larvae, either in the circulatory stage or in the muscle tissue (Marti and Murrell 1986; Madden *et al.* 1990).

The increasing importance of horse meat in the transmission of *Trichinella* to humans, especially in Europe, has prompted several studies on the biological and clinical aspects of this infection. Soule *et al.* (1989) reported transient muscle disorders in horses given 50 000 larvae of *T. spiralis*, along with eosinophilia and increases in serum lactic dehydrogenase, aldolase, and creatine phosphokinase; fever was not observed. Specific antibody responses were detectable 2–5 weeks after exposure. As with swine, the muscle larvae distribution is skewed towards anterior muscles, especially the tongue, facial muscles, masseters, and diaphragm. There is a marked decline in *T. spiralis* muscle larvae burden during the initial year of infection (Soule *et al.* 1989). In pigs, *T. spiralis* muscle larvae may persist considerably longer (Murrell *et al.* 1986).

Experimental infections of other hosts have been reported (Beck 1970; Despommier 1983; Weatherly 1983). There are important differences among host and *Trichinella* species in regard to immune response, clinical signs, and pathological changes.

Diagnosis

Diagnosis of infection is readily made by either direct examination of muscle tissue by microscopy, by recovery of larvae after artificial digestion of muscle samples, or by immunological means (Zimmermann 1983; Madden and Murrell 1990). These procedures are discussed more completely below. It is important to remember that the sensitivity of microscopic and digestion-recovery methods is enhanced when either tongue, masseter, or diaphragm muscle tissue is utilized. Serological tests have been developed for both humans and swine (Oliver *et al.* 1989; Madden and Murrell 1990).

HUMAN

Clinical aspects

The disease caused by *Trichinella* infection in humans is initiated by consuming raw or undercooked meat containing viable larvae. A classification of the severity of the clinical course ranging from asymptomatic to severe trichinellosis has been suggested by Kassur *et al.* (1978). Based on the original number of ingested larvae, symptoms range from asymptomatic to severe. But immune status and prior infection may also modify the outcome. The clinical presentation seems also to differ between the various *Trichinella* species. From the clinical point of view, trichinellosis is divided in two stages, the intestinal and extraintestinal stages.

Intestinal stage

The infected larvae, digested from meat in the stomach, are transferred to the small intestine. There they penetrate the epithelium of the villus, develop through four larval stages, mature, and mate within 2 days. By 5–6 days of infection the female worms begin to deposit live larvae, and in humans deposition of newborn larvae seems to continue for weeks. Most of the newborn larvae migrate into the lamina propria and are subsequently carried to the body tissues through the mesenteric lymphatics and venules.

Symptoms may be absent, but if present they will develop 1–7 days after infection, all of a non-specific nature. Diarrhoea and abdominal cramps predominate, sometimes accompanied by nausea and general malaise. Loss of appetite and weight loss may also occur. Studies indicate that the diarrhoea can be prolonged, lasting for weeks (MacLean *et al.* 1989), but also the opposite has been observed, i.e. hardly any gastro-intestinal symptoms at all (Olaison and Ljungström 1992). These dissimilar responses may be attributed to the species of *Trichinella* (Pozio *et al.* 1993).

Extraintestinal stage

Although adult worms in the small intestine do give rise to some gut damage, the gastrointestinal disorders may be neglected. The main symptoms of the infection in humans are caused by the migrating and encysting larvae. During invasion, the larvae cause damage to cells and a range of allergic reactions. The symptoms normally develop a week or two after penetration of the newborn larvae into muscle fibres.

The main clinical symptoms are fever, often very high; facial oedema, particularly perorbital; muscle tenderness, aching and swelling; weakness, partly due to pain on motion and urticaria. As the larvae normally invade the most active muscles, the patient will experience problems in breathing, chewing, and swallowing. In heavy infections, a diverse range of serious symptoms can arise such as myocarditis, normally seen 3 weeks after infection and pathological damage to the central nervous system, such as petechial haemorrhages causing inflammation. These kind of bleedings are also noted in the conjunctivae and under the finger nails.

A marked eosinophilia appears about 2 weeks after infection, at least 20 per cent, but often over 50 per cent. There is also some degree of leucocytosis and hypoalbuminemia. Elevated levels of creatine phosphokinase and other muscle enzymes are also found.

Diagnosis

The most difficult part in diagnosing trichinellosis, like many other rare infections, is to be aware of the existence of the disease. The infection is usually found as an outbreak, but the first index case has to be identified. Isolated cases are also seen, when the infection has been contracted during a visit to an endemic area, for example as a tourist. Once the diagnosis is suspected there are different tools to confirm the diagnosis.

Clinical signs

High eosinophilia in combination with fever, muscle pain, and orbital oedema should suggest trichinellosis. Usually eosinophilia is the earliest sign with or without gastrointestinal symptoms. During the intestinal stage, the disease is impossible to distinguish from other forms of gastroenteritis. Clinical findings during the extraintestinal stage can be misdiagnosed, e.g. as influenza or exanthematous disease.

History of exposure

It is important to obtain details of consumption of undercooked or raw meat during the preceding 1–3 weeks. In particular, home-made sausages and minced meat should be taken into account. Epidemiological information about similar disease among family members or other groups of people sharing the same kind of food can be of importance.

Parasitological assay

Stool examinations for adult worms are almost always negative as these are few in number and often disintegrated. Newborn larvae may occasionally be found in blood. The definitive test for trichinellosis is muscle biopsy, taken at a site of swelling and tenderness. False-negative biopsies may occur in light infection or if the biopsy is taken too early after infection. Portions of the biopsy can be compressed between glass slides and examined under low power microscopically, or processed for routine histopathological studies. The best time for obtaining a positive biopsy is after 4 weeks of infection. The sensitivity of the test is low, there has to be at least three larvae per gram (Ruitenberg and Kampelmacher 1970). Therefore, it is preferable to subject the tissue to artificial digestion (in pepsin–HCl) because this greatly increases the chances of detecting larvae. The detection of infection would be improved by the development of sensitive PCR-assays (Bandi *et al.* 1993).

Serological assays

Over the years a range of serological assays have been applied for diagnosis of trichinellosis (Ljungström 1983). Common methods used today are enzyme linked immunosorbent assay (ELISA) and indirect immunofluorescense technique (IF). In ELISA various soluble antigens are used. In IF, sections of muscle larvae are employed. The distinct staining pattern, a bright staining of the cuticle and internal organs, is simple to distinguish from non-specific staining.

Antigens

Each stage of the parasite life cycle expresses common antigens, but also exclusively different surface antigens (Philipp *et al.* 1981). Most studied are the antigens derived from the muscle larvae of *Trichinella spiralis*. In 1991, Appleton *et al.* presented a consensus on *T. spiralis* antigens. TSL-1 antigen, stage-specific for the infective larvae, seems to be immunodominant. This antigen, found in granules within specialized cells (the stichocytes), is abundant on the cuticle and in excretory/secretory products. Recently, Wassom *et al.* (1994) decribed a carbohydrate epitope, 3,6-dideoxyhexose, in association with a glycoprotein. It seems to be unique to *Trichinella* and most of the *Trichinella*-specific antibodies recognize this epitope.

Antibody response

A classical antibody response is accompanying the infection. Specific antibodies of IgG, IgM, and IgA class are detected 2–3 weeks after onset of disease (Ljungström 1974). However, a specific IgE response and an increased level of total IgE seem not to be a constant finding (Van Knapen *et al.* 1982; Au *et al.* 1983; Feldmeier *et al.* 1987; Ljungström *et al.* 1988*b*). This may be due to assays used and/or the time after

infection that the sample is taken. The IgG subclasses have a sequential appearance, IgG1 before IgG3 and IgG3 before IgG4, during the course of infection. IgG1 antibodies dominate the immune response. The IgG4 antibodies seem to be related with the chronic stage of infection, measured 1 year after infection. The presence of IgG3, but not IgG4, seems to be correlated with severity of disease (Ljungström *et al.* 1988*b*). The antibody response declines and become negative over the years. In one study, using IF, about 30 per cent of cases had become negative after 2 years (Ljungström 1974).

TREATMENT

In mild cases of trichinellosis there is no need for treatment other then symptomatic. Various benzimidazoles are used for anthelmintic treatment. The drug of choice in humans has been mebendazole as the side-effects are fewer compared to thiabendazole. Over the past few years albendazole has been substituted for mebendazole. Corticosteroid treatment may decrease the severity of the disease. However, it should be noted that corticosteroids in experimental infections prolong the larviposition, resulting in increased larval production. Thus, if these drugs are given during the enteral stage, anthelmintic treatment should also be given.

PROGNOSIS

Muscle pain and muscle weakness persist throughout the period of larval development, but then gradually disappear, although longer persistence has been recorded. After recovery from the acute disease, most of the infected individuals are clinically well. However, the encysted larvae may remain viable for many years, although calcification can occur within less than a year. Death may occur between the third to eight week after infection, as a result of a heavy infection. Immediate causes are exhaustion, pneumonia, or cardiac failure.

EPIDEMIOLOGY

Recent epidemiological evidence indicates that trichinellosis is a cosmopolitan parasitic infection of carrion-feeding carnivores with cannibalistic and scavenger habits (Fig. 60.2) and it has been detected wherever it has been looked for (Pozio *et al.* 1989). The parasite biomass is greater in sylvatic than in domestic cycles (Pozio *et al.* 1989). The spread of the parasite in wild habitats is favoured by its survival in decaying flesh for weeks (protected by the nurse cell) and in living

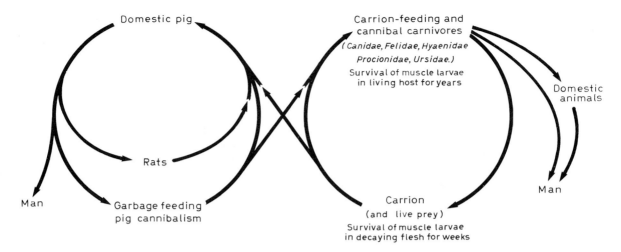

Fig. 60.2   The interaction between the domestic and the sylvatic cycles of *Trichinella*.

host muscle for years (Kumar *et al.* 1990). The epidemiology of trichinellosis is characterized by two main cycles, a synanthropic–domestic cycle (due to *T. spiralis*) and a sylvatic cycle (due to all species and phenotypes, including *T. spiralis*).

Trichinella spiralis is the only species in the genus that is highly infective for infection in swine and rats (Pozio *et al.* 1992*a*). Human beings are responsible for the presence of this nematode in domestic animals (i.e. swine) by housing them in contact with wild hosts or feeding them with uncontrolled food (especially pork scraps; Schad *et al.* 1987). Cannibalistic behaviour, e.g. tail-biting, can also transmit the infection among pigs, and faecal transmission has been demonstrated experimentally, although the epidemiological importance of these routes is problematical. Synanthropic animals (rats and small carnivores) can complicate the epidemiological picture because they can constitute both a reservoir and a link between the domestic and sylvatic habitat (Murrell *et al.* 1987; Leiby *et al.* 1988). However, some authors consider rats as a victim instead of a reservoir of domestic trichinellosis, i.e. infected rats are present because there are infected pigs and not vice versa. *Trichinella spiralis* can also be transmitted to sylvatic mammals and wild carnivores, and omnivorous mammals living far from human habitation can harbour this nematode (La Rosa *et al.* 1991). Domestic trichinellosis is widespread with different degrees of prevalence in pigs of Asia (China, Laos, Russia, Thailand, and Vietnam), of Africa (Egypt), of Europe (Bulgaria, Finland, Lithuania, Poland, Romania, Russia, Spain, Sweden, Ukraine, and former Yugoslavia), of South America (Argentina, Bolivia, Chile, and Uruguay), Central America (Mexico), and

North America (USA and Canada). However, reports of the presence of this parasite in pigs are frequently made in other countries. Although humans primarily acquire this infection by consuming uninspected pork, wild boar, dog (Thailand) and horse meat (France, Italy), sheep and ox (China; Murrell 1994), and even camel meat (from Egypt) have been suspected. Improperly cooked meat (less than 60 °C), raw meat and raw meat products (fresh, smoked, or sausages preserved in oil, salami, fermented pork dishes such as '*labh*' and '*nham*' in Thailand, etc.) are the main sources of infection for man. The drying process of infected meat favours the death of larvae, especially if there is an increase in the salt concentration (Pozio *et al.* 1993).

Four species and three phenotypes, each one characterized by a specific geographical distribution, are responsible for the sylvatic cycle among carnivores. Although these 'sylvatic' parasites can infect domestic swine and synanthropic rats, they produce relatively few larvae which survive for only a few months. Consequently, these sylvatic forms cannot be maintained by a 'domestic' cycle (Bandi *et al.* 1993). Moreover, as reported above, *T. spiralis* which has a cosmopolitan distribution overlapping with the other trichinellas, it can also occur in the sylvatic cycle (Murrell *et al.* 1987). This is an important aspect that has to be kept in mind when control programmes are planned. The distribution of 'sylvatic' trichinellas is correlated with the distribution of sylvatic carnivores. The transmission areas of these parasites are reduced by progressive changes of the natural habitat of these hosts. This is a worldwide phenomenon that should be monitored for its influence on the epidemiology of trichinellosis.

In the arctic and subarctic area of the Holoarctic region, sylvatic trichinellosis is due to *T. nativa*. The isotherm −5 °C in January is probably the southern limit of distribution of this nematode. Wolves, foxes, racoon dogs, and bears represent the main reservoirs. The prevalence of infection reaches 80 per cent in foxes in Finland (Oivanen and Oksanen 1994) and 23 per cent in polar bears in Greenland (Henriksen *et al.* 1994). Sledge dogs are frequently infected (62 per cent). Human infections occur in Inuits (Eskimos) and in other people eating wild animals (e.g. hunters). Bear and walrus flesh are the main source of infection for them. Fatal cases are reported. A biological peculiarity of this species is the high resistance of larvae to freezing in muscles of natural hosts for more than 2 years (Pozio *et al.* 1994*a*). Consequently, freezing cannot be considered a method to make meat safe. In Montana and Pennsylvania (USA), sylvatic carnivores can harbour *Trichinella* T6. Human infections are not documented, but they may occur in people eating improperly cooked game food. Muscle larvae of this parasite are less resistant to freezing than *T. nativa* muscle larvae (Pozio *et al.* 1994*a*).

In the temperate areas of the Palaearctic region sylvatic trichinellosis is due to *T. britovi*. The north border of distribution of this parasite is probably the isotherm −6 °C in January. In the area between the isotherms −5° and −6 °C, both *T. britovi* and *T. nativa* have been found. The south border seems to be the Sahara in Africa and has yet to be established in Asia. The fox and the jackal are the principal reservoirs with a prevalence ranging from 1 to 80 per cent, while the prevalence of infection in the wild boar population is less than 0.1 per cent in areas where 20–25 per cent of foxes are infected. Epidemiological surveys in Italy have shown that this *Trichinella* is present in the fox population living more than 500 m above sea-level (m.a.s.l.), while foxes living below 500 m.a.s.l. are *Trichinella*-free, because, whereas cannibalism is a characteristic of the mountain populations, it is unknown behaviour among foxes living on the plains due to access to other food resources (e.g. garbage dumps) (Rossi and Balbo 1994). In Spain, where both *T. britovi* and *T. spiralis* are present, wild boar populations living above 800 m.a.s.l. were found infected with both species, while only *T. spiralis* was identified in wild boar populations living below 800 m.a.s.l. (Serrano *et al.* 1994). Muscle larvae of *T. britovi* can survive freezing in natural host muscles for some months (Pozio *et al.* 1994*a*). Human infections are caused by the consumption of the meat of wild boars, bears, foxes, free-ranging pigs, and horses. Fatal cases are not documented.

In Africa south of the Sahara only sylvatic trichinellosis due to *T. nelsoni* and *Trichinella* T8 has been documented (Pozio *et al.* 1991). The spotted hyaena (*Crocuta crocuta*) plays the principal role as reservoir. The main sources of human infections are the warthog and the bush pig; however, fewer than 100 human infections have been documented in Kenya, Tanzania, Senegal, and Ethiopia, possibly because it is not customary to eat underdone game food and because of religious practices which avoid the parasite–man contact. Fatal cases are reported (Pozio *et al.* 1994*b*).

In the Palaearctic and Australian regions (Tasmania) the non-encapsulating *T. pseudospiralis* can parasitize both mammals and birds. Four species of marsupials, two of carnivora, one of rodentia, three of raptorial birds, and one of omnivorous birds were found naturally infected (Pozio *et al.* 1992*b*). The first human infection, probably acquired in Tasmania, was recently documented (Andrews *et al.* 1994). However, the human risk related to this species appears very low considering the low infectivity of *T. pseudospiralis* for swine.

Black bears, racoons, red foxes, coyotes, and bobcats of temperate areas of North America (USA) frequently harbour *Trichinella* T5 (Snyder *et al.* 1993). Human infections probably occur among people eating game food. There is, however, only one documented human outbreak, involving 431 patients, two of whom died, and this was due to the consumption of horse meat imported from USA into France, in 1985 (Dupouy-Camet 1993).

Since 1975, nine outbreaks involving 2682 patients who ate raw horse meat have been described in France and Italy (Bouree *et al.* 1979; Mantovani *et al.* 1980; Parravicini *et al.* 1986; Ancelle *et al.* 1988; Pozio *et al.* 1988; Beytout *et al.* 1991; Dupouy-Camet *et al.* 1994; Pozio, unpublished data). The aetiological agents were identified in six epidemics as *T. spiralis*, *T. britovi*, and *Trichinella* T5. Horse meat as a source of human infection was established on the basis of epidemiological investigations. Not until recently it have natural infections of horses with *T. spiralis* been discovered in Mexico (M. G. Ortega Pierres and D. S Zarlenga, personal communication), in spite of thousands of animals having been examined. Consequently, *Trichinella* infection in horses has to be considered a rare event. *Trichinella* transmission to the horse appears to arise from the accidental ingestion of a carcass of an infected rodent or small carnivore present on pastureland. It has also been speculated that infection may occur in horses being ready for slaughter with a mash containing carcasses of infected fur animals or pork scraps.

In conclusion, veterinarians and physicians have to consider trichinellosis as an infection that may occur everywhere when improperly cooked meat or raw meat products of uncontrolled animals are consumed.

CONTROL

PRE-SLAUGHTER PREVENTION

The establishment and maintenance of *T. spiralis*-free pig herds is based on the requirement that pigs be prevented from eating uncooked meat whether it is meat scraps, rodents, other wild animals, or dead pig carcasses. Because *Trichinella* is transmitted only through ingestion of meat, interruption of its transmission can be targeted to this unique pathway. However, the farm management level required to accomplish this is frequently difficult to achieve because of entrenched cultural, socio-economic, and historical conditions. However, the elements of an effective preventive pig management programme are:

1. Strict adherence to garbage feeding regulations, particularly cooking requirements (100 °C for 30 minutes).
2. Stringent rodent control.
3. Preventing exposure of pigs to dead animal carcasses, especially pigs, rats.
4. Prompt and proper disposal of dead pig and other animal carcasses (e.g. burial, incineration, or rendering). This minimizes infection risk for commensal wild animals.
5. Construction of effective barriers between pigs, wild animals, and even domestic pets.

The importance of wild animals in the epidemiology and control of synanthropic (domestic) trichinellosis cannot be over emphasized. There is strong, but indirect, evidence that feral dogs and cats, and farm-associated wild animals may serve as important reservoirs of infection of *T. spiralis* and can re-introduce the parasite into a pig herd unless great care is taken to prevent exposure (Dame *et al.* 1987; Murrell *et al.* 1987; Dobey and Murrell 1989; Bessonov 1992).

Public health and veterinary service authorities have sufficient means to establish and maintain continuous surveillance programmes. Such programmes allow identification of infected herds and make it possible to attempt eradication. National-level surveillance can be carried out using slaughter inspection data coupled with trace-backs to farms of origin (Ruitenberg *et al.* 1983; Murrell 1985*b*). In many developed regions (e.g. European Union, Russia, Chile) inspection at slaughter is mandatory. Those countries not requiring inspection for *Trichinella* (e.g. United States) may survey instead by serological surveys using national statistical sampling methods. Excellent serological tests are now available (Madden and Murrell, 1990).

POST-SLAUGHTER CONTROL

Meat inspection has proved to be a very successful strategy for controlling trichinellosis. Government-organized and supervised inspection has been a crucial factor in many regions (e.g. European Union). Inspection currently is performed by either of two direct methods: microscopical examination or muscle sample digestion (Zimmermann 1983). The trichinoscope method utilizes small pieces of the cura of the diaphragm which are compressed between two glass plates and examined under low microscopical power; often a projection screen is used. This method is expensive and labour-intensive and is not standardized worldwide (i.e. number and sizes of pieces to be examined). The practical limit of sensitivity is about three trichinellae larvae per gram of muscle (Ruitenberg and Sluiters 1974). In the United States, where 60–68 per cent of infected animals harbour less than 1 larvae per gram, the microscopical method has serious drawbacks for an eradication strategy (Zimmermann and Zinter 1971; Schad *et al.* 1985).

The digestion method is rapidly supplanting the trichinoscope procedure in most countries where inspection for trichinellae is practised. This method, introduced about 15 years ago, involves the artificial digestion (pepsin–HCl) of diaphragm tissue pooled into batches in order to reduce the number of samples and time required for examination (Zimmermann 1983). Generally, a pool or batch consists of 1 gram samples from 100 animals. Instruments are now employed (e.g. Trichomatic® 35, Stomacher®) to make the process fast and consistent. If, on examination of a pooled digest, trichinae are observed, the infected animal is identified through first digesting repooled tissue samples divided into 20 groups of five and then each samples from the group of five recognized as positive. The digestion method offers considerable economic advantages because of lower labour demands, especially in abattoirs with high throughputs; the cost may be one-tenth that of trichinelloscopy. Important to eradication efforts is the fact that the digestion method has greater sensitivity and reliability, although dead larvae or calcified cysts may be destroyed by digestion. In the United States and in the European Union, all horse meat for human consumption is inspected by the pooled digestion procedure.

More recently, immunological tests have been developed for use in abattoir testing (Ruitenberg *et al.* 1983). An ELISA test using stichosome antigens (Gamble *et al.* 1983) has been tested under modern high volume slaughter house conditions and found to be highly sensitive and practical (Oliver *et al.* 1989). These results have prompted the US Department of Agriculture to promulgate a regulation permitting the use of immunological tests for slaughterhouse inspection (FSIS 1990). This regulation (9 CFR. Ch. III, 318.10f) allows approval of any test that detects at least 98 per cent of swine bearing trichinellae at larval densities equal to or less than one trichinellae per gram of diaphragm pillar muscle at a 95 per cent confidence interval. As improvements continue to be made in instrumentation and procedures, replacement of the trichinelloscope and digestion tests in large volume abattoirs may be expected.

In countries where meat inspection for *Trichinella* is not mandatory, other strategies for reducing consumer risk are followed. In the United States, for example, consumers are advised on proper meat handling procedures (e.g. cooking, freezing, curing) for killing any *Trichinella* present. Cooking to an internal temperature of 60 °C for at least 1 minute is advised. Consumers are also urged to freeze pork at either –15 °C for 20 days, –23 °C for 10 days, or –30 °C for 6 days if the meat is less than 15 cm thick. These temperatures may not be adequate, however, for wild game meat infected with species such as *T. nativa*. The curing of pork sufficient to kill *Trichinella* is difficult to standardize (Lin *et al.* 1990). The process used must be one that has been demonstrated to be effective (FSIS 1990). Commercial production of ready-to-eat pork products is carried out under scrutiny of regulatory agencies to ensure food safety.

A role for food irradiation in the treatment of meat to reduce the risk of food-borne micro-organisms and parasites is receiving serious consideration (Roberts and Murrell 1988, 1993). Gamma irradiation is highly effective for the devitalization of *T. spiralis* larvae in pork (Brake *et al.* 1985). The Food and Drug Administration in the United States has approved low dose irradiation (up to 1.0 kGy) for the treatment of pork to control trichinellosis.

Because wild game are an important source of infection for humans and pigs, all such meat should be considered as suspect and should only be consumed after either inspection by the trichinoscope on digestion methods or after thorough cooking. Many countries have instituted mandatory inspection of wild boars (e.g. Russia, Estonia, Lithuania, Germany). Others provide educational programmes for hunters and consumers of game foods. For example, in the United States, the Montana Department of Fish, Wildlife, and Parks and the Montana State University Extension Service publish and circulate pamphlets to hunters on the dangers of eating improperly cooked bear meat. The Montana State University Veterinary Laboratory also offers free diagnostic services.

There have been few attempts to eradicate *Trichinella* from wild animal populations. It is well recognized that an important factor in the epidemiology of trichinellosis in wild game populations is the habit of hunters leaving the offal and carcasses of game and fur-bearing animals in the forests, where they serve as a source of infection for other animals (Bessonov 1992). Worley *et al.* (1994) has reported success in reducing the incidence of trichinellosis in a wild boar population in New Hampshire (USA). The primary means of control was enforced safe disposal of offal from wild boars taken by hunters. This suggests that transmission of *T. spiralis* in this game park was maintained primarily by scavenging of boars on discarded carcass remnants.

The idea of a vaccine for the control of trichinellosis in domestic swine herds is attractive. A candidate vaccine has been developed (Marti *et al.* 1987), utilizing antigens of the newborn larval stage. This approach could have value for eradication in herds in which the management strategies (discussed above) have not been completely successful. The costs to produce such a vaccine for such limited use, however, may be high.

REFERENCES

Ancelle, T. *et al.* (1988). Two outbreaks of trichinosis caused by horse meat in France in 1985. *American Journal of Epidemiology*, **127**, 1302–11.

Andrews, J. R. H., Ainsworth, R., and Abernethy, D. (1994). *Trichinella pseudospiralis* in humans; description of a case and its treatment. *Transactions of the Royal Society of Tropical Medicine and Hygiene*, **88**, 200–3.

Appelton, J. A., Bell, R. G., Homan, W., and Van Knapen, F. (1991). Consensus on *Trichinella spiralis* antigens and antibodies. *Parasitology Today*, **7**, 190–2.

Au, A. C. S., Ko, R., Simon, J. W., Ridell, N. J., Wong, F. W., and Templer, M. J. (1983). Study of acute trichinosis in Ghurkas; specificity and sensitivity of enzyme-linked immunosorbent assays for IgM, IgE antibodies to *Trichinella* larval antigens in diagnosis. *Transactions of the Royal Society of Tropical Medicine and Hygiene*, **77**, 412–15.

Bandi, C., La Rosa, G., Comincini, S., Damiani, G., and Pozio, E. (1993). Random amplified polymorphic DNA technique for the identification of *Trichinella* species. *Parasitology*, **107**, 419–24.

Beck, W. J. (1970). Trichinosis in domesticated and experimental animals. In *Trichinosis in man and animals* (ed. S. E. Gould), pp. 61–80. Charles C. Thomas, Springfield, Illinois.

Bessonov, A. S. (1992). Trichinellosis in the USSR (1983–1987): Tendency to spreading. *Wiadomosci Parazytologiczne*, **38**, 147–55.

Beytout, I., Mora, M., Laurichesse, H., Cambon, M., and Rey, M. (1991). Emergence en Auvergne d'une épidémie de trichinose. *Bulletin Epidemiologique Hebdamadaire*, **13**, 53.

Bouree, P., Bouvier, J. B., Passeron, J., Galanaud, P., and Dormont, J. (1979). Outbreaks of trichinosis near Paris. *British Medical Journal*, **1**, 1047–9.

Brake, R. J., Murrell, K. D., Ray, E. E., Thomas, J. D., Muggenberg, B. A., and Savinski, S. (1985). Destruction of *Trichinella spiralis* of low dose irradiation of infected pork. *Journal of Food Safety*, **7**, 127–34.

Britov, V. A. and Boev, S. N. (1972). Taxonomic rank of various strains of *Trichinella* and their circulation in nature. *Vestnik Akademii nauk Kazachskoj SSSR*, **28**, 27–32.

Bruschi, F., Tassi, C., and Pozio, E. (1990). Parasite specific antibody response in *Trichinella* sp. 3 human infection: a one year follow-up. *American Journal of Tropical Medicine and Hygiene*, **43**, 186–93.

Campbell, W. C. (1979). History of trichinosis: Paget, Owen and the discovery of *Trichinella spiralis*. *Bulletin of the History of Medicine*, **53**, 520–52.

Campbell, W. C. (ed.) (1983). *Trichinella and trichinosis*. Plenum Press, New York.

Campbell, W. L. and Cuckler, A. C. (1966). Further studies on the effect of thiabendazole on trichinosis in swine, with notes on the biology of the infection. *Journal of Parasitology*, **52**, 260–79.

Dame, J. B., Murrell, K. D., Worley, D. E., and Schad, G. A. (1987). *Trichinella spiralis*: Genetic evidence for synanthropic subspecies in sylvatic hosts. *Experimental Parasitology*, **64**, 195–203.

Despommier, D. D. (1983). Biology, In *Trichinella and trichinosis*, (ed. W. C. Campbell), pp. 75–151. Plenum Press, New York.

Dobey, P. B. and Murrell, K. D. (1989). Illinois Trichinellosis program. In *Trichinellosis*, (ed. C. E. Tanner, A. R. Martinez-Fernandez, and F. Bolas-Fernandez), pp. 432–8. CSIC Press, Madrid, Spain.

Dupouy-Camet, J. (1993). Caractéres parasitologiques, pathogéniques, antigéniques, isoenzymatiques et génomiques de deux isolats de *Trichinella* d'origine équine. These de doctorat de l'Université Paris XII.

Dupouy-Camet, J., Soulé, Cl., and Ancelle, T. (1994). Recent news on trichinellosis: another outbreak due to horsemeat consumption in France in 1993. *Parasite*, **1**, 99–103.

Feldmeier, H., Fischer, H., and Blaumeiser, G. (1987). Kinetics of humoral response during the acute and the convalescent phase of human trichinosis. *Zentralblatt für Bakteriologie, Mikrobiologie und Hygiene*, **A264**, 221–34.

FSIS (1990). *Approval of other tests for trichinosis in pork*. 9 CFR Ch. III (1-1-90 edition). USDA.

Gabriel, B. W. and Justus D. E. (1979). Quantitation of immediate and delayed hypersensitivity responses in *Trichinella*-infected mice. Correlation with worm expulsion *International Archives of Allergy and Applied Immunology*, **60**, 275–85.

Gamble, H. R., Anderson, W. R., Graham, C. E., and Murrell, K. D. (1983). Diagnosis of swine trichinosis by enzyme-linked immunosorbent assay (ELISA) using an excretory-secretory antigen. *Veterinary Parasitology*, **13**, 349–61.

Garkavi, B. L. (1972). Species of *Trichinella* isolated from wild animals. *Veterinary*, **10**, 90–1.

Gould, S. E. (1945). *Trichinosis*. Charles C. Thomas, Illinois.

Grencis, R. K., Hultner, L., and Else, K. J. (1991). Host protective immunity to *Trichinella spiralis* in mice: activation of Th subsets and lymphokine secretion in mice expressing different response phenotypes. *Immunology*, **74**, 329–32.

Hanbury, R. D., Doby, P. B., Miller, H. O., and Murrell, K. D. (1986). Trichinosis in a herd of swine: canibalism as a major mode of transmission. *Journal of the American Veterinary Association*, **188**, 1155–9.

Henriksen, S. A., Born, E. W., and Eiersted, L. (1994). Infections with *Trichinella* in polar bears (*Ursus maritimus*) in Greenland: prevalence according to age and sex. In *Trichinellosis*, (ed. W. C. Campbell, E. Pozio, and F. Bruschi), pp. 565–8. ISS Press, Rome, Italy.

Herndon, F. J. and Kayes, S. G. (1992). Depletion of eosinophils by anti-IL-5 mAb treatment of mice infected with *Trichinella spiralis* does not alter parasite burden of immunological resistance to reinfection. *Journal of Immunology*, **149**, 3642–7.

Kassur, B., Januszkiewicz, J., and Poznanska, H. (1978). Clinic of trichinellosis. In *Trichinellosis*, (ed. C. W. Kim and Z. S. Pawlowski), pp. 27–44. University Press of New England.

Kumar, V., Pozio, E., De Borchgrave, J., Mortelmans, J., and De Meurichy, W. (1990). Characterization of a *Trichinella* isolate from polar bear. *Annales de la Societé Belge de Médecine Tropicale*, **70**, 131–5.

La Rosa, G., Pozio, E., Barrat, J., and Blancou, J. (1991). Identification of sylvatic *Trichinella* (T3) in foxes from France. *Veterinary Parasitology*, **40**, 113–17.

Leiby, D. A., Schad, G. A., Duffy, C. H., and Murrell, K. D. (1988). *Trichinella spiralis* in an agricultural ecosystem. III. Epidemiological investigations of *Trichinella spiralis* in resident wild and feral animals. *Journal of Wildlife Diseases*, **24**, 606–9.

Leidy, J. (1846). Remarks on trichina. *Proceedings of the Academy of Natural Sciences of Philadelphia*, **3**, 107–8.

Lin, K. W. *et al.* (1990). Bioassay analysis of dry-cured ham processed to affect *Trichinella spiralis*. *Journal of Food Science*, **55**, 289–97.

Ljungström, I. (1974). Antibody response to *Trichinella spiralis*. In *Trichinosis*, (ed. C. W. Kim), pp. 449–60. Intext Educational, New York.

Ljungström, I. (1983). Immunodiagnosis in Man. In *Trichinella and trichinosis*, (ed. W. C. Campbell), pp. 403–4. Plenum Press, New York.

Ljungström, I., Hammarström, L., Kociecka, W., and Smith, C. I. E. (1988a). The response of IgE subclasses and IgE during early and late stages of human *Trichinella spiralis* infection. In *Trichinosis*, (ed. C. E. Tanner, A. R. Martinez-Fernandez, and F. Bolas-Fernandez), pp. 210–17. CSIC Press, Madrid, Spain.

Ljungström, I., Hammarström, L., Kociecka, W., and Smith, C. I. E. (1988b). The sequential appearance of IgG subclasses and IgE during the course of *Trichinella spiralis* infection. *Clinical Experimental Immunology*, **74**, 230–5.

MacLean, J. M. D., Viallet, J., Law, C., and Staudt, M. (1989). Trichinosis in the Canadian Arctic: report of five outbreaks and a new clinical syndrome. *Journal of Infectious Diseases*, **160**, 513–20.

Madden, K. B. and Murrell, K. D. (1990). Immunodiagnosis of nematode infections and prospects for vaccination with special references to *Trichinella spiralis*. *Review Science and Technical Office of International Epizootiology*, **9**, 519–32.

Madden, K. B., Murrell, K. D., and Lunney, J. K. (1990). Trichinella spiralis: major histocompatibility complex-associated elimination of encysted muscle larvae in swine. *Experimental Parasitology*, **70**, 443–51.

Mantovani, A., Filippini, I., and Bergomi, S. (1980). Indagini su un'epidemia di trichinellosi umana verificatasi in Italia. *Parassitologia*, **22**, 107–34.

Marti, H. P. and Murrell, K. D. (1986). Trichinella spiralis: Anti-fecundity and anti-newborn larvae immunity in swine. *Experimental Parasitology*, **62**, 370–5.

Marti, H. P., Murrell, K. D., and Gamble, H. R. (1987). *Trichinella spiralis*: Immunization of pigs with newborn larvae antigens. *Experimental Parasitology*, **63**, 68–73.

Murrell, K. D. (1985a). *Trichinella spiralis*: acquired immunity in swine. *Experimental Parasitology*, **59**, 347–54.

Murrell, K. D. (1985b). Strategies for the control of human trichinosis transmitted by pork. *Food Technology*, **39**, 65–8 and 110–11.

Murrell, K. D. (1994). Beef as a source of trichinellosis. *Parasitology Today*, **10**, 434.

Murrell, K. D., Fayer, R., and Dubey, J. P. (1986). Parasitic organisms. *Advances in Meat Research*, **2**, 311–77.

Murrell, K. D., Stringfellow, F., Dame, J. B., Leiby, D. A., Duffy, C., and Schad, G. A. (1987). *Trichinella spiralis* in an agricultural ecosystem. II. Evidence for natural transmission of *Trichinella spiralis spiralis* from domestic swine to wildlife. *Journal of Parasitology*, **73**, 103–9.

Oivanen, L. and Oksanen, A. (1994). Trichinellosis in domestic swine and wildlife in Finland. In *Trichinellosis* (ed. W. C. Campbell, E. Pozio and F. Bruschi), pp. 569–74. ISS Press, Rome, Italy.

Olaison, L. and Ljungström, I. (1992). An outbreak of trichinosis in Lebanon. *Transactions of the Royal Society of Tropical Medicine and Hygiene*, **86**, 658–60.

Oliver, D. G., Singh, P., Allison, D. E., Murrell, K. D., and Gamble, H. R. (1989). Field evaluation of an enzyme immunoassay for detection of trichinellosis in hogs in a high volume North Carolina abattoir. In *Trichinellosis*, (ed. C. E. Tanner, A. R. Martinez-Fernandez, and F. Bolas-Fernandez), pp. 439–44. CSIC Press, Madrid, Spain.

Olsen, B. S., Villella, J. B., and Gould, S. E. (1964). Distribution of *Trichinella spiralis* in muscles of experimentally infected swine. *Journal of Parasitology*, **50**, 489–95.

Owen, R. (1835). Description of a microscopic enteozoon infecting the muscles of the human body. *Transactions of the Zoological Society of London*, **1**, 315–24.

Parravicini, M., Grampa, A., Salmini, G., Parravicini, V., Dietz, A., and Montanari, M. (1986). Focolaio epidemico di trichinosi da carne di cavallo. *Giornale di Malattie Infettive e Parassitarie*, **38**, 482–7.

Philipp, M., Taylor, P. M., Parkhous, R. M. E., and Ogilvie, B. M. (1981). Immune response to stage-specific surface-antigens of the parasitic nematode *Trichinella spiralis*. *Journal of Experimental Medicine*, **154**, 210–15.

Pozio, E., Cappelli, O., Marchesi, L., Valeri, P., and Rossi P. (1988). Third outbreak of trichinellosis caused by consumption of horse meat in Italy. *Annales de Parasitologie Humaine et Comparée*, **63**, 48–53.

Pozio, E., La Rosa, G., and Rossi P. (1989). *Trichinella* Reference Centre. *Parasitology Today*, **5**, 169–70.

Pozio, E., La Rosa, G., and Verster, A. (1991). Identification by isoenzyme patterns of two gene pools of *Trichinella nelsoni* in Africa. *Annals of Tropical Medicine and Parasitology*, **85**, 281–3.

Pozio, E., La Rosa, G., Rossi, P., and Murrell, K. D. (1992a). Biological characterizations of *Trichinella* isolates from various host species and geographic regions. *Journal of Parasitology*, **78**, 647–53.

Pozio, E., Shaikenov, B., La Rosa, G., and Obendorf, D. L. (1992b). Allozymic and biological characters of *Trichinella pseudospiralis* isolates from free-ranging animals. *Journal of Parasitology*, **78**, 1087–90.

Pozio, E., La Rosa, G., Murell, K. D., and Lichtenfels, J. R. (1992c). Taxonomic revision of the genus *Trichinella*. *Journal of Parasitology*, **78**, 654–9.

Pozio, E., Varese, P., Gomez Morales, M. A., Croppo, G. P., Pelliccia, D., and Bruschi, F. (1993). Comparison of human trichinellosis caused by *Trichinella spiralis* and by *Trichinella britovi*. *American Journal of Tropical Medicine and Hygiene*, **48**, 568–75.

Pozio, E., La Rosa, G., and Amati, M. (1994a). Factors influencing the resistance of *Trichinella* muscle larvae to freezing. In *Trichinellosis*, (ed. W. C. Campbell, E. Pozio, and F. Bruschi), pp. 173–8. ISS Press, Rome, Italy,

Pozio, E., Verster, A., Braack, L., De Meneghi, D., and La Rosa, G. (1994b). Trichinellosis south of the Sahara. In *Trichinellosis*, (ed. W. C. Campbell, E. Pozio, and F. Bruschi), pp. 527–32. ISS Press, Rome, Italy.

Railliet, A. (1896). Quelques rectifications a la nomenclature des parasites. *Recueil de Medicine Veterinaire*, **3**, 157–61.

Roberts, T. and Murrell, K. D. (1988). Foodborne disease in Africa and irradiation as a potential control technique. *Proceedings of Seminar on Food Irradiation for Developing Countries in Africa*, IAEA-TECDOC-576, pp. 145–50. International Atomic Energy Agency, Vienna.

Roberts, T. and Murrell, K. D. (1993). Economic losses caused by foodborne parasitic diseases. *Proceedings of a symposium on Cost-Benefit Aspects of Food Irradiation Processing*, IAEA-SM-328/60, pp. 51–75. International Atomic Energy Agency, Vienna.

Rossi, L. and Balbo, T. (1994). Habitat related differences in the prevalence of vulpine trichinellosis in NW Italy. In *Trichinellosis*, (ed. W. C. Campbell, E. Pozio, and F. Bruschi), pp. 575–80. ISS Press, Rome, Italy.

Ruitenberg, E. J. and Kampelmacher, E. H. (1970). Diagnostische Methoden zur Feststellung der Invasion mit *Trichinella spiralis*. *Fleischwirtschaft*, **50**, 42–44, 47.

Ruitenberg, E. J. and Sluiters, J. F. (1974). *Trichinella spiralis* infection in the Netherlands. In *Trichinellosis* (ed. C. W. Kim), pp. 539–48. Intext, New York.

Ruitenberg, E. J., Van Knapen, F., and Elgersma, A. (1983). Incidence and control of *Trichinella spiralis* throughout the world. *Food Technology*, **37**, 98–100.

Schad, G. A., Kelly, M., Leiby, D. A., Blumrick, K., Duffy, C., and Murrell, K. D. (1985). Swine trichinosis in Mid-Atlantic slaughterhouses: Possible relationships to hog marketing systems. *Preventive Veterinary Medicine*, **3**, 391–4.

Schad, G. A., Duffy, C. H., Leiby, D. A., Murrell, K. D., and Zirkle, E. W. (1987). *Trichinella spiralis* in an agricultural ecosystem: transmission under natural and experimentally modified on-farm conditions. *Journal of Parasitology*, **73**, 95–102.

Schwartz, B. (1937). *Annual Report of Bureau of Animal Industry*, pp. 60–61. Washington.

Schwartz, B. (1938). Trichinosis in swine and its relationship to public health. *Journal of the American Veterinary Medical Association*, **92**, 317–37.

Serrano, F. et al. (1994). Relationship between habitat and *Trichinella* species. In *Trichinellosis*, (ed. W. C. Campbell, E. Pozio, and F. Bruschi), pp. 549–54. ISS Press, Rome.

Snyder, D. E., Zarlenga, D. S., La Rosa, G., and Pozio, E. (1993). Biochemical, biological, and genetic characterization of a sylvatic isolate of *Trichinella*. *Journal of Parasitology*, **79**, 347–52.

Soule, C. et al. (1989). Experimental trichinosis in horses: Biological and parasitological evaluation. *Veterinary Parasitology*, **31**, 19–36.

Van Knapen, F., Franchimont, J. H., Verdonk, A. R., Stumpf, J., and Undeutsch, K. (1982). Detection of specific immunoglobulins (IgG, IgM, IgA, IgE) and total IgE levels in human trichinosis by means of the enzyme-linked immunosorbent assay. *American Journal of Tropical Medicine and Hygiene*, **31**, 973–76.

Virchow, R. (1859). Recherches sur le developpement du *Trichina spiralis. Comptes Rendus des Seances de l'Academie des Sciences*, **49**, 660–62.

Wassom, D. L., Wisniewski, N., McNell, M., and Grieve R. B. (1994). Immunodiagnosis of *Trichinella* infection: Use of unique carbohydrate epitopes as target antigens. In *Trichinellosis*, (ed. W. C. Campbell, E. Pozio, and F. Bruschi), pp. 295–8. ISS Press, Rome, Italy.

Weatherly, N. F. (1983). Anatomical pathology. In *Trichinella and Trichinosis*, (ed. W. C. Campbell), pp. 173–208. Plenum Press, New York.

Worley, D. E., Seesee, F. M., Zarlenga, D. S., and Murrell, K. D. (1994). Attempts to eradicate trichinellosis from a wild boar population in a private game park (USA). In *Trichinellosis*, (ed. W. C. Campbell, E. Pozio, and F. Bruschi), pp. 611–16. ISS Press, Rome, Italy.

Zenker, F. A. (1860). Über die Trichinen-Krankheit des Menschen. *Virchows Archiv für Pathoiogische Anatomie und Physiologie und für Klinische Medizin*, **188**, 561–72.

Zimmermann, W. J. (1983). Surveillances in swine and other animals by muscle examination. In *Trichinella and Trichinosis*, (ed. W. C. Campbell), pp. 515–28. Plenum Press, New York.

Zimmermann, W. J. and Zinter, D. E. (1971). The prevalence of trichinosis in swine in the United States, 1966–1970. *HSMHA Health Reports*, **86**, 937–45.

61 ZOONOTIC HOOKWORM INFECTIONS (ANCYLOSTOMOSIS)

Paul Prociv

SUMMARY

Hookworms are host-specific nematodes of the family Ancylostomatidae, comprising 18 genera that parasitize a wide range of mammals. The common zoonotic species, however, all belong to the genus *Ancylostoma*, and occur in peridomestic animals.

In the definitive host, they attach to and feed on the intestinal mucosa. Some species cause blood loss. Eggs passed in host faeces embryonate in the soil. The third-stage larva infects the next host, either by skin contact or following ingestion. The relative importance to the life cycle of these two routes, or of paratenic hosts, is unknown. Larvae of some species also become hypobiotic in the definitive host, being reactivated by endogenous or host stimuli. This underlies transmammary transmission in at least one species.

Recognized clinical manifestations of human infection involve the skin, intestine, and blood. The most widely distributed hookworm is *Ancylostoma caninum*, a common parasite of dogs that is able to develop in the human gut, sometimes provoking eosinophilic enteritis. *Ancylostoma braziliense*, found in dogs and cats in the tropics, causes human creeping eruption, the most commonly recognized form of cutaneous *larva migrans*. A very close relative, *A. ceylanicum*, can complete its life cycle in humans, to cause abdominal symptoms and anaemia. Little is known about the feline hookworm, *A. tubaeforme*, which might be incapable of infecting people. Rare case reports of infections with other species are not of public health concern. The cold-climate parasite of dogs, *Uncinaria stenocephala*, has been shown only experimentally to cause human skin lesions.

Hookworm infections in their normal hosts respond readily to anthelminthic treatment. Clinical manifestations in people also respond to available therapy. However, human infection can be prevented only by individual hygiene; it is unrealistic to control the parasites in their reservoir hosts.

HISTORY

THE PARASITES

The anthropophilic hookworms, *Ancylostoma duodenale* and *Necator americanus*, are included here because they feature prominently in the major discoveries relating to hookworm infections (Looss 1905, 1911; Grove 1990) and share many characteristics with the zoonotic species (Anderson 1992).

The first recorded description of a hookworm was that of the genus *Uncinaria*, from a fox, by Fröhlich in 1789. In 1800, Zeder described *Strongylus tubaeformis* (now *Ancylostoma tubaeforme*) from a cat in 1783 (Biocca 1954). In 1859, Ercolani published a description of *A. caninum* (as *Strongylus caninum*) and, for the next 100 years, hookworms from both dogs and cats were referred to simply as *A. caninum* (Burrows 1962). Dubini first described *A. duodenale* in 1838, from a human autopsy in Milan. While it had been suspected for many years that at least two species occurred in the human gut, it was not until 1902 that Stiles in the United States distinguished *N. americanus*.

Looss (1905), working in Egypt, described in meticulous detail the anatomy of *A. duodenale*, and reasoned that the ancient Egyptians would not have been aware of hookworms. *Ancylostoma braziliense* was first described in 1910, by Gomes de Faria, from dogs and cats in Brazil. The following year, Looss described *A. ceylanicum* from a civet cat in Ceylon and, in 1913, this species was reported from prisoners in India. However, its subsequent confusion with *A. braziliense* invalidated all later reports of *A. braziliense* from the human gut (Yoshida 1971*a*). The separation of *A. braziliense* and *A. ceylanicum* by Biocca (1951) was not widely recognized until the matter was resolved by cross-breeding experiments (Rep *et al.* 1968), and more detailed work by Yoshida *et al.* (1974). Biocca (1954) also redescribed *A. caninum* and *A. tubaeforme*, confirming them to be distinct species. Burrows (1962) distinguished even further details, to conclude that *A. caninum* occurs only in dogs, and *A. tubaeforme* in cats.

THE LIFE CYCLES

In 1866, Leuckart described the hatching and moulting of *Uncinaria stenocephala* larvae, and infected dogs by giving them larvae in drinking water. Twenty years later, Leichtenstern showed that humans also could be infected by swallowing larvae of *A. duodenale* (Looss 1905).

Looss confirmed the host specificity of *A. duodenale* in 1897, when he fed third-stage larvae (L3) to dogs, cats, and monkeys, and recovered only a few infertile, adult worms from several young animals. Shortly afterwards, accidental self-infection led him to report skin invasion by *A. duodenale* L3 (provoking widespread scepticism) which, as he was able to show in 1902, penetrated hair follicles. In dogs, he then traced the passage of *A. caninum* larvae through lymphatics, blood vessels, lungs, and trachea to the gastrointestinal tract (Looss 1911). Lambinet, in 1905, reported that patent infections in dogs followed oral, subcutaneous, or percutaneous inoculation of L3, with the last route being least efficient (Grove 1990).

Goodey (1925*a*) found that *Uncinaria stenocephala* L3 also penetrate mouse skin, retaining their loose outer sheaths in the process (Goodey 1925*b*). Yokogawa and Oiso (1926) determined that *A. caninum* L3 given by mouth to dogs developed predominantly in the intestine, with very few undergoing tracheal migration, while in rabbits and guinea-pigs fed by mouth, larvae invaded the circulation to pass through the lungs. In 1931, Nakajima reported that L3 migrated into the muscles of rodents, without developing further (Behnke 1990).

Dove (1932) showed that L3 of *A. braziliense* could survive at room temperature for 4 months, and infect both dogs and cats after either oral or percutaneous administration, with a prepatent period of 13–27 days. The oral route was more effective, and dogs seemed more susceptible to infection. A monkey infected percutanously developed itchy skin nodules, with a cough that persisted from 2 to 5 days after exposure. To penetrate human skin, larvae required warmth, humidity, and a surface film of water. Schwartz and Alicata (1934) found that *A. caninum* larvae in guinea-pig lungs had not developed beyond the L3, whereas in dogs 4 days after infection, L4 were already in the gut. This confirmed that pulmonary migration was not necessary for development. Around this time, Maplestone (1933) in India reported that *A. ceylanicum* (mistakenly called *A. braziliense*) infected humans through the skin.

Adler and Clark, in 1922, described what they interpreted as intrauterine acquisition of *A. caninum* by neonatal pups and, for the next 50 years, this mechanism was presumed to account for all maternally transmitted helminthic infections (Miller 1971). The transmammary route was discovered by Olsen and Lyons (1965), working on the life cycle of *Uncinaria lucasi* Stiles, 1901, a hookworm of northern fur seals. Shortly afterwards, a similar path was demonstrated for *A. caninum*, by Enigk and Stoye in Germany and Stone and Girardeau in the United States (Miller 1971). A tissue depot of arrested larvae would seem essential to this route, and Lee *et al.* (1975) were the first to recognize *A. caninum* larvae in canine skeletal muscle. They also demonstrated L3 inside individual muscle fibres of mice, cats, and monkeys, but did acknowledge that Inatome had originally observed this, in mice, in 1932. Earlier reports of *A. caninum* hypobiosis in dogs referred only to larval arrest in the intestine, first recognized by Scott in 1928 (Scott 1930; Behnke 1990). In 1973, Schad *et al.* presented evidence that arrested larval development probably also occurred in humans infected with *A. duodenale.*

THE DISEASES

Cutaneous *larva migrans*

Cutaneous lesions were the first-recognized clinical manifestations of zoonotic hookworm infections. In England, in 1874, Lee coined the term, 'creeping eruption', for advancing, serpiginous skin lesions (Lee 1884) which later were attributed to larvae of the bot-fly, *Gasterophilus* (Tamura 1921). Crocker, in 1892, named the aetiological agent *larva migrans*, a label that was soon being used for the actual lesions (Radcliffe-Crocker 1907). Only after Beaver *et al.* (1952) proposed the term, 'visceral *larva migrans*,' for human-toxocarosis did the skin lesions of larval helminthosis need to be distinguished as 'cutaneous.'

In 1902, Bentley, in India, described ground itch caused by skin-penetrating *A. duodenale* larvae, and distinguished it from creeping eruption. Shortly afterwards, Smith (1904) in the United States found that *N. americanus* also caused ground itch. According to Tamura (1921), van Harlingen in the United States was the first to describe creeping eruption attributed to zoonotic hookworms, in 1902. Tamura discerned several clinical patterns of the disease, indicating diverse causal agents, and reported a distinct form in Japan, resulting from larval *Gnathostoma* infection. This parasite was known to cause human skin nodules in Thailand, but had not been incriminated previously in creeping disease.

In Florida, Kirby-Smith diagnosed 2500 cases of creeping eruption, over 15 years which he distinguished from ground itch caused by *N. americanus*. Most of 300 patients seen in Jacksonville in the summer of 1924 were children who had been exposed at beaches above the tidal zone, but the heaviest infections were seen in adults in contact with damp soil (Kirby-Smith *et al.* 1926). Serial sections of 48 excised lesions revealed five nematode larvae, probably strongle, in the epidermis and hair follicles; one measured 550×20 μm. The disease was acquired in warm, humid conditions, and was not associated with *N. americanus* infection. The authors speculated that hypersensitivity explained individual variation in susceptibility, and that the infection reservoir was in small, peridomestic animals, such as rats, dogs, cats, or chickens. White and Dove (1928) clearly implicated exposure to soil contaminated by dog and cat faeces which, when cultured, yielded nematode larvae that produced skin lesions in human volunteers. From autopsied dogs and cats, they recovered *A. braziliense* and smaller numbers of *A. caninum*, finding that L3 of the former caused classical creeping eruption in humans, while *A. caninum* larvae produced only transient papules of the ground itch pattern.

Shelmire (1928) reconfirmed the differences in cutaneous pathogenicity between these species, as did Heydon (1929), who surmised that the 'sandworm' reported from Australia and South Africa was identical to American creeping eruption. Experimentally exposed dogs and cats developed 'ground itch' rather than linear skin lesions (Dove 1932). In the meantime, Fülleborn in 1927 had infected himself with L3 of *Uncinaria stenocephala* to show that this species could also cause human cutaneous lesions (Grove 1990). Maplestone (1933) suspected geographic variation in *A. braziliense*, because creeping disease was not seen in India, where the local strain caused patent human intestinal infection (see above).

Hunter and Worth (1945) exposed two volunteers to high numbers (1000–1500) of *A. caninum* larvae. One developed numerous, static papules associated with oedema and urticaria, whereas the other, who had a history of allergies, also had short, migratory lesions, which recurred with oedema over 6 months. Wright and Gold (1946) diagnosed Löffler's syndrome (respiratory symptoms, blood eosinophilia and transient, radiological pulmonary opacities) in 26 of 76 patients with creeping eruption. Although unable to detect patent infection or larvae in sputum, they suspected that either migrating larvae or a systemic allergic response accounted for the lung involvement. Then, Muhleisen (1953) identified hookworm larvae in a patient's sputum, from 12 to 36 days after heavy exposure to soil contaminated with dog faeces. While the species was indeterminate, the limited migrations of the skin lesions suggested *A. caninum*.

Anaemia

The implication of hookworm infection in human anaemia was a remarkably tortuous process (Roche and Layrisse 1966; Grove 1990). Subsequently, only one zoonotic species, *A. ceylanicum*, has been incriminated aetiologically.

Wells (1931) was the first to measure blood lost to hookworms, estimating 0.84 ml/worm/day for dogs infected with *A. caninum* (a figure substantially reduced by later workers). Rep (1966) calculated a corresponding loss of 0.014 ml in prepatent *A. ceylanicum* infections. Anten and Zuidema (1964) reported anaemia in Dutch marines heavily infected with *A. ceylanicum* (then thought to be *A. braziliense*) from West New Guinea, finding the species in 9 of 11 men. In total, these patients produced 111 *N. americanus* and 665 specimens of *A. ceylanicum* after treatment (none recalled having skin rashes). Wijers and Smit (1966) then demonstrated that experimental *A. ceylanicum* infection in humans caused severe gastrointestinal symptoms, which was later confirmed by Carroll and Grove (1986).

Eosinophilic enteritis

In 1988, Croese found what he suspected to be a single adult *A. caninum* in one patient among a series of 33 with eosinophilic enteritis from Townsville, in northeastern Australia. Shortly afterwards, he retrieved by colonoscopy an adult *A. caninum* from another patient with the disease (Prociv and Croese 1990). Subsequently, most Australian patients with eosinophilic enteritis were shown to have circulating antibodies to excretory–secretory antigens of adult *A. caninum* (Loukas *et al.* 1992). To date, solitary adult hookworms have been found in 15 patients from the state of Queensland, and serological testing indicates that infection, both clinical and subclinical, is very common (Croese *et al.* 1994a,b). Sporadic human intestinal infections with adult *A. caninum* have been reported previously (Beaver *et al.* 1984), but in obscure publications and without attribution of any clinical significance.

Pathogenesis

For a long time, hookworm secretions have been suspected to play a major role in the pathogenesis of infection. Looss (1905) believed that adult worms fed on the intestinal mucosa rather than blood, and that oesophageal and cephalic gland products helped digest host tissues. The anticoagulant effect of *A. caninum* secretions was already known in 1903, but more than 50 years were to pass before it was localized to the amphidial glands (Thorson 1956b) and subsequently ascribed to a protein of molecular weight 20–50 kDa (Eiff 1966). Thorson (1956a,b) also found that immune dog serum inhibited hookworm oesophageal proteases (but not the anticoagulant activity), and was able to partially immunize pups against *A. caninum* infection with hookworm oesophageal extracts (Thorson 1956*c*). The first specific enzymatic activity found in hookworm L3 was a collagenolytic/gelatinolytic protease from *A. caninum* (Lewert and Lee 1954). Hotez and Cerami (1983) demonstrated elastinolytic as well as anticoagulant properties in a 36 kDa protease, secreted by adult *A. caninum* and also present in homogenates of this species and *A. duodenale*. Carroll *et al.* (1984) detected anticoagulant activity within attachment-sites of *A. ceylanicum* in dog intestinal mucosa. Subsequently, the analysis of secretory products from the common hookworm species has progressed considerably (see pp. 537–38). The major diagnostic antigen in human *A. caninum*-associated enteritis appears to be a 68 kDa protease (Loukas *et al.* 1994).

THE AGENTS

GENERAL DESCRIPTION AND CLASSIFICATION

The order Strongylida comprises four superfamilies of bursate nematodes: Strongyloidea, Trichostrongyloidea, Metastrongyloidea, and Ancylostomatoidea (Beaver *et al.* 1984). Hookworms comprise the last group, which has only a single family (Anderson 1992), Ancylostomatidae. Their name derives not from the hook-like buccal teeth, but from the dorsal bend in the anterior body that enables 'hooking' on to the intestinal mucosa. They are small to medium-sized and thick-bodied, with large, subglobular buccal capsules bearing cutting plates or teeth, but no corona radiata. The male copulatory bursa is symmetrical, comprising a median and lateral lobes, reinforced by seven pairs of rays: two dorsal, three lateral, and two ventral.

The group is divided into two subfamilies, Ancylostomatinae and Bunostominae (Lichtenfels 1980), and classified according to the structure of the buccal capsule, the male copulatory bursa, and the female tail. The Ancylostomatinae, which include the genera *Ancylostoma* and *Uncinaria*, possess a dorsal gutter in the buccal capsule, a dorsal bursal ray with a single main stem for most of its length and a shallow median fissure, a gubernaculum in males, a terminal spine on the female tail, and the vulva in the posterior half of the body. The Bunostominae, which include *Necator* and *Bunostomum*, have a tooth-like dorsal cone supporting the duct of the dorsal oesophageal gland, a dorsal bursal ray usually with two long stems, no gubernaculum in the male or spine on the female tail, and vulva in the anterior half of the body.

While there are 18 genera in the family Ancylostomatidae, all the important zoonotic hookworms belong to the genus *Ancylostoma*. They have a deep buccal capsule with one to three pairs of teeth at the ventro-lateral margin, a notch on the dorsal margin

and two triangular lancets, or dorsal teeth, at the opening of the dorsal oesophageal gland. In females, the vulva is in the posterior third of the body. In the male bursa, the ventral ray is cleft, the dorsal is bifurcate, and each branch is tridigitate. The lateral rays arise from a common trunk, and the externodorsal ray may arise from a common trunk with the dorsal ray. The spicules are equal, and a gubernaculum is present.

HOST RANGE

Hookworms inhabit the small intestines of placental mammals (with one exception, a South American opossum) and generally have a high degree of host specificity. The Ancylostomatinae comprise eight genera which occur in carnivores and omnivores, whereas the 10 genera in the Bunostominae parasitize omnivores and herbivores. They probably evolved with early omnivorous mammals in the Cretaceous period and blossomed with the mammals in the Eocene (Lichtenfels 1980). The genus *Ancylostoma* parasitizes a wide range of hosts, but most species occur in the Carnivora, with secondary colonizers developing in lemurs, primates, edentates, and the aardvark.

ZOONOTIC SPECIES

Human infections have been confirmed with only a small number of zoonotic hookworms that, not surprisingly, parasitize animals closely associated with people. Third-stage larvae of other species may also be able to infect humans, but have little opportunity because of their remote habitats. Only the common species are described here.

Ancylostoma caninum (Ercolani, 1859) Hall, 1913

This is the most widespread and best studied hookworm species. Its relatively stout body narrows gradually anteriorly. Females reach 14–20 mm in length by 0.50–0.56 mm in width, and males 11–13 mm by 0.35–0.40 mm. Living specimens are cream to grey in colour, streaked with red according to the amount of blood ingested. Fixed specimens curve dorsally, with a sharper bend anteriorly, so the mouth faces anterodorsally. The most obvious characteristic, three ventral teeth along the anterior margin of each denticular plate, immediately distinguishes this species from the otherwise almost identical human parasite, *A. duodenale*. Inside the buccal capsule, the dorsal gutter ends in a deep median cleft along the dorsal margin. Pairs of inconspicuous, triangular dorsal and centrolateral teeth occur deep in the cavity. On each side of the stoma, ventrolaterally, are the amphidial (formerly cephalic) gland openings. Internally, the club-shaped, cuticle-lined, tri-radiate oesophagus (or pharynx) extends back from the buccal capsule for about 8 per cent of the body length, to join the intestine through a valvular structure. Each of the three oesophageal segments (one dorsal and two subventral) consists of muscle tissue encapsulating an extensive, single-celled gland. The dorsal gland drains into the dorsal gutter of the buccal capsule, while the subventrals open into the anterior oesophageal lumen. The large, bilateral, single-celled amphidial glands extend posteriorly on each side of the pseudocoelom for 60 per cent of the body length, being most conspicuous in the anterior third. The ultrastructure of *Ancylostoma* has not been examined, but is likely to resemble that of *N. americanus*, where each gland opens anteriorly into the amphidial ampulla, its secretions flowing over the ciliated endings of the amphidial nerves (McLaren 1974). Behind these glands, the genital tract is also clearly visible through the tough cuticle, obscuring most other internal structures. Ventrally, the two single-celled excretory (formerly cervical) glands extend posteriad, from the excretory pore in the midline just behind the nerve-ring, for about 25 per cent of the body length, in intimate association with each lateral hypodermal cord. Glands and oesophagus are held together by a 'mesentery' of connecting membranes. In the female, the tail is conoid and the vulva opens in the ventral midline about one-third the body length from the anus. The amphidelphic reproductive system extends symmetrically posteriorly and anteriorly from the vulva, and the white, thick uteri are clearly discernible among ovarian and tubular coils. In the mid-body of the male is a conspicuous seminal vesicle, located between the single, coiled testis anteriorly and the straight, conspicuous, muscular ejaculatory duct (formerly, prostatic gland) posteriorly, ventral to the intestine. The genital canal continues between a pair of cement glands to open into the cloaca. Extending anteriorly from the cloaca are two, bristle-like, copulatory spicules, controlled by a dorsal gubernaculum, and retractor and extensor muscles. The spicules are 0.73–0.96 mm long (similar to *A. duodenale*, but significantly shorter than in *A. tubaeforme*.) The cloaca opens into the campanulate bursa, which is well developed and supported by fleshy rays in a pattern characteristic of the species. Eggs are 56–75 μm long by 34–47 μm wide, and contain 4–8 cells when freshly passed in faeces.

Ancylostoma tubaeforme (Zeder, 1800) Biocca, 1954

This species is almost identical with *A. caninum*, but slightly smaller (Biocca 1954; Burrows 1962). Females attain 12–15 mm in length by 0.38–0.43 mm in width, and males 9.5–11 mm by 0.30–0.35 mm. In fixed speci-

mens, the mouth turns more dorsad than in *A. caninum*. The three pairs of ventral teeth on the anterior margin of the buccal capsule, and the deep 'oesophageal' teeth, are proportionally larger, and the oesophagus shorter, than in *A. caninum*, but these are not a strong differential features. More distinct is the thicker cuticle of *A. tubaeforme*, at all levels of the body (Burrows 1962). The male bursa is very similar to but slightly smaller than that of *A. caninum*, while the spicules are 50 per cent longer, at 1.10–1.47 mm Eggs of both species are identical.

Ancylostoma braziliense Gomes de Faria, 1910

This species is noticeably smaller than the above two, and is even smaller (by about 20 per cent) in cats than in dogs (Norris 1971a). Heat-fixed female worms bend sharply at the level of the vulva, which distinguishes them from *A. ceylanicum* (Yoshida 1971a). In dogs, females grow to 8.9–10.5 mm by 0.31–0.39 mm, and males 7.1–8.1 mm by 0.25–0.31 mm. In cats, the corresponding dimensions are 6.1–10.6 by 0.18–0.32, and 4.2–7.2 by 0.16–0.24 mm. In the buccal capsule, the prominent anterior edge of each lateral denticular plate bears a minute, inward-pointing, ventral and a large, dorsal-pointing, lateral tooth. The oesophagus is 9–10 per cent of the body length. Spicules in the male are 0.69–1.02 mm long in cats, and 0.85–1.10 mm in dogs.

Ancylostoma ceylanicum (Looss, 1911) Leiper, 1915

This species is almost identical with *A. braziliense* (Biocca 1951). Chief distinguishing features (Yoshida 1971a) are the non-bent fixed females of *A. ceylanicum*, the pattern of copulatory bursal rays in males, and the cuticular striations, which are markedly wider in *A. ceylanicum* at all levels of the body in both sexes. The average distance between striations in the anterior part of *A. braziliense* is 5.1–5.4 μm (males–females) cf. 7.7–8.6 μm in *A. ceylanicum* and, near the tail, 4.6–5.3 μm cf. 8.4–9.8 μm, respectively. Striation intervals are not affected by the method of fixation, nor do they overlap between the two species.

Unusual records

Necator suillus Ackert and Payne, 1922, found in Trinidad and Central America, is a porcine hookworm very similar to *N. americanus*. While the latter does not develop in pigs, it probably evolved from *N. suillus* (Schad 1991) and its L3 can invade pig skin to cause ground itch (Ackert and Payne 1923). Buckley (1933) cultured eggs from adult *N. suillus* and infected himself percutaneously. Lesions developed at the entry site and, 54 days later, hookworm eggs appeared in his stools. Infection remained patent for four months, until treatment with oil of chenopodium expelled three adult *N. suillus*. He did not report abdominal symptoms, but speculated that this species may account for some presumed *N. americanus* infections in people living close to pigs.

Cyclodontostomum purvisi (Adams, 1933) is a parasite of the large intestine of rats in South-East Asia. Two adult specimens, a male and female, were found incidentally in the faeces of a 47-year-old man in Thailand (Bhaibulaya and Indrangarm 1975). No clinical significance could be attached to this case.

Ancylostoma malayanum (Alessandrini, 1905) infects bears in India and South-East Asia, and has a buccal capsule like that of *A. duodenale*. It is the largest member of the genus, with males growing to 15 mm and females 19 mm. One case of human infection has been reported (Beaver *et al.* 1984).

Ancylostoma kusimaense Nayayoshi, 1955, which resembles *A. ceylanicum*, was originally described from a badger in Japan, but has also been found in a dog there (Yoshida 1965). *Ancylostoma paraduodenale* Biocca, 1951 closely resembles *A. duodenale* and occurs in the small intestine of lions and related carnivores in Africa. The infectivity to people of either species is unknown.

Bunostomum phlebotomum occurs in cattle and related ungulates in most warm and temperate regions (Soulsby 1982; Anderson 1992), and can cause human cutaneous infection (Mayhew, 1947).

Uncinaria stenocephala has not been reported to infect humans, except for the cutaneous lesions that Fülleborn induced in himself experimentally.

LIFE CYCLES

General outline

Hookworms are considered to be highly specific for the definitive host, even though few life cycles have been studied (Schad 1991; Anderson 1992). Eggs, usually in the 4–8 cell stage, pass in host faeces and embryonate rapidly in the outside world. Their slight variation only in size is inadequate for speciation. Under suitable conditions, the first-stage larva (L1) hatches within 24–48 hours and feeds on faecal bacteria, prior to moulting 1–2 days later. Both the free-living L1 and L2 have a muscular (rhabditoid) pharynx for ingesting semisolid material. They synthesize and store lipid within intestinal cells and adjacent tissues (Hill and Roberson 1985), presumably as fuel reserves for the infective stage. The rate of development to the L3 varies with species and temperature. The optimum for *A. caninum* is around 30 °C, cf. 20 °C for *Uncinaria stenocephala*, which is adapted to colder climates (Gibbs and Gibbs 1959). Following the second moult, at 5–9 days of embryonation (under optimal conditions), the

infective larva retains the L2 cuticle as a loose sheath, perhaps to reduce water loss. It has a relatively non-muscular (filariform) pharynx and does not feed (until entry to the host), but moves to the surface, moisture levels permitting, to await contact with a new host. Under natural conditions, the L3 of *A. ceylanicum* and *A. caninum* perish if frozen, but in the laboratory they have been successfully resuscitated after long periods of storage in liquid nitrogen (Vetter and Klaver-Wesseling 1977).

L3 require at least a capillary film of water to migrate, moving against the flow in wet soil (Kalkofen 1987). On damp substrates, they 'stand up' on their tails and wave about in response to vibrations, warmth, and carbon dioxide (Granzer and Haas 1991). Transfer to the host, even to a single hair, is by instantaneous adhesion on direct contact. Positive thermotaxis cannot help L3 to seek out suitable hosts, but is probably critical for skin location and penetration in furred animals. Needing traction to penetrate, L3 on intact skin usually invade via hair follicles, which minimize sideslip. Without the pressure of surface tension or overlying clothing, a hookworm larva freely suspended in water cannot penetrate skin (Smith 1904; Looss 1911; Goodey 1922, 1925a; Scott 1930; Dove 1932).

A range of mammalian hosts can be invaded by the L3 of most hookworm species investigated. Evolutionary pressure did not confer selectivity on this stage, whose chances of encounter with any mammal, let alone a definitive host, must be infinitesimal. The need for rapid attachment and invasion leaves no time for deliberation. Most species can invade transdermally and perorally, the predominant natural route determined by ecology and host behaviour (Miller 1971). Experimentally, alimentary inoculation of L3 consistently yields larger worm burdens, but this need not indicate the natural route (Scott 1930). Most free-ranging definitive hosts avoid feeding near sites of faecal contamination. Further, under laboratory conditions, transdermal penetration may be suboptimal and, in most studies, tissues that might have harboured hypobiotic L3 after percutaneous exposure were not examined. In fact, subcutaneous inoculation seems to be the most efficient route of infection.

The loose cuticular sheath is usually, but not always, discarded during skin penetration. Ensheathed L3 may be able to ingest large molecules, which perhaps enter the sheath through a residual mouth pore (Kumar and Pritchard 1994). However, to feed, migrate, and grow, L3 must be activated by host cues and/or nutrients, such as host serum (Hawdon and Schad 1991; Schad 1991). Skin-penetrating L3 enter dermal lymphatics or blood capillaries, are swept into the systemic circulation and, once in the pulmonary capillaries, either proceed into the systemic circulation (somatic migration), or puncture alveoli to then reach the gut by tracheal migration. Larvae of some species accumulate in various tissues and become dormant (hypobiotic), until reactivated by extrinsic or endogenous stimuli. No species uses intermediate hosts. *Ancylostoma braziliense*, *A. tubaeforme*, and *A. caninum* can use paratenic hosts, but their significance is unknown, and L3 vary in invasiveness, tissue distribution, and persistence in different rodents (Norris 1971*b*).

The third moult occurs in transit from the airways to the gut. The L4 is characterized by glandular development and sexual differentiation. A well-formed buccal capsule enables it to attach and feed on the intestinal mucosa. After the final moult, genital tract maturation leads to copulation and egg production. The frequency of copulation is unknown, but it does not interrupt feeding (Wells 1931) and is often observed *in vitro* in hookworms removed from dogs.

To attach, adult worms push forwards to bury their buccal capsules into the intestinal mucosa, explaining their usual location deep in mucosal folds. They feed on the tissues and blood, and change position frequently. In established infections, adult female worms slightly but consistently outnumber males, and congregate higher up the bowel (Behnke 1990). Pre-patent periods range from 2 to 7 weeks, the shorter intervals applying to zoonotic species (Anderson 1992). Egg production increases in the first 1–2 months of patency, plateaus, and then gradually declines with senescence. Zoonotic hookworms are relatively short lived in their normal hosts. Average longevity varies with species, but is generally less than 12 months, and is considerably shorter in abnormal hosts. There is no convincing evidence that host immunity contributes to worm demise, which is probably programmed genetically.

Only two zoonotic hookworms are known to use humans as definitive hosts, *A. ceylanicum* often successfully, and *A. caninum* only occasionally, and without developing to full maturity.

Ancylostoma caninum

Faeces in soil provide the most suitable embryonating conditions for eggs. At optimal temperatures (23–30 °C) and adequate humidity, infective larvae appear at 5 days. Development is faster at higher temperatures, but fewer larvae survive, and for shorter periods. L3 survive for up to 14 months in sterile, phosphate-buffered saline at 10–15 °C (Miller 1978) and at least 7 weeks in coproculture at 25 °C (Hawdon and Schad 1991), but probably considerably shorter under natural conditions. Coprophagic insects, such as dung beetles, may facilitate the dissemination of larvae (Beaver *et al.* 1984), and insects might even serve as paratenic or transport hosts (Little 1961; Anderson 1992), although their significance is unknown.

Both definitive and paratenic hosts can be infected either through the skin or by mouth (Norris 1971*b*; Behnke 1990). In dogs exposed percutaneously, some larvae migrate tracheally, resuming development after leaving the lungs (Looss 1911). In pups, the third moult occurs about 48 hours after infection, in the trachea and pharynx (Matsusaki 1950), and the final moult is completed in the gut by day 6. However, if inoculated intragastrically, some L3 develop directly into adult worms in the intestine (Yokagawa and Oiso 1926; Miller 1971). Eggs appear in faeces as early as 14 days after infection.

Arrested development of *A. caninum* in the dog intestine was first described over 60 years ago (Scott 1930). Some L3 can be induced to arrest by pre-chilling for varying periods, and they become hypobiotic in either the intestine or skeletal muscle (Schad 1977; Schad and Page 1982). However, populations of *A. caninum* are likely to vary geographically (Gibbs 1986), and tropical strains have not yet been tested for cold-induced hypobiosis. Perhaps other factors, such as rainfall or humidity, or cyclical changes within the host, influence L3 development in hot climates. Larvae may even affect each other by secreting pheromone-like substances (Gibbs 1986).

In older dogs, a natural age resistance develops to infection, and is more marked in females (Miller 1971). Fewer invading larvae develop into adults, the remainder probably migrating somatically into skeletal muscle. Age resistance may be strengthened by previous exposure to hookworms, although it is not clear what role immunity plays in larval arrest (Schad and Page 1982; Gibbs 1986).

Larval reactivation in dogs is also poorly understood, but seems unrelated to immunity or the presence of adult worms in the gut (Schad and Page 1982; Soulsby 1982; Behnke 1990). Sporadic larval 'awakening' explains the continued reappearance of infection in dogs which have been successfully treated with anthelminthics and protected from further exposure to L3. In pregnant bitches following parturition, hormonal changes activate hypobiotic larvae to migrate to the mammary glands (Gibbs 1986), presumably via the bloodstream, leading to neonatal infection. Larvae transfer in the milk for up to 20 days post-partum. This need not reflect their prolonged mobilization, for their rates of traversing the mammary glands may vary. Some larvae remain in tissue depots, for a bitch can transmit infection to subsequent litters without further exposure herself. Transplacental transmission of *A. caninum* does not occur (Miller 1971; Burke and Roberson 1985*a,b*).

In rodents and primates exposed orally or cutaneously (Lee *et al.* 1975; Behnke 1990), most L3 migrate somatically, to embed in skeletal muscles mainly of the anterior body, where they can survive for over a year and remain infective to dogs (Miller 1971). In mice, some larvae invade the brain (Nichols 1956). Following percutaneous infection, at least in rats, a proportion of L3 invade directly into the underlying muscle (Matsusaki 1951). In guinea-pigs, L3 can persist in skeletal muscle for 3 years and remain infective to dogs (Stone *et al.* 1979). In pigs, larvae have been recovered from belly fat as well as skeletal muscle 6 months after infection. A single larva, probably of this species, has been found in human muscle 3 months after exposure to infection (Little *et al.* 1983).

L3 ingested by dogs, either from the environment or in paratenic host tissues, may develop directly into adult worms, without tracheal migration. In young pups exposed via milk, the prepatent period is usually 14 days, ranging from 12 to 16 days (Stone and Peckham 1970), cf. 15–18 days after percutaneous infection (Soulsby 1982). Copulating adult worms have been observed as early as 12 days after infection (Scott 1930), and they attain their maximal size at 30 days. The prepatent period in older dogs is 15–26 days (Anderson 1992).

Adult worms live an average of 6 months. They occupy mainly the second and third quarters of the small intestine, aggregating around the central jejunum. They disperse more widely in heavy infections, even into the colon (Krupp 1961; Behnke 1990). The female can produce as many as 28 000 eggs day, but the number is usually much lower and declines in heavy infections (to around 5000) and in ageing worms, e.g. 1500 eggs/day at 8 months (Sarles 1929).

Ancylostoma tubaeforme

Cats can be infected through the skin or by mouth. Oral administration of L3 produces heavier infections than cutaneous exposure, both in cats and in rodent paratenic hosts (Norris 1971*b*). Subcutaneous inoculation is even more efficient (Anderson 1992). Previous assumptions that a lack of enzymes prevented L3 of *A. tubaeforme* from penetrating skin (Matthews 1975, 1977) are questionable (see p. 537). There is no direct evidence, but paratenic hosts may be more important in this life cycle, because cats habitually bury their faeces, are less social animals than dogs, and the prevalence and intensity of natural infections rise with age. Translactational transmission in cats has been neither demonstrated nor supported by epidemiological observations. In mice, L3 undergo somatic migration to accumulate in anterior carcass muscles and the brain, where they can survive for at least 10 months. In a study showing postnatal transfer of L3 to suckling mice (Setasuban 1975), the dams were infected around parturition. Because the larvae would have been migrating through mammary glands during suckling, it

cannot be inferred that hypobiotic L3 are sensitive to hormonal stimuli, or even that they occur in cats. In orally infected cats, the prepatent period is 18 days, and egg output peaks at 4–5 weeks after infection (Onwuliri *et al.* 1981).

Ancylostoma braziliense

L3 can invade both feline and canine definitive hosts, and rodent paratenic hosts, via skin or perorally, although the latter route seems to be more efficient (Norris 1971*b*; Yoshida 1971*b*). Larvae given orally to dogs develop directly in the gut, without tracheal migration. Skin-invading L3 follow the tracheo-oesophageal route, recommencing development on reaching the gastrointestinal tract. In rodents exposed cutaneously, significant numbers of larvae are retarded in the skin for a month or longer, particularly in the rat (although creeping eruption develops only in people). Many of these larvae can be found in the hair follicles and sebaceous glands (Norris 1971*b*). As experimental infections involve unnaturally high doses, it may be that larvae inhibit each other's migration and development, but this has never been investigated. Following either oral or cutaneous infection, L3 in rodents invade local tissues then migrate somatically, to accumulate in the anterior carcass. In mice, larvae survive in the muscles of the head and neck for as long as 18 months (Norris 1971*b*). In pups infected by either route, the prepatent period is 14 days (Yoshida *et al.* 1974), and is similar in cats (Scott 1930). Young cats and dogs are much more susceptible to infection than older animals (Scott 1930), but transmammary transmission has not been demonstrated experimentally (Miller 1971).

Ancylostoma ceylanicum

Given intragastrically to pups, L3 develop into adults in the gut, whereas following cutaneous exposure, they undergo tracheal migration, to recommence development after entering the trachea. The prepatent period by either route is 14 days in dogs (Yoshida *et al.* 1974), compared with 18–26 days in humans (Yoshida *et al.* 1971). In hamsters infected orally with adapted-strain L3, the prepatent period is 13–17 days (Behnke 1990). Age resistance to this species does not seem to occur (Miller 1971). There is no evidence of larval hypobiosis or transmammary transmission, and very little is known of its behaviour in paratenic hosts. In mice, some larvae of hamster-adapted strains can reach the intestine, and a few may even mature into fertile adults with cortisone treatment (Behnke 1990). L3 of dog-adapted strains infect mice much more efficiently by mouth than percutaneously, and some undergo tracheal migration, possibly recycling between gut and lungs. In neonatal mice, occasional adult worms appear but, in older mice, even immunosuppression does not allow further development of the parasite (Carroll *et al.* 1983).

Uncinaria stenocephala

Infection can be acquired through the skin or by mouth. Lactogenic transmission is not indicated by epidemiological or experimental evidence. The pre-patent period in orally infected pups is 15 days, and adult worms aggregate mainly in the third quarter of the small intestine (Anderson 1992).

PHYSIOLOGY

Host invasion

Invasive larvae of different species vary in their secretory and penetrating abilities, but the relationship between enzyme production and skin invasion has not been established.

The host epidermal basement membrane seems to be a major barrier to invading larvae (Vetter and Leegwater-v.d. Linden 1977*a*). L3 of *A. braziliense* appear capable of directly penetrating intact canine skin, and also of burrowing laterally through the epidermis 'in search of' hair follicle systems, while the other species invade only via hair follicles (Vetter and Leegwater-v.d. Linden 1977*a,b,c*). Both *A. caninum* and *A. duodenale* produce a major metalloprotease of 68 kDa and, variably, a minor protease of 38 kDa, which may be involved in ecdysis and histolysis (Hotez *et al.* 1990). The poor skin-penetrability of *A. tubaeforme* L3 cannot be attributed to a lack of secreted enzymes; inappropriate substrates were used in the original studies (Matthews 1975, 1977), and the findings for both *A. tubaeforme* and *A. caninum* were similar. L3 of *A. braziliense, A. caninum*, and *A. tubaeforme* all secrete a hyaluronidase of about 87 kDa, which may facilitate penetration of skin and deeper tissues. *Ancylostoma braziliense* has by far the greatest activity (Hotez *et al.* 1992), perhaps relating to its role in cutaneous *larva migrans*.

Host specificity

The determinants of host specificity are unknown, but act from the moment of L3 invasion. Larval behaviour and development is orchestrated by a complex array of poorly studied receptors, responding to specific host molecular configurations and physiological cues (e.g. hormonal, thermal, pH, and other metabolite gradients), and manifest as differential migration, growth, and maturation in paratenic and definitive hosts. While these responses may be modulated by immune factors, the evidence is lacking. They might simply

require specific nutrient molecules; e.g. adding canine serum to the culture medium extended the *in vitro* survival of adult *A. caninum* to 3 months, with egg production for the first 2 months (Komiya *et al.* 1956).

Populations of parasite (and host) species vary sufficiently to include individuals more tolerant of 'abnormal' hosts (or parasites). Selection of these underlies the establishment of laboratory strains of human hookworms in dogs and rodents. Conversely, occasional *A. caninum* attempt to develop, with varying success, in the human host (see p. 541–2).

Worm feeding

The adult worm maintains its position in the gut by the suction generated by oesophageal pumping. The plug of mucosa within the buccal capsule is a dynamic mass of liquefying tissue, not being 'grasped' by the buccal teeth, but rather being macerated by them and funnelled over deeper structures towards the oesophagus. The parasite depends on efficient and rapid digestion and absorption of nutrients, and cannot risk obstruction to flow by clotted host blood. At the attachment site, histolytic enzymes from the amphidial and perhaps excretory glands (Looss 1905; Eiff 1966; McLaren 1974; Harrop *et al.* 1995) soften the surrounding mucosa, which is drawn into the buccal cavity, injected with dorsal oesophageal gland enzymes, and shredded by the deep teeth. Ventral gland products are added to the food stream in the oesphageal lumen.

Worm feeding is intermittent, involving rapid, wave-like, oesophageal contractions (up to 4/sec) that pump mucosa and blood into the intestine (Wells 1931; Roche and Layrisse 1966; Kalkofen 1970, 1974). Intestinal transit can take as little as 2 minutes. Probably because of tissue depletion at the attachment site, *A. caninum* changes position every 4–6 hours, leaving small ulcers which heal within 6–24 hours. Increased numbers of lymphocytes are evident in the lesions at 2 hours and, by 4 hours, numerous neutrophils and variable numbers of eosinophils may be present (Kalkofen 1970, 1974).

Anticoagulation

Blood loss through the worm's intestine, around its mouth and into the surrounding mucosa may predispose the host to anaemia. In *A. caninum*, anticoagulant activity derives selectively from the amphidial glands (Thorson 1956*b*), and has been detected in canine intestinal mucosa around feeding adult *A. ceylanicum* (Carroll *et al.* 1984). A 37 kDa elastinolytic metalloprotease secreted by adult *A. caninum*, but also found in homogenates of *A. caninum* and *A. duodenale*, has fibrinolytic anticoagulant properties (Hotez and

Cerami 1983; Hotez *et al.* 1985). Closely related, if not identical, enzymes (including a 68 kDa protease) are secreted by L3 of these two species. These proteases may function in ecdysis and histolysis (Hotez *et al.* 1990), although an invasive larva could be protected by anticoagulants or thrombolytics. Soluble extracts of adult *A. caninum* contain an inhibitor of clotting factor Xa (Cappello *et al.* 1993), and recombinant small-protein derivatives from this species are potent inhibitors of factor Xa and factor VIIa/tissue-factor complex (Stanssens *et al.* 1996).

Because not all hookworm species cause host blood loss, it remains unclear whether anticoagulation is a primary goal, or an 'unintentional side-effect', of hookworm proteolytic secretory activity. Furthermore, a copious blood flow might satisfy the worm's oxygen needs (see below) more than its nutritional requirements.

Miscellaneous hookworm secretions

It is very likely that hookworms modulate local inflammatory and perhaps systemic immune responses in the host. A novel 41 kDa glycoprotein from *A. caninum*, neutrophil inhibitory factor (NIF), blocks the adhesion of activated human neutrophils to vascular endothelial cells by binding to the integrin CD11b/CD18 (Moyle *et al.* 1994). Its significance is not yet clear, but it may inhibit white cell infiltration and degranulation and hence damage to the worm during feeding. Immunohistochemical studies indicate that NIF originates from the amphidial and excretory glands (Sawangjaroen 1996). A cysteine protease of unknown function is secreted by adult *A. caninum*, and is also present in the L3 (Dowd *et al.* 1994). Acetylcholinesterase is released from the amphidial and oesophageal glands of the L4 and adult *N. americanus*; it has been speculated to act as a chemical holdfast, by inhibiting local gut peristalsis and/or secretion (McLaren *et al.* 1974, McLaren 1976; Schad 1991), but it probably has other functions. However, this enzyme has not been found in significant quantities in *Ancylostoma* species (McLaren 1976; Pritchard *et al.* 1990; Schad 1991).

Energy metabolism

Very little is known of the metabolism of hookworms. They are extravagant feeders, and nutrient intake seems to exceed their requirements. The colour change in blood passing through the parasite suggests considerable oxygen extraction (Wells 1931; Roche and Layrisse 1966). Host blood may provide as much as 30 per cent of its oxygen needs (Schad 1991), the remainder being absorbed through the cuticle. There is no evidence that carbohydrate is stored as an energy source; host serum glucose is apparently metabolized directly via anaerobic glycolysis. Lipid stores in L3 are abundant, but little is known of their role in adult worms.

THE HOSTS

RESERVOIR HOSTS

Ancylostoma caninum

Penetrating larvae may cause ground itch in dogs, which can be more severe and prolonged in older animals (Scott 1930). Dogs kennelled under poor hygiene can be exposed to large numbers of L3, leading to eczema, ulceration, and secondary infection, especially on the paws. Irritation leads to self-mutilation and lameness. The lesions histologically are characterized by acanthosis and hyperkeratinization, with infiltration by lymphocytes, neutrophils, eosinophils, and mast cells (Kalkofen 1987). Haemorrhagic pneumonia may follow cutaneous infection by massive numbers of larvae. About 4 days after exposure, as L4 arrive in the intestine, diarrhoea commences and blood appears in the faeces at about 8 days (Miller 1971).

Apart from a transient initial decline in circulating eosinophil numbers, blood leucocytosis and eosinophilia follow infection by either the oral or cutaneous routes in dogs (Scott 1930). The clinical outcome depends on worm numbers and host factors, including age, size, nutritional status, iron reserves and acquired resistance (Miller 1971; Kalkofen 1987). In lighter infections, mild enteritis may occur, while the major complication of heavy infections is anaemia, as each adult worm drains an average of 0.08–0.20 ml blood/day. Intraluminal blood loss commences with the fourth moult 8 days after infection, coincident with adult worm feeding (Miller 1971). Initially, anaemia is of the acute haemorrhagic type but, as the dog becomes iron-deficient, a hypochromic, microcytic film develops. Neonatal pups are most susceptible because of heavy maternal infection, and low reserves and dietary intake of iron. In pups below 6 months of age, haemorrhagic diarrhoea and circulatory collapse can result from an LD_{50} of worms as low as 100–150/kg body weight. Older pups, having greater iron reserves, protein intake and bone marrow responsiveness, are more resistant to severe consequences. In well-nourished dogs, hookworm disease tends to be acute, with deaths generally occurring between 10 and 24 days after a heavy, primary infection.

Ancylostoma caninum probably causes canine eosinophilic enteritis, but has evaded incrimination because the inflammatory response eliminates the offending worms before the dog presents for treatment or autopsy, and 'innocent bystanders' such as *Toxocara canis* are frequently blamed.

Ancylostoma tubaeforme

Little is known of this species' pathogenicity in cats under natural conditions (Soulsby 1982). Experimentally, larval doses determine the outcome in young cats inoculated intragastrically (Onwuliri *et al.* 1981). Inocula exceeding 1000 L3 produce clinical signs as early as 3 weeks. Blood haemoglobin begins to decline soon after exposure, and most cats die within 6 weeks, from relentless weight and blood loss (with haemoglobin levels down to 4 gm/100 ml). Doses of 500 L3 or less cause an initial decline in body weight and haemoglobin, which plateau at 6 weeks. The prepatent period is 18 days, regardless of the infective dose, and faecal egg output rises rapidly to plateau at 5–6 weeks. Worm burdens are logarithmically related to the larval dose, although their growth rate seems independent of their numbers. Host demise appears inevitable beyond a 'threshold' adult worm burden of 180–210.

Ancylostoma braziliense

This species causes negligible blood loss; pups infected with 700 adult worms lose less than 1 ml blood daily (Miller 1971). Signs of infection are restricted to gastrointestinal disturbances, such as mild diarrhoea. A protein-losing enteropathy may appear.

Ancylostoma ceylanicum

This species may cause as much blood loss in dogs as does *A. caninum*, but, just as its epidemiology in carnivores is not known, so its clinical significance remains unclear (Miller 1971). Experimentally, young dogs exposed percutaneously to L3 developed diarrhoea between 2 and 3 weeks (Carroll and Grove 1984). Egg output was detected in faeces by 3 weeks, remained steady to 8 weeks, then gradually declined to 2 per cent of the original at 36 weeks; few worms were found at autopsy (averaging 10/dog in four dogs). In dogs receiving more than 4000 L3, the diarrhoea persisted indefinitely, often with large quantities of blood and mucus. At 6 weeks in light infections, adult worms were aggregated in the first half of the small intestine; with increasing numbers (exceeding 1000 L3), they spread thoughout the entire small intestine and into the colon. In dogs given 12 000 L3, 50 per cent of worms were in the appendix/caecum/colon. Faecal egg output, infective dose, and adult worm burden all correlated closely, and individual worm fecundity was independent of numbers. Blood haemoglobin levels continued rising in dogs given less than 500 L3, but

fell in dogs with more than 1300, returning to preinfection levels at 6–12 weeks, and catching up with controls at 20 weeks. However, in dogs given 12 000 L3, the levels plateaued at only 50 per cent of normal, and red cell volumes declined. Sternal marrow iron stores disappeared in the heaviest infections. Total white cell counts rose only in heavier infections, but all dogs developed blood eosinophilia, which was unrelated to the intensity of infection. Blood eosinophils declined in the first 2 weeks, then rose to a plateau at 4–6 weeks (1.2×10^9/l), following which they gradually declined, but never returned to normal. All dogs had circulating IgM and IgG antibodies to larval antigens, and lymphocytes responded to adult worm antigens. IgM antibody levels rose during the first 2 weeks, then declined and vanished within 8 weeks. IgG rose more slowly, levelled off at 4 weeks and persisted throughout the study (36 weeks). Skin testing with L3 and adult antigens produced acute responses at 15 min which persisted beyond 5 hours in heavier infections.

Uncinaria stenocephala

This is not a haematophagous parasite. The major clinical problem in dogs is diarrhoea associated with protein-losing enteropathy in heavy infections (Miller 1971; Walker and Jacobs 1985). Exposure to large numbers of L3, usually in dirty kennels, causes skin lesions at larval penetration sites, sometimes with severe paw damage.

Diagnosis

All these infections in dogs or cats can be diagnosed coprologically. If faecal concentration is required to detect light infections, they are unlikely to be of clinical significance (except in cases of eosinophilic enteritis). As hookworm species cannot be distinguished on egg morphology, speciation requires adult worms, obtained following treatment or necropsy. Cultured larvae of all species are very similar, although some can be differentiated on subtle morphological features and temperature sensitivities (Hill and Roberson 1985). Eventually, DNA probes should simplify species diagnosis, in all parasite stages.

Treatment

Many anthelminthics can remove hookworms from the gastrointestinal tract. Their availability varies internationally, and they are usually presented in broad-spectrum combinations to cover cestodes and sometimes even ectoparasites. Effective agents include the benzimidazole carbamates, such as mebendazole, albendazole and fenbendazole, pyrantel and oxantel, thenium, butamisole, dichlorvos, and nitroscanate. In addition, ivermectin and milbemycin D may affect hypobiotic larvae in canine tissues (Kalkofen 1987), although the evidence is not yet convincing. Dogs and cats should be treated regularly, at intervals of 3-months or less, because of re-exposure to infection, or reactivation of hypobiotic larvae. Bitches should be dosed at least once during pregnancy, and nursing litters at least twice, at 1–2 weeks of age and 2 weeks later, to prevent severe anaemia. In north-eastern Australia and elsewhere, the prevalence of canine hookworms has declined with widespread prophylaxis against *Dirofilaria immitis*. It may be that regular diethylcarbamazine or ivermectin treatment eradicates developing intestinal worms. The first case of drug resistance in *A. caninum*, to an oxantel–pyrantel combination, has been reported in a dog originating from north-eastern Australia (Jackson *et al.* 1987).

Acutely ill or severely debilitated dogs (or, less commonly, cats) may need to receive supportive treatment, such as blood transfusions and iron replacement, in addition to anthelminthic therapy (Kalkofen 1987).

HUMANS

GENERAL

Invasive larvae of all hookworm species potentially can cause skin disease, but this develops infrequently and inconsistently. Sensitization, and the dose of infective larvae, appear to determine its severity. In experimental studies, the number of lesions is generally about 10 per cent of the larval dose. In sufficient numbers (thousands), even species not typically associated with creeping eruption, such as *A. caninum*, may produce recurrent migratory lesions that persist or recur for months. It is possible that unusual host immune responses are involved, or that, at high densities, larvae affect each other via secretions that perhaps accumulate in the skin. Each zoonotic hookworm species causes distinct clinical problems in humans, affecting the skin, intestine, or blood.

Ancylostoma braziliense

This is the only species that consistently causes classical creeping eruption with small numbers of larvae, and only in humans; no other animal has yet been found to develop similar lesions. The explanation may lie in the unique structure of human epidermis, which has far fewer hairs, sebaceous glands, and apocrine sweat glands than canine skin, and more eccrine sweat glands in regions where typical lesions occur, such as the limbs (Vetter and Leegwater-v.d. Linden 1977*a*). Pilosebaceous complexes in dog skin act as conduits for L3 into the dermis, and their scarcity in human

skin may hinder the egress of some larvae from the epidermis.

Larvae can invade skin directly or through sweaty or damp clothing, eliciting a prickling sensation. Local macules appear soon afterwards, and may develop into papules within an hour (Dove 1932), followed by intense, local itching. Occasionally, a single larva will produce a linear lesion, which appears within 1–4 days and then follows a tortuous course lasting up to 3 months or more. Lesions are often multiple, and the tortuous, 2–3 mm wide tracks move about 2–3 cm daily. While larvae may interrupt their movements, sometimes resting for weeks, the lesions are usually continuous. Itching is worse at night, and often prickling pain is felt in the lesion. Vesiculobullous eruptions may develop, and secondary bacterial infection is common. While individual lesions can persist and progress intermittently for months, their total numbers decline spontaneously, about 50 per cent with each passing week (Katz *et al.* 1965).

Staggered tracheal migration of larvae after their protracted escape from skin sites could account for the Löffler's syndrome that is diagnosed rarely (Muhleisen 1953). It may be far more common than reported, perhaps because most cases are subclinical, or full blood counts and chest radiographs are not taken routinely. In 26 (50 per cent) of 52 patients with creeping eruption attributed to *A. braziliense*, transient, migratory infiltrates appeared in chest X-rays 7 or more days after the rash commenced, and persisted for several weeks (in one case, from 59 to 89 days post-exposure) (Wright and Gold 1946). Only nine had mild cough, and none had abnormal chest signs. Blood eosinophilia developed in most, and lasted 4–6 weeks, with eosinophils in the sputum of some.

Cutaneous *larva migrans* caused by *A. braziliense* is becoming more common in travellers returning home from the tropics (Caumes *et al.* 1993, Davies *et al.* 1993). Exposure usually occurs on beaches, and symptoms commence between 1 and 29 days after returning home. Diagnosis rests on clinical recognition of the pathognomonic lesions. Limited unpublished observations suggest that most patients will demonstrate circulating antibodies to hookworm antigens (once serology becomes available), and this could help diagnose atypical cases. The temptation to establish a diagnosis by biopsy should be resisted. Migrating larvae are usually beyond the visible lesion and, should one actually be captured within a biopsy (a rare event), speciation from tissue sections is impossible.

In a unique case, a hookworm larva (species indeterminate) was removed from a patient with focal keratitis who had lived in Jacksonville, Florida (Nadbath and Lawlor 1965). The mode of infection was not explained, but the parasite could have migrated either from adjacent skin or directly into the cornea from contaminated soil or water. The diagnostic biopsy was curative.

Early forms of treatment, such as cautery, or freezing with ethyl chloride or liquid nitrogen, relied on the physical destruction of migrating larvae, and were painful and usually unsuccessful. Thiabendazole, either systemically or topically, has been the mainstay of chemotherapy almost since it was introduced 30 years ago. However, single oral doses are not very effective, while prolonged treatment is poorly tolerated (Caumes *et al.* 1993). Topical thiabendazole, as a 15 per cent cream in water-soluble base, needs to be applied three times daily for 3–5 days (Davies *et al.* 1993). Recently, albendazole has proven far more effective, taken orally as a 400 mg daily dose for 3–5 days; shorter treatment is less successful. In most patients, tracks stop moving and pruritus resolves within 24–48 hours of commencing treatment. Ivermectin, in a single 12 mg oral dose, is even more effective (Caumes *et al.* 1993).

There is no convincing evidence that *A. braziliense* develops in the human gut, but the possibility should not be totally rejected.

Ancylostoma caninum

Infective larvae of this species can also penetrate skin directly or through damp clothing. In sensitized individuals, penetration sites are marked by small papules, which develop within hours of exposure, vesiculate sometimes, and resolve usually within a week. Heavy exposure, perhaps involving thousands of larvae, can produce numerous papules and pustules (Miller *et al.* 1991), some of which may be followed by short, migratory tracks, which can recur at variable intervals and in widely separated sites, for up to 7 months (Hunter and Worth 1945). This is quite distinct from the continuous, intermittently migratory, creeping eruptions of *A. braziliense*, although accompanying, rapidly developing, linear urticarial lesions are sometimes mistaken for creeping eruption or the *larva currens* of strongyloidosis. While the discrepancy between larval dose and number of lesions might suggest that it is cuticular sheaths discarded by larvae in the epidermis that elicit hypersensitivity, this does not reconcile with migrating lesions. Skin biopsy may show eosinophilic folliculitis, with larvae apparently arrested in hair follicles (Miller *et al.* 1991), indicating that many L3 can invade one follicle.

Skeletal muscle is almost certainly the tissue reservoir of hypobiotic L3, even though only one case of myositis has been reported in a patient heavily infected with larvae, presumably of this species (Little *et al.* 1983). A muscle biopsy, taken 3 months after exposure in a man with weakness, tiredness, and painful muscle swelling in one leg, yielded one L3 among 250 stained sections. Cutaneous *larva migrans*, respiratory symptoms, and blood eosinophilia had been documented shortly after exposure. Myositis may be far more common than indicated by this one case, but would be very difficult to diagnose. In another patient heavily infected with *A. caninum* L3 (Miller *et al.* 1991), pain in muscles underlying the skin eruptions responded rapidly to thiabendazole treatment, again suggesting local invasion. It is not known if larvae penetrate muscles only after circulatory dispersal, or, as suspected from experimental rodents, also directly through overlying skin (Matsusaki 1951).

Eosinophilic enteritis (EE), even though recognized only recently, occurs much more frequently than cutaneous lesions in people exposed to *A. caninum* larvae. In north-eastern Australia, where the disease is common and usually caused by the parasite, more than 200 cases have been diagnosed clinically and serologically over 4 years (Croese *et al.* 1994*a,b*). However, adult hookworms (solitary and immature in each case) have been found in only 15 patients (confirmed as *A. caninum* in nine, but probably this species in the others). While most did have EE, one was entirely asymptomatic.

The presentation of EE is variable, and it is impossible to diagnose clinically. Typical manifestations include recurrent abdominal pain, usually central and colicky. Severe cases present with an acute abdomen, sometimes with distal small bowel obstruction, leaving the surgeon little choice but to operate. Most of these patients develop blood eosinophilia, but it may be absent in the early acute phase (Croese *et al.* 1990). High serum IgE levels are another non-specific feature. Radiology, with and without contrast studies, may show small bowel thickening and obstruction. Laparotomy reveals inflamed segments of distal ileum, varying in length from 2 to 100 cm, with intense serositis and, sometimes, turbid (eosinophilic) ascites. Occasionally, colon, caecum, and appendix are involved. Other patients have a milder, intermittent or chronic pattern of illness, which can persist for years. Occult or frank intestinal blood loss can occur, and presentation may be precipitated by rectal bleeding. Colonoscopy often reveals focal inflammation and/or ulceration of the terminal ileum and colon. In subclinical, or chronic, cases, small aphthous-like ulcers of the ileal and caecal mucosa may represent hookworm bite sites (Croese *et al.* 1996). In most cases, symptoms are not severe enough to justify surgery or colonoscopy, but blood eosinophilia suggests the diagnosis.

The histopathology of canine hookworm enteritis is described in detail elsewhere (Walker *et al.* 1995). The ileal segment may appear grossly inflamed and oedematous, and all layers of its wall may be heavily infiltrated with eosinophils. This undoubtedly represents a true allergic response, in people sensitized to secretory products of developing L3, L4 or adult worms. It seems unrelated to the intensity of exposure, although EE has not yet been diagnosed in a patient known to have been exposed to large numbers of L3. In not one case has there been evidence of preceding cutaneous *larva migrans* or Löffler's syndrome.

Patent human infection with *A. caninum* has never been documented, making the diagnosis of EE very difficult, in the absence of a worm or a tissue specimen. Among patients with confirmed EE, or who have typical clinical features and blood eosinophilia, 70 per cent have circulating IgG and IgE antibodies to adult *A. caninum* excretory–secretory antigens (ES Ags) demonstrable by ELISA. In the city of Townsville, 30 per cent of patients who complain of non-specific, recurrent abdominal pain but do not have blood eosinophilia are seropositive, compared with 8 per cent of healthy controls (Croese *et al.* 1994*a*). A Western blot using ES antigens of *A. caninum* is more sensitive and specific than the ELISA; more than 80 per cent of patients with eosinophilic enteritis demonstrate antibodies to a protein fraction of molecular weight 68 kDa (Ac68). Detection of specific IgG4 antibodies by immunoblot may be even more sensitive and specific (Loukas *et al.* 1996). However, it is premature to incriminate Ac68 as the putative allergen, for the correlation between disease severity and specific antibody levels is poor. One of the strongest IgE responses, both in ELISA and immunoblot, was from an asymptomatic man with a solitary adult *A. caninum*, whereas a woman with florid EE and a worm *in situ* was seronegative (Croese *et al.* 1994*b*). Monoclonal antibody studies indicate that Ac68 originates from the excretory glands of adult *A. caninum*, whereas sera from patients often bind more strongly to amphidial gland cytoplasm, suggesting that another molecule is allergenic (Sawangjaroen *et al.* 1995).

Hookworm EE can be diagnosed only if clinicians are aware of the disease. The histopathological diagnosis is confirmed by examining biopsy material, but rarely is a worm found to establish the aetiology. Furthermore, even experienced pathologists can overlook the small, inconspicuous parasite embedded between oedematous mucosal folds (Walker *et al.* 1995). Present serology is neither adequately sensitive nor specific for diagnosing acute cases, and the surgeon may not be able to await test results. Neither the ELISA nor Western blot distinguishes infections with *A. caninum* from those with anthropophilic hookworms (which can be diagnosed coprologically).

Treatment is simple: a single 300 mg dose of mebendazole usually brings about a dramatic resolution of symptoms within 24 hours. In fact, failure of response suggests a mistaken diagnosis. A smaller dose, or another anthelminthic, such as pyrantel, may also prove to be effective, but has not been clinically trialled. Having anti-inflammatory and anti-eosinophil activity, corticosteroids also rapidly suppress the symptoms, but are less specific in their action than anthelminthics. Many patients relapse, weeks or months later, apparently without re-exposure to infection. This, and the seasonal incidence of EE (Croese 1995), suggests that sporadic activation of dormant larvae underlies the intermittent appearance of immature adult worms in the gut, but currently available anthelminthics are unlikely to eradicate hypobiotic L3 sequestered within muscle fibres.

In the cooler parts of Australia, EE is much less common, reflecting both the lower prevalence of *A. caninum* in dogs and human contact with soil. Two likely cases have now been diagnosed in North America (Khoshoo *et al.* 1994, 1995) and, with growing awareness amongst clinicians and pathologists, the disease should eventually be recognized in most parts of the world where *A. caninum* occurs.

Ancylostoma ceylanicum

Occasionally, skin invasion by L3 of this species causes cutaneous lesions that resemble the 'ground itch' of *A. caninum*. Short linear lesions can develop, but not like the creeping eruption of *A. braziliense* (Maplestone 1933; Haydon and Bearup 1963; Wijers and Smit 1966; Bearup 1967). In most cases, recurrent, acute abdominal symptoms (colicky pain, distension, and flatulence) commence 15–20 days after exposure, about 1–2 weeks before eggs appear in stools. The pain can be quite severe, even in light, prepatent infections (Wijers and Smit 1966; Carroll and Grove 1986). The close clinical resemblance to EE caused by *A. caninum* infection suggests underlying intestinal hypersensitivity. In experimental infections, serum IgG and IgM antibodies (measured by ELISA) and lymphocyte responsiveness to *A. ceylanicum* antigens can be detected within 2 weeks of infection, and may be more pronounced in individuals previously exposed to anthropophilic hookworms (Carroll and Grove 1986).

While it could be argued that volunteers in experimental infections received too many infective larvae, suppressing the numbers of developing worms, *A. ceylanicum* under natural conditions causes only light and short-lived human intestinal infections which produce few if any eggs; it behaves as if in an unsuitable host (Chowdhury and Schad 1972; Carroll and Grove 1986). An exception is the West New Guinea (and probably Indonesian) strain, which does cause heavy natural infections, greatly outnumbering *N. americanus* in some individuals and producing anaemia (Anten and Zuidema 1964). No patients infected in New Guinea recalled skin rashes indicative of larval invasion.

Infections causing anaemia should be managed as typical human hookworm disease, with anthelminthics, iron supplementation, and other supportive therapy, as required.

Other species

Nothing is known about the pathogenicity of *A. tubaeforme* to humans. In one recorded study, its L3 failed to invade human skin (Kalkofen 1987).

With *U. stenocephala*, there seem to have been no further reports of cutaneous, or any other, disease in humans since the original experimental self-infection by Fülleborn.

Bunostomum phlebotomum, of bovids, has also been shown, by one case report (Mayhew 1947), to cause human cutaneous *larva migrans*; the larvae may have penetrated skin abrasions, and caused short-lived creeping eruptions (interestingly, calves also seemed to experience discomfort from larval invasion).

EPIDEMIOLOGY

GENERAL CONSIDERATIONS

The common zoonotic hookworms occur over a much wider geographical range than the two anthropophilic species, including many developed regions which were never endemic for the latter. Factors determining the distribution of any species include the presence of suitable hosts and environmental conditions supporting transmission. In addition, human infection requires appropriate human behaviour that ensures exposure to infective larvae.

A common and important misconception held by patients is that infection is acquired from direct contact with dogs. In reality, the source of human infection is usually damp, shady soil or grass that may appear quite innocent, having been contaminated with animal faeces some time previously. While heavy exposure can be an occupational risk in warm, humid conditions, just a single larva of *A. braziliense* may cause creeping eruption, and this may well apply to eosinophilic enteritis caused by *A. caninum*.

ANCYLOSTOMA CANINUM

Human eosinophilic enteritis has been reported from many parts of the world but, with the exception of the two American patients (Khoshoo *et al.* 1994, 1995), all cases attributed to *A. caninum* so far have been diagnosed in northern Australia. Inevitably, both the infection and associated disease will be recognized elsewhere. The geographical distribution of cutaneous lesions cannot be defined, for they occur infrequently and are too non-specific.

The parasite occurs naturally in the small intestine of the dog, fox, coyote, wolf, bear, and other wild carnivores (Levine 1968). Geographically, it is found in most tropical and temperate zones, being recorded between southern Canada and Germany in the north, and the southern extremities of Africa and Australia (excluding the island of Tasmania). In New Jersey, USA, *A. caninum* was found (on faecal examination for eggs) in 24 per cent of 1331 dogs (Burrows 1962). Necropsies of 213 infected dogs showed worm burdens ranging from 1 to 547 (average, 50 worms/dog). While not parasitizing cats, it is easily confused with *A. tubaeforme*.

ANCYLOSTOMA TUBAEFORME

This species coexists with *A. caninum* for most of its range, although its distribution is less fully documented. It is found in cats of all the inhabited continents, extending well beyond the tropics (Levine 1968), but does not infect dogs. In New Jersey, infection was detected coprologically in 37 per cent of 1568 cats (Burrows 1962), with a worm burden ranging from 1 to 124 worms/cat (average 20). Its infectivity to humans is unknown.

ANCYLOSTOMA BRAZILIENSE

Creeping eruption suggestive of *A. braziliense* infection in humans has been reported frequently from the south-eastern United States, the northern half of South America, southern Europe, South Africa, India the Philippines, and Australia (Beaver *et al.* 1984). With larvae requiring higher developmental temperatures, *A. braziliense* is more restricted geographically than the other hookworms of dogs and cats (Miller 1971). It occurs in Africa, southern Asia, tropical Australia, South and Central America, and the Gulf states of the United States. Hookworms, predominantly *A. braziliense*, were found in 26/27 pound dogs necropsied in Jacksonville, Florida (White and Dove 1928).

ANCYLOSTOMA CEYLANICUM

This parasite occurs in Asia, including Indonesia and Japan, Melanesia and parts of South America, where it naturally infects mainly cats and dogs. While it has been reported from humans in most of these regions, only the strain in Western New Guinea (Irian Jaya) and probably Indonesia seems well adapted to this host (Anten and Zuidema 1964).

UNCINARIA STENOCEPHALA

This species requires lower environmental temperatures for larval development. It occurs in dogs, cats, foxes, and wolves outside the tropical hookworm belt (Levine 1968; Miller 1971), extending to the Arctic Circle in northern America and Europe, and in southern Australia.

PREVENTION AND CONTROL

Wherever hookworms are enzootic, it is virtually impossible to prevent infections in dogs and cats unless the animals are severely restricted in their movements (Kalkofen 1987). Hunting and racing dogs are particularly susceptible to heavy infections because of their housing conditions. Even concrete floors do not prevent development and transmission of infective larvae. Floors of kennels and dog runs should be kept as smooth as possible, and dry, preferably in sunlight. Dog faeces should be shovelled out before hosing. If outbreaks occur, treatment of the ground with sodium borate will kill hookworm larvae (and also any grass).

In the general community, control becomes even more problematic, especially where there are sizeable populations of stray animals. Surveys consistently show higher prevalences of hookworm infection in stray than in pet dogs. Legislation to enforce animal control is essential, but politically sensitive and of limited effectiveness, owing to the cost of enforcement and the degree of irrational public resistance, based on the emotional appeal of dogs and cats. Given that environmental control may be unrealistic, the remaining alternative measures for reducing hookworm infection prevalences are vaccination and anthelminthic treatment.

An effective vaccine, based on live, irradiated L3 of *A. caninum*, has been developed (Miller 1971), and variants have also proven successful (Kalkofen 1987). While not completely protecting pups, vaccination did prevent heavy infections and, more significantly, the development of clinical disease. It even protected against infection with related species of hookworms. However, for logistical and, possibly, sociological and commercial reasons, the vaccine did not gain widespread use, and was withdrawn soon after its introduction (Miller 1978). It gained an undeservedly negative reputation because of complications in older, infected dogs, which should not have been vaccinated. Perhaps more importantly, it seems that regular anthelminthic medication of pet dogs is an important foundation of the veterinarian–client relationship.

Anthelminthic chemotherapy is described above. If ivermectin or another drug is confirmed to destroy arrested tissue larvae, and teratogenicity is not a problem, then it will become possible to prevent neonatal infections by treating bitches before conception, or intragestationally. An additional benefit may be the suppression of toxocarosis.

CONCLUSIONS

It seems that more research has been done on *A. caninum* than on all other hookworm species combined, both zoonotic and anthropophilic. The reasons for this are obvious. For the same reasons, *A. caninum* is best placed, of all the zoonotic hookworms, to infect humans. Yet, probably the most common and significant complication of human *A. caninum* infection, eosinophilic enteritis, has been recognized only in the past 7 years, raising many new questions about hookworm biology, physiology, and host–parasite relationships. In enzootic areas, how many of the human population carry hypobiotic larvae of *A. caninum*? How long do larvae survive in human tissues? How many people harbour intestinal *A. caninum* without experiencing symptoms? Why do only a few develop enteritis? Why do even fewer develop cutaneous lesions? Is the disease caused by newly acquired or reactivated dormant larvae? Is a single exposure sufficient to provoke intestinal hypersensitivity? Is the putative allergen also secreted by the anthropophilic hookworms? Do they also cause eosinophilic enteritis? Do other parasites that inoculate antigens into the gut mucosa cause this disease? Does *A. caninum* cause enteritis in dogs?

Our knowledge of other zoonotic species is far more limited. The behaviour in experimental hosts of *A. ceylanicum*, which is known to develop fully in humans, has been surprisingly neglected. We still cannot be certain if *A. tubaeforme*, common in cats throughout much of the world, is capable of infecting people, let alone causing disease. If it has taken so long for us to recognize the most common manifestation of human infection with the most common zoonotic hookworm, will it be just a matter of time before other zoonotic species are also implicated in potentially serious human ailments?

REFERENCES
(* Denotes recommended further reading.)

Ackert, J. E. and Payne, F. K. (1923). Investigations of the control of hookworm disease. XII. Studies of the occurrence, distribution and morphology of *Necator suillus*, including descriptions of the other species of *Necator*. *American Journal of Hygiene*, **3**, 1–25.

*Anderson, R. C. (1992). 3.2 The Superfamily Ancylostomatidae. In *Nematode Parasites of Vertebrates*, pp. 40–61. CAB International, Wallingford.

Anten, J. F. G. and Zuidema, P. J. (1964). Hookworm infection in Dutch serviceman returning from West New Guinea. *Tropical and Geographical Medicine*, **16**, 216–24.

Bearup, A. J. (1967). Correspondence: *A. braziliense*. *Tropical and Geographical Medicine*, **19**, 161–2.

Beaver, P. C., Snyder, C. H., Carrera, G. M., Dent, J. H., and Lafferty, J. W. (1952). Chronic eosinophilia due to visceral larva migrans. *Pediatrics*, **9**, 7–18.

*Beaver, P. C., Jung, R. C., and Cupp, E. W. (1984). *Clinical Parasitology*. Lea and Febiger, Philadelphia.

*Behnke, J. M. (1990). Laboratory animal models. In *Hookworm disease: current status and new directions*, (ed. G. A. Schad and K. S. Warren), pp. 105–28. Taylor and Francis, London.

Bhaibulaya, M. and Indrangarm, S. (1975). Man, an accidental host of *Cyclodontostomum purvisi* (Adams, 1933), and the occurrence in rats in Thailand. *Southeast Asian Journal of Tropical Medicine and Public Health*, **6**, 391–4.

Biocca, E. (1951). On *Ancylostoma braziliense* and its morphological differentiation from *Ancylostoma ceylanicum*. *Journal of Helminthology*, **25**, 1–10.

Biocca, E. (1954). Ridescrizione di *Ancylostoma tubaeforme* (Zeder, 1800) parassita del gatto, considerato erroneamente sinonimo di *Ancylostoma caninum* (Ercolani, 1859), parassita del cane. *Revista Parassitologia*, **15**, 267–8.

Buckley, J. J. C. (1933). *Necator suillus* as a human infection. *The British Medical Journal*, **April 22**, 699–700.

Burke, T. M. and Roberson, E. L. (1985a). Prenatal and lactational transmission of *Toxocara canis* and *Ancylostoma caninum*: experimental infection of the bitch before pregnancy. *International Journal for Parasitology*, **15**, 71–5.

Burke, T. M. and Roberson, E. L. (1985b). Prenatal and lactational transmission of *Toxocara canis* and *Ancylostoma caninum*: experimental infection of the bitch at midpregnancy and parturition. *International Journal for Parasitology*, **15**, 485–90.

Burrows, R. B. (1962). Comparative morphology of *Ancylostoma tubaeforme* (Zeder, 1800) and *Ancylostoma caninum* (Ercolani, 1859). *Journal of Parasitology*, **48**, 715–18.

Cappello, M., Clyne, L. P., McPhedran, P., and Hotez, P. (1993). *Ancylostoma* factor Xa inhibitor: partial purification and its identification as a major hookworm anticoagulant *in vitro*. *Journal of Infectious Diseases*, **167**, 1474–7.

Carroll, S. M. and Grove, D. I. (1984). Parasitological, hematologic, and immunologic responses in acute and chronic infections of dogs with *Ancylostoma ceylanicum*: a model of human hookworm infection. *Journal of Infectious Diseases*, **150**, 284–94.

Carroll, S. M. and Grove, D. I. (1986). Experimental infection of humans with *Ancylostoma ceylanicum*: clinical, parasitological, haematological and immunological findings. *Tropical and Geographical Medicine*, **38**, 38–45.

Carroll, S. M., Grove, D. I., Dawkins, H. J. S., Mitchell, G. F., and Whitten, L. K. (1983). Infections with a Malaysian dog strain of *Ancylostoma ceylanicum* in outbred, inbred and immunocompromised mice. *Parasitology*, **87**, 229–38.

Carroll, S. M., Howse, D. J., and Grove, D. I. (1984). The anticoagulant effects of the hookworm *Ancylostoma ceylanicum*: observations on human and dog blood *in vitro* and infected dogs *in vivo*. *Thrombosis and Haemostasis*, **51**, 222–7.

Caumes, E., Carriere, J., Datry, A., Gaxotte, P., Danis, M., and Gentilini, M. (1993). A randomized trial of ivermectin versus albendazole for the treatment of cutaneous larva

migrans. *American Journal of Tropical Medicine and Hygiene*, **49**, 641–4.

Chowdhury, A. B. and Schad, G. A. (1972). *Ancylostoma ceylanicum*: a parasite of man in Calcutta and environs. *American Journal of Tropical Medicine and Hygiene*, **21**, 300–1.

Croese, T. J. (1988). Eosinophilic enteritis—a recent north Queensland experience. *Australian and New Zealand Journal of Medicine*, **18**, 848–53.

Croese, J. (1995). Seasonal influence on human enteric infection with *Ancylostoma caninum*. *American Journal of Tropical Medicine and Hygiene*, **53**, 158–61.

Croese, J., Prociv, P., Maguire, E., and Crawford, A. (1990). Eosinophilic enteritis presenting as surgical emergencies: a report of six cases. *Medical Journal of Australia*, **153**, 415–17.

Croese, J., Loukas, A., Opdebeeck, J., and Prociv, P. (1994a). Occult enteric infection by *Ancylostoma caninum*: a previously unrecognised zoonosis. *Gastroenterology*, **106**, 3–13.

Croese, J., Loukas, A., Opdebeeck, J., Fairley, S., and Prociv, P. (1994b). Human enteric infection with canine hookworms: an emerging problem in developed communities. *Annals of Internal Medicine*, **120**, 369–74.

Croese, J., Fairley, S., Loukas, A., Hack, J., and Stronach, P. (1996). Ileal ulceration: an index of cryptic infection by *Ancylostoma caninum*. *Gastroenterology and Hepatology*, **11**, 524–31.

Davies, H. D., Sakuls, P., and Keystone, J. S. (1993). Creeping eruption: a review of clinical presentation and management of 60 cases presenting to a tropical disease unit. *Archives of Dermatology*, **129**, 588–91.

Dove, W. E. (1932). Further studies on *Ancylostoma braziliense* and the etiology of creeping eruption. *American Journal of Hygiene*, **15**, 664–711.

Dowd, A. J., Dalton, J. P., Loukas, A. C., Prociv, P., and Brindley, P. J. (1994). Secretion of cysteine proteinase by the human pathogen *Ancylostoma caninum*. *American Journal of Tropical Medicine and Hygiene*, **51**, 341–7.

Eiff, J. A. (1966). Nature of an anticoagulant from the cephalic glands of *Ancylostoma caninum*. *Journal of Parasitology*, **52**, 833–43.

Gibbs, H. C. (1986). Hypobiosis in parasitic nematodes—an update. *Advances in Parasitology*, **25**, 129–74.

Gibbs, H. C. and Gibbs, K. E. (1959). The effects of temperature on the development of the free-living stages of *Dochmoides stenocephala* (Railliet, 1884) (Ancylostomatidae: Nematoda). *Canadian Journal of Zoology*, **37**, 247–57.

Goodey, T. (1922). Observations on the ensheathed larvae of some parasitic nematodes. *Annals of Applied Biology*, **9**, 33–48.

Goodey, T. (1925a). Observations on certain conditions requisite for skin penetration by the infective larvae of Strongyloides and Ankylostomes. *Journal of Helminthology*, **3**, 51–62.

Goodey, T. (1925b). Skin penetration by the infective larvae of *Dochmoides stenocephala*. *Journal of Helminthology*, **3**, 173–6.

Granzer, M. and Haas, W. (1991). Host-finding and host recognition of infective *Ancylostoma caninum* larvae. *International Journal for Parasitology*, **21**, 429–40.

*Grove, D. I., (1990). *A history of helminthology*. CAB International, Oxford.

Harrop, S. A., Sawangjaroen, N., Prociv, P., and Brindley, P. J. (1995). Characterization of cathepsin B proteinase genes expressed by adult *Ancylostoma caninum*. *Molecular and Biochemical Parasitology*, **71**, 163–71.

Hawdon, J. M. and Schad, G. A (1991). Long-term storage of hookworm infective larvae in buffered saline solution maintains larval responsiveness to host signals. *Journal of the Helminthological Society of Washington*, **58**, 140–2.

Haydon, G. A. M. and Bearup, A. J. (1963). *Ancylostoma braziliense* and *Ancylostoma ceylanicum*. *Transactions of the Royal Society of Tropical Medicine and Hygiene*, **57**, 76.

Haydon, G. M. (1929). Creeping eruption or larva migrans in north Queensland and a note on the worm *Gnathostoma spinigerum* (Owen). *Medical Journal of Australia*, i, 583–91.

Hill, R. L. and Roberson, E. L. (1985). Differences in lipid granulation as the basis for a morphologic differentiation between the third-stage larvae of *Uncinaria stenocephala* and *Ancylostoma caninum*. *Journal of Parasitology*, **71**, 745–50.

Hotez, P. and Cerami, A. (1983). Secretion of proteolytic anticoagulant by *Ancylostoma* hookworms. *Journal of Experimental Medicine*, **157**, 1594–603.

Hotez, P. J., Trang, N. L., McKerrow, J. H., and Cerami, A. (1985). Isolation and characterization of a proteolytic enzyme from the adult hookworm *Ancylostoma caninum*. *Journal of Biological Chemistry*, **250**, 7343–8.

Hotez, P. *et al.* (1990). Metalloproteases of infective *Ancylostoma* hookworm larvae and their possible functions in tissue invasion and ecdysis. *Infection and Immunity*, **58**, 3883–92.

Hotez, P. J. *et al.* (1992). Hyaluronidase from infective *Ancylostoma* hookworm larvae and its possible function as a virulence factor in tissue invasion and in cutaneous larva migrans. *Infection and Immunity*, **60**, 1018–23.

Hunter, G. W. and Worth, C. B. (1945). Variations in response to filariform larvae of *Ancylostoma caninum* in the skin of man. *Journal of Parasitology*, **31**, 366–72.

Jackson, R., Lance, D., Townsend, K., and Stewart, K. (1987). Isolation of anthelminthic resistant *Ancylostoma caninum*. *New Zealand Veterinary Journal*, **35**, 215–16.

Kalkofen, U. P. (1970). Attachment and feeding behaviour of *Ancylostoma caninum*. *Zeitschrift fur Parasitenkunde*, **33**, 339–54.

Kalkofen, U. P. (1974). Intestinal trauma resulting from feeding activities of *Ancylostoma caninum*. *American Journal of Tropical Medicine and Hygiene*, **23**, 1046–53.

*Kalkofen, U. P. (1987). Hookworms of dogs and cats. *Veterinary Clinics of North America: Small Animal Practice*, **17**, 1341–54.

Katz, R., Ziegler, J., and Blank, H. (1965). The natural course of creeping eruption and treatment with thiabendazole. *Archives of Dermatology*, **91**, 420–4.

Khoshoo, V., Schantz, P., Craver, R., Stern, G. M., Loukas, A., and Prociv, P. (1994). Dog hookworm: a cause of eosinophilic enterocolitis in humans. *Journal of Pediatric Gastroenterology and Nutrition*, **19**, 448–452.

Khoshoo, V., Craver, R., Schantz, P., Loukas, A., and Prociv, P. (1995). Abdominal pain, pan-gut eosinophilia, and dog hookworm infection. *Journal of Pediatric Gastroenterology and Nutrition*, **21**, 481.

*Kirby-Smith, J. L., Dove, W. E., and White, G. F. (1926). Creeping eruption. *Archives of Dermatology and Syphilology*, **13**, 137–75.

Komiya, Y., Yasuraoka, K., and Sato, A. (1956). Survival of *Ancylostoma caninum in vitro* (I). *Japanese Journal of Medical Science and Biology*, **9**, 283–92.

Krupp, I. M. (1961). Effects of crowding and of superinfection on habitat selection and egg production in *Ancylostoma caninum*. *Journal of Parasitology*, **47**, 957–61.

Kumar, S. and Pritchard, D. I. (1994). Apparent feeding behaviour of ensheathed third-stage infective larvae of human hookworms. *International Journal for Parasitology*, **24**, 133–6.

Lee, K. T., Little, M. D., and Beaver, P. C. (1975). Intracellular (muscle-fiber) habitat of *Ancylostoma caninum* in some mammalian hosts. *Journal of Parasitology*, **61**, 589–98.

Lee, R. J. (1884). Short notice of a second case of creeping eruption similar to that described in vol. III Clinical Society's Transactions. *Transactions of the Clinical Society of London*, **17**, 75–6.

*Levine, N. D. (1968). Hookworms. In *Nematode parasites of domestic animals and man*, pp. 85–115. Burgess Publishing, Minneapolis.

Lewert, R. M. and Lee, C. L. (1954). Studies on the passage of helminth larvae through host tissues. I. Histochemical studies on the extracellular changes caused by penetrating larvae. II. Enzymatic activity of larvae *in vitro* and *in vivo*. *Journal of Infectious Diseases*, **95**, 13–51.

*Lichtenfels, J. R. (1980). No. 8. Keys to the genera of the Superfamilies Ancylostomatoidea and Diaphanocephaloidea. In *CIH Keys to the Nematode Parasites of Vertebrates*, (ed. R. C. Anderson, A. G. Chabaud, and S. Willmott). Farnham Royal, London.

Little, M. D. (1961). Observations on the possible role of insects as paratenic hosts for *Ancylostoma caninum*. *Journal of Parasitology*, **47**, 263–7.

Little, M. D., Halsey, N. A., Cline, B. L., and Katz, S. P. (1983). *Ancylostoma* larva in muscle fiber of man following cutaneous larva migrans. *American Journal of Tropical Medicine and Hygiene*, **32**, 1285–8.

*Looss, A. (1905). The anatomy and life history of *Agchylostoma duodenale* Dub. A monograph. *Records of the Egyptian Government School of Medicine*, Vol III. National Printing Department, Cairo.

*Looss, A. (1911). The anatomy and life history of *Agchylostoma duodenale* Dub. A monograph. *Records of the Egyptian Government School of Medicine*, Vol IV. National Printing Department, Cairo.

Loukas, A., Croese, J., Opdebeeck, J., and Prociv, P. (1992). Detection of antibodies to secretions of *Ancylostoma caninum* in human eosinophilic enteritis. *Transactions of the Royal Society of Tropical Medicine and Hygiene*, **86**, 650–3.

Loukas, A., Croese, J., Opdebeeck, J., and Prociv, P. (1994). Immunologic incrimination of *Ancylostoma caninum* as a human enteric pathogen. *American Journal of Tropical Medicine and Hygiene*, **50**, 69–77.

Loukas, A., Opdebeeck, J., Croese, J., and Prociv, P. (1996). IgG subclass antibodies against excretory/secretory antigens of *Ancylostoma caninum* in human enteric infections. *American Journal of Tropical Medicine and Hygiene*, **54**, 672–6.

McLaren, D. J., Burt, J. S., and Ogilvie, B. M. (1974). The anterior glands of adult *Necator americanus* (Nematoda: Strongyloidea)—II. Cytochemical and functional studies. *International Journal for Parasitology*, **4**, 39–46.

Maplestone, P. A. (1933). Creeping eruption produced by hookworm larvae. *Indian Medical Gazette*, **68**, 251–6.

Matsusaki, G. (1950). Studies on the life history of the hookworm. Part VII: on the development of *Ancylostoma caninum* in the normal host. *Yokahama Medical Bulletin*, **1**, 111–20.

Matsusaki, G. (1951). Studies on the life history of the hookworm. Part VI: on the development of *Ancylostoma caninum* in the abnormal host. *Yokahama Medical Bulletin*, **2**, 154–60.

Matthews, B. E. (1975). Mechanism of skin penetration by *Ancylostoma tubaeforme* larvae. *Parasitology*, **70**, 25–38.

Matthews, B. E. (1977). The passage of larval helminths through tissue barriers. *Symposia of the British Society for Parasitology*, **15**, 93–119.

Mayhew, R. L. (1947). Creeping eruption caused by the larvae of the cattle hookworm, *Bunostomun phlebotomum*. *Proceedings of the Society for Experimental Biology and Medicine*, **66**, 12–14.

McLaren, D. J. (1974). The anterior glands of adult *Necator americanus* (Nematoda: Strongyloidea)—I. Ultrastructural studies. *International Journal for Parasitology*, **4**, 25–37.

McLaren, D. J. (1976). Sense organs and their secretions. In *The Organization of Nematodes* (ed. N. A. Croll), pp. 139–61. Academic Press, London.

Miller, A. C., Walker, J., Jaworski, R., de Launey, W., and Paver, R. (1991). Hookworm folliculitis. *Archives of Dermatology*, **127**, 547–9.

*Miller, T. A. (1971). Vaccination against the canine hookworm diseases. *Advances in Parasitology*, **9**, 153–83.

*Miller, T. A. (1978). Industrial development and field use of the canine hookworm vaccine. *Advances in Parasitology*, **16**, 333–42.

Moyle, M. *et al.* (1994). A hookworm glycoprotein that inhibits neutrophil function is a ligand of the integrin CD11b/CD18. *Journal of Biological Chemistry*, **269**, 10008–15.

Muhleisen, J. P. (1953). Demonstration of pulmonary migration of the causative agent of creeping eruption. *Annals of Internal Medicine*, **38**, 595–600.

Nadbath, R. P. and Lawlor, P. P. (1965). Nematode (Ancylostoma) in the cornea. A case report. *American Journal of Ophthalmology*, **59**, 486–90.

Nichols, R. L. (1956). The etiology of visceral larva migrans. II. Comparative larval morphology of *Ascaris lumbricoides*, *Necator americanus*, *Strongyloides stercoralis* and *Ancylostoma caninum*. *Journal of Parasitology*, **42**, 363–99.

Norris, D. E. (1971*a*). Morphology of a North American strain of *Ancylostoma braziliense* Gomes de Faria, 1910. *Journal of Parasitology*, **57**, 993–7.

Norris, D. E. (1971*b*). The migratory behaviour of the infective larvae of *Ancylostoma braziliense* and *Ancylostoma tubaeforme* in rodent paratenic hosts. *Journal of Parasitology*, **57**, 998–1009.

Olsen, O. W. and Lyons, E. T. (1965). Life cycle of *Uncinaria lucasi* Stiles, 1901 (Nematoda: Ancylostomatidae) of fur seals, *Callorhinus ursinus* Linn., on the Pribilof Islands of Alaska. *Journal of Parasitology*, **51**, 689–700.

Onwuliri, C. O. E., Nwosu, A. B. C., and Anya, A. O. (1981). Experimental *Ancylostoma tubaeforme* infection of cats: changes in blood values and worm burden in relation to single infections of varying size. *Zeitschrift für Parasitenkunde*, **64**, 149–55.

Pritchard, D. I., McKean, P. G., and Schad, G. A. (1990). An immunological and biochemical comparison of hookworm species. *Parasitology Today*, **6**, 154–6.

Prociv, P. and Croese, J. (1990). Human eosinophilic enteritis caused by *Ancylostoma caninum*, a common dog hookworm. *Lancet*, **355**, 1299–302.

Radcliffe-Crocker, H. (1907). *Diseases of the skin*, (3rd edn), Vol. 2. P. Blakiston's Son and Co., Philadelphia.

Rep, B. H. (1966). Pathogenicity of *Ancylostoma braziliense*. IV. Blood loss caused by the worms in the prepatent period. *Tropical and Geographical Medicine*, **18**, 329–52.

Rep, B. H., Vetter, J. C. M., and Eijsker, M. (1968). Cross breeding experiemtns in *Ancylostoma braziliense* de Faria, 1910 and *A. ceylanicum* Looss, 1911. *Tropical and Geographical Medicine*, **20**, 367–78.

*Roche, M. and Layrisse, M. (1966). The nature and causes of 'hookworm anemia'. *American Journal of Tropical Medicine and Hygiene*, **15**, 1031–1102.

Sarles, M. P. (1929). The effect of age and size of infestation on the egg production of the dog hookworm, *Ancylostoma caninum*. *American Journal of Hygiene*, **10**, 658–66.

Sawangjaroen, N. (1996). Studies of excretory–secretory antigens of adult *Ancylostoma caninum*. Ph.D. thesis, The University of Queensland, Brisbane, Australia.

Sawangjaroen, N., Opdebeeck, J. P., and Prociv, P. (1995). Immunohistochemical localization of excretory/secretory antigens in adult *Ancylostoma caninum* using monoclonal antibodies and infected human sera. *Experimental Parasitology*, **17**, 29–35.

Schad, G. A. (1977). The role of arrested development in the regulation of nematode populations. In *Regulation of Parasite Populations*, (ed. G. W. Esch), pp. 111–67. Academic Press, New York.

*Schad, G. A. (1991). The parasite. In *Hookworm infections, human parasitic diseases*, Vol. 4 (ed. H. M. Gilles and P. A. J. Ball), pp. 15–49. Elsevier Science Publishers, Amsterdam.

Schad, G. A., Chowdhury, A. B., Dean, C. G., Kochar, V. K., Nawalinski, T. A., Thomas, J., and Tonascia, J. A. (1973). Arrested development in human hookworm infections: an adaptation to a seasonally unfavorable external environment. *Science*, **180**, 502–504.

Schad, G. A. and Page, M. R. (1982). *Ancylostoma caninum*: adult worm removal, corticosteroid treatment, and resumed development of arrested larvae in dogs. *Experimental Parasitology*, **54**, 303–9.

Schwartz, B. and Alicata, J. E. (1934). Development of *Ancylostoma caninum* following percutaneous infection. *Journal of Parasitology*, **20**, 326.

Scott, J. A. (1930). The biology of hookworms in their hosts. *Quarterly Review of Biology*, **5**, 79–97.

Setasuban, P. (1975). Transmammary transmission of *Ancylostoma tubaeforme* in mice. *Southeast Asian Journal of Tropical Medicine and Public Health*, **6**, 608–9.

Shelmire, B. (1928). Experimental creeping eruption from a cat and dog hookworm (*Ancylostoma braziliense*). *Journal of the American Medical Association*, **91**, 938–43.

Smith, C. A. (1904). Uncinariasis in the South, with special reference to mode of infection. *Journal of the American Medical Association*, **43**, 592–7.

*Soulsby, E. J. L. (1982). *Helminths, arthropods and protozoa of domesticated animals*, (7th edn). Bailliere Tindall, London.

Stanssens, P. *et al.* (1996). Anticoagulant repertoire of the hookworm *Ancylostoma caninum*. *Proceedings of the National Academy of Science of the USA*, **93**, 2149–54.

Stone, W. M. and Peckham, J. C. (1970). Infectivity of *Ancylostoma caninum* larvae from canine milk. *American Journal of Veterinary Research*, **31**, 1693–4.

Stone, W. M., Stewart, T. B., and Smith, F. (1979). Longevity and infectivity of somatic larvae of *Ancylostoma caninum* in guinea and swine. *Journal of Parasitology*, **65**, 460–1.

*Tamura, H. (1921). On creeping disease. *The British Journal of Dermatology and Syphilis*, **33**, 81–102; 138–51.

Thorson, R. E. (1956*a*). Proteolytic activity in extracts of the esophagus of adults of *Ancylostoma caninum* and the effect of immune serum on this activity. *Journal of Parasitology*, **42**, 21–5.

Thorson, R. E. (1956*b*). The effect of extracts of the amhidial glands, excretory glands, and esophagus of adults of *Ancylostoma caninum* on the coagulation of dog's blood. *Journal of Parasitology*, **42**, 26–30.

Thorson, R. E. (1956*c*). The stimulation of acquired immunity in dogs by injections of extracts of the esophagus of adult hookworms. *Journal of Parasitology*, **42**, 501–4.

Vetter, J. C. M. and Klaver-Wesseling, J. C. M. (1977). Unimpaired infectivity of *Ancylostoma ceylanicum* after storage in liquid nitrogen for one year. *Journal of Parasitology*, **63**, 700.

Vetter, J. C. M. and Leegwater-v.d. Linden, M. E. (1977*a*). Skin penetration of infective hookworm larvae. I. The path of migration of infective larvae of *Ancylostoma braziliense* in canine skin. *Zeitschrift fur Parasitenkunde*, **53**, 255–62.

Vetter, J. C. M. and Leegwater-v. d. Linden, M. E. (1977*b*). Skin penetration of infective hookworm larvae. II. The path of migration of infective larvae of *Ancylostoma braziliense* in the metacarpal foot pads of dogs. *Zeitschrift fur Parasitenkunde*, **53**, 263–6.

Vetter, J. C. M. and Leegwater-v. d. Linden, M. E. (1977*c*). Skin penetration of infective hookworm larvae. III. Comparative studies on the path of migration of the hookworms *Ancylostoma braziliense*, *Ancylostoma ceylanicum*, and *Ancylostoma caninum*. *Zeitschrift fur Parasitenkunde*, **53**, 155–8.

Walker, M. J. and Jacobs D. E. (1985). Pathophysiology of *Uncinaria stenocephala* infections of dogs. *Veterinary Annual*, **25**, 263–71.

*Walker, N., Croese, J., Loukas, A., Clouston, A., and Prociv, P. (1995). Eosinophilic enteritis in north-eastern Australia: pathology, association with *Ancylostoma caninum* and implications. *American Journal of Surgical Pathology*, **19**, 328–37.

Wells, H. S. (1931). Observations on the blood sucking activities of the hookworm, *Ancylostoma caninum*. *Journal of Parasitology*, **17**, 167–82.

White, G. F. and Dove, W. E. (1928). The causation of creeping eruption. *Journal of the American Medical Association*, **90**, 1701–4.

Wijers, D. J. B. and Smit, A. M. (1966). Early symptoms after experimental infection of man with *Ancylostoma braziliense* var. *ceylanicum*. *Tropical and Geographical Medicine*, **18**, 48–52.

Wright, D. O. and Gold, E. M. (1946). Löffler's syndrome associated with creeping eruption (cutaneous helminthiasis): report of twenty-six cases. *Archives of Internal Medicine*, **78**, 303–12.

Yokagawa, S. and Oiso, T. (1926). Studies on oral infection with Ancylostoma. *American Journal of Hygiene*, **6**, 484–97.

Yoshida, Y. (1965). *Ancylostoma kusimaense* from a dog in Japan and comparative morphology of related ancylostomes. *Journal of Parasitology*, **51**, 631–5.

Yoshida, Y. (1971*a*). Comparative stages of *Ancylostoma braziliense* and *Ancylostoma ceylanicum*. I. The adult stage. *Journal of Parasitology*, **57**, 983–9.

Yoshida, Y. (1971*b*). Comparative stages of *Ancylostoma braziliense* and *Ancylostoma ceylanicum*. II. The infective larval stage. *Journal of Parasitology*, **57**, 990–2.

Yoshida, Y., Okamoto, K., and Chin, J. K. (1971). Experimental infection of man with *Ancylostoma ceylanicum*. *Chinese Journal of Microbiology*, **4**, 157–67.

Yoshida, Y., Kondo, K., Kurimoto, H., Fukutome, S., and Shirasaka, S. (1974). Comparative stages of *Ancylostoma braziliense* and *Ancylostoma ceylanicum*. III. Life history in the definitive host. *Journal of Parasitology*, **60**, 636–41.

62   ANISAKIOSIS[1]

Thomas C. Cheng

SUMMARY

The zoonotic disease known as human anisakiosis is caused by larval nematodes belonging to the family Anisakidae. Not all anisakids are capable of causing anisakiosis in humans. Only those that normally utilize homeothermic vertebrates as definitive hosts can serve as aetiological agents. Those species that normally utilize poikilothermic vertebrates as definitive hosts cannot survive sufficiently long in the human alimentary tract to cause the disease syndrome. Human anisakiosis involves the penetration of the lining of the alimentary tract with resulting development of a granuloma surrounding the worm.

Ingestion of viable larval nematodes in fish fillet is the primary method for human infection; however, certain marine invertebrates, e.g. cephalopods, scallops, and shrimp can also serve as sources of infection.

The prevention of human anisakiosis is most commonly achieved by candling fish fillet followed by removal of the worms. This also renders the fillet more aesthetically pleasing. There are other methods of controlling human anisakiosis, including heating and refrigeration. These, however, have drawbacks from the standpoint of marketing. Another method is to refrigerate fish aboard fishing vessels as soon as possible after catching. This prevents migration of anisakid larvae into body muscles of the fish.

HISTORY

DISCOVERY OF DISEASE

Prior to 1960, only two references existed to members of the Anisakidae occurring in humans. Hitchcock (1950) reported that 10 per cent of 100 Eskimos she examined in Alaska spontaneously eliminated larval nematodes. One was identified as *Porrocaecum* sp. and another was *Anisakis* sp. Buckley (1951) reported a specimen of *Porrocaecum decipiens* recovered from the mouth of a patient at night.

ORGANISMS

Subsequent to the earlier incidental reports, the major landmark report was that by van Thiel *et al.* (1960). According to these investigators the zoonotic disease known as anisakiosis, sometimes known as the herring or cod worm disease, was initially recognized by M. Straub in The Netherlands.

PATHOGENESIS

Straub had examined a patient suffering from severe abdominal colic and gastrointestinal distress within 24 hours of having eaten lightly salted herring. As a result of laparotomy performed 24 hours after the onset of the symptoms, an ulcer measuring 1.5 cm in diameter was found in the ileal wall, and from it protruded a nematode that measured 1.3 cm in length. The worm was identified as *Eustoma rotundatum* by Kuipers *et al.* (1960). It was subsequently designated by van Thiel *et al.* (1960) as *Anisakis marina*. Detailed information pertaining to the taxonomy of the causative nematodes has been reviewed by Myers (1975) and Cheng (1982), and that pertaining to the epidemiology and pathology of human anisakiosis has been reviewed by Oshima (1972), Jackson (1975), Cheng (1976, 1982), and Higashi (1985). Consequently, only brief reviews are presented herein, with emphasis on what has not been reviewed.

The initial reports of human anisakiosis from The Netherlands stimulated considerable interest worldwide, especially in the Scandinavian countries, Britain, and Japan. Since human infections are derived from ingestion of raw or poorly cooked marine fish, the greatest interest has been in countries where fish constitute a major part of the protein diet. Furthermore, in relatively recent years an increase in the popularity of seafoods has occurred. The main reasons are:

(1)   the increasing popularity on the part of the more urbane segments of advanced societies for exotic foods such as sashimi and sushi, South American ceviche, Scandinavian gravlax, Hawaiian lomi

[1]Contribution No. 4 from the Marine Research Institute.

lomi (raw salmon), Dutch pickled or green herring, smoked salmon, and other raw and undercooked seafoods; and

(2)   the development of mariculture worldwide.

Because of these developments, certain diseases that had been restricted to marine vertebrates have become zoonotic, including anisakiosis.

Interest in human anisakiosis in the United States came into focus with the reporting of increased number of cases (reviewed by Jackson 1975). As a result, Clintwood (1970) conducted a survey of fresh market fish in the Washington, DC area. She reported that species of *Phocanema, Anisakis,* and *Contracaecum* can all cause 'a dangerous parasitic syndrome in man'. This caused considerable concern for that unit within the US Food and Drug Administration responsible for the safety of seafoods, resulting in the conducting of surveys along the Atlantic, Gulf, and Pacific coasts of the United States and experimental infectivity studies. Subsequently, Cheng (1976, 1982) reported that those larval nematodes that have been known to cause human anisakiosis or are potential pathogens have marine mammals or birds as their natural definitive hosts, the reason being that those nematodes utilizing poikilothermic vertebrates as their natural definitive hosts are incapable of surviving at mammalian body temperatures (Cheng 1976).

EPIDEMIOLOGY

Since those species of larval anisakids that can cause human anisakiosis utilize homeothermic vertebrates as the natural definitive hosts, in nature one would expect them to be more abundant in those parts of the seas and oceans where such animals are more numerous. This, however, need not be the case, since fish harbouring infective larvae may migrate, at least periodically, away from areas where homeotherms occur. Nevertheless, since the eggs, L1s, and L2s are essentially sedentary and L3s occur in invertebrates incapable of migrating long distances, one would expect to find areas of greater endemicity, e.g. the North Sea, the North Atlantic, and areas of the Pacific in the vicinity of Japan, Hawaii, Samoa, and Tahiti.

Commercial fishing can contribute to the distribution of anisakids. Cheng (1976) reported that smaller specimens of fish which the fishermen do not choose to retain commonly are permitted to sit on the deck in the sun for at least 3–4 hours before they are thrown back into the sea. As the deck is cleared of fish before the next haul, many discarded fish harbouring anisakid larvae are thrown back into the sea. Such moribund or dead fish are rapidly eaten by larger fish and the parasites are passed on to the predators, and thus these fishing vessels serve as vehicles for the transport of these parasites from one area to another.

THE AGENTS

TAXONOMY

In view of the above pertaining to the survival of anisakid larvae in homeothermic hosts, including humans, it can be concluded that certain members of the genera *Anisakis, Belanisakis, Phocanema, Porrocaecum, Paradujardinia, Pseudoterranova, Cloeoascaris, Phocascaris,* and *Contracaecum* are either actual or potential causative agents of human anisakiosis. All of these nematodes belong to the family Anisakidae of the order Ascarida and suborder Ascaridina (Chitwood 1969).

The morphological basis for specific identification of larval anisakid nematodes is not well established at this time. Furthermore, it is also difficult to distinguish between members of certain closely related genera by examining larvae. Exact identifications are only reliable by examining sexually mature adult worms. Consequently, if specific identification is essential, larvae recovered from fish must be fed to suitable homeothermic hosts and the sexually mature adults recovered from these identified. Nevertheless, anisakids, based on certain morphological characteristics (Fig. 62.1), can be divided into five groups: the *Anisakis, Phocanema, Contracaecum, Raphidascaris,* and *Multicaecum* groups.

Larvae of the *Anisakis* group

Ventriculus present; anteriorly projecting intestinal caecum and posteriorly directed ventricular appendix absent (Fig. 62.2). Includes members of six genera

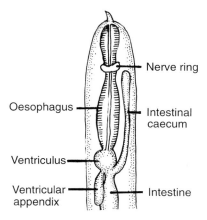

Fig. 62.1   Schematic drawing of anterior portion of a hypothetical anisakid nematode, showing anatomical structures.

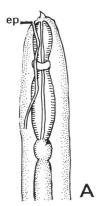

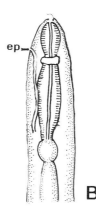

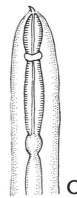

A
Anisakis*
Acanthocheilus
Paranisakiopsis

B
Metanisakis
Paranisakis
Pseudoanisakis

C
Belanisakis*
Heligmus
Ichthyanisakis

Fig. 62.2 Anterior portions of members of those genera belonging to the *Anisakis* group. Those genera marked with an asterisk are real or potential causative agents of human anisakiosis. ep, Excretory pore.

(*Anisakis, Acanthocheilus, Paranisakiopsis, Metanisakis, Paranisakis, Pseudoanisakis*). The excretory pore is situated at the anterior end of the body, at base of lips in members of *Anisakis, Acanthocheilus*, and *Paranisakiopsis* (Fig. 62.2A). Excretory pore situated at the level of the circumoesophageal nerve ring in members of *Metanisakis, Paranisakis*, and *Pseudoanisakis* (Fig. 62.2B).

Among members of the *Anisakis* group, only members of *Anisakis* naturally attain the adult stage in homeothermic vertebrates, in mammals, and hence can cause human anisakiosis. Adults of *Acanthocheilus* and *Paranisakiopsis* are parasites of elasmobranchs and bony fishes, respectively, and hence most probably are incapable of causing human anisakiosis. The adults of *Metanisakis, Paranisakis*, and *Pseudoanisakis* are parasites of fishes, and consequently their larvae are not believed to be involved in human anisakiosis.

In addition to the six genera assigned to the *Anisakis* group, three others (*Belanisakis, Heligmus, Ichthyanisakis*) have been tentatively assigned to this group because all of the new members possess a ventriculus but no intestinal caecum or ventricular appendix (Fig. 62.2C). The position of the excretory pore of members of these genera, however, remains underdetermined and hence their tentative membership in the *Anisakis* group.

Among members of the three genera tentatively assigned to the *Anisakis* group, the adults of *Heligmus* and *Ichthyanisakis* are intestinal parasites of fish, and hence the larvae, if ingested by humans, cannot cause anisakiosis.

Adults of *Belanisakis* are parasites of birds, which are homeotherms; hence, the larvae could cause human anisakiosis.

It is noted that Oshima (1972) has recognized three types of *Anisakis* larvae that can cause human anisakiosis. Type I larvae are characterized by the presence of a prominent anterioventral boring tooth, a short tail, a mucron, and an oesophagus with a long ventriculus that ends obliquely at its junction with the intestine. Type II larvae are characterized by a long tapered tail, short vertriculus, which has a horizontal junction with the intestine, and the presence of a prominent anterioventral boring tooth. These larvae have no caudal mucron. Type III larvae are rarely seen. These are stout larvae, each with a ventriculus similar to that of Type II larvae and a short tail with a tiny mucron.

Larvae of *Phocanema* group

Ventriculus and anteriorly directed intestinal caecum present; ventricular appendix absent; excretory pore situated anteriorly at the base of the lips in members of *Phocanema* and *Terranova* (Fig. 62.3A), at the level of the circumoesophageal nerve ring in members of *Porrocaecum, Paradujardinia, Pseudoterranova*, and *Dujardinascaris* (Fig. 62.3B). The position of the excretory pore in members of *Cloeoascaris*, tentatively assigned to this group, is unknown (Fig. 62.3C).

Adults of the genus *Phocanema* utilize seals as their natural definitive hosts, and hence their larvae can cause human anisakiosis. In fact, human infections with *Phocanema* spp. have been documented (Hayasaka *et al.* 1970; Little and MacPhail 1972; Kates *et al.* 1973; Little and Most 1973). *Terranova* spp., on the other hand, utilize poikilothermic vertebrates, e.g. bony and elasmobranch fishes, and hence usually are not involved in human anisakiosis. However, Oshima (1972) reported that what have been designated as *Terranova* Type A larvae, which occur in squid, may be a possible causative agent of human anisakiosis. This remains to be confirmed.

No human cases of anisakiosis have been reported to be caused by members of *Porrocaecum, Paradujardinia, Pseudoterranova, Dujardinascaris*, or *Cloeoascaris*.

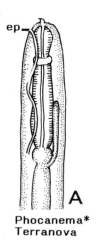

Phocanema*
Terranova

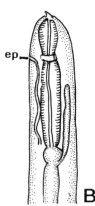

Porrocaecum*
Paradujardinia*
Pseudoterranova*
Dujardinascaris

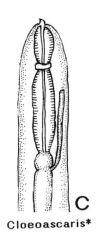

Cloeoascaris*

Fig. 62.3 Anterior portions of members of those genera belonging to the *Phocanema* group. Those genera marked with an asterisk are real or potential causative agents of human anisakiosis. ep, Excretory pore.

In nature, *Porrocaecum* spp. utilize birds and fishes, *Paradujardinia* spp. utilize manatees, *Pseudoterranova* spp. utilize marine mammals, and *Cloeoascaris* spp. utilize semiaquatic mammals as their definitive hosts. Consequently, the larvae of these four genera could theoretically cause human anisakiosis. Adults of *Dujardinascaris* utilize reptiles and fishes, both poikilothermic groups, as their natural hosts and hence the larvae most probably cannot cause human anisakiosis.

Larvae of the *Contracaecum* group

Ventriculus, posteriorly directed ventricular appendix, and anteriorly directed intestinal caecum present; the

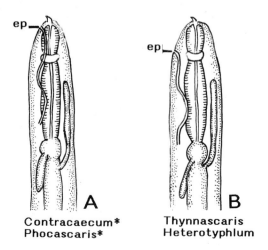

Contracaecum*
Phocascaris*

Thynnascaris
Heterotyphlum

Fig. 62.4 Anterior portions of members of those genera belonging to the *Contracaecum* group. Those genera marked with an asterisk are real or potential causative agents of human anisakiosis. ep, Excretory pore.

excretory pore is anteriorly situated at the base of the lips in members of *Contracaecum* and *Phocascaris* (Fig. 6 2 .4A), and is situated at the level of the circumoesophageal nerve ring in members of *Thynnascaris* and *Heterotyphlum* (Fig. 62.4B).

Adults of *Contracaecum* spp. are intestinal parasites of marine mammals and birds, while adults of *Phocascaris* spp. are parasitic in seals. Consequently, the larvae of both these genera are possible causative agents of human anisakiosis. In fact, Ashby *et al.* (1964) reported human anisakiosis due to *Contracaecum*. Also, Cheng (1982) has reported that *Contracaecum* larvae in the muscle of cod, *Gadus callarias*, caught off the coast of Massachusetts, USA, can cause intestinal anisakiosis in rats.

The definitive hosts of *Thynnascaris* and *Heterotyphlum* are fish. Therefore, human anisakiosis due to the larvae of these nematode genera is unlikely. The reports that larval *Thynnascaris* spp. can cause anisakiosis in humans and in experimentally infected mice (Benatre *et al.* 1968; Petter 1969) are believed to reflect misidentification of *Contracaecum* as *Thynnascaris*. Similarly, a type of *Thynnascaris* from the cutlassfish, *Trichiuris lepturus*, which possibly is identical to that which occurs in brown shrimp, *Penaeus aztecus*, from Florida and the Gulf of Mexico, which can produce gastrointestinal lesions in mice (Norris and Overstreet 1976), is most probably a member of *Contracaecum*.

Larvae of the *Raphidascaris* group

Ventriculus and ventricular appendix present; anteriorly projecting intestinal caecum absent (Fig. 62.5); excretory pore is at the level of the nerve ring.

Raphidascaris and *Raphidascaroides* are the two genera of anisakids that have larvae belonging to this group.

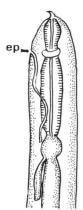

Fig. 62.5 Anterior portion of members of those genera belonging to the *Raphidascaris* group. ep, Excretory pore.

Since the adults of these genera are intestinal parasites of fish, it is doubtful whether they can cause human anisakiosis.

Larvae of the *Multicaecum* group

Ventriculus, multiple ventricular appendixes, and anteriorly projecting intestinal caecum present. The larvae of two genera of nematodes, *Multicaecum* and *Polycaecum*, belong to this group. The adults are parasites of crocodiles, which are poikilotherms, and hence these larvae most probably are incapable of causing human anisakiosis.

As stated, it is not always possible to identify at the generic level those anisakid larvae found in fish that may cause human anisakiosis. Also, even if whole larvae are recovered from a gastric or intestinal lesion in cases of human anisakiosis, it is not always possible to place the specimens in a specific genus or genera. It is possible, however, to place such larvae in one of the groups. The identification of larvae in histopathological sections should be left to experts.

If identification beyond the group level is essential, then viable larvae must be fed to experimental definitive hosts, and if adults are subsequently recovered, they can be identified to the generic level by employing the following diagnostic characteristics. Only those genera the members of which are known or potential causative agents of human anisakiosis are included:

Anisakis Dujardin, 1845

Synonyms: *Stomachus* Goeze (in Zeder, 1800)
　　　　　Filocapsularia Deslongchamps, 1824

Peritrachelius Diesing, 1851
Conocephalus Diesing, 1860

Generic features: three lips, each bearing a bilobed anterior projection which carries a single dentigerous ridge, present; interlabia absent; excretory pore opening at base of subventral lip; oesophagus with anterior muscular portion and posterior ventriculus, the latter being oblong and sometimes sigmoid, or as broad as long; no oesophageal appendix or intestinal caecum; vulva in middle or anterior third of body; spicules of male unequal; preanal papillae numerous; postanal papillae, including a group of three or four pairs, set close to tip of tail on ventral side.

Type species: *A. simplex* (Rudolphi, 1809) Baylis, 1920. Parasites of marine mammals.

Belanisakis Maplestone, 1932

Generic features: cervical alae present; interlabia and dentigerous ridges present; oesophagus with posterior muscular ventriculus; intestinal caecum and ventricular appendix absent; vulva anterior to middle of body; spicules stout, equal; gubernaculum short.

Type species: *B. ibidis* Maplestone, 1932. Parasites of birds.

Phocanema Myers, 1959

Generic features: three prominent, fleshy, well-developed bilobed lips present; dentigerous ridges present; interlabia absent; excretory pore opening at base of subventral lips; oesophagus with anterior muscular portion and posterior ventriculus; vulva opens in anterior third of body; anteriorly projecting intestinal caecum present; spicules subequal; gubernaculum absent; three postanal dentigerous ridges present.

Type species: *P. decipiens* (Krabbe, 1878) Myers, 1959. Parasites of marine mammals.

Porrocaecum Railliet and Henry, 1912

Generic features: three lips, dentigerous ridges, and interlabia present; excretory pore at level of nerve ring; oesophagus with anterior muscular portion and posterior ventriculus of oblong shape (ventriculus short in generotype but in other species bent at an angle so as to open into intestine laterally); intestinal caecum present; vulva near middle of body; spicules equal; gubernaculum usually absent.

Type species: *P. crassum* (Deslongchamps, 1824) Railliet and Henry, 1912. Parasites of birds and fishes.

Paradujardinia Travassos, 1933

Generic features: dorsal lip octagonal in outline, lip pulp gives rise to small conical, anterior processes that project forward and inward; interlabia well developed;

dentigerous ridges absent; excretory pore at level of nerve ring; ventriculus spherical; intestinal caecum narrow; vulva anterior to mid-length of body; spicules short; gubernaculum absent.

Type species: *P. halicoris* (Owen, 1833) Travassos, 1933. Parasites of Sirenia.

Pseudoterranova Mozgovoy, 1950

Generic features: lips similar in shape, internally projecting bilobed part with long teeth in the dentigerous ridges; interlabia absent; excretory pore may be at level of nerve ring; ventriculus present; intestinal caecum only slightly longer than ventriculus; vulva a short distance posterior to oesophagus; spicules small, unequal; gubernaculum present.

Type species: *P. kogiae* (Johnston and Mawson, 1939) Mozgovoy, 1950. Parasites of whales.

Cloeoascaris Baylis, 1923

Generic features: each lip with a pair of large conical teeth on inner surface; interlabia absent; collar-like cuticular fold surrounds neck; area between cuticular fold and bases of lips covered with small spines; oesophagus with small rounded ventriculus; intestinal caecum present; vulva in anterior half of body; spicules short, slender, and equal.

Type species: *C. spinicollis* Baylis, 1923. Parasites of semiaquatic land mammals.

Contracaecum Railliet and Henry, 1912

Synonyms: *Kathleena* Leiper and Atkinson, 1914
             Cerascaris Cobb, 1928
             Amphicaecum Walton, 1929
             Iheringascaris Pereira, 1935

Generic features: lips with anterolateral projections; dentigerous ridges absent; interlabia present, usually well developed; excretory pore at base of subventral lips; oesophagus with anterior muscular portion and reduced posterior ventriculus with posterior appendix; anterior projecting intestinal caecum present; vulva in anterior region of body; male without definite caudal alae; with numerous preanal papillae; spicules long, alate; gubernaculum absent.

Type species: *C. spiculigerum* (Rudolphi, 1809) Railliet and Henry, 1912. Parasites of marine mammals and birds.

Phocascaris Höst, 1932

Generic features: lips with three deep incisions directed toward oral aperture; interlabia absent; dentigerous ridges present; excretory pore opens at level of nerve ring; oesophagus with small ventriculus and ventricular appendix; intestinal caeca absent; vulva

in anterior half of body; spicules equal, alate; gubernaculum absent.

Type species: *P. phocae* Höst, 1932. Parasites of marine mammals.

MOLECULAR BIOLOGY

Nothing is known about the molecular biology of anisakids at this time.

DISEASE MECHANISMS

See p. 566.

GROWTH AND SURVIVAL REQUIREMENTS

Although well over 200 species of anisakid nematodes have been described, there is surprisingly little information pertaining to the life cycles of these nematodes. Drawing upon what is known about the life cycles of anisakids of terrestrial and freshwater vertebrates, and piecing together what has been reported from marine animals, it is generally recognized that the life cycles of marine anisakids involve at least one, more commonly two, intermediate hosts, in addition to the definitive host (Margolis 1970; Oshima 1972) (Fig. 62.6). Furthermore, alternative developmental routes may occur, at least in the case of *Contracaecum spiculigerum*, a parasite of marine piscivorous birds and hence a potential causative agent of human anisakiosis (Huizinga 1966). Paratenic hosts may also be involved (Fig. 62.6).

Adult

Adult marine anisakids are parasites of piscivorous reptiles, fishes, birds, or mammals. These adults usually occur in either the stomach or the small intestine. With those species that parasitize birds, the nematodes usually are buried in the mucosal wall of the proventriculus.

Egg

As eggs are laid, they are passed out into sea water in the host's faeces and, as is the pattern among ascaroids, the L1 undergoes the first moult while still within the egg capsule. Anisakid eggs passed from marine vertebrates are thin-shelled and are non-resistant to desiccation, low temperatures, and chemicals.

L1

After an embryonic developmental period within the egg shell, the L1 is formed. Organogenesis within this stage is rudimentary.

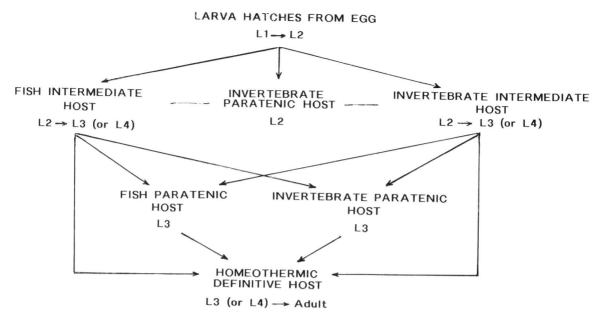

Fig. 62.6 Possible pathways in the life cycles of anisakid nematodes that can cause human anisakiosis.

L2

As the initial ecdysis of anisakid larvae occurs with the egg shell, the stage escaping from the pliable capsule is the L2. It bears a small boring tooth or stylet. Both the oesophagus and ventriculus are distinguishable but the rest of the alimentary tract is not clearly defined. The L2 is sheathed and, at least in the case of *Phocanema decipiens*, Scott (1957) reported that it is very active; wriggling and gyrating about a verticle plane. However, once it becomes attached to the bottom by its posterior end, it remains somewhat sedentary and does not move along the substrate. Similarly, Huizinga (1966) reported that *Contracaecum spiculigerum* L2s are attached to the substrate by the aid of a viscous material; however, it is usually the anterior end that is attached. In either case, the attached L2s undergo a characteristic gyrating movement. Cheng (1976) has speculated that this type of movement could serve as an attraction for the first intermediate host.

L3

Free-living L2s must be ingested by an intermediate host, the first, before further development occurs. From what is known, the first intermediate host is usually an aquatic protostomate invertebrate. Wülker (1930) reported the occurrence of larval *Contracaecum* in *Rhinocalalanus nasutus*, Cobb (1930) described *Paranisakis pectinis* in the visceral mass of a scallop, *Aequipecten*, and Hutton *et al.* (1962) reported larval *Contracaecum* in several species of shrimp. Also, Hutton

(1964), while examining bay scallops, *Aequipecten gibbus*, off the east coast of Florida, found numerous specimens of an immature nematode which he believed to represent Cobb's (1930) species. However, his finding of the presence of a short, anteriorly projecting intestinal caecum caused him to transfer *P. pectinis* to the genus *Porrocaecum*. The same larval worm was reported by Cheng (1973) in 2.3 per cent of 400 specimens of the scallop *Aequipecten irradians* from off the coast of North Carolina. In this pelecypod, this parasite is commonly, although not always, found in the adductor muscle, causing it to become brownish in colour.

Several investigators have reported that planktonic copepods can harbour larval marine anisakids. Included among these is Apstein (1911) who reported larval *Contracaecum* spp. in the coelom of *Calanus finmarchicus*, *Pseudocalanus* sp., and *Euchaeta* sp. from the North Sea. L3s of *Contracaecum* spp. have also been reported in the chaetognath *Sagitta* (Pierantoni 1914; Lebour 1917; Wülker 1929; Ass 1961).

Because of the poorly developed state of larval anisakids, it is not possible to identify with certainty as to whether the larvae found in the marine invertebrates cited above are L2s, L3s, or even L4s. However, Markowski's (1937) report of successful infection of the marine copepods *Eurytemora affinis* and *Ascartia bifilosa* with L2s of *Contracaecum aduncum*; Penner's (1941) report of successfully infecting another marine copepod, *Tigriopus californicus*, with L2s of *Contracaecum* sp. hatched from eggs obtained from sea lions; Valter's (1969) report of successfully infecting isopods with L2s

of *C. aduncum*; and Huizinga's (1966) success at infecting the copepods *Cyclops vernalis* and *T. californicus* with
L2s of *C. spiculigerun* strongly suggest that these marine
invertebrates are true intermediate hosts.

It is noted that in addition to the above, several
Japanese investigators (Ichihara *et al.* 1966; Kobayashi
et al. 1966; Okumura 1967; Otsuru 1968; Kato *et al.*
1968; Kosugi *et al.* 1969, 1970; Saito *et al.* 1970) reported
what was designated as Type I *Anisakis* larvae (most
probably the larvae of *A. simplex*) in the musculature
of the cephalopod *Todarodes pacificus*. Kato *et al.* (1968)
and Kosugi *et al.* (1969) also reported the occurrence
of Type II *Anisakis* larvae (most probably the larvae of
A. physeteris) in another cephalopod, *Doryteuthis bleekeri*.
Although experimental proof is wanting, the general
opinion held by Japanese parasitologists is that the
larval anisakids in cephalopods are L3s, and hence are
infective to the natural definitive host or humans if
ingested in raw or poorly cooked squid. In the same
vein, anisakid L2s developing into L3s in shrimp, scallops, and other edible marine invertebrates are potential causative agents of human anisakiosis if ingested in
insufficiently cooked, cured, or raw seafoods. It is
noted, however, that nematodes other than anisakids
in marine fish and shellfish can cause parasitoses in
humans (see Rodrick and Cheng 1989).

L4

Anisakids found in the stomachs of vertebrates that
serve as definitive hosts are most commonly either L4s
or adults. This is especially true of *Contracaecum* spp.
Thus, it would appear that it is the L3 that is ingested
and the third and fourth moults occur in the alimentary canal of the final host. Huizinga (1966) postulated
that with *Contracaecum spiculigerum*, the avian definitive host becomes infected when fish harbouring
ensheathed L3s are ingested and the nematode larvae
undergo two additional moults in the bird before
becoming adults. Also, Kagei *et al.* (1967) hypothesized
that with *Anisakis simplex* or possibly *A. typica*, the L3s
undergo two moults in the first ventriculus of the blue
white dolphin and in the process metamorphose and
grow into adults. Thus, it would appear that it is the
L3 that is the infective form to the definitive host.

Although what is stated seems reasonable, there are
reports to the contrary. Specifically, Gibson (1970)
observed only one moult for an *Anisakis* larva prior to
attaining the 'pre-adult' form in the stomach of a rat,
and Davey (1965, 1969) reported that *Porrocaecum
decipiens* only moults once in the final host. Thus, as
depicted in Fig. 62.6, it would appear that certain
species enter the definitive host as L3s and undergo
two moults therein, while other species enter as L4s
and only undergo the fourth or final moult within the
definitive host.

Finally, as stated earlier, paratenic hosts are commonly involved in the life cycles of anisakid nematodes. Specifically, as depicted in Fig. 62.6, L3s in the
fish or invertebrate intermediate host, if ingested by a
fish or another invertebrate paratenic host, are conveyed to the vertebrate definitive host as L3s. It is only
after the paratenic host is ingested by a suitable
definitive host that the L3 (or L4) undergoes the
remaining moults and develop into the adult.

In view of the above, it is now apparent that human
anisakiosis can be acquired from the ingestion of L3s
(or L4s) in either fish intermediate or paratenic hosts,
or from ingesting L3s (or L4s) in invertebrate intermediate or paratenic hosts.

THE HOSTS

NON-HUMAN MAMMALS

Incubation period

Nothing is known about the incubation period of
anisakiosis in marine mammals.

Symptoms and signs

Pathological alterations in natural definitive hosts of
anisakids have been studied to some extent. As human
anisakiosis is caused by those species of anisakids that
utilize marine homeothermic vertebrates as natural
definite hosts, the review being presented involves
only information pertaining to mammals and birds.
For those interested in the symptoms and signs of
piscian anisakiosis, the review by Margolis (1970) is
recommended.

According to Rausch (1953) and Schiller (1954),
when L3s of *Porrocaecum decipiens* are ingested by the
otter, *Enhydra lutris*, they become free in the small
intestine and burrow into the mucosa where they
undergo the third moult and develop into L4s. These
larvae migrate away from the host's intestinal mucosa,
up the alimentary tract, and enter the stomach where
they become attached to the gastric mucosa. At this
site, the larvae undergo the fourth moult and mature.
Young adults remain attached to the host's stomach
wall until they reach sexual maturity, at which time
they become lumen parasites.

According to Rausch (1953), there are no externally
visible symptoms in infected otters until they are near
the terminal stages of illness, at which time they
become weak and depressed before dying. As sea otters
do not contain much subcutaneous or abdominal fat,
an overall deteriorating body condition in parasitized
animals is not readily evident. The cause of death of
P. decipiens-infected animals appeared to be a general-

ized peritonitis resulting from penetration of the gut wall by larval parasites.

Diagnosis

Diagnosis of anisakiosis in their natural mammalian hosts has not been addressed in the literature.

Pathology

In the case of the otter infected with *P. decipiens* reported by Rausch (1953), numerous nematodes were found on the surface of the greater omentum and the body cavity contained a thin, blood-stained fluid. The intestinal coils and serous membranes were coated with a fibropurulent exudate. Furthermore, the intestinal coils adhered to one another and to the greater omentum in inflamed areas. Where the omentum was penetrated, it was thickened and often adhered to internal organs that were invaded by larval nematodes. The areas surrounding intestinal perforations were inflamed and greatly congested. The nematodes often protruded into the abdominal cavity and dense aggregations of L3s were found attached to the intestinal wall around the perforations. The stomach included dense aggregations of *P. decipiens* embedded in the mucosa, but no stomach perforations were noted. In the gastric lesions, L4s and immature adults predominated. These could be recognized by their darker colour in contrast to the translucent younger stages.

Microscopically, Rausch (1953) determined that the anterior ends of the nematodes in the stomach were deeply embedded in the gastric mucosa. The gastric mucosa was eroded to the level of the muscularis mucosa in the areas of parasite attachment and occasional invasions into the muscularis externa were noted. The tissues were infiltrated with monocytes, and the general area was hyperaemic.

In the small intestine, these areas showing pathological manifestation were those directly surrounding the sites of invasion. The mucosa in such an area underwent epithelial desquamation, but it was otherwise unaltered. Groups of nematode larvae occurred at each focus which was infiltrated mainly by segmented neutrophils. Some fibroblastic proliferation also occurred.

The omentum near perforations was coated with a fibropurulent exudate, although the serosal epithelium was usually intact. Cellular reaction consisted mainly of infiltration by segmented neutrophils. When nematodes were found embedded in inflammatory tissue, tissue liquefaction around the anterior end of the worm was observed. The invaded spleen showed marked fibrosis, adherent omentum, and hyperaemia in regions where the parasites occurred. The cellular exudate consisted of segmented neutrophils, macro-

phages, and plasma cells in decreasing order of abundance.

Prior to Rausch's (1953) exhaustive study, Hoeppli (1932) had reported an ulcerous lesion in the gastric wall of a walrus, *Rosmarus rosmarus*, infected with *Anisakis* sp. which was subsequently identified by Hsu and Hoeppli (1933) as *A. alata* (= *A. rosmari*). The ulcerous lesion was characterized by host necrotic tissues surrounding the anterior terminal of the worm. Specifically, Hoeppli reported a zone of tissue liquefaction about 0.5 mm in diameter surrounding the anterior end of the parasite. He attributed this liquefaction to oesophageal secretions of the parasite.

An additional pathological study in a marine mammal associated with anisakids is that by Young and Lowe (1969). They described the histopathology in a grey seal, *Halichoerus grypus*, and a porpoise, *Phocaena phocaena*, infected with *Anisakis* sp., *A. simplex*, and *Contracaecum* sp. These mammals were taken in British coastal waters. The lesions produced in these hosts were limited to the stomach. These were characterized as eosinophilic granulomata and there was usually an eosinophilic substance surrounding the anterior ends of the parasites. A zone of necrotic host tissues surrounded the eosinophilic tunic.

Other reports of anisakids in marine mammals include that of Martin *et al.* (1970) who reported invasion of the brain of a Pacific striped dolphin, *Lagenorhynchus obliquidens*, by a nematode which was identified as *Contracaecum* sp. from its eggs. The lesion in the brain measured about 30 mm in diameter. At one corner of this lesion, channels, 2–3 mm in diameter, were noted. The sections of the worm were located in these channels. Also, Florels-Barroeta *et al.* (1961) reported *Contracaecum osculatum* adults from the brains of four California sea lions, *Zalophus californianus*, from Mexico. The resulting pathology, however, was not recorded.

Experimental mammals

In addition to natural anisakid infections in marine mammals, some information is available pertaining to experimental infections in laboratory mammals. Myers (1963) fed an unstated number of '*Anisakis*'-type larvae to guinea-pigs. She reported that the larvae penetrated the stomach wall and then migrated randomly throughout the internal organs. Specifically, larvae were recovered from the stomach, liver, mesenteries, pancreas, small and large intestines, thyroid gland, fatty tissues around the kidneys, and in two cases, larvae were encysted under the skin. No difference in behaviour of the hosts was noted in comparison with the controls. Living larvae were observed in the guinea-pigs for 5 days, but no trace of their presence were found on day 6. The larvae underwent no observable development in the guinea-pigs, and the migrating larvae removed from the body cavity were infectious to other guinea-pigs.

In experimentally infected guinea-pigs, the actively migrating anisakid larvae caused pathological alterations similar to mechanical injury, i.e. only local defence reactions of the involved organs were observed. Microscopically, infiltration by leucocytes and macrophages around the worms occurred. The site in the gastric wall penetrated by each larva appeared as a small haemorrhagic focus at 24 hours and was undetectable at 48 hours.

Kuipers *et al.* (1963) and Kuipers (1964) studied rabbits experimentally infected *per os* with *Anisakis* larvae. They reported that within 24 hours, the larvae had penetrated the mucosal layer of the gastrointestinal wall, causing only a slight reaction with necrosis and some eosinophilic infiltration. After 3–4 days, the larvae apparently died and the lesions had not changed. After several weeks to months, calcified remnants of larvae may be found scattered throughout the gastrointestinal walls, most commonly in the cardiac and pyloric regions of the stomach and the appendix.

In another experiment, Kuipers (1964) sensitized rabbits with lyopholysed *Anisakis* antigen prior to, or at the time of, exposure to *Anisakis* larvae. No differences were noted in the resulting histopathological pictures. In still another experiment, rabbits were fed several sequential doses of *Anisakis* larvae. It was subsequently found that the first-delivered worms became calcified, more recently administered larvae were necrotic, and those fed within 72 hours were viable. If the larvae had not penetrated in the proximity of 1 cm from a previous point of penetration, the host reaction was the same as that of a primary exposure. However, if the site of larval penetration was less than 1 cm from that of a worm from a previous dose, the host reaction was much more severe, being characterized by oedema and diffuse infiltration by eosinophils. When two larvae of the same dosage penetrated the same area, only primary reactions resulted. Similarly, only primary reactions occurred if more than 4 months intervened between penetrations by larvae.

Kuipers *et al.* (1963) examined the serological reaction of experimentally infected rabbits. They found that a complement-fixation test with *Anisakis* antigen changed from negative to positive 3–5 days post-exposure and the titre rose to about 1 : 32 in 2–3 weeks, and subsequently gradually decreased, becoming negative again after 4 months.

Oyanagi (1967), who experimentally infected rabbits and dogs with *Anisakis* larvae, reported a light eosinophilic infiltration around penetrating worms in both hosts upon primary exposure. These reactions receded in about 1 week. Oyanagi (1967), in a second experiment, sensitized rabbits by surgically implanting *Anisakis*-type larvae from the fish *Scomber japonicus*. The sensitized hosts were then given an oral dose of larvae after 2 weeks. The challenge dose resulted in oedema, phlebitis, bleeding, and massive eosinophilic infiltration in the hosts; however, the invasion rate of larvae into the gastrointestinal wall of sensitized rabbits was only about two-thirds of that of the control group and the degeneration of the larvae was more rapid and pronounced in the sensitized group.

Oyanagi (1967) also injected control and sensitized rabbits with physiological saline in which *Anisakis* larvae had moulted. Eosinophilic infiltrations occurred in all cases, but were more pronounced in sensitized rabbits than in the controls.

Asami (1966) studied the infectivity and susceptibility of *Anisakis*-type larvae in guinea-pigs. Each experimental host was fed 10 larvae and was sacrificed 3–4 hours later. No difference was found in the infectivity of encapsulated or unencapsulated larvae from fish. Also, he reported that starvation of hosts and administration of drugs that reduced gastric secretions facilitated penetration of the stomach wall by larvae, while increased gastric secretion to some extent inhibited penetration. Thus, exogenous factors were found to modify infectivity of the parasite. However, when freshly obtained infective larvae were used, no marked differences in infectivity were noted in control and experimental hosts. From these data, Asami concluded that the establishment of the parasite is controlled more by the infectivity of the larvae than the susceptibility of the host. Interestingly, he also reported that the anterior ends of anisakid larvae, even when cut in half, were invasive, but to a lesser degree than whole worms.

Rapidity of the appearance of eosinophilia in experimental anisakiosis is correlated with the site of injection of the antigen(s) in the form of acetone-dried saline extract of *Anisakis* larvae (Iwanaga 1970). When injected intraperitoneally into guinea-pigs, eosinophilia appeared within a day; intradermal injection induced eosinophilia within a few hours; intracardial injection resulted in immediate eosinophilia. Also, sensitized hosts were slower to respond than non-sensitized ones to intracardial injections. Eosinophilia could be induced in non-immunized guinea-pigs by transfer of serum from sensitized animals.

BIRDS

As those species of anisakids that can cause human anisakiosis also include those that utilize birds as natural definitive hosts, a brief review of what is known about the pathology of anisakiosis in avian hosts is being presented.

Rizkova (1953) reported there is depression of the activities of haematopoietic organs and the central nervous system of ducks infected with *Porrocaecum*. These activities could be stimulated by treatment with therapeutic doses of carbon tetrachloride or normal butylidene chloride.

Baer (1961) described the tissue reactions in a young blackbird heavily infected with *Porrocaecum eniscaudatum*. The nematodes had penetrated the intestinal mucosa and were represented by all developmental stages. Although L4s are normally not present in the host's intestinal mucosa, in this case they were, and their presence stimulated the development of fibrous tumours on the peritoneal surface of the intestine. Young adult worms were partially ensheathed by the cuticles of L4s.

HUMANS

Incubation period

The onset of the symptoms of human anisakiosis varies from one to several days when the intestine is involved and one to several months if the stomach is involved.

Symptoms and signs

Detailed reviews of human anisakiosis have been provided by Oshima (1972), Cheng (1982), and others. Presented herein is an abbreviated account.

The clinical symptoms of human anisakiosis include gastric or intestinal pain and vomiting. However, the pressure point is not as sharp as in the case of acute appendicitis. Medium leucocytosis generally occurs although eosinophilia is not always acute. There is no abnormal tension of the abdominal muscles and no fever results. These signs are important in distinguishing anisakiosis from acute appendicitis and internal obstruction (Yoshimura 1966; Ishikura 1969).

Diagnosis

The diagnosis of human anisakiosis, other than finding the worm in histological sections resulting from biopsies, is far from satisfactory at this time. Skin tests involving both crude somatic and metabolic antigens have been tried with limited success (Morishita and Kobayashi 1965; Taniguchi 1966; Hayasaka *et al.* 1968; Kobayashi *et al.* 1968 *a,b*). However, Suzuki *et al.* (1970) reported that the utilization of purified antigens resulted in a higher percentage of positives. Even then, only 43 per cent of cases of mild gastric anisakiosis were diagnosed.

Both complement fixation and immunofluorescence tests have been utilized for the diagnosis of human anisakiosis. These have also met with limited success because of cross-antigenicity with other helminths and the failure to detect light infections (Merkelbach 1964; Yoshimura 1966; Ruitenberg 1970).

Pathology

Surgical findings in all reports are quite similar. Laparotomy usually reveals a clear yellow fluid in the abdominal cavity, the areas of infection are characterized by swelling and hyperaemia, and the serosa in the affected areas are covered with fibrin. Also, the sites of infection are marked by a firm infiltration of about 2.5 cm, and an 'ulcer crater' occurs within the area (van Thiel *et al.* 1960; Asami *et al.* 1965; Yokogawa and Yoshimura 1967).

Macroscopically, foci of nematode invasions in the stomach are usually intact, and occasionally ulceration or haemorrhage occurs in the mucosa. The granulomata are visible or can be felt in the submucosa. In contrast, the foci of nematode invasions in the intestine involve severe pathological changes such as gaseous fullness, redness, perforation, and/or ileus.

Histopathologically, the outstanding features of human anisakiosis are massive eosinophilic infiltration associated with marked oedema, infiltration by histiocytes, neutrophils, plasma cells, and occasional giant cells. The anisakid larvae occur in the eosinophilic abscess or phlegmon in the submucosa. If the larvae have completely penetrated the gut wall, abscesses of similar cellular constituents may occur in the mesenteries (Nishimura 1963).

Anisakiosis-associated granulomata can occur in the gastric, small intestinal, and large intestinal walls, with the stomach being the more frequent site. According to Kojima *et al.* (1966), the histopathological lesions can be classified into four types: phlegmonous, abscess, abscess–granulomatous, and granulomatous. Oshima (1972) added a fifth type, designated as the foreign body response type. This is the least severe of the five types. Brief reviews are presented at this point.

Foreign body response type

The histopathological picture associated with this type of response includes infiltration and proliferation of neutrophils associated with a few eosinophils and giant cells. There is little or no oedema, but fibrin exudation, haemorrhage, and vascular damage usually occur. Moreover, granulomas generally develop around the parasite. This type of response is associated with benign clinical symptoms and does not require surgery. According to Oyanagi (1967), Kikuchi *et al.* (1967), and Miyazato *et al.* (1970), foreign body responses result from primary infections, i.e. without presensitization.

Phlegmonous type

This type of reaction has also been referred to as the arthus type. There is extensive oedematous thickening

accompanied by infiltration by lymphocytes, monocytes, neutrophils, and plasma cells. Moreover, there is
an inflammatory response in the associated blood
vessels, haemorrhage, and exudation of fibrin. The
larval nematode at the centre of the reaction complex
is usually viable and a thin layer of tightly packed
eosinophils, neutrophils, and histiocytes occurs adjacent to the larva. This type of reaction is frequently
associated with acute intestinal anisakiosis within 1
week of infection.

Abscess type

This type of reaction is characterized by the accumulation of numerous eosinophils, histiocytes, and lymphocytes surrounding the worm embedded in the
submucosa. A distinct granulomatous zone is apparent.
Necrosis and haemorrhage with eosinophilic infiltration
and fibrin exudation occur in the inner layer of the
granuloma. Slight phlegmonous changes are present in
the peripheral zone of the granuloma. The cuticle of
the larva at the centre of the reaction complex is
destroyed and degeneration of the internal structures
has commenced. This type of lesion is often associated
with chronic cases of gastric and intestinal anisakiosis.

Abscess–granulomatous type

This type of reaction is associated with the degraded
debris of larval anisakids. The abscess surrounding the
residual debris is reduced; however, it is surrounded
by a conspicuous tunic of granulomatous cells accompanied by some deposition of collagen. There is less
infiltration of eosinophils into the granuloma than in
the case of the abscess type. In some cases, lymphocytes, rather than eosinophils, represent the dominant
cells. Giant cells are commonly present along the
periphery of the decomposed larva. Furthermore,
usually numerous eosinophils have invaded the site
occupied by the remnants of the parasite. This type of
lesion occurs primarily in cases of gastric anisakiosis
that are at least 6 months old.

Granulomatous type

This type of reaction represents an advanced stage of
the abscess–granulomatous type. It is characterized by
the replacement of abscess by granulomatous cells
coupled with the infiltration of eosinophils. By this
stage, the causative parasite is no longer recognizable
since it has either totally or almost totally disintegrated. This type of reaction is occasionally found at
sites in the gastric and intestinal walls of old infections.

The mechanism(s) involved for the development of
lesions associated with larval anisakids remains uncertain. There are two extant theories: the double hit
theory and the exacerbation theory. These are considered at this point.

Double hit theory

According to this theory, penetration of the gastric or
intestinal mucosa by anisakid larva induces a local
hypersensitivity which persists for a period of time. If a
second larva penetrates at about the same site within
this period, an eosinophilic phlegmonous inflammation occurs (van Thiel *et al.* 1960; Kuipers *et al.*
1963; Kuipers 1964; Aréan 1971).

This theory has been criticized since it has been
demonstrated that a severe reaction occurs in the
rabbit stomach as a result of a single infection
(Ruitenberg 1970; Ruitenberg and Loendersloot
1971). None the less, Oyanagi (1967) and Young
and Lowe (1969) reported that the reaction to a
second infection is more severe than that from the
first.

Exacerbation theory

According to this theory, the anisakid larva, after penetrating into the submucosa of the host's alimentary
canal, survives for 2 or 3 weeks. During the seventh to
tenth days post-penetration, granulation appears
around the larva. Subsequently, the living larva sens-
itizes the newly formed granuloma with its metabolic
products. After the worm dies, its cuticle commences
to disintegrate and the cells and fluid exuding from
the dead worm react directly with the sensitized granuloma, resulting in an allergic inflammation around the
dead larva. There is some experimental proof of this
theory (Oyanagi 1967; Hayasaka *et al.* 1968). However,
although this theory effectively explains the abscess
and abscess–granulomatous types of reactions, it does
not explain the phlegmonous type of lesions, i.e. a
living larva remains at the centre of the phlegmon,
and there is severe tissue reaction which develops
within a few days, but not of sufficient duration for the
sensitization of the surrounding tissues.

Treatment

Therapeutic resection, in the case of human anisakiosis, has a 10–20 per cent casualty rate (Kuipers *et al.*
1960; Ashby *et al.* 1964); therefore, conservative treatment, i.e. treatment with antiallergic drugs without
surgery, has been the treatment of choice. Daniels
(1962) treated a patient in this manner after biopsy of
a phlegmon of the small intestine revealed eosinophil
infiltration. However, in 1966 the same patient underwent surgery for stenosis of the small intestine in the
same region that had been biopsied earlier. Because of
the possible correlation between the initial infection
and the subsequent stenosis, Kuipers (1967) recommended long-term monitoring of patients undergoing
conservative treatment due to the possibility of late
manifestations of anisakiosis.

Prognosis

If surgery is not performed and antiallergic drugs have no lasting effect, the prognosis of severe cases of human anisakiosis is not promising.

EPIDEMIOLOGY

OCCURRENCE

Anisakid nematodes are worldwide in their distribution. However, since, as stated, those species that cause human anisakiosis utilize marine birds and mammals as their natural definitive hosts, one would expect the causative species to be more abundant in areas where the natural definitive hosts are more prevalent. However, as stated earlier, fishing practices, host migration, and other exogenous factors do influence the distribution of anisakids.

As to be expected, human anisakiosis is most prevalent in those regions where raw or inadequately cooked seafoods, especially fish, form a part of the daily diet. Thus, the largest number of cases have been reported from Japan, The Netherlands, and Norway. However, with the increased consumption of such dishes as sushi and sashimi, which consist of raw seafood, the disease has been reported from the United States, Great Britain, France, and other affluent countries.

SOURCES

Human anisakiosis can only be acquired from eating raw or poorly treated seafood, primarily fish, including infective larvae. The disease could also be acquired from eating raw shellfish, including shrimp, squid, and scallops, harbouring infective larvae.

TRANSMISSION

See growth and survival requirements presented earlier.

COMMUNICABILITY

Human anisakiosis cannot be transmitted from human to human or from vertebrate definitive hosts to humans.

PREVENTION AND CONTROL

PREVENTION

The best method for preventing human anisakiosis is to abstain from eating raw or poorly cooked fish. Being aware of the problem, the commercial fisheries industry has devised methods to recognize and remove the causative larvae from fillet. This practice was primarily initiated in Canada and has been introduced to the United States and elsewhere. The detection and removal of anisakids are not solely based on disease prevention. These measures, to a greater extent, are based on the aesthetics and market value of fish fillets.

The detection of larval nematodes in fish fillet is still primarily dependent on traditional candling, although some effort has been made to develop methods for improving detection and to facilitate removal of parasites (Anon. 1988).

CONTROL STRATEGIES

At the present, control strategies for human anisakiosis include the identification and removal of anisakid larvae from fish fillet. In addition, cooking, freezing, and other measures are effective. The following is a brief review of these strategies.

Obtaining fish

In order to reduce the prevalence and incidence of nematodes larvae in fish, assessment and documentation of certain factors associated with the occurrence of parasites should be recorded. Such information should include species of fish, fish sizes, locations of fishing grounds, and season. When documented over time, a pattern of high prevalence and incidence (intensity) may become apparent and such information should be shared with fishermen so that problem areas and periods of times can be avoided.

As with any factor related to the quality and wholesomeness of the end product, selection of high quality, fresh fish is the first step in controlling the presence of larval anisakids. Fish that have been held for long periods prior to gutting are more likely to have parasites in their fillets. Thus, procuring fish that have been gutted shortly after capture makes control measures easier; however, this is not always a practical solution.

Candling

As stated, the most commonly employed technique for determining the presence or absence of anisakid nematode larvae in fish fillet is candling. This method involves shining a bright light through a piece of fish muscle and viewing it. Parasites, if present, can usually be spotted by this technique.

Although studies involving testing various spectra of light as sources for detecting parasites have been conducted (Valdimarsson *et al.* 1985), the most effective is a combination of the physical factors proposed by the Canadian Institute of Fisheries Technology (Anon.

1988). It is noted, however, that candling is not effective in the case of dark-fleshed fish.

Lighting

Among the physical factors that favour parasite detection and removal by candling, lighting is of paramount importance. Both lighting in the plant and for candling are important.

In that part of the plant where candling is carried out, overhead lighting with cool, white fluorescent bulbs is ideal. Furthermore, there should be minimal shading and no distinct shadows. The indirect lighting ideally should be between 35 and 50 fc (foot candles) or 375–540 lux measured 13 cm above the working surface. The measurement should be taken with the operator present to account for shading.

The candling light boxes, 30 × 65 × 0.3 cm in size (Fig. 62.7), should have a white plexiglass working surface. The top surface should be 5–6 mm thick and be 45–60 per cent translucent. The light source should be a two-bulb fluorescent fixture (F20-T12 cool white bulbs) with the light intensity adjusted to 300–500 fc (3230–5380 lux) as measured at the table surface. Light adjustment is made by incorporating a filter in the light box. Ambient and table light levels should be matched within the recommended range or detection efficiency will be hampered.

Knives

As stated, the objective of candling is to locate and remove nematode larvae from fish fillet. The Fisheries Development Branch of the Canadian Institute of Fisheries Technology (Anon. 1988) has recommended that for most efficient trimming of fillets the knife blade should be 1–12 cm long and 1.5–2.0 cm wide. The plastic handle, 11–12 cm long, should have a contour suitable for a good grip by the thumb and index finger. The blade should be about 56 'Rockwell C' in hardness and be sharp. Commonly, a crochet hook is employed to remove the worms; however, a hook could be ground at the tip of the trimming knife for removing worms.

Heating

Although elevated temperatures will kill anisakid larvae in fish fillet, heating is not always a desirable or practical method from the standpoint of the wholesaler or retailer, since, as indicated in Table 62.1, 50–60 °C is required to kill these parasites (Bier 1976). Furthermore, dead nematodes still render fillets unsightly at the market place. Also, fillets that had been heated to 50–60 °C have shorter shelf-lives.

Freezing

Normal refrigerator temperatures do not kill anisakid larvae in fillet. As indicated in Table 62.2, it takes refrigeration at –20 °C, even then, it takes at least 52 hours to kill the parasites (Bier 1976).

Smoking and pickling

The effectiveness of smoking and pickling in destroying anisakid larvae in fish fillet has been studied to some extent. In general, smoking and marination are insufficient. The possible exception is dry salting, provided the salt reaches all parts of the muscles in concentrated form (Bier 1976).

Table 62.1   Heat tolerance of anisakid larvae (modified after Bier 1976)

Parasite	Temperature (°C)	Maximum survival time of larvae
Anisakis sp.	50–55	10 sec[a]
Anisakis sp.	50–55	10 sec
Anisakis sp.	60	1 sec
Anisakis sp.	45	78 min
Phocanema sp.	60	1 min[a]
Phocanema sp.	50	10 min[a]
Phocanema sp.	45	30 min[a]
Phocanema sp.	40	57 h[a]
Phocanema sp.	60	1 min
Phocanema sp.	50	10 min
Phocanema sp.	45	30 min
Phocanema sp.	40	57 h

[a] Heat tolerance of larvae embedded in fish fillet. The remaining data pertain to isolated larvae.

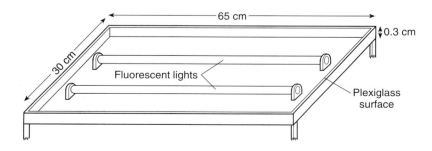

Fig. 62.7   Recommended candling light box.

Table 62.2 Cold tolerance of anisakid larvae in fish (modified after Bier 1976)

Parasite	Temperature (°C)	Maximum survival time of larvae
Anisakis sp.	−5	144 h
Anisakis sp.	−10	288 h
Anisakis sp.	−17	10 h
Phocanema sp.	−5	96 h
Phocanema sp.	−10	17 h
Phocanema sp.	−20	16.5 h
Contracaecum sp.	−20	52 h

Refrigeration aboard the fishing vessel

There is an additional method for eliminating or reducing the number of anisakid larvae in fish fillet. A few preliminary remarks are warranted prior to discussing this method.

Anisakid nematodes found in marine fish are either adults or larvae (Cheng 1976). The adults are limited exclusively to the hosts' alimentary tracts while larvae may occur in various tissues, the coelom, as well as the alimentary tract. It has also been reported that those larvae found in the alimentary tract are primarily L3s that had been recently ingested by the fish host. If the fish is a compatible definitive host, these larvae will develop to maturity; if not, the larvae are either passed out in faeces or may penetrate the fish's gastric or intestinal wall and survive either encapsulated or free in the liver, peritoneum, muscles, or some other tissue. If this occurs, no further development, except for minimal growth, ensues. Thus, the fish must be considered as paratenic hosts for the L3s. If an additional moult occurs, the fish qualifies as a true second intermediate host.

As a result of personal observations aboard fishing vessels in the Atlantic, Cheng (1976) reported that when both the cod, *Gadus callarias*, and the summer flounder, *Paralichthys dentatus*, are removed from the nets and dumped on the deck, there is rapid disintegration of the digestive tract, especially if the ambient temperature is 30 °C or higher. The host's stomach and intestine become greyish black and there is concurrent disintegration of the cells lining these organs. Usually, total disintegration occurs in 6–8 hours. As this decomposition process progresses, the nematodes normally occurring in the stomach and intestine migrate via one of three routes:

(1) some migrate anteriorly; these primarily from the stomach, and exit from the fish host via the gill filaments;

(2) others, primarily these in the intestine, migrate posteriorly and exit from the anus; and

(3) lastly, still others, again primarily from the intestine, burrow through the disintegrating intestinal wall and migrate non-directionally in the body cavity. Some of these come to lie in the mesenteries while others enter the body wall musculature; still others pass through the muscles and protrude from the body surfaces of their fish hosts.

Since the ingestion of anisakid larvae embedded in fish muscle is the primary way human anisakiosis can be acquired, rapid refrigeration (including freezing) aboard fishing vessels, which, in turn, would retard the decomposition of the alimentary tract of captured fish, would partially or totally inhibit the migration of nematodes into the body wall musculature. Thus the incidence of human anisakiosis can be reduced. It is this practice that has all but eliminated the human anisakiosis problem in the Netherlands.

Alternative, or at tandem, the rapid gutting of captured fish aboard fishing vessels prior to refrigeration can also reduce the incidence of human anisakiosis. Unfortunately, in many parts of the world where marine fish comprise a major portion of the protein diet, fishing vessels are such that neither mass gutting nor refrigeration is possible. Hence, it is in such areas that human anisakiosis is most prevalent.

Methods and programmes

The only programmes known to this author to control human anisakiosis are the candling process practices by Canadian fish processors and the ship-board refrigeration (and sometimes gutting) of freshly caught fish in The Netherlands. Additional programmes are the freezing of seafoods required in The Netherlands and the United States targeted at seafoods intended for raw consumption.

Evaluation

As far as this author has been able to ascertain, no formal evaluation programme is under way at this time to determine the effectiveness of candling in controlling human anisakiosis. This practice is intended primarily for marketing more aesthetically pleasing fillets. As this process requires special training and equipment, and is not effective for dark-fleshed fish, the US Food and Drug Administration has rejected it as a control against human anisakiosis.

Legislation

The requirement of rapid refrigeration of fish aboard fishing vessels in The Netherlands has been mentioned. Also, all fish intended for raw consumption are required to be frozen.

In the United States, the Food and Drug Administration has established codes pertaining to the preparation of raw, marinated, or partially cooked fishery products in general. In brief, these state that fisheries products, including fin fish and certain molluscs and crustaceans which had not been cooked throughout to 60 °C or above, must have been blast frozen to −35 °C or below for 15 hours or regularly frozen to −20 °C or below for 168 hours (7 days).

Although no legal requirement for freezing exists in Japan, and freezing is not customary for most species of fish, it is common practice to freeze Pacific salmon in order to kill parasitic helminths.

The regulations and practices summarized above greatly reduce, if not eliminate, the chances of human anisakiosis.

REFERENCES

Anon. (1988). *Improvements in parasite detection and removal.* Report No. 112, Fisher. Dev. Branch, Canadian Institute of Fisheries Technology, Nova Scotia, Canada.

Apstein, C. H. (1911). Parasiten von *Calanus finmarchicus* Kürze Mitteilung. *Wissenschaften Meeresuntersuchen*, **19**, n.s. 13 Abt. Kiel, 205–22.

Aréan, V. M. (1971). Anisakiasis. In *Pathology of protozoal and helminthic diseases*, (ed. S. A. Marcial-Rojas). Williams & Wilkins, Baltimore.

Asami, K. (1966). Larval anisakiasis in Japan. *Fourth Pacific Science Congress, Proceedings Abstracts, and Papers*, **8**, 3.

Asami, L., Watanuki, T., Sakai, H., Imano, H., and Okamoto, R. (1965). Two cases of stomach granuloma caused by *Anisakis*-like larval nematodes in Japan. *American Journal of Tropical Medicine and Hygiene*, **14**, 119–23.

Ashby, B. S., Appleton, P. J., and Dawson, I. (1964). Eosinophilic granuloma of *Eustoma rotundatum*. *British Medical Journal*, **1**, 1141–5.

Ass, M. Y. (1961). [The life cycle of nematodes of the genus *Contracaecum*.] *Trady Karad. Biologischer Stantsii*, **7**, 110–12 [in Russian].

Baer, J. G. (1961). Host reactions in young birds to naturally occurring superinfections with *Porrocaecum ensicaudatum*. *Journal of Helminthology*, (R. T. Leiper Supplement), 1–4.

Benatre, A. *et al.* (1968). Le granulome eosinophilique du tube digestif. *Review de Medicine de Tours*, **2**, 237–43.

Bier, J. W. (1976). Experimental anisakiasis: cultivation and temperature tolerance determinations. *Journal of Milk and Food Technology*, **39**, 132–40.

Buckley, J. J. C. (1951). *Porrocaecum decipiens* in the month of a patient. *Transactions of the Royal Society of Tropical Medicine and Hygiene, Demonstration*, **44**, 362.

Cheng, T. C. (1973). Human parasites transmissible by seafood—and related problems. In *Microbial Safety of Fishery Products*, (ed. C. O. Chichester and H. D. Graham). Academic Press, New York.

Cheng, T. C. (1976). The natural history of anisakiasis in animals. *Journal of Milk and Food Technology*, **39**, 32–46.

Cheng, T. C. (1982). Anisakiasis. In *Handbook of Zoonoses*, Volume II, Section C, (ed. J. H. Steele). CRC Press, Boca Raton, Florida.

Chitwood, M. B. (1969). The systematics and biology of some parasite nematodes. *Chemical Zoology*, Vol. III, (ed. M. Florkin and B. T. Scheer). pp. 223–44. Academic Press, New York.

Chitwood, M. B. (1970). Nematodes of medical significance found in market fish. *American Journal of Tropical Medicine and Hygiene*, **19**, 599–602.

Cobb, N. A. (1930). A nemic parasite of *Pecten. Journal of Parasitology*, **17**, 104–5.

Daniels, J. J. M. H. (1962). De eosinfile flegmone van het masgdarmkanaal veroorzoakt door de haring worm. *Nederlander Tiel Geneeshunde*, **106**, 131–2.

Davey, K. G. (1965). Molting in a parasitic nematode, *Phocanema decipiens*. I. Cytological events. *Canadian Journal of Zoology*, **43**, 997–1003.

Davey, K. G. (1969). Molting in a nematode, *Phocanema decipiens*. V. Timing of feeding during the moulting cycle. *Journal of the Fisheries Research Board of Canada*, **26**, 935–9.

Flores-Barroeta, L., Hidalgo-Escalante, E., and Oleac, P. (1961). Nematodes from birds and mammals IV (1). Erratic parasitosis in *Zalophus californianus* from Asuncion Island, Baja California, Mexico. *Helminthology*. **3**, 112–16.

Gibson, D. I. (1970). Aspects of the development of herring-worm (*Anisakis* sp. larvae) in experimentally infected rats. *Norwegian Journal of Zoology*, **18**, 175–87.

Hayasaka, H., Ishikura, H., and Mizukaki, H., Ueno, T., Utsumi, A., and Saeki, H. (1968). [Studies on anisakiasis. VIII. Experimental studies on granuloma formation.] *Japanese Journal of Parasitology*, **15**, 502–14. [in Japanese with English summary].

Hayasaka, H., Ishikura, H., and Mizukaki, H. (1970). [Anisakiasis-intestinal anisakiasis]. *Hokkaido Journal of Surgery*, 15, 1–7 [in Japanese with English summary].

Higashi, G. I. (1985). Foodborne parasites transmitted to man from fish and other aquatic foods. *Food Technology*, **39**, 69–111.

Hitchcock, D. J. (1950). Parasitological study of the eskimos in the Bethel area of Alaska. *Journal of Parasitology*, **36**, 232–4.

Hoeppli, R. (1932). Tissue reactions due to parasites. *Far East Association of Tropical Medicine Transactions of 8th Congress*, pp. 183–93.

Hsu, H. T. and Hoeppli, R. (1933). On some parasitic nematodes collected in Amoy. *Peking Natural History Bulletin*, **8**, 155–68.

Huizinga, H. W. (1966). Studies on the life cycle and development of *Contracaecum spiculigerum* from marine piscivorous birds. *Journal of the Elisha Mitchell Scientific Society*, **82**, 181–95.

Hutton, R. F., Ball, T., and Eldred, B. (1962). Immature nematodes of the genus *Contracaecum* Raillet and Henry, 1912, from shrimps. *Journal of Parasitology*, **48**, 327–32.

Ichihara, A., Kato, K., Kamegai, S., Kamegai, S., and Nonobe, H. (1966). [On the parasites of fishes and shellfishes in Sagami Bay. IV. Parasites of *Pneumatophorus japonicus japonicus* (Houttuyn)]. *Japanese Journal of Parasitology*, **15**, 345–6 [in Japanese].

Ishikura, H. (1969). [On anisakiasis, its occurrence and clinical observation.] *Nippon Rinsho Geka Igakuno*, **30**, 85–94 [in Japanese].

Iwanaga, H. (1970). [Studies on eosinophilia in the guinea pig sensitized with *Anisakis* saline extract.] *Japanese Journal of Parasitology*, **19**, 207–14. [in Japanese].

Jackson, G. J. (1975). The 'new disease' status of human anisakiasis and North American cases: a review. *Journal of Milk and Food Technology*, **38**, 769–73.

Kagei, N., Oshima, T., Kebayashi, A., Kumada, M., and Komiya, Y. (1967). [Morphological differences in each of the stages of *Anisakis* from a blue white dolphin.] *Japanese Journal of Parasitology*, **16**, 290 [in Japanese].

Kates, S., Wright, K. A., and Wright, R. (1973). A case of human infection with the cod nematode *Phocanema* sp. *American Journal of Tropical Medicine and Hygiene*, **22**, 606–9.

Kato, T., Uminuma, M., Ito, K., and Miura, K. (1968). [On Anisakinae from the marine fishes at The Tokyo Central Fish Market.] *Shokukin Eisei Kenkyu*, **18**, 31–41 [in Japanese].

Kikuchi, Y., Ueda, T., Yoshiki, T., Aizawa, M., and Ishikura, H. (1967). [Experimental studies of the immunopathology of intestinal anisakiasis]. *Igakuno Ayumi*, **62**, 731–8. [in Japanese].

Kobayashi, A., Koyama, T., Kurnada, M., Komiya, Y., Oshima, T., and Kagei, N. (1966). [On the development of *Anisakis* ova.] *Japanese Journal of Parasitology*, **15**, 545–7. [in Japanese].

Kobayashi, A., Koyama, T., Kumada, M., Suguro, T., and Koito, K. (1968a). [Skin test with somatic and ES (excretions and secretions) antigens from *Anisakis* larvae. I. Survey of normal populations on skin sensitivity to different antigens.] *Japanese Journal of Parasitology*, **17**, 407–11 [in Japanese with English summary].

Kobayashi, A., Koyama, T., Kumada, M., Suguro, T., and Koito, K. (1968b). [Skin test with somatic and ES (excretions and secretions) antigens from *Anisakis* larvae. II. Difference of antigenicity between the two antigens. *Japanese Journal of Parasitology*, **17**, 414–19 [in Japanese with English summary].

Kojima, K., Oyanagi, T., and Shiraki, K. (1966). Pathology of anisakiasis. *Nippon Rinsho*, **24**, 2314–18.

Kosugi, L., Kikuchi, S., Hirabayashi, H., and Hayashi, S. (1969). [Seasonal occurrence of the larvae of *Anisakis* and related nematodes in the fishes from Sagami Bay.] *Japanese Journal of Parasitology*, **18**, 352 [in Japanese].

Kosugi, K., Kikuchi, S., Hirabayashi, H., and Hayashi, S. (1970). Seasonal occurrence of the larvae of *Anisakis* and related nematodes in the fishes from Sagami Bay, the results of two years observation, 1968 to 1969. *Japanese Journal of Parasitology*, **19**, 106–7.

Kuipers, F. C. (1964). Eosinophilic phlegmonous inflammation of the alimentary canal caused by a parasite from herring. *Pathology and Microbiology*, **27**, 925–30.

Kuipers, F. C. (1967). Stenose van de dunne darm als laat gevolg van een haringworm flegmone. *Nederlander Tier Geneeskunde*, **111**, 599–601.

Kuipers, F. C., van Thiel, P., Rodenburg, W., Wielinga, W., and Roskam, R. T. (1960). Eosinophilic phlegmon of the alimentary canal caused by a worm. *Lancet*, **2**, 1170–3.

Kuipers, F. C., Kampelmacher, E., and Steenbergen, J. (1963). Ondersoekingen over haringwormsiekte bij konijnen. *Nederlander Tier Geneeskunde*, **107**, 990–5.

Lebour, M. V. (1917). Some parasites of *Sagitta bipunctata*. *Journal of the Marine Biological Association of the United Kingdom*, **11**, 201–6.

Little, M. D. and MacPhail, J. C. (1972). Large nematode larva from the abdominal cavity of a man in Massachusetts. *American Journal of Tropical Medicine and Hygiene*, **21**, 948–50.

Little, M. D. and Most, H. (1973). Anisakid larva from the throat of a woman in New York. *American Journal of Tropical Medicine and Hygiene*, **22**, 609–10.

Margolis, L. (1970). Nematode diseases of marine fishes, In *A Symposium on Diseases of Fishes and Shellfishes*, (ed. S. F. Snieszko). American Fisheries Society Special Publication No. 5, Washington, D. C.

Markowski, S. (1937). Über die Entwicklungsgeschichte und Biologie des Nematodes *Contracaecum aduncum* (Rudolphi, 1802). *Bulletin de International Academies Polonensis de Sciences et Letters, Classe Sciences, Mathematiques, et Nature. Series B. Sciences,* **2**, 227–47.

Martin, W. E., Haun, C. K., Barrows, H. S., and Cravioto, H. (1970). Nematode damage to brain of striped dolphin, *Lagenorhynchus obliguidens*. *Transactions of the American Microscopical Society*, **80**, 200–5.

Merkelbach, J. W. C. (1964). Een visser met herringwormziekte (anisakiasis) van het rectum. *Nederlandica Tijdschrift Geneos*, **108**, 2131–2.

Miyazato, T., Inoue, T., and Hosokawa, S. (1970). Six case reports of human gastric anisakiasis found by surgery. *Japanese Journal of Parasitology*, **19**, 342–5.

Morishita, T. and Kobayashi, M. (1965). [On a trial of the skin test in human anisakiasis.] *Japanese Journal of Parasitology*, **14**, 230–4. [in Japanese with English summary].

Myers, B. J. (1963). Migration of *Anisakis*-type larvae in experimental animals. *Canadian Journal of Zoology*, **41**, 147–8.

Myers, B. J. (1975). The nematodes that cause anisakiasis. *Journal of Milk and Food Technology*, **38**, 774–82.

Nishimura, T. (1963). On a certain nematode larvae found from the abscess of the mesentery of man. *Transaction of the 19th Branch Meetings on Parasitology, Western Division*, Parasitological Society of Japan.

Norris, D. E. and Overstreet, R. M. (1976). The public health implications of larval *Thynnascaris* nematodes from shellfish. *Journal of Milk and Food Technology*, **39**, 47–54.

Okumura, T. (1967). [Experimental studies on anisakiasis.] *Osakashiritsu Daigaku Igakuno*, **16**, 465–97, [in Japanese].

Oshima, T. (1972). *Anisakis* and anisakiasis in Japan and adjacent area. In *Progress in Medical Parasitology in Japan*, Vol. 4, Meguro Parasitological Museum, Tokyo.

Otsuru, M. (1968). [Anisakiasis]. *Niigata Igakkai Zasshi*, **82**, 295–8, [in Japanese].

Oyanagi, T. (1967). [Experimental studies on the visceral migrans of gastrointestinal walls due to *Anisakis* larvae.] *Japanese Journal of Parasitology*, **16**, 470–93. [in Japanese].

Penner, L. R. (1941). The commissary of the zoo-parasitic problems. *Zoonooz*, **13**, 7.

Petter, A. J. (1969). Enquete sur les nématodes des poissons de la région Nantaise. Identification des larves d'ascarides parasitant les sardines (en repport avec les granulomes éosinophiles observés chez l'homme dans la région). *Annals de Parasitologie*, **44**, 559–79.

Pierantoni, C. (1914). Sopra un nematode parasita della *Sagitta* e sul suo probable ciclo evolutivo. *Proceedings of the 9th International Congress of Zoology*, Monaco, 1913, pp. 663–4.

Rausch, R. (1953). Studies on the helminth fauna of Alaska XIII. *Ecology*, **34**, 584–604.

Rizkova, N. P. (1953). [The blood picture of domestic ducks during treatment of disease.] In *Papers on Helminthology Presented to Academician K. I. Skryabin on His 75th Birthday*. Ixdatelstvo Akademii Nauk SSSR, Moscow, pp. 607–610 [in Russian].

Rodrick, G. E. and Cheng, T. C. (1989). Parasites: occurrence and significance is marine animals. *Food Technology*, **43**, 98–102.

Ruitenberg, E. J. (1970). Anisakiasis: pathogenesis, serodiagnosis, and prevention. Ph.D. thesis, University of Utrecht, The Netherlands.

Ruitenberg, E. J. and Loendersloot, J. (1971). Enzymhistochemisch onderzoek van *Anisakis* sp. *Tijdschrift Diergeneeskunde Deel*, **96**, 247–52.

Saito, T., Kitayama, H., and Tankawa, Y. (1970). [Frequency of *Anisakis* larvae in marine fishes and cuttlefishes captured in the area of Hokkaido]. Reports of the Hokkaido Institute of Public Health, **20**, 115–22, [in Japanese].

Schiller, E. L. (1954). Studies on the helminth fauna of Alaska XVII. *Biological Bulletin*, **106**, 107–21.

Scott, D. M. (1957). Records of larval *Contracaecum* sp. in 3 species of mysids from the Bras d'Or Lakes, Nova Scotia, Canada. *Journal of Parasitology*, **43**, 290.

Suzuki, T., Shiraki, T., and Otsuru, M. (1970). [Studies on the immunological diagnosis of anisakiasis, I. Antigenic analysis of *Anisakis* larvae by means of electrophoresis.] *Japanese Journal of Parasitology*, **17**, 213–16 [in Japanese with English summary].

Taniguchi, M. (1966). [Studies on anisakiasis, I. On its antigenicity.] *Japanese Journal of Parasitology*, **15**, 502–4 [in Japanese with English summary].

Valdimarsson, G., Einarsson, H., and King, F. J. (1985). Detection of parasites in fish muscle by candling technique. *Journal of the Association of Official Analytical Chemists*, **68**, 549–55.

Valter, E. D. (1969). [On the participation of isopods in the life cycle of *Contracaecum aduncum* (Ascaridata, Anisakoidea).] *Parazitologiya*, **2**, 521–7 [in Russian].

van Thiel, P. H., Kuipers, F. C., and Roskarn, R. T. (1960). A nematode parasite to herring causing acute abdominal syndromes in man. *Tropical and Geographic Medicine*, **2**, 97–113.

Wülker, G. (1929). Der Wirtswechsel der parasitischen Nematoden von Meeresfischen. *Zoologischer Anzager*, Supplement 4, 147–57.

Wülker, G. (1930). Über Nematoden aus Nordseetieren II. *Zoologischer Anzager*, **88**, 1–16.

Yokogawa, M. and Yoshimura, H. (1967). Clinicopathologic studies on larval anisakiasis in Japan. *American Journal of Tropical Medicine and Hygiene*, **16**, 723–8.

Yoshimura, H. (1966). [Larva migrans by *Anisakis*-like larva causing eosinophilic phlegmon of human digestive tract.] *Minophagen Medical Review*, **11**, 105–11 [in Japanese].

Young, P. C. and Lowe, D. (1969). Larval nematodes from fish of the subfamily Anisakinae and gastro-intestinal lesions in mammals. *Journal of Comparative Pathology*, **79**, 301–13.

63 TOXOCAROSIS

S. Lloyd

SUMMARY

This chapter discusses the role of *Toxocara canis* in the syndromes of visceral, ocular, and covert toxocarosis (VT, OT, CT). While the transmission dynamics of *T. canis* to humans have never been fully elucidated, the potential roles of pet dogs, stray dogs, and foxes, and the influence of their population densities and the age demography of the populations, are compared in relation to contamination of the environment with eggs. Routes of infection for children by geophagia, poor hygiene, fly-borne, and meat-borne ingestion of eggs or larvae are described. The development of prolonged *in vitro* culture and analysis of the excretions/secretions (ES) and surface of *T. canis* larvae have gone a long way to explaining the importance of these ES antigens and their rapid production and shedding in the prolonged course of infection and pathogenesis of disease. ES antigens also have greatly improved the sensitivity and specificity of serodiagnosis. Nevertheless, we still have insufficient understanding as to differences in the aetiology of the larvae or differences in immune responses among individuals to account for development of VT versus CT or OT in different individuals. Our understanding that most of the pathology in toxocarosis is due to the immunopathological response of the host to *T. canis* ES has emphasized the need for vigorous anti-inflammatory therapy in treatment; unfortunately, less information is available as to the true efficacy of the anthelmintics currently available. The complexity of the *T. canis* life cycle in dogs is described and therapeutic regimens to prevent excretion of eggs by pet dogs are given. This, plus adequate control or exclusion of stray or wild canids from a property should prevent most cases of VT. Control of the other sources of infection, free-ranging stray dogs and foxes, will be difficult, and more data are needed to clarify the importance of these and of fly-borne and meat-borne transfer of infection to humans to target these for control.

HISTORY

Toxocara canis was first described as *Ascaris canis* in 1782. Similarly, the clinical entity of visceral larva migrans was initially ascribed in 1947 to *Ascaris lumbricoides*, until Beaver *et al.* (1952) serially sectioned a larva from a patient, identified it as *Toxocara canis* and later reproduced infection in two children. Wilder (1950) reported 24 cases of ocular disease, but it was several years before the larvae were identified as *Toxocara* (Nichols 1956). A milestone in the history of *T. canis* was the prolonged *in vitro* culture of larvae (de Savigny 1975) to produce excretory-secretory antigens (ES), with which diagnosis was developed (de Savigny *et al.* 1979) and a considerable advance made in our understanding of the cuticle of nematodes (Maizels *et al.* 1993). The fact that *T. canis* produces blindness in children created considerable publicity which is out of proportion compared with the importance of many other childhood or tropical parasitic diseases.

THE AGENT AND GEOGRAPHIC DISTRIBUTION

Toxocara canis (Werner 1782) Stiles 1905, is the agent usually considered important in visceral and ocular toxocarosis (larva migrans) and the recently described covert toxocarosis (VT, OT, and CT). Adult *T. canis* occur only in the small intestine of canids; they are cream-white in colour, thick bodied, and the body bends ventrally at the anterior, has cervical alae and reaches 10–18 cm. Eggs, 90×75 μm, have a thick, brown shell with a finely pitted surface; they are single celled when passed in canine faeces. They develop in the environment to what is generally called an infective, second-stage larva (L2). *Toxocara canis* is cosmopolitan in distribution: it seems most prevalent in wet tropical areas; it is absent from the frigid Arctic region although it is found above 60°N; and low prevalences have been recorded in arid and semi-arid desert regions.

A number of other ascarids cause some form of larva migrans; while infections seem to be rare or asymptomatic, they may complicate immunodiagnosis. *Toxocara cati* (Schrank 1788) Brumpt 1927, in the intestine of cats is very similar to *T. canis* and also cosmopolitan in distribution. Its role in visceral and ocular toxocarosis has never been reliably confirmed or refuted. *Baylisascaris procyonis* (Stefanski and Zamowski 1951) Sprent 1958, of racoons has been identified in a few cases of ocular and neurological disease in Europe and North America. *Ascaris suum* Göze 1782, of pigs, and *Toxocara vitulorum* (Göze 1782) Travassos 1927, of cattle and buffalo, can create short-lived infections (Amerasinghe *et al.* 1993) and many other ascarids are proposed, e.g. *Toxocara pteropodis* (bats), *Toxascaris* (dogs, cats), *Lagochilascaris* (opossums), *Porrocaecum* (birds of prey), *Ophidascaris, Polydelphis, Travassoascaris* (snakes), etc., but their role seems extremely limited mainly through lack of human contact with eggs.

THE HOSTS

1. *Toxocara canis*
   definitive host: dog, fox; less prevalent in other canids, e.g. coyote, wolf, jackal
   paratenic host: essentially every species of mammal, and bird
2. *Toxocara cati*
   definitive host: cats and other Felidae
   paratenic host: rodents, birds
3. *Baylisascaris procyonis*
   definitive host: racoons
   paratenic host: rodents, birds

LIFE CYCLE AND EPIDEMIOLOGY

The life cycle of *T. canis* has been described by Lloyd (1987, 1993) and its complexity is depicted in Fig. 63.1. A similar life cycle undoubtedly occurs in other Canidae and infection is probably transmitted freely between canids. Eggs are produced only by Canidae, the highest output coming from the pivotal part of the life cycle—transfer of infection from the pregnant bitch/vixen to her pups/cubs. Adult dogs/foxes also produce eggs, albeit at lower levels.

Infection of dogs

1. When adult dogs ingest eggs the majority of larvae migrate to the somatic tissues. In a proportion of dogs, this possibly related to genetic susceptibility or hormonal effects, such as lactation, metoestrus, some larvae undergo tracheal migration to return to the intestine to develop to adult worms.
2. Larvae remain in the tissues of dogs for several years. If a bitch becomes pregnant, larvae then activate and migrate across the placenta to the fetus. The larvae then complete their migration to the intestine in the newborn pup and develop to produce eggs at about 2.5 weeks. Adult worms in

pups also develop from larvae transferred from the bitch in her milk and from ingested eggs. Pups usually are heavily infected.

3. The lactating bitch is reinfected from her pups while she is cleaning them, in this way eating larvae that are swept out in their faeces. These continue development to adulthood in her intestine so she excretes a significant number of eggs.
4. Larvae in eggs of *T. canis* eaten by any species of mammal or bird (paratenic hosts) hatch, migrate into the tissues, and remain viable for prolonged periods. Stray dogs, foxes, etc., that scavenge rodents, lagomorphs and birds, but potentially also large animals, e.g. sheep, and pets which hunt or are fed raw meat, eat these larvae. Adults develop in the intestine without any further migration.

Eggs in the environment

Adult *T. canis* are extremely fecund. Faecal egg counts in pups can reach 100 000/g of faeces; a female worm can produce more than 100 000 eggs/day; and total daily output from a heavily infected bitch and her pups was recorded as 1.5×10^7 eggs.

Eggs develop only at 10 °C or above and reach L2 in about 2–7 weeks at 15–25 °C, but remain viable through very cold weather if protected by snow or faeces. Only heat, greater than 30–35 °C, and desiccation will kill the thick-shelled eggs. In favourable conditions, eggs remain viable in large numbers for 6–12 months; survive composting for at least a year; and some probably survive in moist, cool conditions for 2–4 years.

Faeces disintegrate with time to release eggs into surrounding soil. This, plus the number produced and their prolonged survival mean there is an ubiquitous reservoir of eggs in the environment. Eggs are common in soil samples (Table 63.1) although many surveys do not differentiate *T. canis* and *T. cati* eggs. Density of eggs is reported as 0.1 to 23 eggs/g soil (Lloyd 1993).

The egg surface is incredibly sticky and so could be carried long distances attached to objects. A number of invertebrates, e.g. earthworms, cockroaches, beetles,

Table 63.1 Percentage egg-positive soil samples

Country	Percentage positive samples in
Jordan	15% playgrounds/public places
Lithuania, Vilnius	8% parks/playgrounds
Japan, Tokushima	63% sandpits
Japan, Hyogo Prefecture	41.9% sandpits/parks
Australia, Brisbane	0% sandpits; 1% parks
USA, St Joseph/ Benton Harbour	19% parks
Germany, Hannover	56% sandpits
Ireland, Dublin	6% parks, 38% gardens
UK, London	66% parks

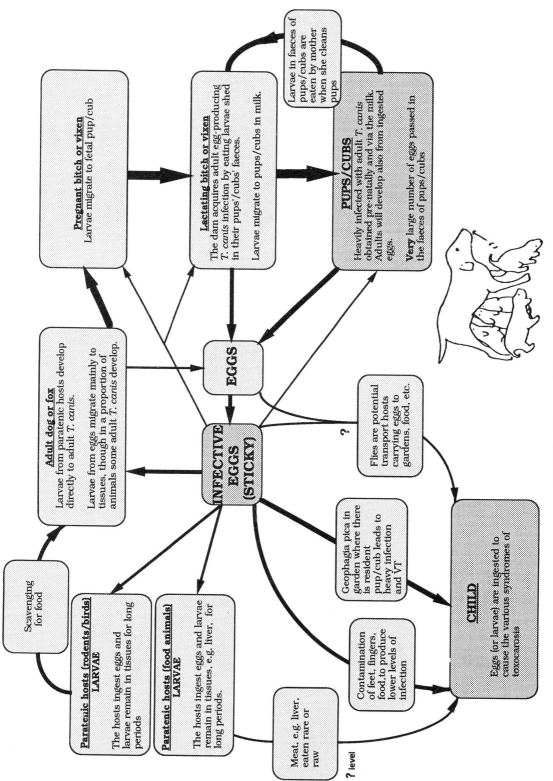

Fig. 63.1 Life cycle of *Toxocara canis*.

slugs, are attracted to faeces to eat and may transport eggs that stick to their bodies for short distances and can ingest eggs which pass intact through their gut (Takahashi *et al.* 1990). There is potential for longer distance transfer by flies. Lawson and Gemmell (1990) showed that *Taenia* eggs are transported over 80 m from dog faeces by flies to be deposited on to pasture for ingestion by sheep. *Toxocara* eggs have been found on and in wild-caught flies (Umeche and Mandah 1989); flies therefore have the potential to transfer eggs to soil/lawns in gardens from faeces in neighbouring areas. In the UK, more than 50 per cent of patients with clinical toxocarosis have never owned a dog or had close contact with one; a role for fly transfer of eggs to them needs evaluation.

Infection in humans

Humans can acquire *T. canis* eggs from canid faeces by a number of routes. Risk factors include:

(1)   geophagia pica,
(2)   poor hygiene,
(3)   contact with dogs, particularly pups and cubs, but also adults, e.g. ownership of a dog or access of dogs/foxes to play areas,
(4)   consumption of raw/undercooked meat or contaminated food.

Socio-economic status will influence all these and the risks, and levels of infection acquired, vary between VT and OT.

An important risk factor for VT is geophagia pica which occurs in most cases. Geophagia is common in about 10–25 per cent of young children, may increase with nutritional deficiency and is most likely to be satisfied where children are outdoors unsupervised; thus, tropical climate, poverty, and low social status all contribute to VT. Large numbers of eggs must be in the soil so a second risk factor for VT is ownership of a puppy(ies) or close contact with pups, e.g. a neighbour's, as pups are the most heavily infected group of dogs. Fox cubs born in urban gardens also could heavily contaminate soil.

Geophagia will induce infection, albeit at lower levels, if there are smaller numbers of eggs in the soil. These eggs might come from even well cared for pet dogs, although there is evidence for a downward trend in prevalence of infection in pet dogs: at Oklahoma State University Veterinary School, prevalence of *T. canis* in dogs of all ages decreased from 8 per cent in 1981 to 4 per cent in 1990; at the University of Pennsylvania school, while 5.5 per cent of dogs were infected, only 1.7 per cent of those older than 2 years were passing eggs; in Dublin Ireland, faecal samples from pet dogs were negative, as were faecal samples

collected from a city park in Cambridge, UK, where pet dogs are walked regularly (Kirkpatrick 1988; Holland *et al.* 1991; Jordan *et al.* 1993; Lloyd, unpublished observations).

Urban foxes are another source of infection, even for fenced gardens. Infection is very prevalent in foxes: in Bristol, UK, Richards *et al.* (1993) found 14–73 per cent of foxes older than 2 years to be infected, while more than 60 per cent rural or mixed urban/rural groups of foxes in Wales and Germany were infected. Stray dogs have access to unfenced gardens and surveys show a higher prevalence of infection in these compared with pet dogs. The high prevalences in stray/wild canid populations undoubtedly are dietary; scavenged paratenic hosts being an important food.

Geophagia is not the only route for human infection. *Toxocara canis* eggs are very sticky and may adhere to fingers, toys, food-stuffs, etc., that are laid on the ground in play areas and then placed in the mouth. This fact has long been used to explain infection in children that have no family pet or direct access to dogs. Regulations requiring leashing/kerbing of dogs, and provision of 'dog toilets', all point to the emphasis given to this route of infection by publicity. An out of court settlement by a Council in the United Kingdom to a child with OT seemed to accept egg contamination in a park as the source of infection. In fact the relative importance of pet dogs versus other canids in contamination of parks has never been ascertained, while other sites and routes of infection are possible.

The relative importance of food-borne infection has never been ascertained. Where canids have access to unfenced vegetable gardens, transfer of eggs from faeces to perhaps salad greens might occur by rain splash, etc. Also, helminth eggs survive many sewage treatment processes: 12–47 *Toxocara* spp. eggs were found in 100 g of dried sludge (Horak 1992), so effluent or sludge used on vegetable crops could transfer low levels of infection.

Finally, food animals, poultry, ruminants, etc., act as paratenic hosts; larvae are found in all tissues, with highest numbers in the liver. Beaver (1956) described transfer of infection to humans through the consumption of raw liver; raw chicken livers and lightly cooked rabbit have been implicated as sources of infection; and, recently, eggs attached to snails collected in a meadow frequented by dogs were suggested as the cause of disease in an adult (Nagakura *et al.* 1989; Romeu *et al.* 1991). Finally, meat can be contaminated with fly-borne taeniid eggs from dog faeces (Lawson and Gemmell 1990), and so possibly with eggs of *T. canis* also.

The relative importance of different canid populations in contaminating the environment will depend not only on the prevalence and intensity of infection within them, but also on the density of that population in a given area. Although information is becoming available, populations have not been studied concurrently. The density of owned dogs in Zimbabwe was calculated as 3.4 dogs/km² rising to 68/km² in urban areas (Brooks 1990). In Lagos, Nigeria, figures for owned dogs were: urban 131/km²; rural 15/km². Dog densities were given as 3000/km² in Sri Lanka, 1922/km² in Dumagueti city, the Philippines, and 100–150 pet dogs/km² in various cities in the United States, United Kingdom, and Germany. Stray dogs were recorded at 330/km² in a high-density housing area in the United Kingdom and at 127–1304/km² in different areas in Valencia, Spain. Fox densities in various cities and rural areas in the United Kingdom are described as 0.2–5.0 family groups (each group being two adults and 4.0–4.5 cubs)/km² (Harris and Rayner 1986; Richards and Lewis 1993).

Age distribution of populations also influences contamination; pups/cubs produce the highest numbers of eggs. Cubs make up a very high proportion of the fox population in the spring and summer months, before they disperse in autumn/winter. In Zimbabwe, puppies were numerous; approximately 20 per cent of the dog population was below 3 months old. However, the percentage of dogs younger than 1 year is lower than this in populations studied in the United Kingdom and United States. The territories used by animals also will influence contamination. Pups/cubs usually remain confined to one area until 2–3 months of age. A lactating bitch, with her own worms, plus the eggs she has acquired from cleaning her pups, will be walked for exercise; the vixen will hunt. Unconfined foxes and dogs can range over a territory of several kilometres.

Toxocara cati is similar to *T. canis* except that transmission is transmammary not prenatal and adult cats are more likely to be infected as they are more susceptible to egg-induced infection and are more likely to be free to hunt. *Toxocara cati* eggs are found in many of the same areas as *T. canis* and cats are considered responsible for the high levels of contamination in childrens' sandpits. However, available data suggest *T. cati* is not as important in toxocarosis, e.g. occupational groups at risk include hydatid control officers and dog breeders but not cat breeders and, in Iceland where dog ownership is controlled, *Toxocara* antibody responses were negative (Woodruff *et al.* 1982). Nevertheless, humans will eat *T. cati* eggs in the same way that they acquire *Toxoplasma gondii* (see Chapter 66) and the infection might stimulate cross-reacting antibodies. Development of a *T. cati*-positive and *T. canis*-negative monoclonal antibody to detect circulating antigen or a species-specific molecular probe is required to determine the importance of *T. cati*.

The risk factor for *B. procyonis* is contact with racoons, more than 70 per cent of which are infected.

Racoons are kept as pets and for rehabilitation. In the wild, racoons contaminate sites, 'racoon latrines' in wooded areas. A child was infected by chewing fallen tree bark from a 'racoon latrine' (Kazacos 1991).

Toxocara vitulorum, common in buffalo and cattle in tropical areas, is transferred to calves only via colostrum and milk. The eggs are ubiquitous in village environments in soil and water and larvae might have a short-lived migration when eaten by children. This migration is unlikely to cause disease, but could induce cross-reacting antibody and perhaps, in repeated infections, an eosinophilia.

Serological examinations in Holland have shown that children are seropositive to *Ascaris* as commonly as to *Toxocara*. As *A. lumbricoides* is uncommon, these probably are *A. suum* infections from pig slurry/sludge that is commonly used as a fertilizer on farms and gardens (van Knapen *et al.* 1992). While a large bolus of *A. suum* eggs given maliciously to students was pathogenic (severe pneumonia; eosinophilia), larvae are short-lived and so unlikely to cause disease in moderate or low numbers. Repeated exposure, e.g. in areas where intensive pig production, with its slurry disposal problems, is common or where free-ranging pigs are reared, might induce an eosinophilia of unknown origin.

MOLECULAR BIOLOGY

The oral and secretory apertures and surface of ascaridoid larvae have been considered important sites for production of antigens since the 1960s. Maizels and colleagues recently have confirmed this and supplied considerable insight into the structure of the nematode cuticle and glycocalyx and into the molecular structure, elaboration, and function of parasite antigens (Meghji and Maizels 1986; Page *et al.* 1992*a,b*; Khoo *et al.* 1993; Maizels *et al.* 1993). These studies were facilitated by the remarkable ability of the L2 to survive *in vitro* in defined medium with a high rate of production of excretions/secretions (ES), an estimated 9 pg to 8 ng protein/larva/day. The ES molecules defined so far are highly glycosylated with 400 μg CHO/mg protein and some lipid. The CHO determinants are immunodominant with the majority of monoclonal antibodies produced recognizing these. Five major groups of molecules with molecular weights of 32, 55, 70, 120, and 400 kDa have been identified; the 120 kDa molecule is the predominant product, at least *in vitro*.

The epicuticle of *T. canis* L2 is lipophilic. About 10 nm from this, and about 10–20 nm wide, is an outer fuzzy glycocalyx that is a mucilaginous, highly glycosylated matrix containing the ES molecules (Maizels and Page 1990; Maizels *et al.* 1993). The sites of glycosylation, and so probably synthesis of the ES molecules, have now been detected (Page *et al.* 1992*a*). The 32 kDa molecule seems to be transported through the cuticle. The others occur in the oesophageal gland and the secretory gland, and all, with the exception of the 400 kDa molecule, are then secreted to form the surface glycocalyx/coat; the 400 kDa molecule is secreted but does not become part of the coat. The glycocalyx/coat then is shed: 25 per cent of surface radiolabelled molecules were released into culture medium within 1 hour, with 80 per cent released over 48 hours.

ES antigen function is being related to the prolonged migration and survival of *T. canis* larvae. The larvae produce their surface antigens in response to the change to parasitism, e.g. they are virtually absent from newly hatched larvae, but develop by 24 h in conditions mimicking the mammalian host (Kennedy *et al.* 1987). Enzymes in ES should aid both migration and survival of the larvae (Robertson *et al.* 1989). There are significant quantities of elastase in ES that can degrade extracellular matrix proteins to aid migration of larvae through connective tissues; these seemed to be related to the 120 kDa molecule. Acetylcholinesterase is prominent, associated probably with the 70 kDa fraction. Superoxide dismutase in ES may protect against reactive oxygen molecules and so cell killing (Maizels *et al.* 1993). ES molecules are shed *in vivo* as they are detectable in serum and tissues (Robertson *et al.* 1988). This could aid larval survival as deposition of ES in granulomata or in immune complexes might divert the immune response from the larvae themselves (Parsons *et al.* 1986). Also, surface antigen is aggregated and shed in response to attack by antibody and/or cells (Smith *et al.* 1981; Badley *et al.* 1987; Page *et al.* 1992*b*), the larva thereby sloughing off and escaping the effector mechanisms of the host.

The molecular structure and stereochemistry of the saccharides, particularly the 400 kDa molecule, are similar to blood group H (O) and A antigens. This accounts for the binding of heterophile antibodies to larvae and the elevated isohaemagglutinin titres seen in some infected persons.

SYMPTOMS AND PATHOLOGY

HUMAN INFECTIONS

Infection with *T. canis* can be divided into four syndromes:

(1)   classic visceral larva migrans/toxocarosis (VT);
(2)   classic ocular larva migrans/toxocarosis (OT);
(3)   the recently described 'covert' toxocarosis (CT); and
(4)   asymptomatic infections.

Visceral toxocarosis

This occurs when a large number of *T. canis* larvae migrate in the tissues. Commonly, but not exclusively, the patient is 2–4 years of age with a history of geophagia and contact with puppies. The classical symptoms and signs are high eosinophilia (usually greater than 30 per cent or greater than 400/mm³), hepatosplenomegaly, fever, respiratory signs (rales with cough and wheezing from bronchitis and pneumonitis), lymphadenopathy, pallor, and skin lesions, and there may be neurological manifestations, e.g. convulsions, strabismus, myocarditis, with heart problems, and, occasionally, ocular lesions. Many patients have an IgG/IgE hypergammaglobulinaemia with globulin levels between 4 and 7 gm/dl and elevated titres of antibody to Forssman antigen and blood group A and B antigens (Zinkham 1978, Lloyd 1987).

Ocular toxocarosis

Loss in visual acuity is the most publicised and emotive manifestation, particularly as many patients come from a non-dog-owning family. Ocular lesions can occur at any age, but most commonly in older children (Gillespie 1993; Gillespie *et al.* 1993). Patients seem to be lightly infected although, occasionally, OT and VT occur concurrently. Visual acuity may be affected directly by the larvae but mainly by the host immunopathological response. The degree of visual loss is variable from blurring of vision through to blindness, usually unilateral, and only rarely (1–3 per cent) bilateral. The inflammatory response is frequently reported as a granuloma on the posterior pole which, on or near the macula, can cause severe visual loss. Granulomata on the peripheral retina now seem equally common and may be associated with pars planitis (Schantz *et al.* 1980). Repair of these peripheral lesions with development of fibrosis can produce chronic damage; fibrous traction bands from the lesion to the posterior pole lead to vitreoretinal traction, retinal detachment and loss of vision (Gillespie *et al.* 1993). Inflammation can be extensive with endophthalmitis and uveitis, also optic neuritis. Despite severe inflammation, only a few patients report ocular pain. *Baylisascaris procyonis* has been positively identified in several OT patients and *Porrocaecum* or *Hexametra* spp. in one.

Covert toxocarosis

There is an increasing trend to recognition of this milder form of toxocarosis. This syndrome was recognized in adult patients in the Midi-Pyrenees (Glickman *et al.* 1987; Magnaval and Baixench 1993) and in children in Ireland (Taylor *et al.* 1987; Gillespie 1993; Taylor 1993) as a variety of non-specific symptoms which, when grouped together and with positive toxocaral antibody and/or eosinophilia, indicated a *T. canis* aetiology. Predominant symptoms vary somewhat between studies: this might relate to adults versus children; to a large proportion of asthmatics in one group studied; and possibly response to questions. Commonly there is weakness/lethargy (in as many as 70 per cent), abdominal pain (30–60 per cent), lymphadenopathy (2–60 per cent), skin lesions or pruritis (5–40 per cent), respiratory features, cough/wheeze (12–70 per cent, highest in the study group containing asthmatics), headache (23–48 per cent), cervical adenitis, fever, anaemia, myalgia (particularly limb pains), nausea, and other signs, including occasionally pica. There can be eosinophilia and increased total IgE. Smith (1993) has postulated that CT patients are less able to develop a protective immune response, permitting unlimited larval migration so that even a small number of larvae induce severe immunopathology.

Asymptomatic

Positive toxocaral antibody and/or eosinophilia can occur in the absence of other symptoms or signs either currently or in the history, e.g. 26 per cent of hydatid control officers in New Zealand tested seropositive, but gave no history of symptoms (Clemett 1985). That asymptomatic infection is common is indicated by high seropositivity of the general population in all countries of the world. Usually, 2–10 per cent of the population in the Western world are seropositive and there is higher seroprevalence in tropical developing communities, and in children. In part these are explained by past infection and light infection, insufficient to cause symptoms or signs, although some might represent cross-reacting, non-pathogenic *Toxocara* infection. Conversely, the proportion of patients in whom toxocarosis goes undiagnosed is unknown. The non-specific features of toxocarosis, particularly covert toxocarosis, are variable in persistence and easily confused with a variety of febrile, asthmatic, or infectious childhood conditions. Also, significant, unilateral loss of vision might go unnoticed and undiagnosed in young children. Further, as positive serology is relatively common, it could mask an alternate diagnosis. For example, a case of retinoblastoma was masked by positive *Toxocara* titres (Pollard 1987).

Encephalitis; behavioural changes; asthma

An association of *T. canis* larvae with encephalitis, meningitis, neuropsychological deficits, epilepsy, and asthma, is not clear-cut (Glickman 1993). In general, all these syndromes and a number of others, e.g. rheumatism, all require cause and effect with *Toxocara* to be demonstrated.

Neurological disease with eosinophilic encephalitis or meningoencephalitis manifest on magnetic resonance imaging as diffuse and circumscribed hyperintense lesions, has been diagnosed and attributed to heavy *T. canis* infection. The signs were associated with positive toxocaral antibody responses and present with or without other symptoms of VT such as myelitis (Mimoso *et al.* 1993; Sommer *et al.* 1994). In addition, although prevalence with *B. procyonis* in man is low, it has a propensity for migration to and in the CNS in paratenic hosts (5–7 per cent of larvae enter the brain) causing at least two cases of fatal eosinophilic meningoencephalitis (Kazacos 1991).

Toxocara canis larvae can accumulate in the brain. In experimental studies in mice, reduced cognisance in mazes, etc., has been described. Some studies in children suggested that *Toxocara*-positive children performed less well in a battery of neurophyschological tests and showed greater hyperactivity, but other studies showed no differences in cognitive function. Similarly, while a relationship between seropositivity and epilepsy was evident in case control studies (Arpino *et al.* 1990), the sequence of events between epilepsy leading to pica, etc., and infection, or the reverse, has not been clarified (Glickman 1993).

Similarly, there is no clear relationship between IgE, asthma, and *Toxocara*. Total IgE often is elevated in toxocarosis patients and an IgE isotype antibody response is common. However, while higher prevalence of IgG and IgE antibodies was found in asthmatics compared to non-asthmatics in a study in Hawaii, this correlation is not always observed. More detailed case-control studies are needed and the results must consider the genetic influence of atopy in this relationship. Nevertheless, acute respiratory failure, bronchospasm, has been recorded as a presenting symptom of toxocarosis.

CANINE INFECTIONS

Clinical signs and pathology are not usually attributed to *T. canis* in adult dogs but *T. canis* can cause illness, even death, in heavily infected pups. Very large numbers of larvae in newborn pups can damage tissue as they migrate through the lungs to produce respiratory signs. Adult *T. canis* in the intestine of pups induce hypertrophy of the tunica muscularis, villous atrophy, malabsorption, and poor growth.

PATHOGENESIS

The pathogenesis of *T. canis* is related to the number of larvae, their migration, their production of antigens, the host response to these, and differences between individual host responses. These have been studied principally in mice, but experimental studies adequately reproduce clinical disease in man.

On initial infection, larvae migrate rapidly, within a week, through the liver and lungs to other tissues. There may be fever, abdominal pain, coughing, and wheezing if a very large bolus of larvae destroys tissue leaving haemorrhagic tracts and necrosis. A host response develops rapidly—eosinophilia, a specific antibody response and, in many patients, an hyperglobulinaemia and heterophile antibody response, all of which can persist for many months, even years. Gradually, larvae become encapsulated in the musculature and liver. In the granuloma, initially there are eosinophils which degranulate; gradually these are replaced by macrophages and mononuclear cells; the centre becomes predominantly macrophages surrounded by fibroblasts and a collagenous capsule.

Specific antibody occurs in all isotypes, IgM, IgA, IgG, and IgE (Bowman *et al.* 1987; Smith 1993). IgM can persist rather than declining, possibly indicating a failure in isotype switching or an unusual configuration of the *T. canis* antigens. Clinical toxocarosis also is associated with a higher than normal proportion of Th2-type cells which produce interleukin (IL)-4 and IL-5 and a lower than normal proportion of Th1-type cells which produce IL-2 and α-interferon (α-IFN) (De Carli *et al.* 1993). IL-4 and IL-5 promote IgE and eosinophil responses, so the abnormal expansion of Th2 cells can account for high levels of IgE, eosinophilia, and eosinophilic granulomata in patients.

Despite specific antibody and cell responses, there is prolonged survival of *T. canis* larvae in the tissues and granulomata and often a long course for toxocarosis This may in part be explained by immune evasion. The presence of sinuous tracts of antigen in tissues; the presence of extracellular antigen within the granulomata; and the presence of granulomata that contain no larva or its remnants, but that do contain ES; all are consistent with active shedding of antigens. In this way larvae would shed the host immune response, escape and re-migrate.

With time, an increasing proportion of larvae is found in the liver. Also, if an initial dose is large enough, an increased proportion of challenge larvae are found in eosinophilic granulomata in the liver, termed liver entrapment (Parsons and Grieve 1990). As the eosinophilic reaction seems to be in response to the presence of the larvae rather than the cause of their entrapment (Grieve *et al.* 1993), the biological significance of larval entrapment in granulomata, in which they do remain viable, is unknown. It might reduce potentially damaging migration to other tissues, or might increase predation through liver disease (Grieve *et al.* 1993).

It is reasonable to accept that symptoms of VT are associated with a large number of larvae migrating and re-migrating through the tissues. The marked cell response and the preponderance of larvae in the liver account for the splenomegaly and hepatomegaly. Large numbers of migrating larvae and the response to them in various tissues can account for the myocarditis, encephalitis, and neurological symptoms, etc., seen in some patients. Lesions would subside as the larvae become encapsulated or are destroyed. In OT, damage and loss of vision can be directly related to the host response to even a single larva. A larva in the eye stimulates a *de novo* IgE response, an eosinophil reaction and a granuloma. The impaired vision is related to the site of the granuloma or the diffuse uveitis and leucoria. Even should the larva leave a granuloma, the continued inflammatory response to ES and then fibrous healing can produce tractional changes in the posterior pole or retinal detachment.

There is some evidence in laboratory animals that larvae can be killed by immune responses; infected rabbits produced antibody that was larvicidal *in vitro*. Smith (1993) also demonstrated that some (11 per cent) VT/OT patients had antibodies that bound to larvae *in vitro* at both 2 °C and 37 °C. Although the antibody was not larvicidal, ES antigen turnover might be metabolically reduced by it to enhance entrapment and killing. From this, Smith has suggested that the unusual clinical presentation of CT may result from a genetically related immune deficiency that allows prolonged migration of possibly only a few larvae in the individual. For example, a high proportion of Irish CT patients exhibited poor antibody binding to larvae and low titres of IgE compared with Scottish VT/OT patients.

DIAGNOSIS

Immunodiagnosis is the most commonly used method to establish aetiology in patients presenting with symptoms and signs of toxocarosis. It is rare to undertake parasitological diagnosis. Biopsy often will not detect larvae and cannot be justified.

An ELISA for antibody to *T. canis* ES is now widely used and is commercially available, although results in different laboratories are difficult to compare, each using different starting dilutions, optical density cut-off points, and/or antigen batches (Taylor 1993). Nevertheless, 91 per cent sensitivity and 86 per cent specificity were ascribed recently to a commercial test in Europe (Jaquier *et al.* 1991). Specificity and the predictive values are high in northern areas of Europe and the United States. Here, cross-reactions to *Ascaris*, *Anasakis*, and blood group antigens are usually ruled out by dilution of antigen and serum (Van Knapen *et al.* 1992; van Knapen and Buijs 1993). The specificity of the test was supported by the evidence that *Toxocara* and *Ascaris* exposure occurred at almost equal levels but in different individuals in Holland (Van Knapen *et al.* 1992). There seems to be no cross-reaction with *B. procyonis*. However, extensive cross-reactions occur between antigens of *T. cati*, *T. vitulorum*, and *T. canis*, so, even though these parasites seem unlikely as causes of disease, they may induce false-positive *T. canis* reactions, although the extent of this is unknown. In tropical populations parasitism is prevalent and Lynch *et al.* (1988) showed that a competitive inhibition ELISA (using a cocktail of soluble heterologous parasite antigens) increased specificity.

The reaction of patient sera with Western blots of ES antigens has not been tested extensively, but may improve specificity where cross-reacting parasitism is prevalent. Magnaval *et al.* (1991) described it as almost as sensitive but more specific and recommended it be used as a confirmatory test after screening by ELISA. Of the pattern that develops, four low molecular weight bands (24, 28, 30, 35 kDa) were recorded as specific for toxocarosis; three high molecular weight bands (132, 147, 200 kDa) indicated cross-reactivity. *Toxocara* radio-allergo-absorbant test and ELISA for IgE were insufficient for diagnosis when used alone (Magnaval *et al.* 1992). Nevertheless, these authors suggest the tests might show promise to record efficacy of treatment manifested by a decline in the IgE titres. IgE ELISA has greater application for diagnosis of OT (below).

An experimental antigen-capture (AG)-ELISA uses the monoclonal antibody Tcn-2 that reacts with a carbohydrate epitope found on all the ES antigens of *T. canis* (Robertson *et al.* 1988; Gillespie *et al.* 1993). Diagnostic efficiency was poor due to immune complex formation and false-positive reactions with several helminth infections, but such a test would be particularly useful in OT.

Other tests that may aid confirmation of VT or CT include γ-glutomyl-tranferase levels reflecting liver damage, e.g. from repeated infection; ecography showing highly reflective areas (granulomata) in the liver that correspond with low density areas on computed tomography (Magnaval and Baixench 1993); and radiography showing focal consolidation in the lungs.

Sensitivity of ELISA is very high in VT; all are usually antibody positive, some with very high levels of antibody accompanying the symptoms and signs of VT. In contrast, the spectrum of serum titres reported in CT has ranged from negative, through low levels (formerly considered light or previous infection), to high levels consistent with VT. The presence of serum antibody in CT therefore must be considered only in the light of the group of symptoms and signs that produce a recognizable syndrome. Taylor *et al.* (1987) consider history taking as important since symptoms often were acknowledged in history, rather than given as presenting complaints.

OT poses additional difficulties for diagnosis, particularly with the need for urgency in differentiation from malignant retinoblastoma. Serology is less effective than for VT as serum titres may be low or absent in many OT patients. Confirmation can be obtained by examination of vitreous and/or aqueous humour, although this is an invasive technique. Antibody, particularly IgE antibody, may be found; the value of this test is that *de novo* antibody production occurs in a *Toxocara* infected eye in the absence of systemic stimulation, while spillover of antibody from serum into normal eyes does not occur (Soulsby *et al.* 1980). Soluble ES antigen has been detected with AG-ELISA. Cytology reveals lymphocytes and eosinophils (often degranulated) in toxocarosis whereas levels of lactic dehydrogenase and phosphoglucose isomerase are normal in toxocarosis but often elevated in retinoblastoma (Shields *et al.* 1977; Dinning *et al.* 1988; Robertson *et al.* 1989).

Ecography has been used to identify *Toxocara* granuloma hidden by active inflammation in the eye (Wan *et al.* 1991). Ecography can reveal a solid highly refractive mass and the vitreal traction band(s) between a peripheral mass and the posterior pole and/or a retinal detachment. These latter would be unlikely with retinoblastoma, often seen as a mass with clumped or dust-like calcifications.

Occasionally migratory tracts may be seen on the retina, or a larva may be visible to be extirpated or photographed for identification. Bowman (1987) has devised keys based on morphological features of whole larvae or larvae in cross-section which will aid differentiation of species in human tissues, including the eye. *Toxocara canis* larvae are $350-450 \times 14-21$ μm; larvae of *T. cati* apparently are slightly smaller in diameter, e.g. 12–16 μm; while *B. procyonis* grows in the host, reaching $1500 \times 70-80$ μm (Kazacos 1991).

TREATMENT

Much of the pathology induced by *T. canis* is due to the immunopathological host response to ES antigens. Therapy for VT and CT therefore concentrates on anti-inflammatory agents. Glucocorticoids, e.g. prednisolone, methylprednisolone, betamethasone, are used systemically. In severe cases cytotoxic immunosuppressants such as azathioprine have been added to the therapeutic regimen (Sommer *et al.* 1994).

Anthelmintic therapy should be included, although evidence for efficacy is only moderate. The difficulties in determining the efficacy of anthelmintics in human toxocarosis lie in:

(1) the relatively small number of cases that are treated;
(2) treatment is begun after variable lengths of infection and disease, and migrating versus 'trapped' larvae may respond differently;
(3) the immunopathological response may vary between patients;
(4) symptoms and signs may undergo remission in both treated and placebo-treated patients; and
(5) the dose rates of drug and length of treatment vary between trials.

Trials have reported efficacy (a reduction in symptoms and signs) in the region of 47–50 per cent for thiabendazole and 53–57 per cent for albendazole and mebendazole (Magnaval and Charlet 1987; Stürchler *et al.* 1989). In a double blind trial, Magnaval *et al.* (1992) found mebendazole had only moderate efficacy or was equivalent to a placebo. Diethycarbamazine has been reported as better than a placebo (Magnaval and Baixench 1993). Diethycarbamazine is usually given at 6 mg/kg/day in three divided doses for 2–3 weeks. Thiabendazole has been extensively used at two times 25 mg/kg/day for 5–10 days and usually is the only drug approved for prescription. However, the newer benzimidazoles are better absorbed. Mebendazole (1 g three times a day for 3 weeks) now seems to be used as frequently as thiabendazole, but albendazole is well tolerated and has proven efficacy against other tissue parasites. A minimum dose of albendazole of 10 mg/kg/day for 5 days has been recommended (Stürchler *et al.* 1989), but a higher and longer regimen might improve efficacy. For example, the drug is prescribed for hydatid disease and *Taenia solium* in many countries at a dose rate of 800 mg/day for 28 days for patients weighting more than 60 kg, or at 10–25 mg/kg/day for 8 days, respectively. In cases of cerebral toxocarosis, albendazole must be the drug of choice with its known pharmacokinetics in the CNS. Patients treated with benzimidazoles must be monitored for liver function as hepatotoxicity is occasionally reported.

In OT, vigorous anti-inflammatory therapy, both systemic and local, for the immunopathological response, is important (Dinning *et al.* 1988). A live larva within the eye could be removed surgically by vitrectomy to prevent further ES antigen production. However, a larva could remain undetected within a granuloma, so anthelmintics, even though their efficacy and their penetration into the eye is unproved, could be useful. Laser coagulation has been used to destroy an intraocular parasite (Fitzgerald and Rubin 1974). Vitrectomy and epiretinal dissection to relieve traction causing macular distortion and retinal detachment often improve vision (Dinning *et al.* 1988).

CONTROL

Infection with *T. canis*, at least from pet dogs, is preventable, although in practice the exact sources and routes of infection for man have not yet been fully determined. Control of *T. canis* is preferable to treatment of infection in humans because, even though the number of human cases is low, the time from infection to diagnosis may be prolonged, and effective therapy is not achieved in all cases. Toxocarosis is not notifiable so numbers of cases/year must be estimated from diagnostic laboratory records. In one 6-month period in England, of 1182 sera 150 were positive, one third being OT patients (Gillespie 1993). Over a 10-year period in the United States, of 2000–3500 samples submitted/year, 25–33 per cent were positive with an estimated 70 per cent OT and 20 per cent VT; 95 per cent of the OT cases had faulty vision, 20 per cent being blind in one or both eyes (Schantz and Stehr-Green 1988). Costs of diagnosis and treatment of CT in adult patients were given as £620/patient by Magnaval and Baixench (1993). Costs for OT are likely to be higher. Furthermore, these costs do not take into account the emotive aspects of disease or loss of vision in a child.

EGGS

Eggs are hard to eliminate because their thick shell confers considerable resistance. On concrete, i.e. dry pavements exposed to sunlight, eggs will desiccate, but those in cracks will be protected. In kennels, while iodine and xylol have some effects, they are impractical. Hypochlorite (bleach) solution poured on flat surfaces can help by decoating the sticky surface of eggs so they can be washed away, but they won't be killed. Only dry heat, e.g. a flame gun, is lethal. In damp, shaded soil eggs potentially will survive for years; detailed studies on length of survival have never been performed. Only drastic measures will clean soil in gardens. Surface soil contaminated heavily with *B. procyonis* or *T. canis* could be broken up, turned and flamed several times or 10–20 cm of top soil removed and replaced (Kazacos 1991). Sand in sand-boxes can be steam sterilized or replaced.

CONTROL OF CONTAMINATION BY PET DOGS

The bitch and her puppies

The clear relationship between pica, puppies, and VT in young children pinpoint the puppy for treatment.

Two therapeutic regimens prevent or markedly reduce the excretion of eggs from puppies and the lactating bitch (Llyod 1985, 1993; Jacobs and Fisher 1993).

1. This destroys larvae in the bitch as they migrate to the fetus/pup. Bitches are treated from 22 days before to 2–20 days after parturition with high-dose fenbendazole (50 mg/kg/day) and this markedly reduces levels of infection in the puppies. The treatment kills only activating larvae, and as not all larvae activate at each pregnancy and as new larvae will accumulate between pregnancies, the bitch needs to be treated at each pregnancy. Each course of treatment is relatively expensive. Shorter periods of treatment with this and other drugs continue to be examined for efficacy.

2. This kills worms as they develop in the intestine. The bitch and pups are treated every 10–14 days from 2 weeks after parturition until 8–12 weeks. Products with high efficacy against intestinal stages of *T. canis* include fenbendazole, mebendazole, pyrantel, febantel, milbemycin, nitroscanate. Ease of administration to the very young puppy, e.g. a liquid, safety and efficacy in a single dose, all are important considerations.

Unfortunately, as the bitch and her pups, unless heavily infected, will appear perfectly healthy, many owners often do not consider anthelmintic treatments. Also, while an increasing number of veterinary surgeons (64 per cent) surveyed in the United States recommended treatment of the nursing bitch, fewer than half administered drugs prophylactically to at least some puppies and these often too late (only 16 per cent at <3 weeks) (Harvey *et al.* 1991).

Newly purchased puppies

A survey recently demonstrated that 12 per cent of puppies sold out of pet stores in Atlanta were infected with *T. canis*. The same undoubtedly is true in other Western countries and for pups sold or given privately. Indeed, a US$1.5 million award was made by a USA court to a child with OT against the vendor of a puppy. Further, while a relatively high proportion of newly purchased pups are likely to be presented to a veterinary surgeon for vaccination, about 25 per cent of the veterinarians surveyed above did not routinely test for intestinal worms in pups and fewer than 50 per cent routinely administered anthelmintics to pups.

Adult dogs

Adult dogs infected with adult egg-laying *T. canis* are perfectly healthy and current parasitological diagnostic techniques have poor sensitivity and are time consuming. Routine anthelmintic treatment therefore is

recommended. Publicity and education for this is important as 29 per cent of the veterinarians surveyed either never discussed the zoonosis with their clients, or only when asked. Unfortunately, studies have not yet investigated the rate of re-infection in dogs so the treatment interval required has not been determined. Nevertheless, even at a low infection pressure dogs were infected within 3 months. Thus, in a study in Germany, nine bitches (3–9 months old) were exposed to infection by being walked for 3 h/day, 5 days/week, for 3 months, in an urban area with 150 dogs/km^2. While none of these dogs proved susceptible to *T. canis* adult infection, they must have acquired tissue larvae as some pups in five litters from these bitches were born infected (Stoye *et al.* 1993). The levels of infection acquired were very low but then the exposure of the dogs was very limited. Recently, the interval recommended in the United Kingdom decreased from 6 to 3 months, but this still is insufficient. In the absence of data on the rate of re-infection, the interval must be based on the pre-patent period of infection with *T. canis* which, although little studied, can be less than 1 month. Since susceptible animals theoretically could be re-infected immediately after treatment, treatments at 1 month intervals must be appropriate (Lloyd 1993). In the United States, treatment of dogs daily or monthly is likely to be recommended for control of heartworm and hookworm diseases, and the programmes usually also have greater than 90 per cent efficacy against *Toxocara*.

LEGISLATION

Legislation has been invoked by many local councils for the restraint of dogs: exclusion of dogs from parks and beaches; requiring owners to collect their dog's faeces; provision of dog 'toilet areas'; and 'leash' laws for dogs. However, such legislation is difficult to administer and often not enforced. Frequently the only persons that obey the restrictions are the most responsible of pet owners whose dogs are least likely to be infected; other owned dogs, stray dogs, and foxes remain uncontrolled. Further, methods for disposal of the faeces require evaluation. Canine faeces would place an additional burden on sewage disposal systems; in the later 1980s there were an estimated 52–54 million dogs in the United States, 29 million in the EC, 7.3 million in the United Kingdom, and 1.3 million in Zimbabwe. *Toxocara* eggs do survive sewage processing although the risk this poses is undetermined.

CONTROL OF CONTAMINATION BY OTHER DEFINITIVE HOSTS

Treatment of stray dogs and foxes is not practical. These populations need to be controlled in number;

control of stray dogs is necessary not only to prevent toxocarosis but also to reduce dog bites. The populations must be excluded from gardens, play areas, and playgrounds by fencing to prevent contamination with faeces. Sandboxes should be covered.

HYGIENE AND FOOD

Good hand washing is necessary. Children at play should be supervised to encourage this and to prevent geophagia. Vegetables to be eaten raw should be well washed, but as the eggs are very sticky, vegetable gardens should preferably be well fenced to exclude all canines. The importance of fly-borne egg contamination of food requires evaluation, but fly control is required for other reasons also. The importance of larvae in meat from food animals is also undetermined; meat, particularly liver, should be thoroughly cooked.

REFERENCES

Amerasinghe, P. H., Rajapakse, R. P. V. J., Lloyd, S., and Fernando, S. T. (1993). Antigen-induced protection against infection with *Toxocara vitulorum* larvae in mice. *Parasitology Research*, **78**, 643–7.

Arpino, C., Gattinara, G. C., Piergili, D., and Curatolo, P. (1990). *Toxocara* infection and epilepsy in children: a case-control study. *Epilepsia*, **31**, 33–6.

Badley, J. E., Grieve, R. B., Rockey, J. H., and Glickman, L. T. (1987). Immune-mediated adherence of eosinophils to *Toxocara canis* infective larvae: the role of excretory-secretory antigens. *Parasite Immunology*, **9**, 133–43.

Beaver, P. C. (1956). Parasitological reviews: larva migrans. *Experimental Parasitology*, **5**, 587–621.

Beaver, P. C., Snyder, C. H., Carrera, G. M., Dent, J. H., and Lafferty, J. W. (1952). Chronic eosinophilia due to visceral larva migrans. *Pediatrics*, **9**, 7–19.

Bowman, D. D. (1987). Diagnostic morphology of four larval ascaridoid nematodes that may cause visceral larva migrans: *Toxascaris leonina, Baylisascaris procyonis, Lagochilascaris sprenti,* and *Hexametra leidyi. Journal of Parasitology*, **73**, 1198–1215.

Bowman, D. D., Mika-Grieve, M., and Grieve, R. B. (1987). Circulating excretory-secretory antigen levels and specific antibody responses in mice infected with *Toxocara canis. American Journal of Tropical Medicine and Hygiene*, **36**, 75–82.

Brooks, R. (1990). Survey of the dog population in Zimbabwe and its level of rabies vaccination. *Veterinary Record*, **127**, 592–6.

Carli, M. de, Romagnani, S., and Del Prete, G. F. (1993). Human T-cell response to excretory-secretory antigens of *Toxocara canis.* A model of preferential *in vitro* and *in vivo* activation of Th2 cells. In Toxocara *and toxocariasis: clinical, epidemiological and molecular perspectives*, (ed. J. W. Lewis and R. M. Maizels), pp. 125–32. Institute of Biology and British Society of Parasitology, London.

Clemett, R. S. (1985). Toxocaral infection in hydatid control officers: diagnosis by enzyme immunoassay. *New Zealand Journal of Medicine*, **98**, 737–9.

Dinning, W. J., Gillespie, S. H., Cooling, R. J., and Maizels, R. M. (1988). Toxocariasis: a practical approach to the management of ocular disease. *Eye*, **2**, 580–2.

Fitzgerald, C. R. and Rubin, M. L. (1974). Intraocular parasite destroyed by photocoagulation. *Archives of Ophthalmology*, **91**, 162–4.

Gillespie, S. H. (1993). The clinical spectrum of human toxocariasis. In Toxocara *and toxocariasis: clinical, epidemiological and molecular perspectives*, (ed. J. W. Lewis and R. M. Maizels), pp. 55–61. Institute of Biology and British Society of Parasitology, London.

Gillespie, S. H., Dinning, W. J., Voller, A., and Crowcroft, N. S. (1993). The spectrum of ocular toxocariasis. *Eye*, **7**, 415–18.

Glickman, L. T. (1993). The epidemiology of human toxocariasis. In Toxocara *and toxocariasis: clinical, epidemiological and molecular perspectives*, (ed. J. W. Lewis and R. M. Maizels), pp. 3–10. Institute of Biology and British Society of Parasitology, London.

Glickman, L. T. *et al.* (1987). Visceral larva migrans in French adults: a new disease syndrome? *American Journal of Epidemiology*, **125**, 1019–34.

Grieve, R. B., Stewart, V. A., and Parsons, J. C. (1993). Immunobiology of larval toxocariasis (*Toxocara canis*): a summary of recent research. In Toxocara *and toxocariasis: clinical, epidemiological and molecular perspectives*, (ed. J. W. Lewis and R. M. Maizels), pp. 117–24. Institute of Biology and British Society of Parasitology, London.

Harris, S. and Rayner, J. M. V. (1986). Urban fox (*Vulpes vulpes*) population estimates and habitat requirements in several British cities. *Journal of Animal Ecology*, **55**, 575–91.

Harvey, J. B., Roberts, J. M., and Schantz, P. M. (1991). Survey of veterinarians recommendations for treatment and control of intestinal parasites in dogs—profilic health implications. *Journal of the American Veterinary Association*, **199**, 702–6.

Holland, C., O'Connor, P., Taylor, M. R. H., Hughes, G., Girdwood, R. W. A., and Smith, H. (1991). Families, parks, gardens and toxocariasis. *Scandinavian Journal of Infectious Diseases*, **23**, 225–31.

Horak, P. (1992). Helminth eggs in the sludge from three sewage treatment plants in Czechoslovakia. *Folia Parasitologia*, **39**, 153–7.

Jacobs, D. E. and Fisher, M. A. (1993). Recent developments in the chemotherapy of *Toxocara canis* infection in puppies and the prevention of toxocariasis. In Toxocara *and toxocariasis: clinical epidemiological and molecular perspectives*, (ed. J. W. Lewis and R. M. Maizels), pp. 111–16. Institute of Biology and British Society of Parasitology, London.

Jaquier, P., Gottstein, B., Stingelin, Y., and Eckert, J. (1991). Immunodiagnosis of toxocariasis in humans: evaluation of a new enzyme linked immunosorbent assay. *Journal of Clinical Microbiology*, **29**, 1831–5.

Jordan, H. E., Mullins, S. T., and Stebbins, M. E. (1993). Endoparasitism in dogs: 21,583 cases (1981–1990). *Journal of the American Veterinary Association*, **203**, 547–9.

Kazacos, K. R. (1991). Visceral and ocular larva migrans. *Seminars in Veterinary Medicine and Surgery (Small Animal)*, **6**, 227–35.

Kennedy, M. W., Maizels, R. M., Meghji, M., Young, L., Qureshi, F., and Smith, H. V. (1987). Species-specific and common antigens of *Toxocara cati* and *Toxocara canis* infective larvae. *Parasite Immunology*, **9**, 407–20.

Khoo, K. -H., Morris, H. R., and Dell, A. (1993). Structural characterization of the major glycans of *Toxocara canis* ES antigens. In *Toxocara and toxocariasis: clinical, epidemiological and molecular perspectives*, (ed. J. W. Lewis and R. M. Maizels), pp. 133–40. Institute of Biology and British Society of Parasitology, London.

Kirkpatrick, C. E. (1988). Epizootiology of endoparasitic infections in pet dogs and cats presented to a veterinary teaching hospital. *Veterinary Parasitology*, **30**, 113–24.

Knapen, F. van and Buijs, J. (1993). Diagnosis of *Toxocara* infection. In *Toxocara and toxocariasis: clinical, epidemiological and molecular perspectives*, (ed. J. W. Lewis and R. M. Maizels), pp. 49–53. Institute of Biology and British Society of Parasitology, London.

Knapen, F. van, Buijs, J., Kortbeek, L. M., and Ljungstrom, I. (1992). Larva migrans syndrome: *Toxocara, Ascaris*, or both? *Lancet*, **340**, 590–1.

Lawson, J. R. and Gemmell, M. A. (1990). Transmission of taeniid tapeworm eggs via blowflies to intermediate hosts. *Parasitology*, **100**, 143–6.

Lloyd S. (1985). *Toxocara canis*: infection, treatment and control. *Veterinary Annual*, **25**, 368–75.

Lloyd S. (1987). Immunobiology of *Toxocara canis* and visceral larva migrans. In *Immune responses in parasitic infections: immunology immunopathology, and immunoprophylaxis*, Vol. I. *Nematodes*, (ed. E. J. L. Soulsby), pp. 299–324. CRC Press, Boca Raton.

Lloyd, S. (1993). *Toxocara canis*: the dog. In *Toxocara and toxocariasis: clinical, epidemiological and molecular perspectives*, (ed. J. W. Lewis, and R. M. Maizels), pp. 11–24. Institute of Biology and British Society of Parasitology, London.

Lynch, N. R., Wilkes, L. K., Hodgen, A. N., and Truner, K. J. (1988). Specificity of *Toxocara* ELISA in tropical populations. *Parasite Immunology*, **10**, 323–7.

Magnaval, J. -F. and Baixench, M. T. (1993). Toxocariasis in the Midi-Pyrenees. In *Toxocara and toxocariasis: clinical, epidemiological and molecular perspectives*, (eds. J. W. Lewis and R. M. Maizels), pp. 63–9. Institute of Biology and British Society of Parasitology, London.

Magnaval, J. -F., and Charlet, J. -P. (1987). Efficacité comparée du thiabendazole et du mebendazole dans la traitement de la toxocarose. *Therapie*, **42**, 541–4.

Magnaval, J. -F., Fabre, J. -P., Maurires, P., Charlet, J. P., and Larrand, B. de. (1991). Application of the western-blotting procedure for the immunodiagnosis of human toxocariasis. *Parasitology Research*, **77**, 697–702.

Magnaval, J. -F., Charlet, J. -P., and Larrard, B. de (1992). Étude double aveugle de l' efficacité du mebendazole dans les formes mineures de la toxocarose humaine. *Therapie*, **47**, 145–8.

Maizels, R. M. and Page, A. P. (1990). Surface associated glycoproteins from *Toxocara canis* L2 parasites. *Acta Tropica*, **47**, 355–64.

Maizels, R. M., Gems, D. H., and Page, A. P. (1993). Synthesis and secretion of TES antigens from *Toxocara canis* infective larvae. In *Toxocara and toxocariasis: clinical, epidemiological and molecular perspectives*, (ed. J. W. Lewis and R. M. Maizels), pp. 141–50. Institute of Biology and British Society of Parasitology, London.

Meghji, M. and Maizels, R. M. (1986). Biochemical properties of larval excretory-secretory (ES) glycoproteins of the parasitic nematode *Toxocara canis*. *Molecular and Biochemical Parasitology*, **18**, 155–70.

Mimoso, M. G., Periera, M. C., Estavao, M. H., Barroso, A. A., and Mota, H. C. (1993). Eosinophilic meningoencephalitis due to *Toxocara canis*. *European Journal of Pediatrics*, **152**, 783–4.

Nagakura, K., Tachibana, H., Kaneda, Y., and Kato, Y. (1989). Toxocariasis possibly caused by ingesting raw chicken. *Journal of Infectious Diseases*, **160**, 735–6.

Nichols, R. L. (1956). The etiology of visceral larva migrans. I. Diagnostic morphology of infective second-stage *Toxocara* larvae. *Journal of Parasitology*, **42**, 349–62.

Page, A. P., Hamilton, A. J., and Maizels, R. M. (1992*a*). *Toxocara canis*: monoclonal antibodies to carbohydrate epitopes of secreted (TES) antigens localize to different secretion-related structures in infective larvae. *Experimental Parasitology*, **75**, 56–71.

Page, A. P., Rudin, W., Fluri, E., Blaxter, M. L., and Maizels, R. M. (1992*b*). *Toxocara canis*: a labile antigenic coat overlying the epicuticle of infective larvae. *Experimental Parasitology*, **75**, 72–86.

Parsons, J. C. and Grieve, R. B. (1990). Kinetics of liver trapping of infective larvae in murine toxocariasis. *Journal of Parasitology*, **76**, 529–36.

Parsons, J. C., Bowman, D. D., and Grieve, R. B. (1986). Tissue localization of excretory-secretory antigens of larval *Toxocara canis* in acute and chronic murine toxocariasis. *American Journal of Tropical Medicine and Hygiene*, **35**, 974–81.

Pollard, Z. F. (1987). Long-term follow-up in patients with ocular toxocariasis as measured by ELISA titers. *Annals of Ophthalmology*, **19**, 167–9.

Richards, D. T. and Lewis, J. W. (1993). Epidemiology of *Toxocara canis* in the fox. In *Toxocara and toxocariasis: clinical, epidemiological and molecular perspectives*, (ed. J. W. Lewis and R. M. Maizels), pp. 25–37. Institute of Biology and British Society of Parasitology, London.

Richards, D. T., Harris, S., and Lewis, J. W. (1993). Epidemiology of *Toxocara canis* in red foxes (*Vulpes vulpes*) from urban areas of Bristol. *Parasitology*, **107**, 167–73.

Robertson, B. D., Burkot, T. R., Gillespie, S. H., Kennedy, M. W., Wambai, Z., and Maizels, R. M. (1988). Detection of circulating parasite antigen and specific antibody in *Toxocara canis* infection. *Clinical and Experimental Immunology*, **74**, 236–41.

Robertson, B. D., Bianco, A. E., McKerrow, J. H., and Maizels, R. M. (1989). Proteolytic enzymes secreted by larvae of the nematode *Toxocara canis*. *Experimental Parasitology*, **69**, 30–6.

Romeu, J., Roig, J., Bada, J. L., Riera, C., and Muñoz, C. (1991). Adult human toxocariasis acquired by eating raw snails. *Journal of Infectious Diseases*, **164**, 438.

Savigny, D. H. de. (1975). *In vitro* maintenance of *Toxocara canis* larvae and a simple method for the production of *Toxocara* ES antigens for use in serodiagnostic tests for visceral larva migrans. *Journal of Parasitology*, **61**, 781–2.

Savigny, D. H. de, Voller, A., and Woodruff, A. W. (1979). Toxocariasis: serological diagnosis by enzyme immunoassay. *Journal of Clinical Pathology*, **32**, 283–8.

Schantz, P. M. and Stehr-Green, J. K. (1988). Toxocaral larva migrans. *Journal of the American Veterinary Medical Association*, **192**, 28–32.

Schantz, P. M., Weis, P. E., Pollard, Z. F., and White, M. (1980). Risk factors for toxocaral ocular larva migrans: a case-control study. *American Journal of Public Health*, **70**, 1269–72.

Shields, J. A., Lerner, H. A., and Felberg, N. T. (1977). Aqueous cytology and enzymes in nematode endophthalmitis. *Annals of Ophthalmology*, **19**, 167–9.

Smith, H. V. (1993). Antibody reactivity in human toxocariasis. In Toxocara *and toxocariasis: clinical, epidemiological and molecular perspectives*, (ed. J. W. Lewis and R. M. Maizels), pp. 91–109. Institute of Biology and British Society of Parasitology, London.

Smith, H. V., Quinn, R., Kusel, J. R., and Girdwood, R. W. A. (1981). The effect of temperature and antimetabolites on antibody binding to the outer surface of second stage *Toxocara canis* larvae. *Molecular and Biochemical Parasitology*, **4**, 183–93.

Sommer, C., Ringelstein, E. B., Biniek, R., and Glockner, W. M. (1994). Adult *Toxocara canis* encephalitis. *Journal of Neurology, Neurosurgery and Psychiatry*, **57**, 229–31.

Soulsby, E. J. L., Stromberg, B. E., Donnelly, J. J., and Rockey, J. H. (1980). Intraocular immunoglobulin E induced by intravitreal infection with *Ascaris* and *Toxocara* spp. larvae. *Ophthalmological Research*, **12**, 45.

Stoye, M., Hesse, A., and Kuschfeldt, S. (1993). Studies on the infection risk for dogs reared helminth-free under conventional conditions in an urban area. *Journal of Veterinary Medicine, B*, **40**, 453–8.

Stürchler, D., Schubarth, P., Gualzata, M., Gottstein, B., and Oettli, A. (1989). Thiabendazole versus albendazole in treatment of toxocariasis. *Annals of Tropical Medicine and Parasitology*, **83**, 473–6.

Takahashi, J., Uga, S., and Matsumura, T. (1990). Cockroach as a possible transmitter of *Toxocara canis*. *Japanese Journal of Parasitology*, **39**, 551–6.

Taylor, M. R. H. (1993). Toxocariasis in Ireland. In Toxocara *and toxocariasis: clinical, epidemiological and molecular perspectives*, (ed. J. W. Lewis and R. M. Maizels), pp. 71–80. Institute of Biology and British Society of Parasitology, London.

Taylor, M. R. H., Keane, C. T., O'Connor, P., Girdwood, R. W. A., and Smith, H. (1987). Clinical features of covert toxocariasis. *Scandanavian Journal of Infectious Diseases*, **19**, 693–6.

Umeche, M. and Mandah, L. E. (1989). *Musca domestica* as a carrier of intestinal helminths in Calabor, Nigeria. *East African Medical Journal* **66**, 349–52.

Wan, W. L., Cano, M. R., Pince, K. J., and Green, R. L. (1991). Ecographic characteristics of ocular toxocariasis. *Ophthalmology*, **98**, 28–32.

Wilder, H. C. (1950). Nematode enophthalmitis. *Transactions of the American Academy of Ophthalmology*, **55**, 99–109.

Woodruff, A. W., de Savigny, D. H., and Hendy-Ibbs, P. M. (1982). Toxocaral and toxoplasmal antibodies in cat breeders and in Icelanders exposed to cats but not to dogs. *British Medical Journal*, **284**, 309–10.

Zinkham, W. H. (1978). Visceral larva migrans. A review and reassessment indicating two forms of clinical assessments: visceral and ocular. *American Journal of Diseases of Childhood*, **132**, 627–33.

64 TRICHOSTRONGYLIDOSIS

T. J. Nolan

SUMMARY

Trichostrongylidosis is an infection involving nematodes of the superfamily Trichostrongyloidea, mainly those of the genus *Trichostrongylus*. Infections are usually asymptomatic, but when heavy a variety of gastrointestinal symptoms, including abdominal pain and diarrhoea, can be present. Infections are initiated by the ingestion of third-stage larvae. There is no parenteral migration and the adults are usually found in the mucosa of the duodenum. Eggs pass out with the faeces, hatch in about 1 day and the larvae develop to the infective stage in 2 or 3 days. Human infections with *Trichostrongylus* spp. have been reported worldwide, and are particularly common in southern Asia. Infections respond well to anthelminitics and periodic dosing of livestock is the chief method of control.

HISTORY

The type species for the genus *Trichostrongylus* (*T. retortaeformis*) was described from rabbits in 1800 and *T. orientalis* was described from man in 1914 (Nagaty 1932). By 1927 human infections with animal-infecting species of *Trichostrongylus* were known well enough for Sandground (1929) to consider them in his differential diagnosis of a nematode infection found in a missionary from Africa.

In 1947 Stoll estimated that there were 5.5 million cases of human trichostrongylidosis in the world, the vast majority of them being in Asia. In 1953 Watson revised Stoll's estimate using new reports of prevalence from India, Indonesia, China, the Middle East, and Africa as well as more up to date population estimates. He estimated that 58 million human cases occurred worldwide, with 30 million being found in Indonesia (based on a 41.2 per cent incidence, more recent estimates of the prevalence (Oemijati 1971) put it in the range of 11 per cent in this region). While Stoll's estimate was probably too conservative and Watson's may be skewed by the one prevalence estimate from Indonesia, the true number of cases today most likely is nearer to Watson's estimate than to Stoll's. With the increase in the human population in the areas with the highest prevalence rates that has occurred since 1953, coupled with the lack of any major change in the risk behaviour of these populations, Watson's estimate of 58 million cases appears reasonable.

Our knowledge of the life cycle parameters of *Trichostrongylus* spp. infections in humans comes from studies by Joe (1947) done in the 1940s. Using human volunteers and *T. colubriformis* and *T. axei* he was able to estimate the prepatent period, some of the clinical signs, and the differences in infectivity of the different species for humans.

THE AGENT

TAXONOMY

Members of the genus *Trichostrongylus* are nematodes of the class Secernentea, order Strongylida, and superfamily Trichostrongyloidea. Adult *Trichostrongylus* spp. are slender, generally under 10 mm in length, and the male has a copulatory bursa at its posterior end. The adult worms lodge in the mucosa of the stomach or small intestine, the exact location varies depending on the species. The female worms lay thin-walled 'strongyle-type' eggs which pass out with the faeces. Eggs hatch in 1 or 2 days in faeces or damp soil and the larvae eventually develop to the infective third-stage, which is enclosed in the cuticle of the second stage. Infection takes place when these third-stage larvae are swallowed by the host. These larvae invade the mucosa of the digestive tract and eventually develop to adults. There is no parenteral migration.

Ten species have been reported to infect humans: *Trichostrongylus axei*, *T. affinis*, *T. brevis*, *T. calcaratus*, *T. capricola*, *T. colubriformis*, *T. orientalis*, *T. probolurus*, *T. skrjabini*, and *T. vitrinus*. With the exceptions of *T. brevis* and *T. orientalis*, all are parasites of domestic and wild ruminants (Acha and Szyfres 1987). Humans are the natural host for *T. orientalis*, although it has also been found in sheep and camels. *Trichostrongylus brevis* is known only from humans. Other trichostrongylids of ruminants that have been found in man are *Haemonchus contortus*, *Ostertagia ostertagia*, *O. circumcincta*, and *Marshallagia marshalli* (Ghadirian and Arfaa 1973). These four nematodes have been reported on only a very few occasions despite their widespread occurrence in domestic livestock.

DISEASE MECHANISMS

The adults of *Trichostrongylus* spp. feed on the mucosal tissue of the gastrointestinal tract. The resulting tissue destruction leads to the symptoms of the disease.

GROWTH AND SURVIVAL REQUIREMENTS

The eggs and larvae of *Trichostronglus* spp. are resistant to cold and desiccation. Third-stage larvae over winter on pasture in Great Britain and in the southern hemisphere, after drought, the desicated third-stage larvae will rehydrate when the rains arrive and are still infective (Soulsby 1982). These parasites may also over winter in the host as hypobiotic third-stage larvae.

THE HOSTS

ANIMAL

Incubation period

In ruminants the time from ingestion of the third-stage larvae to the passage of eggs in the feces ranges from 2 to 3 weeks, depending on the species.

Clinical signs

Ruminants with heavy infections usually have diarrhoea and show a rapid weight loss. Signs in lighter infections range from none to soft faeces and a decline in the rate of weight gain. In most cases ruminants infected with *Trichostrongylus* sp. are also infected with other nematodes and thus the clinical signs will reflect the mix of parasites and may therefore be different from those just described (Soulsby 1982).

Diagnosis

Trichostrongylus sp. infections in ruminants are usually diagnosed by finding the eggs in a faecal flotation using either a saturated sugar or salt solution. Because many ruminant nematode parasites produce 'strongyle-type' eggs a definitive diagnosis may require identification of larvae recovered from a faecal culture. But, because of the availability of broad-spectrum anthelmintics, this larval identification procedure is rarely done.

Pathology

The third-stage larvae penetrate the wall of the abomasum or intestine, depending on the species, and will tunnel within the mucosa. When the worms moult to

the adult stage they break out of these tunnels, resulting in oedema and haemorrhage. Large numbers of adults can lead to erosion of the mucosal surface, with the subsequent development of diarrhoea. The heavily infected animal generally loses weight.

Treatment

Infected animals can be treated with ivermectin, levamisole, or one of the benzimidazoles. Because the pasture is now contaminated with eggs and larvae, treated animals should be moved to new pasture after they are treated or treated prophylactically for the rest of the grazing season.

HUMAN

Incubation period

The time between ingesting the third-stage larva and the development of the mature adult in humans has been reported to be 21 days (for *T. colubriformis*), although it might be expected that this time period will vary depending on the species of *Trichostrongylus* (Joe 1947). The adult worms can live for several years.

Symptoms

The symptoms and their severity depend on the number of worms present. Most infections are asymptomatic, but in heavy infections (over 100 adult worms) diarrhoea (sometimes tinged with blood), abdominal pain, mild anaemia, and weight loss have been reported (Boreham *et al.* 1995). A transient eosinophilia may also be present. An accurate description of the symptoms present in a heavy infection is difficult as most people harbouring many adult *Trichostrongylus* sp. are also infected with other gastrointestinal nematodes.

Diagnosis

Diagnosis is usually made by examining the stools for eggs. The 'strongyle-type' eggs laid by *Trichostrongylus* spp. must be differentiated from hookworm eggs (Webb 1937). *Trichostrongylus* spp. eggs measure 73–95 μm long and 40–50 μm wide. They generally have dissimilar poles, one end is rounded while the other is somewhat pointed. Thus the eggs are larger than those of the hookworms and have a different shape. Hookworm and *Trichostrongylus* spp. infections can also be distinguished by examining the first-stage larvae obtained by faecal culture. The most obvious difference between these first-stage larvae is that those of *Trichostrongylus* spp. will have a bead-like swelling on the caudal tip of the tail while hookworm larvae have a tail that ends in a point. Specific diagnosis can be made by recovering adult male worms from the faeces after treatment. The spicules, gubernaculum, and bursal rays are used in making a species identification.

Pathology

Very little is known about the pathology of these worms in humans although it is thought to be similar to that seen in the animal host. Desquamation with haemorrhage has been reported at the intestinal sites infected by adult worms.

Treatment

Thiabendazole, mebendazole, pyrantel embonate, and bephenium hydroxynaphthoate have successfully cleared *Trichostrongylus* infections from humans (Markell 1968; Bundy *et al.* 1985; Panasoponkul *et al.* 1985; Boreham *et al.* 1995). A follow-up faecal examination should be done 2–4 weeks after treatment to verify that the infection has been cleared.

Prognosis

Patients cured of a *Trichostrongylus* infection make a rapid and complete recovery.

EPIDEMIOLOGY

OCCURRENCE

Members of the genus *Trichostrongylus* are common in ruminants worldwide and human infections have been reported from every continent except, of course, Antarctica. Human infections are common across southern Asia, as well as in Korea and some areas of Japan. Endemic areas are also found in Africa (Egypt, Ethiopia, Zaire, and Zimbabwe).

SOURCES, TRANSMISSION, AND COMMUNICABILITY

Many of the infections in Asia are due to *T. orientalis* and are the result of the use of human faeces as fertilizer. The infection is acquired while eating uncooked plant material on which the larvae are present. Of the remaining infections in these endemic areas the most common source of infection was domestic animals sharing living quarters with humans (Ghadirian and Arfaa 1975). Also, the use of animal faeces as fuel has been implicated in the infection of the people who gather and prepare the faeces for this purpose (Ghardirian and Arfaa 1975). The source of infections in non-endemic areas is most likely the accidental ingestion of larvae acquired from livestock pasture or the ingestion of unwashed vegetables grown with animal manure used as fertilizer (Boreham *et al.* 1995).

The human to human transmission of species of *Trichostrongylus*, other than *T. orientalis* and *T. brevis*, is probably low to non-existent. Even the two species parasitizing humans are transmitted indirectly, and thus are not transmissible to people associated with infected humans, but who do not eat uncooked material from plants fertilized with human faeces.

PREVENTION AND CONTROL

PREVENTION

In areas where *T. orientalis* is prevalent, uncooked plant material should not be eaten, especially vegetables and other crops that might have been fertilized with nightsoil. In endemic areas where other species of *Trichostrongylus* are found, hands should be washed before preparing or eating meals and vegetables should be throughly washed or cooked before eating. The practice of sharing living quarters with domestic livestock should be discouraged.

CONTROL STRATEGIES

Trichostrongylus orientalis can be controlled by proper sanitation (i.e. removal of human faeces from areas where humans may come in contact with it) and the sterilization of nightsoil before its use as a fertilizer. Infections with *Trichostrongylus* spp. of animal origin can be controlled by periodic treatment of domestic livestock with anthelmintics. The time between treatments will depend on the local conditions. Since well-nourished livestock are better able to reduce their parasite burdens, animals should be kept well fed and their diet supplemented with minerals. Particular care should be taken with animals under a year of age as they are still developing an immune response to the worms and therefore have higher worm burdens than older animals.

Since larvae will survive on pasture for about 1 month only, pasture rotation, with a period of greater than 1 month, will help to reduce worm burdens in livestock.

REFERENCES

Acha P. N. and Szyfres, B. (1987). *Zoonoses and communicable diseases common to man and animals*, (2nd edn). Pan American Health Organization, Washington, DC.

Boreham, R. E., McCowan, M. J., Ryan, A. E., Allworth, A. M., and Robson, J. M. (1995). Human trichostrongyliasis in Queensland. *Pathology*, **27**, 182–5.

Bundy, D. A. P., Terry, S. I., Murphy, C. P., and Harris, E. A. (1985). First record of *Trichostrongylus axei* infection of man in the Caribbean region. *Transactions of the Royal Society of Tropical Medicine and Hygiene*, **79**, 562–3.

Ghadirian, E. and Arfaa, F. (1973). First report of human infection with *Haemonchus contortus, Ostertagia ostertagi,* and *Marshallagia marshalli* in Iran. *Journal of Parasitology,* **59,** 1144–5.

Ghadirian, E. and Arfaa, F (1975). Present status of trichostrongyliasis in Iran. *American Journal of Tropical Medicine and Hygiene,* **24,** 935–41.

Joe, L. K. (1947). *Trichostrongylus* infectious in man and domestic animals in Java. *Journal of Parasitology,* **33,** 359–62.

Markell, E. K. (1968). Pseudohookworm infection—trichostrongyliasis. Treatment with thiabendazole. *New England Journal of Medicine,* **278,** 831–2.

Nagaty, H. F. (1932). The Genus *Trichostrongylus* Looss, 1905. *Annals of Tropical Medicine and Parasitology,* **26,** 457–518.

Oemijati, S. (1971). Gastrointestinal infections in Indonesia (a review). In *Proceedings of the seventh southeast Asian regional seminar on tropical medicine and public health. Infectious diseases of the gastrointestinal system in Southeast Asia and the Far East,* (ed. J. Cross), pp. 153–61.

Panasoponkul, C., Radomyos, P., and Singhasivanon, V. (1985). *Trichostrongylus* infection in a Thai boy. *South-East Asian Journal of Tropical Medicine and Public Health,* **16,** 513–14.

Sandground, J. H. (1929). *Ternidens deminutus* (Railliet and Henry) as a parasite of man in southern Rhodesia; together with observations and experimental infection studies on an unidentified nematode parasite of man from this region. *Annals of Tropical Medicine and Parasitology,* **23,** 23–32.

Soulsby, E. J. L. (1982). *Helminths, arthropods and protozoa of domesticated animals,* (7th edn). Lea and Febiger, Philadelphia.

Stoll, N. R. (1947). This wormy world. *Journal of Parasitology,* **33,** 1–18.

Watson, J. M. (1953). Human trichostrongylosis and its relationship to ancylostomiasis in southern Iraq, with comments on world incidence. *Parasitology,* **43,** 102–9.

Webb, J. L. (1937). The helminths of the intestinal canal of man in Mauritius; and a first record of *Trichostrongylus axei* locally. *Parasitology,* **29,** 469–76.

65 SCABIES AND OTHER MITE INFESTATIONS

W. N. Beesley

SUMMARY

Species of mites of animals and birds are considered which affect man either directly by causing primary irritation, hypersensitivity reactions, etc. or as vectors of diseases such as scrub typhus. The most important genera of mites in the two categories are *Sarcoptes* and *Leptotrombidium*. Details are given of the biology, diagnosis, pathology, immunology, and control of these and other mites which transfer from animals to humans.

INTRODUCTION

Most of the many thousands of species of mites do no harm to vertebrates, but some cause the serious skin conditions known as scabies in man or mange in animals. Zoonotic mites which can transfer from animals to man include the sarcoptids, demodicids, and cheyletids. The larvae of a further group of mites, the trombiculids, will feed on man, to whom they may also transmit scrub typhus. It is convenient to consider each of these groups separately.

SARCOPTIC MANGE

HISTORY

Scabies, also known in man as sarcoptic acariasis, crusted scabies, Norwegian itch, seven-year itch, and (in animals) mange, is a severe irritating skin condition caused by the mite *Sarcoptes scabiei*. It is quite likely that the ancient Greeks suffered from skin problems such as scabies, as inscriptions at a newly excavated medical centre in Ephesus show that patients were first screened into those with infectious skin diseases (which would include scabies), those with mild skin diseases, and those with major but non-infectious illnesses. Patients with skin problems were treated by bathing, exposure to sunlight, and treatment with honey or herbs.

The Bible mentions that any 'beeves' (cattle) or sheep which were blind, broken, maimed, had scurvy, or were scabbed should not be offered in sacrifice. Cattle scab and sheep scab disease today, especially in warm countries, include infestation by both *Sarcoptes* and *Psoroptes* mites, which must have affected livestock thousands of years ago. When cattle became domesticated the sarcoptic ingredient of their scab disease was probably recognized as a zoonotic condition, although its counterpart in sheep virtually never affects man.

The first mention of human scabies was about AD 940, and in the seventeenth century the Scottish doctor Thomas Moufet described the mites as 'always lying under the outward skin and creeping under it as do moles, biting it and causing a fierce itching' (Rothschild and Clay 1952), hence the notion of a burrowing parasite had been accepted. Scabies has long been associated with wars and great disasters, when large numbers of people are crowded together in unhygienic conditions. Armies have suffered from scabies over the centuries and in Britain during the Second World War there were up to 6000 new cases among soldiers each month; civilians are likewise badly affected and there were at least 68 000 cases in Norway in 1943, for example. In most industrialized countries skin diseases account for some 6–18 per cent of consultations at primary health care level, and at times scabies can be an important item (Anon. 1991; Cox and Paterson 1991).

Scabies occurs in most countries of world but diagnosis is often made difficult by concurrent skin diseases, such as psoriasis, or secondary bacterial infections. In the tropics, West African 'craw-craw' and New Guinea 'kas kas' are complications of skin infections initiated by *S. scabiei* (Gordon and Lavoipierre 1972).

The human itch mite, *S. scabiei*, was first described in 1758 by Linnaeus, who named it *Acarus siro* var. *scabiei*, to distinguish it from the grain mite, *A. siro* var. *farinae*. De Geer renamed the human itch mite *A. scabiei* in 1778, and in 1802 Latreille erected the genus *Sarcoptes*; *S. scabiei* was also called *S. hominis* by Hering in 1838 and *S. communis* by Delafond and Bourguignon in 1862. During the nineteenth century many new species of *Sarcoptes* were named from domesticated animals, e.g. *S. equi*, *S. bovis*, *S. ovis*, *S. equi*, *S. suis*, etc.

There has been much discussion about the validity of the forms of *Sarcoptes* recovered from animals and man. These have been considered as different physiological races, strains, varieties, subspecies, and full species. It is now generally accepted that there are only about 10 true species, and the styles *S. scabiei* var. *scabiei* (= var. *hominis*), *S. scabiei* var. *bovis*, etc. are now obsolete.

Also included in the family Sarcoptidae are *Knemidokoptes*, which causes mange in birds, and *Notoedres cati*, the face mange of cats. The latter can produce a transient dermatitis in man, following contact with infested cats, rabbits (Zumpt 1961), or lynx (Sequiera and Dowdeswell 1942). The sarcoptids *Chirnyssus* (bats), *Nycteridocoptes* (bats), and *Mysarcoptes* (rodents) do not affect man. The related family Psoroptidae includes *Psoroptes*, *Otodectes*, *Chorioptes*, and *Caparinia*. These show marked host specificity and can be responsible for highly contagious and serious forms of mange in animals (Meleney 1985) but none of them appears capable of transmission to man.

SARCOPTES: BIOLOGY

All sarcoptids are important to man or animals, causing serious skin damage, but we are chiefly concerned with *Sarcoptes*. *Notoedres* and *Knemidokoptes* are generally similar in appearance and biology.

The female *Sarcoptes* mite is disc-shaped and measures 350–450 μm across. This stage is easily identifiable by the prominent dorsal spines and pegs. Male sarcoptic mites measure about 200–250 μm in length, the larvae and nymphs being correspondingly smaller. The life cycle of *S. scabiei* was thoroughly studied by Mellanby (1943) and surprisingly little new information has been added since. The parasite lives in a sinuous tunnel which she has bored in the outer layer of the skin, never penetrating the stratum corneum. Each day the female mite lays 1–4 eggs in her tunnel, where all the motile stages will appear in due course. The reproductive life of the female is about 8 weeks. The burrow is extended by 0.5–5.0 mm each day and the mites are seen on the surface of the skin only while moving from one host to the next or when seeking a mate.

In addition to the motile stages, the tunnels will eventually contain empty egg shells, cuticles of the various developmental stages, and the excretory and secretory (ES) products of the parasites. These substances are strongly antigenic and elicit a strong reaction in the host. The important immunological aspect of scabies received little attention until comparatively recently.

Scabies patients are often unavoidably dirty and former recommendations for the control of the disease usually included a hot bath and a savage scrubbing of the skin. This was intended to reduce the numbers of mites and to improve the efficiency of any available medication. Bathing as such probably has little beneficial effect, and in any case there is often a shortage of washing water in those places where scabies has become a serious problem. After bathing, use of a medicinal soap was suggested, followed by the application of 5–10 per cent sulphur in an ointment or soft paraffin, the use of an organic sulphur preparation or benzyl benzoate lotion. Sulphur ointment is messy, stains, and often has an unpleasant odour. Much more effective acaricides are now available, although for use on infants, children, or pregnant women sulphur preparations have been preferred in the past to lindane, crotamiton, or organophosphorous acaricides (see pp. 000–00).

SCABIES IN ANIMALS

According to Zumpt (1961) and Lapage (1968), most species of *Sarcoptes* are transmissible to man: *S. equi*, *S. bovis*, *S. ovis*, *S. caprae*, *S. suis*, *S. dromedarii*, *S. canis*, *S. vulpis* (fox), *S. leonis* (lion), *S. aucheniae* (alpaca), and *S. wombati*.

Human scabies infections usually involve quite small numbers of *Sarcoptes*, compared with the many hundreds or thousands of the parasites in individual animal hosts. This helps to explain why people who work closely with farm animals can easily become infected. Two species of *Sarcoptes* are usually responsible for human infestations, i.e. apart from his own species, *S. scabiei*. *Sarcoptes bovis* is a frequent parasite of cattle and buffaloes in many parts of the world, mites easily transferring to the operator during hand milking. This gives rise to 'milker's itch' or 'dairyman's itch'. Human infections are generally seen on the arms and across the side of the neck—or on the chest and shoulders in warmer countries when little clothing may be worn.

Sarcoptes equi can also affect man. It was formerly quite common on horses in Britain and the USA, for example, but has now been eradicated. The disease is sufficiently serious and contagious in equines to often merit its own section in national legislation and it remains a 'notifiable' (reportable) condition in many countries. In man, 'horse itch' or 'cavalryman's itch' can occur in people who groom horses, but riders are also at risk, especially if they are involved with brushing or harnessing the animal. Veterinarians can also become infected.

INCUBATION PERIOD

The female mite must first penetrate the skin, which she does in about 30 minutes, and then make a burrow parallel with the surface. In this she lays her eggs, which hatch 3–5 days later. The life cycle from oviposition to adult mite takes about 10–20 days.

SYMPTOMS AND SIGNS

Infection of animals is almost always by contact with other infected animals, including suckling. Mange rarely follows contact with materials which have been contaminated by infected animals, although there are records of survival by *Sarcoptes* for 17 days. Animals are most often in contact with other animals by the head or flank, so that infestations are often first seen in these areas, especially those covered by thin skin and with little hair. Thus *Sarcoptes* in pigs commonly begins on the forehead and ears, while in horses it is seen on the head and neck. In sheep and goats, the mites are rarely found on the woolly areas, but especially in the tropics can produce deeply fissured lesions on the face and pinnae, on the cheeks, and round the eyes. Animals can also reinfect themselves, transferring the mites from one part of the body to another, e.g. in dogs from the muzzle by licking the root of the tail.

The primary lesions of sarcoptic mange consist of red vesicles and papules, with crusting of the dried exudate which leaks from the damaged tissues. The connective tissues of the skin proliferate and keratinization increases so that the skin becomes thickened and wrinkled. The hair follicles are deprived of their blood supply and the hairs fall out, leaving bald patches. Pruritus is caused by the activity of the mites and the sensitization of the skin tissues by mite antigen. There may be secondary bacterial infection, with consequent inflammatory reactions. Presumably, as in man, a non-specific generalized rash is produced as the host becomes sensitized to mite antigen: faecal material, secretions, and fragmented cast cuticles.

DIAGNOSIS

Thick crusty skin lesions are suggestive of sarcoptic mange, although at an early stage in the disease there may be confusion with other mange conditions, e.g. in sheep, *Psoroptes*, mycotic dermatitis (dermatophilosis), and scrapie.

Because such large numbers of mites occur in animal mange, the parasites are usually easier to find than in human scabies. In order to identify the burrowing *Sarcoptes* mites in animals a deep skin scraping is made with the back of a scalpel, just to the point of oozing blood; the blade can be wetted with glycerol to assist collection of the scraping. If the material is first warmed very gently live mites are sometimes seen under the microscope and can then easily be picked up on the point of a moistened needle. Direct microscopic examination of skin scrapings is often a waste of time and workers usually proceed directly to a concentration technique. The scrapings are treated with 10–20 per cent aqueous potassium or sodium hydroxide, either by boiling the material in a wide-mouthed test tube for a few minutes or by leaving the tube in a water bath for 15–30 minutes. Material boiled in KOH in a normal narrow test tube tends to superheat and bubble out of the tube. The scrapings dissolve, leaving the mites clearly visible when the deposit is washed, centrifuged, and examined under the microscope. A variation on this method is to digest the scraping as before and then float up the mites so that they may be pipetted off or taken from the surface film with a coverslip. Female mites are more common than males in skin scrapings, a reflection of their longevity. Empty egg shells of *Sarcoptes* soon disintegrate and are not common in the burrows or scrapings therefore.

The following method was suggested by Pruett *et al.* (1986) for the counting of mites in scab lesions in animals. Skin scrapings are taken from areas of about 6.5 cm^2, using a scalpel as before. Each scraping is washed in a 70 per cent ethanol–eosin solution and after 5–10 minutes filtered through a Buchner funnel on to a 112 μm mesh nylon screen. Eggs and mites are washed from the screen on to black filter paper for microscopic examination. The filtrate which passes through the funnel is also examined for eggs and mites.

In histological sections *Sarcoptes* mites are usually visible, but not necessarily precisely identifiable, by their chitinized exoskeleton (Georgi and Georgi 1985). Fluorescence microscopy may be useful in demonstrating the parasites in tissues.

PATHOLOGY

Small mange lesions may have little effect on the health of the animal host, but large areas of infestation may lead to progressive emaciation, secondary infection, and even death, sarcoptic mange being an acknowledged cause of debilitation, 'toxaemia' and death in camels. In dogs the initial erythema may go unnoticed, but the later papular dermatitis will be evident. The skin becomes dry and thickened, hair is lost and there may be pyoderma and self-mutilation; death can ensue in severe cases.

Sarcoptic mange is a common condition in pigs, although debilitation and weight loss may or may not occur. In this host the mites work their way through the skin during the first 1–2 days of the infestation

(Morsy *et al.* 1989). Increasing numbers of tunnels are made during the next few weeks, but by 4 weeks the openings of the tunnels have become covered with keratinized epidermal crust which increases in thickness and may split, allowing access to pathogenic bacteria. After 7 weeks, the crusts began to fall off, the tunnel mouths reappear and most of the mites leave their tunnels. A humoral immune response is produced in infected pigs, with antibody titres peaking at about 8 weeks. However, no decrease in mitogen-induced lymphocyte blastogenesis was observed between clean pigs and artificial infested animals over a the first 4 weeks (Wooten *et al.* 1986). In dogs attacked by another burrowing mite, *Demodex*, lymphocytic proliferation is suppressed in cases of pyoderma but not in animals with uncomplicated demodicosis. A similar pattern may occur in other animals, including pigs and cattle.

Cattle scabies can be due to *Sarcoptes* or *Psoroptes*, but little has been done on the bovine *Sarcoptes*, despite the fact that this mite can transfer to man. In studies on *P. bovis*, Pruett *et al.* (1986) found that antibody levels rise in relation to the increasing population of mites, while T-cell function is depressed if the cattle are prevented from scratching by being stanchioned. It is thought that a reaginic-type antibody is a component of the developing humoral response and is involved in a type I hypersensitivity reaction with *Psoroptes* antigen (s) in the skin. Accumulation of serous fluid in the skin as a result of this reaction would provide a favourable environment for the increase in the mite population.

Further studies are needed on host immunity in animal mange and ways in which the immune responses of the host may be suppressed in simple and complicated infestations in both immature and adult hosts. Such data would also help in relation to the pathology of human scabies infections.

TREATMENT

Good reviews of the treatment of animal scabies were given by Meleney (1985) and Drummond (1986). Early treatments included arsenical compounds, benzyl benzoate, sulphur, and organic sulphur preparations such as monsulfiram (Manickam and Kathaperumal 1975). Lindane was also used until there was concern about its storage in the fatty tissues of food animals. Later came the organophosphorous (OP) compounds, e.g. coumaphos and propetamphos, the methylmethaniminamide amitraz, synthetic pyrethroids and invermectin. Small animals can be treated individually with a shampoo or dressing, while farm animals are usually plunge dipped or sprayed. Invermectin has proved effective against *S. bovis* by topical application or subcutaneous injection, the active ingredient reaching the parasites from the body tissues.

PROGNOSIS

This is generally good if there is no re-infection. However, sarcoptic mange can be extremely serious in camels, for example, when death may ensue in severe cases.

SCABIES IN MAN

Man is nearly always infested by his own species, *S. scabiei*. *Sarcoptes* of animal origin seem poorly adapted for life on the human host. They will attack the skin superficially, but do not usually tunnel and infestations generally last for only a few days or weeks before regressing. However, daily exposure to mites from infected animals, especially milking cattle or buffaloes, can produce lesions, seeming to indicate a single chronic infection. People can, of course, sometimes be victims of their own human species and one from animals at the same time.

INCUBATION PERIOD

There is usually a 4–6-week period between infection and the onset of symptoms. During this time the female mite has mined her burrow and begun to lay eggs.

SYMPTOMS AND SIGNS

Two types of skin reaction are seen in human scabies: the primary skin penetration lesions, tunnels, and vesicles, and the secondary scabies rash, which occurs away from the primary infection sites and is due to host sensitization.

Some 65 per cent of the mites in human infections are found in the skin of the hands and wrists, especially in the interdigital webs. The remainder of the mite population tends to occur in the skin of the ulnar surface of the forearms, the axillae, elbows, feet, and genital areas. The perineal area, penis, and scrotum may also become infested (Staughton 1985). These are all possible primary infection sites and some will be due to sexual contact. Lesions are particularly thick and crusted in so-called Norwegian scabies, although there is little or no pruritic reaction in this unusual condition.

In small children, scabies lesions are often widespread, and continual scratching may lead to secondary infection, masking the classical appearance of interdigital web lesions. Irritable children with erosions and papules around the napkin (diaper) area may be experiencing scabies, while nursing mothers may be affected by *Sarcoptes* around their nipples and on their breasts, as well as in the more usual sites. It is of interest that the face and palms are affected only in early infancy (Staughton 1985).

The scabies rash, as distinct from the primary lesion, is seen as a follicular papular eruption on those parts of the body which have not been actively attacked by burrowing mites. The rash tends to occur around the waist and shoulders and over the posterior parts of the upper thighs and the buttocks. The arms, calves, and ankles can also be affected, but not the head, centre of the chest or back, palms of the hands, or soles of the feet. It is quite possible for a patient to be unaware of the infection until the scabies rash appears (Service 1986).

The itching associated with scabies is often at its worst during the night, because the mites are stimulated into activity by warmth, as when people sleep together under bedding. *Sarcoptes* mites are virtually immobile at temperatures less than 20 °C and transfer of infection in used blankets, sheets or pillows (fomites) is unlikely (Gordon and Lavoipierre 1962).

DIAGNOSIS

Grossly, a pustular or papular itchy skin eruption affecting any of the areas noted above is suspect, bearing in mind the difference between the sites of primary infection and the occurrence of the scabies rash. Human scabies is generally diagnosed on the basis of the tunnels made by the mites. A punctate rash is often associated with the tunnels, which are easier to see in people with lighter coloured skins. Digests of skin scrapings may demonstrate the mites, but this procedure is not usually carried out in human cases, especially as mites tend to be fewer in number than in animal scabies. It is possible to demonstrate mite tunnels by rubbing Indian ink into the suspected area of skin, when some of the dye will be drawn into the open end of the tunnel, revealing the winding burrow. The faeces left by the mites may be visible through the skin as tiny dark, gritty specks, the tunnel itself ending in a small, pearly object, the egg-laying mite. The roof of the burrow can be raised with a needle and the mite removed for identification, free of debris. Mellanby (1943) found that the average number of mature adult female mites found on an individual is about 11; most patients have up to 15 mites, while only about 3 per cent have more than 50 mites (one individual had 511 mites).

PATHOLOGY

It should be possible for patients to become desensitized to mite antigens and this is what may happen in hyperkeratotic (Norwegian or crusty) scabies, when large numbers of *Sarcoptes* are present in a host who experiences little or no pruritus. This form of scabies may be due to a suppression of the immune response (as can happen in canine demodectic mange: see later). The crusty form of scabies may also occur in patients who have received large doses of corticosteroids. These reduce the irritation and hence the scratching by the patient, so allowing unencumbered increase of the mite population. A related phenomenon has been seen in horses, where dermatosis caused by *D. equi* was found to be associated with glucocorticoid therapy (Scott and White 1983).

The histopathology, immunology, and immunopathology of human scabies infections has been well reviewed by Allen (1987). Patients with active scabies infestations show immediate skin reactions to *Sarcoptes* antigen, and high levels of IgE, IgG, and IgM antibodies specific for scabies mites circulate in the serum. The lesions at first show superficial and deep dermal infiltrations with lymphocytes and histiocytes, with large numbers of eosinophils evident. As the disease progresses plasma cells and atypical mononuclear cells also appear with vasculitis, sometimes associated with thrombosis, in the dermal vessels. The perivascular mononuclear cell infiltrates in the dermis consist mainly of T lymphocytes, with some macrophages and very few B lymphocytes. Studies on the deposition of complement (C3) and immunoglobulins in the skin of scabies patients have led to the suggestion that the deposition of antigen–antibody complexes and complement activation are important in the production of lesions in the infested skin. It may be that the formation of immune complexes may also play some part in the acute glomerulonephritis cases which have been frequently found associated with scabies in the Caribbean.

It is still not clear why such large populations of mites develop in the cases of hyperkeratotic scabies associated with immunological aberrations. Epidermal Langerhans cells may be involved in controlling the mite population within the dermis, and such cells have been shown to affect the protective immunological responses of animals to tick infestation (Nithiuthai and Allen 1984). Recent work by Mollison *et al.* (1993) suggests a link in Australian aborigines between the occurrence of a high seroprevalence of HTLV-I and hyperkeratotic scabies. These authors consider that uncharacterized immunological defects caused by the virus explain the occurrence of this particularly serious form of scabies in these patients, to the extent that the scabies acts as a marker for the virus, just as does infestation with the intestinal nematode *Strongyloides stercoralis*. A similar conclusion was reached by Daisley *et al.* (1993), who reported a young woman patient in Trinidad who presented with *Tinea corporis, T. unguium,* and the generalized exfoliative pruritic rash of hyperkeratotic scabies. The patient was seronegative for HIV but positive for HTLV-I. She was successfully treated for the mycoses and the scabies but eventually died from a T-cell lymphoma. She also had metastatic calcification of the proximal tubules. Again, the fulminating scabies infection appeared to serve as an indicator for the presence of HTLV-I.

Further studies are being carried out on the immunological aspects of scabies and it seems likely that some of the perplexing complications of this disease will soon be solved.

TREATMENT

A useful review of the treatment of mite infestations in man is given by George (1986). Permethrin, malathion, and lindane are in common use for the treatment of human scabies; the older preparations benzyl benzoate and monosulfiram are also used, and will be mentioned first. As a general rule, scabicides should not be applied to very young children, nursing mothers, or pregnant women; neither should they be applied to the head and neck areas, which in any case are rarely affected. Even if scabies tunnels cannot be found, the presence of itchy papular or pustular lesions on the buttocks, for example, could justify use of a scabicide. It should be noted that people who have definitely been cured of scabies by use of a scabicide may retain their sensitivity to mite antigens, so that they often react immediately on reinfection, without any further period of sensitization.

Benzyl benzoate has been used since 1937 for the treatment of scabies. It is a clear, oily, colourless liquid available as 20–35 per cent emulsions. As well as simple application, benzyl benzoate was at one time formulated with disulfiram, DDT and disulfiram, and DDT and benzocaine. In Britain it is used at a concentration of 25 per cent, applied over the whole body excepting the head and neck. Treatment is often applied in the evening, repeated without bathing next day, and the acaricide then washed off 24 hours later. A third application may be necessary. Benzyl benzoate is not generally recommended for use on children, as the necessary 25 per cent concentration may cause irritation in the very young.

Monosulfiram (tetraethylthiuram monosulphide, Tetmosol) is applied as a 25 per cent solution, diluted with 2–3 parts of water. Monosulfiram acts more slowly than benzyl benzoate against *Sarcoptes*, and repeat treatments may be necessary for 2–3 consecutive days. There are sometimes hypersensitive skin reactions. Also, as this scabicide inhibits aldehyde dehydrogenase, required during the oxidation of ethanol in the liver, alcohol should be avoided before and for at least 48 hours after treatment. Monosulfiram can also be used in the form of a soap for washing and bathing, when it shows a slow curative effect and also acts as a prophylactic.

Mitigal is a yellow oily preparation (active ingredient 2, 7-dimethylthianthrene = dimethyl diphenylene disulphide), which contains 25 per cent of organically combined sulphur. It is applied to the whole body apart from the neck and head, and a single treatment usually gives a complete cure; Mitigal may produce a mild dermatitis, although to a less extent than inorganic sulphur; it is also rather expensive.

Crotamiton (N-ethyl-o-crotonyltoluide) is a liquid similar in appearance to benzyl-benzoate and was first used against human scabies in 1946. It has good scabicidal activity, but requires daily application on five occasions. It is preferable to first bathe with soap and warm water, dry the skin and then apply the 10 per cent cream or lotion over the whole body below the neck. The patient should not then wash until the sixth day after treatment. Although it sometimes causes local irritation crotamiton is also used, like calamine lotion, as an antipruritic to help allay the itching after scabies. It seems also to have some activity against the secondary bacterial skin infections commonly associated with scabies in children.

The benzimidazole compound thiabendazole is best known as an effective anthelmintic in man and animals and, in agriculture, as a fungicide, but it cured a stubborn case of scabies in man (Allegré *et al.* 1992). A dose rate of 25 mg/kg body weight daily for 10 days was effective in another group of patients, although this also produced side-effects such as nausea, dizziness, and diarrhoea. An alternative 5 per cent cream formulation used 1–3 times daily for 5 days cured scabies in 73–83 per cent of cases, with only a mild transient dermatitis (Villabos and Neuman 1975).

Lindane (hexachlorocylohexane, HCH, BHC) is an organochlorine compound which is used against scabies in the form of a 1 per cent lotion, applied thinly over the body below the neck; 24 hours later it is washed off with warm soapy water. If necessary, treatment may be repeated after 7 days. Lindane has also been formulated in concentrations of 0.3 per cent (USA) and 2 per cent. Overdosage may be harmful as lindane can be toxic if absorbed through extensively damaged skin. However, after many millions of applications of lindane, only 19 reports have appeared of possibly genuine toxicity, as distinct from inappropriate use of the drug (George 1986). It is perhaps unfair that comparatively little is known about the possible side-effects which may follow the use of alternative scabicides to lindane.

Malathion is an organophospharous (OP) compound available as a 0.5 per cent preparation, for use over the whole body omitting the head and neck; it is washed off after 24 hours. A second OP compound, trichlorphon, cured 29 of 30 cases of scabies which had failed to respond to conventional treatment (Gonzalez *et al.* 1976).

Permethrin, a synthetic pyrethroid, is a new scabicide. It is available as a 5 per cent cream for use over the whole body, avoiding contact with the eyes, and may be washed off after 8–24 hours. A 1 per cent preparation in liquid paraffin has also given good results. The related pyrethroid deltamethrin has proved effective against human scabies, applied in the form of a preparation containing 0.02 per cent deltamethrin plus 2.5 per cent piperonyl butoxide as synergist.

Ivermectin is well known in the successful treatment of human onchocerciasis, and oral doses of 100–200 μg/ kg used for this purpose in Sierra Leone also produced some benefit against head lice, although not in patients suffering from scabies (Dunne *et al.*, 1991). This contrasts with the successful use of ivermectin against *Sarcoptes* in dogs, cattle, sheep, and camels (Campbell, 1989).

Aqueous scabicidal preparations are generally preferred to alcoholic ones, which may irritate excoriated or delicate skin. When applying acaricide, particular attention should be given to the webs of the fingers and toes, and lotion should be brushed under the nails. Providing the applications are carried out carefully, lindane, malathion, and permethrin should clear scabies with one application.

PROGNOSIS

Modern scabicides are generally very effective, but there may be some itching after treatment has been applied, as material from the dead and disintegrating mites continues to react with the tissues of the host. At this stage an antipruritic agent may be useful.

EPIDEMIOLOGY

Human scabies exists in endemic form in many parts of the world and becomes epidemic in times of war, mass movements of refugee populations, etc. There was an epidemic in Britain in 1944–46, at the end of the Second World War, but epidemics may arise for no apparent reason. Changes in life styles, especially among young adults, may have been a factor in the upsurge of scabies in 1963–70 in the USA (Orkin 1971) and in 1990–91 in Britain (Cox and Paterson 1991). During the latter epidemic 10–15 per cent of all patients in out-patient departments had scabies.

PREVENTION AND CONTROL STRATEGIES

Prevention of scabies is theoretically straightforward, by avoiding close contact with infected people, but this may be impossible in conditions of national emergency, when gross overcrowding often occurs. It is important that all members of a family are treated if one has been confirmed as suffering from scabies, and monosulfiram soap can be a useful prophylactic tool. In practice, modern treatment is very satisfactory and specific prophylactic measures are rarely taken. However, no serious efforts have been made to eradicate human scabies from a major geographical area.

DEMODECTIC SCABIES

Demodex is a very highly developed mite which lives in the hair follicles and sebaceous glands of various mammals, causing demodectic or follicular mange. It is rarely of any medical importance but it can be a serious problem in animals. There are conflicting views about its possible natural transmission from animals to man.

DISCOVERY OF THE ORGANISM

The human species, *Demodex folliculorum*, was discovered by Simon in 1842. There are many other species of *Demodex*, and it now appears that most hosts can harbour two species, e.g. *D. brevis* and *D. folliculorum* in man, *D. caballi* and *D. equi* in horses, and *D. bovis* and *D. ghanensis* in cattle.

THE AGENT

Demodex is the sole genus in the family Demodicidae, which belongs to the suborder Trombidiformes (Prostigmata). The mites are elongated, measuring up to 330 μm in length in the female. They have four stumpy legs and a long annulated 'abdomen' which makes them look quite unlike other genera of mites. It is common for each host species to harbour two species of *Demodex*, and in man *D. folliculorum* measures about 255 (200–400) μm in length while *D. brevis* average about 235 (100–250) μm. The life cycle is completed in 18–24 days, and is spent almost entirely in the sebaceous glands or hair follicles, where the female lays 20–25 eggs. Two larval stages and one nymph precede the adult stage.

THE HOSTS—ANIMAL

Demodex has been recovered from most species of mammals, but the most serious skin lesions (mange) occur in dogs, cattle, and goats. Demodectic mange is usually a mild condition in horses, sheep, and pigs.

INCUBATION PERIOD

Transmission between animal hosts probably occurs very early in life, as in suckling. Otherwise infection follows habitual close contact, particularly in younger animals. In dogs the infection is usually apparent at 3–9 months of age.

SYMPTOMS AND SIGNS

Demodex occurs in the skin of perhaps 40–75 per cent of apparently normal dogs, and the development of actual disease is unusual in most species of hosts. The mites invade the hair follicles and sebaceous glands, but in the early stages of the infection the host shows little or no discomfort.

In dogs the skin becomes erythematous, inflamed, and intensely itchy. The skin later becomes wrinkly and scaly, with hair loss (red or squamous mange). In pustular demodectic mange, which generally follows the squamous form of the condition, small pustules initially develop around the muzzle and down the chest, and may spread to the abdomen, flanks, and feet. There are massive and multiple infestations of the sebaceous glands, which often become secondarily infected with staphylococci and other bacteria; large abscesses may be formed and the dog will often have a repulsive smell. Demodectic pyoderma and toxaemia in dogs can be fatal. Pustular demodectic mange can be a serious problem in cattle in Africa.

DIAGNOSIS

It should be remembered that *Demodex* populations form part of the normal skin fauna in many hosts. Deep skin scrapings are necessary in order to prove the presence of mites, using the technique described above under *Sarcoptes* infections.

Bovine demodicosis is usually obvious in the form of skin pustules. These may be 2–3 cm in diameter and are packed full of cheesy material containing thousands of mites, readily expressed when the nodule is nicked with a sharp scalpel. Mites also invade the meibomian sebaceous glands of the eyelids in both cattle and horses. It is not known if the 'skin' and 'eyelid' species of *Demodex* which attack cattle and horses have different forms of pathogenesis.

Demodex in sheep, goats and pigs is associated with the presence of scale or small pustules, but as the parasite is not zoonotic the disease in these animals will not be discussed further.

PATHOLOGY

In the squamous form of demodicosis in dogs, the hair follicles are distended with mites and cellular debris, the follicular epithelium is atrophic, hyperkeratosis develops, and cornified material exfoliates from the skin surface. The sebaceous glands atrophy or hypertrophy and the mites probably feed on the hyperplastic cells. Hyperpigmentation gives the skin a deep red to coppery colour. Eventually much of the body is affected and there is considerable hair loss. The pustular form of demodicosis in dogs usually follows the squamous form of the disease and is accompanied by massive infiltration of the skin with polymorphonuclear leucocytes and lymphocytes.

The immunopathology of demodectic infestations has been investigated in detail only in dogs, where it is thought that appearance of the huge populations of mites is due to an immunosuppressive effect operating through the T cells. Individuals of some breeds, e.g. Dobermans, and some families of dogs seem genetically lacking in immune reponsiveness to *Demodex*, while other animals apparently become immunodeficient following exposure to mite antigen. It was thought that decreased lymphocyte response to mitogen stimulation was due in some way to the suppressive activity of the metabolic products produced by mites themselves. However, Barta *et al.* (1983) have shown that in dogs lymphocytic suppression occurred only in those animals which had demodectic mange complicated by bacterial pyoderma. It is not known why such severe demodectic lesions may develop in dogs and cattle compared with those produced in man, pigs, and horses, for example, and more studies are needed on the immunological responses of the host to *Demodex*. Little is known about mite-specific immunological reactions or the ways in which these could disrupt the feeding and reproductive behaviour of *Demodex* within the hair follicles (Allen 1987).

TREATMENT

Treatment regimes used in animals for the control of demodectic mange are likely to succeed against severe cases only if medication is applied early enough. Well-established bovine demodectic mange may fail to respond to treatment. Unless they have become infected with bacteria, individual nodules may regress after 2–4 months, further nodules often appear.

Recommended acaricides include skin applications of rotenone, lindane, benzyl benzoate, amitraz, pyrethroids, etc. (see p. 000) As with the treatment of *Sarcoptes* infections, it may be difficult to ensure intimate contact between an acaricide applied to the skin and the tunnelling parasites. A systemic approach to dosing is therefore a logical alternative method of application of the acaricide. The oral use of OP acaricides, e.g. 30 mg tablets of cythioate, has cured canine demodicosis and successful results have also been reported with injections of ivermectin, used at 400 or 600 μg/kg (Campbell 1989).

The assessment of acaricidal treatment of *Demodex*, especially in dogs, is notoriously difficult. Apparent clinical improvements may be due simply to cyclical changes in the mite population or to natural regression of the infection (see p. 000). Control measures against demodectic mange are likely to succeed against serious cases only if medication is applied early enough, especially in canine or bovine infections. Unless they have become infected with bacteria, individual nodules may regress after 2–4 months, only to be replaced by further nodules. Control measures against bovine demodectic mange in poorer countries, if affordable at all, are often applied jointly against demodectic, sarcoptic, and psoroptic mange.

PROGNOSIS

In localized canine demodectic mange the lesions tend to be small and circumscribed, resolving within 6–8 weeks. The prognosis is poor in severely debilitated dogs, especially where the condition has progressed to pyoderma. Generalized demodicosis is in any case difficult to eradicate, so that the condition usually regresses, only to reappear at a later date. Demodectic mange in most other hosts usually resolves without further incident.

THE HUMAN HOST

SYMPTOMS AND SIGNS

In man, *Demodex* rarely produces any ill effects or even becomes obvious, but may it may cause or be involved in such skin conditions as granulomatous acne, impetigo, rosacea, pityriasis and blepharitis. The skin of the forehead, nose, cheeks lateral to the nose, and the lips are common infection sites. Comedones, ingrown hairs, and dilated hair follicles can be associated with *Demodex*.

DIAGNOSIS

Mites are most likely to be found in material expressed from comedones or pustules on the face. Ear wax may also contain *Demodex*. *Demodex folliculorum* females measure about 255 (200–400) μm in length, while those of *D. brevis* average about 235 (100–250) μm.

PATHOLOGY

Demodex is a low-grade pathogen and rarely produces any ill effects in humans, but it may sometimes cause or be associated with such skin conditions as acne, impetigo and rosacea, as already mentioned. *Demodex* have occasionally been seen in histological sections of skin tumours—of the nipple, for example, and in the past this has led to claims that *Demodex* may be involved in the pathogenesis of such lesions.

Portions of mites can cause confusion during the interpretation of histological preparations, but at least one of the characteristic stumpy legs or part of the body is usually visible (Georgi and Georgi 1985). Infected sebaceous glands often contain enormous numbers of leucocytes.

TREATMENT

Daily washing with medicated soap containing monosulfiram can reduce infections. A cream incorporating 0.5 per cent lindane (HCH) has proved useful, and the other scabicides already mentioned should also be expected to prove effective. Older alternatives include the application of 10 per cent sulphur or benzyl benzoate preparations, or 0.5 per cent selenium sulphide cream. Acaricides should not be applied directly to the eyelids.

EPIDEMIOLOGY

Demodex is probably a common occupant of the skin, but it is hardly a medical problem, so that virtually no statistical information is available about its incidence or prevalence. It seems less common in young people, and its prevalence has sometimes risen to 100 per cent in the elderly in some parts of the USA. Blepharitis has been recorded in 25 per cent of patients over the age of 20 years, also in the United States. *Demodex* seems rather more common in females. For all practical purposes, there is no question of control strategies and programmes in the human population.

CHEYLETIELLA, *FUR MITE*

Cheyletiella is a member of the superfamily Cheyletoidea, in the suborder Trombidiformes (Prostigmata). It is a non-burrowing mite which lives on the keratin layer of the epidermis of certain mammals. It is an obligate parasite and easily identified by its numerous feathered bristles and the strong comb-like palps, which help the mite to hold on to the hairs of its host. For many years after its first description by Megnin in 1878 only one species, *C. parasitivorax*, the rabbit fur mite, was recognized. It was thought that people developed a dermatitis after contacting infected rabbits, or dogs or cats which had presumably become infested from rabbits. In 1965 Smiley realized that there are five very closely related species: *C. parasitivorax* and

C. furmani of rabbits, *C. strandtmanni* of the hare, *C. yasguri* of dogs, and *C. blakei* of cats. Other species have been described from wild animals. It is now accepted that the cat, dog, and rabbit species can cause dermatitis in man. No work has been done on possible skin conditions which might be caused by the rabbit and hare species.

Female mites attach their eggs to hairs 2–3 mm above the skin surface; all stages are very motile and this aids their rapid spread between hosts if these are in close contact. As the mites stimulate the production of scurfy material, they are often called 'walking dandruff'. Lesions caused by *C. yasguri* in puppies spread along the back and may reach the head, but adult dogs usually have only light infestations. *Cheyletiella blakei* causes a dermatitis in cats, and one infested cat passed mite eggs in its faeces for several weeks, these having been picked up when the animal was grooming itself. *Cheyletiella parasitivorax* can affect the entire back and flanks of rabbits.

Irritation in pet owners usually starts 2–4 days after exposure and is transitory but daily contact with mites from an affected puppy or kitten may give the impression of a single chronic infestation, as with some other species of zoonotic mites. Unpleasant rashes may appear on the front of the chest and abdomen, across the waist and along the forearms in children and elderly people who have cuddled or nursed a pet animal. Such rashes in older people are sometimes dismissed as 'nerves' until it is realized that there is an acariasis originating from the pet. Soothing lotions such as calamine will help the human patient and the usual acaricides will be effective on the pet. An interesting trial of ivermectin for the control of *Cheyletiella* in polar foxes, using two subcutaneous injections of up to 500 μg/kg, with a 6-week interval, was completely successful (Malczewski *et al.* 1984).

TROMBICULID MITES: CHIGGERS, HARVEST MITES, BERRY BUGS

There are more than 1200 species of trombiculid mites, which usually live harmlessly in soil and vegetation, sucking liquid from small arthropods, etc. in the soil. Some 50 species, however, have larval stages which attack man or livestock, feeding on tissue fluids and lymph. The larva then falls to the ground to moult into the nymph and adult stages. Larvae of the European harvest mite or berry bug, *Neotrombicula autumnalis*, and of the genera *Eutrombicula* and *Schoengastia*, which occur across the Americas and Pacific, cause no more than a very irritating itch or dermatitis in man. However, *Leptotrombidium akamushi* and members of the *L. deliense* group of species transmit scrub typhus in various parts of east and South-East Asia, extending to

the Pacific and northern Queensland, Australia. Scrub typhus, caused by *Rickettsia tsutsugamushi*, is dealt with in another part of this volume.

DISCOVERY OF THE MITES

The irritation ('scrub itch') caused by trombiculid mites was known in China at least 400 years ago, when they were associated with 'a prickly sensation and a red rash' (Gordon and Lavoipierre 19.). The relationship between the mites and scrub typhus was not discovered until 1899. The European harvest mite, berry bug, or red itch mite, *Neotrombicula autumnalis*, was named in 1790 and the common American chigger or red bug, *Eutrombicula alfreddugesi*, was described by Oudemans in 1910.

THE MITES

Trombiculids are placed in the family Trombiculidae, in the Trombidiformes (Prostigmata) group of mites. There are four subfamilies in the family, with at least 21 genera/subgenera in the medically important Trombiculinae and a further 14 in the other subfamilies. The Trombiculinae include *Trombicula*, *Neotrombicula*, *Eutrombicula*, *Leptotrombidium*, and *Ascoschoengastia*. As well as infesting man, these genera attack various other mammals, including bats, and several species of birds and snakes. The intense itch caused by trombiculid larvae when they feed on man may be because they are feeding on an atypical mammal host rather than one of their true bird or reptile hosts. However, *Ascoschoengastia aethiopica*, a bat trombiculid, was found infesting the eyelids of a child but caused no irritation (Zumpt 1961).

Only the larval mites have medical and veterinary significance, hence it is of practical interest to note diagnostic features of only this stage in the life cycle. Larval trombiculids are tiny (0.15–3.0 mm) and are quite hairy. The five feathered hairs and two sensillae on the dorsal rectangular or pentagonal scutum are useful in the identification of trombiculid larvae. The larvae are yellow to bright red or orange and they take up lymph and other tissue fluid, not blood, from any suitable mammal. The female mite measures 1–2 mm in length and is covered in tiny hairs, giving her a velvety appearance. Her eggs are laid on damp soil and the hatching larvae are picked up by passing hosts. These are normally small rodents, but the larvae readily feed on man, dogs, cats, and grazing animals; chickens can also be attacked. The bright colour of the larvae fades as they swell while feeding on the host's tissue fluids. The fed larvae fall to the ground to complete their development through the nymphal and adult stages.

DISEASE MECHANISMS

Only the larval trombiculids feed on animals, taking a single meal, so that, in the case of *Leptotrombidium*, only they can pass on the scrub typhus rickettsia. The micro-organisms are transmitted through the ovaries of the female mite (transovarially), she herself playing no inoculative part in the transmission of disease. A larva feeds only once, so that it could theoretically at the same feed both transmit rickettsias taken in a larva of the previous generation and become re-infected its present host.

THE HOST: ANIMALS

Trombiculid larvae normally parasitize rodents, insectivores, and birds, but they also willingly feed on various other warm-blooded animals, including man. The mites are usually found where the skin is soft and moist. In dogs and cats they often attach to the face and pinnae, especially in gun dogs. Horses, sheep, and cattle may be attacked on the lower legs ('itchy heel') and face. The fed larvae fall to the ground to complete their life cycle through the nymph and adult stages.

SYMPTOMS AND SIGNS

The larval mites are usually easily seen attached to the skin, feet (horses and sheep), pinna (game dogs), etc., wherever the body of the host has been in contact with the ground. The parasites cause considerable irritation, with erythema of the skin. Secondary infection may follow the host's scratching. Irritation in dogs may lead to haematomata in the pinnae because of head shaking, while in horses continual stamping may lead to cracking of the hoof.

DIAGNOSIS

The brightly coloured larval mites are usually obvious on the skin and have already indicated their presence by pruritus. They may also stimulate the production of a weeping exudate which may dry to form a crust which hides the mites, so that a simple skin scraping may be needed to demonstrate the parasites.

PATHOLOGY

Trombiculid larvae take several days to attach to the host, and some species may remain there for about a month, although the *Leptotrombidium* vectors of scrub typhus only attach for 2–10 days and their bites are much less irritating. Their saliva partially digests the skin tissues and during this process of hydrolysis a feeding tube (stylostome) is formed within the tissues through which the liquefied cellular material is ingested.

TREATMENT AND CONTROL

Soothing lotions can be useful on dogs, and repellents such as dimethyl phthalate are effective, although these may be uneconomic for use on animals especially as they would frequently require reapplication in hot humid areas. Acaricidal foot baths can be used for horses. The various acaricides already mentioned are effective against the mites.

THE HOST: HUMAN

SYMPTOMS AND SIGNS

In man, trombiculid larvae feed on soft or moist skin, e.g. ankles, groin and armpits, or around the waist, where the clothing is constricted by a belt. They cause extreme irritation and the intense pruritus may last for several days after the mites have been removed.

PATHOLOGY

The lesion is similar to that in animals, although a papule forms at the site of infection, later usually becoming necrotic to form the typical black 'eschar' (Bell 1985). Trombiculid larvae can sensitize people so that they produce an immediate and delayed-type skin hypersensitivity (Allen, 1987).

TREATMENT

Personal prophylaxis and treatment is centered on the use of repellents to treat clothing, particularly socks or stockings, cuffs and collars. Diethyltoluamide, dimethylphthalate, dibutylphthalate, and benzyl benzoate are all effective when used in this way. Repellents can also be sprayed or smeared over the body, paying special attention to areas where the mites tend to attach, such as the ankles, waistline, etc. Spraying the undergrowth with such residual insecticides as HCH, toxaphene, fenthion, malathion, propoxur, or diazinon will reduce the mite population and so help to stop any transmission of scrub typhus.

EPIDEMIOLOGY OF SCRUB TYPHUS

The epidemiology of scrub typhus varies in different parts of the world, i.e. South-East Asia, Oceania, northern parts of Australia and as far as south-eastern Siberia. Transmission sites are often associated with natural vegetational habitats which have been modified by man, as when primeval forest is removed by 'slash and burn' farming procedures. After a few harvests the land is abandoned and becomes colonized by secondary scrub. In this way areas which separate two major vegetational zones, usually forest and farm, are left with large numbers of trombiculid mites and their rodent hosts. These dangerous areas are known as 'mite islands'. All known foci of scrub typhus exist because of changes in the environment and the association between the mites, wild rodents, transitional secondary vegetation, and the scrub typhus rickettsia has been described as 'a zoonotic tetrad of chigger-borne rickettsiosis' (Service 1986).

LARGE-SCALE CONTROL

The overall control of trombiculid mites concentrates on separating infected rodents from the human population by bush clearing. Personal control of the mites has been mentioned above. Mite islands can be eradicated by cutting down the bush and burning it. As the infection is transmitted transovarially by the mites they themselves form the reservoir of infection, and rodent control alone may not have an immediate effect on the prevalence of the disease, as the larval mites will naturally use man as the remaining food source. In this way an apparently good, but in practice incomplete, control scheme may result in a worse itch mite problem than existed previously.

OTHER MITES AFFECTING MAN

DERMANYSSUS AND ORNITHONYSSUS (= LIPONYSSUS, = MACRONYSSUS), POULTRY MITES

Dermanyssus and *Ornithonyssus* belong to the superfamily Dermanyssoidea, suborder Mesostigmata (gamasid mites) in the Parasitiformes. Zumpt (1961) places *Dermanyssus* in its own subfamily and *Ornithonyssus* in the Macronyssinae. However, it is convenient to consider them together as they are both closely involved with poultry and man. The two species are superficially very similar, with long legs, but the anal plate in *Dermanyssus* is triangular, whereas that of *Ornithonyssus* is pear-shaped. *Dermanyssus gallinae* (= *D. avium*), the chicken red mite, was described by Duges in 1834. The northern fowl mite of poultry, *O. sylviarum*, was identified by Canestrini and Fanzago in 1877, and has also been placed at different times in the genera *Macronyssus*, *Liponyssus*, and *Bdellonyssus*. *Dermanyssus gallinae*, *O. sylviarum* and two other species, *O. bursa*, the tro-

pical fowl mite, and *O. bacoti*, the tropical rat mite, can all irritate humans and give rise to various levels of dermatitis.

Dermanyssus gallinae is a blood-sucking mite, and has a pair of very fine chelicerae which together form a sucking tube. Red mites appear coloured only when they have fed recently, the gut darkening as the blood is digested so that mites usually appear black. Poultry can become severely anaemic following the continual attacks of red mites, and really heavy infestations can be fatal. *Dermanyssus gallinae* feeds mainly at night, leaving the host during the day to hide away in cracks and crevices, where it lays its eggs. However, in heavy infestations, 'overspill' populations of mites will be seen on poultry during the day. Apart from the irritation which it causes to people in poultry houses, it has been suggested that *D. gallinae* may transmit St Louis encephalitis but the evidence is conflicting and this mite certainly plays no important part in the epidemiology of the disease.

Ornithonyssus has tiny pincer-like ends to its mouthparts, feeding on the fluid which leaks from the wounds it makes. It can feed at any time of the day or night, so that infested flocks have no rest from the continual irritation of *O. sylviarum*. The eggs of *O. sylviarum* and *O. bursa* are attached to the host, while those of the tropical rat mite are laid in the burrows.

People often become temporarily infested with poultry mites when working in poultry houses. The mites cause an unpleasant 'creepy' sensation and there may be considerable irritation and actual dermatitis, although it is not usually necessary to use a protective repellent as the application of an organophosphorous or pyrethroid acaricide generally gives satisfactory control. Personnel who daily handle infested eggs or birds may develop an allergic respiratory condition following inhalation of *O. sylviarum* allergens (Lutsky and Bar-Sela, 1982).

MACRONYSSUS (= LEIOGNATHUS = LIPONYSSUS) BACOTI, TROPICAL RAT MITE

As this species is in the family Macronyssidae it is very similar in appearance to the two species of poultry mites considered above. *Macronyssus bacoti* normally infests rats, mole-rats, and mice, but has been recorded on several occasions as a cause of dermatitis in man, especially in factories which have heavy infestations of domestic rats. It may play a minor role in the transmission of murine typhus, tularaemia, and plague. It is a useful laboratory vector of the filarial nematode *Litomosoides carinii*, which infects the cotton rat, and which is useful in the screening of candidate filaricides.

PNEUMONYSSUS SPP. AND RHINOPHAGA SPP., LUNG MITES

There are at least 10 species of *Pneumonyssus* and six of *Rhinophaga* (Zumpt 1961). These are all parasites of the lungs (*Pneumonyssus*), nasal passages or frontal sinuses (*Rhinophaga*) of various species of primates and hyraxes. It is quite conceivable that humans may become infested as a result of contact with monkeys or baboons kept as pets.

TRIXACARUS CAVIAE, THE GUINEA-PIG MITE

This is a small burrowing mite with similar habits to *Sarcoptes*. In the guinea-pig it can cause alopecia and crusting over the back. It has been reported on pet owners, where scabies-like lesions may occur on the abdomen, axillae, and groin (Kummel *et al.* 1980).

DERMATOPHAGOIDES PTERONYSSINUS AND D. FARINAE, HOUSE DUST MITES

Dermatophagoides pteronyssinus (= *Mealia pteronyssina* and *D. farinae* normally live on or burrow into the skin of rodents, bats, and birds, but can infest man. *Dermatophagoides pteronyssinus* has been responsible for several chronic cases of scalp infestations (eczema seborrhica), one of which persisted for at least 7 years (Traver 1951). Skin lesions due to these mites have been reported from Europe, North America, and Japan.

PYEMOTES VENTRICOSUS, ACARUS SIRO, ETC., GRAIN MITES

Pyemotes (= *Pediculoides*) *ventricosus*, the grain itch or straw itch mite, and some 10 genera of tyroglyphid mites, e.g. *Acarus*, *Tyrophagus*, *Glycyphagus*, *Rhizoglyphus*, *Caloglyphus*, *Carpoglyphus*, live in stored food, including grain, flour, rice, copra, dried fruit, vanilla pods, cheese, etc. The white or cream-coloured adult mites measure about 0.2–0.6 mm and have long body hairs, which often equal the length of the body itself. They do not parasitize vertebrates but can be troublesome accidental pests to people who work in dock warehouses, farm stores, grain silos, etc., causing various allergic dermatitis conditions, the so-called grain itch, millers' itch, bakers' itch, copra itch, vanilla workers' rash, etc. As these mites are no more likely to affect animals than man they will not be considered in any detail.

REFERENCES

Allegré, T. *et al.* (1992). Use of thiabendazole in an HIV-positive patient with scabies resistant to local treatment. *Presse Médicale*, **21**, 1821–2.

Allen, J. R. (1987). Immunology, immunopathology and immunoprophylaxis of tick and mite infestations. In *Immune responses in parasitic infections. Vol IV: Protozoa, arthropods and invertebrates*, (ed. E. J. L. Soulsby), pp. 141–74. CRC Press, Boca Ratan, Florida.

Anon. (ed.) (1991). Skin diseases and public health medicine. *Lancet*, **337**, 1008–9.

Barta, O., Waltman, C., Oyekan, P., McGrath, R. K., and Hribernik, T. N. (1983). Lymphocytic transformation suppression caused by pyoderma—failure to demonstrate it in uncomplicated demodectic mange. *Comparative Immunology, Microbiology and Infectious Diseases*, **6**, 9–17.

Bell, D. R. (1985). *Lecture notes on tropical medicine*, (2nd edn). Blackwell Scientific Publications, Oxford.

Campbell, W. C. (1989). *Ivermectin and abamectin*. Springer-Verlag, New York.

Cox, N. H. and Paterson, W. D. (1991). Epidemiology of scabies: the new epidemic. *Lancet*, **337**, 1547–8.

Daisley, H., Charles, W., and Suite, M. (1993). Crusted (Norwegian) scabies as a pre-diagnostic indicator for HTLV-I infection. *Transactions of the Royal Society of Tropical Medicine and Hygiene*, **87**, 295.

Drummond, R. O. (1986). Acarine infestations of domestic animals. In *Chemotherapy of parasitic diseases*, (ed. W. C. Campbell and R. S. Rew), pp. 566–83. Plenum Press, New York.

Dunne, C. L., Malone, C. J., and Whitworth, J. A. G. (1991). Ivermectin in man. *Transactions of the Royal Society of Tropical Medicine and Hygiene*, **85**, 550–1.

George, J. G. (1986). Acarine infestations of man. In *Chemotherapy of parasitic diseases*, (ed. W. C. Campbell and R. S. Rew) pp. 541–50. Plenum Press, New York.

Georgi, M. E. and Georgi, J. R. (1985). Histopathological diagnosis. In *Parasitology for veterinarians*, (J. R. Georgi), pp. 301–30. W. B. Saunders, Philadelphia.

Gonzalez, D., Trujillo, V. M., Salazar, M., and Ortega, O. (1976). Treatment of scabies disease resistant to medication. *Medicina Cutanea Ibero Latino-Americano*, **4**, 149–52.

Gordon, R. M. and Lavoipierre, M. M. J. (1972). *Entomology for students of medicine*. Blackwell Scientific Publications, Oxford.

Kummel, B. A., Estes, S. A., and Arlian, L. G. (1980). *Trixacarus caviae* infestation of guineapigs. *Journal of the American Veterinary Medical Association*, **177**, 903–7.

Lapage, G. (1968) *Veterinary parasitology*, (2nd edn). Oliver and Boyd, London.

Lutsky, I. and Bar-Sela, S. (1982). Northern fowl mite in occupational asthma of poultry workers. *Lancet*, **323**, 874–5.

Malczewski, A., Kopczewski, A., Malczewski, M., and Zielinski, J. (1984). Mange due to *Cheyletiella blakei* in polar foxes in Poland. *Zentralblatt für Bakteriologie, Mikrobiologie and Hygiene*, **258**, 412–13.

Manickam, R. and Kathaperumal, V. (1975). Efficacy of tetraethylthiuram monosulphide and benzyl benzoate against sarcoptic mange in pigs. *Journal of Veterinary Science*, **5**, 150–3.

Meleney, W. P. (1985). Mange mites and other parasitic mites, In *World Animal Science*. Vol. B2: *Parasites, pests and predators*, (ed. S. M. Gaafar, W. E. Howard, and R. E. Marsh). pp. 317–46. Elsevier, Amsterdam.

Mellanby, K. (1943). *Scabies: Oxford War Manuals*. Oxford University Press, London.

Mollison, L. C., Lo, S. T., and Marning, G. (1993). An association between HTLV-I and Norwegian scabies in aborigines in Australia. *Lancet*, **341**, 1281–2.

Morsy, G. H., Turek, J. J., and Gaafar, S. M. (1989). Scanning electron microscopy of sarcoptic mange lesions in swine. *Veterinary Parasitology*, **31**, 281–8.

Nithiuthai, S. and Allen, J. R. (1984). Significant changes in epidermal Langerhans cells of guineapigs infested with ticks. *Immunology*, **51**, 133–9.

Orkin, M. (1971). Resurgence of scabies. *Journal of the American Medical Association*, **217**, 593–7.

Pruett, J. H., Guillot, F. S., and Fisher, W. F. (1986). Humoral and cellular immunoresponsiveness of stanchioned cattle infested with *Psoroptes ovis*. *Veterinary Parasitology*, **22**, 121–33.

Rothschild, M. and Clay, T. (1952). *Fleas, flukes and cuckoos*. New Naturalist Library Collins, London.

Scott, D. W. and White, K. K. (1983). Demodicosis associated with systemic glucocorticoid therapy in two horses. *Equine Practice*, **5**, 31–5.

Sequiera, J. H. and Dowdeswell, R. M. (1942). 'Cat itch' from a pet lynx. *East African Medical Journal*, **18**, 345–7.

Service, M. W. (1986). *Lecture notes on medical entomology*. Blackwell Scientific Publications, Oxford.

Staughton, R. C. D. (1985). Vesicles. In *French's Index of differential diagnosis*, (ed. F. Dudley Hart), pp. 877–81. Wright, Bristol.

Traver, J. R. (1951). Unusual scalp dermatitisin human caused by the mite *Dermatophagoides*. *Proceedings of the Entomological Society of Washington*, **53**, 1–25.

Villabos, D. and Neuman, V. (1975). Studies on the scabicidal action of 5 per cent thiabendazole used topically. *Boletino Chileno Parasitologia*, **30**, 2–5.

Wooten, E. L., Blecha, F., Broce, A. B., and Pollmann, D. S. (1986). The effect of sarcoptic mange on growth performance, leukocytes and lymphocyte proliferative responses in pigs. *Veterinary Parasitology*, **22**, 315–24.

Zumpt, F. (1961). *The arthropod parasites of vertebrates in Africa south of the Sahara*. Vol. I: *Chelicerata*. South African Institute for Medical Research, Johannesburg.

66 INFESTATION BY FLEAS

W. N. Beesley

SUMMARY

The most important fleas which attack man to be considered are: *Pulex irritans*, *Tunga penetrans*, *Ctenocephalides felis/canis*, and *Xenopsylla cheopis*; also included are *Ceratophyllus gallinae* and *Echidnophaga gallinacea*. Biology, pathology, immune reactions, disease transmission, and control are discussed.

INTRODUCTION

There are perhaps 3000 species and subspecies of fleas, belonging to about 200 genera in 15 families, but fortunately very few are of medical or veterinary importance. Some 95 per cent of all species feed on mammals, the others attacking birds and even lizards. Fleas irritate the host when they take their blood feeds and they may stimulate serious hypersensitivity reactions, but their prime importance is in the transmission of various diseases to man and animals. Medically, the key species are *Xenopsylla cheopis*, which transmits plague and murine typhus, *Ctenocephalides* spp., the dog and cat fleas, which may transmit certain tapeworms to man, and the sand flea or chigoe, *Tunga penetrans*, which buries itself in the skin of the toe or foot, causing boil-like lesions.

HISTORY

Fleas are tiny ectoparasites which have evolved in close association with their hosts in nests, burrows, and lairs, hence the frequency with which they occur in birds' nests, rat burrows, etc. Fossil fleas closely resembling today's species have been found in Baltic amber dating back 50 million years and it is likely that flea–mammal associations are very much older.

The most important zoonotic relationship between fleas and man involves *Yersinia pestis*, the plague bacillus (Chapter 26). The Bible indicates that the Israelites realized the connection between bubonic plague and rats, although they did not suspect the part played by rat fleas in the transmission of the disease. The great Black Death (bubonic plague) pandemics reached Europe in AD 543, AD 1348, and then at frequent intervals through the following centuries, at one time exterminating one-quarter of the population of Europe. The plague bacillus was identified in 1894 and 4 years later Simond suggested that fleas transmitted the disease. In 1903 the principal rat flea vector, *X. cheopis*, was described by Rothschild, and it is now known that at least 30 species of fleas from various genera can transmit plague.

Aristotle knew nothing of the life cycle of fleas, but believed that dung was a necessary ingredient for their development. John Donne, the future Dean of St Paul's Cathedral, London, wrote 400 years ago that the flea 'sucked me first and now sucks thee, and in this flea our two bloods mingled be', an observation only one step away from realization that disease could be transmitted by insects. Robert Hooke, the seventeenth-century English naturalist, knew fleas as 'small brown skipping animals', but it was only in 1694 that the Dutch microscopist Leeuwenhoek suggested that pigeon fleas fed on blood—a view disputed by others who felt that fleas fed only on dead flies, dung, and the sawdust left in spittoons (Rothschild and Clay 1957). Fleas certainly commanded the interest of the population, as noted by an unknown writer: 'The arithmetic flea adds to your misery, subtracts your pleasure, divides your attention and multiplies like the devil!' (cited by Burns 1991). In 1758 Linnaeus named the first two species of fleas, *Pulex irritans* and *Tunga penetrans*. Since that time many new species have been described. The most credit for the taxonomy and naming of new fleas must go to Hopkins and Rothschild (see Smit 1973), who took 18 years to catalogue most of the flea species of the world, filling five volumes, totalling 2500 pages.

Medieval flea-killing preparations included mare's urine and various herbs, such as wormwood (*Artemisia absinthium*). In the nineteenth century, wooden or ivory flea-trap phials, baited with honey, were fashionable. These were hung over the chest from a cord and were supposed to attract the parasites from the skin of the victim. Later came sulphur and organic sulphur soaps incorporating monosulphiram, etc., also various soothing creams, followed by DDT, the first of the organochlorine insecticides. Last on the scene were the organophosphorus and pyrethroid insecticides (see p. 720).

THE PARASITES

Fleas occupy the order Siphonaptera, a name which describes their method of feeding through thin capillary-like mouthparts, and their lack of wings. The laterally compressed adults measure 1–5 mm in length and have a covering of bristles and small spines. They are usually dark brown in colour. They may or may not have individually distinctive comb-like frills (ctenidia) on the head and thorax (p. 718). The species in which we are interested all belong to the family Pulicidae, with the exception of the chicken flea, *Ceratophyllus gallinae*, in the family Ceratophyllidae.

Both sexes feed on blood, the female taking such large meals that she often evacuates undigested blood. This rich excrement provides valuable protein food for the larval fleas. Individual fleas can feed for 4 hours, and one which weighed only 0.6 mg had a stomach volume of 0.5 mm^3 (Rothschild and Clay 1957). Adult fleas feed on the host several times during their life, which may last 1–2 years.

The fertilized female may produce up to 1000 eggs, laying 2–20 each day in dirt and dust, floor cracks, and the dens, nests or bedding of the host. The emerging larvae are very active and feed on organic debris, including the blood or semi-digested blood passed in the faeces of the adult fleas. The larvae take 2–3 weeks to several months to complete their development through usually three instars, although *Tunga penetrans* has only two larval stages. The final larval stage spins a sticky coat to which dirt adheres, forming an excellent camouflage. The pupal stage normally lasts 10–17 days but may be much longer, and the adult female, whether fed or unfed, can survive for many months. Unfed fleas kept in high humidity conditions can live for as long as 18–20 months.

PULEX IRRITANS, THE HUMAN FLEA

There are six species of *Pulex*, three each in the nominate subgenus *Pulex* and in *Juxtapulex*. The female of *Pulex* (*P.*) *irritans* is dark brown and 3.0–4.0 mm in length. It has no ctenidia. As well as being a widespread and common nuisance flea of man, this species also feeds on various coarse-coated mammals such as the pig, badger, dog, deer, and peccary. In other words, the so-called human flea is an indiscriminate feeder which happens to include man among its hosts.

Pulex (*P.*) *irritans* can transmit plague from person to person, although *P.* (*P.*) *simulans*, which occurs in parts of North America, may be more important in this form of transmission of the disease (Smit 1973). *Pulex* (*P.*) *irritans* can also transmit to man murine typhus, erysipeloid, and *Dipylidium caninum*, the dog and cat tapeworm.

XENOPSYLLA CHEOPIS, RAT FLEA

The female is about 2.0 mm in length; like *P. irritans* it has no ctenidia. It feeds primarily on murid rodents but in their absence will readily attack man. At least 220 species of rodent fleas of various genera have been found to harbour plague bacilli, and 30 of these can transmit the disease. In practice, *X. cheopis* is the usual vector of plague in Asia, Europe, Africa, and the Americans; it also transmits murine typhus, melioidosis and erysipeloid. Sixteen other species of *Xenopsylla*, e.g. *X. brasiliensis* in Africa and *X. astia* in South-East Asia, can transmit plague, and at least one, *X. conformis*, can act as a vector of brucellosis (Smit 1973). The role of fleas in the transmission of plague and other diseases is discussed later.

TUNGA PENETRANS—SAND FLEA, CHIGOE, OR JIGGER FLEA

Tunga is usually placed in the family Pulicidae, although some authors allocate it to its own family, the Tungidae. The nine species of *Tunga* may be divided into the *penetrans* and *caecator* groups, and they occur in the warmer areas of the Americas, Africa, China, and Japan.

Tunga penetrans is the most notorious species because of its unpleasant habit of burrowing to feed within the skin of the toes or foot of the human host. As well as 'sand flea' and 'chigoe', it is also known in the Americas as 'chigger', which is also the name commonly used there for trombiculid mites.

The adult *T. penetrans* is only 1–1.2 mm in length and lacks ctenidia. It was one of the first two fleas to be described by Linnaeus. Historically, it seems to have figured on ancient Peruvian pottery, and was well known to the early Spanish colonists. *Tunga penetrans* infests people in Central and South America, the West Indies, and across Africa to Madagascar. A few cases of tungosis have also occurred in persons returning to India from infested areas, but this species does not occur naturally in any part of Asia. *Tunga penetrans* was originally a parasite of pigs, which may act as a reservoir for the human infection, especially if these animals are kept near the house. The usual hosts are man, pigs, and other domestic animals, armadilloes and murid rodents. *Tunga penetrans* does not transmit any diseases to man.

The female is agile but has a limited range of jump and once she has attached to a suitable host soon burrows into the skin, remaining there for up to 2 weeks. The male does not attack man. The body of the female distends by the extreme stretching of the intersegmental unchitinized membrane between abdominal segments II and III. She begins to produce eggs 5 days after attachment to the host and after 7–10 days the flea is 5–6 mm long and contains several thousand eggs, up to 200 of which escape from the flea and fall to the ground inside or outside houses. Meanwhile the legs of the flea have begun to disintegrate. The pupal period lasts 5–14 days, and the life cycle may be complete in as little as 18 days.

The foot is the usual site of infestation in man, following the habit of going barefoot. The condition usually presents as a painful swelling of the underside of the toe, between the toes, or under a toe nail, and the lesions may become septic. The hands, arms, and buttocks may also be infested, especially in babies and beggars. Severe infestations have also been recorded from leprosy patients (Service 1986). Heavy infestations can be quite crippling and the consequent damage to the skin may lead to secondary infection, ulceration, and even tetanus or gangrene. There is concern about the sand flea in Trinidad, where 7.0 per cent of males and 3.4 per cent of females in the south of the island were found to be infested; one 7-year-old boy had 15 sand flea lesions (Chadee *et al.* 1991).

The appearance of the infected toe in endemic areas is diagnostic. The bloated egg-filled body of the female flea is demonstrated by removing the surface of the lesion. It is remarkable that the female flea can feed on blood and leucocytes, living in close but static contact with the host tissues for 8–10 days despite the immune response. This peculiar host association is unique among the fleas, corresponding to the furuncular myiasis caused by larvae of *Dermatobia hominis* and *Hypoderma* spp. It represents a greater physical and immunological feat than that of a very mobile calliphorid larva which feeds for several days on cellular exudate in the tissues of a sheep.

Treatment of the sand flea lesion is straightforward, as the investigative action of removing the roof of the lesion with a clean needle exposes the female flea, which can then be lifted out intact. This should be done carefully, or sepsis or tetanus may follow. A suitable dressing should be applied in order to prevent secondary bacterial infection.

The life cycle of *T. penetrans* has an interesting counterpart in Australia, where the flea *Uropsylla tasmanica* attacks marsupials (Kettle 1990). The eggs are glued to the hairs of the host, from where the larvae burrow into the skin. These steadily mature, then fall to the ground and develop into pupae and adult fleas. They do not attack man.

CTENOCEPHALIDES FELIS AND CT. CANIS, THE CAT AND DOG FLEAS

Ctenocephalides canis was described by Curtis in 1826 and *Ct. felis* by Bouche 9 years later; the genus now contains a total of 12 'forms' i.e. species and subspecies (Smit 1973). *Ctenocephalides felis* itself has at least four subspecies: *felis, strongylus, damarensis,* and *orientalis. Ctenocephalides felis* has much wider tastes than the name suggests, and in most countries dogs are more likely to be infested with *Ct. felis* than *Ct. canis*, an exception being Ireland (Baker and Elharam 1992). The dog flea appears to have quite precise host needs, and larvae originating from females which had fed on cats fail to develop to the pupal stage. The dog and cat fleas will be discussed together, for convenience.

Female cat and dog fleas measure 2.0–3.25 mm and when fed can survive for up to 234 days. They often lay their eggs on the host as well as in corners of rooms, cracks in flooring, etc. Thus eggs, larvae, and adults can be found in the coat of the host.

It is rare for fleas to cause really severe clinical symptoms or death in animals, but this has happened when large numbers of *Ct. felis* have fed on lambs and kids (Yeruham *et al.* 1989). *Ctenocephalides felis* and *Ct. canis* can act as vectors for plague and Boutonneuse fever (*Rickettsia conorii*), but are important principally as intermediate hosts for the cestode *Dipylidium caninum*, a common intestinal parasite of dogs and cats. The mammal host becomes infected by ingesting a flea which contains the larval cysticercoid stage of the tapeworm. The adult flea cannot take in tapeworm eggs as it has only very fine sucking mouthparts, so that the infection enters the flea cycle when the chewing flea larvae ingests tapeworm eggs. The cysticercoid then develops inside the larval stages of the flea and is confined there through the pupal and early adult stages. The infected adult flea is then swallowed during grooming. Infection of man is very uncommon but can occur in children if they happen to show undue curiosity about a flea moving over the floor, cushions etc., catching and then eating the infected parasite.

CERATOPHYLLUS GALLINAE, THE CHICKEN FLEA

This species is 3.0–3.5 mm in length and is the commonest bird flea likely to be found on man. It also occurs on rodents. There are specific fleas named for sparrows, house martins, etc. but *C. gallinae* is the species which usually invades bedrooms or hospital wards from the vacated nests of wild birds in the eaves of buildings. This also happens with *Dermanyssus gallinae*, the poultry red mite. *Ceratophyllus gallinae* has also attacked people out of doors (Kettle 1990).

ECHIDNOPHAGA GALLINACEA, THE CHICKEN STICKTIGHT FLEA

This species is only about 1.5 mm in length. It has an angular shape to its head but no ctenidia. It is very prolific, laying up to 20 eggs each day. It is restricted to warm countries, attacking primarily poultry and wild birds, but also dogs, cats, horses, rabbits, rodents, pigs, and occasionally man. On birds it usually attaches itself to the combs and wattles and sometimes around the cloaca. Its semi-permanent mode of parasitism resembles that of *Tunga penetrans* although it does not burrow into the skin. *Echidnophaga gallinacea* can transmit plague and murine typhus and the related species *E. larina* can act as intermediate host for the dog and cat tapeworm *Dipylidium caninum* (Smit 1973).

DIAGNOSIS

Fleas are are easily identified as 1–5 mm long, bilaterally compressed arthropods, usually dark brown in colour, with a range from yellow-brown to almost black. Dog and cat fleas have sets of spines arranged in ctenidia ('combs') attached to the head and pronotum, while in the chicken flea there is only a pronotal comb. There are no ctenidia at all in the three other species which commonly attack man, *Pulex irritans*, *Xenopsylla cheopis*, and *Tunga penetrans*. Details of diagnostic features such as the ctenidia, mesopleural rods, spermathecae, and the various arrangements of spines and setae are given in Smit (1973). Precise specific and subspecific identification is often a task for the specialist.

In man fleas often bite during the day on the ankles and legs, although at night they can attack anywhere on the body. Their eggs are always laid off the host. Occasionally the flea-bite rash goes by a particular name, such as the Mexican 'Hebra's prurigo', which can be simulated by the intradermal inoculation of an extract made from human, dog, and cat fleas (Almeida and Croce 1990).

In dogs and cats, fleas are most commonly found attached to the skin under the fur of the neck, abdomen, and other thin-skinned areas. After their feed they may lay eggs in the coat, but usually leave to lay eggs in the carpet, cracks in the floorboards, etc. 'Flea dirt', the faecal pellets of the adults, appears as black gritty material on the surface of the skin. Flea faeces are suitably demonstrated as such by placing them on damp filter paper, when a reddish halo of haemoglobin will appear.

SYMPTOMS, HISTOPATHOLOGY AND IMMUNOPATHOLOGY OF THE FLEA BITE LESIONS

The very first flea bite in an unsensitized individual causes no visible lesion (the induction period), but as further bites follow and sensitivity gradually builds up there is intense itching for one or more days, with a 1–4 mm diameter area of swollen and erythematous skin. A moderate urticaria is the usual sign of flea activity once the initial wheals have subsided.

The first bite stimulates little response because this is the first exposure to saliva which contains anticoagulant but no immunogenic protein. The low molecular weight proteins which will be responsible for a later reaction as the host becomes sensitized are haptens (incomplete antigens), which become immunogenic by fixation to collagen in the skin. After a period of about 5 days of unreactive flea bites the accumulated hapten has had time to combine with skin collagen, making the hapten immunogenic (Hopla 1982; Nelson 1987), stimulating the host to produce antibody. Because antibody is now available, conjugated hapten from any future flea bites can be immediately targetted by host antibody.

In practice, there is a sequence of host skin reactions of the type seen in response to biting flies. This begins with stage I (induction: no visible reaction), to stage II (delayed response), stage III (immediate response followed by a delayed response), stage IV (immediate-type reaction only), and finally stage V—in which the host has become desensitized and therefore nonreactive. It was formerly considered that delayed and immediate type reactions were due to different antigens, but it is now realized that the two types of reaction are immunologically related and are both part of the normal immune response (Nelson 1987)

The following description of the histopathological reaction to flea bites relates to precise experiments carried out on guinea-pigs and is summarized from Nelson (1987), although it is accepted that such reactions may differ in different species of hosts. In guinea-pigs there is virtually no dermal cellular response until several hours into stage II, when there is a strong infiltration of mainly monocytes and lymphocytes. Stage III (immediate then delayed response) begins some 9 days after the first exposure to fleas. At about 20 minutes after feeding there is a heavy infiltration of eosinophils; this gives way to a dominance of monocytes and lymphocytes after 24 hours. Some 7 weeks after the first exposure stage IV (immediate reactivity) begins, when eosinophils predominate in the skin and mononuclear cells disappear from the infiltrate. After a further 4 weeks all reactivity ends and the animal enters stage V—desensitization.

The involvement of the basophil in skin reactions following tick bites (cutaneous basophil hypersensitivity) is now recognized and this type of cell has also been identified in flea bite reactions. Basophilic leucocytes appear in the skin rather slowly, along with a strong immediate response of circulating eosinophils.

One way in which skin reactions to flea bites in dogs differ from those in guinea-pigs seems due to the marked erythematous and papular reactions which often develop in dogs, aggravated by scratching in response to intense pruritus. This leads to oedema of the upper corium with a heavy infiltration of eosinophils with neutrophils, mast cells, and lymphocytes. Delayed responses to flea feeding may or may not be observed in dogs, and seem rare in cats and rabbits. There is no comparable information on the histopathology of the skin in humans bitten by fleas.

Flea allergy dermatitis of dogs and cats is most usual in animals which have become naturally infested with fairly small numbers of fleas and then been 'defleaed' at frequent intervals. Similarly, dogs exposed to fleas only once, twice or three times each week become strongly allergic to further bites after 8 weeks, with higher levels of IgE and decreased IgG than dogs continuously exposed to large populations of fleas. The act of feeding by even single fleas on sporadically challenged but sensitized hosts often stimulates quite severe reactions, while the heavily infested but desensitized animals show a delayed, weak and short-lived allergic response (Halliwell 1982). These results help to explain the sudden severe reactions against flea bites observed in hypersensitive individuals experiencing 'summer eczema' (dogs) or miliary dermatitis (cats) in the southern USA (Harman *et al.* 1987). These studies may also help to explain human papular urticaria.

Theoretically it should be possible to artificially desensitize humans and animals against flea bites, and some success has been obtained using extracts of *Ct. felis* in dogs. Attempts to produce desensitization in humans, however, have so far given inconsistent results. Immunization of animals against the bites of blood-sucking arthropods, including fleas, may be possible in order to allow the parasite to penetrate the skin with its mouthparts while preventing it from actually taking blood. A successful vaccine has been reported against the East African cattle tick, *Rhipicephalus appendiculatus*, which is of course much more sedentary than the temporarily parasitic flea. Progress against other blood-sucking parasites will probably be very slow indeed.

Flea dermatitis can occur regardless of whether the flea species is the one appropriately named for that host. For example, along the Mediterranean coasts sheep and goats can be severely irritated by cat fleas, as can cattle and buffaloes in India.

Following the attacks of (usually) cat fleas or human fleas, some people develop a mental condition known as delusory parasitosis, in which they imagine that they are continually attacked by large numbers of unseen external parasites at all times of the day.

There is a relationship between the breeding of rabbit fleas and the level of hormones during the pregnancy of the host, such that the newborn rabbits are available as a source of food for their parasites, which in turn then have plenty of faecal blood available for their own larvae (Rothschild and Clay 1957). Flea

infestations of cattle can likewise be affected by the hormone state of the host, high parasite populations having been observed on pregnant cows and low numbers on bullocks. It is quite possible that similar parallel cycles occur in other species of hosts, including man.

DISEASES TRANSMITTED TO MAN BY FLEAS

PLAGUE (*YERSINIA PESTIS*)

Plague is principally a disease of wild animals, especially rodents, which is transmitted by their fleas. In the so-called urban cycle man becomes infected incidentally to the normal animal to animal transmission. This is most likely to happen when rats are in close association with people, as in very poor areas of large cities. It is rare for fleas to become infected on one human and then transmit the disease to another person. The most important vector of human plague is *X. cheopis*, although *X. astia, X. brasiliensis*, and other species maintain the disease in various species of rats. Some 220 species of rodent fleas can harbour the bacilli and approximately 30 species can transmit the disease (Service 1986). The pneumonic form of plague is not transmitted by insects.

Rats infected with plague develop an acute and fatal septicaemia. The fleas leave the host as it dies and cools, and some of these parasites may attack man. The bubonic form of plague is transmitted by regurgitation of some of the mass of plague bacilli contained in the proventriculus of the flea, the organ having become temporarily blocked by the rapidly reproducing bacteria. Blood meals in fleas whose alimentary canals have become blocked cannot pass down to the stomach. The flea then starves and bites repeatedly in order to take up blood.

Man can also become infected following a direct bite from the freshly contaminated mouthparts of the flea. Another method of infection is by contaminated faeces of the flea being rubbed into abrasions or mucous membranes. Flea faeces can remain infective for up to 3 years. This mode of transmission is similar to that of *Trypanosoma cruzi* in the faeces of triatomid bugs.

Cavanaugh and Randall (1959) demonstrated that *Y. pestis* transmitted by blocked fleas is of the non-capsulated phagocytosis-susceptible type. The bacteria which escape phagocytosis and destruction by the neutrophils find a favourable environment within the monocytes in which they can multiply. On release from the monocytes the plague organisms are encapsulated and are then resistant to phagocytosis. Within 24 hours in animals which are sensitive to flea bites, *Y. pestis* at the site are surrounded by monocytic skin infiltrations and destroyed.

The control of fleas is discussed below. Both rats and their fleas have unfortunately shown resistance to insecticides and rodenticides in some parts of the world.

OTHER DISEASES TRANSMITTED BY FLEAS

Rickettsia mooseri (*R. typhi*) causes a milder form of typhus (murine typhus; flea-borne endemic typhus) than the louse-borne epidemic typhus, due to *R. prowazecki*, but can still produce a significant death rate, e.g. 5 per cent (Kettle 1990). In the period 1931–46 there were at least 42 000 reported cases of murine typhus in the United States, and the actual total may have exceeded 200 000 (Kettle 1990). At least seven species of fleas, of six genera, have been found to be infected with *R. mooseri*, but *X. cheopis* is the major vector of the disease.

Rickettsia mooseri organisms are ingested with the blood meal of the flea and multiply rapidly in the cells of the midgut. Unlike *Y. pestis* bacteria, the rickettsiae do not block the gut. Man can only be infected when flea faeces containing the rickettsiae are accidentally rubbed into abrasions or contact mucous membranes. This rather negative mode of transmission is compensated for by the extreme virulence of *R. mooseri*, an infective dose for man being only one-fifth of the single excrement of one infected flea (Bibikova 1977). The flea faeces remaining infective for up to 9 years (Service 1986). The disease is spread between rats and other rodents by various species of fleas and also by rat lice. Man usually becomes infected following bites by *X. cheopis*, although dog and cat fleas and human fleas can also transmit the infection.

Boutonneuse fever (*Rickettsia conorii*) is normally transmitted by the dog tick, *Rhipicephalus sanguineus*, but dog fleas have also been incriminated as vectors. Mansueto *et al.* (1989) found that 20.8 per cent of *Ctenocephalides* (species not recorded) collected from dogs in Palermo, Sicily, harboured rickettsiae similar to *R. conorii*. The characteristic black eschar which forms in man at the site of the bite of the infecting tick may be absent in patients who subsequently develop boutonneuse fever, and this may be because the infecting bite was due to a flea rather than a tick.

Other human diseases which are less commonly transmitted by fleas include tularaemia, Q fever, pseudotuberculosis, erysipeloid, and listeriosis (Smit 1973; Service 1986).

DOMESTIC CONTROL OF FLEAS

A flea problem in human dwellings commonly originates with a pet dog or cat. This should be bathed in an appropriate insecticide formulation, such as one containing a pyrethroid, an organophosphorus compound, or a carbamate. An alternative is to spray the animal or treat it with an aerosol. This may need to be done twice a week, while at the same time the house, particularly the indoors living area of the animal is thoroughly cleaned with a vacuum cleaner. This should remove most of the immature stages of the fleas, when an insecticide dust or spray can be used to complete the eradication procedure. For the more general control of fleas, insecticide powders can be applied to the floors of dwelling houses and rat runs.

Methoprene is an insect growth regulator (IGR) which acts on the developing stages of several species of arthropods, including fleas. It is effective mainly against the third stage larvae, but female fleas exposed to methoprene lay eggs which either fail to hatch or which produce larvae destined to die in the first instar, a delayed lethal effect.

Oral tablet preparations of organophosphorous insecticides such as cythioate have been used for the control of fleas on dogs, as for demodectic mange (see also Chapter 62). The insecticide affects feeding fleas after they have taken in blood containing the active ingredient in a sufficient concentration.

Plastic insecticidal collars, which usually contain an organophosphorous insecticide such as 15 per cent diazinon or 5–20 per cent dichlorvos, should kill the fleas on the host within a few hours and provide 4–5 months' protection against a new flea challenge.

Reasonable personal protection against fleas will be provided by the application of repellents such as dimethyl phthalate ('dimp'), diethyltoluamide ('deet'), or benzyl benzoate.

Unfed fleas can survive for long periods in empty houses, so that they are unlikely to starve to death in vacant property. Hungry adult fleas are stimulated into activity by vibration and an apparently flea-free dwelling or chicken house which has been empty for a year can reveal its population of hungry fleas soon after people have walked across the floorboards.

Even the most thorough application of insecticide cannot guarantee that a pet dog or cat will remain uninfested when it returns to its outdoors territory. This is an important practical point for the owner, who may be surprised to see tapeworm segments passed by a pet within a few weeks of treatment, despite the use of an anthelmintic against the worms and insecticide against the fleas. Reinfestation of pets by fleas harbouring tapeworm cysticercoids is always likely.

FLEA CONTROL PROGRAMMES

Large programmes will be necessary for the urban control of outbreaks of plague or murine typhus.

These will probably involve the use of both insecticides and rodenticides, e.g. the anticoagulants warfarin, furmarin, or bromadiolone. Insecticidal fogs and aerosols can also be used. It is important to apply the insecticide against the fleas before using the rodenticide, as otherwise the fleas will leave the dead rodents to bite man, with possible accelerated disease transmission.

REFERENCES

Almeida, F. A. and Croce, J. (1990). Study of flea-bite hypersensitivity in patients with Hebra's prurigo. *Medicina Cutanea Ibero-Latino-America*, **43**, 132–7 [cited in *Review of Medical and Veterinary Entomology*, **81**, item 748].

Baker, K. P. and Elharam, S. (1992). The biology of *Ctenocephalides canis* in Ireland. *Veterinary Parasitology*, **45**, 141–6.

Bibikova, V. A. (1977). Contemporary views on the interrelationships between fleas and the pathogens of human and animal disease. *Annual Review of Entomology*, **22**, 23–32.

Burns, D. A. (1991). A potpourri of parasites in poetry and proverb. *British Medical Journal*, **303**, 1611–12.

Cavanaugh, D. C. and Randall, R. (1959). The role of multiplication of *Pasteurella pestis* in mononuclear phagocytes in the pathogenesis of flea-borne plague. *Journal of Immunology*, **83**, 348–58.

Chadee, D. D., Furlonge, E., Narynsingh, C., and Maitre, A. Le (1991). *Tunga penetrans* in the south of Trinidad. *Transactions of the Royal Society of Tropical Medicine and Hygiene*, **85**, 549.

Halliwell, R. E. W. (1982). The immune response to flea antigen in different dog populations. *Journal of the American Veterinary Medical Association*, **181**, 274.

Harman, D. W., Halliwell, R. E., and Greiner, E. C. (1987). Flea species of dogs and cats in north-central Florida. *Veterinary Parasitology*, **23**, 135–40.

Hopla, C. E. (1982). Arthropodiases, in *CRE Handbook Series in Zoonoses, section C: Parasitic Zoonoses*, Vol. III, (ed. G. V. Hillyer and C. E. Hopla). CRC Press, Boca Raton, Florida, USA.

Kettle, D. S. (1990). *Medical and veterinary entomology*. Commonwealth Agricultural Bureaux, Wallingford, Oxford.

Mansueto, S., Vitale, G., Lavagnino, A., Di Rosa, S., and Merulla, R. (1989). Rickettsiae of the spotted fever group in dog fleas (*Ctenocephalides* spp.) in Western Sicily. *Annals of Tropical Medicine and Parasitology*, **83**, 325.

Nelson, W. A. (1987). Blood-sucking and myiasis-producing arthropods. In *Immune responses in parasitic infections: immunology, immunopathology and immunoprophylaxis. Vol. IV Protozoa, arthropods and invertebrates*, (ed. E. J. L. Soulsby), pp. 175–209. CRC Press, Boca Raton, Florida.

Rothschild, M. and Clay, T. (1957). *Fleas, flukes and cuckoos*, (3rd edn.), New Naturalist Series. Collins, London.

Service, M. W. (1986). *Lecture notes on medical entomology*. Balckwell Scientific, Oxford.

Smit, F. G. A. M. (1973). Siphonaptera (Fleas), in *Insects and other arthropods of medical importance*, (ed. K. G. V. Smith). British Museum (Natural History), London.

Yeruham, I., Rosen, S., and Hadani, A. (1989). Mortality in calves, lambs and kids caused by severe infestation with the cat flea, *Ctenocephalides felis felis*, in Israel. *Veterinary Parasitology*, **30**, 351–6.

67 THE MYIASES

W. N. Beesley

SUMMARY

The larvae of some 50 species of Diptera can produce myiasis in man. Most species are of little medical importance, but several can be responsible for serious lesions. Damage is usually caused to the skin, which may or may not need to have been damaged in some way in order to facilitate the entry of the first-instar larvae. Myiasis may also affect the eyes, ears, nose, urogenital tract or, rarely, the alimentary canal. The condition may be due to larvae acting either as obligatory or facultative parasites, although none use man as their exclusive host. Outstanding examples of serious damage include that caused by the calliphorines (*Cochliomyia*, *Chrysomya*, *Cordylobia*, *Auchmeromyia*), cuterebrids (*Dermatobia*), and oestrids (*Oestrus*, *Hypoderma*).

Myiasis species are distributed worldwide, but are a problem mainly in the warmer countries. Large-scale eradication programmes have been successfully carried through only against the cattle warble fly, *Hypoderma* spp. and New World screwworm fly, *Cochliomyia hominivorax*. The latter has now been cleared from the USA and Mexico and its recent eradication from Libya is described.

INTRODUCTION

Myiasis may be defined as the infestation of live human or other vertebrate animals with larvae of Diptera (true flies), the larvae feeding for at least some period upon the host's living or locally necrotic tissue, liquid body substances, or ingested food. Zumpt (1965) lists over 50 dipteran species which can cause myiasis in man in the Old World alone.

The species which cause myiasis may be classified in terms of the site affected (Table 67.1) or on the basis of their obligatory or facultative parasitism (Table 67.2). Obligatory myiasis parasites are usually host-specific, penetrate unbroken skin, feed on internal tissues, and are migratory in the first instar. The facultative species are less host-specific, may infest several host species, often use already damaged skin and are sessile and subcutaneous in their feeding habits

Table 67.1 Classification of human myiases

Type of myiasis	Examples
Dermal/subdermal	*Cordylobia anthropophaga*
	Cordylobia rodhaini
	Cochliomyia hominivorax
	Chrysomya bezziana
	Lucilia sericata, L. cuprina
	Dermatobia hominis
Creeping subdermal	*Hypoderma bovis, H. lineatum*
	Gasterophilus haemorrhoidalis
	G. pecorum, G. inermis
Sanguinivorous	*Auchmeromyia luteola*
	(= *A. senegalensis*)
Nasopharyngeal	*Oestrus ovis*
Ophthalmomyiasis	*Oestrus ovis*
	Wohlfahrtia magnifica
Aural	*Wohlfahrtia magnifica*
	Coch. hominivorax
	Oestrus ovis
	Musca domestica
Urinogenital	*Calliphora vicina*
	Fannia canicularis
Intestinal/enteric (pseudomyiasis)	*Fannia canicularis*
	Musca domestica
	Calliphora vicina
	Sarcophaga haemorrhoidalis

(Nelson 1987). The sites of infestation and feeding habits of the various myiasis species differ greatly. Some myiasis larvae burrow into the skin and produce boils or migration tracks (dermal and subdermal myiases); others suck blood, invade the cavities and tissues of the head (nasopharyngeal, aural, or ophthalmomyiases), feed in the gut (intestinal or enteric myiasis), or parasitize the urogenital system, usually the urethra or vagina. The excretory and secretory (ES) products of myiasis larvae are often strongly antigenic and current work demonstrates that their immunology is quite complex.

The condition of 'pseudomyiasis' is a special category of myiasis, when the gut of a living host contains live or dead larvae which have been accidentally swallowed, for example when larvae of *Drosophila* are eaten with ripe fruit. Apparent enteric infestation may also be recorded when larvae are found in fresh human or

Table 67.2 Examples of obligatory and facultative myiasis species with their usual location in the human host

Obligatory myiasis
  Species which can complete their larval development in man

Species	Site
Auchmeromyia luteola (= senegalensis)	Skin – bloodsucking
Cordylobia anthropophaga	Dermal furunculosis
Cordylobia (= Stasisia) rodhaini	Dermal furunculosis
Cochliomyia hominivorax	Wounds
Chrysomya bezziana	Wounds
Wohlfahrtia magnifica	Wounds, ears, nose
Wohlfahrtia vigil	Dermal
Dermatobia hominis	Dermal

  Species which cannot complete their development in man

Oestrus ovis	Eye, ear, nose
Gasterophilus haemorrhoidalis	Dermal
Hypoderma lineatum, H. bovis	Dermal, eye
Oedemagena tarandi	Dermal

Facultative myiasis
  Species which can complete their development in man (note: the references to 'alimentary tract' myiasis do not represent true invasive myiasis)

Musca domestica	Wounds, intestine
Lucilia sericata, L. cuprina	Wounds
Calliphora vicina	Wounds, intestine
Wohlfahrtia nuba	Wounds
Chrysomya megacephala	Wounds

  Species which seem unable to complete their development in man

Fannia canicularis, F. scalaris	Urinogenital, intestine
Musca crassirostris	Intestine
(also various syrphids, psychodids, piophilids, etc.)	

animal faeces, but have developed from eggs laid in that material. This can easily happen in warm countries, where larvae can hatch only 7–8 hours after oviposition. True intestinal myiasis does not ocur in man, although there are examples from animals, e.g. the infestation of the stomach and intestines by *Gasterophilus* in equines.

THE AGENTS

No myiasis species is exclusive to man, so that none would die out if man were to leave a locality permanently. Several species, however, will readily invade his tissues, e.g. *Wohlfahrtia magnifica*, *Auchmeromyia luteola* (= *senegalensis*), *Cordylobia anthropophaga*, and *Cochliomyia hominivorax*.

It is convenient to consider the Diptera which cause myiasis on the basis of their taxonomy. There are occasional instances of human myiasis among the Nematocera and the phorids, syrphids, and piophilids but in practical terms human myiasis is confined to the Muscidae, Calliphoridae, Sarcophagidae, Gasterophilidae, Cuterebridae, Oestridae, and Hypodermatidae. As the life cycles, types and severity of lesions, and control measures can all vary considerably, the various features of each species will be examined as each is dis-

cussed. Although some taxonomic details are given, full descriptions of the adult flies and their larvae are provided in Zumpt's classic reference (1965).

MUSCIDAE

Musca domestica, **the common housefly**

Musca domestica was one of the original insects described by Linnaeus in his Systema Naturae in 1758. The female is 6.5–7.5 mm in length, with a grey-olive thorax bearing four dark stripes; the abdomen has a yellowish ground colour and median black stripe; the most obvious wing vein has a prominent sharp elbow.

Musca domestica breeds in a wide range of decomposing organic material, including animal and human faeces and vegetable refuse, and its main importance lies in its mechanical transmission of viruses, bacteria, protozoa, and (in animals) helminths. Despite its close relationship with humans and their houses, only a few cases of urogenital, dermal, nasopharyngeal, or skin myiasis in man have been recorded. Larvae which hatch from eggs laid in or near wounds produce little or no irritation. However, in one well-documented case of urinary myiasis from Romania, *M. domestica* larvae were seen crawling from the urethra of a young man who had certainly been infected with larvae hatched from eggs laid at night on his body or clothing (Zumpt 1965). Larvae of *M. domestica* can appear in the faeces after their accidental ingestion with food. Myiasis in animals due to any species of *Musca* is uncommon. Rare cases of traumatic tissue myiasis in man due to larvae of *M. sorbens* and of 'pseudomyiasis' due to *M. crassirostris* have been reported.

Fannia canicularis, the lesser housefly

This species, as *Musca canicularis*, was first described by Linnaeus in 1761, although the genus *Fannia* was erected by Robineau-Desvoidy. *Fannia* is only about 4–6 mm in length and is grey to almost black in colour; it lacks the angular wing vein of *M. domestica*. Its mature larvae have fleshy lateral processes by which the various species may be identified. Five species of *Fannia* have been incriminated in mild cases of human myiasis, the most important being *F. canicularis* and *F. scalaris*. *Fannia canicularis* has generally similar habits to *M. domestica*, but tends to be more frequently associated with human myiasis, despite the fact that it is exophilic, i.e. tends to keep outside buildings and so make less contact with people and their food. As with *M. domestica*, larvae of *F. canicularis* can cause urogenital myiasis and its larvae may also be passed in the faeces, usually after eating infested fruit or vegetables.

Fannia scalaris shows an even greater preference for human and animal excrement than does *F. canicularis*, visiting latrine pits and earth and chemical closets. Its larvae can appear in the faeces if contaminated fruit or vegetables have been eaten or of course if eggs were laid in the excrement soon after defaecation. This latter may have been the origin of a chronic case of supposedly 'intestinal myiasis' due to *Fannia* larvae, recorded in Cambridge in 1836, and one of the first observations of human infestation with fly larvae. It was stated that 'the chamber vessel was sometimes half-full of these animals' (Jenyns 1839). Genuine but short-lived rectal myiasis has been recorded for both *F. canicularis* and *F. scalaris*.

CALLIPHORIDAE: NON-METALLIC SPECIES

Auchmeromyia luteola (= *senegalensis*), the Congo floor maggot

There are five species of *Auchmeromyia* but only *A. luteola* causes myiasis in man. *Auchmeromyia luteola* was originally considered a *Musca* by Fabricius in 1805, but in 1907 the Liverpool workers Newstead, Dutton and Todd transferred it to *Auchmeromyia*. *Auchmeromyia luteola* is 8–13 mm in length and has a yellow-brown body with weak thoracic stripes and a deep second abdominal segment. *Auchmeromyia luteola* is restricted to Africa south of the Sahara, including the Cape Verde Islands, west of Senegal, and the specific name *senegalensis* used by Macquart in 1851 is now replacing *luteola*.

Larvae of *A. luteola* are unusual in that they suck blood from their hosts, which include domestic pigs, wart hogs and ant bears, as well as man. It was previously thought that larvae of *A. luteola* fed only on man, but this is quite incorrect. The adult flies feed on excrement, particularly human faeces, and rotting fruit and vegetables. Batches of about 50 eggs are laid on sand or soil and the emerging larvae hide in cracks and crevices in the floor of dwelling houses or under the sleeping mats of the occupants. Unfed newly hatched larvae can survive for up to 37 days and the maggots can become permanent inhabitants of the soil floors of primitive dwellings. The larvae are obligatory parasites of mammals and at night crawl on to the skin to feed, a process which lasts 10–20 minutes, depending on the size of the larva. Fed larvae are pink and when fully mature measure up to 18 mm. Larvae can feed every night, but because they can starve for long periods they may take blood only about every 5 days under natural conditions. They will probably take 5–20 feeds during their minimum 3–4 week development, although they may not reach the pupal stage for 12 weeks, depending upon the availability of food.

Human hosts feel a slight prick as the larva begins to feed, and there may be a second prick as the maggot withdraws its mouthparts. Some people feel pain and experience swelling after the feed. The larvae may become a serious nuisance, and in any case it is best to sleep on a bedstead rather than directly on the ground. Larvae are unable to climb more than a few centimetres although of course bedding must not be allowed to touch the soil. The Congo floor maggot was formerly quite a common pest in some parts of Africa, but improved standards of hygiene have now made it rather unusual. At one time *A. luteola* was thought to be a possible mechanical vector of *Trypanosoma*, but this is most unlikely.

Congo floor maggots were formerly thought to infest only man, but most individuals are found in and around the burrows of warthogs and ant bears. In the absence of man, suids can provide 98 per cent of the blood source of the larvae; hyenas can also be attacked. Other hosts may exist, and it would be useful to investigate this, using modern blood identification techniques.

Cordylobia anthropophaga, tumbu fly or mango fly

Cordylobia was named by Grunberg in 1903, and has three species. One of these, *C. rodhaini*, was formerly placed in the genus *Stasisia*, but it is preferable to keep all three species in *Cordylobia* (Zumpt 1965). *Cordylobia anthropophaga* resembles *A. luteola* but has a much shallower second abdominal segment. *Cordylobia anthropophaga* and *A. luteola* have both been confused in the past with another calliphorid, *Bengalia depressa*, which does not cause myiasis. *Cordylobia anthropophaga* occurs widely in sub-Saharan Africa and in some areas can be a common cause of human myiasis. The adult flies feed on fermenting fruit and vegetables and animal excreta, hence they are often attracted into houses.

There are now several reports of tumbu infestations acquired by tourists and others who have recently visited endemic areas in Africa. The normal hosts of *C. anthropophaga* are dogs, particularly puppies, and various species of rats, but cats, goats, mice, monkeys, chimpanzees, and chickens are also attacked. Of some interest is the recent first record of *C. anthropophaga* infestation seen in a quarantine dog in England (Fox *et al.* 1992). The animal had a total of 10 larvae, which were all successfully expressed manually.

Cordylobia anthropophaga lay batches of 100–300 eggs in shaded sandy soil contaminated by rat or human urine or faeces. A common alternative is provided by soiled laundry, as when inadequately washed children's clothes are hung out to dry—although the flies tend to avoid strong sunlight. The flies never deposit their eggs on the bare skin or attach them to hairs. If the surface of the sand or soil containing larvae is touched the parasites will emerge and actively attempt to attach themselves to the skin. Using their mouthhooks and salivary enzymes, the larvae can burrow completely into the skin in less than a minute, although they may take 30 minutes to do so. They can remain for some time on soiled laundry until the clothes are worn next to the skin. Newly emerged larvae can survive for up to 2 weeks on the ground.

The penetration of the first instar larvae is normally hardly noticed, but there may be an intense local reaction. Later there is itching and a pricking sensation, and the papule which has been formed becomes red. Soon the itching and discomfort increase, with induration of the surrounding tissues and leakage of serous fluid.

Infestations are characterized by multiple 'blind boils', 1–2 cm in diameter, usually across the back and buttocks, although the thighs, abdomen, and arms may also be affected. There may be up to 60 lesions in the back of a child, although 5–10 is more usual. The larvae complete their development in about 8–12 days. If undisturbed, as can happen in children or neglected adults, the mature larvae fall to the ground, pupate and develop into mature flies within 10–20 days, longer in cool weather.

Any furuncular swelling seen in children or adults where *C. anthropophaga* is common should be regarded as a possible tumbu fly lesion. The swelling is tender and has a small central breathing hole through which weeps serous fluid and sometimes a little blood, but not pus. Larvae can be removed intact after sealing the boil with a material such as medicinal paraffin, petroleum jelly, or glycerin. The larva soon becomes very active, begins to emerge from its burrow and can be squeezed out or withdrawn with forceps. It is important not to tear the larva or pull it apart, as a severe reaction could follow; the way would also be open to secondary bacterial infection.

As people often become infested with larvae of *C. anthropophaga* from the sand in latrines, or by contact with contaminated laundry, shoes should be worn and clothing or bedding not spread out to dry on the ground or on hedges. Larvae are killed when laundered clothing is ironed. It may or may not be economic to exclude flies from houses using fine wire mesh.

Cordylobia anthropophaga gained notoriety in the first report of an immune response by a mammal host to invasion by an arthropod parasite (Blacklock and Gordon 1927). It was shown that a complete but localized skin immunity, lasting for 3 months, developed in guinea-pigs which had been infested with *C. anthropophaga*. In man and dogs the protective immunity lasts for about 1 year. Sixty years later these observations were expanded in work on the immune responses stimulated by the myiasis parasites *Lucilia* (sheep) and *Hypoderma* (cattle), and by *Rhipicephalus* ticks on cattle. These studies have culminated in the development of serological diagnostic tests for hypodermosis in man and animals and in promising trials of vaccines against infestations by *Lucilia* and *Rhipicephalus*. Nelson (1987) has given an excellent review of the immunology and immunopathology of infestations by calliphorid and other myiasis species.

Cordylobia rodhaini, formerly known as *Stasisia rodhaini*, is closely related to *C. anthropophaga*. In 1905 Gedoelst named as *C. rodhaini* a fly larva taken from the arm of a Commandant Lund in the Belgian Congo. 'Lund's fly' was moved into the genus *Stasisia* by Surcouf in 1914, but is now recognized as a *Cordylobia*. Like *C. anthropophaga*, it occurs in much of tropical Africa, especially in forest areas. It is a larger fly than *C. anthropophaga*, and its correspondingly larger and more destructive larvae can take 12–15 days to develop within their boils, at least in the laboratory on the African giant rat, one of the principal hosts. *Cordylobia rodhaini* is much less common in man than *C. anthropophaga*, but the larval lesions are more painful. Usually only 1–5 boils are seen but infestations with 87 and 92 larvae have been recorded. Several species of wild animals serve as hosts, particularly the African giant rat and various duikers (antelopes); other hosts include shrews, monkeys, gerbils, and rats.

CALLIPHORIDAE: METALLIC SPECIES

Cochliomyia hominivorax, New World screwworm (NWS)

The adult flies are 10–15 mm long, metallic green to bluish-green with three distinct dark longitudinal stripes down the thorax. The face is orange to reddish, with deep red eyes. In the larvae the tracheal breathing vessels are clearly seen in the posterior part of the parasite, being dark coloured in the last three segments of the larva; in the other North American screwworm fly, *C. macellaria,* the tracheal trunks are unpigmented.

Cochliomyia hominivorax is found from Belize and Guatemala to Uruguay and northern Chile, also including the West Indies; human cases of myiasis are quite common in these areas. *Cochliomyia hominivorax,* previously known as *Callitroga americana,* is an extremely destructive species whose larvae normally feed only on live hosts, although they can be cultured artificially under highly specific conditions. The female lays her batches of 10–500 eggs at the edge of any type of skin wound, no matter how small. These include tick bites, barbed wire cuts, castration and dehorning wounds, fresh brand sites, navels of newborn animals, the exposed tissues in broken horns, etc. Eggs may be laid on healthy mucous membranes, such as the vagina, especially after birth, and in the nasal passages and mouth. Carcasses are not used as a food source by NWS larvae, but because the adult flies commonly visit decaying material and faeces, they are able to transmit several pathogens. Cattle are the prime host for the larvae, but all warm-blooded animals seem at risk, including chickens. *Cochliomyia hominivorax* larvae were originally described from human cases in Cayenne, South America, the infestations leading to the death of three of the six men involved. Human infestations usually involve the ears, nose, mouth, and orbit; as with animals, the newborn infants can develop NWS myiasis and lesions may occur on the umbilicus. A total of 385 larvae were removed over a period of 9 days from a patient who had an infestation of the nasal passages.

Deep lesions are rapidly produced as the larvae invade the skin and excavate large holes up to 4–5 cm deep. The gregarious parasites embed themselves in the flesh, using their spines as anchors, and can be difficult to remove. The smell of the lesion attracts further ovipositing females, and a heavily infested wound may contain as many as 2000–3000 larvae. Foul-smelling discharges and bloody exudates often flow out of the wounds. Antibodies to the screwworm larvae can be detected after 7 days, peaking at 3 weeks and persisting for about 8 weeks (Thomas and Pruett 1992). The larvae feed for 4–8 days, after which they fall from the host to pupate in the soil. The life cycle takes about 3 weeks but may extend to 2–3 months in cool weather.

Control of C. hominivorax and the sterile insect technique

The wounds caused in man by New World screwworm—or any other dermal myiasis species—can be treated by first cleaning them, then dusting or packing with antibiotic powder. Serious healing problems are rare unless the people who have been infested are far from medical help. Lesions on animals are usually dusted or sprayed with an organophosphorous (OP) insecticide such as coumaphos; synthetic pyrethroids are also very effective. Adult screwworm fly populations have also been effectively reduced using the so-called screwworm adult suppression system (SWASS). This involves the distribution of pellets containing a mixture of dried blood, sugar, corn cob grits, dichlorvos OP insecticide, and the insect attractant Swormlure-2. The technique proved useful in the USA and northern Mexico, although less so in more humid areas. Much greater success was obtained with the sterile male or sterile insect technique (SIT), a form of birth control. Huge numbers of flies are reared artifically, their larvae allowed to develop to the early pupal stage, then sterilized by radiation from caesium-137. The pupae are then dropped by air in the target area, so that overwhelming numbers of sterile male flies emerge to mate with the existing females. Each NWS female mates only once so that each mating effectively ends her reproductive life, and no eggs will be laid if she pairs with a sterile male. The massive numbers of sterile male flies introduced into the target area can lead to the eradication of the original population within a few months. SIT eradicated NWS from the southern USA and Mexico and it is hoped to clear the pest from Central America during the next few years.

The most recent example of the SIT eradication of *C. hominivorax* from an entire country took place in Libya in 1991. Cases of NWS myiasis had suddenly appeared in sheep in Libya March 1988 (Gabaj and Beesley 1989), following a year when there had already been a large number of myiasis problems in farm livestock. The 1988 screwworm infestations probably originated in a consignment of Uruguayan sheep. The outbreak of disease posed an enormous threat to both livestock and man in North Africa, and it was quite likely that the pest would spread to much of Africa. Cases of human infestation were soon added to those on animals, but the main worry centred on the livestock, and by the end of the outbreak in April 1991 more than 14 400 cases of NWS myiasis in animals had been identified and treated. As in all warm countries, several other species of myiasis larvae were involved with the livestock in addition to NWS.

In 1988 the UN Food and Agriculture Organization (FAO) decided to set up a programme for the control of the screwworm outbreak in North Africa.

Preliminary work occupied most of 1989–90 and the actual SIT operation was carried out during the first 4 months of 1991. The operation was completely successful. It was also one of the most outstanding examples of international collaboration in animal health ever organized. The $80 million cost of the programme involved Libya (over $25m), the USA, Mexico, Australia, and most European countries, as well as multi-donor institutions such as UNDP, the UN International Atomic Energy Agency, the European Community, and OPEC (Food and Agriculture Organization 1992).

Cochliomyia macellaria is the 'secondary screwworm' and occurs from south-east Canada to Argentina. It is not an obligatory myiasis fly and tends to be much more common than *C. hominivorax*. It lays 25–500 eggs at each oviposition and completes its life cycle in only half the time taken by *C. hominivorax*.

It is possible that other species of screwworm, such as *C. minima* and *C. aldrichi*, presently known only from South and Central America, may move in to fill the ecological niches left by the eradication of *C. hominivorax* and appropriate surveillance is being carried out by FAO.

Chrysomya bezziana, Old World screwworm (OWS)

Some 10 species of *Chrysomya* (sometimes incorrectly spelled as (*Chrysomyia*) can cause myiasis in man, but only *C. bezziana*, the Old World screwworm, is medically important. *Chrysomya bezziana* adults measure 6–12 mm and are metallic green or blue, with dark legs. For several years it was confused with *C. megacephala* (see next species), the correct name being allocated by Villeneuve in 1914. Like *Cochliomyia hominivorax* its larvae cause an obligatory and extremely destructive myiasis, while the larvae of other *Chrysomya* species usually develop in carcasses and decomposing material. *Chrysomya bezziana* occurs in many African and Asian countries, from India and China to Papua New Guinea, and a few cases in animals have been reported from the Middle East, e.g. Bahrein. A wide range of host species can be infested, including man, cattle, buffaloes, sheep, horses, dogs, camels, antelopes, elephants, and rhinoceros, although infestations are most usual in animals. *Chrysomya bezziana* was first described from cattle in the Congo in 1910 but human infestations were not seen until 1920, in India. The first cases seen in Africa involved a man who had 163 larvae in a facial wound. The overriding concern with *C. bezziana* is that it may arrive in northern Australia, either in the form of adult flies blown by wind from Papua New Guinea or as larvae in the wounds of imported animals.

The adult female lays batches of 150–600 eggs in wounds, ulcers, scratches, and mucous membranes,

much as does *C. hominivorax*. The larvae complete their development in about 5–6 days, then fall from the wound to pupate on the ground. The entire life cycle can be as short as 20 days. Severe and multiple lesion can lead to the death of livestock. Adult flies will feed on dead animals, decaying material, cow dung, etc. Individual lesions in man may contain many hundreds of larvae and, all parts of the body are at risk, especially soft skin soft or mucous tissue. Leg ulcers and discharging wounds are likewise attractive sites for ovipositing flies. A mixed infection of *C. bezziana* and a *Sarcophaga* species was recorded in a bone-deep non-healing leg ulcer of a drug addict in India (Fotedar *et al.* 1991). The lesion had expanded largely because of the relative unresponsiveness to pain of the patient.

Treatment of OWS lesions is similar to that used for NWS myiasis; it is of interest that *C. bezziana* larvae are killed following the injection of ivermectin so long as the lesions are not too well established.

Chrysomya megacephala

Chrysomya megacephala, the oriental latrine fly, was originally described by Fabricius in 1794 as *Musca megacephala*. Until Villeneuve in 1914 was able to separate it from *Chrysomya bezziana* many cases of myiasis in man and animals were wrongly attributed to '*C. dux*', one of the previous names for *C. megacephala*. Morphological details of the two species are given in Zumpt (1965). It is now established that *C. megacephala* breeds mainly in faeces and carrion, the larvae only occasionally being found in wounds as a facultative myiasis species. As well as man, it can infest existing wounds of cattle, sheep, and equines in Asia and Australia, and larvae were collected from sheep in Libya during the New World screwworm control programme. Other species of *Chrysomya* which can cause human myiasis are *C. chloropyga*, *C. mallochi*, *C. putoria*, and *C. inclinata*.

Lucilia sericata and *L. cuprina*, greenbottles, sheep blowflies

Lucilia sericata was first described, as *Musca sericata*, by Meigen in 1826; in 1830 it was moved by Robineau-Desvoidy to his new genus *Lucilia*. In the same year Wiedemann named *Musca cuprina* from a specimen collected in China, and this species was renamed *L. cuprina* in 1928. Both species were allocated to the genus *Phaenicia* and *L. sericata* is often known as *P. sericata* in the USA today. Interestingly enough, Linnaeus named only one *Lucilia*, which he called *Musca caesar*, in his 1758 Systema Naturae. *Lucilia sericata* is shiny green while *L. cuprina* is copper coloured; both have prominent spines on the thorax.

Lucilia sericata is often known as the European sheep blowfly, but its distribution extends to the USA ('fleeceworm'), South Africa and the Antipodes. *Lucilia cuprina* is common in many parts of Africa, and probably spread from that continent to Asia. It also seems to have moved from South Africa to Australia in the late nineteenth century, and has become a very important pest of sheep in that country. Another name for both species is sheep strike fly, strike being a term for myiasis and fleeceworms (USA). The involvement of the larvae of greenbottle flies in myiasis wounds in sheep was recorded in England in 1534 by J. Fitzherbert in his 'Bookes on Husbandry', and there is no doubt that the condition had already been known to farmers for hundreds of years.

The females feed and lay their eggs on fresh or decaying meat, fish, and carcasses but will also oviposit on live animals, usually sheep, when their larvae can cause serious myiasis. It is possible that only certain strains of both species cause myiasis. *Lucilia sericata* and *L. cuprina* are both primary strike flies, i.e. their larvae can penetrate intact as well as damaged skin. Myiasis lesions are most commonly seen on the hindquarters and loins, although sheep shearing wounds, barbed wire cuts, damaged horns, tick-bites, and the umbilical area in the newborn are all attractive to ovipositing females. Weakened, sick or neglected people or animals are at risk from blowfly myiasis. An elderly debilitated patient admitted to a a London hospital presented with several third instar *L. sericata* larvae feeding in an existing lesion on his leg.

Lucilia larvae spend about 5 days feeding on the sheep, creating lesions which are usually shallow rather than deep, but which can lead to 'toxaemia', loss of skin insulation and secondary bacterial infection. The larvae have the advantage of living in warm tissues under the protection of the fleece, whereas those which are feeding on carrion, abattoir refuse, etc. may take 11 days to complete their development. The pupal period lasts 4–25 days, and the entire life cycle can be completed in 9 days if myiasis forms a part of development.

The lesions do not usually lead to the death of the sheep, but in very severe cases sheep can die in only 5–10 days. The larvae can even penetrate through the body wall into the abdominal cavity (personal observation). More usually the sheep becomes very irritable, the lesion(s) eventually occupying an area of several square centimetres. This encourages further oviposition by other species of *Lucilia*, as well as by *Calliphora* and *Protophormia*, both facultative myiasis genera.

Sheep are dipped, sprayed, or high-power jetted to protect them against blowfly myiasis (Beesley 1985, 1986). Good hygiene and, if necessary, the treatment of breeding sites with persistent insecticides will help to reduce the numbers of blowflies.

Human infestations with *L. sericata* and *L. cuprina* are rare, but eggs can be laid in wounds and ulcers, especially when these are foul-smelling and purulent. The larvae may be seen in the soiled dressings of patients and can invade the covered wounds. Paracelsus noticed in the early sixteenth century that wounds which had become infested with 'fly maggots' healed more quickly than those kept free of larvae, and this formed the basis of a cleaning and healing treatment. Blowfly larvae ingest necrotic and secondarily infected tissue, leaving a base of healthy pink tissue. The beneficial effect of the larvae is due partly to their mechanical scavenging activity and partly to their secretion of a collagenase. Unfortunately, the larvae may go on to attack healthy tissue if there is insufficient necrotic material available. *Lucilia sericata* larvae were used to help heal tissues damaged by osteomyelitis, amputation, shell splinters, etc. during the Napoleonic wars and into the First World War, when W. S. Baer found badly wounded men in surprisingly good condition despite infestation of their wounds with thousands of *Lucilia* larvae. It was shown that larvae of *L. sericata* are superior in healing activity to those of other species and as late as 1934 at least 5800 cases were recorded where surgeons in the USA and Canada had used *L. sericata* maggot therapy with great success. Georgi (1985) cites a case of an American prisoner of war in Vietnam who treated his wounds with blowfly larvae, flushing them out with his own urine 'once the maggots had done their work to his satisfaction'.

The reaction by the sheep host to invasion by larvae of *L. cuprina* involves a massive cellular immune response within 48 hours, mainly by the migration of neutrophils (Bowles *et al.*, 1992). The cellular infiltration which follows both primary and secondary invasion suggests polyclonal activation of T cells and their selective recruitment to the lesion site. Studies along these lines are part of a research programme which it is hoped will eventually yield a vaccine sutable for the protection of sheep against blowfly myiasis (see Nelson 1987).

Calliphora spp., bluebottle flies

These are large, robust flies, usually bluish or blue-black and with a very hairy appearance. As with *Lucilia* there are strong black bristles on the thorax. The life cycle is similar to that of *Lucilia*, but species can be oviparous or ovoviviparous, in which case the eggs hatch immediately. *Calliphora stygia* is oviparous in Australia, but lays first instar larvae in warm weather. In sheep, *C. augur*, *C. albifrontalis*, *C. stygia*, and *C. nociva* can cause severe myiasis, often penetrating unbroken skin (primary myiasis). Other species, such as *C. vomitoria*, are involved in secondary myiasis, occurring only in lesions already created by accidental cuts, etc., or produced by the larvae of other species of blowflies. Wounds in man have been found infested with larvae of *C. vicina*, *C. vomitoria*, and *C. croceipalpis*, and *C. vicina* has also been found in human urogenital myiasis. As with *Lucilia*, *Calliphora* larvae may appear in the faeces following the ingestion of contaminated food.

Protophormia (=*Phormia*) *terraenovae* and *Phormia regina*, the black blowflies

These species have a shiny black or purplish-black thorax and abdomen. *Protophormia terraenovae* is common in countries outside the tropics, its range extending to within 1000 km of the North Pole (Oldroyd and Smith 1973). It is normally saprophytic but can cause primary or secondary myiasis in sheep in Europe and North America. It has also been recovered from sores and wounds in people in the USA. Larvae of *P. regina* are also usually saprophytic, feeding on carrion, but they can cause myiasis in sheep as well as being responsible for dermal or enteric myiasis in man in North America but not apparently in the Old World (Zumpt 1965).

SARCOPHAGIDAE, FLESHFLIES

The sarcophagids, *Sarcophaga* and *Wohlfahrtia*, are large, hairy and non-metallic flies which have three black or dark-brown stripes down the thorax. The abdomen of *Sarcophaga* has a heavy black on grey chess board pattern, while *Wohlfahrtia* usually has a less dense but clearer pattern of spots and triangles. Most sarcophagids reduce the length of their life cycle by depositing very active first-instar larvae, rather than eggs, although *S. crassipalpis* lays eggs which contain fully developed first-stage larvae, ready for immediate hatch. Thus the sarcophagids have a great advantage over calliphorids breeding on carrion, as larvae of the latter may have to wait more than 24 hours before emerging from the egg. Sarcophagid larvae take only 3–4 days to complete their development. Myiasis due to *Sarcophaga* is less common than that involving *Wohlfahrtia*. In contrast to calliphorid larvae, the posterior spiracles of sarcophagid larvae are hidden, recessed in a deep pit.

Sarcophaga haemorrhoidalis

Sarcophaga is associated with man throughout the world and many species have been incriminated as facultative myiasis flies. Twenty of these affect man (Zumpt 1965), mainly by pseudomyiasis of the alimentary tract but sometimes by lesions of the ear, etc. *Sarcophaga* larvae are commonly deposited by the female fly during the act of defaecation. Contaminated food containing newly hatched or mature larvae may

be swallowed, giving rise to pain, digestive disturbances or nervous disorders. Live or dead larvae may be passed. In wounds, *S. haemorrhoidalis* is the usual species observed, although it tends to follow some other calliphorid which has acted as the primary parasite, e.g. *Lucilia sericata* or *Wohlfahrtia magnifica*. In Libya, *S. tibialis* was found in scalp lesions associated with ringworm disease (*Microsporum audouini*).

Wohlfahrtia magnifica, Wohlfahrt's wound myiasis fly

In 1770, Dr J. A. Wohlfahrt, a physician in Halle, near Leipzig, Germany, extracted a fly larvae from the eye of a patient. One hundred years later Schiner named this species *Sarcophila magnifica* and in 1916 it became *Wohlfahrtia magnifica* (Zumpt 1965). This is the most important species, the others being *W. nuba* and the North American *W. vigil*. All are obligatory parasites of warm-blooded animals, including man.

Wohlfahrtia magnifica occurs all round the Mediterranean and through the Middle East to Asiatic Russia and China. It seems able to attack all species of domesticated animals, especially sheep, cattle and camels, and also geese. Oddly enough, although it must surely parasitize wild animals, no such records are available. In both man and animals the larvae may be deposited in wounds, cuts, and sores; in humans they often infest the ear, nose, or orbit, causing great pain as they do so. In the ear they may penetrate as far as the ear drum, leading to deafness, while in the eye there may be destruction of the eyeball. Severe damage may be caused to the nasal tissues and this may even be fatal. Nevertheless, myiasis due to *Wohlfahrtia* hardly ever compares with the damage caused by screwworm larvae.

Larval development takes 5–8 days, the adults emerging from the puparia after 8–15 days. Of interest is the great resilience of *W. magnifica* larvae, which have produced normal adult flies after exposure to 95 per cent ethanol for 1 hour (Kettle 1990).

Wohlfahrtia nuba, a smaller version of *W. magnifica*, occurs from West Africa to Pakistan. It causes a traumatic wound myiasis in man and animals; it is also said to have been reared from dead locusts.

Wohlfahrtia vigil occurs in North America from Alaska and Nova Scotia to approximately 35°N in the western USA (subspecies *opaca*) and 40°N in the east (subspecies *vigil*). Larvae are dropped on to the skin, but penetrate only if it is tender so that infants and young children are the principal targets. Small, boil-like lesions reminiscent of tumbu fly lesions are produced, usually on the neck, chest or navel. There are usually 12–14 lesions, rarely up to 20 (Kettle 1990) The lesions caused by *W. vigil* are shallower than those produced by the other two species, which eat further into the tissues.

As *Wohlfahrtia* is not attracted to carcasses, good garbage hygiene has little effect on its activity. Adult rats, and possibly other rodents and lagomorphs, seem to be important hosts, and their control can help to reduce the population of *Wohlfahrtia*. Larvae are removed by simply squeezing them out, followed by suitable treatment of the lesions.

GASTEROPHILIDAE

Gasterophilus, horse bot fly

Linnaeus named *G. haemorrhoidalis* and *nasalis* in 1758, de Geer following with *G. intestinalis* in 1776. Various generic names have since been applied to *Gasterophilus*, including the incorrect *Gastrophilus* and the quite descriptive *Stomachobia*. *Gastetrophilus* was originally placed in the Oestridae, but this family has now been split into several much more valid family divisions (see later). The family Gasterophilidae includes six genera which cause myiasis, but only *Gasterophilus* itself affects man. Its nine species all parasitize equines and at least four of these can affect man: *G. pecorum*, *G. nigricornis*, *G. haemorrhoidalis*, and *G. inermis*. *Gasterophilus intestinalis* is very common but is not a proven human myiasis species (Zumpt 1965).

The adult fly resembles a large hairy bee, but it does of course differ in having only one pair of wings and no mouthparts. During its short life span the female fly will hope to lay 160–2400 eggs, depending on its size. The female flies irritate horses by their persistent attacks while attempting to stick their eggs to the hairs of the host. In most species the eggs are attached to hairs, the first instar larvae usually remaining within the egg until stimulated to emerge by warmth and friction. In practice this is caused by the licking action of the host's tongue. In some species the eggs hatch and the larvae can penetrate unbroken skin. In *G. pecorum* the eggs are laid on the leaves of plants and are ingested as the host feeds. First—instar larvae of *Gasterophilus* penetrate the tongue, lips or inside of the cheek and begin a migration which may leave microabscesses in its tunnels and which ends when the spiny red third instar larvae firmly attach to the wall of the stomach, intestine, or rectum of the equine, depending upon the species.

First-instar larvae of *G. pecorum* and *G. haemorrhoidalis* can penetrate human skin and cause a creeping myiasis as they move along just under the skin. This may leave a prominent indurated track in its wake. The first-instar larvae cannot develop to the second instar in man.

CUTEREBRIDAE

Dermatobia hominis (=*cyaniventris*), human bot fly

This species was originally named *Oestrus hominis* by 'Linnaeus junior' in 1781, i.e. 3 years after the death of his systematist father. It seems likely therefore that at least one of the species of animals and plants described by Carl Linnaeus was named posthumously by his son.

Dermatobia hominis is a little larger than the housefly, with a yellow head, grey thorax and shiny dark blue abdomen It occurs in moist, cool tropical highlands up to about 2000 metres above sea-level, from Mexico to northern Chile and Argentina, and also in the West Indies. It can be a problem in coffee areas. The larvae are obligatory parasites of man and many other mammal hosts, also chickens and turkeys. Cattle are probably a significant host for this parasite. The female flies are peculiar in that they do not feed. They also attach their eggs to the bodies of 'slave flies' such as mosquitoes, muscids, etc., a total of some 50 species of phoresy flies being used in this way. The larvae develop within the eggs in 4–9 days but hatch only when the 'host' fly begins to feed on an animal or man. The warmth of that host stimulates the larvae to emerge from their egg shells and invade the skin, using the puncture made by the blood-feeding carrier fly or penetrating the unbroken skin. They can bury themselves in 5–15 minutes.

The larvae burrow into the subdermis and grow within boil-like swellings, growing to the 20–25 mm third instar in 4–12 weeks, although this stage of development may occupy 18 weeks. The second-stage larvae are pear-shaped, while the third stage are grub-like and have a pair of stout mouth hooks. Myiasis lesions may appear on almost any part of the body, often becoming infected with bacteria and causing much pain. Animals are usually infested on the back and flanks. In man the orbit, scalp, nose, arms, abdomen, buttocks, genitals, etc. may be attacked, the site of the lesion depending entirely upon the original site used by the fly which carried the *Dermatobia* eggs. One enterprising entomologist, August Busck, deliberately reared *D. hominis* in his arm and described the succeeding events (Busck 1912). There are two records of fatalities, in a 5-month-old and an 18-month-old child, in which a larva penetrated the soft bone of the skull and entered the brain.

In cattle in particular several boils may be confluent and often attract screwworm flies, sarcophagids, etc., so that the ultimate lesion can be extremely unpleasant. Young animals in particular may become so badly affected as to die from tissue destruction and 'toxaemia'. The larvae complete their development in 5–10 weeks, after which they fall to the ground and pupate for a similar time before emergence of the adult fly.

Larvae may be encouraged to withdraw from their lesions by the application of grease, fat, or vaseline, which clogs the posterior respiratory spiracles. Surgical removal of the larvae may be necessary, especially if the eye is affected. Suitably treated lesions heal after a week or so.

In animals the use of organophosphorous and synthetic pyrethroid insecticidal dips, sprays and dressings is effective against *Dermatobia*. Ivermectin, given to cattle by subcutaneous injection, has also given satisfactory results.

Cuterebra, the type genus of the family, occurs in North America and has four species. It very rarely acts as a human parasite, normally causing myiasis in rodents and rabbits. Eggs are laid near the entrance to the burrow and the larvae penetrate the skin to form cyst-like subcutaneous swellings. In *C. emasculator* the larvae parasitize the scrotum and can castrate the host. Cats and dogs may become infected with other species, as may man, who may suffer dermal or nasal myiasis.

OESTRIDAE

'Oestrids' formerly included all those species now classified in the families Gasterophilidae, Cuterebridae, Oestridae, and Hypodermatidae. It is now accepted that the Oestridae *sensu strictu* contain some 20 genera (Zumpt 1965); only *Oestrus ovis* itself is of some importance as a cause of human myiasis.

The Oestridae have relatively wide and large heads and rather stout bodies. They are all obligatory myiasis species, attacking man and his livestock. All have vestigial mouthparts, and although they have an alimentary tract seem able to take little if any sustenance. The same peculiarity occurs in some species of moths. Oestrid flies can live for only a few days, during which time they must mate and oviposit—or larviposit, in the case of *Oestrus ovis*.

Oestrus ovis

There are at least six species of *Oestrus*, of which the most important is *O. ovis*, the sheep nasal bot fly. This is also the only species to attack man. *Oestrus ovis* occurs throughout the world in sheep- and goat-farming areas. Adults have black tubercles on the head and thorax and a patterned black and grey abdomen. Larvae and adults of the sheep nasal fly were already known to Redi in 1686 and to Réaumur in 1734, before Linnaeus fully described it in 1758 in his *Systema Naturae*. Portchinsky (1913) eventually showed that the female fly hatches her eggs within her body, then flicks the first-instar larvae into the nasal orifices of sheep. As with *Gasterophilus* laying their eggs on horses, the female *O. ovis* flies irritate the sheep as they continually fly around the head attempting to deposit their larvae. The young larvae then climb up the nasal passages, developing through the three instars and causing much pain and distress to the host as they grow and feed. The fully mature spiny larvae are 25 mm in length. As many as 138 mature larvae have been recovered from a single infested host. Individual larvae from the same larviposition may take 1–9 months before they are mature. They

are eventually sneezed or snorted out from the nasal passages, pupating on the ground for 1–2 months.

Human infestation with *O. ovis* is quite common along the Mediterranean coast, the Middle East, and India, and presents a minor problem in some parts of Russia, South Africa, the United States, and the Pacific. In people, usually shepherds and goatherds, the tiny first-instar larvae produce irritation in the eye, the usual site in man; the infestation may be quite painful. The adult flies are obviously attracted to herdsmen who have fed on fresh milk or cheese from their sheep or goats and who carry the corresponding aroma. *Oestrus ovis* larvae can infest other parts of the human host as well as the nose: five Iraqi patients had larvae in their ears, nose, or throat. The larvae were 2–8 mm in length and were all in their first instar (Al-Dabagh *et al.* 1980). Dogs, usually those used as guard animals around the flock, can also become infested with larvae of *O. ovis*.

Rhinoestrus purpureus is the horse nasal bot fly. Like *O. ovis*, it was originally confined to the palaearctic region, but has spread with equines to many areas of Africa and the east. It is not unlike *O. ovis* in appearance and its biology is similar, using its ovipositor to flick first-stage larvae into the nose of the host. Up to 200 larvae have been recovered from the nasal and pharyngeal passages, throat, and base of the tongue, so that this is a serious veterinary problem in Russia and elsewhere. There have been several records of human ocular myiasis due to *R. purpureus*.

HYPODERMATIDAE

Hypoderma lineatum and H. bovis, cattle grubs or warbles

The hypodermatids share with *Oestrus* the oestrid characters of vestigial mouthparts in the adult and obligatory myiasis in the larvae, but they are hairy and quite unlike the tuberculate adults of the true Oestridae, so that they merit their own family, the Hypodermatidae. *Hypoderma* itself is confined to the temperate regions of the northern hemisphere, where its larvae parasitize mainly bovids and cervids. *Hypoderma lineatum* and *H. bovis* very rarely affect man; *H. diana* of red deer is an even rarer species in man.

The irritating effect of warble flies on cattle and the serious economic effects of their larvae on the skins intended for leather manufacture has been known since Roman times, but the first scientific paper on the subject was that by Vallisnieri in 1710. *Hypoderma bovis* was described as *Oestrus bovis* by Linnaeus in 1758 and '*O. lineatus*' by De Villers in 1798. Because the second and third larval stages of *Hypoderma* live in cysts under the skin of cattle, it was originally thought that the larvae hatched from eggs injected subcutaneously by the female fly, hence the generic name. It was next erroneously believed that the eggs or larvae were licked from the skin and swallowed, as happens with the horse bot fly, *Gasterophilus*. It is now known that the eggs of *Hypoderma* are attached to the hairs of the underside of the body, the young larvae then spiralling down the hair to penetrate the skin via the hair follicles. After a 5–6 month migration, through the connective tissues and the oesophagus (*H. lineatum*) or epidural fat (*H. bovis*) the larvae reach the skin of the back, where they rest and feed for a further 4–6 weeks while they moult into the second and third instars. These are encysted by the host and the 25 mm third-stage stage larva later falls to the ground to pupate.

Infections of people and horses usually involve only single larvae, in contrast to the 20–30 which commonly occur in cattle. *Hypoderma* myiasis in man nearly always involves *H. lineatum* and tends to occur in farm children. *Hypoderma* eggs are laid on the hairs of the body, probably the legs or arms, but larvae are not noticed until they surface, usually in the gum or on the scalp and still in their first instar. Larvae may also appear in skin of the back, abdomen, chest, or genital region. Third-stage larvae can reach 20 mm in length but in man are usually no more than 5–12 mm long. In one case in England a boy of 7 years had a larva which broke the surface of the skin just above the right eyebrow. A 3-year-old Belgian girl was affected by three *Hypoderma* larvae which surfaced in the parietal and temporal regions of her head (Leclerq 1969). A Norwegian surgeon described 22 cases of human myiasis with *Hypoderma* larvae, often causing painful swellings and abscesses (Zumpt 1965) Extensive intra-cranial haematomata due to migrating *Hypoderma* larvae have been recorded in man and horses, while larvae of the closely related reindeer warble fly, *Oedemagena tarandi*, can cause ophthalmomyiasis in people in Scandinavia. The larval migrations sometimes seen in man and horses would seem to mimic the extensive travels of the larvae in cattle.

Antibodies are produced against the first-stage larvae while they are actively migrating through the tissues, and serological tests have been devised for the detection of infestations both in cattle and man. Antibodies continue to circulate for up to 6 months after the-first-stage larvae have died or been killed with insecticide. At least three larval proteins, one a collagenase, are immunogenic. The early crude gel diffusion precipitin tests used in cattle have given way to ELISA and micro-ELISA techniques, which reveal the presence of infestation well before the larvae arrive in the skin of the back.

Because of the importance of warble grub damage to the leather industry, strenuous attempts have been made in many countries to eradicate the pest. This has been almost completely successful in Britain and Ireland, using organophophorous insecticides and ivermectin.

REFERENCES

Al-Dabagh, M., Al-Mufti, N., Shafiq, M., Al-Rawas, A.Y., and Al-Safar, S. (1980). *Annals of Tropical Medicine and Parasitology*, **74**, 73–7.

Beesley, W. N. (1985). Flies and myiasis. In *Parasites, pests and predators*, (ed. S. M. Gaafar), pp. 299–315. Elsevier, Amsterdam.

Beesley, W. N. (1986). Insect infestations of domestic animals. In *Chemotherapy of parasitic diseases*, (ed. W. C. Campbell and R. S. Rew) pp. 551–66. Plenum Press, New York.

Blacklock, B. and Gordon, R. M. (1927). Experimental production of immunity against metazoan parasites and an investigation of its nature. *Annals of Tropical Medicine and Parasitology*, **21**, 181–224.

Bowles, V. Grey, S. T., and Brandon, M. R. (1992). Cellular immune responses in the skin of sheep infected with larvae of Lucilia cuprina. *Veterinary Parasitology*, **44**, 151–62.

Busck, A. (1912). On the rearing of *Dermatobia hominis*. *Proceedings of the Entomological Society of Washington*, **14**, 9–12

Food and Agriculture Organization (1992). *The New World Screwworm eradication programme*. FAO, Rome.

Fotedar, R., Banergee, U., and Verma, A. K. (1991). Human cutaneous myiasis due to mixed infestation in a drug addict. *Annals of Tropical Medicine and Parasitology*, **85**, 339–40.

Fox, M. T., Jacobs, D. E., Hall, M. J. R., Bennett, M. P. (1992). Tumb fly (*Cordylobia anthropophaga*) myiasis in a quarantined dog in England. *Veterinary Record*, **130**, 100–101.

Gabaj, M. M. and Beesley, W. N. (1989). American screwworm fly in Libya. *Veterinary Record*, **124**, 152.

Georgi, J. R. (1985). *Parasitology for veterinarians*, (4th edn). Saunders, Philadelphia.

Jenyns, L. (1839). Note of a case in which *Fannia canicularis* larvae were expelled from the human intestine. *Transactions of the Royal Entomological Society of London*, **11**, 152–6.

Kettle, D. S. (1990). *Medical and veterinary entomology*. Commonwealth Agricultural Bureaux (CAB) International, Wallingford, Oxford.

Leclercq, M. (1969) *Entomological parasitology*. Pergamon, Oxford.

Nelson, W. A. (1987). Blood-sucking and myiasis-producing arthropods. In *Immune responses in parasitic infections: immunology, immunopathology and immunoprophylaxis, vol. IV: Protozoa, arthropods and invertebrates*, (ed. E. J. L. Soulsby) pp. 175–209. CRC Press, Boca Raton, Florida.

Oldroyd, H. and Smith, K. G. V. (1973). Eggs and larvae of flies, In *Insects and arthropods of medical importance*, (ed. K. G. V. Smith) pp. 269–323. British Museum (Natural History), London.

Thomas, D. B. and Pruett, J. H. (1992). Kinetic development and decline of antiscrewworm antibodies in the sera of infested sheep. *Journal of Medical Entomology*, **29**, 870–3.

Zumpt, F. (1965) *Myiasis in man and animals in the Old World*. Butterworths, London.

FURTHER READING

James, M. J. (1947). *The flies that cause myiasis in man*. United States Department of Agriculture, Miscellaneous Publication No. 631. USDA, Washington.

Smith, K. G. V. (1973). *Insects and other arthropods of medical importance*. British Museum (Natural History), London.

Soulsby, E. J. L. (1982). *Helminths, arthropods and protozoa of domesticated animals*, (7th edn). Baillière Tindall, London.

68   HISTOPLASMOSIS

K. D. Clinkenbeard

SUMMARY

The dimorphic fungus *Histoplasma capsulatum* is a facultative intracellular pathogen of the mononuclear phagocytic system of human beings and animals and causes disease with high morbidity but low mortality. *Histoplasma capsulatum* var. *capsulatum* is a saprophytic soil fungus of temperate climates, particularly North America. High levels of soil contamination with *Histoplasma* organisms is associated with bird roosting areas and bat-infested caves. Infection is by inhalation of microconidia or mycelial fragments resulting in a clinically inapparent pulmonary infection or a transient 'flu-like' pneumonitis. More severe disseminated histoplasmosis can be a sequela to pulmonary histoplasmosis in immunocompromised hosts or from high exposure to *Histoplasma* organisms. Two other variants, *Histoplasma capsulatum* var. *farciminosum* and *Histoplasma capsulatum* var. *duboisii* cause epizootic lymphangitis in horses and African histoplasmosis in human beings, respectively. Histoplasmosis caused by variants *capsulatum* and *duboisii* are infectious, non-contagious diseases in which control consists of reducing exposure to dusts from highly contaminated environments, whereas epizootic lymphangitis is contagious via insect or arthropod vectors in which control of vector and quarantine and depopulation are employed.

HISTORY

The initial recognition of infection by the yeast organism which was subsequently classified as *Histoplasma capsulatum* was by Rivolta in 1873 from lymphocutaneous lesions in a horse (Rivolta 1873). He named the budding yeast *Cryptococcus farciminosum*. The disease entity produced was called pseudoglanders and is currently termed epizootic lymphangitis.

More than 30 years elapsed before recognition of the first case of infection by *Histoplasma* in a human being. In 1905, Samuel T. Darling, a US Army pathologist in the Panama Canal Zone, identified what he thought was a *Leishmania*-like protozoan parasite, while examining microscopic smears of lung, spleen, and bone marrow of a patient suspected of succumbing to miliary tuberculosis (Darling 1906). He named the organism *Histoplasma capsulatum*, because it appeared to be an encapsulated protozoan-like organism associated with the reticuloendothelial system.

The identity of Darling's *Histoplasma* organism as a fungi was not made until 1912 when the mycologist Henrique da Rocha-Lima (1912) reviewed some of Darling's slides. Da Rocha-Lima noted the cytological similarities between the Darling's *Histoplasma* organism and *Cryptococcus farciminosum*. Ironically, the misnomer *Histoplasma* was retained for these fungi when Redaelli and Ciferri (1934) reclassified *Cryptococcus farciminosum* as *Histoplasma farciminosum* in 1934. *Histoplasma farciminosum* was again reclassified as a variant of *Histoplasma capsulatum* (var. *farciminosum*) in 1985 (Weeks *et al.* 1985).

A larger yeast species of *Histoplasma* was recognized in 1943 by J. T. Duncan (1947) on histopathological examination of a skin lesion from an English mining engineer residing in Ghana. Several other cases of infection by this species, termed African histoplasmosis, were described before case material shared by A. Dubois with Vanbreusent in 1952 was studied, and the organism classified as *Histoplasma duboisii* (Dubois *et al.* 1952). In 1957, *Histoplasma duboisii* was again reclassified as *Histoplasma capsulatum* var. *duboisii* (Drouhet, 1957).

Between 1906 and 1932, several additional cases of Darling's histoplasmosis were identified at necropsy in Panama and in the US, before the first ante-mortum case was recognized by Edna H. Tompkins at Vanderbilt University on a blood smear from a child suffering from an unexplained febrile disease (Dodd and Tomkins 1934). *Histoplasma capsulatum* was cultured from this case and demonstrated to be a dimorphoric fungus by William A. De Monbreum and subsequently confirmed by others (Ciferri and Redaelli 1934; De Monbreum 1934; Conant 1941).

The initial recognized cases of human histoplasmosis were severe, systemic forms typically diagnosed at necropsy, but in 1939 De Monbreum, Goodpasture, and collaborators diagnosed ante-mortum a natural case of histoplasmosis in a dog (De Monbreum 1939). Subsequently, De Monbreum was able to demonstrate experimentally that clinically inapparent histoplasmosis occurred in dogs. Based on these observations and at that time recent characterization of the severe and mild forms of coccidiomycosis, De Monbreum speculated that histoplasmosis was more common than recognized and that natural clinically inapparent infections also occurred.

De Monbreum (1939) and others had speculated that animals might represent the source of infection for man. Several epizootics in dogs suggested a common source exposure, and the route of exposure was speculated to be inhalation of air-borne organisms (Menges 1951). C. W. Emmons (1949) was able to demonstrate that *Histoplasma capsulatum* was a soil saprophyte and that inhalation of aerosolized microconidia and mycelial fragments was the source of infection. Menges and co-workers were able to document a point source epizootic of histoplasmosis in dogs and human beings involving exposure to a *Histoplasma*-contaminated chicken coop (Menges *et al.* 1954). This work was expanded by Ajello, Emmons, and others to demonstrate that aerosolized soils contaminated with bird or bat guano are primary potential sources of *Histoplasma capsulatum* exposure (Ajello and Zeidberg 1951; Emmons 1958).

By 1945, 71 cases of severe human histoplasmosis, termed disseminated histoplasmosis, had been reported (Parsons and Zarafonetis 1945), but in that year Christie and Peterson (1945) used a delayed-type hypersensitivity skin test to extracted *Histoplasma* antigen to demonstrate that asymptomatic pulmonary histoplasmosis was common in human beings. They were able to show that asymptomatic pulmonary histoplasmosis was the cause of non-tuberculous pulmonary calcification common in human beings in the midwestern United States. The high prevalence of asymptomatic pulmonary histoplasmosis was confirmed by Palmer (1945) in a large survey of histoplasmin skin reactivity, and Edwards *et al.* (1969) and co-workers were able in a study of histoplasmin skin reactivity in naval recruits with life-long, one-county residents to delineate the river basins of the Mississippi River system as the endemic region for histoplasmosis in the United States.

In contrast to the non-contagious mode of transmission for infection by *Histoplasma capsulatum* var. *capsulatum*, Singh and co-workers studying outbreaks of epizootic lymphangitis in military horses and mules in India following the Second World War could not identify the environmental source for *Histoplasma capsulatum* var. *farciminosum* infection. However, the seasonal incidence, identification of the organism in the gut of biting flies, and demonstration of fomite transmission support a contagious mode of transmission by biting insects for epizootic lymphangitis (Singh, 1965, 1966; Singh *et al.*, 1965).

The clinicopathological manifestations of histoplasmosis have been compiled since the 1920s by many talented physicians, veterinarians, mycologists, and others. The work culminated in descriptions of the various clinical forms of epizootic lymphangitis in horses (Singh 1966), the clinical syndromes of African histoplasmosis in human beings (Cockshott and Lucas 1964), and the complex clinical entities comprising disseminated histoplasmosis for human beings, dogs, and cats (Goodwin *et al.* 1980; Clinkenbeard *et al.* 1987, 1988*a*) as well as manifestation of disseminated histoplasmosis in immunocompromised patients (Wheat *et al.* 1985). Numerous excellent reviews of histoplasmosis are available (Schwarz and Baum 1957, 1981; Domer and Moser 1980; Goodwin *et al.* 1980, 1981; Rippon 1988*a*,*b*; Maresca and Kobayashi 1989; Wu-Hsieh and Howard 1989).

THE AGENT

Three variants of *Histoplasma capsulatum* have been recognized: *Histoplasma capsulatum* var. *capsulatum*, *Histoplasma capsulatum* var. *duboisii*, and *Histoplasma capsulatum* var. *farciminosum*. *Histoplasma capsulatum* exists in the environment as a filamentous heterothallic ascomycete. The teleomorph is *Ajellomyces capsulatum* (formerly *Emonseilla capsulatum*) classified in the family Arthrodermataceae, order Onygenales of the Ascomycotina (Know-Chung 1972; Rippon 1988a). However, ubiquinone metabolite classification suggests that the *Histoplasma* teleomorphs belong to the genera *Emonseilla* rather than to *Ajellomyces* (Fukushima *et al.* 1991).

Several subclasses of *Histoplasma capsulatum* var. *capsulatum* are distinguished by restriction mapping nuclear, mitochondrial, or ribosomal DNA length pleomorphisms (Vincent *et al.* 1986; Spitzer *et al.* 1989; Keath *et al.* 1992). Polymerase chain reaction-based DNA fingerprinting using arbitrary primers can distinguish isolates within subclasses, suggesting that considerable genetic diversity may exist within subclasses (Kersulyte *et al.* 1992). Restriction fragment length polymorphisms of a *Histoplasma capsulatum*-specific nuclear gene *yps-3* can be used to distinguish *Histoplasma capsulatum* from morphologically or serologically similar fungal species: *Blastomyces dermatiditis*, *Candida* spp., *Chrysosporium keratinophilum*, and *Sepedonium chrysospermum* (Keath *et al.* 1992). In addition, chemiluminescent single-stranded DNA probes can be used to differentiate rRNA in lysates of clinical cultures of all variants of *Histoplasma capsulatum* from those of *Blastomyces dermatiditis*, *Coccidioides immitis*, *Paracoccidioides brasiliensis*, and morphologically related saprophytic fungi (Padhye *et al.* 1992; Stockman *et al.* 1993).

In laboratory culture at temperatures of less than 30 °C, *Histoplasma capsulatum* from infected tissues grows as white type A (albino) or brown type B (brown) mould colonies. Microscopically, septate hyphae produce 8–14 μm *Chrysosporium*-type tuberculate macroconidia similar to *Renispora flavissima* (Rippon 1988a). Microconidia of 2–4 μm are also produced. At temperatures above 30 °C, the filamentous form converts via pseudohyphae to a yeast form. Yeast cells are round to oval with a distinct single nucleus and form narrow-based buds.

In infected tissue, the yeast form of *Histoplasma capsulatum* is a facultative intracellular parasite of the mononuclear phagocyte system (MPS). The yeast cells are similar to that described for the yeast form in culture except for the appearance of a thin, nonstaining halo surrounding the yeast cells. This halo appears to be a capsule, and hence the name '*capsulatum*', but this halo has been attributed to 'drying artefacts' of the staining process (Larsh and Hall 1987). The yeast can be present extracellularly as well as intracellularly in the cytoplasm of macrophages (histiocytes) or circulating monocytes and are best visualized on cytological preparations stained with Romanoskytype stains. Occasionally, *Histoplasma* organisms are observed in neutrophils and rarely in eosinophils or megakaryocytes of infected hosts (Clinkenbeard *et al.* 1988a; Ferry *et al.* 1991). The yeast form of *Histoplasma capsulatum* var. *duboisii* are larger than *Histoplasma capsulatum* var. *capsulatum* or var. *farciminosum*. The variants can also be distinguished using monoclonal antibodies (Hamilton *et al.* 1990).

The dimorphoric conversion of inhaled microconidia and mycelial fragments to pseudohyphae and then to the yeast form is a complex process which can be triggered by temperatures above 30 °C and possibly other tissue environmental factors (Maresca and Kobayashi 1989). This conversion requires 6–8 days to occur and results in major changes in gene expression, cellular metabolism, and composition and structure of cellular organelles. Expression of heat-shock proteins (hsp) is required for yeast-phase transition, but heat-shock proteins may not be the signal, but rather they may mediate morphogenesis (Lambowitz *et al.* 1983). Temperatures above 30 °C are required for yeast-phase growth, but are also permissible for mycelial-phase growth, suggesting that other environmental conditions in addition to heat shock are required (Maresca and Kobayashi 1989). Reduced oxygen tension and intracellular redox potential are required for yeast-phase growth. Extracellular cysteine can elicit reduced intracellular redox potential and mediate phase transition (Scherr 1957). Reduced oxygen tension results in an initial resting state in morphogenesis in which markedly reduced mitochondrial

oxidative phosphorylation, ATP depletion, and uncoupling of oxidative phosphorylation occur (Medoff *et al.* 1986a). This stage is followed by induction of a unique cysteine oxidase and increased oxidative metabolism (Sacco *et al.* 1983).

In addition to changes in expression of heat-shock proteins, intracellular concentrations of cyclic adenosine 3′,5′-monophosphate (c-AMP) are high during mycelial growth, but decrease during the yeast-phase transition (Medoff *et al.* 1981). Phase transition can be effected by changing the extracellular c-AMP concentration in the absence of a temperature shift, suggesting that c-AMP is an important second messenger (Maresca and Kobayashi 1989). Tubulin expression and assemble is important in yeast-phase morphogenesis and may be regulated by c-AMP (Harris *et al.* 1989; Maresca and Kobayashi 1989).

Total ribonucleic acid synthesis decreases during the initial resting stage of yeast-phase transition, and then increases during the later morphogenic stage. A protein factor termed histin may regulate RNA synthesis during phase transition, and new RNA polymerases may be expressed (Cheung *et al.* 1974; Boguslawski *et al.* 1975). Three particular mRNA species not present in mycelial phase, termed yeast-phase specific-3 (yps-3) mRNA, are synthesized within 24 hours of temperature upshift (Keath *et al.* 1989).

Changes also occur during morphogenesis in cell wall and plasma membrane composition. The basic biochemical composition of the cell wall for mycelium and yeast is similar, e.g. both contain chitins, glucans, proteins and lipids, but the exact chemical composition, e.g. percentage of particular glycosyl residues in glucans, changes during morphogenesis (Domer and Moser 1980). Likewise, the membrane protein composition changes during morphogenesis with expression of yeast-phase specific membrane proteins, (Kumar and Maresca 1988). The relationship between these changes and structural and architectural form of the yeast versus the mycelial forms are complex and are not well understood. However, some of these changes in cell wall and plasma membrane structure may be important for survival of *Histoplasma capsulatum* in the host.

Although *Histoplasma capsulatum* is classified as a pathogenic rather than an opportunistic fungus, no well-defined virulence factors have been identified. Yeast-phase *Histoplasma capsulatum* secrete elastolytic and collagenolytic proteinases, but their role in pathogenesis is uncertain (Okeke and Muller 1991a,b). Virulence is correlated with increased thermal sensitivity of yeast-phase transition, expression of *hsp 70* and *yps-3*, and α-1,3 glucan cell wall content, but *Histoplasma capsulatum* appears to be atoxogenic (Medoff *et al.* 1986b; Caruso *et al.* 1987; Klimpel and Goldman 1988; Keath *et al.* 1989; Eissenberg *et al.* 1991).

It appears that rather than producing 'offensive' type virulence factors, the ability of *Histoplasma capsulatum* to proliferate in the host MPS and evade host general immunity is its major mechanism of virulence. *Histoplasma* organisms are facultative intracellular parasites of the MPS cells, composed of circulating monocytes, macrophages, and tissue histiocytes. The factors responsible for intracellular survival of *Histoplasma* organisms has not been clearly established. Unopsonized *Histoplasma* organisms are phagocytosed by a leucocyte adherence-promoting glycoprotein (CR3/LFA-1, p150, 95 and CD18)-mediated mechanism (Bullock and Wright 1987; Newman *et al.* 1990). However, phagocytosed *Histoplasma* organisms fail to elicit release of reactive oxygen metabolites and moderate phagolysosomal acidification by as yet unidentified mechanisms (Wolf *et al.* 1987; Eissenberg *et al.* 1993). In contrast to naive macrophages, mononuclear phagocytes from immunized animals can restrict growth of *Histoplasma capsulatum*, suggesting that these survival factors are not sufficient to overcome acquired host immunity (Howard 1973).

THE HOST

ANIMALS

Both natural and experimental histoplasmosis have been described in a variety of animals comprising mammalian and avian species. The natural disease caused by *Histoplasma capsulatum* var. *capsulatum* is most adequately described in dogs and cats. The prevalence of clinically inapparent histoplasmosis is high as indicated by the high numbers of dogs and cats in endemic areas that harbour *Histoplasma* organisms in their lungs or associated lymph nodes (Emmons *et al.* 1955; Turner *et al.* 1972a/b). Clinically apparent pulmonary histoplasmosis is less common. The incubation period is 7–14 days (Menges *et al.* 1954; Ward *et al.* 1979). In dogs, pulmonary histoplasmosis can resolve with no sequelae, with calcification of interstitial lung nodules and tracheobronchial lymph nodes, or with development of clinically apparent disseminated histoplasmosis (Burk *et al.* 1978). In contrast, calcified pulmonary lesions typically do not develop in cats. Most cats with clinically apparent disseminated histoplasmosis present with respiratory signs, suggesting that clinically apparent pulmonary infection precedes disseminated infection (Clinkenbeard *et al.* 1987; Wolf and Green 1987).

Clinically apparent disseminated histoplasmosis in cats is typically a fulminating systemic disease of young cats with signs of anaemia, weight loss, lethargy, fever, anorexia, and interstitial lung disease (Wolf and Belden 1984; Clinkenbeard *et al.* 1987, 1989a). Lameness, skin lesions, oral ulcers, ocular discharge and blindness, and diarrhoea are signs arising from focal organ dysfunction associated with disseminated histoplasmosis in less than 10 per cent of affected cats (Clinkenbeard *et al.* 1989a). The clinical course of the disease is 1–2 months often resulting in death, euthanasia, or treatment failure (Clinkenbeard *et al.*, 1987). This severe fulminating form of disseminated histoplasmosis is similar to that seen in infants and young children (Goodwin *et al.* 1980).

In contrast, clinically apparent disseminated histoplasmosis in dogs is typically a subacute to chronic diarrhoeal disease of young to middle-aged dogs (Mitchell and Stark 1980; Clinkenbeard *et al.* 1988b, 1989b). Weight loss and anaemia are also common signs, but fever, lymphadenopathy, hepatomegaly, splenomegaly, and respiratory signs are seen in 50 per cent or fewer of the cases (Clinkenbeard *et al.* 1989b). Focal sign other than diarrhoea which can develop in 10 per cent of dogs with disseminated histoplasmosis are lameness, oral ulcers, ocular discharge and blindness, and CNS signs (Clinkenbeard *et al.* 1989b). The course and progression of disseminated histoplasmosis in dogs is similar to that of subacute to chronic disseminated histoplasmosis in adult human beings (Goodwin *et al.*, 1980; Clinkenbeard *et al.* 1989b). The clinical course of the disease is 2–12 months, often resulting in euthanasia or death (Clinkenbeard *et al.* 1989b).

The diagnostic approach is similar for disseminated histoplasmosis in dogs and cats. Cytological or histopathological detection of *Histoplasma* infection is the most common method, but mycotic culture is also used. Rectal mucosa and bone marrow are the most productive sampling sites for diagnosis of disseminated histoplasmosis in dogs and cats, respectively (Clinkenbeard *et al.* 1987, 1988b). Serological tests consisting of serum antibody titres or skin-delayed type hypersensitivity testing have not proved useful for diagnosis of disseminated histoplasmosis in dogs or cats. Serology has suffered from cross-reactions with antigens from other fungal organisms, high basal titres in *Histoplasma* endemic areas, and anergy (Turner *et al.* 1972b; Clinkenbeard *et al.* 1989b).

Disseminated histoplasmosis in both dogs and cats is associated with widespread *Histoplasma* infection of tissues. *Histoplasma* organisms were identified in 62 and 76 per cent of tissues examined histologically at necropsy in dogs and cats, respectively (Clinkenbeard *et al.* 1987, 1988b). Small and large intestine, liver, lungs, lymph nodes, and spleen are infection in most cases in dogs, and lungs, liver, lymph nodes, spleen, bone marrow, and eyes are most often involved in cats. Organ enlargement, granulomas, mucosal erosions, and focal haemorrhage and necrosis are common lesions in dogs and cats.

Similar treatment regiments of amphotericin B or ketoconazole, employed separately, combined, or sequentially, have been used for disseminated histoplasmosis in dogs and cats (Clinkenbeard *et al.* 1989*a,b*). Amphotericin B resolves infection more quickly than ketoconazole, but it is also potentially nephrotoxic. However, with adequate fluid therapy support and monitoring of renal function, the incidence of amphotericin-induced renal failure appears to be low (Mitchell and Stark 1980). Ketoconazole has the advantage of oral administration, but prolonged treatment periods are required to resolve *Histoplasma* infection. Ketoconazole causes vomition and anorexia in some cats. Itraconazole and fluconazole have been recently been advocated for the treatment of disseminated histoplasmosis in both dogs and cats (Wolf 1990). Despite adequate treatment regiments, prognosis for recover (without relapse) is poor, particularly in cats (Clinkenbeard *et al.* 1989*a,b*).

Histoplasma capsulatum var. *farciminosum* infects primarily horses and donkeys. A lymphocutaneous form is most common, but ocular, pulmonary, gastrointestinal, and disseminated forms also occur (Singh 1965*a*; Gabal *et al.* 1983; Soliman *et al.* 1991). Incubation time is 4 to 72 days and may vary by the form of the disease observed (Singh 1965*b*). Clinically, the lymphocutaneous form resembles infection by the dimorphoric fungus *Sporothrix schenckii* in cats (Dunstan *et al.* 1989; Clinkenbeard 1991). Nodules and cords form along the course of lymphatic spread with subsequent ulceration of nodules and exudation (Gabal *et al.* 1983). The course of infection is typically 6 months, at which time a quiescent stage is reached. Morbidity is low, but loss of usefulness or epizootic control programme result in destruction of many infected horses (Gabal *et al.* 1983). Horses are also susceptible to infection by *Histoplasma capsulatum* var. *capsulatum*, but the disease produced, i.e. pulmonary or disseminated histoplasmosis, is similar to the disease produced by the var. *capsulatum* organism in other hosts (Rezabek *et al.* 1993).

HUMAN BEINGS

The course of histoplasmosis in human beings is complex and is related to the level of exposure and the immunocompetence of the individual (Goodwin *et al.* 1980). The incubation period for pulmonary histoplasmosis is 3–30 days with means of 7 days for heavy exposure and 14 days for light exposure. Mild exposure in immunocompetent individuals results in asymptomatic histoplasmosis (Goodwin *et al.* 1981). The prevalence of asymptomatic histoplasmosis may reach more than 90 per cent of inhabitants in endemic areas or in point-source epidemics in non-endemic areas (Goodwin *et al.*

1981; Wheat 1992). Asymptomatic infections are associated with conversion to positive histoplasmin skin reactivity and positive serum antibody titres to histoplasmin (Wheat 1992).

Heavy exposure in normal individuals results in symptomatic pulmonary histoplasmosis. The most common symptoms are fever, headache, cough, chills, and chest pain, and are associated with conversion to positive histoplasmin skin reactivity and positive serum antibody titres to histoplasmin (Goodwin *et al.* 1981; Wheat 1992). However, the high prevalence of positivity of these tests in endemic areas limits their utility in diagnosis (Jordan *et al.* 1990). The duration of illness may be related to level of exposure and varies from 1 to 21 days.

Histoplasma infection is cleared by development of cell-mediated immunity, but this immunity is not permanent. Skin reactivity to histoplasmin parallels development of cell-mediated immunity, and can also wane following resolution of infection (Zeidberg *et al.* 1951). Asymptomatic reinfection can occur and is detected by reactivation of histoplasmin skin reactivity (Goodwin *et al.* 1981). Symptomatic re-infection is likely to be uncommon. The calcified pulmonary lesions commonly observed in *Histoplasma* endemic regions likely develop by recurrent re-infection over the lifetime of the individual (Goodwin *et al.* 1981).

Disseminated histoplasmosis is thought to be a sequela of pulmonary histoplasmosis in immunocompromised individuals (Goodwin *et al.* 1980). Dissemination of infection beyond the lungs and their associated lymph nodes to spleen, liver, and extrapulmonary lymph nodes develops not only in progressive systemic infection, but it is the normal course of asymptomatic or symptomatic pulmonary histoplasmosis. In the normal host, cell-mediated immunity develops, and the extrapulmonary infection is cleared (or limited) along with the pulmonary infection. In immunocompromised individuals, effective cell-mediated immunity is not developed, and the extrapulmonary extension of infection persists and becomes progressive (Payan *et al.* 1984; Clapp *et al.* 1987).

Goodwin and collaborators have recognized several clinical forms of disseminated histoplasmosis in human beings (Goodwin *et al.* 1980). A fulminating systemic form of disseminated histoplasmosis occurs in infants and children below 2 years of age. In many of these individuals, onset of progressive, systemic disease developed 2 months to 2 years following acute pulmonary histoplasmosis. The most frequent symptoms are fever, malaise, cough, and weight loss. As the infection progresses, diarrhoea, vomiting, and anaemia often develop. Severe systemic inflammatory disease and haematological disturbances result in death in 1–2 months in untreated cases (Goodwin *et al.* 1980).

Subacute disseminated histoplasmosis is similar to acute disseminated disease and exhibits systemic inflammatory symptoms of weight loss, weakness, fever, and malaise, but also develops destructive focal lesions of the intestines or oropharynx, adrenal glands, heart, or CNS. Adults as well as children and infants can be affected with subacute disease. Severe effects of the focal lesions such as intestinal perforation, Addison's disease, endocarditis, and CNS disease in subacute disseminated histoplasmosis can progress to death after 10–12 months (Goodwin *et al.* 1980).

Chronic disseminated histoplasmosis occurs in adults and is associated with only mild, intermittent, or no systemic inflammatory (constitutional) symptoms (Goodwin *et al.* 1980). When fully developed, symptoms associated with focal lesions of oropharyngeal ulcers, adrenal gland destruction, endocarditis, or CNS disease are prominent. Haematological changes are minimal. The course of disease may take years to develop critical illness.

Histopathology, fungal culture, and cytology are commonly employed for diagnosis of human disseminated histoplasmosis. Blood culture or cytology, urine culture, and ascitic fluid cytology are useful for diagnosis of acute disease; buffy coat smear cytology or blood or urine culture and liver biopsy histopathology are useful for diagnosis of subacute disease; and oropharyngeal ulcer, liver, or other organ biopsy histopathology are useful for diagnosis of chronic disease (Goodwin *et al.* 1980).

Skin testing is negative in most cases of disseminated histoplasmosis, and positivity of complement fixation serology is likely influenced more by the antecedent pulmonary infection rather than by disseminated disease (Goodwin *et al.* 1980). Detection of *Histoplasma capsulatum* polysaccharide antigen in sera or urine is useful for diagnosis of disseminated histoplasmosis (Wheat *et al.* 1989).

The clinical syndromes in human beings caused by *Histoplasma capsulatum* var. *duboisii* differ from those of *Histoplasma capsulatum* var. *capsulatum* (Rippon 1988*b*). The portal of entry for *Histoplasma capsulatum* var. *duboisii* has not been conclusively demonstrated, but it is assumed to be inhalation. However, acute pulmonary disease is typically absent. Focal infection of skin, lymphocutaneous tissues, subcutis, or bone appears to be the common disease form, but multiorgan disseminated disease also occurs (Cockshott and Lucas 1964). Natural infection and clinical disease by *Histoplasma capsulatum* var. *duboisii* also occur in baboons (Butler and Hubbard 1991).

Antifungal therapy in human beings utilizes amphotericin B, ketoconazole, itraconazole, and fluconazole (Mabey and Hay 1989; Negroni *et al.* 1989, 1992). No antifungal treatment is recommended for symptomatic pulmonary histoplasmosis, except in immunocompromised individuals or those with disease predisposing to development of chronic pulmonary histoplasmosis (Wheat 1992). As with treatment of disseminated histoplasmosis in dogs and cats, amphotericin B is more useful for individuals with severe *Histoplasma* parasitism, whereas ketoconazole acts to clear infection more slowly (Wheat 1992). Itraconazole and fluconazole may be more efficacious than ketoconazole with fewer untoward effects, but like ketoconazole, these newer azoles require prolonged treatment regiments (Dismukes *et al.* 1992). *Histoplasma* polysaccharide antigen levels can be used to assess treatment course (Wheat *et al.* 1989). Treatment failure is associated with chronic cavitary pulmonary disease, HIV infection, and other severe systemic diseases (Dismukes *et al.* 1992; Wheat *et al.* 1993).

Immunity

Histoplasma capsulatum appears to evade general host immunity by escaping killing by host phagocytes. Although neutrophils are capable of phagocytosing *Histoplasma capsulatum*, the yeast are resistant to killing by human neutrophils for exposure times of less than 24 hours (Schaffner *et al.* 1986). The survival of *Histoplasma capsulatum* in neutrophils does not appear to correlate with the level of micro-organism catalase production or resistance to *in vitro* killing by reactive oxygen intermediates (Schaffner *et al.* 1986; Kurita *et al.* 1991). At longer exposure times, neutrophils are fungistatic, and this activity is mediated by components of the azurophilic granules (Newman *et al.* 1993).

Likewise, acquired humoral immune response is insufficient by itself to limit infection by *Histoplasma capsulatum* (Wu-Hseieh and Howard 1989). Experimental pulmonary histoplasmosis in mice elicits clonal selection of B-lymphocytes and CD3+, CD4– and CD8– T lymphocytes in pulmonary lymph nodes and high IgG, but low IgM anti-*Histoplasma* antibodies (Fojtasek *et al.* 1993). Passive transfer of humoral immunity is not effective in limiting *Histoplasma* infection, and in fact, high antibody levels and circulating immune complexes may immunosuppress infected individuals (Cox 1979; Taylor *et al.* 1984).

In contrast, acquired cell-mediated immunity is able to limit infection by *Histoplasma capsulatum* (Wu-Hseieh and Howard 1989). Delayed-type hypersensitivity reaction is associated with resolution of infection in healthy human beings (Goodwin *et al.* 1980). Adoptive transfer of protective immunity in animals is affected by lymphoid cells rather than with humoral factors (Khardori *et al.* 1983). In mice, adoptive transfer of CD4+ helper T-lymphocytes elicits protection against persistent *Histoplasma* infection (Allendoerfer *et al.*

1993). *Histoplasma* cell wall, membrane, cytosolic antigens, and heat-shock proteins stimulate T-cell reactivity, and some of these antigens elicit protective cell-mediated immune response in mice (Deepe and Brunner 1990; Gomez *et al.* 1991, 1992).

Histoplasma infection elicits changes in lymphokine levels. Tumour necrosis factor-α (TNF-α) in bronchoalveolar lavage fluid of experimentally infected mice increases during the first 24 hours following infection and then declines (Smith *et al.* 1990). Antibody neutralization of TNF-α activity in these mice accelerates mortality (Smith *et al.* 1990). Splenocyte interleukin (IL-1 and IL-2) production decreases during the peak of experimental *Histoplasma* infection in mice (weeks 1–3 of infection) (Watson *et al.* 1985).

Lymphokines from immune T lymphocytes can activate naive macrophages to kill *Histoplasma capsulatum*. Early activation of splenic macrophages by TNF-α limits experimental histoplasmosis in mice (Wu-Hsieh *et al.* 1992). Macrophages expressing defensin are also able to limit intracellular yeast multiplication, and macrophages activated by γ-interferon are capable of killing *Histoplasma* yeast by superoxide anion-dependent and nitric oxide-dependent mechanisms as well as by iron limitation (Brummer *et al.*, 1991; Lane *et al.*, 1991; Couto *et al.*, 1994; Nakamura *et al.*, 1994).

Persistent *Histoplasma* infection in human beings is associated with suppression of cell-mediated immunity (Clapp *et al.* 1987). In these patience, CD8+ T-lymphocyte numbers are high and CD4+ T-lymphocyte numbers are low (Payan *et al.* 1984). T-lymphocyte anergy and an increase in γ/δ T-lymphocyte numbers as well as CD3+, CD2–, CD4–, and CD8– T lymphocytes has been observed in an individual with disseminated histoplasmosis (Lehman *et al.* 1989). T-lymphocyte subpopulation counts return to normal with recovery from persistent *Histoplasma* infection (Payan *et al.*, 1984).

EPIDEMIOLOGY

The prevalence of human asymptomatic pulmonary histoplasmosis in endemic regions is estimated to be more than 50 per cent based on positive skin tests for histoplasmin (Leggiadro *et al.* 1991; Wheat 1992). The prevalence of clinically inapparent pulmonary histoplasmosis in dogs and cats in endemic regions is estimated to be 36–50 per cent and 18–44 per cent, respectively, based on culture at necropsy of healthy animals (Rowley *et al.* 1954; Emmons *et al.* 1955). The incidence of symptomatic or clinically apparent versus asymptomatic or clinically inapparent pulmonary histoplasmosis likely depends on the level of environmental exposure, such that incidence may be affected by

locale and other variables. The incidence rates for symptomatic pulmonary and disseminated histoplasmosis in human beings during two large urban epidemics were 1–50/100 and 1/2000 infected individuals, respectively (Wheat 1992). In endemic regions, case rates of 0.2 to 46 cases of human disseminated histoplasmosis per 100 000 infected persons per year has been estimated (Goodwin *et al.* 1980; Wheat *et al.* 1982). The case prevalence of disseminated histoplasmosis at a veterinary teaching hospital in an endemic region of the mid-western United States of 185 cases in cats and 62 cases in dogs per 100 000 hospital records per year has been estimated (Clinkenbeard *et al.* 1987). If these rates are comparable, then disseminated histoplasmosis appears to be more common in cats and dogs than in human beings.

Proximity to bird roosts is a significant factor in determining exposure level. Exposure level in schoolchildren as reflected by skin reactivity to histoplasmin is related to the proximity of the school to bird roosts (Chin *et al.* 1970). Blackbirds and starlings are the avian species most often associated with epidemics of histoplasmosis, because their habit of roosting in large flocks can result in high levels of environmental contamination. The growth of *Histoplasma capsulatum* is enhanced in droppings-enriched soil (Schwarz *et al.* 1957*b*). Disturbance of the soil of bird roosts by demolition or other activities is associated with epidemics of symptomatic pulmonary histoplasmosis (Chin *et al.* 1970). However, *Histoplasma* organisms are also present in soils of endemic areas in the absence of obvious bird roosts, and in three recent epidemics in Indianapolis, Indiana, no historical evidence of bird roosts was found (Ajello 1967; Wheat 1992).

Human and animal exposure to microfoci of heavily contaminated soil can result in point source epidemics and epizootics. Numerous incidences of point-source outbreaks from chicken and pigeon coops, bird roosting areas, and bat-invested caves or buildings contaminated with *Histoplasma* organisms have been described (Menges *et al.* 1954; Ajello *et al.* 1960; Di Salvo and Johnson 1979; Ward *et al.* 1979). Although avian species are not infected by *Histoplasma capsulatum*, feathers and chicken manure in potting soil can act as fomites for *Histoplasma* infection. Bats can be infected by *Histoplasma* organisms, and bat guano can also serve as a fomite (Diercks *et al.* 1965; Klite and Young 1965).

The geographic distribution of *Histoplasma* endemic regions consists of river basins with temperate climates with moderate to high humidity. These conditions are also those at which *Histoplasma capsulatum* growth is best in soil cultures (Ajello 1967). However, particular ranges of temperature and moisture alone are not sufficient to explain the geographic distribution of *Histoplasma* endemicity. Several workers have speculated on particular environmental attributes and soil composition which may be important growth determinants, thereby determine the geographic pattern of *Histoplasma* endemic regions (Zeidberg and Ajello 1954; Stotzky and Post 1961; Lavie and Stotzky 1986).

For *Histoplasma capsulatum* var. *capsulatum*, the Missouri, Mississippi, and Ohio River basins in the United States may be the most heavily endemic region (Edwards *et al.* 1969). This region is coincidentally heavy populated by starlings, which may enhance the other environmental factors of this region for *Histoplasma* soil contamination. In addition to the Mississippi River basin, local areas of endemicity for *Histoplasma capsulatum* var. *capsulatum* are present in Central and South America, Africa, Asia, Australia, and Europe. In contrast, the endemic area for *Histoplasma capsulatum* var. *duboisii* is limited to equatorial Africa, and that for *Histoplasma capsulatum* var. *farciminosum* extends from Scandinavia, central and southern Europe, Russia, northern Africa, to India and southern Asia, with the heaviest endemic regions in Egypt and India (Gabal *et al.* 1983; Rippon 1988*a*).

Some regions with conditions unfavourable for *Histoplasma capsulatum*, such as deserts or arid plains, can contain microcosums of suitable environments for *Histoplasma capsulatum* proliferation. This is particularly true when factors such as irrigation or poultry production modify an otherwise unfavourable environment into a favourable one (Kabli *et al.* 1986). Histoplasmosis encountered distant to endemic regions may represent sporadic infections or the infected individuals may have contracted the infection in an endemic region and then moved to a non-endemic region prior to disease development or diagnosis (Oddo *et al.* 1990).

Human beings, most domestic and feral mammalian species appear to be susceptible to natural or experimental *Histoplasma capsulatum* var. *capsulatum* infection resulting in asymptomatic or clinically inapparent pulmonary as well as disseminated histoplasmosis (Ajello 1967). It has been proposed that infection with *Histoplasma capsulatum* only progresses to clinically apparent disseminated disease in immunocompromised hosts (Goodwin *et al.* 1980). Risk factors for disseminated histoplasmosis in human beings are young age, infection with human immunodeficiency virus (HIV), treatment with immunosuppressive medications for neoplasia, immune-mediated mediated diseases, or organ transplantation, and neoplasia (particularly lymphomas) (Goodwin *et al.* 1980; Wheat *et al.* 1982, 1985; Toloff-Rubin and Rubin 1992). HIV-infected individuals may be susceptible to infection by less virulent, temperature-sensitive strains of *Histo-*

plasma capsulatum var. *capsulatum* (Spitzer *et al.* 1990). These factors support the hypothesis that immunocompromise is important for development of disseminated histoplasmosis; however, these risk factors are identified in a minority of cases (Goodwin *et al.* 1980).

Risk factors for disseminated histoplasmosis identified in dogs and cats are young age and treatment with immunosuppressive doses of corticosteroids (Clinkenbeard *et al.* 1989*a,b*). Interestingly, infection of cats with feline leukemia virus (FeLV), which elicits immunocompromise in cats, appears not to be associated with development of disseminated histoplasmosis (Clinkenbeard *et al.* 1987).

Inhalation of microconidia and mycelial fragments is the route of natural *Histoplasma capsulatum* var. *capsulatum* infection. Direct infection can also occur by traumatic implantation of laboratory cultures or necropsy material or by long-term peritoneal dialysis (Tosh *et al.* 1964; Tesh and Schneidau 1966; Lim *et al.* 1991). Oral inoculation has been considered as a potential route of infection, particularly in dogs with disseminated histoplasmosis presenting with primarily or exclusive gastrointestinal disease (Menges 1951). However, the widespread infection by *Histoplasma* organisms of extragastrointestinal tissues in these dogs and the difficulty of establishing experimental infection by gastric route in dogs does not support an oral route of infection (Farrell and Cole 1968; Da Costa *et al.* 1981).

Infection by *Histoplasma capsulatum* var. *capsulatum* is not contagious except in unusual situations. Rare cases of horizontal transmission have been reported. Horizontal transmission is associated with conjugal contraction of individuals with cutaneous lesions of the genitalia and by solid organ transplantation of infected organs (Sills *et al.* 1973; Gottesdiener 1989; Cohen *et al.* 1991; Sridhar *et al.* 1991; Wong and Allen 1992). No documented cases of vertical transmission from animals to human beings or vice versa have been reported (Sills *et al.* 1973). This is in contrast to the significant vertical transmission of the related dimorphoric fungus *Sporothrix schenckii* from cats to human beings (Dunstan *et al.* 1989, Clinkenbeard 1991). In contrast to *Histoplasma capsulatum* var. *capsulatum*, equine infection by *Histoplasma capsulatum* var. *farciminosum* is contagious and is transmitted by bites of contaminated flies or ticks as well as through skin traumatized with contaminated tack (Singh 1965).

PREVENTION AND CONTROL

Several aspects of histoplasmosis caused by *Histoplasma capsulatum* var. *capsulatum* and var. *duboisii* make institution of preventative or control strategies difficult. The exposure levels to *Histoplasma capsulatum* var. *capsulatum* vary with locale within the endemic regions, and identification of the numerous heavily contaminated sites is not practical in most situations. However, an attempt to identify sites should be made for sites with a high historical or scientific potential for heavy *Histoplasma* contamination and where earth moving or demolition will likely expose large populations to dust from the site. Recurrent epidemics of histoplasmosis have resulted from disturbance of the same contaminated site (Chin *et al.* 1970; Wheat 1992). Large bird roosts, poultry operations, or bat habitats are candidates for heavily contaminated sites (Weeks and Stickley 1984).

Bird roosts in use for 3 or more years are typically contaminated (Chick *et al.* 1981; Weeks and Stickley 1984). Preventing long-term use of roosting areas can decrease environmental contamination (D'Alessio *et al.* 1965). Methods for managing bird roosts employ dispersion or killing of birds (Weeks and Stickley 1984). The efficacy of dispersion techniques has been questioned (Weeks and Stickley 1984). In addition to controlling use of roosts, soil decontamination has also been advocated (Weeks and Tosh 1971). Physical removal of the contaminated top soil layer or covering of the contaminated top soil layer with additional soil reduces environmental contamination from problem sites (Weeks and Tosh 1971). Spraying of *Histoplasma* contaminated soil with 3 per cent formalin also reduces contamination, although the volume required (330 000 gallons for 7.5-acre site) is troublesome (Tosh *et al.* 1966; Weeks and Tosh 1971).

Physical removal of downed trees or thickets without hazardous exposure of personnel to *Histoplasma* has proved difficult. The high exposure of heavy equipment operators and others during clearing bird roosts has resulted in fatal acute pulmonary histoplasmosis (Chin *et al.* 1970). Even when precautions are taken, high exposure to both workers and surrounding residence can occur (Tosh *et al.* 1967). Use of respirators during removal of contaminated soil, trees, or bat guano is advised (Tuttle and Kern 1981).

Persons at high risk for histoplasmosis need to be informed of the probability of high exposure in certain environments. In this regard, health-care workers need to be educated of the increased risk for contraction of histoplasmosis posed to individuals with HIV infection or neoplasia, as well as those on immunosuppressive therapies. Unfortunately, in many instants the avoidance of insidious exposure by high-risk individuals may not be possible (Wheat 1992), but, advising high-risk individuals to avoid areas of probable high *Histoplasma* contamination, e.g. bat-infested caves, is warranted.

In contrast to the difficulty of devising control strategies for histoplasmosis, several control strategies are available for equine epizootic lymphangitis. These strategies consist of control of biting flies and ticks, practice of general hygiene and disinfection, and quarantine of infected animals (Radostits *et al.* 1994). Destruction of infected horses in non-enzootic areas has been recommended. In some Middle Eastern countries, veterinary rules mandate that infected animals be condemned (Gabal *et al.* 1983).

REFERENCES

Ajello, L. (1967). Comparative ecology of respiratory mycotic disease agents. *Bacteriological Reviews*, **31**, 6–24.

Ajello, L. and Zeidberg, L. D. (1951). Isolation of *Histoplasma capsulatum* and *Allescheria boydii* from soil. *Science*, **113**, 662–3.

Ajello. L., Manson-Bahr, P. E. C., and Moore, J. C. (1960). Amboni caves, Tanganyika, a new endemic area for histoplasmosis. *American Journal of Tropical Medicine and Hygiene*, **9**, 633–8.

Allendoerfer, R., MaGee, D. M., Deepe, G. S., and Graybill, J. R. (1993). Transfer of protective immunity in murine histoplasmosis by CD4 positive T-cell clone. *Infection and Immunity*, **61**, 714–18.

Boguslawski, G., Medoff, G., Schlessinger, D., and Kobayaski, G. S. (1975). Histin, an RNA polymerase inhibitor from *Histoplasma capsulatum*. *Biochemical and Biophysical Research Communications*, **64**, 625–32.

Brummer, E., Kurita, N., Yoshida, S., Nishimura, K., and Miyaji, M. (1991). Killing of *Histoplasma capsulatum* by gamma-interferon-activated human monocyte-derived macrophages: Evidence for a superoxide anion-dependent mechanism. *Journal of Medical Microbiology*, **35**, 29–34.

Bullock, W. E. and Wright, S. D. (1987). Role of the adherence-promoting receptors, CR3, LFA-1 and p150,95, in binding of *Histoplasma capsulatum* by human macrophages. *Journal of Experimental Medicine*, **165**, 195–210.

Burk, R. L., Cornley, E. A., and Corwin, L. A. (1978). The radiographic appearance of pulmonary histoplasmosis in the dog and cat: A review of 37 case histories. *American Veterinary Radiological Society Journal*, **19**, 2–6.

Butler, T. M. and Hubbard, G. B. (1991). An epizootic of *Histoplasma capsulatum* var. *duboisii* (African histoplasmosis) in an American baboon colony. *Laboratory Animal Sciences*, **41**, 407–10.

Caruso, M., Sacco, M., Medoff, G., and Maresca, B. (1987). Heat shock 70 gene is differentially expressed in *Histoplasma capsulatum* strains with different levels of thermotolerance and pathogenicity. *Molecular Microbiology*, **2**, 151–8.

Cheung, S. C., Kobayaski, G. S., Schlessinger, D., and Medoff, G. (1974). RNA metabolism during morphogenesis in *Histoplasma capsulatum*. *Journal of General Microbiology*, **82**, 301–7.

Chick, E. W. *et al.* (1981). Hitchcock's birds, or the increase rate of exposure of *Histoplasma* from blackbird roost sites. *Chest*, **80**, 434–8.

Chin, T. D. Y., Tosh, F. E., and Weeks, R. J. (1970). Ecological and epidemiological studies of histoplasmosis in the United States of America. *Mycopathologia et Mycologia*, **41**, 35–44.

Ciferri, R. and Redaelli, P. (1934). *Histoplasma capsulatum* Darling's agent of 'histoplasmosis', systematic position and characterization. *Journal of Tropical Medicine and Hygiene*, **37**, 278–80.

Clapp, D. W., Kleiman, M. B., and Brahmi, Z. (1987). Immunoregulatory lymphocyte populations in disseminated histoplasmosis of infancy. *Journal of Infectious Diseases*, **156**, 687–8.

Clinkenbeard, K. D. (1991). Diagnostic cytology: Sporotrichosis. *Compendium of Continuing Education in Veterinary Practice*, **13**, 207–11.

Clinkenbeard, K. D., Cowell, R. L., and Tyler, R. D. (1987). Disseminated histoplasmosis in cats: 12 cases (1981–1986). *Journal of the American Veterinary Medical Association*, **190**, 1445–8.

Clinkenbeard, K. D., Cowell, R. L., and Tyler, R. D. (1988a). Disseminated histoplasmosis in dogs: 12 cases (1981–1986). *Journal of the American Veterinary Medical Association*, **193**, 1443–7.

Clinkenbeard, K. D., Cowell, R. L., and Tyler, R. D. (1988b). Identification of intracellular *Histoplasma* organisms in circulating eosinophils of a dog. *Journal of the American Veterinary Medical Association*, **192**, 217–18.

Clinkenbeard, K. D., Wolf, A. M., Cowell, R. L., and Tyler, R. D. (1989a). Feline disseminated histoplasmosis. *Compendium of Continuing Education in Veterinary Practice*, **11**, 1223–33.

Clinkenbeard, K. D., Wolf, A. M., Cowell, R. L., and Tyler, R. D. (1989b). Canine disseminated histoplasmosis. *Compendium of Continuing Education in Veterinary Practice*, **11**, 1347–59.

Cockshott, W. P. and Lucas, A. O. (1964). Histoplasmosis duboisii. *Quarterly Journal of Medicine*, **33**, 223–38.

Cohen, P. R., Held, J. L., Grossman, M. E., Ross, M. J., and Silvers, D. N. (1991). Disseminated histoplasmosis presenting as an ulcerative verrucous plaque in a human immunodeficiency virus-infected man. Report of a case possibly involving human-to-human transmission of histoplasmosis. *International Journal of Dermatology*, **30**, 104–8.

Conant, N. F. (1941). A cultural study of the life-cycle of *Histoplasma capsulatum* Darling 1906. *Journal of Bacteriology*, **41**, 563–79.

Couto, M. A., Liu, L., Lehner, R. I., and Ganz, T. (1994). Inhibition of intracellular *Histoplasma capsulatum* replication in murine macrophages that produce human defensin. *Infection and Immunity*, **62**, 2375–8.

Cox, R. A. (1979). Immunologic studies of patients with histoplasmosis. *American Review of Respiratory Diseases*, **120**, 143–9.

Christie, A. and Peterson, J. C. (1945). Pulmonary calification in negative reactors to tuberculin. *American Journal of Public Health*, **35**, 1131–47.

Da Costa, E. O. *et al.* (1981). Experimental histoplasmosis I. Puppies exposed to a natural reservoir of *H. Capsulatum*. **8**, 77–84.

D'Alessio, D. J., Heeren, R. H., Hendricks, S. L., Ogilvie, P., and Furcolow, M. L. (1965). A Starling roost as the source of urban epidemic histoplasmosis in an area of low incidence. *American Review of Respiratory Diseases*, **92**, 725–31.

Darling, S. T. (1906). A protozoon general infection producing pseudotuberculosis in the lungs and focal necrosis in the liver, spleen, and lymphnodes. *Journal of the American Medical Association*, **46**, 1283–5.

Da Rocha-Lima, H. (1912). Beitrag zur Kenntnis der blastomykosen, lymphangitis epizootica und histoplasmosis. *Zentralblatt für Bakteriologie, Parasitenkunde Infetionskrankheiten und Hygiene, I Orig.*, **67**, 233–49.

Deepe, G. S. and Brunner, G. D. (1990). Functional analysis of *Histoplasma capsulatum*-reactive T-cell hybridomas. *Infection and Immunity*, **58**, 1538–44.

De Monbreum, W. A. (1934). The cultivation and cultural characteristics of Darling's *Histoplasma capsulatum*. *American Journal of Tropical Medicine*, **14**, 93–125.

De Monbreum, W. A. (1939). The dog as a natural host for *Histoplasma capsulatum*. *American Journal of Tropical Medicine*, **14**, 565–87.

Diercks, F. H., Shacklette, M. H., Kelley, H. B., Klite, P. D., Thompson, S. W., and Keenan, C. M. (1965). Naturally occurring histoplasmosis among 935 bats collected in Panama and the Canal Zone, July 1961–February 1965. *American Journal of Tropical Medicine and Hygiene*, **14**, 1060–72.

Di Salvo, A. F. and Johnson, W. M. (1979). Histoplasmosis in South Carolina: Support for the microfocus concept. *American Journal of Epidemiology*, **109**, 480–92.

Dismukes, W. E., Bradsher, R. W., Cloud, G. C., Kauffman, C. A., Chapman, S. W., and George, R. B. (1992). Itraconazole therapy for blastomycosis and histoplasmosis. NIAID Mycoses Study Group. *American Journal of Medicine*, **93**, 489–97.

Dodd, K. and Tomkins, E. H. (1934). A case of histoplasmosis of Darling in an infant. *American Journal of Tropical Medicine*, **14**, 127–37.

Domer, J. E. and Moser, S. A. (1980). Histoplasmosis—a review. *Review of Medical and Veterinary Mycology*, **15**, 159–81.

Drouhet, E. (1957). Quelques aspects biologiques et mycologiques de l'histoplasmose. *Pathologic Biologic (Paris)*, **33**, 439–461.

Dubois, A., Janssens, P. G., and Brutsaert, P. (1952). Un cas d'histoplasmose africaine, avec une note mycologique sur *Histoplasma duboisii* n. sp. par R. Vanbreuseghem. *Annales de la Société Belge de Médecine Tropicale*, **32**, 569–84.

Duncan, J. T. (1947). A unique form of *Histoplasma*. *Transactions of the Royal Society of Tropical Medicine and Hygiene*, **40**, 364–5.

Dunstan, R. W., Reimann, K. A., and Langham, R. F. (1989). Feline sporotrichosis. *Journal of the American Veterinary Medical Association*, **189**, 880–3.

Edwards, L. B., Acquqviva, F. A., Livesay, V. T., Cross, F. W., and Palmer, C. E. (1969). An atlas of sensitivity to tuberculin, PPD-B, and histoplasmin in the United States. *American Review of Respiratory Diseases*, **99**, 1–132.

Eissenberg, L. G., West, J. L., Woods, J. P., and Goldman, W. E. (1991). Infection of P388D1 macrophages and respiratory epithelial cells by *Histoplasma capsulatum*: Selection of avirulent variants and their potential role in persistent histoplasmosis. *Infection and Immunity*, **59**, 1639–46.

Eissenberg, L. G., Goldman, W. E., and Schlesinger, P. H. (1993). *Histoplasma capsulatum* modulates the acidification of phagolysosomes. *Journal of Experimental Medicine*, **177**, 1605–11.

Emmons, C. W. (1949). Isolation of *Histoplasma capsulatum* from soil. *Public Health Reports*, **64**, 892–6.

Emmons, C. W. (1958). Association of bats with histoplasmosis. *Public Health Reports*, **73**, 590–5.

Emmons, C. W. *et al.* (1955). Histoplasmosis, proved occurrence of inapparent infections in dogs, cats, and other animals. *American Journal of Hygiene*, **61**, 40–4.

Farrell, R. L. and Cole, C. R. (1968). Experimental canine histoplasmosis with acute fatal and chronic recovered courses. *American Journal of Pathology*, **53**, 425–45.

Ferry, J. A., Pettit, C. K., Rosenberg, A. E., and Harris, N. L. (1991). Fungi in Megakaryocytes. *American Journal of Clinical Pathology*, **96**, 577–81.

Fojtasek, M. F., Sherman, M. R., Garringer, T., Blair, R., Wheat, L. J., and Schnizlein-Bick, C. T. (1993). Local immunity in lung-associated lymph nodes in a murine model of pulmonary histoplasmosis. *Infection and Immunity*, **61**, 4607–14.

Fukushima, K., Takeo, K., Takizawa, K., Nishimura, K., and Miyaji, M. (1991). Reevaluation of the teleomorph of the genus *Histoplasma* by ubiquinone systems. *Mycopathologia*, **116**, 151–4.

Gabal, M. A., Hassen, F. K., Siad, A. A., and Karim K. A. (1983). Study of equine histoplasmosis farciminosi and characterization of *Histoplasma farciminosum*. *Saboraudia*, **21**, 121–7.

Gomez, F. J., Gomez, A. M., and Deepe, G. S. (1991). Protective efficacy of a 62-kilodalton antigen, HIS-62, from the cell wall and cell membrane of *Histoplasma capsulatum* yeast cells. *Infection and Immunity*, **59**, 4459–64.

Gomez, F. J., Gomez, A. M., and Deepe, G. S. (1992). An 80-kilodalton antigen from *Histoplasma capsulatum* that has homology to heat shock protein 70 induces cell-mediated immune responses and protection in mice. *Infection and Immunity*, **60**, 2565–71.

Goodwin, R. A., Shapiro, J. L., Thurman, G. H., Thurman, S. S., and Des Prez, R. M. (1980). Disseminated histoplasmosis: clinical and pathologic correlations. *Medicine*, **59**, 1–33.

Goodwin, R. A., Loyd, J. E., and Des Prez, R. M. (1981). Histoplasmosis in normal hosts. *Medicine*, **60**, 231–66.

Gottesdiener, K. M. (1989). Transplanted infections: Donor-to-host transmission with the allograft. *Annals of Internal Medicine*, **110**, 1001–16.

Hamilton, A. J., Bartholomew, M. A., Fenelon, L., Figueroa, J., and Hay, R. J. (1990). Preparation of monoclonal antibodies that differentiate between *Histoplasma capsulatum* variant *capsulatum* and *H. capsulatum* variant *duboisii*. *Transactions of the Royal Society of Tropical Medicine and Hygiene*, **84**, 425–8.

Harris, G. S., Keath, E. J., and Medoff, J. (1989). Expression of alpha- and beta-tubulin genes during dimorphic-phase transition of *Histoplasma capsulatum*. *Molecular and Cell Biology*, **9**, 2042–9.

Howard, D. H. (1973). Further studies on the inhibition of *Histoplasma capsulatum* within macrophages from immunized animals. *Infection and Immunity*, **8**, 577–81.

Jordan, M. M., Chawla, J., Owens, M. W., and George, R. B. (1990). Significance of false-positive serologic tests for histoplasmosis and blastomycosis in an endemic area. *American Review of Respiratory Diseases*, **141**, 1487–90.

Kabli, S., Koschmann, J. R., Robertstad, G. W., Lawrence, J., Ajello, L., and Redetzke, K. (1986). Endemic canine and feline histoplasmosis in El Paso, Texas. *Journal of Medical and Veterinary Mycology*, **24**, 41–50.

Keath, E. J., Painter, A. A., Kobayashi, G. S., and Medoff, G. (1989). Variable expression of yeast-phase-specific gene in *Histoplasma capsulatum* strains differing in thermotolerance and virulence. *Infection and Immunity*, **57**, 1384–90.

Keath, E. J., Kobayaski, G. S., and Medoff, G. (1992). Typing of *Histoplasma capsulatum* by restriction fragment length polymorphisms in a nuclear gene. *Journal of Clinical Microbiology*, **30**, 2104–7.

Kersulyte, D., Woods, J. P., Keath, E. J., Goldman, W. E., and Berg, D. E. (1992). Diversity among clinical isolates of *Histoplasma capsulatum* detected by polymerase chain reaction with arbitrary primers. *Journal of Bacteriology*, **174**, 7075–9.

Khardori, N., Chaudhary, S., McConnachie, P., and Tewari, R. P. (1983). Characterization of lymphocytes responsible for protective immunity to histoplasmosis in mice. *Mykosen*, **26**, 523–32.

Klimpel, K. R. and Goldman, W. E. (1988). Cell walls from avirulent variants of *Histoplasma capsulatum* lack alpha-(1,3)-glucan. *Infection and Immunity*, **56**, 2997–3000.

Klite, P. D. and Young, R. V. (1965). Bats and histoplasmosis. A clinico-epidemiologic study of two human cases. *Annals of Internal Medicine*, **62**, 1263–71.

Know-Chung, K. J. (1972). Sexual stage of *Histoplasma capsulatum*. *Science*, **175**, 326.

Kumar, B. V. and Maresca, B. (1988). Purification of membranes and identification of phase specific proteins of the dimorphoric fungus *Histoplasma capsulatum*. *Archives of Biochemistry and Biophysics*, **261**, 212–21.

Kurita, N., Terao, K., Brummer, E., Ito, E., Nishimura, K., and Miyaji, M. (1991). Resistance of *Histoplasma capsulatum* to killing by human neutrophils. Evasion of oxidative burst and lysosomal-fusion products. *Mycopathologia*, **115**, 207–13.

Lambowitz, A. L., Kobayashi, G. S., Painter, A., and Medoff, G. (1983). Possible relationship of morphogenesis in pathogenic fungus, *Histoplasma capsulatum*, to heat shock response. *Nature (London)*, **303**, 806–8.

Lane, T. E., Wu-Hsieh B. A., and Howard, D. H. (1991). Iron limitation and the gamma interferon-mediated anti-histoplasma state of murine macrophages. *Infection and Immunity*, **59**, 2274–8.

Larsh, H. W. and Hall, N. K. (1987). *Histoplasma capsulatum*. In *Infectious Diseases and medical microbiology* (ed. A. Braude), pp. 580–3. WB Saunders, Philadelphia.

Lavie, S. and Stotzky, G. (1986). Interaction between clay minerals and siderophores affect the respiration of *Histoplasmosis capsulatum*. *Applied Environmental Microbiology*, **51**, 74–9.

Leggiadro, R. J., Luedtke, G. S., Convey, A., Gibson, L., and Barrett, F. F. (1991). Prevalence of histoplasmosis in a mid-southern population. *Southern Medical Journal*, **84**, 1360–1.

Lehman, P. F., Sawyer, T., and Donabedian, H. (1989). Novel abnormality in subpopulations of circulating lymphocytes. T-γ/δ and CD2-, 3+,4-,8- lymphocytes in histoplasmosis-associated immunmodeficiency. *International Archives of Allergy and Applied Immunology*, **90**, 213–18.

Lim, W., Chau, S. P., Chan, P. C., and Cheng, I. K. (1991). *Histoplasmosis capsulatum* infection associated with continuous ambulatory peritoneal dialysis. *Journal of Infection*, **22**, 179–82.

Mabey, D. C. and Hay, R. J. (1989). Further studies on the treatment of African histoplasmosis with ketoconazole. *Transactions of the Royal Society of Tropical Medicine and Hygiene*, **83**, 560–2.

Maresca, B. and Kobayashi, G. S. (1989). Dimorphism in *Histoplasma capsulatum*: A model for the study of cell differentiation in pathogenic fungi. *Microbiology Reviews*, **53**, 186–209.

Medoff, J., Jacobson, E., and Medoff, G. (1981). Regulation of dimorphorism in *Histoplasma capsulatum* by cyclic AMP. *Journal of Bacteriology*, **145**, 1452–5.

Medoff, G. *et al.* (1986*a*). Irreversible block of the mycelial to yeast phase transition of *H. capsulatum*. *Science*, **231**, 476–9.

Medoff, G. *et al.* (1986*b*). Correlation between pathogenicity and temperature in different strains of *H. capsulatum*. *Journal of Clinical Investigation*, **78**, 1638–47.

Menges, R. W. (1951). Canine histoplasmosis. *Journal of the American Veterinary Medical Association*, **119**, 411–15.

Menges, R. W., Furcolow, M. L., and Habermann, R. T. (1954). An outbreak of histoplasmosis involving animals and man. *American Journal of Veterinary Research*, **15**, 520–4.

Mitchell, M. and Stark, D. R. (1980). Disseminated canine histoplasmosis: A clinical survey of 24 cases in Texas. *Canadian Verterinary Journal*, **21**, 95–100.

Nakamura, L. T., Wu-Hsieh, B. A., and Howard, D. H. (1994). Recombinant murine gamma-interferon stimulates macrophages of the RAW cell line to inhibit intracellular growth of *Histoplasma capsulatum*. *Infection and Immunity*, **62**, 680–4.

Negroni, R., Robles, A. M., Arechavala, A., and Taborda, A. (1989). Itraconazole in human histoplasmosis. *Mycoses*, **32**, 123–30.

Negroni, R., Taborda, A., Robles, A. M., and Arechavala, A. (1992). Itraconazole in treatment of histoplasmosis associate with AIDS. *Mycoses*, **35**, 281–7.

Newman, S. L., Bucher, C., Rhodes, J., and Bullock, W. E. (1990). Phagocytosis of *Histoplasma capsulatum* yeast and microconidia by human cultured macrophages and alveolar macrophages. Cellular cytoskeleton requirement for attachment and ingestion. *Journal of Clinical Investigation*, **85**, 223–30.

Newman, S. L., Gootee, L., and Gabay, J. E. (1993). Human neutrophil-mediated fungistasis against *Histoplasma capsulatum*. Localization of fungistatic activity to the azurophilic granules. *Journal of Clinical Microbiology*, **92**, 624–31.

Oddo, D., Etchart, M., and Thompson, L. (1990). *Histoplasma duboisii* (African histoplasmosis). An African case reported from Chile with ultrastructural study. *Pathology Research Practice*, **186**, 514–17.

Okeke, C. N. and Muller, J. (1991*a*). Production of extracellular collagenolytic proteinase by *Histoplasma capsulatum*. var. *duboisii* and *Histoplasma capsulatum* var. *capsulatum* in the yeast phase. *Mycoses*, **34**, 453–60.

Okeke, C. N. and Muller, J. (1991*b*). *In vitro* production of extracellular elastolytic proteinase by *Histoplasma capsulatum* var. *duboisii* and *Histoplasma capsulatum* var. *capsulatum* in the yeast phase. *Mycoses*, **34**, 461–7.

Padhye, A. A., Smith, G., Mclaughlin, D., Standard, P. G., and Kaufman, L. (1992). Comparative evaluation of a chemiluminescent DNA probe and an exoantigen test for rapid identification of *Histoplasma capsulatum*. *Journal of Clinical Microbiology*, **30**, 3108–11.

Palmer, C. E. (1945). Nontuberculous pulmonary calification and sensitivity to histoplasmin. *Public Health Reports*, **60**, 513–20.

Parsons, R. J. and Zarafonetis, C. J. D. (1945). Histoplasmosis in man. Report of 7 cases and review of 71 cases. *Archives of Internal Medicine*, **75**, 1–23.

Payan, D. G. *et al.* (1984). Changes in immunoregulatory lymphocyte populations in patients with histoplasmosis. *Journal of Clinical Immunology*, **4**, 98–107.

Radostits, O. M., Blood, D. C., and Gay, C. C. (1994). Epizootic lymphangitis. In *Veterinary medicine: A textbook of the diseases of cattle, sheep, pigs, goats, and horses*, (8th edn), pp. 1167–9. Bailliere Tindall, London.

Redaelli, P. and Ciferri, R. (1934). Affinite entre less agents d'histoplasmose humaine, du farcin equin et d'une mycose spontanee des murides. *Bolletino della Sezione Italiana della Societa Internazionale della Microbiologia*, **6**, 376–9.

Rezabek, G. B. (1993). Histoplasmosis in horses. *Journal Comparative Pathology*, **109**, 47–55.

Rippon, J. W. (1988*a*). Histoplasmosis. In *Medical mycology*, pp. 381–423. WB Saunders Philadelphia.

Rippon, J. W. (1988*b*). Histoplasmosis duboisii. In *Medical mycology*, pp. 424–32. WB Saunders, Philadelphia.

Rivolta, S. (1873). *Dei parassiti vegetale con intro duzione allo studio delle malattie parassitarie e delle alterazioni dell' alimento degli animale domestici*, pp. 592. Torino.

Rowley, D. A., Haberman, R. T., and Emmons, C. W. (1954). Histoplasmosis: Pathologic study of fifty cats and fifty dogs from Loudoun County, Virginia. *Journal of Infectious Diseases*, **95**, 98–108.

Sacco, M., Medoff, G., Lambowitz, A. L., Kumar, B. V., Kobayaski, G. S., and Painter, A. (1983). Sulphydryl-induced respiratory pathway and their role in morphogenesis in the fungus *Histoplasma capsulatum*. *Journal of Biological Chemistry*, **258**, 8223–30.

Schaffner, A., Davis, C. E., Schaffner, T., Market, M., Douglas, H., and Braude, A. I. (1986). *In vitro* susceptibility of fungi to killing by neutrophil granulocytes discriminates between primary pathogenicity and opportunism. *Journal of Clinical Investigation*, **78**, 511–24.

Scherr, G. H. (1957). Studies on the dimorphism of *Histoplasma capsulatum*. *Experimental celi Research*, **12**, 92–107.

Schwartz, J. (1981). *Histoplasmosis*. Praeger Publishers, New York.

Schwartz, J. and Baum, G. L. (1957). The history of histoplasmosis 1906–1957. *New England Journal of Medicine*, **256**, 253–8.

Schwartz, J., Baum, G. L., Baum, C. J. K., Bingham, E. L., and Rubel, H. (1957). Successful infection of pigeons and chickens with *Histoplasma capsulatum*. *Mycopathologia*, **8**, 189–93.

Sills, M., Schwartz, A., and Weg, J. G. (1973). Conjungal histoplasmosis. A consequence of progressive dissemination in the index case after steroid therapy. *Annals of Internal Medicine*, **79**, 221–4.

Singh, T. (1965). Studies on epizootic lymphangitis. I. Modes of infection and transmission of equine histoplasmosis. *Indian Journal of Veterinary Science*, **35**, 102–10.

Singh, T. (1966). Studies on epizootic lymphangitis. Study of clinical cases and experimental transmission. *Indian Journal of Veterinary Science*, **36**, 45–59.

Singh, T., Vermani, B. M. L., and Bhalla, N. P. (1965). Studies on epizootic lymphangitis. I. Pathogenesis and histopathology of equine histoplasmosis. *Indian Journal of Veterinary Science*, **35**, 111–20.

Smith, J. G., Magee, D. M., Williams, D. M., and Graybill, J. R., (1990). Tumor necrosis factor-alpha plays a role in host defense against *Histoplasma capsulatum*. *Journal of Infection Diseases*, **162**, 1349–53.

Soliman, R., Ebeid, M., Essa, M., Abd-el-Hamid, M., Khamis, Y., and Said, A. H. (1991). Ocular histoplasmosis due to *Histoplasma farciminosum* in Egyptian donkeys. *Mycoses*, **34**, 261–6.

Spitzer, E. D., Lasker, B. A., Travis, S. J., Kobayaski, G. S., and Medoff, G. (1989). Use of mitochondrial and ribosomal DNA polymorphisms to classify clinical and soil isolates of *Histoplasma capsulatum*. *Infection and Immunology*, **57**, 1409–12.

Spitzer, E. D., Keath, E. J., Travis, S. J., Painter, A. A., Kobayaski, G. S., and Medoff, G. (1990). Temperature-sensitive variants of *Histoplasma capsulatum* isolated from patients with acquired immunodeficiency syndrome. *Journal of Infectious Diseases*, **162**, 258–61.

Sridhar, N. R., Tchervenkov, J. I., Weiss, M. A., Hijazi, Y. M., and First, M. R. (1991). Disseminated histoplasmosis in a renal transplant patient: A cause of renal failure several years following transplantation. *American Journal of Kidney Diseases*, **17**, 719–21.

Stockman, L., Clark, K. A., Hunt, J. M., and Roberts, G. D. (1993). Evaluation of commercially available acridinium ester-labeled chemiluminescent DNA probes for culture identification of *Blastomyces dermatiditis*, *Coccidioides immitis*, *Cryptococcus neoformans*, and *Histoplasma capsulatum*. *Journal of Clinical Microbiology*, **31**, 845–50.

Stotzky, G. and Post, A. H. (1961). Soil minerals as possible factors in geographic distribution of *Histoplasma capsulatum*. *Canadian Journal of Microbiology*, **13**, 1–7.

Taylor, M. L., Diaz, S., Gonzalez, P. A., Sosa, A. C., and Toriello, C. (1984). Relationship between pathogenesis and immune regulation mechanisms in histoplasmosis: A hypothetical approach. *Review of Infectious Diseases*, **6**, 775–82.

Tesh, R. B. and Schneidau, J. C. (1966). Primary cutaneous histoplasmosis. *New England Journal of Medicine*, **275**, 597–9.

Toloff-Rubin, N. E. and Rubin, R. H. (1992). Opportunistic fungal and bacterial infection in the renal transplant recipient. *Journal of the American Society of Nephrology*, **2**, S264–269.

Tosh, F. E., Balhuizen, J., and Yates, J. L. (1964). Primary cutaneous histoplasmosis. *Archives of Internal Medicine*, **114**, 118–19.

Tosh, F. E., Weeks, R. J., Pfeiffer, F. R., Hendricks, S. L., and Chin, T. D. Y., (1966). Chemical decontamination of soil containing *Histoplasma capsulatum*. *American Journal of Epidemiology*, **83**, 262–70.

Tosh, F. E., Weeks, R. J., Pfeiffer, F. R., Hendricks, S. L., Greer, D. L., and Chin, T. D. Y. (1967). The use of formalin to kill *Histoplasma capsulatum* at a epidemic site. *American Journal of Epidemiology*, **85**, 259–65.

Turner, C., Smith, C. D., and Furcolow, M. L. (1972*a*). Frequency of isolation of *Histoplasma capsulatum* and *Blastomyces dermatitidis* from dogs in Kentucky. *American Journal of Veterinary Research*, **33**, 137–41.

Turner, C., Smith, C. D., and Furcolow, M. L. (1972*b*). The efficiency of serologic and cultural methods in detection of infections with *Histoplasma* and *Blastomyces* in mongrel dogs. *Sabouraudia*, **19**, 1–5.

Tuttle, M. D. and Kern, S. J. (1981). *Bats and public health*, Milwaukee Public Museum, Milwaukee.

Vincent, R. D., Goewert, R., Goldman, W. E., Kobayaski, G. S., Lambowitz, A. M., and Medoff, G. (1986). Classification of *Histoplasma capsulatum* isolates by restriction fragment polymorphisms. *Journal of Bacteriology*, **165**, 813–18.

Ward, J. I., *et al.* (1979). Acute histoplasmosis: Clinical, epidemiologic and serologic findings of an outbreak associated with exposure to a fallen tree. *American Journal of Medicine*, **66**, 587–95.

Watson, S. R., Schmitt, S. K., Hendricks, D. E., and Bullock, W. E. (1985). Immunoregulation in disseminated murine histoplasmosis: Disturbances in the production of interleukins 1 and 2. *Journal of Immunology*, **135**, 3487–93.

Weeks, R. J. and Stickley, A. R. (1984). *Histoplasmosis and its relation to bird roosts: A review*. US Fish and Wildlife Service, Denver.

Weeks, R. J. and Tosh, F. E. (1971). Control of epidemic foci of *Histoplasma capsulatum*. In *Histoplasmosis, Proceedings of the Second National Conference*, (ed. L. Ajello, E. W. Chick, and M. L. Furcolow), pp. 184–9. Charles C. Thomas, Springfield, IL.

Weeks, R. J., Padhye, A. A., and Ajello, L. (1985). *Histoplasma capsulatum* var *farciminosum*: A new combination for *Histoplasma farciminosum*. *Mycologia*, **77**, 964–70.

Wheat, L. J. (1992). Histoplasmosis in Indianapolis. *Clinical Infections Diseases*, **14**, s91–99.

Wheat, L. J., *et al.* (1982). Risk factors for disseminated or fatal histoplasmosis: Analysis of a large urban outbreak. *Annals of Internal Medicine*, **96**, 159–63.

Wheat, L. J., Slama, T. G., and Zeckel, M. L. (1985). Histoplasmosis in the acquired immune deficiency syndrome. *American Journal of Medicine*, **78**, 203–10.

Wheat, L. J., Connolly-Stringfield, P., Kohler, R. B., Frame, P. T., and Gupta, M. R. (1989). *Histoplasma capsulatum* polysaccharide antigen detection in diagnosis and management of disseminated histoplasmosis in patients with acquired immunodeficiency syndrome. *American Journal of Medicine*, **87**, 396–400.

Wheat, J. *et al.* (1993). Prevention of relapse of histoplasmosis with itraconazole in patients with the acquired immunodeficiency syndrome. The National Institutes of Allergy and Infectious Diseases Clinical Trials and Mycoses Study Group Collaborators. *Annals of Internal Medicine*, **118**, 610–16.

Wolf, A. M. (1990). Histoplasmosis. In *Infectious diseases of the dog and cat* (ed. C. E. Greene), pp. 679–86. WB Saunders, Philadelphia.

Wolf, A. M. and Belden, M. N. (1984). Feline histoplasmosis: A literature review and retrospective study of 20 new cases. *Journal of the American Animal Hospital Association*, **20**, 995–8.

Wolf, A. M. and Green, R. W. (1987). The radiographic appearance of pulmonary histoplasmosis in the cat. *Veterinary Radiology*, **28**, 34–7.

Wolf, J. E., Kerchberger, V., Kobyaski, G. S., and Little, J. R. (1987). Modulation of macrophage oxidative burst by *Histoplasma capsulatum*. *Journal of Immunology*, **138**, 582–6.

Wong, S. Y. and Allen, D. M. (1992). Transmission of disseminated histoplasmosis via cadaveric renal transplantation: Case report. *Clinical Infectious Diseases*, **14**, 232–4.

Wu-Hsieh, B. and Howard, D. H. (1989). Histoplasmosis. In *Immunology of fungal disease*, (ed. R. A. J. Cox), pp. 199–225. CRC Press, Boca Raton, Florida.

Wu-Hsiesh, B. A., Lee, G. S., Franco, M., and Hofman, F. M. (1992). Early activation of splenic macrophages by tumor necrosis factor alpha is important in determining the outcome of experimental histoplasmosis in mice. *Infection and Immunity*, **60**, 4230–8.

Zeidberg, L. D. and Ajello, L. (1954). Environmental factors influencing the occurrence of *Histoplasma capsulatum* and *Microsporum gypseum* in soil. *Journal of Bacteriology*, **68**, 156–9.

Zeidberg, L. D., Dillion, A., and Gass, R. S. (1951). Some factors in the epidemiology of histoplasmin sensitivity in Williamson Country, Tennessee. *American Journal of Public Health*, **41**, 80–9.

69 RINGWORM (DERMATOPHYTOSIS)

A. H. Sparkes

SUMMARY

Ringworm or dermatophytosis is an infection of the keratinized tissues (stratum corneum, hair, or nails) with a fungus from the *Epidermophyton*, *Microsporum*, or *Trichophyton* genera. Around 40 indivdual dermatophyte species are recognized and classified as antropophilic, zoophilic, or geophilic, depending on their major reservoir in nature (humans, animals, and soil, respectively). Zoophilic dermatophytes may result in zoonoses when humans are exposed to these organisms, and dermatophytosis is considered to be one of the most common zoonotic diseases. The majority of zoonotic dermatophytoses are caused by three species: *M. canis* (usually derived from pet animals, particularly cats and dogs), *T. verrucosum* (usually derived from cattle), and *T. mentagrophytes* var *mentagrophytes* (a cosmopolitan organism with a wide host range, including rodents, farm animals, and pets). Infection may be acquired through direct contact with an infected animal, or indirectly through contact with a contaminated environment. While clinical disease is rarely serious, the lesions can result in disfigurement and pain, although zoophilic dermatophyte infections in man are generally self-limiting and respond well to treatment. Control of infection from domestic animals is problematic as identification and treatment of infected individuals is not always easy, and there is frequently heavy contamination of the environment with infectious material. Immunoprophylaxis is an attractive means of controlling infection in animals, and the development and widespread use of efficacious *T. verrucosum* vaccines in certain countries has already proved valuable in the management of cattle ringworm.

HISTORY

Dermatophytes have probably been in existence for millions of years, although the first recorded descriptions of the disease only go back as far as AD 30. Dermatophytosis has a distinguished history though, in being the first human disease for which a microorganism was identified as the cause when Remark found fungal elements in crusts from an affected patient (Ajello 1974). Since that time numerous mycologists have contributed to our current understanding of a complex disease.

THE AGENT

The dermatophytes are a highly specialized group of related, filamentous, pathogenic fungi that share the unusual ability to digest and derive nutrition from keratin (Ajello 1974). The term dermatophyte is restricted to those members of the three genera of *Microsporum*, *Trichophyton*, or *Epidermophyton* that cause disease by parasitizing the keratinized tissues (skin, hair, and nails) of man and animals (Ajello 1974; Matsumoto and Ajello 1987; Muller *et al.* 1989). Some fungi classified in these genera are simply saprophytes existing in the soil (geophilic) without causing disease, while certain keratinophilic fungi from other genera (e.g. *Aphanoascus* and *Chrysosporium* spp.) may at times cause disease of the keratinized tissues, but by the above definition, in neither of these cases can the fungi be referred to as dermatophytes and in the latter instance the infection is referred to as a dermatomycosis (ISHAM 1980; Matsumoto and Ajello 1987).

TAXONOMY

The taxonomy of the dermatophytes has been reviewed by Ajello (1975) and Matsumoto and Ajello (1987). The three main divisions of the higher fungi are the Ascomycota, the Basidiomycota, and the Deuteromycota. Although the Deuteromycetes may be regarded as a provisional taxonomic grouping for those fungi in which a sexual reproductive cycle has not been observed, the anamorph or asexual ('imperfect') stages of many fungi in this group (including dermatophytes) predominate in nature, and thus even when a sexual stage is found, the anamorphs are usually still classified as Deuteromycetes with the sexual ('perfect' or teleomorph) forms classified in a

Table 69.1 Anamorph and teleomorph classification of the dermatophytes

	Anamorph	Teleomorph
Kingdom	Fungi	Fungi
Division	Deuteromycota	Ascomycota
Genera	*Epidermophyton*	*Arthroderma*
	Trichophyton	(*Nannizzia*)
	Microsporum	

Table 69.2 Ecological classification of dermatophytes into geophilic, zoophilic, and anthropophilic species

Geophilic	Zoophilic	Anthropophilic
		E. floccosum
M. gypseum	*M. canis*	*M. audouinii*
M. fulvum	*M. canis* var.	*M. ferrugineum*
M. cookei	*distortum*	
M. nanum	*M. equinum*	
M. praecox	*M. gallinae*	
M. racemosum	*M. persicolor*	
T. vanbreuseghemii		
T. simii	*T. verrucosum*	*T. mentagrophytes*
T. terrestre	*T. equinum*	var. *interdigitale*
T. phaseoliforme	*T. mentagrophytes* var.	*T. rubrum*
T. vanbreuseghemii	*mentagrophytes*	*T. tonsurans*
T. ajelloi	*T. mentagrophytes* var.	*T. violaceum*
	erinacei	*T. concentricum*
	T. mentagrophytes var.	*T. gourvilii*
	quinckeanum	*T. megninii*
		T. schoenleinii
		T. soudanense
		T. yaoundei

separate appropriate taxonomic group (Table 69.1). The three genera, *Trichophyton*, *Microsporum*, and *Epidermophyton* contain around 40 recognized dermatophyte species, although in *Epidermophyton* only one validated dermatophyte species (*E. floccosum*) has been described (Table 69.2).

Where sexual reproduction has been observed in the dermatophytes, their teleomorph states have been classified in the *Arthroderma* genus of the Ascomycotina subphylum. Teleomorphs of *Microsporum* species were previously classified in the *Nannizzia* genus but this has now been shown to be congeneric with *Arthroderma* (Weitzman *et al.* 1986). The systematic classification of individual dermatophytes is based primarily on their morphology in clinical specimens and culture, their mating behaviour, and their physiologicalcharacteristics.

The dermatophytes are almost exclusively heterothallic fungi, with individual isolates being designated as either the '+' or '−' mating type, sexual reproduction therefore requires the presence of a compatible opposite mating type. The teleomorphs of most geo-

philic dermatophytes have been identified, but sexual reproduction has not been observed in a number of zoophilic and anthropophilic species, where isolates have either been exclusively of one mating type, or of a non-reactive nature. Even where telemorphs have been identified, in some species clinical isolates tend to be of a single mating type, for example the '−' type for *M. canis* which may, at least in some cases, be due to differences in the pathogenicity of the mating types (Rippon and Garber 1969).

Based on their ecology (natural habitat and primary source of nutrition), dermatophytes may conveniently be classified as geophilic (predominantly found in soil), zoophilic (predominantly found on animals), or anthropophilic (predominantly found on man) (Table 60.2), with zoophilic and anthropophilic dermatophytes displaying varying degrees of host–species specificity.

DISEASE MECHANISMS

Dermatophytes produce one of two types of asexual spores (conidia) depending on whether they are growing under saprophytic or parasitic conditions. During saprophytic growth (in the environment or in laboratory culture), macroconidia (multicellular) and/or microconidia (unicellular) are produced which are valuable in the laboratory identification of individual species (Rebell and Taplin 1970). However, the production of these spores is suppressed during parasitic growth on humans or animals, and instead arthroconidia are produced which arise from segmentation and fragmentation of hyphae. During parasitic growth, vast numbers of these resistant spores may be produced, and they are considered to be the main infectious particles of dermatophytes (Hashimoto 1991). The widespread dissemination of infected material from patients with dermatophytosis into the environment has been well documented (MacKenzie 1961; Shirouchi and Murata 1987), and this material may remain viable for many years (Dvorak *et al.* 1968) acting as a major source of infection. Material in hairs and/or scale from animals infected with *M. canis* or *T. mentagrophytes* var. *mentagrophytes* has been shown to remain viable for up to 18 months or more (Dvorak *et al.* 1968; Sparkes *et al.* 1994a), while *T. verrucosum*-infected material has been shown to remain viable for between 18 months and 5 years (McPherson 1957; Dvorak *et al.* 1968). However, the survival times depend on a number of factors, including the nature of the infected material and the conditions of storage. Arthrospores contained within hair, skin, or crusts are protected from the lethal effects of ultraviolet radiation (McPherson 1957), and these materials are likely to be the major source of persistent environmental contamination.

Arthrospores adhere strongly to keratin, and the presence of keratinocytes along with appropriate temperature, humidity, pH, and organic compounds, such as certain amino acids and sugars, produces favourable conditions for germination which can occur within a few hours. Nevertheless, dermatophytes are thought unable to penetrate a normal intact epidermis (DeVroey 1985), where the physical barrier of cornified epithelium, the fungistatic activity of saturated fatty acids in sebum and sweat, and normal epidermopoiesis provide a hostile environment (Kligman and Ginsberg 1950). When infection does occur, dermatophytes invade the zone of differentiating or newly differentiated keratin at the base of the stratum corneum or hair (Evans and Gentles 1985), and a number of predisposing factors, including maceration of the skin, mild trauma induced by rubbing or abrasion, occlusion, and increased hydration of the skin, will predispose to disease by facilitating penetration of the fungal elements. Hyphae invade keratinized tissue by a combination of physical pressure and production of a wide range of extracellular enzymes, including keratinases, peptidases, and lipases. In addition to facilitating penetration of keratinized tissues, these enzymes may be important in providing nutrition and provoking inflammation (Minocha et al. 1972).

Most dermatophytes infect both stratum corneum and hairs (and sometimes nails), but in three species (T. concentricum, E. floccosum, and M. persicolor) hair parasitism has not been observed (Rebell and Taplin 1970). Of those species that do infect hairs, most, including all the zoophilic species, produce an ectothrix infection with spore formation occurring outside and around the hair cortex. As with healthy intact stratum corneum, properties of the mature hair normally prevent fungal invasion in vivo, and thus only hairs in anagen are parasitized and fungal invasion only occurs deep in the hair follicle (Kligman 1955) where the keratin is immature. After penetration of the hair shaft, the hyphae grow down to the upper limit of the keratogenous zone, with some hyphae penetrating deeper towards the base of the keratogenous zone. In both stratum corneum and hair, infection is only maintained by active downward growth of hyphae occurring at the same rate as new keratin is produced, the growth of the stratum corneum or hair carrying the older parts of the fungal thallus upwards.

Although dermatophytes invade keratinized tissues and are able to use these tissues as a source of nutrition, their keratinophilic nature is primarily determined by host factors which prevent invasion and proliferation in deeper, living tissues. The temperature-sensitive nature of the dermatophytes may be one factor restricting invasion to superficial sites (Richardson 1990), but potent fungistatic substances are present in serum (principally unsaturated transferrin) that prevent deeper penetration of the organism (King et al. 1975). α_2-macroglobulin may also contribute to this inhibitory effect by antagonism of dermatophyte keratinases (Yu et al. 1972).

In both animals and man, dermatophytosis results in the development of both a humoral and cell-mediated immune response, and the latter is considered crucial to the natural resolution of disease and the development of acquired immunity (Grappel et al. 1974; Calderon and Hay 1984; Svejgaard 1985). The effector mechanisms by which cell-mediated immunity leads to elimination of the organism are not fully understood, but appear to involve disruption of the normal epidermal barrier, allowing penetration of serum inhibitory factors to the site of infection, the fungicidal activity of neutrophils and monocytes recruited to the site of the infection (Calderon 1989), and increased epidermal turnover leading to shedding of the organism (Berk et al. 1976; Tagami 1985)

The duration of infection in both animals and man varies considerably between individuals. In some, short-lived self-limiting infections occur, whereas in others infection may be chronic, lasting many months or years, and may also be recalcitrant to therapy. It has been observed that the duration of infection is generally inversely related to the degree of inflammation induced, and thus the administration of corticosteroids in doses sufficient to suppress the inflammatory response leads to more severe and more prolonged infections (Abu-Samra and Ibrahim 1988). The poor inflammatory response in chronic infections may also be related to the development of an inadequate cell-mediated immune response in these individuals (Hay 1986).

THE HOSTS

INCUBATION PERIOD

Under natural and experimental conditions, the incubation period for dermatophytosis in humans and animals is typically several days to 3 weeks. However, due to the keratinophilic nature of the spores, passive contamination of the skin or hair may occur and both animals and man may thus carry spores asymptomatically if they have contact with an infected individual or contaminated environment. In some cases, such individuals may later go on to develop clinical disease.

SYMPTOMS AND SIGNS

Humans

In man, the clinical presentation of dermatophytosis varies according to the site of infection (Evans and

Gentles 1985), and is typically described as tinea capitis (infection of the scalp), tinea barbae (infection of the beard), tinea corporis (infection of the body or glabrous skin), tinea cruris (infection of the groin), tinea pedis (infection of the foot), and tinea unguium (infection of the nail) (ISHAM 1980). Tinea manuum and tinea faciei (infections of the hand, and glabrous skin of the face, respectively) are additional terms used by some to identify these forms of tinea corporis. There is a complex host–parasite relationship in dermatophytosis, and clinical disease shows a spectrum between lesions demonstrating vary little inflammation, through to highly inflamed and sometimes painful lesions. The factors responsible for the wide variation in clinical presentation are not fully understood; however, important determinants include the site of the infection, with infections of the soles and palms often being chronic with little inflammation; the immune response; and the species of dermatophyte involved. In man, up to 90 per cent of chronic dermatophyte infections are caused by *T. rubrum* (Hay 1982), whereas human infection with zoophilic dermatophyte species tends to result in more inflammatory lesions that undergo spontaneous remission after a period of weeks to months.

The classical ringworm lesions occur in tinea capitis, tinea corporis, and tinea barbae, which are the most common sites for zoophilic dermatophyte infections. The typical lesions are centrifugally growing, circumscribed, roughly circular areas of variable erythema, scaling, and desquamation, often having raised borders and either with or without a central healing area (Evans and Gentles 1985; Hay *et al.* 1992; Weedon 1992). Alopecia accompanies infection due to the increased fragility of infected hairs. The lesions vary in size and may be singular or multiple, and in the latter case affected areas may coalesce, giving irregular patches of infection. In areas such as the foot and in body folds lesions may be less circumscribed, and in tinea pedis and tinea manuum diffuse scaling is often

the major sign, whereas tinea unguium usually leads to dystrophic nails.

The three zoophilic dermatophytes that most commonly cause human dermatophytosis (*M. canis*, *T. verrucosum*, and *T. mentagrophytes* var. *mentagrophytes*) tend to produce different degrees of inflammation. Infections with *M. canis* although variable, are generally moderately inflammatory and only rarely result in very severe inflammation (Marples 1956). In contrast, both *T. verrucosum* and *T. mentagrophytes* var. *mentagrophytes* frequently cause highly inflammatory lesions, which in tinea capitis and tinea barbae may be frequently accompanied by kerion formation—a suppurating, boggy, highly inflamed area of folliculitis (Hay *et al.* 1992, Weedon 1992).

Other distinct lesions associated with dermatophytes are seen occasionally (ISHAM 1980; Evans and Gentles 1985; Weedon 1992) including favus (chronic tinea capitis in which large crusts form over an erythematous base), granulomatous dermatophytia (including Majocchi's and Wilson's granulomata; circumscribed, nodular granulomatous perifolliculitis due to rupture of infected hair follicles), and dermatophytic pseudomycetoma. Pseudomycetomas are rare lesions resembling true enumycotic mycetomas (discharging subcutaneous swellings containing granules or microcolonies of the aetiological agent in the pus), and may result from rupture of hair follicles followed by limited growth of the dermatophyte in the subcutaneous tissues, resulting in a severe host response with the formation of pseudogranules (Ajello *et al.* 1980).

Animals

As in humans, the clinical appearance of dermatophytosis in animals is highly variable. In most domestic animals the classical ringworm lesion is similar to tinea capitis in man, with a circular or irregular patch of alopecia, scaling and crusting, with central healing. Other common clinical signs include folliculitis, furun-

Table 69.3 Major dermatophytes of the domestic animals, and their reservoirs

Dermatophyte	Reservoir	Cat	Dog	Horse	Cattle	Sheep/ goats	Pigs	Poultry
M. canis	Cats	F	F	O	R	O	R	
M. gypseum	Soil	O	F	F	R	R	R	
M. nanum	Pigs		R				F	
M. equinum	Horses			F				
T. mentagrophytes var. *mentagrophytes*	Rodents	F	F	O	O	O	O	
T. verrucosum	Cattle	R	R	R	F	O	R	
T. equinum	Horses		R	F				
T. gallinae	Fowl	R	R					F

F, frequent; O, occasional; R, rare.

culosis, generalized alopecia with scaling, and (particularly in cats with *M. canis* infection) a chronic infection with minor lesions discernible only on close examination. Kerion formation in cattle with *T. verrucosum* infection is also seen frequently (Scott 1988). In cats, dermatophytosis may occasionally present as 'miliary dermatitis' (Scott 1980), and infections of the nails, granulomatous dermatophytia, and pseudomycetoma have also been described (Scott 1980). The zoophilic dermatophytes show variable host-specificity, and a wide range of species have at times been isolated from most animal hosts (Table 69.3).

DIAGNOSIS

A diagnosis of dermatophytosis cannot be made on the basis of clinical signs alone, and the three tests most widely used for the confirmation of a diagnosis are examination of hairs under ultraviolet light (Wood's lamp); direct microscopic examination of hairs, nails or scale; and fungal culture.

Under Wood's lamp illumination, hairs infected with *M. canis*, *M. audouinii*, *T. schoenleinii*, or *M. ferrugineum* may produce a characteristic yellow-green fluorescence (Rebell and Taplin 1970) and thus examination of lesions, or hairs plucked from lesions, can be valuable. The fluorescence induced by these dermatophytes is only present in the cortex and medulla of hairs infected *in vivo*, being absent from invading hyphae and arthrospores, infected scales and crusts, and from *in vitro* cultures including hairs infected *in vitro*. The fluorescent material appears to be identical in most or all of the dermatophytes involved (Chattaway and Barlow 1958), but its precise nature is unknown and it is uncertain whether the material is an excreted fungal metabolite or an altered substance present in the hair shaft. Not all infections caused by these dermatophytes result in fluorescence of hairs, and in both man and animals, a variable proportion of *M. canis* infections have been reported where fluorescence was not observed. The reasons for the sometimes wide variation in the prevalence of fluorescence between different reports are not known, but may include factors such as the stage of infection (McAleer 1980), differences in the use of the Wood's lamp (Moriello 1991), pathogenic differences in *M. canis* (Rebell *et al.* 1956), and differences in the host–parasite relationship (Sparkes *et al.* 1993). Although fluorescence is only observed in a limited number of dermatophyte infections, examination under Wood's lamp is nevertheless very valuable as a rapid screening test in tinea capitis in man, and in canine and feline dermatophytosis where *M. canis* is the major casual organism. Care should be taken during examination with a Wood's lamp to distinguish the true fluorescence associated with dermatophyte infections from the bluish fluorescence often produced by the topical use of various ointments or the presence of scales and crusts.

Direct microscopic examination of hair and/or scale is a simple but important technique, and has the advantages of being both rapid and providing unequivocal evidence of dermatophytosis if parasitized hair or skin scales are found, although considerable expertise is required to reliably identify fungal elements, and to distinguish these from artefacts. Examination of material is usually performed after keratinous debris has been cleared by the addition of 10–20 per cent potassium hydroxide and with experience, in human dermatophytosis, direct microscopy may yield positive results in a very high proportion of cases, whereas in veterinary medicine positive diagnoses are typically achieved in around 40–60 per cent of samples from which dermatophytes are cultured. The sensitivity and ease of interpretation of direct microscopy can be enhanced in both human and veterinary medicine by the use of fluorescent microscopy in combination with fluorescent dyes that bind to fungal elements such as calcofluor white (Hageage and Harrington 1984; Sparkes *et al.* 1994*b*).

Fungal culture is generally regarded as the most reliable diagnostic test for dermatophytosis, and culture of representative material on defined media such as Sabouraud's dextrose agar has the advantages of being both a sensitive technique, and one that allows identification of the infecting dermatophyte by virtue of the macroscopic and microscopic morphology of the colony (Rebell and Taplin 1970). However, in some situations, such as tinea unguium, results of fungal culture are often negative, emphasizing the importance of other additional diagnostic techniques such as direct microscopy. Cultures are normally maintained at 25–30 °C and colonies will often appear within 7 days, although cultures are typically maintained for 2–3 weeks before being discarded. The growth of most dermatophytes is inhibited at higher temperatures, but in the case of *T. verrucosum*, culture at 37 °C is optimal for growth. Dermatophyte test medium (DTM) was described by Taplin *et al.* (1969) and incorporates phenol red in the culture medium as a pH indicator. The medium works on the principle that fungal utilization of proteins results in the production of alkaline metabolites (turning the medium red in colour) whereas utilization of carbohydrates results in acidic metabolites (maintaining or turning the medium yellow in colour). Dermatophytes generally utilize proteins in the medium first, resulting in red coloration, before later using carbohydrates and causing a return to yellow coloration. In contrast, most other fungi utilize carbohydrates first, thus maintaining the yellow colour of the medium, and only later use proteins.

Dermatophyte test medium was therefore designed to allow an evaluation of the colour change in the medium in relation to the appearance of fungal colonies for the diagnosis of dermatophytosis without the need for detailed knowledge of fungal morphology (Taplin *et al.* 1969). However, as DTM may alter the characteristic growth of dermatophytes, including suppression of conidia production, subculture on Sabouraud's dextrose agar may sometimes be required for confirmation of the nature of an isolate and identification of the species. Additionally, some dermatophytes, perhaps metabolically atypical strains, have been found not to cause an early colour change on DTM (Moriello and DeBoer 1991). Thus results of culture on DTM require careful interpretation, and this medium does not preclude the need for some mycological knowledge.

TREATMENT

Treatment of infections in man

Treatment of dermatophytosis is altered according to the clinical syndrome and the response to therapy. In general, recent focal lesions of the glabrous skin may be treated topically, whereas systemic treatment is recommended for chronic or widespread infections and in cases of tinea capitis and tinea unguium. Where systemic treatment is used, topical therapy may also be a useful adjunct and, for example in tinea capitis, topical therapy may help reduce dissemination of infectious particles in the environment. To further reduce environmental contamination in tinea capitis, clipping of hair around the lesion has been advocated. Table 69.4 lists some of the agents commonly used in the treat-

Table 69.4 Some topical and systemic agents widely used in the treatment of dermatophytosis

Class of drug	Topical preparations	Systemic preparations
Azoles		
Triazoles		Fluconazole
		Itraconazole
Imidazoles	Clotrimazole	
	Miconazole	
	Econazole	
	Enilconazole	
	Ketoconazole	Ketoconazole
Morpholines	Amorolfine	
Allylamines	Terbinafine	Terbinafine
	Naftifine	
Miscellaneous		Griseofulvin
	Chlorhexidine	
	Lime sulphur	
	Povidone-iodine	

ment of dermatophytosis. Specific antifungal therapy should be combined with appropriate antibiotic therapy where secondary bacterial infection accompanies the dermatophytosis.

Until recently, the imidazoles were generally considered to be the most effective of the available topical agents, although they did not always give results superior to traditional topical treatments such as benzoic acid compound ointment (which combines keratinolytic and mild antifungal properties) (Clayton and Conner 1973). However, newer topical preparations containing the allylamine antifungal agents naftifine or terbinafine have proved at least as effective as the imidazoles, with some studies showing a more rapid response time and/or a higher response rate.

A wide range of systemic antifungal agents are available for the treatment of dermatophytosis, including griseofulvin, azoles, and allylamines (Table 69.4). Griseofulvin is derived from *Penicillium griseofulvum* and was the first systemic antifungal agent, being used in both man and animals from 1958. It exhibits fungistatic properties against the dermatophytes and, although the mechanism of action is incompletely understood, it appears to interfere with intracellular spindle formation, inhibit cell wall synthesis, and inhibit binding of DNA and RNA. Short-term responses to griseofulvin are generally good, but relapses after cessation of treatment may occur Legendre and Steltz 1980; Hay 1990) and additionally there is evidence that relative or absolute resistance to griseofulvin may occur in some cases and contribute to poor success with this drug.

The azoles are generally considered to be fungistatic drugs and exert their effect by interfering with the cytochrome P450 enzymes, thereby inhibiting ergosterol synthesis, inhibiting cell proliferation, and affecting membrane permeability. Ketoconazole was the first systemic agent used as an alternative to griseofulvin for dermatophyte treatment, but despite showing equivalent or superior activity, the occurrence of hepatotoxicity and endocrine disturbances (due to interference with mammalian P450 activity) limits the value of this drug. The newer triazoles, and especially itraconazole, show a much greater specificity for fungal P450 and are safer, better tolerated, and free of the adverse endocrinological effects of ketoconazole. Compared to griseofulvin, the triazoles have shown superior results in clinical trials, which is assisted by the persistence of itraconazole at therapeutic levels in the skin for several weeks after cessation of treatment.

The allylamines, like the azoles, interfere with ergosterol biosynthesis, but through blocking squalene epoxidation rather than cytochrome P450. There is a very narrow margin between the fungistatic and fungicidal concentration of terbinafine, and in clinical usage this is regarded as a fungicidal agent. Results of trials with terbinafine have generally shown an excellent cure rate with superior activity compared to griseofulvin and a low prevalence of side-effects (Hay 1990; Elewski 1993). As with itraconazole, therapeutic concentrations may remain in the skin for more than 3 weeks after cessation of treatment. The trizoles and/or allylamines are likely to replace griseofulvin as the treatment of choice for dermatophytosis (Roberts 1991; Elewski 1993).

Treatment of infections in animals

Although many infections will be self-limiting, treatment of dermatophytosis in animals is usually recommended to prevent spread of the disease and reduce the zoonotic potential, following the same general pattern as that in man.

In farm animals and horses, topical therapy alone is frequently used for treatment, including iodophors, lime sulphur, natamycin, and imidazoles (e.g. enilconazole). Although topical therapy may be successfully combined with systemic griseofulvin treatment, this is often not economically viable when dealing with dermatophytosis in cattle. In canine and feline dermatophytosis, topical therapy with azoles, combined with clipping hair around the lesion, may be adequate for small focal lesions, but if a rapid response is not achieved systemic therapy is indicated. For generalized or recalcitrant localized dermatophytosis a combination of systemic and topical treatment is usually indicated. Total body clipping of hair has been advocated in long-or medium-haired animals to facilitate topical treatment and reduce the environmental contamination of spores (Medleau and White-Weithers 1992), but this procedure may increase the severity of the lesions, presumably through trauma to the skin facilitating spread of the disease. While creams may be applied to focal lesions, more extensive disease will require the use of dips, sprays, or shampoos, but little critical information is available on the most appropriate preparations. In one study, 0.2 per cent enilconazole and lime sulphur (3 per cent dilution from concentrate) dips showed greater fungicidal activity against arthrospores in dog and cat hairs than 0.1 per cent chlorhexidine or 0.8 per cent providone–iodine dips, which in turn showed greater activity than a 0.5 per cent sodium hypochlorite dip or ketoconazole shampoo (White-Weithers 1993). Lime sulphur or 1 per cent chlorhexidine (Moriello 1991) may be the most appropriate dips for use in cats, as enilconazole is not licensed for use in this species.

The only systemic agent currently licensed for use in animals is griseofulvin. On an empirical basis, the initial dose of this drug administered to dogs and cats is usually around 50 mg/kg daily, but this is doubled if response is poor (Medleau and White-Weithers 1992). As in humans, infections recalcitrant to griseofulvin are encountered, and treatment during pregnancy is contra-indicated due to the teratogenic nature of the drug (Scott *et al.* 1975). Other serious side-effects occasionally reported with griseofulvin use in cats include ataxia, anaemia, neutropenia, bone marrow hypoplasia, and hepatopathy (Helton *et al.* 1986; Levy 1991; Rottman *et al.* 1991). Initial reports suggest ketoconazole at 10 mg/kg once or twice daily (Medleau and Chalmers 1992) and itraconazole at 10 mg/kg daily or every other day (Medleau and White-Weithers 1992) are efficacious in the treatment of feline dermatophytosis, and the latter drug in particular may have the advantage of producing fewer side-effects.

PROGNOSIS

Dermatophytosis is a common disease in man but rarely serious, with infections generally being restricted to the stratum corneum where they may cause disfigurement, pruritus and pain. In many cases of dermatophytosis the disease is self-limiting, and humans infected with zoophilic dermatophyte species tend to undergo spontaneous resolution after a period of weeks to months. A good response to appropriate antimycotic therapy can generally be expected with these infections. In contrast, chronic dermatophyte infections, and particularly tinea unguium, do not always respond well to therapy, but these infections are usually produced by anthropophilic species. Spontaneous resolution of disease (due to the development of acquired immunity) is also typical of dermatophytosis in many animals, although as in man, chronic infections may occur in some cases.

EPIDEMIOLOGY

OCCURRENCE

Dermatophytosis is the most common cutaneous fungal infection in man and most, if not all the dermatophyte species have been implicated as human pathogens at some time (Rebell and Taplin 1970). In an extensive worldwide review of the literature (DeVroey 1985), the major causal organisms of human dermatophytosis were found to be *T. rubrum* (40.6 per cent), *T. violaceum* (21.5 per cent), *T. mentagrophytes* (14.4 per cent), and *M. canis* (9.6 per cent). None of the other species reported were responsible for more than 4 per cent of the total isolates. However, the species of dermatophyte involved and pattern of infection varies greatly between different countries,

Table 69.5 Prevalence (%) of dermatophytes isolated from humans—UK studies

Source	Walker (1950)	Beare and Cheeseman (1953)	Carlier (1963)	MacKenzie and Rusk (1964)	Greatorex (1978)	English and Lewis (1974)	Murray (1966)	Fleming (1975)	Gentles and Scott (1981)
Location	UK	N. Ireland	Birmingham	N. Ireland	Somerset	S. West	UK	N. Ireland	Scotland
Period	1946–49	1949–51	1945–62	1959–63	1953–75	1960–70	1962–65	1967–73	1960—79
Total isolates	2473	584	1507	981	485	3518	1523	1699	4423
Anthropophilic/geophilic									
M. audouinii	57.9	73.6	19.4	0	0.6	1.3	1.2	0	0.1
T. rubrum	3.9	0.2	1.2	9.2	21.4	42.4	47.7	17.5	59.9
E. floccosum	2.1	0.2	1.7	8.7	8.9	11.8	7.9	12.4	7.0
T. ment. var. *interdigitale*	4.9	0.2	[a]	5.1	[a]	16.4	[a]	11.9	13.9
T. tonsurans	1.6	5.0	5.6	13.3	0	1	2.4	6.2	2.1
M. gypseum	0.3	0	0.1	0.5	0.2	0.3	0	0	0.1
Others	2.5	0.2	7.1	0.9	0	1.0	2.4	0.3	1.2
Zoophilic									
M. canis	22.0	12.0	48.8	14.2	4.5	4.7	4.4	10.9	5.0
T. verrucosum	2.1	6.0	1.5	36.0	25.2	15.9	9.3	28.9	8.5
T. ment. var. *mentagrophytes*	2.1	2.7	[a]	12.0	[a]	3.4	[a]	11.9	1.8
T. ment. var. *quinckeanum*	0.1	0	[a]	0.1	[a]	<0.1	[a]	0	0
T. ment. var. *erinacei*	0	0	[a]	0	[a]	1.8	[a]	0	0.3
T. equinum	0.3	0	0	0.1	0	0.1	[a]	0	0
T. mentagrophytes	–	–	14.6[a]	–	39.2[a]	–	24.6[a]	–	–

[a] Varieties of *T. mentagrophytes* not specified.

Table 69.6 Prevalence (%) of dermatophytes isolated from humans—European and American studies

Source	Miguens et al. (1991)	Neves (1966)	Corallini de Bracalenti (1980)	Mantovani and Morganti (1977)	Londero and Ramos (1980)	Sinski and Flouras (1984)	Bienias and Wlodarczyk (1990)	Sinski and Kelley (1991)	Terragni et al. (1993)
Location	Spain	Portugal	Argentina	Italy	Brazil	USA	Poland	USA	Italy
Period	1951–87	1959–61	1959–78	1966–76	1970–79	1979–81	1982–85	1985–87	1970–89
Total isolates	3351	2345	998	1342	2862	6502	657	14 696	12 266
Anthropophilic/geophilic									
M. audouinii	0.2	0.1	0	1.1	0	0.3	0	0.1	0
T. rubrum	24.6	5.2	27.8	8.1	53.2	53.7	0	54.9	30.4
E. floccosum	11.8	4.6	6.2	10.7	14.8	4.4	15.8	2.0	8.5
T. ment. var. *interdigitale*	[a]	[a]	[a]	0	[a]	[a]	30.1	[a]	[a]
T. tonsurans	4.0	11.8	0.5	2.8	0	27.9	11.4	31.3	0.5
T. violaceum	1.2	39.2	0	6.1	0	0.2	0	0.1	1.6
M. gypseum	5.2	<0.1	3.0	5.7	0.8	0.9	0	0.7	2.9
Others	3.0	9.9	0.5	4.3	0.2	0.1	6.3	0 1	0.5
Zoophilic									
M. canis	25.5	22.5	55.0	46.7	3.8	3.7	2.7	4 2	49.0
T. verrucosum	3.1	<0.1	0	4.8	0.5	0.3	0	0.2	1.5
T. ment. var. *mentagrophytes*	[a]	[a]	[a]	9.6	[a]	[a]	31.5	[a]	[a]
T. ment. var. *quinckeanum*	[a]	[a]	[a]	0	[a]	[a]	2.6	[a]	[a]
T. mentagrophytes	21.4[a]	6.6[a]	7.0	–	26.7[a]	8.6	–	6.4[a]	5.2[a]

[a] Varieties of *T. mentagrophytes* not specified.

different regions, and with the passage of time (DeVroey 1985; Rippon 1985; Tables 69.5 and 69.6).

Although human dermatophytosis tends to be dominated by infection with anthropophilic species, zoophilic infections do form a substantial proportion of cases, and dermatophytosis is considered to be one of the most common zoonoses, with *M. canis*, *T. verrucosum* and *T. mentagrophytes* var. *mentagrophytes* most commonly implicated (Tables 69.5, 69.6 and 69.7). Infections with these three dermatophyte species occur throughout the world (DeVroey 1985; Rippon 1985). Although the prevalence of many zoophilic infections

in man is relatively stable, some countries and regions have experienced a marked rise in the incidence of zoophilic tinea capitis infections in recent years due to *M. canis* and, to a lesser extent, *T. mentagrophytes* var. *mentagrophytes* (Rippon 1985). *Microsporum canis* is now the most common cause of tinea capitis in South America, Australia, New Zealand, the Middle East, and many European countries including Great Britain, Italy, Spain, Portugal, and Scandinavia (DeVroey 1985; Rippon 1985; Lunder and Lunder 1992; Table 69.6).

Worldwide, the vast majority of tinea capitis cases due both to *M. canis* and other dermatophyte species

Table 69.7   Major dermatophytes of the domestic animals and their reservoirs

Dermatophyte	Main animal reservoir(s)	Frequency in humans	Geographical distribution
M. canis	Cats, dogs	Common	Worldwide
T. verrucosum	Cattle	Common	Worldwide
T. ment. var. mentagrophytes	Rodents, domestic animals	Common	Worldwide
T. ment. var. erinacei	Hedgehogs	Occasional	Europe, New Zealand
T. ment. var. quinckeanum	Mice	Occasional	Worldwide
T. equinum	Horses	Occasional	Worldwide
T. simii	Monkeys, chickens	Rare	India
M. equinum	Horses	Rare	Worldwide
T. gallinae	Chicken	Rare	Worldwide
M. persicolor	Voles	Rare	Europe, USA
M. nanum	Pigs	Rare	Worldwide

occur in children, which may relate to lower levels of fungal-inhibitory fatty acids present in this age group (Kligman and Ginsberg 1950). A sex predisposition towards both males and females has been reported, while others have suggested no sex predilection. Cultural differences between regions and over time may explain this, as it has been suggested that longer hair may help protect against infection by making penetration of infective spores to the scalp more difficult (McAleer 1980; DeVroey 1985). Although *M. canis* is the most common cause of tinea capitis in many countries, tinea corporis is often a more common manifestation of infection with this organism, with the exposed areas of the body most often affected. The predisposition towards juvenile infections is much less pronounced with tinea corporis and a sex predisposition towards females has been reported. *Microsporum canis* rarely causes lesions other than tinea capitis and tinea corporis.

In man, *T. verrucosum* and *T. mentagrophytes* var. *mentagrophytes* infections are mainly a cause of tinea corporis but they are also the main causal agents of tinea barbae, and less commonly a cause of tinea capitis. Infections are seen in both children and adults and although some studies suggest a predisposition amongst children, no consistent sex predisposition has been reported.

Human to human transmission of zoophilic dermatophytes is generally limited so that these species rarely cause major outbreaks of human dermatophytosis, although several cases may occur within a single family due to shared contact with a common source (Marples 1956; Carlier 1963).

In addition to *M. canis*, *T. verrucosum*, and *T. mentagrophytes* var. *mentagrophytes*, many other zoophilic dermatophytes have also been reported to cause disease in man, some of which show marked geographical restriction which is often related to the natural reservoir of the organism. These dermatophytes are generally a cause of tinea corporis or more rarely tinea capitis and they are summarized in Table 69.7.

SOURCES AND TRANSMISSION

Human infection with zoophilic dermatophytes requires either direct contact with an infected animal, or indirect transmission through fomites and parasitized skin scales or hair shed into the environment. Although the former may be a more efficient means of transmission, the extensive contamination of the environment from clinical cases and the prolonged survival time of dermatophytes in infected material is of considerable epidemiological importance, and may be a more common source of infection. Zoophilic dermatophytes apparently lose pathogenicity during serial passage in humans, and thus most infections are acquired directly from the animal or the environment rather than from human contact (Marples 1956).

The major hosts and the geographical occurrence of the zoophilic dermatophytes is shown in Table 69.7, and the frequency of different dermatophytes infecting domestic animals is shown in Table 69.3. A different pattern of zoophilic infections is encountered in rural and urban populations which relates to the source of the infections. Infections with *T. verrucosum* or *T. mentagrophytes* are usually seen in rural populations, with *T. verrucosum* occurring almost exclusively in these areas, being acquired directly or indirectly from infected cattle (Georg 1960; Chmel 1980). The source of infection with *T. mentagrophytes* is often more difficult to determine. While the occasional infections with *T. mentagrophytes* var. *erinacei* can usually be traced to contact with a hedgehog, *T. mentagrophytes* var. *mentagrophytes* is a cosmopolitan species infecting many domestic animals (Table 69.3) as well as rodents which are considered to be the reservoir for this dermatophyte. Environmental contamination from infected rodents around feed and bedding stores on farms probably represents an important source of human infection. In urban populations, infection is more usually acquired from pet animals, and *M. canis* is most frequently implicated (Georg 1960; Chmel 1980), with cats considered the major reservoir for this species. Pet rodents such as guinea-pigs, rabbits, and mice may also act as a potential source of dermatophytosis, most commonly with either *T. mentagrophytes* var. *mentagrophytes* or *T. mentagrophytes* var. *quinckeanum*. The variation in the relative prevalence of *M. canis* and *T. verrucosum* infections in the different surveys shown in Tables 69.5 and 69.6 largely reflects the different populations from which the patients were drawn.

Particularly with dermatophytes well adapted to infecting certain species (e.g. *M. canis* with cats), some infections may remain chronic and localized and thus an affected animal may not necessarily show obvious lesions. However, these chronic localized infections should be distinguished from passive carriage of dermatophyte spores in the hair-coat. Due to the keratinophilic nature of arthrospores, if animals or humans are exposed to a heavily contaminated environment, cultures of hair-brushings frequently yield dermatophytes due to passive contamination of the hair-coat or scalp. In general, the infection to inoculation ratio for dermatophytes is considered to be low, so passive asymptomatic carriers should not present a major risk either to other animals or to man, although if clinical disease occurs as a result of their carriage, they may then become a significant source of infectious material.

PREVENTION AND CONTROL

The prevention and control of zoonotic dermatophyte infections is far from simple. While there is little realistic prospect of controlling infections acquired from wild animals (e.g. *T. mentagrophytes* or *M. persicolor* from hedgehogs and rodents), measures can be taken to reduce the risks from domestic animals.

Not infrequently, human dermatophyte infections may be diagnosed and an animal origin suspected. Co-operation between the medical and veterinary professions is required in this situation, and it is important to confirm the diagnosis and identify the causal agent by fungal culture. The likely sources of infection can be identified once the dermatophyte species is known, and appropriate investigations of contact animals can be carried out to detect infected individuals. A planned and co-ordinated approach to the investigation is required though, so that pet animals are neither incorrectly blamed for human disease, nor overlooked as possible sources. As not all cats will show gross lesions when infected with *M. canis* careful clinical examination is necessary in suspected individuals, which may have to be combined with examination under Wood's lamp illumination and fungal cultures of hair brushings.

When dermatophytosis is suspected in animals, again confirmation of disease should be sought using appropriate diagnostic tests, and owners should be made aware of the potential zoonotic risks. Appropriate treatment of the affected animal(s) should be implemented immediately but the precise nature of the therapy will vary according to the circumstances.

In large animals (most commonly cattle and horses) there is little information from controlled studies on which to base treatment recommendations, but topical therapy using sprays or dips are most frequently used (see above). Clipping of the hair around lesions is impractical when dealing with a large herd of infected animals, but is often feasible in equine dermatophytosis where clipped hairs should be collected and disposed of by burning. Treatment of dermatophytosis should also include consideration of environmental and fomite contamination with infective material. Where feasible this should involve burning of disposable material which is likely to be the most reliable method of destroying arthrospores. Disinfectants and antifungals recommended for fomite and environmental decontamination include 5 per cent lime sulphur, 0.5–5 per cent sodium hypochlorite, 5 per cent formalin, 3 per cent cresol, 2 per cent glutaraldehyde, 1–2 per cent chlorhexidine, 0.1 per cent natamycin, 0.2 per cent enilconazole, and formaldehyde gas although, again, with many of these agents there have been few or no appropriate controlled studies to confirm their efficacy against dermatophytes in the environment. With widespread dissemination of infective material, effective environmental decontamination may be difficult to achieve in many situations, and repeated outbreaks of ringworm amongst successive batches of housed calves, for example, are common on individual farms.

Suspected cases of canine and feline dermatophytosis should again be confirmed by appropriate diagnostic tests, and owners should be warned of the zoonotic risk. Unless small focal lesions are present, treatment will usually be based on a combination of topical and systemic therapy, and the hair should be clipped around individual lesions to enhance topical therapy and again reduce environmental contamination. It is advisable to clip the hair with scissors rather than electric clippers so that skin trauma with subsequent exacerbation of the lesions can be avoided, and clipped hairs should be destroyed by burning. With very extensive lesions, careful total body clipping (with electric clippers) is advisable to reduce environmental contamination. The use of environmental disinfectants will have a more limited role where the animal is an indoor pet, but wherever feasible the environment and fomites should be treated and this should be combined with thorough and regular vacuum cleaning of carpets and furnishings to reduce the burden of infection. Special consideration needs to be given to multi-cat households where dermatophytosis is identified. In addition to careful environmental decontamination, attempts may be made to separate infected from uninfected cats, with topical prophylactic treatment for the uninfected group provided by regular use of dips or shampoos and additional systemic treatment provided for the infected cats (Carney and Moriello 1993).

PROPHYLAXIS AGAINST DERMATOPHYTOSIS IN DOMESTIC ANIMALS

Control of the spread of dermatophytosis is difficult due to the movement of animals and the shedding of infectious particles from infected individuals. Maintaining animals in isolation is rarely practical and could not be justified simply as a measure to prevent dermatophytosis. However, the possibility of protection of individuals by immunoprophylaxis was suggested by the observation of acquired resistance to natural and experimental infections. In 1950, Wharton *et al.* demonstrated complete resistance to experimental infection with *T. rubrum* in rabbits following repeated vaccination with a saline suspension of killed mycelium emulsified in oil with tubercle bacilli. Subsequently, Keeney and Huppert (1959) induced complete or partial protection to *T. mentagrophytes* infection in guinea-pigs by repeated daily topical application of lyophilized, powdered mycelium suspended in polyethylene glycol and, using a similar technique, these investigators also produced local protection in humans by application of the antigenic material between the toes (Huppert and Keeney 1959).

On a commercial basis, cattle vaccines have been developed against *T. verrucosum* and have found widespread use, primarily in Scandinavian and eastern European countries. The vaccines employed have been based on either live attenuated strains of *T. verrucosum* (Gudding and Naes 1986), or formalin-inactivated fungus (Wawrzkiewicz and Wawrzkiewicz 1992). Lyophilized vaccine is administered by intramuscular injection after reconstitution with water, and two injections are administered 10–14 days apart. The success of these vaccines has been demonstrated by experimental challenge studies, and also the results of extensive field trials (Tornquist *et al.* 1985; Gudding and Naes 1986; Gudding *et al.* 1991; Wawrzkiewicz and Wawrzkiewicz 1992). Other similar products have been developed including a *T. mentagrophytes* vaccine for use in fox farms to prevent dermatophytosis by this agent, which is reported to be widespread in the USSR (Rybnikar *et al.* 1991*a*); and a *T. equinum* vaccine for horses (Rybnikar *et al.* 1991*b*), but these have not been widely used. Most recently, a commercial *M. canis* vaccine has been marketed in the USA for use in cats.

If dermatophyte vaccines are able to exhibit high efficacy, there is no doubt that their widespread use could have a significant impact on the incidence of dermatophytosis in domestic animals, and thereby zoophilic dermatophytosis in man.

REFERENCES

Abu-Samra, M. T. and Ibrahim, K. E. E. (1988). The effect of 9a-fluoroprednisolone on the pathogenicity of *Microsporum canis* and *Trichophyton violaceum* to horses. *Mycoses*, **31**, 71–9.

Ajello, L. (1974). Natural history of the dermatophytes and related fungi. *Mycopathologia et Mycologia Applicata*, **53**, 93–110.

Ajello, L. (1975). Taxonomy of the dermatophytes: A review of their imperfect and perfect states. In *Recent advances in medical and veterinary mycology*, (ed. K. Iwata), pp. 289–97. University Park Press, Baltimore.

Ajello, L., Kaplan, W., and Chandler, F. W. (1980). Dermatophyte mycetomas: fact or fiction? In *Proceedings of the fifth international conference of the mycoses—superficial, cutaneous and, sub-cutaneous infections*, pp. 135–140. Pan American Health Organization, Scientific Publication No. 396, Washington.

Beare, J. M. and Cheeseman, E. A. (1953). The problem of ringworm in Northern Ireland. *Ulster Medical Journal*, **22**, (Suppl. 1), 1–43.

Berk, S. H., Penneys, N. S., and Weinstein, G. D. (1976). Epidermal activity in annular dermatophytosis. *Archives of Dermatology*, **112**, 485–8.

Bienias, L. and Wlodarczyk, W. (1990). Dermatomycoses and their etiology in the material of the dermatological department in Lodz, Poland. *Mycoses*, **33**, 581–6.

Calderon, R. A. (1989). Immunoregulation of Dermatophytosis. *CRC Critical Reviews in Microbiology*, **16**, 339–68.

Calderon, R. A. and Hay, R. J. (1984). Cell-mediated immunity in experimental murine dermatophytosis II. Adoptive transfer of immunity to dermatophyte infection by lymphoid cells from doners with acute or chronic infections. *Immunology*, **53**, 465–72.

Carlier, G. I. M. (1963). A seventeen year survey of the ringworm flora of Birmingham. *Journal of Hygiene (Cambridge)*, **61**, 291–305.

Carney, H. C. and Moriello, K. A. (1993). Dermatophytosis: cattery management plan. In *Current Veterinary Dermatology*, pp. 34–43. (ed. C. E. Griffin, K. W. Kwochka, and J. M. MacDonald. Mosby Year Books, St. Louis.

Chattaway, F. W. and Barlow, A. J. E. (1958). Fluorescent substances produced by dermatophytes. *Nature*, **181**, 281.

Chmel, L. (1980). Zoophilic deramtophytes and infection in man. In *Medical Mycology*, (ed. H. Preusser) pp. 61–6. Zentralblatt fur Bakteriologie, Parasitenkunde, Infektionskrankheiten und Hygiene, Supplement 8. Gustav Fischer Verlag, Stuttgart.

Clayton, Y. C. and Conner, B. L. (1973). Comparison of clotrimazole cream, Whitfield's ointment and nystatin ointment for topical treatment of ringworm infections, pityriasis versicolor, erythrasma and candidiasis. *British Journal of Dermatology*, **89**, 297–303.

Corallini de Bracalenti, B. J. (1980). A modern laboratory for diagnosing dermatomycoses. In *Proceedings of the fifth international conference on the mycoses—superficial, cutaneous, and subcutaneous infections*, pp. 178–87. Scientific Publication No. 396, Pan American Health Organisation, Washington.

DeVroey, C. (1985). Epidemiology of ringworm (dermatophytosis). *Seminars in Dermatology*, **4**, 185–200.

Dvorak, J., Hubalek, Z., and Otcenasek, M. (1968). Survival of dermatophytes in human skin scales. *Archives of Dermatology*, **98**, 540–2.

Elewski, B. E. (1993). Mechanisms of action of systemic antifungal agents. *Journal of the American Academy of Dermatology*, **28**, S28–S34.

English, M. P. and Lewis, L. (1974). Ringworm in the South-West of England, 1960–1970, with special reference to onychomycosis. *British Journal of Dermatology*, **90**, 67–75.

Evans, E. G. V. and Gentles, J. C. (1985). *Essentials of medical mycology*. Churchill Livingstone, Edinburgh.

Fleming, W. A. (1975). Dermatophyte isolations in Northern Ireland 1967–1973. *Ulster Medical Journal*, **44**, 44–7.

Gentles, J. C. and Scott E. (1981). Superficial mycoses in the West of Scotland. *Scottish Medical Journal*, **26**, 328–35.

Georg, L. K. (1960). Epidemiology of the dermatophytoses sources of infection, modes of transmission and epidemicity. *Annals of the New York Academy of Sciences*, **89**, 69–77.

Grappel, S. F., Bishop, C. T., and Blank, F. (1974). Immunology of dermatophytes and dermatophytosis. *Bacteriological Reviews*, **38**, 222–50.

Greatorex, F. B. (1978). Mycology in Somerset 1953–75. *Medical Laboratory Sciences*, **35**, 75–80.

Gudding R. and Naess, B. (1986). Vaccination of cattle against ringworm caused by *Trichophyton verrucosum*. *American Journal of Veterinary Research*, **47**, 2415–17.

Gudding, R. Naess, B., and Aamodt O. (1991). Immunisation against ringworm in cattle. *Veterinary Record*, **128**, 84–5.

Hageage, G. J. and Harrington, B. J. (1984). Use of calcafluor white in clinical mycology. *Laboratory Medicine*, **15**, 109–12.

Hashimoto, T. (1991). Infectious propagules of dermatophytes. In *The fungal spore and disease initiation in plants and animals*, (ed. G. T. Cole and H. C. Hoch. pp. 181–202. Plenum Press, New York.

Hay, R. J. (1982). Chronic dermatophyte infections I. Clinical and mycological features. *British Journal of Dermatology*, **106**, 1–7.

Hay, R. J. (1986). Chronic dermatophyte infections. In *Superficial fungal infections*, (ed. J. L. Verbov), MTP Press, Lancaster. pp. 21–33.

Hay, R. J. (1990). Antifungal drugs in dermatology. *Seminars in Dermatology*, **9**, 309–17.

Hay, R. J., Roberts, S. O. B., and MacKenzie, D. W. R. (1992). Mycology. In *Textbook of Dermatology*, Vol. 2, (ed. R. H. Champion, J. L. Burton, and F. J. G. Ebling, pp. 1127–216. Blackwell Scientific Publications, Oxford.

Helton, K. A., Nesbitt, G. H., and Caciolo, P. L. (1986). Griseofulvin toxicity in cats: literature review and report of seven cases. *Journal of the American Animal Hospital Association*, **22**, 453–8.

Huppert, M. and Keeney, E. L. (1959). Immunization against superficial fungous infection II. Studies on human volunteer subjects. *Journal of Investigative Dermatology*, **32**, 15–19.

ISHAM, (International Society for Human and Animal Mycology) (1980). Nomenclature of mycoses. *Sabouraudia*, **18**, 78–84.

Keeney, E. L. and Huppert, M. (1959). Immunization against superficial fungous infection I. Studies on experimental animals. *Journal of Investigative Dermatology*, **32**, 7–13.

King, R. D., Khan, H. A., Foye, J. C., and Greenberg, J. H. (1975). Transferrin, iron, and dermatophytes. I. Serum dermatophyte inhibitory component definitively identified as unsaturated transferrin. *Journal of Laboratory and Clinical Medicine*, **86**, 204–12.

Kligman, A. M. (1955). Tinea capitis due to *M. audouini* and *M. canis* II. Dynamics of the host-parasite relationship. *Archives of Dermatology*, **71**, 313–37.

Kligman, A. M. and Ginsberg, D. (1950). Immunity of the adult scalp to infection with *Microsporum audouini*. *Journal of Investigative Dermatology*, **14**, 345–58.

Legendre, R. and Steltz, M. (1980). A multi-centre, double-blind comparison of ketoconazole and griseofulvin in the treatment of infections due to dermatophytes. *Reviews of Infectious Diseases*, **2**, 586–91.

Levy, J. K. (1991). Ataxia in a kitten treated with griseofulvin. *Journal of the American Veterinary Medical Association*, **198**, 105–6.

Londero, A. T. and Ramos, C. D. (1980). A twenty-year (1960–1979) survey of dermatophytes in the state of Rio Grande do Sul, Brazil. In *Proceedings of the fifth international conference on the mycoses—superficial, cutaneous, and subcutaneous infections*. pp. 188–92. Scientific Publication No. 396, Pan American Health Organisation, Washington.

Lunder, M. and Lunder, M. (1992). Is *Microsporum canis* infection about to become a serious dermatological problem? *Dermatology*, **184**, 87–9.

McAleer, R. (1980). Fungal infections of the scalp in Western Australia. *Sabouraudia*, **18**, 185–90.

MacKenzie, D. W. R. (1961). The extra-human occurrence of *Trichophyton tonsurans* var. *sulfureum* in a residential school. *Sabouraudia*, **1**, 58–64.

MacKenzie, D. W. R. and Rusk, L. W. (1964). The mycological diagnostic service: a five year survey (1959–1963). *Ulster Medical Journal*, **33**, 94–100.

McPherson, E. A. (1957). The influence of physical factors on dermatomycosis in domestic animals. *Veterinary Record*, **69**, 1010–13.

Mantovani, A. and Morganti, L. (1977). Dermatophyto-zoonoses in Italy. *Veterinary Science Communications*, **1**, 171–7.

Marples, M. J. (1956). The ecology of *Microsporum canis* Bodin in New Zealand. *Journal of Hygiene (Cambridge)*, **54**, 378–87.

Matsumoto, T. and Ajello, L. (1987). Current taxonomic concepts pertaining to the dermatophytes and related fungi. *International Journal of Dermatology*, **26**, 491–9.

Medleau, L. and Chalmers, S. A. (1992). Ketoconazole for treatment of dermatophytosis in cats. *Journal of the American Veterinary Medical Association*, **200**, 77–8.

Medleau, L. and White-Weithers, N. E. (1992). Treating and preventing the various forms of dermatophytosis. *Veterinary Medicine*, **87**, 1096–100.

Miguens, M. P., Pereiro, M., and Pereiro, M. (1991). Review of dermatophytoses in Galacia from 1951 to 1987, and comparison with other areas of Spain. *Mycopathologia*, **113**, 65–78.

Minocha, Y., Pasricha, J. S., Mohapatra, L. N., and Kandhari, K. C. (1972). Proteolytic activity of dermatophytes and its role in the pathogenesis of skin lesions. *Sabouraudia*, **10**, 79–85.

Moriello, K. A. (1991). The management of dermatophytosis in catteries. In *Consultations in feline internal medicine*, (ed. J. R. August), pp. 89–94. WB Saunders, Philadelphia.

Moriello, K. A. and DeBoer, D. J. (1991). Fungal flora of the haircoat of cats with and without dermatophytosis. *Journal of Medical and Veterinary Mycology*, **29**, 285–92.

Muller, G. H., Kirk, R. W., and Scott, D. W. (1989). Fungal diseases. In *Small animal dermatology*, (4th edn). WB Saunders, Philadelphia., pp. 295–346.

Murray, I. G. (1966). The changing pattern of dermatophyte infections in the British Isles. *Monthly Bulletin of the Ministry of Health and Public Health Laboratory Service*, **25**, 210–14.

Neves, H. (1966). Unitary concepts of ringworm. *Mycopathologia et Mycologia Applicata*, **30**, 1–18.

Rebell, G. and Taplin, D. (1970). *Dermatophytes: Their recognition and identification*. University of Miami Press, Florida.

Rebell, G., Timmons, H. F., Lamb, J. H. Hicks, P. K., and Groves, F., and Coalson, R. E. (1956). Experimental *Microsporum canis* infection in kittens. *American Journal of Veterinary Research*, **57**, 74–8.

Richardson, M. D. (1990). Diagnosis and pathogenesis of dermatophyte infections. *British Journal of Clinical Practice*, **71**, (Symposium Supplement), 98–102.

Rippon, J. W. (1985). The changing epidemiology and emerging patterns of dermatophyte species. In *Current topics in medical mycology*, Vol. 1, (ed. M. R. McGinnis), pp. 208–34. Springer-Verlag, New York.

Rippon, J. W. and Garber, E. D. (1969). Dermatophyte pathogenicity as a function of mating type and associated enzymes. *Journal of Investigative Dermatology*, **53**, 445–8.

Roberts, M. M. (1991). Developments in the management of superficial fungal infections. *Journal of Antimicrobial Chemotherapy*, **28**, (Suppl. A), 47–57.

Rottman, J. B., English, R. V., Breitschwerdt, E. B., and Duncan, D. E. (1991). Bone marrow hypoplasia in a cat treated with griseofulvin. *Journal of the American Veterinary Medical Association*, **198**, 429–31.

Rybnikar, A. Chumela, J., Vrzal, V., Krys, F., and Janouskovcova, H. (1991*a*). Prophylactic and therapeutic use of a vaccine against trichophytosis in a large herd of silver foxes and arctic foxes. *Acta Veterinaria Brno*, **60**, 285–8.

Rybnikar, A., Chumela, J., Vrzal, V., Lysak, J., and Petras, J. (1991*b*). Vaccination of horses against trichophytosis. *Acta Veterinaria Brno*, **60**, 165–89.

Scott, D. W. (1980). Feline dermatology 1900–1978: a monograph. *Journal of the American Animal Hospital Association*, **16**, 331–459.

Scott, D. W. (1988). Fungal diseases. In *Large animal dermatology*, pp. 168–202. WB Saunders, Philadelphia.

Scott, F. W., de LaHunta, A., Schultz, R. D., Bistner, S. I., and Riis, R. C. (1975). Teratogenesis in cats associated with griseofulvin therapy. *Teratology*, **11**, 79–86.

Shirouchi, Y. and Murata J. (1987). Transition of isolation ratios of dermatophytes from house dust of patients with tinea. *Journal of Dermatology*, **14**, 15–19.

Sinski, J. T. and Flouras, K. (1984). A survey of dermatophytes isolated in human patients in the United States from 1979 to 1981 with chronological listings of worldwide incidence of five dermatophytes often isolated in the United States. *Mycopathologia*, **85**, 97–120.

Sinski, J. T. and Kelley, L. M. (1991). A survey of dermatophytes from human patients in the United States from 1985 to 1987. *Mycopathologia*, **114**, 117–26.

Sparkes, A. H., Gruffydd-Jones, T. J., Shaw, S. E., Wright, A. J., and Stokes, C. R. (1993). Epidemiological and diagnostic features of canine and feline dermatophytosis in the United Kingdom from 1956 to 1991. *Veterinary Record*, **133**, 57–61.

Sparkes, A. H., Werrett, G., Stokes, C. R., and Gruffydd-Jones, T. J. (1994*a*). *Microsporum canis*: Inapparent carriage by cats and the viability of arthrospores. *Journal of Small Animal Practice*, **35**, 397–401.

Sparkes, A. H., Werrett, G., Stokes, C. R., and Gruffydd-Jones, T. J. (1994*b*). Improved sensitivity in the diagnosis of dermatophytosis by fluorescence microscopy with calcofluor white. *Veterinary Record*, **134**, 307–8.

Svejgaard, E. (1985). Immunological investigations of dermatophytes and dermatophytosis. *Seminars in Dermatology*, **4**, 201–21.

Tagami, H. (1985). Epidermal cell proliferation in guinea pigs with experimental dermatophytosis. *Journal of Investigative Dermatology*, **85**, 153–5.

Taplin, D., Zaias, N., Rebell, G., and Blank, H. (1969). Isolation and recognition of dermatophytes on a new medium (DTM). *Archives of Dermatology*, **99**, 203–9.

Terragni, L., Lasagni, A., and Oriani, A. (1993). Deramtophytes and dermatophytoses in the Milan area between 1970 and 1989. *Mycoses*, **36**, 313–17.

Tornquist, M., Bendixen, P. H., and Pehrson, B. (1985). Vaccination against ringworm of calves in specialized beef production. *Acta Veterinaria Scandinavica*, **26**, 21–9.

Walker, J. (1950). The dermatophytes of Great Britain. Report of a three years' survey. *British Journal of Dermatology and Syphilology*, **62**, 239–251.

Wawrzkiewicz, K. and Wawrzkiewicz, J. (1992). An inactivated vaccine against ringworm. Comparative Immunology. *Microbiology and Infectious Diseases*, **15**, 31–40.

Weedon, D. (1992). Mycoses and algal infections. In *The skin; systematic pathology*, Vol. 9, In (ed. D. Weedon) pp. 639–76. Churchill Livingstone, Edinburgh.

Weitzman, I. McGinnis, M. R., Padhye, A. A., and Ajello, L. (1986). The genus *Arthroderma* and its later synonym *Nannizzia*. *Mycotaxon*, **25**, 505–18.

Wharton, M. L., Reiss, F., and Wharton, D. R. A. (1950). Active immunization against *Trichophyton purpureum* infection in rabbits. *Journal of Investigative Dermatology*, **14**, 291–303.

White-Weithers, N. (1993). Evaluation of topical therapies for the treatment of dematophytosis in dogs and cats. *Proceedings of the Annual Members Meeting of the American Academy of Veterinary Dermatology and the American College of Veterinary Dermatology*, pp. 29–30.

Yu, R. J., Grappel, S. F., and Blank, F. (1972). Inhibition of keratinases by alpha2-macroglobulin. *Experientia*, **28**, 886.

Sheelagh Lloyd

A variety of organisms are presented, that either are not closely related to a group already described, are free-living and accidentally infect man and animals, or are of tenuous 'parasitic' or zoonotic origin.

NEMATODES

LARVAE IN NODULES AND ADULT *OESOPHAGOSTOMUM* SPP. AND ADULT *TERNIDENS DEMINUTUS* IN THE INTESTINE

HOSTS AND GEOGRAPHIC DISTRIBUTION

These are parasites of non-human primates in Africa and Asia and humans can be definitive hosts. Humans are infected with *Oesophagostomum bifurcum* (Creplin, 1849) in Africa, *O. aculeatum* (Linstow, 1879), (= *O. apiostomum*) in Asia and Africa (particularly Uganda, China, the Philippines), and *O. stephanostomum* Railliet and Henry, 1909 in Brazil, Surinam, East and West Africa. A focus of high prevalence (often >20–50 per cent) with *O. bifurcum* exists in north-eastern Ghana/north-western Togo (Polderman and Blotkamp 1995). *Ternidens deminutus* (Railliet and Henry, 1905) Railliet and Henry, 1909 has been described primarily in Zimbabwe, but also sporadically in East and Central Africa and recently in Surinam.

INFECTION IN HUMANS

Most sporadic human infections were presumed to be accidental oral ingestion of L3 on vegetation from eggs in non-human primate faeces. Human–human transmission seems likely in the foci of infection in West Africa and Zimbabwe.

Oesophagostomum larvae induce eosinophilic tumour-like nodules in the serosa of the intestinal wall or omentum. There may be many 2–3 cm nodules on the colon or ileocaecal region or isolated 'abscesses' or 'tumours' with a purulent or caseous content. Each may contain an immature worm. Abdominal symptoms are varied but, characteristically, *O. bifurcum* presents as a hard epigastric or periumbilical mass (Polderman and Blotkamp 1995). Occasionally there is intestinal occlusion. Immature *Oesophagostomum* can emerge into the lumen while *T. deminutus* develops only in the lumen to lay eggs. Adult infections cause little harm.

DIAGNOSIS

Immatures often are identified after surgical removal of a nodule. Eggs are easily overlooked as they resemble hookworm eggs. *Ternidens deminutus* eggs are in fact larger, 70–94 by 40–60 μm. *Oesophagostomum* is diagnosed on cultured L3 (Blotkamp *et al.* 1993) which are 700–950 μm (larger than *Necator*) with prominent intestinal cells and a long 'hair-like' tail to the transversely striated sheath. Adults are about 1 cm long: *T. deminutus* has a globose buccal capsule, mouth collar, and leaf crown (Goldsmid and Lyons 1973); *Oesophagostomum* a cylindrical buccal capsule, double leaf crown, cephalic vesicle, and distinct ventral groove. An IgG4 ELISA for *Oesophagostomum* is under experimental evaluation.

TREATMENT

Surgery may be necessary for large abscesses. Pyrantel, albendazole, ivermectin, and other broad-spectrum anthelmintics kill adults. Polderman and Blotkamp (1995) question whether treatment of immature *Oesophagostomum* in the nodules could aggravate the pathology.

INTESTINAL ACANTHOCEPHALA ('THORNY HEADED WORMS')

HOSTS AND GEOGRAPHIC DISTRIBUTION

Moniliformis moniliformis (Bremser 1811) Travassos, 1915 (normal hosts, rodents, particularly *Rattus* spp.) and *Macracanthorhynchus hirudinaceus* (Pallas 1781) Travassos, 1917 (of domestic and wild pigs) sporadically infect man worldwide. Other species are very rare in humans: *Macracanthorhynchus ingens* (Von Linstow, 1879) Meyer 1932 (racoon and skunk) in the southern USA; *Corynosoma strumosum* (Rudolphi 1802) Lühe 1904 and a related *Bolbosoma* spp. Porta, 1908 (Cetacea, particularly seals) in Alaska and Japan, respectively; *Pseudoacanthocephalus bufonis* (Shipley 1903) Petrochenko, 1956 (widely distributed in toads in South-East Asia); and *Acanthocephalus rauschii* (Schmidt, 1969) (probably of marine fish) in the peritoneum of an Eskimo in Alaska.

INFECTION IN HUMANS

Eggs are ingested by arthropod intermediate hosts (beetles, cockroaches, millipedes, for acanthocephalans parasitic in land animals; crustaceans for those in aquatic vertebrates) and an infective cystacanth develops. Adult parasites develop in the intestines of humans that swallow these. In China and South-East Asia, infection is related to the habit of eating beetles (Leng *et al.* 1983). However, cystacanths re-encyst if eaten by vertebrates other than the definitive host, so snake or frog paratenic hosts could be important as are fish paratenic hosts for aquatic species.

Weakness and abdominal pain or intestinal perforation by the proboscis have led to diagnosis of the worm but many infections do little obvious harm.

DIAGNOSIS

Faecal eggs are ellipsoid or spindle-shaped, dark brown and measure 80–100 by 45–65 μm (*M. hirudinaceus*) and 110–120 by 56–60 μm (*M. moniliformis*). They have four membranes of which, in terrestrial species, one is very thick and may be pitted. Eggs contain an 'acanthor' larva provided with an anterior circlet of hooks. Adults are cylindrical and 1–1000 cm long with a 'thorny head'—a cylindrical or oval, invaginable proboscis armed with hooks.

TREATMENT

There is no evidence for high efficacy by any anthelmintic.

LARYNX AND TRACHEA—ADULT *MAMMOMONOGAMUS* SPP

HOSTS AND GEOGRAPHIC DISTRIBUTION

Over 100 human infections with *Mammomonogamus laryngeus* (Railliet 1899) Ryzhikov 1948 and *M. nasicola* (von Linstow 1899) Ryzhikov 1948 are recorded, primarily in the Caribbean and Brazil, but also in Mexico. Patients in Western countries have a recent history of travel in the Caribbean. Definitive hosts are ruminants in these areas plus much of Central and South America, South-East Asia, the Indian subcontinent, and tropical Africa.

INFECTION IN HUMANS

Eggs in bovine faeces embryonate to L3. Probably, eggs, or L3 that hatch, are ingested accidentally on vegetables. A paratenic host might be involved, e.g. earthworm, snail, as the related *Syngamus trachea* uses an earthworm.

Patients have a chronic, non-productive cough with a 'crawling sensation' or 'lump in the throat'. The cough may be paroxysmal with haemoptysis or vomiting. Some have severe 'asthma' symptoms because of obstruction of air passages.

DIAGNOSIS AND TREATMENT

Eggs in sputum or faeces are ellipsoid and average 82 × 42 μm (*M. laryngeus*) or 93 × 50 μm (*M. nasicola*) (larger than hookworm eggs) with a thicker shell and initially two cells. Males and females (up to 2 cm) live in permanent copulation in a 'Y' configuration and are described by Euzeby *et al.* (1987). They can be visualized and removed by bronchoscopy from the larynx, trachea, and sometimes bronchi, but their red colour is difficult to discern against an inflamed mucosa. The newer benzimidazoles and avermectins should be effective.

CONJUNCTIVAL SAC—ADULT *THELAZIA* SPP

HOSTS AND GEOGRAPHIC DISTRIBUTION

Thelazia callipaeda Railliet and Henry, 1910 and *Thelazia californiensis* Price, 1930 are common parasites of the conjunctiva of dogs and also cats and rabbits in Asia and western USA, respectively. Both have been described in the conjunctival sac of humans.

INFECTION IN HUMANS

Thelazia are transmitted by various muscid flies which acquire L1 by lapping secretions from the eyes of dogs.

L3 develop and migrate out of the mouthparts of a fly feeding around the eye. Human infection occurs at any age but is most common in young children, including babies. The parasites cause pain, conjunctivitis, and excess lachrymation. Often one, but as many as eight adults may be present.

DIAGNOSIS AND TREATMENT

Larvae grow from 500 μm to 1–1.5 cm. They can be removed physically with fine forceps. Avermectins at 200 μg/kg are more than 99 per cent effective in animals.

KIDNEY—ADULT *DIOCTOPHYMA RENALE* ('RED SCOURGE')

HOSTS AND GEOGRAPHIC DISTRIBUTION

Fewer than 20 human cases of *Dioctophyma renale* (Goeze 1782) Stiles, 1901 are described, most in North America, but also Russia, Iran, South-East Asia. Australia, and Spain, and the parasite occurs in South America. Normal hosts are piscivorous mammals, mainly mink in North America, but also other mustelids and canids.

INFECTION IN HUMANS

Eggs passed in urine develop in water and hatch when swallowed by an aquatic oligochaete annelid intermediate host. Annelids in drinking water are infective, uncooked fish and probably frogs that serve as paratenic hosts. Infective larvae penetrate the gut and develop in the peritoneal cavity and then kidney.

The adult worm in a thick-walled cyst containing haemorrhagic debris usually is found in or on the right kidney and has been confused with a tumour. Some are asymptomatic but symptoms include loin pain, haematuria, and worms have been expelled from the urethra. In one case, the lesion abscessed through the skin over the kidney. In two cases, a dioctophymid L3 was found in a subcutaneous nodule on the chest. Identity of the larva was not completely confirmed and could be a related *Eustrongylides* spp. of piscivorous birds. One *Eustrongylides* infection has been described in Maryland.

DIAGNOSIS

At least one *D. renale* infection was detected by eggs in the urine. Eggs are 70–80 by 40–50 μm, barrel-shaped, brownish yellow with a thick, pitted shell and clear areas at the poles. Ultrasound reveals echo-dense masses (the same echo-density as renal parenchyma). The blood-red worm reaches 1 m by 1 cm but seems to disintegrate after 1–3 years or more. Eggs remain in the granuloma-

tous tissue of the cyst wall but the 'double-walled rings' of eggs can easily be confused with radially striated Liesegang-like rings (Tuur *et al.* 1987).

TREATMENT

The cyst and kidney (if atrophied) are removed surgically.

NODULES IN ORAL OR SUBCUTANEOUS TISSUES CONTAINING ADULT *GONGYLONEMA PULCHRUM*

HOSTS AND GEOGRAPHIC DISTRIBUTION

Gongylonema pulchrum Molin, 1857 adults lie in a zipper fashion in the oesophageal wall of ruminants, pigs, and other vertebrates, in most countries. Worldwide, fewer than 50 human cases have been described.

INFECTION IN HUMANS

Beetle and cockroach intermediate hosts ingest eggs in ruminant faeces and humans presumably acquire infection eating these. Also, L3 are said to emerge from cockroaches in water, and contaminated water has been implicated in human infection. In man, *G. pulchrum* is found coiled in a painful, tumour-like mass in the oral epithelium or subcutaneously.

DIAGNOSIS AND TREATMENT

The worm is extracted surgically, possibly after anti-inflammatory therapy. Worms are recognized, whole or in cross-section, by asymmetrical alae and cuticular bosses that lie in eight longitudinal series on the anterior of the body (Chitwood and Lichtenfels 1972).

NECK ABSCESSES CONTAINING *LAGOCHILASCARIS MINOR*

HOSTS AND GEOGRAPHIC DISTRIBUTION

Although only 50–100 cases of *Lagochilascaris minor* Leiper, 1909 have been described, infection may be more common as all are in rural people in the neotropical forest areas of Brazil, Surinam, Costa Rica, Mexico, Trinidad and Tobago. The normal hosts seem to be sylvatic Canidae, Felidae, and opossums.

INFECTION IN HUMANS

Adults mature in the rhino-oro-pharynx of cats. Mice eating early L3 in eggs from their faeces are intermediate hosts (Campos *et al.* 1992). In man, parasites mature and eggs develop in the tissues. Infection probably is acquired through eating larvae in rodents, agouti, etc. Self-infection in lung and cervical tissues has been suggested.

Patients present with a persistent, purulent, discharging abscess in the soft tissues of the neck and throat. A rare fatal encephalopathy or lung infection has occurred.

DIAGNOSIS

Adult worms and eggs found in the lesion and discharges are described by Sprent (1971). Adult females reach 1–2 cm long with three ascarid lips and small lateral alae over most of the body. Eggs are spherical to oval, 60–85 μm long and the thick shell has a reticulate pattern of ridges surrounding saucer-like pits.

TREATMENT

Surgical debridement and excision usually have a favourable outcome. As many parasite stages are present, anthelmintics should be given. Although used only in individual patients, prolonged courses of ivermectin, levamisole, and albendazole are described as effective.

SKIN BLISTERS AND ULCERS—*DRACUNCULUS* SPP

HOSTS AND GEOGRAPHIC DISTRIBUTION

Dracunculus medinensis (Linneaus 1758) Gallandant, 1773, 'the guinea worm' is one of the oldest known worms, probably depicted as the staff and serpent of Aesculapius, the Roman god of medicine. Formerly a scourge in arid and semiarid areas of Asia, the Middle East, and northern Africa, this parasite is the subject of an intensive campaign for global eradication. The dog and other mammals occasionally are infected but seem incidental to the epidemiology. In North America, however, rare human *Dracunculus* is due to *Dracunculus insignis* (Leidy 1858) Chandler, 1942 from racoons, mink, and other carnivores.

INFECTION IN HUMANS

Females protrude from skin ulcers on racoons to lay L1 in water. *Cyclops* are intermediate hosts, and tadpoles and frogs suitable paratenic hosts. In racoons, parasites migrate through the peritoneal cavity and subcutaneous musculature for many months before moving to the extremities. Human infection probably is acquired through drinking *Cyclops* in dirty water.

The female emerging in summer induces an allergic rash, red papule, then blister on an extremity. The long female is coiled near this. Secondary infection or worms that fail to emerge and degenerate cause severe abscessation.

DIAGNOSIS AND TREATMENT

L1 (500–760 μm with a very striated cuticle and long pointed tail) may be obtained after placing cold water on a ruptured blister. The worm is surgically excised or extracted. Histology reveals the female worm amid an inflammatory reaction. For worms that are difficult to remove, corticosteroid therapy, perhaps with accompanying albendazole or ivermectin, might be helpful, though conclusive efficacy has not been demonstrated.

MIGRATING CUTANEOUS SWELLINGS AND EOSINOPHILIC MENINGITIS— *GNATHOSTOMA* SPP

HOSTS AND GEOGRAPHIC DISTRIBUTION

Gnathostoma spinigerum Owen, 1836, found in gastric nodules of wild and domestic Canidae, Felidae, and other carnivores, is the main species infecting man. It is particularly common throughout South-East Asia, China, Japan, also India and Pakistan, and is present in Mexico, Ecuador, and Australia, and probably elsewhere in Central and South America. *Gnathostoma hispidum* Fedtchenko, 1872, *Gnathostoma doloresi* Tubangui, 1925 (both parasites of pigs in Asia) and *Gnathostoma nipponicum* Yamaguti, 1941 (in weasels, etc., in Japan) are also being reported.

INFECTION IN HUMANS

L1 hatch in water. First intermediate hosts are freshwater copepods. Second intermediate hosts are fish with L3 in the muscles. Several fish are involved, though loach is common for *G. spinigerum*, *G. hispidum* and *G. nipponicum* and brook trout for *G. doloresi*. L3 occur also in amphibians, reptiles, rodents, pigs, and fowl infected either as intermediate hosts from copepods or as paratenic hosts from predation (Ando *et al.* 1992). In the definitive host the immatures migrate in the connective tissue and muscles but return to the stomach to mature.

Humans acquire infection primarily from raw fish in ethnic dishes such as '*Hu-sae*'; outbreaks of disease after a festival have occurred. Infection might arise from eating raw frogs, snakes, wild boar, etc., and through drinking copepods in water. Skin penetration by L3 in food handlers and occasional prenatal infections are described. Cases in emigrants and travellers from South-East Asia are increasing in frequency, while imported, chilled fish poses a threat. Infection with *G. hispidicum* in urban Japan was attributed to loach from Taiwan, Korea, or China, and a case of gnathostomiosis in The Netherlands to imported trout.

In man, larvae migrate primarily in the subcutaneous tissues but also CNS and other organs (Migasena *et al.*, 1991; Rusnak and Lucey 1993). In heavy infections, transient gastrointestinal symptoms may occur within 24–48 hours. Migration though the liver and chest can induce mild chest pain, cough, fever. Cutaneous gnathostomiosis develops within 3 weeks to several months or longer and manifests as eosinophilia and episodes of migrating, sometimes pruritic swelling(s) lasting 1–2 weeks. Although intermittent, these signs can persist for 8–12 years. Occasionally an abscess develops.

CNS gnathostomiosis develops in some patients and causes significant mortality from intracranial necrotic tracks and haemorrhage. A series of 162 patients showed acute, radicular nerve root pain from the spine to the extremities and/or trunk, often rapidly followed by paralysis or severe headache, neck stiffness, vomiting, impairment of senses and convulsions, with or without weakness or paralysis of the limbs (Punyagupta *et al.* 1990). Occasional pulmonary migration produces non-specific respiratory signs. Gastrointestinal gnathostomiosis is rare but has been confused with appendicitis or carcinoma. In ocular gnathostomiosis, the worm produces uveitis, haemorrhage, and iris holes.

DIAGNOSIS

Migrating swellings and eosinophilia, with or without eosinophilic myelitis, history of residence/travel in South-East Asia, and dietary preferences are suggestive. The worm can be very difficult to recover from CNS or cutaneous lesions. It may be visible in the eye. Larvae are 2 or 3–15 mm long, colourless to rust coloured, with a characteristic head bulb bearing 3–4 or more rows of hooklets. The cuticle has several rows of spines anteriorly.

CNS gnathostomiosis is differentiated from other eosinophilic meningitides by the characteristic acute nerve root pain plus bloody or xanthochromic CSF (Punyagupta *et al.* 1990). Larger parasites and their damage might be visible on CT scan. Difficulties in diagnosis have led to experimental identification of specific antigens, e.g. a 24 kDa antigen (Nopparatana *et al.* 1991) with potential for diagnosis.

TREATMENT

Spontaneous recovery from cutaneous and even CNS gnathostomiosis is possible, although patients are usually left with partial neurological defects. However, cutaneous migration, facial in particular, could lead to CNS or ocular complications and there is 12 per cent mortality from CNS infection. The parasite can be removed surgically from an accessible abscess, or from a digit or the eye. Blind excision of a migratory lesion is not normally successful as the parasite is reported to move as fast as 1 cm/hour, the oedema and inflammation indicating its previous location. Albendazole (400 mg once or twice daily) proved 94 per cent effective (Kraivichian *et al.* 1992) and could be useful in cerebral gnathostomiosis. Single or repeated ivermectin had 70–80 per cent efficacy experimentally (Anantaphruti *et al.* 1992).

MENINGOENCEPHALITIS—*MICRONEMA DELETRIX*

HOSTS AND GEOGRAPHIC DISTRIBUTION

Micronema (syn. *Halicephalobus*) *deletrix* Anderson and Bemrick, 1965 belongs to a group of usually free-living nematodes. The only descriptions of it come from occasional infections with females, larvae and eggs in horses and a few human cases in the USA, Europe, Japan, Egypt, and Columbia. Males and a free-living habitat are unknown.

INFECTION IN HUMANS

Halicephalobus deletrix presents as a non-suppurative meningoencephalitis with a rapid, fatal progression. There are multifocal necrotizing granulomata containing macrophages, multinucleate giant cells, lymphocytes, eosinophils, and the parasites. Infection is thought to be through oral and nasal wounds, though other mucosa and the skin could be involved. Haematogenous spread is suggested as parasites frequently are found in and near blood vessels in the brain. Infections in other tissues occur in horses.

DIAGNOSIS AND TREATMENT

Nematodes are identified in sections or teased from tissues. Females are 15–20 μm wide by 250–390 μm long, with a rhabditiform oesophagus, an ovary reflected dorsally, and uterus reflected ventrally in the region of the vulva. Eggs, 40×15 μm, have flattened sides. The presence of females and eggs rather than just larvae differentiate *H. deletrix* from the closely related *Strongyloides*. Treatment has not been successful. CNS involvement suggests albendazole should be tried.

PENTASTOMIDA (ARTHROPODS)

PENTASTOMID NYMPHS IN THE NASOPHARYNX AND VISCERA

HOSTS AND GEOGRAPHIC DISTRIBUTION

Human infection with *Linguatula serrata* Froelich, 1789 is sporadic, but cosmopolitan. Incidence is higher where definitive host dogs are fed viscera of ruminants, e.g. the Middle East, Turkey, parts of North Africa, the Indian subcontinent, and some Mediterranean countries. *Armillifer armillatus* Wyman, (1847?5) Sambon, 1910 in tropical and subtropical Africa is more common in man than *Armillifer grandis* (Hett 1915) in Africa and *Armillifer moniliformis* (Deising 1836) in Asia, primarily South-East Asia. Adults normally occur in the trachea and lungs of large snakes, *Python, Bitis* spp. There is an unconfirmed report of infection with *Leiperia cincinnalis* of crocodiles (Africa) and a subcutaneous creeping eruption from *Raillietella hemidactyli* of lizards (South-East Asia) and one report of *Sebekia* spp.

INFECTION IN HUMANS

Man is an intermediate host for the *Armillifer* spp. and *L. serrata*. Eggs are infective when laid. The clawed, four to six-legged, oval larva develops to a nymph (5–6 mm long) in the MLN, liver, and occasionally peritoneum, omentum, and lungs of rodent and lagomorph or ruminant intermediate hosts, respectively. As eggs are already infective in the female worm, heavy infections in people in western and central Africa have been related to trapping snakes for skins and eating snake meat containing many eggs or an adult female worm. Water, food, and soil contaminated with dog or snake faeces are sources of infection. There is potential for infection when cleaning aquaria of pet snakes of unknown origin.

Nymphs are found on the peritoneum, mesenteries, on and in the liver, abdominal lymph nodes, pleura, and lungs. Most human infections are asymptomatic. Some heavy infections have been correlated with prolonged abdominal pain and acute fatal cases have involved massive infection, including the brain.

Man also is a temporary definitive host for *L. serrata*. The nymph, acquired from eating raw liver or lymph nodes of domestic ruminants and lagomorphs, attaches on to the nasopharyngeal mucosa and causes severe irritation with coughing (perhaps paroxysmal) and sneezing. Symptoms (called 'halzoun' or 'marrara' in the Middle East and Sudan) are self-limiting after 1–7 or 14 days. Very rarely, parasites develop to adulthood. In some patients, possibly sensitized by previous adult or larval infection. acute congestion and oedema of the nasopharynx and larynx mucosae have more severe consequences.

DIAGNOSIS AND TREATMENT

Nymph(s) (tongue-shaped, slightly flattened anteroventrally, annulated, with two pairs of cranial hooks and up to 6–10 mm) are best revealed and physically removed by endoscopy. In visceral infection, radio-

graphy reveals crescent-shaped calcifications, 0.5–2 cm across. Calcification may occur by 2 years but can be delayed. The nymph, if still present, assumes a curled or crescent shape similar to *L. serrata* above. Histology reveals the annulated cuticle with sclerotized openings in it (Chitwood and Lichtenfels 1972; Drabick 1987). Ocular infection is reported occasionally. Ivermectin might be useful in an acute infection with large numbers of nymphal stages. Advice must be given on dietary habits, contact with dogs and snakes, and their treatment, perhaps with avermectins, attempted.

PROTOZOA

INTESTINE—CILIATED *BALANTIDIUM COLI*

HOSTS AND GEOGRAPHIC DISTRIBUTION

Balantidium coli (Malmsten 1857) Stein, 1862 is a cosmopolitan parasite in pigs. It infects captive and free-living non-human primates and occasionally other animal species. Human infection usually is sporadic, but worldwide, and occasionally relatively common in farm workers and rural dwellers.

INFECTION IN HUMANS

Infection is by oral ingestion of cysts excreted in pig faeces, either directly or via contaminated food/water. Infection from captive non-human primates and human–human transmission in institutions have been reported.

Normally only 1 in 5 human infections is symptomatic. In primates, including man, *B. coli* invades the large intestine mucosa to produce an ulcer. There is diarrhoea or dysentery indistinguishable from amoebic dysentery. Intestinal perforation has been reported.

DIAGNOSIS

Cysts, 40–60 µm, or trophozoites, 60–70 µm long, are shed irregularly in the faeces. They have a large, kidney-shaped macronucleus, cilia, contractile vacuoles and large funnel-shaped peristome. Barium defines the ulcer and biopsy will reveal trophozoites invading tissues.

TREATMENT

Treatment is necessary as infection can be fatal. Metronidazole at 750 mg to 1.25 g (for adults) daily in three doses for 10 days is effective (Garcia-Laverde and de Bonilla 1975). Other 5-nitroimidazoles could be used. Prolonged, 10–20 day courses of tetracycline or iodoquinol are described.

AMOEBIC DYSENTERY AND LIVER ABSCESSES—*ENTAMOEBA HISTOLYTICA*

HOSTS AND GEOGRAPHIC DISTRIBUTION

Man is the principal host of *Entamoeba histolytica* (Schaudinn 1903) Walker, 1911. The world prevalence of 10 per cent requires re-examination as Brumpt's observation of a morphologically identical, but non-pathogenic species has been confirmed. *Entamoeba dispar* Brumpt, 1925 can be differentiated by analyses of isoenzymes, surface antigens, restriction fragment length polymorphisms, sequences of single copy genes, and small subunit rRNA sequences. It is more common, by some tenfold, than *E. histolytica.*

Entamoeba histolytica has a yearly incidence of about 40–50 million cases and 40 000–100 000 deaths. It is cosmopolitan, but much more common in hot countries of low socio-economic stature. In Western patients, foreign travel, particularly of a month or more, is an important risk factor. Although human–human transmission is paramount, *E. histolytica* is widespread in many non-human primates. Infection is reported in dogs and cats but these do not excrete cysts and are unlikely to infect man, the reverse being the case.

INFECTION IN HUMANS

Urban overcrowding and poor sanitation favour amoebiosis. Water, raw fruit, and vegetables contaminated with cysts from faeces are the most important sources of infection. Flies are implicated in transmission. Examples exist of hand-borne transmission, i.e. from an infected maid or cook preparing food (Gatti *et al.* 1995).

Entamoeba histolytica is very cytotoxic. It adheres to cells by a galactose-specific lectin and destroys target cells within 5 min.

Intestinal

The incubation period is 8–10 days to several months. Minute, yellow nodules penetrate into and undermine the mucosa and submucosa, causing flask-shaped ulcers. Erosion of blood vessels gives intraluminal bleeding. Patients may be asymptomatic or the diarrhoea may be relatively mild, with flecks of mucus containing blood and organisms. In severe infections there are abdominal cramps, straining, painful spasms of the rectal sphincter, and very liquid faeces with blood and mucus. Intestinal perforation occurs in about 1 per cent of cases. On recovery from severe erosion, fibrosis can produce intestinal stricture.

Occasionally a large, protruding mass (amoeboma) of necrotic granulation and fibrous tissue develops at the colon flexures, caecum, or retrosigmoid junction.

Visceral, usually hepatic

Haematogenous spread to the liver occurs in about 5–8 per cent of symptomatic patients. A sterile abscess, usually near the surface in the right liver, contains a cream to brown viscous pus of necrosed liver cells. Surrounding liver cells are relatively normal interspersed with multiplying trophozoites.

There is liver tenderness or severe, continuous pain, fever, and weight loss. Occasionally a liver abscess will penetrate the diaphragm causing pulmonary signs, or discharge into the peritoneum, or through the skin inducing cutaneous amoebiasis. Cerebral amoebiasis is rare.

DIAGNOSIS

Endoscopy can detect an ulcer to obtain a smear. Faecal or biopsy smears, stained with iron haematoxylin, trichrome, etc., show 10–40 μm trophozoites with a vesicular nucleus of 3–5 μm (a small central karyosome and chromatin lining the nuclear membrane). On haematoxylin and eosin stain, the nucleus and cytoplasm of trophozoites are eosinophilic and basophilic, respectively, the opposite to host cells. Cysts average 10–15 μm, contain four nuclei, chromatoid bodies with rounded ends, and possibly a glycogen vacuole. Sensitivity will be increased by culture in Robinson, Dobell-Leidlaw, etc., media (Robinson 1968). Red cell ingestion only by pathogenic *E. histolytica* is highly specific, although only 53 per cent sensitive in cases with dysentery (Gonzalez-Ruiz *et al.* 1994). Cultured *Entamoeba* can be identified by distinct zymodemes (patterns of isoenzymes) in the different species (see Sargeaunt and Williams 1978, 1979).

Immunological tests also differentiate *E. histolytica* and *E. dispar*. There is a faecal capture test for histolysain, a proteinase enzyme produced only by pathogenic *E. histolytica* (Luaces *et al.* 1993). Several faecal antigen capture ELISAs, in particular one that detects the pathogen-specific galactose adhesin of *E. histolytica*, have good sensitivity and specificity compared with isoenzyme analysis (Haque *et al.* 1995). Further field evaluation of these is required.

Indirect haemagglutination, latex agglutination, or ELISA are 95–99 per cent sensitive in detecting antibodies in liver amoebiasis (Rosenblatt *et al.* 1995). Ultrasound reveals an oval or round lesion, frequently hypoechoic and heterogeneous and without wall structure. The CT image has a round or oval enhancing rim and low density centre (Vassiliades *et al.* 1992).

TREATMENT

Drugs have luminal, visceral, or mixed efficacy. Commonly, intestinal infection is treated with diloxanide furoate, 500 mg orally three times a day for 10 days. Other products are iodoquinol or paromomycin. For invasive intestinal and hepatic disease this is combined with metronidazole, 800 and 400 mg three times a day for 5 and 10 days, respectively. Other 5-nitroimidazoles (tinidazole, ornidazole) are available. Emetine hydrochloride or the less toxic dehydroemetine are alternatives in monitored intestinal patients. Recent strain variation or resistance to metronidazole has been suggested, so some give chloroquine concurrently. Vaccines, possibly incorporating the adhesin or other surface molecules, are under study.

INTESTINE—*ENTAMOEBA POLECKI*

HOSTS AND GEOGRAPHIC DISTRIBUTION

Entamoeba polecki von Prowazek, 1912, a parasite of pigs and monkeys, has foci of infection in man in South-East Asia and Papua New Guinea. Infection is recorded sporadically in emigrants and in other countries, e.g. Venezuela, India, France, Tasmania.

INFECTION IN HUMANS

Where sanitation is poor, direct pig faecal contamination of water and food is the most likely route of infection. Subsequent human–human transmission is probable and infections have been derived from captive monkeys (Sargeaunt *et al.* 1992).

Infection normally is asymptomatic, although rare reports of abdominal cramps, diarrhoea, and nausea were coincident with excretion of large numbers of cysts.

DIAGNOSIS AND TREATMENT

Cysts are uninucleate, 14–16 μm in diameter, with a larger, 3–4 μm, nucleus and diffuse but central karyosome. Diloxanide furoate and metronidazole are used.

INTESTINE—NON-INVASIVE AMOEBAE

Other amoebae live harmlessly in humans. Some also infect animals, particularly pigs and monkeys. Most are common worldwide. *Entamoeba coli* has large (10–30, usually 20–30 μm) cysts with eight nuclei. The karyosome is eccentric and the chromatin coarse. Chromatoid bodies have a splintered, not rounded shape. *Entamoeba hartmanni* has small cysts (5–10 μm) with

four nuclei and chromatoid bars of the *E. histolytica* type. *Endolimax nana* has a small oval cyst with small curved chromatoid bars and four nuclei. The karyosome is large, often eccentric, usually irregular, and sometimes fragmented. *Iodamoeba bütschlii* is uninucleate with a large vacuole containing glycogen that stains brown with iodine. *Dientamoeba fragilis* is binucleate and occasionally has been associated with abdominal pain. *Entamoeba gingivalis* is a non-encysting amoeba, 10–20 μm, with a central karyosome, in the mouth.

AMOEBIC MYELOENCEPHALITIS— FREE-LIVING AMOEBAS

HOSTS AND GEOGRAPHIC DISTRIBUTION

Naegleria, *Acanthamoeba*, and the Leptomyxida occur worldwide as free-living predators controlling soil bacterial populations, and are found also in warm or thermally heated water (ponds, lakes, domestic, pools, spas, sewage, cooling towers, heating, air conditioning, contact lens solutions, contraceptive IUDs, etc.). *Naegleria* is rare in healthy humans but *Acanthamoeba* can be cultured from the nasopharynx of 1–24 per cent.

Naegleria fowleri Carter, 1970 causes acute, rapidly fatal primary amoebic meningoencephalitis (PAM). *Naegleria australiensis* (de Jonckheere 1981) might have disease potential. *Acanthamoeba culbertsoni* (Singh and Das 1970) and *A. castellanii* (Douglas 1930) emend. Volkovsky, 1931 and some leptomyxid amoebae, e.g *Balamuthia mandrillaris* Visvesvara, Schuster and Martinez, 1993, cause subacute granulomatous amoebic encephalitis (GAE). Fewer than 200, 100, and 50 cases are recorded worldwide for these groups, respectively. They also occasionally infect domestic and wild animals and birds (Visvesvara and Stehr-Green 1990).

INFECTION IN HUMANS

Naegleria infection is not uncommon, with 100 per cent seropositive in some surveys. Disease usually occurs in young, healthy persons. There is a history of swimming or contact with water. Parasites, acquired by inhalation or ingestion, gain access to the brain via the cribiform plate. Parasites are highly destructive, producing haemorrhagic and necrotic meningoencephalitis involving particularly the olfactory and fronto-temporal regions. After incubation lasting a few days to 2 weeks, there are CNS signs of headache, fever, nausea, vomiting, and changes in mental status. The condition is rapidly fatal in 2–10 days.

Acanthamoeba and leptomyxid amoebae produce a more disseminated, slowly progressive and fatal infection, most commonly in immunosuppressed patients.

Parasites are inhaled or ingested but also gain entrance through skin, mucosal, and corneal abrasions. Seventy five per cent of AIDS patients manifest cutaneous lesions (Murakawa *et al.* 1995). Skin granulomata occur on the extremities and face, ulcerate and become pustules. GAE is seen in a minority of patients (most non-HIV patients and <50 per cent of AIDS patients). Organisms reach the CNS in the same way as *Naegleria* but also by haematogenous spread. Multifocal (occasionally one) necrotizing granulomas containing parasites, including cysts, and multinucleate giant cells develop deeper in the midline and fronto-temporal region. There is confusion, dizziness, drowsiness for a week to several months before coma and death. Occasionally multifocal lesions occur in the lungs, presenting as pneumonitis, and in other organs.

When *Acanthamoeba* enters corneal abrasions, the keratitis, although not common, can have severe consequences. Risk factors are use of contact lens (daily use, soft disposable lens), the use of home-made saline or chlorine disinfectants, swimming in lenses, and irregular use of lens disinfectants (Radford *et al.* 1995). There is severe pain (absent in herpes keratitis) while a pathognomonic sign is radial neuritis around the corneal nerve (McCulley *et al.* 1995).

DIAGNOSIS

CSF analysis usually shows elevated neutrophils (*Naegleria*) or monocytes (*Acanthamoeba*) and increased protein. *Naegleria* can be detected and cultured in CSF but antibodies have not been produced. *Acanthamoeba* can only be cultured from biopsy material but antibodies have been demonstrated in patients, at least experimentally. Recent developments of monoclonal antibodies, DNA probes, and a *Naegleria* species-specific PCR will aid diagnosis (Kilvington and Beeching 1995). Allozyme and isoenzyme analyses differentiate species and pathogenic organisms in environmental isolations (Moss *et al.* 1988; Badenoch *et al.* 1995).

Pathogenic species grow at 33–44 °C on agar seeded with enterobacteriaceae or other complex media and are cytopathic for mammalian cells and virulent in mice. *Balamuthia* does not grow on agar, but does on mammalian cells and in mice. Iron haematoxylin will stain trophozoites; methenamine silver staine cysts. *Naegleria* trophozoites are elongate, averaging 22 by 7 μm, with usually a single, occasionally four nuclei. They exhibit cytoplasmic extensions of the surface, amoebostomes for feeding, and monopodial locomotion. Cysts, 15–18 μm, round and double walled, develop on agar. In non-nutrient liquids, amoebae transform to flagellates. *Acanthamoeba* are larger than *Naegleria*, with variable pseudopodia and needle-like projections acanthopodia. Cysts are 15–28 μm with a polygonal arrangement of an exo and endocyst and

opercula for excystation. *Balamuthia* cysts have a tripartite wall. In histological sections and corneal smears amoebae are easily overlooked as they resemble macrophages. *Acanthamoeba* cysts may be present. Immunofluorescent testing has been used retrospectively to identify human cases (Visvesvara *et al.*, 1993).

TREATMENT

There are very few recoveries. *Naegleria* is sensitive to amphotericin B *in vitro*; doses of 1 mg/kg/day intravenously reached by the second day have been recommended. There is no therapy for systemic *Acanthamoeba*. Fluconazole, flucytosine, sulphadiazine have been tried. In contrast, rapid diagnosis and treatment of *Acanthamoeba* keratitis gives good prognosis for visual recovery. Treatment involves chlorhexidine, diamidines (propamidine isethionate, but hexamidine and other superior analogues show greater activity), neomycin sulphate, or clotrimazole, although additional evaluation of all these products is needed. Keratoplasty or, in severe untreated cases, corneal transplantation may be needed.

The *Acanthamoeba* are ubiquitous in soil, dust, and tap water, so disinfection of lenses must be thorough and lens cases cleaned and replaced regularly. Solutions containing hydrogen peroxide or chlorhexidine-thimerosal kill trophozoites and cysts. However, *Acanthamoeba* produces catalase and breaks down hydrogen peroxide so a two-step system is needed (Gray *et al.* 1995).

MYCOSES

PNEUMONIA IN IMMUNODEFICIENT PERSONS—*PNEUMOCYSTIS CARINII*

HOSTS AND GEOGRAPHIC DISTRIBUTION

Pneumocystis carinii was assigned to the Protozoa by Chagas, 1906 and Delanöe, 1912. Recently, it has been reclassified with the fungi, based on ribosomal RNA and other gene sequence homologies. It is cosmopolitan and common in the lungs of man, a wide variety of wild mammals, and domestic animals also. In studies in the USA more than 80 per cent of people were seropositive and infection had occurred by 2–3 years (Hopewell and Masur 1995). Lower animals were considered to act as a reservoir of infection for man but a revised nomenclature based on genotype differences of *Pneumocystis* in different host species was developed in 1994 (Wakefield 1995), i.e. *P. carinii* special form *carinii* in rats; *P. carinii* sp. f. *hominis* in humans, etc. There also is some strain variation in the same host species.

INFECTION IN HUMANS

Experimental rat infection is acquired by inhalation of air from rooms containing infected rats or environmental air. Presumably carrier humans are important. The infective stage is not known but *Pneumocystis* DNA sequences have been detected in air from animal rooms, a patient's room and in an open, rural location (Bartlett *et al.* 1994; Wakefield 1995). A life cycle in the environment might be possible, but its potential structure is unknown.

Disease is not expressed unless the patient is immunosuppressed, inducing activation of existing infection or new infection (Keely *et al.* 1995). *Pneumocystis carinii* pneumonia used to occur in individual or clusters of patients who were on immunosuppressive/cytotoxic therapy or were malnourished. It is now the most frequent index diagnosis for AIDS in the USA and Europe. For reasons unknown, frequency of disease is lower in Africa.

Pneumocystis carinii proliferates over 8–12 weeks. Trophozoites attach to type 1 alveolar epithelial cells, mediated by their major surface glycoprotein, fibronectin, and other host proteins, and kill them (Hopewell and Masur 1995; de Stefano and Walzer 1995). Alveolar/capillary membranes are breached and a frothy exudate containing parasites, fibrin, and dead cells collects in alveoli. Decreased lung surfactant seems important. There is some interstitial pneumonitis.

The few symptoms early in the course of disease are non-specific with fever, tiredness, weight loss for days to months before the pneumonia, represented by a cough and shortness of breath, develops. Pneumonia may be quite advanced before treatment is sought. Radiographs may vary from normal, early in the disease, to a diffuse, bilateral, finely granular or reticular infiltration. Cystic 'pneumatocoeles' and cavitation might be present especially after treatment. In some patients dermal infection occurs, seen commonly as a polyploid lesion at the auditory canal but occasionally nodules over the body. Brain, eye, and other organs occasionally are involved (Raviglione 1990). Disease may develop more acutely in those undergoing immunosuppressive therapy.

DIAGNOSIS

Any pulmonary abnormalities plus a CD4 + count of less than $300/mm^3$ must include *P. carinii* in the differential diagnosis (Hopewell and Masur 1995). Confirmation involves morphological identification of life cycle stages in induced sputum or bronchoalveolar lavage cytospun on to slides. A minimum of 10^4 organisms/ml is required, but sensitivities of 70–90 or 95 per cent in patients with symptoms are described (Hopewell and Masur 1995). Methenamine silver and toluidine blue O stain the cyst wall; Wright–Giemsa is required for the

sporozoites and trophozoites, the latter outnumber cysts greatly. Immunofluorescent antibodies are available. All the stains seem to produce equally good results. Cysts are oval or cup-shaped, 5–6 μm long with eight sporozoites of 1–2 μm. Trophozoites are 2–6 μm with an eccentric nucleus and reticular cytoplasm. A number of simple and nested PCRs have been developed in various laboratories. All show good sensitivity and specificity, and greater relative sensitivity compared with microscopic techniques (Evans *et al.* 1995; Lu *et al.* 1995; Moonens *et al.* 1995). However, there still is variation between different PCR tests and the clinical relevance of a positive result still needs evaluation.

TREATMENT

The clinical management and prophylaxis of *P. carinii* infections are reviewed in many articles (Hopewell and Masur 1995; Jolley and Hastings 1995; Sattler and Walzer 1995. Simonds *et al.* 1995). There are several regimens but most commonly trimethoprim—sulphamethoxazole (5 and 25 mg/kg, respectively) is given every 6–8 h orally or, in moderate to severe cases, intravenously. Adverse reactions are common, especially in the second week. For intolerant patients, the alternates are less effective. Dosages may be reduced or trimethoprim/dapsone, pentamidine (itself producing adverse reactions in many patients), or atovaquone (well tolerated) are useful (Spencer and Goa 1995). Concurrent prednisone or prednisolone therapy (40 mg every 12 for 5 days) can reduce early deterioration in oxygenation from inflammation in response to dead organisms. Complications of treatment include respiratory failure and pneumothorax.

Prophylaxis and maintenance, not 100 per cent effective, usually are considered for HIV patients with CD4+ counts below $200/mm^3$ or $200-400/mm^3$. As many as 65 per cent of patients relapse or are reinfected within 12 months of initial treatment. Trimethoprim–sulphamethoxazole is the most effective and most commonly used, with the advantage of activity against *Toxoplasma gondii* and some bacterial pathogens. Aerosol pentamidine is not quite as effective and has no reactivity against the other infections. A recent trial examined roxithromycin, but this and atovaquone need further evaluation.

MENINGITIS—*CRYPTOCOCCUS NEOFORMANS*, AN OPPORTUNISTIC FUNGUS

HOSTS AND GEOGRAPHIC DISTRIBUTION

At least 6 per cent of AIDS patients develop cryptococcosis in the USA; more in Africa. *Cryptococcus neoformans*. (Sanfelice 1894) Vuillemin, 1901 is an encapsulated yeast divided into two varieties and four serotypes. *Cryptococcus neoformans* var *neoformans* (serotypes A and D) is found worldwide, primarily (90 per cent) in immunosuppressed individuals. It reproduces in soils and debris enriched with pigeon droppings, but other birds could be involved. For example, 27 per cent of pet canaries in two Italian towns, and 10 per cent of wild birds, particularly parrots, in Mexico, were infected. *Cryptococcus neoformans* var *gatti* (serotypes B and C) is found in debris associated with red river gum trees, so patients reside in rural districts in Africa, Australia, South-East Asia, southern California, and occasionally Europe. Disease is most frequent in immunocompetent persons (Speed and Dunt 1995). Both varieties have caused disease in dogs, cats, and other animals.

INFECTION IN HUMANS

Basidiospores (0.6–11 μm) are airborne and inhaled but cutaneous implantation also can initiate disease. Close human transfer must be possible as organisms can be in sputum in large numbers in patients with respiratory disease. Also, disease in lower animals manifests primarily as lesions of the nasal cavities and head and neck, so affected pets have a public health risk.

The yeast multiplies in small air passages and compresses tissue but induces little host response. Infection usually goes no further and remains asymptomatic, but spread, primarily to the CNS but also to other tissues, occurs. Most patients present, not with respiratory signs, but with CNS signs of severe headache, fever, nausea, vomiting, altered mental status, decline in health, etc. Virulence is aided by the polysaccharide capsule which strongly inhibits phagocytosis and complement activation (Kozel 1995). There is chronic basal meningitis or focal brain lesions, the latter being more common with *C. n.* var. *gatti*. Increased intracranial pressure may in part be related to yeasts or capsules blocking CSF uptake by arachnoid villi. Also, the yeasts produce mannitol which may osmotically contribute to cerebral oedema. About 20–50 per cent of patients show pulmonary disease at the time of diagnosis and there can be involvement of other tissues (joints, heart, skin, genitourinary tract). The skin (nodules, ulcers, molluscan-type lesions or cellulitis) is involved in about 10 per cent of patients.

DIAGNOSIS

Diagnosis has been reviewed by Saag (1995). CT or MRI scans show ventricular enlargement and cerebral atrophy although, occasionally, the ventricles are small and there is cerebral oedema or a *Cryptococcus* mass. Patients can be screened for serum antigen before inva-

sive procedures are undertaken. Diagnosis is confirmed by lumbar puncture for culture of CSF (>2 ml) and antigen capture tests. Immunosuppressed patients also often have positive blood and urine cultures and *Cryptococcus* can be cultured from tissues, e.g. skin nodules. Indian ink or Nigrosin stains may reveal roundish, budding yeasts, 5–15 μm with a birefringent, polysaccharide capsule that stains red with mucicarmine. The yeast grows at 37 °C, pseudohyphae are absent, it produces urease and phenyloxidase and a brown melanin-like pigmentation on medium containing diphenolic compounds. When other organs are involved, methenamine silver and PAS-stained histological sections are useful. The sensitivity of Latex agglutination and ELISA antigen detection tests is 93–99 per cent in patients with culture-confirmed cryptococcal meningitis. PCR and other methods are under investigation.

TREATMENT

Amphotericin B is administered intravenously at 0.5 mg/kg/day for 2–4 weeks (renal toxicity is important after 4 weeks). This frequently is accompanied by 5-flucytosine at 100 mg/kg/day in four divided doses, but flucytosine has higher toxicity in AIDS patients (Saag 1995). Alternates are fluconazole or itraconazole. Lumbar puncture can relieve increased intracranial pressure. Subsequent maintenance therapy is important as a high percentage, 50–70 per cent of AIDS patients and a lower percentage of non-HIV patients, will relapse (Saag 1995). Prophylaxis with fluconazole remains controversial. (Pinner *et al.* 1995; Saag 1995), considerations being cost-effectiveness and the development of drug resistance (Saag 1995). Vaccines and monoclonal antibody therapy are under study, as are other drugs and combinations.

REFERENCES

Anantaphruti, M. T., Nuamtanong, S., and Waikagul, J. (1992). Effect of ivermectin on experimental gnathostomiasis in rabbits. *Tropical Medicine and Parasitology*, **43**, 65–7.

Ando, K., Tokura, H., Matsuoka, H., Taylor, D., and Chinzei, Y. (1992). Life cycle of *Gnathostoma nipponicum* Yamaguti, 1941. *Journal of Helminthology*, **66**, 53–61.

Badenoch, P. R., Adams, M., and Coster, D. J. (1995). Corneal virulence, cytopathic effect on human keratocytes and genetic characterization of *Acanthamoeba*. *International Journal of Parasitology*, **25**, 229–39.

Bartlett, M. S. *et al.* (1994). *Pneumocystis carinii* detected in air. *Journal of Eukaryotic Microbiology*, **41**, (suppl.), S75.

Blotkamp, J., Krepel, H. P., Kumar, V., Baeta, S., van T Noordende, J. M., and Polderman, A. M. (1993). Observations on the morphology of adults and larval stages of *Oesophagostomum* sp. isolated from man in northern Togo and Ghana. *Journal of Helminthology*, **67**, 49–61.

Campos, D. M. B., Filha, L. G. F., Vieira, M. A., Paco, J. M., and Maia, M. A. (1992). Experimental life cycle of *Lagochilascaris minor* Leiper, 1909. *Revista Institute Medicine Tropical Saode Paulo*, **34**, 227–87.

Chitwood, M. and Lichtenfels, J. R. (1972). Identification of parasitic metazoa in tissue sections. *Experimental Parasitology*, **32**, 407–519.

Drabick, J. J. (1987). Pentastomiasis. *Reviews of the Infectious Diseases*, **9**, 1087–94.

Evans, R., Joss, A. W. L., Parratt, D., Pennington, T. H., and Hoyden, D. O. (1995). The role of a nested polymerase chain reaction in the diagnosis of *Pneumocystis carinii* pneumonia. *Journal Clinical Pathology and Clinical Molecular Pathology*, **48**, M347–M350.

Euzeby, J., Gevrey, J., Graber, M., and Mejia-Garcia, A. (1987). Mammomonogamosis. In *Helminth zoonoses*, (ed. S. Geerts, V. Kumar, and J. Brandt). pp. 225–7. Nijhoff, Dordrecht.

Garcia-Laverde, A. and de Bonilla, L. (1975). Clinical trials with metronidazole in human balantidiasis. *American Journal Tropical Medicine and Hygiene*, **24**, 781–3.

Gatti, S., Cevini, C., Bruno, A., Novati, S., and Scaglia, M. (1995). Transmission of *Entamoeba histolytica* within a family complex. *Transactions of the Royal Society of Tropical Medicine and Hygiene*, **89**, 403–5.

Goldsmid, J. M. and Lyons, N. F. (1973). Studies on *Ternidens deminutus* Railliet and Henry, 1909 (Nematoda) I. External morphology. *Journal of Helminthology*, **47**, 119–26.

Gonzalez-Ruiz, A. *et al.* (1994). Value of microscopy in the diagnosis of dysentery associated with invasive *Entamoeba histolytica*. *Journal of Clinical Pathology*, **47**, 236–9.

Gray, T. B., Cursons, R. T., Sherwan, J. F., and Rose, P. R. (1995). *Acanthamoeba*, bacterial, and fungal contamination of contact lens storage cases. *British Journal of Ophthalmology*, **79**, 601–5.

Haque, R., Neville, L. M., Hahn, P., and Petri, W. A. (1995). Rapid diagnosis of *Entamoeba* infection using *Entamoeba* and *Entamoeba histolytica* stool antigen detection kits. *Journal of Clinical Microbiology*, **33**, 2558–61.

Hopewell, P. C. and Masur, H. (1995). *Pneumocystis carinii* pneumonia: current concepts. In *The medical management of AIDS*, (ed. M. A. Sande and P. A. Volbereding). pp. 367–99. W. B. Saunders, Philadephia.

Jolley, A. E. and Hastings, J. G. M. (1995). Therapeutic progress. 4. Treatment and prophylaxis of *Pneumocystis carinii*. *Journal Clinical Pharmacy and Therapeutics*, **20**, 121–30.

Keely, S. P., Stronger, J. R., Baughman, R. P., Linke, M. J., Walzer, P. D., and Smulian, A. G. (1995). Genetic variation among *Pneumocystis carinii* isolates in recurrent pneumocystosis. *Journal of Infectious Diseases*, **172**, 595–8.

Kilvington, S. and Beeching, J. (1995). Development of a PCR for identification of *Naegleria fowleri* from the environment. *Applied and Environmental Microbiology*, **61**, 3764–7.

Kozel, T. R. (1995). Virulence factors of *Cryptococcus neoformans*. *Trends in Microbiology*, **3**, 295–9.

Kraivichian, P., Kulkumthorn, M., Yingyourd, P., Akarabovorn, P., and Paireepai, C. C. (1992). Albendazole for the treatment of human gnathostomiasis. *Transactions of the Royal Society of Tropical Medicine and Hygiene*, **86**, 418–21.

Leng, Y. J., Huang, W. D., and Liang, P. N. (1983). Human infection with *Macracanthorhynchus hirudinaceus* Travassos, 1916 in Guangdong Province, with notes on its prevalence in China. *Annals of Tropical Medicine and Parasitology*, **77**, 107–9.

Lu, J. J., Chen, C. H., Bartlett, M. S., Smith, J. W., and Lee, C. H. (1995). Comparison of 6 different PCR methods for detection of *Pneumocystis carinii*. *Journal of Clinical Microbiology*, **33**, 2785–8.

Luaces, A. L., Osorio L. M., and Barrett, A. J. (1993). A new test for infection by *Entamoeba histolytica*. *Parasitology Today*, **9**, 69–71.

McCulley, J. P., Alizadeh, H., and Niederkorn, J. Y. (1995). *Acanthamoeba* keratitis. *CLAO. Journal*, **21**, 73–6.

Migasena, S., Pitisuttihum, P., and Desakorn, V. (1991). *Gnathostoma* larva migrans among guests at a New Year party. *Southeast Asian Journal of Tropical Medicine and Public Health*, **22**, (Suppl) 225–7.

Moonens, F., Liesnard, C., Brancart, F., Vanvooren, J. P., and Serruys, E. (1995). Rapid simple and nested polymerase chain reaction for the diagnosis of *Pneumocystis carinii* pneumonia. *Scandinavian Journal of Infectious Diseases*, **27**, 358–62.

Moss, D. M., Brandt, F. H., Mathews, H. M., and Viscesara, G. S. (1988). High resolution polyacrylamide gradient gel electrophoresis (PGGE) of isoenzymes from five *Naegleria* species. *Journal of Protozoology*, **35**, 26–31.

Murakawa, G. J. *et al.* (1995). Disseminated acanthamebiasis in patients with AIDS. A report of five cases and review of the literature. *Archives of Dermatology*, **131**, 1291–6.

Nopparatana, C., Setasuban, P., Chaicumpa, W., and Tapchaisri, P. (1991). Purification of *Gnathostoma spinigerum* specific antigen and diagnosis of human ganthostomiasis. *International Journal of Parasitology*, **21**, 677–87.

Pinner, R. W., Hajjeh, R. A., and Powderly, W. G. (1995). Prospects for preventing cryptococcosis in persons infected with human immunodeficiency virus. *Clinics in Infectious Diseases*, **21**, (Suppl. 1), S103–S107.

Polderman, A. M. and Blotkamp, J. (1995). *Oesophagostomum* infections in humans. *Parasitology Today*, **11**, 451–6.

Punyagupta, S., Bunnag, T., and Juttijudata, P. (1990). Eosinophilic meningitis in Thailand. Clinical and epidemiological characteristics of 162 patients with myeloencephalitis probably caused by *Gnathostoma spinigerum*. *Journal of Neurological Science*, **96**, 241–56.

Radford, C. F., Bacon, A. S., Dart, J. K., and Minassian, D. C. (1995). Risk factors for acanthamoeba keratitis in contact lens users: a case-control study. *British Medical Journal*, **310**, 1567–70.

Raviglione, M. C. (1990). Extrapulmonary pneumocystosis: the first 50 cases. *Reviews of the Infectious Diseases*, **12**, 1127–38.

Robinson, G. L. (1968). The laboratory diagnosis of human parasitic amoebae. *Transactions of the Royal Society of Tropical Medicine and Hygiene*, **62**, 285–94.

Rosenblatt, J. E., Sloan, L. M., and Bestrom, J. E. (1995). Evaluation of an enzyme-linked immunoassay for the detection of serum antibodies to *Entamoeba histolytica*. *Diagnostic Microbiology and Infectious Disease*, **22**, 275–8.

Rusnak, J. M. and Lucey, D. R. (1993). Clinical ganthostomiasis–case report and review of the English language literature. *Clinics in Infections Diseases*, **16**, 33–50.

Saag, M. S. (1995). Cryptococcosis and other fungal infections (histoplasmosis, coccidioidomycosis). In *The medical management of AIDS*, (ed. M. A. Sande and P. A. Volbereding), pp. 437–59. W. B. Saunders, Philadephia.

Sargeaunt, P. G. and Williams, J. E. (1978). Electrophoretic isoenzyme patterns of *Entamoeba histolytica* and *Entamoeba coli*. *Transactions of the Royal Society Tropical Medicine and Hygiene*, **72**, 164–6.

Sargeaunt, P. G. and Williams, J. E. (1979). Electrophoretic isoenzyme patterns of the pathogenic and nonpathogenic intestinal amoeba of man. *Transactions of the Royal Society of Tropical Medicine and Hygiene*, **73**, 225–7.

Sargeaunt, P. G., Patrick, S., and O'Keefe, D. (1992). Human infections of *Entamoeba chattoni* masquerade as *Entamoeba histolytica*. *Transactions of the Royal Society of Tropical Medicine and Hygiene*, **86**, 633.

Sattler, F. R. and Walzer, P. D. (ed.) (1995). *Pneumocystis carinii*. In Pneumocystic carinii, (ed. F. R. Sattler and P. D. Walzer). *Baillière's Clinical Infectious Diseases*, **2**, (3), 576.

Simonds, R. J., Hughes, W. T., Feinberg, J., and Navin, T. R. (1995). Preventing pneumocystis pneumonia in persons infected with human immunodeficiency virus. *Clinics in Infections Diseases*, **21**, (suppl. 1), S44–S48.

Speed, B. and Dunt, D. (1995). Clinical and host differences between infections with the two varieties of *Cryptococcus neoformans*. *Clinics in Infectious Diseases*, **21**, 28–34.

Spencer, C. M. and Goa, K. L. (1995). Atovaquone—a review of its pharmacological properties and therapeutic efficacy in opportunistic infections. *Drugs*, **50**, 176–96.

Sprent, J. F. A. (1971). Speciation and development in the genus *Lagochilascaris*. *Parasitology*, **62**, 71–112.

de Stefano, J. A. and Walzer, P. D. (1995). New Biological insights. In *Pneumocystis carinii*, (ed. F. R. Sattler and P. D. Walzer). *Baillière's Clinical Infectious Diseases*, **2**, (3), 415–30.

Tuur, S. M., Nelson, A. M., Gibson, D. W., Neafie, R. C., Johnson, F. B., Mostofi, F. K., and Connor, D. H. (1987). Leisegang rings in tissue: how to distinguish Leisegang rings from the giant kidney worm, *Dioctophyma renale*. *American Journal of Surgical Pathology*, **11**, 598–605.

Vassiliades, V. G., Bree, R. L., and Korobkin, M. (1992). Focal and diffuse benign hepatic disease: correlative imaging. *Seminars in Ultrasound, CT and MRI*, **13**, 313–35.

Visvesvara, G. S. and Stehr-Green, J. K. (1990). Epidemiology of free-living ameba infections. *Journal of Protozoology*, **37**, (Suppl.), 25S–33S.

Visvesvara, G. S., Schuster, F. L., and Martinez, A. J. (1993). *Balamuthia mandrillaris*, n.g., n.sp., agent of amebic meningoencephalitis in humans and other animals. *Journal of Eukaryotic Microbiology*, **40**, 504–14.

Wakefield, A. E. (1995). Re-examination of epidemiological concepts. In *Pneumocystis carinii*, (ed. F. R. Sattler and P. D. Walzer). *Baillière's Clinical Infectious Diseases*, **2**, (3), 431–48.

INDEX

Note: References in **bold** indicate chapter headings.
Where a genus name appears alone, references are to unspecified members of that genus or to the genus as a whole.